ROCKWOOD AND GREEN'S

FRACTURES IN ADULTS

SIXTH EDITION

ROCKWOOD AND GREEN'S

FRACTURES IN ADULTS

VOLUME 1

SIXTH EDITION

EDITORS

Robert W. Bucholz, MD
Professor and Chairman
Department of Orthopaedic Surgery
University of Texas Southwestern Medical School
Dallas, Texas

James D. Heckman, MD
Editor-in-Chief
The Journal of Bone and Joint Surgery
Needham, Massachusetts
Visiting Clinical Professor
Department of Orthopedic Surgery
Harvard Medical School
Visiting Orthopaedic Surgeon
Department of Orthopaedic Surgery
Massachusetts General Hospital
Boston, Massachusetts

Charles M. Court-Brown, MD
Professor of Orthopaedic Trauma
Royal Infirmary of Edinburgh
Edinburgh, United Kingdom

ASSOCIATE EDITORS

Kenneth J. Koval, MD
Director, Orthopaedic Trauma Service
Dartmouth Hitchcock Medical Center
Lebanon, New Hampshire

Paul Tornetta III, MD
Professor
Department of Orthopaedic Surgery
Boston University School of Medicine
Director of Orthopaedic Trauma
Boston University Medical Center
Boston, Massachusetts

Michael A. Wirth, MD
Professor of Orthopaedics
The Charles A. Rockwood Jr., MD Chair of the
Department of Orthopaedics
University of Texas Health Science Center
Chief of Shoulder Surgery
South Texas Veteran Health Care System
San Antonio, Texas

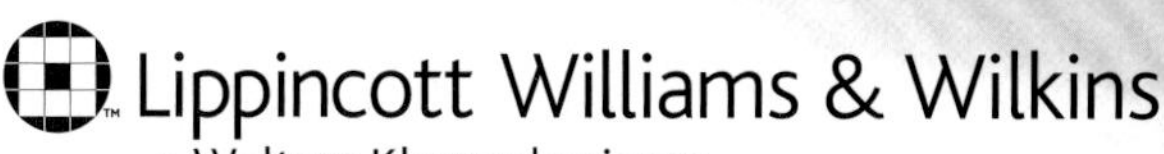

a Wolters Kluwer business
Philadelphia • Baltimore • New York • London
Buenos Aires • Hong Kong • Sydney • Tokyo

Acquisitions Editor: Robert Hurley
Developmental Editor: Keith Donnellan, Dovetail Content Solutions
Managing Editor: Jenny Kim
Project Manager: Alicia Jackson
Senior Manufacturing Manager: Benjamin Rivera
Director of Marketing: Sharon Zinner
Creative Director: Doug Smock
Cover Designer: Mike Pottman
Production Service: Maryland Composition
Printer: RR Donnelley-Willard

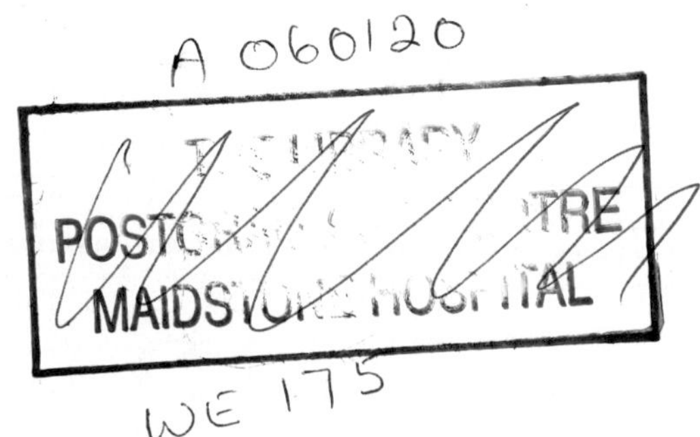

530 Walnut Street
Philadelphia, PA 19106 USA
LWW.com

5th Edition, ©2001 Lippincott Williams & Wilkins

Printed in the USA

Library of Congress Cataloging-in-Publication Data

Rockwood and Green's fractures in adults. — 6th ed. / editors, Robert W. Bucholz ... [et al.]
p. ; cm.
Includes bibliographical references and index.
ISBN 0-7817-4636-1
1. Fractures. 2. Dislocations. I. Rockwood, Charles A., 1936- II. Green, David P. III. Bucholz, Robert W. IV. Title: Fractures in adults.
[DNLM: 1. Fractures. 2. Dislocations. WE 175 R684 2006]
RD101F739 2006
617.1′5—dc22

2005028856

Care has been taken to confirm the accuracy of the information presented and to describe generally accepted practices. However, the authors, editors, and publisher are not responsible for errors or omissions or for any consequences from application of the information in this book and make no warranty, expressed or implied, with respect to the currency, completeness, or accuracy of the contents of the publication. Application of the information in a particular situation remains the professional responsibility of the practitioner.

The authors, editors, and publisher have exerted every effort to ensure that drug selection and dosage set forth in this text are in accordance with current recommendations and practice at the time of publication. However, in view of ongoing research, changes in government regulations, and the constant flow of information relating to drug therapy and drug reactions, the reader is urged to check the package insert for each drug for any change in indications and dosage and for added warnings and precautions. This is particularly important when the recommended agent is a new or infrequently employed drug.

Some drugs and medical devices presented in the publication have Food and Drug Administration (FDA) clearance for limited use in restricted research settings. It is the responsibility of the health care provider to ascertain the FDA status of each drug or device planned for use in their clinical practice.

To purchase additional copies of this book, call our customer service department at (800) 638-3030 or fax orders to (301) 223-2320. International customers should call (301) 223-2300.

Visit Lippincott Williams & Wilkins on the Internet: at LWW.com. Lippincott Williams & Wilkins customer service representatives are available from 8:30 am to 6 pm, EST.

10 9 8 7 6 5 4 3 2 1

We dedicate this Sixth Edition of *Rockwood and Green's Fractures in Adults* to Charles A. Rockwood, Jr, MD and David P. Green, MD, who served as our inspiration and mentors for carrying on the revision and update of this textbook.

To our wives, (Marybeth, Susan, and Jacqui) who supported us and graciously forgave our many absences from family activities so that we could complete the project.

CONTENTS

SECTION TWO: UPPER EXTREMITY

VOLUME 2

SECTION THREE: SPINE

SECTION FOUR: LOWER EXTREMITY

Charles M. Court-Brown, MD, FRCS Ed(Orth) Professor of Orthopaedic Trauma, Royal Infirmary of Edinburgh, Edinburgh, United Kingdom

Douglas R. Dirschl, MD Frank C. Wilson Distinguished Professor and Chairman of Orthopaedics, University of North Carolina at Chapel Hill, Chapel Hill, North Carolina

Paul J. Dougherty, MD Chief, Orthopaedic Trauma, Program Director, Orthopaedic Surgery Residency, Department of Orthopaedic Surgery, Henry Ford Hospital, Bloomfield, Michigan

John S. Early, MD Clinical Professor of Orthopaedics, University of Texas Southwestern Medical Center, Presbyterian Hospital of Dallas, Texas Orthopaedic Associates, Dallas, Texas

Robert K. Eastlack, MD Chief Resident of Orthopaedic Surgery, University of California, San Diego, California

Kenneth A. Egol, MD Chief of Trauma Service, New York University Hospital for Joint Diseases, Department of Orthopaedic Surgery, New York, New York

Thomas A. Einhorn, MD Professor and Chairman of Orthopaedic Surgery, Boston University Medical Center, Boston, Massachusetts

Christian Gaebler, MD, PhD Professor of Traumatology, University of Vienna Medical School, Vienna, Austria

Leesa M. Galatz, MD Assistant Professor of Orthopaedic Surgery, Washington University, Shoulder and Elbow Service, Department of Orthopaedic Surgery, Barnes Jewish Hospital, St. Louis, Missouri

Christian Gerber, MD Professor and Chairman of Orthopaedics, Balgrist University Hospital, Zürich, Switzerland

Peter V. Giannoudis, BSc, MB, MD, EEC(ortho) Professor of Trauma and Orthopaedic Surgery, University of Leeds, St. James University Hospital, Leeds, United Kingdom

Gregory J. Gilot, MD Assistant Professor of Orthopaedic Surgery, Indiana University School of Medicine, Indianapolis, Indiana

Thomas Gösling, MD General Surgeon, Trauma and Orthopaedic Trauma Surgeon, Hannover Medical School, Hannover, Germany

Robert M. Harris, MD Orthopaedic Program Director, Department of Orthopaedic Surgery, Atlanta Medical Center, Atlanta, Georgia

Lior Heller, MD Clinical Instructor of Plastic Surgery, MD Anderson Cancer Center, Houston, Texas

Mark H. Henry, MD Clinical Assistant Professor of Orthopaedic Surgery, University of Texas, Houston, Texas

Ralph Hertel, MD Professor of Orthopaedic Surgery, University of Bern, Department of Orthopaedic Surgery, Lindenhofspital, Bern, Switzerland

Per Olof Josefsson, MD, PhD Associate Professor of Orthopaedics, Malmv University Hospital, University of Lund, Malmv, Sweden

Leo Joskowicz, PhD Associate Professor of Computer Science, Head of Computer-Aided Surgery Laboratory, Director, Leibniz Center for Research in Computer Science, School of Engineering and Computer Science, The Hebrew University of Jerusalem, Jerusalem, Israel

Sanjeev Kakar, BSc(Hons), MD, MRCS Orthopaedic Research Fellow, Department of Orthopaedic Surgery, Boston University School of Medicine, Boston, Massachusetts

Kerry M. Kallas, MD Musculoskeletal Radiologist, Consulting Radiologists, LTD, Minneapolis, Minnesota

Magnus K. Karlsson, MD, PhD Associate Professor, Clinical and Molecular Osteoporosis Research Unit, Department of Clinical Sciences, Lund University, Department of Orthopaedics, Malmö, Sweden

Kenneth J. Koval, MD Professor of Orthopaedics, Director, Orthopaedic Trauma Service, Dartmouth-Hitchcock Medical Center, Lebanon, New Hampshire

Christian Krettek, MD, FRACS Trauma Department, Hannover Medical School, Hannover, Germany

Young W. Kwon, MD, PhD Assistant Professor of Orthopaedic Surgery, New York University School of Medicine, Shoulder and Elbow Service, Department of Orthopaedic Surgery, New York University for Joint Disease, New York, New York

Mark D. Lazarus, MD Shoulder and Elbow Service, The Rothman Institute at Jefferson, Associate Professor of Orthopaedic Surgery, Thomas Jefferson University, Philadelphia, Pennsylvania

Ross K. Leighton, MD, FRCS(C), FACS Associate Professor of Surgery, Division of Orthopaedics, Dalhousie University, QEII Health Sciences Centre, Halifax, Nova Scotia, Canada

Kwok-sui Leung, MB.BS, MD, FRCS Ed, FHKCOS, FACS Chairman, Consultant in Traumatology, Departments of Orthopaedics and Traumatology, Prince Wales Hospital, The Chinese University of Hong Kong, China

L. Scott Levin, MD, FACS Chief of Surgery, Division of Plastic and Reconstructive Surgery, Duke University Medical Center, Durham, North Carolina

Meir Liebergall, MD Associate Professor in Orthopaedic Surgery, Hebrew University, Chairman, Department of Orthopaedic Surgery, The Hadassah-Hebrew University Medical Center, Jerusalem, Israel

Jay D. Mabrey, MD, FAAOS Chief, Department of Orthopaedics, George Truett Orthopaedics Institute, Baylor University Medical Center, Dallas, Texas

A. Steven Malekzadeh, MD Department of Orthopaedic Surgery, University of Texas Southwestern Medical Center, Dallas, Texas

William A. Marinelli, MD Associate Professor of Medicine, University of Minnesota, Pulmonary and Critical Care Staff Physician, Director of Respiratory Care, Hennepin County Medical Center, Minneapolis, Minnesota

J.L. Marsh, MD Professor of Orthopaedics and Rehabilitation, University of Iowa Hospitals and Clinics, Iowa City, Iowa

Michael D. McKee, MD, FRCS(C) Associate Professor of Orthopaedic Surgery, University of Toronto, St. Michael's Hospital, Toronto, Ontario, Canada

Margaret M. McQueen, MD, FRCS Ed(Orth) Consultant Orthopaedic Trauma Surgeon, Edinburgh Orthopaedic Trauma Unit, Royal Infirmary of Edinburgh, Edinburgh, United Kingdom

Robert N. Meek, MD Clinical Professor of Orthopaedics, University of British Columbia, Vancouver, British Columbia, Canada

Sohail K. Mirza, MD Associate Professor of Orthopaedic Surgery, Department of Orthopaedics and Sports Medicine, University of Washington Medical School, Director of Spine Trauma Research, University of Washington, Seattle Washington

Kirti D. Moholkar, FRCSI (TR & Ortho), MCh Consultant Orthopaedic Surgeon, The Royal Orthopaedic Hospital NHS Trust, Birmingham, United Kingdom

Bernard F. Morrey, MD Professor of Orthopaedics, Mayo Medical School, Consultant, Department of Orthopaedics, Mayo Clinic, Rochester, Minnesota

Rami Mosheiff, MD Associate Professor in Orthopaedic Surgery, Hebrew University, Head of Orthopaedic Trauma Center, The Hadassah-Hebrew University Medical Center, Jerusalem, Israel

Sean E. Nork, MD Associate Professor of Orthopaedic Surgery, Harborview Medical Center, University of Washington, Seattle, Washington

Karl Obrant, MD Professor of Orthopaedics, Department of Clinical Sciences, Lund University, Malmö, Switzerland

Peter J. O'Brien, MD, FRCS(C) Associate Professor of Orthopaedics, University of British Columbia, Vancouver Acute Hospital, Vancouver, British Columbia, Canada

Shawn W. O'Driscoll, PhD, MD Professor of Orthopaedics, May Medical School, Consultant, Department of Orthopaedics, May Clinic, Rochester, Minnesota

Steven A. Olson, MD, FACS Associate Professor of Orthopaedic Surgery, Chief, Orthopaedic Trauma Service, Duke University Medical Center, Durham, North Carolina

Hans-Christoph Pape, MD Professor of Orthopaedics and Trauma, Hannover Medical School, Hannover, Germany

Edward A. Perez, MD University of Tennessee Campbell Clinic, Department of Orthopaedic Surgery, Memphis, Tennessee

Mark C. Reilly, MD Assistant Professor, Co-Chief Orthopaedic Trauma Service, New Jersey Medical School, Department of Orthopaedics, Newark, New Jersey

David Ring, MD Instructor of Orthopaedics, Harvard Medical School, Hand and Upper Extremity Service, Department of Orthopaedic Surgery, Massachusetts General Hospital, Boston, Massachusetts

C. Michael Robinson, BMedSci, FRCS Ed(Orth) Consultant and Senior Lecturer of Orthopaedics and Trauma, Edinburgh Orthopaedic Trauma Unit, New Royal Infirmary of Edinburgh, Edinburgh, United Kingdom

Charles A. Rockwood, Jr., MD Professor and Chairman Emeritus of Orthopaedics, University of Texas Health Science Center at San Antonio, University Hospital, San Antonio, Texas

Dominique A. Rothenfluh, MD Laboratory for Regenerative Medicine and Pharmacobiology, Integrative Biosciences Institute, Swiss Federal Institute of Technology, Lausanne, Switzerland

David S. Ruch, MD Professor of Orthopaedic Surgery, Duke University Medical Center, Durham, North Carolina

Charles L. Saltzman, MD Professor of Orthopaedics and Rehabilitation, Engineering, Physical Therapy and Rehabilitations Sciences, University of Iowa, Iowa City, Iowa

David W. Sanders, MD, MSc, FRCS(C) Assistant Professor of Orthopaedic Surgery, London Health Sciences Centre, University of Western Ontario, London, Ontario, Canada

Roy W. Sanders, MD Chief of Orthopaedics, Tampa General Hospital, Director of Orthopaedic Trauma Services, Florida Orthopaedic Institute, Tampa, Florida

Robert C. Schenck, Jr., MD Professor and Division Chief of Sports Medicine, Department of Orthopaedics and Rehabilitations, University of New Mexico School of Medicine, Head Team Physician, University of New Mexico-Lobos, Albuquerque, New Mexico

Andrew H. Schmidt, MD Associate Professor of Orthopedic Surgery, University of Minnesota, Faculty, Department of Orthopedic Surgery, Hennepin County Medical Center, Minneapolis, Minnesota

Carl Seon, MD Clinical Assistant Professor, Joan C. Edwards School of Medicine, Marshall University, Huntington, West Virginia, Bone and Joint Surgeons, Charleston, West Virginia

John W. Sperling, MD Associate Professor of Orthopaedic Surgery, Mayo Medical School, Orthopaedic Surgeon, Mayo Clinic, Rochester, Minnesota

James P. Stannard, MD Associate Professor of Orthopaedic Surgery, Chief, Section of Orthopaedic Trauma, University of Alabama at Birmingham, Birmingham, Alabama

Adam J. Starr, MD Associate Professor of Orthopaedic Surgery, University of Texas Southwestern Medical Center, Dallas, Texas

David C. Teague, MD, FACS Associate Professor, Henry James Freede Chair in Orthopaedic Surgery, Interim Chairman, Department of Orthopaedic Surgery and Rehabilitation, University of Oklahoma College of Medicine, Oklahoma City, Oklahoma

David C. Templeman, MD Assistant Professor of Orthopaedic Surgery, University of Minnesota, Department of Orthopaedics, Hennepin County Medical Center, Minneapolis, Minnesota

Alan F. Tencer, PhD Professor of Orthopaedics and Sports Medicine, Orthopaedic Science Laboratory, Harborview Medical Center, University of Washington, Seattle, Washington

Paul Tornetta III, MD Professor of Orthopaedic Surgery, Boston University School of Medicine, Director of Orthopaedic Trauma, Boston University Medical Center, Boston, Massachusetts

Eleftherios Tsiridis, MD, FRCS Orthopaedic Research Fellow, Department of Orthopaedic Surgery, Boston University School of Medicine, Boston, Massachusetts

Jon J.P. Warner, MD, BA Chief, The Harvard Shoulder Service, Professor of Orthopaedic Surgery, Harvard Medical School, Massachusetts General and Brigham and Women's Hospitals, Boston, Massachusetts

Daniel C. Wascher, MD Professor of Sports Medicine, Department of Orthopaedics and Rehabilitation, University of New Mexico, University of New Mexico Hospital, University of New Mexico Health Sciences Center, Albuquerque, New Mexico

J. Tracy Watson, MD Professor of Orthopaedic Surgery, Chief, Division of Orthopaedic Traumatology, Saint Louis University School of Medicine, St. Louis, Missouri

Kristy L. Weber, MD Associate Professor of Orthopaedic Surgery, Johns Hopkins University, Baltimore, Maryland

Gerald R. Williams, Jr., MD Professor of Orthopaedic Surgery, Chief, Shoulder and Elbow Service, University of Pennsylvania, Chief, Orthopaedic Surgery, Presbyterian Medical Center, Philadelphia, Pennsylvania

Mark C. Willis, Jr., MD Assistant Professor of Orthopaedic Surgery, Director of Trauma Surgery, Virginia Commonwealth University, Richmond, Virginia

Michael A. Wirth, MD Professor of Orthopaedics, The Charles A. Rockwood, Jr, MD, Chair of Orthopaedics, University of Texas Health Science Center, Chief of Shoulder Service, South Texas Veterans Health Care System—Audie L. Murphy Division, University Hospital, San Antonio, Texas

Bruce H. Ziran, MD Associate Professor of Orthopaedic Surgery, Northeast Ohio Universities College of Medicine, Director of Orthopaedic Trauma, St. Elizabeth Health Center, Youngstown, Ohio

Joseph D. Zuckerman, MD Professor and Chairman of Orthopaedic Surgery, New York University Hospital for Joint Diseases, New York, New York

PREFACE

The original edition of *Rockwood and Green* listed several defined goals which the subsequent four editions maintained and met. Drs. Rockwood and Green were keen to present the historical context and pathological anatomy of all fractures and dislocations and to provide a comprehensive discussion of the different management alternatives as well as the "author's preferred treatment," a phrase that has become synonymous with the text. This format has been maintained in the 6th edition, although the historical sections in many of the chapters have been condensed. However, in many other aspects this edition marks a turning point in the history of the book itself.

When the original edition was published in 1975, it is unlikely that many surgeons realized just how much the management of orthopaedic trauma was destined to evolve and change over the next 30 years. The management of the multiply injured patient was just beginning to improve but most fractures were treated nonoperatively, and fracture union, rather than optimal patient outcome, was the yardstick of success. Later editions have documented the expansion of operative fracture fixation, but the pace of change has accelerated and this is reflected in the 6th edition.

There are five more chapters than in the 5th edition, and nearly two-thirds of the authors are new to *Rockwood and Green*. All have been chosen because of their expertise in a particular field of skeletal trauma and most represent the younger generation of orthopaedic trauma surgeons. The new chapters reflect new trends. There are chapters on epidemiology and osteoporotic fractures which reflect a rapidly changing patient population and the rising power of the grey vote! Chapters dealing with the enhancement of fracture healing, outcome studies, imaging, and surgical navigation demonstrate the importance of new techniques, whereas a number of chapters such as those dealing with the multiply injured patient, war wounds and limb salvage, compartment syndrome, periprosthetic fractures, and complications have been significantly altered in response to changing new surgical technology. We believe that they all enhance the quality of this edition. Two CDs have also been included in the book. These contain narrated videos of upper and lower limb surgical approaches performed on cadavers. They demonstrate the anatomy and safety zones during tissue dissection. We believe that they will prove helpful to surgeons and have set an icon on pages to indicate a correlation between text and video.

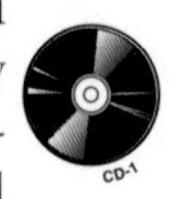

We are conscious of the difficulty of producing the definitive text on skeletal trauma without increasing the size of the book. We have attempted to expand the use of tables and to condense the text and references where possible. Pearls and pitfalls of care, a popular addition to the 5th edition, has been maintained and expanded.

The most obvious change is that this edition has a distinctly international flavor. Skeletal trauma is an international discipline, and surgeons from many parts of the world have contributed to the new ideas and techniques detailed in this book. Much of the current cutting edge research and technology changing the face of orthopaedic trauma care originates from Europe, Australia, Asia, and South America. Nineteen of the authors (from eight different countries) are based outside the United States. We believe that this broadens and improves the scope of the book. It will also ensure that *Rockwood and Green* remains the first reference for orthopaedic trauma care for the estimated 175,000 practicing orthopaedic surgeons in the world.

Keeping up with the pace of change gets more difficult and the editorial board of the 6th edition has been expanded to include associate editors Paul Tornetta, Michael Wirth, and Ken Koval. Their industry has been impressive and we are grateful to them.

Robert W. Bucholz
James D. Heckman
Charles M. Court-Brown

ROCKWOOD AND GREEN'S

FRACTURES IN ADULTS

SIXTH EDITION

SECTION

ONE

GENERAL PRINCIPLES

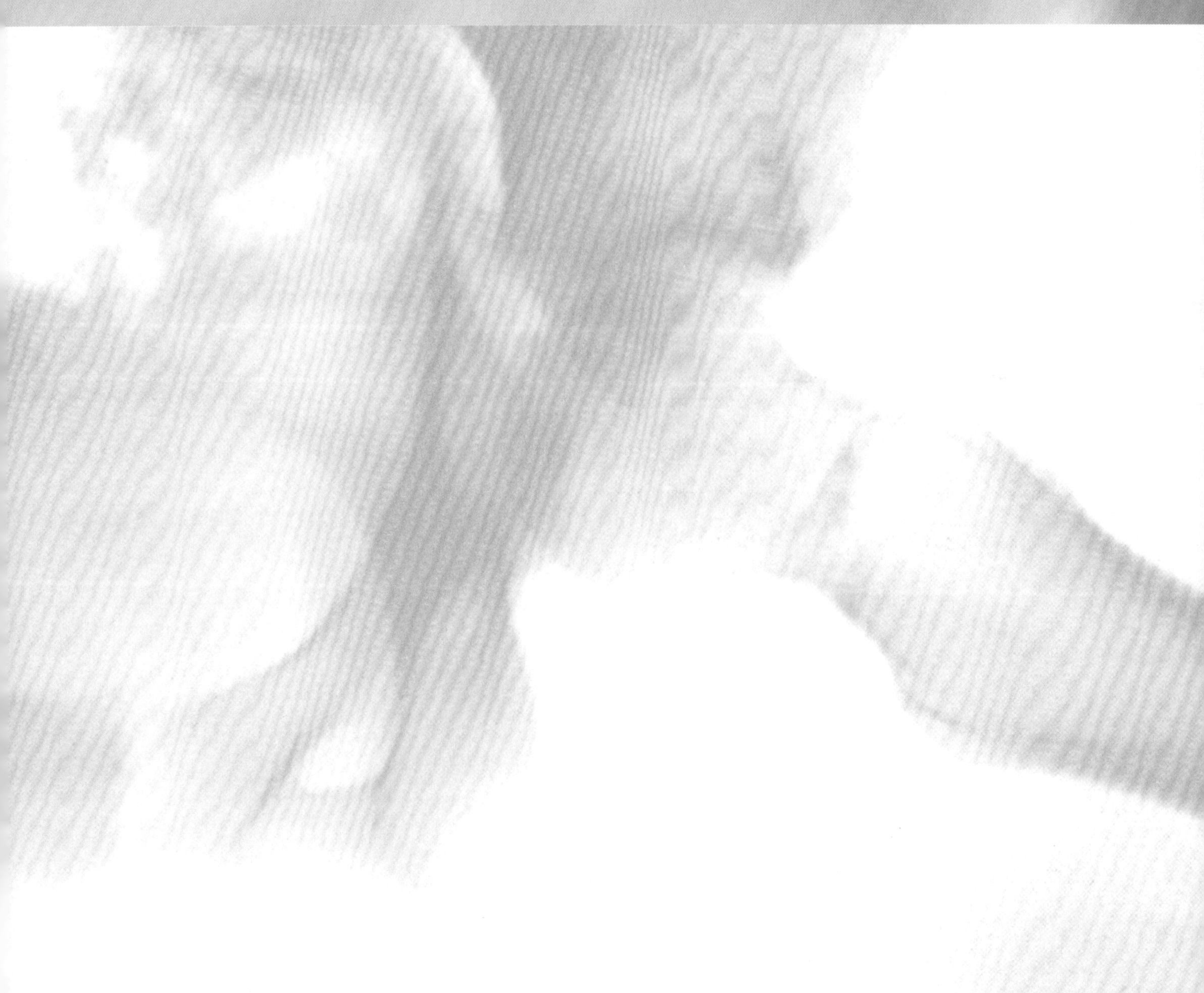

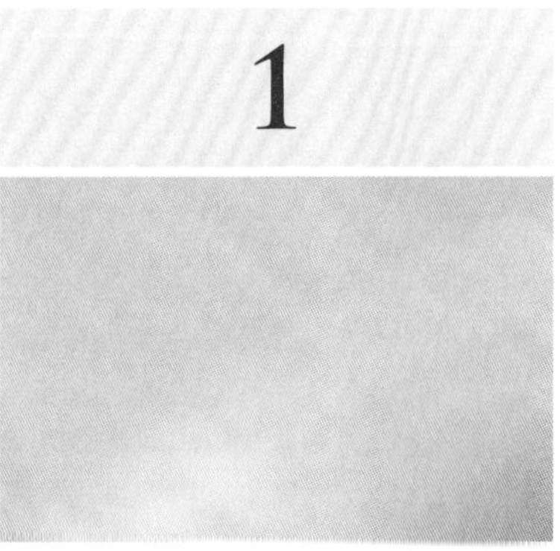

BIOMECHANICS OF FIXATION AND FRACTURES

Allan F. Tencer

This chapter provides a fundamental discussion of the concepts of biomechanics, demonstrates how these ideas describe the basic functions of fixation devices, and illustrates how they can be used to avoid clinical problems associated with the mechanics of fracture fixation. Emphasis has been placed on addressing practical problems. First, fundamental concepts of mechanics as they apply to the practice of orthopaedic fractures are explained. This section is followed by a short discussion on the mechanical organization of bone, its ability to carry load, and the relationship of applied forces and specific fracture patterns. A discussion of bone injury mechanisms, including specific mechanisms observed in car crashes, is next presented. Description of the mechanics of healing bone follows, which is relevant to understanding the timing of applying load to healing fractures in patients. Finally, the performance of various types of fixation systems is discussed, with emphasis on fixation of difficult fractures, such as the femoral neck, and those involving osteoporotic bone. The focus of the discussion is not on comparing the myriad number of specific devices available, but rather on demonstrating the common mechanical principles involved in fracture fixation, so that potential problems common to various devices can be recognized and avoided.

In the study of biomechanics as it relates to fracture fixation, the fundamental mechanical question remains: Is the fixation system stiff and strong enough to allow the patient early mobility, before bony union is complete, without delaying healing, creating bone deformity, or damaging the implant, and yet flexible enough to stimulate union? The issue of which brand of fixation is strongest or stiffest is not specifically addressed because that is not the standard by which different devices should be judged. Within a range of fixation stiffness it has been shown that bone will heal, and the amount of stabilizing callus depends on the stiffness of the fixation.

BASIC CONCEPTS

Before describing the performance of fracture fixation systems, some basic concepts used in biomechanics will be introduced. As Figure 1-1 demonstrates, loads in many different directions may act on a fixed fracture, including body weight and forces induced by muscle contraction and ligament tension. A *force* causes an object to either accelerate or decelerate. It has *magnitude* (strength) and acts in a specific direction; therefore, it is termed a *vector*. However complex the system of forces acting on a bone, each force may be separated into its vector components, and any number of components acting in the same direction can be summed to yield the net or *resultant force*. For example, consider the force acting at the shoe/floor interface during ambulation. It can be separated into a vertical force due to body weight and a horizontal frictional force, which produces the forward thrust. Similarly, muscle forces can be separated in the same manner—one force along the axis of the long bone, and one perpendicular. The components of the different forces, which act in the same direction, can be added, and the resultant force acting on the bone can then be found. This concept is important when designing fracture fixation systems because it allows the designer to size the implants so that they can withstand the mechanical loads applied without failure.

The two major loads acting on a long bone are those that cause it to displace in a linear direction (translation), and those that cause it to rotate, typically around a joint center. Muscles typically cause a bone to rotate (e.g., the biceps causes the forearm to rotate, the anterior tibialis causes the foot to dorsiflex). When a force causes rotation, it is termed a *moment* and has a *moment arm*. The moment arm is the lever arm against which the force acts to cause rotation. It is the perpendicular distance of the muscle force from the center of rotation of the joint. As shown in Figure 1-2, the moment or rotary force is affected not only by the magnitude of the force applied, but also by its distance from the center of rotation. In the example, two moments act on the outstretched arm. The weight carried in the hand rotates the arm downward, while the balancing muscle force rotates the arm upward. Equilibrium is reached by balancing the moments so that the arm does not rotate and the weight can be carried. Note that to achieve this, the muscle force must be eight times as large as the weight of the object, arm, and hand because its moment arm or distance from the center of the joint is only one-eighth as long.

The basic forces—compression, transverse loading, torsion, and bending, cause bone to behave in predictable ways. A *compressive force* (Fig. 1-3) results in shortening the length of the bone, while *tension* elongates it. *Torsion* causes twisting of the bone about its long axis, whereas *bending* causes it to bow at the center. The forces and moments that act on a long bone during functional use produce three basic stresses on the healing fracture region: tension, compression, and *shear* (because all forces can be combined to their basic components as shown previously). *Stress*, as shown in Figure 1-4, is simply the force divided by the area over which it acts. This is a convenient way to express how the force affects a material locally. For example, comparing two bones, one with half the cross-sectional area of the other, if the smaller bone is subjected to half the force of

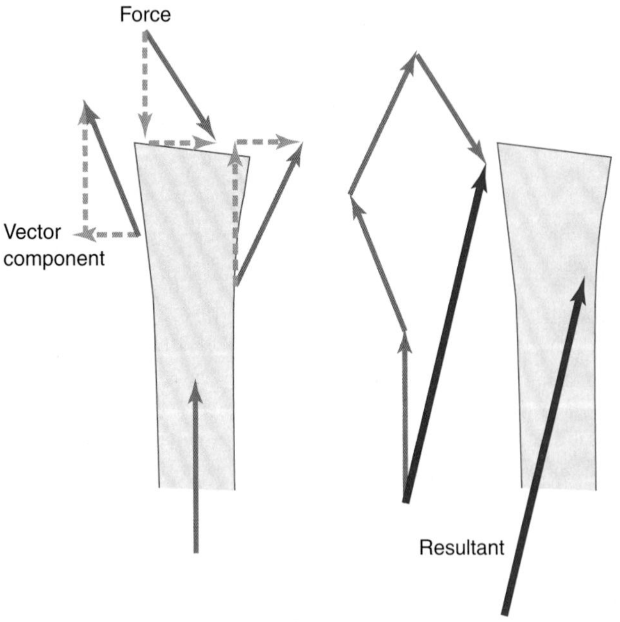

FIGURE 1-1 Forces acting on a long bone during functional use. A vector indicates that the force has both magnitude and direction. The complex system of forces can be split into components acting perpendicular and parallel to the ground, or the axis of the bone.

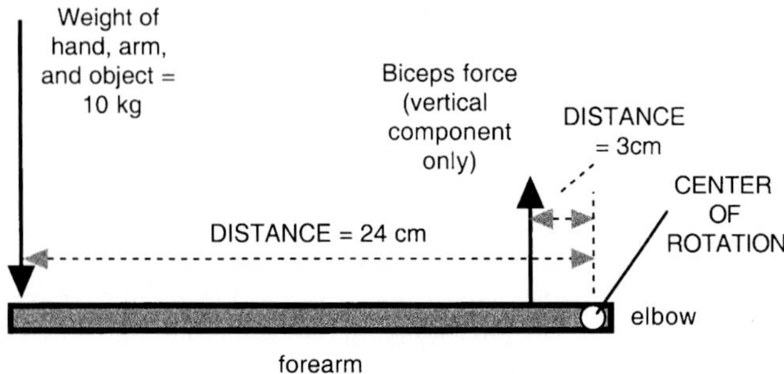

Balance moments to hold arm steady:
24 cm x 10 N = 3 cm x Biceps force
Biceps force = 80 N

FIGURE 1-2 In this example, the outstretched arm is a lever. The moment or load that rotates the arm downward around the elbow, the center of rotation, is defined as the product of the weight of the object arm and hand × distance from the elbow (in this example for simplicity, the center of gravity of the hand, arm, and object are combined). This moment must be counteracted by a moment in the opposite direction, due to the vertical component of the biceps muscle acting through its lever, which is smaller than the lever arm of the weight arm and hand. The biceps force is then calculated from (10 kg × 24 cm)/3 cm = 80 kg. The biceps force is much greater than the weight of the object arm and hand because its lever arm is smaller.

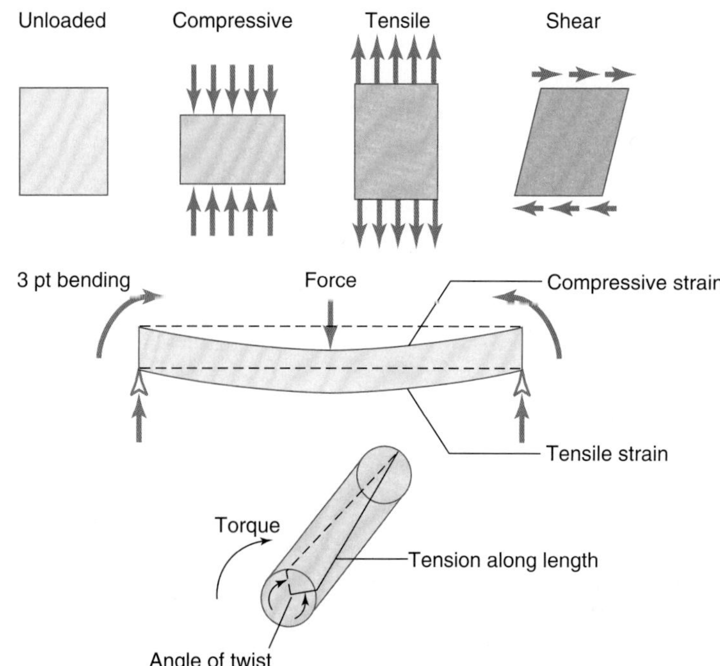

FIGURE 1-3 Basic forces acting on a long bone and the deflection of the bone in response **(top)**. Compression shortens the length, tension increases the length, shear distorts the length **(middle),** bending causes the bone to bow, and **(bottom)** torsion results in twisting about the long axis.

the larger bone, the stress experienced by each bone would be the same. Therefore, a smaller woman with less weight has proportionally smaller bones to keep the stresses on the bone tissue similar to that of a larger and heavier man. The stresses acting on fracture callus as a result of the different forces, in an idealized case, are shown in Figure 1-5. Just as stress is normalized force (force per unit area), length changes can also be normalized. *Strain* is simply the change in height or length that a bone undergoes during loading divided by its original height or length, as shown in Figure 1-4. Under the same force, a bone twice as long will have twice the length change, but dividing the length change by the original length of the bone

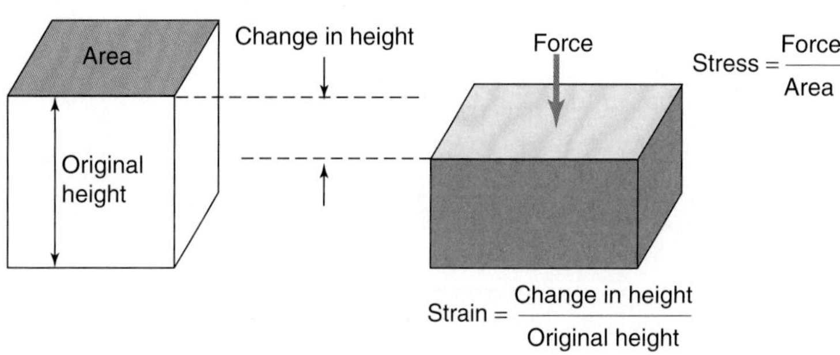

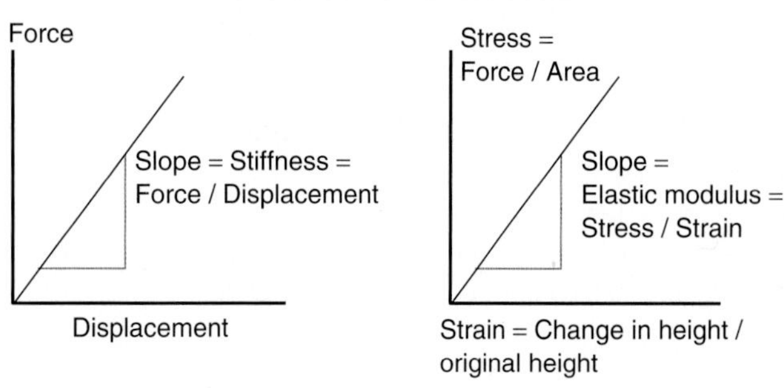

FIGURE 1-4 The stress is defined as the force acting on a surface divided by the area over which it acts. Strain is the change in height or length of the object under load divided by its original height or length. Stiffness is defined as the slope of a force versus displacement graph, i.e., the change in force divided by the corresponding change in displacement. Elastic modulus is the corresponding slope, but of a stress versus strain graph.

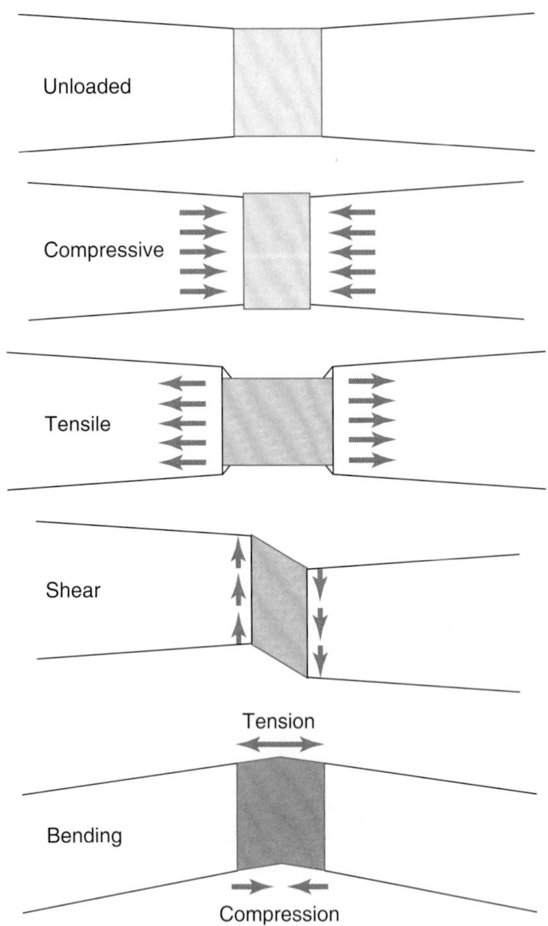

FIGURE 1-5 Resulting stresses acting in fracture callus in a idealized case with each of the basic forces applied (top to bottom): unloaded, compressive stresses along the bone axis and expansive stresses perpendicular to the bone axis due to compression, tensile and contraction stresses due to tension, distortion due to shearing and tension on the convex side, compression on the concave side, and internal shearing due to bending.

shows that the strain is the same in both cases. (If both bones are composed of the same materials, they should both have approximately the same strain under a given stress.)

Mechanical testing of fractured long bones with fixation devices applied demonstrates a specific type of behavior, as shown in Figure 1-6. This diagram represents the data measured in an experimental test of the *structural properties* of the bone-fixation construct—that is, the properties of the fixation device and bone combined. *Material properties* relate to the properties of the substances that make up each component (bone, stainless steel, titanium). As load is applied to the construct in a testing machine, the construct deforms. This deformation is termed *elastic* because when the load is removed, the construct will return to its original shape (an important consideration in preventing malalignment of the bone fracture components). At some loads, however, the construct becomes overloaded, entering the *plastic* range. If the load is released after loading in the plastic range but before failure, some *permanent deformation* remains in the construct. Practically, this represents a bent plate, fixator, or rod with a malaligned fracture. The point at which elastic behavior changes to plastic is termed the *yield point*. The elastic range represents the working range for the fixation construct. Its two most important properties are its yield point, which defines its safe functional load and its stiffness, or the amount it deforms under load in the elastic range. (A third very important property, fatigue, will be discussed later.) Note that a fixation construct may have different yield points and degrees of stiffness for loads acting in different directions. An example is a half-pin external fixator construct applied to a tibia, with the pins oriented anteriorly-posteriorly. The stiffness is much greater in anterior-posterior bending than medial-lateral bending for this construct. Another property to consider is the *work done* in deforming a fixation construct. The product of the force applied and the distance the construct bends is defined as the work done, and is represented by the area under the force-displacement graph of Figure 1-6. *Toughness* can be defined as the work carried out to fracture a construct or material, including both the elastic and plastic regions of deformation. A material may be flexible and tough (e.g., rubber, or a child's bone that deforms but is difficult to break) or stiff but *brittle* (e.g., glass, elderly bone), if it cannot absorb much deformation without fracturing.

The factors that govern stiffness and yield point are the material from which the fixation device is made and its shape (considering an ununited fracture in which the fracture callus contributes little to structural properties). A construct made of higher elastic modulus materials will be stiffer (e.g., stainless steel as compared to titanium). Stiffness of a construct is found by dividing the force applied by the deformation that the construct exhibited. The *elastic (or Young's)* modulus is determined by dividing the stress applied by the resulting strain. Unlike whole constructs, where it is difficult to determine stress (because it is hard to define the area over which the force is applied and at least two different materials are involved), uniform blocks of materials can be characterized by their elastic modulus. The moduli of some common orthopaedic materials are given in Table 1-1. As shown, the elastic modulus of titanium alloy is about one-half that of stainless steel so, given two plates of the same size and shape, the one made of titanium would be expected to have about one-half the stiffness of the stainless steel plate.

The shape of the implant is important in determining the loads that it can support. As shown in Figure 1-7, the same wooden 2 × 4 beam that bends easily when load is applied to its wider surface, becomes much stiffer when load is applied to its narrower surface. This is because, in the latter case, the material of the 2 × 4 resisting the load is distributed farther away from the center of the beam (note that in this example, the material of the beam did not change, just its orientation relative to the load applied). This concept of distribution of material is reflected in the shape property, *moment of inertia*. The moment of inertia provides a measure of how the material is distributed in the cross section of the object relative to the load applied to

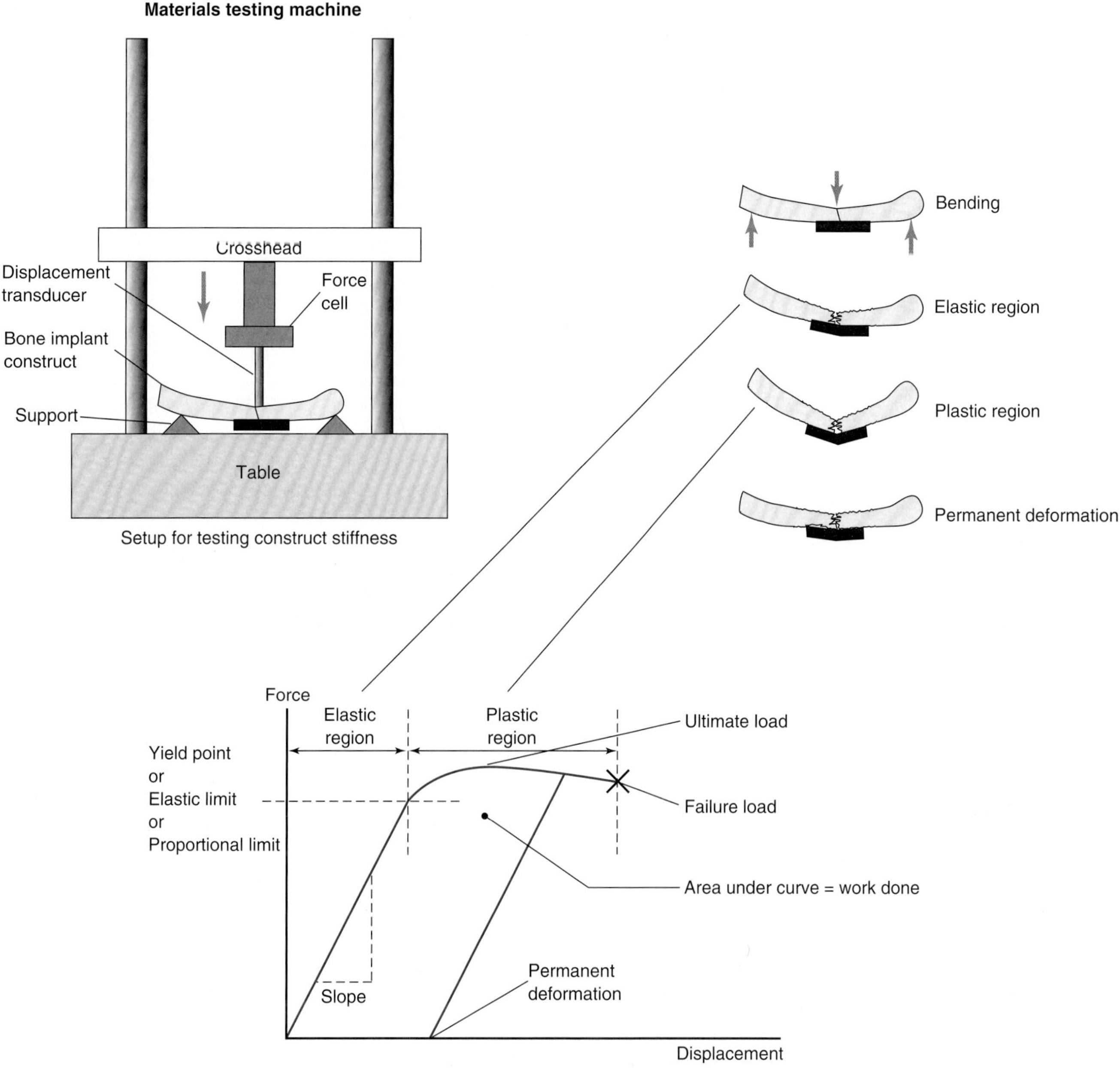

FIGURE 1-6 **Top left.** A fixation construct (bone-fixation-bone) set up in a mechanical testing machine. In this example, a long bone is fixed with a plate and subjected to bending. **Top right.** The construct during loading in the elastic region, plastic region, and with permanent deformation. **Bottom.** The resulting measurements from the testing machine that measures force applied and displacement at the point of the applied load. The graph demonstrates the elastic region where the construct acts like a spring, returning to its original shape after the load is released, the plastic region where the plate may have permanently bent, and the failure load where the fixation fails.

it. The farther away the material is from the center of the beam, the greater its stiffness will be. Steel I beams were developed to take advantage of this concept—greater stiffness using less material. For cylindrical objects like rods, pins, or screws, their stiffness is related to the fourth power of their diameter. This is why, as shown in Figure 1-7, for rods made of the same materials and of similar thickness, a 16-mm-diameter intramedullary (IM) rod is 1.7 times as stiff as a 14-mm rod $[(16/14)^4]$, and a 7-mm-diameter pedicle screw is 1.85 times as stiff as a 6-mm-diameter screw.

TABLE 1-1 Basic Engineering Properties of Common Engineering Materials

Material	Ultimate Strength Tensile (MPa)	Ultimate Strength Compressive (MPa)	Yield Strength 0.2% Offset (MPa)	Elastic Modulus (MPa)
Muscle	0.2			
Skin	8			50
Cartilage	4	10		20
Fascia	10			
Tendon	70			400
Cortical bone	100	175	80	15,000
Cancellous bone	2	3		1,000
Plaster of paris	70	75	20	
Polyethylene	40	20	20	1,000
PTFE Teflon	25			500
Acrylic bone cement	40	80		2,000
Titanium (pure, cold worked)	500		400	100,000
Titanium (Al-4V) (alloy F 136)	900		800	100,000
Stainless steel (316 L) (annealed)	>500		>200	200,000
Stainless steel (cold worked)	>850		>700	200,000
Cobalt chrome (cast)	>450		>50	20,000
Cobalt chrome (wrought, annealed)	>300		>300	230,000
Cobalt chrome (wrought, cold work)	1,500		1,000	230,000
Super alloys (CoNiMo)	1,800		1,600	230,000

MPa, megapascal.
(Ultimate tensile strength or maximum force in tension, yield strength at 0.2% offset, the strength at which the strain in the material [change in length/original length] is 0.2%, a usual standard for metals, elastic modulus or stress/strain).

A third important property of a fracture fixation construct is its ability to resist *fatigue* under cyclic loading. A load can be applied below the yield point of the construct, yet progressively create a crack that grows until the local force in the region of the crack is above yield and the construct fails. Some materials have an endurance limit below which they can support loads indefinitely without failure. An important aspect to fatigue performance of a fixation construct is the effect of a *stress concentrator*. In completely uniform materials, the stresses, in tension for example, will be almost identical throughout the material. Fixation devices have holes, screw threads, and other features where shape changes occur. In a very radical change in shape, for example, as shown in Figure 1-8, the sharp corner between threads of a different diameter in a fixation screw causes a stress concentrator at the corner. This explains why the base of a screw thread, where it meets the shaft of the screw, has rounded corners. The stresses on a fracture construct are increased when applied in heavier patients, with poor bone-to-bone contact

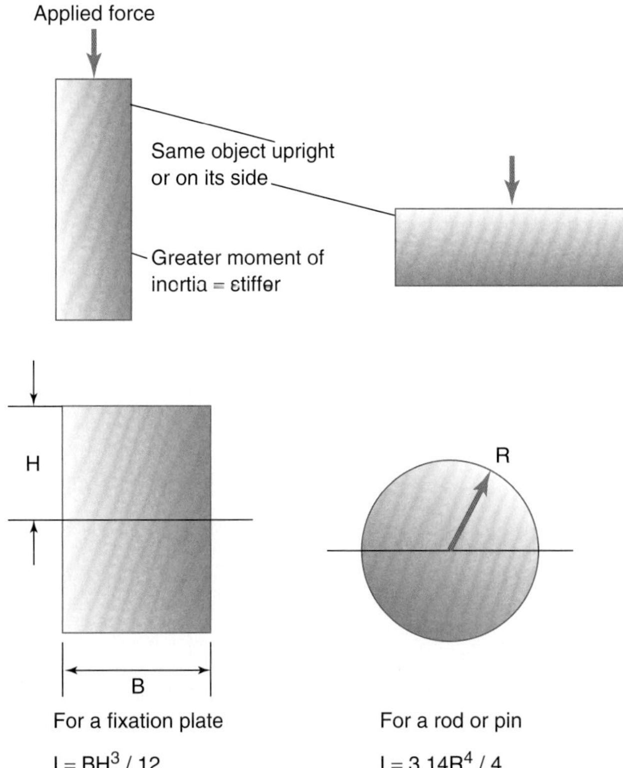

FIGURE 1-7 Concept of moment of inertia or the effect of the geometry of an object on its stiffness. **Top.** Looking at the edge of a wood 2 × 4 (used in home building), left, the 2 × 4 with the load applied on the shorter side is stiffer than the same 2 × 4 with the load applied on its long edge. The area of the 2 × 4 is farther away from the central axis when the load is applied on the short edge. **Bottom.** The *moment of inertia* is a term used to describe how the material is distributed within an object. Left, for a plate, looking at its edge, the moment of inertia and the stiffness increase directly with the plate's width and the cube of its height. For a tube, such as an IM rod, the moment of inertia increases with the fourth power of its diameter. Therefore, a 16-mm-diameter IM rod is 1.7 times as stiff as a 14-mm rod and 2.3 times as stiff as a 13-mm rod, if all the rods have the same thickness and are made of the same material.

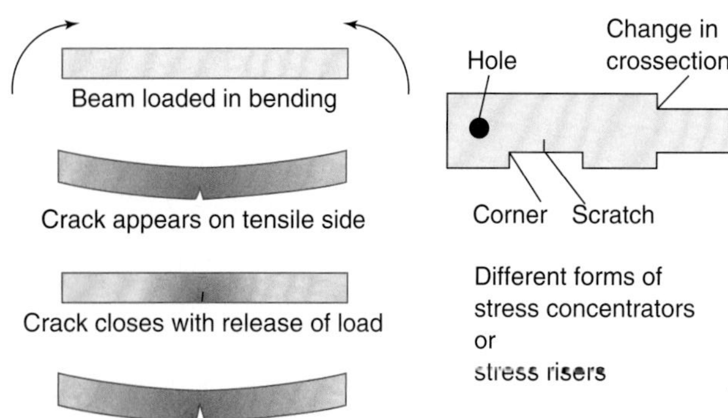

FIGURE 1-8 A stress concentrator is a region of an object where stresses are higher than in the surrounding material. **Left.** Taking the example of a fracture plate subjected to bending, the bottom surface elongates under load. In the region of highest tensile forces, a scratch starts to grow into a crack that closes when the load is released, then reopens slightly larger with the next load cycle, eventually growing to a point where the plate fails. Crack growth is accentuated by stress corrosion, poor bone-to-bone contact at the fracture, and by loads applied by heavier patients. **Right.** Stress concentrators (sometimes referred to as *stress risers*) occur around holes, sharp corners, scratches, and at corners from changes in cross section.

across the fracture site, delayed union, early weight bearing before the fracture has united, and when smaller low-profile fixation devices are used. For these circumstances, consider the use of larger implants, taking care not to create stress concentrators by scuffing or scratching the implant, and delay weight bearing until some fracture consolidation is apparent. These steps can increase the number of load cycles that the implant can bear without failure.

A scratch can also cause a local small stress concentrator. When immersed in the saline environment of the body, *stress corrosion* can occur. Stress corrosion combines the effects of the local growth of the crack due to cyclic loading with galvanic corrosion. A *galvanic cell* describes a local environment where electrons flow from the more negative to the more positive material when immersed in a liquid conductor (saline, in this case) (Fig. 1-9). Material is actually removed from the more negative electrode, such as the surface of the plate during galvanic corrosion. In a fixed fracture, the dissimilar materials are the surface of the plate, for example, stainless steel, which has an oxide surface coating and the same material within the just-opening crack that has not yet developed the oxide film. The conductive fluid is the blood and saline found in the surrounding tissues. Galvanic corrosion can accelerate the failure of an implant, even when the implant is loaded well below its yield point, by increasing the rate at which the crack grows, because along with yielding at the site of the crack, material at the crack is being removed by the corrosion process. Another mechanism of corrosion, termed *fretting*, results when the surfaces of two implants rub together—for example, the head of a screw against the surface of the plate through which it passes. *Crevice corrosion*, not common in modern orthopaedic materials, results from small galvanic cells formed by impurities in the surface of the implant, causing crevices as the material corrodes (1).

A final basic property is *viscoelasticity*. Biologic materials do not act as pure springs when load is applied to them. For example, if a load is applied to a tendon, and the load is maintained for a period of time, the tissue will continue to deform or *creep*. This is the basic principal behind stretching exercises. Under a constant load, a metal fixation plate will deform and remain at that deformation until the load is removed (elastic behavior). In contrast, the tendon both deforms elastically and creeps, exhibiting both viscous and elastic behavior. This property has important implications for certain types of fixation, especially those that rely on loading of soft tissues, such as in certain types of spinal fixation (to be discussed later in this chapter).

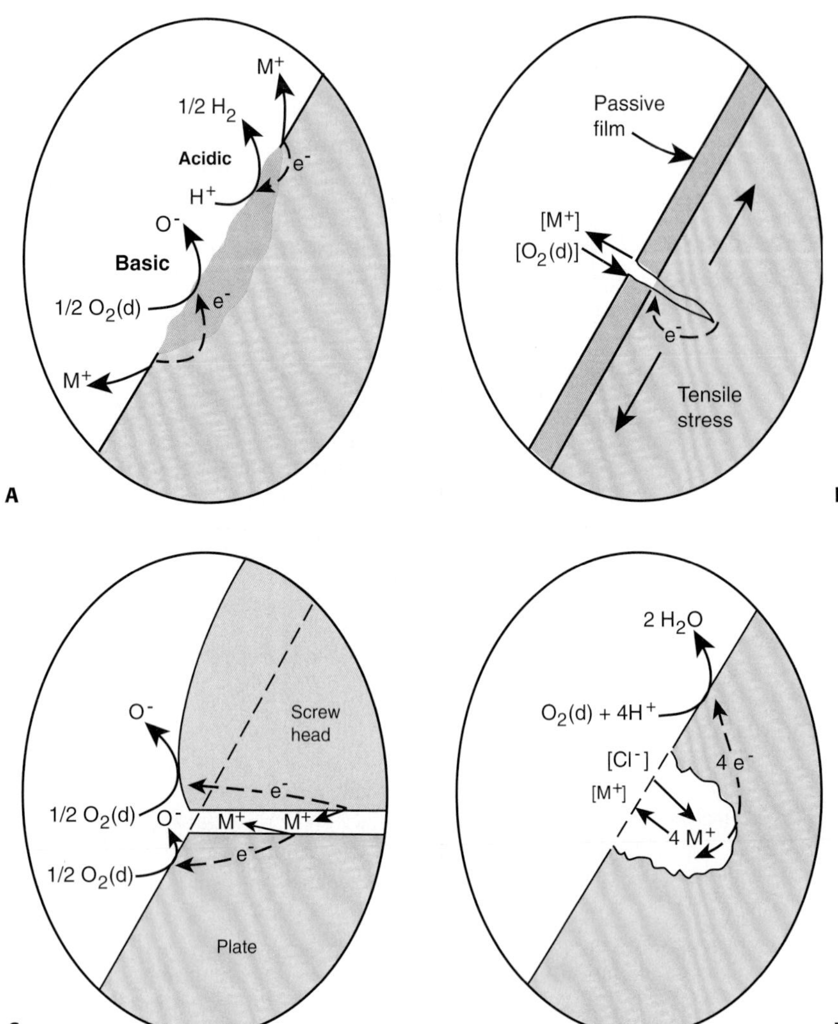

FIGURE 1-9 **A.** Illustration of crevice corrosion with a local galvanic cell caused by an impurity in the surface of a plate and ions, M +, being released, resulting in loss of material and formation of a crevice. **B.** Stress corrosion occurs by a local galvanic cell setup between the material at the tip of the crack, which just opened and has not oxidized and the remaining oxidized surface of the plate. The released ions enhance crack growth occurring from loading. **C.** Fretting corrosion caused by the loss of the oxide layer on the plate's surface due to rubbing of the base of the screw against the plate. **D.** Galvanic corrosion around a scratch or pit in the plate (1).

A second property is *loading rate dependence*. In simple terms, stretching a soft tissue can be thought of as stretching two components, one elastic and one viscous, which make up that tissue. For example, consider a spring connected in a series to the handle of a syringe (Fig. 1-10). When a compressive force is applied, the spring instantly compresses, representing the elastic response of the tissue. The syringe plunger starts to displace and continues as it pushes fluid through the orifice. If the force is held constant, the plunger will continue to move, representing the viscous creep of the tissue. If the compressive force is applied slowly, the syringe handle offers little resistance. As the rate of force application increases, the resistance of the syringe to motion increases. This represents the increase in stiffness of the tissue at higher loading rates. That is, the stiffness of the tissue depends on the rate at which the load is applied. A well-known example of loading rate dependence relates to ligament and bone failure. At low loading rates, ligament is weaker than bone, and the ligament fails generally in midsubstance. At higher loading rates, the ligament becomes stiffer, and failure may occur by avulsion of the bony attachment of the ligament. *Stress relaxation* occurs if the applied force, instead of increasing, is held constant. As the fluid flows out of the syringe, without further movement of the plunger, the internal force decreases. These three properties, creep, stress relaxation, and load rate dependence, make up the basic tissue viscoelastic properties. Keep in mind that the model used in this discussion is a simple linear series model, for explanation purposes only. More complex models using combinations of these basic components have successfully described the observed tissue properties. Another example of tissue viscoelasticity, besides tendon and other soft tissues, is found in trabecular bone, e.g., spinal vertebrae. In this case, the trabecular structure acts as the spring component, while forcing the interstitial fluid through the porous matrix, as the trabeculae deform represents the viscous component. Under higher loading rates, there is resistance to flow, increasing the internal pressure, and therefore, the stiffness of the structure. These effects have been observed at high loading rates, such as during fracture, as shown in Figure 1-11 (2).

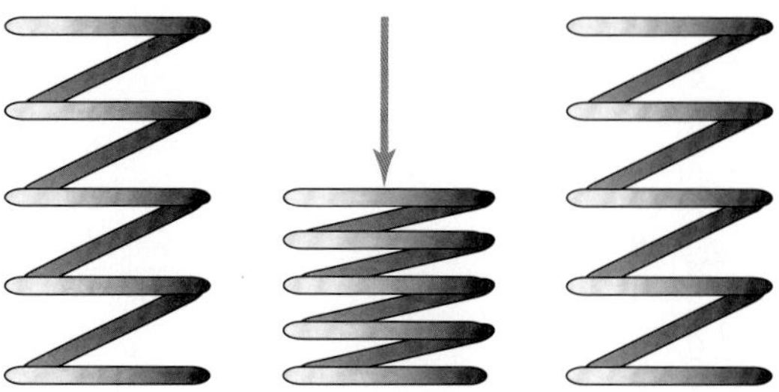

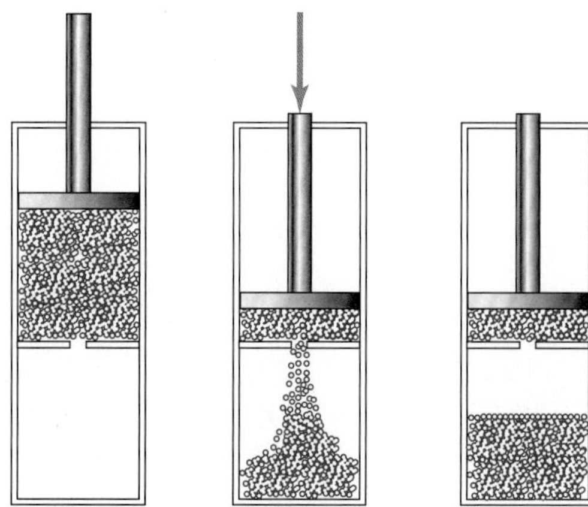

FIGURE 1-10 Viscoelastic response is explained in this simple model consisting of an elastic or spring component that instantly compresses when a load is applied to it, connected in series with a viscous component, modeled here as a syringe, through which a fluid is forced. Loading the syringe's handle with a constant force causes it to continue to creep or displace, in contrast with the spring, which reaches its final displacement instantly. Further, if the force is applied to the syringe handle more rapidly, there is greater resistance to motion, explaining the increased stiffness of tissue to increased rates of loading.

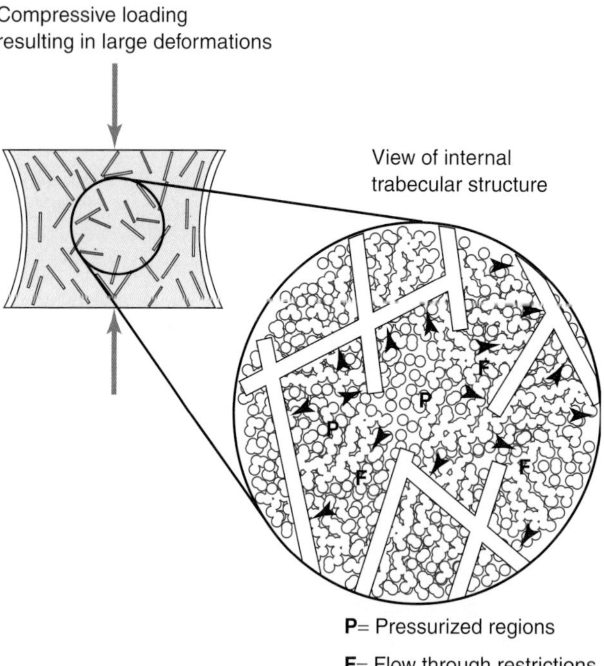

FIGURE 1-11 Trabecular bone possesses some features of the spring and syringe viscoelastic model described in Figure 1-10, although it should be appreciated that this is an idealized model. The trabecular structure acts as the spring element. At higher loading rates, the interstitial fluid resists flowing through the trabecular spaces, causing increased internal pressure, and therefore, long bone stiffness. This anatomical feature allows vertebrae and the metaphyseal ends of long bones to resist dynamic loads caused by rapidly applied forces (2).

In summary, bones and joints can be subjected to a wide variety of forces, but these forces can be resolved into basic components that create tension, compression, shearing, twisting, and bending. These forces cause internal, compressive, tensile, and shear stresses in the tissue. The stiffness of a fixation construct used to stabilize a fracture describes how much it deforms under a given load acting in a specific direction. Stiffness may vary with direction and is highly dependent on the shape of the fixation construct. The effect of shape is described by the moment of inertia. In combination with the moment of inertia, the elastic modulus of the material describes how stiff the fixation will be under load and its ability to withstand the forces of, for example, the patient's weight during ambulation. Failure of fixation can come not only from loading above its yield point but also as a result of repetitive stress. Repetitive loading can cause growth of a crack at a stress concentrator and can be significantly accentuated by corrosion when the implant is immersed in bodily fluids. Biologic tissues behave viscoelastically and can creep under constant load, stress relax when the elongation is fixed, and increase stiffness as the rate of load application increases. In this chapter, these mechanical properties are described in basic units of measurements, defined in Table 1-2.

TABLE 1-2 Definitions of the Units Used to Describe the Basic Properties of Fracture Constructs

Force, newtons (N) 1 N ~ 0.254 lb

Displacement, millimeters (mm)

Stress, pressure, modulus, megapascals (MPa) where 1 MPa = force of 1 N/area of 1 mm^2

Modulus = stress/strain, where stress units are MPa, strain has no units

Strain (no units), strain = change in length (mm)/original length (mm)

BIOMECHANICS OF INTACT AND HEALING BONE

Bone can be considered to have a hierarchical structure. As shown in Figure 1-12, the lowest level of the structure consists of single collagen fibrils with embedded apatite crystals. At this level of structure, changing the collagen-to-mineral ratio has a significant effect on the elastic modulus of bone (2–4), as it decreases with loss of mineral (Fig. 1-13). This is important from a fracture healing perspective because mineralizing healing callus goes through phases of increasing mineral density and corresponding increased modulus as healing occurs. At the next level of structural organization, the orientation of the collagen fibrils is important (5–11). As demonstrated in Figure 1-14, the orientation of its fibers affects the ability of bone to support loads in specific directions. During fracture healing, the callus initially starts as a disorganized random array of fibers, which progressively reorganizes to become stiffest along the directions of the major applied loads (body weight and muscle forces) that the bone is exposed to. At the next level, the density of the haversion systems affects bone strength. It has been repeatedly demonstrated that there is a power law relationship between bone density and strength at this level of structure (Fig. 1-15). This means that as bone density decreases, its strength decreases as the square of its density (as density decreases by half, strength decreases by a factor of 4). This forms the basis for predicting changes in bone strength due to osteoporosis, for example. Sim-

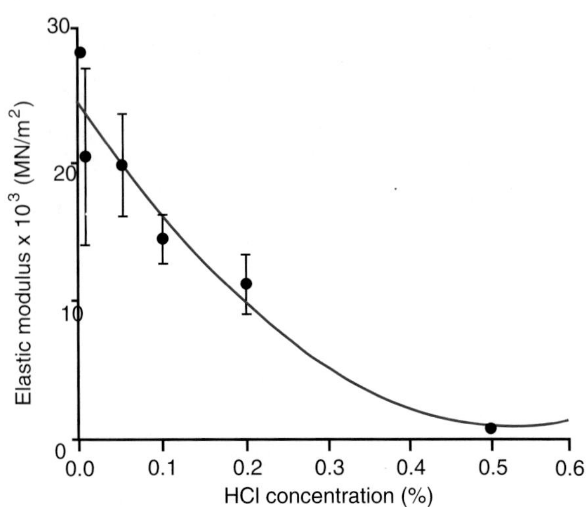

FIGURE 1-13 Elastic modulus of bone samples tested in tension after exposure to different concentrations of HCl. Greater HCl concentration progressively demineralizes bone, leaving ultimately, only collagen. This diagram illustrates the contribution of bone mineral to the tensile elastic modulus of whole bone (3).

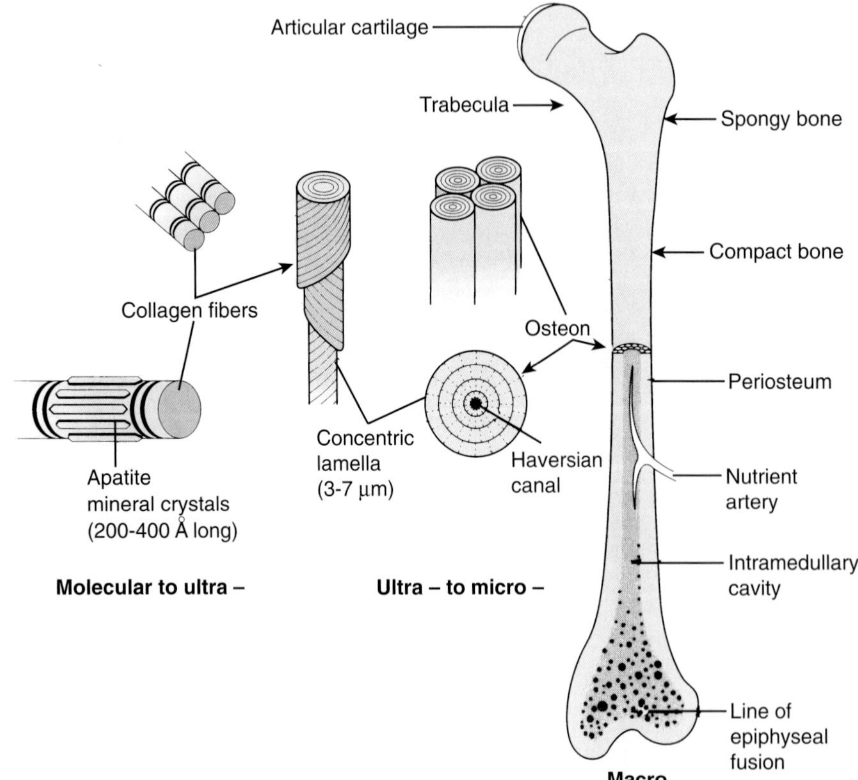

FIGURE 1-12 The hierarchical structure of bone is demonstrated. At the lowest level of organization, the ratio of mineral crystals to collagen fibrils determines elastic modulus of the combined material, as shown in Figure 1-13. At the next level, the fiber orientation is important in determining the difference in bone strength in various directions. At the final level, the lamellae of bone fibers form haversian systems, which particularly in trabecular bone, are oriented in the direction of the major loads that the bone must support.

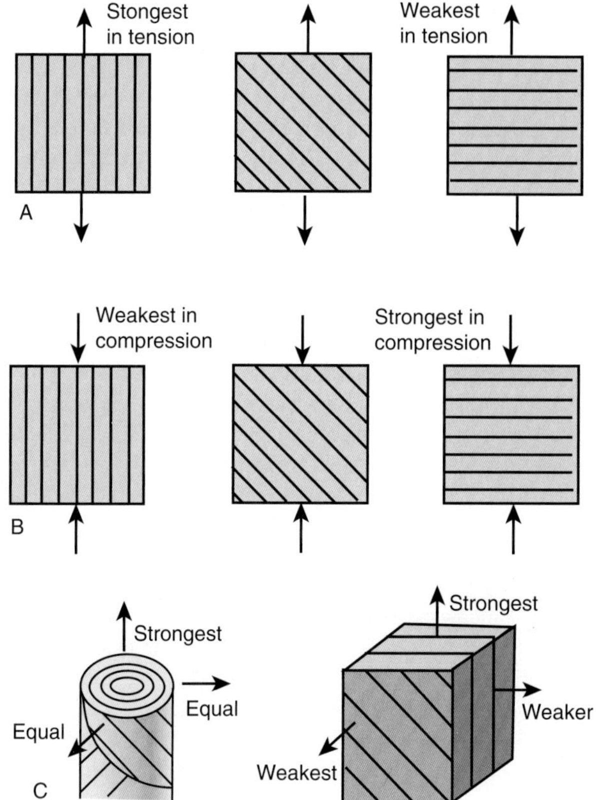

FIGURE 1-14 Effects of collagen fibril direction on the resistance to loads applied in different directions. The weakest directions in relation to a given load are those in which the fibers separate along their cement (bonding) lines during loading (11).

ilarly, the modulus changes with bone density by a power of between 2 and 3 (12,13,43,117). Noninvasive measures of bone density such as quantitative computed tomography (qCT) have been shown to have a significant predictive relationship to bone strength (17,18).

Several additional factors can affect bone strength. As discussed previously, bone is a viscoelastic material with strength and modulus that both increase as loading rate increases (e.g., in fracture impact loading vs. normal ambulation) (2,19–23). Age also affects bone properties. The bending strength and modulus increase as bone mineralizes and matures from childhood to adulthood and slowly decrease thereafter (24–26), and impact energy absorbed decreases with age (27) as bone becomes more brittle. Defects or holes in bone (e.g., from drilling for screws) affect its strength (28–32). The torsional strength of bone decreases as the diameter of the hole or defect increases (Fig. 1-16). As the hole increases to 30% of the bone's diameter, bone strength decreases to about 50% of that of the intact bone without a defect. An important consideration, applicable in the resection of bone (such as in removal of a tumor), is the shape of the hole or defect left after tumor removal. Leaving a hole with square corners significantly decreases strength, compared to the same hole with rounded corners, because the square corner is a large stress concentrator. Although oval or circular holes are still stress risers, they do not have the additional effect of the sharp corner (29). Table 1-3 summarizes the strength of cortical and cancellous bone material as well as the ultimate strengths of various whole bones.

As a fracture heals, its strength is affected by changes in its mineral content, callus diameter, and fiber organization, as was discussed previously. The initial callus forms from the periosteal surface outward, which is beneficial mechanically, because as the outer diameter of the healing area enlarges, its moment of

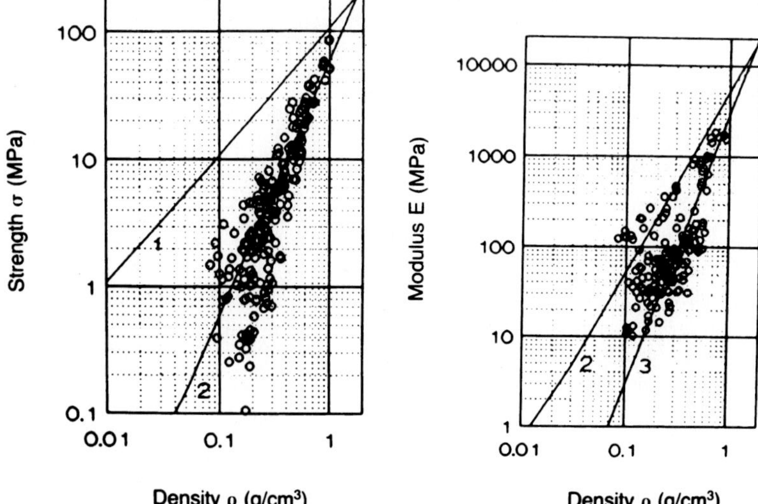

FIGURE 1-15 The relationship of trabecular bone density to compressive strength and modulus demonstrates a power-law relationship, so that these properties decrease by a factor of about four when density decreases by half (2).

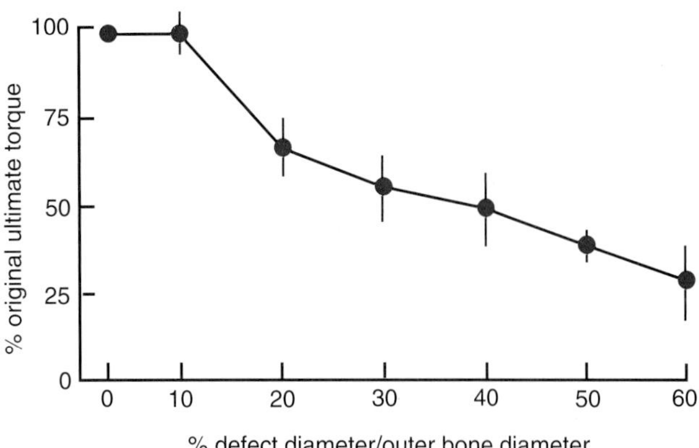

FIGURE 1-16 The relationship of ultimate torque (failure torque) of a long bone to the diameter of the hole divided by the outer diameter of the bone. There is no change in ultimate torque until the defect size increases beyond greater than 10% of the bone's diameter (30).

inertia, and therefore, its initial stiffness both increase, as shown in Figure 1-17 (33). The cross-sectional area increases progressively, as shown in Figure 1-18, as does the mineral content of the callus (34). The mechanical results of these changes to bone as the fracture heals are shown in Figure 1-19. From torsional tests of healing rabbit long bones, progressive increases were observed in stiffness and peak torque to failure with time (35). Interestingly, in that experiment, the stiffness appeared to gain normal values, while the peak torque to failure lagged behind. Figure 1-18 shows that beyond 4 weeks (in rats, whose bones heal rapidly), the cross-sectional area starts to decrease as the bone remodels to normal shape, while the bone tissue continues to mineralize.

The mechanical environment created by the fixation system along with the available blood supply affects the type of tissue formed in a healing fracture. The theory of interfragmentary strain attempts to relate the types of tissues formed to the amount of strain experienced by the tissue between the healing bone fragments (33). This theory is a simple depiction and cannot represent the complex stresses that the healing tissue is exposed to during actual healing. Nonetheless, within the limitations of the theory, as shown in Figure 1-20, when large strains occur in the tissues between healing bone surfaces, granulation tissue is formed. Intermediate level strains produce cartilage, and small strains result in primary bone healing, or direct deposition of bone tissue with limited callus formation.

Among the limitations of this theory, recognize that it does not follow that zero strain will result in maximum bone formation. Load and some resulting strain are necessary within the healing fracture to stimulate bone formation. In a study in which controlled daily displacements in a specific direction were applied to healing long bones using an external fixator, and the bone mineral within the healing fracture was measured with time, there was an optimal displacement above or below where less mineral was created in the fracture callus (Fig. 1-21) (36). Fracture fixation constructs of different stiffnesses, within a certain range, produce healed fractures with similar mechanical properties; however, they may reach this endpoint by different routes. In a study of femoral fixation using IM rods of either 5% or 50% of the torsional stiffness of the intact femur, the femurs fixed with the lower stiffness rods produced an abundance of stabilizing callus, as opposed to the femurs with more rigid fixation (Fig. 1-22), because with more rigid fixation, there was less necessity for biological fracture stabilization. In both cases, however, the mechanical properties of the healed fractures were ultimately similar (37). These studies demonstrate that some strain due to loading of the fracture stimulates healing and that bone will adapt and heal within a relatively wide range of mechanical stabilization environments.

In summary, a number of factors affect bone strength, and similarly, a healing fracture. Increasing mineral content increases fracture stiffness. Callus that forms on the periosteal surface is beneficial in increasing the moment of inertia and, therefore, the stiffness of the fractured region. Healing fractures exhibit a number of stages, with stiffness returning to normal followed later by peak load to failure. Bone will heal within a range of mechanical environments. To a certain extent, healing bone will compensate for more flexible fixation by forming a greater quantity of fracture callus; however, there is an optimal range of displacement of a healing callus within which significantly greater mineral can be shown to form in the same time.

BIOMECHANICS OF BONE FRACTURE

To appreciate why bone fractures in certain patterns, one must understand that, as shown in Table 1-3, bone is weakest in tension and strongest in compression. Therefore, when a force creates tensile stresses in a particular region of a loaded bone, failure will occur first in that region. The simplest example, shown in Figure 1-23, is the transverse fracture created in a long bone subjected to pure bending. Because in this example, the upper, convex surface undergoes the greatest elongation, it is subjected to the largest tensile stresses, and failure (indicated by a crack) initiates here. The crack then progresses transversely through the material, and layers just below the outer layer become subjected to high tensile stress, until they crack as well. In this manner, the crack progresses through the bone transversely until it fails. The concave surface is subjected to compression, so the crack does not initiate there. A second example is the fracture line or crack that occurs when a bone is subjected to torsion or axial twisting. In that case, a spiral fracture results. Consider, as shown in Figure 1-23, a rectangular area on the surface of a long bone that is loaded in torsion. The rectangle distorts as the bone twists, with one diagonal of the rectangle elongating and the other shortening, depending on the direction of twist. A crack will form perpendicular to the diagonal that is elongating, and it progresses around the perimeter of the bone resulting in a spiral fracture. The region of bone with the smallest diameter usually has the greatest distortion, as it allows

TABLE 1-3 **Mechanical Properties of Bone Material and Whole Bones in Different Loading Directions**

Bone Type	Load Type	Elastic Modulus (X10 E9 N/m^2)	Ultimate Stress (X10 E6 N/m^2)	Reference
Cortical	Tension	11.4–19.1	107–146	Crowninshield Ann Biomed Eng 1974;2:217 Evans Acta Anat 1958;35:285 Evans Am J Anat 1967;120:79 Wright Med Biol Eng 1976;14:671 Reilly J Biomech 1974;7:271
	Compression	15.1–19.7	156–212	Curry 1984, Princeton University Press
	Shear		73–82	Yamada 1970, Williams and Wilkins, Baltimore
Cancellous	Tension	~0.2–5.0	~3–20	Curry J Biomech 1979;12:459
	Compression	0.1–3	1.5–50	Carter J Bone Jt Surg; 1977;59A:954 Weaver J Bone Jt Surg 1966;48A:289 Galante Calcif Tissue Res 1970;5:236
	Shear		6.6 +/− 1.7	Stone J Biomech 1983;16:743

Bone Type	Loading Direction and Type	Ultimate Strength	Reference
Cervical spine	Axial compressive impact	980–7,400 N	Yoganandan J Spinal Disorders 1991;4:73 McElhaney Soc Auto Eng 1983;83:1615 Nusholtz 25th STAPP car crash conf 1981;1197
Cervical spine	Extension	57 N-m	Nahum Accidental Injury 1993, Springer-Verlag
Cervical spine	Flexion	120 N-m	Nahum Accidental Injury 1993, Springer-Verlag
Cervical spine	Lateral bending	54 N-m	Nahum Accidental Injury 1993, Springer-Verlag
Lumbar spine	Axial compressive impact	1,400–9,000 N	Cody Spine 1991;16:146 Bell Calcif Tissue Res 1967;1:75 Brassow Eur J Radiol 1982;2:99 Hansson Spine 1980;5:46 Halton J Anat 1979;129:753 Tran Spine 1994;20:1984
Sacroiliac Joint	Axial compressive impact	3,450–3,694 N	Fasola 1955; Wright Patterson AFB
Femoral neck	Lateral to medial at trochanter	1,000–4,000 N	Smith J Bone Jt Surg 1953;35A:367
Femoral neck	Vertical impact at femoral head	725–10,570 N	Alho Clin Orthop 1988;227:292 Leicher Clin Orthop 1982;163:272 Stankewitz J Orthop Res 1996;14:786
Femur	Torsion	183 N-m	Martens J Biomech 1980;13:667
Femur	from impact at knee along axis	6,230–17,130 N	Patrick 9th STAPP car crash conf 1966:237 Viano J Biomech 1980;13:701
Femur	Three point bending, posterior	21.2–31.3 Nm	Mather J Biomech 1968;1:331
Patella	Impact perpendicular to anterior	6,900–10,012 N	Patrick 9th STAPP car crash conf 1966:237
Tibia	Axial torsion	101 +/− 35 Nm	Martens J Biomech 1980;13:667
Foot and ankle	Impact perpendicular to sole	4,107–6,468 N	Assal 46th AAAM 2002;273 Yoganandan 1996; Soc Auto Eng 962426 Schueler In 1996; Soc Auto Eng PT-56, 551 Kitagawa 1998; Soc Auto Eng 983145 Funk 2000; Soc Auto Eng; 2000–01–0155 McMaster 2000; STAPP car crash conf 44:357

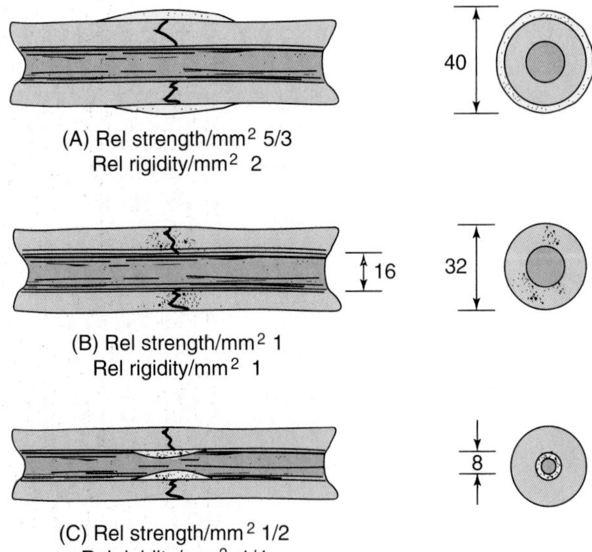

FIGURE 1-17 A comparison of the moments of inertia and resulting strengths when fracture callus is located **(A)** on the outer surface, **(B)** on the bone surfaces, or **(C)** in the medullary canal. The strength and rigidity are significantly increased when callus is located over the periosteal surface, compared to within the medullary canal (33).

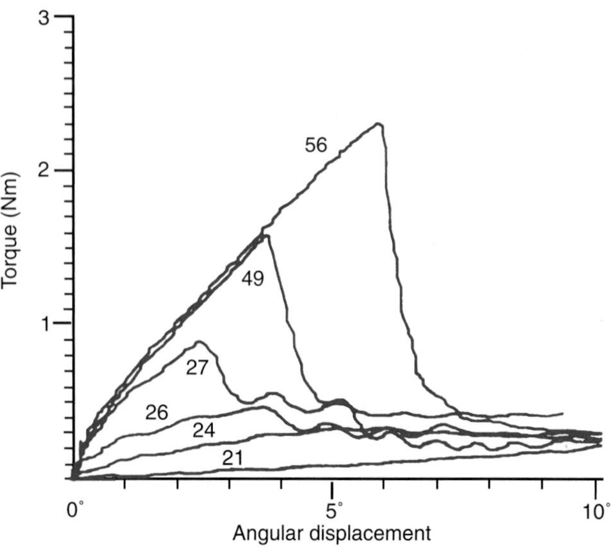

FIGURE 1-19 A comparison of superimposed torque-angular displacement plots taken from experimental long bones at different stages of healing, shows the significant increase in both stiffness and peak torque to failure with increased duration of healing. Numerical values are time in days postfracture in rabbits (35).

the largest amount of twist. This explains why torsional fractures of the tibia often occur in the narrow distal third (Fig. 1-24).

A compressive load results in failure of cortical bone by shear, indicated by slippage along the diagonal, because bone is weaker in shear than in compression (Fig. 1-25). (The stresses 45° to the compressive force within the material are shear stresses.) In this case, compression causes the surfaces of the bone at 45° to the applied load to slide along an oblique surface. At very high loads, such as during impact fractures, crushing or comminution of bone also occurs, especially at the weaker

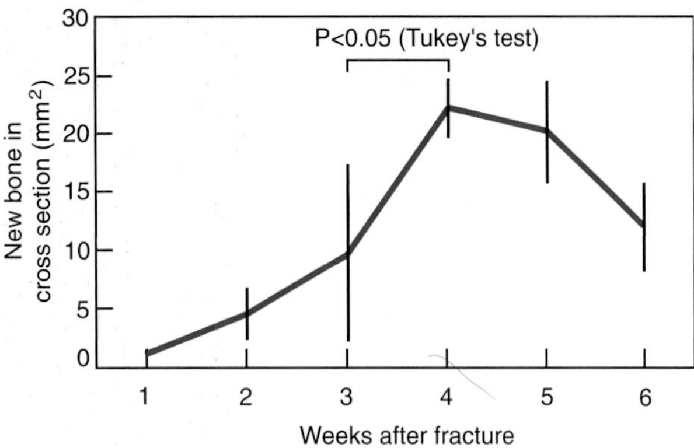

FIGURE 1-18 Changes in the cross-sectional area of a healing femoral fracture, which peaks and slowly decreases. There is a similar increase in the mineral content. (The data come from rats that heal more rapidly than humans, indicated by the 4-week time to peak mineralization [34].)

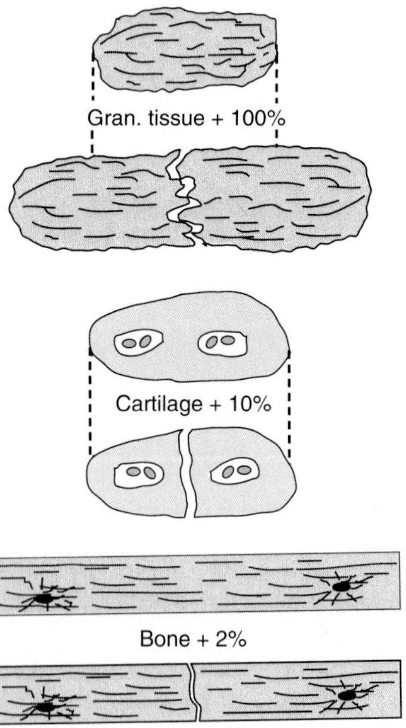

FIGURE 1-20 The theory of interfragmentary strain estimates that large strains (>100%) resulting from very flexible fixation produce granulation tissue within the fracture site, whereas smaller strains (<10%) result in cartilage, and very small strains (<2%), produce bone (33).

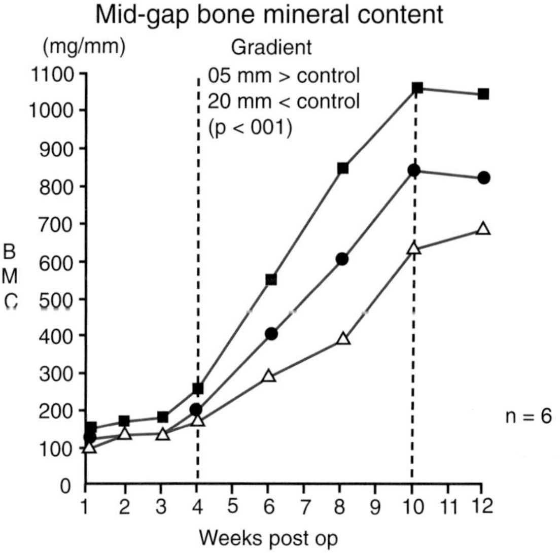

FIGURE 1-21 The effect on bone mineral within a healing fracture of different cyclic displacements applied daily (*upper curve*, 0.5 mm; *middle curve*, 1.0 mm; *lower curve*, 2.0 mm for 500 cycles/day). This shows that there is an optimal longitudinal displacement below or above where less mineral is created within the healing fracture (36).

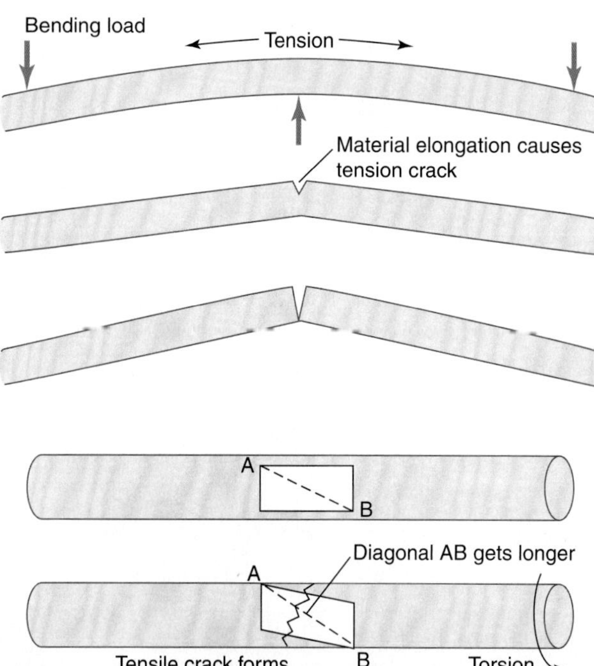

FIGURE 1-23 **Top.** A transverse fracture is created by the progressive tensile failure of bone material starting from the convex surface where elongation, and therefore, stress is greatest, with the crack progressing to the concave side. **Bottom.** A spiral fracture is created by the progressive failure in tension of fibers on the bone surface along the diagonal that elongates as the material on the surface distorts when torque is applied. (A rectangle on the surface becomes a parallelogram, with one diagonal elongating. The crack will be transverse to the diagonal.)

metaphyseal ends of a long bone. The trabecular bone at the metaphyseal ends is weaker in compression than the diaphyseal cortical bone is in shear. Because of this, it is unlikely that shearing failure will occur in the diaphysis due to pure compressive forces. The butterfly fracture (Fig. 1-25) results from combined bending and compression. Bending load causes the fracture to start to fail in tension producing a transverse crack, but as the crack progresses and the remaining intact bone weakens, it starts to fail in compression, causing an oblique (shear) fracture line. As the ends of the failing bone are driven together, a third fragment, the butterfly, may result as the oblique fragment splits off. The production of a butterfly fragment probably depends on the timing and magnitude of the two basic applied loads, compression and bending.

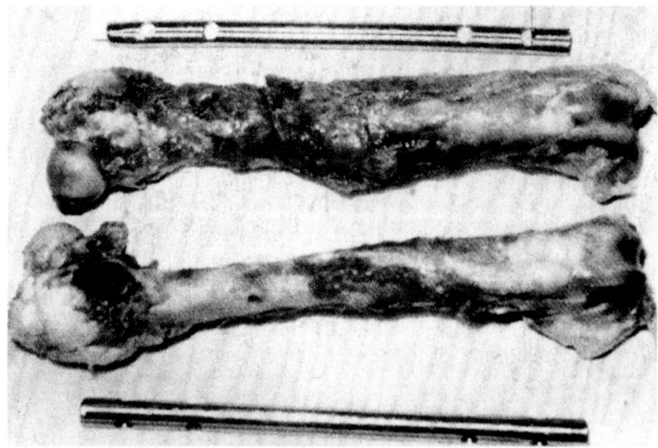

FIGURE 1-22 A comparison of the different healing responses of dog femurs with midshaft fractures fixed with IM rods of 5% **(top)** or 50% **(bottom)** of the torsional stiffness of the intact femur. Although the femurs fixed with rods of lower stiffness produced more callus as additional stabilization against functional loads, there was ultimately no difference in mechanical properties between the femurs fixed with rods of different stiffnesses (37).

Aging, especially with osteoporosis, changes the force required to fracture and the types of fractures that occur. As shown in Figure 1-15, trabecular bone stiffness varies with the cube (third power) of its density and strength approximately with the square of its density (2). Bone mass normally peaks around age 25 to 30 and decreases up to 1% thereafter. If the density of trabecular bone is decreased by 30%, in a 60- to 70-year-old due to osteoporosis, the compressive strength is about half of that of a 30-year-old. Typical fractures due to osteoporosis occur in the vertebrae, the distal radius, and the femoral neck. In addition, osteoporosis changes the cross-sectional shape of long bones, decreasing thickness by increasing the endosteal diameter, while causing the periosteal diameter to increase. If cortical outer diameter—for example, in the femur—increased and cortical thickness decreased at the same rate, the moment of inertia of the bone cross section would be larger. That is

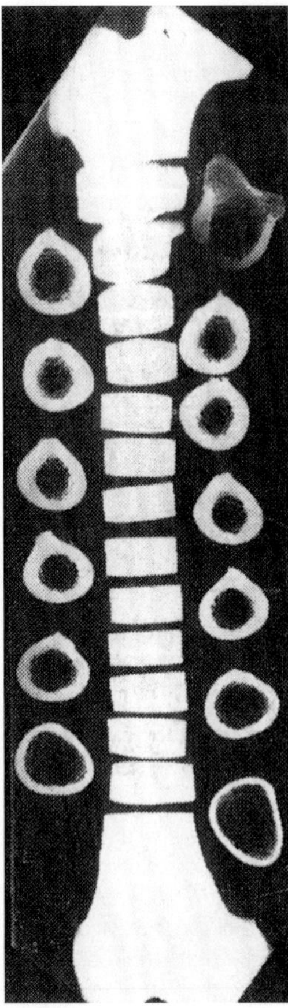

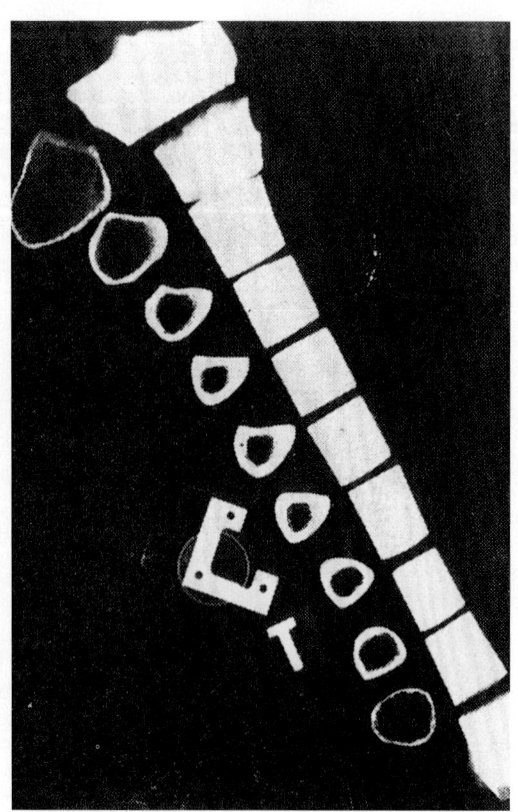

FIGURE 1-24 Cross sections through a femur **(left)** and a tibia **(right)**. The small cross section of the distal third of the tibia results in more distorsion and higher stresses and explains why torsional failure often occurs in this area.

why large-diameter thin tubing can be substituted for smaller-diameter thicker tubing in structures (e.g., sailboat masts), saving weight while not sacrificing strength. In the femur, however, the inner surface of the cortex also becomes more irregular and porous, decreasing material strength. A common result of loss of femoral bone mass combined with other factors is a hip fracture usually resulting from a fall. The most likely scenario related to femur fracture was reported to include female gender, patients older than 80 years of age, falling while ambulating indoors, and falling during the afternoon hours (38).

Auto crashes account for many fractures. Some particular mechanisms have been observed. Fracture of the calcaneus or the malleoli of the foot and ankle can occur through a combination of the foot being forced against the brake pedal by the weight of the occupant during a high-speed frontal collision, or in combination with the floor pan of the auto crushing into the space where the foot resides. Drivers who were braking during a crash were shown to be much more likely to injure their right foot compared with their left foot (39). If the Achilles' tendon applies load to resist the forced dorsiflexion of the foot on the brake pedal, the combination of these two loads cause three-point bending loading of the calcaneus, with the posterior facet of the talus as the fulcrum. A crack initiates on the plantar or tensile side of the calcaneus, and a tongue-type calcaneus fracture can occur. Inversion or eversion combined with compression is likely to result in a malleolar fracture (40), although the forces causing these high-energy fractures are not entirely predictable.

A major mechanism of midshaft femur fractures is impact with the dashboard of the vehicle in a frontal collision, especially unrestrained drivers who submarine or slide forward in the seat. Tensing the quadriceps and hamstrings muscles during a crash applies significant additional compression along the femur (41). Its anterior bow causes external compressive force from contact of the knee with the dashboard, and internal muscle forces to bend the femur, resulting in transverse or oblique fractures. If the femur of the occupant hits the dashboard in an adducted orientation, the femur can be displaced from the acetabulum, causing a fracture of the acetabular roof and dislocation of the hip joint. Pelvic fractures result from loading in side impact crashes, where the door punches inward against the hip and pelvis. The actual fracture pattern (symphysis, sacroiliac joint, or both) is probably the result of the specific alignment of the pelvis and the location of the applied loads at impact. Pelvic fracture classifications are based on the presumed mechanism of injury and specific forces applied (42). Bilateral hip fractures have been found to occur in crashes when the vehicle has a large center console that tends to trap the pelvis as force is also

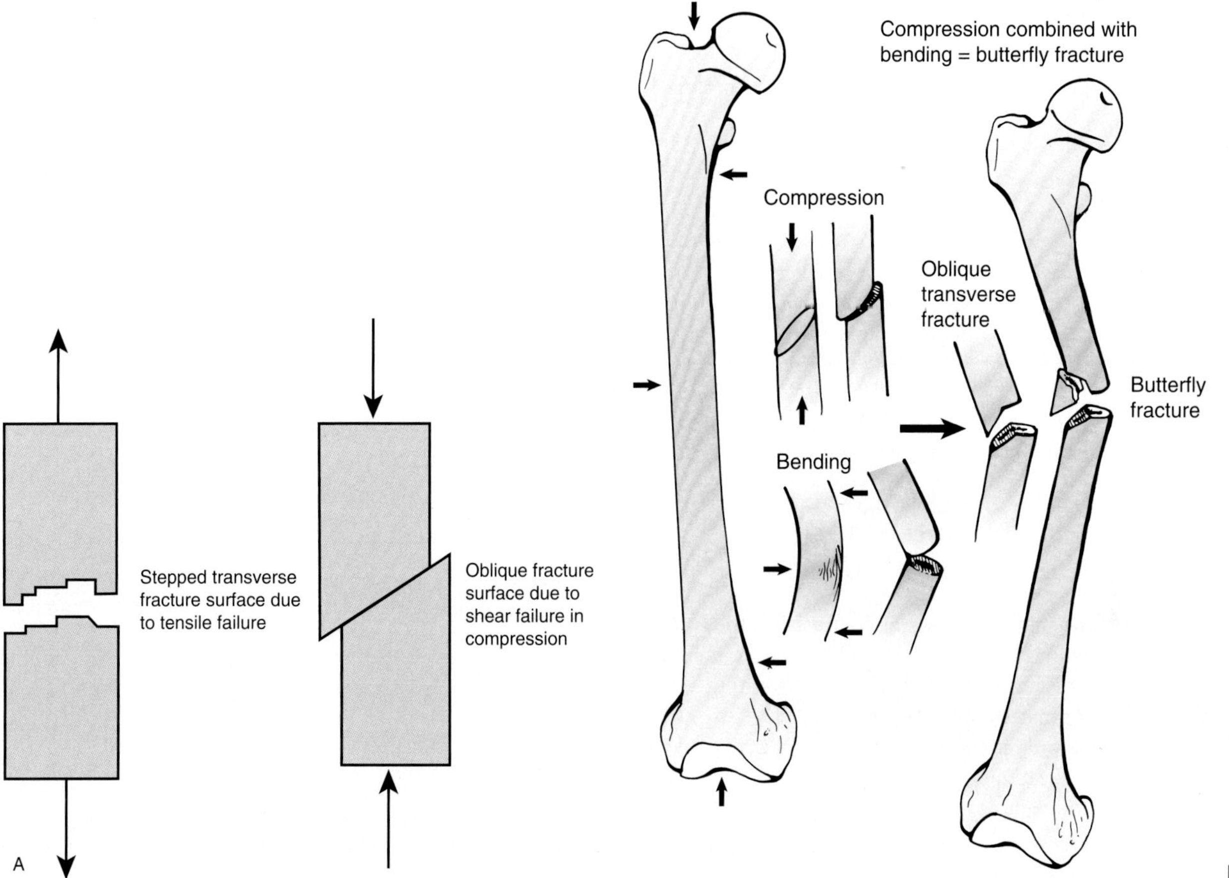

FIGURE 1-25 **A.** Tensile fracture (*left*) causes a stepped surface as fibers pull apart. The crack progresses, then steps to an adjacent region where failure continues. Pure compression (*right*) of cortical bone results in failure by shearing or sliding along oblique surfaces. In reality, pure compression of a long bone (in a fall, for example) results in crushing of the much weaker metaphyseal trabecular bone with a pilon fracture of the distal tibia or a tibial plateau fracture as the result. **B.** Some fractures that combine bending and compression demonstrate transverse cracking due to bending followed by an oblique crack characteristic of compressive failure. The butterfly fracture with additional splitting of the fragment secondary to the initial fracture is an example.

applied on the hip opposite that which contacts the door. In crashes in which occupants have lap but not shoulder belts, torso forward motion creates the classic "chance fracture," which is combined compression and flexion failure of a lumbar vertebra, usually at the level where the lap belt forms a fulcrum.

BIOMECHANICS OF FRACTURE IMPLANTS

Avoiding Mechanical Problems With Fracture Fixation Devices

This section discusses the function of commonly used fixation devices for skeletal fracture fixation. Observed fixation problems with devices such as wire, cable, screws, plates, IM rods, and external fixators are explained with the objective of reducing the potential for mechanical damage or failure of these devices during use.

Cerclage Wire Breakage

The tensile strength of surgical wire has been shown to increase directly with its diameter, and when twisted, the optimal number of turns is between four and eight. Solid wire is very sensitive to notches or scratches, however. Testing shows that notches as small as 1% of the diameter of the wire can reduce its fatigue life by 63%. For this reason, cable has been introduced for cerclage applications. Cable has significantly better fatigue performance compared to wire, as shown in Figure 1-26 (43).

Screw Breakage by Shearing During Insertion

A screw is a mechanical device that is used to convert rotary force (torque) into compression between a plate and bone, or

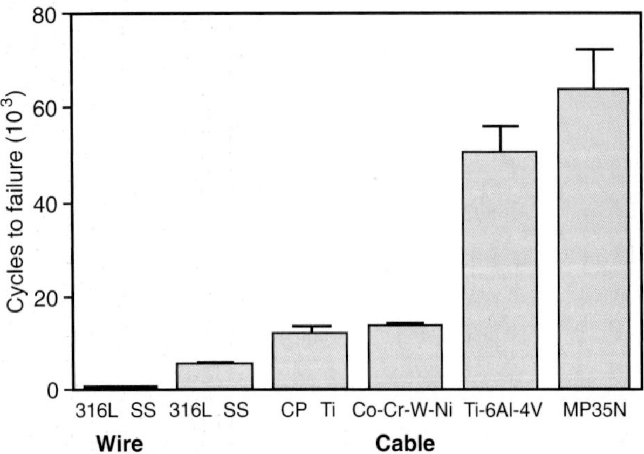

FIGURE 1-26 A comparison of the fatigue resistance of wire and cables made of the indicated materials. Wire, 316 SS (stainless steel); cable, 316 SS; Cp Ti, commercially pure titanium; Co-Cr-W-Ni, cobalt chrome; Ti 6Al 4V, titanium alloy; MP35N, nickel alloy (43).

between bone fragments. As shown in Figure 1-27, the thread of a screw if unwound from the shaft is really a ramp or inclined plane that pulls, for example, underlying bone toward the fixation plate, causing compression between them. The basic components of a screw are shown in Figure 1-28. Because of its function, the screw head and shaft must be free to turn in the plate; otherwise, the compressive force generated may be limited. (This does not apply to screws that are designed to be threaded into the plate holes in locking plates.) One common problem is that sometimes threads are tapped into both bone components. The bone component in which the screw head will rest should be drilled oversize to allow the shaft of the screw to turn freely, and only the other should be tapped. Tapping is necessary in cortical bone so that the torque applied can be used to create compression instead of cutting threads and overcoming friction between the screw thread and bone that it is being driven into (Fig. 1-29) (44). With cancellous bone, as discussed later, tapping is less advantageous, unless the bone is very dense. One common problem during screw placement is shear failure of the screw, typically the head twisting off, leaving the shaft embedded in bone and difficult to remove. This can occur especially when using smaller (less than 4 mm in diameter) screws in dense bone, especially without tapping. The stiffness and strength of a screw are related to the fourth power of its diameter (the effect of moment of inertia, for screws of the same material). A 6-mm-diameter screw is approximately five times as stiff as a 3-mm-diameter screw and 16 times as resistant to shear failure by over-torquing the screw during insertion.

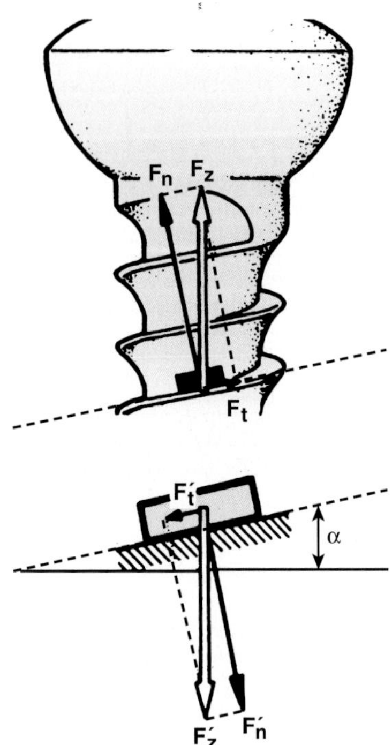

FIGURE 1-27 A screw is a mechanical device that converts torque into compression between objects. The screw thread is actually an inclined plane that slowly pulls the objects it is embedded into together. For this reason, the head and screw shaft in one part must be free to rotate. If this part of the screw is threaded into the hole of the first part (for example, the plate), it will not allow the surfaces to compress. (Fn, normal or compressive force acting against the screw head; Ft, tangential or frictional force acting along the screw thread; Fz, resultant of the two forces; α, angle of the screw thread. The smaller the angle α (finer thread) is, the lower the frictional force will be.

Screw Pullout

Particularly in cancellous bone, the maximum force that a screw can withstand along its axis, the pullout force, depends on the size of the screw and the density of the bone it is placed into. As shown in Figure 1-30, when the force acting on the screw exceeds its pullout strength, the screw will pull or shear out of the hole, carrying the sheared bone within its threads, because it is usually the bone that fails and not the screw. The maximum pullout force increases with larger screw diameter, a longer length embedded, and greater density of the bone it is placed into (45–48). The diameter and length of the embedded screw can be thought of as defining the outer surface of a cylinder along which the screw shears. Given the maximum stress that bone of a particular density can withstand, increasing the surface area of the screw cylinder increases the pullout force (force = stress × area over which it acts). To enhance screw purchase, consider embedding the largest-diameter screw possible into bone of the greatest density, over as long a purchase length as possible (45,46). Pullout strength also increases significantly if the screw is placed through both bone cortices.

In cancellous bone, screw pullout becomes a more significant problem because the porosity of cancellous bone reduces its density and, therefore, its shear strength (49). Hole preparation, specifically drilling but not tapping, improves the pullout strength of screws placed into cancellous bone (such as pedicle

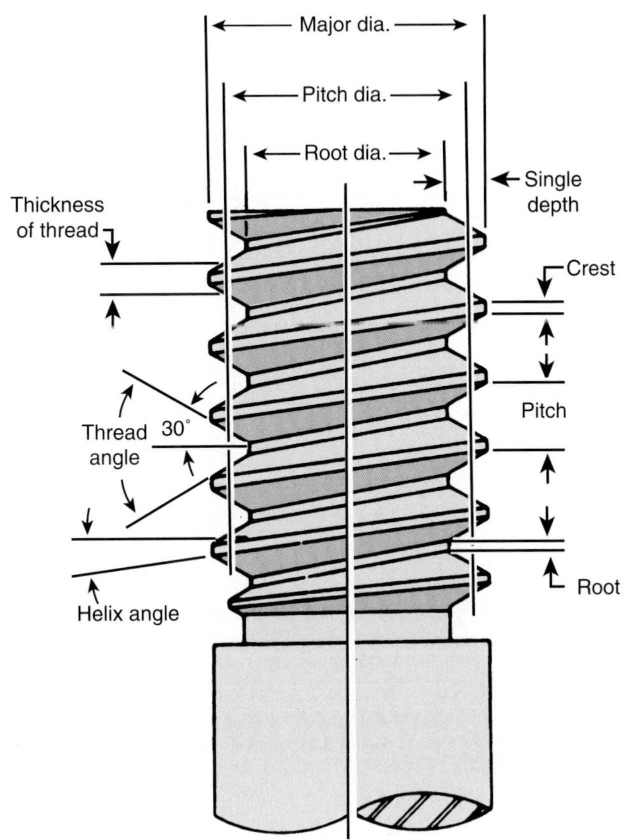

FIGURE 1-28 Nomenclature of screws. The root diameter is the inner diameter of the screw, and the pitch defines the distance between threads.

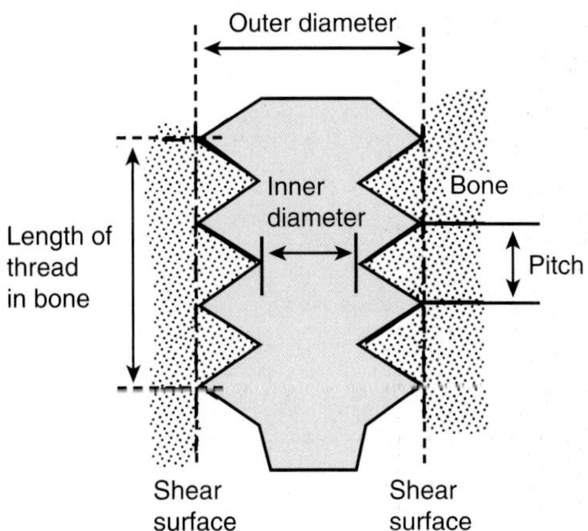

FIGURE 1-30 The factors that determine the pullout strength of a screw are its outer diameter and length of engagement (this defines the dimensions of a cylinder of bone that carried in the threads and is sheared out as the screw is pulled out of bone) and the shear strength of bone at the screw/bone interface, which is directly related to its density. A finer-pitch screw produces a small gain in purchase (45).

screws in the vertebral body) (47). The reason that tapping reduces strength, as shown in Figure 1-31, is that running the tap in and out of the hole removes bone, effectively increasing the diameter of the hole and reducing the amount of bone material that interacts with the screw threads. Tapping has more effect as bone density decreases and can reduce the pullout strength from 10% to as much as 30%. It should also be noted that the findings of studies related to pullout strength relate to the time immediately after insertion. As the bone heals, it also

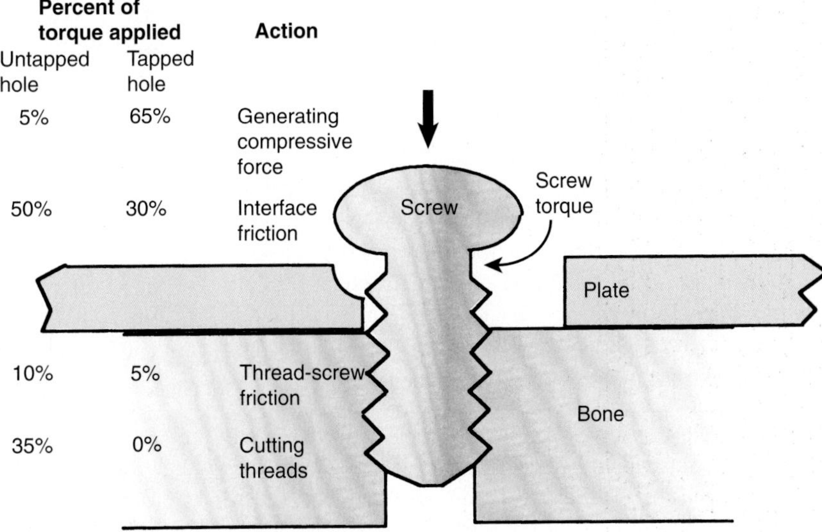

FIGURE 1-29 Schematic diagram showing the approximate distribution of torque acting on screw placed into cortical bone. With a pretapped hole, about 65% of the applied torque produces compression, and 35% goes to overcome the friction associated with driving the screw. When the hole is not tapped, only about 5% of the torque is used to produce compression; the rest goes to overcome friction and to cut threads in bone. These observations do not apply in cancellous bone (44).

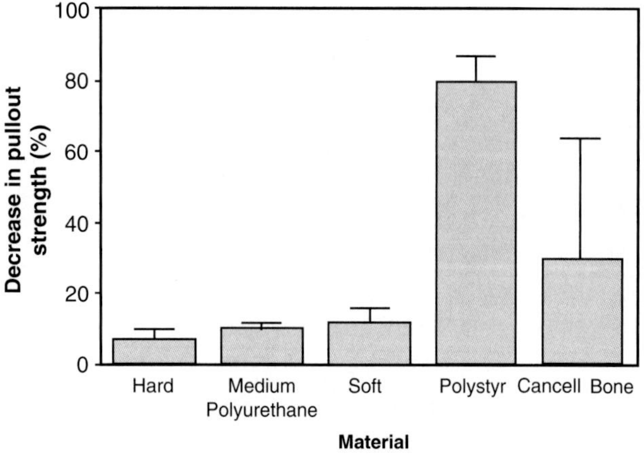

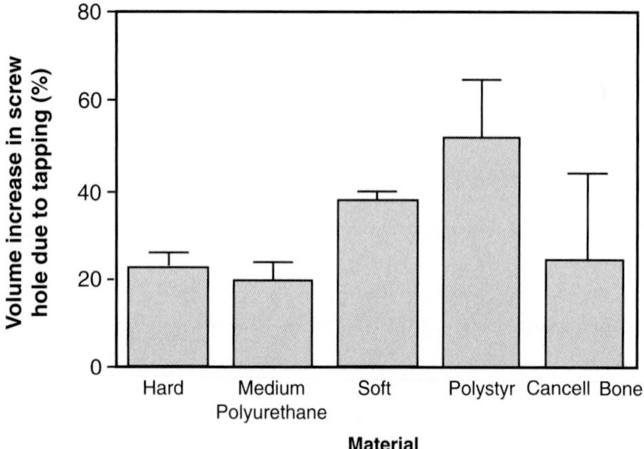

FIGURE 1-31 **Top.** The decrease in pullout strength in various types of foam used to test bone screws demonstrating the percentage in decrease of pullout strength between screws placed into holes that were either drilled only or drilled and tapped. **Bottom.** The percentage in increase in volume comparing holes that were drilled only and those that were drilled and tapped. Tapping in cancellous bone increases hole volume, which decreases pullout strength (45).

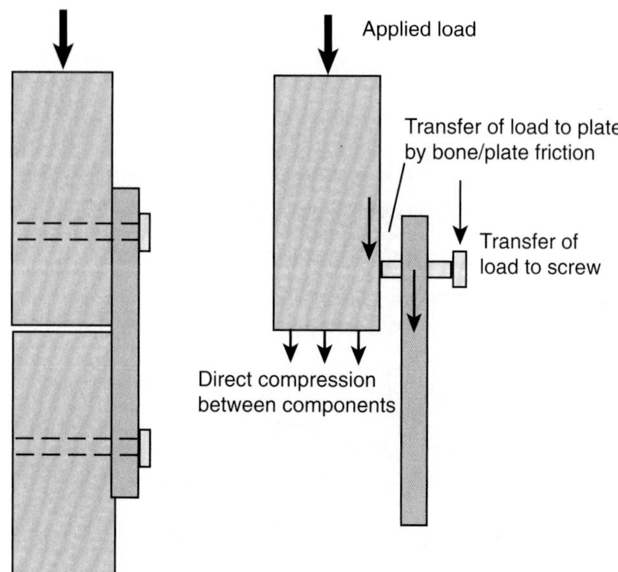

FIGURE 1-32 A mechanism for rapid failure of screws in cyclic bending occurs when the screw has not been tightened sufficiently to keep the plate from sliding along the bone surface (the plate-bone gap shown here is exaggerated for clarity). The result is that bending loads are applied transverse to the long axis of the screw which, in combination with fretting corrosion caused by the screws rubbing against the plate, results in early failure of the screw (51).

remodels around the screw, possibly doubling its initial pullout strength (50).

Screw Breakage by Cyclic Loading

A mechanism exists through which cortical screws can fail due to cyclic bending, shown in Figure 1-32. This mode of loading could occur during functional use. It is important that the screw is tightened against the plate to the maximum extent possible, and the tightening torque must be effectively transferred to compressive force between plate and bone (Fig. 1-29). The screw holds the plate against bone partly by frictional contact, which depends on the frictional force generated between the undersurface of the plate and bone. The frictional force depends directly on the compressive force generated by the screws. If any sliding occurs between the plate and bone, the bending load will be transferred from the head of the screw into the plate, where screw-plate contact occurs. Bending loads perpendicular to the axis of the screw, along with possible stress corrosion and fretting corrosion, may cause the screws to fail rapidly in fatigue. Zand et al (51) showed that screws tightened against a plate with only 10% to 15% less force than the maximum possible failed in fewer than 1,000 loading cycles, by bending fatigue, compared with fully tightened screws that were able to sustain over 2.5 million loading cycles. Screws that screw into and lock to the plate reduce this problem.

Cannulated screws are commonly used for fixation, as they have the significant advantage that they can be precisely guided into position over a guidewire, which may aid in reducing a fracture fragment. Cannulated screws follow the same mechanical principles as solid screws, discussed previously; however, to create the central hole, material must be removed from the center of the screw. Manufacturers commonly increase the minor diameter (the diameter of the screw at the base of the thread) to accommodate loss of this material. The same size cannulated screws usually have less thread depth compared with solid screws. The result is, depending on the screw size, less pullout strength. For 4-mm-diameter screws, cannulated screws, of the same outside diameter had about 16% lower pullout strength (52). Alternatively, to keep the same thread depth, the outer diameter of the screw may be increased.

Breakage of Fracture Fixation Plates

The fracture fixation plate is designed to stabilize a fracture by driving the ends of the fracture together, compressing them.

This is beneficial to fracture healing because it improves stability, opening the possibility for primary bone healing with minimal callus formation, and by enhancing the resistance of the plate to bending fatigue failure. Observing the cross section of an oval hole in a dynamic compression fracture plate, Figure 1-33 shows that one border of the hole actually has an inclined surface. When the head of the screw displaces downward toward the bone surface, the screw and the fragment of bone it is attached to slide toward the center of the plate. This action, which occurs for both fracture components, causes the fracture surfaces to be driven together (53), and it creates significant compressive forces across the ends of the fracture (54). Compressing the ends of the fracture significantly improves the stability of the construct and reduces bending and torsional stresses applied to the plate, increasing its life. Stability is improved because the bone ends resist bending forces that close the fracture gap, and torsional loads are resisted by the frictional force and interlock between the ends of the fracture components. Also, the fracture gap that must be healed is smaller.

It is important to appreciate that the plate is vulnerable to bending failure, as plates are thin, relatively easy to bend (compared to bone), and have low moments of inertia. They are designed to apply compressive force to the ends of the fracture, and the stabilized bone can then resist the bending loads applied during functional use. If a gap is left on the side opposite the plate (Fig. 1-34), the fracture site becomes a fulcrum around which the plate bends under combined compressive and bending loads such as those which occur during ambulation (if the compressive force is not located directly down the tibial shaft, which occurs during heel strike and toeoff, then bending loads will be applied along with the compressive force). Gapping can also occur when a segment of bone is missing at the fracture site, or if the plate is not properly contoured during application. Figure 1-35 demonstrates how a flat, noncontoured plate tightened against a flat bone surface will cause a gap to appear on the opposite cortex (55,56). This is why a plate is prebent suffi-

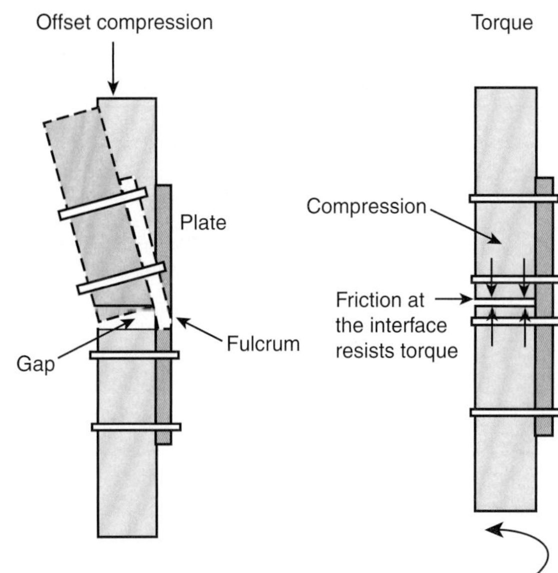

FIGURE 1-34 **Left.** When a gap is left on the cortex opposite that to which the plate is attached, bending of the plate at the fracture site can cause the plate to fail rapidly in bending. **Right.** Compressing the fracture surfaces not only allows the bone cortices to resist bending loads, but the frictional contact and interdigitation helps to resist torsion.

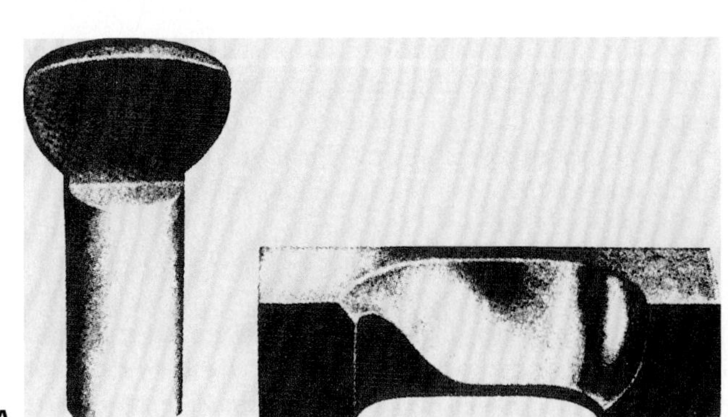

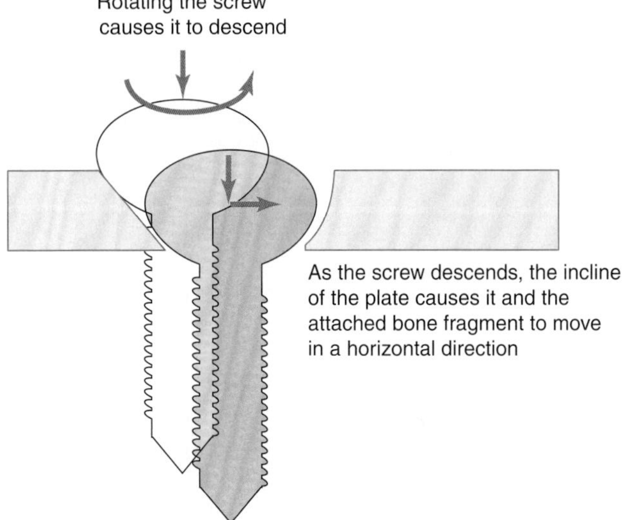

FIGURE 1-33 **A.** Cross section through the head of a bone screw and the hole in a fracture plate showing the geometry. **B.** As the screw is tightened, the head slides down the inclined border of the plate, which displaces the screw sideways, and therefore, the screw and the bone fragment to which the screw is attached are displaced toward the opposite fragment (53).

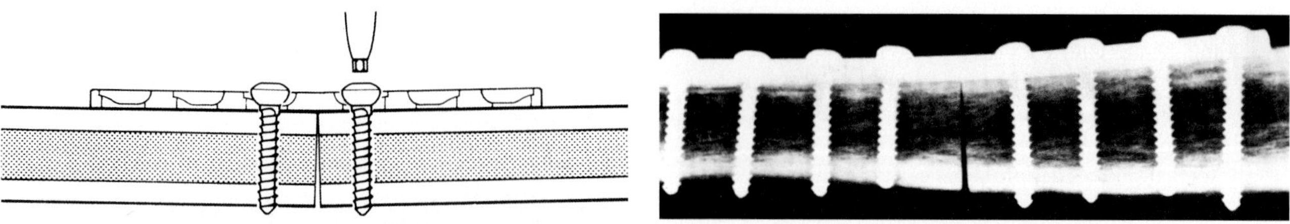

FIGURE 1-35 A demonstration of the gapping that occurs on the opposite cortex when a flat plate is applied to a flat bone surface. Slightly prebending the plate causes the ends of the opposite cortices to be driven together when the plate is applied (58).

ciently to create an initial gap between it and the bone surface that it will be applied to (56–58). Gapping also occurs when the plate is applied to the predominantly compressive instead of the tension side of a long bone during functional loading, which causes bending. Figure 1-36 shows that placing the plate on the compressive side will cause a gap to open under load.

Plate stresses are significantly increased by gapping at the fracture (55). In comminuted fractures where it is difficult to approximate the fracture ends, screws should be placed as close as possible across the fracture gap to reduce strains in the plate (59). Torsional and bending stiffness of a fracture construct can be significantly increased and, therefore, plate strain can be reduced by increasing the number of cortices of fixation (i.e., screw-cortex contact). As shown in Figure 1-37, however, there is an optimum number of cortices—eight for dynamic compression plates (DCP) and nine for limited contact dynamic compression plates (LC-DCP)—beyond which there is little additional gain in torsional stiffness (60). Figure 1-38 shows several interesting aspects related to plate fixation with screws. First, plate strains are highest at the two holes adjacent to the fracture gap and become very small, five holes away. Second, this occurs regardless of whether the screws were placed near the fracture (locations 2, 3, 4, 5), far from the fracture (locations 7, 8, 9, 10), or mixed (locations 2, 6, 9) (59). These data also indicate that not all holes of the plate need to be filled with screws in order to provide similar fixation stiffness.

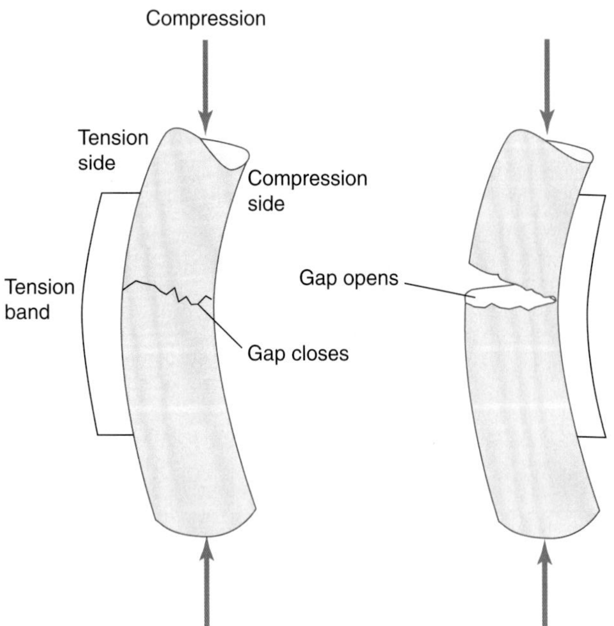

FIGURE 1-36 The application of a plate on the compressive as opposed to the tensile side of a bone subjected to bending causes a gap to open on the opposite side of the plate during functional loading.

A significant recent development in plate design is the locking or less-invasive stabilization system (LISS) plate, also called the *noncontact plate* or *internal fixator* (61). The screw head has a machine thread, separate from the bone thread, which locks it to the plate. The screws and plate form a rigid connection. In addition, the screws have been designed with a finer thread for unicortical fixation (61). The LISS plate functions differently biomechanically from the DCP. The DCP is compressed against the bone fragments by the screws and requires bone-to-plate contact to produce a stable fracture construct. Buttressing of the opposite cortex is important in maintaining fracture stability and reducing plate stresses with the DCP. Bending loads applied to the screws in the nonlocking DCP cause the screws to rotate within the plate resulting in fracture fragment motion, higher plate stresses, and reduced stability at the fracture site (62).

The LISS plate acts conceptually like an external fixator (62), where the pins are rigidly connected to the side bar and bone-to-fixator contact is minimized. This produces less interference with the biological processes of fracture healing, especially helping to preserve the blood supply near the fracture site. Also, the LISS plate provides more stability in comminuted fractures where cortical buttressing and compression are difficult to achieve, and fracture mechanical stability occurs mainly through the hardware. LISS plates do not allow the screws to be directed obliquely, except when specifically designed into the implant, and they do not permit interfragmentary compression at the fracture site. Bending loads applied to the screws from bone are resisted by the locking interface between the screw head and the threads in the plate. Therefore, these plates are not as dependent on cortical buttressing for stability as the DCP. Dynamic fatigue testing has shown that LISS plates have fatigue strengths similar to other systems and are able to support

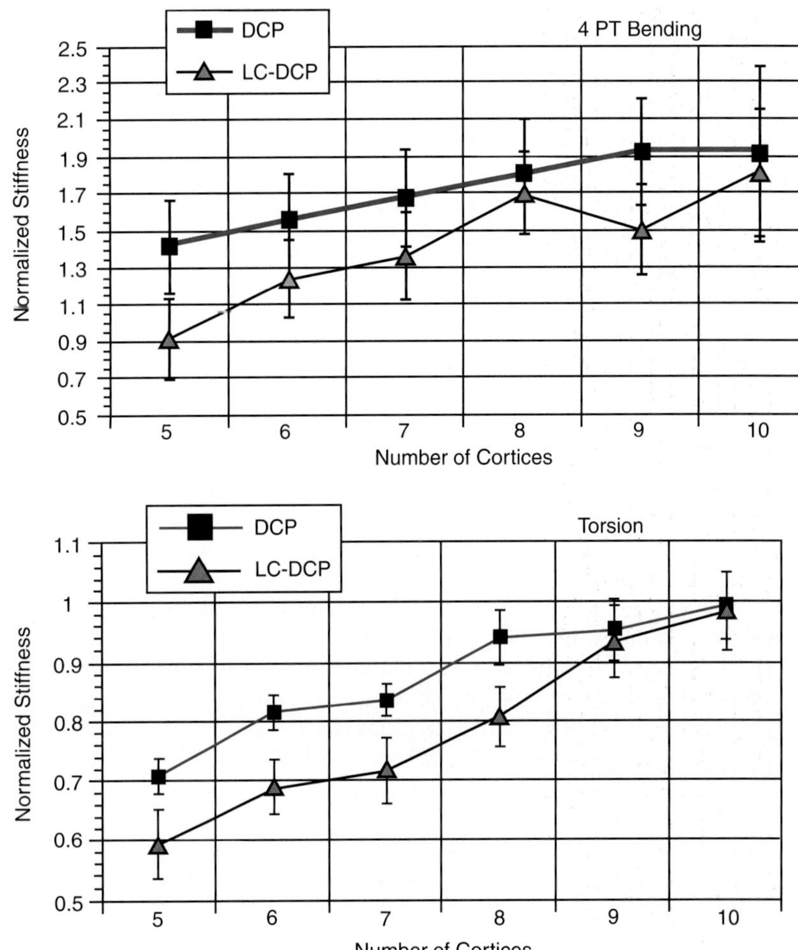

FIGURE 1-37 Relative stiffness of a plate-bone construct in torsion **(top)** and bending **(bottom)** as a function of the number of cortices through which screws have been placed (DCP, dynamic compression plate; LC-DCP, limited contact dynamic compression plate) (60).

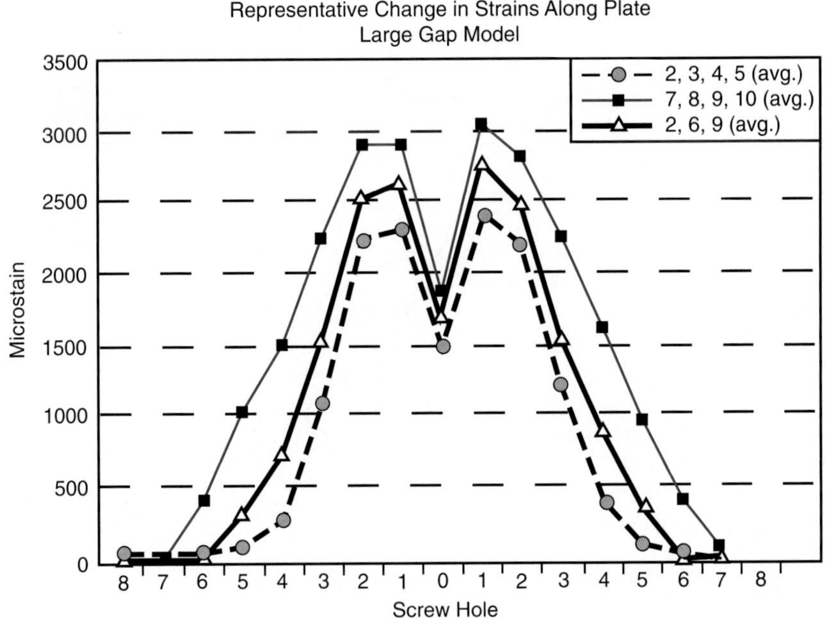

FIGURE 1-38 Distribution of strain (measured in microstrain or strain $\times$ 10^{-6}) at various locations along a plate regardless of screw placement in different locations (holes 2, 3, 4, and 5; holes 7, 8, 9, and 10; holes 2, 6, and 9) (59).

loads comparable to one body weight for 2 million cycles, which should be sufficient for normal fracture healing (61). Because screw pullout strength is related directly to the length of screw purchase in bone cortex, the unicortical screws, used in some systems, have lower pullout strength than bicortical screws. More screws must be used to compensate for the inherent lower pullout strength of the unicortical screw.

Plate Failure Through a Screw Hole

Many plates are long with multiple screw holes to provide flexibility of fixation of bone fractures with complex geometries. It is not necessary to place screws in every hole in the plate (59), but the effects of screw placement on fixation stiffness should be understood. The screw hole will be an area of elevated stresses on the plate, unless the plate is made thicker near the holes to compensate, as is the case with some plates. Placing the plate so that an empty screw hole is located over the fracture will significantly increase the potential for fatigue fracture of the plate. The plate material around the holes will have higher material stresses than occurs in the solid regions of the plate. Around the holes, the force acts through a smaller cross-sectional area, so the material stresses must be higher. A second consideration related to multihole plates is that separating the screws so that there is a greater distance between them across the fracture site results in lower stiffness of the plate-fracture construct (31). As with any beam (plate) (Fig. 1-39), the greater the distance between the supports (screws), the greater the bending displacement and the higher the stresses will be for the same applied load. It is best to avoid placing screw holes over or near the fracture site, and it is beneficial, in terms of improving fixation stiffness, to place screws as close together across the fracture site as possible.

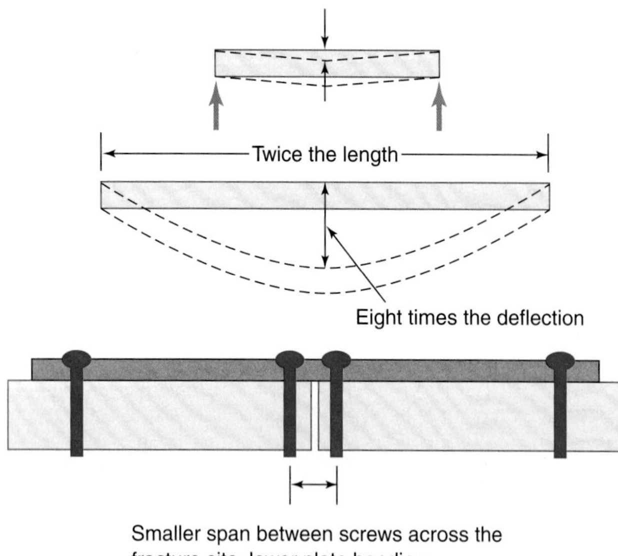

FIGURE 1-39 The greater the span or distance of a beam is between its supports, the lower its stiffness will be, and the more it will deform under load in bending and torsion. For this reason, screws should be placed as close together across the fracture site as possible.

The Problem With Fully Threaded Lag Screws

The lag screw is a very effective device for generating large compressive forces across fracture fragments, and these forces are applied directly across the fracture site. The head and upper part of the shaft of the screw must be allowed to glide in one fracture component so that it pulls the other fracture component toward it to create compression across the two. As shown in Figure 1-40, a fully threaded lag screw blocks the gliding action between the two components. Comparing the compressive forces across the fracture site using fully and partly threaded lag screws demonstrated that the average compressive force at the opposite cortex (i.e., the force in the screw itself) was about 50% greater when a partly threaded screw was used (63).

Femoral Splitting Due to IM Rod Insertion

Insertion of an IM rod into the femur can lead to difficulties because the femur has a significant anterior curvature (64), as shown in Figure 1-41. The rod, which also has a curved shape to accommodate the femoral bow, must conform to the curvature of the femur as insertion progresses. Placing a rod, which is essentially a steel curved spring, down the femur causes the rod to bend, because the femur is generally much stiffer than the rod. Figure 1-42 shows that rod contact with the internal surfaces of the femur generates forces with resist insertion. These rod-femur contact forces, directed perpendicular to the surface of the medullary canal cause the femur to expand and will result in splitting if they become too large (65). The factors

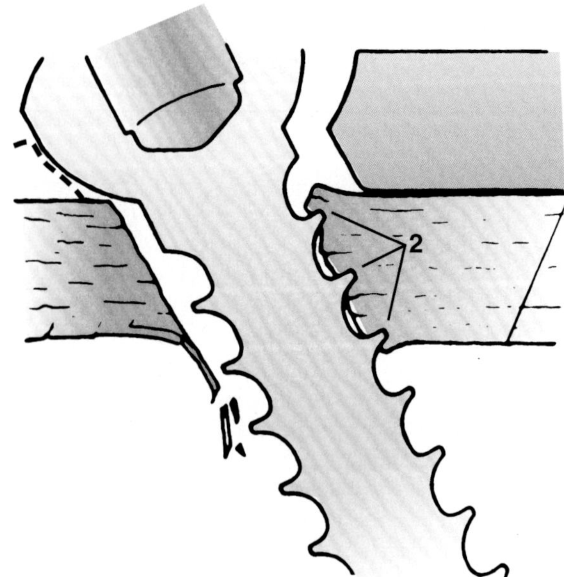

FIGURE 1-40 Using a fully threaded lag screw causes the threads to engage in bone on both sides of the fracture. This inhibits the screw from compressing the bone fragments together (63).

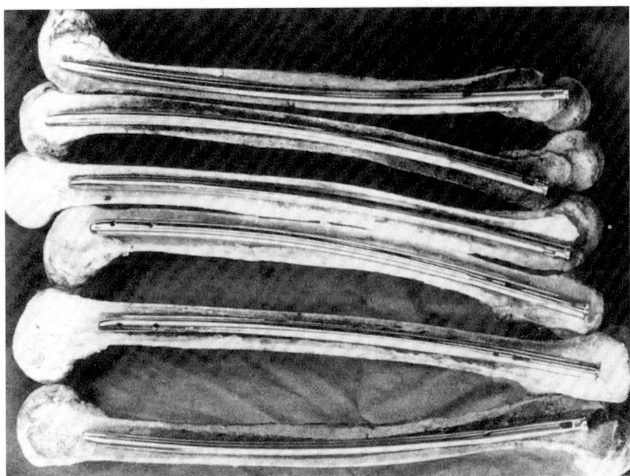

FIGURE 1-41 These cross sections of various femora demonstrate the curvature that an IM rod must conform to when it is fully inserted (64).

that govern the amount of bending of the rod during insertion and the resulting internal forces acting within the femur are the proximal starting hole position, the length of the proximal fragment, the initial curvature of the IM rod compared with the curvature of the femur, and the rod bending stiffness. Rod stiffness can vary considerably (66). Figure 1-43 demonstrates examples where rod proximal starting hole position resulted in femoral splitting during rod insertion (65). Some newer IM nails employ a valgus bend to be used with a femoral trochanteric entry portal. The basic principles regarding nail geometry, entry portal location, and excessive nail bending resulting in femoral splitting remain the same, however.

IM Rod and Locking Screw Breakage

Fractures of IM rods and locking screws occur occasionally during healing. The worst mechanical situation for IM rod fixation of the femur or tibia occurs when the fracture is very distal. Figure 1-44 compares the forces acting on idealized femora with more proximal and more distal fractures. For a specific location of the external load (muscle load or body weight), the more distal fracture results in a longer moment arm (the perpendicular distance from the load to the fracture site), creating a greater moment, and therefore, higher stresses in the rod. The highest stresses in the rod occur near the fracture site. With a distal fracture, in addition to the greater moment, the locking holes, significant stress risers, are usually located just distal to the fracture site. It has been shown that the maximum stresses acting in the rod increase rapidly once the distance between the fracture and the most superior of the distal screw holes is reduced to less than about 4 cm (67). In addition, placing the distal locking screws can be difficult because they must be inserted freehand under fluoroscopic guidance. It is possible to nick the corner of the screw hole of the rod with the drill or while driving the screw, creating an additional stress riser, which can accentuate the fatigue process. Awareness of these

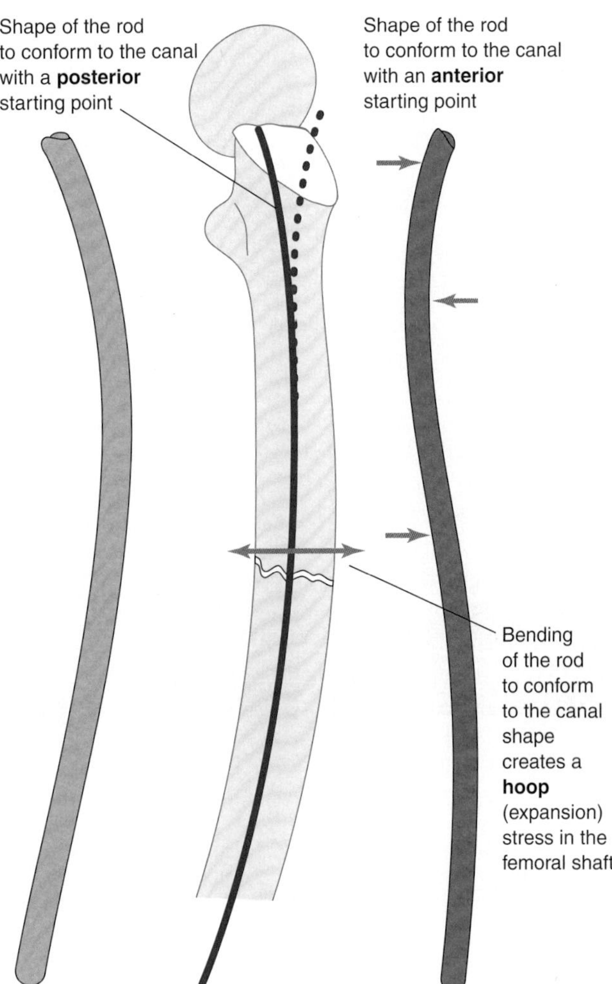

FIGURE 1-42 Mismatch of the curvature between the IM rod and the medullary canal results in bending stresses that could cause splitting of the femur during insertion (65).

potential problems has led to design changes such as closing the proximal section of the rod, increasing material thickness around the screw holes, and cold forming, which increases the material's strength.

Screw bending and breakage can also occur. When distal screws are placed into bone with relatively low bone density, the cortices essentially support the screw. The distal end of the femur widens rapidly (Fig. 1-45), so the length of the screws can be quite variable. For the same diameter and material, the stiffness and strength of a screw subjected to bending decreases as the third power of its length (the distance between cortices). If one screw is twice as long as the other, and assuming that the trabecular bone does not contribute to support of the screw, one can expect the stiffness and strength of the longer screw to be eight times less than the shorter screw and the deformation to be eight times greater under the same load. This creates a trade-off in fixation of these fractures with respect to screw

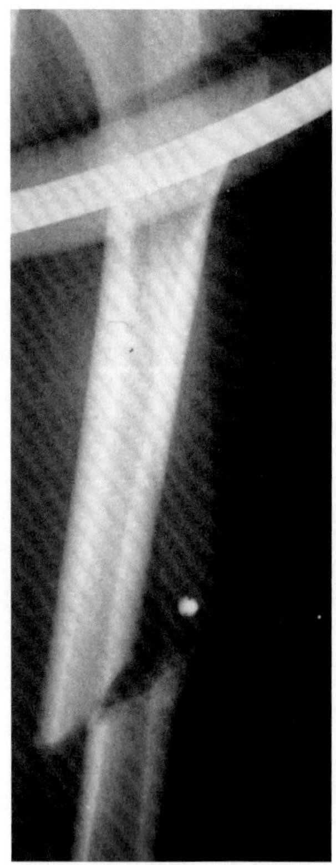
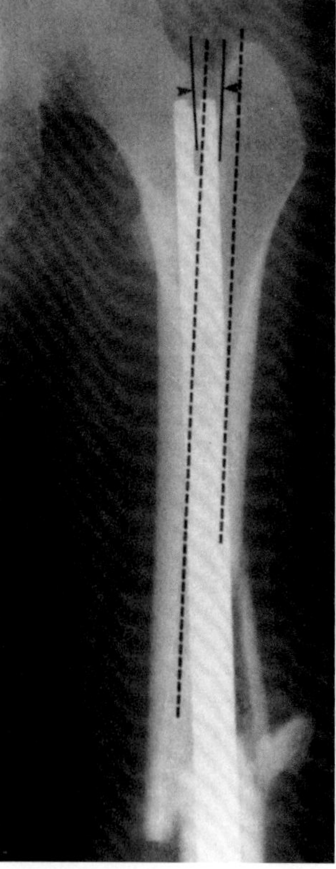
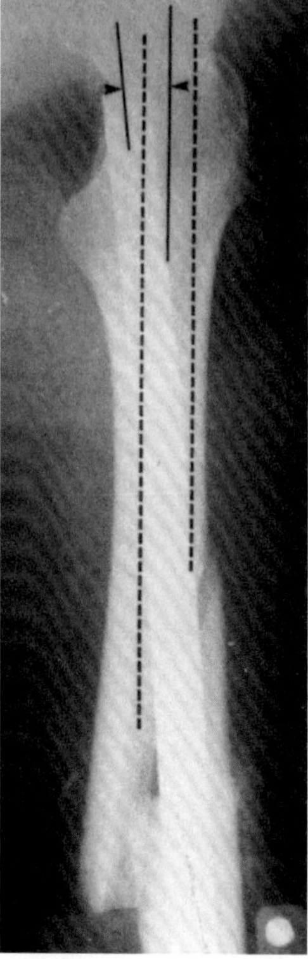

FIGURE 1-43 The starting position selected for rod entry into the medullary canal affects the degree to which it must bend and, therefore, the internal forces generated in the femur. A starting position offset from the axis of the medullary canal, coupled with a stiff rod and a longer proximal segment, which requires the rod to bend more during insertion, generate higher insertion forces and internal femoral forces. In this example of a midshaft femoral fracture **(left)**, the starting hole was selected medial relative to the axis of the medullary canal **(middle)**, and posterior **(right)**. The medullary canal is outlined in dashed lines. Therefore, the rod must bend both medially and posteriorly as it is inserted into the canal and has created internal stresses, which have split the midshaft end of the femur (65).

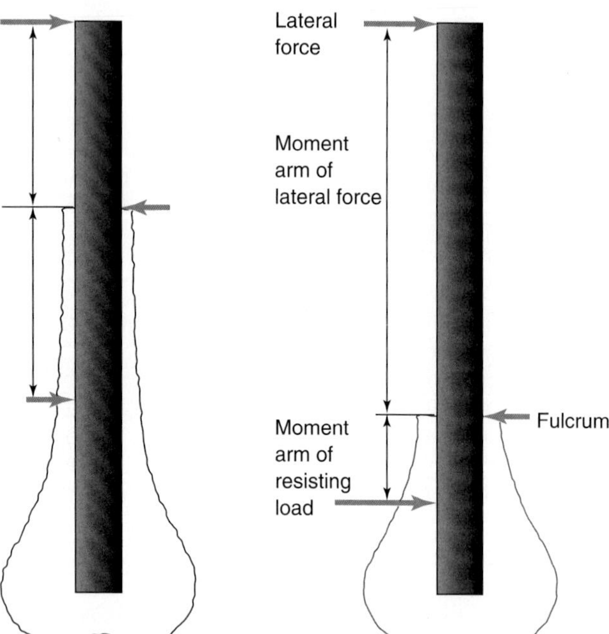

FIGURE 1-44 If the same force acts on IM rods placed in femora with more proximal **(left)** or more distal **(right)** fractures, the moment arm of the force will be longer in the case of the more distal fracture, and therefore the moment, acting at the fracture site, on the implant, will be larger. For the more distal fracture, the high stress region, close to the fracture site, is also significantly closer to the distal locking screw holes, which are significant stress risers.

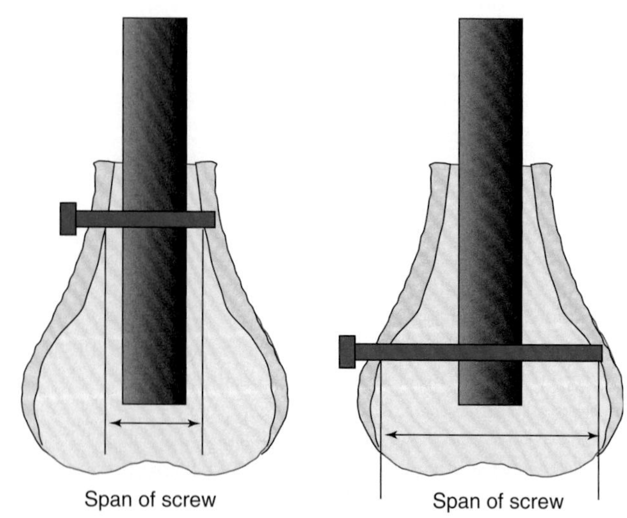

FIGURE 1-45 Because the distal end of the femur flares rapidly, the length of the locking screw required to cross lock the rod can be quite variable. If the screw is not well supported by trabecular bone but mainly by cortex, then its stiffness and strength decrease with the third power of its length between cortices. If the screw length doubles, the deformation of the screw under the same load increases by a factor of eight.

placement. If the screws are too close to the fracture, the stresses in the rod increase, whereas if they are within the flair of the metaphysis, with poor trabecular bone, their length increases, decreasing screw stiffness and strength.

Loosening of External Fixator Pins

Loosening of fixator pins in bone is thought to result from several causes. Because the shape of the end of the pin is self-tapping, it can affect the local heat generated in bone during insertion, potentially causing thermal necrosis around the pin-hole site (68), along with bone microcracking. In addition, high local stresses can occur in the pins and bone if the hole through which the pin is inserted is undersized (69). A third mechanism (Fig. 1-46) is micromotion, which induces bone resorption at the pin/bone interface if the pin is a loose fit in the hole. To reduce these problems, slight undersizing of the bone hole, by approximately 0.1 mm in diameter, has been advocated. If the bone hole is undersized by 0.3 mm in diameter, the yield strength of bone may be exceeded when the pin is inserted (69).

Excessively Flexible External Fixation

An external fixator is an assembly of pins attached to bone fragments, along with clamps and sidebars that couple the pins. This assembly allows considerable variation in frame construction to accommodate the fracture. Although the optimal stiffness of a fixator is not specifically known, and the stiffness necessary to stabilize the fracture and create healing changes as the fracture consolidates, it must be rigid enough to initially support the forces applied by the patient during ambulation without causing malalignment of the fracture. On the other hand, the fixator should not be so stiff that the fracture is shielded from the stresses required to stimulate healing. Some basic mechanical guidelines in frame construction will ensure that frames are adequately constructed for the loads they are subjected to. Figure 1-47 demonstrates that when the diameter of a pin or sidebar increases, its stiffness and strength increase to the fourth power of the relative change in diameter (actually the ratio of the larger to the smaller diameter), and as its length (distance between bone surface and sidebar) decreases, stiffness and strength increase to the third power of the length change. This principle also holds for the pins spanning the fracture, which affect the unsupported length of the sidebar across the fracture. In construction of a frame, it is beneficial to decrease the sidebar to bone distance, which decreases the unsupported lengths of the pins to increase the pin diameter, and decrease the distance between the pins that span the fracture. Increasing the number of pins applied also increases frame stiffness (70,71). Using a partly threaded pin and burying the pin thread completely within the cortex enhances the stiffness of the pin, as the smaller diameter of the root of the pin thread is not exposed.

The previous comments pertain to uniplane fixators, which are constructed to resist the major loads, axial compression, and anterior-posterior bending, acting on a long bone such as the tibia during walking, with the sidebar usually aligned with the anterior-posterior plane. To resist torsion and out-of-plane (medial-lateral) bending, the fixator can be assembled with additional

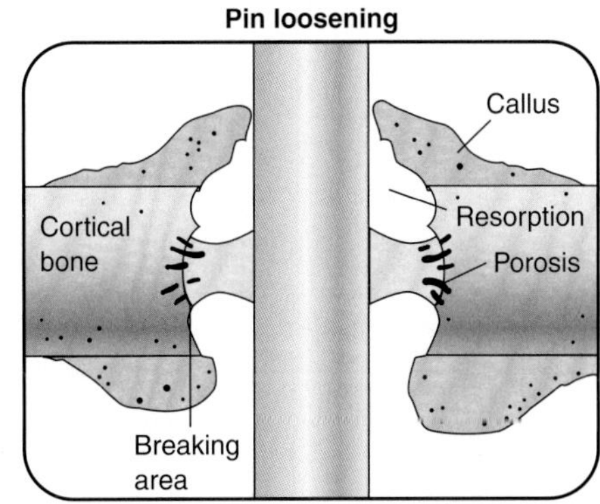

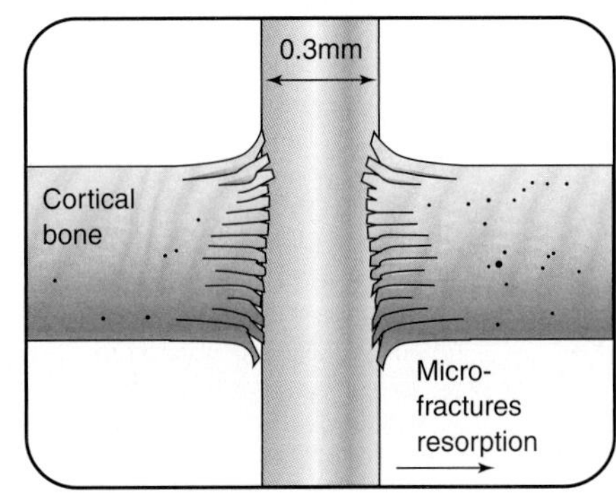

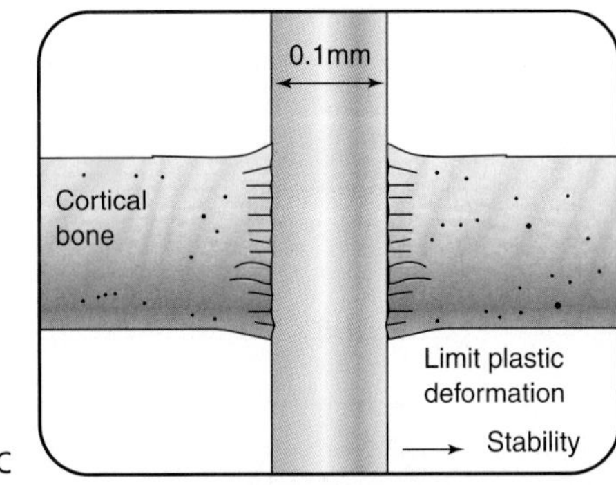

FIGURE 1-46 A proposed mechanism for loosening external fixation pins involves under- or oversizing the diameter of the pin relative to the bone hole. **A.** If the pin and bone hole are the same diameter, micromotion can occur with bone resorption. **B.** If the pin is more than 0.3 mm smaller in diameter than the hole in bone, microfracture may occur during insertion. **C.** If the bone hole diameter is about 0.1 mm smaller than the pin diameter, the bone is prestressed but does not fracture, micromotion is eliminated, and pin stability is maintained (56).

pins and sidebars in other planes. A comparison of the relative stiffnesses of different fixator assemblies is given in Figure 1-48. The unilateral half pin frame with sidebars mounted at right angles provides overall, the greatest resistance to bending, compression, and torsional loads (72). Hybrid fixation devices have adopted components of both unilateral bar fixators and ring fixators with wire transfixing pins. Both axial compression and tor-

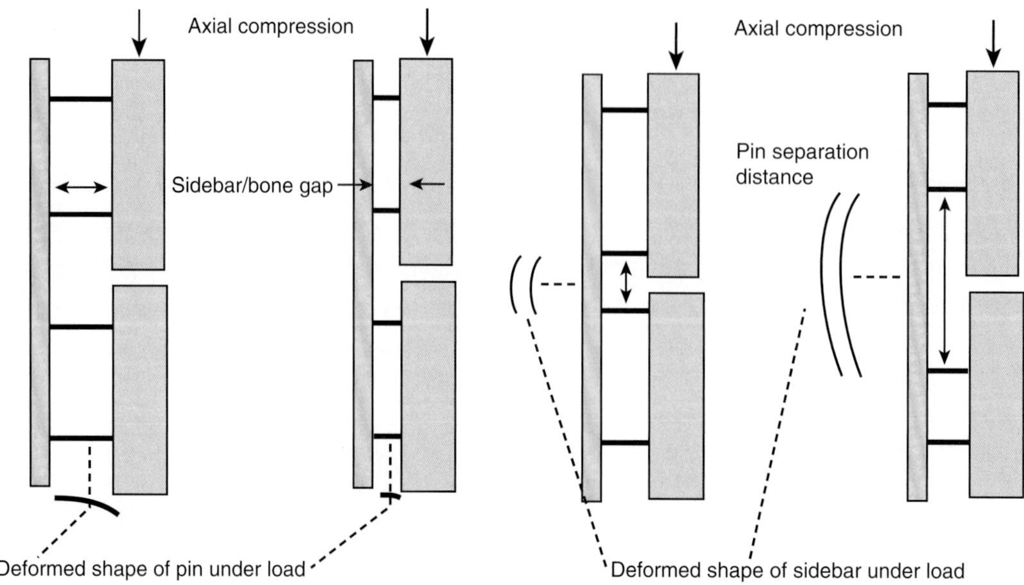

FIGURE 1-47 To produce more rigidity in construction of an external fixator, the basic principles that should be considered are that for pin-and-rod-type sidebars; stiffness increases with the fourth power of the cross-sectional area (the moment of inertia, Fig. 1-7) and decreases with the third power of their span or unsupported length (Fig. 1-45). This explains why it is beneficial to decrease sidebar to bone distance, increase pin diameter, place pins as close together across the fracture site as possible, and use larger-diameter or multiple sidebars in frame construction (70,71).

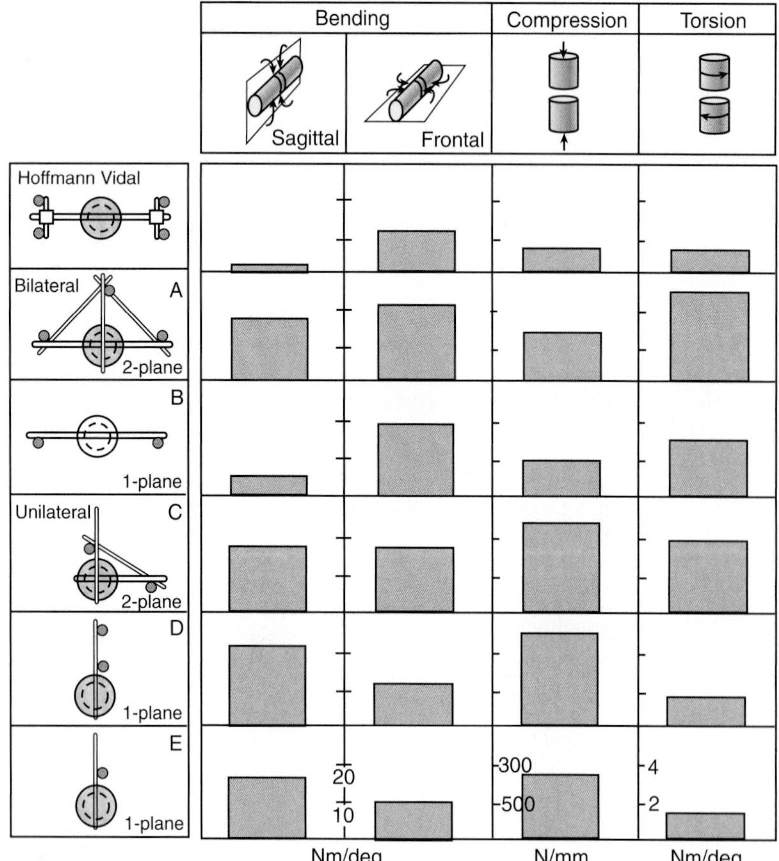

FIGURE 1-48 A comparison of the bending, compression, and torsional stiffnesses of different external fixation constructs for multiplane load resistance (72).

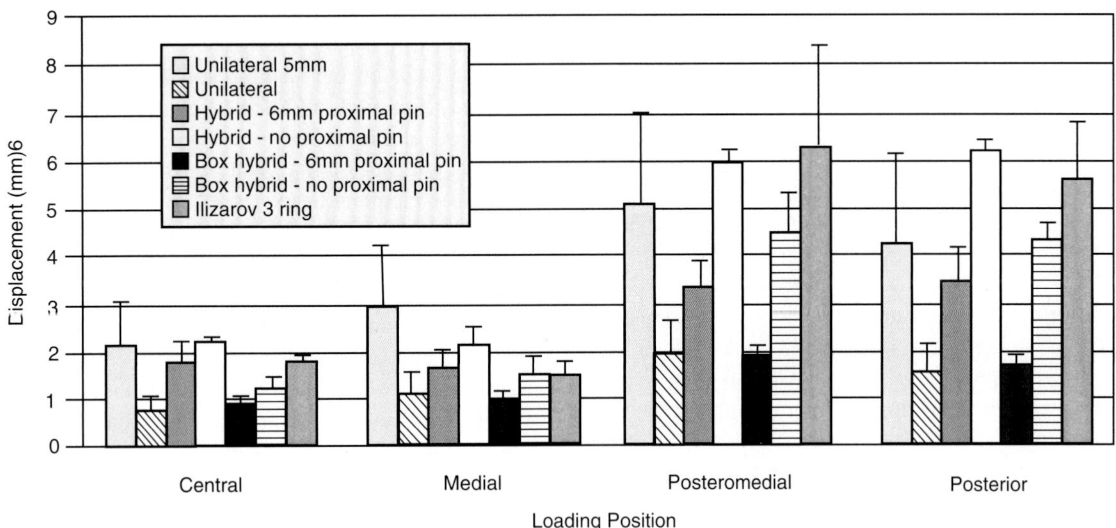

FIGURE 1-49 A comparison of displacement of the proximal fragment in a simulated tibia fracture under 100 N load with various unilateral and hybrid external fixators (the box type uses both a large unilateral frame connecting bar and two smaller-diameter connecting rods) (75).

sional stiffnesses have been found to increase significantly with increases in the number and diameter of the transfixing wires, and pretensioning the wires (73). More anterior wire placement or adding an anteromedial half pin has been found to increase anterior-posterior bending stiffness (74). Testing a number of different configurations (Fig. 1-49) showed that the box type (two rings above and two below the fracture, along with anterior half pins, two connecting rods, and a unilateral bar) was the stiffest configuration, compared with a unilateral frame alone or a unilateral frame with rings only proximal to the fracture site. Adding an anterior half pin significantly increased fixation stiffness (75).

Fixation in Osteoporotic Bone

Because attachment to bone, by a screw for example, is directly related to bone density, and a dominant mechanical characteristic of osteoporotic bone is low density, several strategies can be used when osteoporotic bone is encountered. These approaches include cortical buttressing by impaction, wide buttressing, which spreads the load over a larger surface area, long splintage, improved anchoring, and increasing the local bone density by injection of, for example, hydroxyapatite or methylmethacrylate (Fig. 1-50) (76). Impaction can be applied to fractures of the distal radius, femoral neck, and lumbar vertebrae. The dynamic

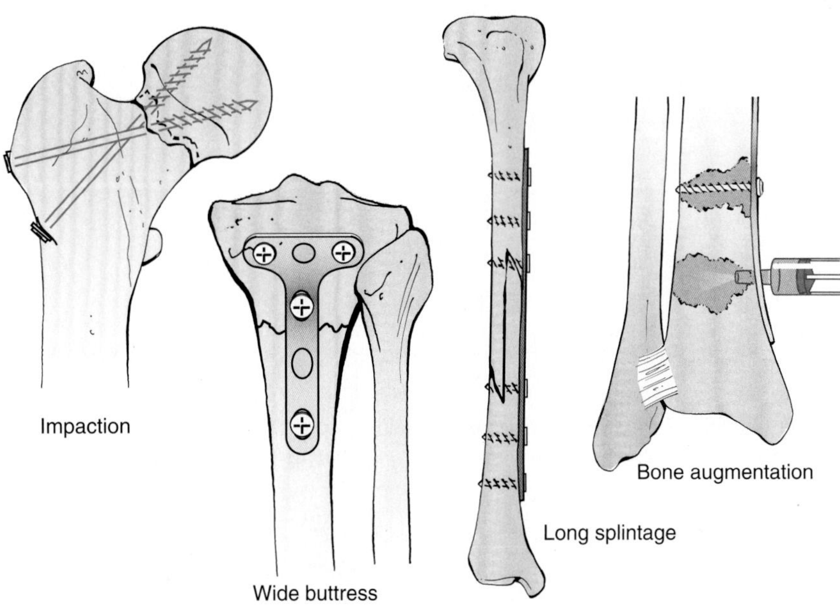

FIGURE 1-50 Some basic strategies to augment fixation strength in osteoporotic bone including impaction of the fracture components using a device that allows sliding, buttressing with a wide plate, increasing the plate length, and augmenting the bone locally by injection of methymethacrylate or a calcium phosphate cement (58).

hip screw is an example of a device that allows controlled fracture impaction of the femoral neck. An angled blade plate applied to supracondylar femur fractures, as compared with a condylar screw, provides wider buttressing; that is, a larger surface area of contact with bone. The rafter plate that permits placement of numerous cancellous screws for tibial plateau fractures is another example of the application of this principle (77). Long splinting with a longer, more flexible plate has been applied in humerus fractures, and the interlocked IM rod is a second example of long splinting. Enhanced anchoring of pedicle screws using augmenting laminar hooks is an example of augmentation of anchoring (78). The locking plate, where the screws are threaded into the plate and fixed so they cannot rotate, can be useful for stabilizing osteoporotic fractures where cortical buttressing is not practical because of low bone density, and the fixation hardware must support more of the load. Hydroxyapatite-coated external fixation pins have been shown to enhance the screw-bone interface (79). Interlocking screws, where a standard screw has a 45° hole drilled into the shaft to accept an interlocking pin, can be used to reduce screw backout (80).

Enhancement of local bone density using either polymethylmethacrylate (PMMA) or more recently, absorbable hydroxyapatite cement, has been studied, particularly in relation to fixation of femoral and vertebral osteoporotic fractures. PMMA injection has been widely employed in vertebroplasty through a transpedicular approach (81) and has been shown to restore stiffness of fractured vertebrae to intact levels. Biomechanical studies have shown significantly improved strength of the fixation of femoral neck fractures, up to 170% (82), and similar findings, including decreased shortening and greater stability were noted when hydroxyapatite cement was applied to unstable three-part intertrochanteric fractures fixed with a dynamic hip screw (83). Calcium phosphate cements used in vertebroplasty instead of PMMA also restored the stiffness of fractured vertebrae to intact levels (84). Calcium phosphate cement injection into the pedicle (85) has been shown to improve the bending stiffness of pedicle screws by up to 125%.

BIOMECHANICAL ASPECTS OF FRACTURE FIXATION IN SPECIFIC LOCATIONS

In the previous discussion, common problems such as screw pullout and plate breakage (common to fracture fixation, mainly in the long bones) were discussed. In this section, the focus is placed on specific challenging problems in fixation, including the femoral neck, tibial plateau, pelvis, and spine.

Fixation of the Proximal Femur

Fixation of proximal femoral fractures is particularly challenging because the compressive force acting through the femoral head can range from four to eight times the body weight during normal activities (86). This force acts through a significant moment arm (the length of the femoral neck), which causes large bending loads on the fixation hardware. In addition, many of these fractures occur in the elderly who are likely to have trabecular bone of low density and poor mechanical quality (87). Also, it is not possible to gain screw purchase in the cortical bone of the femoral head.

The major force acting in, for example, a basicervical fracture of the femoral neck, fixed with a sliding hip screw is the joint reaction force through the femoral head, which derives from body weight and forces generated by muscle action during ambulation. The joint reaction force can be divided into two components. One (Fig. 1-51) is perpendicular to the axis of the sliding screw and causes shearing of the fracture surfaces along the fracture line, which results in inferior displacement and varus angulation of the femoral head, and increases the resistance of the screw to sliding. The other component is parallel to the screw, driving the surfaces together, enhancing stability by frictional and mechanical interlocking of the fracture. The aim of femoral neck fixation systems is to use the parallel component of the joint force to allow the surfaces to slide together. This is the basic principle behind selecting a higher-angle hip screw when possible. The actual stiffness provided by the sliding hip screw, the reconstruction nail, and multiple pin constructs are quite similar, except that the reconstruction nail offers significantly greater torsional stiffness than the other forms of fixation, because of its tubular shape (88–91).

When using the compression (or sliding) hip screw, or a nail with a sliding lag screw, it is important to ensure that the

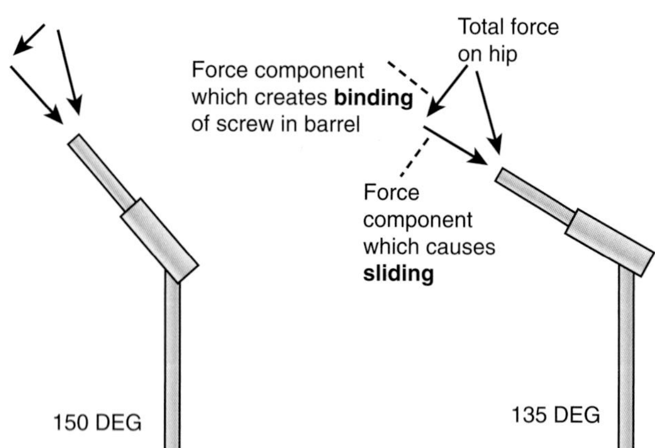

FIGURE 1-51 The joint reaction force in the femoral head can be divided into two major components. The component that is parallel to the axis of the femoral neck produces sliding and impaction of the fracture components and the other, transverse to the femoral neck, causes the screw component of the femoral hip screw to bind and resist sliding. The higher-angle hip screw has a screw axis more closely aligned with the joint reaction force so the force component that produces sliding is larger, while the transverse force component that resists sliding is smaller.

screw can slide freely in the barrel of the side plate or the hole in the nail. The following comments related to sliding hip screws apply as well to nail/lag screw constructs. When screw sliding occurs, the barrel supports the screw against inferior bending of the femoral head because the construct is buttressed by fracture interdigitation. Adherence to two basic mechanical principles will enhance the screw's ability to slide in the side plate or nail. As mentioned, the higher-angle hip screw is more effective at accommodating sliding. Also, the screw should be engaged as deeply as possible within the barrel. For the same force acting at the femoral end of the screw, the internal force where the screw contacts the barrel is increased if less of the screw remains in the barrel. This occurs because the moment (bending load) caused by the force transverse to the axis of the screw (Fh in Fig. 1-52) (at the femoral head) acts over a longer moment arm

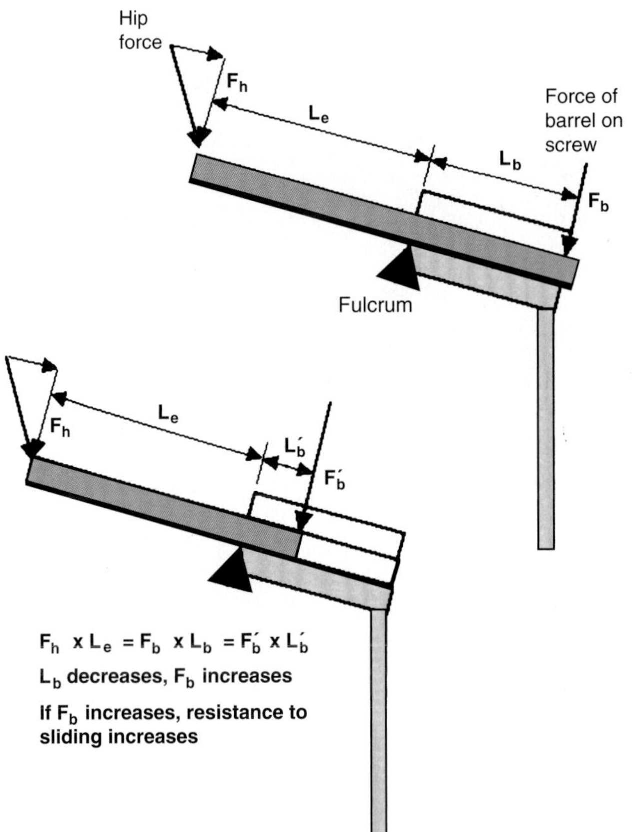

FIGURE 1-52 The greater the length of the sliding screw within the barrel is, the lower its resistance to sliding will be. In this diagram, Fh is the component of the joint reaction force perpendicular to the axis of the screw. The inferior edge of the proximal end of the barrel is the location of the fulcrum in bending. An internal force, Fb, from the surface of the barrel acts against the screw to counteract Fh. For equilibrium, the moments produced by Fh (Fh × Le) and Fb (Fb × Lb) must be equal. If Lb, the distance from the point of application of internal force Fb to the fulcrum decreases, Fb must increase to produce the same moment. If Fb is larger, the frictional force and, therefore, the resistance to screw sliding will increase (128). (Le is the length of the screw beyond the barrel.)

or perpendicular distance (Le) (force × perpendicular distance to the edge of the barrel, which is the fulcrum). The balancing moment arm, Lb, is shorter because less of the screw remains in the barrel. Because Fh acts over a longer moment arm while Fe acts over a shorter moment arm, Fb increases. The internal force, Fb, where the screw contacts the barrel, causes a greater frictional resistance force that requires more force to overcome in order to permit sliding (92). Sliding hip screws with either two- or four-hole side plates appear to provide equivalent resistance to physiologic compressive loading (93).

Several factors affect the strength of femoral neck fixation using multiple screws. The number of screws used (three or four) is not a significant factor (91). Factors that do increase the strength of this type of fixation include a more horizontal fracture line with respect to the long axes of the screws (94), placement of the screws in areas of greater femoral head bone density (90,95), fractures with less comminution (95,96), and a shorter moment arm for the joint load (shorter distance from the center of the femoral head to the fracture line) (95). The most important factor has been found to be the quality of the reduction due to the importance of cortical buttressing in reducing fracture displacement (97). Under physiological load, several mechanisms of fixation failure have been observed (Fig. 1-53). In some cases, the screws bend inferiorly, especially if buttressing of the fracture surfaces inferior to the screws is not possible because of fracture comminution. If no washers are used to distribute the screw load against bone, the fixation screw heads have been found to pull through cortex near the greater trochanter, when the cortex is thin. Finally, if the screws are not well supported inferiorly where they cross the fracture, they may rotate inferiorly carrying the femoral head into a varus orientation (82). Supporting at least one screw against the inferior cortex may help prevent this occurrence.

Fixation Around the Metaphyseal Region of the Knee

Both supracondylar femur and tibial plateau fractures are challenging to stabilize because they may involve fixation of multiple small fragments of primarily cancellous bone. Supracondylar fixation alternatives have been mechanically compared, including condylar plates, plates with lag screws across the fracture site, and blade plates. All devices tested appeared to provide similar construct stiffnesses. The most important factor identified was maintaining contact at the cortex opposite that on which the fixation device was applied. Fixation constructs without cortical contact were only about 20% as stiff as those with cortical buttressing (98). The retrograde IM supracondylar nail was found to 14% less stiff in axial compression and 17% less stiff in torsion, compared with a fixed-angle side plate (99). Several newer fixation systems have been described for femoral supracondylar fracture stabilization. One system consists of a blade plate with

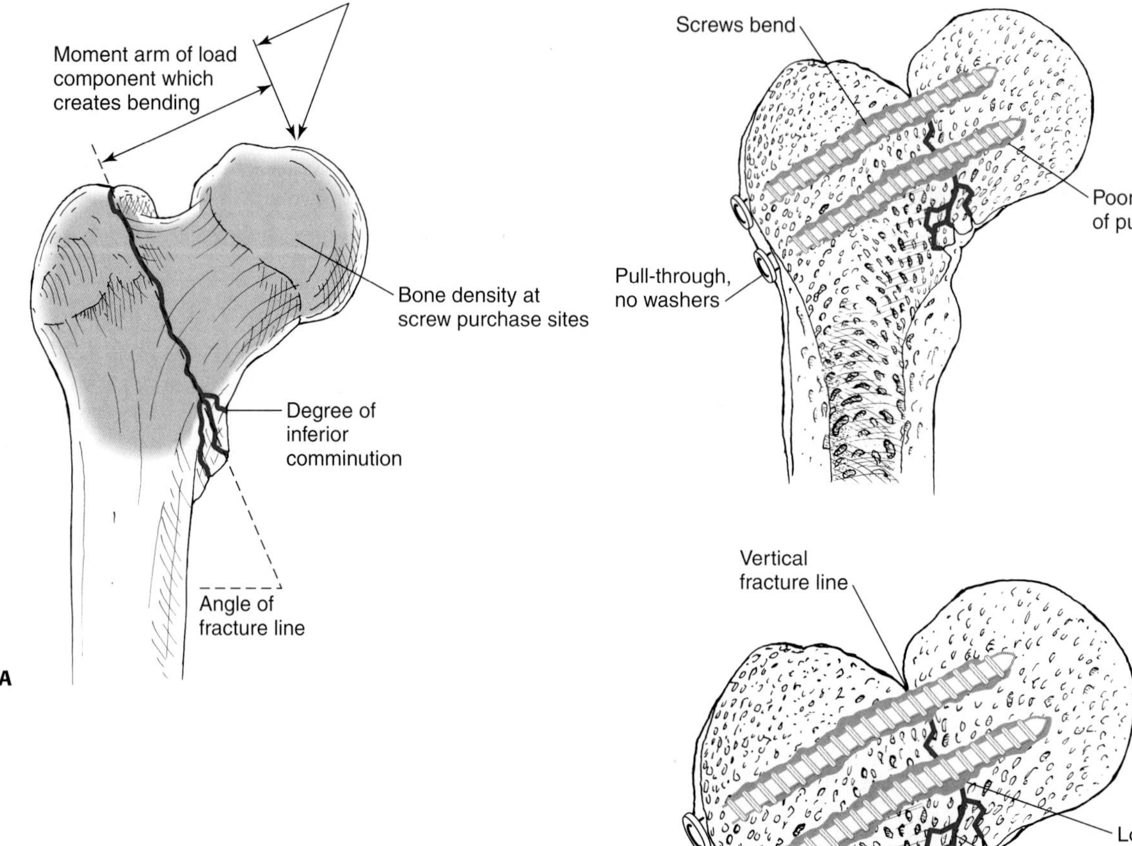

FIGURE 1-53 **A.** Some factors that decrease the strength of femoral neck fracture fixation include decreased bone density, a more vertical fracture surface that facilitates sliding of the fracture components, comminution at the inferior cortex that reduces buttressing against bending, and a longer moment arm or distance of the center of the femoral head to the fracture line. **B.** Observed mechanisms of failure of femoral neck fixation using screws include bending of the pins, displacement of the screw heads through the thin cortex of the greater trochanter, especially if washers are not used, and rotation of the screws inferiorly through the low-density cancellous bone of the Ward's triangle area until they settle against the inferior cortex (95).

a screw threaded through the plate to triangulate it (Fig. 1-54). This has been found to be significantly stiffer than conventional constructs (100). The LISS uses a low-profile plate with monocortical screws distally, which also lock to the plate. LISS plates have more elastic deformation and less subsidence than a condylar screw or buttress plate (101).

Tibial plateau fractures are challenging to fix for the same reasons that make supracondylar fractures difficult. Different fixation methods include screws alone or screws placed through an L- or T-shaped plate that buttresses the cortex. Fixation with T-plates and screws has been found to provide the greatest resistance to an axial compressive load (102). As Figure 1-55 shows, fixation with screws alone requires that the screw resist bending forces, as the tibial fragment is loaded distally in compression through the joint. With the addition of a plate, not only is the load distributed to the plate, but additional screws can be placed in the stronger cortical bone distal to the metaphysis of the tibia. The disadvantage of adding a buttressing plate is the greater invasiveness that it requires for installation. An alternative to tibial fracture fixation with screws is multiple Kirschner wires, which in essence form a raft under the fragment. Various configurations have been tested (103) and show that the construct's stiffness is most increased by adding more wires, regardless of their specific orientations.

The fractured patella is challenging to stabilize because of

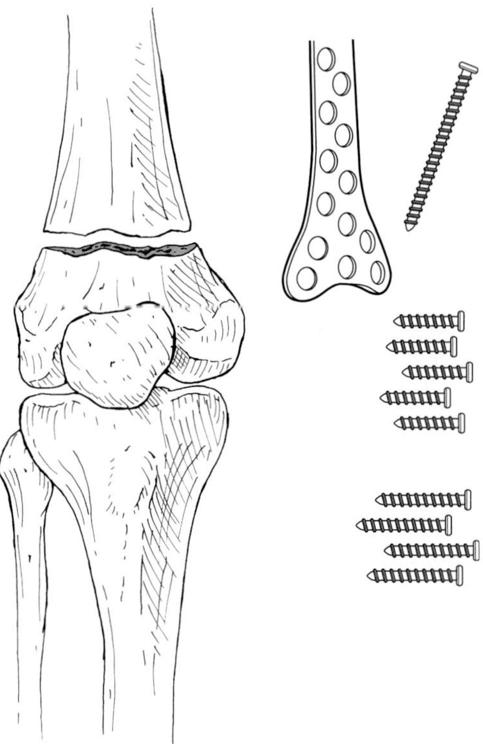

FIGURE 1-54 The triangulated blade plate is a simple construct that has been shown to significantly improve the stiffness of supracondylar fractures (100).

the large tensile and bending forces generated by contracting the quadriceps muscles (104). The tensile force causes significant bending in the patella with the knee flexed, which tends to open the anterior surface of the fracture. A variety of screw, wire, or combination screw and wire fixation constructs have been developed. Screw fixation can generate greater compression across the fracture site, but wire can withstand higher tensile forces because it does not depend upon the purchase of threads in the cancellous bone of the patella for fixation as do screws (105).

Fixation of Pelvic Fractures

The pelvis can be considered, in general terms, as the structural base of the spinal column, with a flexible anterior joint, the symphysis pubis, and two semirigid posterior hinges, the sacroiliac joints, which are subjected to large bending loads. The major external loads include the weight of the torso acting through the sacrum, the abductor and gluteus muscle forces, and the joint reactions acting through the acetabuli. Because these force vectors do not align, both anterior-posterior and medial-lateral bending loads act on the pelvis along with compression through the sacrum and tensile stresses around the pelvic ring that tend to open the symphysis. When the sacroiliac (SI) joint is not completely disrupted, anterior plating of the symphysis pubis alone provides stability similar to anterior plating combined with posterior fixation using as an SI plate or iliac screws (106,107). With complete disruption of the SI joint or with fracture through the sacrum, using a single-legged stance model, the use of two anterior plates combined with a single SI screw was most effective at reducing SI joint gapping, rotation, and pubis symphysis gapping. This construct was followed in order of increased joint motions by two SI screws, two anterior SI plates, and various combinations of posterior tension band plates, sacral bars, and iliosacral screws (108,109). Another construct that might be considered for sacral fractures is a triangulated combination of a sacroiliac screw, a screw placed into the iliac wing, and a vertical bar attached to the iliac screw with fixation into L5. This setup resists the vertical compression component of the loads applied through the spine into the sacrum (110).

Fixation of the Spine

The halo apparatus is an external fixation device for cervical spine injuries with specific mechanical characteristics that

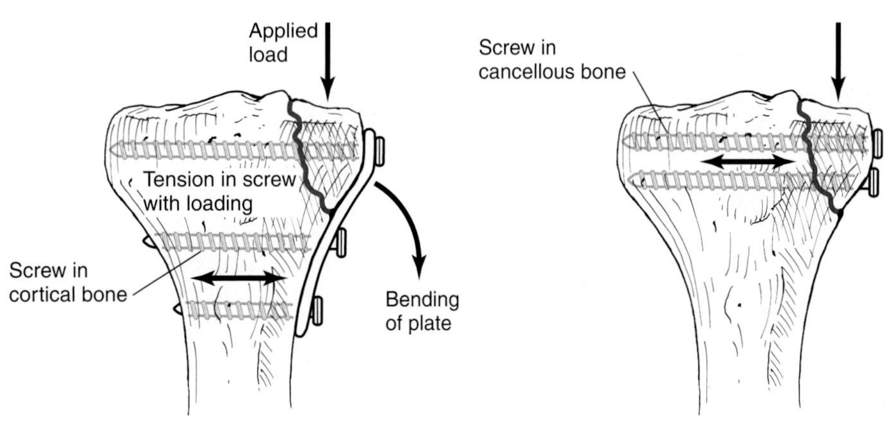

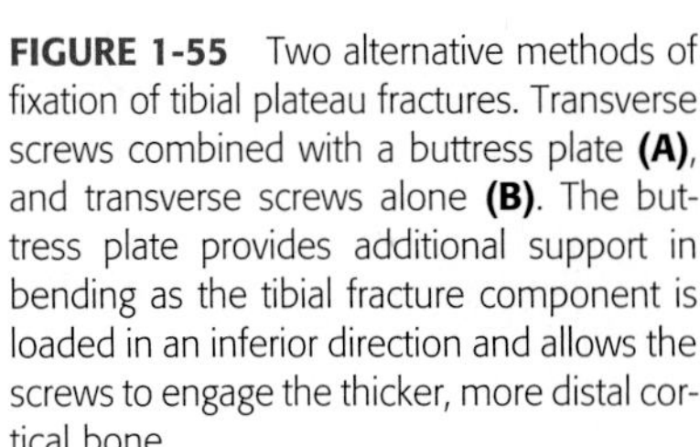

FIGURE 1-55 Two alternative methods of fixation of tibial plateau fractures. Transverse screws combined with a buttress plate **(A)**, and transverse screws alone **(B)**. The buttress plate provides additional support in bending as the tibial fracture component is loaded in an inferior direction and allows the screws to engage the thicker, more distal cortical bone.

allow it to stabilize the injured cervical spine against bending, but not compressive loads. These features include the fit of the jacket on the torso and the frictional characteristics of the lining (Fig. 1-56). High-friction linings decrease slip at the vest lining/torso interface, more rigid vests reduce deflection under loads, and less-flexible superstructures all decrease cervical spine motion at the injury level. Although stiffening the vest enhances its ability to stabilize the injury, this property must be balanced with enough flexibility to provide reasonable comfort for the wearer and to accommodate chest expansion and contraction. The injured cervical segment is relatively distant from the vest, so small motions of the vest can result in relatively large displacements at the injury site (111). A very rigid halo superstructure attaching the vest to the halo ring may not increase injury stability if it is connected to a poorly fitting vest.

A number of methods are available to reconstruct cervical spine injuries. The major differences between these approaches relate to the location of the fixation (either anterior, lateral, or posterior) and to the method by which the fixation is attached to bone. Generally, the most rigid fixation is the one with the longest moment arm from the center of rotation of the injured segment. For a specific applied moment (e.g., flexion), posterior fixation, being located further from the center of rotation, results in greater rigidity. Figure 1-57 shows the approximate locations of the centers of rotation at different cervical spine levels when the posterior elements have been disrupted (112). After corpectomy, testing has shown that posterior rods provide the greatest stability, which is unchanged after augmentation with an anterior plate, whereas anterior plating alone offers the least stability (113). Similarly, another test showed that after corpectomy, sagittal plane motion was most rigid after supplementation with lateral mass plates, was less rigid with an anterior plate alone, and

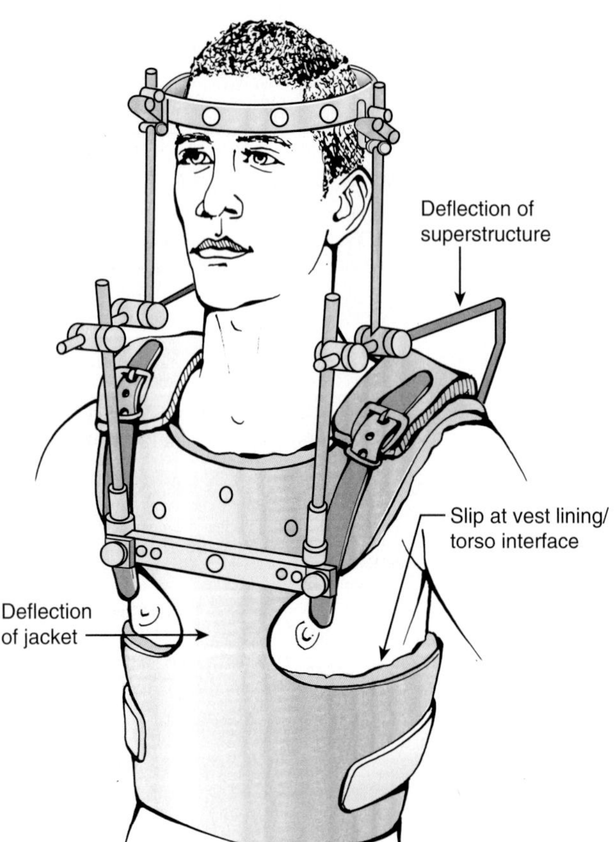

FIGURE 1-56 A schematic diagram showing possible sources of deformation in the halo apparatus. The large distance from the vest-to-chest contact points to the cervical injury site results in relatively large motions at the injury site for small motions of the vest (111).

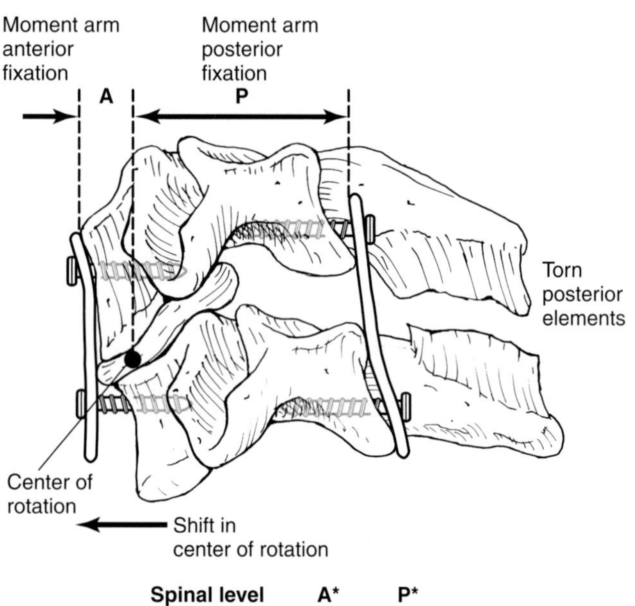

Spinal level	A*	P*
C2-3	0.27	0.73
C3-4	0.32	0.68
C4-5	0.36	0.64
C5-6	0.39	0.61
C6-7	0.44	0.56

*In % of anterior-posterior diameter of vertebra

FIGURE 1-57 The ratios, in terms of anterior-posterior vertebra diameter of the location of the center of rotation at each vertebral level, from the anterior and posterior surfaces. A fixation device must resist bending moments caused by flexion, extension, lateral bending, and torsion. The resisting moment in the fixation is the product of the force acting in the fixation (e.g., at the screw-plate junction) and the distance of that point on the fixation to the center of rotation of the motion segment. The longer the moment arm for the same bending load is, the smaller the force on the fixation components will be. Posterior fixation, by its location, will have lower moments in its components (112).

least rigid with strut grafting alone (114). Anterior plates provide relatively similar stability, especially if augmented with a bone graft; however, with multilevel corpectomy, anterior plate constructs were more prone to fatigue loosening than single level corpectomies (115). Some of the newer semiconstrained anterior plates allow screw rotation that results in more load sharing with the graft. By comparison, the compressive load estimated to be transmitted through the graft increased from about 40% with a fully constrained device to about 80% when a semiconstrained device was used (116). Wiring or plating with lateral mass screws generally reduces anterior-posterior motion across the fixed segment by 20% to 70%, so none of the techniques can be considered as entirely rigid (117).

The type of attachment of the fixation system to the vertebra is fundamental to its performance. Wires, hooks, screws, or combinations of these three items all produce different types of force transfer between the fixation and the vertebra (Fig. 1-58) (118). A wire can resist only tension, whereas a screw can resist forces in all directions (tension, compression, bending transverse to the axis of the screw), except for rotation about its longitudinal axis. A hook only resists forces that drive its surface against bone and depends also on its shape and the bone surface it rests against. For this reason, screws are biomechanically superior to other forms of vertebral attachments.

In general, pedicle screws resist pullout in the same manner as bone screws described elsewhere; therefore, pullout strength increases with increased density of the bone it is embedded into (45–48,119,120), a greater insertion depth (121), engagement of the anterior cortex (122), and a larger screw diameter. Single screws placed into pedicles and loaded in a caudal-cephalad direction, which occurs during flexion and extension of the vertebra, are vulnerable to toggling and eventual loosening, even under relatively small forces. As shown in Figure 1-59, the screw tends to toggle about the base of the pedicle, which is the stiffest region and is mainly composed of cortical bone. Toggling tends to open the screw hole in a "windshield wiper" fashion (123,124). Toggling can be reduced if the screw head is locked to the plate or rod and if the plate or rod contacts the vertebra over a wide area (124).

Consider some fundamental principles when applying lumbar spinal fixation. Longer fixation, attached to a greater number of vertebrae reduces forces acting on the screws, because of the effect of the greater lever arm of a longer plate or rod. A longer fusion, although biomechanically advan-

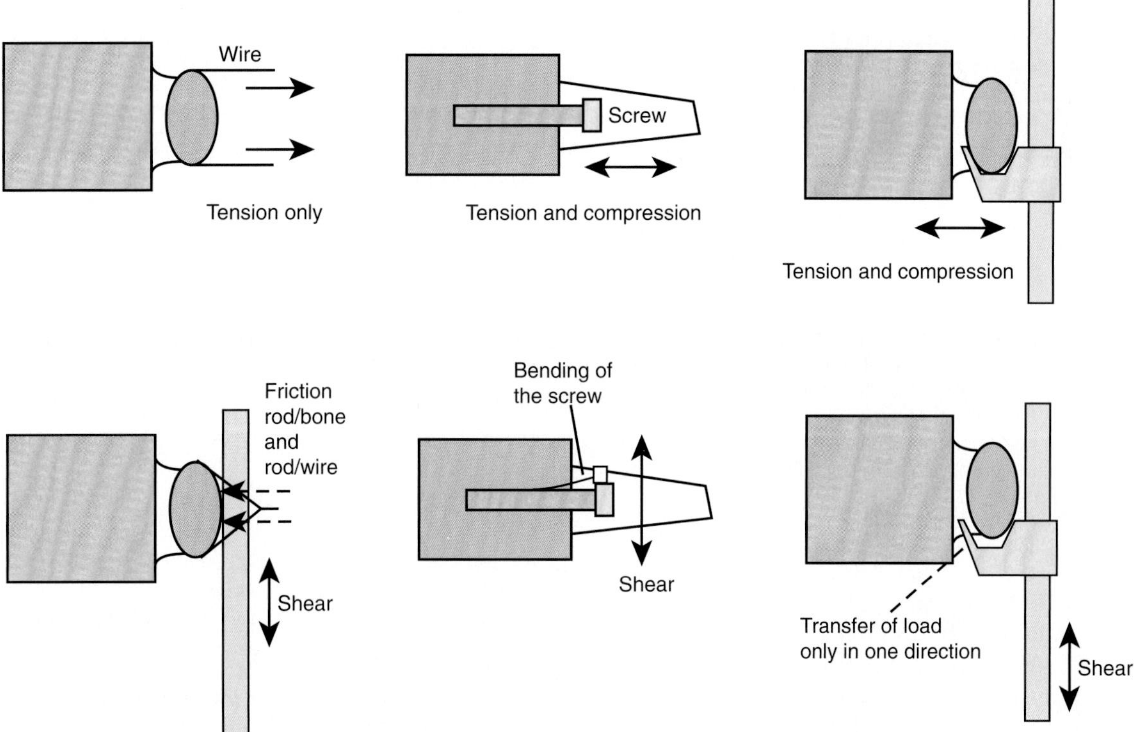

FIGURE 1-58 Comparisons of the forces that can be resisted by different methods of attachment of the fixation to the vertebra. A sublaminar wire resists only tension, whereas a screw can resist forces in all directions except for rotation about its long axis. A hook resists only forces that drive it against the bone surfaces.

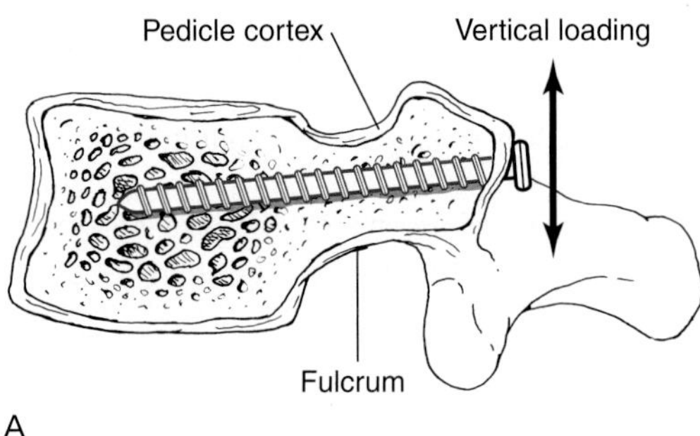

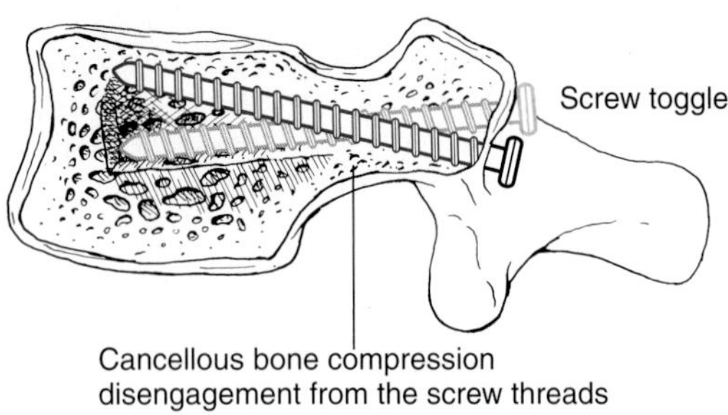

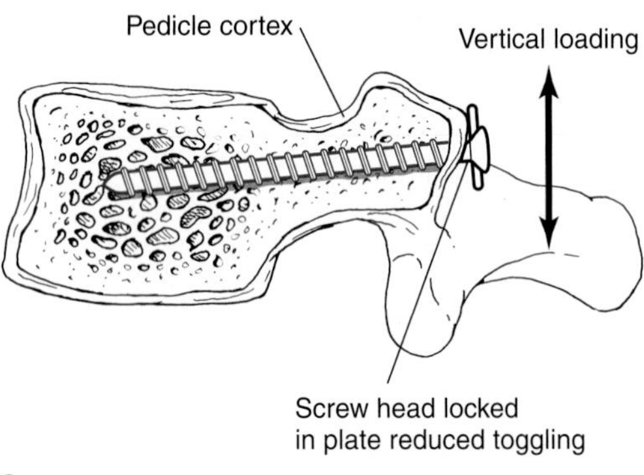

FIGURE 1-59 **A.** The mechanism of toggling of a single pedicle screw subjected to a caudocephalad loading. **B.** The fulcrum is at the base of the pedicle, the narrowest region with little cancellous bone. The screw toggle compresses bone within the vertebral body. **C.** Toggling is reduced if the plate or rod to which the screw connects contacts the vertebra over a wide surface, which prevents it from rotating while the screw head is locked to the plate or rod (124).

tageous, is not necessarily beneficial from a clinical perspective. Adding an anterior strut graft or a fusion cage is important, as it buttresses a posterior fixation system against flexion moments, reducing forces in the fixation (125,126). Coupler bars, which connect the fixation rods to form an H configuration, prevent the rods from rotating medial and lateral when torsion is applied to the motion segment (Fig. 1-60). This construct significantly enhances the implant's torsional and lateral bending stability.

Extensive testing has been performed on a variety of posterior and anterior thoracolumbar fixation devices as they continue to be developed. Testing anterior fixation systems with and without an augmented strut graft showed that load sharing with the graft ranged from 63% to 89% for six systems tested—three were plates and three were based on locked rods. These tests demonstrated the significant effect of the graft in sagittal plane stability of the fixation. The most rigid systems, not significantly different in performance, relied on either a thick rigid plate or large rods (127). In cases of delayed or nonunion, the cyclic performance of the implant can be very important, more so than its static stiffness or maximum load to failure. A comparison test of 12 fixation systems showed that only three could withstand 2 million load cycles with 600 N of compressive force. The two fixations with greatest bending strength also did not fail after cycling; however, there was no correlation between bending strength and cyclic failure for the other 10 systems, indicating that particular design aspects could cause fatigue failure, regardless of static strength (128). Three devices failed in less than 10,000 cycles. Currently, most posterior devices use essentially the same principles: pedicle screws, an adjustable screw to rod or plate interface to enhance fixation assembly, interconnecting rods, (or less frequently, plates), a low-profile assembly, and crosslinks. These components provide similar fixation stiffness. Lumbosacral fixation using sacral screws was most rigid, demonstrated the least screw strain when supplemented with iliac screws, and was more effective than using screws at S1 supplemented with screws at S2 (129).

The biomechanical properties of fusion cages have been investigated. A fusion cage is a hollow threaded insert that can be applied from anterior, lateral, or posterior directions in single or double units. A wide variety of fusion cages are available for the cervical spine. The devices fall into one of three categories: screw designs with a horizontal cylinder and external threads, box shapes, and vertical cylinders. In general, all cage designs increased flexion stiffness by 130% to 180%. Only a few box or cylinder designs increased extension stiffness, and box designs were most effective in increasing axial rotation and lateral bending stiffnesses, ranging from 140% to 180% of intact values (126). Testing lumbar fusion cages has shown that placing fusion cages in lateral, posterolateral, or posterior orientations had little effect on stiffness, except for the effect of posterior placement in torsional loading, as insertion damaged the lamina or facets, reducing the motion segment's inherent torsional stability. Fixation with cages alone did not significantly increase lumbar motion segment stability, so augmentation with posterior fixation in cases of motion segment instability is necessary. Because cage fixation relies on the combination of soft tissue distraction and the strength of the vertebral cancellous bone, the properties of these tissues will have a significant effect on the performance of cage implants (130).

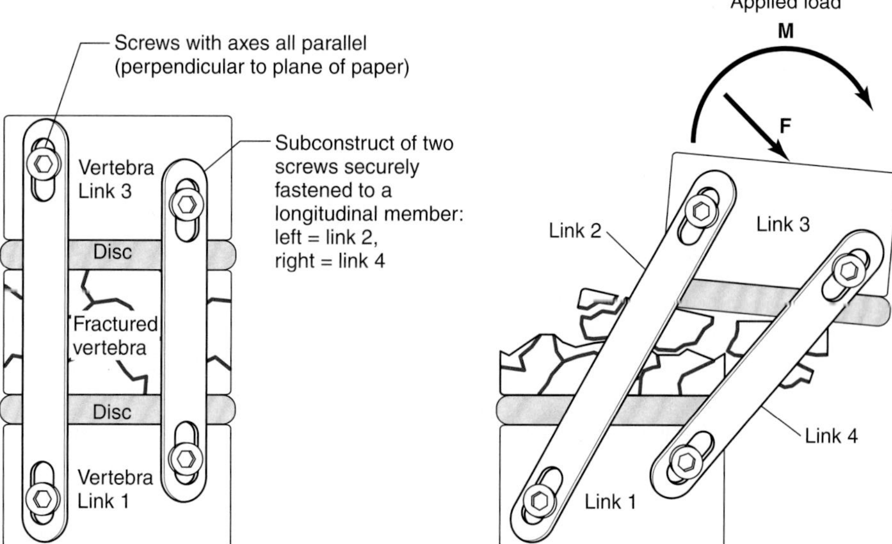

FIGURE 1-60 Without a coupler bar between two longitudinal rods **(left)**, they can rotate when a lateral moment or axial torsion is applied **(right)**. A coupler connecting the rods to form an H configuration reduces this effect.

SUMMARY

Effective fracture fixation requires a biomechanical appreciation of the forces applied to a damaged bone or joint and the basic mechanisms by which these loads are transferred through the bridging fixation and at the implant-bone interface. In particular, the importance of the contribution of cortex-to-cortex contact across the fracture site in resisting both compressive and bending forces must be emphasized. This buttress contributes significantly to the construct's stability and the implant's functional life. Many of the observations used to formulate these basic principles have been made using cadaveric bone in experimental simulations. It is important to correlate these findings to clinical observations of the mechanics of fixation during fracture healing.

REFERENCES

1. Black J, *Orthopedic Biomaterials in Research and Practise*. Churchill Livingstone: New York, 1988.
2. Carter DR, Hayes WC. The compressive behavior of bone as a two-phase porous structure. *J Bone Jt Surg* 1977:59A:954–962.
3. Burstein AH, Zika IM, Heiple KG, Klein L. Contribution of collagen and mineral to the elastic-plastic properties of bone. *J Bone Jt Surg* 1975;57A:956–961.
4. Currey JD. The mechanical consequences of variation in the mineral content of bone. *J Biomech* 1969;2:1–11.
5. Ascenzi A, Bonucci E. The compressive properties of single osteons. *Anat Rec* 1968; 161:377–392.
6. Ascenzi A, Bonucci E. The shearing properties of single osteons. *Anat Rec* 1972;172: 499–510.
7. Ascenzi A, Bonucci E. The tensile properties of single osteons. *Anat Rec* 1967;158: 375–386.
8. Ascenzi A, Bonucci E, Simkin A. An approach to the mechanical properties of single osteonic lamellae. *J Biomech* 1973;6:227–235.
9. Evans FG. Relations between the microscopic structure and tensile strength of human bone. *Acta Anat* 1958;35:285–301.
10. Evans FG, Bang S. Differences and relationships between the physical properties and the structure of human femoral, tibial, and fibular cortical bone. *Am J Anat* 1967;120: 79–88.
11. Evans FG, Vincentelli R. Relation of collagen fiber orientation to some mechanical properties of human cortical bone. *J Biomech* 1969;2:63–71.
12. Bartley MH Jr, Arnold JS, Haslam RK, et al. The relationship of bone strength and bone quantity in health, disease, and aging. *J Gerontol* 1996;21:517–521.
13. Bell GH, Dunbar O, Beck JS, Gibb A. Variations in strength of vertebrae with age and their relation to osteoporosis. *Calcif Tissue Res* 1967;1:75–86.
14. Cody DD, Goldstein SA, Flynn MJ, Brown EB. Correlations between vertebral regional bone mineral density (rBMD) and whole bone fracture load. *Spine* 1991;16:146–154.
15. Galante J, Rostoker W, Ray RD. Physical properties of trabecular bone. *Calcif Tissue Res* 1970;5:236–246.
16. Alho A, Husby T, Hoiseth A. Bone mineral content and mechanical strength. An ex-vivo study on human femora at autopsy. *Clin Orthop Rel Res* 1988;227:292–297.
17. Lotz JC, Gerhart TN, Hayes WC, Mechanical properties of trabecular bone from the proximal femur by single-energy quantitative computed tomography. *J Computer Assisted Tomogr* 1990;14:107–114.
18. Dalen N, Hellstrom LG, Jacobson B. Bone mineral content and mechanical strength of the femoral neck. *Acta Orthop Scand* 1976;47:503–508.
19. Crowninshield RD, Pope MH. The response of compact bone in tension at various strain rates. *Ann Biomed Eng* 1974;2:217–225.
20. Currey JD. The mechanical adaptation of bones. Princeton, NJ: Princeton University Press, 1984.
21. Currey JD. The effects of strain rate, reconstruction, and mineral content on some mechanical properties of bovine bone. *J Biomech* 1975;8:81–86.
22. McElhaney JH. Dynamic response of bone and muscle tissue. *J Appl Physiol* 1966;21: 1231–1236.
23. Wright TM, Hayes WC. Tensile testing of bone over a wide range of strain rates: Effects of strain rate, microstructure and density. *Med Biol Eng* 1976;14:671–680.
24. Burstein AH, Reilly DL, Martens M. Aging of bone tissue: Mechanical properties. *J Bone Jt Surg* 1976;58A:82–86.
25. Currey JD, Butler G. The mechanical properties of the bone tissue in children. *J Bone Jt Surg* 1975;57A:810–814.
26. Weaver JK, Chalmers J. Cancellous bone: Its strength and changes with aging and an evaluation of some methods for measuring its mineral content 1. Age changes in cancellous bone. *J Bone Jt Surg* 1966;48A:289–299.
27. Currey JD. Changes in the impact energy absorption of bone with age. *J Biomech* 1979; 12:459–469.
28. Brooks DB, Burstein AH, Frankel UH. The biomechanics of torsional fractures. *J Bone Jt Surg* 1970;52A:507–514.
29. Clark CR, Morgan C, Sonstegard DA, Matthews LS. The effect of biopsy-hole shape and size on bone strength. *J Bone Jt Surg* 1977;59A:213–217.
30. Edgarton BC, An K-A, Morrey BF. Torsional strength reduction due to cortical defects in bone. *J Orthop Res* 1990;8:851–855.
31. Laurence M, Freeman MA, Swanson SA. Engineering considerations in the internal fixation of fractures of the tibial shaft. *J Bone Jt Surg* 1969;51B:754–768.
32. McBroom RJ, Cheal EJ, Hayes WC. Strength reductions from metastatic cortical defects in long bones *J Orthop Res* 1988;6:369–378.
33. Perren SM. Physical and biological aspects of fracture healing with special reference to internal fixation. *Clin Orthop Rel Res* 1975;138:175–194.
34. Aro HT, Wippenman BW, Hodgson SF, et al. Prediction of properties of fracture callus by measurement of mineral density using micro-bone densitometry. *J Bone Jt Surg* 1989; 71A:1020–1030.
35. White III AA, Panjabi MM, Southwick WO. The four biomechanical stages of fracture repair. *J Bone Jt Surg* 1977;59A:188–192.
36. White III AA, Panjabi MM, Southwick WO. Effects of compression and cyclical loading on fracture healing—A quantitative biomechanical study. *J Biomech* 1977;10:233–239.

37. Woodard Pl, Self J, Calhoun JH, et al. The effect of implant axial and torsional stiffness on fracture healing. *J Orthop Trauma* 1987;1:331–340.
38. Aharonoff GB, Dennis MG, Elshinawy A, et al. Circumstances of falls causing hip fractures in the elderly. *Clin Orthop Rel Res* 1998;348:10–14.
39. Assal M, Huber P, Rohr E, et al. Are drivers more likely to injure their right or left foot in a frontal car crash: A car crash and biomechanical investigation. 46th Annual Proceedings, Association for the Advancement of Automotive Medicine. 2002;273–288.
40. Funk JR, Tourret LJ, George SE, Crandall JR. The role of axial loading in malleolar fractures. *SAE Trans* 2000-01-0155, 2000.
41. Tencer AF, Kaufman R, Ryan K, et al. Estimating the loads in femurs of occupants in actual motor vehicle crashes using frontal crash test data. *Accident Analysis and Prevention* 2002;34(1):1–11.
42. Young JWR, Burgess AR, Brumback RJ. Lateral compression fractures of the pelvis: The importance of plain radiographs in the diagnosis and surgical management. *Skeletal Radiol* 1986;15:103–109.
43. Georgette FS, Sander TW, Oh I. The fatigue resistance of orthopedic wire and cable systems. Washington, DC: Second World Congress on Biomaterials, 1984:146.
44. Hughes AN, Jordan BA. The mechanical properties of surgical bone screws and some aspects of insertion practise. *Injury* 1972;4:25–38.
45. Chapman JR, Harrington RM, Lee KM, et al. Factors affecting the pullout strength of cancellous bone screws. *ASME J Biomech Eng* 1996;118:391–398.
46. DeCoster TA, Heetderks DB, Downey DJ, et al. Optimizing bone screw pullout force. *J Orthop Trauma* 1990;4:169–174.
47. Finlay JB, Jarada I, Boune RB, et al. Analysis of the pull-out strength of screws and pegs used to secure tibial components following total knee arthroplasty. *Clin Orthop Rel Res* 1989;247:220–231.
48. Wittenberg RH, Shea M, Swartz DE, et al. Importance of bone mineral density in instrumented spinal fusions. *Spine* 1991;16:648–652.
49. Stone JL, Beaupre GS, Hayes WC. Multiaxial strength characteristics of trabecular bone. *J Biomech* 1983;16:743–752.
50. Schatzker J, Sanderson R, Murnaghan JP. The holding power of orthopedic screws in vivo. *Clin Orthop Rel Res* 1975;108:115–126.
51. Zand MS, Goldstein SA, Matthews LS. Fatigue failure of cortical bone screws. *J Biomech* 1983;16:305–311.
52. Tencer AF, Asnis SE, Harrington RM, et al. Biomechanics of cannulated and noncannulated screws. In: Asnis SE, Kyle RF, eds. *Cannulated Screw Fixation, Principles and Operative Techniques*. New York: Springer-Verlag, 1996.
53. Allgower M. Cinderella of surgery-fractures? *Surg Clin N Am* 1978;58:1071–1093.
54. Cordey J, Florin P, Klaue K, Perren SM. Compression achieved with the dynamic compression plate: Effects of the inclined sloping cylinder and inclination of the screw. In: Uhthoff HK, ed. *Current Concepts of Internal Fixation of Fractures*. Berlin: Springer-Verlag, 1980:192–200.
55. Askew MJ, Mow VC, Wirth CR, et al. Analysis of the intraosseous stress field due to compression plating. *J Biomech* 1975;8:203–212.
56. Muller ME, Allgower M, Schneider R, et al. *Manual of Internal Fixation*. Berlin: Springer Verlag, 1979:85–96.
57. Nunamaker DM, Perren SM. A radiological and histological analysis of fracture healing using prebending of compression plates. *Clin Orthop Rel Res* 1979;138:167–174.
58. Gotzen L, Hutter J, Haas N. The prebending of AO plates in compression osteosynthesis. In: Uhthoff HK, ed. *Current Concepts of Internal Fixation of Fractures. Berlin:* Springer-Verlag, 1980:201–210.
59. Ellis T, Bourgeault CA, Kyle RF. Screw position affects dynamic compression plate strain in an in vitro fracture model. *J Orthop Trauma* 2001;15:333–337.
60. ElMaraghy AW, ElMaraghy MW, Nousiainen M, et al. Influence of the number of cortices on the stiffness of plate fixation of diaphyseal fractures. *J Orthop Trauma* 2001; 15:186–191.
61. Frigg R, Appenzeller A, Christensen R, et al. The development of the distal femur: Less Invasive Stabilization System (LISS). *Injury* 2001;32:S-C-24–31.
62. Karnezis IA, Miles AW, Cunningham JL, Learmonth ID. Biological internal fixation of long bone fractures: A biomechanical study of a noncontact plate system. *Injury* 1998; 29:689–695
63. Klaue K, Perren SM, Kowalski M. Internal fixation with a self-compressing plate and screw: Improvements of the plate hole and screw design, I. Mechanical investigation. *J Orthop Trauma* 1991;5:280–288.
64. Zuber K, Schneider E, Eulenberger J, et al. Form und Dimension der Markhohle menschlicher Femora in Hinblick auf die Passung von Marknagelimplantaten. *Unfallchirurg* 1988;91:314–319.
65. Johnson KD, Tencer AF, Sherman MC. Biomechanical factors affecting fracture stability and femoral bursting in closed intramedullary nailing of femoral shaft fractures, with illustrative case presentations. *J Orthop Trauma* 1987;1:1–11.
66. Russell TA, Taylor JC, LaVelle DG, et al. Mechanical characterization of femoral interlocking intramedullary nailing systems. *J Orthop Trauma* 1991;5:332–340.
67. Bucholz RW, Ross SE, Lawrence KL. Fatigue fracture of the interlocking nail in the treatment of fractures of the distal part of the femoral shaft. *J Bone Jt Surg* 1987;69A: 1391–1399.
68. Wikenheiser MA, Lewallen DG, Markel MD. In vitro mechanical, thermal, and microstructural performance of five external fixation pins. 38th Annual Meeting of the Orthopedic Research Society, 1992;17:409.
69. Huiskes R, Chao EYS, Crippen TE. Parametric analyses of pin-bone stresses in external fracture fixation. *J Orthop Res* 1985;3:341–349.
70. Huiskes R, Chao EYS. Guidelines for external fixation frame rigidity and stresses. *J Orthop Res* 1986;4:68–75.
71. Tencer AF, Claudi B, Pearce S, et al. Development of a variable stiffness fixation system for stabilization of segmental defects of the tibia. *J Orthop Res* 1984;1:395–404.
72. Behrens F, Johnson WD. Unilateral external fixation: Methods to increase and reduce frame stiffness, *Clin Orthop Rel Res* 1989;241:48–56.
73. Calhoun JH, Li F, Ledbetter BR, et al. Biomechanics of Ilizarov for fracture fixation. 37th Annual Meeting of the Orthopedic Research Society, 1991;16:439.
74. Geller J, Tornetta III P, Tiburzi D, et al. Tension wire position for hybrid external fixation of the proximal tibia. *J Orthop Trauma* 2000;14:502–504.
75. Roberts CS, Dodds JC, Perry K, et al. Hybrid external fixation of the proximal tibia: Strategies to improve frame stability. *J Orthop Trauma* 2003;17:415–420.
76. Hertel R, Jost B. Basic principles and techniques of internal fixation in osteoporotic bone. In: An YH, ed. *Internal Fixation in Osteoporotic Bone*. New York: Thieme, 2002: 108–115.
77. Benirschke SK, Swiontkowski MF. Knee. In: Hansen ST, Swiontkowski MF, eds. *Orthopedic Trauma Protocols*. New York: Raven Press, 1993.
78. Ayerby SA, Ehteshami JR, McLain RF. Offset laminar hooks decrease bending moments of pedicle screws during in situ contouring. *Spine* 1997;22:376–381.
79. Moroni A, Aspenberg P, Toksvig-Larsen S, et al. Enhanced fixation with hydroxyapatite-coated pins. *Clin Orthop Rel Res* 1998;346:171–177.
80. McKoy BE, Conner GS, An YH. An interlocking screw for fixation in osteoporotic bone. In: An YH, ed. *Internal Fixation in Osteoporotic Bone*. New York: Thieme, 2002:237–241.
81. Liebschner MAK, Rosenberg WS, Keaveny TM. Effects of bone cement volume and distribution on vertebral stiffness after vertebroplasty. *Spine* 2001;26:1547–1554.
82. Stankewich CJ, Swiontkowski MF, Tencer AF, et al. Augmentation of femoral neck fracture fixation with an injectable calcium-phosphate bone mineral cement. *J Orthop Res* 1996;14:786–793.
83. Elder S, Frankenberg E, Yetkilner DN, et al. Biomechanical evaluation of calcium phosphate cement augmented fixation of unstable intertrochanteric fractures. 43rd Annual Meeting of the Orthopedic Research Society, 1998;23:432.
84. Lim TH, Breback GT, Renner SM, et al. Biomechanical evaluation of an injectable calcium phosphate cement for vertebroplasty. *Spine* 2002;27:1297–1302.
85. Bai B, Kummer FJ, Spivak J. Augmentation of anterior vertebral body screw fixation by an injectable biodegradable calcium phosphate bone substitute. *Spine* 2001;24: 2679–2683.
86. Paul JP. Approaches to design. Force actions transmitted by joints in the human body. *Proc Roy Soc London*. B 1976;192:163–172.
87. Leicher I, Margulies JY, Weinreb A, et al. The relationship between bone density, mineral content, and mechanical strength in the femoral neck. *Clin Orthop Rel Res* 1982;163:272–281.
88. Goodman SB, Davidson JA, Locke L, et al. A biomechanical study of two methods of internal fixation of unstable fractures of the femoral neck, *J Orthop Trauma* 1992;6: 66–72.
89. Russell TA, Dingman CA, Wisnewski P. Mechanical and clinical rationale for femoral neck fracture fixation with a cephalomedullary interlocking nail. 37th Annual Meeting of the Orthopedic Research Society, 1992;17:177.
90. Swiontkowski MF, Harrington RM, Keller TS, et al. Torsion and bending analysis of internal fixation techniques for femoral neck fractures: The role of implant design and bone density. *J Orthop Res* 1987;5:433–444.
91. Van Audekercke R, Martens M, Mulier JC, et al. Experimental study on internal fixation of femoral neck fractures. *Clin Orthop Rel Res* 1979;141:203–212.
92. Kyle RF, Wright TM, Burstein AH. Biomechanical analysis of the sliding characteristics of compression hip screws. *J Bone Jt Surg* 1980;62A:1308–1314.
93. McLoughlin SW, Wheeler DL, Rider J, et al. Biomechanical evaluation of the dynamic hip screw with two- and four-hole side plates. *J Orthop Trauma* 2000;14:318–323.
94. Edwards WT, Lewallen DG, Hayes WC. The effect of pin number and fracture pattern on immediate mechanical fixation of a subcapital hip fracture model. 31st Annual Meeting of the Orthopedic Research Society, 1985;10:219.
95. Stankewitz CJ, Chapman J, Muthusamy R, et al. Relationship of mechanical factors to the strength of proximal femur fractures fixed with cancellous screws. *J Orthop Trauma* 1996;10:248–257.
96. Rubin R, Trent P, Arnold W, et al. Knowles pinning of experimental femoral neck fractures: A biomechanical study. *J Trauma* 1981;21:1036–1039.
97. Spangler L, Cummings P, Tencer AF, et al. Biomechanical factors and failure of transcervical hip fracture repair. *Injury* 2001;32:223–228.
98. Frankenburg EP, Robinson AP, Urquhart AG, et al. Supracondylar femur fractures: A biomechanical analysis of four fixation devices. 38th Annual Meeting of the Orthopedic Research Society, 1992;17:413.
99. Meyer RW, Plaxton NA, Postak PD, et al. Mechanical comparison of a distal femoral side plate and a retrograde intramedullary nail. *J Orthop Trauma* 2000;14:398–404.
100. Simonian PT, Thomson GT, Emley W, et al. Angled screw placement in the lateral condyle buttress plate for supracondylar femur fractures. 43th Annual Meeting of the Orthopedic Research Society, 1998.
101. Marti A, Fankhauser C, Frenk A, et al. Biomechanical evaluation of the less invasive stabilization system for the internal fixation of distal femur fractures. *J Orthop Res* 2001; 15:482–487.
102. Denny LD, Keating EM, Engelhardt JA, et al. A comparison of fixation techniques in tibial plateau fractures. 30th Annual Meeting of the Orthopedic Research Society, 1984; 9:314.
103. Beris AE, Glisson RR, Seaber AV, et al. Load tolerance of tibial plateau depressions reinforced with a cluster of K-wires. 34th Annual Meeting of the Orthopedic Research Society, 1988;13:301.
104. Hungerford DS, Barry M. Biomechanics of the patellofemoral joint. *Clin Orthop Rel Res* 1979;144:9–15.

105. Benjamin J, Bried J, Dohm M, et al. Biomechanical evaluation of various forms of fixation of transverse patellar fractures. *J Orthop Trauma* 1987;1:219–222.
106. Simonian PT, Routt ML, Harrington RM, Tencer AF. The unstable iliac fracture: A biomechanical evaluation of internal fixation. *Injury* 1997;28:469–475.
107. Simonian PT, Schwappach JR, Routt Jr MLC, et al. Evaluation of new plate designs for symphysis pubis internal fixation. *J Trauma* 1996;41:498–502.
108. Leighton RK, Waddell JP, Bray TJ, et al. Biomechanical testing of new and old fixation devices for vertical shear fracture of the pelvis. *J Orthop Trauma* 1991;5:313–317.
109. Yinger K, Scalise J, Olson SA, et al. Biomechanical comparison of posterior pelvic ring fixation. *J Orthop Trauma* 2003;17:481–487.
110. Schildhauer TA, LeDoux WR, Chapman JR, et al. Triangular osteosynthesis and iliosacral screw fixation for unstable sacral fractures: A cadaveric and biomechanical evaluation under cyclic loads. *J Orthop Trauma* 2003;17:22–31.
111. Mirza SK, Moquin RR, Anderson PA, et al. Stabilizing properties of the halo apparatus. *Spine* 1997;22:727–733.
112. Amevo B, Aprill C, Bogduk N. Abnormal instantaneous axes of rotation in patients with neck pain. *Spine* 1992;17:748–756.
113. Singh K, Vaccaro AR, Kim J, et al. Biomechanical comparison of cervical spine reconstructive techniques after a multilevel corpectomy of the cervical spine. *Spine* 2003; 28:2352–2358.
114. Kirkpatrick JS, Levy JA, Carillo J, et al. Reconstruction after multilevel corpectomy in the cervical spine. *Spine* 1999;24:1186–1191.
115. Isomi T, Panjabi MM, Wang J-L, et al. Stabilizing potential of anterior cervical plates in multilevel corpectomies. *Spine* 1999;24:2219–2223.
116. Rapoff AJ, Conrad BP, Johnson WM, et al. Load sharing in Premier and Zephir anterior cervical plates. *Spine* 2003;28:2648–2651.
117. Mihara H, Cheng BC, David SM, et al. Biomechanical comparison of posterior cervical fixation. *Spine* 2001;26:1662–1667.
118. Coe JD, Herzig MA, Warden KE, et al. Load to failure of spinal implants in osteoporotic spines: A comparison of pedicle screws, laminar hooks, and spinous process wires. 35th Annual Meeting of the Orthopedic Research Society, 1989;14:71.
119. Mann KA, Bartel DL. A structural analysis of the fixation of pedicle screws to vertebrae. 36th Annual Meeting of the Orthopedic Research Society, 1990:15:611.
120. Wu S-S, Edwards WT, Zou D, et al. Transpedicular vertebral screws in human vertebrae: Effect on screw-vertebra interface stiffness. 38th Annual Meeting of the Orthopedic Research Society, 1992;17:459.
121. Krag MH, Beynnan BD, Pope MH, et al. An internal fixator for posterior application to short segments of the thoracic, lumbar or lumbosacral spine. Design and testing. *Clin Orthop Rel Res* 1986;203:75–98.
122. Misenhimer GR, Peek RD, Wiltze LL, et al. Anatomic analysis of pedicle canal and cancellous diameter related to screw size, *Spine* 1989;14:367–372.
123. Ashman RB, Galpin RD, Corin JD, et al. Biomechanical analysis of pedicle screw instrumentation in a corpectomy model. *Spine* 1989;14:1398–1405.
124. Law M, Tencer AF, Anderson PA. Caudo-cephalad loading of pedicle screws: Mechanisms of loosening and methods of augmentation. *Spine* 1993;18:2438–2443.
125. Krag MH. Biomechanics of thoracolumbar spinal fixation. A review. *Spine* 1991;16: S85–S98.
126. Kandziora F, Pflugmacher R, Schafer J, et al. Biomechanical comparison of cervical spine interbody fusion cages. *Spine* 2001;26:1850–1857.
127. Brodke DS, Gollogly S, Bachus KN, et al. Anterior thoracolumbar instrumentation: Stiffness and load sharing characteristics of plate and rod systems. *Spine* 2003;1794–1801.
128. Kotani Y, Cunningham BW, Parker LM, et al. Static and fatigue biomechanical properties of anterior thoracolumbar instrumentation systems. *Spine* 1999;24:1406–1413.
129. Lebwohl NH, Cunningham BW, Dmitriev A, et al. Biomechanical comparison of lumbosacral fixation techniques in a calf spine model. *Spine* 2002;27:2312–2320.
130. Tencer AF, Hampton D, Eddy S. Biomechanical properties of threaded inserts for lumbar interbody spinal fusion. *Spine* 1995;20:2408–2414.

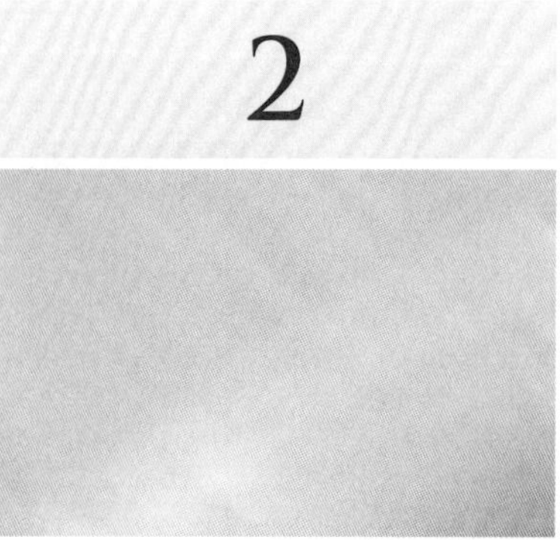

CLASSIFICATION OF FRACTURES

Douglas R. Dirschl and Lisa K. Cannada

Fracture classification systems have existed for nearly as long as people have identified fractures; they certainly predate the advent of radiography. Even in the earliest written surviving medical text, the Edwin Smith Papyrus, there was a rudimentary classification of fractures. If a fracture could be characterized as "having a wound over it, piercing through" (an open fracture), it was determined to be an "ailment not to be treated." This provides an example of one of the earliest fracture classification systems, which served to characterize the fracture and to guide the treatment.

Throughout the ages, all fracture classification systems have been used to serve numerous purposes: to characterize fractures as to certain general and specific features, to guide treatment, and to predict outcomes. This chapter reviews the purposes and goals of fracture classification, the history of using these systems, and the general types of fracture classification systems in common use today. This chapter also provides a critical analysis of the effectiveness of fracture classification systems, as well as some of these systems' limitations. Finally, this chapter will comment on the possible future of fracture classification systems.

PURPOSES OF FRACTURE CLASSIFICATION SYSTEMS

Taxonomy, or the naming and categorization of items, is not unique to orthopaedics or to fractures. Taxonomy is a universal phenomenon that occurs in all fields of science and art. One clear and simple example is the system of taxonomy that has been used to divide the natural world into three kingdoms: animals, plants, and bacteria (Fig. 2-1). This taxonomy, although simple, is a perfect example of the types of classification that permeate the world of arts and sciences—and the first general purpose of classifications systems—to name things.

A second function of classifications systems in general has been to describe things according to characteristics and to provide a hierarchy of those characteristics. A group of common descriptors are created, so that individual items can be classified into various groups. Groups are then ordered into a hierarchy according to some definition of complexity. A simple example of this is the phylogeny used to describe the animal kingdom. This system describes and groups animals according to common characteristics, and then orders those groups in a hierarchy ac-

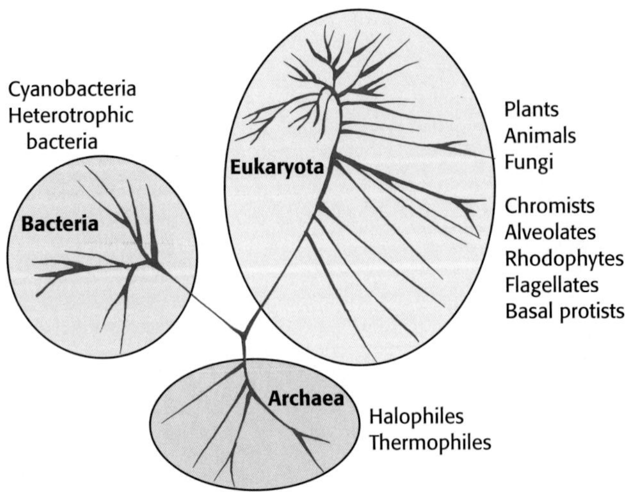

FIGURE 2-1 Balloon diagram showing taxonomy of the natural world.

cording to the complexity of the organism. This is, in principle, analogous to many fracture classification systems, which provide a group of common descriptors for fractures that are ordered according to complexity.

A third purpose of classification systems is to guide action or intervention. This feature of classification systems is not universally seen, and it is generally present only in classification systems that are diagnostic in nature. This fact introduces one of the key distinctions among classification systems—that between systems used for description and characterization and those used to guide actions and predict outcomes. For example, the classification system for the animal kingdom names and classifies animals, but it is descriptive only, as it does not guide the observer in any suggested action. In orthopaedic practice, however, physicians use fracture classification systems to assist in making treatment decisions. In fact, many fracture classification systems were designed specifically for the purpose of guiding treatment. We should have higher expectations of the validity and integrity of systems that are used to guide actions than of those used purely as descriptive tools.

The fourth purpose of classification systems is to assist in predicting outcomes of an intervention or treatment. The ability to reliably predict an outcome from a fracture classification alone would be of tremendous benefit, for it would allow physicians to counsel patients beginning at the time of injury as to the expected outcome. This ability would also assist greatly in clinical research, as it would allow comparison of one clinical study's results of a particular fracture to that of another. Note that for a classification system to reliably predict outcomes, a rigorous analysis of the reliability and validity of the classification system is necessary. Table 2-1 summarizes the purposes of classification systems, along with the level of reliability and validity necessary for high performance of the system.

TABLE 2-1 Purposes of Classification Systems

To name	High validity and reliability not required
To describe and compare	
To guide action	High validity and reliability recommended
To predict outcomes	

HISTORY OF FRACTURE CLASSIFICATION

Fracture classifications have existed much longer than radiographs. Although the Edmund Smith Papyrus did not make a clear distinction between comminuted and noncomminuted fractures, it clearly classified fractures as open or closed and provided guidelines for treatment based on that classification. Open fractures, for example, were synonymous with early death in ancient Egypt, and these fractures were "ailments not to be treated."

In the 18th and 19th centuries, still before the discovery of radiographs, there were fracture classification systems that were based on the clinical appearance of the limb alone. The Colles fracture of the distal radius, in which the distal fragment was displaced dorsally—causing the dinner fork deformity of the distal radius—was a common fracture. Any fracture with this clinical deformity was considered a Colles fracture and was treated by correcting the deformity and immobilizing the limb (1). The Pott fracture, a fracture of the distal tibia and fibula with varus deformity, was likewise a fracture classification that was based only on the clinical appearance of the limb (2). These are just two examples of a fairly large number of fracture classifications that were accepted and in widespread use before the development of radiographic imaging.

After the advent of radiography, fracture classification systems expanded in number and came into common usage. Radiography so altered the understanding of fractures and the methods of fracture care, that nearly all fracture classification systems in use today are based solely on a characterization of the fracture fragments on plain radiographs. Most modern fracture classification systems are based on a description of the location, number, and displacement of fracture lines viewed on radiographs, rather than on the clinical appearance of the fractured limb. Although countless fracture classification systems based on radiographs have been described in the past century for fractures in all parts of the skeleton, only the most enduring classification systems remain in common usage today. Examples of these classification systems are the Garden (3) and Neer (4) classification systems of proximal femoral and proximal humeral fractures, respectively. These, and other commonly used classification systems, will be discussed in more detail in a later part of this chapter.

Nearly all fracture classification systems in use today are based on having observers (usually orthopaedic physicians) make judgments and interpretations based on analyzing plain radiographs of the fractured bone. Usually, anteroposterior and lateral radiographs are used, although some fracture classification systems allow for or encourage the use of additional radiograph views, such as oblique radiographs, or internal and external rotation radiographs. Each decision made in the process of classifying a fracture is based on a human's interpretation of the often-complex patterns of shadows evident on a plain radiograph of the fractured limb. This, in turn, requires that the observer have a detailed and fundamental understanding of the osteology of the bone being imaged and of the fracture that is classified. The observer must be able to accurately and completely identify all of the fracture lines, understand the origin and nature of all fracture fragments, and delineate the relationship of all the fracture fragments to one another. Finally, the procedure of fracture classification requires that the observer very accurately quantify the amount of displacement or angulation of each fracture fragment from the location in which it should be in the nonfractured situation.

More recently, many investigators have added CT scanning to assist in classifying fractures. In most cases, the CT scan data have been used and applied to a classification system that was devised for use with plain radiographs alone. There are a few classification systems that are specifically designed for use with CT imaging data. The most well-known example of such a system is the Sanders classification system for fractures of the calcaneus (5), which was designed for use with a carefully defined semicoronal CT sequence through the posterior facet of the subtalar joint.

Until very recently, most fracture classification systems relied solely on radiographs in order to classify the fracture, guide treatment, and predict outcome. It has become increasingly appreciated, however, that nonradiographic factors such as the extent of soft tissue injury, the presence of other injuries (skeletal or nonskeletal), the presence of medical comorbidities, and a variety of other nonradiographic factors have a large effect on treatment decisions and on the outcomes of fracture treatment (6,7). These factors, however, are not accounted for in radiographic systems for fracture classification.

In reviewing a radiograph of a fracture, it is difficult to fully appreciate the extent of soft tissue damage that has occurred, and it is impossible to glean the patient's medical history from the radiograph alone. For example, if one views a radiograph of the transverse tibial shaft fracture shown in Figure 2-2, one may conclude that this is a simple, low-energy injury. In this example, however, the fracture occurred as a result of very high energy, and the patient sustained extensive soft tissue damage. In addition, the patient was an insulin-dependent diabetic with severe peripheral neuropathy and skin ulcerations on the fractured limb. From the view of the plain radiographs or application of a fracture classification based on radiographs alone, there is no way to account for these additional factors. The patient in this example required amputation, a treatment that would not be predicted by review of the radiographs alone. A discussion of the role of classifying the soft tissue injury in characterizing fractures will take place later in this chapter.

TYPES OF FRACTURE CLASSIFICATION SYSTEMS

Classification systems used to characterize fractures can be divided into three broad categories: (a) those that are fracture

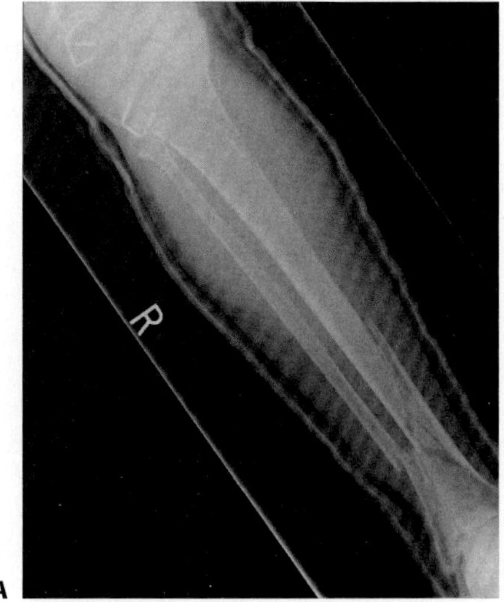

A

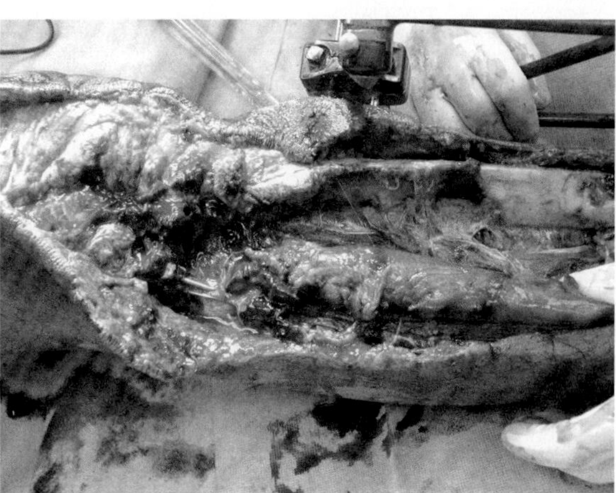
B

FIGURE 2-2 Tibial fracture as seen on radiograph **(A)** and intraoperatively **(B)**. The radiograph appearance greatly underestimates the overall severity of the injury.

specific, which evolved around and were generated for classifying a single fracture in a single location in the skeleton; (b) those that are generic or universal fracture classification systems, which apply a single, consistent methodology to the classification of fractures in all parts of the human skeleton; and (c) those that attempt to classify the soft tissue injury. It is beyond the scope of this chapter to discuss individually all the fracture classification systems now in common usage, but it is important to understand the differences between the general types of classification systems. For this reason, some examples of each of the three fracture classification system types will be discussed.

Examples of Fracture-Specific Classification Systems

The Garden classification of femoral neck fractures (3) is a longstanding fracture classification system that describes femoral head displacement and angulation on anteroposterior and lateral hip radiographs (see Fig. 44-15). The classification is essentially descriptive, describing the location and displacement of the fractured femoral neck and head. The fracture types are ordered, however, to indicate increasing fracture severity, greater fracture instability, and higher risk of complications with attempts at reduction and fracture stabilization. This feature of ordering fracture types by severity takes the classification system from a nominal system to an ordinal system. Garden types 1 and 2 fractures are considered to be stable injuries and are frequently treated with percutaneous internal fixation. Garden 3 and 4 fractures have been grouped as unstable fracture patterns and, although closed reduction and internal fixation is used in some circumstances, most Garden type 3 and 4 fractures in elderly patients are treated with arthroplasty.

The Schatzker classification of proximal tibia fractures (8,9) is an example of another descriptive classification system that has been widely used and is based on the location of the major fracture line in the proximal tibia as well as the presence or absence of a depressed segment of the proximal tibia's articular surface (see Fig. 50-6). This fracture classification does not depend on the amount of displacement or depression of the articular fractures, but only on the location of the fracture lines. The Schatzker classification seems very simple, but it also demonstrates some areas of confusion that can result from fracture classifications. For example, Schatzker type V and VI fractures are distinct fracture types in the system, but observers have a great deal of difficulty in distinguishing these two fracture types from one another when viewing fracture radiographs. Also, the Schatzker VI fracture group includes fractures classified as type C1 and C3 by the AO/OTA system (description to follow), thus demonstrating an area of inconsistency between two commonly used but different systems for classifying the same fracture that can lead to confusion among observers.

The Neer classification system for proximal humeral fractures (4) is a descriptive fracture classification system that has been widely used and extensively taught (Fig. 2-3). It is based on the number of fracture "parts;" a part is defined as a fracture fragment that is either displaced more than 1 cm or angulated more than 45 degrees. The Neer classification groups fractures into nondisplaced (one-part), two-part, three-part, or four-part fractures. Nondisplaced fractures in the Neer system involve any number of fracture lines, none of which meet the displacement or angulation criteria to be considered a "part." Two-part fractures in the Neer system can represent either a fracture across the surgical neck of the humerus or a greater tuberosity fracture that is displaced. Three-part fractures classically involve the humeral head; greater or lesser tuberosity fragments are displaced or angulated. Four-part fractures involve displacement or angulation of the humeral head and greater and lesser tuberosities. Note that in addition to correctly identifying the fracture fragments, this classification system requires the observer to make careful and accurate measurements of fragment displacement and angulation to determine if a fragment constitutes a part.

The Lauge-Hansen classification of malleolar ankle fractures (10) is an example of a widely used system that is based primarily on the mechanism of injury. The system makes use of the fact that particular mechanisms of injury to the ankle will result in predictable patterns of fracture to the malleoli. The fracture's appearance on the radiographs is used to infer the mechanism of the injury. The injuries are classified according to the position of the foot at the time of injury and the direction of the deforming force at the time of fracture. The position of the foot is described as pronation or supination, and the deforming force is categorized as external rotation, inversion, or eversion. This creates six general fracture types, which are essentially nominal—they are not ordered into increasing injury severity. Within each fracture type, however, there is an ordinal scale, with varying degrees of severity being assigned to each type (1–4) according to the fracture pattern. With this classification system, correct determination of the fracture type can guide the manipulations necessary to affect fracture reduction, as the treating physician must reverse the direction of the injuring forces to achieve a reduction. For example, internal rotation is required to achieve reduction of a supination external rotation fracture pattern.

Generic or Universal Classification Systems

The AO/OTA (Orthopaedic Trauma Association) fracture classification (11) is essentially the only generic or universal system in wide usage today. It is universal in the sense that the same fracture classification system can be applied to any bone within the body. This classification system was devised through a consensus panel of orthopaedic traumatologists who were members of the OTA, and it is based on a classification system initially developed and proposed by the AO/ASIF group in Europe (12, 13). The OTA believed there was a need for a detailed universal system for fracture classification to allow for standardization of research and communication among orthopaedic surgeons. The AO/OTA fracture classification system is an alphanumeric system that can be applied to most bones within the body.

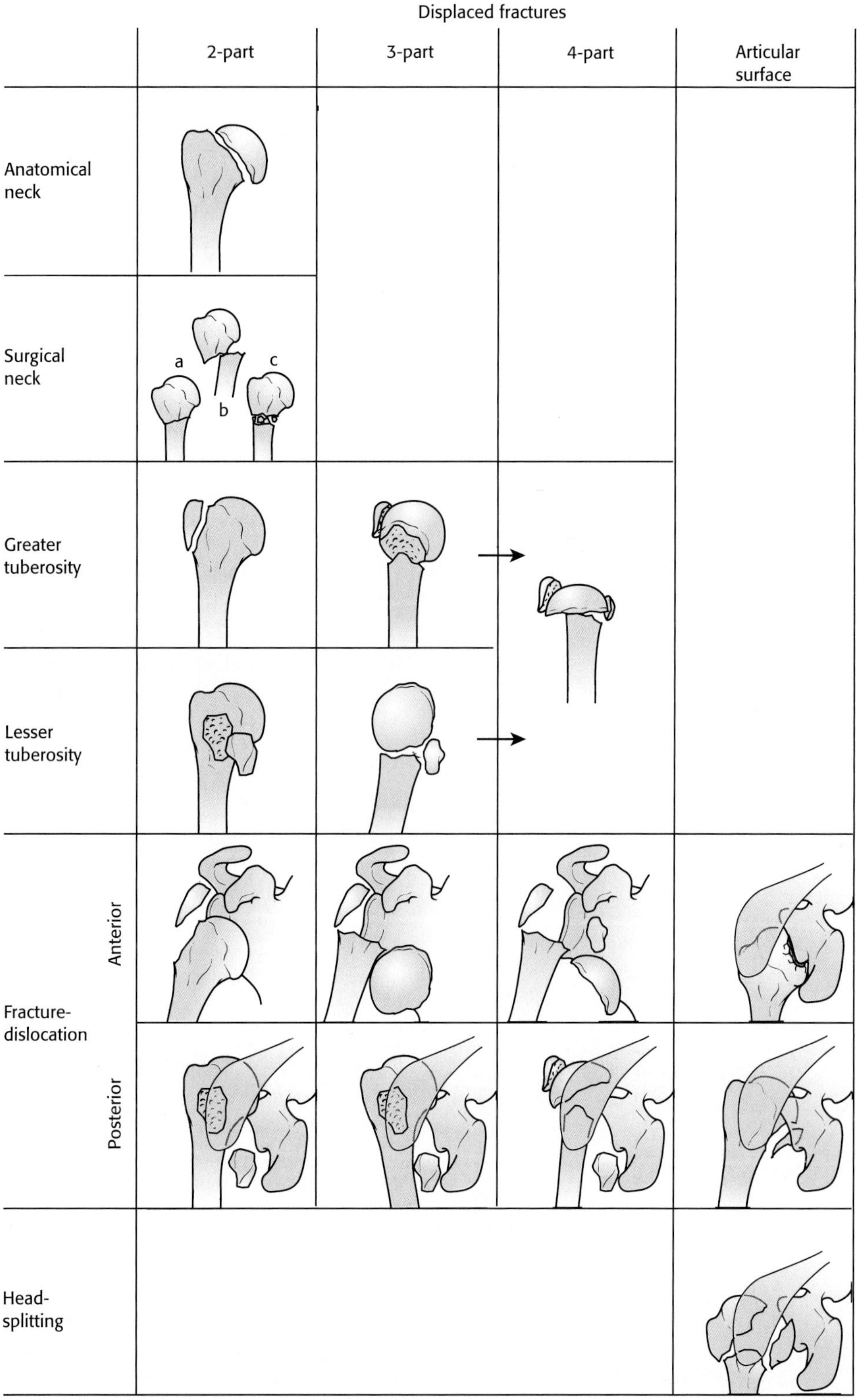

Displaced fractures

	2-part	3-part	4-part	Articular surface
Anatomical neck				
Surgical neck	a b c			
Greater tuberosity				
Lesser tuberosity				
Fracture-dislocation — Anterior				
Fracture-dislocation — Posterior				
Head-splitting				

FIGURE 2-3 The Neer four-part classification of proximal humerus fractures. A fracture is displaced if the fracture fragments are separated 1 cm or greater, or if angulation between the fracture fragments is more than 45 degrees. A displaced fracture is either a two-part, a three-part, or a four-part fracture. (Reprinted with permission from Neer CS. Displaced proximal humeral fractures: I. Classification and evaluation. *J Bone Joint Surg* 1970;52A:1077–1089.)

In applying the OTA fracture classification system, there are five questions that must be answered for each fracture:

1. **Which bone?** The major bones in the body are numbered: the humerus is No. 1, the forearm is No. 2, the femur No. 3, the tibia No. 4, and so on (Fig. 2-4).
2. **Where in the bone is the fracture?** The answer to this question identifies a specific segment within the bone. The second number of the coding system is applied to the location in the bone. In most long bones, the diaphyseal segment (2) is located between the proximal (1) and distal (3) segments. The dividing lines between the shaft segment and the proximal and distal segments occur in metaphysis of the bone. The tibia is assigned a fourth segment, which is the malleolar segment. An example of the application of answering the first two questions of the AO/OTA classification, a midshaft femoral fracture will be given a numeric classification of 32 (3 for femur, 2 for the diaphyseal segment) (Fig. 2-4).

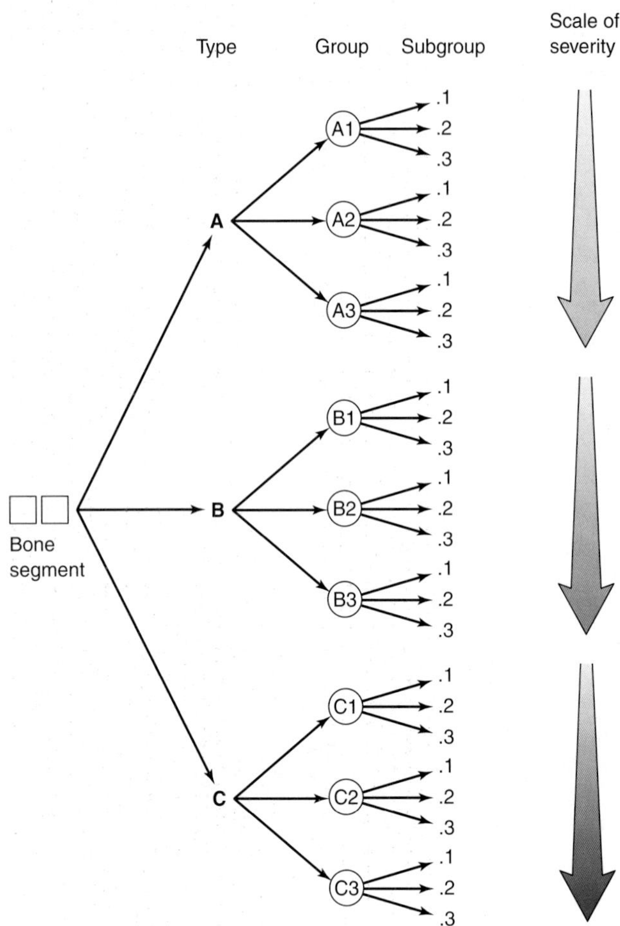

FIGURE 2-4 The AO/ASIF comprehensive long bone classification applied to proximal humeral fractures. This system describes three types of proximal humerus fractures (types A, B, and C). Type A fractures are described as unifocal extra-articular (two-segment) fractures, type B as bifocal extra-articular (three-segment) fractures, and type C fractures are described as anatomic neck or articular segment fractures. Each type includes three fracture patterns, with nine subgroups for each type of fracture. The subgroup classification indicates the degree of displacement. (Adapted and reprinted with permission from Müller ME, Allgower M, Schneider R, et al. *Manual of internal fixation.* New York: Springer-Verlag, 1991.)

3. **Which fracture type?** The fracture type in this system can be A, B, or C, but these three types are defined differently in diaphyseal fractures and fractures at either end of the bone. For diaphyseal fractures, the type A fracture is a simple fracture with two fragments. The type B diaphyseal fracture has some comminution, but there can still be contact between the proximal and distal fragments. The type C diaphyseal fracture is a highly comminuted or segmental fracture with no contact possible between proximal and distal fragments. For proximal and distal segment fractures, type A fractures are considered to be extra-articular, type B fractures are partial articular (there is some continuity between the shaft and some portion of the articular surface), and type C fractures involve complete disruption of the articular surface from the diaphysis. An example of this portion of the classification system is shown in Figure 2-4.
4. **Which group does the fracture belong to?** Grouping further divides the fractures according to more specific descriptive details. Fracture groups are not consistently defined; that is, fracture groups are different for each fracture type. Complete description of the fracture groups is beyond the scope of this chapter.
5. **Which subgroup?** This is the most detailed determination in the AO/OTA classification system. As is the case with groups, subgroups differ from bone to bone and depend on key features for any given bone in its classification. The intended purpose of the subgroups is to increase the precision of the classification system. Discussion of this fracture classification in this amount of depth is beyond the scope of this chapter, and the reader is referred to the references for a more detailed description of this universal fracture classification system.

The AO/OTA classification system is an evolving system. It is continually evaluated by a committee of the OTA and is open for change where appropriate. Note that the AO/OTA fracture classification system, and its precursor, the AO/ASIF system, were designed for delineation and recording of the maximum possible amount of detail about the individual fracture pattern and appearance on radiographs. The assumption made during the development of these classification systems is that, with specific definitions/diagrams and a high degree of detail will come greater accuracy and a superior fracture classification system that could be applied by any orthopaedic surgeon. It was believed such a system could potentially result in better prognostic and research capabilities. As will be discussed later in the chapter, greater specificity and detail in a fracture classification system does not necessarily correlate well with good performance of the classification system.

Classifications of Soft Tissue Injury Associated with Fractures

The skin and soft tissue represent an organ system. The energy of the injury may be reflected in the soft tissue damage to the extremity involved. If one sees a radiograph demonstrating a comminuted fracture, it is often thought that is a high-energy injury, but there may be other patient factors that come into consideration, which may lead to a comminuted fracture from a lower-energy mechanism. This may be evident in an elderly patient with ground-level falls who has a significantly comminuted distal humerus fracture. The energy of the injury itself resulted only from a ground-level fall, but led to a complex fracture type due to underlying osteoporotic bone. Some of the value in the soft tissue classification system is in planning the treatment and also in predicting the outcome.

The clearest example of a fracture with an associated soft tissue injury is the open fracture. Early classification systems for open fractures focused only on the size of the opening in the skin. With time, however, it was recognized that the extent of muscle injury, local vascular damage, and periosteal stripping are also of paramount significance. Gustilo et al (14,15) developed the classification system now used by most North American orthopaedists to describe open fractures. This classification system takes into account the skin wound, the extent of local soft tissue injury and contamination, and the severity of the fracture pattern (see Table 12-2). The Gustilo classification system originally included type I, type II, and type III fractures. This system was modified later to expand the type III open fractures into subtypes A, B, and C. It is important to note that the type III-C fracture is defined as any open fracture in which there is an accompanying vascular injury that requires repair. The Gustilo classification system has been applied to open fractures in nearly all long bones. It is important to recognize that this classification system only can be applied fully after surgical debridement of the open fracture has been performed. This system has proven useful in predicting risk of infection in open tibial fractures (14).

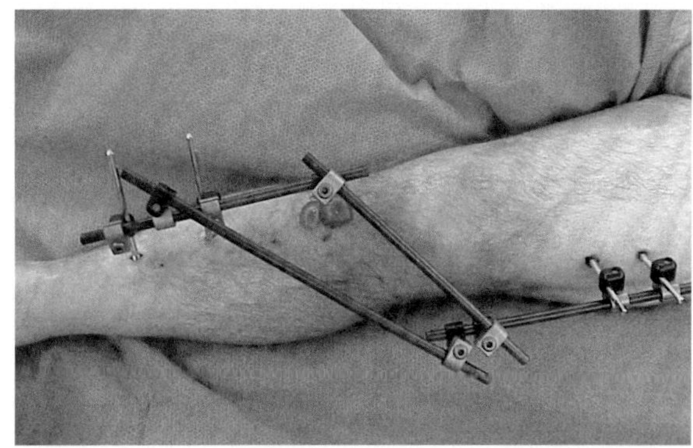

FIGURE 2-5 Example of a Tscherne type II fracture of the proximal tibia.

Interobserver agreement in grading open tibial fractures according to the classification of Gustilo was investigated by Brumback and Jones (16), who presented radiographs and videotapes of surgical debridements to a group of orthopaedic traumatologists who classified the fractures. They reported an average interobserver agreement of 60%. The range of agreement, however, was wide, ranging from 42% to 94%. Percentage agreement was best for the most severe and the least severe injuries, and was poorer for fractures in the middle range of the classification system. That the classification system did not have similar reliability across the spectrum of injury severity has been a criticism of this classification system as a prognostic indicator for any but the least severe and most severe injuries.

The classification of Oestern and Tscherne can be used to characterize the severity of closed fractures (17) (Table 2-2). This system remains the only published classification system for the soft tissue injury associated with closed fractures. Fractures are assigned one of four grades, from 0 to 3. Figure 2-5 is an example of a patient with a Tscherne grade 2 closed tibial plateau fracture. The presence of deep skin abrasions, muscle contusion, fracture blisters, and massive soft tissue swelling, as

TABLE 2-2 Oestern and Tscherne Classification of Closed Fractures

Grade	Soft Tissue Injury	Bony Injury
Grade 0	Minimal soft tissue damage Indirect injury to limb	Simple fracture pattern
Grade 1	Superficial abrasion/contusion	Mild fracture pattern
Grade 2	Deep abrasion with skin or muscle contusion Direct trauma to limb	Severe fracture pattern
Grade 3	Extensive skin contusion or crush Severe damage to underlying muscle Subcutaneous avulsion Compartmental syndrome may be present	Severe fracture pattern

in this patient, may lead the surgeon away from immediate articular stabilization and toward temporary spanning external fixation. No studies have been done to determine the interobserver reliability of the Tscherne system for the classifying soft tissue injuries associated with closed fractures.

The value of a classification system is greatly enhanced if it can assist in predicting outcome. A prospective study completed by Gaston et al (18) assessed various fracture classification schemes against several validated functional outcome measures in patients with tibial shift fractures. The Tscherne classification system of closed fractures was better able to predict outcome than the other classification systems used. The Tscherne system was most strongly predictive of time to return to prolonged walking or running.

LIMITATIONS OF FRACTURE CLASSIFICATION SYSTEMS

To be successful and valuable as a predictive tool, a classification system must be both reliable and valid (19–21). Reliability reflects the ability of a classification system to return the same result for the same fracture radiographs over multiple observers or by the same observer when viewing the fracture on multiple occasions. The former is termed *interobserver reliability*, or the agreement between different observers using the classification system to assess the same cases. The latter is termed *intraobserver reproducibility*, the agreement of the same observer's assessment, using the classification system, for the same cases on repeated occasions. The validity of a classification system reflects the accuracy with which the system describes the true fracture entity. A valid classification system would correctly categorize the fracture in a large percentage of cases, when compared to a "gold standard." Unfortunately, there is no such gold standard for fracture classification—not even observation at surgery can be considered infallible—so assessing the performance of fracture classification systems must be confined to evaluating interobserver reliability and intraobserver reproducibility.

There has been discussion over the appropriate use of the terms *agreement* and *accuracy* in reference to the performance of fracture classification systems, as well as which of these terms is the best measure of a system's performance. The term *accuracy* implies that there is a correct answer or a gold standard against which comparisons can be made, validated and determined to be true or false. The term *agreement*, however, indicates that there is no defined gold standard and that unanimous agreement among all individuals that might classify a given fracture is the highest measure of a classification system's performance. These two terms are not congruent, and they are not interchangeable. Each is tested by a vastly different statistical method, and to optimize each term would require a radically different method for generating and validating a fracture classification system. It has been unclear at times whether individuals developing and applying classification systems today are expecting the classification to serve as a gold standard or if they are attempting to develop the classification to achieve optimal agreement among observers.

In the late 1980s and early 1990s, studies began to appear in the orthopaedic literature assessing the interobserver reliability of various fracture classifications systems (22–29). In 1993, Albert Burstein, PhD, published a controversial editorial entitled "Fracture Classification Systems: Do They Work and Are They Useful?" In this article, he arrayed some important issues and considerations for fracture classification systems (19). He stated that classification systems are tools, and that the measure of whether such a tool works is if it produces the same result, time after time, in the hands of any individual who employs the tool. Dr. Burstein went on to say that "any classification scheme, be it nominal, ordinal, or scalar, should be proved to be a workable tool before it is used in a discriminatory or predictive manner." He emphasized that the key distinction for a classification system was between its use to describe and characterize fractures and its use to guide treatment or predict outcomes. This latter use requires a system to be proven as a valid tool; the minimum criteria for acceptable performance of any classification system, then, should be demonstration of a high degree of interobserver reliability and intraobserver reproducibility.

A number of studies have been published since Dr. Burstein's editorial appeared and nearly all concluded that fracture classification systems had substantial interobserver variability. Classification systems for fractures of the proximal femur (22,24,26,29–31), proximal humerus (25,28,32–34), ankle (27,29,31,35,36), distal tibia (21,37,38), and tibial plateau (39–43), among others, were all shown to have poor-to-slight interobserver reliability. The earliest of these studies looked only at the observed percentage of agreement, that is, the percentage of times that individual pairs of observers categorized fractures into the same category. Subsequent studies, however, have most frequently used a statistical test known as the *kappa statistic*, a test that analyzes pair-wise comparisons between observers applying the same classification system to a specific set of fracture cases. Originally introduced by Cohen in 1960 (44), the kappa statistic and its variants are the most recognized and widely used methods for measuring reliability of fracture classification systems. The kappa statistic adjusts the proportion of agreement between any two observers by correction for the proportion of agreement that could have occurred by chance alone. Kappa values can range from $+1.0$ (perfect agreement) to 0.0 (chance agreement) to -1.0 (perfect disagreement) (Table 2-3).

The original kappa statistic is appropriate when there are only two choices of fracture categories or when the fracture classification system is nominal—all categorical differences are equally important. In most situations, however, there are more than two categories into which a fracture can be classified, and fracture classification systems are ordinal, as the categorical differences are ranked according to injury severity, treatment method, or presumed outcome. In these cases, the most appropriate variant of the kappa statistic to be used is the weighted kappa statistic, described by Fleiss (45,46), in which some

TABLE 2-3 Range of the Kappa Statistic

Value of Kappa Statistic	Level of Agreement
+1.00	Perfect agreement
0.00	Agreement equal to chance
−1.00	Perfect disagreement

credit is given to partial agreement and not all disagreements are treated equally. For example, in the Neer classification of proximal humeral fractures, disagreement between a nondisplaced and a two-part fracture has far fewer treatment implications than disagreement between a nondisplaced and a four-part fracture. By weighting kappa values, one can account for the different levels of importance between levels of disagreement. The most appropriate use of the weighted kappa statistic should include a clear explanation of the weighting scheme selected, because the results of the kappa statistic will vary (even with the same observations) if the weighting scheme varies (20). Thus, without specific knowledge of the weighting scheme used, it is difficult to compare the results of fracture classification system reliability across different studies.

In most studies, the guidelines proposed by Landis and Koch (47) have been used to categorize kappa values. Values less than 0.00 indicate poor reliability, 0.01 to 0.20 indicate slight reliability, 0.21 to 0.40 indicate fair reliability, 0.41 to 0.60 indicate moderate reliability, 0.61 to 0.80 indicate substantial reliability, and 0.81 to 1.00 indicate nearly perfect agreement. Although these criteria have gained widespread acceptance, the values were chosen arbitrarily and were never intended to serve as general benchmarks. A second set of criteria, also arbitrary, have proposed by Svanholm et al (48): less than 0.50 indicate poor reliability, 0.51 to 0.74 indicate good reliability, and greater than 0.75 indicate excellent reliability.

Observer variability, using the kappa statistic, has been found to be a limitation of many fracture classification systems. A large number of studies have documented only fair-to-poor intraobserver reliability for a wide range of fracture classification systems. Systems tested have included, among others, the Neer fracture classification system of proximal humeral fractures (25,28,32,49), the Garden classification systems of proximal femoral fractures (22,24,26,30,31), the Rüedi and Allgöwer and AO classification systems of distal tibial fractures (21,37,38), the Lauge-Hansen and Weber classification of malleolar fractures (29,35,36,50), and the Schatzker and AO fracture classification system of proximal tibial fractures (39–43). Even the Gustilo-Anderson classification system for classifying open fractures has been shown to have only fair interobserver reliability (16). Additionally, studies have shown observer variability in classifying a variety of other orthopaedic injuries, such as fractures of the acetabulum (51–53), the distal radius (23,54,55), the scaphoid (56), the spine (57), and gunshot fractures of the femur (58).

More recent studies have attempted to isolate the sources of this variability, but the root cause for the variability has not been identified. It remains unknown if any system for the fracture classification can perform with excellent intraobserver reliability when it will be used by a large number of observers. A methodology of validating fracture classification systems has been purposed, but it is highly detailed, extremely time-consuming, and it is unknown whether it can be practically applied (59).

The use of the weighted kappa statistic in studies assessing the reliability of fracture classification systems should clearly state the weighting scheme used. Methodological issues such as this were evaluated in a systematic review of 44 published studies assessing the reliability of fracture classification systems (59). A variety of methodological issues were identified, including a failure to ensure that the study sample of fracture radiographs represented the spectrum and frequency of injury severity seen for the particular fracture in 61% of studies, a failure to justify the size of the study group in 100% of the studies, and inadequate statistical analysis of the data in 61% of studies. Although the investigators in this study used very rigid and, some would argue, unfairly rigorous criteria to evaluate these studies, their conclusion that reliability studies of fracture classification cannot be easily compared one to another is valid and appropriate. The creation and adoption of a systematic methodological approach to developing and validating new fracture classification systems seems appropriate and is needed.

To date, only one study has attempted to validate whether a fracture classification scheme correlates well with outcomes after fracture care (60). In a prospective, multicenter study, 200 patients with unilateral isolated lower-extremity fractures (acetabulum, femur, tibia, talus, or calcaneus) underwent a variety of functional outcome measurements at 6 and 12 months, including the Sickness Impact Profile and the AMA Impairment rating. The AO/OTA fracture classification for each of these patients was correlated with the functional outcome measures. The study indicated some significant differences in functional outcome between type C and type B fractures, but there was no significant difference between type C and type A fractures. The investigators concluded that the AO/OTA code for fracture classification might not be a good predictor of 6- and 12-month functional performance and impairment for patients with isolated lower-extremity fractures.

Additional, deeper research has attempted to elucidate some of the reasons for interobserver variation in fracture classification. These studies have generally focused on a few specific variables or tasks involved in the fracture classification process. Some of these reports that have been investigated are discussed in the following paragraphs.

Quality of Fracture Radiographs

The quality of the radiographs varies normally in clinical practice and may affect the observer's ability to accurately or reproducibly identify and classify the fracture. Physicians have attributed observed intraobserver variability in fracture classification systems to variations in the quality of radiographs (24,25, 28,32,54,55). Studies looking specifically at this variable however, have not shown it to be a significant source of intraobserver variability (35,21). In one such study involving classification of tibial plafond fractures using the Rüedi and Allgöwer system, observers were asked to classify the fractures, but were also asked to determine whether the radiographs were of adequate quality to classify the fracture (37). In that study, observers did not agree as well on the quality of the radiographs (mean kappa 0.38 ± 0.046) as on the classification of the fractures themselves (mean kappa 0.43 ± 0.048). In addition, the extent of interobserver agreement on the quality of the radiographs had no correlation with the extent of agreement in classifying the fractures. The investigators concluded that, based on the results of their study, it appeared that improving the quality of plain radiographic images would be unlikely to improve the reliability of fracture classification of the tibial plafond.

Further studies using advanced imaging modalities, such as CT or MRI scanning, in which high-quality images should always be obtained, have generally not demonstrated improved intraobserver reliability over studies that have used plain radiographs alone. Bernstein et al found that CT scans did not improve interobserver agreement for the Neer classification of proximal humerus fractures (32). In a study of a CT scan's impact on determining treatment plan and fracture classification for tibial plateau fractures, Chan et al found that viewing the CT scans did not improve interobserver agreement on classification, but did increase agreement regarding treatment plan (39). Two studies investigating the effect of adding CT information to plain radiographs on the interobserver agreement in classifying fractures of the tibial plateau and tibial plafond failed to show a significant improvement in agreement after adding CT scan information (21,39,40). Katz et al (61), studying distal radius fractures, found that the addition of a CT scan occasionally resulted in changes in treatment plans and also increased agreement among observers on the surgical plan in treating these injuries. These investigators, and others, have concluded that CT scan information may be a useful adjunct in surgical planning for a severe articular fracture, but is probably not required for the purpose of fracture classification.

Some contradictory data were recently published in the German literature (62). Thirty-five distal radius fractures that had been classified as AO/OTA A2 and A3 (extra-articular types) after radiographic review underwent CT scanning. The scans revealed that 57% of the fractures had an intra-articular component and had been inappropriately classified as AO/OTA type A fractures. This study did not attempt to determine interobserver reliability of the classification; a single observer reviewing the CT scans disagreed with the original fracture classification in 57% of cases. It remains unproven whether CT scanning is a useful adjunct to improve interobserver agreement in the classification of fractures.

A recent study reported on the impact of MRI scanning on the interobserver reliability of classifying tibial plateau fractures according to the Schatzker classification system (43). Three orthopaedic trauma surgeons classified tibial plateau fractures first with plain radiographs, and then with either the addition of a CT and an MRI scan. Kappa values averaged 0.68 with plain radiographs alone, 0.73 with the addition of a CT scan, and 0.85 with addition of an MRI scan. No statistical analysis was reported to indicate whether adding CT and MRI information resulted in a statistically significant improvement in reliability.

Difficulty Identifying Fracture Lines on Radiographs

All fracture classification systems require the use of a diagnostic image, usually a radiograph, on which the investigator must make observations, measurements, or both. Even with high-quality radiographs, however, overlapping osseous fragments or densities can make it difficult to accurately identify each fracture fragment. Osteopenia can also increase the difficulty in accurately classifying fractures. Osteopenic bone casts a much fainter "shadow" on radiographic films, making the delineation of fine trabecular or articular details a much more difficult task for the observer. Osteopenia represents a physiologic parameter that may affect treatment plans and outcomes, but it is not mentioned in any classification system.

Periarticular fractures may also be difficult to accurately classify with plain radiographs. Articular fractures tend to occur in areas of the skeleton with complex 3-D osteology, may be highly comminuted, and the classification systems used for these fractures are predicated on the accurate identification of each fracture fragment and determining its relationship to the other fragments and/or its position in the nonfracture situation. Observer variability in identifying these small fracture fragments in complex fractures would be expected to lead to poorer interobserver reliability of the fracture classification system. Dirschl et al investigated the observers' ability to identify small articular fragments in classifying tibial plafond fractures according to the Rüedi and Allgöwer classification (37). Observers classified 25 tibial plafond fractures on radiographs and then on line drawings that had been made from those radiographs by the senior investigator; interobserver reliability was no different in the two situations. At a second classification session, observers were asked to mark the articular fragments first on the fracture radiographs and then to classify the fractures. In a final session, the observers classified the radiographs after the fracture fragments had been premarked by the senior investigator. Having observers mark the fracture fragments resulted in no improvement in interobserver reliability of the fracture classification system. When identification of the articular fragments was removed from the fracture classification process, however, by having the fragments premarked by the senior investigator, the interobserver reliability was significantly improved (mean kappa value increased from 0.43 to 0.54; $p < .025$). The investigators believed the results of this study indicated that observers classifying tibial plafond fractures have great difficulty identifying the fragments of the tibial articular surface on radiographs. They went on to postulate that fracture classification systems based on identification of the number and displacement of small articular fragments may inherently perform poorly on reliability analyses, due to observer difficulty in reliably identifying the fracture fragments.

Variability Making Measurements on Radiographs

The amount of displacement of fracture fragments, particularly articular fragments, has long been felt to be important in characterizing fractures and has been used by many physicians to make decisions regarding treatment. Additionally, some fracture classification systems are predicated on the observer accurately identifying the amount of displacement and/or angulation of fracture fragments (e.g., the Neer classification system for proximal humeral fractures). Finally, the quality of fracture care has frequently been judged by measuring the amount of displacement of articular fracture fragments on posttreatment radiographs.

Numerous studies have shown, however, that there is inconsistency among observers in making measurements on radiographs and that this may be a source for variability in fracture classification. One such study assessed the errors in measuring articular incongruity of tibial plateau fractures (40). In this study, five orthopaedic traumatologists measured the maximum articular depression and the maximum condylar widening on 56 sets of tibial plateau fracture radiographs. For 38 of the cases, the observers also had a CT scan of the knee to assist in making measurements. The results of the study indicated that the 95% tolerance limits for measuring maximum articular depression were ± 12 mm, and for measuring maximum condylar widening, the tolerance limits were ± 9 mm. This result indicates that there is substantial unpredictability in making these seemingly simple measurements.

Tolerance limits, of course, will decrease as the range of measurements decreases (the range of articular depression in the study in the previous paragraph was 35 mm). Thus, it would be expected that lower tolerance limits would result from the measurement of reduced tibial plateau than those observed in the reported study, which measured injury films. However, in a study examining the tolerance limits for measuring articular congruity in healed distal radial fractures, tolerance limits of ± 3 mm were identified, when the range of articular congruity measurements was only 4 mm (7).

It has been suggested that CT scanning may improve the reliability of measuring articular fracture displacements. In one study of intra-articular fractures of the distal radius, there was poor correlation between measuring gap widths or step deformities on plain radiographs as compared to CT scans (63). Nearly one-third of measurements made from plain radiographs were significantly different than those made from CT scans. Another study extended these findings by examining known intra-articular displacements made in the hip joints of cadaveric specimens (49). The investigators observed that CT-generated data were far more accurate and reproducible than were data obtained from plain films. Moed et al reported on a series of posterior wall acetabular fractures treated with open reduction and internal fixation where reduction was assessed on both plain radiographs and on CT scans (64). Of 59 patients who were graded as having an anatomic reduction based on plain radiographs and for whom postoperative CT scans were obtained, 46 had a gap or step-off greater than 2 mm. These results may not be characteristic of all fractures, because the posterior wall of the acetabulum may be more difficult to profile using plain radiographs than most areas of other joints.

From this work, it appears that there is significant observer variability in the routine measurement of articular incongruity on radiographs. It also seems highly unlikely that observers using plain radiographs can reliably measure small amounts of incongruity. This suggests that it is necessary to improve our ability to reliably assess the displacement of fracture fragments in order to reduce variability in articular fracture assessment.

Complexity of Decision Making in Applying a Fracture Classification

Some fracture classification systems are quite complex, requiring the observer to choose between a large number of possible categories in characterizing a fracture. The AO/OTA system, for example, has up to 27 possible classifications for a fracture of a single bone segment (there are three choices each for fracture type, group, and subgroup). It seems reasonable that observers would find it easier to classify a fracture if there were a smaller number of choices to be made, and studies of the AO/OTA fracture classification system have confirmed this. In nearly all cases, for a variety of fractures, classification as to type can be performed much more reliably than classification into groups or subgroups (21,30,35,38,41,55,65). These studies concluded that, for optimal reliability, using this classification beyond characterization as to type was not recommended.

It has also been proposed that limiting observers' choices to no more than two for any step in classifying fractures would improve the ability of the observer to classify the fracture and would improve interobserver reliability. In 1996, the developers of the AO/ASIF comprehensive classification of fractures (CCF) modified that system to incorporate binary decision making (13). The reasoning was that, if observers could answer a series of yes or no questions about the fracture, they could more precisely and reliably classify the fracture. The modification was planned, announced, and implemented without any sort of validation that the modification would achieve the desired outcomes or that binary decision making would improve reliability in fracture classification.

Since 1997, however, two investigations of specific fracture types have evaluated whether binary decision making improves reliability in fracture classification. The first of these studies developed a binary modification of the Rüedi and Allgöwer classification of tibial plafond fractures and had observers classify 25 fractures according to the original classification system and the binary modification (37). The binary modification was applied rigidly in fracture classification sessions that were proctored by the investigator; observers were forced to make binary decisions about the fracture radiographs, and were not permitted to jump to the final fracture classification. The results of this study indicated that the binary modification of this classification system did not perform with greater reliability than the standard classification system (mean kappa 0.43 ± 0.048 standard and 0.35 ± 0.038 binary). Another investigation compared the interobserver reliability of classification of malleolar tibial fractures (segment 44) according to the classic and binary modification of the AO/ASIF CCF (35). Six observers classified 50 malleolar fractures according to both the standard and binary systems, and no difference in interobserver reliability could be shown between the two systems (mean kappa 0.61 standard and 0.62 binary). The investigators concluded that strictly enforced binary decision making did not improve reliability in the classification of malleolar fractures according to the AO/ASIF CCF. The results of these two studies cast doubt on the effectiveness of binary decision making in improving interobserver reliability in fracture classification.

Categorization of a Continuous Variable

All fracture classification systems in common use today are categorical; regardless of the classification system's nature or complexity, each groups fractures into discreet categories. Injuries to individual patients, however, occur on a continuum of energy and severity of injury; fractures follow this same pattern, occurring on a spectrum of injury severity. The process of fracture classification, then, can be said to be a process by which a continuous variable, such as fracture severity, is made a categorical one. This "categorization" of a continuous variable may be a source of intraobserver variability in fracture classification systems (20,65). One recent study concluded that "it has become clear that these deficiencies are related to the fact that the infinite variation of injury is a continuous variable and to force this continuous variable into a classification scheme, a dichotomous variable, will result in the discrepancies that have been documented" (20). The investigators further suggested that "multiple classifiers, blinded to the treatment selected and clinical outcomes, and consensus methodology should be used to optimize the utility of injury classification schemes for research and publication purposes."

In an effort to address this issue, some investigators have proposed that, instead of classifying fractures, perhaps fractures should merely be rank ordered from the least severe to the most severe. This system would serve as a means to preserve the continuum of fracture severity and has been proposed as a way of potentially improving interobserver reliability. An initial study using this methodology in tibial plafond fracture showed promise (66). Three orthopaedic traumatologists ranked 25 tibial plafond fractures from the least severe to the most severe, and the group demonstrated outstanding interobserver reliability, with a Cronbach's alpha statistic (67) of 0.94 (nearly perfect agreement). In a subsequent study, the rank order concept was expanded, and 69 observers ranked a series of 10 tibial plafond fractures (68). The intraclass correlation coefficient was 0.62, representing substantial agreement, but also represented some deterioration from the results with only three observers. Based on these results, which are superior to those of most categorical fracture classification systems that have been evaluated, further study of this sort of classification system appears to be warranted.

It has been postulated that one means of implementing a fracture classification system that ranks cases on a continuum of injury severity would be to approach the matter in the same way as clinicians determine bone age in children (68). A series of radiographs would be published that represent the spectrum of fracture severity, from the least severe to the most severe, and then an observer would simply review these examples and determine where the fracture he was assessing lay on this spectrum of severity. This concept is markedly different from any scheme used to date to classify fractures, it would be unlikely to completely replace other fracture classification systems, and may have a variety of weaknesses that have not yet been determined. Such a system will require extensive testing and validation before it could be widely used.

Poor Attention to Classification of Nonradiographic Factors

Measuring the injury severity and predicting the outcome after a fracture depends on much more than radiographic factors (6,7,69). Recently, physicians have come to question whether any system for fracture classification that relies solely on radiographic data will be highly reliable or highly predictive of outcome of severe fractures. There is strong evidence that the extent of injury to the soft tissues (cartilage, muscle, tendon, skin, etc), the magnitude and durations of the patient's physiologic response to injury, the presence of comorbid conditions, and the patient's socioeconomic background and lifestyle may all play critical roles in influencing outcomes following severe fractures.

As an example, it is well recognized that injury to articular cartilage is a critical and significant contributor to the overall severity of an articular fracture, as evidenced by studies documenting poor outcomes after osteochondritis dissecans and other chondral injuries. The information in the orthopaedic clinical literature indicates that the severity of injury to the articular surface during fracture has an important bearing on outcome and the eventual development of posttraumatic osteoarthrosis. A better understanding of the impaction injury to the articular cartilage and the prognosis of such injury will be critical to improving our assessment and understanding of severe intra-articular fractures. Unfortunately, there are no imaging modalities that have been validated to indicate the extent of injury to the cartilage of the articular surface and/or the potential for repair or the risk of posttraumatic degeneration of the articular cartilage. Plain radiographs and CT scans provide very little information about the current and future health of the articular cartilage in a joint with a fracture.

Inherent Variability in Human Observations

It is to be expected that human observers, no matter how well trained, will have some level of variability in applying any tool—no matter how reliable—in classifying fractures. It is entirely unknown what is the magnitude of the "baseline" level of inherent human variability in fracture classification. As such, it is extremely difficult for investigators to know with precision what represents excellent interobserver reliability in fracture classification. There is disagreement over what is the best statistical analysis that should be used in assessing reliability or what level of agreement is acceptable in studies on fracture classification. Statistics such as the intraclass correlation coefficient are very good as indicators of when a laboratory test, such as the hematocrit or serum calcium level, has acceptable reliability and reproducibility. Whether the same threshold level of reliability should be applied to a process such as fracture classification is unknown. Similarly, the interpretation of the weighted kappa statistic for fracture classification is somewhat difficult, as there are few guidelines to aid in interpreting their results. Landis and Koch admit that their widely accepted reference intervals for the kappa statistic were chosen arbitrarily. Additionally, a recent investigation seemed to indicate that using the kappa statistic with a small number of observers introduces the possibility of "sampling error," causing an increased variance in the kappa statistic itself (52,59). Having a large number of observers causes stabilization of the kappa value around a "mean value" for the agreement among the observers. Invariably, however, a larger number of observers results in a lower mean kappa value, indicating poorer interobserver reliability of the classification system being tested. This seems to mean that studies of small numbers of observers reporting excellent reliability in fracture classification systems may be reporting spuriously high results for the kappa statistic, results that would be much lower if a large number of observers were used instead. Unfortunately, there are currently no better or more reliable methods for reporting and interpreting interobserver reliability than the use of the intraclass correlation or the kappa statistic.

CURRENT USEFULNESS OF FRACTURE CLASSIFICATION SYSTEMS

Fracture classification systems are highly useful for describing fractures; this has been one of the best uses for fracture classification systems. Using a well-known fracture classification to describe a fracture to an orthopaedist or colleague who cannot view the fracture radiographs immediately provides the orthopaedist with a visual image of the fracture. This visual image, even if it is not highly reliable to statistical testing, enhances communication between orthopaedic surgeons.

Fracture classification systems are also useful as educational tools. Educating orthopaedic trainees in systems of fracture classification is highly valuable, for many systems are devised from the mechanism of injury or from the anatomical alignment of the fracture fragments. These are important educational tools to assist orthopaedic trainees in understanding the osteology of the skeleton and in understanding the various mechanisms of injury that can result in fractures. Educational systems using fracture classification methodologies can assist orthopaedic trainees in formulating a context in which to make treatment decisions and can also provide an important historical context of fracture care and fracture classification in orthopaedics.

Fracture classification systems have been said to be useful in guiding treatment, and it is clearly the intent of many fracture classification systems to guide treatment based on fracture classification. It is unclear, however, from much of the literature that has been published, whether fracture classification systems have been proven to be valid tools to guide treatment. The fact that there is so much observer variability in fracture classification makes the reader skeptical of comparative clinical studies that have used fracture classification as a guide to treatment.

Fracture classification systems have also been said to be useful in predicting outcomes after fracture care. The orthopaedic literature to date, however, does not seem to clearly indicate that fracture classification systems can be used to predict patient outcomes in any sort of valid or reproducible way. The interobserver variability of many fracture classification systems is one of the key reasons that the literature cannot clearly show this correlation. One exception to this, however, is that most fracture classification systems have good reliability in characterizing the most severe and least severe injuries—those that correlate with the best and worst outcomes. Classification systems demonstrate the poorest reliability and the poorest ability to predict outcomes in the midrange of injury severity.

THE FUTURE OF FRACTURE CLASSIFICATION SYSTEMS

In the future, there will be a more comprehensive determination of injury severity than merely classifying a fracture according to plain radiographs. It has become clear in recent years that variables other than radiograph appearance of the fracture play a huge role in determining patient outcome. These variables will be used in new systems of determining injury severity in patients with fractures. Objective measures of energy of injury using CT scans, finite element models or volumetric measures, measures of the extent of injury to soft tissues, objective measures of the patient's physiologic reserve and response to injury, such as serum lactate levels, will become available. An assessment of patients' overall health status and the existence of comorbid conditions are some examples of items that may be used in the future to make determination of fracture severity more comprehensive. These factors will likely be combined with the radiographic appearance of the fracture to better guide treatment and to better predict fracture care outcomes.

Better imaging modalities will also assist us in more reliably determining and characterizing the injury severity in patients with fractures. Newer uses for CT scanning, MRI, and ultrasound will all be instrumental in providing the treating surgeon with more information about the extent of soft tissue injury, the health of the bone and cartilage, and the biology at the fracture site. We may also gain additional information about the patient's ability to heal well. All of these aspects will advance the orthopaedist's ability to determine injury severity. For example, it is possible with very high-energy MRI scans to determine the proteoglycan content of articular cartilage. Because articular cartilage is not imaged on CT or plain radiographic imaging, its health has been generally excluded from the classification of fractures. The long-term health of the articular cartilage, however, is crucial to the patient's outcome after a severe articular injury. Our ability in the future to use advanced imaging modalities to better characterize the health and predict the future health of the articular cartilage will be a great advancement in our ability to accurately classify fractures and to use fracture classification as a predictive measure.

Newer fracture classification methods will be devised. These systems will better ensure that fractures can be measured and characterized on a continuum, which is how they occur. These new classification systems will better represent the continuum of injury severity than do systems in use today—many of which were based simply on anatomical considerations rather than on injury severity. Ideas such as rank ordering fractures, putting fractures on a continuum, and sending fractures to a fracture classification clearing house (for classification by a single or a small number of observers) are a few possible future approaches to advancing and making fracture classification more reproducible.

There will be improved agreement regarding what sort of validation process a fracture classification system should undergo before becoming available for general use. Most classification systems in general use have had no formal validation. Most of the systems have come into general use due to the reputation or influence of the individual or group that devised them, or perhaps because the system has been in use so long that it has simply become part of the vernacular in fracture classification and fracture care. One study has proposed a formal, detailed, and very time-consuming methodology for validating all fracture classification systems, very similar to that which was performed for patient-based outcome measures, such as the short form 36 and the musculoskeletal functional assessment (59). At this time, it is unclear whether such validation methods would improve the interobserver reliability of fracture classification systems. Such methods would be exhaustive and very time consuming, and many orthopaedic surgeons do not believe that such detailed validation is necessary for fracture classification systems.

The use of imaging processing and analysis techniques will advance our understanding and ability to classify fractures. Advances in imaging processes, image analysis, perhaps when coupled with neural nets and other learning technologies, may make it possible in the future for computers to be taught to classify fractures with a high degree of reliability and reproducibility. One could envision a system by which digital images of a fracture are classified according to any number of classification systems and that this is done automatically by a computer system at the time the radiographs are obtained, much as a computer generates EKG readings at the time the patient's cardiac tracing is obtained, even today.

Finally, there will be more precise validation of fracture classification systems. Rigorous statistical methods or at least consensus statistical methodologies will be developed and will be implemented that while detailed, time consuming, and involved, will result in greatly improved validation of many fracture classification systems.

REFERENCES

1. Colles A. On the fracture of the carpal extremity of the radius. *Edinb Med Surg J* 1814; 10:182–186.
2. Pott P. Some few general remarks on fractures and dislocations. Hanes L, Clarke W, Callius R, eds. London, 1765.
3. Garden RS. Low angle fixation in fractures of the femoral neck. *J Bone Joint Surg (Br)* 1961;43:647–663.
4. Neer CS. Displaced proximal humeral fractures. Part I: classification and evaluation. *J Bone Joint Surg (Am)* 1970;52:1077–1089.
5. Sanders R. Displaced intra-articular fractures of the calcaneus. *J Bone Joint Surg (Am)* 2000;225–250.
6. Dirschl DR, Dawson PA. Assessment of injury severity in tibial plateau fractures. *Clin Orthop Rel Res* 2004;423:85–92.
7. Marsh JL, Buckwalter J, Gelberman RC, et al. Does an anatomic reduction really change the result in the management of articular fractures? *J Bone Joint Surg* 2002;84A: 1259–1271.
8. Schatzker J. Fractures of the tibial plateau. In Schatzker M, Tile M, eds. *Rationale of operative fractures care.* Berlin: Springer-Verlag, 1988:279–295.
9. Schatzker J, McBroom R. Tibial plateau fractures: the Toronto experience 1968–1975. *Clin Orthop Rel Res* 1979;138:94–104.
10. Lauge-Hansen N. Fractures of the ankle III: genetic roentgenologic diagnosis of fractures of the ankle. *AJR* 1954;71:456–471.
11. Orthopaedic Trauma Association Committee for Coding and Classification. Fracture and dislocation compendium. *J Orthop Trauma* 1996;10(Suppl 1).
12. Muller ME. The comprehensive classification of fractures of long bone. In: Muller ME, Allgower M, Schneider R, Willenegger H, eds. *Manual of internal fixation: techniques recommended by the AO-ASIF group*, 3rd ed. Heidelberg: Springer-Verlag, 1991.
13. Muller ME, Nazarian S, Kack P. *CCF: Comprehensive classification of fractures*. Bern: Maurice E. Muller Foundation, 1996.
14. Gustilo RB, Anderson JT. Prediction of infection in the treatment of one thousand and twenty-five open fractures in long bones. *J Bone Joint Surg* 1976;58A:453–458.
15. Gustilo RB, Mendoza RM, Williams DN. Problems in the management of type III (severe) open fractures: a new classification of type III open fractures. *J Trauma* 1984;24(8): 742–746.
16. Brumback RJ, Jones AL. Interobserver agreement in the classification of open fractures of the tibia. *J Bone Joint Surg (Am)* 1994;76:1162–1166.
17. Oestern HJ, Txcherne H. Pathophysiology and classification of soft tissue injuries associated with fractures. In: Tscherne H, ed. *Fracture with soft tissue injuries*. New York: Springer-Verlag, 1984:1–9.
18. Gaston P, Will R, Elton RA, et al. Fractures of the tibia: can their outcome be predicted? *J Bone Joint Surg* 1999;81B:71–76.
19. Burstein AH. Fracture classification systems: do they work and are they useful? *J Bone Joint Surg (Am)* 1993;75:1743–1744.
20. Garbuz DS, Masri BA, Esdaile J, et al. Classification systems in orthopaedics. *J Am Acad Orthop Surg* 2002;10:290–297.
21. Martin JS, Marsh JL, Bonar SK, et al. Assessment of the AO/ASIF fracture classification for the distal tibia. *J Orthop Trauma* 1997;11:477–483.
22. Andersen E, Jorgensen LG, Hededam LT. Evans classification of trochanteric fractures: an assessment for the interobserver reliability and intraobserver reproducibility. *Injury* 1990;21:377–378.
23. Anderson GR, Rasmussen JB, Dahl B, et al. Older's classification of Colle's fractures: good intraobserver and interobserver reproducibility in 185 cases. *Acta Orthop Scand* 1991;62:463–464.
24. Frandsen PA, Andersen E, Madsen F, et al. Garden's classification of femoral neck fractures: an assessment of inter-observer variation. *J Bone Joint Surg (Br)* 1988;70:588–590.
25. Kristiansen B, Andersen ULS, Olsen CA, et al. The Neer classification of fractures of the proximal humerus: an assessment of interobserver variation. *Skeletal Radiol* 1988;17: 420–422.
26. Oakes DA, Jackson KR, Davies MR, et al. The impact of the Garden classification on proposed operative treatment. *Clin Orthop Rel Res* 2003;409:232–240.
27. Rasmussen S, Madsen PV, Bennicke K. Observer variation in the Lauge-Hansen classification of ankle fractures: precision improved by instruction. *Acta Orthop Scand* 1993;64: 693–694.
28. Sidor JL, Zuckerman JD, Lyon T, et al. The Neer classification system for proximal humeral fractures: an assessment of interobserver reliability and intraobserver reproducibility. *J Bone Joint Surg (Am)* 1993;75:1745–1750.

29. Thomsen NOB, Overgaard S, Olen LH, et al. Observer variation in the radiographic classification of ankle fractures. *J Bone Joint Surg (Br)* 1991;73:676–678.
30. Pervez H, Parker MJ, Pryor GA, et al. Classification of trochanteric fracture of the proximal femur: a study of the reliability of current systems. *Injury* 2002;33:713–715.
31. Schipper IB, Steyerberg EW, Castelein RM, et al. Reliability of the AO/ASIF classification for peritrochanteric femoral fractures. *Acta Orthop Scand* 2001;72:36–41.
32. Bernstein J, Adler LM, Blank JE, et al. Evaluation of the Neer system of classification of proximal humeral fractures with computerized tomographic scans and plain radiographs. *J Bone Joint Surg (Am)* 1996;78:1371–1375.
33. Brorson S, Bagger J, Sylvest A, et al. Low agreement among 24 doctors using the Neer classification; only moderate agreement on displacement, even between specialists. *International Orthop* 2002;26:271–273.
34. Siebenrock KA, Gerber C. The reproducibility of classification of fractures of the proximal end of the humerus. *J Bone Joint Surg (Am)* 1993;75:1751–1755.
35. Craig WL III, Dirschl DR. An assessment of the effectiveness of binary decision-making in improving the reliability of the AO/ASIF classification of fractures of the ankle. *J Orthop Trauma* 1998;12:280–284.
36. Nielsen JO, Dons-Jensen H, Sorensen HT. Lauge-Hansen classification of malleolar fractures: an assessment of the reproducibility of 118 cases. *Acta Orthop Scand* 1990;61: 385–387.
37. Dirschl DR, Adams GL. A critical assessment of methods to improve reliability in the classification of fractures, using fractures of the tibial plafond as a model. *J Orthop Trauma*, 1997;11:471–476.
38. Swiontkowski JF, Sands AK, Agel J, et al. Interobserver variation in the AO/OTA fracture classification system for pilon fractures: is there a problem? *J Orthop Trauma* 1997;11: 467–470.
39. Chan PSH, Klimkiewicz JJ, Luchette WT, et al. Impact of CT scan on treatment plan and fracture classification of tibial plateau fractures. *J Orthop Trauma* 1997;11:484–489.
40. Martin J, Marsh JL, Nepola JV, et al. Radiographic fracture assessments: which ones can we reliably make? *J Orthop Trauma* 2000;14(6):379–385.
41. Walton NP, Harish S, Roberts C, et al. AO or Schatzker? How reliable is classification of tibial plateau fractures? *Arch Orthop Trauma Surg* 2003;123:396–398.
42. Wicky S, Blaser PF, Blanc CH, et al. Comparison between standard radiography and spiral CT with 3D reconstruction in the evaluation, classification and management of tibial plateau fractures. *Eur Radiol* 2000;10:1227–1232.
43. Yacoubian SV, Nevins RT, Sallis JG, et al. Impact of MRI on treatment plan and fracture classification of tibial plateau fractures. *J Orthop Trauma* 2002;16:632–637.
44. Cohen J. A coefficient of agreement for nominal scales. *Educational and Psychological Measurement* 1960;20:37–46.
45. Fleiss JL. In: *Statistical methods for rates and proportions*, 2nd ed. New York: John Wiley & Sons, 1981:218.
46. Fleiss JL, Stakter MJ, Fischman SL, et al. Interexaminer reliability in caries trials. *J Dent Res* 1979;58:604–609.
47. Landis JR, Koch GG. The measurement of observer agreement for categorical data. *Biometrics* 1977;33:159–174.
48. Svanholm H, Starklint H, Gundersen HJ, et al. Reproducibility of histomorphologic diagnoses with special reference to the kappa statistic. *APMIS* 1989;97:689–698.
49. Borrelli J Jr, Goldfarb C, Catalano L, et al. Assessment of articular fragment displacement in acetabular fractures: a comparison of computed tomography and plain radiographs. *J Orthop Trauma* 2002;16:449–456.
50. Thomsen NOB, Olsen LH, Nielsen ST. Kappa statistics in the assessment of observer variation: the significance of multiple observers classifying ankle fractures. *J Orthop Sci* 2002;7:163–166.
51. Beaule PE, Dorey FJ, Matta JM. Letournel classification for acetabular fractures: assessment of interobserver and intraobserver reliability. *J Bone Joint Surg (Am)* 2003;85: 1704–1709.
52. Petrisor BA, Bhandari M, Orr RD, et al. Improving reliability in the classification of fractures of the acetabulum. *Arch Orthop Trauma Surg* 2003;123:228–233.
53. Visutipol B, Chobrangsin P, Ketmalasiri B, et al. Evaluation of Letournel and Judet classification of acetabular fracture with plain radiographs and three-dimensional computerized tomographic scan. *J Orthop Surg* 2000;8:33–37.
54. Andersen DJ, Blair WF, Steyers CM, et al. Classification of distal radius fractures: an analysis of interobserver reliability and intraobserver reproducibility. *J Hand Surg* 1996; 21A:574–582.
55. Kreder HJ, Hanel DP, McKee M, et al. Consistency of AO fracture classification for the distal radius. *J Bone Joint Surg (Br)* 1996;78:726–731.
56. Desai VV, Davis TRC, Barton NJ. The prognostic value and reproducibility of the radiological features of the fractured scaphoid. *J Hand Surg (Br)* 1999;5:586–590.
57. Oner FC, Ramos LMP, Simmermacher RKJ, et al. Classification of thoracic and lumbar spine fractures: problems of reproducibility. *Eur Spine J* 2002;11:235–245.
58. Shepherd LE, Zalavras CG, Jaki K, et al. Gunshot femoral shaft fractures: is the current classification system reliable? *Clin Orthop Rel Res* 2003;408:101–109.
59. Audige L, Bhandari M, Kellam J. How reliable are reliability studies of fracture classifications? A systematic review of their methodologies. *Acta Orthop Scand* 2004;75:184–194.
60. Swiontkowski JF, Agel J, McAndrew MP, et al. Outcome validation of the AO/OTA fracture classification system. *J Orthop Trauma* 2000;14:534–541.
61. Katz MA, Beredjiklian PK, Bozentka DJ, et al. Computed tomography scanning of intra-articular distal radius fractures: does it influence treatment? *J Hand Surg (Am)* 2001; 26(3):415–421.
62. Dahlen HC, Franck WM, Sabauri G, et al. Incorrect classification of extraarticular distal radius fractures by conventional radiographs: comparison between biplanar radiologic diagnostics and CT assessment of fracture morphology. *Unfallchirurg* 2004;107(6): 491–498.
63. Cole RJ, Bindra RR, Evanoff BA, et al. Radiographic evaluation of osseous displacement following intraarticular fracture of the distal radius: reliability of plain radiographs versus computed tomography. *J Hand Surg (Am)* 1997;22:792–800.
64. Moed RB, Carr SEW, Watson JT. Open reduction and internal fixation of posterior wall fractures of the acetabulum. *Clin Orthop and Rel Res* 2000;377:57–67.
65. Martin JS, Marsh JL. Current classification of fractures; rationale and utility. *Radiol Clin N Am* 1997;35:491–506.
66. DeCoster TA, Willis MC, Marsh JL, et al. Rank order analysis of tibial plafond fracture: does injury or reduction predict outcome? *Foot and Ankle International* 20: 44–49, 1999.
67. Cronbach LJ. Coefficient alpha and the internal structure of tests. *Psychometrika* 1951; 16:297–334.
68. Dirschl DR. Reliability and General Applicability of Classification of Fractures of the Tibial Plafond According to a Rank Order Method. Proceedings of the 15th Annual Meeting of the Orthopaedic Trauma Association, Charlotte, NC, 1999;383–384.
69. Dirschl DR, Marsh JL, Buckwalter J, et al. The clinical and basic science of articular fractures. *J Am Acad Orthop Surg* 2004;12:416–423.

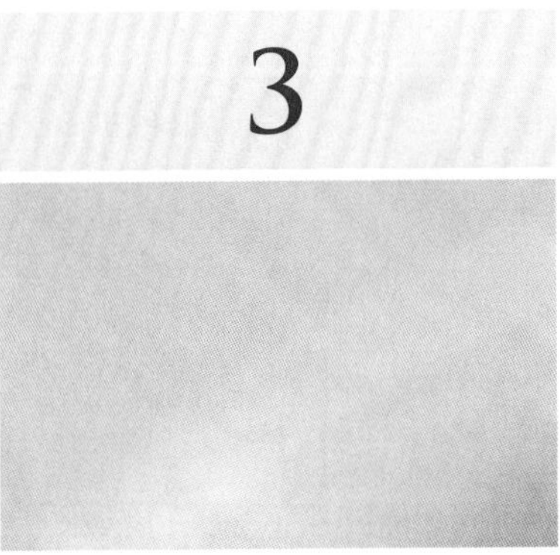

MANAGEMENT OF THE MULTIPLY INJURED PATIENT

Hans-Christoph Pape and Peter V. Giannoudis

DEFINITIONS OF POLYTRAUMA: INCIDENCE, INJURY DISTRIBUTION, AND MORTALITY

Trauma is a major health problem and a leading cause of death, particularly in younger adults and adolescents. The severity of consequent illness and the resulting disability is high compared with other disease processes (1). Yet it fails to attract the kind of research and clinical funding given to other major pathological processes. In some countries trauma services continue to be poorly coordinated and steps to remedy this are only beginning (2). As such, it has been considered the "neglected disease of the modern society." In 1998 it was estimated that 5.8 million people died worldwide from accidental injuries (3). In the United States, 12,400 people die each month following trauma (4). According to data from major trauma registries, the mean age of patients with polytrauma is 29 to 34 years and the males are affected in 60% to 80% of the cases. Thus, the burden on society due to lost earnings and long-term disability of young, able people is huge (5).

Over the years, several studies have been published concerning the epidemiology of major injuries, although these are by no means homogenous and comparable. One of the main limitations has been the lack of clear and accepted definitions especially in the presence of multiple injuries. The definition of multiple trauma varies among surgeons from different specialties and between different centers and countries. This has led to the development of standardized scoring systems to allow comparable stratification of injuries between centers and to aid prediction of morbidity and mortality.

Trauma scoring systems have been developed to convert the severity of injury into numeric values, allowing clinicians to communicate by means of quality assurance and quality control programs. In order for a scoring system to be considered as rational, it should fulfill such requirements as accuracy, reliability, and specificity. The Injury Severity Score (ISS), an anatomical scoring system that provides an overall score for patients with multiple injuries, is still one of the most widely employed methods (6). This is based on the Abbreviated Injury Scale (AIS), a standardized system of classification for the severity of individual injuries from 1 (mild) to 6 (usually fatal). Each injury is assigned an AIS score and is allocated to one of six body regions: head, face, chest, abdomen, extremities (including pelvis), and external structures. The total ISS score is calculated from the sum of the squares of the three worst regional values. It is important to emphasize that only the worst injury in each body region is used. The ISS ranges from 1 to 75, with any region scoring 6 automatically given a score of 75. The ISS limits the total number of contributing injuries to three only, one each from the three most injured regions, which may result in underscoring the degree of trauma sustained if a patient has more than one significant injury in more than three regions. More importantly perhaps, the ISS only takes into account one injury per body region resulting in inability to account for multiple injuries to the same body region. This is particularly troublesome in patients with multiple extremity trauma. To address some of these limitations, Osler et al proposed a modification to the system which they termed the New Injury Severity Score (NISS) (7). This is defined as the sum of squares of the AIS scores of each of a patient's three most severe injuries regardless of the body region in which they occur. Both systems have been shown to be good predictors of outcome in multiple trauma patients (7–10).

Anatomical injury distribution is not the only factor which will determine outcome in traumatized patients. A number of other systems have been introduced which use initial vital signs to determine the degree of physiological response to injury. For example, the Revised Trauma Score (RTS) uses values based on the Glasgow Coma Scale (GCS), systolic blood pressure and respiratory rate to give a total score (11). This is combined using a complex weighted method with the ISS and the age of the patient in the Trauma Injury Severity Score (TRISS) (12). Though such systems improve upon the anatomic systems alone in prediction of morbidity and mortality, they become increasingly complex and unwieldy, making bedside estimation impossible. Other systems exist, such as those based on the International Classification of Diseases (ICD). These have been shown to have greater accuracy in predicting outcome, though again many have found them too complex to be practical. The selection of scoring systems for use in different situations remains a controversial and keenly debated topic (13).

In general terms, polytrauma can be defined as injury to at least two organ systems that causse a potentially life-threatening condition. In practical terms this has been represented as those patients with an ISS of 16 or above, and it has been proposed that all such patients should be cared for in a designated trauma center (14). Recently data published from the Trauma Audit and Research Network for the epidemiology of trauma in the United Kingdom revealed that of a total 159,746 patients, 18.2% had an ISS greater or equal to 16 (15). The overall mortality rate was 6.6%. Analysis of survivors versus nonsurvivors revealed a significantly higher ISS, incidence of systolic blood pressure below 90 mm Hg, GCS less than 15, and higher fluid resuscitation requirements in the nonsurvivor group of patients. Nonsurvivors had also a significantly higher prevalence of chest trauma, head injuries, solid abdominal organ injury or fracture of more than one long bone.

The prevalence of polytrauma (ISS >16) in the elderly has been given only cursory attention in the literature. Analysis of data from major trauma centers revealed an incidence of 1.94%. The mean age of the patients was 75.7 years (range 65–100 years) and the mean ISS 25.3 points (range 16–75 points). Head injury was sustained by 73.6% of the patients, 35.4% had an injury to the thorax, 33.5% lower extremity injuries, 27.7% injuries to the upper extremities, 19.1% had spinal injuries, 18.2% had an injury to the face, 12.8% had an injury to their pelvis and abdomen, and 5.9% had sustained burns. The overall mortality rate was 42.3%, significantly higher than the reported incidence of mortality in younger patients with similar injuries. Increased age, the presence of physiological derangement on admission, higher incidence of lower limb injuries, and more severe head or chest injuries were independently predictive of reduced survival rates. Diminished physiologic reserve, preexisting comorbid conditions, and deficiencies in management may contribute to the higher rates of morbidity and mortality in the elderly patient with trauma as compared with the young patient with equivalent trauma. Age should therefore be considered as an important factor in contemporary scoring systems and treatment algorithms.

STAGED APPROACH TO CARE

Primary care of severely injured patients depends on knowledge of typical posttraumatic courses. This allows anticipation of potential problems and sensible decision making regarding the timing of interventions using a systematic approach (16). Four different phases of the posttraumatic course can be differentiated.

1. Acute "reanimation" period (1–3 hours)
2. Primary "stabilization" period (1–48 hours)
3. Secondary "regeneration" period (2–10 days)
4. Tertiary "reconstruction and rehabilitation" period (weeks to months after trauma)

Acute "Reanimation" Period

This phase includes the time from admission to the control of the acute life-threatening conditions. More recently with increased emphasis on prehospital care this phase can be extended to the first point of contact with medical service at the scene. Rapid systematic assessment is performed to immediately identify potentially life-threatening conditions. Diagnosis should be followed by prioritized management of the airway and any breathing disorders followed by circulatory support as set down in Advanced Trauma Life Support (ATLS) (17) and prehospital care guidelines (18). This may involve rapid institution of various emergency procedures, including airway control, thoracocentesis, rapid control of external bleeding, and vigorous fluid and/or blood replacement therapy.

This is followed by the "secondary survey," a complete acute diagnostic checkup, but this should only be undertaken if there is no acute life-threatening situation, which would make immediate surgery necessary. In these cases this secondary assessment intended to identify all injuries sustained should be delayed until the patient is properly stabilized.

Primary "Stabilization" Period

This phase begins when any acute life-threatening situation has been remedied and there is complete stability of the respiratory, hemodynamic, and neurologic systems of the patient. This is the usual phase where major extremity injuries are managed, including acute management of fractures associated with arterial injuries or the presence of acute compartment syndrome. Fractures can be temporary stabilized with external fixation and the compartments released where appropriate. The primary period should not exceed 48 hours.

Secondary "Regeneration" Period

In this phase the general condition of the patient is stabilized and monitored. It is vital to regularly re-evaluate the constantly evolving clinical picture to avoid harmful impact from intensive care treatment or the burden of complex operative procedures. Unnecessary surgical interventions should not be performed during the acute response phase following trauma. Physiological and intensive care scoring systems may be employed to monitor clinical progress. In the presence of systemic inflammation and multiple organ dysfunction syndrome (MODS), appropriate supportive measures should be undertaken in an intensive care environment.

Tertiary "Reconstruction and Rehabilitation" Period

This final rehabilitation period is accompanied by any necessary surgical procedures, including final reconstructive measures. Only when adequate recovery is demonstrated should complex surgical procedures be contemplated. Such interventions include the definitive management of complex midface fractures, spinal or pelvic fractures, or joint reconstruction.

IMPACT OF RESCUE CONDITIONS ON THE CLINICAL COURSE

The trimodal distribution of deaths following severe injury has been well described. Early death rates from remediable causes have been reduced by the implementation of ATLS protocols and the centralization of trauma services. Improvements in critical care have reduced late death from sepsis and multiple organ failure, although understanding of these phenomena is far from complete (19). Immediate and very early deaths are on the whole only reduced by improvements in safety and accident prevention. However, it is increasingly recognized that interventions such as endotracheal intubation at a very early stage can influence the later clinical course. To this end, progressively more interest is being directed to prehospital care of polytrauma patients. Studies have demonstrated that early access by trained emergency medical physicians capable of delivering advanced life support on scene can increase survival (20–23). Procedures such as endotracheal intubation, thoracic drainage, sedation, and resuscitation can be provided as appropriate (18,24). Subsequent evacuation by air ambulance to a designated trauma center can further improve long-term outcome (25,26).

Entrapment

Motor vehicle accidents with entrapment are particularly challenging to emergency systems because of the severity of the ensuing trauma and the inherent complexity of rescue procedures. The extrication procedure of entrapped trauma patients after motor vehicle accidents requires close cooperation between the medical and the technical rescue team. A practical approach to extrication consists of initial assessment, rapid access for a single person, extended access for advanced life support where necessary, and the extrication itself. During the extrication process the trauma victim is at high risk of additional injury or of the aggravation of existing lesions. Improper handling during extrication without consideration of the ongoing resuscitation process may increase the time spent at the scene and expose the patient to unnecessary risks. Earlier studies report a significant number of neurologic injuries that appear to be a result of the extrication process or of inadequate immobilization during transport. Recent work also underlines the need for appropriate and situation adapted Advanced Life Support (ALS) procedures to improve outcome after prehospital trauma resuscitation (27). Ensuring an unobstructed airway and adequate oxygenation are first priorities in the resuscitation of the entrapped trauma patient; a high proportion of patients may have to be intubated while still entrapped. Conventional intubation by use of the laryngoscope is the golden standard using rapid sequence intubation. However, this access might be impossible in case of entrapment. Other techniques include ventral intubation, blind endotracheal intubation, laryngeal mask airway, retrograde intubation, and emergency cricothyroidotomy (28,29).

Aggressive prehospital resuscitation is commenced at initial access to the patient, including basic monitoring, airway management, hemorrhage control, fluid infusion, analgesia, and cervical spine stabilization. If the patient deteriorates, rapid extrication procedures have to be performed. Aggressive field resuscitation and immediate transport to a level 1 trauma center is associated with mortality lower than that predicted by TRISS and ASCOT (A Severity Characterization of Trauma) scores in spite of the prolonged prehospital time (23,30).

Hypothermia

Trauma patients are inherently predisposed to hypothermia from a variety of intrinsic and iatrogenic causes. In contrast to the perceived benefits in elective surgery, clinical experience with trauma patients has identified hypothermia as a significant contributing factor to subsequent morbidity and mortality (31,32). A core temperature below 34°C is associated with a significantly increased mortality (33). It is hypothesized that this diverse effect of hypothermia is related to depletion of high-energy phosphates like adenosine-triphosphate (ATP) in trauma patients (34). Furthermore, hypothermia has been demonstrated to induce coagulopathic states by disordered enzymatic function, reduced platelet activity, and altered fibrinolysis (35,36).

Coagulation and cardiac sequelae are the most pertinent physiological concerns in hemorrhagic models of hypothermic shock despite adequate volume replacement (37,38). Hypothermia and coagulopathy often mandate a simplified approach to complex surgical problems. There are few controlled investigations, but clinical opinion strongly supports the active prevention of hypothermia in the acutely traumatized patient. Both passive and active rewarming techniques, including the use of warming blankets and other conductive heat devices, preclinical use of fluid warmers, and extracorporeal devices in severe cases, have been successfully utilized (39). The ideal method of rewarming is unclear but must be individualized to the patient and it is institution specific. Conversely, hypothermia has selected clinical benefits when appropriately used in cases of trauma under clinical conditions. Severe hypothermia has allowed remarkable survivals in the course of accidental circulatory arrest. The selective application of mild hypothermia in severe traumatic brain injury is an area with promise, though existing studies are somewhat contradictory and work is ongoing (40).

INITIAL ASSESSMENT AND EARLY MANAGEMENT

The next phase in patient management is acute treatment in the emergency department at the primary hospital. The trauma team has to quickly ascertain the extent of the injury as well as assess the pulmonary and hemodynamic status of the patient. Carefully planned diagnostic and operative tactics should be applied and coordinated to avoid mistakes that could impact negatively on the patient's prognosis. The decisions made depend on the level of expertise of the treating surgeon and the trauma team and their experience of managing trauma cases. During the treatment course, the clinical scenario can change rapidly and management plans must be able to adapt accordingly.

Management by inexperienced surgeons can lead to inefficient handling of the changing situation and negatively impact on patient prognosis (41). Use of standardized care protocols has been shown to improve timing, process and outcome (42). Because of logistical restraints, significant numbers of traumatized patients are still initially managed by inexperienced personnel. In these situations, a structured approach or algorithm to guide management has proven to be of increased benefit. A systematic, problem solving approach is directed with proper guidance as to initial assessment and therapeutic procedures in different situations, while minimizing unnecessary and prolonged diagnostic pursuits (43). This approach has proved invaluable in saving time, minimizing mistakes, and guiding inexperienced personnel to providing better care (44–46). It has been demonstrated that the use of the algorithm has especially reduced mortality in patients with moderately severe polytrauma, represented by an ISS of 20 and 50 (47). For patients with an ISS above 50, however, the algorithm did not influence their clinical outcome (47). These patients usually have life-threatening conditions, where the severest prognosis is given. Patients with less severe injuries are likely to have good outcomes even where initial management is suboptimal.

The primary goal of initial management is to rapidly diagnose and immediately treat life-threatening conditions. These include:

- Airway obstruction or injury and asphyxia (e.g., laryngeal trauma)
- Tension pneumothorax or hemothorax
- Open thoracic injury and flail chest
- Cardiac tamponade
- Massive internal or external hemorrhage

In these situations accurate rapid diagnosis, together with immediate administration of life saving procedures, is necessary. This may necessitate that the patient be taken urgently to the operating room without further investigations. Again, good knowledge of treatment algorithms is of paramount importance in achieving this goal to avoid distraction from occult immediately threatening problems to obvious or spectacular but less dangerous secondary lesions. A pertinent example would be neglect of intra-abdominal exsanguination while attempting to deal with severe extremity injury.

Respiratory Function

Management of the airway and breathing systems should be prioritized as they represent the most rapid threat to survival. Airway obstruction may be a result of

- Midfacial fractures with obstruction of the nasopharynx
- Mandibular fractures with the obstruction of the pharynx by the base of the tongue
- Direct laryngeal or tracheal injury
- Blood or vomit aspiration
- Foreign bodies (e.g., dentures)

Treatment should prioritize removal of any airway obstruction. If the obstruction is subglottic, emergency cricothyroidotomy or tracheostomy can be lifesaving. Obstruction of the trachea in the region of the mediastinum can cause severe respiratory impairment. This can lead to severe mediastinal emphysema and perforation of the endotracheal tube.

The next priority is to maintain respiration, which could be compromised by thoracic or central nervous dysfunction. Disorders of the respiratory system can be diagnosed clinically from symptoms and signs, including dyspnea, cyanosis, stridor, depressed conscious level, abnormal chest expansion and the presence of major thoracic injuries. Thoracic injury might cause acute respiratory derangement, including lung contusion, tension pneumothorax, and hemothorax. Tension pneumothorax is a life-threatening condition and should be diagnosed clinically and treated without delay. The management of pneumothorax and hemothorax should include the insertion of a chest drain to decompress the chest.

Pulmonary edema can be caused by cardiac dysfunction, occurring as a consequence of direct cardiac trauma (48,49) or secondary myocardial infarction. Alternatively, isolated blunt thoracic trauma may cause high-pressure edema, which has been observed following thoracic compression. Management of these two conditions differs—one requiring fluid replacement therapy and the other the use of diuretics. However, the initial management of both types of edema involves continues suction and the use of positive end-expiratory pressure (PEEP).

Severe head injury can cause central respiratory impairment, which can be best verified through the use of a physical component summary. Severe shock may result in severe cerebral hypoxia and subsequent respiratory impairment. It is important that the emergency physician does not underestimate the effect of hemorrhagic shock. Continuous observation of the spontaneously breathing patient with minor injuries in these cases can be justified. In the severely or multiple injured patient, immediate intubation and ventilation for adequate oxygenation is indicated. A tidal volume of 8 to 10 mL/kg body weight, PEEP of 5 mL, and 50% O_2 saturation are prerequisites for adequate ventilation.

Cardiovascular Function

Following assessment of the respiratory system, investigation of the cardiovascular system is necessary in the presence of shock. Hemorrhagic shock should be distinguished from other causes, such as cardiogenic and neurogenic shock. The presence of flat jugular veins might indicate the presence of hemorrhagic shock. An elevated jugular venous pressure can be diagnostic of cardiogenic shock, caused by coronary heart disease, myocardial infarction (MI), cardiac contusion, tension pneumothorax, or cardiac tamponade. To establish this diagnosis the insertion of a pulmonary artery catheter may be necessary.

Neurogenic Shock

Relative hypovolemia is the cause of neurogenic shock, usually due to spinal injury. Loss of the autonomic supply leads to a decrease in vascular tone with blood pooling in the periphery. This can occur without significant blood loss. The resultant increase in skin perfusion lead to warm periphery and a decrease in central blood delivery. This type of shock may be difficult to distinguish from hypovolemia.

Cardiogenic Shock

Cardiogenic shock requires immediate attention and frequently immediate surgery. The heart can be impaired by cardiac tamponade, tension pneumothorax, and hemothorax, or in rare cases by intra-abdominal bleeding. These pathologies may necessitate immediate surgical intervention, including placement of a chest drain, pericardiocentesis, and emergency thoracotomy. If there is indirect impairment of cardiac function, medical treatment should be introduced and normovolemia should be restored. Raised jugular venous pressure in cardiogenic shock may be the result of right-sided heart failure. This should be confirmed through measurement of the central venous pressure. Right heart failure may result in blood pooling in the pulmonary system. This can be difficult to distinguish from peripheral blood loss. The two can coexist and may impair cardiac function. These conditions include:

- Cardiac tamponade
- Tension pneumothorax
- Myocardial infarction
- Cardiac contusion

The presence of penetrating cardiac trauma associated with an elevated central pressure and a decreased peripheral systemic pressure should alert the treating doctor to the possibility of cardiac tamponade. A normal chest x-ray may not rule out this possibility, but ultrasound should provide an immediate diagnosis. The treatment of this condition should include emergency pericardiocentesis. Following aspiration of 10 mL of fluid from the pericardial sac, an immediate improvement of the heart stroke volume is seen with an increase in the peripheral systemic perfusion. Emergency thoracotomy is rarely indicated. If required it can be performed through an incision between the fourth and fifth ribs on the left side, followed by opening the pericardium in a craniocaudal direction to avoid injury to the phrenic nerve. One or two transmural stitches allow temporary cardiac closure and cardiac massage can then be conducted.

Tension pneumothorax causes rapidly increasing cyanosis, a rapid deterioration of respiratory function and can cause acute right ventricular failure. As the condition progresses, raised intrathoracic pressure causes reduced right-sided venous return to the heart. As mediastinal shifting occurs, kinking or obstruction of the venacaval system can lead to complete obstruction resulting in cardiac arrest. Rapid diagnosis followed by immediate decompression is a lifesaving measure.

Cardiac failure may cause MI independent from the trauma. This diagnosis should be considered in elderly people following road traffic accidents. In these patients MI may have been caused by hypovolemia, hypoxia, or the acute release of catecholamines in the blood stream at the time of the accident or alternatively occurred incidentally causing the accident. A diagnosis of MI can be confirmed from acute changes on electrocardiography and an increase of blood markers (creatine kinase MB). The treatment of MI should include medical therapy to control arrhythmias. Patients with MI should be treated in the intensive care unit (ICU) with continuous monitoring from the medical team.

Cardiac contusion can be difficult to differentiate from MI. Contusion is usually seen following blunt anterior thoracic wall trauma associated with a fracture of the sternum. Differentiating this condition from MI in the acute setting is of secondary importance to the initial management as both diagnoses require similar management, including control of cardiac arrhythmias and heart failure with continuous invasive monitoring.

Hypovolemic/Hemorrhagic Shock

Hemorrhagic shock can be diagnosed through classical clinical parameters though physiological reserve can mean that alterations in pulse and blood pressure are a relatively late sign. The extent of hypovolemia is often underestimated. Perhaps the most sensitive indicator of intravascular volume is peripheral capillary blood flow, evaluated by assessing the nail beds and conjunctiva. Urine output is also a sensitive parameter that can be used for the diagnosis of shock, to determine severity and monitor the response to treatment. As a rough estimate, normal urine output should exceed 1 mL/kg/hr or 30 mL in 30 minutes. Anuria is extremely unusual and often indicates obstruction. This should be investigated by imaging the renal tract as a matter of urgency, though in the face of ongoing deterioration of other parameters hypovolemia should be assumed in the trauma patient until this can be undertaken.

Measurements of the right-sided filling pressure can be achieved using subclavian or jugular central venous catheters. The central venous pressure is likely to increase where there is an increase in the intrathoracic pressure (e.g., in thoracic trauma or mechanical ventilation with PEEP) and thus is often of little value when initially assessing shock. Use of a pulmonary arterial catheter (Swan-Ganz catheter) allows much more accurate and reliable estimation of cardiac function in complex cases. However, Swan-Ganz catheter insertion is a skilled procedure, particularly in the acute setting and certainly requires ICU monitoring.

Laboratory parameters provide further information when evaluating shock status and can be especially useful in assessing response to therapy. In particular, the arterial pH, base excess, and plasma lactate levels have been used. Abnormal values reflect ongoing tissue ischemia and various clinical and experimental studies have shown a correlation between these parameters and the grade of shock (50–52). Furthermore, abnormality—particularly where it is ongoing and fails to correct with therapy—has been shown to correlate with poor outcome (53,54). These parameters indicate generalized or local tissue ischemia and give no information regarding the etiology of the condition.

The general management of shock includes rapid and adequate restoration of the hemodynamic status of the patient through the use of fluid and blood concentrate replacement therapy; this is detailed below. Blood should be ordered immediately when shock has been diagnosed clinically. If the rescue team has indicated the possibility of massive bleeding, erythrocyte concentrate should be available when the patient arrives in the emergency room. Once volume restoration has been started, any external or internal bleeding should be identified. External blood loss is usually obvious though the volume lost prior to admission is usually unclear. Furthermore, the identification of external sites of hemorrhage should not distract from a rigorous search for internal bleeding, the identification of which can be more problematic. Internal blood loss should be suspected in all patients, particularly where shock is recalcitrant. This usually occurs in one of three body regions—the thorax, abdomen, or pelvis.

Differentiation of the site of internal bleeding can usually be made by using a combination of clinical judgment, thoracic and pelvic anterior-posterior radiographs and abdominal ultrasonography. Abdominal ultrasound should be conducted in the first few minutes of the patient's arrival to the emergency room where this is available. Increasingly emergency department and trauma personnel are being trained in ultrasound examination and appropriate equipment is being made available.

Neurologic Status

If a patient has to be intubated and sedated, it is important for the emergency doctor to fully evaluate the neurological status prior to this. The size and reaction of the pupils are important indicators of the presence of any central impairment (abnormal pupillary reaction and size). The light reflex reflects the function of the second and third cranial nerves, oculocephalic reflex depends on the integrity of the third and fourth cranial nerves, and the corneal reflex represents intact fifth and seventh cranial nerves. The GCS also provides important information regarding the neurological status of patients, particularly when serial measurements are possible and can provide a useful aid in clinical decision making. It is argued that computed tomography (CT) should be performed if the GCS is less than 10; and where the GCS is less than 8, continuous intracranial pressure monitoring may be necessary. These figures only act as a guide; however, trauma severity and overall clinical condition should also be taken into account.

Management of Hemorrhagic Shock

Using a parallel approach it is usual to commence immediate management of posttraumatic shock while full evaluation of respiratory, neurologic, and cardiovascular status is ongoing. Prolonged shock can lead to further posttraumatic complications and therefore impact negatively on the patient's prognosis. Two large bore intravenous cannulae should be inserted during the preclinical phase and rapid fluid replacement therapy should commence as soon as possible. The cannulae are usually placed in the antecubital fossae and fastened securely to prevent dislodgement.

On arrival in the emergency room, further IV lines can be inserted as appropriate. Single internal jugular or subclavian vein lines have the disadvantage of not allowing rapid transfusion of large amounts of fluid. If lines in the peripheral veins are not feasible, venous cutdowns can be conducted by using the long saphenous vein around the ankle.

The choice of fluid for trauma resuscitation remains a controversial issue (55). Historically, crystalloid solutions were considered unsuitable as they were rapidly lost from circulation with plasma or serum being preferred. Work in the 1960s, however, revealed that resuscitation with crystalloid led to lower rates of renal impairment and mortality. It was considered that during hemorrhage, fluid is redistributed to the circulation from the extracellular compartment and these losses must also be replaced. Therefore infusion of a combination of crystalloid and blood at a 3:1 ratio was recommended. However, widespread application of these principles, particularly in military conflict, coincided with the emergence of adult respiratory distress syndrome or shock lung as a clinical entity in survivors of major trauma. Whether this was a consequence of large volume crystalloid infusion was unclear. Interest in the use of colloid products was therefore renewed, but early results were conflicting, partly due to shortcomings in trial design. Meta-analysis of these smaller studies revealed no overall difference in the rate of pulmonary insufficiency following resuscitation with either fluid type. Moreover, when final mortality was considered, particularly in the subgroup of trauma patients, a significant improvement in the overall survival rate was observed in the group administered crystalloid (56,57). Crystalloid fluid is therefore considered to be the first treatment choice in most centers and is particularly favored in US trauma centers. Ringers lactate has various theoretical advantages over isotonic saline though clinical trials have not shown differences in outcome. Research into fluid selection for resuscitation is ongoing, particularly as much early evidence is based on the use of albumin as a colloid. Since then, newer products with higher molecular weights have become available that should be more efficient in maintaining fluid in the intravascular space. There is further evidence however that in cases of severe hemorrhagic shock, increased capillary permeability allows these molecules to leak into the interstitium, worsening tissue edema and oxygen delivery (55).

Animal studies demonstrating that small bolus administration of hypertonic saline was as effective as large volume crystalloid have provoked considerable interest in potential clinical applications (58). This effect was enhanced by combination with dextran (59). Though improvements in microvascular circulation were observed, this also appeared to increase bleeding. Meta-analysis of early clinical trials revealed that hypertonic saline offered no advantage over standard crystalloid resuscitation though hypertonic saline dextran might (60). This effect was particularly striking in patients with closed head injury, and further animal studies have revealed that hypertonic saline can increase cerebral perfusion while decreasing cerebral edema (61).

Blood Replacement

Secondary to maintaining intravascular volume, preservation of the patient's oxygen carrying capacity is essential. In cases of massive hemorrhage this will inevitably require the replacement of red blood cells. Furthermore, lost, depleted, and diluted components of the coagulation cascade will also require replacement. It is becoming increasingly apparent, however, particularly in young healthy trauma victims, that much lower hemoglobin concentrations than previously thought optimal are tolerated and indeed may be beneficial (62). Not only is blood a precious resource, but transfusion also carries the risk of various complications, including the transmission of infective agents. Traditionally, target hemoglobin concentrations of 10 g/L have been advocated, but it has recently been shown that concentrations as low as 5 g/L are acceptable in normovolemic healthy volunteers (63). Randomized trials in selected normovolemic intensive care patients showed that maintenance of hemoglobin concentrations between 7 and 9 g/L resulted in equivalent and perhaps superior outcome to maintenance above 10 g/L (64) and transfusion requirement has been shown to constitute an independent risk factor for mortality in trauma (65). This may be related to the potential of blood products to cause an inflammatory response in the recipient (66,67).

In cases with severe blood loss, transfusion is currently unavoidable and indeed, there is no clear point where continued administration becomes futile (68). Ideally, fully crossmatched blood should be used but in an emergency universal donor O-negative blood can be used immediately. A sample should be drawn for crossmatch prior to administration as the transfusion of O-negative blood can interfere with subsequent analysis. The blood bank should be able to deliver type-specific blood within 15 to 20 minutes of the patient's arrival in the emergency room. This blood is not fully crossmatched and therefore still carries a relative risk of transfusion reaction. Crossmatched blood should be available within 30 to 40 minutes in most cases.

Coagulopathy should be anticipated in the victims of severe trauma as a result of hemodilution, hypothermia, consumption, and disseminated intravascular coagulation. Correction and avoidance of hypothermia and the administration of warmed fluids is of utmost importance. The administration of platelets, fresh frozen plasma and other blood products should be guided by laboratory results alongside clinical judgment. Expert hematological advice is often required (69,70). Procoagulant therapy for severe coagulopathy remains experimental, though early results are promising. For example, recombinant activated factor VII has shown the potential to activate clotting cascades at sites of injury without inducing excessive systemic coagulability (55,71,72).

With the cost and potential adverse effects of autologous blood transfusion becoming increasingly relevant, interest in alternatives continues. Hemoglobin-based oxygen carrying fluids have been under investigation since the 1930s. Modern solutions using tetrameric polymerized human hemoglobin have been shown to be safe and phase III clinical trials are underway (55).

Monitoring Response to Fluid Replacement Therapy

Response to volume replacement therapy is initially usually monitored using the clinical response of the patient and simple measurements, including pulse, blood pressure, capillary refill, and urine output. Urinary catheterization is mandatory. In the severely injured or complex patient, invasive techniques, including arterial monitoring and central venous or pulmonary artery pressure recording should be considered at an early stage. Though controversy still exists in specific situations, current goals include normalization of vital signs and maintenance of central venous pressure between 8 and 15 mm Hg. Serial recording of acid-base parameters, the base excess and serum lactate in particular, have been shown to be particularly useful in assessing response to therapy and detecting the presence of occult hypoperfusion in apparently stable patients (53,54,73). Ongoing requirement for blood transfusion should be monitored by regular measurement of the hemoglobin concentration. This can be rapidly estimated where necessary using most bedside arterial blood gas analyzers. Ongoing excessive fluid or blood requirement should always prompt a repeated search for sources of hemorrhage. Shock treatment is a dynamic process and in cases where there is ongoing bleeding, surgical intervention is often indicated.

More recently, several methods for improved monitoring of cardiovascular status and tissue perfusion have been introduced, including gastric tonometry, near infrared spectroscopy, transthoracic impedance cardiography, central venous oximetry, and skeletal muscle acid-base estimation. Many of these techniques remain experimental and are not available on a widespread basis. They may be available in certain centers and expert advice is essential.

Secondary–Tertiary Survey

As discussed previously it may be necessary to postpone a full head to toe examination until life-threatening problems have been remedied and the patient has been stabilized. A systematic secondary survey should never be omitted, however. Missed comparatively minor injuries which subsequently receive suboptimal treatment can cause long-term loss of function and considerable morbidity. Such incidents have been the subject of successful litigation despite lifesaving therapy for other more serious injuries. Moreover, it is sensible to repeat the secondary survey, once the immediate danger has passed, away from the busy emergency department. This way omissions and missed opportunities to prevent long-term problems should be minimized. For similar reasons, a thorough, systematic approach should always be employed, with each patient being examined in the same manner, proceeding in a craniocaudal direction and including all body regions. A low threshold for x-ray examination of peripheral injuries should be employed particularly in the presence of major trauma. As an absolute minimum, x-rays of the chest, pelvis, and cervical spine should be obtained as advocated in ATLS teaching. Only through the use of such a structured approach will the morbidity and mortality of patients be decreased.

Diagnostic errors have been shown to occur frequently when treating isolated injuries (74). In polytrauma patients, the clinical picture is more complex and it is more likely that some injuries may be missed or overlooked. A retrospective analysis of diagnostic omission following polytrauma described 327 patients documenting the type and incidence of missed injuries (75). The majority of patients had suffered road traffic accidents in which 50% were car drivers, 24% motorcycle riders, and 26% pedestrians. The overall incidence of missed injuries was 12%; that is, 4% of the total 1205 injuries were missed. The most common type of overlooked injuries were fractures, particularly around large joints. The majority of missed injuries were picked up within 3 days following admission, though longer intervals have also been reported.

The reasons for overlooking injuries usually relate to poor primary assessment and are significantly more common with the less experienced physician. It was found that mistakes in the initial clinical examination were based on insufficient or nonsystematic examination or misinterpretation of the injury site (75). The initial examination is more difficult in unconscious or sedated patients with major injuries. In these cases the usual indicator of pain cannot reliably be used to direct examination. Signs such as crepitus, deformity, hematoma, swelling, or joint effusion must be used to direct investigation. Poor x-ray quality, misinterpretation of x-rays, admission, and the total number of injuries present were also important factors in the incidence of missed injuries.

The tertiary survey provides another opportunity to evaluate any newly discovered physical findings and diagnose any missed injuries. It also consists of a repeated head-to-toe evaluation of the trauma patient. Daily laboratory data and new radiological examination in the form of plain x-rays, CT, or magnetic resonance imaging (MRI) should be considered along with the clinical signs. Repeated physical examination is of paramount importance and contributes favorably to the patient's long-term outcome.

DEFINITION OF THE PATIENT'S CONDITION

Once initial assessment and intervention is complete patients should be placed into one of four categories in order to guide the subsequent approach to their care. This is done on the basis of overall injury severity, the presence of specific injuries and current hemodynamic status as detailed above (73). Any deterioration in clinical state or physiological parameters should prompt rapid reassessment and adjustment of management approach as appropriate (76). Achieving the end points of resuscitation is of paramount importance for the stratification of the patient into the appropriate category. End points of resuscitation include stable hemodynamics, stable oxygen saturation, lactate level below 2 mmol/L, no coagulation disturbances, normal temperature, urinary output above 1 mL/kg/hr, and no requirement for inotropic support.

Stable

Stable patients have no immediately life-threatening injuries, respond to initial therapy, and are hemodynamically stable without inotropic support. There is no evidence of physiologic disturbance such as coagulopathy or respiratory distress nor ongoing occult hypoperfusion manifesting as abnormalities of acid base status. They are not hypothermic. These patients have the physiological reserve to withstand prolonged operative intervention where this is appropriate and can be managed using an ETC approach, with reconstruction of complex injuries.

Borderline

Borderline patients have stabilized in response to initial resuscitative attempts but have clinical features or combinations of injury, which have been associated with poor outcome and put them at risk of rapid deterioration. These have been defined as follows (126):

- ISS <40
- Hypothermia <35°
- Initial mean pulmonary arterial pressure >24 mm Hg or a >6–mm Hg rise in pulmonary artery pressure during intramedullary nailing or other operative intervention
- Multiple injuries (ISS >20) in association with thoracic trauma (AIS >2)
- Multiple injuries in association with severe abdominal or pelvic injury and hemorrhagic shock at presentation (systolic BP <90 mm Hg)
- Radiographic evidence of pulmonary contusion
- Patients with bilateral femoral fracture
- Patients with moderate or severe head injuries (AIS ≥3)

This group of patients can be initially managed using an ETC approach but this should be undertaken with caution and forethought given to operative strategy should the patient require a rapid change of treatment rationale. Additional invasive monitoring should be instituted and provision made for ICU admission. A low threshold should be used for conversion to a damage control approach to management as detailed below at the first sign of deterioration.

Unstable

Patients who remain hemodynamically unstable despite initial intervention are at greatly increased risk of rapid deterioration, subsequent multiple organ failure and death. Treatment in these cases has evolved to use a "damage control" approach. This entails rapid lifesaving surgery only as absolutely necessary and timely transfer to the ICU for further stabilization and monitoring. Temporary stabilization of fractures using external fixation, hemorrhage control, and exteriorization of gastrointestinal injuries where possible is advocated. Complex reconstructive procedures should be delayed until stability is achieved and the acute immunoinflammatory response to injury has subsided. This rationale is intended to reduce in magnitude the "second hit" of operative intervention or at least delay it until the patient is physiologically equipped to cope.

In Extremis

These patients are very close to death having suffered severe injuries and often have ongoing uncontrolled blood loss. They remain severely unstable despite ongoing resuscitative efforts and are usually suffering the effects of a "deadly triad" of hypothermia, acidosis, and coagulopathy. A damage control approach is certainly advocated, and only lifesaving procedures should be attempted so as not to drive this process further. The patients should then be transferred directly to intensive care for invasive monitoring and advanced hematological, pulmonary, and cardiovascular support. Orthopedic injuries can be stabilized rapidly in the emergency department or intensive care unit using external fixation and this should not delay other therapy. Any reconstructive surgery is again delayed and can be performed if the patient survives.

SURGICAL PRIORITIES IN POLYTRAUMA: WHAT COMES FIRST?

In patients with polytrauma, decision making as to which injury to address first can be difficult, particularly if they appear imminently dangerous or may be contributing to hemodynamic instability. With different injuries falling under the remit of different surgical specialties, disagreements as to surgical priority can occur and it is of utmost importance that a cooperative multidisciplinary approach is adopted. Epidemiological mortality studies and clinical experience reveal that certain injuries can be rapidly fatal and should be considered in precedence to others, although careful individual decision making must be used as every case is different.

Rarely, early operative treatment without prolonged diagnostic procedures may be lifesaving. These include penetrating thoracic injuries resulting in cardiac tamponade, open arterial injuries, and pelvic trauma. Continuous bleeding with shock resistant to supportive therapy in the thoracic, abdominal, or pelvic regions are primary indicators for surgical intervention. With the use of thoracic and pelvic radiographs and abdominal sonography 95% of sources of major bleeding should be identified immediately.

Urgent Lifesaving Surgery

Hemothorax

Hemothorax is usually easily diagnosed from the chest x-ray; however, in the presence of extensive lung contusion or atelectasis the diagnosis can be difficult. Ultrasound examination has shown the potential to identify free thoracic fluid though CT remains the gold standard and often reveals the source of any bleeding (77).

Significant bleeding into the pleural space and resultant hemothorax is treated during the primary survey by a chest tube. Usually, the indication comes from the chest x-ray, and only occasionally are clinical findings the sole basis for chest tube insertion, as chest x-ray can usually be performed very rapidly. It is standard practice to insert the chest tube in the mid-axillary line at the fifth intercostal space Lower insertion risks injury to the diaphragm or intra-abdominal organs. Blunt dissection should prevent structural injury and is important even where the operator is confident of positioning as intra-abdominal injuries may lead to increased intra-abdominal pressure and diaphragmatic elevation or even rupture.

A traditional chest tube of at least 28-gauge should be used to drain a hemothorax; modern percutaneous drains used in thoracic medicine are not sufficient for this indication. A large diameter reduces the danger of coagulation, allows rapid blood evacuation, and allows relative confidence that drained contents are representative of thoracic blood loss. It is usual to direct the tube cordally to drain blood and cranially in the presence of a pneumothorax.

The presence of a hemothorax is not diagnostic of major thoracic hemorrhage. In most cases, bleeding is the result of injury to an intercostal vessel, and this will usually arrest spontaneously. Emergency department thoracotomy remains controversial, although recognized indications include traumatic arrest or recalcitrant profound hypotension in penetrating trauma, rapid exsanguination (>1,500 mL initially or 250 mL/hr), and unresponsive hypotension in blunt thoracic trauma. As a last resort to control catastrophic subdiaphragmatic hemorrhage, the aorta can be cross-clamped. These interventions are regarded as futile in patients with blunt thoracic trauma in cardiac arrest where there has been no witnessed cardiac output and in patients with severe head injuries. There is recent evidence that increased caution should be employed before undertaking emergency thoracotomy in blunt trauma patients for all indications, particularly in the emergency department, due to a relatively high rate of nontherapeutic procedures and poor outcome (78,79).

Mediastinal Hemorrhage and Thoracic Aortic Injury

Mediastinal hemorrhage due to injury to the thoracic aorta is commonly diagnosed erroneously due to poor quality chest radiography obtained in emergency situations with a supine position and insufficient inspiration. Mediastinal enlargement observed on plain chest radiography is rather nonspecific. In this context, one should pay careful attention to the presence of dilated jugular veins, which offer some differentiation of cardiac from aortic injuries. Nonetheless, further imaging should be rapidly obtained in the hemodynamically stable patient by contrast-enhanced thoracic CT. Although traditional CT scanning sometimes lead to false-positive results and angiography has been regarded as the gold standard in diagnosis, many centers believe that contrast-enhanced high-resolution spiral CT is preferable (80–82).

Free intrathoracic rupture in injury to the thoracic aorta is exceedingly rare in patients surviving long enough to reach the emergency room alive. In most cases, the adventitia is preserved and further intrathoracic blood loss is prevented by the parietal pleura. Furthermore there is increasing evidence that repair can be delayed in the presence of other life-threatening injuries and occasionally conservative management can be successful (83–85). These patients should, however, always be treated in a center with an acute thoracic surgical service. Nonoperative treatment of incomplete aortic ruptures in hemodynamically stable patients consists of a controlled hypotension or active reduction of blood pressure while controlling for a difference in blood pressure between the upper and lower parts of the body. Indications for immediate intervention include the development of hemodynamic instability without alternate explanation, hemorrhage via the chest tubes (>500 mL/hr), or a blood pressure gradient between upper and lower extremities leading to an impaired perfusion of the lower limbs (difference of mean blood pressure >30 mm Hg). Given the high mortality rate associated with emergency repair in cases of traumatic aortic injury, there is increasing interest in the use of endovascular stenting in such situations (86–88).

If the clinical situation arouses the suspicion of cardiac injury in the presence of radiological mediastinal abnormality, the diagnosis is generally cardiac tamponade. Pericardiocentesis should be performed. If there is acute decompensation, an emergent thoracocentesis is indicated. Further diagnostics are too time-consuming in this immediately life-threatening situation. If the patient is still hemodynamically stable, a very sensitive and readily available test is the transthoracic echocardiogram.

Severe Pelvic Trauma and Packing

Pelvic fracture is often seen in conjunction with multisystem trauma and can lead to rapid occult hemorrhage. Treatment should be thought of as part of the resuscitative effort and early intervention can be life saving (89). Bleeding is commonly from multiple small sites rather than injured major vessels and, due to the large volume of the retroperitoneum, in severe cases spontaneous arrest is unlikely (90). Furthermore, it is common for the retroperitoneum to be breached during the injury further decreasing the barrier to ongoing hematoma expansion. Treatment with the pneumatic antishock garment or pelvic beltstraps can give some temporary stabilization (91), but results are inconclusive and severe complications have been reported in relation to their use.

Although there has been increasing interest in the use of selective angiography in these cases to embolize bleeding vessels, this intervention is often time consuming to organize and perform. Patients must be relatively stable and careful selection is crucial. Embolization can be used as an adjunct to other interventions where continued arterial hemorrhage is suspected. In severe injuries with profound hemodynamic instability, external fixation with a pelvic C-clamp, and open tamponade by packing is recommended (Fig. 3-1) (92,93). With the patient supine, preparation from the subcostal margin to the pubic symphysis is performed with the abdomen and pelvis completely exposed. If a C-clamp has already been applied for posterior pelvic instability, it should be loosened. In vertical pelvic instability (C-type injury), the leg should be accessible to allow reduction where required.

Following application of an external fixation device, if there is prior evidence of free intraperitoneal fluid a midline laparotomy should be performed and the intra-abdominal organs examined for bleeding following standard management protocols for blunt abdominal trauma. If, however, initial diagnostic imaging has shown no evidence of intra-abdominal fluid and a major source of pelvic hemorrhage is suspected a lower midline laparotomy can be employed. Initial attention should be directed to the retroperitoneum. Following skin incision ruptured pelvic soft tissues are usually readily visible. Any hematoma is evacuated and the paravesical space explored for bleeding sources. Major bleeding vessels should be ligated where possible; in diffuse bleeding, well-directed packing with external stabilization is most recommended.

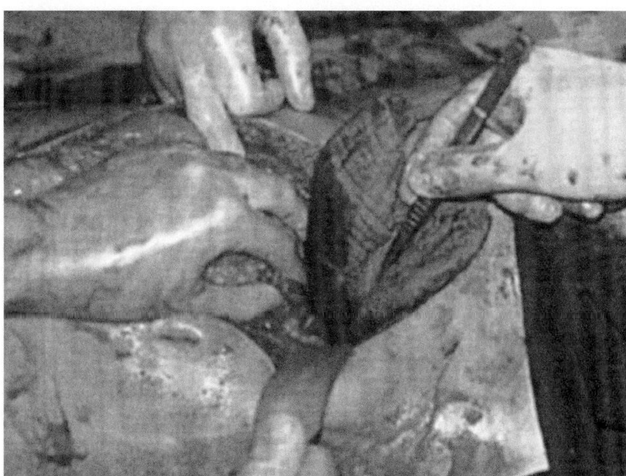

FIGURE 3-1 Application of pelvic packing in a patient with hemodynamic instability.

If hemorrhage is obviously originating from a deep dorsal source, particularly in cases of posterior pelvic instability, attempts at further extraperitoneal exploration should be made in the presacral region. Major bleeding sources can be identified and treated appropriately. In cases of catastrophic arterial hemorrhage, temporary control can be achieved by cross-clamping the aorta. In venous hemorrhage, often no single bleeding source is identifiable. Usually, bleeding originates from disruption of the presacral venous plexus or the fracture site itself. Again, well-directed packing can often adequately control bleeding.

Following this intervention, temporary abdominal closure is performed and correction of physiological abnormalities should be undertaken without delay, with particular regard to coagulopathy and hypothermia. Packing is left in situ and changed routinely at 24 to 48 hours, though in cases of suspected ongoing hemorrhage and recalcitrant shock, earlier reintervention should be considered. At planned revision the cavity should be thoroughly examined for sites of ongoing hemorrhage following debridement as necessary and removal of hematoma. Further bleeding points can be dealt with, but if diffuse hemorrhage persists, further packing with subsequent surgical revision is required. A staged approach to the management of pelvic fractures is shown in Figure 3-2.

Treat Exsanguinating Abdominal Hemorrhage or Expanding Intracranial Hematoma First?

Controversy remains over such difficult situations with compelling arguments being presented for each case. There is increasing evidence for conservative management of abdominal injuries except in the most unstable patients, and apparent intra-abdom-

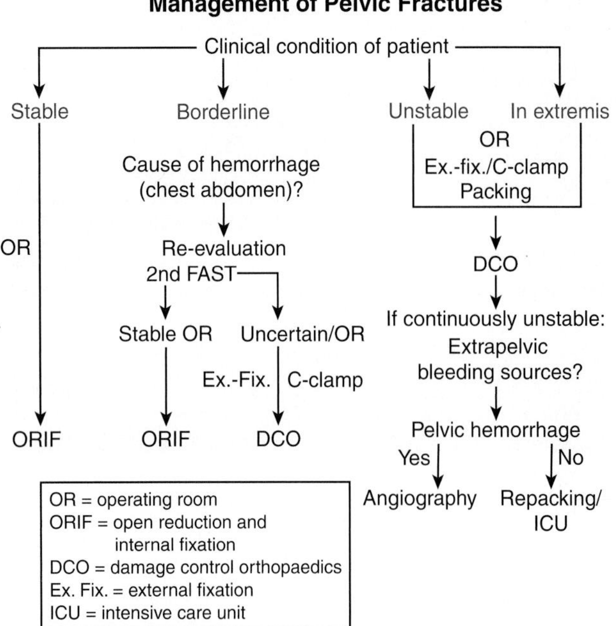

FIGURE 3-2 Algorithm of management of pelvic fractures.

inal hemorrhage is often pelvic in origin. Evacuating an intracranial hematoma if the patient exsanguinates is obviously futile. However, there is equally little benefit in saving a patient's life if the result is profoundly disabling brain injury or death from tentorial herniation. Once compensatory autoregulatory mechanisms are overwhelmed, intracranial pressure rapidly increases. There is evidence that in patients with head injury, death from extracranial causes alone is unusual. In a study of almost 50,000 trauma patients 70% of deaths were attributed to the head injury alone and only 7% to extracranial trauma, with the rest caused by a combination of both (94). However, craniotomy should not be undertaken without imaging to confirm a surgically treatable lesion except in the rarest of circumstances. CT scanning is time-consuming and can cause a significant delay in treatment. This time might be better spent rapidly attempting hemodynamic stabilization. There is also evidence that in hypotensive patients undergoing head CT, emergency laparotomy is required far more frequently than craniotomy (21% vs. 2.5%) (95). Furthermore, inferior outcome has been demonstrated in head injured patients with shock, suggesting that early correction of hypotension may protect against secondary brain injury (96).

It is clear that in these patients, rapid complex management decisions must be made and clinical experience is essential. Thankfully, such dilemmas seldom occur. In a review of 800 patients with significant head and abdominal injuries, 52 required craniotomy, 40 laparotomy, and only 3 required both (97).

MOLECULAR ASPECTS OF TRAUMA

Trauma and surgery induce changes in the inflammatory immunological and coagulatory cascades. The availability of techniques to measure biological markers of immune reactivity has vastly expanded our knowledge of the events that occur at the cellular level. Before referring to the immunologic events occurring following trauma, it is essential to understand the pathogenesis of the most severe posttraumatic complications, adult respiratory distress syndrome (ARDS) and MODS in these circumstances. MODS is characterized by generalized inflammation and tissue damage. In the early 1970s Tilney et al (98) were given credit for first describing sequential failure of multiple organs in 18 consecutive patients with ruptured abdominal aortic aneurysm who required postoperative hemodialysis. These authors concluded that this was the result of a combination of preexisting disease and hemorrhagic shock. Eisman et al (99) introduced the term *multiple-organ failure* to describe the clinical course of 42 patients with progressive organ failure; half of these patients had an intra-abdominal abscess implicated as the inciting event. Thus, sepsis was added to the list of risk factors for MODS. Subsequently, Fry et al (100) retrospectively reviewed 553 patients who required emergency operations; two thirds had sustained major trauma. Thirty-eight (7%) patients developed MODS and 90% were septic. The authors proposed that MODS was a fatal expression of uncontrolled infection. This led to an aggressive policy of mandatory laparotomy to rule out intra-abdominal abscess (100).

Faist et al (101) published a review of 433 trauma patients who required emergency operations (99% blunt mechanism); 50 (12%) developed ARDS and 34 (8%) developed MODS. The authors described two distinct patterns of MODS: rapid single-phase MODS due to massive tissue injury and shock or delayed two-phase MODS due to moderate trauma and shock followed by delayed sepsis. Goris et al (102) reviewed 92 MODS patients who had clinical signs of sepsis. They separated these patients into two groups: 55 trauma patients (all blunt mechanism) versus 37 nontrauma patients who had undergone emergency laparotomy. Bacterial sepsis was confirmed in only 33% of the trauma-related MODS patients, compared with 65% of the nontrauma patients (102). In addition, a provocative report by Norton (103) showed that drainage of an abdominal abscess reverses MODS in a disappointingly small proportion of patients. Thus, the above clinical observations suggested that MODS frequently may occur in the absence of infection and the inflammatory system was implicated as a causative factor. It is known today that the activation of the inflammatory system is the norm after traumatic injury and this leads to the development of the systemic inflammatory response syndrome (SIRS).

This is followed by a period of recovery mediated by a counterregulatory anti-inflammatory response (104). It appears that the key players in this host inflammatory response are the cytokines, the leukocytes, the endothelium, and subsequent leukocyte–endothelial cell interactions. Reactive oxygen species, eicosanoids, and microcirculatory disturbances also play pivotal roles (105).

Within this inflammatory process, a fine balance exists between the beneficial effects of inflammation and the potential for the process itself to cause and aggravate tissue injury leading to ARDS and MODS. If this inflammatory response is exaggerated or perpetuated, patients enter a state of malignant systemic inflammation (moderate or severe SIRS) that can evolve into overt ARDS or MODS. In these patients, pulmonary failure occurs first, then the other organs fail because the lungs are either more vulnerable or our clinical tools to detect lung failure are more sensitive. Proposed mechanisms for the nonseptic (inflammatory) development of MODS include the following:

- **Macrophage theory**—increased production of cytokines and other inflammatory mediators by activated macrophages
- **Microcirculatory theory**—prolonged hypovolemic shock promotes MODS through inadequate global oxygen delivery and ischemia reperfusion phenomena
- **Endothelial cell**—leukocyte interactions leading to remote organ injury
- **Gut hypothesis**—gut origin bacteria or their products contribute to MODS. It has been used to explain why no obvious site of infection can be found in as many as 30% of the bacteremic patients who die from MODS.
- **One- and two-hit theories**—In the one-hit model the initial injury and shock give rise to an intense systemic inflammatory response with the potential for remote organ injury. In the two-hit model, the initial stimulus is less intense and normally resolves but the patient is vulnerable to a secondary inflammatory insult that can reactivate the systemic inflammatory response and precipitate late multiple organ dysfunction. Secondary insults to the inflammatory system in the two-hit model can be caused by factors such as surgical procedures and sepsis (Fig. 3-3)

It is believed that significant overlap exists in the different inflammatory theories of the development of MODS. In most patients, irrespective of the triggering event, MODS follows a predictable course, generally beginning with the lungs and progressing to liver, gastrointestinal tract, and kidney. The mortality rate progressively rises from 20% with one failed organ system to 100% when four systems fail (100).

Lately, increased knowledge of posttraumatic immunological responses has resulted in a clearer appreciation of these processes (106,107). Specific markers of the systemic inflammatory response have been identified and can now be included in the assessment of these patients (108). The clinical course of the patient following polytrauma therefore is primarily determined by three factors: the initial trauma ("first hit"); the patient's biological constitution; and the timing and quality of any medical intervention, which can be thought of as additional trauma ("second hit") if the procedure is large enough. The treating physician can modulate only the medical interventions. The more severely traumatized the patient is, the more critical the strategy becomes.

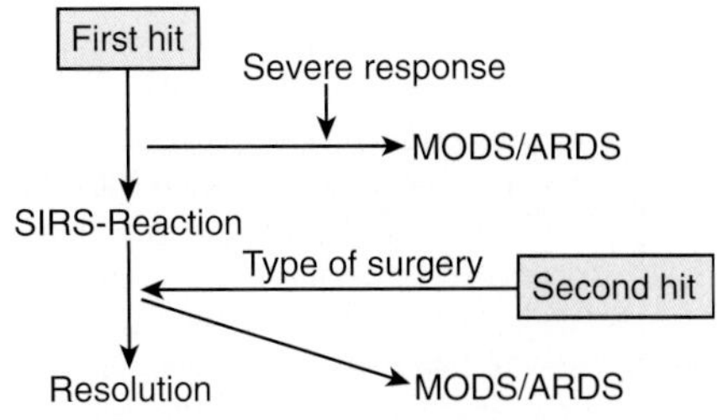

FIGURE 3-3 One and two hit inflammatory models.

Systemic Impact of Trauma ("First Hit")

The development of a trauma-induced inflammatory response is recognized as a part of the physiologic reaction after trauma (109). The extent of this inflammation is influenced by external (injury severity) as well as internal factors (individual genetic predisposition) and can be quantified by specific markers such as cytokines (Table 3-1). An injured or a surgical patient is a veritable stew of cytokines. An overwhelming systemic inflammation (SIRS) has been attributed to a state that predisposes to further posttraumatic complications (MODS) (110).

Certain injuries have been observed to occur more frequently in patients who go on to develop these complications in the posttraumatic course. Among the extremity injuries, femoral shaft fracture has been associated with an increased risk of adverse outcome (111). This appears to be based on the fact that a femoral fracture is associated with significant soft tissue damage and blood loss in view of the fact that the largest soft tissue envelope of any long bone surrounds the femoral shaft (112). Osseous and soft tissue injuries initiate a local inflammatory response with increased systemic concentrations of proinflammatory cytokines. These cytokine levels correlate with the degree of tissue damage and the severity of fracture. These findings support our understanding that inflammatory mediators are locally generated (113,114).

Several studies have demonstrated the biological profile of the first hit in trauma patients and have shown a direct correlation between the level of the release of the inflammatory (stimulation) and anti-inflammatory mediators (suppression) and the degree of injury (115–117). The development of a massive immune reaction by a patient with bilateral femoral fractures who

TABLE 3-1 Variety of Defined Cytokines

Group	Examples
Interleukins (IL)	IL-1, IL-2, IL-3, IL-4, IL-5, IL-6, IL-7, IL-8, IL-10, IL-11, IL-12, IL-13, IL-18
Tumor necrosis factors (TNF)	TNF, lymphotoxin (LT)
Interferons (IFN)	IFN-α, INF-β, INF-γ
Colony stimulating factors (CSF)	G-CSF, M-CSF, GM-CSF

showed a massive inflammatory reaction and his inflammatory profile was subsequently hyperstimulated by the surgical procedure itself (bilateral reamed femoral nailing) further supports the importance of the first hit (118). Although there was no obvious additional risk factor (no chest injury) the patient died from full-blown ARDS 3 days after injury. This case clearly not only illustrates the existence of biological variation in the inflammatory response to injury but also confirms the importance of the degree of response to the first hit and the response to the second hit (surgical) that created the final fatal event (Fig. 3-4). The above studies suggest that the degree of the initial injury is important in determining a patient's susceptibility to posttraumatic complications.

Comparison of different inflammatory markers has demonstrated that measurement of proinflammatory cytokines appears to be most useful for routine clinical work (Table 3-2). Roumen et al (119,120) reported that levels of the primary inflammatory cytokines, tumour necrosis factor-α (TNF-α) and interleukin-1β (IL-1β) had a good correlation with the initial degree of hemorrhage and nonsurvival after ARDS and MODS. This finding is, however, not consistent (121,122). Previous results from our group demonstrated that the reliability of both TNF-α and IL-1β concentrations as acute markers for trauma and surgery is low. In other clinical studies, the use of TNF-α as a marker has been disappointing. This is in part due to its pharmacokinetics: TNF-α has a short plasma half-life of 14–18 minutes. Binding to soluble TNF-α receptors and natural TNF-α–binding proteins can also interfere with measured plasma levels (123).

In contrast, IL-6 appears to be a more reliable marker. A clinical study confirmed early elevation of IL-6 levels immediately after trauma; patients with the most severe injuries had the highest IL-6 concentrations (124). The association between early elevations in IL-6 plasma concentrations, high ISS, and late adverse outcome is well established (125). Levels remained elevated for more than 5 days in patients with a high ISS (124). An early rise of IL-6 exceeding 800 pg/mL on admission was able to discriminate trauma patients who later developed MODS (124).

Systemic Impact of Operative Procedures ("Second Hit")

The "second hit" is observed to be compounded by factors such as the type of surgical procedure, blood loss, sepsis, and ischemia, all of which will heighten the inflammatory response (126). Furthermore, one can consider any subsequent physiological stresses as serial subsequent "hits," including septic episodes, blood transfusion, dehydration, and surgical intervention. When considered in these terms it becomes easy to understand how, even in a patient with only a moderate first hit, the clinical situation can rapidly deteriorate if further insults are allowed to take place. The overriding principle of damage control surgery is therefore to minimize subsequent stresses subjected on unstable patients at high risk for posttraumatic complications.

In trauma patients undergoing orthopedic procedures, subsequent increases in IL-6 plasma levels were proportional to the magnitude of the operation. Most investigations examining quantification of the second hit response induced by orthopedic surgery deal with the stabilization of long bone fractures. Femoral nailing was found to have a significant impact on inflamma-

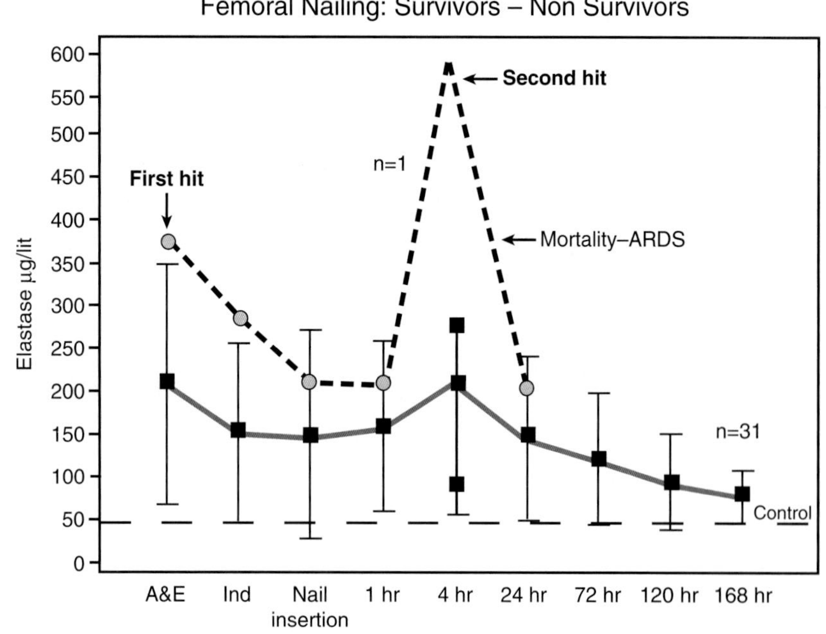

FIGURE 3-4 Plasma elastase levels illustrating the 1st and 2nd hit phenomenon following femoral nailing. The *dashed line* represents the patient who developed adult respiratory distress syndrome (ARDS) and died. (From Giannoudis PV. Stimulation of the inflammatory system by reamed and undreamed nailing an analysis of the second hit. Thesis, University of Leeds, 1999.)

TABLE 3-2 **Type, Source, and Common Actions of the Relevant Cytokines**

Cytokine	Source	Actions
Pro-inflammatory release	Macrophages/monocytes	Promotes muscle metabolism, cachexia, apoptosis, and ICAM
TFN-α	T Lymphocytes/macrophages	Cardio depressant
IL-1	Macrophages/monocytes	Expression of COX-2, iNOS, ICAM 1
IL-6	Macrophages/monocytes	Endogenous pyrogen
IL-8	Macrophages	Synergizes with TNF-α
IL-12	T-lymphocytes	Mediates acute hepatic phase response
IL-18	T-lymphocytes, NK cells	Activates HPA axis
IFN-γ	T-lymphocytes	Pyrogen and downregulates TNF-α and IL-1 (anti-inflammatory)
Fas ligand	T-lymphocytes	
Anti-inflammatory	T-lymphocytes	Chemoattractant
		Recruits neutrophils, releases superoxides and proteases
IL-4		Associated with IL-6
IL-10		Differentiation of T cells
IL-13		Promotes neutrophil and coagulation activation
		Synergistic with IL-18
		Induces IFN-γ
		Synergizes with IL-1 and IL-12
		Downregulates Fas ligand and TNF-α
		Promotes IL-2, IL-12, IL-18
		Activates macrophage-acute lung injury
		Induces apoptosis, tumor surveillance
		Control of hyper-inflammation
		Growth factor for T cells, NK cells
		Downregulates IL-1, TNF, IL-6, IL-8
		Increases effects of glucocorticoids
		Suppression of TNF, IL-1, and IL-18
		Promotes production of TNF-receptor-1
		Downregulates TNF-α and IL-1-β and IL-8.
		Inhibits the antibody dependent cellular cytotoxicity and LPS-induced IL-6 secretion.

tory response, and lead to a marked increase in IL-6 concentrations (127,128). Our recent clinical findings support these results, demonstrating that IL-6 concentrations varied according to the type of orthopedic surgery performed. The inflammatory response induced by femoral nailing was comparable to that induced by uncemented total hip arthroplasty (110).

After the initial proinflammatory response, a secondary immune suppressive effect of operative treatment is described. This was characterized by raised concentrations of the anti-inflammatory IL-10 and reduced class II human leukocyte antigen (HLA) expression on peripheral blood mononuclear cells. Again, the effect of femoral nailing was investigated, demonstrating that reamed femoral nailing was associated with greater impairment of immune reactivity than the unreamed nailing technique (129).

The second hit appears to be additive to the primary insult, and if the combination is sufficiently severe, the patient's physiological reserve is overcome. The result is either rapid deterioration, or a prolonged clinical course characterized by systemic inflammation. The inflammatory response ultimately results in microvascular damage. This process is mediated in part by activated polymorphonuclear leukocytes. A crucial pathophysiological step in this process is neutrophil adherence to capillary endothelial cells and subsequent extravasation (130). The neutrophils are then stimulated to release oxygen-free radicals and proteases, resulting in injury to the vessel wall (131). This contributes to increased capillary permeability, leading to interstitial edema. All these factors are known to be involved in the development of MODS.

MANAGEMENT OF SKELETAL INJURIES

Evolution of Treatment of Major Fractures: Historical Perspective

Until the middle of the last century, early definitive fracture stabilization was performed only as an exception, as it was believed that multiply injured patients were too unstable to survive surgical intervention. Complex laboratory investigations and monitoring facilities were not available. Consequently estimation of the patient's status was, on the whole, performed by clinical assessment only. Thus, complications were usually identified only in their late stages. Signs of MODS in the first posttraumatic week were similar to those caused by fat embolism syndrome, which was due to unstabilized fractures. This syndrome is characterized by hypoxia, cerebral depression (coma), coagulopathy (petechial bleeding), and renal failure (anuria). Embolism was thought to be directly related to the release of fat and intramedullary content from the fracture site by fracture or early surgical treatment (132,133). It was also believed, however, that pathological movements of the fracture might be responsible for further liberation of intramedullary contents into the bloodstream.

Early fracture stabilization was then performed, as more advanced techniques for the postoperative care were available, with improved outcome observed (134). This methodology was not widely accepted initially, however, since it seemed to be common sense that surgical fracture stabilization should be performed only in patients who were in a stable condition (i.e., without signs of fat embolism syndrome). Furthermore, rapid fracture healing was observed when operations were performed later in the posttraumatic course. Therefore, a great number of patients were subjected to prolonged skeletal traction (135,136). Not until the early 1980s was the first meaningful study published, showing that early, definitive stabilization of long bone fractures reduced the incidence of the fat embolism syndrome compared with traditional nonsurgical treatment (137).

As further clinical studies demonstrated the benefit of early, definitive fracture stabilization, acceptance of this treatment method became more widespread (138,139). Early operative treatment implied stabilization within 24 hours (137). It was reported that the effect of early fracture stabilization became more evident with increasing injury severity (140). The first prospective, randomized trial was published by Bone et al (141) and demonstrated the advantages of early fracture stabilization (ETC). Patients with delayed fracture stabilization had a prolonged duration of ventilatory therapy and stayed longer in both critical care and hospital (137,140).

An essential prerequisite for ETC was an optimization of rescue conditions and a reduction of the rescue time. Furthermore, the improvements in intensive care medicine with improved cardiovascular monitoring and facilities for prolonged ventilatory support facilitated the development of a more aggressive surgical approach (142,143).

Consequently, early definitive fracture stabilization represented a significant progress, resulting in pain reduction, early mobilization, and the associated reduction in thromboembolic and infective complications. The advantages gained by countless patients who were able to mobilize early are well described (144). Some patients with a very high ISS did not appear to benefit from this procedure, however. Even with excellent rescue conditions, an unacceptably high number of complications were observed.

Several studies supported the previous findings of Ecke et al (145) that a higher incidence of complications were observed in patients with severe thoracic injuries or hemorrhagic shock and in unstable patients who underwent surgical procedures (146–148). The dynamic nature of parenchymal lung injuries and the difficulty in early determination of injury severity are still significant problems in the decision making process for the timing of fracture stabilization. Unexpected complications after ETC were observed in those patients whose severity of chest injuries was initially underestimated (111).

Concerns have also been raised about polytraumatized patients with associated head trauma. It was thought, that prolonged surgery could cause intraoperative hypotension, hypoxia, and coagulopathy in combination with increased blood loss and fluid requirements during and after the orthopedic operation. This would be detrimental to cerebral perfusion and would be an additional insult to the already injured brain, thus outweighing the benefits of early fracture stabilization (149).

The strict application of ETC, even in patients with a high ISS, brain injury, or severe chest trauma, limited discussion of best management for these polytraumatized patients. Patients submitted to ETC during the last three decades have demonstrated a progressively lower ISS (Table 3-3). It could be concluded that a more cautious approach regarding surgical treatment has been chosen.

As it became evident that these specific subgroups of polytraumatized patients do not benefit from ETC, the "borderline patient" was identified. These patients were demonstrated to be at particular risk of late, poor outcome. Description of the clinical and laboratory characteristics of the borderline patient has been previously described.

The concept of "damage control" provided a solution to the management of borderline patients and those in an unstable or extremis condition. The term *damage control* was initially described by the US Navy as "the capacity of the ship to absorb damage and maintain mission integrity." In the polytraumatized patient, this concept of surgical treatment intends to control but not to definitively repair the trauma-induced injuries early after trauma. After restoration of normal physiology (core temperature, coagulation, hemodynamics, respiratory status), definitive management of injuries is performed (150). Specific criteria have been developed, which should be fulfilled to apply this new concept (DCO) (150). Indications for damage control in abdominal surgery include inability to achieve hemostasis due to coagulopathy, inaccessible major venous injury, time-consuming procedure in a patient with suboptimal response to resuscitation, management of extra-abdominal life-threatening injury, reassessment of intra-abdominal contents, and inability to reapproximate abdominal fascia due to visceral edema. The concept of temporary control of hemorrhage by compression, as undertaken in abdominal damage control, has a long tradition. In 1908, Pringle described for the first time the principles of compression via packing in order to control hepatic bleeding. This maneuver was modified by others and gained widespread use in severe abdominal injuries (150,151). The damage control concept consists of three separate components:

1. Resuscitative surgery for rapid hemorrhage control
2. Restoration of normal physiologic parameters
3. Definitive surgical management

Based on the concepts of damage control surgery, the application of the same principles to the management of multiply injured patients with associated long bone and pelvic fractures was named "damage control orthopedics" (DCO) and was again separated into three stages. The first stage involves early temporary stabilization of unstable fractures and the control of hemorrhage. The second stage consists of resuscitation of the patients in the intensive care unit and optimization of their condition. The third stage involves delayed definitive fracture management when the patient's condition allows. The favorite tool of the trauma surgeon to achieve temporary stabilization of the fractured pelvis or a long bone fracture is the application of an external fixator. External fixation is an expedient and minimally invasive method of providing stabilization and can be used efficiently to accomplish early fracture stabilization but postpone the additional biological stresses posed by prolonged surgical procedures. The delayed definite procedure to stabilize long bone fractures, and in particular femur fractures, is most fre-

TABLE 3-3 ISS of Patients Submitted to ETC in the Last Three Decades

Author (Ref.)	Year	Inclusion Criteria	Range of Injury Severity Score (ISS)	Mean ISS Primary Definitive Surgery	Mean ISS Secondary Definitive Surgery	ARDS Incidence (%)	Mortality (%)
Johnson (140)	1985	ISS >18	38	38.2	38.0	7–39	4.5
Bone (141)	1989	–	31–32	31.8	31.3	0.6–3.3	1.2
Pape (111)	1993	ISS >18	34–55	52.2	55.2	7–33	2–21
Van Os (225)	1994	?	29–38	–	–	20–26	5.3
Charash (226)	1994	ISS >18	25–29	27	29	0–10	8–60
Bone (227)	1995	ISS >18	26–29	–	–	0–33	8.2
Bosse (228)	1997	ISS >17	23–30	–	–	1–3	2.7
Carlsson (229)	1998	?	18–34	–	–	21–72	0–6

quently intramedullary nailing and is carried out when the condition of the patient allows. Two studies recently have reported that the damage control orthopedics approach was a safe treatment method for fractures of the shaft of the femur in selected multiply injured patients (152,153). The application of DCO in multiply injured patients is illustrated in Table 3-4.

The practice of delaying the definitive surgery in DCO attempts to reduce the biological load of surgical trauma on the already traumatized patient. This hypothesis was assessed in a recent prospective randomized study by means of measuring proinflammatory cytokines. Clinically stable patients with an ISS greater than 16 and a femoral shaft fracture were randomized to early total care (ETC; primary intramedullary nailing of the femur within 24 hours) and damage control orthopedics (initial temporary stabilization of the femur with external fixator and subsequent intramedullary nailing). A sustained inflammatory response (higher levels of IL-6) was measured after primary (<24 hours) intramedullary femoral instrumentation, but not after initial external fixation or after secondary conversion to an intramedullary implant. The authors concluded that DCO appears to minimize the additional surgical impact induced by the acute stabilization of the femur (154).

Other issues that have been discussed with regard to the DCO concept include the ideal time to perform the secondary definitive surgery and whether it is safe to convert an external fixator to an intramedullary nail or is thus associated with an unacceptably high infection rate.

It has been shown that days 2 to 4 do not offer optimal conditions for definitive surgery. In general during this period, marked immune reactions are ongoing (155) and enhanced generalized edema is observed (156). Nevertheless, these patients represent a highly diverse group and individual clinical judgment is more reliable, especially when combined with information from the newer laboratory tests. In a retrospective analysis of 4314 patients treated in our clinic, it was found that a prolonged secondary procedure was associated with the development of MODS. Also the patients who developed complications had their surgery performed between day 2 and 4, whereas patients who did not go on to develop MODS were operated between day 6 and 8 (157).

The measurement of inflammatory mediators has been shown to be sensitive in gauging the ongoing response in recovering patients (158). A prospective study has recently shown that polytraumatized patients submitted to secondary definitive surgery at day 2 to 4, developed a significantly increased inflammatory response, compared to those operated at day 6 to 8. It was concluded that, in different posttraumatic periods, a variable inflammatory response to comparable stimuli is observed. This may contribute to variations in clinical outcome that have been observed, e.g., the higher incidence of MODS (124). Based on this concept, the following recommendations can be made for specific groups of patients (Fig. 3-5).

With this evidence, early major surgery has to be judged as too great a burden for polytraumatized patients. Primary procedures of greater than 6 hours duration and major surgical procedures at day 2 to 4 should be avoided. Increased knowledge and advances in the field of molecular biology and genetics may lead to new parameters, helping to select patients with a high risk for adverse outcome.

Regarding the issue whether external fixation can be converted safely to an intramedullary nail, the infection rates reported in the literature are low, ranging from 1.7% to 3%

TABLE 3-4 Classification of Fractures with Open and Closed Soft Tissue Injury

Closed	Open	Gustillo Classification	Simple Fractures, No Further Injury Complex Fractures
C1	O1	II, IIIa	Superficial contusion by fragments Simple transverse or oblique fracture
C2	O2	IIIb	Deep, contaminated wound, limited soft tissue contusion by direct trauma, including potential compartment syndrome, multiple bony fragments
C3	O3	IIIc	Extensive soft tissue damage (contusion, degloving) with loss of periosteum, including compartment syndrome, crush fracture and bone loss
C4	O4		O3 + vascular injury requiring operation
	O5		Complete or incomplete amputation with complete ischemia, no more than 1/4 of circumferential soft tissues preserved

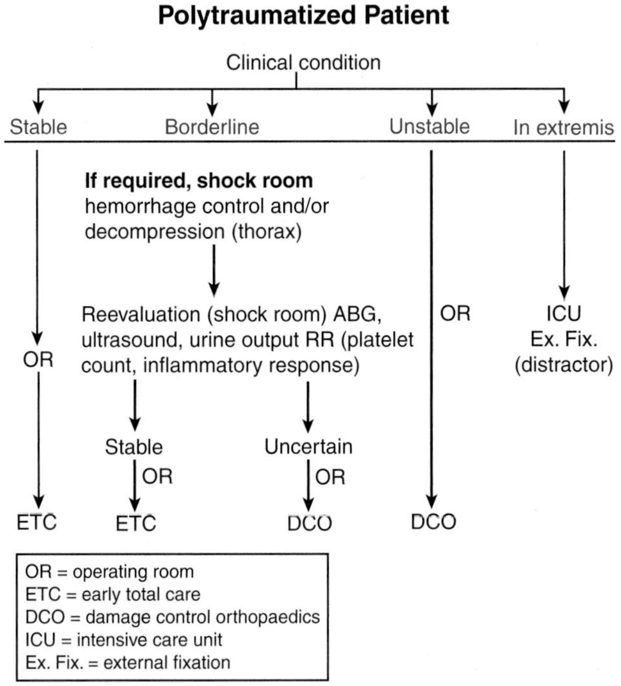

Polytraumatized Patient

Clinical condition

Stable | Borderline | Unstable | In extremis

If required, shock room
hemorrhage control and/or
decompression (thorax)

Reevaluation (shock room) ABG, ultrasound, urine output RR (platelet count, inflammatory response)

Stable — OR — ETC

Uncertain — OR — DCO

Stable — OR — ETC

Unstable — OR — DCO

In extremis — ICU Ex. Fix. (distractor)

OR = operating room
ETC = early total care
DCO = damage control orthopaedics
ICU = intensive care unit
Ex. Fix. = external fixation

FIGURE 3-5 Treatment protocol based on patients' clinical condition (234).

(152,153). According to these reports conversion of the external fixator to a nail should be done the first 2 weeks, thus minimizing the risk of developing deep sepsis.

In summary, initial temporary fracture stabilization appears to be an advantageous treatment strategy in patients with severe polytrauma who are at high risk for development of systemic complications, such as MODS.

Priorities in Fracture Care

The sequence of fracture treatment in multiply injured patients with serial injuries to an extremity is a crucial part of the management concept. Some body sections are prone to progressive soft tissue damage because of their anatomy. Therefore, the recommended sequence of treatment is tibia, femur, pelvis, spine, and upper extremity.

In this context, the simultaneous treatment of different extremity injuries should be considered. Yet, certain logistic requirements should be met for simultaneous trauma surgery. To fulfill the priorities of fracture care, the sequence of treatment in serial extremity injury and the management strategy of contralateral fractures of both upper and lower extremities should be followed.

The type of osteosynthesis in multiply injured patients depends not only on the local bony and soft tissue situation but much more on the general, pulmonary, and hemodynamic status of the patient. Again, a priority oriented management strategy is usually extremely valuable.

Management of Unilateral Fracture Patterns

In serial injuries of the upper extremity, the surgeon should rather be aware of the overall fracture pattern than consider each fracture as an isolated problem. Even though early definitive osteosynthesis would be preferred in all fractures, often the general status of the multiply injured patient or the local conditions do not allow for lengthy procedures. In these cases, careful immobilization of shaft fractures is recommended as the first step of fracture management.

If there are periarticular fractures of the large joints and immediate open reduction and fixation is impossible, transarticular external fixation should be performed (e.g., transfixation of the elbow). Furthermore, in any case with concomitant vascular injury or any evidence of a developing compartment syndrome, a fasciotomy of the forearm should not be delayed.

In serial injuries of the lower extremity (e.g., distal femoral and proximal tibial fractures on the same side, "floating knee"), a flexible but structured and priority oriented management should be applied (159). Again, the general status of the patients is crucial to the concept. In our example of a floating knee in a stable patient, starting from a small incision at the 30° flexed knee joint, a retrograde distal unreamed femoral nail is inserted. Then, an antegrade tibia nail is inserted through the same incision. In the same fracture pattern in an unstable patient, a closed reduction by extension and external fixation (transfixation of the knee joint) is performed as a temporarily stabilizing procedure to minimize additional damage, especially to the soft tissues. A secondary definitive osteosynthesis then can be done, when the patient has safely recovered from the initial potentially life-threatening injuries. During the whole procedure, good communication between the anesthesiologist and the surgeon is highly important, since the procedure may have to be adapted to any change in the patient's vital parameters.

In coexisting diametaphyseal and periarticular fractures, the priorities of treatment are dictated by the extent of bone and soft tissue damage. High priority is given to femoral head fractures (Pipkin I–III) and fractures of the talus. Other periarticular fractures are of lower priority, particularly if other complications—such as compartment syndrome, a pulseless extremity, or an open fracture—are present.

Just as important are the "little" injuries to the hand, fingers, tarsus, or toes. They should be considered in the overall management concept as well and possibly anatomically reduced and fixed, at least temporarily.

Management of Bilateral Fracture Patterns

In bilateral fractures, simultaneous treatment is an attractive concept. Especially in bilateral tibial fractures, both legs are surgically cleaned and draped at the same time. The operative procedure is performed sequentially because of the fluoroscopy (space, handling). If the vital signs of the patient deteriorate during the operation the second leg may just be temporarily stabilized using an external fixator (e.g., the pinless fixator;

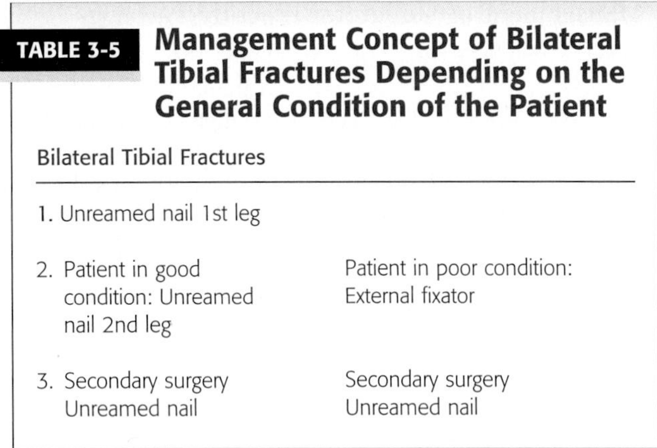

TABLE 3-5 Management Concept of Bilateral Tibial Fractures Depending on the General Condition of the Patient

Bilateral Tibial Fractures	
1. Unreamed nail 1st leg	
2. Patient in good condition: Unreamed nail 2nd leg	Patient in poor condition: External fixator
3. Secondary surgery Unreamed nail	Secondary surgery Unreamed nail

Table 3-5). The definitive osteosynthesis then may be delayed until the general status of the patient is stabilized again.

The priorities in with worse being treated injuries first.

Upper Extremity Injuries

The management of upper extremity fractures in multiply injured patients is usually secondary to injuries to the head and trunk or to the lower extremity. If there is a closed fracture to the upper extremity without any associated injury (vascular or nerve damage or compartment syndrome), the proximal fractures (shoulder, proximal humerus, and humerus shaft) are fixed by a shoulder body bandage (Gilchrist bandage). The definitive osteosynthesis may be performed during the secondary management, possibly after further imaging. Any humerus fracture should be fixed with the elbow in full extension if the duration of the intensive care period is going to be prolonged. This way of splinting seems advantageous because of the decreased muscular tension pulling the joint into a varus position. Alternatively, this fracture may be fixed by an external fixator.

In fractures about the elbow, a transarticular external fixation should be used, if the definitive osteosynthesis has to be delayed.

Besides the traditional cast, the external fixator is also useful in managing injuries to the forearm, wrist, and hand if the patient is unstable or a reduction of the operation time is necessary.

Lower Extremity Injuries

In our experience, long bone fractures associated with a severe head injury or chest trauma (lung contusions) require a specially modified strategy. We strongly recommend the extended monitoring of respiratory function, ventilation (capnography), and pulmonary hemodynamics. Additionally, intracranial pressure monitoring is mandatory in patients with a severe head injury (160).

Unstable Pelvic Injuries

Essential for the assessment of pelvic injuries is a thorough clinical and radiologic examination. This examination is usually done during the initial checkup. In consequence, the pelvic injury may be classified roughly with these data and with the history of the accident. The simple classification by the AO-ABC system (Fig. 3-6) can assist in the decision-making process (134). Here, type A injuries include stable fractures such as fractures of the pelvic rim, avulsion fractures, and undisplaced anterior pelvic ring fractures. The posterior rim is not injured at all. Type B injuries comprise fractures with only partially intact posterior structures and rotational dislocations may be possible. Sometimes, this injury may initially be an internal rotation dislocation, resulting in excellent bony compression and stabilization of the pelvis. Moreover, they still carry an increased risk of intra-abdominal injuries (161). If the injury results in the open book type of fracture with both alae externally rotated, urogenital lesions and hemorrhagic complications are much more common.

Since the differentiation of type B and C injuries may be difficult, a CT scan of the pelvis is recommended. If there is no CT available diagonal x-rays (inlet and outlet) may serve as an alternative. In C type injuries, the pelvis shows translational instability of the dorsal pelvic ring, (i.e., the stabilizing structures are all severed; Fig. 3-7). One or both pelvic halves are separated from the trunk. This injury is associated with an ex-

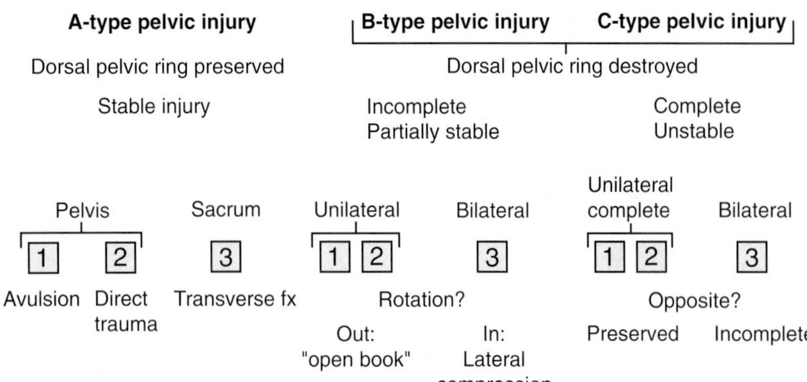

FIGURE 3-6 Classification of pelvic ring fractures in A-, B-, C-type fracture similar to the AO classification.

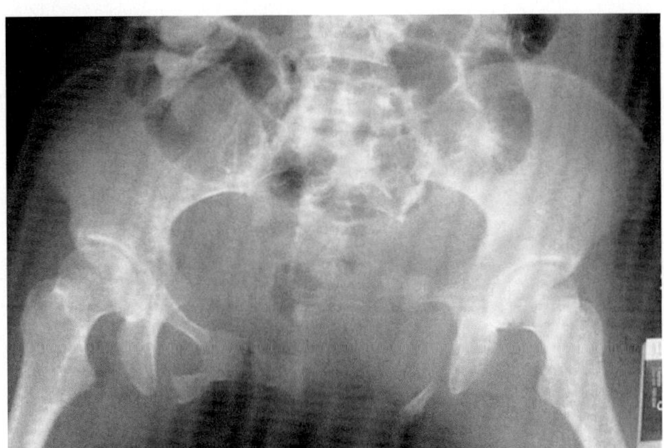

FIGURE 3-7 Type C pelvic fracture.

tremely high rate of hemorrhagic complications and other pelvic injuries.

This simple classification has significant therapeutic implications:

- In type A injuries, operative treatment is generally not required.
- Type B injuries are sufficiently stabilized by osteosynthesis of the anterior pelvic ring allowing only for early mobilization.
- Type C injuries require anterior and posterior osteosynthesis for adequate stability.

Additionally, the differentiation of several sectors of injury proved useful. Transsymphysis, transpubic, transacetabular, and transiliac fractures are differentiated from the transiliosacral and transsacral fractures. This process is easy to memorize and requires a structured analysis of the x-rays. For each of the injured regions, we have standardized the recommendations for osteosynthesis.

Since more than 80% of unstable pelvic injuries are associated with multiple injuries, the supine position is preferred during the primary treatment period. The supine position also allows reconstruction of the symphysis and sacroiliac joint. Generally speaking, we recommend early stabilization ofr fractures of the pelvic ring to avoid ongoing blood loss and to simplify ICU care and early ambulation (89).

Complex Pelvic Injuries

Pelvic injuries associated with any other injury to local pelvic organs are called complex pelvic injuries (162). These injuries comprise about 10% of pelvic injuries and show a significantly higher mortality (30% to 60%) in comparison to simple pelvic injuries. During the early phase, hemorrhage is the most common cause of death. Later on, ARDS and multiple organ dysfunction syndrome (MODS) are the sequelae of the blood loss and initially persistent shock determine the further course and eventual outcome of the patient.

During acute therapy, only immediate, priority-guided management concepts save the lives of these severely injured patients and improve the prognosis. A variety of methods for hemorrhage control in pelvic injuries are discussed in the literature. With these techniques several very complex therapeutic protocols have been developed. Our own experience has resulted in a rather simple algorithm requiring three decisions within the first 30 minutes after admission. The therapeutic goal is based on a combined strategy of intensive shock treatment, early stabilization of the pelvic ring, and potential operative hemorrhage control and packing rather than a single treatment option. After hemorrhage control is achieved, the associated urogenital and intestinal injuries should be treated to avoid septic complications.

In urogenital injuries, the primary goal is reliable urine drainage. During the first laparotomy, intraperitoneal ruptures of the bladder are repaired. In injuries of the urethra, the recommendations are to splint the urethra using a transurethral catheter, and the definitive procedure is done during the secondary period to reduce the rate of late strictures. If early realignment is not possible, then a suprapubic catheter should be inserted.

In injuries to the rectum or anus (open pelvic fractures), a temporary colostomy of the transverse colon guarantees proper excretion and maintains a low contamination. At the end of the procedure, an extensive antegrade washout of the distal part is undertaken to reduce the microbial load. Any potential muscular or skin necrosis is primarily radically debrided to minimize activation of the immune system. A highly active surgical management of planned revisions, extensive lavage/jet lavage and debridement reduces the rate of pelvic sepsis to a minimum.

Unstable Injuries of the Spine

Generally, operative treatment of unstable spine injuries is mandatory, if only for intensive care nursing purposes. Nonoperative treatment (e.g., jacket, Halo fixator) is unsuitable in multiply injured patients, because the immobilization of the patients carries a high risk. Not only are the intensive care nursing procedures much easier after internal stabilization, but the time of immobilization and time of intensive care stay are also significantly reduced.

Spine injuries with neurologic symptoms usually are stabilized in the same procedure as the spinal cord decompression. However, in recent years, unstable injuries of the spine even without neurologic symptoms are much more often stabilized during the acute period, because of the reasons mentioned earlier.

In our experience, after diagnosing an unstable injury of the spine without neurologic symptoms, a closed reduction is advised in the following situations:

- Fractures of the cervical spine
- Rotational injury of the lower thoracic or lumbar spine (AO classification type C injury)

In any other injury, the reduction is performed in the operating room just before the actual procedure. If there is but a slight suspicion of a fracture fragment or a protruding intervertebral disc narrowing the spinal canal after closed reduction, further imaging (e.g., CT, MRI) are required. In multiply injured patients in particular, closed reduction may be difficult because of concomitant extremity injuries. In these cases, proper correction of rotation and axis can be only managed intraoperatively.

In the case of interposition of a bone fragment or intervertebral disc, open reduction is always indicated following extraction of the impediment to avoid spinal cord compression.

The ventral approach is our standard procedure for operative management of the upper (Cl to C3) and lower (C4 to C7) cervical spine. Therefore, the patient's head is fixed to a special reduction apparatus using the rim of the halo fixator. In the case of thoracic or lumbar spine injuries, the associated injuries to the trunk (chest, abdomen) have to be considered. Nonetheless, in our experience, injuries requiring dorsal and ventral stabilization may usually be fixed using at least a dorsal internal fixator in the acute management period. Depending on the general status of the patient, the ventral stabilization may be performed during the secondary period. Even intrathoracic or intra-abdominal injuries are not necessarily a contraindication for the required prone position for dorsal instrumentation. The prone position has been successfully used as a therapeutic strategy in severe lung injury. Other authors have found no contraindications to the prone position or thoracocentesis in multiply injured patients (163).

Assessment of Fracture Severity

Closed Fractures

In our experience, there are many difficulties in properly diagnosing and assessing the true soft tissue damage in closed fractures. A skin contusion at an otherwise closed fracture site may raise more therapeutic and prognostic problems than an inside-out puncture wound in an open fractures. This type of blunt injury implies significant weakening of the natural skin barrier. Skin necrosis secondary to contusion is often the entry point for infections, especially in the ICU environment. This issue has been addressed with the development of a classification system to allow the clinician to decide the appropriate therapeutic approach that would be beneficial to the patients' overall condition.

Soft tissue injuries therefore can be classified as follows (164):

Closed fracture C0: No injury or very minor soft tissue injury. The C0 classification covers simple fractures (i.e., fractures caused by indirect mechanisms of injury).

Closed fracture C1: Superficial abrasions or contusions from internal fragment pressure along with simple to moderate fracture types are included.

Closed fracture C2: Deep, contaminated abrasions or local dermal and muscular contusions due to tangential forces are included here. Also, the threatening compartment syndrome is classified as G2. These injuries usually are caused by direct forces, additionally resulting in moderate to severe fracture types. The closed bisegmental tibial fracture after a typical bumper impact is an illustrative example.

Closed fracture C3: Extensive skin contusions or muscular destruction, subcutaneous degloving and obvious compartment syndrome combined with any closed fracture are graded C3. In this subgroup of the classification, there are severe fracture types and comminuted fractures.

Closed fracture C4: The same injuries as in C3 closed fractures associated with a significant vascular damage requiring operative treatment form the C4 closed fractures group.

Open Fractures

Open fracture care is an essential part of primary management. Primary care of open fractures consists of radical debridement, extensive irrigation, assessment of the damage to the soft tissues, and finally stable fracture fixation.

A careful assessment of the injury severity is the first step in the development of a treatment strategy. Here, time and mechanism of injury, the energy of the causative force, and the severity of the fracture should be considered. Additionally, with respect to the preservation of an injured extremity, the extent of vascular and nerve damage, and the general condition of the patient are of great importance. In high-energy trauma, soft tissues may be severely damaged, requiring careful evaluation and extensive debridement during the initial assessment.

Open fractures from low-energy trauma are usually associated with less soft tissue damage and may almost be treated like closed injuries. After the initial debridement, the fracture may be stabilized with the most suitable implant and method of fixation.

Open fractures from high-energy trauma represent a unique problem—that is, a combination of considerable soft tissue damage and extensive bone destruction. This injury requires a graded concept of care (Table 3-6). A sophisticated treatment plan should be established, adequately considering the important aspects of sufficient debridement, temporary stabilization with respect to the secondary definitive stabilization as well as the closure of the wound. Our experience with this type of injury shows an almost individual "personality" of each fracture requiring "personal" treatment. In multiply injured patients, the overall injury severity has to be considered as well as the extent of the shock and the initial blood loss. Taking these factors into account, a clear therapeutic concept should be established for each patient individually.

Classification of Soft Tissue Damage

Several classifications have been proposed over the years for the grading of open fractures but the standard system of classifying the soft tissue component of a fracture remains that of Gustilo et al (165). Despite the doubts that have been raised over its reliability, it seems likely to remain in common usage as it is fairly simple to remember and to apply.

A thorough assessment of the soft tissue damage is even more

TABLE 3-6 Protocol of Management of Open Fractures

Emergency room	Clinical examination Classify soft tissue damage Doppler examination Neurologic examination Antibiotics/ tetanus prophylaxis
Primary Operation	Adequate debridement (Vascular reconstruction) Fasciotomy >6 h of ischemia Fracture stabilization Transfixation if joint injury
Intensive care unit	Continuous monitoring: Peripheral perfusion Compartment pressure Transcutaneous pO2
Secondary operation	Operative revision (~48 h) Soft tissue (<72 h) reconstruction Joint reconstruction
Tertiary operation	Mesh graft transplantation Bone grafts

crucial in multiply injured patients. In this group, the prognosis of the soft tissue damage depends on a multitude of parameters potentially ending up in a vicious circle. Besides the overall tissue hypoxia and acidosis, there is a general hypoperfusion of the extremities due to the hemorrhagic shock. All these factors should be taken into account in the clinical decision making and planning.

Reconstruction Versus Amputation

As a result of new microsurgical techniques, new methods of bone reconstruction and more skillful application of the Ilizarov technique, the preservation of a limb, especially in grade IIIb and IIIc fractures of the lower extremity, is more commonly attempted nowadays. Reconstructive bone and soft tissue surgery usually requires repeated operations, long-term hospital stays, and prolonged periods of treatment implicating considerable social and economic effects for the patient and his or her family that have to be appreciated by the responsible surgeon. Several authors therefore have looked into criteria to guide surgeons in their decision for preservation or amputation of a severely injured extremity. From the surgical point of view, the attempt to preserve the limb seems to be the best decision for the patient. But from a socioeconomic point, the prolonged hospital stay may have severe effects for the patient: the financial loss for the patient from prolonged hospital stays and loss of time at work was proven to be higher than in a primary amputation. Even more, in patients with preserved limbs, there is a low probability for these patients to get back to their jobs. Furthermore, many attempts at reconstruction leave the patients incapable of earning a living for more than 2 years (166).

If a severely injured patient survives after primary amputation, the question is, whether the amputation was unavoidable or the reconstruction was possible. If the patient dies, the question is, whether the severity of the injuries was underestimated initially and an early amputation would have saved the patient's life. Last, if the patient survives after primary reconstruction but suffers from complications requiring prolonged treatment, the question is, whether the bad outcome justified the expended resources.

In order therefore to define a clear, unmistakable and acceptable guideline for the treatment of severe injuries to the extremities, we are obliged to consider these problems and include them in our decision-making process.

Guiding Aid: Orientation at Primary Clinical Findings

In 1985, Gregory et al (167) analyzed 60 patients with open fractures and developed a scoring system classifying severe injuries to the lower extremities. Seventeen patients were categorized into the most severe group, the "mangled extremity syndrome" (MES). The patients were classified retrospectively by analysis of the extent of the soft tissue injury, the severity of the fracture, and injury of major anatomic structures such as nerves and vessels. Additionally, age, preexisting comorbidities, potential prolonged shock, and the time to treatment were included in the assessment.

Additionally, the overall injury severity was estimated using the ISS and included in the scoring system. The resulting score was published as the "mangled extremity syndrome index" (MESI). In this retrospective analysis, a score of 20 points was found to be the "cutoff" point for amputation. In 7 out of these 17 patients, the preservation of the limb was attempted. Each patient in this group scored below 20 points. In the remaining ten cases, amputation was performed. Each patient in this second group scored above 20 points in the MESI. The assessment term "extensive trauma of an anatomic structure" was found to be a major problem. Nerve injuries that are known to be crucial for the prognosis of the extremity are supposed to be so categorized. But in doing so, some specialists argued, the effect of nerve damages was possibly underestimated (167).

Another retrospective analysis was published by Howe et al in 1987 (168). A new scoring system was developed, the "predictive salvage index." This score showed a high positive predictability (sensitivity 78%, specificity 100%) for the benefits of amputation. Timing and technique of vascular reconstruction were considered as independent parameters. The calculated score divided dermal, muscular, and bony damage into slight, moderate, or severe and counted one to three points, respectively. For the score, the four suitable parameters were summarized. When a total of more than eight points was calculated, primary amputation was recommended. Using this cutoff, a high positive predictability for the functional outcome was found (78% sensitivity, 100% specificity).

A third retrospective study of 26 injuries to the lower extremities with vascular lesions included the extent of the soft tissue damage, the time of ischemia, the duration of prolonged shock, and the age of the patient as predictive items for an amputation. Starting from here, the authors developed a score with the soft tissue damage showing the highest positive predictability for the outcome. A cumulative analysis of variances showed this soft tissue damage to be as predictive as the sum of all of the four parameters. Using their population, Lange et al (169) also defined guiding parameters for the development of a therapeutic strategy in extremity injuries. They showed that in patients with similar local injuries, the age, comorbidities, and the social environment of the patients play an important role in the outcome. The authors stressed the crucial role of the posterior tibial nerve and suggested that intraoperative exploration with exclusion of a posterior tibial nerve lesion compulsory. In multiply injured patients the difficulties in assessing any kind of score and estimating the predictability are discussed (169).

In 1990, Helfet et al (170) found Lange's absolute indications for amputation difficult to determine in certain patients. In an overview of the literature, Helfet et al found 59% of third-degree open tibial fractures (Gustilo grade IIIc) being amputated. Half of these procedures were secondary amputations, at least 24 hours after the trauma. They concluded that obviously the valid criteria in decision making at that time were insufficient, resulting in delayed amputation. Consequently, from the retrospective analysis of 26 severe injuries to the lower extremity with vascular injuries (Gustilo grade IIIC) four parameters were significant: extent of the bone and soft tissue damage, time of ischemia, initial shock, and age of the patient. The resulting score gave the cutoff for amputation as seven points (Table 3-7). In a prospective multicenter study, this score was verified. It was shown that in patients with a score of more than seven points, there was a 100% probability of amputation.

Most recently, McNamara et al (171) evaluated the MESS by retrospectively studying 24 patients with grade IIIc injuries. The results confirmed the high predictability. To improve the predictive value, nerve damage and a detailed assessment of the bone and soft tissue damage were included. The newly formed score wad called the NISSSA score and showed a sensitivity of 81.8% and a specificity of 92.3% (171).

TABLE 3-7 The Mangled Extremity Severity Score (MESS)

1.	**Bone and soft tissue injuries**	
	Type-A fractures: 1° open or closed	1
	Type-B fractures: 1° open or closed	2
	Type-C fractures: 3° open or closed	3
	Amputating injury	4
2.	**Time of ischemia**	
	Peripheral pulses palpable	0
	Peripheral pulses not palpable but capillary pulse normal	1*
	No pulse in Doppler, refill >3 sec, paresis incomplete	2*
	No pulse, cold extremity, paresis complete	3*
3.	**Circulation**	
	Systolic blood pressure always >90 mm Hg	0
	Unstable circulation until admission to ER	1
	Unstable circulation until end of surgery	2
4.	**Age**	
	<30 years	0
	30–50 years	1
	>50 years	2
	TOTAL:	

* Double points if time of ischemia >6 hours.
Helfet DL, Howey T, Sanders R, Johansen K. Limb salvage versus amputation. Preliminary results of the Mangled Extremity Severity Score. *Clin Orthop Relt Res* 1990;256:80–86.

Comparison of Upper and Lower Extremities

In severe open fractures of the upper extremity different principles are applied to develop the proper treatment strategy: The sensitivity of the foot, the continuity of all large nerves, maintenance of proper length, are of less consequence in the treatment plan for the arm (172). However, the prosthetic care of the lower extremity is much more sophisticated than of the upper extremity, especially in below knee amputations. This is why the different scoring systems should be used with caution in injuries of the upper extremity.

Debridement

After deciding to salvage the limb, extensive and critical debridement forms the first step in the operative treatment plan. Here all components of the soft tissues have to be regarded. Being too cautious with the debridement, especially with nonvital tissue in multiply injured patients has been demonstrated to lead to a deterioration of the patient's condition and even organ failure. Clearly, an easy compromise should be avoided. Sufficient surgical exposure of the injury is essential to assess and to treat the soft tissue damage. The possibility of extensive degloving has to be kept in mind. The mechanism of injury and a thorough clinical exam provide key information for the assessment of such an injury.

In multiply injured patients, there is a high risk of increasing soft tissue necrosis due to impaired soft tissue perfusion (e.g., in posttraumatic edema, increased capillary permeability, massive volume resuscitation, unstable circulation). Therefore, in many patients regular operative revisions need to be scheduled. These second-look surgeries allow repeated assessment of the soft tissues. This strategy enables the surgeon to do a timely redebridement if required (e.g., with high-pressure irrigation). These operative revisions of soft tissue injures should be scheduled every 48 hours as long as there is an impaired perfusion of the damage zone. The recent introduction of vacuum therapy may save the patient some of the planned second-look surgeries but will not replace repeat exploration.

Following successful debridement, vascular reconstruction, and stabilization of the fracture, the soft tissue repair should be planned meticulously.

Operative Strategy Depending on Overall Injury Severity

The question of the multiply injured patient needing and tolerating reconstructive surgery is dictated by the overall condition and the extent of the accompanying injuries than by the local situation alone (Fig. 3-8). A lengthy reconstruction or replantation procedure may harm the patient and put him into a life-threatening situation. Additionally, attention has to be paid to the general long-term prognosis of an open injury in the multiply injured patient. To establish a therapeutic plan, all these parameters need to be considered.

Patients of ISS Groups (1–15 points and 16–25 points) and Grade IIIa–c Soft Tissue Injuries. In this subgroup of multiply injured patients, there is an indication for reconstruction. The surgery is largely standardized. Following extensive and radical debridement, in the case of a vascular injury, the second step consists of vascular repair, sometimes requiring the interposition of a venous graft. Next, fractures should usually be stabilized using intramedullary osteosynthesis. This type of implants is much less damaging to the soft tissues than any direct osteosynthesis. There is less soft tissue damage and only minimal impairment of the circulation of the bone (173).

The covering and closure of any soft tissue defect depends on the extent of the injury. In most cases, the wound will be covered temporarily using synthetic skin grafts or vacuum systems, before final cover by plastic reconstructive surgery. In general, the expected result of a reconstruction or limb saving strategy should outweigh the result of an amputation and fitting of a good prosthesis.

Patients of ISS Groups (1–15 points and 16–25 points) With Complete and Incomplete Amputations. In terms of the surgical management, these injuries are very similar. Replantation as an option has to be considered with referral to a specialized center. Before this, hemorrhage may be stopped by elevation and application of a pressure bandage. The conservation of the amputated limb follows clear emergency medicine guidelines (174).

Amputation injuries in children always have to be considered for replantation. Children, with their better tissue regenerative ability, show better functional outcome than similarly injured adults.

Patients of ISS Groups (26–50 points and >50 points). In recent years, level one trauma centers have improved their critical care and osteosynthesis treatment and increasingly succeeded in saving the most severely traumatized extremities.

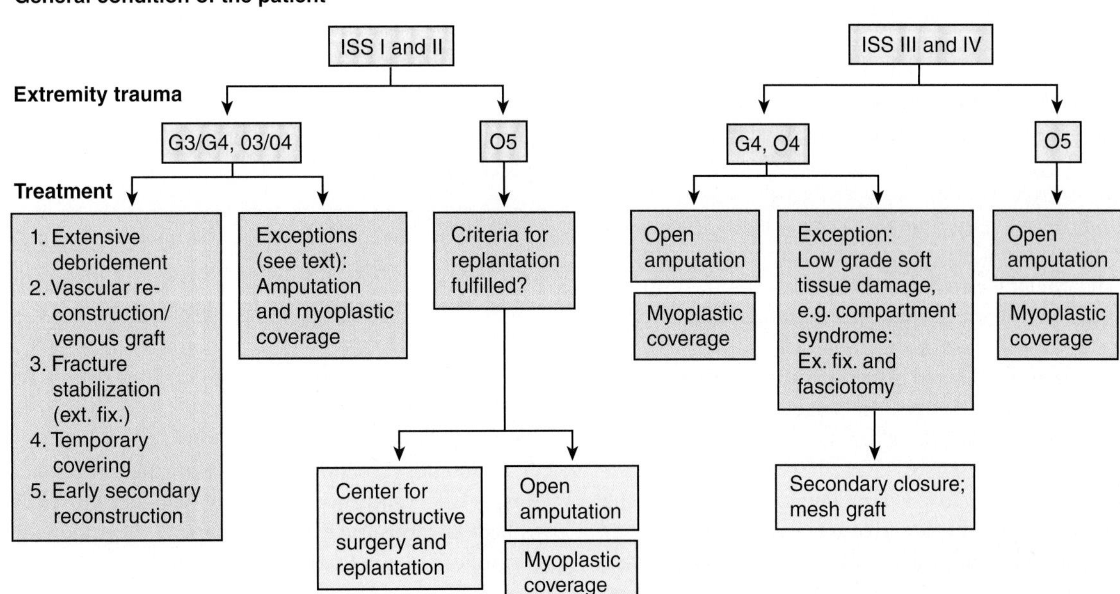

FIGURE 3-8 Algorithm for "reconstruction/amputation" in open fracture care depending on the overall injury severity. ISS group I: ≤15; ISS II: 16–25; ISS III: 26–50; ISS IV: ≥50 points. (Modified from Sudkamp N, Haas N, Flory PJ, et al. Criteria for amputation, reconstruction and replantation of extremities in multiple trauma patients. *Chirurg* 1989;60:774–781.)

Nevertheless, these limbs often require secondary amputation (175).

In this subgroup of most severely injured patients with extremity injuries the preservation of the extremity should not be attempted at all. The principle "life before limb" should absolutely hold true, and the indication for amputation may be widened. If the decision for amputation is made, it should be performed by open or guillotine amputation. Primary closure of the wounds is associated with a high risk for complications, because the overall extent of the soft tissue damage and the posttraumatic edema is difficult to estimate.

Intra-Articular Open Fractures

Today, most surgeons prefer a two-step strategy in the management of open intra-articular fractures. First, the injury is debrided, the joint surface is reconstructed using a minimal invasive osteosynthetic (MIO) technique and the joint is immobilized by transarticular external fixation. The minimally invasive osteosynthesis comprises the reconstruction of the joint itself, temporary stabilization with K-wires, and stabilization with lag screws and adjusting or set screws. Plate osteosyntheses is contraindicated in these injuries, because of the extensive soft tissue damage (176). So, the definitive osteosynthesis is carried out secondarily following consolidation of the soft tissues. In this procedure, the initially reconstructed block of articular bone fragments is attached to the metaphysis. Sometimes, shortening of the fractured bone has to be accepted at least temporarily to close potential bony or soft tissue defects.

The Ilizarov fixator is widely appreciated as a good alternative to conventional transfixation technique (transarticular external fixation). The Ilizarov method allows for stabilization in the damage zone by K-wires inserted in the metaphyseal area and connected by ring fixators.

Timing of Soft Tissue Reconstruction

In many multiply injured patients, primary wound closure is bad practice. The relative hypoxia of the tissues may lead to impaired and delayed wound healing and a higher risk of wound infection. In small soft tissue injuries, we recommend secondary closure of the wound after covering the wound with artificial skin until the swelling decreases. An absolute prerequisite for wound closure is to completely cover the implants with vital and well-perfused soft tissues. In these defects, artificial skin replacements are used first and afterwards the wound is closed progressively over several days. In some cases, continuous wound closure may be an option also.

In medium-sized soft tissue defects, secondary closure is often achieved by local transposition after mobilization of the surrounding soft tissues. In extensive soft tissue defects associated with significant periosteal damage, the soft tissue covers require excellent perfusion. The covering procedure should be done within 72 hours of the trauma. Otherwise, the complete section of the extremity is in danger of further damage.

Large posttraumatic soft tissue defects are challenging for the surgeon and require a well-defined therapeutic strategy. The overall concept of soft tissue coverage depends on the extent of uncovered bone, tendons and nerves. To achieve satisfactory results, early communication and cooperation between the trauma surgeon and the plastic surgeon is recommended.

Soft Tissue Reconstruction. To cover wound defects, there are numerous local and distant flaps described in the literature.

Local Flaps. Rotational flaps are used to cover small and medium-sized soft tissue defects. These flaps consist of different combinations of muscle, fascia, and skin. They allow closure of defects and should be applied without any tension at all. Nonetheless, there are also disadvantages associated with local flaps. On one hand, obtaining flaps from the local soft tissues may be difficult in multiply injured patients because of other injuries. On the other hand, the flap procedure is prevented by the preexisting soft tissue damage. Even more, the perfusion of muscular or myocutaneous flaps must be considered. Often, the real extent of the required transposition is underestimated compared to the actual permitted options. Therefore, a meticulous preoperative plan is mandatory. For the most common defects on the anteromedial tibial surface, gastrocnemius or soleus flaps are useful.

Distant Flaps. The indication for distant flaps is common in multiply injured patients. Microvascular flaps, such as the radial forearm or latissimus dorsi flap, are increasingly used. The indication for a distant flap has to be discussed, however. On one hand, the local situation requires urgent treatment; on the other hand, a prolonged surgical procedure represents a considerable traumatic load for the severely injured patient. Therefore, careful timing of the operation is required. Local as well as systemic complications are common in this patient population.

INTENSIVE CARE UNIT ASPECTS OF MANAGEMENT

The management of the polytrauma patient in the intensive care unit has been the cornerstone of treating complications and improving survival rates. This has been attributed to technological advances and a better understanding of MODS at the molecular level.

Ventilation Strategies

It is widely accepted that early ventilation leads to improvement of pulmonary function and reduces the incidence of ARDS. Among the ventilation strategies, volume and pressure controlled methods have to be separated. Traditionally, volume controlled, low-frequency ventilation using high tidal volume and PEEP have been preferred. However, high tidal volumes may induce high airway pressures, thus causing overstretching of healthy areas of the lung. This may lead to secondary iatrogenic structural damage and formation of scar tissue (177).

Currently, a pressure-controlled ventilation mode, using low tidal volume, is generally preferred. Oxygenation can be additionally improved by a prolonged inspiration time compared with expiratory time. Inversed ratio ventilation induces a higher mean airway flow, thereby improving oxygenation. With prolonged inspiration time, even multiple divided lung compartments that require a long time to be reached can take part in the gas exchange. A shorter expiratory time leads to incompletely evacuated lung areas. In the regional compartments, intrinsic PEEP develops. Therefore, the inversed ratio ventilation enlarges the area which takes part in the gas exchange and reduces intrapulmonary shunt volume. Pressure-controlled ventilation should be combined with PEEP, increasing the functional residual capacity. Thus, the pulmonary areas taking part in the gas exchange could be improved. The optimal height of the PEEP level is still under discussion (178). Using increased PEEP, the pulmonary compliance improves until a critical point is reached ("best PEEP best compliance") (179) but cardiovascular side effects have to be considered.

Modern ventilation strategies with low tidal volume (4–8 mL/kg), best PEEP, low airway pressures (<35 cm H_2O), and an inspiratory oxygen concentration of 55% to 60% are often ideal. Also, hypercapnia may be allowed up to a certain degree (permissive hypercapnia; PHC) (180). It is well tolerated in patients with ARDS and a P_{CO_2} of 60 to 120 mm Hg. Clinical experience shows, that pressure-controlled ventilation with inversed ratio ventilation (I:E [1:1 to 4:1]), low tidal volumes (4–8 mL/kg), frequencies of 10–15/min, permissive hypercapnia (PHC [P_{CO_2} ~70 mm Hg]) and individual PEEP (5–12 cm H_2O), high oxygen concentration (FiO_2 <0.5), and high airway pressure can prevent the lung from further ventilation damage (181). Early experiences using other ventilation strategies (e.g., bilevel positive airway pressure; BIPAP) demonstrated that they are also feasible, although there may be problems with BIPAP in cases in which long-term sedation is required. One of the most recent concepts developed for the prevention of pulmonary failure is the recruitment of alveoli by temporary increase in positive end expiratory pressure (open lung concept) (182). It does not cause sustained cardiovascular side effects and also does not lead to the development of bronchopleural fistulae. Yet, the clinical relevance of this new concept has to be proven in larger series (183).

Adult Respiratory Distress Syndrome

In polytrauma patients, a special situation occurs in two ways: First, there is often a concomitant pulmonary parenchymal lesion, such as a lung contusion. This may lead to worsening of pulmonary function within days after injury. Second, there is a generalized permeability defect due to the initial hemorrhagic shock. The lungs of a polytrauma patient therefore have a pathological water content and inflation by artificial ventilation is a challenging task. The sum of the factors discussed above (e.g., hemorrhagic shock, lung contusions) induces a situation where pulmonary failure may occur.

In the clinical course, the lung is the first organ to fail and it also represents the most frequent organ system developing dysfunction (101). Among the reasons for lung failure during the course of MODS, the theory of the "first filter" also has to be taken into consideration. Activated blood cells, cytokines, toxins and cell debris, often deriving from the areas of injury are directly transported into the lung via the blood stream.

Historically, three phases of ARDS have been differentiated, the third leading to a state of scarring of pulmonary tissue and often irreversible loss of organ function. According to our current knowledge, the formation of scar tissue has often been the result of high intraalveolar pressures due to inadequate ventilation techniques. Because of the improved ventilation strategies described above, the late form is usually not seen now (184). Within days after the injury, changes in vascular permeability with albumin extravasation into the interstitial room have been shown (185). Consequently, an increase in extravascular lung water has been observed, which may result in decompensation of lymph drainage pulmonary interstitial edema. These mechanisms are maintained by inflammatory reactions, such as activation of monocytes and polymorphonuclear leukocytes, thus inducing a release of proteases and cytokines. All these mechanisms may also contribute to the vicious cycle leading to organ failure during the late course after injury.

Multiple Organ Dysfunction Syndrome

The pathophysiology of MODS is defined as an excessive immunoinflammatory reaction (positive amplification of shock mediators) after traumatic hemorrhagic shock and tissue damage, which is followed by systemic tissue damage and permeability leading to specific organ disorder (186). Typically, after a latency period, sequential dysfunction of several organ systems occur (187). The sequence of organ failures is variable, as described below.

Sequence of Organ Failure

This syndrome typically presents with sequential failure of various organ failures (188). Some combinations of isolated organs, such as lung and liver failure are associated with poor outcome (189). It can be difficult to analyze the normal sequence of MODS in severe trauma patients, because of the definition of the isolated organ failure and the sensitivity and the specification of the parameters used. During the course of MODS, 50% of patients develop lung failure followed by liver dysfunction (Table 3-8) (190). As previously described, two forms of the syndrome are described. A one-phase organ failure as a rapid form and a two-phase organ failure as delayed form (101). A correlation between the number of failing organs and mortality during the course of MODS has been seen in many cases. If more than three organ systems fail, the subsequent mortality rate is almost 100%. These results illustrate yet again the importance of multiple organ failure as the most severe complication after severe trauma.

TABLE 3-8 Sequence of Organ Failure

Author (Ref.)	1. Organ	2. Organ	3. Organ
Baue 1975 (230)	Lung	Kidney	Liver
Border 1976 (231)	Lung	Heart	Kidney
Cerra 1987 (232)	Lung	Liver	Intestine
Deitch 1993 (190)	Lung	Liver	Intestine
Fry 1980 (100)	Lung	Liver	Intestine
Goris 1985 (102)	Lung	Liver	Intestine
McMenamy 1981 (233)	Lung	Liver	Heart
Regel 1995 (144)	Lung	Heart	Liver

Pulmonary Failure

While the early phase of lung failure may occur as described above, a late phase has also been described. This occurs in association with MODS, and the pathogenesis of the late lung failure continues to be unclear. It has been associated with immune dysfunction. Also, infective complications have been claimed to play a major role. Typically, late ARDS develops after about 2 to 3 weeks and is the hallmark of organ failure, often irreversible and leading to death. Thus, it must be viewed as part of late MODS.

Liver Failure

The liver is constantly described as the second organ system with dysfunction (Table 3-8). The liver demonstrates deterioration of all three functions, synthesis, excretion, and the reticular endothelial system. First there is a worsening in the reticuloendothelial system. This leads to a decrease in the clearance function even though there is a compensatory increase in the measurable clearance (191). The clearance function of the liver is bypassed and cell debris may be transported into the lung. Some clinical investigations show that the protein synthesis and the excretion of the liver are undergo early dysfunction but late total failure. The exact mechanisms that lead to this course are still being discussed. Obviously, changes of the reticuloendothelial system in the liver are associated with the integrity of the liver cells.

Cardiovascular Failure

Dysfunction of the cardiovascular system occurs at a later stage. Once this complication develops, the mortality rate is very high. The function of the cardiovascular system is well known, with the blood pressure adapted heart rate (192).The heart index reflects the circulating amount of blood per unit time. Obviously, the failure of the cardiovascular system is the terminal variable, which will lead to death, independent of therapeutic interventions. The medications acting on the cardiovascular system usually do not show a clinical response, which has been attributed to a palsy-like reaction of the arterial vascular system.

Renal Failure

Isolated renal failure has become very rare today because early fluid replacement is usually undertaken (193). One of the rare reasons for dysfunction is initial ischemia of the renal parenchyma—that is, direct injury. One of the general responses to trauma is disturbances in the area of the renal tubuli, which might lead to an interstitial edema and a transient dysfunction in excretion and resorption (187). Renal failure usually becomes relevant only if it occurs late after trauma and if it is associated with MODS. In this case, the pathogenesis continues to be unexplained.

Treatment Options for MODS and ARDS

Numerous attempts have been made in the past few decades to develop an effective treatment for both ARDS and MODS. Some workers have tried to reduce the degree of the endothelial leakage by using steroid hormones. However, immunologic side effects have been claimed to prevent this strategy from providing any clinically relevant positive effects (194). Others have tried to lower the pathologically increased pulmonary arterial pressure associated with the syndrome. For this, prostaglandins have been used (195). These did lower the pulmonary arterial pressure in some studies, but were either not associated with a reduction in ARDS or were associated with side effects (e.g., decrease in systemic arterial pressure). In cases of acute worsening of pulmonary failure, nitric oxide was used. It has been shown to exert positive effects in patients with ischemia/reperfusion injury (lung transplant), and there are some reports about its effectiveness in lung contusion. Its use usually has been limited to a few days after trauma only, however, and the effects have to be weighed against possible side effects in every case (195). Likewise, some authors have claimed that the treatment of intestinal failure associated with the development of MODS would provide a causative treatment for MODS. Selective intestinal decontamination by antibiotics was used but failed to provide an improvement of the clinical status. Early enteral feeding has been shown to have positive effects on intestinal function (196). Yet, its use for the development of organ failure has not been proven to date.

L-selectin has been used as a single agent to reduce the degree of adhesion to the endothelial layer. However, a clinical study documenting the effectiveness of L-selectin has not become available (197). Some authors have recently argued that a combination of several immunologically active substances may provide beneficial effects. However, there is a known sustained heterogeneity of pathogenetic pathways, which may not allow a clinical breakthrough in the near future.

Once MODS has developed, symptomatic treatment is the

only treatment option. It consists of adequate ventilation strategies as described above. In cases of severe lung contusions, some authors have favored bronchoalveolar lavage to diagnose the degree of inflammatory change and to assess possible worsening. However, bronchoalveolar lavage does not represent a routine measure for the determination of these pulmonary changes. In addition, there may be temporary worsening of pulmonary function after a lavage has been performed. This is due to the alveolar collapse after suction has been performed. Among the other symptomatic measures, cardiovascular support with inotropic substances is the rule. The support of liver and intestinal dysfunction is usually unable to improve the clinical condition and to reverse the organ failure. Most authors agree that it merely prolongs the time until a lethal outcome is reached (198).

Crush Syndrome

The crush syndrome develops in cases of severe soft tissue trauma and is associated with earthquakes or other conditions in which patients are buried under solid material (199). The destruction of soft tissues represents the major problem, leading to an often devastating intravasation of debris from muscle and fatty tissue (200). Rhabdomyolysis is one of the most feared complications of this syndrome (201). The subsequent clinical presentation is a state of latent shock and subsequent renal failure secondary to direct obstruction of renal tubules (202). Timely dialysis is crucial in these cases. Unless this can be provided, patients succumb within 2 or 3 days after the injury. Even if dialysis is performed early, the patient is at high risk for further complications, mainly due to sepsis deriving from secondary infection of necrotic tissue (203). From the surgical standpoint, debridement is the crucial treatment to avoid secondary complications. Whenever positive swabs are cultured from the injured tissue, antibiotic treatment should be initiated. Some authors have advocated the use of hyperbaric oxygen therapy for these cases. This has been supported by several reports. Although larger or randomized studies are not available, the use of this method appears to be justified in view of the high mortality (204). More importantly, repeated revisions and debridements are required to minimize the area of necrosis and the risk of secondary infection (205).

REHABILITATION

Aftercare in polytrauma patients has to start during the immediate postoperative period. This implies mobilization of the extremities during the course of the intensive care treatment. Among the measures to be undertaken is passive continuous motion. Moreover, mobilization of all major joints may be performed and should be part of a standardized rehabilitation program.

During treatment on the regular ward, these measures are maintained and may be accompanied by active exercises by the patient. These should be performed under the supervision of a trained physiotherapist. Also, the modes of mobilization and the degree of weightbearing should be carefully discussed between the treating surgeon and the physical therapist. From the point of view of the patients, a tendency exists to perform mobilization in a cautious way. Most often, there is a fear of undertaking too much weightbearing. This can often be explained by the severe psychological impact induced by the traumatic insult. Reassurance of the patient represents an important additional factor to ascertain adequate mobilization. These factors are relevant not only in regard to the maintenance of the joint mobility but also in preventing osteoporosis induced by immobility. Careful explanation is crucial so that patients realize the importance of muscular activities, joint mobility and weightbearing. Only then can a joint effort toward rapid mobilization be achieved.

Patients With Head Trauma

During the treatment of patients who have significant head trauma, special care must be taken to avoid the development of secondary brain damage. These patients profit from early rehabilitation measures. Thus, a timely transfer to a rehabilitation center is advisable to facilitate a stimulation of the cognitive functions. Although it may be considered to commence treatment in the primary center, the patients are often still under the influence of sedative drugs or withdrawal symptoms from these drugs. In this situation, a thorough work-up cannot be performed and cognitive training is useless. In an ideal situation, transfer to a specialized facility may overlap with the normalization of the withdrawal symptoms and thus forms the basis of a timely beginning of the rehabilitation program.

OUTCOME STUDIES

General Outcome

Over the past few decades, improved preclinical and clinical emergency care has led to a sustained improvement in the survival rate of multiply injured patients. Therefore, the major treatment goals have changed toward achieving optimal results in terms of rehabilitation and return of the patient to a productive lifestyle (206–208).

In order to judge the true clinical outcome, follow-up studies are required that provide data independent from the subjective view of the treating physician, who may not be able to judge the true outcome. Several factors may be responsible for this fact:

1. The mobility of modern Western societies prevents patients' availability for follow-up.
2. Patients may have a different view on which criteria are important to judge the "outcome" in comparison with doctors (e.g., range of motion versus subjective ability to maintain certain motor skills).
3. Social and psychological aspects may cause a more sustained impairment of the subjective outcome than assessed by the clinical examination performed by an orthopedic surgeon.

The measurement of outcome largely depends on measurements such as the quality of life, employment status, or residual subjective complaints. These variables have to be investigated carefully for several reasons:

1. A detailed analysis of the long-term results following polytrauma provides important information for the development or improvement of treatment guidelines and the allocation of resources.
2. A broad knowledge about long-term outcomes following polytrauma will help trauma surgeons to better manage and advise their patients regarding discharge planning, rehabilitation plans, or career planning. Therefore, patients certainly benefit from a thorough consultation.
3. The length of rehabilitation, physical disability, and employment status following polytrauma are of economic interest.

Trauma patients continue to improve after discharge. Recovery is often prolonged, however, and up to now, the completeness of this recovery has remained uncertain. The outcome following polytrauma has been investigated in previous studies and the following demographic variables were reported to be associated with a poor outcome:

- Female gender (209)
- Old age (210–212)
- ISS (211)
- MAIS (213)
- Head injuries (209,211,214)
- Workers' compensation (215)
- Lower educational level (216)

A long-term study from Germany aimed to evaluate the long-term subjective and objective outcome of patients with multiple blunt injuries (217). In that study, an adequate follow-up period and a combination of subjective evaluation, and an examination performed by a physician were presented. The overall outcome in this patient population was favorable. More than three fourths of the patients graded their overall outcome as satisfactory, good, or very good. The younger patient population trended toward superior results. The most limiting factors for a successful rehabilitation were injuries to the head and the lower extremities (Figs. 3-9 and 3-10).

These results were consistent with previous studies, reporting superior results in young patients (210–212). A very important outcome measurement for polytrauma patients is the economic status and the return to work following the injury. These results have to be viewed in the context of specifics of the German healthcare system. German residents have universal insurance to health care and can receive significant social welfare payments. Despite this apparently favorable situation, significant financial losses due to injury were indicated by 36.9% of the patients and retirement or permanent disability due to physical disability was found in 26.9% of the patients (217).

MacKenzie et al (216) found that 56% of those working full-time before multiple trauma had returned to work 1 year after injury. The group that returned to work was more likely to have had lower severity injury, higher educational level, white collar occupation, and higher preinjury income. Rhodes et al (214) documented a 75% rate of return to preinjury work status in trauma patients. Morris et al (218) reported that 55% of trauma patients had returned to productivity during an average follow-up interval of 2.6 years.

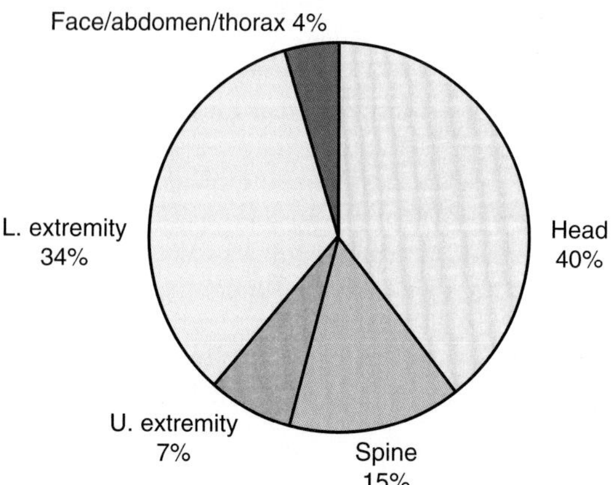

FIGURE 3-9 Injuries responsible for physical disability determined at a 10-year minimum time point after trauma.

It appears from the literature that head injuries and injuries to the lower extremities have been reported to be a limiting factor for a successful rehabilitation process (214,219). Therefore, the outcome of lower extremity injuries requires close attention and is discussed below.

Outcome After Lower Extremity Injuries

Lower extremity injuries are a well-known limiting factor for successful rehabilitation (220,221). In addition, some authors

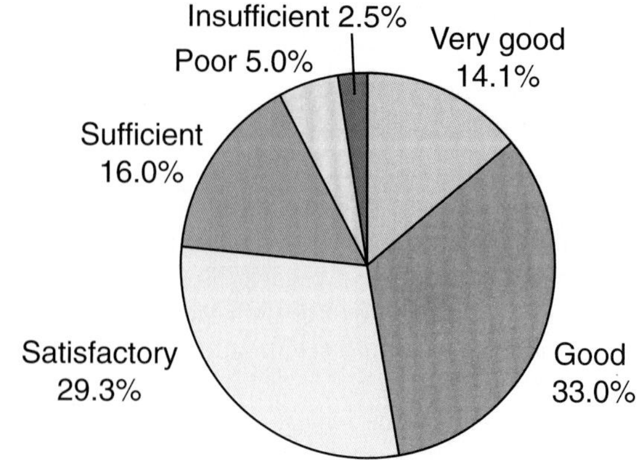

FIGURE 3-10 Overall rehabilitation status as graded by the patients.

have suggested that distal lower extremity injuries represent a particular problem for the functional recovery after polytrauma (222,223). These previous studies have mainly focused on the outcome within the first 2 years postinjury. The recovery in this subset of patients, however, is often prolonged and requires long-term data for evaluation. Social variables such as return to work must be considered in the long-term. Although some polytrauma patients achieve maximum physical restoration within the first few months postinjury, in most cases a longer follow-up is necessary to develop a better understanding of the permanent consequences of the injury. Butcher et al (221) were able to show that in patients with lower extremity trauma the cumulative percentage of first return to work continuously increased until the study end point at 30 months postinjury. Therefore, their study indicates that the posttraumatic recovery in this patient population is continuous. Most previous reports based their hypotheses mainly on subjective outcome measurements.

In a study investigating polytrauma patients at a minimum of 10 years after trauma, combined injuries had poorer outcomes than the two other groups (217). However, the comparison between combined injuries and above-knee injuries demonstrated that all but one tested item showed significantly worse outcomes for combined injuries, whereas the comparison between combined injuries and below-knee injuries showed no significant difference regarding range of motion, limping gait, and weightbearing status. It was believed that this finding further proves the significant impact of below-knee injuries for the functional outcome of the polytrauma patient. It was speculated that various factors played a role in these findings. First, it was argued that the life-threatening injuries are frequently the focus of treatment on their admission to the hospital, and therefore in some cases, the diagnosis and treatment of relatively subtle distal lower extremity injuries may be delayed, resulting in inferior outcomes in this subset of patients. Second, the thin soft tissue envelope below the knee joint may limit the healing potential of injuries below the knee joint as compared with injuries above the joint (217).

These assumptions are in association with the results of Stiegelmar et al, who speculated that in polytrauma patients, foot and ankle injuries are more likely to be a consequence of direct impact and high-energy trauma; and therefore these injuries may be associated with increased soft tissue damage and neurovascular compromise (223).

Moreover, in polytrauma patients, several conditions such as hypotension or hypothermia may result in decreased peripheral blood supply; therefore, the soft tissues of the distal lower extremities are more likely to be compromised by these general insults than proximal injuries. The increased incidence of complex foot and ankle injuries such as pilon, talus, and calcaneus fractures or Lisfranc lesions when compared with isolated injuries may also be relevant. In addition, the rehabilitation process of patients with combined injuries to the extremities may be less favorable than the rehabilitation for an isolated injury (213,215).

Another question that may not be able to be answered is the indication for amputation. The most extensive and demanding study has been performed as a multicenter study among several centers in North America (LEAP study) (206). In this study, patients were investigate specifically in regard to their long-term outcomes after limb reconstruction or amputation. In an observational setup, functional outcomes of 569 patients with severe leg injuries resulting in reconstruction or amputation were evaluated. The authors found no significant difference in scores for the Sickness Impact Profile between the amputation and reconstruction groups at 2 years. The authors concluded that the characteristics of the patients and their injuries should be adjusted and patients who underwent amputation had functional outcomes similar to those of patients who underwent reconstruction. In general, a less favorable outcome was measured in cases of lower educational level, nonwhite race, poverty, lack of private health insurance, poor social support network, low self-efficacy (the patient's confidence in being able to resume life activities), smoking, and involvement in disability compensation litigation. Reconstruction was associated with a higher rate of rehospitalization than primary amputation. Although these results are expected for the population of isolated extremity injuries, they may not be transferable to the more complex situation seen in patients with multiple injuries (206). Similarly, the LEAP study demonstrated a similar return to work by 2 years in patients who underwent amputation and patients who underwent reconstruction (224). Thus, the decision making in polytrauma patients may have to be adjusted to the individual situation. In these patients, amputation of a limb may represent a lifesaving procedure in the early stage after injury. Therefore, factors other than the mere feasibility of limb reconstruction and the local tissue situation have to be considered.

REFERENCES

1. Holbrook TL, Anderson JP, Sieber WJ, et al. Outcome after major trauma: 12-month and 18-month follow-up results from the Trauma Recovery Project. *J Trauma* 1999; 765–771.
2. Gwinnutt CL, Driscoll PA, Whittaker J. Trauma systems–state of the art. *Resuscitation* 2001;48:17–23.
3. Krug E. *Injury: A leading cause of the global burden of disease*. Geneva: World Health Organization, 1999: WHO/HSC/P VI/99.11.
4. MacKenzie EJ, Fowler CJ. Epidemiology. In: Mattox KL, Feliciano DV, Moore EE, eds. *Trauma 4th emergency department*. New York: McGraw-Hill, 2000:21.
5. Zhou Y, Baker TD, Rao K, Li G. Productivity losses from injury in China. *Inj Prev* 2003; 9:124–127.
6. Baker SP, O'Neill B, Haddon W Jr, et al. The injury severity score: a method for describing patients with multiple injuries and evaluating emergency care. *J Trauma* 1974;14:187–196.
7. Osler T, Baker SP, Long W. A modification of the injury severity score that both improves accuracy and simplifies scoring. *J Trauma* 1997;43:922–925.
8. Balogh Z, Offner PJ, Moore EE, et al. NISS predicts postinjury multiple organ failure better than the ISS. *J Trauma* 2000;48:624–627.
9. Balogh ZJ, Varga E, Tomka J, et al. The new injury severity score is a better predictor of extended hospitalization and intensive care unit admission than the injury severity score in patients with multiple orthopaedic injuries. *J Orthop Trauma* 2003;17: 508–512.
10. Jamulitrat S, Sangkerd P, Thongpiyapoom S, et al. A comparison of mortality predictive abilities between NISS and ISS in trauma patients. *J Med Assoc Thai* 2001;84: 1416–1421.
11. Champion HR. A revision to the trauma score. *J Trauma* 1989;29:623–629.
12. Boyd CR, Tolson MA, Copes WS. Evaluating trauma care: The TRISS method. *J Trauma* 1987;27:370–378.
13. Chawda MN, Hildebrand F, Pape HC, et al. Predicting outcome after multiple trauma; which scoring system? *Injury* 2004;35:347–358.

14. Long WB, Bachulius BL, Hynes GD. Accuracy and relationship of mechanism of injury, trauma score and injury severity in identifying major trauma. *Am J Surg* 1986;151: 581–584.
15. Giannoudis PV, Bouamra O, Lecky F. Prevalence of pelvic ring disruptions, associated injuries and mortality in the United Kingdom. OTA Proceedings 2004;412–413.
16. Tscherne H, Oestern HJ, Sturm J. Osteosynthesis of major fractures following poly-trauma. *World J Surg* 1983;7:80–87.
17. Various authors. Initial assessment and management. In: Weigelt JA, ed. *Advanced trauma life support for doctors*. Chicago: American College of Surgeons, 1997:21–49.
18. Kanz KG, Sturm JA, Mutschler W. [Algorithm for prehospital blunt trauma management]. *Unfallchirurg* 2002;105:1007–1014.
19. Regel G, Lobenhoffer P, Lehmann U, et al. Results of treatment of poly-traumatized patients. A comparative analysis of 3406 cases between 1972 and 1991. *Unfallchirurg* 1993;96:350–362.
20. Osterwalder JJ. Mortality of blunt poly-trauma: A comparison between emergency physicians and emergency medical technicians: prospective cohort study at a level I hospital in eastern Switzerland. *J Trauma* 2003;55:355–361.
21. Schmidt U, Muggia-Sullam M, Holch M, et al. Primary management of poly-trauma. Comparison of a German and American air rescue unit. *Unfallchirurg* 1993;96: 287–291.
22. Oppe S, De Charro FT. The effect of medical care by a helicopter trauma team on the probability of survival and the quality of life for hospitalised victims. *Accid Annal Prev* 2001;33:129–138.
23. Sanson G, Di Bartolomeo S, Nardi G, et al. Road traffic accidents with vehicular entrapment: incidence of major injuries and need for advanced life support. *Eur J Emerg Med* 1999;6:285–291.
24. Schlechtriemen T, Schefer S, Stolpe E, et al. Preclinical care of trauma patients in air rescue. Results of the medical quallity management for patients with severe head injury and poly-trauma in the years 2000 and 2001. *Unfallchirurg* 2002;105:974–985.
25. Haas NP, Hoffmann RF, Mauch C, et al. The management of poly-traumatized patients in Germany. *Clin Orthop Relat Res* 1995;318:25–35.
26. Biewener A, Aschenbrenner U, Rammelt S, et al. Impact of helicopter transport and hospital level on mortality of poly-trauma patients. *J Trauma* 2004;56:94–98.
27. Ersson A, Lundberg M, Wramby CO, et al. Extrication of entrapped victims from motor vehicle accidents: the crew concept. *Eur J Emerg Med* 1999;6:341–347.
28. Mahoney PF, Carney CJ. Entrapment, extrication and immobilization. *Eur J Emerg Med* 1996;3:244–246.
29. Gerich TG, Schmidt U, Hubrich V, et al. Prehospital airway management in the acutely injured patient: the role of surgical cricothyroidotomy revisited. *J Trauma* 1998;45: 312–314.
30. Osterwalder JJ. Can the "golden hour of shock" safely be extended in blunt poly-trauma patients? Prospective cohort study at a level I hospital in eastern Switzerland. *Prehospital Disaster Med* 2002;17:75–80.
31. Tsuei BJ, Kearney PA. Hypothermia in the trauma patient. *Injury* 2004;35:7–15.
32. Kirkpatrick AW, Chun R, Brown R, et al. Hypothermia and the trauma patient. *Can J Surg* 1999;42:333–343.
33. Jurkovich GJ, Greiser WB, Luterman A, et al. Hypothermia in trauma victims: an ominous predictor of survival. *J Trauma* 1987;27:1019–1024.
34. Seekamp A, Van Griensven M, Hildebrand F, et al. Adenosine-triphosphate in trauma-related and elective hypothermia. *J Trauma* 1999;47:673–683.
35. Watts DD, Trask A, Soeken K, et al. Hypothermic coagulopathy in trauma: effect of varying levels of hypothermia on enzyme speed, platelet function, and fibrinolytic activity. *J Trauma* 1998;44:846–854.
36. Wolberg AS, Meng ZH, Monroe DMI, et al. A systematic evaluation of the effect of temperature on coagulation enzyme activity and platelet function. *J Trauma* 2004;56: 1221–1228.
37. Krause KR, Howells GA, Buhs CL, et al. Hypothermia induced coagulopathy during hemorrhagic shock. *Am Surg* 2000;66:348–354.
38. Mizushima Y, Wang P, Cioffi WG, et al. Should normothermia be restored and maintained during resuscitation after trauma and hemorrhage? *J Trauma* 2000;48:58–65.
39. Gentilello LM, Jurkovich GJ, Stark MS, et al. Is hypothermia in the victim of major trauma protective or harmful? A randomized, prospective study. *Ann Surg* 1997;226: 439–447; discussion 447–449.
40. Marion DW. Moderate hypothermia in severe head injuries: the present and the future. *Curr Opin Crit Care* 2002;8:111–114.
41. Oestern HJ. [Management of poly-trauma patients in an international comparison]. *Unfallchirurg* 1999;102:80–91.
42. Ruchholtz S, Zintl B, Nast-Kolb D, et al. [Quality management in early clinical poly-trauma management. II. Optimising therapy by treatment guidelines.] *Unfallchirurg* 1997;100:859–866.
43. Nerlich ML, Tscherne H. A trauma algorithm–a decision tool in first aid for severely injured patients. *Zentralbl Chir* 1987;112:1465–1472.
44. Ruchholtz S, Zintl B, Nast-Kolb D, et al. Improvement in the therapy of multiply injured patients by introduction of clinical management guidelines. *Injury* 1998;29:115–129.
45. Waydhas C, Kanz KG, Ruchholtz S, et al. [A time and priority-oriented algorithm]. *Langenbecks Arch Chir Suppl Kongressbd* 1997;114:966–969.
46. Waydhas C, Kanz KG, Ruchholtz S, et al. Algorithms in trauma management. *Unfallchirurg* 1997;100:913–921.
47. Bishop M, Shoemaker WC, Avakian S, et al. Evaluation of a comprehensive algorithm for blunt and penetrating thoracic and abdominal trauma. *Am Surg* 1991;57:737–746.
48. Tsoukas A, Andreade A, Zacharogiannis C, et al. Myocardial contusion presented as acute myocardial infarction after chest trauma. *Echocardiography* 2001;18:167–170.
49. Nagy KK, Krosner SM, Roberts RR, et al. Determining which patients require evaluation for blunt cardiac injury following blunt chest trauma. *World J Surg* 2001;25:108–111.
50. Rixen D, Raum M, Holzgraefe B, et al. Shock and Trauma Study Group. A pig hemorrhagic shock model: oxygen debt and metabolic acidemia as indicators of severity. *Shock* 2001;16:239–244.
51. Rixen D, Siegel JH. Metabolic correlates of oxygen debt predict posttrauma early acute respiratory distress syndrome and the related cytokine response. *J Trauma* 2000;49: 392–403.
52. Siegel JH, Rivkind AI, Dalal S, et al. Early physiologic predictors of injury severity and death in blunt multiple trauma. *Arch Surg* 1990;125:498–508.
53. Blow O, Magliore L, Claridge JA, et al. The golden hour and the silver day: detection and correction of occult hypoperfusion within 24 hours improves outcome from major trauma. *J Trauma* 1999;47:964–969.
54. Claridge JA, Crabtree TD, Pelletier SJ, et al. Persistent occult hypoperfusion is associated with a significant increase in infection rate and mortality in major trauma patients. *J Trauma* 2000;48:8–14; discussion 14–15.
55. Moore FA, McKinley BA, Moore EE. The next generation in shock resuscitation. *Lancet* 2004;363:1988–1996.
56. Schierhout G, Roberts I. Fluid resuscitation with colloid or crystalloid solutions in critically ill patients: a systematic review of randomised trials. *Br Med J* 1998;69: 961–964.
57. Choi P-L, Yip G, Quinonez LG. Crystalloids vs. colloids in fluid resuscitation: a systematic review. *Crit Care Med* 1999;27:200–210.
58. Moore EE. Hypertonic saline dextran for post-injury resuscitation: Experimental background and clinical experience. *Aust N Z J Surg* 1991;61:732–736.
59. Smith GJ, Kramer GC, Perron P. A comparison of several hypertonic solutions for resuscitation of bled sheep. *J Surg Res* 1985;39:517–528.
60. Wade CE, Kramer GC, Grady JJ. Efficacy of hypertonic 7.5% saline and 6% dextran-70 in treating trauma: a meta-analysis of controlled clinical studies. *Surgery* 1997;122: 609–616.
61. Shackford SR. Effects of small-volume resuscitation on intracranial pressure and related cerebral variables. *J Trauma* 1997;42:S48–S53.
62. Practice guidelines for blood component therapy: a report by the American Society of Anaesthesiologists Task Force on Blood Component Therapy. *Anaesthesiology* 1996;84: 732–747.
63. Weiskopf RB, Viele MK, Feiner J. Human cardiovascular and metabolic response to acute, severe isovolaemic hemorrhage. *JAMA* 1998;279:217–221.
64. Herbert PC, Wells G, Blajchmann MA. A multicentre randomized controlled clinical trial of transfusion requirements in critical care. *N Engl J Med* 1999;54:898–905.
65. Malone DL, Dunne J, Tracy JK, et al. Blood transfusion, independent of shock severity, is associated with worse outcome in trauma. *J Trauma* 2003;54:898–905.
66. Hensler T, Heinemann B, Sauerland S, et al. Immunologic alterations associated with high blood transfusion volume after multiple injury: effects on plasmatic cytokine and cytokine receptor concentrations. *Shock* 2003;20:497–502.
67. Aiboshi J, Moore EE, Ciesla DJ, et al. Blood transfusion and the two-insult model of post-injury multiple organ failure. *Shock* 2001;15:302–306.
68. Vaslef SN, Knudsen NW, Neligan PJ, et al. Massive transfusion exceeding 50 units of blood products in trauma patients. *J Trauma* 2002;53:291–295.
69. Hardy JF, De Moerloose P, Samama M. Groupe d'interet en Hemostase Perioperatoire. Massive transfusion and coagulopathy: pathophysiology and implications for clinical management. *Can J Anaesth* 2004;51:293–310.
70. DeLoughery TG. Coagulation defects in trauma patients: etiology, recognition and therapy. *Crit Care Clin* 2004;20:13–24.
71. Schrieber MA, Halcomb JB, Hedner U. The effect of recombinant factor VIIa on coagulopathic pigs with grade V liver injuries. *J Trauma* 2002;53:252–259.
72. Martinowitz U, Halcomb JB, Pusateri AE. Intravenous rFVIIa administered for hemorrhage control in hypothermic coagulopathic swine with grade V liver injuries. *J Trauma* 2001;50:721–729.
73. Meregalli A, Oliveira RP, Friedman G. Occult hypoperfusion is associated with increased mortality in hemodynamically stable, high risk, surgical patients. *Crit Care* 2004;8:R60–65.
74. Chan RN, Ainscow D, Sikorski JM. Diagnostic failures in the multiple injured. *J Trauma* 1980;20:684–687.
75. Tscherne H. Hazards of osteosynthesis: indication errors. *Langenbecks Arch Chir* 1971; 329:1136–1143.
76. Giannoudis PV. Surgical priorities in damage control in poly-trauma. *J Bone Joint Surg Br* 2003;85:478–483.
77. Abboud PA, Kendall J. Emergency department ultrasound for hemothorax after blunt traumatic injury. *J Emerg Med* 2003;25:181–184.
78. Hoth JJ, Scott MJ, Bullock TK, et al. Thoracotomy for blunt trauma: traditional indications may not apply. *Am Surg* 2003;69:1108–1111.
79. Balkan ME, Oktar GL, Kayi-Cangir A, et al. Emergency thoracotomy for blunt thoracic trauma. *Ann Thorac Cardiovasc Surg* 2002;8:78–82.
80. Cardarelli MG, McLaughlin JS, Downing SW, et al. Management of traumatic aortic rupture: a 30-year experience. *Ann Surg* 2002;236:465–469; discussion 469–470.
81. Schoder M, Prokop M, Lammer J. Traumatic injuries: imaging and intervention of large arterial trauma. *Eur Radiol* 2002;12:1617–1631.
82. Downing SW, Sperling JS, Mirvis SE, et al. Experience with spiral computed tomography as the sole diagnostic method for traumatic aortic rupture. *Ann Thorac Surg* 2001; 72:495–501; discussion 501–502.
83. Symbas PN, Sherman AJ, Silver JM, et al. Traumatic rupture of the aorta: immediate or delayed repair? *Ann Surg* 2002;235:796–802.
84. Holmes JH, Bloch RD, Hall RA, et al. Natural history of traumatic rupture of the thoracic aorta managed nonoperatively: a longitudinal analysis. *Ann Thorac Surg* 2002;73: 1149–1154.
85. Langanay T, Verhoye JP, Corbineau H, et al. Surgical treatment of acute traumatic

rupture of the thoracic aorta: a timing reappraisal? *Eur J Cardiothorac Surg* 2002;21: 282–287.
86. Iannelli G, Piscione F, Di Tommaso L, et al. Thoracic aortic emergencies: impact of endovascular surgery. *Ann Thorac Surg* 2004;77:591–596.
87. Kwok PC, Ho KK, Chung TK, et al. Emergency aortic stent grafting for traumatic rupture of the thoracic aorta. *Hong Kong Med J* 2003;9:435–440.
88. Sam A 2nd, Kibbe M, Matsumura J, et al. Blunt traumatic aortic transection: endoluminal repair with commercially available aortic cuffs. *J Vasc Surg* 2003;38:1132–1135.
89. Giannoudis PV, Pape HC. Damage control orthopaedics in unstable pelvic ring injuries. *Injury* 2004;35:671–677.
90. Grimm MR, Vrahas MS, Thomas KA. Pressure-volume characteristics of the intact and disrupted pelvic retroperitoneum. *J Trauma* 1998;44:454–459.
91. Ward LD, Morandi MM, Pearse M, et al. The immediate treatment of pelvic ring disruption with the pelvic stabilizer. *Bull Hosp Jt Dis* 1997;56:104–106.
92. Gansslen A, Giannoudis P, Pape HC. Hemorrhage in pelvic fracture: who needs angiography? *Curr Opin Crit Care* 2003;9:515–523.
93. Thannheimer A, Woltmann A, Vastmans J, et al. [The unstable patient with pelvic fracture.] *Zentralbl Chir* 2004;129:37–42.
94. Gennarelli TA, Champion HR, Sacco WJ, et al. Mortality of patients with head injury and extracranial injury treated in trauma centers. *J Trauma* 1989;29:1193–1201; discussion 1201–1202.
95. Wisner DH, Victor NS, Holcroft JW. Priorities in the management of multiple trauma: intracranial versus intra-abdominal injury. *J Trauma* 1993;35:271–276; discussion 276–278.
96. Wald SL, Shackford SR, Fenwick J. The effect of secondary insults on mortality and long-term disability after severe head injury in a rural region without a trauma system. *J Trauma* 1993;34:377–381; discussion 381–382.
97. Thomason M, Messick J, Rutledge R, et al. Head CT scanning versus urgent exploration in the hypotensive blunt trauma patient. *J Trauma* 1993;34:40–44; discussion 44–45.
98. Tilney NL, Bailey GL, Morgan AP. Sequential system failure after rupture of abdominal aortic aneurysms: An unsolved problem in postoperative care. *Ann Surg* 1973;178: 117–122.
99. Eisman B, Beart R, Norton L. Multiple organ failure. *Surg Gynaecol Obstet* 1977;144: 323–325.
100. Fry DE, Pearlstein L, Fulton RL, et al. Multiple system organ failure: the role of uncontrolled infection. *Arch Surg* 1980;115:136–144.
101. Faist E, Baue AE, Dittmer H, et al. Multiple organ failure in poly-trauma patients. *J Trauma* 1983;23:775–787.
102. Goris JA, Boekhoerst TP, Nuytinck JK, et al. Multiple organ failure. *Arch Surg* 1985; 120:1109–1115.
103. Norton LW. Does drainage of intra-abdominal pus reverse multiple organ failure? *Am J Surg* 1985;149:347–350.
104. Smith RM, Giannoudis PV. Trauma and Immune Response. *J R Soc Med* 1998;91: 417–420.
105. Cipolle MD, Pasquale MD, Cerra FB. Secondary organ dysfunction: from clinical perspectives to molecular mediators. *Crit Care Clin* 1993;9:261–297.
106. Ogura H, Tanaka H, Koh T, et al. Priming, second hit priming, and apoptosis in leukocytes from trauma patients. *J Trauma* 1999;46:774–783.
107. Giannoudis PV, Smith RM, Banks RE, et al. Stimulation of inflammatory markers after blunt trauma. *Brit J Surg* 1998;85:986–990.
108. Giannoudis PV, Hildebrand F, Pape HC. Inflammatory serum markers in patients with multiple trauma. Can they predict outcome? *J Bone Joint Surg Br* 2004;86:313–323.
109. Giannoudis PV. Current concepts of the inflammatory response after major trauma: an update. *Injury* 2003;34:397–404.
110. Pape HC, Schmidt RE, Rice J, et al. Biochemical changes after trauma and skeletal surgery of the lower extremity: quantification of the operative burden. *Crit Care Med* 2000;28:3441–3448.
111. Pape HC, Auf'm Kolk M, Paffrath T, et al. Primary intramedullary femur fixation in multiple trauma patients with associated lung contusion: a cause of post-traumatic ARDS? *J Trauma* 1993;34:540–548.
112. Giannoudis PV, Pape HC, Cohen AP, et al. Review: systemic effects of femoral nailing: from Kuntscher to the immune reactivity era. *Clin Orthop Relat Res* 2002;404:378–386.
113. Hauser CJ, Joshi P, Zhou X, et al. Production of interleukin-10 in human fracture soft-tissue hematomas. *Shock* 1996;6:3–6.
114. Hauser CJ, Zhou X, Joshi P, et al. The immune microenviroment of human fracture/soft-tissue hematomas and its relationship to systemic immunity. *J Trauma* 1997;42: 895–903.
115. Perl M, Gebhard F, Knöferl MW, et al. The pattern of preformed cytokines in tissue frequently affected by blunt trauma. *Shock* 2003;19:299–304.
116. Giannoudis PV, Smith RM, Perry SL, et al. Immediate IL-10 expression following major orthopaedic trauma: relationship to anti-inflammatory response and subsequent development of sepsis. *Intensive Care Med* 2000;26:1076–1081.
117. Giannoudis PV, Smith RM, Ramsden CW, et al. Molecular mediators and trauma: effects of accidental trauma on the production of plasma elastase, IL-6, sICAM-1 and sE-selectin. *Injury* 1996;27:376–377.
118. Giannoudis PV, Abbott C, Stone M, et al. Fatal systemic inflammatory response syndrome following early bilateral femoral nailing. *Intensive Care Med* 1998;24:641–642.
119. Roumen RM, Hendriks T, van de Ven-Jongekrijk M, et al. Cytokine patterns in patients after major vascular surgery, hemorrhagic shock, and severe blunt trauma. Relation with subsequent adult respiratory distress syndrome and multiple organ failure. *Ann Surg* 1993;218:769–776.
120. Roumen RM, Redl H, Schlag G, et al. Inflammatory mediators in relation to the development of multiple organ failure in patients after severe blunt trauma. *Crit Care Med* 1995;23:474–480.
121. Riche F, Pani Y, Laisne M. High tumor necrosis factor serum levels is associated with increased survival in patients with abdominal septic shock: A prospective study in 59 patients. *Surgery* 1996;120:801–807.
122. Casey LC, Balk RA, Bone RC. Plasma cytokine and endotoxin levels correlate with survival in patients with sepsis syndrome. *Ann Intern Med* 1993;119:771–778.
123. Tarn LR, Waxman K, Scannell G, et al. Trauma causes early release of soluble receptors for tumor necrosis factor. *J Trauma* 1993;34:634–647.
124. Gebhard F, Pfetsch H, Steinbach G, et al. Is interleukin-6 an early marker of injury severity following major trauma in humans. *Arch Surg* 2000;135:291–295.
125. Pape HC, van Griensven M, Rice J, et al. Major secondary surgery in blunt trauma patients and perioperative cytokine liberation: determination of the clinical relevance of biochemical markers. *J Trauma* 2001;50:989–1000.
126. Pape HC, Tscherne H. Early definitive fracture fixation, pulmonary function and systemic effects. In: Baue AE, Faist E, Fry M, eds. *Multiple organ failure*. New York: Springer, 2000.279–290.
127. Giannoudis PV, Smith RM, Bellamy MC, et al. Stimulation of the inflammatory system by reamed and unreamed nailing of femoral fractures. An analysis of the second hit. *J Bone Joint Surg Br* 1999;81:356–361.
128. Ertel W, Keel M, Bonaccio M, et al. Release of anti-inflammatory mediators after mechanical trauma correlates with severity of injury and clinical outcome. *J Trauma* 1995; 39:879–887.
129. Smith RM, Giannoudis PV, Bellamy MC, et al. Interleukin-10 release and monocyte human leukocyte antigen-DR expression during femoral nailing. *Clin Orthop Relat Res* 2000;73:233–240.
130. McIntyre TM, Modur V, Prescott SM, et al. Molecular mechanisms of early inflammation. *Thromb Haemost* 1997;77:302–309.
131. Anderson BO, Harken AH. Multiple organ failure: inflammatory priming and activation sequences promote autogenous tissue injury. *J Trauma* 1990;30:S44–S47.
132. Bradford DS, Foster RR, Nossel HL. Coagulation alterations, hypoxemia, and fat embolism in fracture patients. *J Trauma* 1970;10:307–321.
133. Renne J, Wuthier R, House E, et al. Fat macroglobulemia caused by fractures or total hip replacement. *J Bone Joint Surg Am* 1978;60:613–618.
134. Mueller ME, Allgower M, Schneider R, et al. *Manual of osteosynthesis*. Berlin, Heidelberg, New York: Springer-Verlag, 1970.
135. Smith JEM. The results of early and delayed internal fixation of fractures of the shaft of the femur. *J Bone Joint Surg Br* 1964;46:28–32.
136. Wickstrom J, Corban MS. Intramedullary fixation for fractures of the femoral shaft. A study of complications in 298 operations. *J Trauma* 1967;7:551–583.
137. Riska EB, von Bonsdorff H, Hakkinen S, et al. Primary operative fixation of long bone fractures in patients with multiple injuries. *J Trauma* 1977;17:111–121.
138. Talucci RC, Manning J, Lampard S, et al. Early intramedullary nailing of femoral shaft fractures: a cause of fat embolism syndrome. *Am J Surg* 1983;46:107–111.
139. Goris RJ, Gimbrere JS, van Niekerk JL, et al. Early osteosynthesis and prophylactic mechanical ventilation in the multitrauma patient. *J Trauma* 1982;22:895–903.
140. Johnson K, Cadami A, Seibert G. Incidence of ARDS in patients with multiple musculoskeletal injuries: effect of early operative stabilisation of fractures. *J Trauma* 1985;25: 375–384.
141. Bone L, Johnson K, Weigelt J, et al. Early versus delayed stabilisation of femoral fractures. A prospective randomised study. *J Bone Joint Surg Am* 1989;71:336–340.
142. Tscherne H, Oestern HJ, Sturm J. Osteosynthesis of major fractures in poly-trauma. *World J Surg* 1983;7:80–87.
143. Jansson I, Eriksson R, Liljedahl SO, et al. Primary fracture immobilization as a method to prevent post-traumatic pulmonary changes: an experimental model. *Acta Chir Scand* 1982;148:329–338.
144. Regel G, Lobenhoffer P, Grotz M, et al. Treatment results of patients with multiple trauma: An analysis of 3406 cases treated between 1972 and 1991 at a German level I center. *J Trauma* 1995;38:70–78.
145. Ecke H, Faupel L, Quoika P. Gedanken zum Zeitpunkt der Operation bei Frakturen des Oberschenkelknochens. *Unfallchirurg* 1985;11:89–93.
146. Nast-Kolb D, Waydhas C, Jochum M, et al. [Is there a favorable time for the management of femoral shaft fractures in poly-trauma?] *Chirurg* 1990;61:259–265.
147. Reynolds MA, Richardson JD, Spain DA, et al. Is the timing of fracture fixation important for the patient with multiple trauma? *Ann Surg* 1995;222:470–478.
148. Schüller W, Gaudernack T. Lungenkomplikationen nach Oberschenkelmarknagelung. *Hefte Unfallheilkd* 1996;182:273–278.
149. Giannoudis PV, Veysi V, Pape HC, et al. When should we operate on major fractures in patients with severe head injuries? *Am J Surg* 2002;183:261–267.
150. Shapiro MB, Jenkins DH, Schwab CW, et al. Damage Control: Collective review. *J Trauma* 2000;49:969–978.
151. Pringle J. Notes on the arrest of hepatic hemorrhage due to trauma. *Ann Surg* 1908; 48:541–549.
152. Scalea TM, Boswell SA, Scott JD, et al. External fixation as a bridge to intramedullary nailing for patients with multiple injuries and with femur fractures: damage control orthopedics. *J Trauma* 2000;48:613–621.
153. Nowotarski PJ, Turen CH, Brumback RJ, et al. Conversion of external fixation to intramedullary nailing for fractures of the shaft of the femur in multiply injured patients. *J Bone Joint Surg Am* 2000;82:781–788.
154. Pape HC, Grimme K, Van Griensven M, et al. EPOFF Study Group. Impact of intramedullary instrumentation versus damage control for femoral fractures on immunoinflammatory parameters: prospective randomized analysis by the EPOFF Study Group. *J Trauma*. 2003;55:7–13.

155. Waydhas C, Nast-Kolb D, Trupka A, et al. Posttraumatic inflammatory response, secondary operations, and late multiple organ failure. *J Trauma* 1996;40:624–631.
156. Staub NC. Pulmonary edema. *Physiol Rev* 1974;54:678–811.
157. Pape HC, Stalp M, Griensven M, et al. [Optimal timing for secondary surgery in polytrauma patients: an evaluation of 4,314 serious-injury cases]. *Chirurg* 1999;70:1287–1293.
158. Colligan N, Giannoudis PV, Kourgeraki O, et al. Interleukin 13 and inflammatory markers in human sepsis. *Br J Surg* 2004;91:762–768.
159. Krettek C, Schandelmaier P, Lobenhoffer P, et al. [Complex trauma of the knee joint. Diagnosis–management–therapeutic principles]. *Unfallchirurg* 1996;99:616–627.
160. Bulger EM, Nathens AB, Rivara FP, et al. Brain Trauma Foundation. Management of severe head injury: institutional variations in care and effect on outcome. *Crit Care Med* 2002;30:1870–1876.
161. Burgess AR, Eastridge BJ, Young JW, et al. Pelvic ring disruptions: effective classification system and treatment protocols. *J Trauma* 1990;30:848–856.
162. Bosch U, Pohlemann T, Tscherne H. [Primary management of pelvic injuries]. *Orthopade* 1992;21:385–392.
163. Trentz O. [Management of patients with multiple injuries] *Ther Umsch* 1993;50:491–499.
164. Oestern HJ, Tscherne H. Pathophysiology and classification of soft tissue injuries associated with fractures. In: Tscherne H, Gotzen L, eds. *Fractures with soft tissue injuries.* Berlin: Spinger-Verlag, 1984:1–9.
165. Gustilo RB, Mendoza RM, Williams DN. Problems in the management of type III (severe) open fractures: A new classification of Type III open fractures. *J Trauma* 1984;24:742–746.
166. Seekamp A, Regel G, Bauch S, et al. Long-term results of therapy of poly-trauma patients with special reference to serial fractures of the lower extremity. *Unfallchirurg* 1994;97:57–63.
167. Gregory RT, Gould RJ, Peclet M, et al. The mangled extremity syndrome (M.E.S.): A severity grading system for multisystem injury of the extremity. *J Trauma* 1985;25:1147–1150.
168. Howe HR Jr, Poole GV Jr, Hansen KJ, et al. Salvage of lower extremities following combined orthopedic and vascular trauma. A predictive salvage index. *Am Surg* 1987;53:205–208.
169. Lange RH, Bach AW, Hansen ST Jr, et al. Open tibial fractures with associated vascular injuries: prognosis for limb salvage. *J Trauma* 1985;25:203–208.
170. Helfet DL, Howey T, Sanders R, et al. Limb salvage versus amputation. Preliminary results of the Mangled Extremity Severity Score. *Clin Orthop Rel Res* 1990;256:80–86.
171. McNamara MG, Heckman JD, Corley FG. Severe open fractures of the lower extremity: a retrospective evaluation of the Mangled Extremity Severity Score (MESS). *J Orthop Trauma* 1994;8:81–87.
172. Zhong-Wei C, Meyer VE, Kleinert HE, et al. Present indications and contraindications for replantation as reflected by long-term functional results. *Orthop Clin North Am* 1981;12:849–870.
173. Krettek C, Schandelmaier P, Rudolf J, et al. [Current status of surgical technique for unreamed nailing of tibial shaft fractures with the UTN (unreamed tibia nail)]. *Unfallchirurg* 1994;97:575–599.
174. Sudkamp N, Haas N, Flory PJ, et al. [Criteria for amputation, reconstruction and replantation of extremities in multiple trauma patients]. *Chirurg* 1989;60:774–781.
175. Johansen K, Daines M, Howey T, et al. Objective criteria accurately predict amputation following lower extremity trauma. *J Trauma* 1990;30:568–572; discussion 572–573.
176. Bastian L, Blauth M, Thermann H, et al. [Various therapy concepts in severe fractures of the tibial pilon (type C injuries). A comparative study]. *Unfallchirurg* 1995;98:551–558.
177. Lachmann B, Jonson B, Lindroth M, et al. Modes of artificial ventilation in severe respiratory distress syndrome. Lung function and morphology in rabbits after wash-out of alveolar surfactant. *Crit Care Med* 1982;10:724–732.
178. Varpula T, Valta P, Niemi R, et al. Airway pressure release ventilation as a primary ventilatory mode in acute respiratory distress syndrome. *Acta Anaesthesiol Scand* 2004;48:722–731.
179. Nieszkowska A, Lu Q, Vieira S, et al. Incidence and regional distribution of lung overinflation during mechanical ventilation with positive end-expiratory pressure. *Crit Care Med* 2004;32:1496–1503.
180. Tuxen DV. Permissive hypercapnic ventilation. *Am J Respir Crit Care Med* 1994;150:870–874.
181. Wolter TP, Fuchs PC, Horvat N, et al. Is high PEEP low volume ventilation in burn patients beneficial? A retrospective study of 61 patients. *Burns* 2004;30:368–373.
182. Agro F, Barzoi G, Doyle DJ, et al. Reduction in pulmonary shunt using the Open Lung Concept. *Anaesthesia* 2004;59:625–626.
183. Miranda DR, Gommers D, Struijs A, et al. The open lung concept: effects on right ventricular afterload after cardiac surgery. *Br J Anaesth* 2004;Jul 9 [Epub ahead of print].
184. Plotz FB, Slutsky AS, Van Vught AJ, et al. Ventilator-induced lung injury and multiple system organ failure: a critical review of facts and hypotheses. *Intens Care Med* 2004;Jun 24 [Epub ahead of print].
185. Sturm JA, Wisner DH, Oestern HJ, et al. Increased lung capillary permeability after trauma: a prospective clinical study. *J Trauma* 1986;26:409–418.
186. Baue AE. A debate on the subject "Are SIRS and MODS important entities in the clinical evaluation of patients?" *Shock* 2000;14:590–593.
187. Regel G, Sturm JA, Pape HC, et al. Multiple organ failure. Reflection of generalized cell damage of all organs following severe trauma. *Unfallchirurg* 1991;94:487–497.
188. Grotz M, von Griensven M, Stalp M, et al. Scoring multiple organ failure after severe trauma. Comparison of the Goris, Marshall and Moore scores. *Chirurg* 2001;72:723–730.
189. Matuschak GM, Rinaldo JE. Organ interactions in the adult respiratory distress syndrome during sepsis. Role of the liver in host defence. *Chest* 1988;94:400–406.
190. Deitch EA. Multiple organ failure. *Adv Surg* 1993;26:333–356.
191. Pape HC, Remmers D, Grotz M, et al. Reticuloendothelial system activity and organ failure in patients with multiple injuries. *Arch Surg* 1999;134:421–427.
192. Marshall JC, Cook DJ, Christou NV, et al. Multiple organ dysfunction score: a reliable descriptor of a complex clinical outcome. *Crit Care Med* 1995;23:1638–1652.
193. Pape HC, Regel G, Sturm JA, et al. [Can post-traumatic renal failure be modified therapeutically?] *Unfallchirurg* 1992;95:419–425.
194. Thompson BT. Glucocorticoids and acute lung injury. *Crit Care Med* 2003;31(4 Suppl):S253–S257.
195. Lohbrunner H, Deja M, Busch T, et al. [Inhaled nitric oxide for the treatment of ARDS. *Anaesthesist* 2004; Jul 15 [Epub ahead of print].
196. Bastian L, Weimann A. Immunonutrition in patients after multiple trauma. *Br J Nutr* 2002;Suppl 1:S133–S134.
197. Donnelly SC, Haslett C, Dransfield I, et al. Role of selectins in development of adult respiratory distress syndrome. *Lancet* 1994;23;344:215–219.
198. Sakamoto S, Matsubara J, Matsubara T, et al. Clinical effects of percutaneous cardiopulmonary support in severe heart failure: early results and analysis of complications. *Ann Thorac Cardiovasc Surg* 2003;9:105–110.
199. Sever MS, Erek E, Vanholder R, et al. Lessons learned from the catastrophic Marmara earthquake: factors influencing the final outcome of renal victims. *Clin Nephrol* 2004;61:413–421.
200. Hope MJ, McQueen MM. Acute compartment syndrome in the absence of fracture. *J Orthop Trauma* 2004;18:220–224.
201. Malinoski DJ, Slater MS, Mullins RJ. Crush injury and rhabdomyolysis. *Crit Care Clin* 2004;20:171–192.
202. Fujita M, Yokoyama K, Nakamura K, et al. Tibial fractures associated with crush injuries to the soft tissues of the dorsal foot in children. *Injury* 2004;35:272–277.
203. Greaves I, Porter K, Smith JE. Consensus statement on the early management of crush injury and prevention of crush syndrome. *J R Army Med Corps* 2003;149:255–259.
204. Saunders PJ. Hyperbaric oxygen therapy in the management of carbon monoxide poisoning, osteoradionecrosis, burns, skin grafts, and crush injury. *Int J Technol Assess Health Care* 2003;19:521–525.
205. Smith J, Greaves I. Crush injury and crush syndrome: a review. *J Trauma* 2003;54(Suppl):S226–S230.
206. Bosse MJ, MacKenzie EJ, Kellam JF, et al. An analysis of outcomes of reconstruction or amputation after leg-threatening injuries. *N Engl J Med* 2002;347:1924–1931.
207. Grotz M, Hohensee A, Remmers D, et al. Rehabilitation results of patients with multiple injuries and multiple organ failure and long-term intensive care. *J Trauma* 1997;42:919–926.
208. Stalp M, Koch C, Regel G, et al. Development of a standardized instrument for quantitative and reproducible rehabilitation data assessment after poly-trauma. *Chirurg* 2001;72:312–318.
209. Holbrook TL, Hoyt DB, Anderson JP. The importance of gender on outcome after major trauma: functional and psychologic outcomes in women versus men. *J Trauma* 2001;50:270–273.
210. Anke AGW, Stanghelle JK, Finset A, et al. Long-term prevalence of impairments and disabilities after multiple trauma. *J Trauma* 1997;42:54–61.
211. Brennemann FD, Redelmeier DA, Boulanger BR, et al. Long-term outcomes in blunt trauma: who goes back to work? *J Trauma* 1997;42:778–781.
212. Lehmann U, Gobiet W, Regel G, et al. Functional, neuropsychological and social outcome of multiple trauma patients with severe head injury. *Unfallchirurg* 1997;100:552–560.
213. MacKenzie EJ, Burgess AR, McAndrew MP, et al. Patient oriented outcome after unilateral lower extremity fracture. *J Orthop Trauma* 1993;7:393–401.
214. Rhodes M, Aronson J, Moerkirk G, et al. Quality of life after the trauma center. *J Trauma* 1988;28:931–938.
215. Holbrook TL, Anderson JP, Sieber WJ, et al. Outcome after major trauma: discharge and 6-month follow-up results from the trauma recovery project. *J Trauma* 1998;45:315–323.
216. MacKenzie EJ, Morris JA, Jurkovich GJ, et al. Return to work following injury: the role of economic, social, and job-related factors. *Am J Pub Health* 1998;88:1630–1637.
217. Pape HC, Zelle B, Sittaro NA, et al. The objective and subjective outcome after polytrauma–a reexamination 10 years after the initial injury. 70th Annual Meeting of the American Academy of Orthopaedic Surgeons (AAOS), February 5–9, 2003, New Orleans, LA.
218. Morris JA, Sanchez AA, Bass SM, et al. Trauma patients return to productivity. *J Trauma* 1991;31:827–833; discussion 833–834.
219. Seekamp A, Regel G, Tscherne H. Rehabilitation and reintegration of multiply injured patients: an outcome study with special reference to multiple lower limb fractures. *Injury* 1996;27:133–138.
220. Turchin DC, Schemitsch EH, McKee MD, et al. Do foot injuries significantly affect the functional outcome of multiply injured patients? *J Orthop Trauma* 1999;13:1–4.
221. Butcher JL, MacKenzie EJ, Cushing B, et al. Long-term outcomes after lower extremity. *J Trauma* 1996;41:4–9.
222. Tran T, Thordarson D. Functional outcome of multiply injured patients with associated foot injury. *Foot Ankle Int* 2002;23:340–343.
223. Stiegelmar R, McKee MD, Waddell JP, et al. Outcome of foot injuries in multiply injured patients. *Orthop Clin North Am* 2001;32:193–204.

224. McCarthy ML, MacKenzie EJ, Edwin D, et al. LEAP study group. Psychological distress associated with severe lower-limb injury. *J Bone Joint Surg Am* 2003;85-A:1689–1697.
225. Van Os JP, Roumen RMH, Schoots FJ, et al. Is early osteo-synthesis safe in multiple trauma patients with severe thoracic trauma and pulmonary contusion? *J Trauma* 1994; 36:495–499.
226. Charash WE, Fabian TC, Croce MA. Delayed surgical fixation of femur fractures is a risk factor for pulmonary failure independent of thoracic trauma. *J Trauma* 1994;37: 667–671.
227. Bone LB, Babikian G, Stegemann PM. Femoral canal reaming in the polytrauma patient with chest injury: a clinical perspective. *Clin Orthop Rel Res* 1995;318:91–94.
228. Bosse MJ, MacKenzie EJ, Riemer BL, et al. Adult respiratory distress syndrome, pneumonia, and mortality following thoracic injury and a femoral fracture treated either with intramedullary nailing with reaming or with a plate: a comparative study. *J Bone Joint Surg Am* 1997;79:799–809.
229. Carlson DA, Rodman GH, Kaehr D, et al. Femur fractures in chest-injured patients: is reaming contraindicated? *J Orthop Trauma* 1998;12:164–168.
230. Baue AE. Multiple, progressive or sequential systems failure: a syndrome of the 1970s. *Arch Surg* 1975;110:779–781.
231. Border JR, Chenier R, McManamy RH, et al. Multiple systems organ failure: muscle fuel deficit with visceral protein malnutrition. *Surg Clin North Am* 1976;56:1147–1166.
232. Cerra F, Siegel J, Coleman B, et al. Septic autocannibalism: a failure of exogenous nutritional support. *Ann Surg* 1980;192:570–580.
233. McMenamy RH, Birkhahn R, Oswald G. Multiple organ systems failure: the basal state. *J Trauma* 1981;21:99–114.
234. Pape H-C, Giannoudis P, Krettek C. The timing for fracture treatment in polytrauma patients: relevance of damage control orthopaedic surgery. *Am J Surg* 2002;183: 622–629.

THE EPIDEMIOLOGY OF FRACTURES

Charles M. Court-Brown and Kenneth J. Koval

PART 1
OVERVIEW OF EPIDEMIOLOGY

CHARLES M. COURT-BROWN AND BENJAMIN C. CAESAR

Several generations of orthopaedic surgeons have understandably given most of their attention to the constantly evolving treatment methods in orthopaedic trauma. Change has been swift, and as surgeons' primary interest is the optimal care of their patients, their focus has often been on advances in treatment methods, rather than any change in patients or their fractures. There have been considerable changes not only in the type of patient presenting to orthopaedic surgeons, but also in the health systems of most countries, as well as in the economic ability of many countries to finance health. Because orthopaedic trauma absorbs a considerable proportion of most countries' health budgets, it is important to understand the frequency of musculoskeletal injury, the environment in which it occurs, and the treatment costs.

This is the first chapter on fracture epidemiology in six editions of Bucholz's *Rockwood and Green's Fractures in Adults* and, given the enormous scope of musculoskeletal trauma, an attempt has been made to define the process of change and to highlight its effect on health care systems. It is divided into two sections. In the first section, the epidemiology of a well-defined population is presented with a view to determine the incidence of various fractures and define which section of the population presents with different fracture types. The importance of osteopenic or osteoporotic fractures is highlighted, as are the changing trends. It is shown that a number of fractures that were commonly thought of as affecting young people 15 to 20 years ago should now be considered as mainly osteopenic fractures.

In the second part of the chapter, there is an in-depth analysis of the epidemiology of fractures in the United States. This information highlights the scale of the problem as it draws attention to the huge numbers of patients that present with musculoskeletal injury and the considerable strain that they place on the health care system. The requirement for hospitalization is analyzed, as is the associated disability that injury causes. There are also data on the different types of treatment employed in the many parts of the US. The next stage may be to find out why surgeons in different parts of one country use radically different treatment methods.

Both sections of the chapter draw attention to the various modes of injury and how they may be directly affected by legislation and public behavior. In some parts of the world, the incidence of serious injury after motor vehicle accidents is falling because of improved legislation regarding speeding and alcohol use. Combined with improved industrial safety legislation, this may change the spectrum of injury seen by orthopaedic surgeons, although increasing leisure time may merely increase the number of sports-related injuries

It is important that surgeons understand the epidemiology of the fractures that they treat. They often have a skewed view of which fractures are common and which fractures are merely commonly discussed. Much of the literature concerns the management of difficult fractures such as complex pelvic injuries, unstable spinal fractures, four-part proximal humeral fractures, open tibial fractures or hindfoot fractures, and it is easy to assume that surgeons will generally be required to treat these fractures. Many orthopaedic trauma surgeons work in specialized hospitals where fractures such as distal radial fractures, two-part proximal humeral fractures, ankle fractures, metacarpal and metatarsal fractures are rarely seen. As a result, they assume that these fractures are less important, easy to treat, and of little importance to the surgical community. This chapter seeks to define the incidence of different fractures and to detail the changing trends in fracture epidemiology, particularly with regard to the increasing incidence of osteopenic or osteoporotic fractures.

There is no doubt that fracture epidemiology is changing rapidly. In many countries, improvements in social conditions and general health have led to an increasingly elderly population with higher demands and greater political influence. Improvements in workplace legislation and automobile safety have led to a decline in serious fractures in younger patients. This has been helped in many countries by improved road safety legislation and stricter firearm laws. The overall effect is that osteoporotic fractures are rapidly increasing in incidence in many parts of the world to the extent that orthopaedic trauma surgeons are increasingly treating complex fractures in poor-quality bone. In a relatively short space of time, the young femoral diaphyseal fracture has given way to the periprosthetic femoral fracture, industrial injuries have declined in incidence, and grandmothers are consulting the Internet to see how their distal radial fractures should be treated.

The fracture population used in this chapter is from the Royal Infirmary of Edinburgh, Scotland, which is the only hospital dealing with orthopaedic trauma in a well-defined population. All outpatient and inpatient fractures in adults over the age of 12 years during the year 2000 were analyzed. Patients from out of the catchment area and patients who died prior to orthopaedic treatment were excluded. The clinical records and radiographs of all fractures were analyzed to exclude incorrect diagnoses and to document the mode of injury and type of fracture. During the year 2000, there were 5,953 fractures in a population of 534,715.

It is accepted that fracture epidemiology fluctuates in different parts of the world and that the spectrum of fractures presenting to different hospitals may vary considerably, but it is likely that the overall population of the Edinburgh area reflects the overall population of many European and North American areas. It is suggested that the data presented in this chapter can be extrapolated for use in other areas, although it is accepted that there will be differences based mainly on the socioeconomic status of the particular area. It is likely, however, that the trends in fracture epidemiology are broadly similar in many parts of the world.

FRACTURE INCIDENCE

The overall fracture incidence is 11.13 in 1,000 per year. The fracture incidence in males is 11.67 in 1,000 per year, and in females, it is 10.65 in 1,000 per year. These figures are similar

TABLE 4-1 The Fracture Incidences in Different Studies

	Males/1,000 Per Year	Females/1,000 Per Year	Combined/1,000 Per Year
Norway (3)	22.9	21.3	22.8
USA (4)	26	16	21
England (5)	23.5	18.8	21.1
England (4)	10.0	8.1	9.0
Malta (8)	10.0	8.0	9.0
Scotland	11.67	10.65	11.13

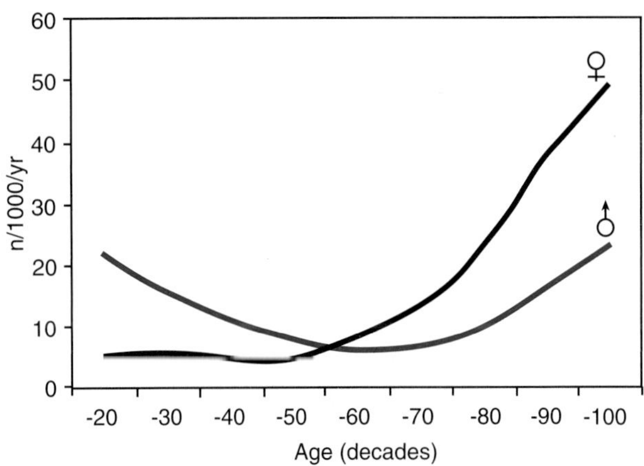

FIGURE 4-1 The age- and gender-specific incidence of fractures.

to some other studies but are less than the incidence of fractures recorded in Norway, the US, and England (Table 4-1). It is difficult to know why the incidences shown in Table 4-1 vary so considerably, and it is also difficult to explain why there is such a discrepancy between the incidence of males and females in some of the studies. A number of reasons may well influence the results of the studies shown in Table 4-1. These factors are the changing epidemiology of fractures in different parts of the world, the socioeconomic status of the areas in which the studies were undertaken, and the methodology that was used. In the Edinburgh study, all of the fractures were checked by reviewing the radiographs. In other studies, the data have been taken from emergency department records, and the incidence of some fractures may well have been overestimated. It is also important to review both in-patient and outpatient records if a true incidence is to be obtained. It is of interest that the incidence of fractures in the population over 65 years of age in Edinburgh is 23.3 in 1,000 per year, which compares with results from England and Australia (1,2). The incidence of fractures in patients aged 12 to 19 years is 13.5 in 1,000 per year, and the incidence in patients aged 40 to 49 years is 6.1 in 1,000 per year. The low incidence of fractures in middle age is also shown in Figure 4-1, which shows the age-related incidence for both men and women for all fractures. Female fracture distribution is unimodal; the peak in incidence starts about the time of menopause and rises consistently in later decades. The highest incidence is 49.7 in 1,000 per year between the ages of 90 to 99 years. In males, the fracture distribution is different. It is bimodal with peaks between 12 to 19 years (21.9 in 1,000 per year) and between 90 to 99 years (23.2 in 1,000 per year). The rise to the second peak begins later than in females, usually starting between 60 to 69 years of age. The later male peak has become more obvious in recent years because males are now living longer, and they are at greater risk of osteopenic or osteoporotic fractures.

Analysis of individual fracture incidence shows that there are eight basic distribution curves (Fig. 4-2). Most fractures have a unimodal distribution affecting either younger or older patients. Some fractures, however, have a bimodal distribution whereby young and older patients are affected, but there is a lower incidence in middle age. If one analyzes males and females separately, the distribution curves shown in Figure 4-2 can be constructed. The eight distribution curves define all fractures. The relative heights of the curves' peaks differ, but the curves remain appropriate for the overall fracture population. A type A curve is often thought of as a typical fracture curve. Both genders show a unimodal distribution, and the fractures are most commonly seen in young males and older females. Generally, the young male peak is higher than the older female peak although, not in all fractures; an example is metatarsal fractures in which the younger male peak is at a similar height to the older female peak. This type of curve is seen in fractures of the scapula, tibial diaphysis, distal radius, ankle, and metatarsus. In type B curves, there is also a young male unimodal distribution, but fractures in females occur in smaller numbers throughout the decades. Type B fractures are generally seen in the hand affecting the fingers, metacarpus, and carpus. They are usually the result of a direct blow or punch.

In type C fractures, both males and females show a unimodal distribution; fractures are rare after middle age. The incidence is less in females than males. These fractures tend to occur in the foot and affect the toes, midfoot, and talus. In type D fractures, there is a young male unimodal distribution, but the female distribution is bimodal affecting younger and older females. Generally, the second female peak starts around the time of menopause. Type D curves are seen in proximal forearm fractures, fractures of the forearm diaphyses, and tibial plafond fractures.

Type E fractures are the opposite of type B fractures. There is a unimodal female distribution affecting older females with a relatively constant, lower incidence of fractures in males throughout the decades. The type E pattern is seen in pelvic fractures, distal humeral fractures, distal radius fractures, and distal femoral fractures. This pattern may be surprising to a

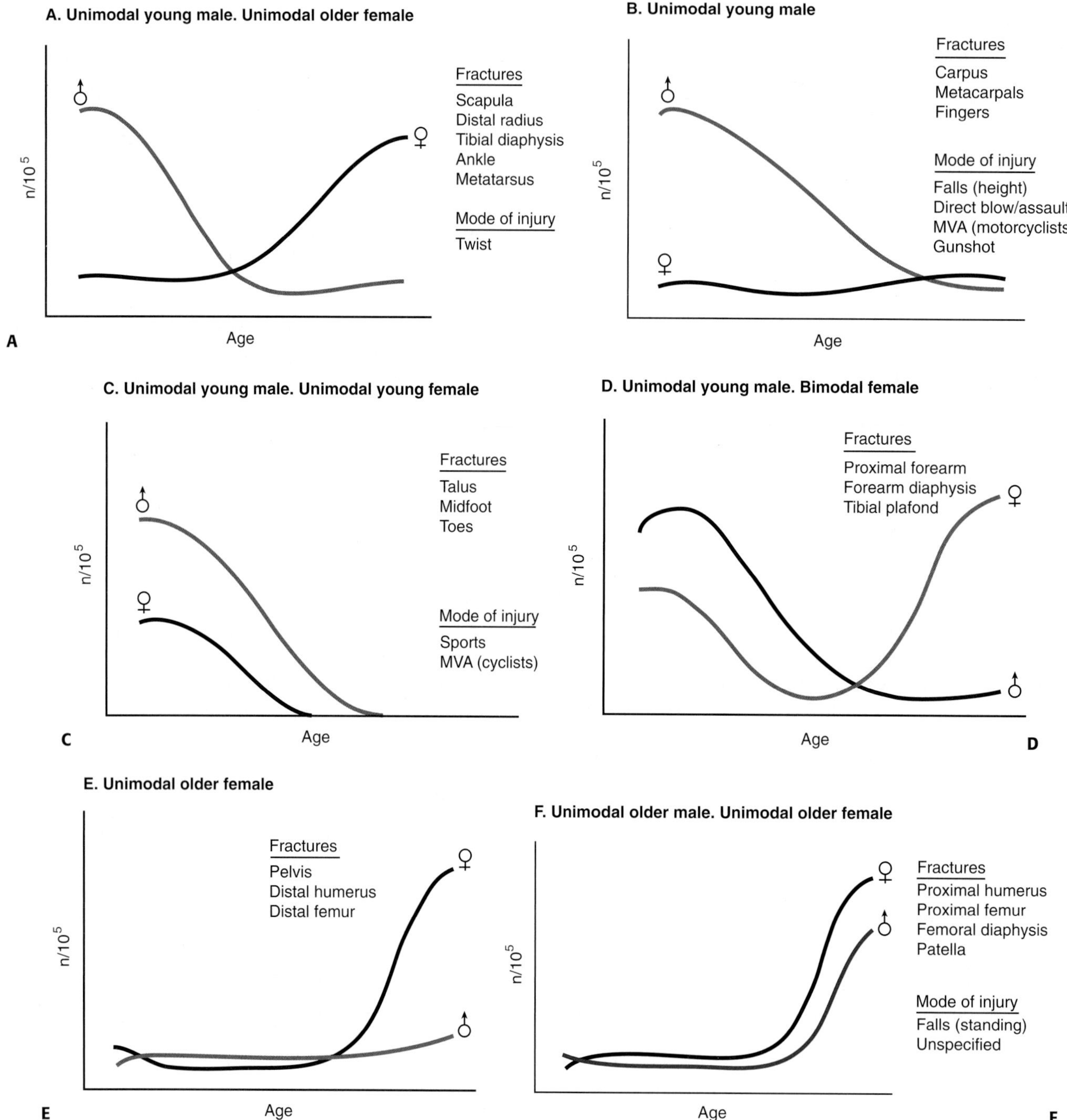

FIGURE 4-2 A–I. The distribution curves for different fractures and causes of fracture (*continues*).

number of surgeons who believe that they see a large number of young male patients with pelvic fractures, distal humeral fractures, and distal femoral fractures; but if the incidence across the community is analyzed, a type E distribution is obtained. Type F fractures are the opposite of type C fractures. In type F fractures, both males and females show a unimodal distribution affecting older patients, and the incidence is higher in females than in males. This pattern is characteristic of fractures of the proximal humerus, humeral diaphysis, proximal femur, femoral diaphysis, and patella. There is some variation regarding when the rise in fracture incidence occurs. Generally, it is earlier in females than in males and usually occurs around the time of

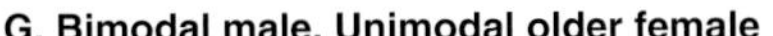

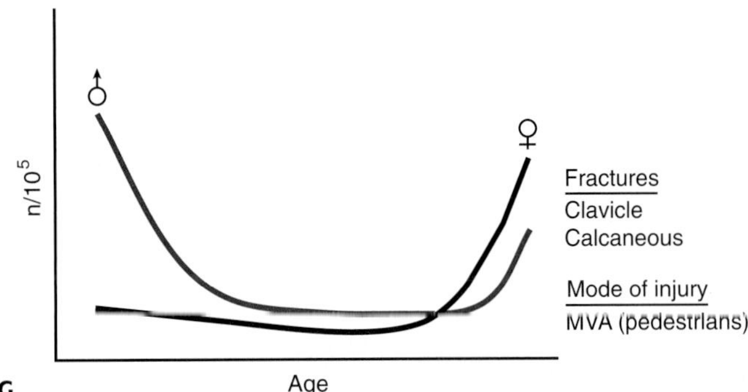

G

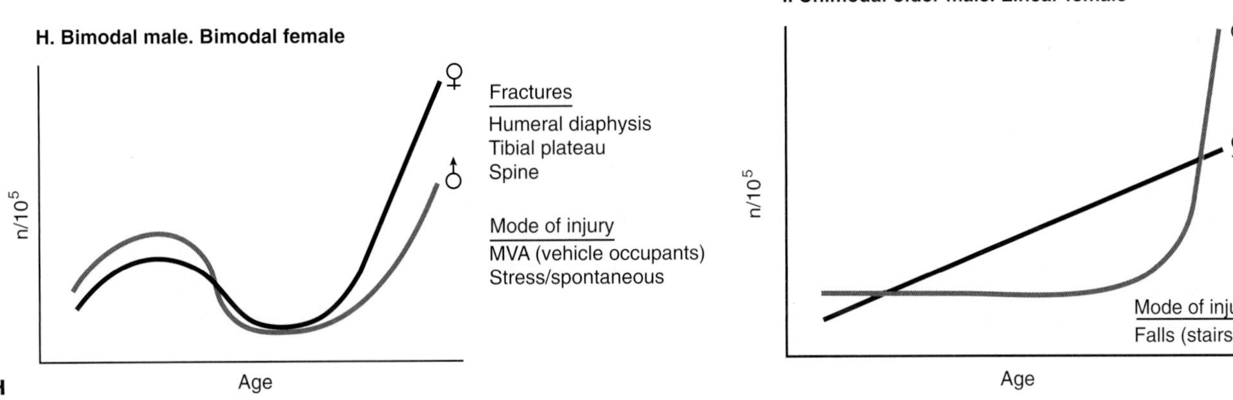

H I

FIGURE 4-2 *(continued.)*

menopause in proximal humeral fractures, humeral diaphyseal fractures, and patellar fractures, but later in femoral diaphyseal fractures and proximal femoral fractures.

In type G fractures, females show a unimodal distribution affecting older females, and males show a bimodal distribution affecting both younger and older males (although the incidence is higher in younger males). The two fractures that show this distribution are those of the calcaneus and clavicle. Type H fractures are unusual in that both males and females show a bimodal distribution. This distribution is seen in fractures of the humeral diaphysis, tibial plateau, and spine.

HOW COMMON ARE DIFFERENT FRACTURES?

There is debate about how common different fractures actually are. Studies that only examine inpatient data will obviously overestimate the frequency with which some fractures occur, and will tend to overestimate the frequency of fractures in males. Table 4-2 shows the relative frequencies of different fractures. It is obvious that fractures of the distal radius are by far the most common, and fractures of the metacarpals and proximal femur occur in approximately equal numbers. Fractures of the distal humerus, distal femur, scapula, talus, and midfoot are rare, and as a result, many surgeons will have little experience in their management. It is interesting to note that if all fractures are considered, the gender ratio is 50/50 despite many fractures having a marked male or female predominance. If the gender ratio in Table 4-2 is compared with the average patient age of the different fractures shown in Table 4-3, it can be seen that fractures with a high female predominance tend to be in patients with an older average age.

WHICH FRACTURES ARE RELATED TO OSTEOPENIA?

Analysis of the fracture distribution curves shown in Figure 4-2 shows that only types B and C are not associated with an increased incidence in older patients. Fractures related to osteopenia or osteoporosis are becoming more frequent. Traditionally, these fractures were always assumed to be those of the proximal femur, distal radius, proximal humerus, or vertebrae, but it is obvious from Table 4-3 that the pattern of osteopenic or osteoporotic fractures in the population is changing. Table 4-3 shows the different fractures listed by age with percentages of patients aged more than 65 and 75 years. The results for vertebral fractures should be ignored, as it was impossible to calculate an accurate figure for their frequency in the popula-

TABLE 4-2 Fractures Arranged in Order of Decreasing Incidence

	No.	%	$n/10^5$	Gender/Ratio
Distal Radius	1,044	17.5	195.2	31/69
Metacarpal	697	11.7	130.3	85/15
Proximal Femur	692	11.6	129.4	26/74
Finger Phalanx	574	9.6	107.3	68/32
Ankle	539	9.0	100.8	47/53
Metatarsal	403	6.8	75.4	43/57
Proximal Humerus	337	5.7	63.0	30/70
Proximal Forearm	297	5.0	55.5	46/54
Toe Phalanx	212	3.6	39.6	66/34
Clavicle	195	3.3	36.5	70/30
Carpus	159	2.7	29.7	72/28
Tibial Diaphysis	115	1.9	21.5	61/39
Pelvis	91	1.5	17.0	30/70
Forearm	74	1.2	13.8	64/36
Calcaneus	73	1.2	13.7	78/22
Proximal Tibia	71	1.2	13.3	54/46
Humeral Diaphysis	69	1.2	12.9	42/58
Patella	57	1.0	10.7	44/56
Femoral Diaphysis	55	0.9	10.3	36/64
Distal Tibia	42	0.7	7.9	57/43
Spine	40	0.7	7.5	62/38
Distal Humerus	31	0.5	5.8	29/71
Midfoot	27	0.4	5.0	48/52
Distal Femur	24	0.4	4.5	33/67
Scapula	17	0.3	3.2	59/41
Talus	17	0.3	3.2	82/18
Sesamoid	1	0.01	0.2	100/0
	5,953	100	1113.3	50/50

The incidence per 100,000 of the population is shown as is the gender ratio of males to females.

TABLE 4-3 **Fractures Arranged in Order of Decreasing Age**

	No.	Average Age (yrs)	> 65 Yrs (%)	> 75 Yrs (%)
Proximal Femur	692	80.5	91.2	78.9
Pelvis	91	69.6	72.5	57.1
Femoral Diaphysis	55	68.0	69.1	58.2
Proximal Humerus	337	64.8	57.0	36.2
Distal Femur	24	61.0	50.0	41.7
Sesamoid	1	58.0	0	0
Patella	57	56.5	49.1	22.8
Distal Humerus	31	56.4	45.2	29.0
Distal Radius	1,044	55.5	45.8	28.2
Humeral Diaphysis	69	54.8	40.5	17.4
Scapula	17	50.5	41.2	29.4
Proximal Tibia	71	48.9	23.9	12.7
Ankle	539	45.9	20.8	10.2
Proximal Forearm	297	45.7	24.2	13.5
Spine	40	43.5	17.5	12.5
Metatarsal	403	42.8	14.2	5.7
Calcaneus	73	40.4	12.3	4.1
Tibial Diaphysis	115	40.0	17.4	11.3
Distal Tibia	42	39.1	14.3	7.1
Clavicle	195	38.3	17.4	12.3
Finger Phalanges	574	36.2	10.6	5.1
Midfoot	27	36.0	0	0
Toe Phalanges	212	35.3	6.5	4.6
Forearm	74	34.6	13.5	12.2
Talus	17	30.5	0	0
Metacarpals	697	29.9	5.5	3.6
	5,953	49.1	33.0	22.6

The percentages of patients over 65 and 75 years of age are also shown.

tion. It is often difficult to age a vertebral fracture, and many patients with osteoporotic vertebral fractures never present to a hospital. The literature indicates that vertebral fractures are common (3), however, and it seems likely that their incidence may be similar to that of distal radius fractures.

If fractures of the proximal radius and proximal humerus are taken as representative of osteoporotic fractures, we can see from Table 4-3 that today many fractures that were formerly thought to occur in younger patients can now be thought of as osteopenic or osteoporotic. Table 4-3 shows that fractures of the pelvis, femoral diaphysis, distal femur, patella, distal humerus, humeral diaphysis, and scapula all have descriptive indices that suggest that they are osteopenic. The percentage of patients over 65 and 75 years of age is similar to fractures of the proximal humerus or distal radius. Table 4-3 confirms the very rapid change in the epidemiology of fractures and indicates that fractures that many surgeons now treat occur in older patients as a result of age-related osteopenia rather than in younger patients as a result of high-energy injury.

OPEN FRACTURES

The incidence of open fractures in the Edinburgh population during the year 2000 is shown in Table 4-4. This shows that open fractures most commonly occur in the leg and foot, and the tibial diaphysis and the distal tibia are most commonly affected. Open fractures of the fingers are also fairly common but are rarely severe. This is in contrast to most of the open fractures of the thigh, leg, and foot, which are associated with a high incidence of Gustilo type III open fractures. Table 4-4 also shows that a number of fractures were not associated with an open wound during the year of the study. This is not to suggest that open fractures in these areas do not occur, but they are clearly very rare, and when they do occur are often associated with very significant soft tissue damage and other musculoskeletal injuries.

ASSOCIATED INJURIES

The 5,953 fractures occurred in 5,545 patients. Isolated fractures occurred in 94.4% of the patients, and 4.6% presented with two fractures. The remaining 1% presented with more than two fractures (range, three to nine fractures). Table 4-5 shows the numbers of other fractures that were associated with each index fracture. The ratio of other fractures to the index fracture is also shown. When this is one, it means that on average, the index fracture is associated with one other fracture. Table 4-5 lists the fractures according to the average number of other fractures that are associated with the index fracture. It is obvious that foot fractures are associated with the highest incidence of other fractures, but that spinal fractures, pelvic fractures, fractures around the knee, distal tibial fractures, and fractures of the humeral diaphysis and distal humerus are associated with a significant number of other fractures. Table 4-5 also lists the

TABLE 4-4 Fractures Arranged in Order of Decreasing Incidence of Open Fractures

	No.	Open (%)	Gustilo III (%)
Tibial Diaphysis	115	19.1	54.5
Distal Tibia	42	16.6	71.3
Finger Phalanges	574	12.5	2.8
Talus	17	11.8	100
Midfoot	27	11.1	100
Forearm	74	9.5	0
Distal Femur	24	8.3	100
Femoral Diaphysis	55	7.2	75
Toe Phalanges	212	6.6	28.6
Humeral Diaphysis	69	4.3	33.3
Patella	57	3.5	50
Metatarsal	403	3.5	21.4
Proximal Tibia	71	2.8	50
Calcaneus	73	2.7	50
Ankle	539	1.7	33.3
Proximal Forearm	297	1.3	0
Pelvis	91	1.1	100
Metacarpals	697	1.0	0
Distal Radius	1,044	0.7	14.3
Spine	40	0	0
Clavicle	195	0	0
Scapula	17	0	0
Proximal Humerus	337	0	0
Distal Humerus	31	0	0
Carpus	159	0	0
Proximal Femur	692	0	0
Sesamoid	1	0	0
	5,953	3.1	22.8

The incidence of Gustilo type III open fractures is also shown in this table.

TABLE 4-5 The Numbers of Index Fractures, Associated Fractures, and the Ratio of the Two

	Index Fracture	Other Fractures	Ratio of Other Fractures/Index	
Talus	17	48	2.82	Calcaneus (19.4%) Metatarsal (12.9%) Spine (6.4%)
Midfoot	27	41	1.52	Metatarsal (24.4%) Calcaneus (9.8%) Spine (5.9%)
Spine	40	48	1.2	Calcaneus (13.0%) Distal Radius (13.0%) Proximal Forearm (9.3%)
Calcaneus	73	31	0.68	Spine (14.6%) Metatarsal (14.6%) Talus (14.6%)
Distal Femur	24	14	0.58	Proximal Tibia (21.4%) Patella (14.3%) Spine (14.3%)
Distal Tibia	42	17	0.41	Tibia Diaphysis (41.2%) Distal Radius (17.6%) Proximal Tibia (11.8%)
Pelvis	91	37	0.40	Distal Radius (21.6%) Spine (13.5%) Proximal Humerus (13.5%)
Proximal Tibia	71	28	0.39	Spine (17.9%) Calcaneus (14.3%) Distal Femur (10.7%)
Humeral Diaphysis	69	22	0.32	Spine (13.6%) Distal Radius (13.6%) Proximal Radius (13.6%)
Distal Humerus	31	10	0.32	Proximal Forearm (40%) Distal Radius (20%) Spine (20%)
Femoral Diaphysis	55	15	0.27	Forearm Diaphysis (11.8%) Distal Radius (11.8%) Patella (11.8%)
Forearm Diaphysis	74	19	0.26	Metacarpal (26.3%) Clavicle (10.5%) Humerus Diaphysis (10.5%)
Scapula	17	4	0.23	Proximal Humerus (50.0%) Proximal Femur (25.0%) Distal Radius (25.0%)
Patella	57	13	0.23	Distal Femur (15.4%) Other Patella (15.4%) Spine (15.4%)
Tibial Diaphysis	115	21	0.18	Distal Tibia (33.3%) Other Tibia Diaphysis (19.0%) Metatarsal (9.5%)

(Continued)

TABLE 4-5 Continued

	Index Fracture	Other Fractures	Ratio of Other Fractures/Index	
Proximal Forearm	297	50	0.17	Proximal Humerus (16.0%) Proximal Forearm (12.0%) Distal Radius (10.0%)
Proximal Humerus	337	48	0.14	Proximal Femur (18.7%) Proximal Forearm (16.7%) Distal Radius (14.6%)
Carpus	159	16	0.10	Distal Radius (22.2%) Proximal Radius (22.2%) Metacarpal (11.1%)
Metatarsal	403	64	0.11	Other Metatarsals (31.2%) Calcaneus (10.9%) Talus (9.4%)
Distal Radius	1044	92	0.09	Other Distal Radius (20.6%) Proximal Femur (13.0%) Proximal Humerus (7.6%)
Clavicle	195	15	0.08	Metatarsal (26.7%) Proximal Humerus (20%) Spine (13.3%)
Proximal Femur	692	46	0.07	Distal Radius (26.1%) Proximal Humerus (19.6%) Proximal Forearm (8.7%)
Metacarpals	697	131	0.04	Other Metacarpals (79.4%) Phalanges (6.9%) Forearm Diaphysis (3.8%)
Finger Phalanges	574	100	0.04	Metacarpal (76.0%) Distal Radius (9.0%) Proximal Humerus (4.0%)
Ankle	539	24	0.04	Calcaneus (12.5%) Distal Radius (12.5%) Metatarsal (12.5%)
Toe Phalanges	212	2	0.01	Distal Radius (100%)
Sesamoid	1	0	0	
	5953	973	0.16	

Note that any ratio >1 means that there are as many associated fractures as index fractures. The table also shows the three most common associated fractures for each index fracture.

three fractures that are most commonly associated with each index fracture. It shows that associated fractures are usually situated near to the index fracture, but that several fractures are associated with spinal fractures. Table 4-5 shows that that the relationship between spinal and calcaneal fractures is important, but also shows that spinal fractures are associated with fractures of the talus, midfoot, distal femur, proximal tibia, patella, and pelvis, in particular.

MODE OF INJURY

There were 12 categories of modes of injury, which were recorded during the study period (Table 4-6). Gunshot fractures are uncommon in Scotland, and only one occurred in the study period. All other common modes of injuries were seen. The section labelled "Other" in Table 4-6 contains the patients who could not or would not remember the cause of injury.

By far, the most common cause of fracture is a fall from a standing height. About 45% of patients sustained a fracture in this way, and Table 4-6 shows that they are generally elderly, and about 70% are female. The other common causes of fracture are a direct blow, an assault, or a sports injury. Direct blows are the opposite of standing falls in that they mainly affect young males. Sports injuries contain a heterogeneous group of injuries caused by twists, falls, and direct blows, but they also predominantly affect young males. Motor vehicle accidents were surprisingly uncommon, causing only 7.2% of the fractures. The United Kingdom has the one of the lowest incidences of mortality related to motor vehicle accidents in the world, and it is likely that the morbidity of motor vehicle accidents in the United Kingdom is also low. It is possible to construct age and gender curves for modes of injury in the same way as can be done for individual fractures. There are nine such curves (Fig. 4-2).

Twisting Injuries

These are relatively infrequent (Table 4-6), and tend to affect young males or older females. Thus, they have a type A distribution (Fig. 4-2). Table 4-7 shows that twisting injuries usually cause lower limb fractures, and most upper limb twisting fractures occur in the fingers. The spectrum of fractures caused by twisting injuries is similar in the three age ranges shown in Table 4-8. Metatarsal and ankle fractures are most common,

TABLE 4-6 The Average Age, Incidence, and Gender Ratio for Each Mode of Injury

	Average Age (yr)	Incidence (%)	Gender Ratio (%)
Twist	45.0	6.5	36/64
Fall from standing height	64.6	45.3	29/71
Fall down stairs or slope	49.1	4.1	40/60
Fall from height	38.2	5.8	72/28
Direct blow/assault/crush	32.3	14.1	79/21
Sport	25.6	12.8	83/17
MVA (vehicle occupant)	37.5	1.8	49/51
MVA (pedestrian)	48.3	1.7	52/48
MVA (motorcyclist)	31.2	1.4	89/11
MVA (cyclist)	29.5	2.3	76/24
Stress/spontaneous	58.9	0.5	30/70
Others	56.9	3.7	46/54

Abbreviation: MVA, motor vehicle accident.

TABLE 4-7 The Relative Frequencies of Upper Limb, Lower Limb, and Axial Skeleton Fractures for Each Mode of Injury

	Upper Limb (%)	Lower Limb (%)	Axial Skeleton (%)
Twist	2.7	97.3	0
Fall (standing)	58.7	40.0	2.3
Fall (stairs/slope)	45.6	51.9	2.5
Fall (height)	40.8	51.5	7.7
Direct blow/assault	79.9	19.8	0.3
Sport	78.7	20.9	0.2
MVA (occupant)	42.4	48.5	9.1
MVA (pedestrian)	34.3	55.5	10.1
MVA (motorcyclist)	65.8	32.9	1.3
MVA (cyclist)	90.2	8.3	1.5
Stress/spontaneous	13.3	80.0	6.6

MVA, motor vehicle accident.

TABLE 4-8 The Distribution of the Three Most Common Fractures for Each Mode of Injury

	12 to 39 years	40 to 59 years	60 to 99 years
Twist	Metatarsal (42.2%) Ankle (41.1%) Toe (3.8%)	Metatarsal (48.3%) Ankle (46.0%) Calcaneus (1.6%)	Ankle (51.1%) Metatarsal (37.2%) Proximal Tibia (2.1%)
Fall (standing)	Distal Radius (20.7%) Metacarpal (17.0%) Proximal Forearm (12.0%)	Distal Radius (25.1%) Ankle (15.9%) Proximal Forearm (10.3%)	Proximal Femur (33.1%) Distal Radius (25.7%) Proximal Humerus (8.3%)
Fall (stairs/slopes)	Ankle (22.5%) Metacarpal (15.7%) Proximal Forearm (11.2%)	Metatarsal (20.3%) Ankle (14.5%) Distal Radius (10.1%)	Distal Radius (22.8%) Proximal Humerus (11.4%) Metatarsal (11.4%)
Fall (height)	Calcaneus (14.1%) Metatarsal (13.1%) Distal Radius (11.6%)	Distal Radius (22.1%) Calcaneus (13.9%) Ankle (7.0%)	Distal Radius (20.7%) Proximal Forearm (11.3%) Calcaneus (9.4%)
Direct blow/assault	Metacarpal (53.7%) Finger (17.4%) Toe (6.2%)	Finger (37.7%) Metacarpal (16.0%) Toe (15.1%)	Finger (47.1%) Toe (11.8%) Distal Radius (11.8%)
Sports	Distal Radius (17.5%) Metacarpal (15.6%) Clavicle (9.0%)	Finger (29.0%) Distal Radius (14.5%) Proximal Humerus (11.6%)	Distal Radius (35.0%) Ankle (15.0%) Finger (10.0%)
MVA (occupants)	Femoral Diaphysis (13.8%) Distal Radius (12.3%) Metatarsal (9.3%)	Distal Femur (11.1%) Proximal Tibia (11.1%) Ankle (11.1%)	Distal Radius (21.1%) Spine (10.5%) Ankle (10.5%)
MVA (pedestrians)	Tibial Diaphysis (28.6%) Ankle (9.5%) Spine (9.5%)	Tibial Diaphysis (19.0%) Proximal Tibia (14.3%) Ankle (14.3%)	Proximal Tibia (21.1%) Metatarsal (15.8%) Tibial Diaphysis (10.5%)
MVA (motorcyclist)	Distal Radius (20.6%) Clavicle (14.3%) Metacarpal (11.1%)	Finger (40.0%) Distal Radius (20.0%) Tibial Diaphysis (6.6%)	
MVA (cyclist)	Proximal Forearm (23.3%) Clavicle (17.5%) Distal Radius (11.6%)	Clavicle (23.1%) Finger (19.2%) Proximal Humerus (15.4%)	
Stress/ spontaneous	Metatarsal (50.0%) Proximal Femur (25.0%) Tibial Diaphysis (12.5%)	Metatarsal (60.0%) Proximal Femur (20.0%) Finger (20.0%)	Proximal Femur (66.6%) Femoral Diaphysis (16.6%) Metatarsal (16.6%)

Note that the fractures are separated by age.
MVA, motor vehicle accident.

representing 80% to 90% of twisting fractures in all three age categories.

Falls From a Standing Height

This is the most common mode of injury, and a Scandinavian study shows that fractures related to falls from a standing height are increasing in frequency (4). About 45% of injuries are caused by a simple fall, and about 70% occur in older females. These injuries have a type F distribution pattern. The age and gender incidences are very similar to those of the proximal humerus with a rise in the incidence of fall-related fractures in females at about the time of menopause (40 to 49 years of age) with a later rise in males (60 to 69 years). Table 4-7 shows that the upper limb is more commonly affected than the lower limb, and that fractures of the axial skeleton are rare. Table 4-8 shows that in younger and middle-aged patients, fractures of the distal radius are most common, although in older patients, proximal femoral fractures are the most common fracture to be caused by a fall from a standing height.

Falls Down Stairs or Slopes

These fractures are unusual in that they do not correspond to types A through H (Fig. 4-2). Females present with a linear distribution, whereas males show a unimodal pattern with a rise in incidence at about 70 years of age. This pattern has been designated as type I. Fractures down stairs or slopes are relatively uncommon compared with falls from a standing height, and slightly more females than males are affected. There is a similar distribution of upper and lower limb fractures, although there are few fractures in the axial skeleton. Table 4-8 shows that there is a different distribution of fractures depending on the age of the patient; ankle fractures are common in younger patients, and distal radial fractures are common in older patients.

Direct Blows or Assaults

Predictably, these are common in young males (Table 4-6) and show a type B pattern (Fig. 4-2). Fractures following direct blows are relatively common, with only falls from a standing height producing more fractures. Most direct blows are either punches or kicks, which accounts for the high incidence of metacarpal, finger, and toe fractures detailed in Table 4-8. The distribution of fractures is similar in the three age categories listed in Table 4-8, although it is interesting to note that finger fractures, rather than metacarpal fractures, become more common in older patients.

Falls From a Height

This category contains all falls from more than 6 feet, so the type of injury will vary, depending on the height from which the patient falls. Overall, these account for approximately 6% of all fractures (Table 4-6) and have a type B distribution that is more common in younger males (Fig. 4-2). The fractures caused by falls from a height tend to be more severe than those produced by twists, standing falls, or a direct blow, but Table 4-8 shows that the most common fractures that are caused by falls from a height are in the feet, ankle, and forearms. Falls from a height are the principal cause of calcaneal fractures, and Table 4-7 shows that they are associated with a significant incidence of fractures to the pelvis and spine.

Sports Injuries

This is a very heterogeneous group of patients who present after twisting injuries, falls, direct blows, motor vehicle accidents, and cycling accidents. They can also present with stress fractures. It could be argued that it is, in fact, the least worthwhile category, but sports injuries are common (Table 4-6). In general, they show a type C pattern, and young males and females are mainly affected, although Table 4-6 shows that overall more males than females sustain sports-related fractures. Table 4-7 shows that almost 80% of sports fractures are in the upper limb, and Table 4-8 indicates that almost all of the common sports-related fractures are in the upper limb, with ankle fractures occurring more commonly in older sportsmen and women.

Motor Vehicle Accidents

It is often assumed that motor vehicle accidents cause most fractures, but Table 4-6 shows that this is not the case. As has already been pointed out, the United Kingdom has a low mortality rate related to motor vehicle accidents, and it may well also have a low morbidity rate. Other countries have less stringent legislation concerning speeding and alcohol abuse and may have a higher incidence of motor vehicle accidents, although, as in Scotland, it is still probably falls, direct blows, and sports that will cause most fractures.

Vehicle Occupants

Table 4-6 shows that there is an equal gender distribution in fractures seen in vehicle occupants. Both males and females show a bimodal distribution with younger and older vehicle occupants being affected, which is a type H pattern. There is a high incidence of pelvic and spinal fractures (Table 4-7), and slightly more lower limb fractures are seen than upper limb fractures. Table 4-8 indicates that the fractures tend to be severe with a high incidence of femoral diaphyseal fractures, distal femoral fractures, and proximal tibial fractures.

Pedestrians

Pedestrians tend to be older than vehicle occupants (Table 4-6). There is an approximately equal gender ratio, and a review of the distribution of fractures shown in Table 4-7 shows that pedestrians have the highest incidence of pelvic and spinal fractures. Lower limb fractures are more common than upper limb fractures. As with vehicle occupants, the fractures are often severe, with a high incidence of tibial diaphyseal fractures and proximal tibial fractures.

Motorcyclists

Predictably, motorcyclists have a type B distribution predominantly affecting young males. Table 4-6 shows that about nine males are injured for every female. The incidence of pelvic and spinal fractures is low, and it is interesting to observe that the incidence of upper limb fractures is consistently higher than the incidence of lower limb fractures. This is probably because motorcyclists that have spinal, pelvic, and/or a severe lower limb injury often die at the scene of the accident. Motorcyclists over the age of 60 are relatively uncommon, but analysis of the common fractures in the two younger age groups shows a fairly widespread spectrum of injuries.

Cyclists

As with motorcyclists, cycle injuries mainly affect young males, but about 25% of the injuries are in young females; therefore, the distribution is type C. The majority of fractures are in the upper limb, and fractures of the axial skeleton are very rare. Table 4-8 shows a similar distribution of fracture in younger and middle-aged patients. There were insufficient elderly cyclists to justify an analysis of their injuries.

Stress/Spontaneous Fractures

These have been combined, as many spontaneous fractures are actually insufficiency fractures occurring in older patients. The combined fracture groups have a type H distribution with a bimodal distribution in both males and females. Fatigue fractures have a type C distribution with younger males and females being affected, and insufficiency fractures have a type E pattern mainly affecting older females. The fractures are usually in the lower limb, and Table 4-8 shows that the proximal femur, metatarsus, and femoral and tibial diaphyses are commonly affected.

Other Modes of Injury

Approximately 4% of patients either had a different mode of injury or had no definite history, usually because of dementia, intoxication, or epileptic fits. There were 41 (19.4%) finger fractures secondary to hyperextension or cutting injuries. Most of the rest of the unspecified mode of injury group probably sustained their fracture in simple falls, and 25.9% of the patients presented with distal radial fractures, 19.9% with proximal femoral fractures, and 5.1% presented with proximal humeral fractures.

GUNSHOT INJURIES

Information regarding the epidemiology of fractures caused by firearms is sparse. They are relatively uncommon in Europe, but the North American literature strongly suggests that they have a type B distribution and are the most common in young males. Gunshot mortality and morbidity rates are greatest in the US where the large urban level I trauma centers see a disproportionate number of fractures caused by firearms. In one level I trauma center, a 1-year analysis showed that firearms caused 15% of all fractures requiring surgical intervention (5). Most fractures involved the femur (22%), hand (18%), tibia (14%), forearm (14%), and humerus (10%). It would seem that the problem of firearm-related fractures is worsening.

TABLE 4-9 Descriptive Indices for the Different Types of Clavicle Fracture

	%	Average Age (yrs)	Gender Ratio (M/F)	Distribution Curve
Medial	4.1	53.5	75/25	Type A
Diaphyseal	68.2	33.2	70/30	Type G
Lateral	27.7	48.6	68/32	Type A

SPECIFIC FRACTURE TYPES

Clavicle

Fractures of the clavicle are most commonly seen in young males, but they are increasingly seen in older patients, and overall, clavicle fractures actually have a type G distribution with an increasing incidence in older males and females. Clavicle fractures are usually subdivided according to their location, and the different characteristics of fractures of the diaphysis and medial and lateral ends of the clavicle are shown in Table 4-9. This shows that medial clavicle fractures are uncommon, and that both medial and lateral clavicle fractures have a type A pattern affecting younger males and older females. Diaphyseal fractures predominantly occur in young males, but there is a late increase in incidence in older males and females. They therefore show a type G pattern. Clavicle fractures usually follow low-energy injuries with 31% caused by falls from a standing height, 31% by sports injuries, and 12% in cycling accidents.

Scapula

These are very rare fractures and have a type A distribution. In young males, they tend to be high-energy injuries, and in older females, they usually follow low-energy injuries. Table 4-10 shows the descriptive indices for extra-articular scapular fractures and for intra-articular fractures involving the glenoid. It shows that both fracture types have a type A pattern affecting young males and older females, but extra-articular fractures are

TABLE 4-10 Descriptive Indices for Extra- and Intra-articular Scapular Fractures

	%	Average Age (yrs)	Gender Ratio (M/F)	Distribution Curve
Extra-articular	64.7	44.2	73/27	Type A
Intra-articular	35.3	62.0	50/50	Type A

more common. The majority of glenoid fractures actually occur in older females following low-energy injuries.

Proximal Humerus

These are common fractures (Table 4-2) that usually occur in older females and have a type F distribution. Most are low-energy injuries, and if it is assumed that the unspecified modes of injuries were mainly falls from a standing height, it is likely that about 78% of proximal humeral fractures are caused by simple falls.

Humeral Diaphysis

Humeral diaphyseal fractures also have a type H distribution mainly with a bimodal distribution in both males and females. The peaks in older patients are higher than those in younger patients, and Table 4-3 indicates that a high proportion of patients are over 65 years of age at the time of fracture. About 62% of these fractures are caused by falls from a standing height, and approximately 4% are pathological, secondary to a metastatic deposit.

Distal Humerus

Distal humeral fractures are relatively uncommon. Surgeons may be surprised that they have a type E distribution mainly affecting older females, but there is a high incidence of OTA type A transcondylar distal humeral fractures in this age group. The type C bicondylar fracture is rare in comparison. Table 4-3 shows a high incidence of fractures in patients over the age of 65 years, and the distal humerus must be regarded as an osteopenic fracture, as its age distribution is very similar to that of the distal radius. About 68% of distal humeral fractures are caused by falls from a standing height. A further 13% are sports-related injuries occurring in younger patients.

Proximal Forearm

These common fractures comprise 5% of all fractures. Overall, they show a type D distribution, but Table 4-11 shows that if they are subdivided into their different fracture types, their distribution changes. Olecranon fractures and fractures affecting both the proximal radius and ulna occur more commonly in older patients, and therefore have a type F pattern. Radial head fractures have a type H pattern with bimodal curves for both males and females, and radial neck fractures show a type A pattern with younger males and older females being affected. Table 4-11 also shows that radial head fractures account for about 56% of all proximal forearm fractures, with olecranon and radial neck fractures occurring in about 20% of patients. Fractures of both the proximal radius and ulna are relatively unusual.

Forearm Diaphysis

Fractures of the diaphysis of the radius and ulna account for 1.2% of all fractures. Overall, they have a type D pattern. Analysis of the three different forearm fractures, the isolated ulna, isolated radius, and both radius and ulna shows that each has a different fracture pattern (Table 4-12). Isolated ulna fractures have a type H pattern with a bimodal distribution in both males and females, whereas isolated radial fractures have a type A pattern with young males and older females presenting with these injuries. Fractures of both the radius and ulna occur mainly in young males, and they show a type B pattern. Sports injuries are the most common cause of forearm fractures (26%) followed by a direct blow to the forearm (20%) and falls from a standing height (19%).

Distal Radius and Ulna

These are the most common fractures encountered by orthopaedic surgeons (Table 4-2), and they have a Type A pattern. Level I trauma centers will see a number of young males with high-energy distal radial fractures, but most occur in older females. Altogether, approximately 75% of distal radial fractures occur in falls from a standing height with about 13% occurring in sports injuries.

TABLE 4-11 Descriptive Indices for the Different Types of Proximal Forearm Fractures

	(%)	Age (yrs)	Gender Ratio (M/F)	Distribution Curve
Olecranon	19.9	59.1	47/53	Type F
Radial Head	56.2	40.5	46/54	Type H
Radial Neck	19.9	48.5	44/56	Type A
Radius and Ulna	4.0	61.3	36/64	Type F

TABLE 4-12 Descriptive Indices for the Different Types of Forearm Diaphyseal Fracture

	(%)	Average Age (yrs)	Gender Ratio (M/F)	Distribution Curve
Ulna	51.3	39.0	45/55	Type H
Radius	23.0	36.1	76/24	Type A
Radius and Ulna	25.7	24.7	63/37	Type B

TABLE 4-13 Descriptive Indices for Carpal Fractures

	%	Average Age (yrs)	Gender Ratio (M/F)	Distribution Curve
Scaphoid	82.4	30.1	72/28	Type B
Non-scaphoid	17.6	46.7	71/29	Type A

Carpus

Most carpal fractures involve the scaphoid (carpal navicular) bone. Table 4-13 shows a breakdown of carpal fractures according to whether or not they involve the scaphoid. It can be seen that patients with scaphoid fractures tend to be younger than those with other carpal fractures. The gender ratio is similar, but scaphoid fractures have a type B pattern with a unimodal young male distribution, whereas nonscaphoid carpal fractures show a type A pattern with fractures also occurring older females.

Metacarpal Fractures

Metacarpal fractures are the second most common fractures seen by orthopaedic surgeons (Table 4-2). They have a type B distribution, and most fractures occur in young men. About 55% occur as a result of a punch or direct blow to the hand. About 6% of patients have multiple metacarpal fractures, and the rest have isolated fractures. Sixty percent of the fractures are in the little finger, 15% in the ring finger, 7% in the middle finger, 8% in the index finger and 10% are in the thumb.

Finger Fractures

As with metacarpal fractures, these are common fractures with a type B pattern. Most finger fractures present in young males. About 34% occur following a punch or direct blow to the fingers, and 21% occur in a fall from a standing height. As with metacarpal fractures, 6% of these fractures are multiple, and the rest are isolated. Thirty percent occur in the little finger, 22% in the ring finger, 18% in the middle finger, 12% in the index finger, and 18% occur in the thumb.

Proximal Femoral Fractures

These are common fractures, and it is generally accepted that, as with other osteopenic fractures, they are increasing in frequency in many parts of the world. The fractures have been subdivided into femoral head fractures, subcapital fractures, and intertrochanteric fractures. Basicervical fractures are included in the subcapital group, and subtrochanteric fractures are combined with femoral diaphyseal fractures.

Femoral head fractures are extremely rare, and the average age and gender ratio shown in Table 4-14 have been taken from the literature. The literature also suggests that femoral head fractures have a type B pattern, but there are insufficient data to measure these statistics precisely. Both subcapital and intertrochanteric fractures have a type F pattern with an increasing incidence in both older males and females. Until relatively recently, proximal femoral fractures were assumed to be a problem predominantly in females, but with increasing male life expectancy, the incidence in older males is now higher and likely to become greater in years to come. Analysis of the data indicates that about 92% of proximal femoral fractures occur as a result of a fall from a standing height.

TABLE 4-14 Descriptive Indices for the Different Types of Proximal Femoral Fracture

	%	Average Age (yrs)	Gender Ratio (M/F)	Distribution Curve
Femoral Head	0.3	40.5	73/27	Type B
Sub-capital	46.3	77.9	27/73	Type F
Inter-trochanteric	53.4	82.1	25/75	Type F

The average, gender ratio, and distribution curve for femoral head fractures has been taken from the literature.

Femoral Fractures

This category includes both subtrochanteric fractures and femoral diaphyseal fractures. Their descriptive indices are shown in Table 4-15. Subtrochanteric fractures affect older males and females, are similar to subcapital and intertrochanteric fractures, and have a type F pattern. Falls from a standing height cause 70% of subtrochanteric fractures.

Femoral diaphyseal fractures have a type A pattern mainly affecting young males and older females. The early male peak is not very pronounced, and there seems no doubt that the epidemiology of femoral diaphyseal fractures is changing rap-

TABLE 4-15 Descriptive Indices for Femoral Diaphyseal Fractures

	%	Average Age (yrs)	Gender Ratio (M/F)	Distribution Curve
Sub-trochanteric	30.1	76.5	47/53	Type F
Diaphysis	69.9	62.4	32/68	Type A

idly. Table 4-15 shows that the average age of patients with femoral diaphyseal fractures is 62.4 years and that the majority of patients are female. This is because periprosthetic and insufficiency femoral fractures are becoming common and are tending to replace the young femoral fracture, which is declining in incidence in many parts of the world due to improved car design and better road safety legislation. Clearly, this does not apply uniformly throughout the world, but presumably many countries that currently have a high incidence of femoral fractures in younger patients will experience change over the next few decades. The mode of injury in younger patients remains motor vehicle accidents; falls from a standing height cause the majority of femoral diaphyseal fractures in the elderly.

Distal Femoral Fractures

Distal femoral fractures are relatively uncommon and, as with femoral diaphyseal fractures, they now tend to occur in older patients. Table 4-3 shows that 50% occur in patients over 65 years of age. The age-related descriptive indices are very similar to those of the proximal humerus, and the distal femoral fracture must now be regarded as an osteopenic fracture. They have a type E pattern. About 50% are caused by falls, but in younger patients, motor vehicle accidents and sports accidents cause distal femoral fractures.

Patella Fractures

Table 4-3 shows that patellar fractures should also be regarded as osteopenic fractures. Approximately 50% of patellar fractures occur in patients over 65 years of age, although the gender ratio is more even than in most osteopenic fractures. They have a type F pattern, and patellar fractures present in both older males and females. About 75% of patellar fractures are caused by falls from a standing height. The majority of the rest are caused by falls down stairs or from a height.

Tibial Plateau Fractures

Tibial plateau fractures have a type H pattern with a bimodal distribution in both male and female patients. They account for 1.2% of all fractures. In younger patients, they are usually high-energy injuries caused by motor vehicle accidents, falls from a height, or sports injuries. In older patients, the most common cause of tibial plateau fractures is a motor vehicle accident when the patient is a pedestrian struck by an automobile.

Tibial Diaphyseal Fractures

Despite the considerable number of articles written about the management of tibial diaphyseal fractures, they are comparatively uncommon, accounting for only 1.9% of all fractures. They do have the highest incidence of open fractures, however (Table 4-4). They have a type A pattern that is more common in younger males and older females. The young male peak is higher than the older female peak, and the fracture is therefore more common in males. In younger patients, tibial fractures are usually caused by motor vehicle accidents and sports injuries, and in older patients, they often occur in pedestrians or as a result of a fall from a standing height. The epidemiology of tibial diaphyseal fractures is discussed in more detail in Chapter 52 where data from the Edinburgh Unit collected between 1988 to 1999 are shown. The incidence of tibial fractures has decreased in the last decade because of a decrease in the incidence of tibial fractures in young men. Otherwise, the earlier data are very similar.

Distal Tibial Fractures

Distal tibial fractures are comparatively unusual fractures accounting for only 0.7% of all fractures. They are common in younger patients, but have a type D pattern indicating that there is a second peak in older female patients. As with tibial diaphyseal fractures, there is a high incidence of open fractures, and the majority are Gustilo type III in severity. Distal tibial fractures are usually the result of high-energy injuries. In younger patients, they are caused by falls from a height, sports injuries, or motor vehicle accidents. In older patients, they are caused by falls from a standing height or motor vehicle accidents.

Ankle Fractures

Ankle fractures are very common, accounting for 9% of all fractures. Overall, they have a type A pattern, but conventionally, ankle fractures are classified according to the number of malleoli involved and the location of the fibular fracture. Table 4-16 shows the descriptive indices of medial malleolar, lateral malleolar, bimalleolar, trimalleolar, and suprasyndesmotic fractures. They are somewhat different, and only the lateral malleolar fractures have a type A pattern affecting young males and older females. Medial malleolar fractures have a type D pattern affecting younger adults of both genders, with a higher incidence in young males. There is, however, a second peak in older females.

TABLE 4-16 Descriptive Indices for the Different Types of Ankle Fractures

	%	Average Age (yrs)	Gender Ratio (M/F)	Distribution Curve
Medial Malleolus	4.9	34.0	64/36	Type D
Lateral Malleolus	63.5	44.4	52/48	Type A
Bimalleolar	11.6	43.1	29/71	Type E
Trimalleolar	7.3	52.7	33/67	Type E
Suprasyndesmotic	7.6	39.0	66/34	Type C

Note that fractures with a posteromedial tibial component have not been included.

TABLE 4-17 Descriptive Indices for Calcaneal Fractures

	%	Average Age (yrs)	Gender Ratio (M/F)	Distribution Curve
Intra-articular	60.1	45.6	73/27	Type G
Extra-articular	39.9	34.4	75/25	Type B

Both bimalleolar and trimalleolar fractures have a type E pattern affecting older females in particular. Table 4-16 shows that the average age of patients with trimalleolar fractures is higher than those who have bimalleolar fractures. Suprasyndesmotic fractures have a type C pattern affecting young males and females, with a higher incidence in young males. The majority of ankle fractures are caused by twisting injuries (31%), falls from a standing height (37%), or sports injuries (10%).

Calcaneal Fractures

Calcaneal fractures account for 1.2% of all fractures. They have a type G pattern with a bimodal male curve and a unimodal curve in older women. Table 4-17 shows the descriptive indices for intra-articular and extra-articular calcaneal fractures. Both occur mainly in males, but the average age of patients with intra-articular fractures is higher. The intra-articular fractures show a type G pattern, but the extra-articular fractures have a type B pattern that is more common in younger males. Falls from a height are the most common cause of both types of calcaneal fracture and occur in 64% of intra-articular fractures and 47% of extra-articular fractures.

Talar Fractures

Talar fractures are very rare. They have a type C pattern mainly affecting young males. They can be subdivided into neck, body, and head fractures, although the latter are extremely rare and none was encountered during the study period. Table 4-18 gives the descriptive indices for talar neck and body fractures. They are both seen in young adults and both have a type C pattern. Talar body fractures are rare in females. Most talar fractures occur as a result of a fall from a height (59%).

Midfoot

Midfoot injuries are rare and involve the cuboid (44.4%), the navicular (48.1%), or the cuneiform bones (7.4%). Like the talus, they have a type C pattern mainly affecting young males. Table 4-4 shows that they are associated with a high incidence of open fractures, which tend to be very severe. Most cuboid fractures are caused but low-energy injuries but cuneiform, and navicular fractures tend to be caused by high-energy injuries such as falls from a height or motor vehicle accidents.

Metatarsus

These are common injuries showing a type A pattern that is more common in younger males and older females. Nine percent of fractures involve more than one metatarsal, but of the isolated metatarsal fractures, 75% involve the fifth metatarsal, 3% the fourth metatarsal, 5% the third metatarsal, 6% the second metatarsal and only 1% involve the hallux metatarsal. The most common cause is a twisting injury (40%), followed by a fall from a standing height (13.6%), and a direct blow to the foot (11.7%).

Toes

Toe fractures are relatively common and have a type C pattern affecting young males and females. About 57% of these fractures are caused by a kick or direct blow to the foot.

Pelvis

Table 4-2 shows that pelvic fractures are relatively uncommon. Due to the difficulty of treating these fractures, they have received considerable attention in the literature, and the implication is that they occur more frequently than they actually do. Patients with pelvic fractures tend to be referred to specialist centers, but if the true incidence is calculated for the overall population, it becomes clear that they occur infrequently. Most pelvic fractures are pubic rami fractures in elderly patients, and comparatively few young patients present with unstable pelvic or acetabular fractures. Table 4-3 shows that if all pelvic fractures are considered, the average age is about 70 years, and more than 70% of patients are at least 65 years of age. Table 4-19 shows the separate descriptive indices for pelvic and ace-

TABLE 4-18 Descriptive Indices for Talar Fractures

	%	Average Age (yrs)	Gender Ratio (M/F)	Distribution Curve
Neck	29.4	28.4	60/40	Type C
Body	70.6	32.1	92/8	Type C

TABLE 4-19 Descriptive Indices for Pelvic and Acetabular Fractures

	%	Average Age (yrs)	Gender Ratio (M/F)	Distribution Curve
Pelvis	92.3	78.3	74/26	Type E
Acetabulum	7.7	59.1	71/29	Type G

tabular fractures and that the average age of patients with pelvic fractures is, in fact, similar to the average age of patients with proximal femoral fractures. These fractures show a type E pattern. About 67% of pelvic fractures occur in simple falls, but in younger patients, they are high-energy fracture usually occurring in motor vehicle accidents and falls from a height.

Acetabular fractures are uncommon. The Edinburgh Unit, like other major trauma units, admits patients with acetabular fractures from a wide area, but if the population is accurately defined, it becomes clear that they are relatively rare injuries. They have a type G distribution with a bimodal male distribution and unimodal older female distribution. In younger patients, pelvic fractures are high-energy injuries usually caused by motor vehicle accidents or falls from a height, whereas in older patients, these fractures frequently follow a fall from standing height.

Spine

Table 4-20 shows the descriptive indices for spinal fractures. These are only traumatic fractures resulting from a well-defined injury. It is accepted that most thoracolumbar fractures are probably osteoporotic in origin, but it is often difficult to know just how old the fracture is when seen on a radiograph. It is also likely that many, if not most, osteoporotic vertebral fractures remain undetected in the community, and it has been estimated that less than 10% of vertebral fractures necessitate hospital admission (3). It has been estimated that the age- and gender-adjusted incidence of clinically diagnosed vertebral fractures is 117 per 100,000 per year (3), but figures vary in different parts of the world.

If osteoporotic vertebral fractures are not considered, Table 4-20 shows that cervical fractures are most common. They have a type H pattern with a bimodal male and female distribution.

TABLE 4-20 Descriptive Indices for the Different Types of Spinal Fractures

	%	Average Age (yrs)	Gender Ratio (M/F)	Distribution Curve
Cervical	51.3	43.4	58/42	Type H
Thoracolumbar	48.7	43.5	66/33	Type B

It is probable that if osteoporotic thoracolumbar fractures are included, the distribution curve is type A.

In younger patients, spinal fractures tend to be the result of high-energy injuries, mainly motor vehicle accidents (47%) and falls from a height (21%). In the elderly, they usually occur as a result of simple falls such as falls down stairs. Thoracolumbar fractures tend to occur in young males and have a type B distribution. If osteoporotic thoracolumbar fractures are included, the distribution is type A.

REFERENCES

1. Jones G, Nguyen PN, Sambrooke PN, et al. Symptomatic fracture incidence in elderly men and women: The Dubbo Osteoporosis Epidemiology Study (DOES). *Osteoporos Int* 1994;4:277–281.
2. O'Neill TW, Cooper C, Finn JD, et al. Incidence of distal forearm fracture in British men and women. *Osteoporos Int* 2001;12:555–558.
3. Cooper C, Atkinson EJ, O'Fallon WM, et al. Incidence of clinically diagnosed vertebral fractures: a population-based study in Rochester, Minnesota, 1985-1989. *J Bone Miner Res* 1992;7:221–227.
4. Kannus P, Niemi S, Parkkari J, et al. Epidemiology of adulthood injuries: a quickly changing injury profile in Finland. *J Clin Epidemiol* 2001;54:597–602.
5. Brown TD, Michas P, Williams RE, et al. The impact of gunshot wounds on an orthopaedic surgical service in an urban trauma center. *J Orthop Trauma* 1997;11:149–153.

PART 2
EXPERIENCE IN THE UNITED STATES

KENNETH J. KOVAL AND MICHAEL COOLEY

Musculoskeletal injuries—including fractures, dislocations and sprains, crushing injuries, open wounds, contusions, and other injuries—occur frequently, resulting in substantial morbidity and use of health care resources. There are categorical differences for each musculoskeletal injury type, and they reveal differences in gender and age groups afflicted, setting in which the injury occurred, mechanism of injury, treatment and recovery times, and associated mortality rates. Furthermore, epidemiological data demonstrate that considerable regional variation exists across the US in treatment philosophy, particularly regarding the use of surgical intervention. This chapter reviews data on current epidemiological trends in musculoskeletal injury from the *National Trauma Data Bank Report 2003* (1), American Academy of Orthopaedic Surgeons (2), and *The Dartmouth Atlas of Musculoskeletal Health Care* (3). Enhanced understanding of current musculoskeletal injury patterns is necessary to facilitate improved allocation of health care resources and to achieve better outcomes.

DATA FROM THE AMERICAN ACADEMY OF ORTHOPAEDIC SURGEONS

Overview

In 1995, the incidence rate for musculoskeletal injuries was 109.2 injuries per thousand persons (Table 4-21), totaling more than 28 million injuries in the US. Men had a higher incidence rate than women, and age correlated inversely with injury rate for musculoskeletal injuries. Sprains or dislocations, the most common category of musculoskeletal injury, accounted for 44% of musculoskeletal injuries and serve as a model of general epidemiological trends. The highest incidence rates occurred in persons aged 18 to 44 and 45 to 64, reflecting the inverse relation of age and injury rate that, at least in this injury category, may be partially influenced by occupational injuries that occur in the younger, employed, age groups. Fractures, the second most common injury, comprised 22% of musculoskeletal injuries, and also had a declining incidence rate as age increased. This, however, was true only to age 65, at which point incidence rates again rose, likely reflecting the increasing rate of hip fracture in the elderly.

Inpatient hospitalization, a measure of the use of health care resources, was required for 3 million musculoskeletal conditions in 1995, approximately 11.1% of all hospital stays. Trauma—resulting in musculoskeletal injury including fractures, dislocations and sprains, and other musculoskeletal injury—accounted for 40% of the musculoskeletal conditions requiring hospitalization. Fractures, the leading category of musculoskeletal injury resulting in hospitalization, accounted for 896,000 inpatient stays, while dislocations or sprains and other injuries caused an additional 306,000 hospitalizations.

By age, the distribution of musculoskeletal conditions result-

TABLE 4-21 Incidence of Persons Injured by Gender and Age: US, 1995

	Persons Injured per 1,000 Population			
	All Injuries	Musculoskeletal Injuries	Fractures	Sprains and Dislocations
Male	228.5	128.5	28.2	52.6
Female	168.7	90.9	20.3	43.0
Less than 18 years	241.1	124.8	29.9	45.9
18–44 years	202.0	118.0	21.2	57.8
45–64 years	165.9	93.1	22.1	46.0
65 years and over	139.0	70.7	24.7	19.6
Total	197.9	109.2	24.2	47.7

All injuries include ICD-9-CM 800–999.
Musculoskeletal injuries include ICD-9-CM 805–829, 831–847, 848.3–848.9, 874–877, 879.2–884, 885–897, 922–924, 926–928, 954–956, 957.1–957.9, and 959.
Fractures include ICD-9-CM 805–829.
Sprains and dislocations include ICD-9-CM 831–847 and 848.3–848.9.
Source: National Center for Health Statistics, National Health Interview Survey, 1995.
(Reprinted with permission from Praemer A, Furner S, Rice D. *Musculoskeletal Conditions in the United States*. Rosemont: American Academy of Orthopaedic Surgeons, 1999.)

TABLE 4-22 Hospitalizations Resulting from Musculoskeletal Conditions by Age Groups: US, 1995*

	Distribution by Age Group (in percents)							
	<18	18–44	45–64	65 & Over	65–74	75–84	85 & Over	Total
Musculoskeletal Diseases and Connective Tissue Disorders	27.7	48.0	59.7	47.9	60.2	46.5	27.3	49.2
Fractures	37.2	26.0	19.6	36.3	20.6	38.1	61.6	29.8
Dislocations and Sprains	4.9	7.2	5.4	2.7	3.6	2.1	2.5	4.6
Other Musculoskeletal Injuries	13.1	10.9	3.2	2.8	2.7	2.2	3.9	5.6
Complications or Reactions**	1.1	2.0	4.2	4.3	4.0	4.0	2.5	3.7
Congenital Malformations	8.6	0.7	0.3	0.1	0.2	—	—	0.9
Neoplasms	1.5	2.1	5.1	3.9	5.0	3.9	1.7	3.5
Other Musculoskeletal Conditions	5.9	2.4	2.6	2.3	2.8	2.4	0.5	2.7

* First listed diagnosis for inpatients discharged from short-stay hospitals.

** Mechanical or other complication or infection and inflammatory reaction to internal orthopaedic or prosthetic device, implant or graft.

— Estimate does not meet standards of reliability or precision.

Source: National Center for Health Statistics. National Hospital Discharge Survey, 1995.

(Reprinted with permission from Praemer A, Furner S, Rice D. *Musculoskeletal Conditions in the United States*. Rosemont: American Academy of Orthopaedic Surgeons, 1999.)

ing in hospitalizations varied as seen in Table 4-22. Among those under 18, trauma (fractures, dislocations and sprains, and other musculoskeletal injuries) encompassed 55% of hospitalizations for musculoskeletal conditions, while in those age 18 to 44, trauma accounted for only 44% of hospitalizations. In persons 45 to 65 years old, trauma accounted for 28% of hospitalizations. The inverse relation between age and injury rate no longer was valid among those 65 and older, however, where fractures accounted for an increasing proportion of musculoskeletal hospitalizations. Thirty-six percent of musculoskeletal-related hospitalizations in those 65 years of age and older were fracture related. Within the 65 and older group, 38.1% of hospitalizations in those 75 to 84 years old were fracture related and in the 85 and older age group, 61.6% resulted from fracture. Given the bimodal distribution of musculoskeletal injury, as well as predictions that the percent of the population age 65 and over will increase from 12.8% to 20.0% over the next 30 years, it is probable that the impact of musculoskeletal injury in the US will continue to increase dramatically.

Frequency of Musculoskeletal Injury

From 1992 to 1994, the average annual number of persons injured in the US was 57.9 million, and is displayed categorically by age, gender, and type of injury in Tables 4-23 and 4-24. Compared with women, men had a higher total injury rate (16.4 vs.12.7 per 100 persons), a higher rate of dislocations and sprains (5.7 vs. 5.1 per 100 persons), and a higher rate of fracture (2.7 vs. 2.0 per 100 persons) (Table 4-24). Figures 4-3 through 4-5 further demonstrate the effect of gender and age on the average annual rate of persons injured for all musculoskeletal injuries, dislocations and sprains, and fractures. Young men had higher rates than young women (those under age 45) in all musculoskeletal injuries, a differential that equalized in the 45 to 64 age category. After age 65, women surpassed men as the predominant victims of injury (Fig. 4-3). A subcategory of musculoskeletal injury, fractures, had similar trends, with male rates clearly higher than female rates for those under age 45. Comparable rates were seen between the ages of 45 and 64. Men had substantially lower rates than women in persons 65 years of age and older (Fig. 4-4), a pattern that reflects the higher incidence of osteoporosis-related fractures in older women. For dislocations and sprains, there was virtually no difference by gender in more elderly age groups, although males under age 45 had higher rates (Fig. 4-5).

Place of Occurrence

As illustrated in Figure 4-6, the most frequently reported place for fractures to occur from 1992 to 1994 was inside and outside

TABLE 4-23 Average Annual Number of Episodes of Persons Injured by Type of Injury: US, 1992 to 1994

	Average Annual Episodes (in thousands)						
	Male	Female	Less than 18 Years	18–44 Years	45–64 Years	65 Years & Over	Total
Fractures	3,321	2,625	1,921	2,344	777	904	5,946
Neck and Trunk	362	333	0	253	*198	243	695
Humerus, Radius, and Ulna	232	238	253	*78	*18	*122	471
Femur	*46	*100	0	0	*17	*129	*146
Tibia, Fibula, and Ankle	320	262	*152	300	*85	*45	581
Other Limbs	1,760	1,331	1,314	1,198	348	230	3,091
Dislocations and Sprains	7,121	6,663	2,746	7,850	2,174	1,014	13,784
Crushing Injury	*241	*102	*53	*229	*61	0	343
Open Wound	5,060	2,492	2,152	3,983	1,009	408	7,552
Contusions	2,928	3,103	1,659	2,635	751	986	6,032
Other Musculoskeletal Injuries	1,628	1,616	919	1,363	584	378	3,244
Total Musculoskeletal Injuries**	20,299	16,601	9,450	18,404	5,356	3,690	36,901
Total Injuries†	31,159	26,726	17,117	26,922	8,034	5,808	57,885

* Estimate does not meet standards of reliability or precision.

** Musculoskeletal injuries include ICD-9-CM 805–829, 831–847, 848.3–848.9, 874–877, 879.2–884, 885–887, 890–894, 895–897, 922–924, 926–928, 954–956, 957.1–957.9, and 959.

† Totals do not add up, due to other categories of fractures not included in the subgroups listed.

Source: National Center for Health Statistics, National Health Interview Survey, 1992–1994.

(Reprinted with permission from Praemer A, Furner S, Rice D. *Musculoskeletal Conditions in the United States*. Rosemont: American Academy of Orthopaedic Surgeons, 1999.)

the home (22.5% and 19.1%, respectively). Fracture occurrence was also commonly reported in streets and highways (12.7%), sports and recreational facilities (12.2%), and schools (11.3%). Industrial settings accounted for only 9.5% of fractures, but were associated with a relatively higher proportion of other musculoskeletal injuries. For example, 11.4% of all injuries, 13.6% of musculoskeletal injuries, and nearly 14% of dislocations and sprains occurred in an industrial setting.

Occupational Injury

Occupational injury, defined by the Bureau of Labor Services, is any injury that results from a work-related accident or exposure involving a sudden event in the workplace. The workplace is a common site of injury, and these events result in substantial illness and disability. In 1997, there were 6.1 million occupational injuries and illnesses reported, resulting in a rate of 7.1 cases per 100 full-time equivalent workers. Ninety-three percent, or 5.7 million cases, resulted from occupational injury, while the remaining 7%, or 430,000 cases, resulted from occupational illness.

Of the injuries and illnesses resulting in lost workdays, those affecting the musculoskeletal system accounted for the majority of lost workdays in both men and women. The most frequent injury to result in work loss, accounting for 43.6% of cases, was injury related to sprains and strains (Table 4-25). Other musculoskeletal injury categories resulting in work loss included fractures, causing 6.4% of cases; dislocations, 1.0%; tendonitis, 0.9%; and amputations, 0.5%. Crushing injuries, lacerations, contusions and other injuries also accounted for some work loss.

When gauging morbidity using median number of work loss days, dislocations resulted in the greatest loss (28 days). Other injuries associated with substantial work loss days were carpal tunnel syndrome (25 days), amputations (20 days), and fractures (17 days). Sprains and strains, with a median work loss of 6 days, was associated with fewer lost days, but still exceeded the median for all occupational injuries and illnesses.

Average workers' compensation claims, an indication of the costs associated with occupational injuries and illnesses, were highest for amputations ($19,272) and fractures ($15,528). The

TABLE 4-24 Average Annual Number of Episodes of Persons Injured by Type of Injury: US, 1992 to 1994

	Average Annual Episodes (rate per 100 persons)			
	All Injuries	Musculoskeletal Injuries	Dislocations and Sprains	Fractures
Male	25.1	16.4	5.7	2.7
Female	20.4	12.7	5.1	2.0
Less than 18 years	25.2	13.9	4.0	2.8
18–44 years	25.3	17.2	7.4	2.2
45–64 years	16.2	10.8	4.4	1.6
65 years & over	18.7	11.9	3.3	2.9
65–74 years	14.9	*	3.6	2.3
75 years & over	24.8	*	2.8	3.9
Total	22.7	14.5	5.4	2.3

* Information not available.

Source: National Center for Health Statistics, National Health Interview Survey, 1992–1994.

(Reprinted with permission from Praemer A, Furner S, Rice D. *Musculoskeletal Conditions in the United States*. Rosemont: American Academy of Orthopaedic Surgeons, 1999.)

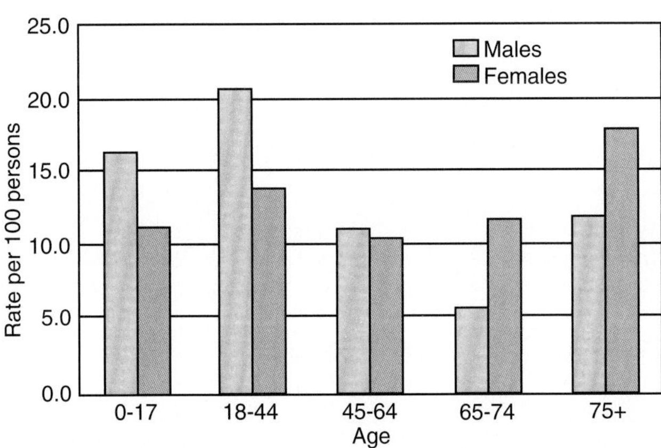

Source: National Center for Health Statistics, National Health Interview Survey, 1992-1994

FIGURE 4-3 Average annual rate of episodes of persons injured by age and gender, all musculoskeletal injuries: US, 1992 to 1994. (Reprinted with permission from Fildes J, et al. *National Trauma Data Bank Report 2003, Version 3.0*. American College of Surgeons, 2003. Available at: http://www.facs.org/trauma/ntdbannualreport2003.pdf.)

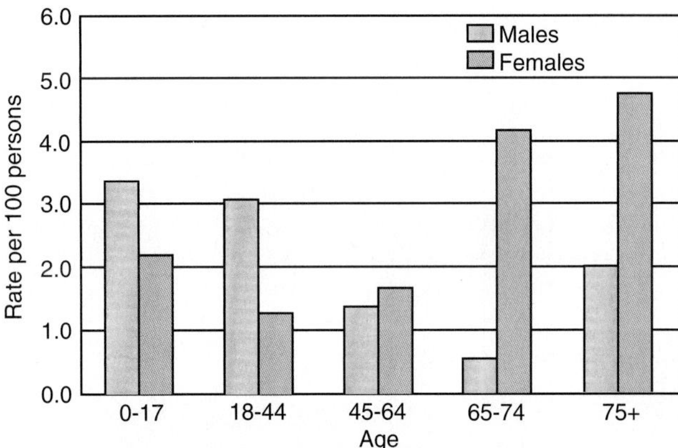

Source: National Center for Health Statistics, National Health Interview Survey, 1992-1994

FIGURE 4-4 Average annual rate of episodes of persons injured by age and gender, fractures: US, 1992 to 1994. (Reprinted with permission from Fildes J, et al. *National Trauma Data Bank Report 2003, Version 3.0*. American College of Surgeons, 2003. Available at: http://www.facs.org/trauma/ntdbannualreport2003.pdf.)

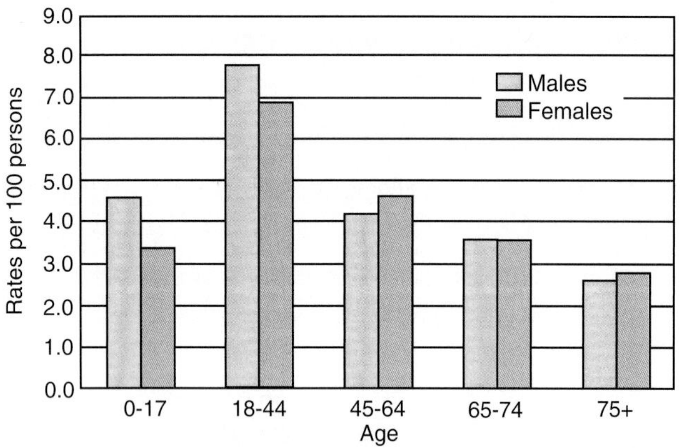

FIGURE 4-5 Average annual rate of episodes of persons injured by age and gender, dislocations and sprains: US, 1992 to 1994. (Reprinted with permission from Fildes J, et al. *National Trauma Data Bank Report 2003, Version 3.0*. American College of Surgeons, 2003. Available at: http://www.facs.org/trauma/ntdbannualreport2003.pdf.)

average cost per workers' compensation claim filed in 1995 to 1996 was $11,033.

Motor Vehicle Accidents

Motor vehicle accidents are a substantial source of trauma to the musculoskeletal system. In 1996, the police reported approximately 6.8 million motor vehicle accidents (US Dept. of Transportation), resulting in death or injury of 3.6 million motor vehicle occupants, and 147,000 pedestrians and cyclists.

The percentage of musculoskeletal injuries resulting from motor vehicle accidents from the 1992 through 1994 National Health Interview Surveys are shown by type of injury in Table 4-26. Injuries resulting from motor vehicle accidents accounted for 11.6% of all injuries; men reported that their injury involved a motor vehicle more often (13.1%) than women (9.9%). Reporting of musculoskeletal injuries resulting from motor vehicle involvement (13.7%) was comparable to that reported for all injuries resulting from motor vehicle involvement (11.6%), with men, again, reporting motor vehicle involvement more often than females (15.1% vs. 11.9%). Overall, it is apparent that men reported higher incidence rates for all injuries related to motor vehicle accidents than women, with an even higher differential for musculoskeletal injuries than women. In addition, there was substantial variability among injury types. The greatest difference occurred with fractures—men reported sustaining a motor vehicle-related fracture more than twice as often as women. Dislocations and sprains also had gender differences, although it was minimal (13.6% for men and 12.0% for women).

Associated Disability

Of the 36.9 million annual musculoskeletal injuries reported between 1992 and 1994, 33.1 million received medical treatment; over half resulted in activity restriction (defined as one-half day of a reduction in a person's normal activity level following injury) and one-fifth resulted in bed-disability (defined as at least one-half day of bed-disability resulting from injury). The categories of injury most likely to be treated were fractures and open wounds (97.4% and 94.5%, respectively). Fracture, which was also the injury most likely to result in bed-disability (27.5%) or activity restriction (64%), had a varying impact on

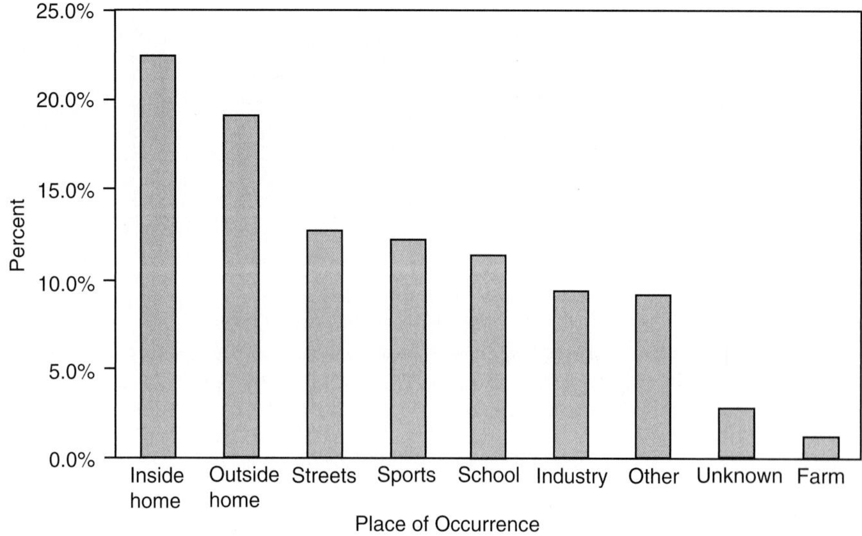

FIGURE 4-6 Percent distribution of fracture location: US, 1992 to 1994. (Reprinted with permission from Fildes J, et al. *National Trauma Data Bank Report 2003, Version 3.0*. American College of Surgeons, 2003. Available at: http://www.facs.org/trauma/ntdbannualreport2003.pdf.)

TABLE 4-25 Distribution of Type of Occupational Injury or Illness by Gender and Median Days Away from Work per Injury or Illness, 1996

	Injuries or Illnesses (percents)			
	Male	Female	Total	Median Work-Loss Days
Dislocation	1.2	0.7	1.0	28
Fracture	7.2	4.9	6.4	17
Sprains & Strains	42.1	46.6	43.6	6
Amputation	0.7	0.2	0.5	20
Crushing Injuries	1.5	0.6	1.2	7
Cuts, Lacerations	8.6	4.1	7.1	3
Bruises, Contusions	8.6	10.8	9.3	3
Heat Burns	1.5	1.7	1.5	4
Tendinitis	0.5	1.7	0.9	9
Carpal Tunnel Syndrome	0.7	3.3	1.6	25
Multiple Injuries	3.3	3.1	3.2	8
All Other	24.1	22.3	23.7	–
	100.0	100.0	100.0	5

Source: Department of Labor, Bureau of Labor Statistics, Case and Demographic Characteristics for Workplace Injuries and Illnesses Involving Days Away From Work, 1996; Supplemental Tables, 1998.
(Reprinted with permission from Praemer A, Furner S, Rice D. *Musculoskeletal Conditions in the United States*. Rosemont: American Academy of Orthopaedic Surgeons, 1999.)

activity restriction based on anatomic site. Fractures of the tibia, fibula, and ankle resulted in both the most activity restriction and the most bed-disability, whereas fractures of the humerus, radius, and ulna were more likely to result in activity restriction, though were less likely to result in bed-disability. After fracture, the second greatest impact on activity restriction occurred with dislocations and sprains, resulting in activity restrictions in 59.4% of patients and bed-disability in 26.9%.

Duration of restricted activity days was also greatest for fracture, which accounted for 145.6 million days of restricted activity and the longest duration of restricted activity per episode among all injury categories (24.5 days). Patient age was an important factor in determining the length of restricted activity. Persons under the age of 65 had 107.3 million restricted-activity days associated with fracture, with duration of 21.3 days per fracture. Among those 65 and older, the number of restricted-activity days was far less (38.3 million), but the duration was significantly greater (42.3 days). These trends are likely due to the higher incidence in younger populations, and the slower recovery time associated with older age. By gender, women with fractures reported 75.1 million days of restricted activity for an average of 28.6 days per fracture, while men had less morbidity using this measure, with corresponding numbers of 70.4 million days and 21.2 days per fracture.

The proportion of total restricted-activity days due to musculoskeletal injury was highest for dislocations and sprains, not fractures. Forty-one percent of the total restricted-activity days were due to dislocations and sprains, compared to 26.6% for fractures. Contusions accounted for 13.4% of total restricted-activity days and smaller percentages were attributable to open wounds, other musculoskeletal injuries, and crushing injuries.

Substantial work-loss and school-loss days were associated with musculoskeletal injury. Among those currently employed, more than 147 million work-loss days were attributable to musculoskeletal injuries. As percentages of work-loss days by injury category, fractures caused 24.7% of work-loss days, and open

TABLE 4-26 Percentage of Injuries with Motor Vehicle Involvement by Type of Injury and Gender: US, 1992 to 1994

	Injuries with Motor Vehicle Involvement (percent)		
Injury	Male	Female	Total
All Injuries	13.1	9.9	11.6
Fractures	16.6	6.8	12.3
Neck and Trunk	*27.3	0	*14.2
Tibia, Fibula, and Ankle	*22.9	0	*12.6
Humerus, Radius, and Ulna	0	*7.5	*3.8
Other Fractures	15.1	*10.9	13.3
Dislocations and Sprains	13.6	12.0	12.9
Open Wounds	8.1	*3.3	6.5
Contusions	25.1	20.7	22.8
Other Injuries	20.5	14.6	17.6
All Musculoskeletal Injuries	15.1	11.9	13.7

* Estimate does not meet standards of reliability or precision.
Source: National Center for Health Statistics, National Health Interview Survey, 1992–1994.
(Reprinted with permission from Praemer A, Furner S, Rice D. *Musculoskeletal Conditions in the United States.* Rosemont: American Academy of Orthopaedic Surgeons, 1999.)

wounds were responsible for 11.8% of work-loss days. Among school children ages 5 to 17, 21.2 million school-loss days resulted from musculoskeletal injuries, whereas fractures accounted for 34.7% of school-loss days, dislocations and sprains resulted in 27.9% of school-loss days, and open wounds caused 21.3% of school-loss days. Overall, fracture was the number one cause of activity restriction, bed-disability, and duration of restricted-activity days, as well as the leading cause of work loss and school loss.

Health Care Utilization

Musculoskeletal injury is a substantial burden on health care resources and accounts for 40.8% of hospitalizations due to musculoskeletal conditions. From 1993 through 1995, almost 1.3 million inpatient hospitalizations, averaging 6.0 days each, occurred annually in the US for all types of musculoskeletal injuries (Table 4-27), resulting in more than 7.5 million patient days per year.

By injury type, fracture dominated the use of inpatient services compared with other categories of musculoskeletal injury, requiring the longest average stay (7.0 days) and 84.9% of patient days (Tables 4-27 and 4-28). As a result, 71.9% of hospitalizations for musculoskeletal injuries in short-stay hospitals were due to fractures, with an average of 906,000 hospitalizations occurring each year (Table 4-28).

Fractures also led to a substantial differential in the overall utilization of inpatient resources by gender (Table 4-27). Epidemiological data indicate that women utilize inpatient services much more than men for musculoskeletal injuries. This is likely due to two main factors, both related to fracture epidemiology. First, the majority of hospitalizations resulted from fractures and occurred predominantly among women (59.5%); and second, women had a longer length of stay following fractures (7.5 days) than men (6.5 days). When these two factors were combined, patient days resulting from fractures accounted for 89.3% of the patient days associated with musculoskeletal injuries among women, compared with 78.2% among men. This was the dominant factor contributing to the overall greater utilization of inpatient resources by females.

Selected anatomic sites of fractures and sprains or dislocations resulted in hospitalization as displayed in Tables 4-29 and 4-30. The fractures are most likely to lead to hospitalizations involving the neck of the femur, ankle, vertebral column, and the tibia and fibula. Women (primarily 65 and older) sustained the majority of fractures of the neck of the femur, as well as the pelvis and the humerus, a disproportional representation that likely reflects

TABLE 4-27 Average Annual Hospitalizations Resulting from Musculoskeletal Injuries, by Age and Gender: US 1993 to 1995

	Gender	Number of Hospitalizations[1]						
		<18	18–44	45–64	65 & Over	Total[3]	Number of Patient Days[2]	Average Length of Stay (days)
Fractures		87,000	203,000	137,000	478,000	906,000	6,402,000	7.1
	Male	55,000	137,000	64,000	110,000	367,000	2,374,000	6.5
	Female	32,000	66,000	72,000	368,000	539,000	4,028,000	7.5
Dislocations		6,000	21,000	9,000	7,000	42,000	120,000	2.8
	Male	4,000	15,000	6,000	2,000	27,000	74,000	2.7
	Female	2,000	5,000	3,000	4,000	15,000	46,000	3.1
Sprains and Strains		9,000	48,000	35,000	29,000	122,000	341,000	2.8
	Male	5,000	33,000	20,000	11,000	69,000	171,000	2.5
	Female	4,000	15,000	16,000	18,000	53,000	170,000	3.2
Crushing Injuries		53,000*	3,000	*	*	53,000	23,000	4.7
	Male	*	3,000	*	*	4,000	20,000	4.7
	Female	*	*	*	*	*	*	*
Contusions		2,000	13,000	8,000	23,000	47,000	195,000	4.1
	Male	1,000	6,000	4,000	8,000	20,000	77,000	3.9
	Female	*	7,000	5,000	15,000	27,000	118,000	4.3
Open Wounds		14,000	59,000	13,000	8,000	94,000	331,000	3.5
	Male	11,000	49,000	10,000	5,000	75,000	252,000	3.4
	Female	4,000	10,000	3,000	3,000	19,000	79,000	4.1
Other		6,000	21,000	9,000	8,000	44,000	132,000	3.0
	Male	3,000	13,000	6,000	3,000	25,000	67,000	2.6
	Female	3,000	8,000	3,000	5,000	19,000	65,000	3.5
Total, All Musculoskeletal Injuries		126,000	368,000	213,000	554,000	1,260,000	7,544,000	6.0
	Male	80,000	257,000	110,000	140,000	588,000	3,035,000	5.2
	Female	46,000	111,000	102,000	414,000	672,000	4,509,000	6.7

[1] First listed diagnosis for inpatient discharged from short-stay hospitals.
[2] Annual average.
[3] Because of rounding, totals may not equal sum of the individual components.
* Estimate does not meet standards of reliability or precision.
(Reprinted with permission from Praemer A, Furner S, Rice D. *Musculoskeletal Conditions in the United States*. Rosemont: American Academy of Orthopaedic Surgeons, 1999.)

both the larger female population among the elderly and the susceptibility to fracture of these bones among the older, more osteoporotic female population. The best example occurred in fractures of the neck of the femur: 90.1% of fractures occurred in patients 65 and older, 78.0% of which were in women.

For fractures, the average length of hospital stay was affected most by injury site (Table 4-29). Hospital stays were generally shorter for fractures in the upper extremity than for fractures of the trunk or lower extremities. The longest lengths of stay occurred in patients with femoral fractures other than the neck of the femur (10.3 days), fractures of the neck of the femur (9.4 days), fractures of the vertebral column (8.1 days), and fractures of the pelvis (7.9 days). Of note, average lengths of stay reflect both the seriousness of the injury as well as the comorbidities of the persons most at risk for sustaining the injury.

Hospitalizations for dislocations were generally shorter, and were predominantly due to dislocations of the knee (22,000) or shoulder (6,000), with respective lengths of stay of 2.1 and 2.3 days (Table 4-30). Hip dislocations, although less frequent (4,000), had a longer average length of stay of 4.7 days.

In addition to hospitalizations, musculoskeletal injuries also resulted in a large number of outpatient physician visits. From 1993 through 1995, there were more than 38.7 million annual visits to physicians in office-based practice as a result of musculoskeletal injuries. The distribution of injury types in outpatient practices differed from that seen at the inpatient care level, and

TABLE 4-28 Distribution of Hospitalizations and Patient Days Resulting From Musculoskeletal Injuries, by Age and Gender: US, 1993 to 1995

	Distribution (in percent)	
	Hospitalizations*	Patient Days†
Fractures	71.9	84.9
Dislocations	3.3	1.6
Sprains and Strains	9.7	4.5
Crushing Injury	0.4	0.3
Contusions	3.7	2.6
Open Wound	7.5	4.4
Other Injury	3.5	1.7

* First listed diagnosis for inpatients discharged from short-stay hospitals.
† Annual average.
Source: National Center for Health Statistics, National Hospital Discharge Survey, 1993–1995.
(Reprinted with permission from Praemer A, Furner S, Rice D. *Musculoskeletal Conditions in the United States*. Rosemont: American Academy of Orthopaedic Surgeons, 1999.)

sprains and strains, not fractures, were the most frequently occurring musculoskeletal injury category. Sprains and strains caused approximately 16.1 million physician visits per year, whereas fractures (still the second most frequent category) resulted in 9.4 million visits, followed by open wounds (3,796,000), contusions (3,148,000), and dislocations (1,993,000).

Financial Costs

The cost of musculoskeletal injuries, including injuries related to fractures, dislocations and sprains, open wounds, crushing injury, traumatic amputation, and other selected injuries affecting the musculoskeletal system, amounted to $41.3 billion in 1995. Seventeen percent ($7.1 billion) were indirect costs, with morbidity costs related to reduced or lost productivity amounting to $2.7 billion, and mortality costs related to the loss of expected earnings in an individual's future totalling $4.4 billion. The remaining 83% of total costs were direct costs related to health care.

Fractures, a costly category of musculoskeletal injuries, were estimated to have utilized $19.3 billion in 1995. Direct costs comprised more than two-thirds of this figure, in large part due to lengthy hospitalizations. Almost 900,000 persons were hospitalized with fractures and the average length of stay was 6.5 days, giving a total of 5.8 million days. As a result, hospital inpatient costs amounted to $7.0 billion and made up the majority of the $13.2 billion in direct costs related to fracture. Indirect costs were $6.2 billion, of which $3.8 billion were mortality costs and $2.4 billion were morbidity costs.

NATIONAL TRAUMA DATA BANK 2003

The National Trauma Data Bank (NTDB) is a trauma registry that contains 731,824 records from 268 US trauma centers. The Annual Report 2003, consisting of 548,735 records from 255 US trauma centers, reviews the combined data set for the period 1997 to 2002 and evaluates the NTDB data, giving insight into the state of trauma care and general characteristics of patients treated at trauma centers in the US (1). Specifically, it contains detailed epidemiological data on age and gender distributions, mechanisms of injury, and mortality.

National Trauma Data Bank Hospitals

Two hundred and sixty-eight hospitals submitted data to the NTDB, 223 (83%) of which met the American College of Surgeons Committee on Trauma criteria to be verified as a trauma center. Sixty-nine hospitals were designated as Level I, 71 as Level II, 34 as Level III, and 49 were either Level IV or V. Sixty-five (24%) were university hospitals and 144 (54%) were community teaching hospitals.

Patient Characteristics

From 1997 to 2002, 548,735 trauma cases were submitted to The NTDB, contributing to the data bank's accrued total of 731,824 records. Persons 17 to 24 years old represented the peak age group of patients in the NTDB, with men injured in motor vehicle accidents and by violence (gunshots, shotguns, stabs, and fights) predominating (Figs. 4-7 and 4-8). A second peak in the age distribution occurred in patients 35 to 44 years old, again including mostly males injured in motor vehicle accidents. A smaller third peak occurred between ages 72 and 85, representing mostly women injured in falls and motor vehicle accidents. Overall, the gender pattern observed was that by ages 20 to 24, men outnumbered women by 3:1 in the trauma registry until after age 40. Men thereafter continued to represent the majority of victims through age 68, at which point women sustained the majority of trauma.

Mechanism of Injury

The most prevalent mechanism of injury in the registry was motor vehicle accidents, which accounted for 39% of cases in the data bank (Fig. 4-9), was responsible for 39.5% of mortalities (Figure 4-10), and was associated with the greatest number of hospital (Fig. 4-11) and ICU days (Fig. 4-12). Younger age groups were most affected, with a dramatic rise in motor vehicle accident cases observed beginning at age 14 and peaking at age 20.

Falls, the second most prevalent source of trauma, accounted

TABLE 4-29 Average Annual Hospitalizations Resulting from Fractures at Selected Anatomic Sites, by Age and Gender: US, 1993 to 1995

	Gender	Number of Hospitalizations[1] <18	18–44	45–64	65 & Over	Total[3]	Number of Patient Days[2]	Average Length of Stay
Fracture of Hand		2,000	11,000	4,000	2,000	18,000	46,000	2.6
	Male	2,000	9,000	3,000	*	14,000	32,000	2.3
	Female	*	2,000	*	*	4,000	15,000	3.6
Fracture of Carpals		*	1,000	1,000	7,000	3,000	14,000	4.6
	Male	*	*	*	*	2,000	7,000	3.8
	Female	*	*	*	*	1,000	7,000	5.9
Fracture of Radius and Ulna		15,000	17,000	12,000	15,000	59,000	185,000	3.1
	Male	9,000	13,000	5,000	3,000	29,000	88,000	3.0
	Female	5,000	5,000	7,000	13,000	30,000	97,000	3.2
Fracture of Humerus		15,000	9,000	9,000	27,000	61,000	254,000	4.2
	Male	9,000	5,000	3,000	6,000	22,000	79,000	3.5
	Female	6,000	4,000	6,000	22,000	38,000	175,000	4.6
Fracture of Clavicle or Scapula		*	4,000	2,000	1,000	7,000	26,000	3.6
	Male	*	3,000	*	*	4,000	14,000	3.4
	Female	*	*	1,000	*	3,000	12,000	3.9
Fracture of Ribs and Sternum		1,000	11,000	10,000	19,000	42,000	233,000	5.6
	Male	1,000	7,000	6,000	7,000	21,000	109,000	5.2
	Female	*	3,000	4,000	13,000	21,000	124,000	5.9
Fracture of Vertebral Column		5,000	24,000	10,000	35,000	74,000	604,000	8.1
	Male	2,000	19,000	6,000	11,000	37,000	315,000	8.4
	Female	3,000	5,000	5,000	25,000	37,000	298,000	7.8
Fracture of Pelvis		3,000	11,000	6,000	35,000	55,000	431,000	7.9
	Male	1,000	6,000	4,000	8,000	19,000	176,000	9.1
	Female	1,000	4,000	3,000	27,000	35,000	255,000	7.2
Fracture of Neck of Femur		3,000	6,000	20,000	273,000	303,000	2,831,000	9.4
	Male	1,000	4,000	10,000	60,000	77,000	710,000	9.3
	Female	1,000	1,000	10,000	213,000	226,000	2,122,000	9.4
Other Fracture of Femur		18,000	15,000	6,000	23,000	62,000	633,000	10.3
	Male	12,000	10,000	3,000	4,000	28,000	273,000	9.6
	Female	6,000	4,000	3,000	20,000	33,000	360,000	10.9
Fracture of Tibia and Fibula		12,000	29,000	17,000	15,000	72,000	476,000	6.6
	Male	8,000	22,000	9,000	4,000	42,000	270,000	6.4
	Female	4,000	7,000	8,000	12,000	30,000	206,000	6.8
Fracture of Ankle		9,000	47,000	31,000	21,000	108,000	454,000	4.2
	Male	6,000	25,000	11,000	4,000	46,000	179,000	3.9
	Female	3,000	22,000	20,000	17,000	62,000	275,000	4.4
Fracture of Foot		2,000	14,000	6,000	2,000	24,000	114,000	4.7
	Male	1,000	11,000	4,000	*	17,000	77,000	4.6
	Female	*	4,000	2,000	*	8,000	37,000	4.9
Fracture of Other and Unspecified Sites		1,000	6,000	4,000	8,000	18,000	101,000	5.6
	Male	*	3,000	1,000	3,000	8,000	45,000	5.5
	Female	*	2,000	2,000	5,000	10,000	55,000	5.6

[1] First listed diagnosis for inpatients discharged from short-stay hospitals.

[2] Annual average.

[3] Because of rounding, totals may not equal sum of the individual components.

* Estimate does not meet standards of reliability or precision.

Source: National Center for Health Statistics, National Hospital Discharge Survey, 1993 to 1995.

(Reprinted with permission from Praemer A, Furner S, Rice D. *Musculoskeletal Conditions in the United States*. Rosemont: American Academy of Orthopaedic Surgeons, 1999.)

TABLE 4-30 Average Annual Hospitalizations Resulting from Sprains or Dislocations at Selected Anatomic Sites, by Age and Gender: US, 1993 to 1995

	Gender	Number of Hospitalizations[1] <18	18–44	45–64	65 & Over	Total[3]	Number of Patient Days[2]	Average Length of Stay
Sprains								
Ankle and Foot		*	4,000	2,000	1,000	8,000	22,000	2.7
	Male	*	3,000	*	*	5,000	8,000	1.8
	Female	*	*	1,000	1,000	4,000	14,000	3.9
Knee and Leg		6,000	18,000	4,000	2,000	30,000	68,000	2.3
	Male	3,000	13,000	2,000	*	19,000	41,000	2.2
	Female	3,000	5,000	2,000	2,000	11,000	27,000	2.5
Shoulder		*	9,000	21,000	15,000	45,000	92,000	2.0
	Male	*	7,000	13,000	7,000	27,000	54,000	2.0
	Female	*	7,000	4,000	5,000	17,000	79,000	2.2
Back		2,000	15,000	7,000	8,000	30,000	134,000	4.4
	Male	1,000	8,000	2,000	3,000	13,000	55,000	4.1
	Female	*	7,000	4,000	5,000	17,000	79,000	4.6
Other and Unspecified Sites		*	2,000	2,000	3,000	8,000	24,000	3.0
	Male	*	2,000	1,000	1,000	5,000	13,000	2.8
	Female	*	*	1,000	2,000	3,000	11,000	3.3
Dislocations								
Shoulder		*	3,000	1,000	1,000	6,000	14,000	2.3
	Male	*	3,000	*	*	4,000	7,000	1.6
	Female	*	*	*	1,000	2,000	7,000	4.1
Knee		4,000	1,000	5,000	2,000	22,000	47,000	2.1
	Male	2,000	8,000	3,000	*	14,000	32,000	2.2
	Female	1,000	3,000	2,000	2,000	8,000	15,000	1.9
Hip		1,000	*	*	*	4,000	17,000	4.7
	Male	*	1,000	*	*	2,000	9,000	4.0
	Female	*	*	*	*	1,000	8,000	5.9
Other and Unspecified Sites		1,000	4,000	3,000	2,000	10,000	42,000	4.1
	Male	1,000	3,000	2,000	1,000	7,000	26,000	4.0
	Female	*	1,000	1,000	1,000	4,000	16,000	4.2

[1] First listed diagnosis for inpatients discharged from short-stay hospitals.
[2] Annual average.
[3] Because of rounding, totals may not equal sum of the individual components.
* Estimate does not meet standards of reliability of precision.
Source: National Center for Health Statistics, National Hospital Discharge Survey, 1993–1995.
(Reprinted with permission from Praemer A, Furner S, Rice D. *Musculoskeletal Conditions in the United States*. Rosemont: American Academy of Orthopaedic Surgeons, 1999.)

for an additional 27% of cases in the NTDB (Fig.4-9). Peak incidence occurred at age 81 (Fig. 4-13), a factor that likely contributed to the high mortality rate (18.3% of total deaths). Falls were also associated with the second largest number of hospital (Fig. 4-11) and ICU days (Fig. 4-12), partly reflecting the increased comorbidities in the elderly.

Gunshot wounds, the third most common injury category (6.5%), accounted for 20.7% of mortalities (Figures 4-9 and 4-10). The number of gunshot wound cases increased abruptly at age 12, but peaked earlier than motor vehicle accident at 19 years, then steadily decreased. Violent injuries overall, including gunshot wounds, stab wounds and assaults/fights, accounted

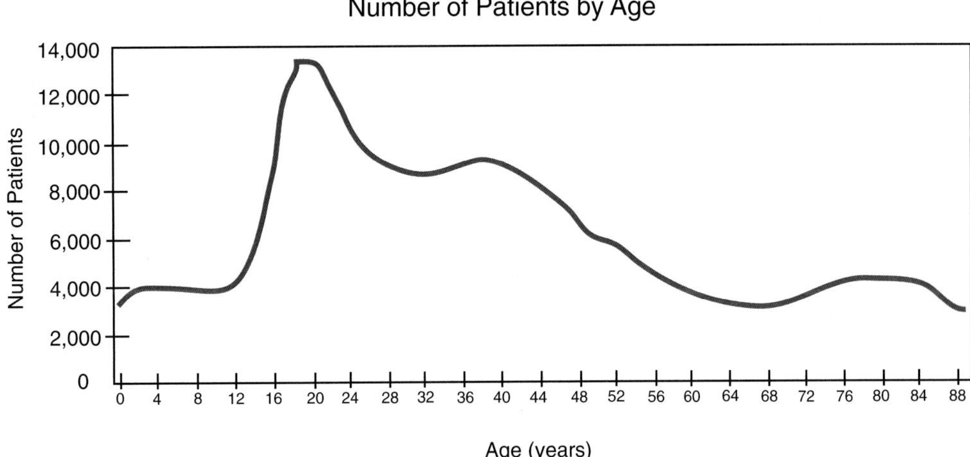

FIGURE 4-7 Number of patients at each age from 0 to 89 in the NTDB. Total N = 548,735. (Reprinted with permission from Praemer A, Furner S, Rice D. *Musculoskeletal Conditions in the United States*. Rosemont: American Academy of Orthopaedic Surgeons, 1999.)

for 13.4% of hospital days (Fig. 4-11) and 13.1% of ICU days (Fig. 4-12).

Mortality

The greatest number of deaths in the NTDB resulted from motor vehicle accidents, followed by gunshot wounds and falls (Fig. 4-10). Death occurred in 5% of motor vehicle crashes in the data bank; crash rates rose dramatically in victims 12 to 20 years old. Deaths from motor vehicle accidents, however, remained relatively stable until age 75, after which they declined (Fig. 4-13), possibly due to infrequent driving among the very elderly. Gunshot wound injuries, although less prevalent than motor vehicle accidents, were associated with death in 16.71% of cases, the highest percentage of any penetrating injury. Falls, the second most prevalent source of trauma and third most common cause of death, resulted in death in 3.6% of cases, a slightly lower percentage than for motor vehicle accidents. Other injuries with high mortality rates included pedestrian injuries, which were associated with death in 8.56% of cases, and burns, which were associated with death in 5.93% of cases.

Regarding age, the percentage of death was highest in those aged 65 to 89 years, due largely to deaths after falls or motor vehicle accident in the elderly. A bimodal distribution was noted in the number of deaths, however, with peaks at 20 and 80 years (Fig. 14). Men who died in motor vehicle accidents and by gunshot wounds, stabbings, assaults, and fights, contributed to the first peak, with the prevalence of violent deaths rising dramatically among those 12 to 20 years old and peaking at 25 to 30 years.

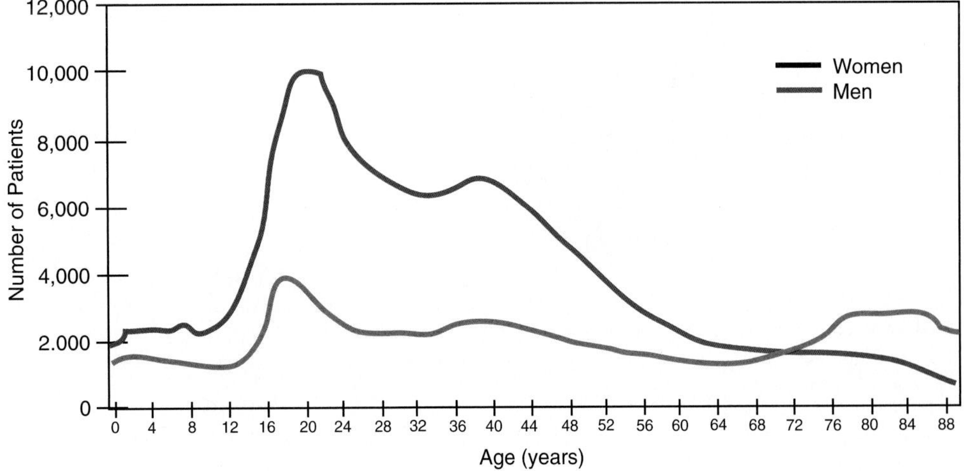

FIGURE 4-8 Number of men and women at each age from 0 to 89 in the NTDB. Total N = 548,735. (Reprinted with permission from Praemer A, Furner S, Rice D. *Musculoskeletal Conditions in the United States*. Rosemont: American Academy of Orthopaedic Surgeons, 1999.)

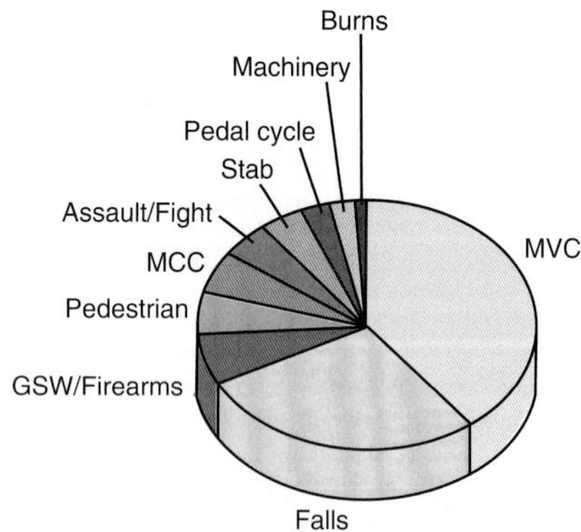

FIGURE 4-9 Proportional distribution of patients, grouped by mechanism of injury in the NTDB. Total N = 453,806. MVC, motor vehicle crash; GSW, gunshot wound; MCC, motorcycle crash. (Reprinted with permission from Praemer A, Furner S, Rice D. *Musculoskeletal Conditions in the United States*. Rosemont: American Academy of Orthopaedic Surgeons, 1999.)

MEDICARE DATA FROM THE DARTMOUTH ATLAS

The Dartmouth Atlas, an analysis of Medicare data (3) from 1996 to 1997, documents regional variation in the rates of fracture and operative treatment for different musculoskeletal conditions. Various databases were analyzed to determine health care demands and utilization across the US. Databases, including the Denominator File, were provided through the Health Care Financing Administration and were analyzed to determine the number of possible Medicare beneficiaries in a designated region, as well as demographic data for these individuals (age, gender, and race). The MEDPAR File (hospital claims data) contained data on the rates of hospital services usage. Physician visit rates and the rates of certain diagnostic procedures and preventative services were obtained from analyzing the Part B Standard Analytical Variable Length File.

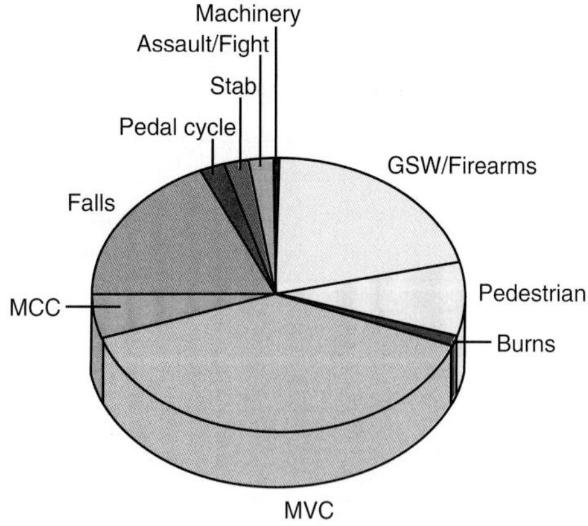

FIGURE 4-10 Proportional distribution of deaths, grouped by mechanism of injury in the NTDB. Total N = 23,730. MVC, motor vehicle crash; GSW, gunshot wound; MCC, motorcycle crash. (Reprinted with permission from Praemer A, Furner S, Rice D. *Musculoskeletal Conditions in the United States*. Rosemont: American Academy of Orthopaedic Surgeons, 1999.)

To define regions of health care delivery, 3,436 hospital service areas were defined, each comprising a region in which an acute care health facility was located with inpatient capabilities. These facilities were identified through the American Hospital Association Annual Survey of Hospitals and the Medicare Provider of Services files. Hospital referral regions were also defined according to the 1996–1999 Dartmouth Atlas of Health Care guidelines, and represent tertiary care facilities in which there was delivery of specific cardiovascular and neurosurgical procedures. All hospital service areas were then assigned to a specific hospital referral region based on the greatest proportion of patients in a designated hospital service area utilizing service in that hospital referral region. Some hospital service areas were reassigned to achieve geographic contiguity, a minimum population size of 120,000, or a high localization index.

The most common musculoskeletal condition requiring hospitalization in the Medicare population was fracture—more than 450,000 patients sustained fractures in 1996 alone. Among fracture types, the most common were hip fractures (femoral neck and intertrochanteric) (45%), followed by fractures of the wrist (20%), ankle (10%), proximal humerus (9%), forearm (5%), femur (thigh bone) (4%), distal humerus/shaft (upper arm) (4%), and proximal tibia/shaft (lower leg) (4%) (Fig. 4-15).

Hip Fracture

Fracture of the proximal femur was the most common fracture type. Incidence increased with age and was highest in white women, likely due to the higher prevalence of osteoporosis in this group. From 1996 to 1997, hip fracture occurred in approximately 420,000 Medicare patients, 98% of whom were treated surgically. The average hip fracture rate was 7.7 per 1,000 Medicare enrollees from 1996 to 1997, but varied twofold, from 4.9 per 1,000 Medicare enrollees in Honolulu to 10.5 in Rome, Georgia. Other hospital referral regions where hip fracture rates were substantially higher than average included Lubbock, Texas (10.0); Nashville, Tennessee (9.5); Winston-Salem, North Carolina (9.5); Chattanooga, Tennessee (9.2); and Cincinnati (9.1) (Fig. 16). In addition to Honolulu, hospital referral regions where hip fracture rates per 1,000 Medicare enrollees were substantially lower than average included San Francisco (5.6); Eugene, Oregon (5.9); San Jose, California (6.0); Newark, New Jersey (6.0); and Manhattan (6.3).

Wrist Fracture

Wrist fracture, the second most common fracture type, occurred in approximately 96,000 Medicare patients in 1996, 85% of whom were women. Wrist fracture rates varied almost fourfold, from 1.5 per 1,000 Medicare enrollees to 5.7. Hospital referral regions with high rates of wrist fracture per 1,000 Medicare enrollees were Huntsville, Alabama (5.7); Tuscaloosa, Ala-

Total Hospital Length of Stay by Mechanism of Injury
Hospital LOS in Days
1,200,000
1,000,000
800,000
600,000
400,000
200,000
0
MVC
Falls
Pedestrian
GSW/Firearms
MCC
Assault/Fight
Stab
Pedal cycle
Machinery
Burns

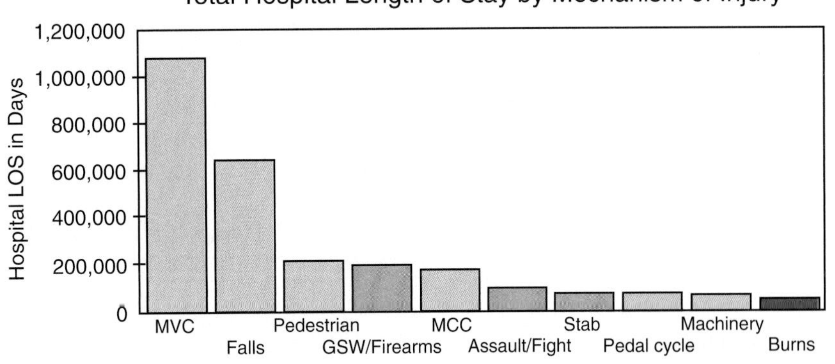

FIGURE 4-11 Hospital length of stay grouped by mechanism of injury in the NTDB. Total N = 453,806. Total hospital length of stay = 2,562,282 days. Blue bars represent blunt mechanism of injury. Green bars represent violent mechanisms of injury. Red bar represents burns. MVC, motor vehicle crash; GSW, gunshot wound; MCC, motorcycle crash. (Reprinted with permission from Praemer A, Furner S, Rice D. *Musculoskeletal Conditions in the United States*. Rosemont: American Academy of Orthopaedic Surgeons, 1999.)

Total ICU length of Stay by Mechanism of Injury
ICU LOS in Days
350,000
300,000
250,000
200,000
150,000
100,000
50,000
0
MVC
Falls
Pedestrian
GSW/Firearms
MCC
Assault/Fight
Pedal cycle
Burns
Stab
Machinery

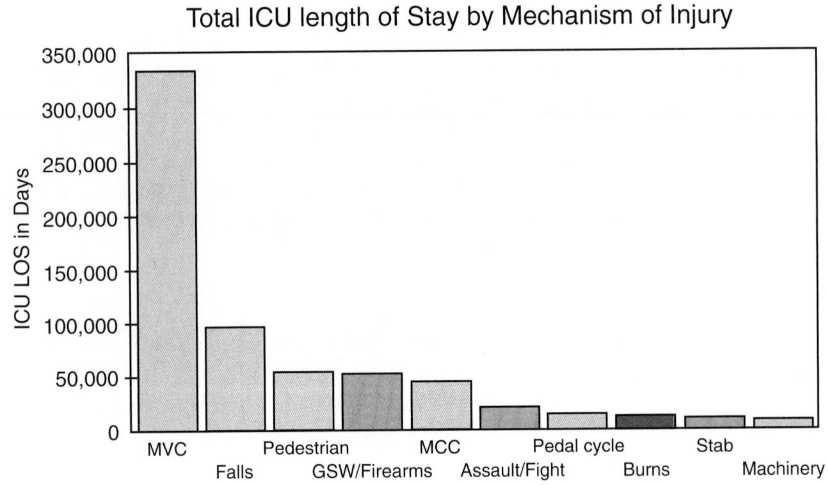

FIGURE 4-12 Total ICU length of stay grouped by mechanism of injury in the NTDB. Total N = 412,687, total ICU length of stay = 644,627 days. Blue bars represent blunt mechanism of injury, green bars represent violent mechanism of injury, and red bars represent burns. MVC, motor vehicle crash; GSW, gunshot wound; MCC, motorcycle crash. (Reprinted with permission from Praemer A, Furner S, Rice D. *Musculoskeletal Conditions in the United States*. Rosemont: American Academy of Orthopaedic Surgeons, 1999.)

Deaths by Mechanism and Age
Number of Patients
1,600
1,400
1,200
1,000
800
600
400
200
0
MVC
Violence
Fall
<1
1-4
5-9
10-14
15-19
20-24
25-34
35-44
45-54
55-64
65-74
75-84
85-89
Age (years)

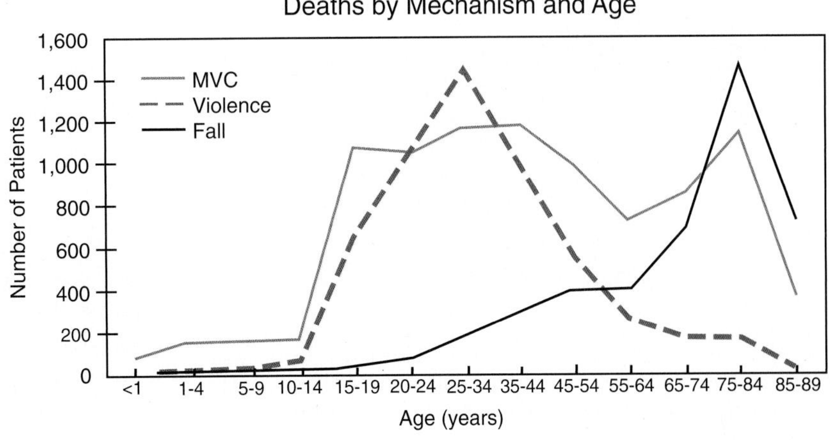

FIGURE 4-13 Number of deaths due to injuries from the most common mechanism of injury categories at each age from 0 to 89 in the NTDB, total N = 18,902. MVC, motor vehicle crash. (Reprinted with permission from Praemer A, Furner S, Rice D. *Musculoskeletal Conditions in the United States*. Rosemont: American Academy of Orthopaedic Surgeons, 1999.)

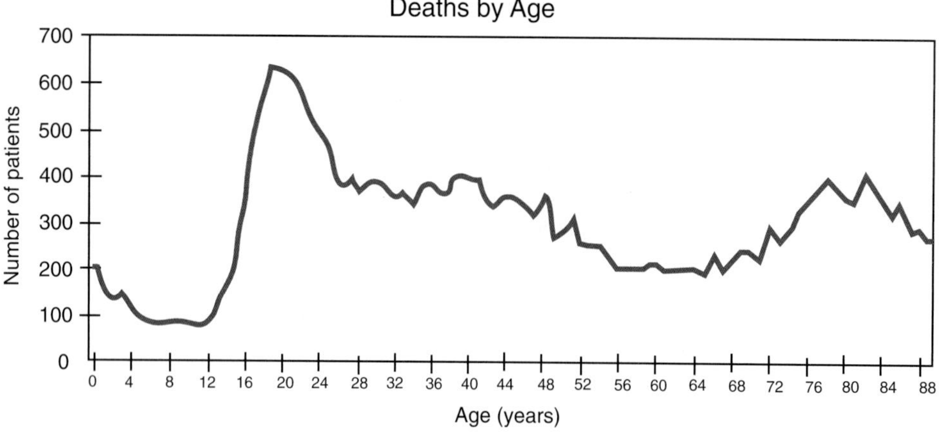

FIGURE 4-14 Number of deaths at each age from 0 to 89 in the NTDB, total N = 27,052. (From Praemer A, Furner S, Rice D. *Musculoskeletal Conditions in the United States*. Rosemont: American Academy of Orthopaedic Surgeons, 1999.)

bama (5.6); Birmingham, Alabama (5.4); Philadelphia, Pennsylvania (5.0); Winston-Salem, North Carolina (4.9); and Ann Arbor, Michigan (4.7) (Fig. 4-17). Hospital referral regions with lower than average rates per 1,000 Medicare enrollees were Everett, Washington (1.5); San Francisco, California (1.6); Stockton, California (1.7); San Jose, California (1.8); Portland, Oregon (1.9); and Sacramento, California (2.0).

Surgical repair rates of wrist fracture varied almost tenfold, as a proportion of all wrist fractures, from 5.1% of all wrist fractures to 50.7% (Fig. 4-18). The US average was 16.5%.

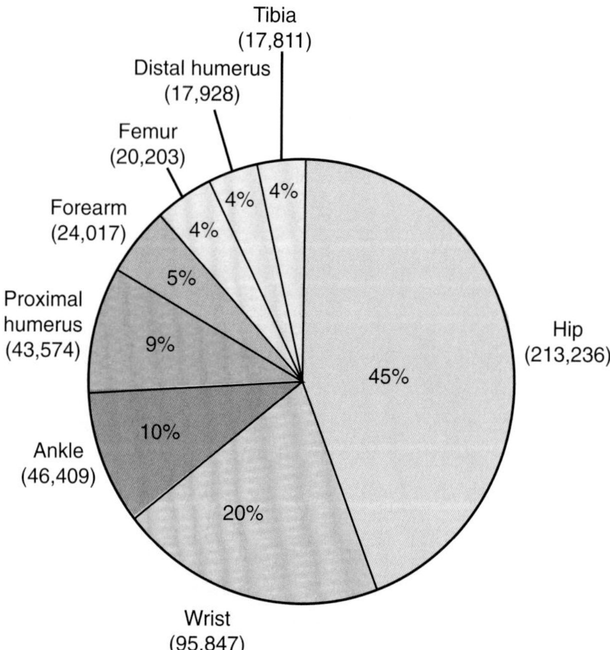

FIGURE 4-15 The relative frequency of eight different types of fractures in Medicare patients. The number of Medicare enrollees with each fracture is in parentheses. (Reprinted with permission from Wennberg J, Cooper MC, eds. *The Dartmouth Atlas of Musculoskeletal Health Care*. Chicago: American Hospital Association Press, 2000.)

Hospital referral regions with relatively high rates of surgical repair of wrist fractures included Olympia, Washington (50.7%); Casper, Wyoming (48.3%); Joplin, Missouri (41.3%); Little Rock, Arkansas (38.2%); Anchorage, Alaska (36.7%); and Seattle, Washington (36.0%). Hospital referral regions with lower than average surgical repair rates were Greenville, North Carolina (5.1%); White Plains, New York (6.4%); Detroit, Michigan (7.7%); Hackensack, New Jersey (7.9%); Morristown, New Jersey (8.6%); and Royal Oak, Michigan (9.1%).

Ankle Fracture

Rates of ankle fracture, the third most common fracture type, varied almost sixfold in 1996 and 1997, from 0.5 to 3.1 per 1,000 Medicare enrollees. The US average rate of ankle fracture was 1.7 per 1,000 Medicare enrollees. Hospital referral regions where rates of ankle fracture per 1,000 Medicare enrollees were higher than the national average included Danville, Pennsylvania (3.1); Altoona, Pennsylvania (2.9); Reading, Pennsylvania (2.8); Allentown, Pennsylvania (2.7); Birmingham, Alabama (2.5); Ann Arbor, Michigan (2.5); and Cincinnati, Ohio (2.4) (Fig. 4-19). Hospital referral regions where rates per 1,000 Medicare enrollees were lower than the national average included Honolulu, Hawaii (0.5); San Jose, California (0.7); New Orleans, Louisiana (0.8); Los Angeles, California (0.8); Sacramento, California (0.8); and Phoenix, Arizona (0.9).

The US average for the proportion of ankle fractures repaired surgically in 1996 and 1997 was 37.2%, and varied from 20.8% to 77.1% (Fig. 4-20), a greater than threefold difference. Hospital referral regions where the proportion of surgical repair of ankle fracture was higher than average included Chico, California (77.1%); Tacoma, Washington (71.4%); Spokane, Washington (70.9%); Eugene, Oregon (69.7%); Little Rock, Arkansas (68.1%); and Phoenix, Arizona (67.9%). Hospital referral regions with a lower than average proportion of ankle fractures treated surgically included Altoona, Pennsylvania (20.8%); Buffalo, New York (21.9%); Charleston, South Carolina (23.1%); White Plains, New York (23.4%); Philadelphia, Pennsylvania

(text continues on page 134)

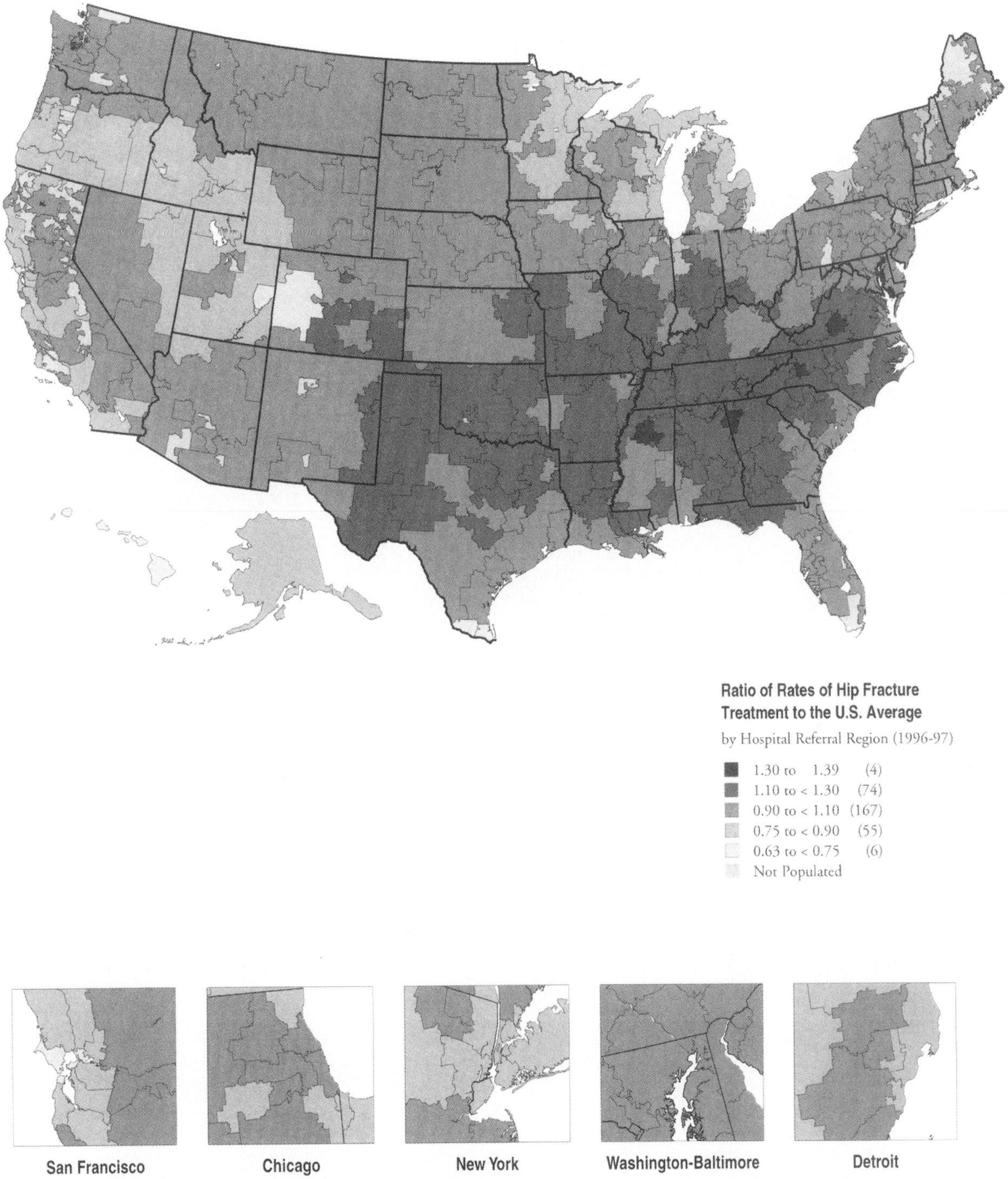

Ratio of Rates of Hip Fracture Treatment to the U.S. Average
by Hospital Referral Region (1996-97)

1.30 to 1.39 (4)
1.10 to < 1.30 (74)
0.90 to < 1.10 (167)
0.75 to < 0.90 (55)
0.63 to < 0.75 (6)
Not Populated

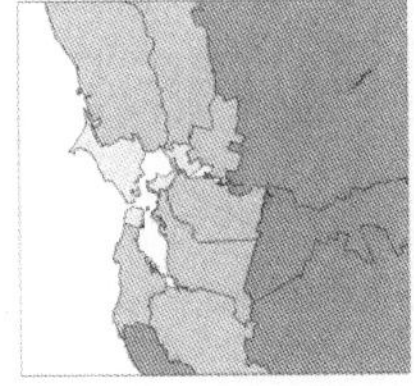

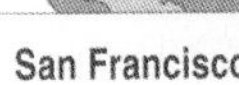
San Francisco

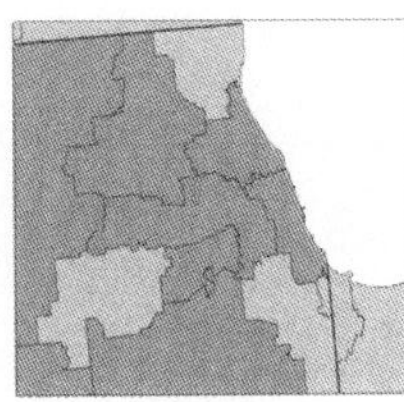
Chicago

New York

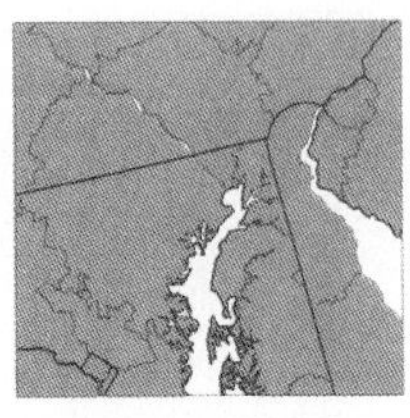
Washington-Baltimore

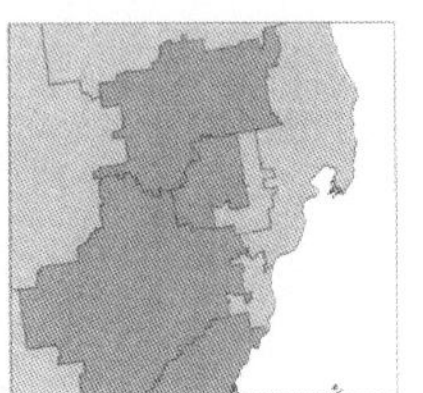
Detroit

FIGURE 4-16 Ratio of rates of hip fracture treatment to the US average by hospital referral region (1996 to 1997). (Reprinted with permission from Wennberg J, Cooper MC, eds. *The Dartmouth Atlas of Musculoskeletal Health Care*. Chicago: American Hospital Association Press, 2000.)

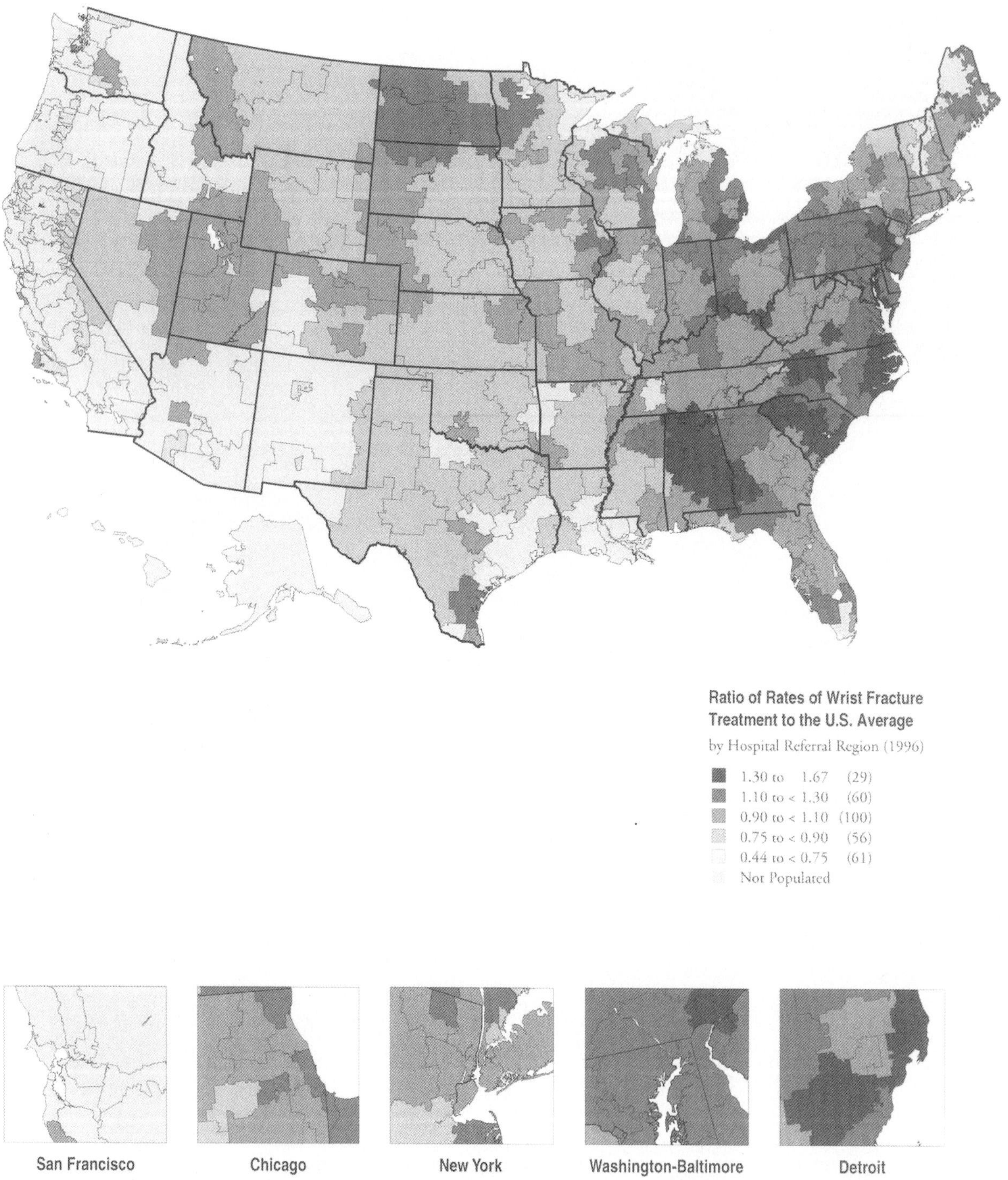

Ratio of Rates of Wrist Fracture Treatment to the U.S. Average

by Hospital Referral Region (1996)

- 1.30 to 1.67 (29)
- 1.10 to < 1.30 (60)
- 0.90 to < 1.10 (100)
- 0.75 to < 0.90 (56)
- 0.44 to < 0.75 (61)
- Not Populated

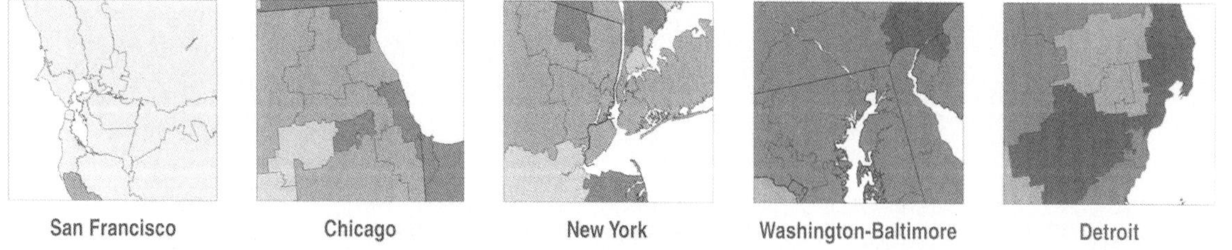

FIGURE 4-17 Ratio of rates of wrist fracture treatment to the US average by hospital referral region (1996 to 1997). (Reprinted with permission from Wennberg J, Cooper MC, eds. *The Dartmouth Atlas of Musculoskeletal Health Care*. Chicago: American Hospital Association Press, 2000.)

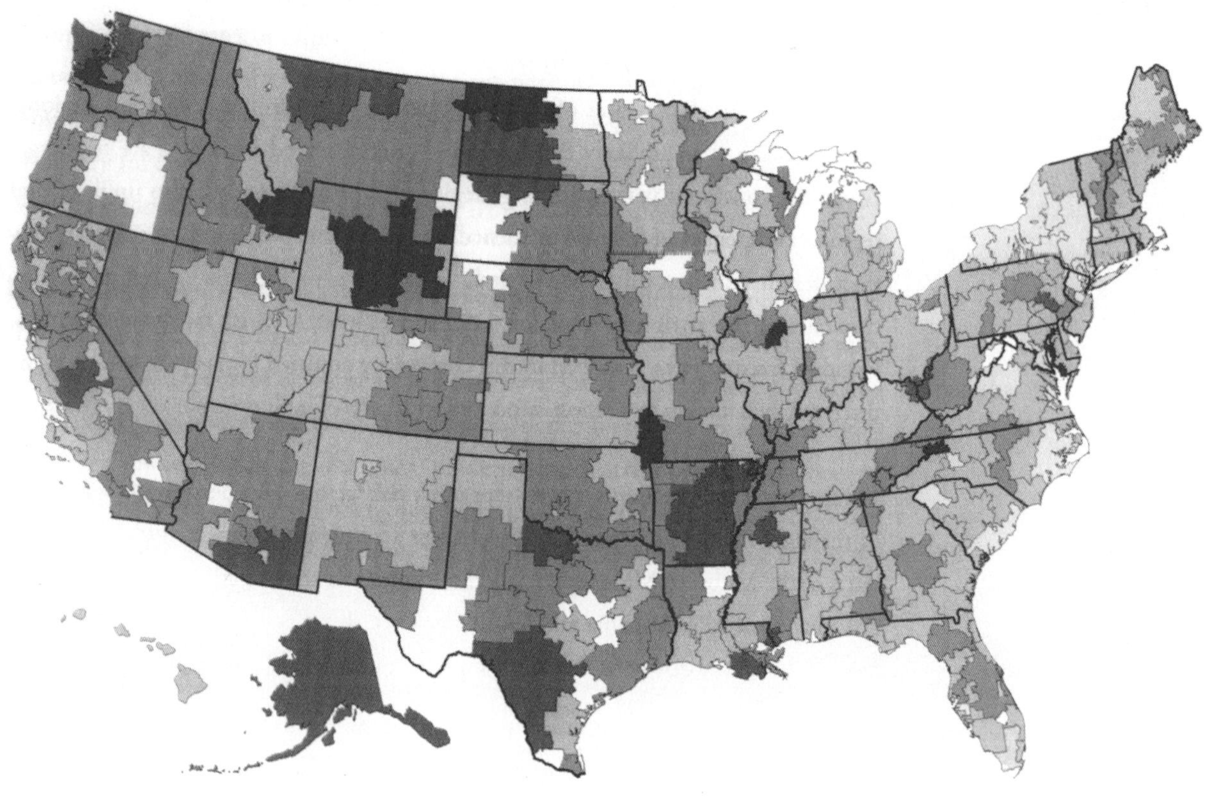

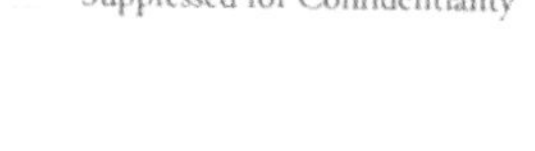

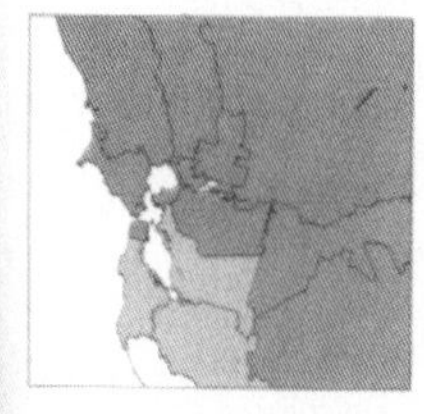

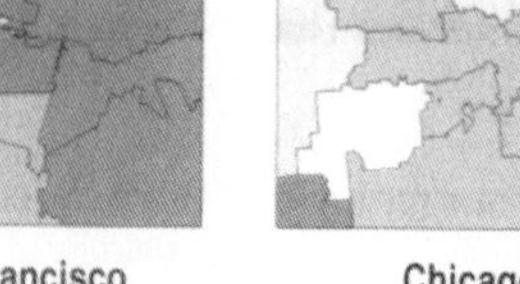

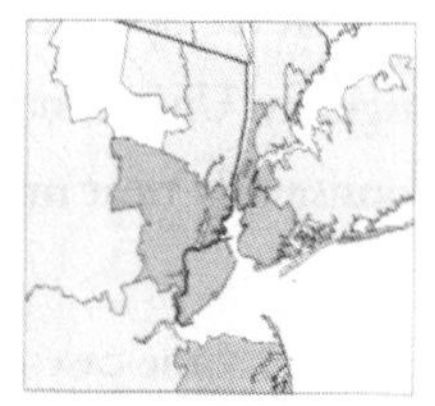

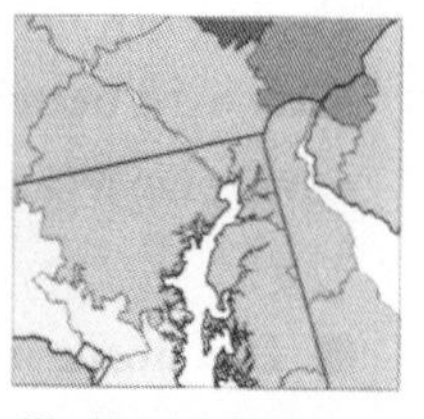

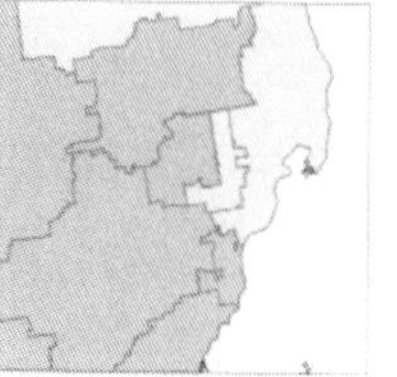

FIGURE 4-18 Proportion of wrist fractures treated surgically by hospital referral region (1996 to 1997). (Reprinted with permission from Wennberg J, Cooper MC, eds. *The Dartmouth Atlas of Musculoskeletal Health Care*. Chicago: American Hospital Association Press, 2000.)

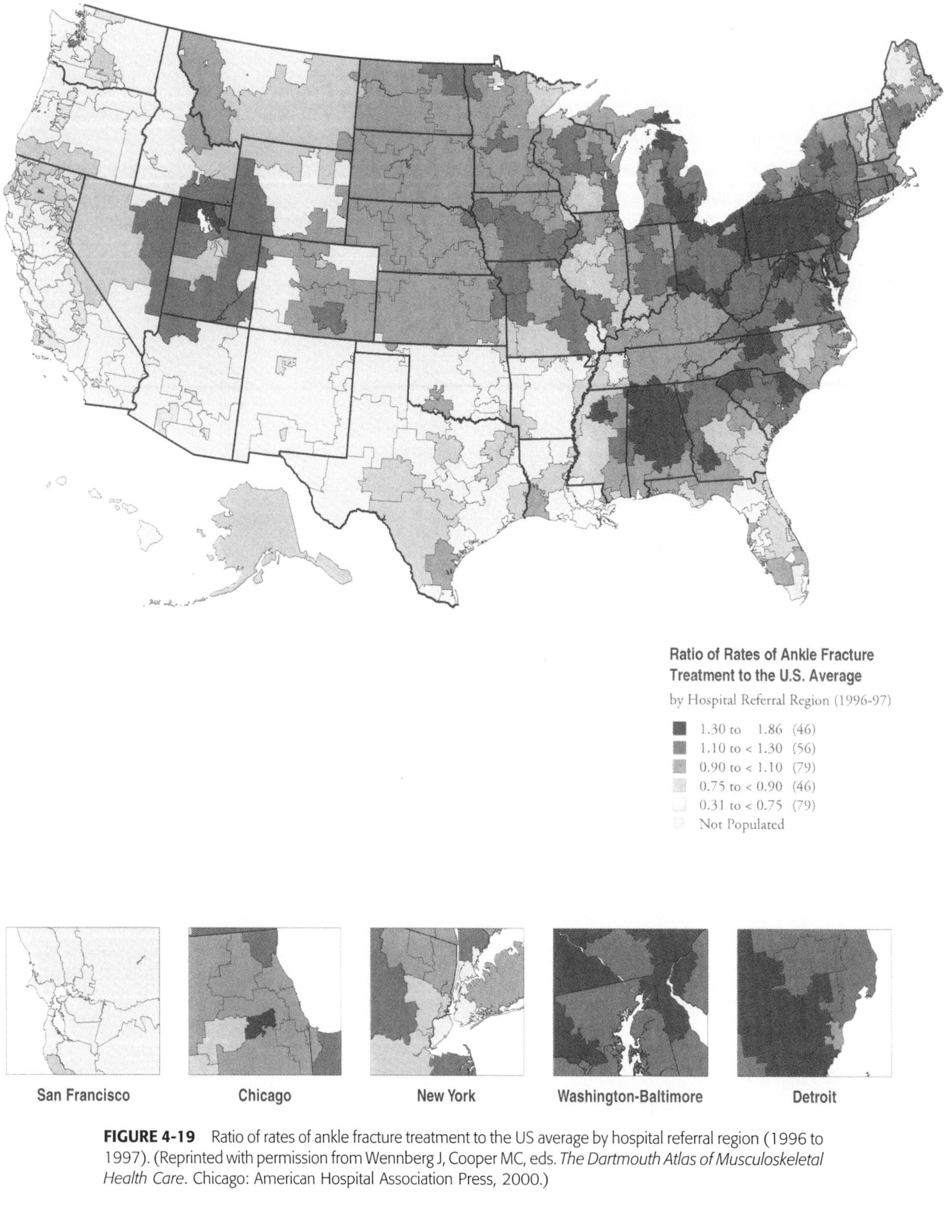

Ratio of Rates of Ankle Fracture Treatment to the U.S. Average
by Hospital Referral Region (1996-97)

1.30 to 1.86 (46)
1.10 to < 1.30 (56)
0.90 to < 1.10 (79)
0.75 to < 0.90 (46)
0.31 to < 0.75 (79)
Not Populated

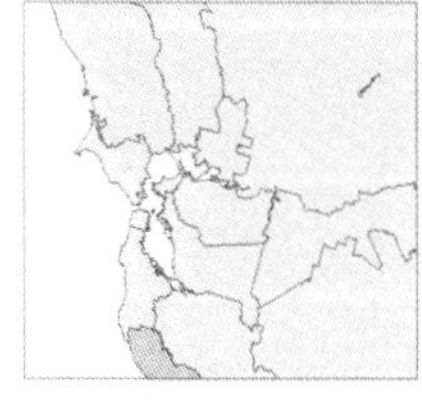

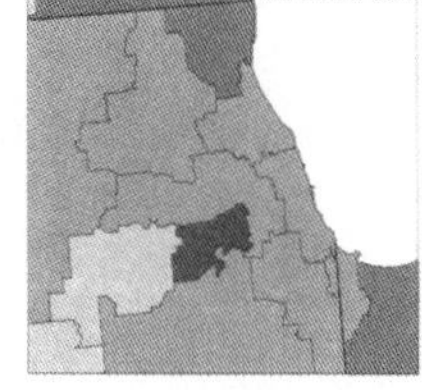

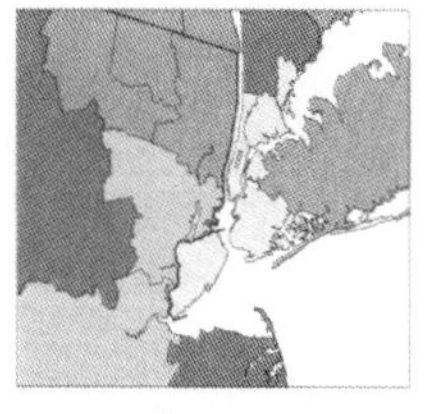

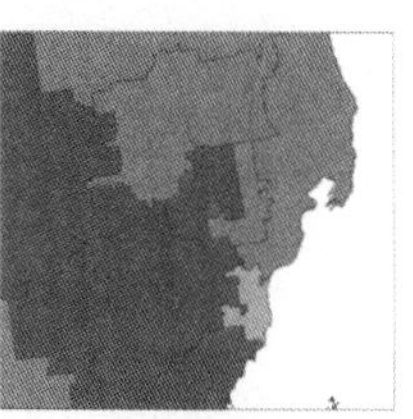

FIGURE 4-19 Ratio of rates of ankle fracture treatment to the US average by hospital referral region (1996 to 1997). (Reprinted with permission from Wennberg J, Cooper MC, eds. *The Dartmouth Atlas of Musculoskeletal Health Care*. Chicago: American Hospital Association Press, 2000.)

Proportion of Ankle Fractures Treated Surgically
by Hospital Referral Region (1996-97)

- 60 or More (32)
- 50 to < 60 (50)
- 40 to < 50 (65)
- 30 to < 40 (109)
- Less than 30 (50)
- Not Populated

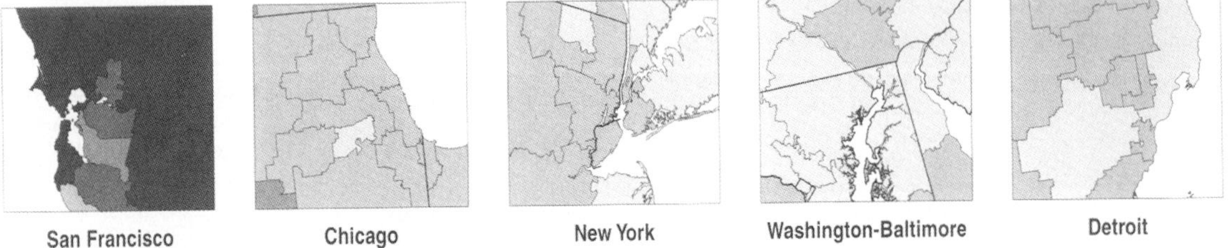

FIGURE 4-20 Proportion of ankle fractures treated surgically by hospital referral region (1996 to 1997). (Reprinted with permission from Wennberg J, Cooper MC, eds. *The Dartmouth Atlas of Musculoskeletal Health Care*. Chicago: American Hospital Association Press, 2000.)

(24.6%); Detroit, Michigan (24.7%); and Albany, New York (25.6%).

Proximal Humerus Fracture

The fourth most common fracture type, proximal humerus fracture, had rates that varied by a factor of 10 in 1996 and 1997, from 0.3 per 1,000 Medicare enrollees to 3.4. The US average was 1.6 per 1,000 Medicare enrollees. Substantially higher than average rates per 1,000 Medicare enrollees were observed among the following hospital referral regions: Covington, Kentucky (3.4); Allentown, Pennsylvania (2.8); Philadelphia, Pennsylvania (2.8); Harrisburg, Pennsylvania (2.5); Columbia, South Carolina (2.5); Cincinnati, Ohio (2.4); and Baltimore, Maryland (2.3) (Fig. 4-21). Hospital referral regions with proximal humerus fracture rates lower than average per 1,000 Medicare enrollees were Jackson, Tennessee (0.3); Honolulu, Hawaii (0.4); Tacoma, Washington (0.5); San Jose, California (0.6); Spokane, Washington (0.6); San Francisco, California (0.7); and San Bernardino, California (0.8).

Surgical repair of proximal humerus fracture in 1996 and 1997 varied tenfold, from 6.4% of all proximal humerus fractures to 60.0%. The US average was 14.3% (Figure 4-22). Hospital referral regions with higher than average surgical repair rates included Tacoma, Washington (60.0%); Little Rock, Arkansas (34.8%); Spokane, Washington (33.3%); Phoenix, Arizona (29.8%); San Diego, California (27.5%); and Minneapolis, Minnesota (22.9%). Hospital referral regions where the proportion of proximal humerus fractures treated surgically was lower than average were Takoma Park, Maryland (6.4%); Detroit, Michigan (8.5%); Buffalo, New York (8.8%); East Long Island, New York (8.9%); Cleveland, Ohio (9.3%); and Milwaukee, Wisconsin (9.8%).

Proximal Forearm and Shaft Fracture

Rates of proximal forearm and shaft(s) fracture varied sixfold in 1996, from 0.3 per 1,000 Medicare enrollees to 1.8. The US average was 0.9 per 1,000 Medicare enrollees. Hospital referral regions where rates of proximal forearm and shaft(s) fracture were substantially higher than this average included Binghamton, New York (1.8); Takoma Park, Maryland (1.4); Detroit, Michigan (1.4); Philadelphia, Pennsylvania (1.3); Providence, Rhode Island (1.2); and Cleveland, Ohio (1.2) (Fig. 4-23). Hospital referral regions where rates were lower than average per 1,000 Medicare enrollees included Honolulu, Hawaii (0.3); Seattle, Washington (0.4); Portland, Oregon (0.4); Little Rock, Arkansas (0.5); Knoxville, Tennessee (0.5); and Spokane, Washington (0.6).

Femur Fracture

Forty thousand Medicare patients sustained a femur fracture in 1996 and 1997, making it the sixth most common fracture type. In the US, the average rate of femur fracture per 1,000 Medicare enrollees was 0.7, and rates varied fourfold from 0.3 to 1.2. Seventy-three percent of these patients were treated surgically. Hospital referral regions where the rate of femur fracture per 1,000 Medicare enrollees was substantially higher than the national average included Tuscaloosa, Alabama (1.2); Lubbock, Texas (1.1); Cincinnati, Ohio (1.0); Toledo, Ohio (1.0); Atlanta (1.0); Kansas City, Missouri (0.9); and Philadelphia, Philadelphia (0.9) (Fig. 4-24). Rates per 1,000 Medicare enrollees were substantially lower than average in the hospital referral regions of Salem, Oregon (0.3); San Francisco, Californai (0.4); Lebanon, New Hampshire (0.4); Boise, Idaho (0.5); Sacramento, California (0.5); and New Brunswick, New Jersey (0.5).

Humeral Shaft and Distal Humerus Fracture

Medicare enrollees experienced 35,000 fractures of the humeral shaft or distal humerus from 1996 to 1997, giving an average rate in the US of 0.6 per 1,000 enrollees, making it the seventh most common fracture category. A sixfold difference in incidence was observed among hospital referral regions. Hospital referral regions where rates of humeral shaft and distal humerus fracture were higher than the US average per 1,000 Medicare enrollees included Hinsdale, Illinois (1.4); Takoma Park, Maryland (1.2); Corpus Christi, Texas (1.1); Tuscaloosa, Alabama (1.1); Norfolk, Virginia (0.9); and Philadelphia, Pennsylvania (0.9) (Fig. 4-25). Hospital referral regions with lower than average rates of humeral shaft and distal humerus fracture per 1,000 Medicare enrollees were San Angelo, Texas (0.3); Eugene, Oregon (0.3); San Francisco, California (0.3); Portland, Oregon (0.3); Seattle, Washington (0.3); and Tucson, Arizona (0.4).

Surgical intervention was used in 38.7% of Medicare patients with fractures of the humeral shaft and distal humerus in 1996 and 1997, with the proportion undergoing surgical repair varying almost fourfold, from 18.6% to 70.1% of all proximal humerus fractures (Fig. 4-26). Hospital referral regions with relatively high surgery rates for humeral shaft and distal humerus fracture included San Francisco, California (70.1%); Seattle, Washington (64.1%); Little Rock, Arkansas (63.6%); Los Angeles, California (55.3%); Knoxville, Tennessee (53.2%); and Peoria, Illinois (50.9%). Hospital referral regions with a low proportion of humeral shaft and distal humerus fractures treated surgically included Paterson, New Jersey (18.6%); Hartford, Connecticut (22.9%); Buffalo, New York, (25.6%); Evanston, Illinois (27.0%); Milwaukee, Wisconsin (27.3%); Washington, D.C. (27.7%); and East Long Island, New York (28.7%).

Lower Leg Fracture

In 1996 and 1997, the average rate of lower leg fracture in the US was 0.6 per 1,000 Medicare enrollees, with rates varying from 0.2 per 1,000 Medicare enrollees to 1.1, more than a fivefold variation. Among hospital referral regions where rates of lower leg fracture per 1,000 Medicare enrollees were higher than average included Spartanburg, South Carolina (1.1); Cincinnati, Ohio (1.1); Toledo, Ohio (1.0); Philadelphia, Pennsylvania (1.0); Pittsburgh, Pennsylvania (0.9); and Birmingham, Alabama (0.9) (Fig. 4-27). Hospital referral regions where rates

(text continues on page 143)

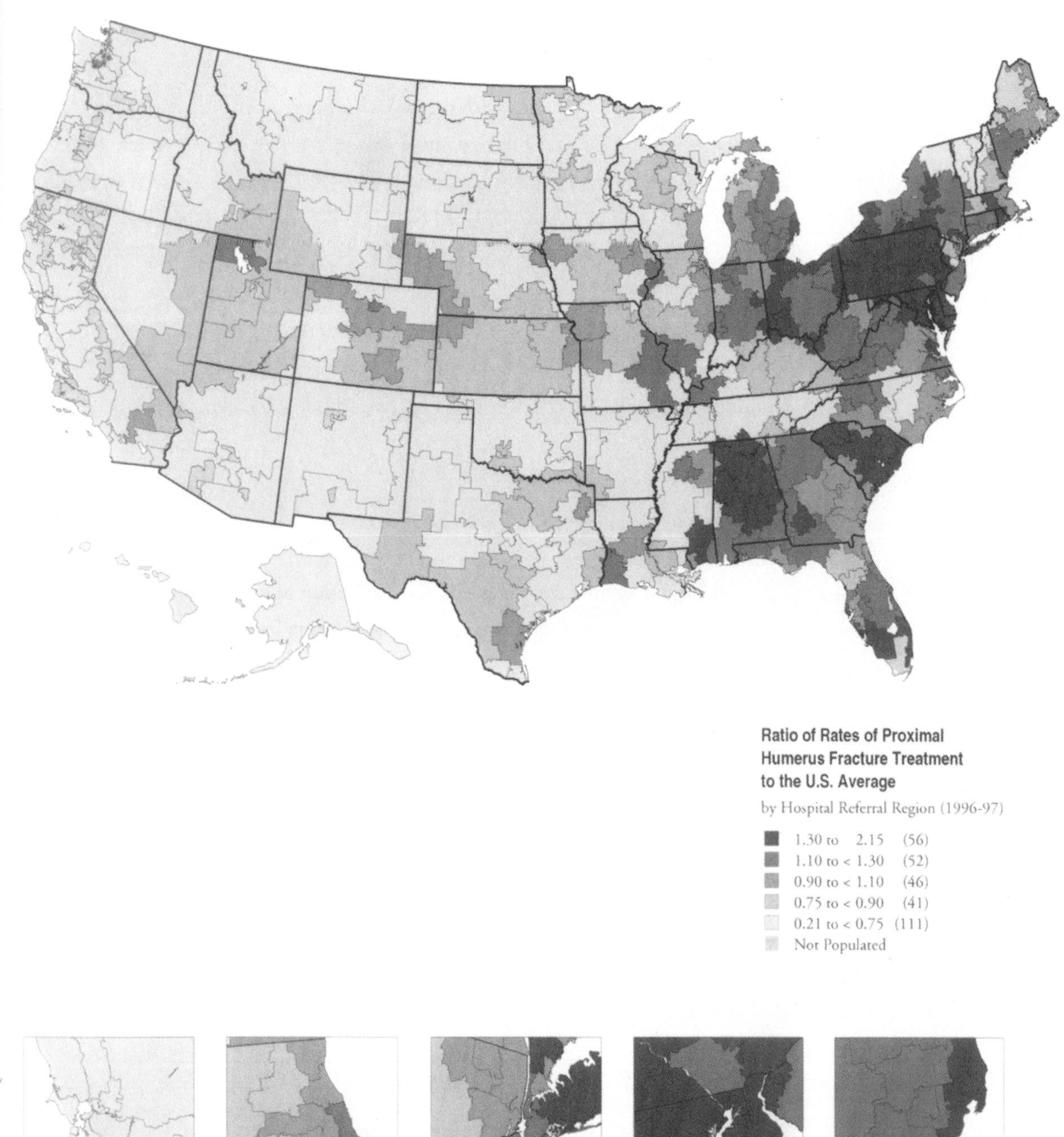

FIGURE 4-21 Rates of proximal humerus fracture treatment to the US average by hospital referral region (1996 to 1997). (Reprinted with permission from Wennberg J, Cooper MC, eds. *The Dartmouth Atlas of Musculoskeletal Health Care*. Chicago: American Hospital Association Press, 2000.)

Proportion of Proximal Humerus Fractures Treated Surgically

by Hospital Referral Region (1996-97)

- 40 or More (8)
- 30 to < 40 (11)
- 20 to < 30 (63)
- 10 to < 20 (144)
- Less than 10 (35)
- Not Populated
- Suppressed for Confidentiality

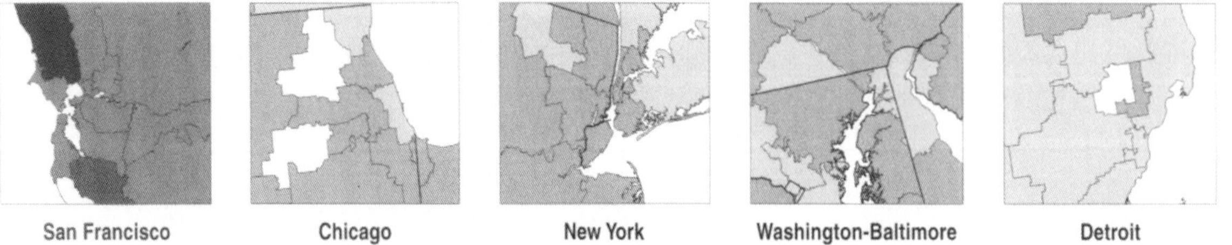

FIGURE 4-22 Proportion of proximal humerus fractures treated surgically by hospital referral region (1996 to 1997). (Reprinted with permission from Wennberg J, Cooper MC, eds. *The Dartmouth Atlas of Musculoskeletal Health Care*. Chicago: American Hospital Association Press, 2000.)

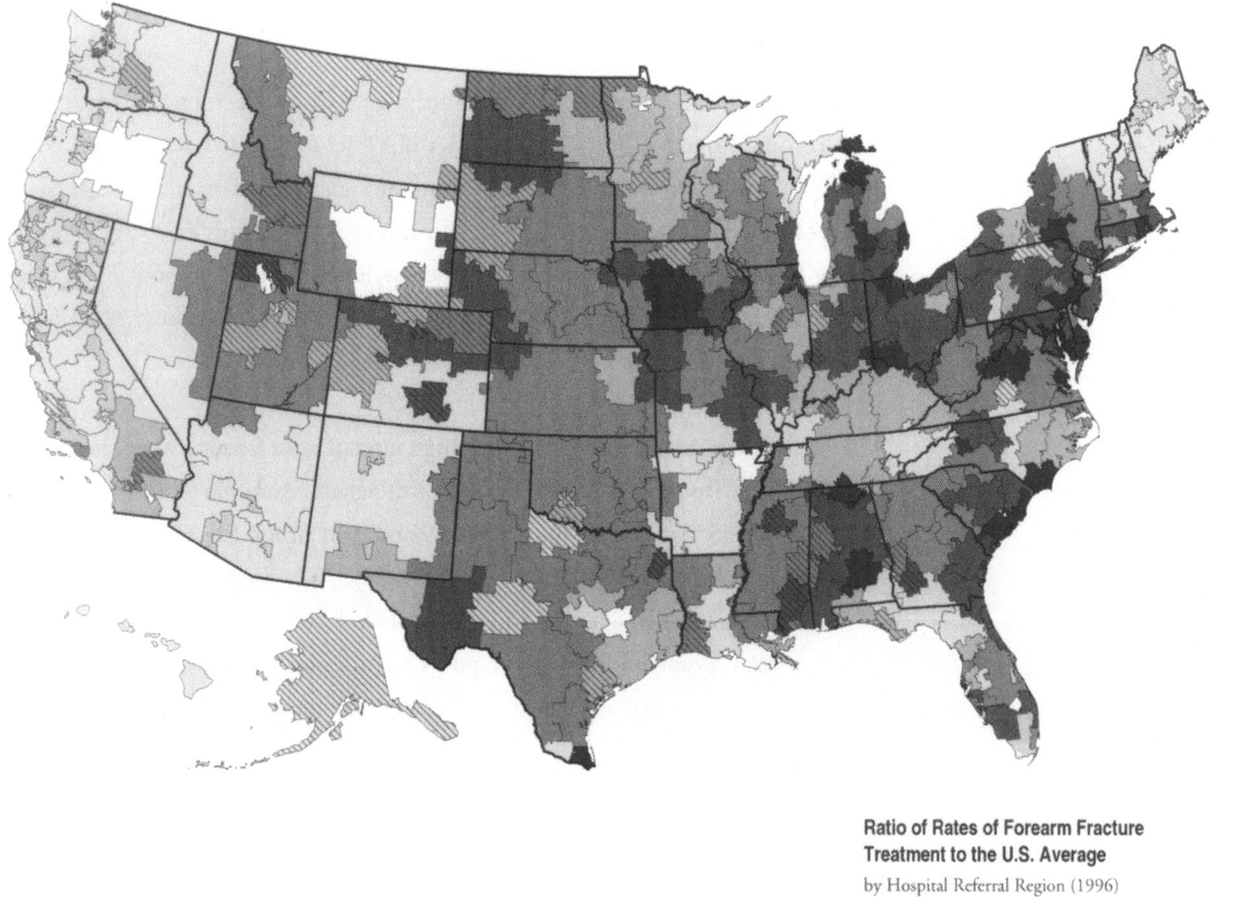

Ratio of Rates of Forearm Fracture Treatment to the U.S. Average

by Hospital Referral Region (1996)

- 1.30 to 2.07 (28)
- 1.10 to < 1.30 (65)
- 0.90 to < 1.10 (87)
- 0.75 to < 0.90 (50)
- 0.34 to < 0.75 (70)
- Not Populated
- Statistically Imprecise
- Suppressed for Confidentiality

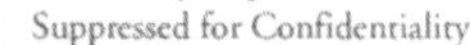

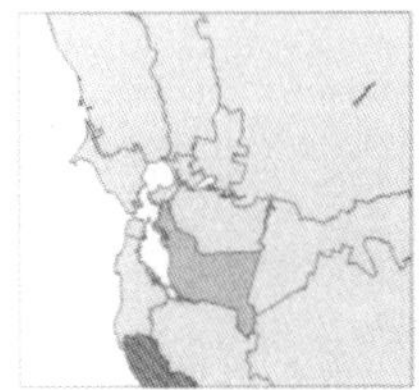

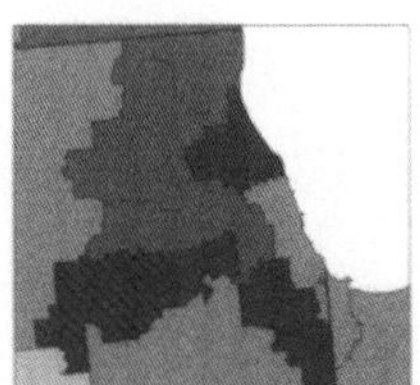

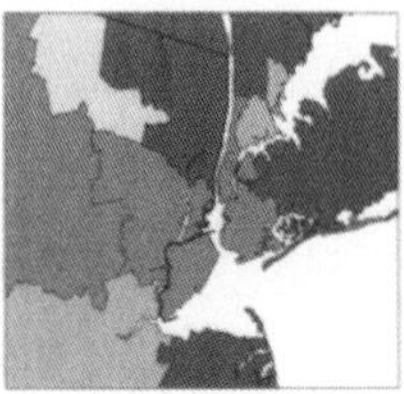

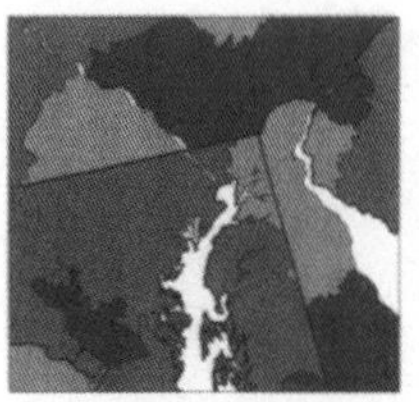

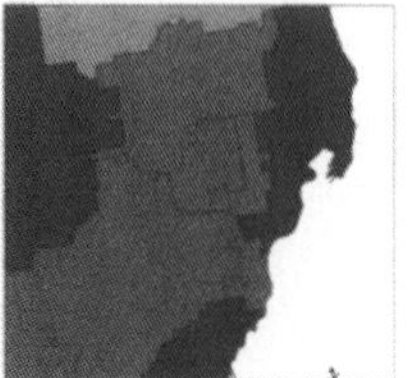

FIGURE 4-23 Ratio of forearm fracture treatment to the US average by hospital referral region (1996 to 1997). (Reprinted with permission from Wennberg J, Cooper MC, eds. *The Dartmouth Atlas of Musculoskeletal Health Care*. Chicago: American Hospital Association Press, 2000.)

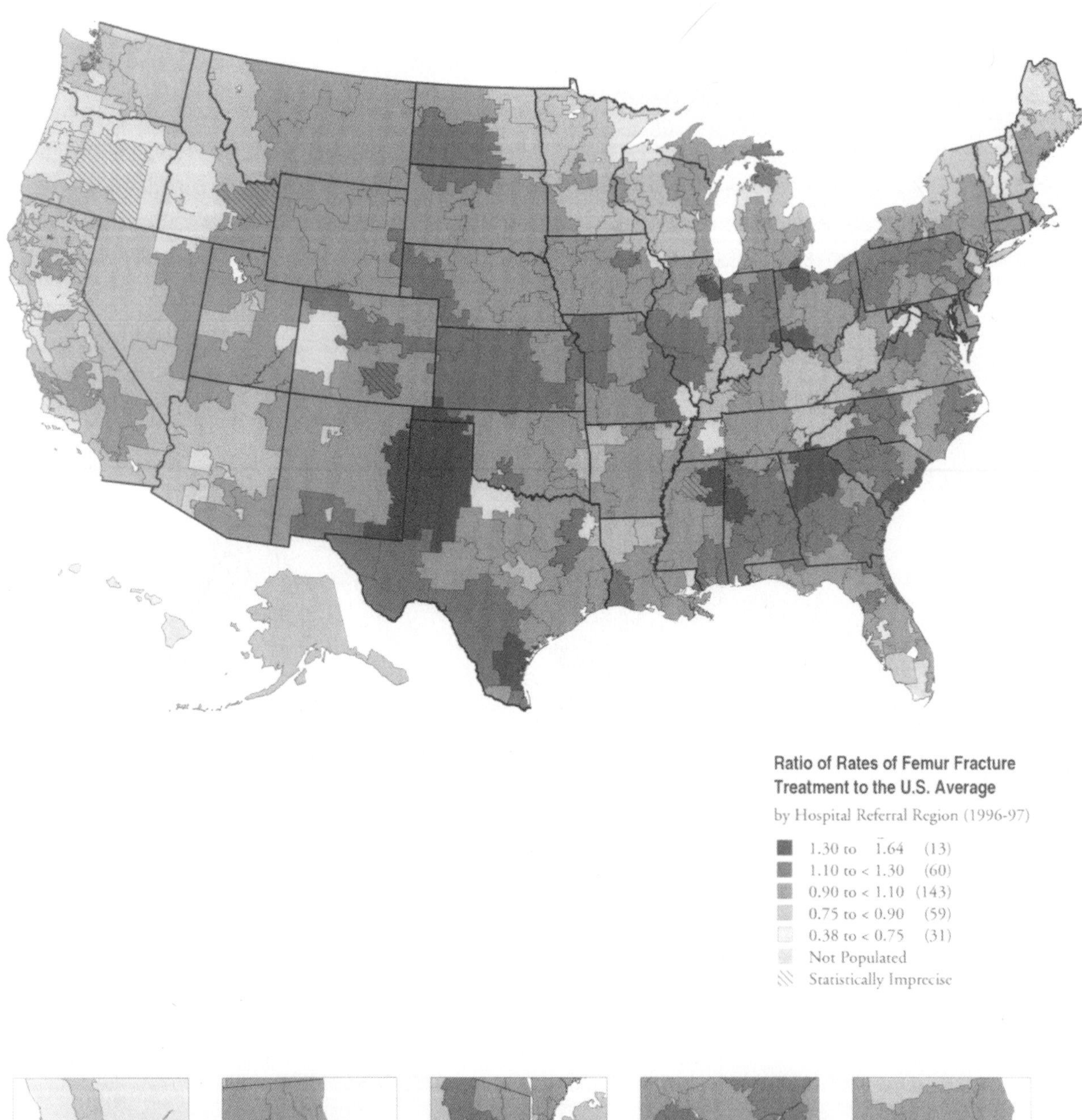

FIGURE 4-24 Ratio of rates of femur fracture treatment to the US average by hospital referral region (1996 to 1997). (Reprinted with permission from Wennberg J, Cooper MC, eds. *The Dartmouth Atlas of Musculoskeletal Health Care*. Chicago: American Hospital Association Press, 2000.)

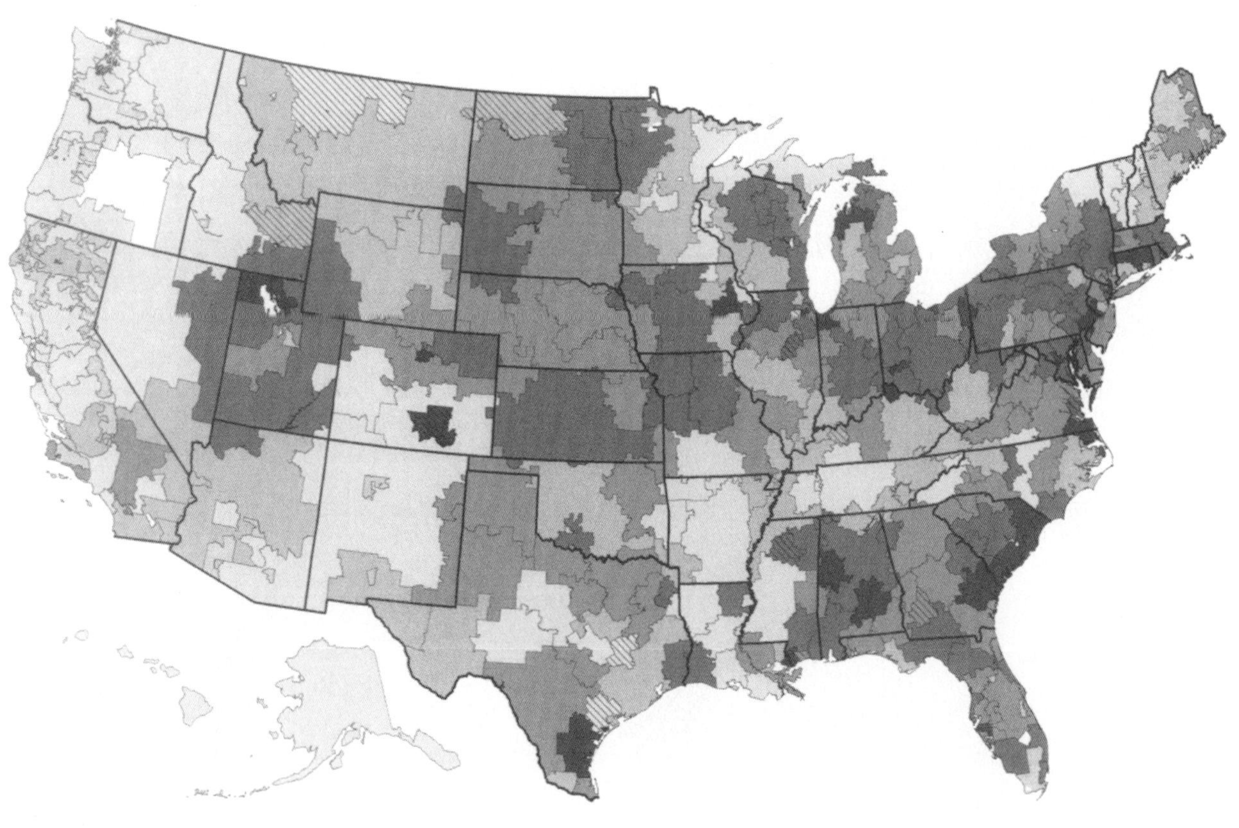

Ratio of Rates of Humeral Shaft/ Distal Humerus Fracture Treatment to the U.S. Average

by Hospital Referral Region (1996-97)

- 1.30 to 2.23 (24)
- 1.10 to < 1.30 (81)
- 0.90 to < 1.10 (84)
- 0.75 to < 0.90 (50)
- 0.39 to < 0.75 (65)
- Not Populated
- Statistically Imprecise
- Suppressed for Confidentiality

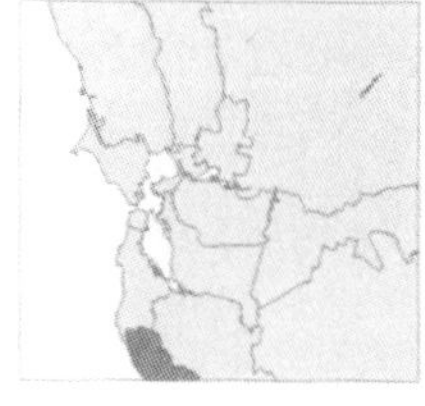

San Francisco

Chicago

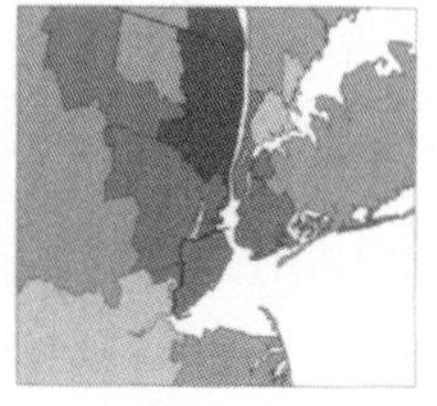

New York

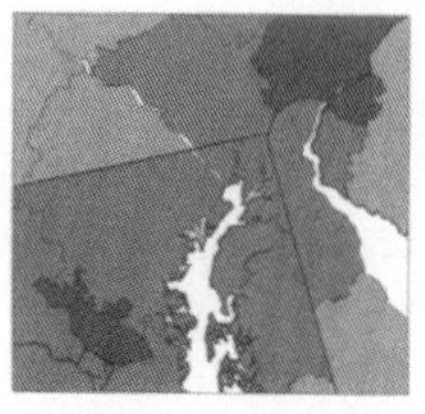

Washington-Baltimore

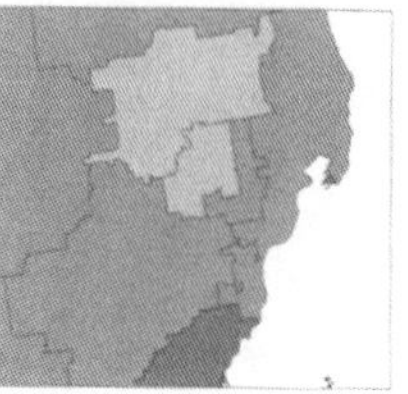

Detroit

FIGURE 4-25 Ratio of rate of humeral shaft/distal humerus fracture treatment to the US average by hospital referral region (1996 to 1997). (Reprinted with permission from Wennberg J, Cooper MC, eds. *The Dartmouth Atlas of Musculoskeletal Health Care*. Chicago: American Hospital Association Press, 2000.)

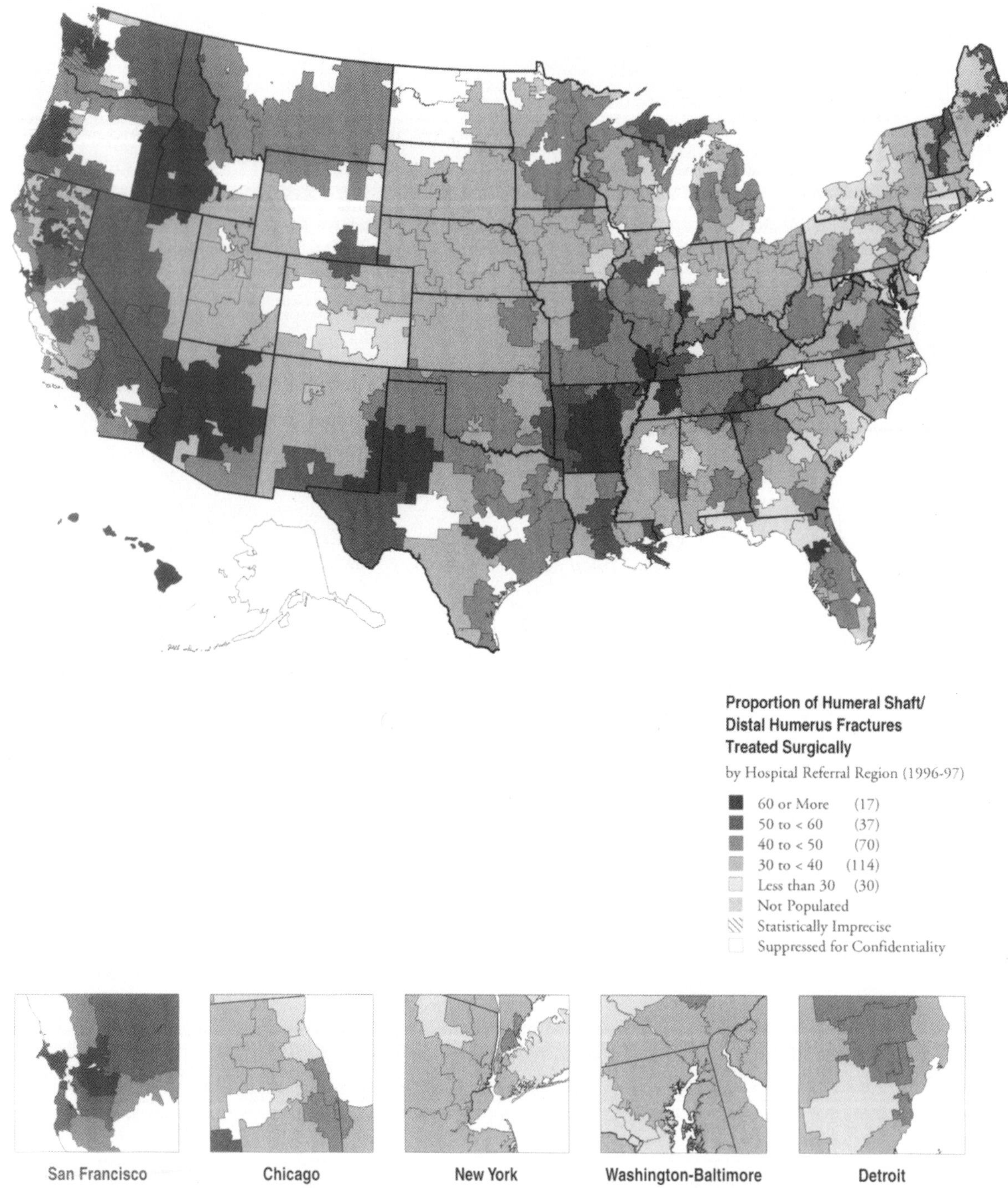

FIGURE 4-26 Proportion of humeral shaft/distal humerus fractures treated surgically by hospital referral region (1996 to 1997). (Reprinted with permission from Wennberg J, Cooper MC, eds. *The Dartmouth Atlas of Musculoskeletal Health Care*. Chicago: American Hospital Association Press, 2000.)

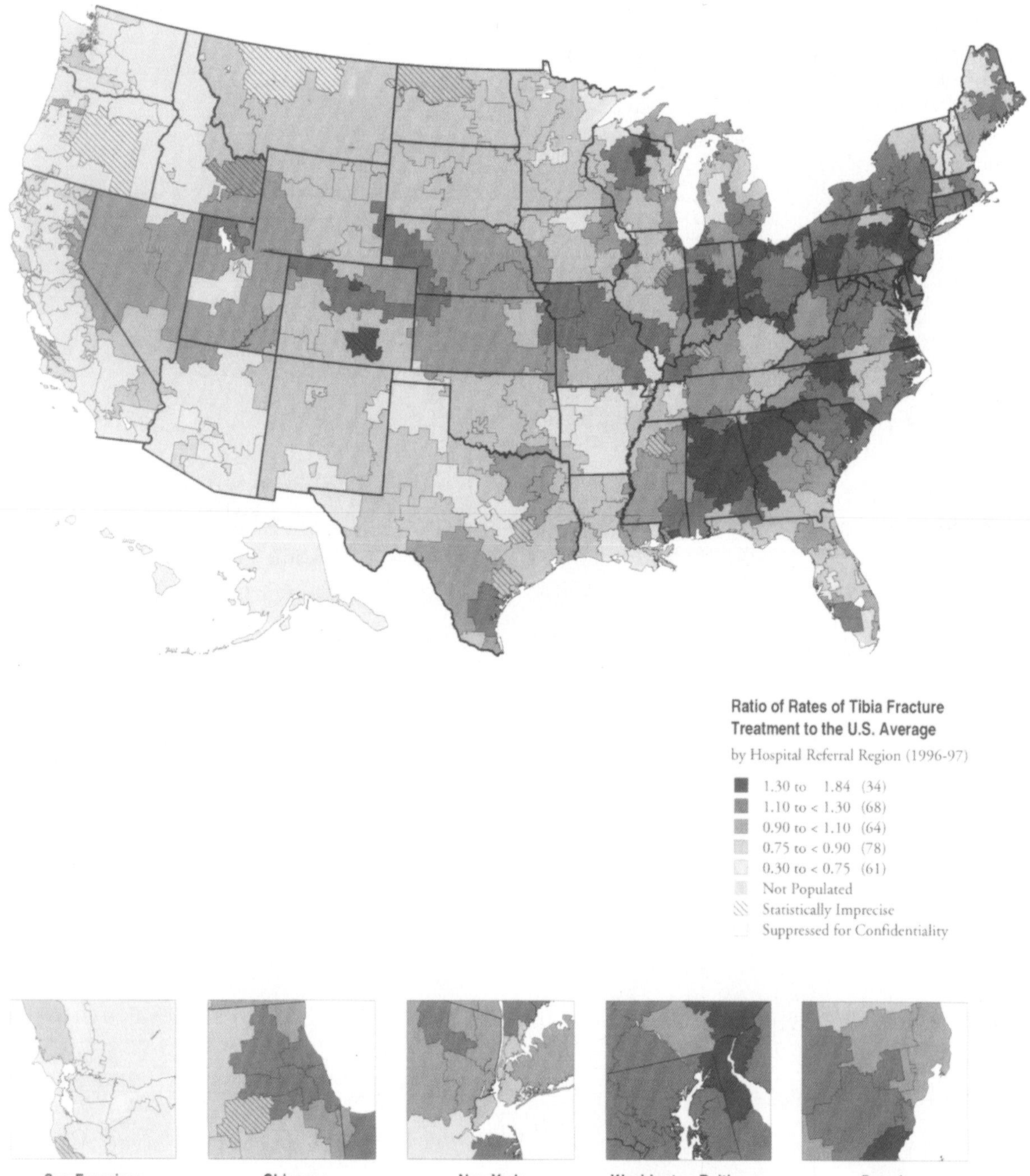

FIGURE 4-27 Ratio of rates of tibia fracture treatment to the US average by hospital referral region (1996 to 1997). (Reprinted with permission from Wennberg J, Cooper MC, eds. *The Dartmouth Atlas of Musculoskeletal Health Care*. Chicago: American Hospital Association Press, 2000.)

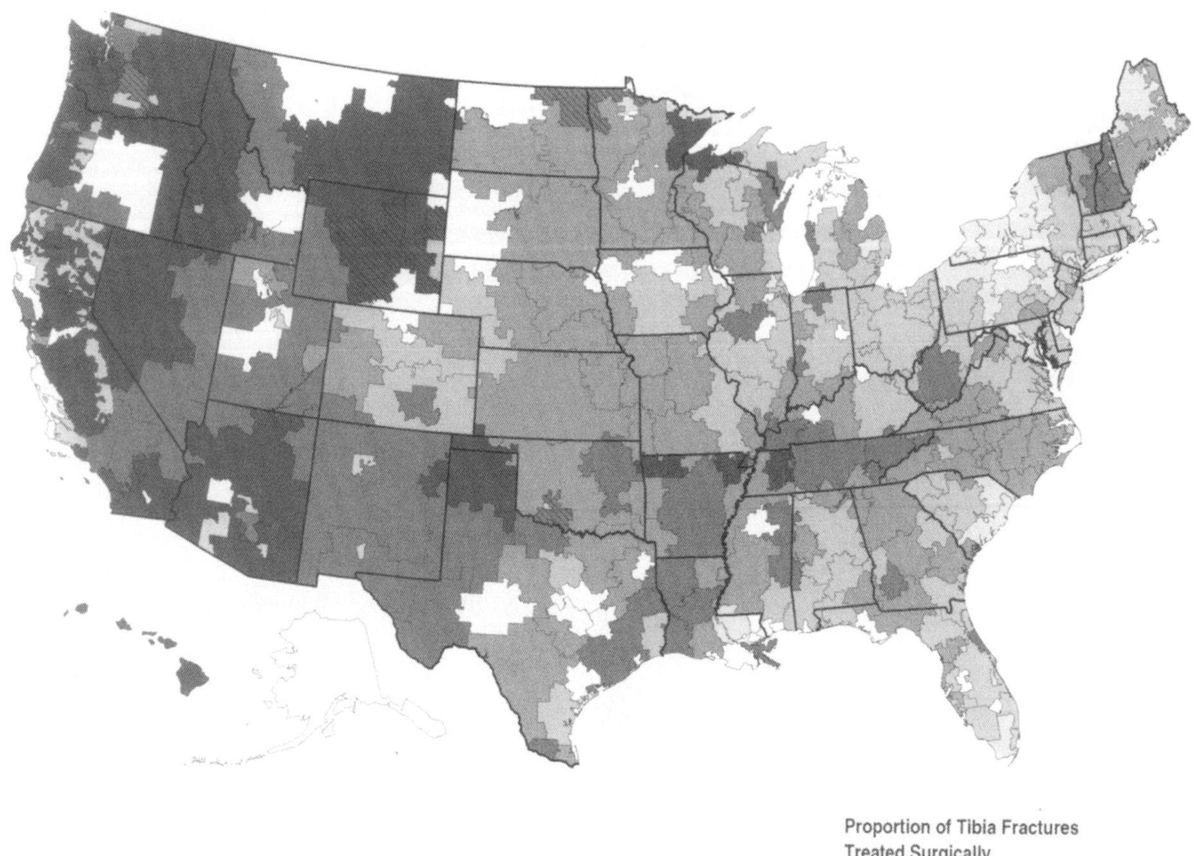

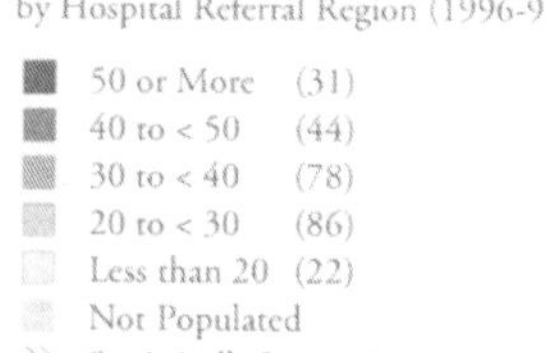

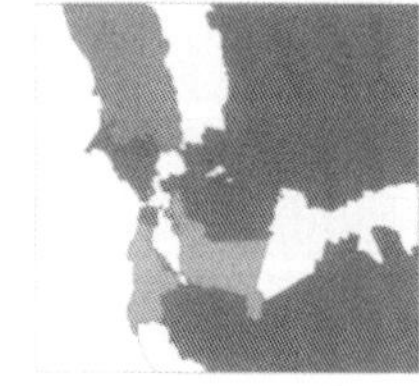

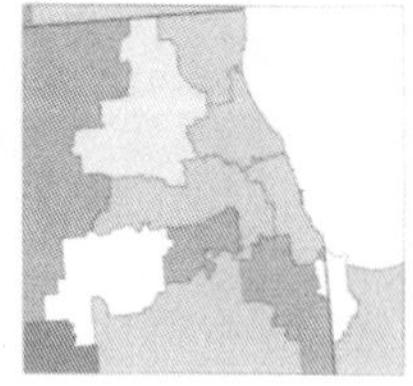

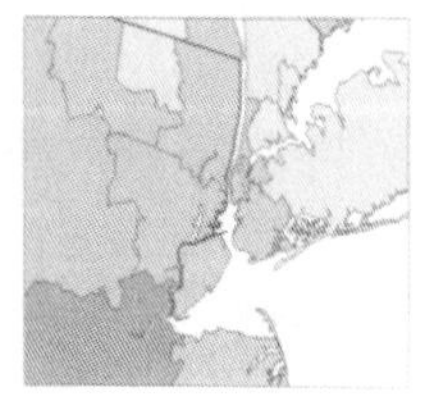

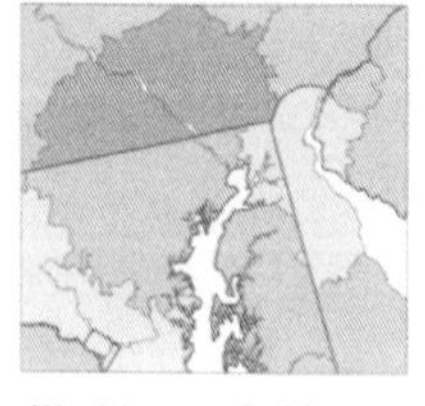

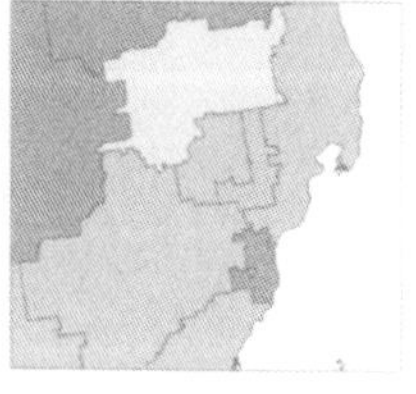

FIGURE 4-28 Proportion of tibial fractures treated surgically in the US by hospital referral region (1996 to 1997). (Reprinted with permission from Wennberg J, Cooper MC, eds. *The Dartmouth Atlas of Musculoskeletal Health Care*. Chicago: American Hospital Association Press, 2000.)

of proximal tibia and tibia shaft fracture were lower than average per 1,000 Medicare enrollees included Honolulu, Hawaii (0.2); Sun City, Arizona (0.2); San Francisco, California (0.2); Eugene, Oregon (0.3); Seattle, Washington (0.3); and Orange County, California (0.3).

Surgical repair of tibia fracture in the US averaged 30.3% from 1996 to 1997. Great variation was observed across hospital referral regions in the proportion of patients treated surgically (Fig. 4-28), however, with the proportion ranging from 13.7% to 69.4%. Hospital referral regions where the proportion of surgical repair of tibia fracture was significantly higher included Duluth, Minnesota (69.4%); San Francisco, California (68.6%); Seattle, Washington (58.3%); Billings, Montana (56.7%); Phoenix, Arizona (53.3%); Los Angeles, California (45.3%); and Houston, Texas (41.7%). Hospital referral regions where the proportion of surgical repair of tibia fracture was significantly lower than average were Buffalo, New York (13.7%); Rochester, New York (14.9%); Syracuse, New York (16.2%); Washington, D.C. (17.4%); Allentown, Pennsylvania (19.5%); and Fort Lauderdale, Florida (21.7%).

CONCLUSION

Musculoskeletal injury is a substantial source of morbidity and financial burden. To optimize treatment and health care resource allocation, study of demographic and epidemiological trends in musculoskeletal injury will continue to be necessary. Improved understanding of injury victim characteristics, as well regional outcome variation, is necessary to enhance future prevention and treatment programs, allowing specific populations to be addressed separately to improve overall outcomes. Furthermore, the differing proportions of injury treated surgically across the country warrant future study and may provide pertinent data on how to minimize morbidity of injury while optimizing both direct and indirect costs.

REFERENCES

1. Fildes J, et al. *National Trauma Data Bank Report 2003, Version 3.0*. American College of Surgeons, 2003. Available at: http://www.facs.org/trauma/ntdbannualreport2003.pdf.
2. Praemer A, Furner S, Rice D. *Musculoskeletal Conditions in the United States*. Rosemont: American Academy of Orthopaedic Surgeons, 1999.
3. Wennberg J, Cooper MC, eds. *The Dartmouth Atlas of Musculoskeletal Health Care*. Chicago: American Hospital Association Press, 2000.

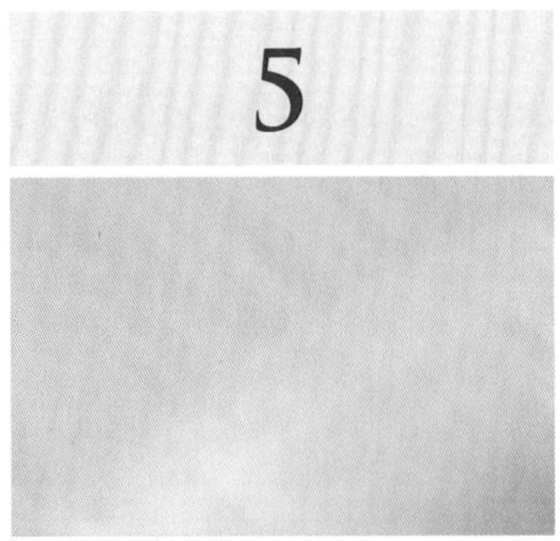

NONOPERATIVE FRACTURE TREATMENT

John F. Connolly

EFFECT OF TREATMENT ON SKELETAL REPAIR PROCESSES

We vertebrates have survived and flourished briefly by evolving efficient processes of skeletal repair and remodeling. They provide us not only with biomechanically ingenious support structures for upright locomotion but also serve as dynamic hemopoietic and osteogenic production and storage centers. Such advantages evolved eons before fracture surgeons came on the scene.

Ossification is not petrification. The skeletal system is very active metabolically with a turnover rate of 3% per year of cortical and 25% per year of cancellous bone (1). This turnover controls repair and maintenance of the matrix of skeletal support and also helps regulate the critical levels of calcium in tissue fluids. In addition, the skeletal marrow system provides a hemopoietic inductive microenvironment for the active production of 300 to 400 billion red cells and 100 to 200 billion white cells daily (2,3). This incredible productivity is increased significantly in response to blood loss or infection. It also depends on the variable half-life of RBCs and WBCs. Marrow stem cells are the seeds not only for hemopoiesis but also for skeletogenesis. Hemopoietic and stromal stem cells have been found escaping continuously into the bloodstream to replace senescent cells throughout the body (4). They are thought to contribute significantly to the maintenance and integrity of connective tissues throughout the body including bone and muscle (2,5,6).

The physician who treats patients with fractures should keep in mind the effect of such treatment, either operative or nonoperative, on the physiologic mechanisms of skeletal maintenance and repair derived from creative vertebrate evolution (7) over at least 250 million years. For instance, repair of fractures has evolved to accommodate for motion of the fracture fragments. For many fractures, this motion between fragments appears to stimulate the early repair processes (8). Rib and clavicle fractures are classic examples of the prompt healing that usually occurs despite, or possibly because of, interfragmentary motion. Fixation techniques, either operative or nonoperative, which eliminate this stimulus of motion (9,10), can sacrifice the gift of evolution-tested callus for the possibility of better cosmesis or function. For some fractures this sacrifice may be unrewarded or even counterproductive. Consequently, surgeons must keep in mind that the treatment we select for the fracture is never a neutral factor in the outcome (11,12).

The mechanisms by which functional motion stimulates callus formation and remodeling are known to be several, including vascular, bioelectric, and biochemical. Some degree of motion at the fracture site stimulates vascular ingrowth from soft tissue as well as from the medullary canal (13–15). This vascular ingrowth carries an invasion of cells as well as nutrients to fuel the hypermetabolic response of fracture healing. Additionally, intermittent loading of the fracture site, either with weightbearing or by muscle activity shifts the piezoelectric balance of the collagen-crystalline matrix. This appears to be the switch that turns on the bioelectric signals for osteoblasts to form new bone. Shear and compressive motion between the fracture fragments also break down bone matrix thereby releasing significant amounts of stimulatory factors from their skeletal storehouse and promoting bone formation (16).

A BRIEF HISTORY OF THE EVOLUTION OF FRACTURE TREATMENT

In contrast to the evolution of biologic processes of vertebrate repair occurring over millions of years, orthopaedic surgical repair of fractures has evolved quite briefly and rapidly. The primary surgical treatment of many open fractures in the Civil War era, for example, was amputation. Operative treatment of fractures, and indeed surgery on all previously inviolate body structures, was made possible by Lister's 1865 development of antiseptic techniques to treat open tibial and patella fractures (Table 5-1). Prior to Lister's development of safe antiseptic surgical techniques the main emphasis for thousands of years was on nonoperative methods for fracture treatment using a variety of splints, traction, or casts. A major objective was to find a

TABLE 5-1 Chronology of Nonoperative Fracture Treatment

Date	Originator	Contribution
3000 BC	Imhotep	Possible Egyptian author of the Edwin Smith Papyrus describing reduction of fractures, and immobilization with wood splints and bandages.
400 BC	Hippocrates	Greek medical icon who described mechanical aids to reduce fractures and dislocations as well as innovative bandaging techniques.
160 AD	Galen	Roman physician and anatomist who described a wide variety of bandages including a spica (wrapped with turns crossing like ear of grain).
1000 AD	Albucasis	Arab physician who advocated reducing femoral fracture with the knee flexed. This remained the position of choice for many hundreds of years. He also described plaster splints using flower, egg white, and other ingredients to support the fractured limb. These dressings were changed infrequently.
1363	de Chauliac	French cleric and surgeon who prescribed isometric traction to the fractured leg by weight attached to a cord and passing through a pulley.
1540	Pare	French military surgeon and unsurpassed innovator who described the differential diagnosis and treatment of hip fractures and dislocations along with many other classic works.
1765	Pott	London surgeon who described types of ankle fractures and the mechanics of reducing fractures to counteract muscle force.
1819	Dupuytren	Parisian surgical giant who among other works performed studies of experimental fractures in cadavers to illustrate mechanisms of injury and techniques of reduction.
1821	Barton	U.S. surgeon who described the treatment of greenstick fractures in children and the fracture-dislocation of radio carpal joint that bears his name.
1847	Smith	Dublin surgeon and pathologist who clarified the differential diagnosis and treatment of wrist fractures including the Colles and Smith fracture.
1852	Mathijesen	Dutch army surgeon who reported the use of plaster-of-paris bandages to immobilize fractures.
1852	Pirogov	Russian military surgeon who refined plaster bandage techniques and emphasized splinting fractures before moving the injured.
1860	Hamilton	New York surgeon and author who collected statistical tables detailing end results of a large number of patients with a wide variety of fractures. This represented the first outcome study to establish standard of care. An important influence on the result of malpractice suits, which were prevalent in this country even in the 19th century.
1861	Buck	U.S. military surgeon who popularized skin traction for femoral fractures with the knee extended.
1863	Hodgen	U.S. physician who modified the leg splint for applying skin traction to femur fractures.
1865	Lister	Glasgow, Scotland, surgeon who first applied antiseptic principles to the treatment of open tibial fractures, which allowed not only the successful treatment of these injuries without amputation but also gave birth eventually to the entire field of operative surgery.
1875	Thomas	Liverpool, England, bracemaker who developed the Thomas splint for immobilizing tuberculosis knees and fractures. This splint was credited for saving many lives of World War I soldiers with femur fractures that had been left unstabilized. Thomas promoted the treatment of fractures by "rest—absolute, uninterrupted, and prolonged." This was adopted for treatment of infections as well as fractures and influenced several generations of English and U.S. orthopaedic surgeons.

(*continued*)

TABLE 5-1 Continued

Date	Originator	Contribution
1876	Championniere	French surgeon who opposed the Thomas advocacy of treating fractures by rest and advocated mobilization and massage of muscles particularly around joints. He emphasized that restoration of function was not related to restoration of shape or length of the limb. These two contrasting approaches to fracture treatment by either rest or active motion remained a source of debate for the next century between Continental and Anglo-American orthopaedic surgeons.
1907	Steinmann	Berlin surgeon who described type of traction using a pin in the distal femur, which has become the standard for femoral fractures.
1919	Pearson	Utilized an ice-tong caliper inserted in the distal femur for traction and also devised an attachment to the Thomas splint to allow knee flexion.
1920	Delbet	French orthopaedic surgeon who described techniques of closed reduction of tibial fractures and application of plaster splints to permit weightbearing treatment of these fractures.
1921	Russell	Australian surgeon who devised a technique of skin traction for the femoral and hip fractures, which allowed flexion of the hip and knee using a double pulley system for mechanical advantage.
1927	Kirschner	Developed skeletal traction using a thin wire drilled through the femur and a tension bow to maintain rigidity of the wire.
1929	Böhler	Austrian surgeon who published a classic text on nonoperative treatment of fractures and particularly emphasized organized trauma centers to care for industrial and other injuries. He further popularized the use of skeletal traction for tibia fractures and skintight walking plaster after the fracture had partially healed.
1950	Charnley	Liverpool, England, orthopaedic surgeon whose text on the closed treatment of common fractures reflected the teaching of H. O. Thomas and Robert Jones. This leading orthopaedic innovator emphasized both the biomechanics and the techniques of fracture reduction as well as the advantages of nonoperative treatment of fractures.
1959	Dehne	U.S. military orthopaedic surgeon who popularized Böhler's weightbearing technique for treatment of tibia fractures in the United States.
1967	Sarmiento	Miami orthopaedic surgeon who applied the principles of prosthetics and orthotics to develop many innovative systems of fracture bracing for both the lower and upper extremity.
1970	Mooney	U.S. surgeon who utilized a combination of plaster cast and knee braces at Rancho Los Amigos Hospital in Los Angeles to treat fractures of the distal femur and proximal tibia encouraging functional weightbearing.
1936	Crutchfield	Developed skull tongs to permit skeletal traction for cervical spine fractures.
1959	Perry	Rancho Los Amigos surgeon who introduced the halo for skeletal traction and fixation of spinal fractures and dislocations.
1973	Gardner	A neurosurgeon who developed the principle of spring-loaded points for skull tongs to simplify application of acute traction for cervical injuries.

Modified from Peltier L. *Fractures: a history and iconography of their treatment*. San Francisco: Norman Publishing, 1990.

material that would allow immobilization of the fracture without requiring daily changes of the immobilizing splint. It was not until military surgeons Mathijesen and Pirogov in 1852 utilized plaster-of-paris techniques to immobilize fractures that this objective was achieved.

Skin and skeletal traction for fracture immobilization only became accepted for general use during the past 100 years based on the techniques of Buck, Kirschner, Steinmann, and others. Thus, in contrast to biologic processes of repair that evolved over eons to allow healing in response to fracture fragment motion, our mechanical methods of fracture immobilization have developed in relatively a few seconds on the evolutionary time scale.

The Anglo-American concept during the past century, as advocated by H. Owen Thomas, Robert Jones, and Watson Jones, was that continuous, uninterrupted rest and immobilization (without allowing fracture motion) were essential for fracture union. This concept was based particularly on experience in treating the then-common problems of tuberculosis and other infections of bone. In contrast, the prevailing concept in the European continent fostered by Lucas-Championnière was that "life is motion." Active, early restoration of muscle and joint function with closed, or if necessary, operative techniques, became the goal of European followers of Lucas-Championnière and others. The consequence has been that European surgeons such as Küntscher, as well as the AO group, have led the development of effective operative fixation techniques. Many of the innovations from the Anglo-American school have, until recently, been directed at nonoperative techniques, particularly casting and bracing of fractures.

SELECTION OF FRACTURES FOR NONOPERATIVE TREATMENT AND ACCEPTABILITY OF REDUCTION

Every student physician learning the art of closed, nonoperative management first desires straightforward guidelines to decide what fractures to treat nonoperatively and what is an acceptable reduction. Perhaps the first rule should be that virtually every fracture can be treated and has been treated nonoperatively. The question in regard to selecting treatment should be: Why can't this particular fracture be treated nonoperatively? As our techniques, surgical skills, and eagerness to treat fractures operatively increase, the answers to this key question can be multiple.

Many patients are more comfortable with operative treatment and return to relative independent function more readily (17). This is particularly true for patients with multiple fractures or systemic injuries from violent mechanisms of the type seen in many trauma centers. However, most patients sustain an isolated fracture that does not usually require the "high powered" care of trauma centers. These isolated fractures may do just as well with nonoperative management without the risk of surgery. Just as the frequency of many procedures such as laminectomies and total joint replacements varies with the concentration and philosophy of surgeons (18), the indications for operative treatment of fractures often depend primarily on the training and biases of that community's fracture surgeons. However, as Keller and co-workers (19) have emphasized, physicians cannot assume that their outcomes will be the same as others and therefore they need to evaluate their own results.

The usual criteria for selecting treatment and evaluating outcome tend to be based on the radiographic characteristics of the fracture (20). Unfortunately, classification of fractures and outcome assessments that rely on these criteria can be misleading and vary from one observer to the next (21,22). Also, the concept that less than anatomic alignment of the fracture leads inevitably to malunion, arthritis, and unsatisfactory function has proven, in general, to be incorrect in long-term studies (23–28). Studies have shown that some shortening and limited fracture angulation do not impair function and may actually speed up fracture healing and restoration of bone strength (27,29). However, failure to achieve perfect reduction naturally creates a question in the mind of any student or patient who looks at an x-ray of a fracture with slight shortening or overriding of fragments and feels that an unsatisfactory result is being accepted. The answer to these concerns is that it is the appearance of the limb, not the x-ray, that counts (see Figs. 5-2, 5-3, 5-4). The natural processes of repair can remodel and restore normal anatomy quite effectively but not if they are impeded by malpositioned internal or external fixation devices (Fig. 5-1). This is even more important for children with growth potential where remodeling permits a wider range of what can be considered an acceptable reduction (30).

The key determinant of the acceptability of reduction is that the patient's fractured limb looks normal clinically. If one in-

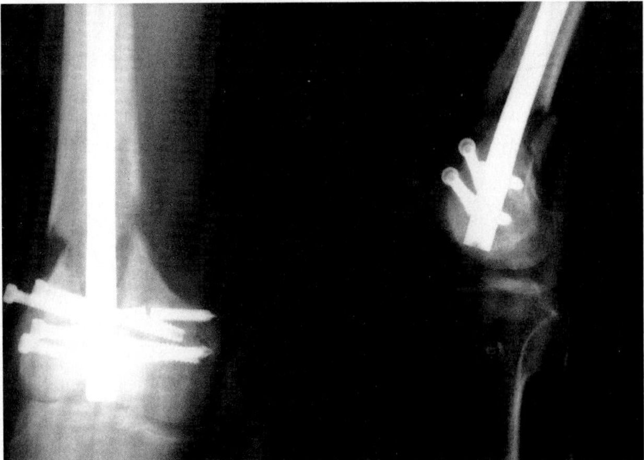

FIGURE 5-1 This distal femoral fracture demonstrates that loose internal fixation may impede processes of fracture repair and lead to bone resorption and a bone gap rather than bone formation and fracture union.

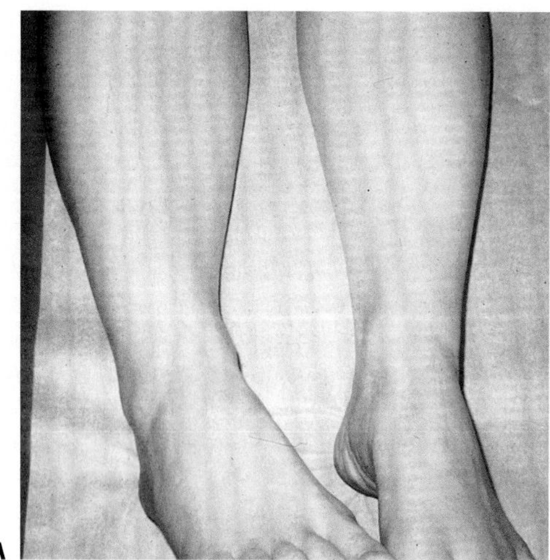

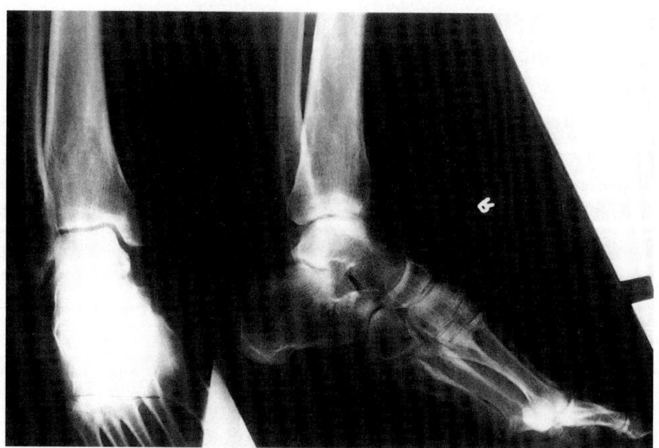

FIGURE 5-2 **A.** This patient's leg demonstrates an internal rotation and varus angulation 1 year after her fractured tibia was considered to have healed satisfactorily by x-ray. The distal torsional angulation of the limb caused the patient discomfort from walking on the lateral aspect of her inverted foot. In reducing a fracture the clinical three-dimensional appearance of limb alignment is a primary determinant of an "acceptable" reduction. **B.** Anteroposterior and lateral x-rays of this patient's healed fracture were considered to show satisfactory alignment but unfortunately the two-dimensional x-ray images did not show the three-dimensional torsional malunion that was causing the patient to invert her foot and produce very painful symptoms with weightbearing.

spects a limb, it is usually possible to determine if it is angulated, malrotated, or shortened (Fig. 5-2). Radiographs are most useful in evaluating the reduction of fractures involving joint surfaces. Also, radiographs are useful in determining that the reduction has restored the joints above and below the fracture to a normal relationship. It is axiomatic that an x-ray of any fracture prior to reduction should include the joints proximal and distal. The same rule holds in order to evaluate the reduction of a fracture adequately. Joint alignment is best assessed on a single x-ray. For example, the tibial fracture particularly requires that the x-ray show both the knee and ankle, obtained, if necessary, by placing the limb diagonally across the cassette. This view should confirm a satisfactory relationship with the knee and ankle despite the presence of slight fracture overriding or shortening.

Slight limb shortening is desirable with closed fracture management, and in fact the creation of a fracture gap by unstable internal fixation techniques has been one of the prime avoidable causes of nonunion in this author's review of 200 osseous healing problems (11) (Fig. 5-1). Fracture shortening or overriding promotes a stronger callus with a wider surface area. This is a classic demonstration of Wolff's law that "bone responds to the need for it" and is consistent with the way in which bone and soft tissues heal in response to applied stresses (31,32) (Fig. 5-3).

In summary, nonoperative treatment can be usually selected for most fractures despite significant and enthusiastic advocacy for operative treatment of all fractures. The treatment chosen should be tailored to the needs of the patient rather than the patient being fitted to the needs of the therapy. The main determinant of an acceptable closed reduction is that the limb appears normal by clinical evaluation to allow prompt restoration of function with healing. Restoration of length of the fractured limb is more important in the weightbearing bones of the lower limb than it is in the upper limb. However, even in weightbearing bones slight shortening from some fracture overriding is preferable to the creation of fracture gaps by unstable internal fixation techniques (33). Consequently, to answer the question of what is an acceptable reduction, one must focus on the appearance and function of the patient's fractured limb and not merely on the x-ray (Figs. 5-2 and 5-3).

OPTIONS IN NONOPERATIVE MANAGEMENT OF FRACTURES

The basic methods of nonoperative fracture management include reduction by traction and manipulation of the fracture followed by immobilization of the reduced fracture using casts, splints, braces, or other techniques. However, a number of common fractures require no reduction and may be effectively treated by providing pain relief, a minimal period of immobilization, and prompt restoration of function. Pain relief is best accomplished using local methods including the technique of rest, ice, compression, and elevation (RICE). The patient should also be prescribed sufficient analgesics to relieve the acute pain of the fracture, which can be quite severe.

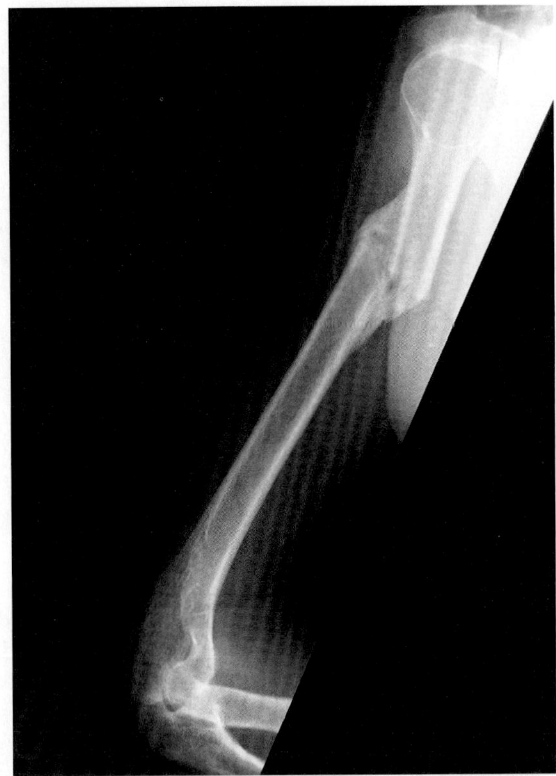

FIGURE 5-3 This humeral shaft fracture was treated with a fracture brace and healed in bayonet apposition, primarily by forming external callus. The massive amount of new bone formed on the circumference of the humerus increased the structural moment of inertia, which is proportionate to the radius to its 4th power (R4). Anatomic realignment is not the *sine qua non* of an "acceptable" reduction.

A whole variety of factors influence the selection of treatment options. For many common fractures, an objective analysis of risks and benefits will strongly favor nonoperative treatment (11,34). This is especially true for fractures that can be effectively and safely treated without reduction as illustrated by the following examples.

UPPER EXTREMITY FRACTURES COMMONLY TREATED NONOPERATIVELY WITHOUT MANIPULATIVE REDUCTION

Clavicle Fracture

Clavicle fractures are very common and archaeologic skeletal remains show a high frequency of these fractures sustained by prehistoric man that healed without benefit of orthopaedic treatment (35). Clavicle fracture in the child heals promptly when splinted in a figure-of-8 harness for 2 to 3 weeks. In the adult, the clavicle fracture is different. Often it is the result of a violent injury, which can comminute and displace the fracture fragments significantly. In a review of the long-term consequences of clavicle fractures (36), we found the frequency of nonunion to be about the same as other fractures (3% to 5%). Splinting of the adult's fractured clavicle with a figure-of-8 harness is often ineffective and uncomfortable. Nonoperative management can often be accomplished best by supporting the weight of the arm in a sling and swath to prevent downward pull on the lateral fragment. Usually satisfactory clinical alignment can be achieved. However, persistent displacement of the adult's clavicle fracture can lead to malunion and prolong symptoms from thoracic outlet compression (36) (Fig. 5-4). Limb threatening ischemia from compression of the subclavian artery may develop long after the displaced clavicle fracture is healed (37). Also, unrecognized subclavian vein thrombosis may lead to repeated pulmonary emboli and even fatal pulmonary failure (the Paget-Von Schroetter syndrome) (38).

Fractures of the lateral third of the clavicle, although not as common as those of the middle third, can present difficulties of management. Operative fixation has been associated with complications including infection, failure of fixation, and persistent nonunion (39). Robinson and Cairns (40) have demonstrated successful results with nonoperative treatment of most displaced lateral fractures of the clavicle, particularly, in middle age and elderly patients. They evaluated over 100 patients so treated by sling immobilization and early range of motion therapy who usually discarded the sling by 2 weeks after the injury. This protocol resulted in an initial 37% nonunion rate, and these nonunions were mostly asymptomatic. Only 11% of the patients required surgery for their nonunions. The authors felt that an asymptomatic fibrous union or nonunion after a displaced lateral clavicle fracture may be analogous to a pain free displaced acromioclavicular separation.

Many of these lateral clavicle fractures, which can be difficult to fix operatively, may be better treated by sling immobilization and early range of motion therapy. The method is usually quite acceptable for the majority of fractures in middle-aged and elderly individuals. Surgical reconstruction can be reserved for the minority of usually younger patients with persistent discomfort or significant disruption of the shoulder suspensory complex.

Fractures of the Scapula

Fractures of the scapula usually result from a severe direct injury to the posterior aspect of the shoulder, and almost all are associated with rib fractures, pulmonary contusion, pneumothorax, or hemopneumothorax (41,42). They may be associated with vascular injuries or injuries to the brachial plexus and these associated problems should be carefully evaluated and treated prior to treatment of the fracture.

Because of the associated injuries, the usual treatment of a scapula fracture is bed rest, application of ice, and analgesics. As the patient becomes ambulatory, the limb is supported in a sling and swath with the arm supported firmly against the chest

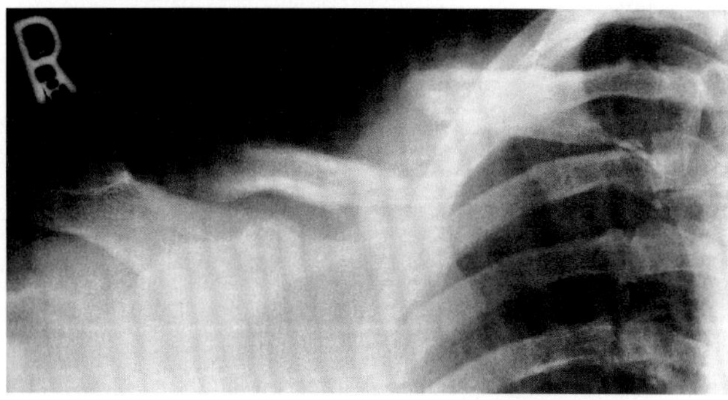

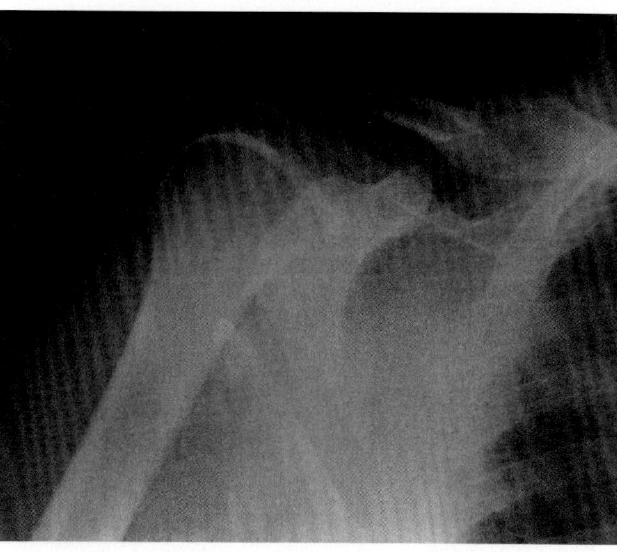

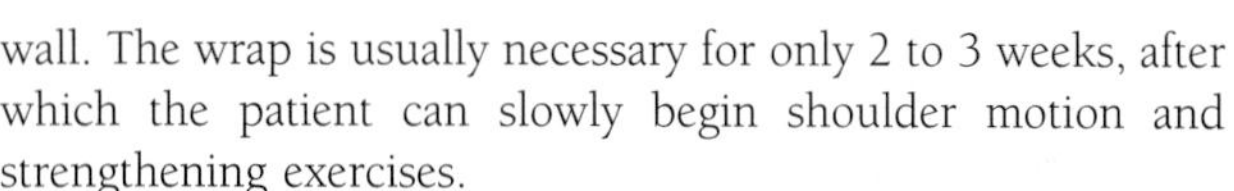

FIGURE 5-4 **A.** This x-ray shows the significant displacement that can occur particularly in the adult's fractured clavicle when the weight of the arm pulls the lateral fragment downward. **B.** This fracture healed with overriding of the fragments and compression of the thoracic outlet particularly when the arm was elevated. Symptoms persisted for 10 years until the malunion was corrected surgically.

wall. The wrap is usually necessary for only 2 to 3 weeks, after which the patient can slowly begin shoulder motion and strengthening exercises.

Intraarticular glenoid fractures can usually be treated nonoperatively unless there is significant displacement of fracture fragments or dislocation of the joint. Fractures of the scapula neck when associated with a fractured clavicle as well as other injuries may require reduction or even operative fixation to prevent drooping of the shoulder and weakness of shoulder muscles (43,44). However, they usually can be reduced by lateral traction for a period of 1 to 2 weeks in bed with the patient in the supine position (45,46) (Fig. 5-5). Edwards and co-authors (47) have found that nonoperative treatment of floating shoulder injuries, especially those with less than 5 mm of fracture displacement, can achieve satisfactory results that are probably equal or superior to those reported with operative treatment. The method that these authors recommend for the relatively undisplaced fractures is the use of a shoulder immobilizer or a sling for a period of 3 to 8 weeks. Physical therapy to regain shoulder motion is prescribed as soon as the associated injuries allow, usually within the first 2 weeks.

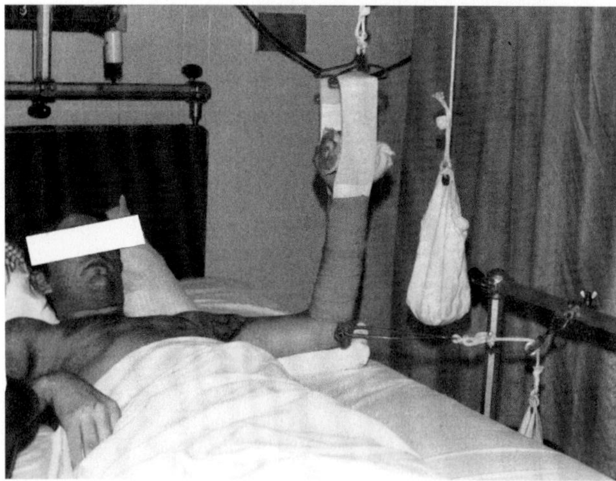

FIGURE 5-5 Fractures of the clavicle and scapula may require olecranon pin traction as illustrated here, particularly for the head injured patient. The pin is inserted through the ulnar shaft distal to the olecranon, taking care to avoid the ulnar nerve. The forearm and hand are supported by skin traction. However, for most fractures of the clavicle and scapula, treatment with a shoulder immobilizing harness or sling and swathe is usually effective.

Proximal Humeral Fractures

A number of investigators have demonstrated that there is little evidence that operative treatment of 2 or 3 part fractures confers benefit on the usual elderly patient who sustains this injury. The usual 2 or 3 part fracture of the surgical neck of the humerus in an osteoporotic elderly patient can be consistently and effectively treated by support in a sling, until initial symptoms subside (48,49). Early gentle range of shoulder motion at 1 to 2 weeks, followed by progressively more vigorous exercise at 3 to 5 weeks, can reliably lead to fracture union and restoration of satisfactory function without necessarily achieving anatomic reduction of these fractures (Fig. 5-6). Clinical stability and union of the fracture usually precedes radiographic union by several weeks (50).

Fracture of the proximal humerus is often associated with a temporary inferior subluxation of the head due to hemorrhage into the joint or the loss of static rotator cuff muscle support. It also may be due to loss of negative intra-articular pressure, which resists gravity forces and normally holds the humeral head in articulation with the glenoid (51,52). This pseudosubluxation disappears with active range of motion and the initial healing of the capsule (53) (Fig. 5-7).

In contrast to inferior subluxation, which is temporary, a superior migration of the humeral head after a fracture usually

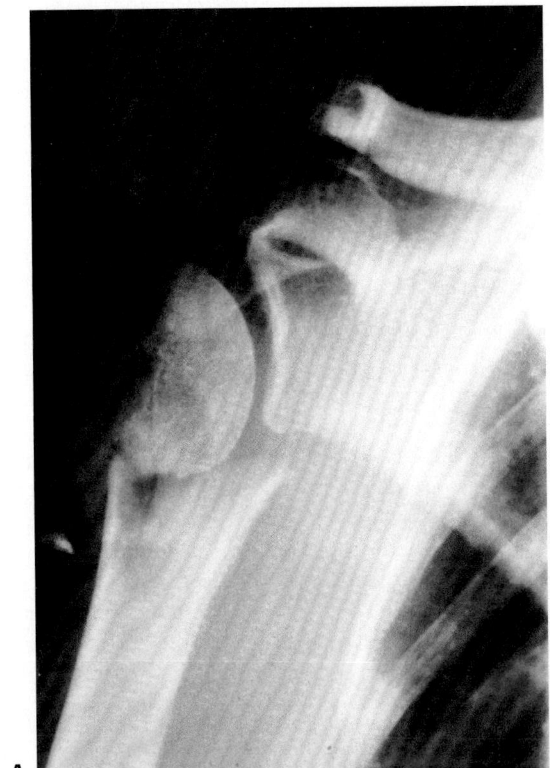

A

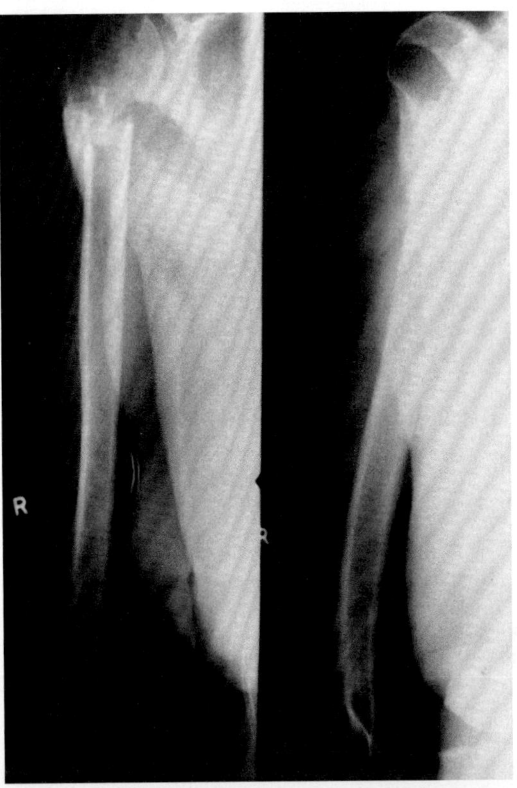

B

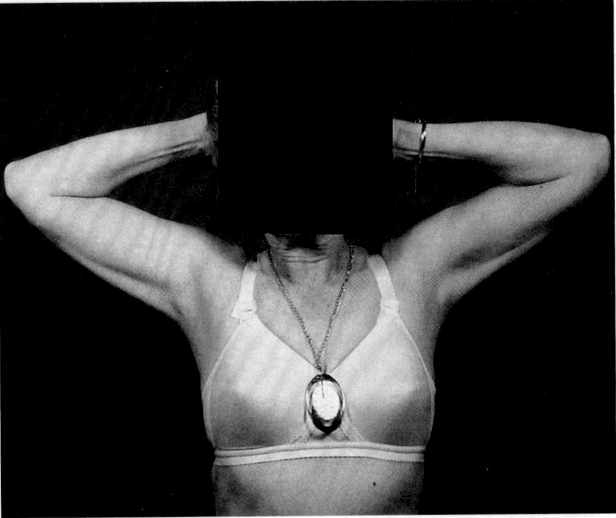

C

FIGURE 5-6 A. Initial x-ray shows a pronounced displacement of the humeral surgical neck fracture resulting from an internal torsional mechanism. **B.** The patient was treated by allowing early external rotational exercises of the shoulder. A satisfactory callus formed and the fracture healed with satisfactory, but nonanatomic, alignment as shown on these x-rays 12 weeks after injury. **C.** The clinical photograph of this patient at 12 weeks postfracture shows the range of motion possible when the emphasis was placed on functional early exercises while the fracture was healing rather than waiting for the fracture to heal radiographically before allowing functional exercises.

indicates loss of rotator cuff function and the need for operative repair (54) (Fig. 5-8). Superior migration of the humeral head results from upward pull of the deltoid muscle unopposed by the rotator cuff forces, which normally maintain the humeral head against the glenoid during shoulder abduction.

Closed reduction of surgical neck fractures is usually unnecessary as well as ineffective. The compulsion to reduce these fractures anatomically is difficult but important to repress (55). One should rather allow the normal forces of shoulder motion and muscle function to align the fracture and anticipate that some degree of remodeling will occur. Furthermore, over forceful manipulation, particularly if resisted by tight muscles, can completely displace the humeral head fragment (56,57).

The shoulder is the most mobile joint in the body and it demands considerable flexibility to maintain its near global range of motion. Therefore, management of fractures about the shoulder should incorporate a program of early exercises to

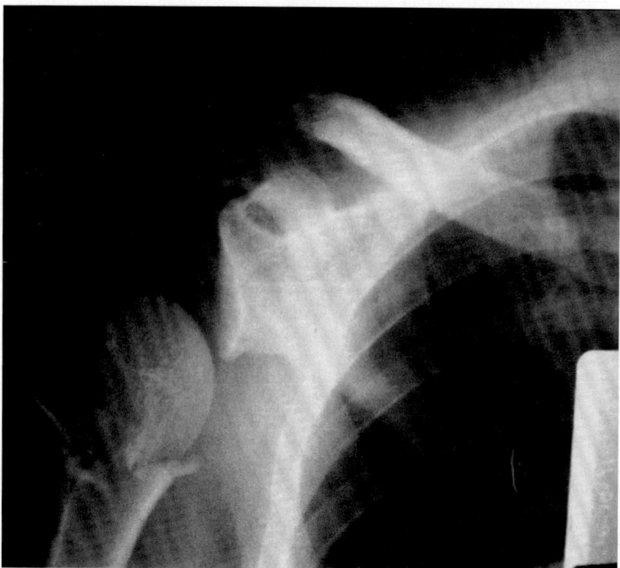

FIGURE 5-7 A fracture of the proximal humerus treated with prolonged immobilization may demonstrate inferior subluxation of the head of the humerus if the patient does not actively exercise the shoulder. This is due to a combination of loss of negative pressure within the joint as well as loss of rotator cuff and deltoid muscle support. It can be overcome by allowing the patient to exercise actively.

maintain motion. Otherwise the shoulder capsule can become progressively stiffer (58,59).

To prevent this rather common problem, which is essentially an adduction contracture of the gleno-humeral capsule, it is essential to incorporate a program of early passive range of motion exercises as soon as the fracture shows early clinical stability. Waiting for complete radiographic healing for 6 to 8 weeks is one of the main causes of nonunion sometimes attributed to "nonoperative treatment." Persistent immobilization of the shoulder may cause the fracture gap to widen due to the pull of the dead weight of the arm and the lack of muscle function impacting the fracture fragments. Prolonged immobilization of the fracture also leads to loss of functional motion, particularly abduction and external rotation of the shoulder. By 2 weeks, gravity-assisted exercises with circumduction or pendulum motions should be encouraged. These can progress by 4 to 6 weeks to passive stretching of the shoulder in abduction and external rotation (59). In doing this the patient braces the scapula against the wall and attempts to bring their clasped hands up behind the head. The shoulders are then abducted and externally rotated, usually with the assistance of a family member, until the individual can bring both elbows back to the wall. This exercise may initially be somewhat painful, but by 8 to 10 weeks it is usually possible to achieve close to full abduction. In using these exercises for most fractures of the surgical neck of the humerus and basing progress toward healing on clinical rather than radiographic criteria, one can minimize long-term consequences of the injury while encouraging healing of the fracture (50).

Humeral Shaft Fractures

Fractures of the humeral shaft provide excellent demonstrations of how well-intentioned but misdirected efforts at fracture reduction and immobilization can be detrimental to healing (60). In the 1930s and 1940s, when management of the humeral shaft fracture emphasized techniques such as abduction "airplane" splints or shoulder spica casts, the humeral fracture became a prime candidate for nonunion. As the failure of these approaches became evident and fracture surgeons became aware that humeral fractures heal with minimal immobilization, techniques such as hanging casts improved results (61). Unfortunately, they often cause patient discomfort and have a tendency to cause fracture angulation and distraction due to the assumed necessity of immobilizing the elbow.

Subsequently, in the last two to three decades Sarmiento and colleagues (28,62,63) have demonstrated that humeral fracture braces, by allowing elbow motion, can realign the axis of the elbow joint, reduce the fracture, and promote healing. This technique has significantly improved results to the point that the humeral shaft fracture treated in this way rarely fails to heal. Fracture brace treatment emphasizes reduction by the force of gravity and functional muscle activity. A well-vascularized muscle envelope surrounds the humeral shaft. This envelope helps to control the alignment of the fracture in the brace and stimulates callus formation. Isometric muscle contraction in the fracture brace does not deform the fracture; rather, it aligns it. Muscle function and elbow motion actually serve to align the humeral fracture by restoring the axis of elbow motion to a normal relationship with the humeral shaft (Fig. 5-9).

Initially, the fracture should be immobilized to make the patient comfortable, preferably with a Velpeau type of dressing. This includes an axillary pad, a sling to support the weight of the arm against the patient's chest, and a circumferential wrap around the chest. The use of "gutter" splints for humeral shaft fractures should generally be discouraged since they tend to be uncomfortable for the patient and angulate the fracture (Fig. 5-9).

The usual treatment is Velpeau immobilization until the swelling subsides by 1 to 2 weeks, when the fracture brace may be applied. This is usually a polypropylene prefabricated brace, which wraps around the arm while allowing elbow flexion and extension. During the initial week or two after application of the brace, the patient generally requires sling support of the arm. Subsequently, active flexion and extension of the elbow is allowed to encourage both alignment of the fracture and to promote a callus response. By 10 to 12 weeks there is usually adequate clinical and radiographic healing to discard the fracture brace.

Fractures of the Head of the Radius

The common undisplaced fractures of the radial head or neck can be treated by aspiration of the hemarthrosis followed by temporary sling support. Holdsworth and co-workers (64) have shown the benefit of aspirating the elbow and instilling a local

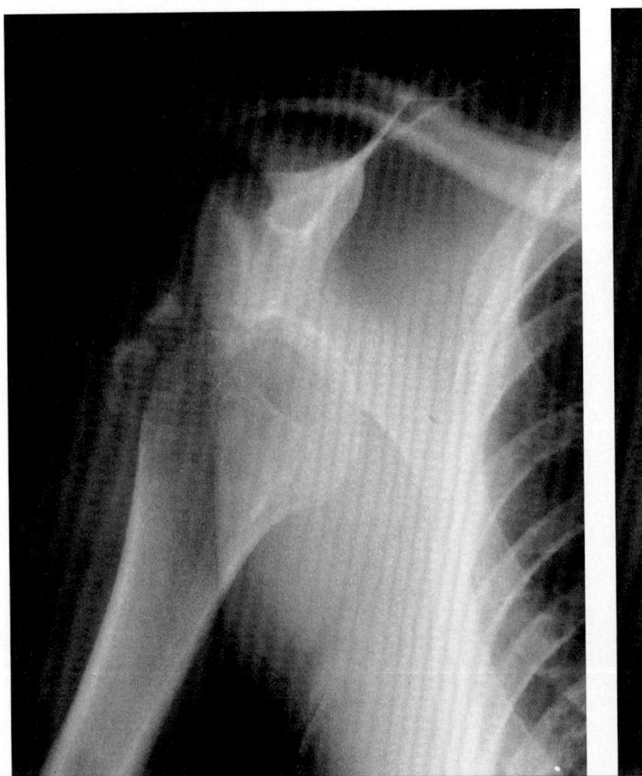

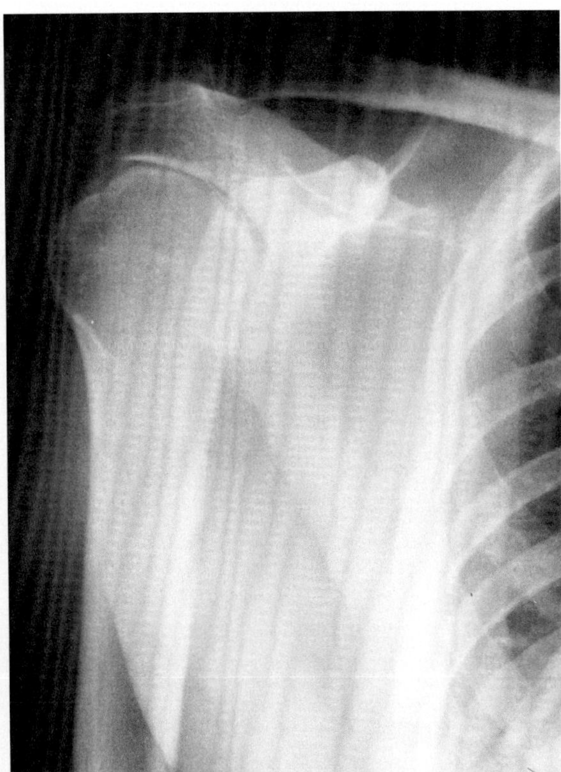

FIGURE 5-8 **A.** A patient in his 40s sustained this fracture dislocation of the shoulder with evidence of rotator cuff disruption. The shoulder was reduced but the rotator cuff was not repaired. **B.** X-rays 3 months after the dislocation show superior migration of the humeral head up toward the acromion as a result of loss of the rotator cuff.

anesthetic to relieve the acute pain and permit early range of motion. Active flexion and extension of the elbow can be started as soon as the acute swelling and pain subside usually within 2 to 3 days. Prolonged elbow immobilization in a sling will inhibit returning motion particularly to full extension (65).

Slight displacement of these fractures can occur and block elbow motion. To determine if this is a problem, the fracture hematoma should be aspirated and a local anesthetic injected (66,67). Elbow range of motion can then be evaluated to determine if the radial head fracture blocks either flexion/extension or supination/pronation. If there is evidence of a mechanical block to elbow motion the fracture fragment should be either excised or reduced and fixed operatively (68). If it is decided that the fragment is not an obstruction to motion, the elbow can be immobilized temporarily in a sling for 48 hours while ice is applied to the elbow. Subsequently, when the pain subsides, the patient begins active forearm rotation and flexion/extension exercises of the elbow. Nearly full range of motion should return by 4 to 6 weeks. Nonunion of nonoperatively treated fractures of the radial head are rare. Even when the fracture line is still apparent months after the injury, healing may still occur.

Operative treatment of such apparent delayed unions or nonunions is rarely necessary since the patient is usually asymptomatic. Broberg and Morrey (69) have shown that for fractures that remain symptomatic, delayed excision of the fractured radial head can achieve satisfactory results. This was true in their experience with 21 patients who had excision of the radial head from 1 month to more than 20 years after fracture.

Isolated Fractures of the Ulna

Like the fracture of the clavicle the isolated fracture of the ulna has been found to be among the commonest in skeletal remains of prehistoric man (35). The classic mechanism of this injury is a direct blow to the forearm occurring when the forearm is raised to protect the head. Most commonly the isolated ulnar fracture is relatively undisplaced. The isolated fracture usually does not present with more than 10 to 20 degrees of angulation and 50% displacement and can be treated without reduction.

Paradoxically, it seems that the more one tries to immobilize the isolated ulnar fracture in a long arm cast, the more likely it is that the fracture will be slow to heal or not heal (70). Functional bracing as developed by Sarmiento and co-workers (63,71), has yielded surprisingly good fracture healing and functional results, often better than even operative techniques (73). The reason for these excellent results is uncertain but it

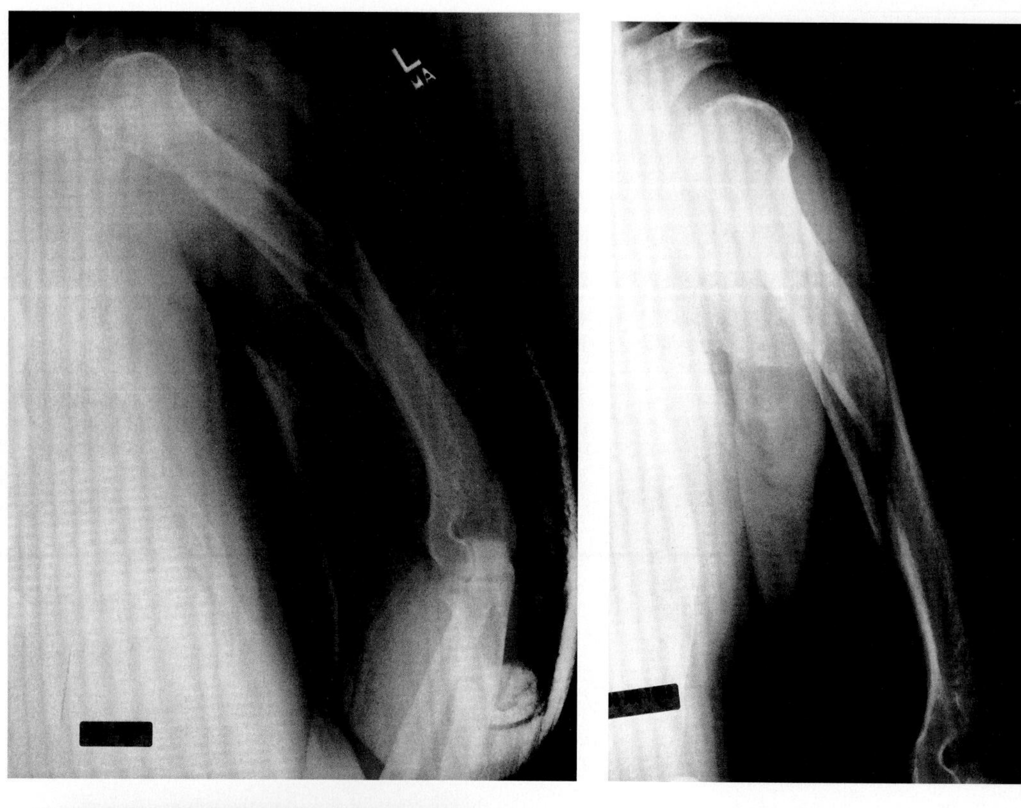

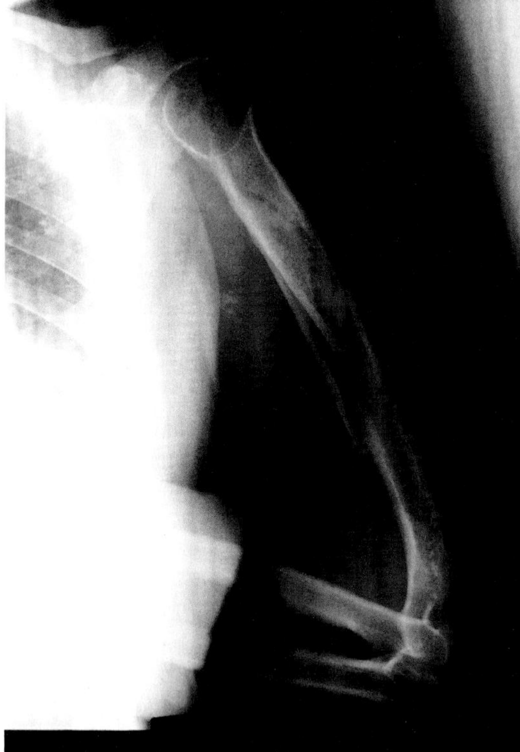

FIGURE 5-9 **A.** This fracture of the humeral shaft was temporarily splinted with a "gutter splint" that actually made the patient uncomfortable due to the plaster rubbing in the axilla. It also produced the unacceptable angulation evident here. **B.** The patient was transferred to a fracture brace and sling within the first week after injury. Active flexion and extension of the elbow permitted gravity and muscle function to align the fracture and restore the axis of elbow motion to normal. **C.** Early fracture union was evident at 8 weeks when the patient had close to normal motion of the elbow and shoulder. *(continues)*

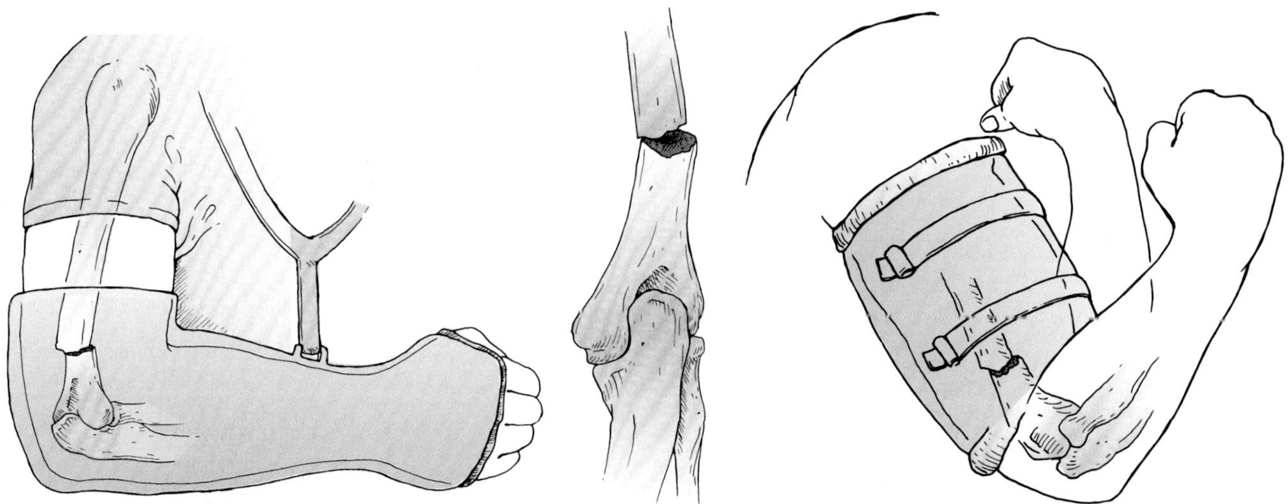

FIGURE 5-9 *(continued)* **D.** Fractures of distal humerus treated in a hanging arm cast without allowing elbow motion may heal with an internal rotation-varus angulation. **E.** A humeral fracture brace or sleeve is effective in aligning the humeral shaft or distal humeral fracture through functional motion of the elbow. This fracture sleeve may be applied to the arm in the early phases of healing as the pain and swelling from the fracture subside. Flexion and extension restore the normal alignment of the elbow axis of motion. (Modified from Connolly J. *Fractures and dislocations. Closed management.* Philadelphia: WB Saunders, 1995, with permission.)

appears that the method improves circulation and promotes early production of external callus. This results from an emphasis on functional muscle activity encouraged by allowing elbow and wrist motion.

The fracture should be immobilized with a splint or cast for the first 3 to 5 days until the swelling and discomfort subside. Subsequently, a prefabricated brace or cast can be applied to support the fracture but allow the elbow and wrist to function freely (Fig. 5-10). The fracture brace has Velcro straps to permit tightening as the swelling subsides. It may be removed for personal hygiene.

In evaluating the progress of healing, most ulnar fractures heal clinically (as evidenced by absence of pain either on direct palpitation or forearm rotation), several weeks or even several months before radiographic healing is complete. However, fractures that achieve clinical union eventually heal radiographically. Therefore, prolonged immobilization preventing the patient from returning to work until there is complete radiographic union is both unnecessary and undesirable for most patients (73).

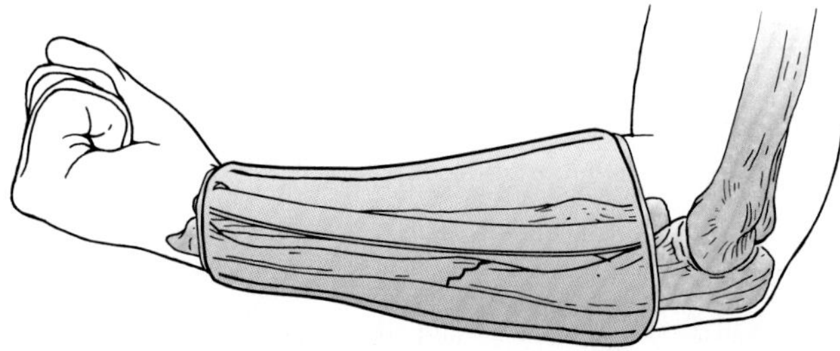

FIGURE 5-10 A fracture brace can be applied to the fractured ulna by 3 to 5 days when swelling and discomfort have subsided. This should permit free elbow, wrist, and finger motion which in turn encourages early clinical union of the fracture. (Modified from Connolly J. *Fractures and dislocations. Closed management.* Philadelphia: WB Saunders, 1995, with permission.)

Fractures of the Carpal Scaphoid

Undisplaced fractures of the mid scaphoid occur commonly and often are not even diagnosed (74). Asymptomatic ununited fractures of the scaphoid have been reported in boxers as well as in other individuals who use their hands for arduous work (75–77). The usual fracture line that runs transversely or slightly obliquely across the longitudinal axis of the scaphoid tends to be compressed by the surrounding muscles of the fingers (Fig. 5-11). This type of fracture is stable and will heal quite quickly and consistently with closed nonoperative treatment (78).

Although there is a trend toward internal screw fixation of the scaphoid fracture, a recent analysis (79) searching for evidence-based data has found no significant benefit from operative fixation for the common undisplaced mid third scaphoid fracture. Internal fixation does result in a significantly earlier return to work compared with casting. However, casting and internal fixation do not differ significantly in clinically relevant outcomes such as grip strength, range of motion, or risk of nonunion (79).

The undisplaced scaphoid fracture does not require reduc-

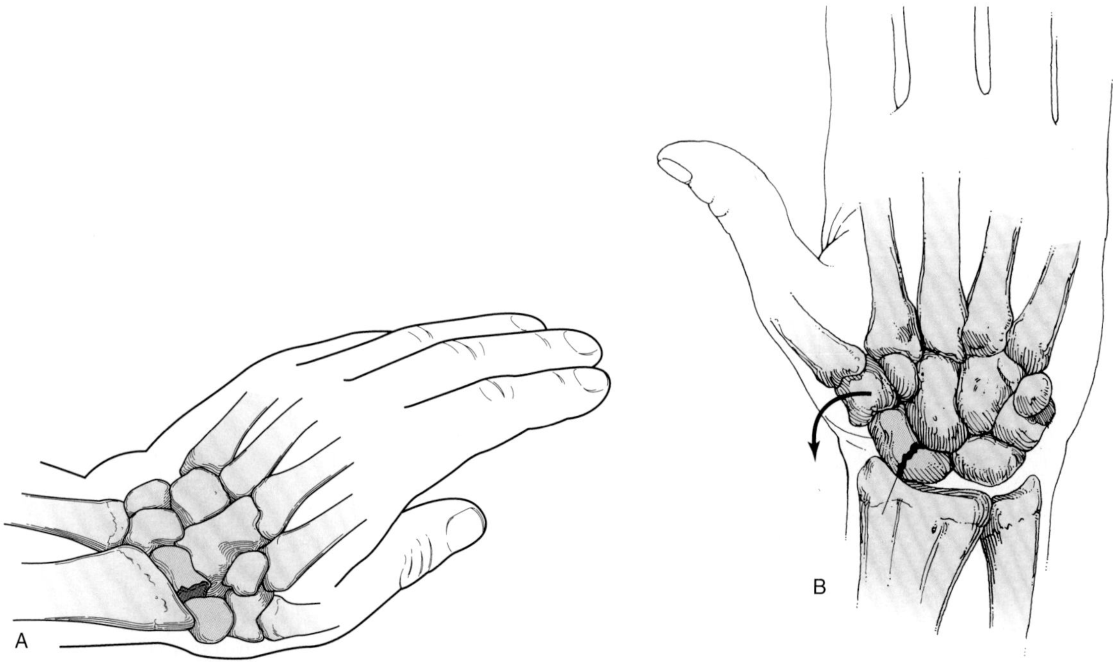

FIGURE 5-11 A. A typical fracture of the carpal scaphoid occurs as the result of a fall on the outstretched hand producing forceful dorsiflexion of the wrist. **B.** An undisplaced scaphoid fracture does not usually require reduction and can be immobilized by radial deviation of the wrist. Ulnar deviation tends to open up the fracture site and should be avoided. (Modified from Connolly J. *Fractures and dislocations. Closed management.* Philadelphia: WB Saunders, 1995, with permission.)

tion and can be immobilized if seen acutely in a cooperative patient using a short arm thumb spica cast extending from below the elbow to the metacarpal heads. A position of wrist dorsiflexion and radial deviation permits compression of the transverse scaphoid fracture and is the position of choice for immobilization. The thumb should be in a grasping position with the cast extending across the interphalangeal joint of the thumb (80,81). If the scaphoid fracture is diagnosed a week or two after injury or occurs in the patient who may not be overly cooperative, a long arm thumb spica cast is preferable to the short arm thumb spica cast and may decrease the risk of delayed or nonunion (82).

The cast should be inspected every 2 weeks, and if it becomes loose, a new snugly fitting cast should be applied. At the end of 8 weeks the cast is removed and the patient evaluated carefully. If the wrist is pain free and a reasonable range of motion is evident, the wrist can be protected in a simple wrist splint. If the patient has persistent discomfort, weakness, pain, or tenderness in the snuff box region, the cast is reapplied for 4 to 6 more weeks. In general, cast immobilization should be continued for no longer than 3 months. If the fracture is still clinically symptomatic after this time, treatment with internal fixation and bone graft should be considered (78,81,83,84).

The strongest case against pessimism in managing the broken scaphoid nonoperatively was that presented in 1961 by P. S. London (85) in a review of 300 cases from the Birmingham accident hospital. London's approach was at variance with the pessimistic thinking of his time, which still seems to prevail today. Using the simple cast immobilization technique described above, 90% to 95% of scaphoid fractures (including those not treated for 3 to 4 weeks after injury) healed.

As with many other fractures, clinical evidence of union of the scaphoid fracture precedes radiographic evidence. There is no conclusive evidence that prolonged immobilization does in fact prevent nonunion (84). Bony union can occur without it, and fibrous union can occur in spite of it. Even though the fracture line is still faintly visible when the plaster is discarded, it usually becomes obliterated during the ensuing 6 to 12 months. Even if fibrous union develops, it is not usually disabling. The fibrous union is most often diagnosed only at the time of some later injury, and these new symptoms often subside within a month of plaster immobilization.

Phalangeal and Metacarpal Fractures

Torsional or twisting mechanisms are fairly common causes of phalangeal and metacarpal fractures. Persistent malrotation with overlapping of the injured finger during grasp can impair function of the hand. This deformation can be corrected not by manipulative reduction but by maintaining joint alignment through functional motion. To prevent malrotation, the preferred method of immobilizing phalangeal fractures is by buddy taping, or splinting, the finger to the adjacent uninjured finger (Fig. 5-12). This allows one to evaluate the rotational alignment of the fingers and correct any malrotation overlap by active flexion and extension of the finger joints.

Among the more difficult fracture problems are those involving the proximal phalanx, the so-called no-man's-land fracture, identical anatomically to Bunnell's no-man's-land in tendon surgery. Multiple metacarpal fractures also provide difficult challenges to reduction and fixation techniques. Burkhalter, Reyes, and Latta (23,86) have demonstrated effective alignment of these problem fractures by maintaining maximum flexion of the metacarpophalangeal (MP) joints and encouraging early finger motion in this position. Burkhalter has pointed out that absolute anatomic restoration of extraarticular fractures is not necessary in the hand, but early motion is essential to avoid stiffness and malfunction. Shortening within reasonable limits will not result in functional loss provided there is no loss of joint motion. Particularly of concern is loss of flexion of the MP joint and secondarily loss of motion in the interphalangeal joints. Burkhalter points out that the major deformities with transverse or oblique fractures include flexion and overriding of the distal fragment as well as abnormal rotation. The key to correcting both of these problems is to place the MP joint in maximum flexion of 70 to 90 degrees. Doing this utilizes the intact dorsal hood as a tension band (Fig. 5-13). The effect of the dorsal tension band is to compress the palmar cortices of the fracture as the finger is flexed. The tension band produced by the extensor mechanism is critical not only for volar cortical compression but also for reduction of the fracture and stabilization of the MP joint in a flexed position. If the extensor tendon is destroyed by the injury, this method of management will become completely ineffective, and internal stabilization becomes necessary.

The technique involves first applying a short arm cast with the wrist in 40 degrees of extension. The distal palmar crease should be free of padding or plaster. After the cast hardens, a well-padded dorsal slab is added, and as this plaster hardens, direct pressure over the distal portion of the proximal phalanx is used to push the MP joint into 70 to 90 degrees of flexion. After the cast is completed, flexion and extension of the proximal interphalangeal (PIP) joint is encouraged. The patient should be instructed to close all fingers simultaneously without allowing overlapping. As the swelling subsides the cast is replaced with a new one. The key is to maintain the MP joint flexion by maintaining pressure over the proximal phalanx (Fig. 5-13).

With this method it is difficult and probably unnecessary to check alignment by standard x-rays because superimposition of multiple skeletal structures in the cast makes assessment quite difficult. One or two linear tomograms may be used if there is any question about reduction. However, the main determinant of the adequacy of alignment is clinical. The advantage with this technique is that with the MP joints flexed almost 90 degrees, no rotation occurs unless it is mirrored in the fingertips. With all the fingers flexed simultaneously to 90 degrees, adjacent digits without fracture will help to de-rotate the fractured one. In addition, the effect of the extrinsic extensors of the metacarpal phalangeal joint is reduced by dorsiflexing the wrist to 45 degrees.

Similar mechanical analysis applies to the difficult fracture of the proximal phalanx, the so-called no-man's-land fracture. To align this fracture, the MP joint is stabilized in maximum flexion. It is this joint that is capable of motion in multiple directions including rotation, abduction, adduction, flexion, and extension. However, the rotational and abduction/adduction motions are eliminated as the MP joint is flexed maximally.

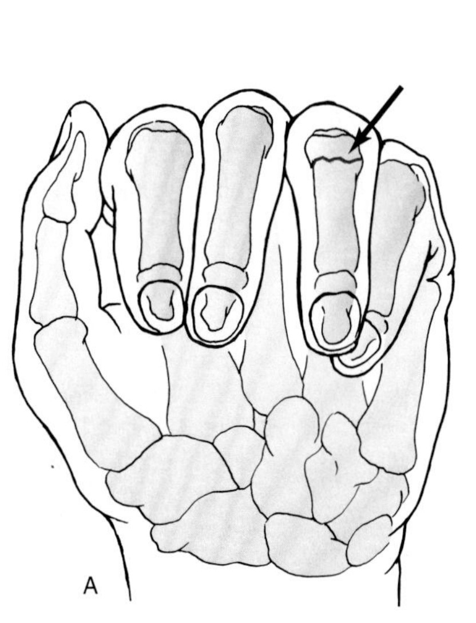

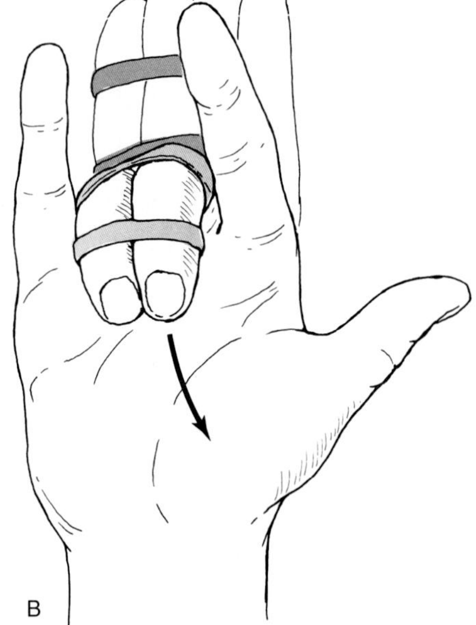

FIGURE 5-12 **A.** A fracture of the phalanx or metacarpal may heal with overlapping fingers if the fractured digit is not held in proper rotational alignment. **B.** The preferred method of immobilizing an isolated phalangeal fracture or metacarpal fracture is by splinting the injured finger to the adjacent finger to aid in proper rotational realignment of the fracture (buddy taping). (Modified from Connolly J. *Fractures and dislocations. Closed management.* Philadelphia: WB Saunders, 1995, with permission.)

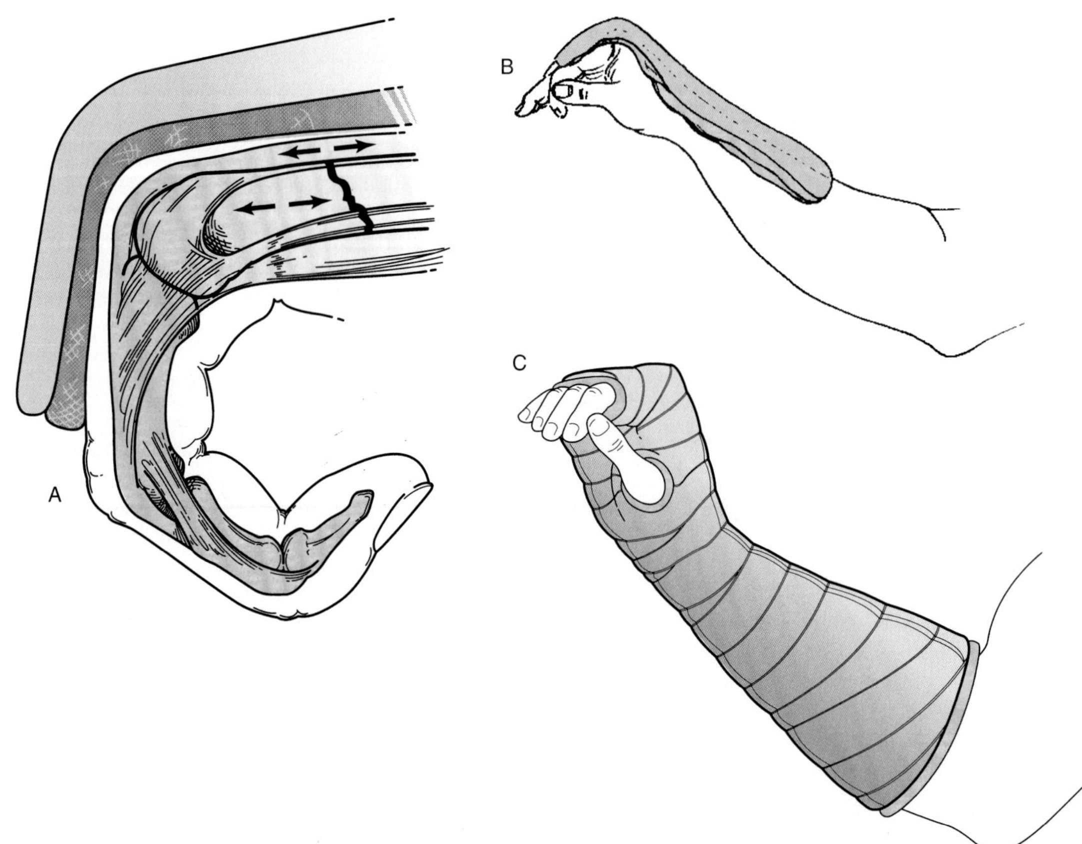

FIGURE 5-13 **A.** The key to correcting flexion and overriding of proximal phalangeal or metacarpal fractures is to place the metacarpophalangeal (MP) joint in maximum flexion of 70 to 90 degrees. This utilizes the intact dorsal hood as a tension band. This dorsal tension band compresses the palmar cortices of the fracture as the finger is flexed. **B.** To maintain this tension band effect of the dorsal mechanism, the fracture is treated with the wrist extended, and a splint is applied to the dorsal surface of the forearm and wrist. Plaster is molded to maintain the MP joints in maximum flexion. To achieve this, the palm should not be heavily padded. The interphalangeal (IP) joints are allowed to flex and are held in the position of function. **C.** The splint is incorporated in a short arm cast, and as the acute swelling subsides the patient is encouraged to actively flex the fingers. Extension should be avoided until the fracture heals, by 3 weeks, when the cast is removed. (Modified from Connolly J. *Fractures and dislocations. Closed management.* Philadelphia: WB Saunders, 1995, with permission.)

There are pitfalls in the closed treatment of any fracture, and the method described here requires attention to detail both acutely and on follow-up. It also requires willingness to abandon the method if alignment is not achieved. The method, however, does not reduce vascularity to the fracture site or produce additional injury to tendons or joints that may cause loss of motion. As Burkhalter and Reyes (23) point out, it would be a hollow victory for the surgeon to obtain an anatomic reduction with solid osseous union but with significant extensor lag of the PIP joint.

Fifth Metacarpal Fractures

In a classic clinical study of the fifth metacarpal fractures in a compensation clinic population in 1970, Hunter and Cowen (87) pointed out the advantage of not over treating these fractures by vigorous attempts at closed or open reduction. My experience has also been that most of these fractures do not warrant any method of reduction that may prolong or create permanent disability. Some shortening and angulation of the fifth metacarpal shaft and neck fractures are compatible with excellent function. Accepting up to 40 degrees of palmar angulation of a metacarpal neck fracture (and up to 20 degrees in a shaft fracture) has not resulted in any functional disability in studied compensation populations (87). The absence of symptoms from palmar angulation of the metacarpal is due to the fact that the fifth carpal-metacarpal joint is quite mobile. There is about 30 degrees of motion in this joint as opposed to the carpal-metacarpal joints of the index or long fingers, in which there is virtually no motion, and thus residual angulatory deformity in these metacarpals is not tolerated as well and must be corrected.

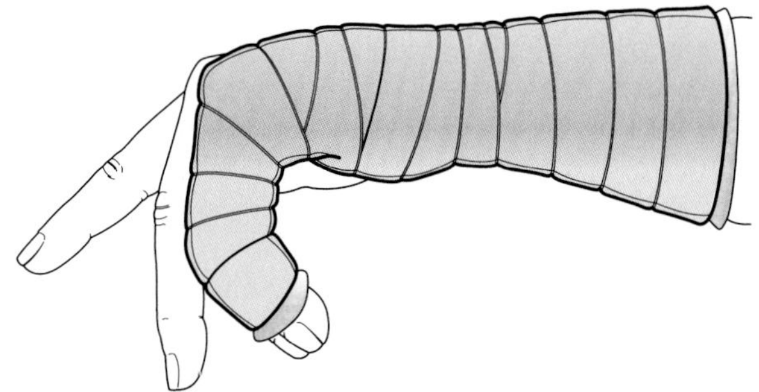

FIGURE 5-14 For fractures of the 4th and 5th metacarpals, a simple lateral splint may be applied. This splint immobilizes both the fractured and the adjacent uninjured finger. The MP joint is flexed 70 to 90 degrees and the IP joints are flexed slightly. The fingertips are directed toward the scaphoid tuberosity to insure rotational alignment. (Modified from Connolly J. *Fractures and dislocations. Closed management.* Philadelphia: WB Saunders, 1995, with permission.)

Rather than attempting a variety of maneuvers to correct the very common angulated fracture of the fifth metacarpal, it is recommended that the hand be splinted in a functional position for 10 days. This position includes maximum flexion of the MP joint and slight flexion of the interphalangeal joints to maintain the extensor hood and capsule of these joints under maximum tension. This is similar to Burkhalter's technique described in the preceding section, but it may be accomplished by a simple lateral gutter splint (Fig. 5-14). Angulation up to 40 degrees may be accepted provided no excessive rotation exists.

With this approach, patients are usually fully recovered by the end of 4 weeks and able to return to full vocational and avocational activities. On returning to work a few patients may temporarily lack full extension of the PIP or MP joint, but these deficits usually disappear quickly.

Previously described methods of closed reduction of fifth metacarpal fractures recommended manipulation followed by maintenance of the hand in a variety of awkward positions. These approaches tend to be associated with complications that are not seen with the Hunter-Cowen approach.

One should be careful to distinguish the metacarpal shaft fracture from a fracture involving the proximal carpal-metacarpal joint. Displaced articular fractures in this area can cause prolonged disability and are best treated by open reduction and internal fixation.

LOWER EXTREMITY FRACTURES COMMONLY TREATED NONOPERATIVELY WITHOUT MANIPULATIVE REDUCTION

Fractures of the Forefoot

The majority of fractures of the forefoot including phalangeal and metatarsal fractures can be treated by closed nonoperative methods consisting primarily of a compression dressing with a subsequent short leg walking cast or brace (88,89). Exceptions to this general rule include multiple fractures or fracture dislocations, and selected fractures in zone III of the fifth metatarsal (90) (Fig. 5-15). Fractures in zone II or I are stable and can usually be treated symptomatically. The treatment initially is with a short leg walking cast, although many patients, particularly with zone I fractures, are more comfortable with an elastic wrap and a functional metatarsal brace. This brace has been developed by Raibel and Colditz and consists of a 1/8-inch thick moldable plastic material applied directly over the metatarsals (90). The brace has an opening on the medial side and a curved shape molded around the fifth metatarsal to prevent movement of the metatarsals while withstanding the force of ambulation. Dameron (90) has found this brace effective in treating acute fractures after a short period of immobilization and elevation to reduce edema. It can be used in any patient with a zone I or II fracture. Zone III fractures tend to be stress fractures in young individuals involved in athletics. When discovered early,

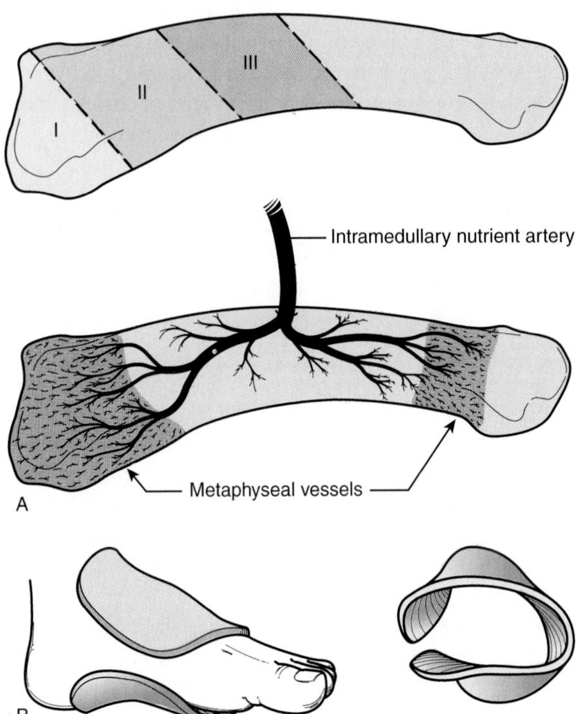

FIGURE 5-15 **A.** Dameron and others have pointed out that there are three anatomic zones at the base of the fifth metatarsal that are important for treatment of the fractures of this bone. The first zone includes the articular surface of the fifth metatarsal-cuboid joint. The second zone encompasses the articulation of the proximal fourth and fifth metatarsals. The third zone extends 1.5 cm distal to the second zone. **B.** A functional brace may be applied for fractures of the proximal fifth metatarsal (zones I and II). This can avoid the need of a cast or operative fixation for the usual fracture in this location. (Modified from Dameron T. Fractures of the proximal fifth metatarsal: Selecting the best treatment option. *J Am Acad Orthop Surg* 1995;3:110–114, with permission.)

fifth metatarsal stress fractures can be treated nonoperatively by modification of activity and use of the functional metatarsal brace. However, when the fracture becomes complete, active athletic individuals prefer operative fixation to allow earlier resumption of their lifestyle.

With most metatarsal fractures, the type of treatment does not seem to have any direct effect on the length of time until symptoms subside. As with other fractures, such as ulnar or scaphoid fractures, radiographic evidence of healing is slower than is clinical union. In a general orthopaedic practice Dameron found more than 90% of the fifth metatarsal fractures occur in zone I and can be treated symptomatically and functionally; 7% to 10% occur in zones II and III and these may be generally slower to heal than the more common zone I fractures (88).

Calcaneal Fractures

The usual mechanism producing a calcaneal fracture is a fall onto the heel from a height, resulting in both extraarticular and intraarticular fractures. Most extraarticular fractures can be treated symptomatically. If the patient is minimally symptomatic, the foot is first managed by the RICE technique, followed by early mobilization. Cast immobilization may be considered, but generally it is best to keep immobilization to a minimum because stiffness of the foot from prolonged immobilization during treatment can be a source of long-term functional impairment.

Many intraarticular calcaneal fractures can also be treated nonoperatively using early mobilization methods. A multicenter study done by the Canadian orthopaedic trauma study group (91,92) showed that most patients with a displaced intraarticular calcaneal fracture treated nonoperatively will not need surgery at all. Approximately 20% will have a less than satisfactory outcome and require a subtalar arthrodesis. This study demonstrated that there is a select patient group with displaced intraarticular calcaneal fractures that do poorly relative to other patients. This group includes young males, workman compensation board patients, heavy laborers, or those patients with a fracture pattern with a Böhler angle of less than 0% and a Sanders-type IV fracture. These patients with fractures that involve the intraarticular surface of the calcaneus are prime candidates for initial open reduction and internal fixation to decrease the possibility of the future need for subtalar fusion.

If the patient is to be treated nonoperatively, in many instances no attempt at reduction is necessary. However any clinical deformity, particularly heel valgus or any lateral or plantar bony prominences require correction.

Even if reduction of the fracture is necessary, mobilization is helpful to diminish edema and prevent stiffness of the joints. A calcaneal fracture, which involves a large amount of cancellous bone, usually achieves stability immediately due to impaction of the fragments at the time of the injury. Therefore, to achieve fracture immobilization one need only eliminate weightbearing stresses (93).

Lance and co-workers (94) found that, in selecting candidates for early mobilization without fracture reduction, there should be a near normal clinical appearance of the heel without peroneal tendon impingement, and the x-rays should show maintenance of reasonable congruity between the posterior articular facet of the talus and the calcaneus. Age and general health status also influence the selection. Patients who are older than 60 years or who are chronically ill generally tend to do best with early active mobilization.

The technique of nonreduction with early mobilization consists of simply elevating the injured foot for 2 to 3 days in a compression dressing and applying cold packs. By the third day the patient should begin to exercise the toes, tarsal joints, and ankle systematically on an hourly basis within the limits of pain. After 3 or 4 days, the patient may be up on crutches, but should be cautioned against weightbearing or dependency of the foot. At the end of the first week, the foot is reexamined for any clinical deformity or area of bony protrusion on the lateral or plantar surface. X-rays are taken to determine that the fracture has maintained an acceptable position. If heel widening or deformity is evident, closed reduction by the Omoto (95) technique, described below in the section on manipulative reduction of fractures, or open reduction should be considered (see Fig. 5-49). Weightbearing is deferred for 6 to 8 weeks with linear fractures and for 10 to 12 weeks for fractures with comminution. If displacement becomes evident during treatment, it is possible still to reduce the calcaneal fracture by operative methods. Pozo et al (93) and others have found that maximum recovery after calcaneal fractures may require 2 to 3 years and that soft tissue injuries are a significant cause for residual symptoms.

Fractures of the Lateral Malleolus

The sequence of injury to the supinated externally rotated ankle, as described by Lauge-Hansen, begins usually with a tear of the anterior tibiofibular ligament followed by a fracture at varying levels of the lateral malleolus or fibula (96). Often the anterior tibiofibular ligament stretches but remains intact. The fracture of the lateral malleolus then occurs at the level of the ankle joint (Fig. 5-16). This type of fracture is quite stable provided the torsional injury did not advance further to involve the posterior tibiofibular ligament or the medial malleolus. For the most part the undisplaced or minimally displaced lateral malleolus fracture is quite analogous to an ankle sprain but often heals more rapidly than does a severely sprained ankle. It can be treated with either a short leg walking cast or an air splint. It should be protected for a period of 1 to 2 weeks with partial weightbearing followed by full weightbearing in the cast or air splint. Walking without external support is usually possible in 3 to 6 weeks.

It is important to distinguish the common fracture of the lateral malleolus at the ankle joint (97) from those fractures of the fibula above the syndesmosis, which are unstable due to shortening and external rotation. Yablon et al (98) and others (99–104) have demonstrated the importance of adequate closed or open reduction to restore both length and rotational alignment of this type of fractured fibula. Failure to restore the fibu-

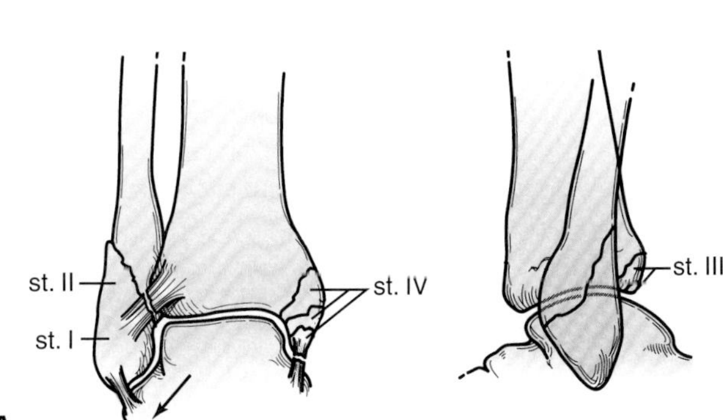

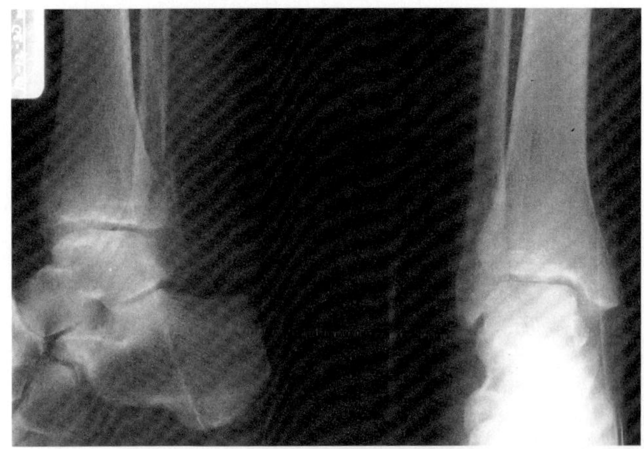

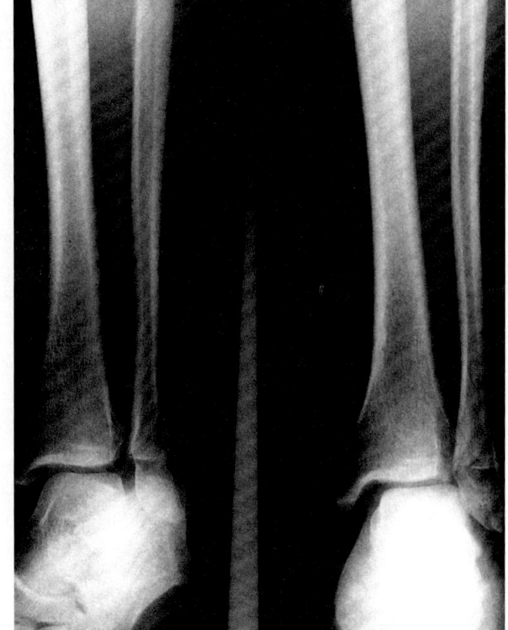

FIGURE 5-16 **A.** The commonest type of ankle fracture involves the lateral malleolus at or slightly above the mortise. This is a spiral oblique fracture that may or may not be associated with a tear of the anterior tibiofibular ligament (stage I and stage II). If the supination external rotation injury rotates circumferentially around the mortise, the posterior malleolus or posterior tibiofibular ligament will be injured (stage III). In stage IV the deltoid ligament or medial malleolus will be injured and the fracture may become unstable. **B.** This stable fracture without shortening or malrotation of the fibula can be treated much like a sprain without reduction. An air brace support is helpful for early functional recovery. **C.** If the lateral malleolus is shortened or malrotated, a more unstable ankle is the result and it generally requires operative treatment. In evaluating the common fracture of the lateral malleolus one should carefully examine for disruption of the tibiofibular as well as the deltoid ligaments. (Modified from Connolly J. *Fractures and dislocations. Closed management.* Philadelphia: WB Saunders, 1995, with permission.)

la's length and rotation can result in abnormal loading of the talus and posttraumatic arthritis (105) (Fig. 5-17).

Fibula Shaft Fractures and the Maisonneuve Fracture

An isolated fracture of the fibula, without a tibial fracture, can occur from a direct impact, such as a kick. These fractures are comminuted and contrast with the usual fibular fracture occurring from an indirect mechanism, which tends to be oblique or spiral. The comminuted, isolated fracture of the fibula can be treated symptomatically. This may require a short leg-walking cast for 4 weeks, after which full weightbearing is usually possible.

This fracture should not be confused with the isolated fibula fracture in the upper third of the bone, which is produced by a torsional injury to the ankle, the so-called Maisonneuve fracture. Pankovich (106) and others have pointed out the common mechanism of this injury in which torsion of the ankle with the foot slightly pronated or supinated is transmitted along the interosseous ligament to the proximal fibula. In most instances the injury also produces disruption of the anterior tibiofibular ligament and/or fracture of the medial malleolus, tear of the deltoid ligament, or an anteromedial joint capsular tear. This injury can lead to a wide diastasis of this distal tibiofibular articulation with difficulty in reduction and internal fixation. Although Pankovich (104,106) pointed out that most Maisonneuve fractures of the proximal fibula with or without diastasis of the ankle can be treated by cast immobilization for 3 to 5 weeks, the more advanced stages of this lesion require repair of the ankle ligaments. Yablon et al (98) as well as Weber and Simpson (105) have shown that restoration of length and rotation of the fibular fracture is sometimes key to correcting diasta-

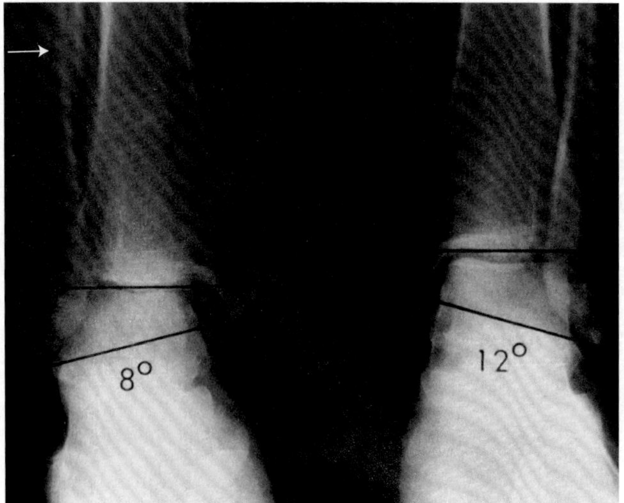

FIGURE 5-17 This anteroposterior x-ray of both ankles shows a proximal fibula fracture that has healed with shortening and malrotation, resulting in malalignment of the ankle mortise and a loss of the normal talocrural angle compared to the opposite side. This usually results in persistent symptoms, which can be alleviated by corrective realignment of the fibula and ankle mortise.

sis of the distal ankle joint and correctly restoring the ankle mortise.

Stress Fractures and Other Undisplaced Tibial Fractures

Undisplaced tibial fractures require no reduction and can generally be managed with a functional brace or a weightbearing cast. It should be remembered that fractures in the distal tibia associated with an intact fibula can develop a varus-internal rotation deformity in the cast. This may be combated by externally rotating the distal fragment with the ankle at the time of cast application. This shifts the floor reaction force lateral to the fracture thereby diminishing the tendency to varus angulation.

Management of tibial stress fractures has been problematic because they most often occur in active young individuals such as military recruits and athletes (107,108). The earliest symptoms are pain and swelling localized typically to the middle of the tibia, within 6 to 12 weeks after beginning vigorous running or forced marching. The patient presents with a slight limp and has tenderness to palpation. This condition has been called a stress reaction or stress process rather then a complete fracture at this point because it begins with an area of hyperemia of the bone before the x-ray shows a fracture line (109). The diagnosis is made at this stage by either a radionuclide bone scan or more likely by magnetic resonance imaging (MRI) of the bone.

The primary treatment is to avoid continued repetitive loading of the bone stressed by running or marching. This usually requires modified activity and rest with the avoidance of running.

Conditioning can be maintained by exercises such as swimming, bicycling, or stretching, but repetitive loading activity should be avoided for 6 to 10 weeks.

The athlete with symptoms of stress fracture (sometimes called "shin splints") of the lower leg involving the tibia or the fibula can be treated by a semirigid pneumatic leg brace (107). This allows the individual to continue playing the sport until the symptom subsides. However, for a complete fracture through the tibia, more supportive treatment is usually necessary, such as a fracture brace or cast.

Intertrochanteric and Femoral Neck Fractures

Although a displaced intertrochanteric fracture in an elderly patient is most efficiently fixed internally (110), an undisplaced intertrochanteric fractures in the young adult need not necessarily require internal fixation. The strong cortical bone of the intertrochanteric region in the younger patient often minimizes comminution of the fracture and thereby prevents shortening or varus angulation. This allows for treatment by a brief period of bed rest (1 to 2 days), symptomatic pain relief, and partial weightbearing on crutches (Fig. 5-18). Most patients can return to work in 2 to 3 weeks. Operative fixation, in contrast, may actually slow down the return to full weightbearing and to work for the younger patient.

Nonoperative treatment of femoral neck fractures in senile patients has also been advocated (111,112) as a reasonable alternative to the frequently complicated operative treatment. Nonoperative treatment may be most humane for the elderly bedridden patient who has been nonambulatory prior to the hip fracture. Emphasis should be placed on avoiding pressure sores using special mattresses, heel protectors, and frequent turning. For such patients who are unlikely to walk again, nonoperative management is a reasonable alternative, which avoids the mental anguish, expense, and hospitalization of surgery, provided good nursing care is available (113). A key factor in deciding about operative versus nonoperative treatment for the elderly bedridden patient should be the clinical examination of how painful the affected hip is when internally or externally rotated. If the patient seems to be in considerable pain, which is more often the case with extracapsular intertrochanteric fractures as compared with intracapsular femoral neck fractures, operative treatment should be seriously considered.

Stress fractures of the femoral neck may also occur in active young individuals. They may or may not require internal fixation (114–116). The usual recommendation is for internal fixation of fatigue or stress fractures that involve the superolateral aspect of the femoral neck. These fractures are subjected to tensile loads, and theoretically may displace, leading to a varus deformity and nonunion. In contrast, incomplete fractures that involve the inferomedial aspect of the femoral neck are subjected to compressive loading and can be treated by nonweightbearing with crutches and careful follow-up. However, if there is any question about the stability of the fracture or the ability of the patient to use crutches properly, the preferable

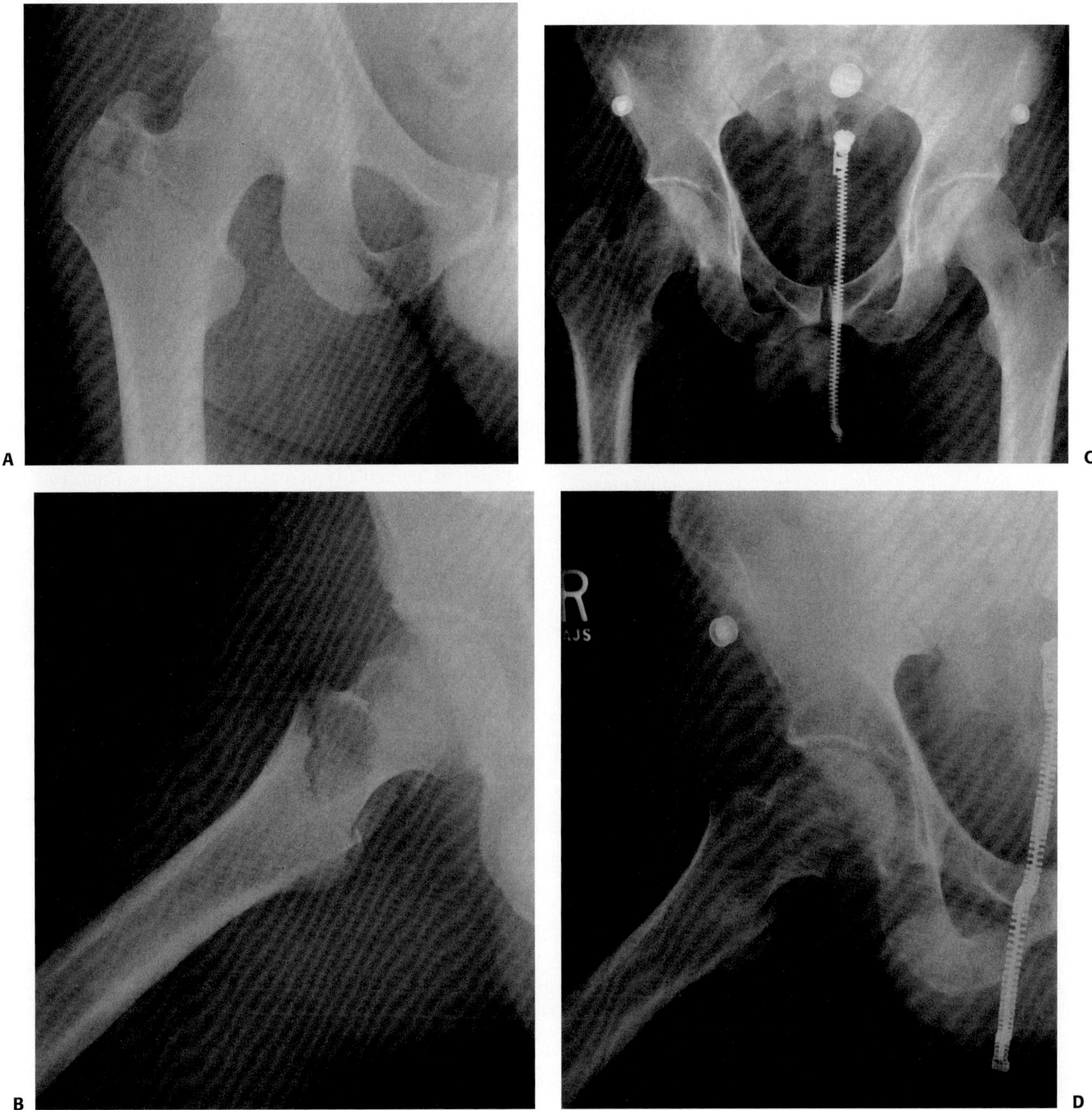

FIGURE 5-18 A,B. Anteroposterior (AP) and lateral x-rays showing an undisplaced intertrochanteric fracture in a 30-year-old laborer who fell 12 feet onto his hip while at work. He was treated symptomatically with bed rest for 2 days and then was up on crutches and out of the hospital. **C,D.** AP and lateral x-rays show healing evident at 4 weeks when the patient was able to return to work on a full-time basis. It is questionable whether this would have been likely if he had been treated with open reduction and internal fixation of this completely undisplaced fracture.

approach is to fix the undisplaced femoral neck stress fracture with multiple pins.

In a prospective study of 170 cases of impacted femoral neck fractures, Raaymakers and Marti (117) found that functional treatment was justified in both young and old patients. This approach consisted of a period of a few days of bed rest in a splint until the acute pain from the fracture subsided. By the end of the first week the majority of patients could be allowed to bear weight partially with the help of crutches. Partial weightbearing was continued for an average of 8 weeks with eventual union in 86% of the patients. The only patients who demonstrated instability of the impacted fracture were those over 70 years of age and younger patients with serious illnesses. Functional, nonoperative treatment in most patients with impacted femoral neck fractures seems to be justified based on these and other reports (114,115,118–122) (Fig. 5-19).

Pelvic Fractures

Approximately half of pelvic fractures result from severe trauma such as motor vehicle accidents or falls from a height (123,124). The other half are caused by moderate trauma such as a fall from a standing height. Most consistently, the less severe mechanism occurs in the older age group and results in fractures of one or both rami (125). Many of these can be treated symptomatically without hospitalization (126). Consequently, in the study by Melton et al (127), which included all of the pelvic fractures occurring in Olmsted County, Minnesota, over a 10-year period, 80% were considered minor.

In a separate series of cases from the Mayo Clinic by Mucha and Farnell (128), 36% were classified as complicated or severe injures. This reflects the difference from the community wide study of Melton's compared with a selective study from the perspective of a trauma center. Melton et al's study was based in the Midwest community of Rochester, Minnesota, with a unique record keeping and retrieval system, and reflects the full spectrum of pelvic fractures seen in one community. It portrays the pelvic fracture demographics seen by most practicing orthopaedic surgeons. Overall, a minority of pelvic fractures (10% to 20%) are the result of significant injury, such as auto versus pedestrian, that is likely to threaten life or the functional recovery of the patient. When these injuries do present, however, the potential for complications is high and should be recognized early to ensure prompt and appropriate management (129–132). Temporary resuscitation aids such as circumferential wrapping of the unstable pelvis with sheeting as described by Routt et al (133) is an effective method of stabilizing the unstable pelvic ring and the hemodynamically unstable patient.

A number of excellent investigators have classified pelvic fracture patterns in order to assess how unstable the injury might be. These classifications are discussed elsewhere in the text and are particularly pertinent to operative management. However, it should be kept in mind that the main morbidity and mortality from pelvic fractures come from associated head, cardiovascular, and abdominal injuries rather than from the pelvic fracture itself.

Clinical assessment of pelvic fracture instability is especially important if one is considering nonoperative treatment. Nonoperative treatment of unstable injuries using external fixators has been reported to be ineffective (134). More often, closed treatment of a displaced fracture requires temporary skeletal traction to correct shortening and torsional deformity of the pelvis. For the most common pelvic fracture without shortening or torsional deformity, involving either the anterior or posterior ring, nonoperative symptomatic treatment can be quite effective (135).

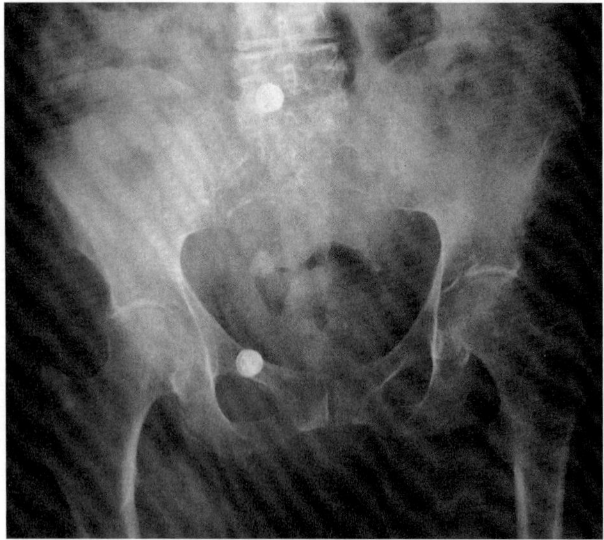

FIGURE 5-19 An impacted femoral neck fracture was treated with a brief period of bed rest followed by protected ambulation with crutches and healed without further displacement of the fracture.

Anterior Pelvic Ring Injuries

Open treatment of symphysis pubis separation has been advocated but rarely is necessary, even with wide separation, which can be closed by external fixation (136) and does not ordinarily cause long-term problems. Indeed, symphysis pubis separation may often spontaneously close as the patient is allowed to bear weight and correct the rotational alignment of the limb (Fig. 5-20). Also, pregnancy following traumatic pubic symphysis separation is more likely to be a problem if the original injury was treated surgically than if it was allowed to heal without reduction (137).

Separation of the pubic symphysis in association with pregnancy, labor, and delivery is rare but may be associated with acute pain, particularly with weightbearing or flexion of the hip. Lindsey and co-authors (138) reviewed this problem and reported that simply placing the patient in a lateral decubitus position, which permits spontaneous reduction of the diastasis, can relieve the symptoms. A well-padded pelvic binder may be applied and the patient can be treated symptomatically with bed rest until the pain subsides. In general the separation of the

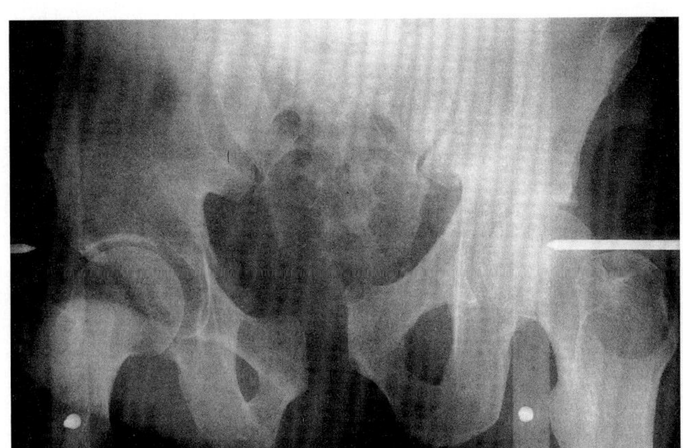
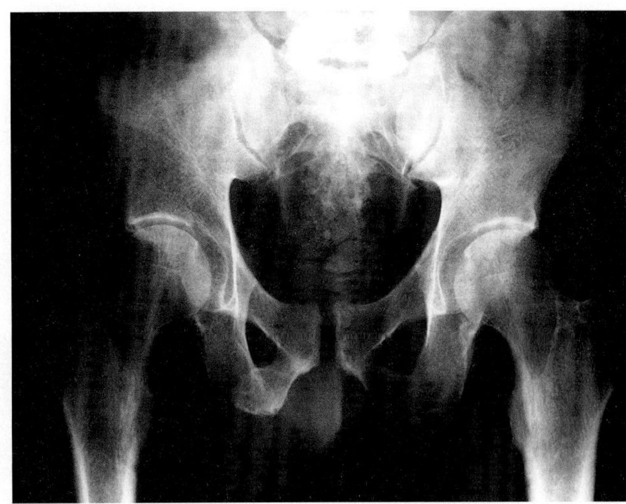

FIGURE 5-20 **A.** Anteroposterior x-rays of a pelvic injury show initial separation of the symphysis pubis and sacroiliac joint. The patient was treated symptomatically with partial weightbearing on crutches within 1 week after injury. **B.** The separated symphysis pubis was seen to be closed spontaneously on this x-ray 1 month after the original injury.

symphysis pubis is less than 1 cm, and nonoperative treatment allows complete functional recovery.

Operative fixation of the symphysis pubis or anterior pelvic ring may be necessary occasionally in conjunction with repair of genitourinary injuries. Displaced pubic ramus fractures in women particularly should be carefully evaluated since they may be associated with vaginal lacerations. These can require operative fixation to avoid or treat complications including vesicovaginal fistulas or chronic infection (Fig. 5-21).

Operative external or internal fixation of the anterior pelvic ring should also be considered when the fracture demonstrates clinical instability, as evidenced by shortening and rotational deformity of the limb or palpable motion of the iliac wing (Fig. 5-21). In such cases stabilization of both the anterior and pelvic rings are generally indicated.

Posterior Pelvic Ring Injuries

The main residual orthopaedic problem from pelvic fracture is pain from a separated or fractured sacroiliac joint (139,140). Many patients complain of sacroiliac joint pain for 6 months to a year after the pelvic fracture, whether the joint had been treated operatively or nonoperatively (139,141).

Sacroiliac symptoms from pelvic injury, due to either fracture or ligament disruption, will generally heal spontaneously. However, healing of the ligamentous injury can take a good deal longer than does healing of the fractured sacrum or ilium (141). Nevertheless, ligaments do heal spontaneously with time (142). Consequently, acute fixation of every separated sacroiliac joint does not seem warranted since in most cases the symptoms subside or diminish (Fig. 5-22). This has been shown in a number of studies analyzing long-term residual problems from major pelvic fractures treated nonoperatively (135,139,143). Henderson (135), in reviewing results from the University of Iowa, found that many patients with major anterior or posterior pelvic disruption did have at least some degree of disability, but 62% had no disability. If the pelvic fracture was measurably unstable initially, the chances of long-term disability increased significantly. Most disability was associated with the amount and severity of vertical displacement through the sacroiliac joint. Although back pain was a fairly common complaint in patients followed up for pelvic fracture, it was not considered particularly severe. The pelvic fracture patients were no more likely to have visited a doctor or been hospitalized for low back symptoms than were normal control patients in the Iowa population. Further support of the Iowa study comes from a number of case reports of patients with bilateral sacroiliac dislocations (24,144–147). These indicated that even the unique bilateral injuries can be treated nonoperatively with surprisingly good functional outcome despite complete displacement of the sacroiliac joints.

Other investigators who have been advocates of operative fixation of the sacroiliac joint have determined that anatomic reduction of the sacroiliac joint is important to correct pelvic obliquity and restore leg length (126,140). But even with anatomic reduction of the sacroiliac joint many patients will still experience some degree of posterior pelvic symptoms (148,149).

SPINAL INJURIES

Cervical Spine Fractures

It has been said that the ease with which a cervical spine fracture can be sustained is exceeded only by the ease with which the diagnosis may be missed. Any patient with neck pain after a direct blow to the head or neck should be carefully evaluated for cervical spine fractures. This is particularly true for the elderly

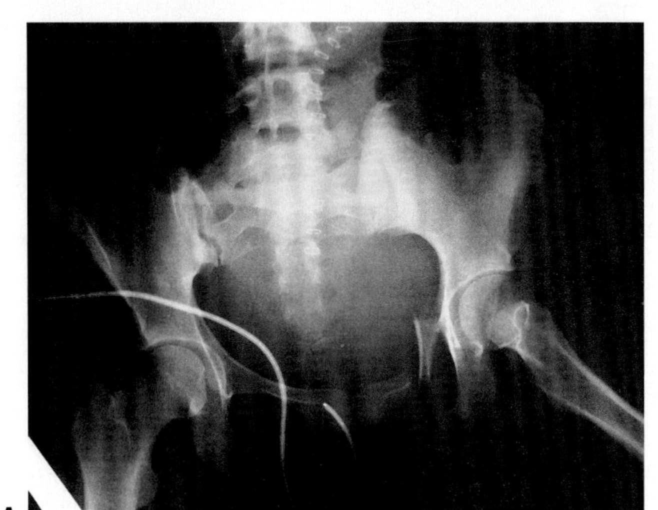

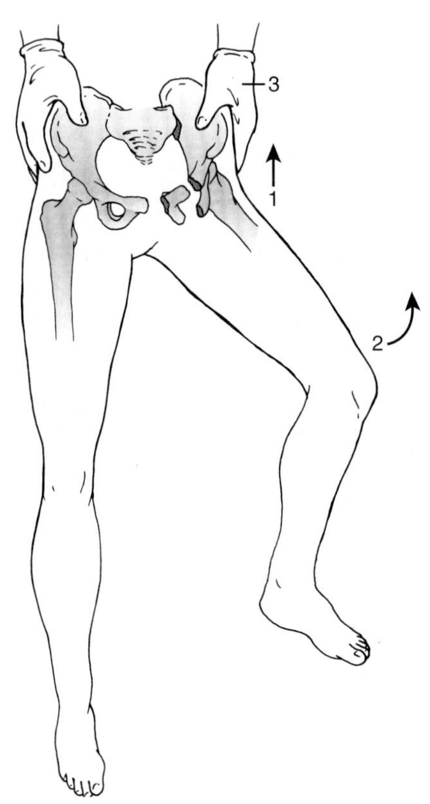

A B

FIGURE 5-21 **A.** Although most pubic ramus fractures do not require operative fixation, this displaced fracture penetrated the patient's vagina and resulted in a vaginal laceration and a subsequent vesicovaginal fistula. Displaced pubic ramus fractures in women should be evaluated carefully for associated gynecologic injuries. **B.** Clinical assessment of pelvic instability is based on evidence of shortening and external rotation of the limb (*1, 2*) as well as a palpable sensation of motion when an internal or external rotation force is applied to the iliac wing (*3*). These findings generally confirm the need for external or internal fixation of the pelvic injury. If closed treatment is dictated by other injuries, the external rotation and shortening of the limb can be corrected by distal femoral traction until early healing occurs. (Modified from Connolly J. *Fractures and dislocations. Closed management.* Philadelphia: WB Saunders, 1995, with permission.)

patient with osteoarthritis or ankylosing spondylitis who sustains a "minor" hyperextension injury to the neck (150) (Fig. 5-23). The general ossification of the arthritic or ankylosed spine causes it to fracture readily, like chalk, with minimal injury (151).

Slucky and Eismont (152) have recommended that treatment of acute injuries of the cervical spinal cord should stress patient resuscitation, spinal immobilization, and skeletal traction for fracture reduction and alignment. In their experience approximately 40% of these injuries have been appropriately treated nonoperatively. Operative treatment does play a role in decompressing and stabilizing the cervical spine electively after the patient is acutely stabilized (153–159).

Central Cord Injuries

Although most cervical spine fractures with spinal cord injury require prompt stabilization, some conditions are prime candidates for nonoperative treatment without reduction. These include cervical spine injuries producing a central cord syndrome (160,161). Most often these patients present with incomplete paralysis and a puzzling lack of evidence of either a fracture or dislocation. This can occur in approximately 15% of patients with significant neurologic injury. The classic mechanism is a hyperextension of the cervical spine in an older patient with arthritis, disk disease, or spondylitis (Fig. 5-23) (162). This sudden hyperextension causes hemorrhage into the central portion of the cord, resulting in upper extremity paralysis greater than the paralysis of the lower extremities. The corticospinal tract (motor tract) and spinothalamic tract (pain and temperature) may be spared or just partially involved.

The central cord lesion can be confirmed by an MRI scan that shows hemorrhage into the central portion of the cord. Management of the patient with a central cord lesion, which is an incomplete neural injury, does not require surgical treatment. In fact, operative treatment may occasionally interfere

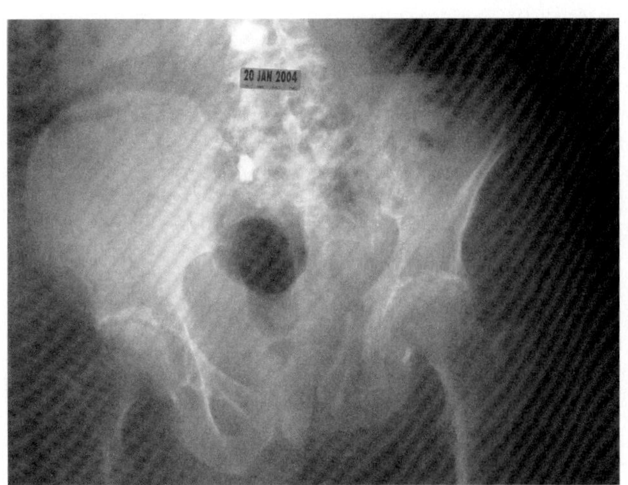

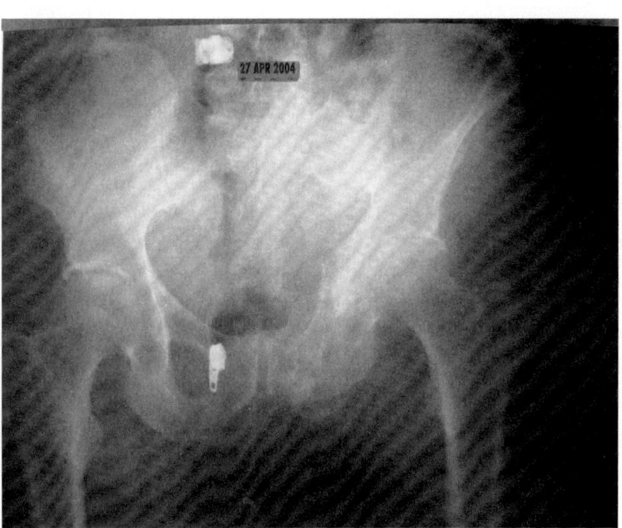

FIGURE 5-22 **A.** A 90-year-old male pedestrian sustained this fracture of the anterior and posterior pelvic rings when he was struck by an automobile. There is x-ray evidence of instability with widening of the sacroiliac joint and displaced fractures of the pubic rami. The patient's pelvis was stable on clinical testing. Consequently, the fracture was treated symptomatically in this elderly gentleman who was permitted to walk with a walker and was discharged from the rehabilitative service 7 days after fracture. **B.** The patient was minimally symptomatic and fully weightbearing at 3 months. Follow-up x-rays showed that the position of the pelvic fractures remained unchanged. This illustrates that careful evaluation of the clinical stability of the pelvis is a key determinant in selecting appropriate management.

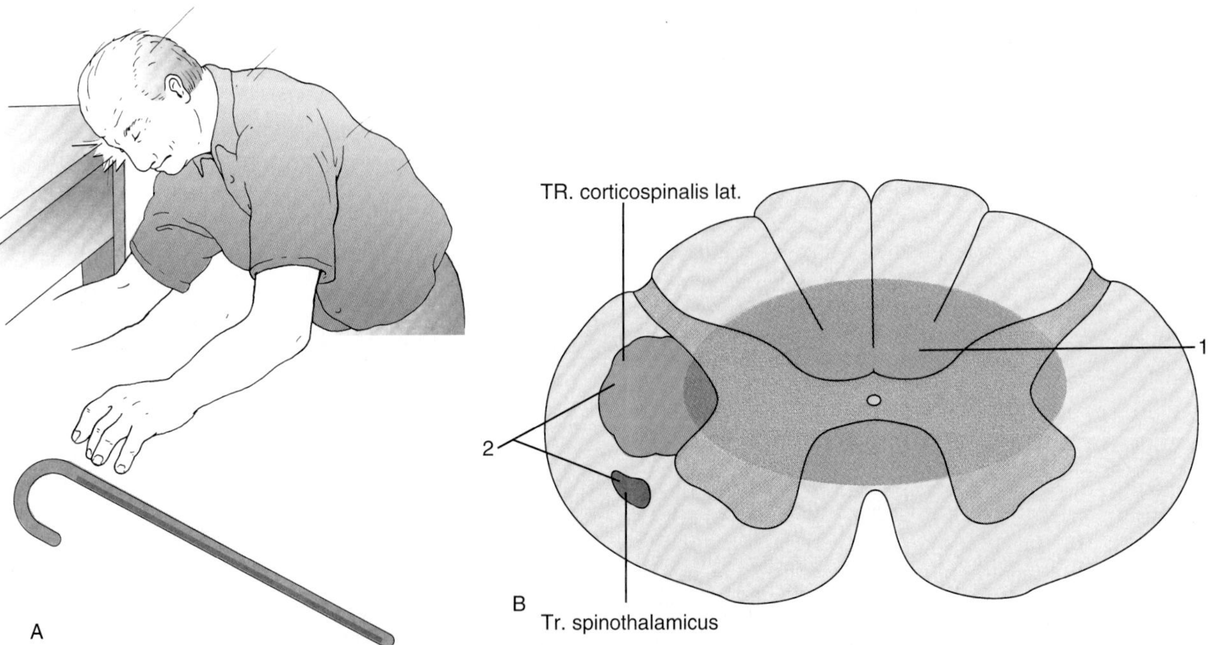

FIGURE 5-23 **A.** The classic mechanism of injury in the elderly patient with long-standing cervical arthritis or ankylosing spondylitis is a hyperextension blow to the head. **B.** The extension injury can cause hemorrhaging into the central portion of the cord (*1*), resulting in central cord syndrome. This generally damages the central portion of the gray matter, resulting in upper extremity paralysis that may or may not be greater than lower extremity involvement. The corticospinal tract (motor tract) and the spinothalamic tract (pain and temperature) may be spared or only partially involved (*2*). (Modified from Connolly J. *Fractures and dislocations. Closed management.* Philadelphia: WB Saunders, 1995, with permission.)

with circulation to the cord and diminish the chances of recovery. Heavy traction on the neck should also be avoided since this may distract the injured cord and worsen the neurologic deficit (163–165). The primary treatment is to protect the spine with a cervical orthosis to prevent recurrent hyperextension and advise the patient and family that chances for some recovery are usually fairly good. Ishida and Tominaga (166) have shown that if a patient has only involvement of the upper extremities with normal strength in the legs prognosis for recovery at about 6 weeks is almost 100%. Motor recovery occurs before sensory recovery. This is particularly true for patients without abnormal MRI signal intensity in the spinal cord. Outcomes are not as favorable for patients with initially severe neurologic damage and older age.

Ankylosing Spondylitis

Another prime candidate for nonoperative treatment of a cervical spine fracture is the patient suffering from ankylosing spondylitis (167–169). These fractures frequently occur as a result of minimal trauma and are associated with severe neurologic deficit in approximately 75% of cases. Fractures are often unstable, but nonoperative treatment is almost uniformly successful in achieving union (168). Although the mortality rate in patients treated nonoperatively is high, the rate of mortality among patients undergoing surgical treatment is considerably higher (50% or more). Nonoperative management also is not without complications since these patients tolerate both bed rest and brace treatment poorly because of significant pulmonary insufficiency. The compromise treatment includes a brief period of halo or skull traction followed by immobilization in a cervical-thoracic brace (Fig. 5-24) adjusted specifically to accommodate the kyphosis that usually results from the ankylosis (167). Management within a specialized spinal cord injury unit probably facilitates and optimizes this form of management. The important point to keep in mind in treating any of these patients is the ease with which the spine can be fractured after minor injury such as a blow to the head, and the significant complications that follow operative as well as nonoperative treatment of this lesion (162,168,169).

Bracing of Cervical Spine Injuries

Patients with cervical (C) spine fractures without neurologic deficit require careful and critical consideration of management options (170). The standard option has been with halo brace immobilization, but this technique has been found to have a number of drawbacks (171–175), especially in elderly patients (150,151,176). Even light traction intentionally or inadvertently applied through the halo can distract the fracture producing nonunion, particularly of odontoid fractures (165,177). Several studies (178–180) have shown that immobilization of the cervical spine fracture with a rigid Philadelphia collar or a cervical-thoracic brace can be as effective as a halo for many cervical fractures. Polin and co-workers (178) have shown that odontoid fractures may be treated with a rigid Philadelphia collar or a cervical-thoracic brace (Fig. 5-24). The type III fractures at the base of the odontoid heal consistently with this method. The majority of the more unstable type II fracture in the middle of the odontoid may also heal satisfactorily. Particularly in the elderly, it is not always necessary to achieve bony union for fractures of the odontoid (176). Stable fibrous union can be an acceptable outcome, provided there is no myelopathy and the elderly patient is a poor candidate for the surgical fusion (181).

Thoracic and Thoracolumbar Fractures

One of the problems in evaluating management approaches to spine fractures is that we obtain most of our reports today from spine centers to which injured patients are referred specifically because of complex problems. This has produced what might be considered a distorted perspective and inconsistent data. Saboe and co-workers (182) for example, in reporting experience from a single tertiary care spinal unit, indicated that approximately 38% of spine trauma patients were referred to their center with neurologic involvement. In contrast a large demographic study by Riggins and Kraus (183) found the overall frequency of nerve injury with spine fractures was 14%. In general the frequency of neurologic deficit can be expected to range from 40% for patients with cervical spine fractures to be 10% with thoracic spine fractures, 4% with thoracolumbar spine fractures-dislocations, and 3% with lumbar spine fractures (183,184).

Other population studies indicate that thoracic and thoracolumbar compression fractures without a history of injury are quite frequent and can be seen in about 1% of patients under the age of 30 but in more than 3% of patients older than 80 years of age. The frequency of asymptomatic fractures of the thoracic vertebrae in elderly osteoporotic patients can exceed 20% (185–187).

In the elderly osteoporotic patient, as soon as the pain symptoms from the thoracic fracture subside, the patient can be started on a program of extension exercises to regain paraspinal muscle function and prevent kyphotic deformity. These include strengthening the upper thoracic paraspinal muscles by doing wall push-ups. Lumbosacral and pelvic muscles can also be strengthened to avoid long-term symptoms. Such an approach is most readily accepted by the elderly patients subject to the problem. Prolonged bedrest or any type of spinal supports tend to worsen symptoms and should be avoided. These patients do not tolerate braces or corsets very well (188). Any evidence of neurologic involvement warrants an evaluation for tumor, either metastatic or primary, as the underlying cause of the fractures.

Some patients with osteoporotic vertebral fractures may occasionally experience persistent pain and functional impairment despite several months of the usual nonoperative treatment. A technique of balloon kyphoplasty has been found effective and safe in relieving pain, restoring vertebral body height, and patient quality of life (189). Kyphoplasty is a minimally invasive surgical procedure which is guided by x-ray images. It consists

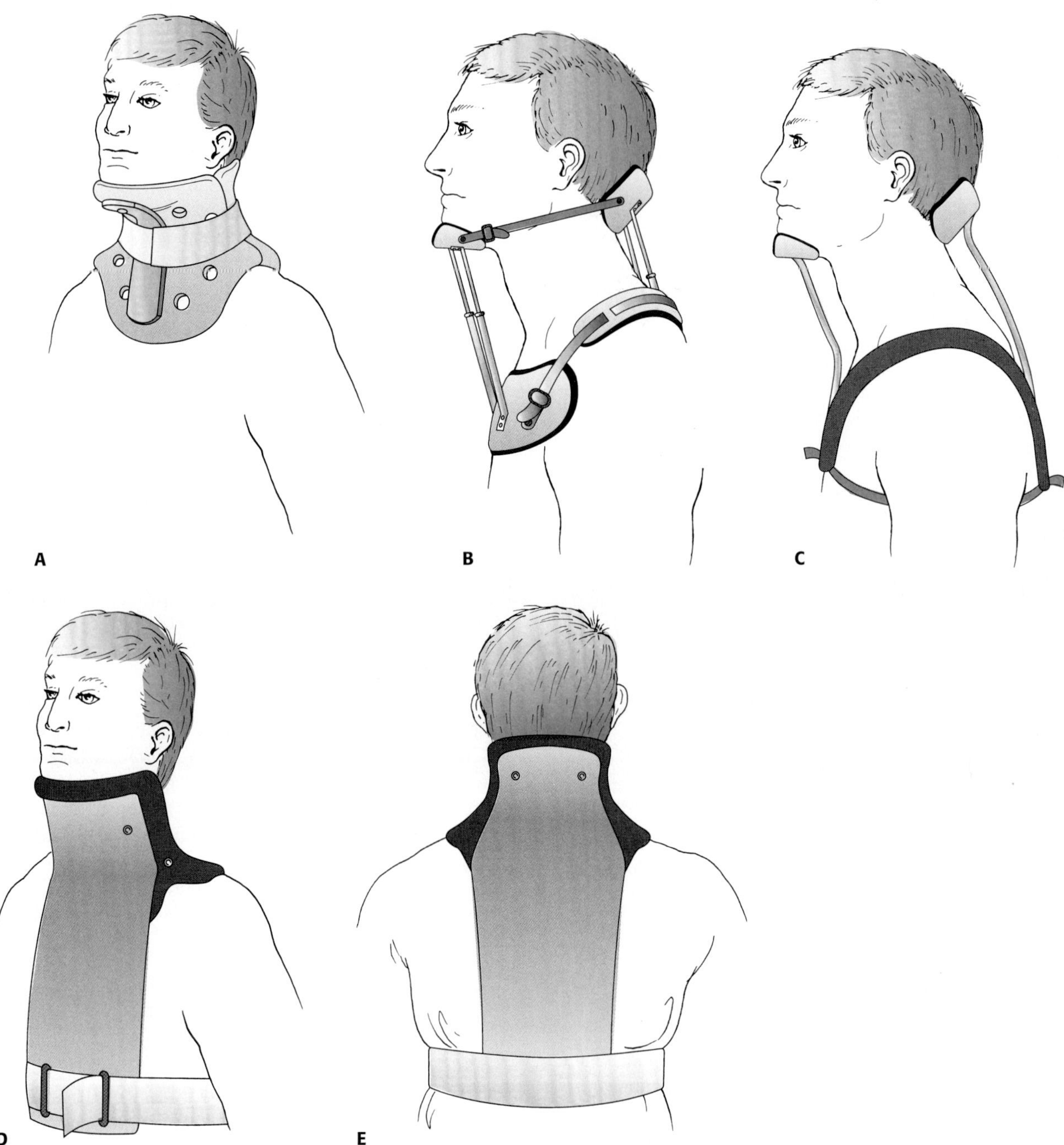

FIGURE 5-24 Cervical bracing. Because of the problems frequently associated with the use of a halo, recent studies indicate that a stable upper cervical spine can be treated with a Philadelphia collar **(A)**, or a four-poster brace **(B)**, or a sternal occipital mandibular immobilization (SOMI) type of brace **(C)**. Stabilization of odontoid fractures as well as lower cervical spine fractures may be possible using a combined Philadelphia collar with a molded fiberglass extension that fits on the chest **(D,E)**. Patients in any of these cervical orthoses should be followed carefully by radiographic and clinical evaluation to detect any delayed displacement of the fracture. (Modified from Connolly J. *Fractures and dislocations. Closed management.* Philadelphia: WB Saunders, 1995, with permission.)

of an inflatable bone tamp being directed into the fractured vertebral body to restore the body height. Fixation is then done by filling the void with viscous cement under volume control. The method has been effective in relieving symptoms both from osteoporotic fractures and pathologic fractures of the thoracolumbar spine. However, the optimal time interval for intervening with this method still needs to be determined (189,190). Injecting cement too soon after an acute vertebral body fracture can lead to cement leakage and serious neurologic complications (191). Consequently, it is recommended to wait at least several months while the vertebral body has gone through a phase of healing to achieve the maximum effect from the percutaneous vertebroplasty or kyphoplasty

In the younger patient, management of thoracic fractures introduces more potential problems (182,192,193) than does the simple wedge fracture in osteoporotic bone. Fredrickson, Yuan, and co-workers (26,194) have carefully reviewed indications for nonoperative treatment in younger patients who sustain more violent and unstable fractures than are seen in the elderly patients. Careful assessment is required particularly in the upper thoracic spine to determine the stability of the injury (195). In general, most of the fractures of the thoracic spine down to T-10 obtain support from the rib cage. If there is any doubt about stability, a period of bed rest for 4 to 6 weeks followed by immobilization in a brace support is generally indicated in the patient who is neurologically intact. If there is evidence of lateral displacement or loss of rib cage support, operative fixation is warranted.

The advent of computed tomography (CT) to evaluate spine fractures has created concern that bone fragments pushed from the vertebral body into the canal may cause progressive neurologic loss. This has led to a number of attempts to define the amount of canal impingement (50% to 60% or more?) that mandates operative intervention (196,197). On critical analyses and follow-up of patients it appears that the primary determinant of neurologic injury is the amount of direct damage sustained at the time of the initial fracture (198–203).

Operative fixation on the basis of arbitrary interpretation of the size of the canal fragments has not been validated (204). In fact, long-term studies indicate that fracture fragments that burst from the vertebral body into the canal remodel quite consistently and the canal can decompress spontaneously (194,205).

The use of CT to determine treatment of spine fractures seems analogous to using only high-powered microscopy to diagnose and treat bone tumors. Both modalities can make the condition look more malignant than it truly is (206). The fact that burst fractures can best be treated symptomatically by relieving pain, restoring paraspinal muscle strength with exercise, and returning the patient to as normal function as possible was first demonstrated by Nicoll (207) in studies of British coal miners. Subsequently, other investigators of patients with work-related fractures of the spine have reinforced Nicoll's observation (208–210). For many patients with compression fractures of the vertebral body, the residual symptomatic impairment is related to the duration and intensity of treatment and not necessarily to the amount of the fracture comminution. This is particularly true in workmen's compensation patients treated for vertebral fractures without neurologic injury (211).

The large number of fractures of the thoracic and lumbar spine seen in minimally symptomatic patients supports the general rule that closed management is the treatment of choice (212–214). Unfortunately, with the development of multiple internal fixation techniques and a massive spinal implant industry, many patients undergo open treatment of thoracic or thoracolumbar fractures for questionable indications (215–217). The use of such technology should not exceed the guidelines supported by common sense (218). A number of careful follow-up studies of injuries treated by closed methods indicate that stable fractures do not require further stabilization or even reduction (154,208–210). Such fractures include the common wedge flexion fracture as well as various fractures in the thoracic spine down to T-10. These undisplaced injuries are usually intrinsically stable because of rib cage support and may be treated adequately by a brief period of bed rest to alleviate pain symptoms followed by early mobilization and exercises (210). Spinal bracing may be prescribed selectively depending on the concerns of the patient. Ideally, use of such bracing should be kept to a minimum (188,219) since it is generally biomechanically ineffective.

Fractures Below T-10

Closed treatment is generally indicated for most flexion-compression fractures in the thoracolumbar region below T-10 without nerve injury (214,220). However, because these fractures no longer have the support of the rib cage they can displace, particularly if they result from flexion-rotation injuries. Internal fixation then would be indicated (202,222,223).

Most (70%) of these thoracolumbar injuries with no or minimal neurologic deficit, such as temporary ileus, bladder weakness, or isolated partial nerve root deficit, can be safely and effectively treated by relatively simple and time-proven methods of closed management (208,209,214,223–226). Closed management, however, should not be equated to management by neglect (226). If bladder or bowel weakness (cauda equina syndrome) is suspected, careful testing for perianal sensation and bladder catheterization and/or urodynamic studies are indicated. Symptomatic relief is obtained by a brief period of bed rest followed by exercises of the spinal support muscles. The patient should be followed closely (202,218,227,228) for any clinical or radiographic changes to detect unanticipated instability of the fracture. For patients who present with multiple nerve root paralysis, operative decompression, including anterior decompression would be indicated (229).

MANIPULATIVE REDUCTION

Mechanics of Reduction Based on Reversing the Original Mechanisms of Injury

Although a number of fractures, as discussed in the preceding section, can be treated by simply allowing muscle and joint function to achieve alignment, many require manipulative reduction to correct or prevent deformity. Closed reduction methods rely on two basic techniques. First, skeletal and soft tissue traction are required to restore length. Rotational manipulation then is necessary to correctly realign joint axes of motion. Understanding mechanisms and potential problems is as important for closed nonoperative reduction as it is for operative techniques (34,230–232).

Reduction of Fractures by Traction or Ligamentotaxis

Fractures result from direct or indirect mechanisms. The majority of fractures produced by high-speed injuries common today result from a direct impact against the bone and soft tissues. These fractures are characterized by comminution of the fragments, shortening, and angulation determined by the direction of the impact. To reduce these and many other such comminuted and shortened fractures requires traction using the principle of ligamentotaxis. *Ligamentotaxis* is the term used to emphasize that, to be effective, traction must be balanced by countertraction provided by the ligaments and soft tissue surrounding the bone. This pull and counterpull restores length and guides alignment of the fracture fragments. Thus, traction relies heavily on the soft tissues that are usually attached to at least some of the fracture fragments unless there is extreme stripping (233) as in a grade III open fracture or an unstable disrupted fracture-dislocation of the spine. In these circumstances traction should be applied carefully to avoid complications associated with overdistracting the injury (165,199,234).

In the past, traction was usually applied directly to the soft tissues and skin, as with Buck's traction on the lower leg. A preferable method now in most instances is with some type of skeletal traction. Skeletal traction restores limb length and aligns the fracture fragments close to normal when it is counterbalanced by the soft tissues still attached to the fragments. Traction can be accomplished also with external fixators that span the fracture site or even span joints. Supplemental fracture fragment fixation by percutaneous pins or screws can also be used to protect against fracture redisplacement as the ligaments stretch out over time. Such techniques are particularly used for comminuted fractures about the knee, the ankle, and the wrist joint (235–237). Ligamentotaxis has also been utilized to reduce fractures in the cervical, thoracic, and lumbar spine by means of halo or other skull traction techniques.

Initial Steps in Acute Reduction of Fractures

Direct application of traction is among the first essential steps to reduce a deformed fractured limb. Temporary splinting combined with traction can be effected by a variety of splinting techniques. One historic method has been with a Thomas splint, which was developed by H. Owen Thomas in England and introduced during World War I by Sir Robert Jones. This simple technique of splinting resulted in lowering the mortality rate of gunshot wound femur fractures from well over 50% to approximately 20% under those wartime circumstances. Subsequently, a wide variety of other splints have been developed to apply traction in order to stabilize the injured limb. A Hare splint is commonly used by rescue squad personnel since it can splint a deformed femur and/or tibia and maintain stability by direct traction (Fig. 5-25). The patient then can be transported in reasonable comfort to the emergency facility. It is axiomatic that in the emergency center fracture stability must be continuously maintained during acute assessment and management of the injured patient. Unfortunately, this axiom is sometimes forgotten in the rush to resuscitate the injured patient.

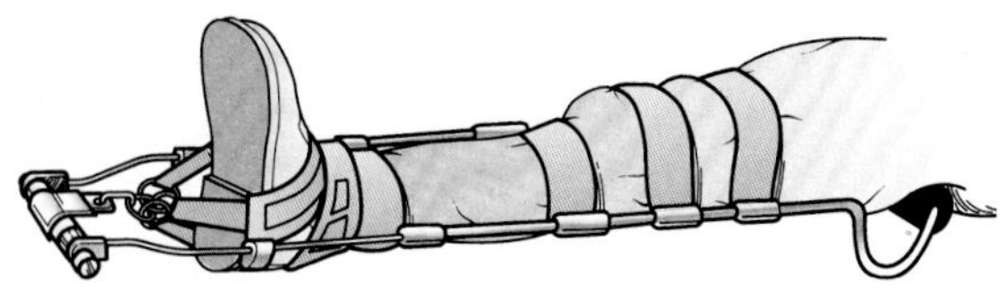

FIGURE 5-25 A Hare splint is useful as a temporary means of immobilizing a fracture of the femur or tibia by direct traction. It should be used only as a temporary splint and replaced by skeletal or skin traction when the patient has been stabilized. (Modified from Connolly J. *Fractures and dislocations. Closed management.* Philadelphia: WB Saunders, 1995, with permission.)

Skin Traction

The use of skin traction to align a fracture, particularly of the femur, has been common since it was popularized by Buck in the Civil War (238). Skin traction is still used today but only as a temporary means of stabilizing adult hip fractures or occasionally the femur fracture in a child's leg. Skin is unable to tolerate more than approximately 6 to 8 pounds of traction for a brief length of time. Heavier or prolonged traction tends to pull off the superficial layers of the skin and can cause pressure necrosis of soft tissues (Fig. 5-26) (239).

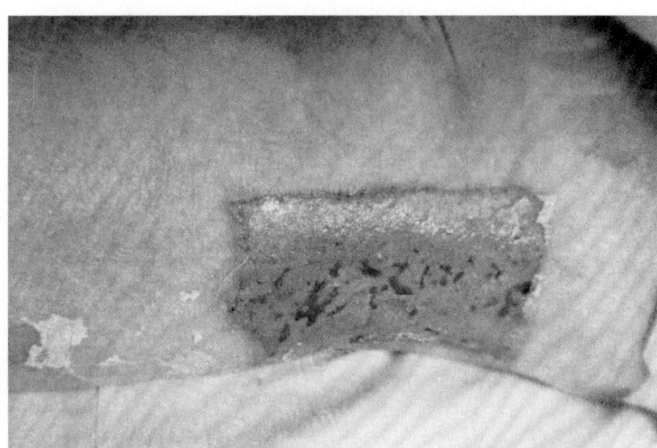

FIGURE 5-26 Skin traction can cause irritation of the skin, allergic reactions, or avulsion of the superficial layers of the dermis. Standard adhesive tape should be avoided since skin irritation as illustrated here is fairly common.

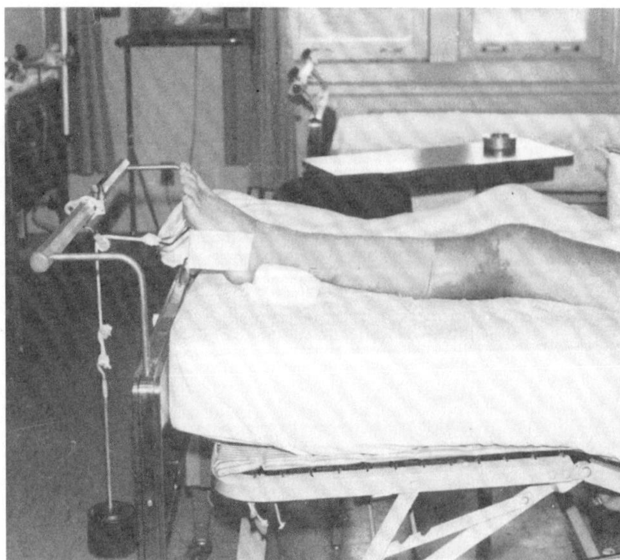

FIGURE 5-27 Skin traction should be applied only as a temporary measure. The traction is applied superior to the malleoli with traction tapes and an elastic bandage wrapped from the ankle to the knee. Avoid more than 6 to 8 pounds of traction since it can produce skin irritation or skin necrosis.

The basic technique of Buck's skin traction is to apply padding around bony prominences of the malleoli. Traction tapes are then applied to the skin and an elastic bandage is wrapped from the ankle to the knee. The end of the tape is then attached to the traction apparatus (Fig. 5-27). Most commonly now a prepackaged type of skin traction is available. It can be applied quickly and easily using sponge-rubber material that can be removed and reapplied often without peeling off the skin.

Application of Skeletal Traction

The preferred method of applying traction for most fractures is by inserting a threaded Steinmann or Bonnell pin into the distal fracture fragment and then applying traction weights directly to it. In inserting any skeletal traction pin the skin must be prepped as with any surgical procedure. Gloves are worn and the area is isolated with towels and sterile precautions are taken. Usually the pin can be inserted under local anesthetic but often the patient is under general or spinal anesthetic. If a local anesthetic is used, the anesthesia should be infiltrated down thoroughly to the sensitive periosteum. The skin should be incised prior to inserting the traction pin to avoid irritation from the pin.

A wide variety of traction techniques are available that allow treatment of fractures from the cervical spine down to the foot (Fig. 5-28).

Once the pin is inserted, the limb is immobilized on some type of support. For the femur, this is most often a Harris modification of a Thomas splint with a Pearson attachment (Fig. 5-29). The splint and traction weight are counterbalanced by a weight at the head of the bed. The foot is kept out of equinus by a plantar support. The Achilles tendon must be well padded, and any bony prominences as well as the peroneal nerve should be protected. For fractures at a proximal level of the femur, traction can be most effective if the limb is held in a 90°–90° position, which maintains both the hip and the knee flexed 90 degrees to correct the tendency of the proximal femur to externally rotate and flex (Fig. 5-30).

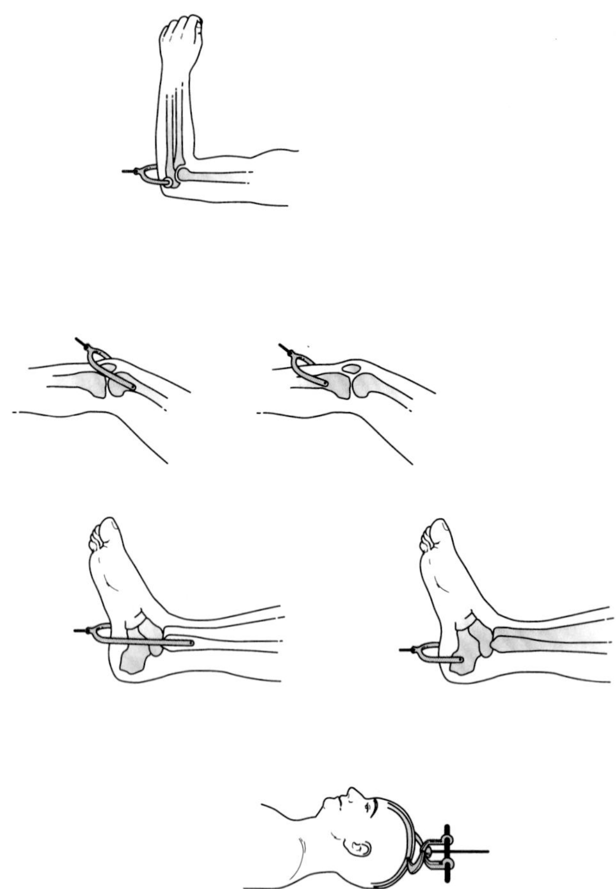

FIGURE 5-28 Skeletal traction sites. A variety of sites for skeletal traction are available. The techniques range from traction in the olecranon to skull traction as illustrated here. (Modified from Connolly J. *Fractures and dislocations. Closed management.* Philadelphia: WB Saunders, 1995, with permission.)

Hazards of Skeletal Traction

Although skeletal traction has been proven to be a very reliable and useful method of reducing and maintaining alignment of many different fractures, it can occasionally be associated with complications. Pins that are left in for more than a few weeks can become sources of infection or mechanical irritations of nearby nerves and vessels (240). Pin tract infection can be managed by (a) having the pin pass through the least amount of soft tissue possible, (b) minimizing movement of joints adjacent

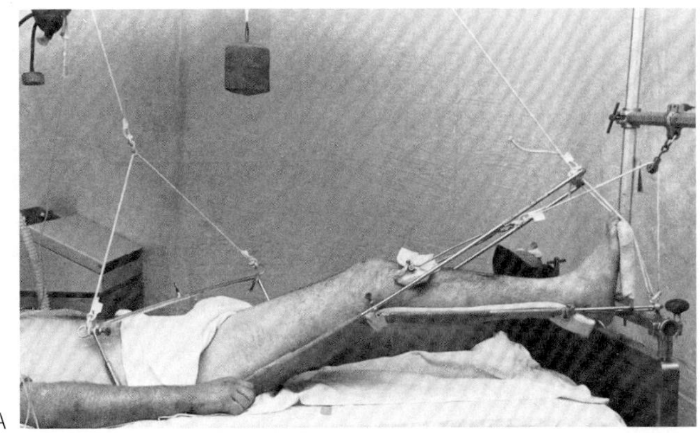
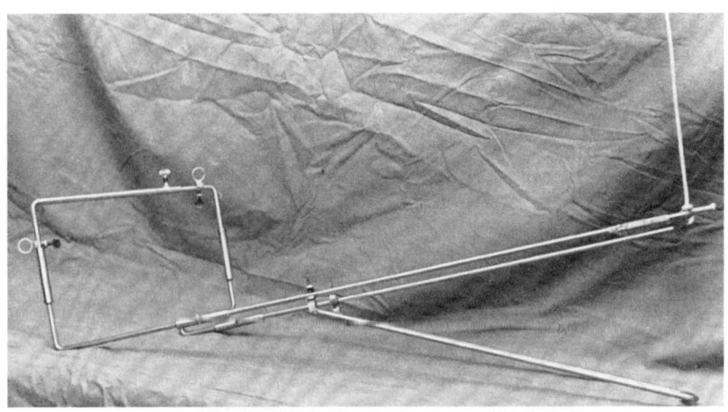

A B

FIGURE 5-29 A,B. Fractures of the femur can be treated in a Harris splint. The entire system is counterbalanced with weights proximally and distally of approximately 10 pounds. Longitudinal skeletal traction is applied through the tibia or occasionally through the distal femur. The foot is held out of equinus by a plantar support to avoid creating a tight heel cord. The Achilles tendon is well padded and all bony prominences are protected especially around the peroneal nerve. The Pearson attachment to the splint allows flexion and extension of the knee.

to the traction pin, and (c) cleansing the skin-pin interface with peroxide and applying an antibiotic ointment.

One of the most common complications from skeletal traction is overdistracting the fracture. This has been found to occur particularly in fractures of the distal radius where ligamentotaxis from external fixation can be exerted too vigorously. Overdistraction of the radiocarpal joint then leads to stiffness and even causalgia of the fingers and hand (241). The technique of skeletal traction for cervical spine injuries can also overdistract if the method is applied too vigorously or without careful monitoring of its effect (161,162,229).

FIGURE 5-30 A 90°–90° system of traction is quite useful for reducing fractures of the proximal femur. The limb can be positioned to correct the tendency of the proximal femoral fragment to flex and externally rotate. It illustrates the principle that traction should bring the distal fragment into alignment with the proximal fragment of a fracture. (Modified from Connolly J. *Fractures and dislocations. Closed management.* Philadelphia: WB Saunders, 1995, with permission.)

Techniques of Cast Application

A plaster-of-paris cast is useful to immobilize most fractures, whether treated nonoperatively or operatively. Complications that can be associated with cast application range from loss of limb to itchy skin. Infections (including gas gangrene), ischemic muscle necrosis from compartment syndrome, and unrecognized vascular injuries can be hidden under a cast and lead to loss of limb (242). One should be particularly cautious in applying casts to patients with loss of protective sensation due to conditions such as diabetes or a head injury. This can lead to rapid skin breakdown from pressure necrosis (Fig. 5-31) (243,244).

Before applying a cast, the circulatory, motor, and sensory status of the limb should be checked to document if the patient has any evidence of neurologic injury. If there is any question of circulatory loss, the cast should not be applied until the circulatory status is clarified and circulation is restored.

Since the limb swells after the fracture, it is important to elevate it in the cast to allow drainage from the extremity. If the patient complains of pain from the cast being too tight the cast should be bi-valved and the cast padding released down to the skin to relieve the tightness.

Edema fluid that persists in the hand or the foot can produce a glue-like effect, impeding the synchrony of motion between tendons, bones, and joints. Encouraging active motion of the fingers, toes, and any muscles in the injured extremity is the most effective method of minimizing functional impairment and preventing "cast disease."

The plaster-of-paris bandage consists of a roll of muslin stiffened by a starch and impregnated with a hemihydrate of calcium sulfate. When water is added, the calcium sulfate crystallizes ($CaSO_4 \cdot H_2O + H_2O = CaSO_4 \cdot 2H_2O$ + heat). The setting

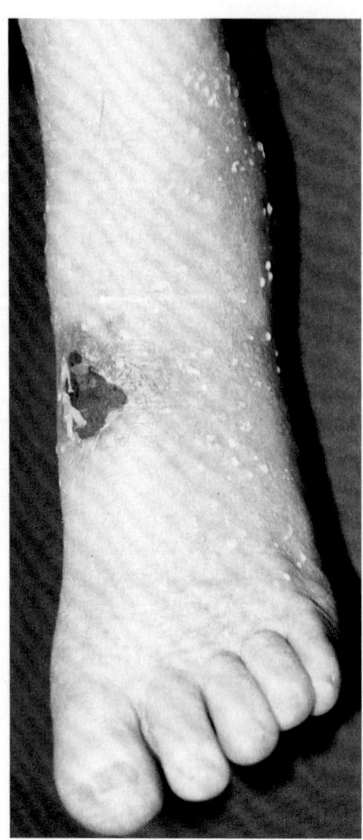

FIGURE 5-31 A cast was applied for an ankle sprain in this patient with long-standing diabetes. Breakdown of the skin and surrounding soft tissues was evident when the cast was removed at 1 week. The loss of protective sensation in this patient was not appreciated, and the cast treatment considerably lengthened the treatment, although fortunately the outcome was satisfactory.

of this material may be accelerated by increasing the temperature of the water or slowed by cooling the water. The crystallization of plaster-of-paris is an exothermic reaction (245).

The plaster cast is applied in layers by molding with the base of one's hand (Fig. 5-32). As the cast is applied and the plaster-of-paris crystallizes, the heat given off can be enough to burn the skin (246). This is especially likely if the water used to soak the plaster was hot to the touch (Fig. 5-33). The plaster bandage should be immersed in a water bath that is at room temperature or at least comfortable to the touch of the person who is applying it. This is true whether one is applying a circular cast or a longitudinal splint. In fact, many thick splints may produce even higher exothermic temperatures than do circular casts.

A number of serious problems can develop whenever an injured or even uninjured limb is immobilized in a cast or any device. One should particularly avoid prolonged use of antishock garments, or applying casts that are likely to produce ischemic injury to underlying structures including skin, nerves and vessels (Fig. 5-34).

Casts and splints that immobilize limbs in a nonfunctioning position, should be avoided, especially for minor injuries. For example, a posterior splint applied for an ankle sprain should not leave the foot and ankle in the equinus position. This makes it impossible for the patient to bear any weight on the limb, promotes edema, and delays recovery from the minor injury (Fig. 5-35). Prolonged lack of function can result in disuse osteoporosis of the foot and subsequent pain with weightbearing (247,248). Casts applied to the upper limb should allow motion of the joints of the fingers. Similarly casts on the lower limb should not impinge on or block toe motion.

The patient's complaints of a painful cast should be heeded and the cast changed promptly. Often this may reveal an area of early skin pressure or irritation that might well advance to full-thickness skin loss. Some patients who repeatedly request cast changes might be better treated by operative fracture fixation.

A variety of casting products have become available as a substitute for the classic plaster-of-paris cast (249,250). The most widely used is a knitted fiberglass fabric, which is impregnated with polyurethane resin. Exposure of this product to water initiates a chemical reaction, which causes the tapes to become rigid. These materials have the advantage over plaster of being relatively lightweight, strong, radiolucent, and, when properly used, resistant to water. The major clinical disadvantage of fiberglass is that it cannot be molded to the limb as well as can plaster. A second disadvantage is that the polyurethane resin will adhere firmly to unprotected skin and to clothing. Therefore, protective gloves should be worn while handling the material, and care should be exercised to avoid contacting unprotected areas of the patient's skin during application. Swabbing lightly with alcohol or acetone may help in removing uncured resin from the skin. If the patient is likely to immerse the cast in water, the extremity should be first wrapped in a water-shedding stockinette. Otherwise the underlying cast padding material will remain soggy under the cast and cause skin irritation.

The fiberglass cast material is applied after fracture reduction is accomplished. One or two layers of stockinette are applied over the limb and cast padding is added over bony prominences. The cast tape is immersed one roll at a time in water at room temperature and carefully applied using gloves to protect the skin. The usual setting time for the material is approximately 3 minutes. This can be lengthened by removing the roll without squeezing it or by using cooler water. The cast is wrapped spirally, overlapping each turn one half to two thirds the width of the tape. The material is less flexible than the usual plaster-of-paris and therefore less moldable around the limb, but still is suitable for most stable fractures that do not require that the cast be closely contoured. The fiberglass material sets faster than plaster-of-paris, and weightbearing may usually be allowed once the cast has dried thoroughly. If the patient complains of any discomfort following cast application, it is best to remove it to check for pressure sores or other problems. The cast may be bi-valved to accommodate for acute swelling, and then a new cast applied once the swelling subsides.

Fiberglass cast removal requires an oscillating type of saw that generates dust that is lower in quantity and larger in particle size than the dust generated on removal of plaster-of-paris casts. This dust usually consists of glass fibers embedded in cured

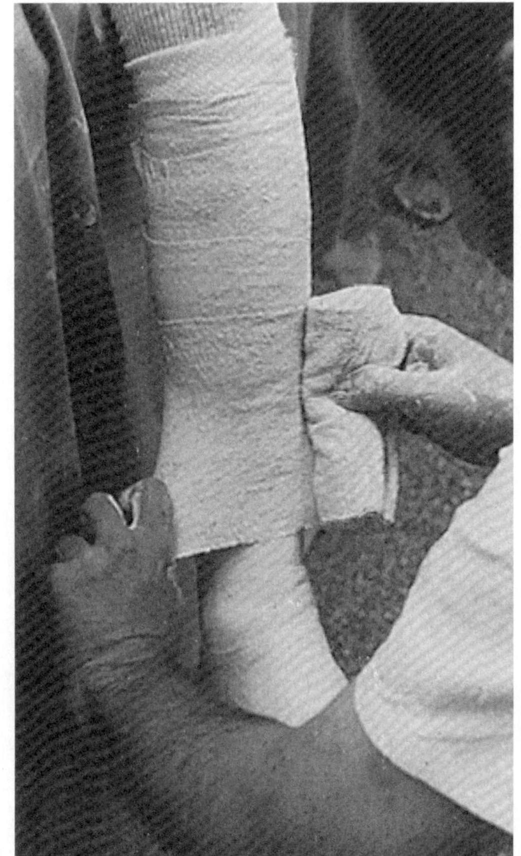
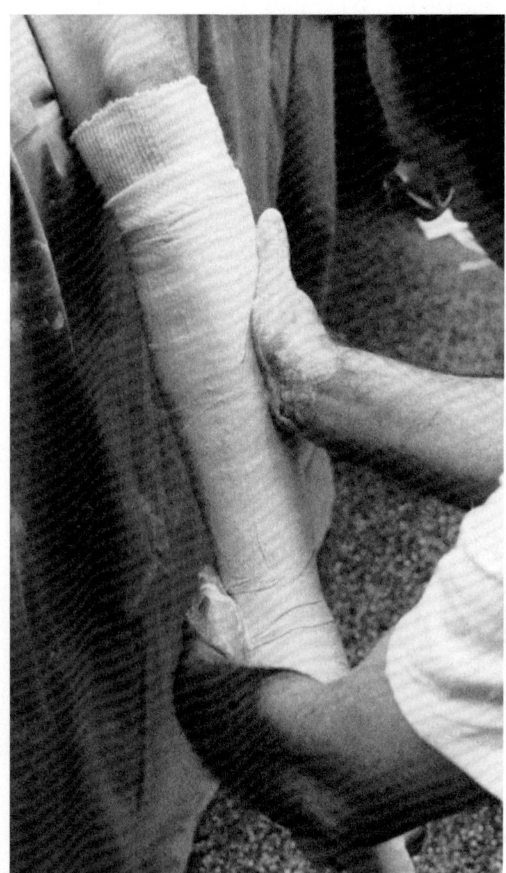

FIGURE 5-32 A. A plaster-of-paris bandage is applied carefully over the cast padding. The roll is applied by the fingertips with the bandage conforming to the circumference of the arm or leg. The roll may be redirected by taking tucks as illustrated with the left hand of the cast technician in this demonstration. **B.** When the cast is completed and the plaster is still wet the structure of the cast is molded to the contour of the leg using the palms of the hands. Avoid any fingertip pressure that can cause pressure points under the cast and subsequent skin necrosis.

polyurethane with a minor amount of glass fiber dust. They are not considered to be respirable-sized particles and fall well below the permissible occupational exposure limits for nuisance dusts. The cast saw must be used carefully to avoid lacerating the skin under the cast. It is best to support the cast with the thumb held against the cast in order to avoid pushing the blade through the patients' skin (Fig. 5-36).

The underlying cast padding is cut down to the skin using bandage scissors while a cast spreader spreads the cast edges (Fig. 5-37).

Reduction by Restoring Joint Axis of Motion

Fractures occur by either direct or indirect mechanisms (34,109,230,232,251). Examples of indirect mechanisms include the patient who falls on the outstretched hand fracturing the shoulder or the skier who twists the leg fixed in the snow and fractures the tibia (252). Direct mechanisms are typified by the motorcyclist who sustains a comminuted open tibial fracture from a direct blow to the leg at high speeds. Reduction techniques should reverse the mechanisms producing the original deformity rather than accentuate them.

The skeleton is least able to resist torsional loading (231,251). Yamada (253) found that the ultimate torsional strength of bone is only one third that of its compressive strength and one half that of its tensile strength. When a uniform skeletal specimen is subjected to torsional testing, it fails in a consistent pattern. The most significant determinant of this fracture pattern is the direction of loading. The patterns of torsional failure are completely predictable and reproducible. Failure occurs first in the cortex, which is subjected to maximum tensile loading. The fracture then spirals over to the opposite cortex in a clockwise or counterclockwise direction. Reversing this mechanism of failure can often restore alignment to a displaced fracture (232,254).

Rotational deformities may be cosmetically unsatisfactory, but, more importantly, they are often detrimental to function because they create a misalignment of the joint axes of motion. Reduction techniques should first recognize the torsional mech-

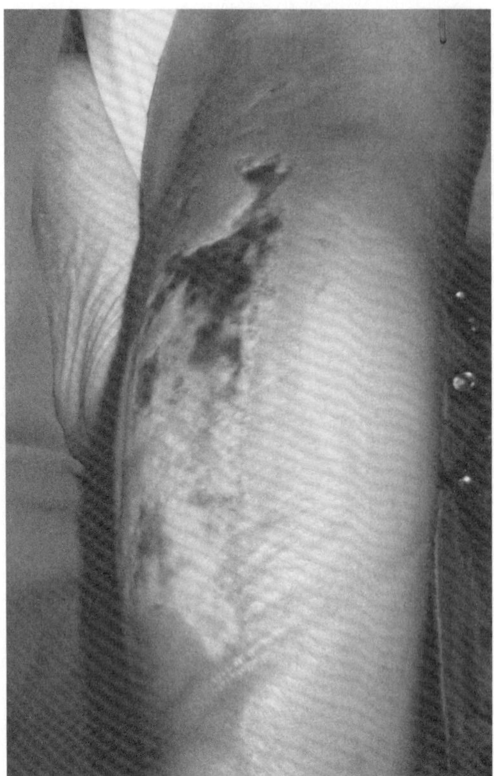

FIGURE 5-33 When plaster is applied it produces an exothermic release of heat. If the water in which the plaster is soaked is too hot, this combination can burn the patient's skin. This illustration shows a third-degree burn of a patient after a cast was applied with water that was well above room temperature. Even plaster splints have been associated occasionally with this complication if the water used to set the material is uncomfortably hot.

anisms that produced the fracture and distort joint alignment. The techniques of reduction should be directed at reversing these torsional mechanisms, particularly in order to restore alignment of the joint axis of motion.

A typical example of a fracture produced by indirect loading is seen in the patient who falls on the outstretched hand, internally twisting the arm while loading the shoulder. This produces a fracture of the proximal humerus with a fairly consistent spiral oblique pattern. The fracture line runs from the distal lateral cortex to the proximal medial cortex due to the internal torsion of the humerus fixed in the glenoid (Fig. 5-38). Immobilizing such a fracture, which was produced by internal rotation, in a sling, which further internally rotates the distal fragment, reproduces the original mechanism and tends to displace the shaft fragment medially (Fig. 5-6). A humeral fracture of this type is reduced by rotating the shaft fragment outward. One can then emphasize early mobilization of the shoulder and arm rather than immobilization of the arm against the chest. Conversely, the humeral fracture resulting from an external torsional load on the extended arm has the opposite mirror image fracture pattern: the fracture line runs from the distal medial cortex upward to the proximal lateral cortex. This externally rotated fracture is best reduced by immobilizing the shoulder with internal rotation and a sling. Following a brief period of immobilization, a humeral fracture sleeve can be applied to allow active elbow motion and utilize function of the muscles and joints around the fracture to maintain the normal axis of the elbow joint.

Forearm Fractures Reduced by Reversing the Mechanism of Injury

Forearm fractures result from failure in compression or tension or both. Compression failure produces the characteristic torus fracture of the child's distal radius, or the impacted Colles fracture in the older adult. Both types of compression fractures occur in relatively undermineralized bone in these age groups. Torsional, indirect loading is also a frequent cause of forearm fractures including the greenstick fracture in the child and the displaced radial shaft fracture in the adult. Here the mechanism is a fall on the outstretched arm twisting the forearm bones, which fail in torsion. The usual position of the forearm at the time of fracture is in supination (Fig. 5-39). This causes the greenstick fracture as well as the adult shaft fracture to angulate in a volar direction. If the fall occurs with the forearm pronated, the torsional mechanism produces a fracture that angulates dorsally.

To reduce these fractures, the torsional mechanism should be reversed. This is done not by hyperextending or hyperflexing the deformity but reversing either the supinated or pronated forearm. Thus, the fracture with volar angulation is usually corrected by pronation. The fracture with dorsal angulation is corrected with supination.

The majority of forearm fractures are produced by direct trauma, which can be quite violent. The function that is most significantly impaired with forearm fractures is the unique rotatory motion (supination/pronation) necessary for positioning of the hand. This requires rotation of the radius and not of the ulna. Fortunately, loss of forearm pronation can be compensated by shoulder abduction. Loss of supination, however, is poorly compensated by the shoulder.

The forearm normally is able to rotate 120 to 140 degrees. The normal lateral bow of the radius permits it to clear the soft tissues of the forearm as it rotates around the ulna. It is important to maintain the normal radial bow and the interosseous space required for rotation of the radius. A fracture that produces loss of the normal radial bow can lead to loss of rotation. It is also important to remember that the interosseous space is greatest in neutral rotation and narrowest in full pronation (255,256). Maintaining extreme pronation during fracture healing can cause some permanent stiffening of the muscles and interosseous ligaments, which in turn will limit supination of the forearm. Therefore, forearm fractures should usually be immobilized in either supination or in neutral rotation.

Closed reduction is the treatment of choice for fracture of the forearm of the child except for the occasional Monteggia

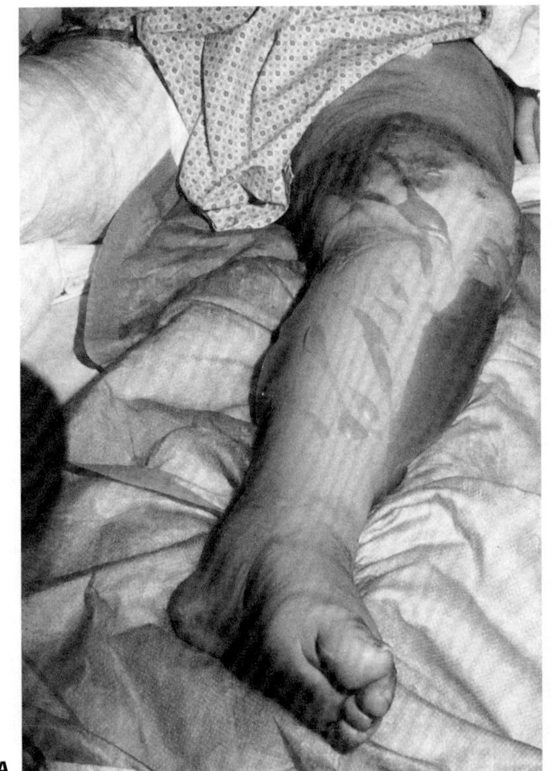

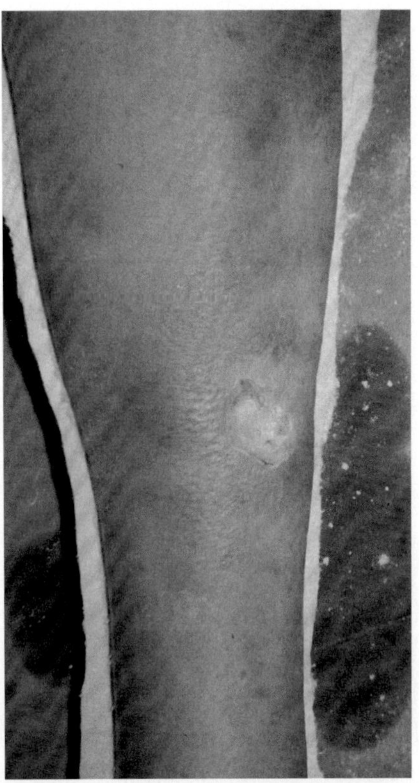

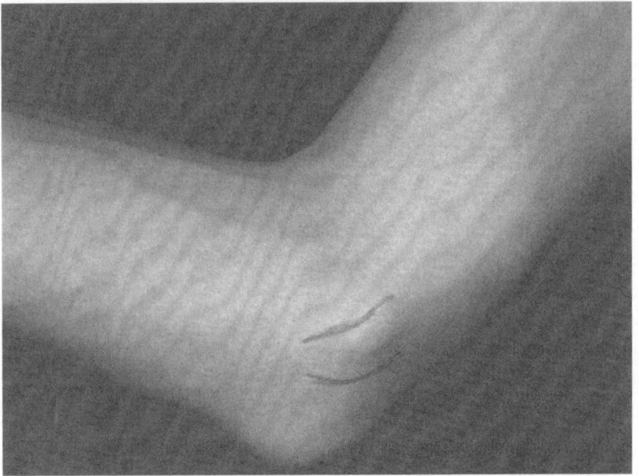

FIGURE 5-34 A variety of problems can develop after application of any type of immobilization device to an injured limb. **A.** Patients should be carefully monitored for the problems illustrated here, including a compartment syndrome after prolonged use of an antishock garment in this patient with multiple fractures. **B.** Pressure necrosis after a cast application with excessive pressure over the bony prominence of the proximal fragment converted a closed tibial fracture to an open fracture. **C.** Ulnar nerve palsy resulted from cast immobilization of a fractured forearm with the elbow flexed beyond 90 degrees. This caused the patient's mobile ulnar nerve to ride over the humeral epicondyle resulting in ischemic neuropathy of the nerve with loss of intrinsic function of the hand. An important principle to follow when immobilizing the elbow is to avoid positioning it beyond a right angle, which increases the risk of ischemic ulnar neuropathy.

fracture-dislocation of the elbow. Closed reduction of adult forearm fractures has also been standard for thousands of years. Shang et al (256) and others (255) in China have shown that traditional bonesetter methods of reducing the forearm fractures in adults can be quite safe and effective. However, because closed reduction is considered somewhat demanding and unpredictable, most orthopaedic surgeons prefer open reduction and internal fixation of fractures of both bones of the forearm (257,258). Nevertheless, it is still worth considering closed methods that can avoid complications such as infections, painful scars, and the need to subsequently remove plates, with the possibility of refracture (10,259–262). Patients with relatively thin forearms as well as young women who do not desire a scar on the forearm may be offered a trial of closed reduction. It should be understood that if reduction is lost or angulation is unacceptable, delayed open reduction can be performed without affecting good results from operative treatment (258).

Technique of Closed Reduction of Forearm Fractures

Closed reduction of the forearm fracture is performed with the patient under either a general or regional anesthetic. The patient

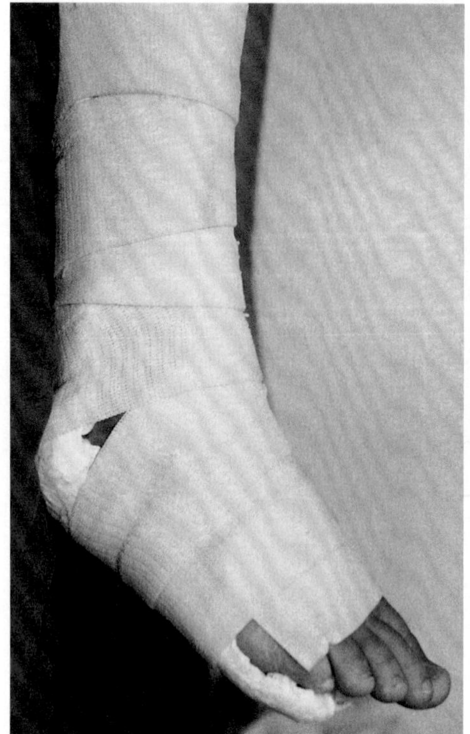

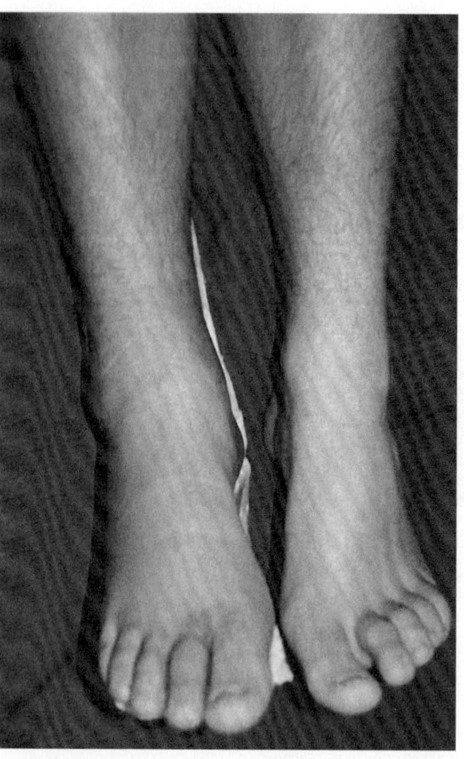

A B

FIGURE 5-35 **A.** Avoid immobilizing limbs in malfunctioning positions especially after minor injuries to the foot or ankle. This illustration shows a fairly typical ankle sprain that was referred from the emergency department in a posterior splint. It failed to support the ankle and allowed it to drift into equinus. **B.** Swelling and disuse changes were evident when the patient returned for follow-up at 1 week.

lies supine with fingers on the fractured side supported in a finger traction apparatus (Fig. 5-40). Countertraction is applied with a weighted sling pulling on the arm. The elbow is flexed 90 degrees and the forearm supinated. The traction is maintained for 5 to 10 minutes to regain the necessary length of the forearm and to correct angular deformity. After the length is restored, the surgeon reduces the fracture by squeezing on the volar and dorsal muscle masses between the radius and ulna, forcing these two bones apart (Fig. 5-41). The forearm is rotated slightly to promote interlocking of the fracture fragments, and correct rotational alignment is judged radiographically by comparing the width of the cortices of the proximal and distal fragments (263).

The goal of closed or open reduction is to restore the skeletal anatomy of the forearm as completely as possible. However, the forearm can accommodate a moderate amount of structural alteration since shortening of the upper extremity is generally tolerated more and is less functionally significant than is shortening in the lower limb. This is true for fractures of both the humerus and the forearm. If the radius shortens more than 5 to 7 mm, it is likely to be associated with disruption of the distal radioulnar articulation. Although some angulation of the forearm fractures can be accepted without impairing rotation, angulation of greater than 15 degrees can limit rotation and may also be cosmetically unacceptable.

The radial bow should be restored to allow the normal return of rotation. The ulnar fracture is usually reduced end to end, although slight overriding is acceptable. Angulation of either the ulna or the radius of less than 10 degrees dorsally or volarly has not been found to affect functional outcome (264).

Schemitsch and Richards (265) devised a method of directly measuring the maximum radial bow (Fig. 5-42) and demonstrated that even with the use of plate fixation malunion can be a problem if the radial bow is not corrected. They reported that restoration of the normal radial bow is particularly important to a good functional outcome. More than 80% return of normal rotation of the forearm was associated with the restoration of the radial bow. Also, restoration of grip strength was associated with the restoration of the radial bow toward normal. This radiographic technique of measuring the normal radial bow in terms of magnitude and location of the maximum bow compared with that of the opposite normal forearm should be kept in mind with either nonoperative or operative treatment (Fig. 5-43). When the radial bow is restored close to that of the uninjured extremity, the range of motion of the forearm and grip strength are also close to normal. An alteration of the normal radial bow therefore appears to be of greater functional significance than is dorsal or volar angulation of less than 10 or 15 degrees (264).

Once satisfactory alignment is achieved, a long arm cast is

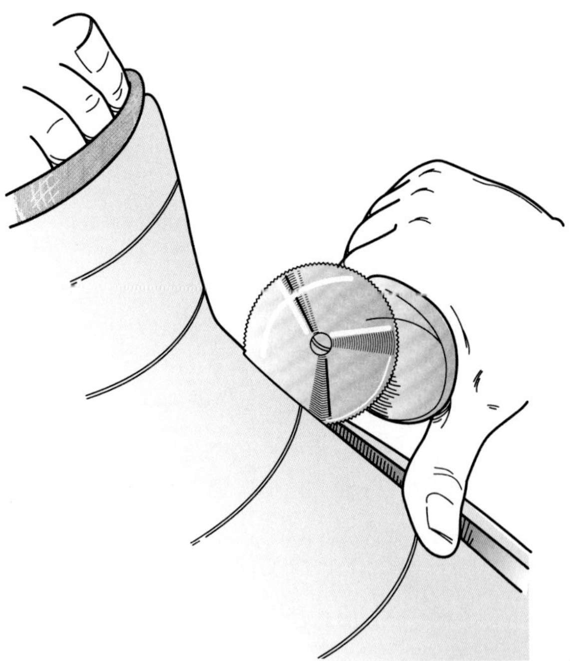

FIGURE 5-36 If a patient complains of any discomfort from a cast, it is best to remove it and check for pressure sores and other problems. The cast saw that is commonly used for cutting plaster is generally safe but can cut skin. The cast saw should be supported with the thumb against the cast to prevent the blade being pushed through the patient's skin and causing a deep laceration. (Modified from Connolly J. *Fractures and dislocations. Closed management.* Philadelphia: WB Saunders, 1995, with permission.)

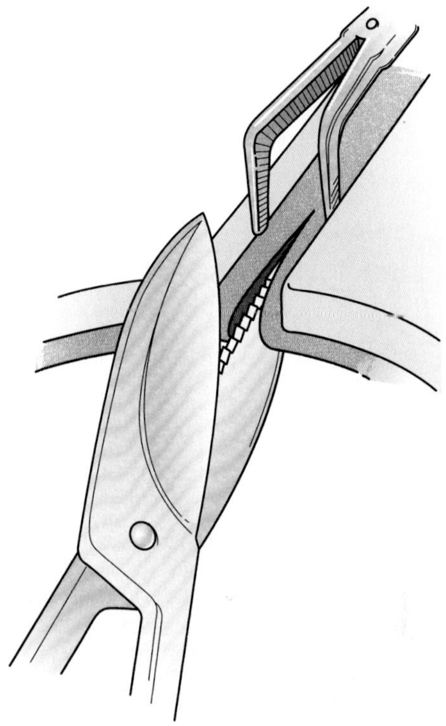

FIGURE 5-37 Once the external plaster is cut the underlying cast padding is also cut using a safety bandage scissors and spreading the cast edges with a cast spreader as illustrated here. (Modified from Connolly J. *Fractures and dislocations. Closed management.* Philadelphia: WB Saunders, 1995, with permission.)

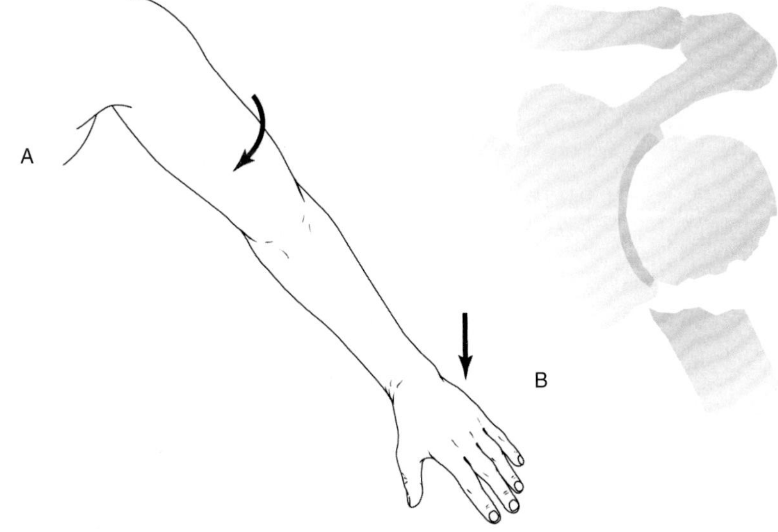

FIGURE 5-38 **A.** A common mechanism producing a fracture of the humerus is a fall on the outstretched hand, which locks the humeral head in the shoulder and internally rotates the arm. **B.** The result is a failure of the proximal humerus with the fracture line running from the distal lateral to the proximal medial cortex. The shaft fragment tends to displace medially (see Fig. 5-6). (Modified from Connolly J. *Fractures and dislocations. Closed management.* Philadelphia: WB Saunders, 1995, with permission.)

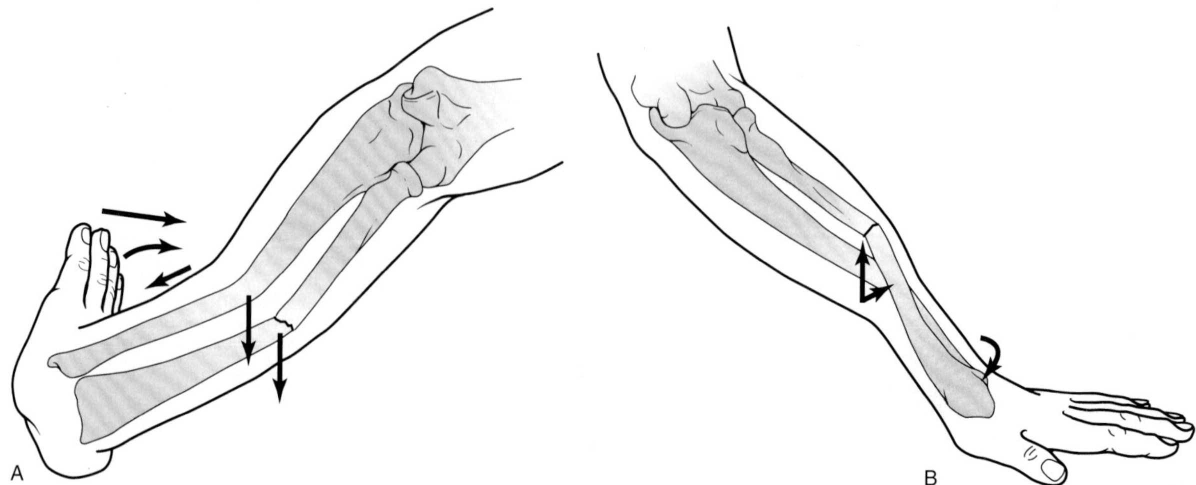

FIGURE 5-39 **A.** A frequent indirect mechanism fracturing the forearm is a fall on the outstretched arm with forceful supination. This produces a fracture with volar angulation due to vectors from the floor reaction force that move up the forearm dorsally. **B.** If the forearm is forcefully pronated at the time of injury, a fracture results that angulates dorsally due to vectors from the floor reaction force that move up the forearm volarly. (Modified from Connolly J. *Fractures and dislocations. Closed management.* Philadelphia: WB Saunders, 1995, with permission.)

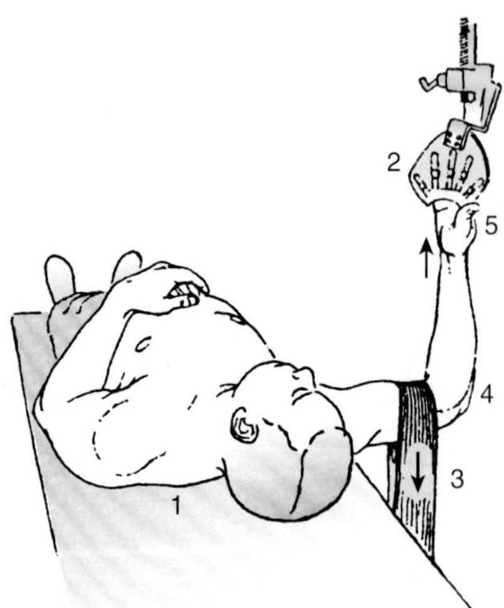

FIGURE 5-40 The technique of closed reduction of forearm fractures under a regional or general anesthetic utilizes traction applied distally and proximally to the forearm. The patient lies supine on a fracture table (*1*) with the fingers held in a finger traction apparatus (*2*). Countertraction is applied with weight on the upper arm (*3*). The elbow is flexed 90 degrees (*4*). The forearm is supinated usually to achieve rotational realignment (*5*). Traction is maintained for 5 to 10 minutes to regain length. (Modified from Connolly J. *Fractures and dislocations. Closed management.* Philadelphia: WB Saunders, 1995, with permission.)

applied. While applying the cast, it is key to maintain the reduction by molding in the interosseous space between the radius and ulna. The forearm is maintained in supination or neutral rotation. This keeps the interosseous space and ligament at maximum width and tension. Reduction is considered inadequate if the radial bow is lost, the interosseous space becomes narrowed, or angulation of the forearm bones exceeds 15 degrees. If the reduction is lost after cast application, the fracture can be remanipulated or open reduction and internal fixation can be carried out.

The cast may have to be changed several times as the patient is followed carefully postreduction. If adequate reduction cannot be maintained during the early stages of treatment, surgical intervention should be recommended. However, slight loss of reduction in the cast may be accepted (Fig. 5-44). During this healing time a wrist brace may be incorporated into the long arm cast to encourage active finger and wrist functional motion while preventing forearm rotation (258). At 4 to 6 weeks, the cast may be replaced by a functional brace.

The average time for healing of displaced two-bone fractures of the forearm by closed method is 15 weeks. Clinical union, evidenced by absence of pain and fracture stability, usually occurs before radiographic healing. A cast or brace should be continued until the fracture is consolidated on the x-ray. The patient should be encouraged to actively exercise the fingers and muscles of the forearm during the period of healing to minimize soft tissue scarring and muscle contracture. This also minimizes the resultant functional impairment when immobilization is discontinued.

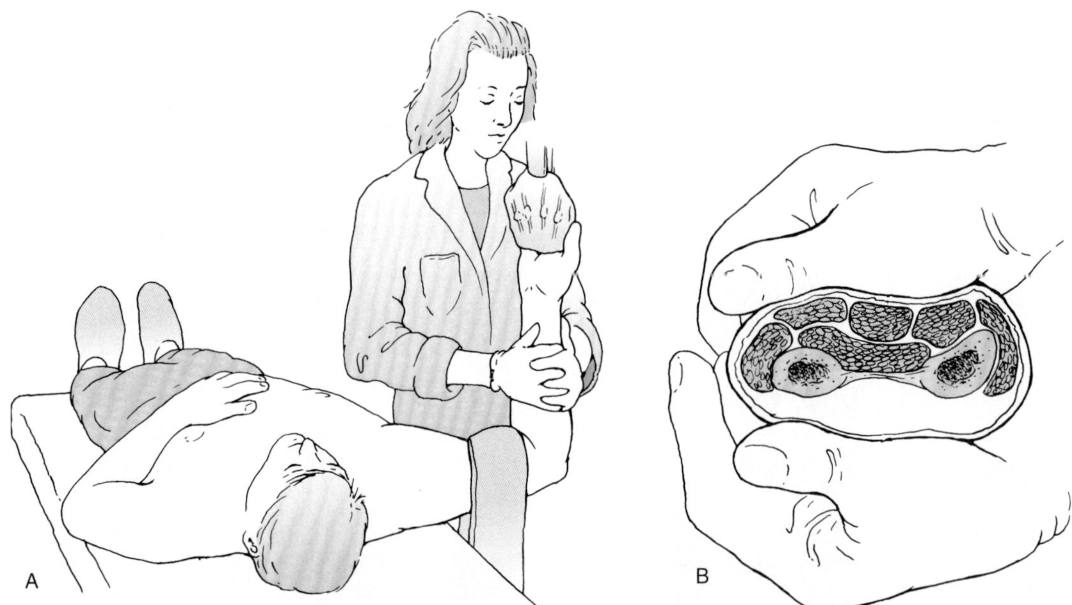

FIGURE 5-41 **A.** After the traction has restored the length of the forearm, the reduction is achieved by directly manipulating and rotating the forearm to interlock fracture fragments in a correct rotational alignment. **B.** The surgeon applies a cast and molds or compresses the interosseous space to maintain the interosseous ligament at maximum tension. This provides important support for the fracture fragments proximally and distally. (Modified from Connolly J. *Fractures and dislocations. Closed management.* Philadelphia: WB Saunders, 1995, with permission.)

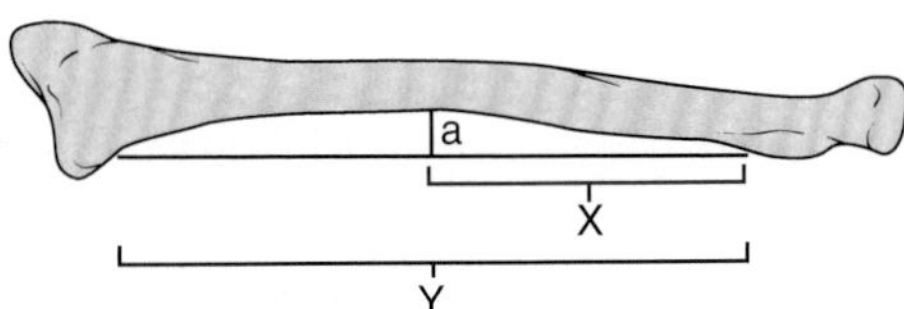

FIGURE 5-42 According to Schemitsch and Richards, to measure the radial bow a line is drawn from the bicipital tuberosity to the most ulnar aspect of the radius at the wrist. A perpendicular line (*a*) is then drawn from the point of maximum radial bow to this line. The height of the perpendicular line (the maximum radial bow) is measured in millimeters. The distance from the bicipital tuberosity to the previously measured perpendicular line at the point of maximum radial bow is then measured. It is recorded as a percentage of the length of the entire bow. This measurement is termed the location of the maximum radial bow. The measurement X/Y × 100 is compared with the same measurement on the opposite uninjured arm. Patients with less than 80% of normal value were found to have diminished rotation and grip strength. Restoration of normal radial bow is related to restoration of forearm rotation and grip strength. (Modified from Schemitsch E, Richards R. The effect of malunion on functional outcome after plate fixation of fractures of both bones of the forearm in adults. *J Bone Joint Surg* 1992;74A:1068–1078, with permission.)

Closed Treatment of Isolated Distal Radial Fractures

An isolated distal radial shaft fracture may be produced by a direct blow to the radius, a common mechanism also for isolated fractures of the ulna. In the early 20th century these were called "chauffeur's fractures" because they were most commonly sustained when the forearm was struck while cranking a motor car.

Isolated distal radial shaft fractures from a direct blow usually are not associated with disruption of the interosseous membrane or injury to the distal radioulnar joint. These fractures are usually stable and can be treated effectively by closed methods. Initially the fracture is managed by immobilization in a long arm cast in neutral rotation for 2 to 3 weeks. This maintains the interosseous space and allows the fracture to begin healing with minimal limitation of pronation or supination. Following the initial period of long arm cast immobilization, the fracture is then held in a fracture brace that should allow the patient to begin some wrist and hand function. The usual time for healing of the isolated fracture of the distal radius without distal radioulnar joint injury is between 10 and 12 weeks.

Colles and Other Fractures of the Distal Radius Produced by Indirect Mechanisms

Colles fracture is typical of the pattern of fracture of osteoporotic bone in postmenopausal women (266). The same hyperexten-

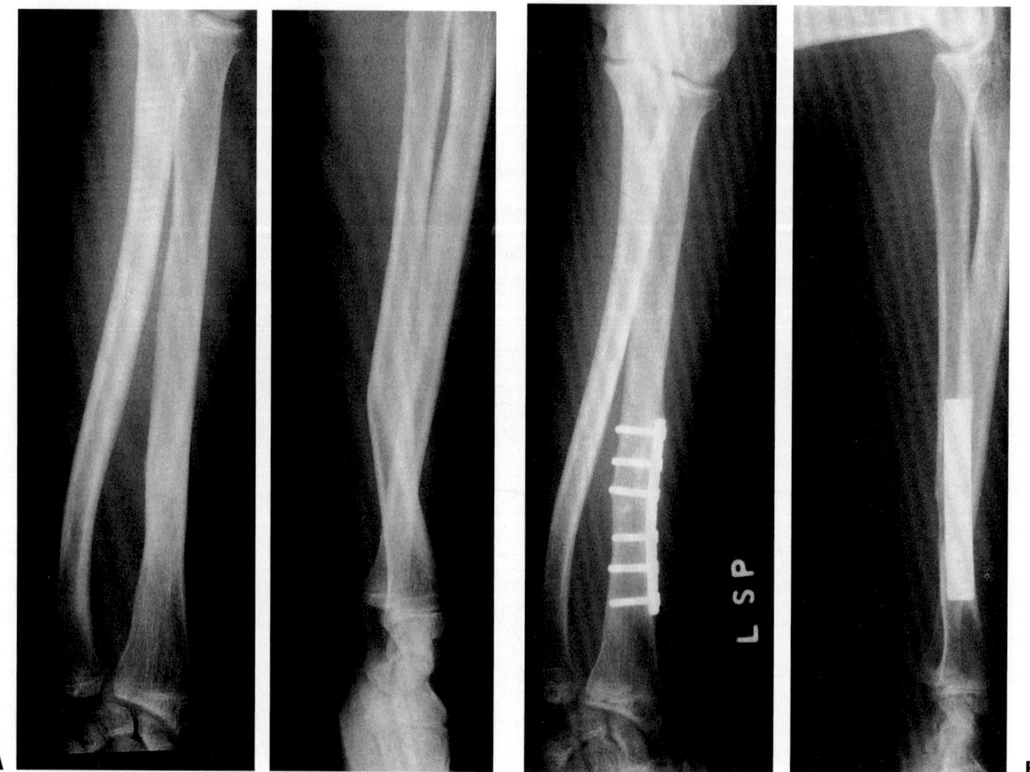

FIGURE 5-43 **A.** Anteroposterior and lateral x-rays show malunion of a fracture of the radius for which corrective osteotomy was recommended. Many such angulatory deformities can be corrected by simple drill osteoclasis and closed re-reduction of the fracture. **B.** X-rays after corrective osteotomy and plate fixation show that volar angulation was corrected but the radial bow was decreased. This left persistent impairment of rotation of the forearm.

sion mechanism producing a Colles fracture in the older woman is likely to produce a fracture of the carpal scaphoid in the young man. Similarly, hyperextension injury to the child's wrist produces a fracture of the distal radial epiphyses or a torus fracture of the radial metaphysis. This variation is due to the differences in bone density among these groups.

Hyperextension-compression injury usually produces a typical dinner-fork deformity, including an abrupt dorsal prominence of the distal radius and carpus and a rounded volar prominence from the proximal radial fragment. Widening of the wrist is a result of a relative displacement of the ulna and radial deviation of the hand. The reduction maneuver should be directed at correcting these problems (Fig. 5-45).

The method of reducing the fracture is to reverse the original mechanism of injury (which was usually hyperextension and supination of the wrist). After adequate anesthesia is achieved, an assistant holds the elbow and offers countertraction while the surgeon, holding the injured hand, as if shaking hands, applies traction and also direct pressure with the thumb and hand on the distal fragment. The forearm is supinated and held with the surgeon's opposite hand. Increasing the dorsal angulation while maintaining the supinated position disimpacts the fracture fragments. Following disimpaction the reduction is achieved by pronating the forearm and wrist. The wrist is then directed into ulnar deviation and slight flexion (Fig. 5-46).

Because a common complication of Colles fractures is wrist swelling, it is best to avoid immediate application of a cast until this swelling subsides. The preferred initial immobilization is with a sugar-tong splint wrapped circumferentially while the assistant holds the wrist in flexion and ulnar deviation (Fig. 5-47). Once the sugar-tong splint is applied, x-rays are taken to evaluate the reduction. If the reduction is not satisfactory, a second manipulation may be carried out, but repeated manipulations should be avoided (267). The splint allows for swelling, which might otherwise compromise circulation. If there is any evidence of circulatory impairment, the splint should be loosened and the padding removed down to the skin. The patient is advised to keep the arm elevated and apply ice to the wrist. A follow-up evaluation should be carried out in 1 to 2 days to ensure that the patient is comfortable and the splint has not become excessively tight. In 7 to 14 days the fracture can be re–x-rayed and a short arm cast can usually be applied. After

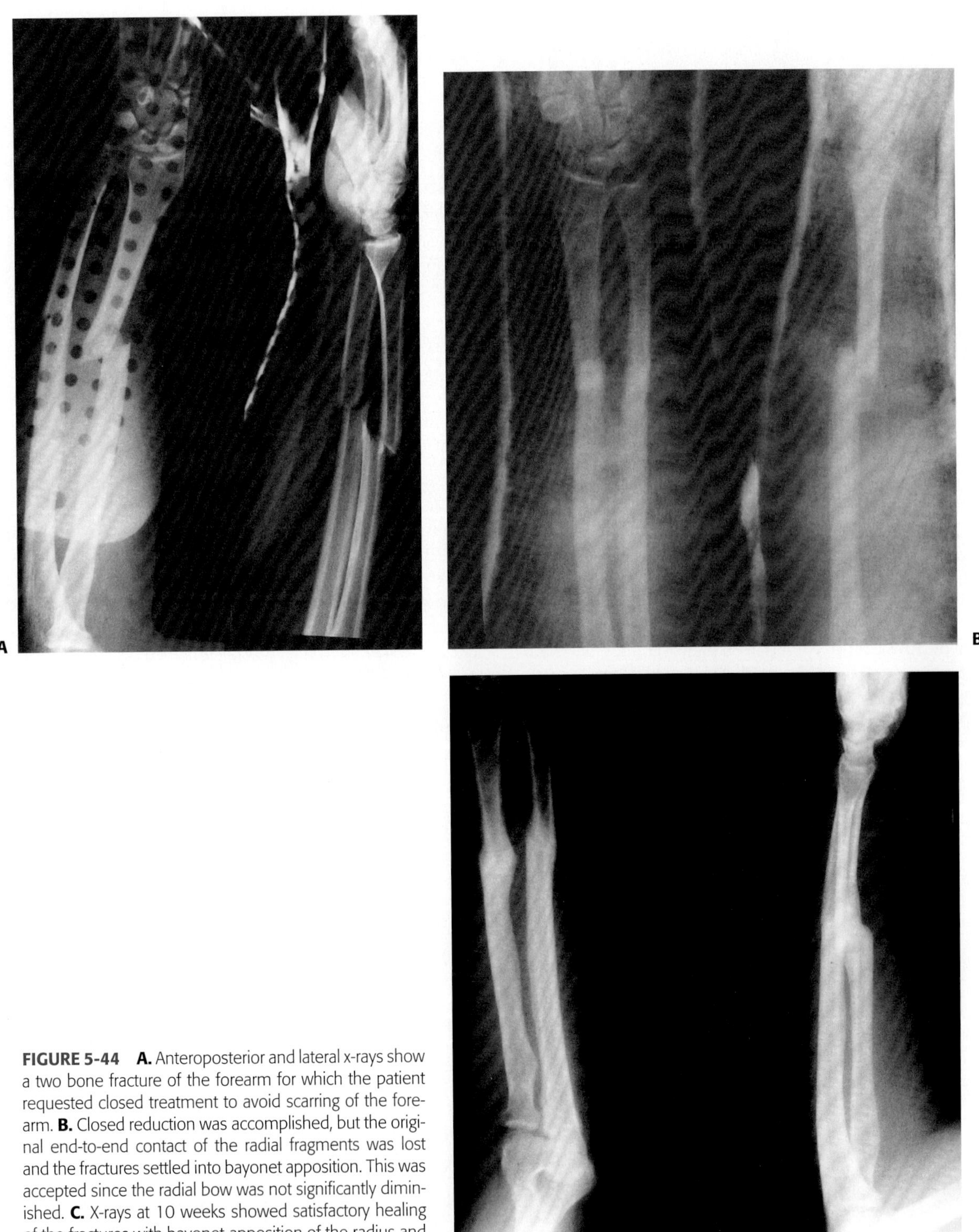

FIGURE 5-44 **A.** Anteroposterior and lateral x-rays show a two bone fracture of the forearm for which the patient requested closed treatment to avoid scarring of the forearm. **B.** Closed reduction was accomplished, but the original end-to-end contact of the radial fragments was lost and the fractures settled into bayonet apposition. This was accepted since the radial bow was not significantly diminished. **C.** X-rays at 10 weeks showed satisfactory healing of the fractures with bayonet apposition of the radius and end-to-end apposition of the ulna. *(continues)*

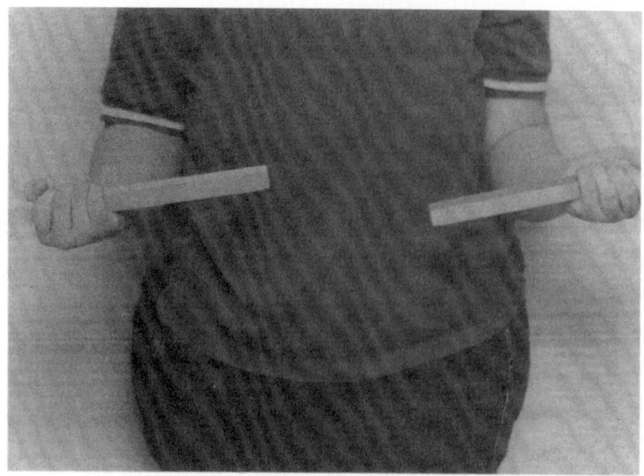

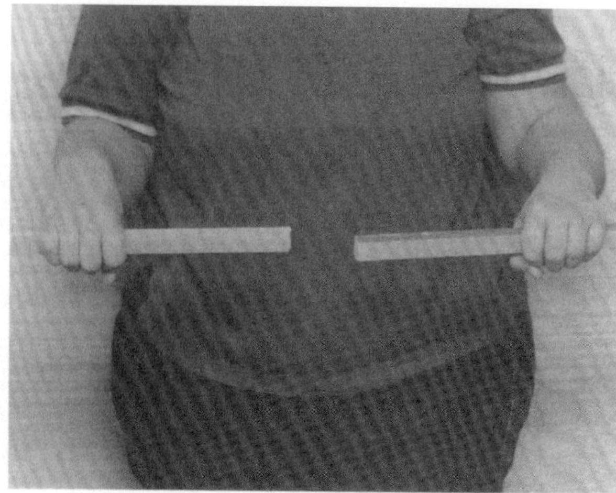

FIGURE 5-44 *(continued)* **D,E.** Follow-up clinical photographs at 16 weeks show the patient with essentially full supination and slight limitation of pronation 6 weeks after the cast was removed.

6 weeks, clinical healing is usually present or at least sufficient to allow a change from a cast to a commercial wrist splint. During the recovery period, the patient is encouraged to actively exercise the fingers and shoulder on the injured side to avoid stiffness. Prolonged use of a sling for more than 1 week should also be avoided since this tends to stiffen the shoulder and inhibit restoration of hand function. Prolonged failure of the patient to resume active hand and shoulder function can lead to sympathetic dystrophy (241,247,268).

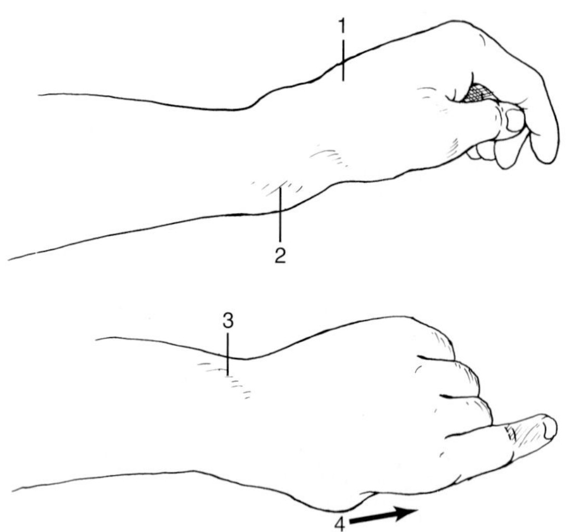

FIGURE 5-45 The Colles fracture produces a typical dinner-fork deformity, which includes an abrupt prominence of the distal radius and carpus (*1*), and a rounded volar prominence from the proximal radial fragment (*2*). Widening of the wrist results from a displacement of the ulna and radial deviation of the hand (*3, 4*). (Modified from Connolly J. *Fractures and dislocations. Closed management.* Philadelphia: WB Saunders, 1995, with permission.)

While more unstable fractures, particularly intraarticular fractures, of the distal radius may require more than closed reduction and splint application to avoid settling and displacement of the joint surface (236,269–272), the vast majority of Colles fractures in elderly patients can be managed by this standard closed reduction technique followed by a minimum period of cast immobilization.

The technique is not complication free, and the patient should be carefully monitored for problems such as median neuropathy, recurrence of the deformity, stiffening of the hand, and sympathetically mediated pain problems (248,266,267, 273). Early decompression of the median nerve in symptomatic patients and the use of immobilization techniques that do not inhibit function of the hand and shoulder may prevent the most frequent of these problems. The problem of loss of, or incomplete, reduction (272) has prompted a number of innovative attempts to improve alignment by external fixation or internal fixation methods. Ironically, as the treatment of Colles fractures has become more intense, problems of pin tract infection, fracture through pin sites, stiffening, and even causalgia of the limb have increased (241), particularly when the techniques overdistract the fractured radius and wrist.

CLOSED REDUCTION OF LOWER LIMB FRACTURES

Closed Reduction of Calcaneal Fractures

Intraarticular calcaneal fractures have frustrated orthopaedic surgeons' attempts to find reliable methods of treatment. Some authors have recommended passive acceptance of the fact that results are "rotten" or even "disastrous" (274).

Of the many problems with treating the comminuted fracture, the most challenging may be to identify what deformities must be corrected to achieve a satisfactory functional outcome.

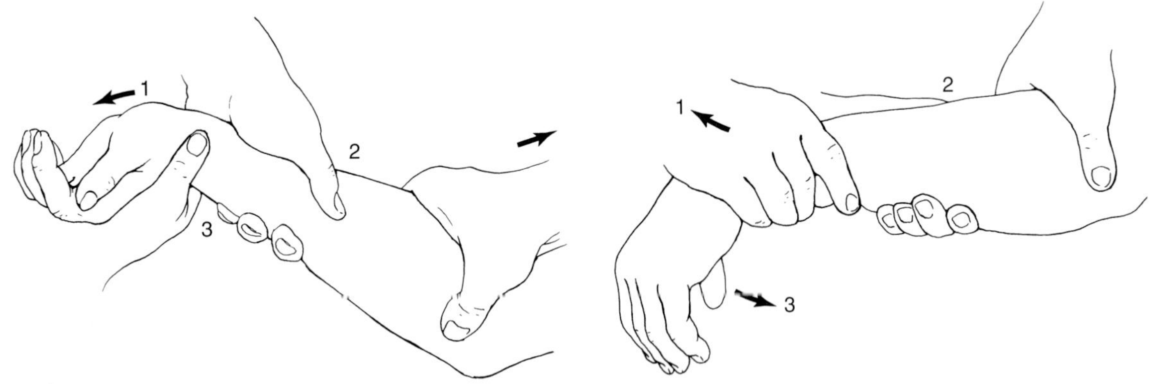

FIGURE 5-46 A. The method of reducing Colles fracture or any fractures is to reverse the original mechanism of injury. With adequate anesthesia an assistant holds the elbow and provides countertraction. (*1*) The surgeon applies traction with one hand and thumb to the distal fragment. (*2*) The forearm is supinated and held with the surgeon's opposite hand. (*3*) The fracture is then disimpacted to allow dorsal angulation while supination is maintained. **B.** (*1*) The reduction is then held by pronating the forearm and wrist. (*2*) The surgeon's left hand remains stationary while pronation is accomplished by the right hand. (*3*) The wrist is directed ulnarward to correct radial deviation as well as dorsal angulation of the distal fragments. (Modified from Connolly J. *Fractures and dislocations. Closed management.* Philadelphia: WB Saunders, 1995, with permission.)

In the era of plain radiographic assessment, a main objective had been to restore Böhler's angle to normal. As CT has provided us with better three-dimensional assessment of the fracture, other investigators have demonstrated the importance of restoring the posterior articular facet in order to achieve a successful outcome (275–277).

Factors other than articular surface congruity also may be important influences on the results. Shortening of the heel weakens the gastrocnemius power, leading to a calcaneus gait after the fracture heals (278,279). Widening and decreased height of the heel will often produce lateral impingement on the sural nerve and peroneal tendons, causing persistent pain particularly with flexion and extension of the ankle. An impact that is sufficient to crush the calcaneus will also produce extensive damage to the important heel pad. Pain symptoms can persist if the bone fragments remain protruding into the heel pad. Swelling of the whole foot and limb also contributes to permanent stiffening, particularly if the limb is immobilized in a cast for a prolonged period of time without functional stimulation (93).

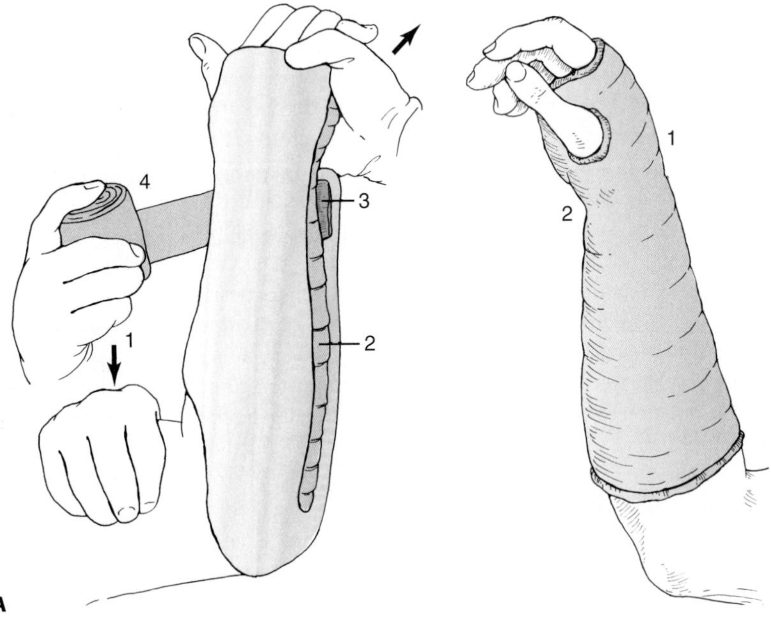

FIGURE 5-47 A. Because of the tendency for swelling in this area, the preferred initial immobilization of a Colles fracture is with a sugar-tong splint. The position of the wrist is maintained by an assistant using steady traction on the elbow and hand (*1*). Cast padding is applied from the metacarpal heads to above the elbow (*2*). A felt pad is applied to the lower surface of the proximal fragment (*3*). A sugar-tong plaster splint is wrapped around the elbow and forearm and held using a circumferential gauze bandage. It should extend from the dorsal surface of the MP joints to the volar surface of the fracture site to maintain the distal fragments in volar angulation (*4*). **B.** The sugar-tong splint can usually be changed to a short-arm cast as the swelling subsides 1 to 2 weeks after the original injury. The cast should be molded firmly on the dorsal surface of the hand and wrist (*1*) and should maintain the wrist in a moderate amount of flexion (*2*). Extremes of flexion should be avoided since this can produce a median neuropathy or impair function of the intrinsic muscles of the hand. (Modified from Connolly J. *Fractures and dislocations. Closed management.* Philadelphia: WB Saunders, 1995, with permission.)

The general objectives of treatment should include not only restoration of the posterior facet articulation or Böhler's angle but also correction of the height, length, and width of the heel. In addition, the treatment should avoid immobilization of the foot and encourage active functional motion.

These goals may be achieved by operative intervention, but a number of comparative studies of operative versus nonoperative treatment have shown no significant benefit from surgery unless normal anatomy can be restored (91,278, 280,281). Unfortunately, operative treatment with wide soft tissue dissection risks wound slough, infection, and even amputation (282,283). Buckley and Tough (92) point out that surgery should not be recommended to patients when the literature suggests it might result in only marginally better outcomes and frequent complications. Generally older sedentary patients and those with nondisplaced or with minimally displaced fractures may be treated successfully with nonsurgical management. Traits which they feel are strongly predictive of satisfaction with surgery include an age younger than 40 years, simple fracture pattern, and accurate reduction.

A reasonable compromise between passive acceptance of deformity without reduction and the complication-prone open reduction is manual reduction of the intraarticular fragments using ligamentotaxis as described by Omoto et al (95). Ligaments important for calcaneal fracture stability include the lateral and medial talocalcaneal and interosseus ligaments. Especially important are the tibiocalcaneal fibers of the deltoid, which attach to the sustentaculum tali and the calcaneofibular ligament, which attaches to the tuberosity fragment. These two ligaments should be intact if manual reduction by ligamentotaxis is to be successful (Fig. 5-48 and 5-49) (284).

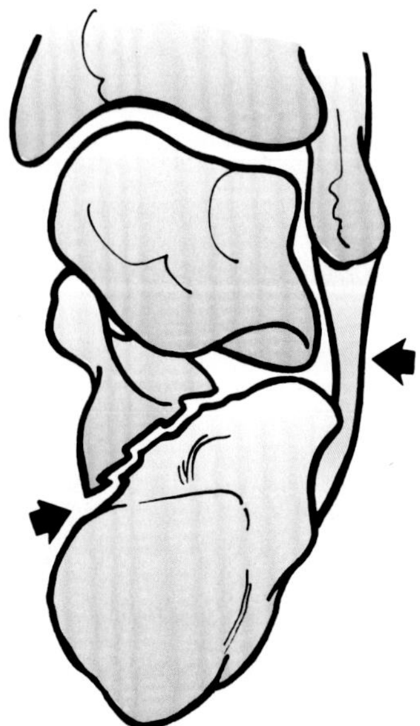

FIGURE 5-48 The lateral fibulocalcaneal ligaments as well as the talocalcaneal ligaments are important in supporting the calcaneus fracture. If the medial and lateral calcaneal ligaments are torn, the entire tuberosity fragment may displace producing essentially a fracture-dislocation of the calcaneus. Closed reduction by the Omoto technique depends on ligamentotaxis and requires intact ligament attachments to be successful.

Omoto Technique of Reduction

Reduction of the acute calcaneal fracture is carried out with the patient prone and under adequate spinal or general anesthesia. The knee is flexed 90 degrees to relax the gastrocsoleus muscle. An assistant holds the leg in this position while the operating surgeon stands at the patient's feet (Fig. 5-49). The surgeon then molds the medial and lateral sides of the calcaneus with both palms while crossing the fingers of both hands around the heel. In this way the calcaneal tuberosity can be squeezed upward toward the sole. Simultaneously, strong traction is applied to lift the thigh off the table while the assistant exerts counterforce. The heel is then rotated into a varus or valgus position depending on whether the injury had displaced the tuberosity fragment into varus or valgus. Traction and heel support are continued while the tuberosity fragment is manipulated. During the manipulation some crepitation may be felt. Roentgenograms are then obtained to confirm the adequacy of the reduction.

A compression dressing is then applied along with ice to the foot to diminish swelling. Active range of motion of the foot and ankle is emphasized on an hourly basis while the foot remains elevated. Subsequently, the patient may walk with crutches without bearing weight on the fractured side. By 2 months after the reduction the patient is allowed to slowly increase weightbearing on the injured foot. By 3 to 4 months the patient should be able to walk without external support.

Closed Reduction of Tibial Fractures

Biomechanics of Injury

As discussed with fractures in the upper limb, the biomechanics of injury of the tibia include direct and indirect mechanisms. The consistent pattern of a tibial fracture sustained by an indirect torsional mechanism failure is a fracture line through the isthmal section of the tibia (252). Here the bone is weakest and here is the area most often subjected to torsional loading. The pattern of failure is very consistent. The proximal fragment displaces medially and anteriorly relative to the distal fragment.

An important consideration in reducing tibial shaft fractures is whether or not the fibula is also fractured (285,286). When intact, the fibula, to some extent, supports the tibial fracture but also may tend to cause a certain amount of internal rotational deformity of a distal fracture. When managing fractures of the distal tibia by casts or fracture brace technique or even by closed nailing, one should pay special attention to the rotational alignment of the fracture (287,288). One must especially avoid an internal rotational displacement of the ankle mortise, which can result in varus positioning of the foot. This positions the foot in a "turned in" relationship to the floor, which cannot be overcome by subtalar motion. As a consequence the patient is forced to bear weight on the lateral aspect of the foot producing perma-

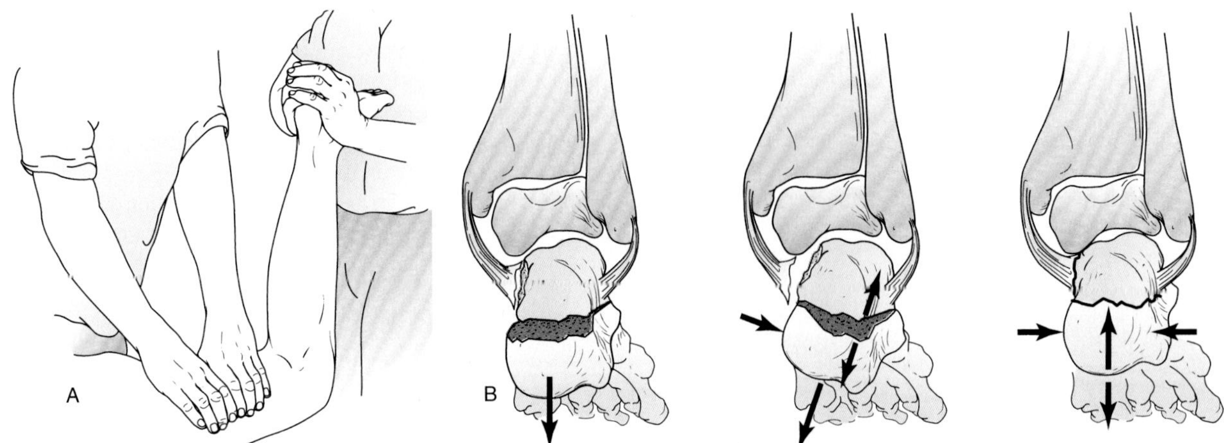

FIGURE 5-49 **A.** Reduction of the acute calcaneal fracture by the Omoto technique is done with the patient under adequate anesthesia. The knee is flexed 90 degrees and the assistant holds the leg in this position. The operating surgeon stands at the patient's feet molding the medial and lateral sides of the calcaneus with the palms of both hands. Simultaneously, strong traction is applied to lift the thigh off the table. **B.** With traction applied to the calcaneal fracture, the heel is rotated into varus or valgus depending on the original tuberosity displacement. The tuberosity fragment is thereby moved closer to the sustentaculum fragment and out of varus or valgus position. A compression dressing is then applied and the foot is elevated to decrease the swelling. Active motion of the foot and ankle are begun within the first or second day. (Modified from Connolly J. *Fractures and dislocations. Closed management.* Philadelphia: WB Saunders, 1995, with permission.)

nent discomfort in the foot and ankle (Fig. 5-2). This problem can be anticipated and prevented by immobilizing the fracture with the foot and ankle in slight external rotation. This shifts the floor reaction force laterally, so that weightbearing produces a valgus rather than a varus moment at the fracture site.

Techniques of Closed Reduction and Cast Application for Fractures of the Tibia

In applying a cast to a fractured tibia, it is important that both the patient and the person applying the cast be comfortable. The patient should be sitting or lying supine on a stable cast table and not leaning forward from a wheelchair or some other similar mobile support (Fig. 5-50). One of the many reasons that this is very important is that it is much harder to apply a cast on a moving target. Also, most people have never had a cast applied before, and a few unexpectedly pass out from the experience.

The initial cast should be applied as soon as possible after the injury. A posterior splint provides inadequate immobilization of the acute fracture and does little to relieve the patient's discomfort. If most patients are given an adequate explanation and the reduction is done gently, the cast can be applied without anesthetic and with minimal narcotics (289,290).

As the patient sits on the edge of an orthopaedic table with the legs hanging down, most shortening can be corrected by the use of gravity and gentle traction on the distal fragment and foot (28). Malrotation can be corrected by comparing the torsion of the fractured leg with the unfractured leg (Fig. 5-50).

Two to three layers of cast padding are first applied from the toes to above the knee. Subsequently, a 4-inch roll of plaster

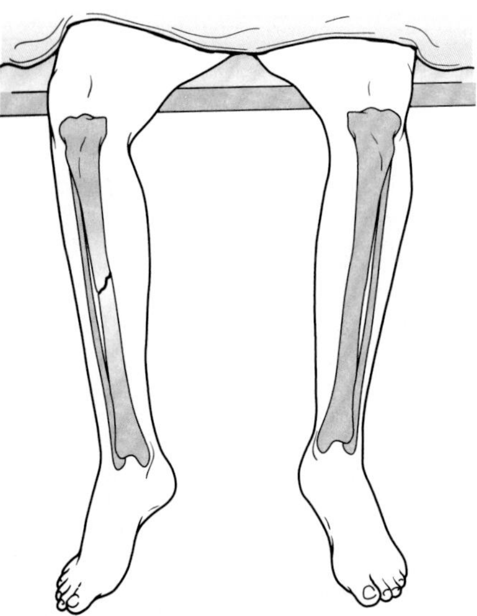

FIGURE 5-50 Cast application for a fractured tibia is done with the patient sitting on a fracture table. The legs hang over the table to allow fracture realignment with gravity. The correct rotation is estimated by comparing the fractured leg with the opposite unfractured leg. (Modified from Connolly J. *Fractures and dislocations. Closed management.* Philadelphia: WB Saunders, 1995, with permission.)

is applied to the foot and ankle with care taken to contour the arch of the foot. A 6-inch roll of plaster is then rolled from the foot up to the knee. The fracture is aligned by molding the plaster to correct any varus or valgus tendency. When the lower leg plaster has hardened, the knee is extended fully and the cast is applied above the knee (Fig. 5-51).

Postreduction x-rays are then taken to evaluate fracture alignment. It is more important to restore the axis of motion of the knee to a normal relationship with the ankle than it is to achieve perfect alignment of the fracture fragments. However, good cortical contact is important to prevent displacement of the fracture fragments in the cast (Figs. 5-52 and 5-53). X-rays should be taken of the patient in the cast showing the alignment of the knee and ankle on the same cassette (Fig. 5-54). This may require that the cassette be placed diagonally for tall patients so that both joints can be visualized on the same film. Shortening

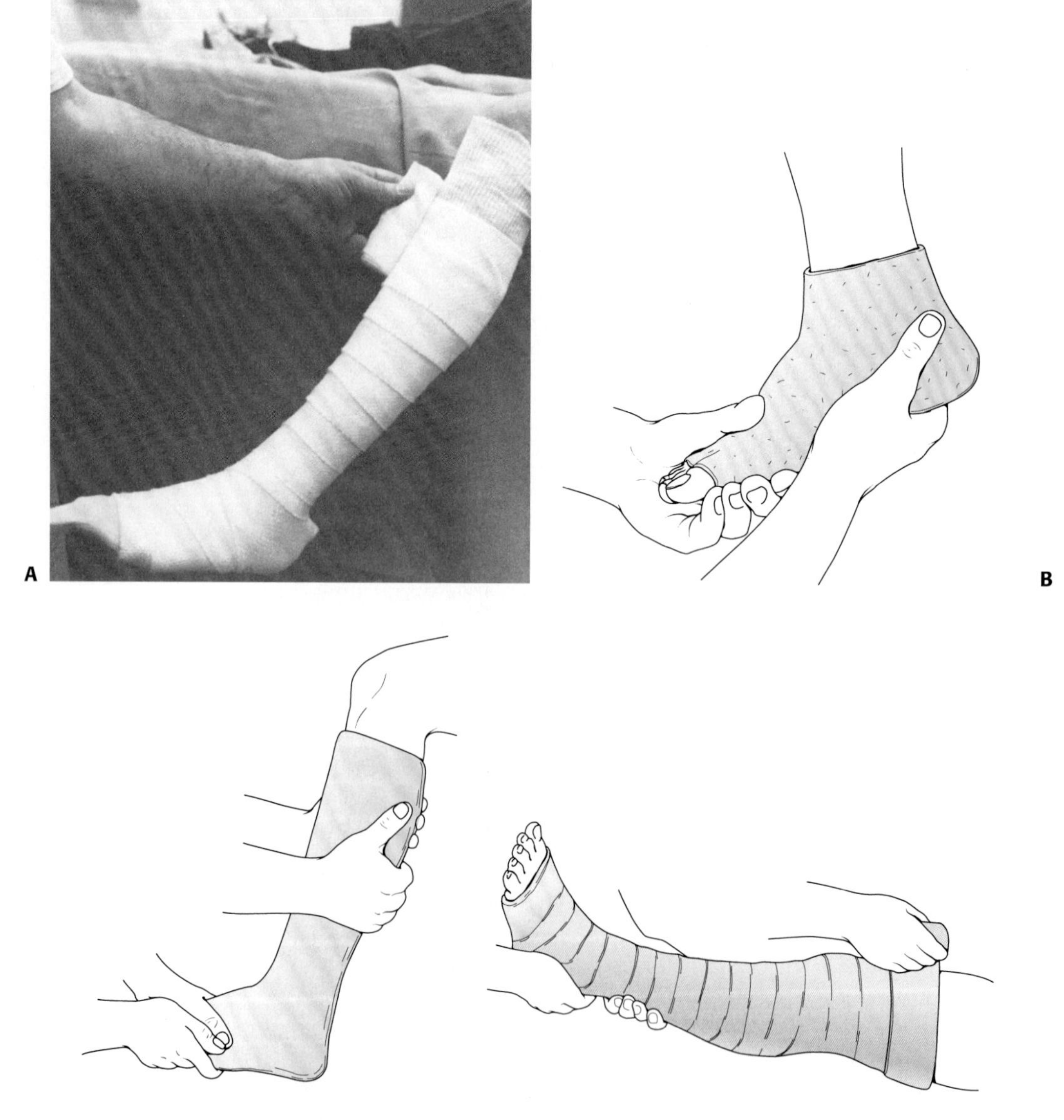

FIGURE 5-51 **A.** Cast padding is applied to the fractured limb over a stockinette, and the leg is padded up to approximately 6 to 8 inches above the knee. **B.** Plaster is applied over the cast padding and molded firmly around the foot and ankle using the palm of the hand and not the fingers. **C.** The cast is then extended over the fracture site up to the knee and the fracture is reduced as the plaster sets by molding firmly around the calf muscles and along the fracture itself. **D.** The cast is then extended above the knee with the knee close to full extension. The patient may be up partially weightbearing with crutches when the plaster has hardened. The leg should be elevated continuously when the patient is not ambulating. (Modified from Connolly J. *Fractures and dislocations. Closed management.* Philadelphia: WB Saunders, 1995, with permission.)

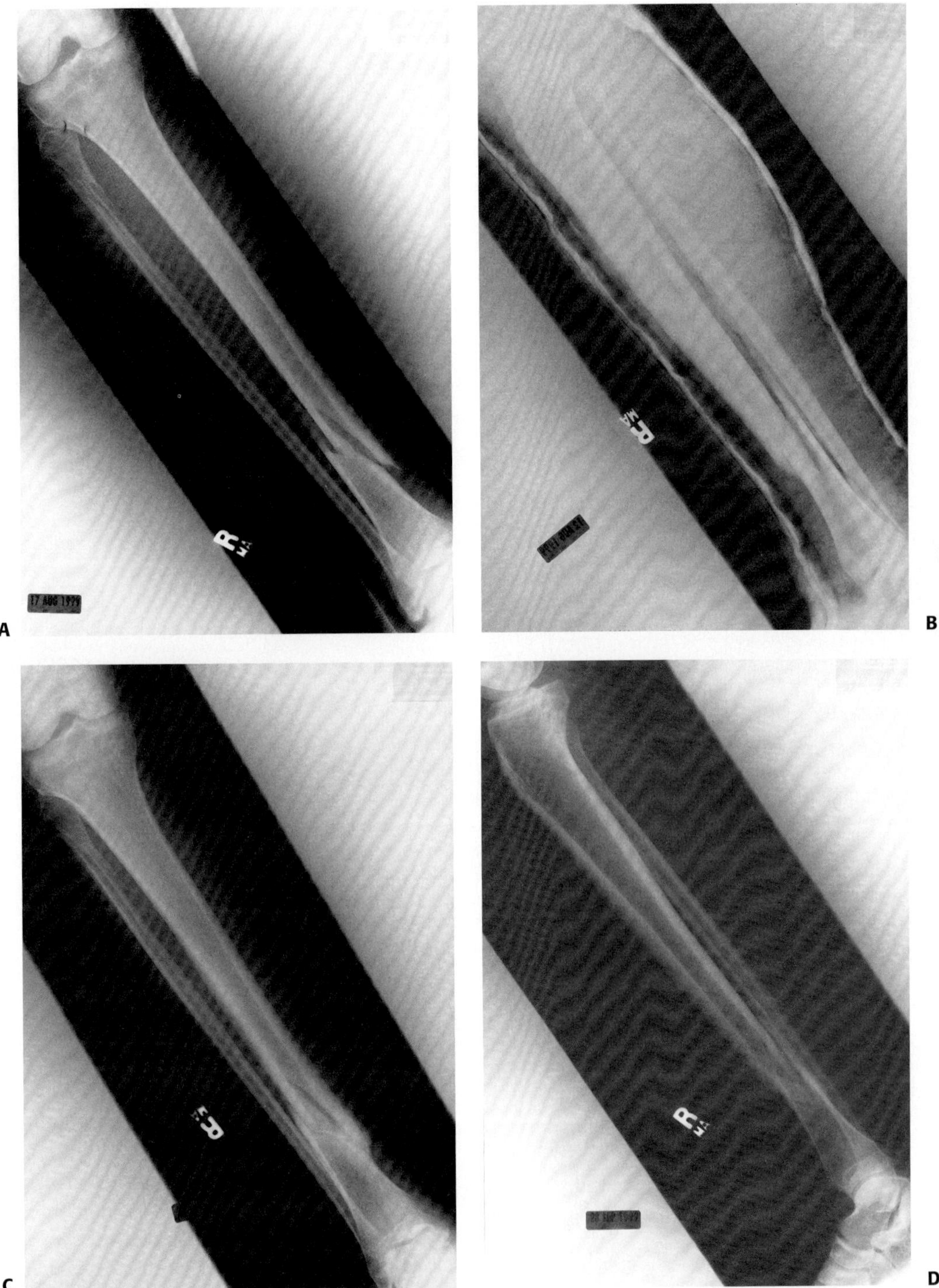

FIGURE 5-52 A,B. Anteroposterior (AP) x-ray of a typical tibia and fibula fracture sustained in a characteristic indirect torsional injury to the leg. The patient's fractures resulted from the foot and ankle being fixed while the upper body twisted about the tibia, resulting in the classic spiral oblique fracture from the distal medial cortex up to the superior lateral cortex of the tibia. The characteristic displacement of the proximal fragment anteromedially was accepted when the patient was treated in the cast as illustrated on these x-rays. **C,D.** With early weightbearing in a fracture cast or brace the fracture heals with periosteal and endosteal callus as illustrated on these AP and lateral x-rays at 12 weeks. Slight shortening was accepted and felt to be helpful to achieve early healing of the fracture and excellent functional recovery of the ankle and knee. Note that the x-rays evaluating alignment of the fracture were taken to include the knee and ankle on the one cassette to be certain that both proximal distal joints were properly aligned.

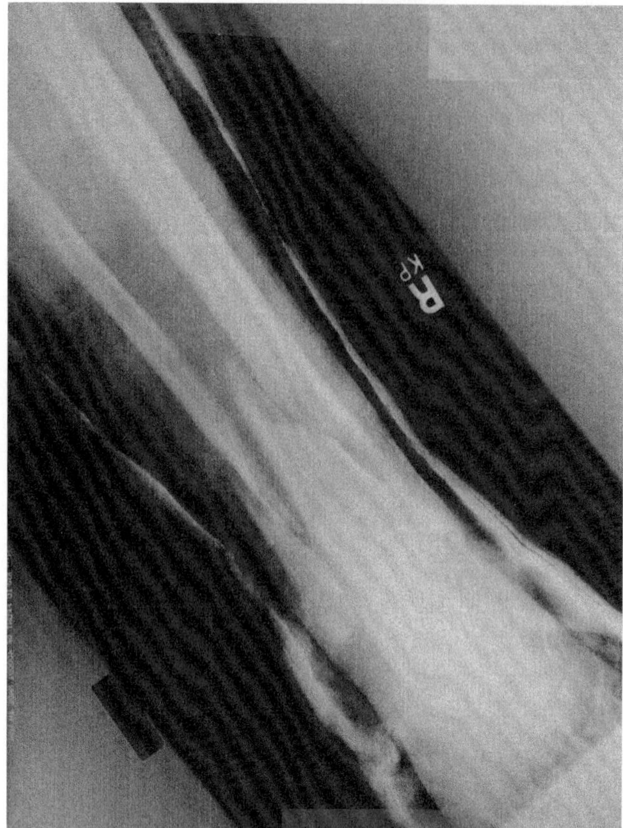

A

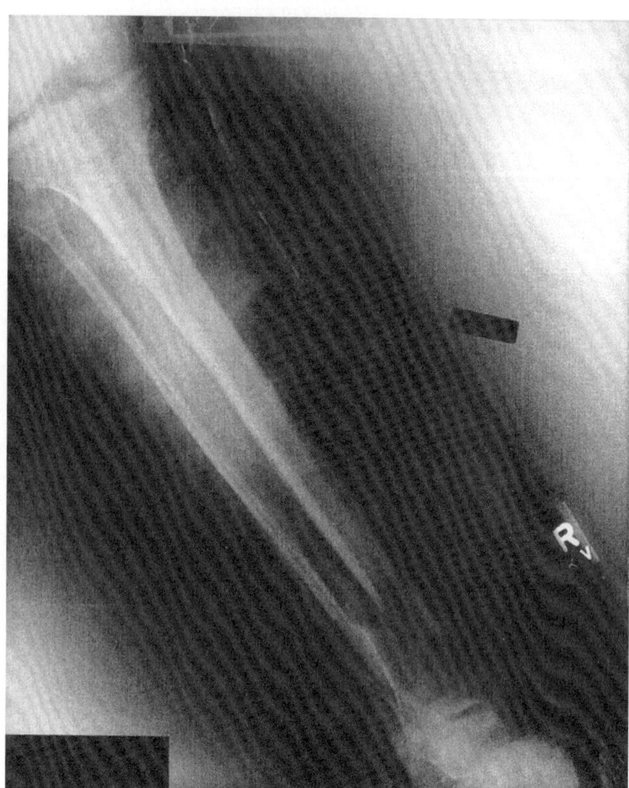

B

FIGURE 5-53 **A.** Although slight displacement of a tibial fracture persisting after closed reduction may be accepted, one should not accept less than 50% apposition of the bone fragments. The malreduction illustrated by this spiral oblique distal tibial fracture is unacceptable since it lacks even minimal bony contact. It only displaced further when the patient began weightbearing in the heavily padded cast. **B.** X-ray at 3 weeks shows displacement of the tibia and fibula and valgus tilt of the ankle. The fracture was then treated by open reduction and internal fixation to correct the shortening and angulation. Fractures that are treated by closed functional methods demand adequate reduction just as do fractures treated by open reduction and internal fixation.

of 1.5 cm or less is quite acceptable provided that the knee and ankle axes are returned to normal alignment. Anterior angulation of the proximal fragment should be avoided since it can lead to skin slough from cast pressure (Fig. 5-54B). Posterior angulation of the distal fragment should also be avoided by allowing the foot to maintain a slight equinus position in the cast (Fig. 5-54C). After the reduction, the patient is usually admitted to the hospital to ensure that the leg is elevated using an overhead suspension. The patient is encouraged to actively exercise the toes.

Three-point weightbearing using crutches is started the day after the cast is applied (12). The patient should be advised there will be some discomfort and possibly some fracture motion felt in the first few weeks. The importance of elevating the leg when not walking should be emphasized to avoid excessive swelling and tightening in the cast. However, any complaints of painful tightness under the cast warrant splitting the cast and cast padding to alleviate the symptoms and prevent any problems such as compartment syndrome.

By 2 to 3 weeks the long leg cast may be changed to a short leg patella tendon–bearing (PTB) cast or a fracture brace (28,63). While the long leg cast may continue to be used, the major advantage of the short leg PTB cast or a fracture brace is that the patient is usually able to return to work or school more rapidly and have a sense of being able to function more normally (Fig. 5-55).

The majority of low-energy tibial fractures can be treated by closed reduction and a functional weightbearing cast or fracture brace (285). Usually, these fractures are supported by the intact interosseous membrane (233) as well as by the surrounding calf muscles. In addition, if the fibula is not fractured, it may also have a stabilizing affect. Severe displacement of the tibial fracture can occur when there is complete disruption of the interosseous membrane and surrounding muscle. This causes signifi-

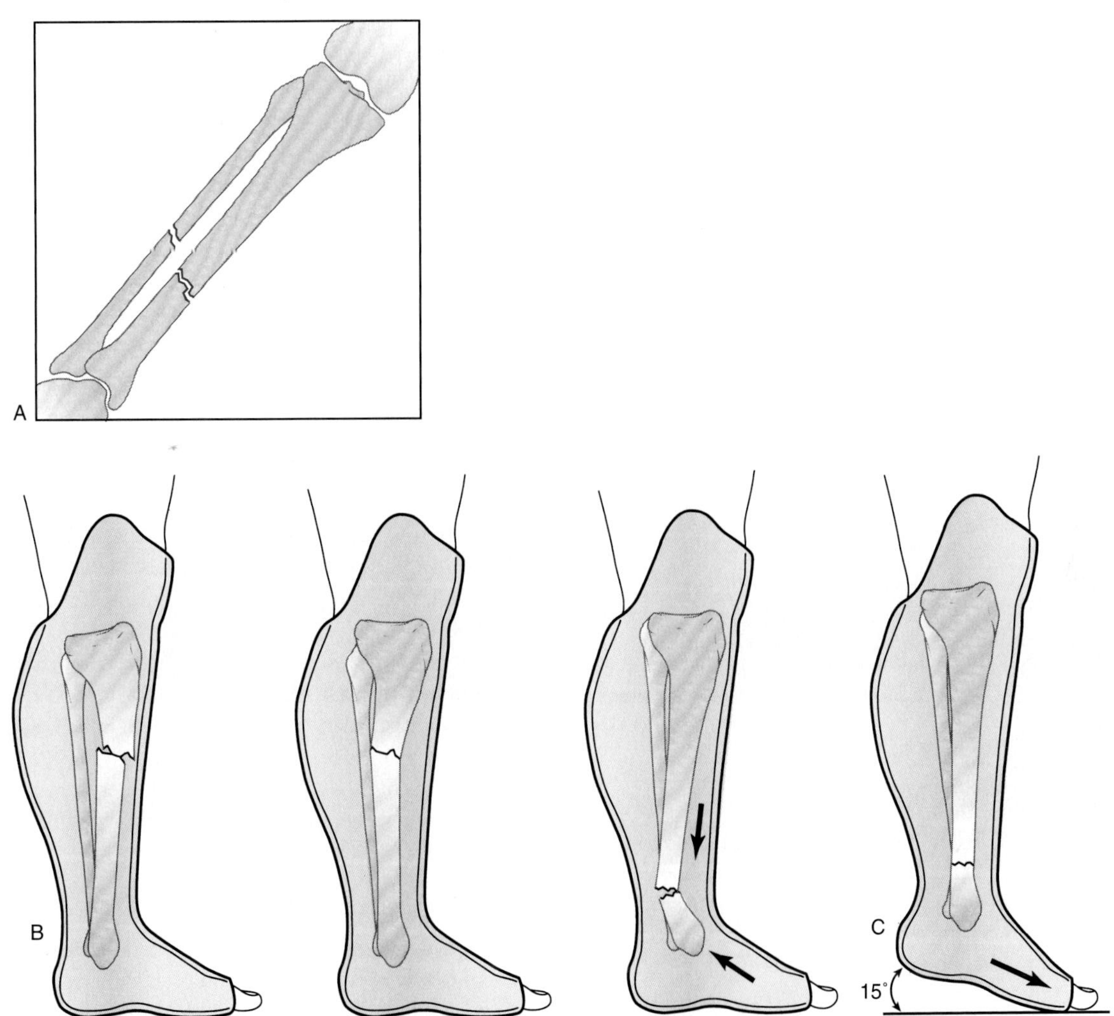

FIGURE 5-54 **A.** Postreduction x-rays should be taken with the patient in the cast to show alignment of the knee and ankle as well as the fracture. This may require placing the x-ray cassette diagonally to visualize the proximal and distal joints. **B.** Anterior angulation of the proximal fragment of the tibia can cause sloughing of the skin if it produces pressure necrosis under the cast (*left*). This can be corrected by allowing slight recurvatum of the fracture as the cast is being applied (*right*). **C.** Posterior angulation of the distal tibial fragment can occur with attempts to dorsiflex the ankle during cast application (*left*). Allowing slight equinus to position the foot will partially correct this tendency (*right*). (Modified from Connolly J. *Fractures and dislocations. Closed management.* Philadelphia: WB Saunders, 1995, with permission.)

cant shortening and instability of the fracture and requires either external fixation or internal stabilization of the tibia (17,63, 288,291,292).

Closed Reduction of Proximal Tibial Plateau Fractures—Influence of the Fibula on the Mechanics of Proximal Tibial Fractures

The usual proximal tibial fracture is the result of a direct blow to the lateral aspect of the leg or knee, the so-called car bumper injury (293). This usually produces a lateral plateau fracture that may or may not be associated with a fibular fracture. If the fibula is intact, the injury can be considered stable. The fibula supports the lateral plateau and prevents it from displacing significantly (294).

One should be alert to the difference between the classic lateral tibial plateau fracture sustained with the knee in extension and the injury sustained with the knee in a flexed position. The latter injury produces a much greater amount of knee instability (Fig. 5-56). The tendency is for this fracture to create a displaced posteromedial fragment that can allow the medial

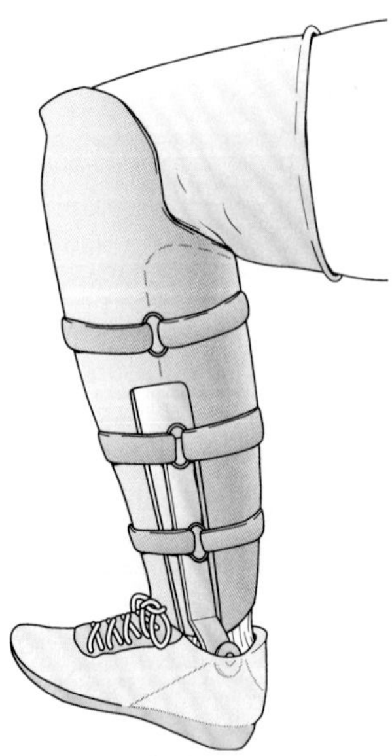

FIGURE 5-55 By 2 to 3 weeks the cast may be replaced by a fracture brace. This is applied over a stockinette and consists of a prefabricated plastic shell attached with Velcro straps. A heel cup and ankle joint are attached to allow ankle dorsiflexion. The patient should wear a tennis shoe and actively use the knee and ankle as the fracture heals. (Modified from Connolly J. *Fractures and dislocations. Closed management.* Philadelphia: WB Saunders, 1995, with permission.)

femoral condyle to subluxate into the defect (243). This causes considerable instability of the knee and a tendency for the deformity to recur even with attempted internal fixation. These different mechanisms of injury must be considered in order to choose treatment based on reversing the mechanism of injury.

While many lateral tibial plateau fractures can be treated symptomatically as previously described above, the majority require some type of reduction with or without internal fixation. Indications for either operative or nonoperative treatment are clinical as well as radiographic. The most extensive long-term studies on the subject have been carried out by Rasmussen (293,296) and by Lansinger and associates (297), who demonstrated that the outcome of these fractures can be predicted by stressing the knee in full extension. Knees with a lateral tibial plateau fracture that are stable in the fully extended position generally heal well without the need for exact anatomic reduction. For this reason it is often not essential in these cases to achieve perfect joint anatomy by open surgical procedures (25).

Technique of Closed Reduction

With the patient under general anesthesia on a fracture table, traction is maintained while an assistant applies direct manual manipulation to correct any tendency to valgus angulation (243). This combination of traction and varus manipulation elevates the plateau fracture using the ligamentous pull of soft tissue attachments (Figs. 5-57 and 5-58). The effect of this manipulation can be assessed immediately by image intensified fluoroscopy. Widening of the condyles can be reduced by direct manual compression along with percutaneous screw insertion.

Arthroscopic assessment of the articular surface has been recommended (298), but can be difficult, and additional swelling of the joint can be produced by the arthroscopic procedure itself. In our opinion, arthroscopy of the acute fracture is more likely to complicate than it is to aid reduction.

After alignment is determined to be satisfactory by x-ray, a cast brace can be applied with the patient still on the fracture table. Hinges are incorporated to allow 40 to 50 degrees of knee motion (Fig. 5-59). The patient subsequently is allowed to bear partial weight in the cast brace and encouraged to actively exercise the knee. The cast brace is maintained for 6 to 8 weeks. Many of these fractures will heal within 6 weeks, after which immobilization in the cast brace may be discontinued. Occasionally, if the fracture is not reduced by manipulation, open reduction and percutaneous fixation with cannulated screws can be used (25,299). This is particularly likely if the fracture has involved the posteromedial aspect of the tibial condyle producing a subluxation of the knee joint in the flexed position (Fig. 5-60).

On long-term follow-up (25) of patients whose fractures have been reduced by these techniques, results have been considered satisfactory particularly when based on functional outcome. Radiographic changes of sclerosis and what might be interpreted as osteoarthritis may be seen after these injuries; however, we have not found a correlation between the radiologic findings and the general clinical result. This contrasts with other joints such as the ankle or the hip where radiographic changes of posttraumatic arthritis usually correlate closely with clinical and functional outcome. The knee, and particularly the lateral plateau, is protected to some extent by the lateral meniscus, which maintains a significant weightbearing function despite fractures involving the articular surface of the lateral plateau.

Femoral Fractures Reduced Nonoperatively by Skeletal Traction and Cast-Bracing

The most widely accepted and usually reliable method of managing femoral shaft fractures is with closed reduction and closed intramedullary nailing (300). This can usually be accomplished as soon as the patient's overall status allows, preferably within the first 24 to 48 hours after injury.

Occasionally femoral fractures require alternate nonoperative methods (301). Typical indications for nonoperative treatment include comminuted fractures of the distal third of the femur, open femoral shaft fractures, infected fractures, and those in which internal fixation may be tenuous and supplemental external support is required (302). In addition, closed intramedullary nailing technique may not be available in some communities or countries because the equipment is inordinately expensive. Under these circumstances the nonoperative technique can produce excellent results (303).

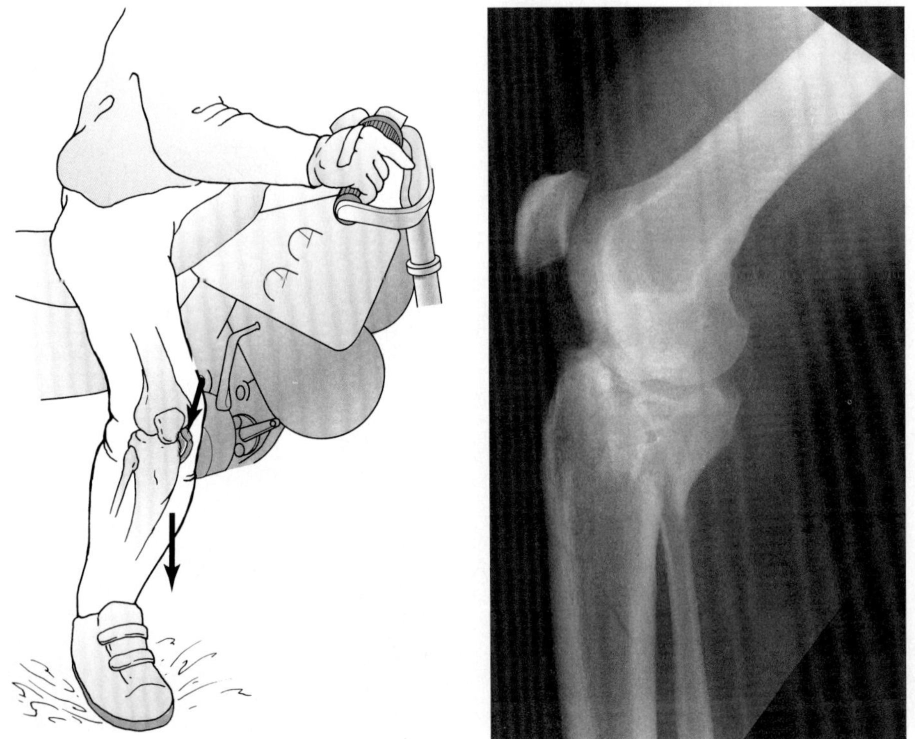

FIGURE 5-56 **A.** Tibial plateau fractures sustained in flexion are generally more unstable than those sustained with the knee in extension. The flexion injury frequently causes the medial femoral condyle to impact on the posteromedial condyle of the tibia, resulting in a tendency for posterior subluxation. **B.** The fracture produced with the knee in flexion tends to result in a posteromedial instability and persistent subluxation of the femoral condyle posteriorly. This requires reduction by realigning the displaced posteromedial fragment of the tibial condyle with the knee in extension, thereby reversing the mechanism of injury. (Modified from Connolly J. *Fractures and dislocations. Closed management.* Philadelphia: WB Saunders, 1995, with permission.)

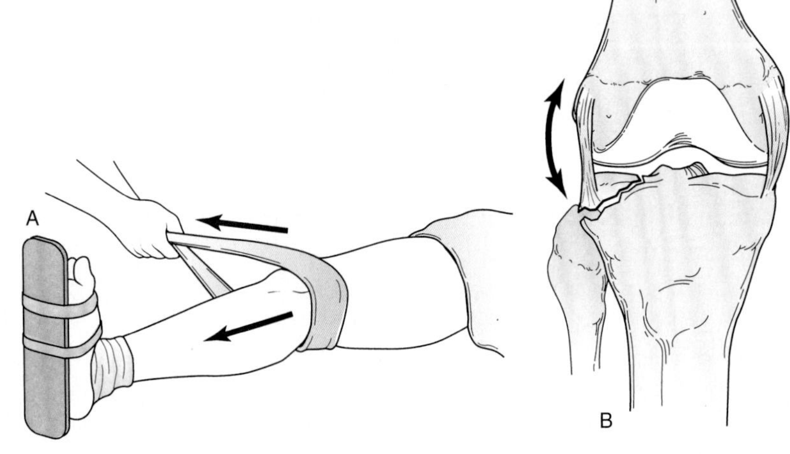

FIGURE 5-57 **A.** The technique of closed reduction of a tibial plateau fracture sustained in flexion is to reverse the mechanism of injury. Traction is applied to the extended knee using a fracture table with the patient under adequate anesthetic. A varus or valgus load can be applied to correct the deforming tendency of the knee. **B.** In this case the longitudinal traction on the extended knee elevates the lateral plateau fragment using ligamentotaxis. (Modified from Connolly J. *Fractures and dislocations. Closed management.* Philadelphia: WB Saunders, 1995, with permission.)

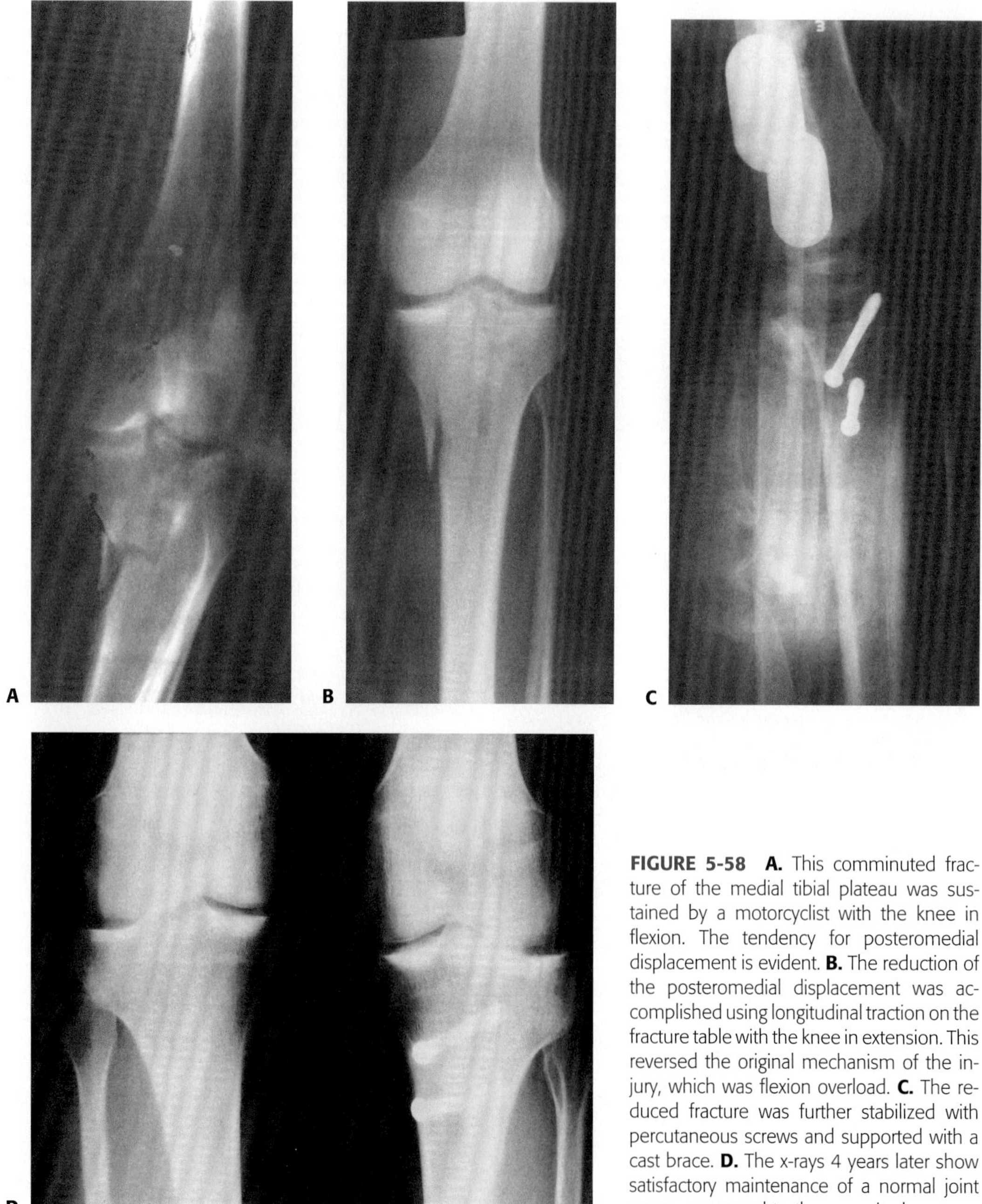

FIGURE 5-58 **A.** This comminuted fracture of the medial tibial plateau was sustained by a motorcyclist with the knee in flexion. The tendency for posteromedial displacement is evident. **B.** The reduction of the posteromedial displacement was accomplished using longitudinal traction on the fracture table with the knee in extension. This reversed the original mechanism of the injury, which was flexion overload. **C.** The reduced fracture was further stabilized with percutaneous screws and supported with a cast brace. **D.** The x-rays 4 years later show satisfactory maintenance of a normal joint space, compared to the opposite knee.

Technique of Inserting a Pin for Distal Femoral Skeletal Traction

The traction pin inserted in the distal femur gives better control of the fracture than a pin in the proximal tibia. This is generally the preferred location for most femoral shaft fractures except very distal ones. The pin is inserted from the medial side under local anesthetic, taking care to avoid the neurovascular structures in the posteromedial aspect of the knee. A hand drill is used to insert a 3-mm Steinmann pin. Stellate incisions around the pin at the entrance and exit sites prevent pinching of the skin (Fig. 5-61). Padding is placed around the pin, a traction bow is attached, and the limb is suspended in balanced traction in a Harris or similar splint using a Pearson attachment to allow knee flexion (Fig. 5-29).

For fractures in the proximal femur, 90°–90° traction is preferred. After the pin is inserted in the distal femur, the hip is flexed 90 degrees and abducted to align the distal fragment with the proximal fragment. The knee is kept flexed at 90 degrees and the leg is supported in a cast (Fig. 5-30).

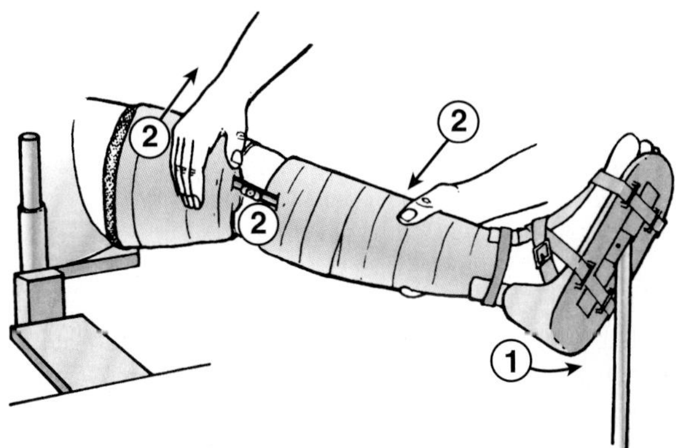

FIGURE 5-59 A cast brace is applied to support the tibial plateau fracture after closed reduction or with internal fixation with the patient still on the fracture table (*1*). The hinges of the cast brace are incorporated so as to apply a valgus load on the knee to unload the medial tibial condyle (*2*). (Modified from Connolly J. *Fractures and dislocations. Closed management.* Philadelphia: WB Saunders, 1995, with permission.)

Initially 15 to 20 pounds of traction are applied to distract the fracture slightly. If necessary, this weight can be increased to 30 pounds. The foot of the bed should be elevated 30 degrees to provide countertraction against the pull of the traction apparatus.

Technique of Closed Reduction and Cast-Brace Application

The cast-brace technique was introduced by Mooney and coworkers (301,305). It permits a fracture to be reduced by closed means and then held in alignment while the patient becomes ambulatory and is able to flex and extend the knee. This method is felt to maximize the natural healing processes since external callus forms quite quickly, particularly in the first 6 weeks after the injury. It minimizes disuse atrophy of joints and muscles, which has followed other nonoperative methods. The method does require skill as well as careful follow-up to avoid excessive angulation or shortening of the fracture site. However, for certain fractures, particularly comminuted distal femoral fractures, the method in our hands has sometimes proven more effective mechanically than the less stable intramedullary nailing by ret-

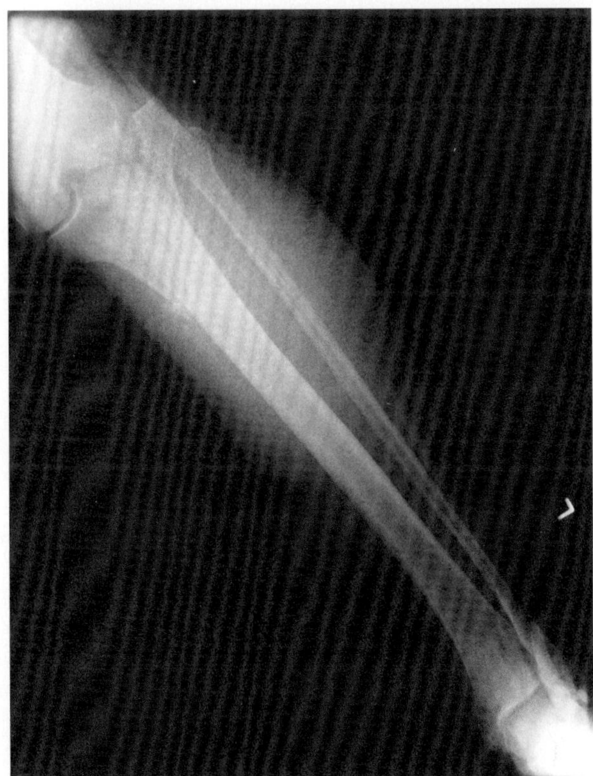

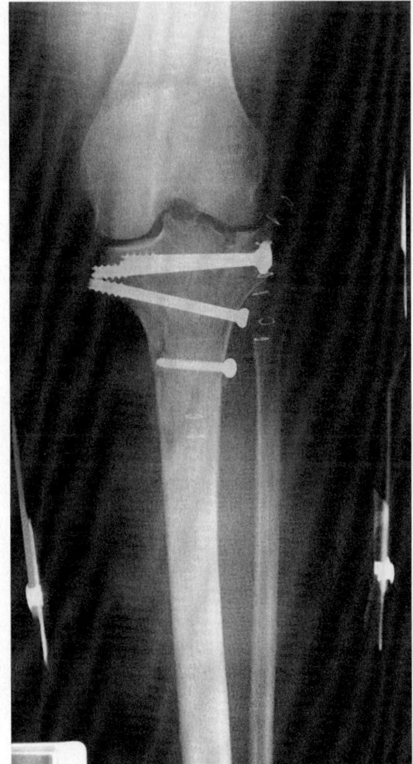

A B

FIGURE 5-60 **A.** This comminuted bicondylar fracture of the tibia with extension into the tibial metaphysis was reduced by longitudinal traction applied to the knee in extension. Because of the comminution, percutaneous screw fixation was used to hold the reduction, permitting a minimally invasive technique for dealing with this unstable injury. **B.** Reduction after longitudinal traction to the extended knee and percutaneous screw fixation was supplemented with cast-brace support. This technique avoids the necessity of wide dissection of the bicondylar fracture, which carries the risk of devascularizing comminuted bone fragments and probably increases the risk of infection.

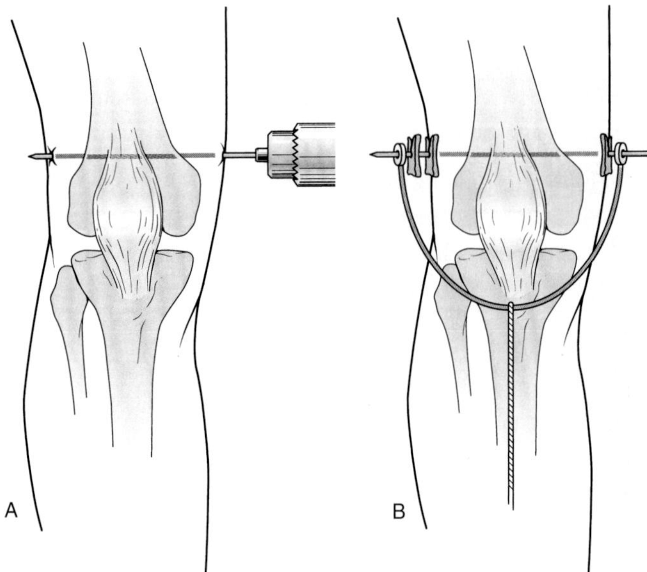

FIGURE 5-61 **A.** Technique of inserting skeletal pins for femoral traction. A skeletal traction pin is inserted in the distal femur from the medial to the lateral side. Local anesthetic is infiltrated down to the periosteum, and care is taken to avoid the neurovascular structures in the posteromedial aspect of the knee. A hand drill is used to insert the 3-mm Steinmann pin, and care is taken to avoid pinching of the skin, which can be painful. **B.** The pin is padded and a traction bow is attached to apply 15 to 20 lbs to the fracture in a Harris splint. (Modified from Connolly J. *Fractures and dislocations. Closed management.* Philadelphia: WB Saunders, 1995, with permission.)

rograde or other techniques (302,304). It is also useful for elderly osteoporotic patients who sustain a supracondylar distal femoral fracture from a fall. The patient can usually adjust to a cast brace and ambulate for functional purposes during the 8 to 10 weeks required for healing.

In most instances a cast brace can be applied with the patient in bed and lightly sedated. The femoral shaft fracture should have been aligned and pulled out to length by the traction technique prior to the cast-brace application (243). The duration of skeletal traction may vary from a few days to 3 or 4 weeks depending on the initial stability of the fracture (301,304) (Fig. 5-62).

Fractures in the distal third of the femoral shaft that are relatively undisplaced at the time of presentation can be managed by early cast-brace application in the first few days after injury. Other, more unstable or open femoral shaft fractures require longer periods for the initial stability of the fracture to develop.

With the patient in bed, an assistant maintains steady traction on the distal femoral pin. A Spandex stockinette is rolled over the leg and across the pin. The assistant continues to support the leg while a 6-inch role of plaster is applied snugly to the thigh. Fractures in the distal third are best reduced with the knee in extension and the leg in external rotation to correct varus deformity (Fig. 5-63). The lower leg portion is applied next, followed by the knee hinges, which should allow knee motion of at least 30 to 40 degrees to maintain the quadriceps and hamstring function. Having some knee motion also eliminates torsion on the fracture site that would be produced by a long leg cast with the knee in extension.

The distal femoral traction pin is left in place below the end of the thigh cast until x-rays have demonstrated satisfactory reduction in the cast brace. The pin actually may be left in for several days more while the patient becomes ambulatory to protect against delayed displacement.

It is important in applying the cast brace to mold over the femoral condyles to provide adequate support to the distal femoral fracture; 1 to 2 cm of shortening of the fracture may be accepted, and in fact, is encouraged in order to close down the fracture gap.

The closed method of treating these fractures has an advantage of not disturbing the fracture milieu, and the early mobilization of the patient with partial weightbearing promotes an abundant external callus. Healing becomes fairly stable by about 6 weeks, at which time the cast brace may be changed. Generally, 12 to 16 weeks are required for the fracture to heal sufficiently to remove the cast brace. During this recovery period the patient should be encouraged to work vigorously to maintain quadriceps and hamstring function and range of motion of the knee from full extension to at least 30 to 40 degrees of flexion.

Nonoperative Treatment of Acetabular Fractures

In his review of the classic literature on acetabular fractures, Tile (126,306) pointed out the importance of distinguishing apples from oranges, that is, distinguishing the relatively undisplaced acetabular fracture produced by low-energy injury from the grossly displaced high-energy acetabular fracture with pelvic disruption. Low-energy injuries produce the majority of acetabular fractures, particularly in the elderly. These usually nondisplaced, or minimally displaced stable fractures can be treated nonoperatively with very satisfying results, provided the fracture is recognized and the patient is maintained on a walker to prevent displacement (307–309). Even some displaced fractures can be reduced by closed means and treated nonoperatively.

In his original classic study on the subject, Letournel (310) cautioned about significant complications from open reduction of acetabular fractures including extensive ectopic bone formation, infection, sciatic nerve injury and vascular injury which occurred in 28% of patients treated operatively. These statistics have not changed significantly in over 20 years since operative treatment of acetabular fractures has improved technically (311). Tornetta (312) has pointed out that clinical results after surgery are better in younger patients than in older patients. Older patients are more likely to have poor bone stock and suffer loss of reduction when treated operatively. Consequently, many such patients would be better candidates for total joint replacement once some fracture healing has occurred rather

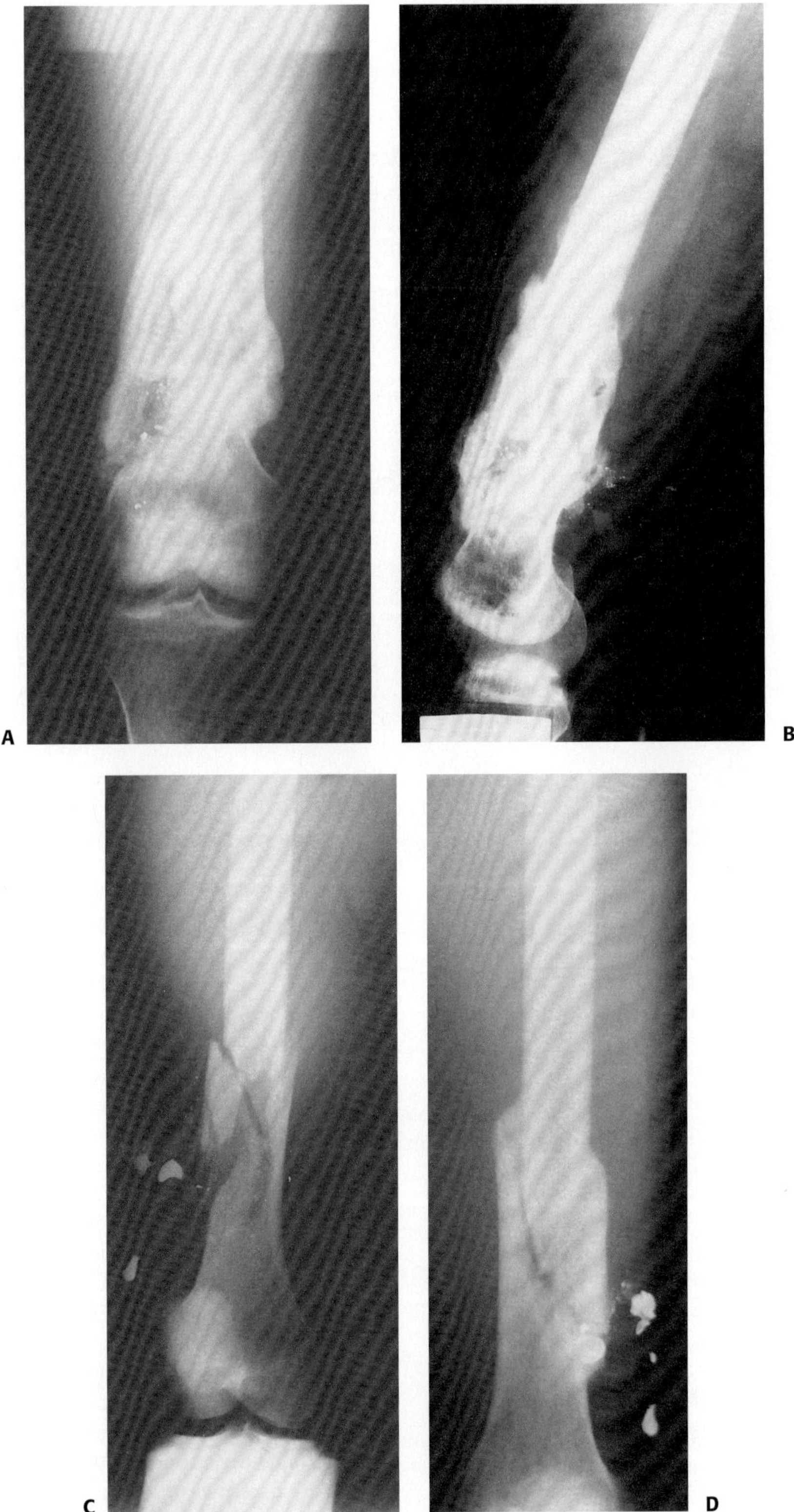

FIGURE 5-62 **A,B.** These anteroposterior lateral x-rays are taken of a comminuted distal third femoral fracture that was treated with approximately 2 weeks of traction followed by cast-bracing application. Fracture healing is evident on the anteroposterior lateral x-rays at 14 weeks, when the cast-brace was removed. **C.** This gunshot fracture of the distal femur was sufficiently stable without traction to permit cast-brace application within 1 week. **D.** Fracture union was evident when the cast-brace was removed at 12 weeks.

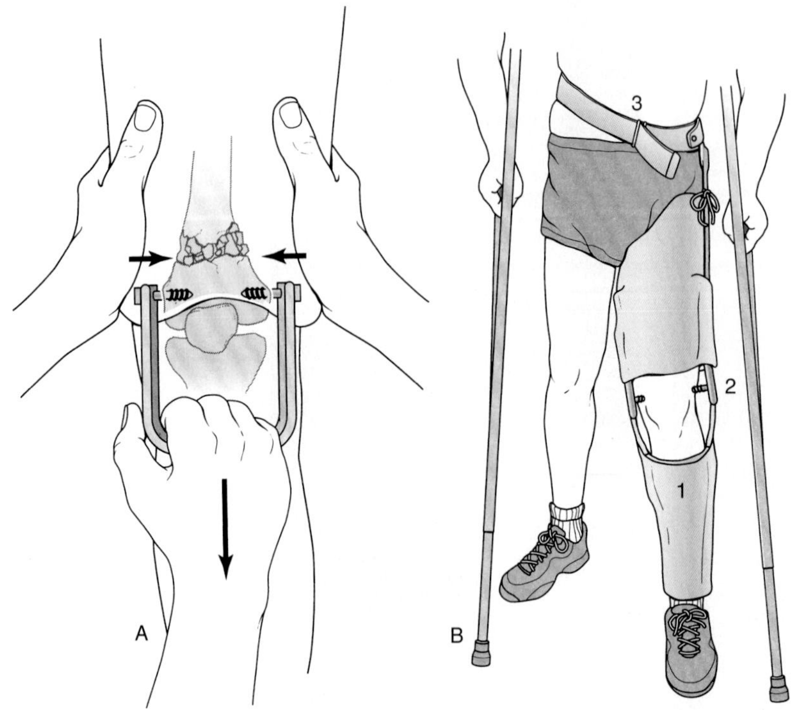

FIGURE 5-63 **A.** Comminuted fractures of the distal femur can be adequately aligned by distal femoral traction. When the initial swelling subsides, a cast brace is applied with an assistant maintaining traction. The surgeon applies the cast, molding over the fracture site. The knee is held in extension and the leg is slightly externally rotated to correct any tendency to varus angulation of the fracture. **B.** The cast is attached by hinges to a knee cast below (*1*). The distal femoral traction pin is left in place until the stability of the fracture is ascertained by x-ray once the patient has become ambulatory (*2*). If the stability of the fracture is in question, a pelvic band with a hinge or a pelvic mini-spica can be attached to the cast to provide hip stability (*3*). (Modified from Connolly J. *Fractures and dislocations. Closed management.* Philadelphia: WB Saunders, 1995, with permission.)

than undergoing an attempted acute open reduction and internal fixation. In addition, because of the need for special reduction clamps, special traction tables, neurologic monitoring apparatus, and qualified assistants many institutions are really not equipped to properly support this type of surgery. This must be seriously considered by any individual surgeon making the decision whether to operate or transfer the patient to a center specializing in care of these fractures or treat the fracture nonoperatively (312).

Consequently, closed nonoperative management of many acetabular fractures is still an important skill for the fracture surgeon to maintain. Closed reduction can be applied to many displaced acetabular fractures including the centrally protruded femoral head, commonly found in osteoporotic patients. The objective is to restore joint congruity without necessarily requiring operative invasion. Rowe and Lowell (313), Lowell (314), and others (315–318) have described the technique of manipulative reduction of acetabular fractures. The typically displaced acetabular fracture with protrusion of the femoral head centrally and superiorly should be reduced as early as possible if the closed attempt is to succeed. As soon as the patient's condition is stabilized sufficiently to allow adequate anesthesia, manipulation is carried out to disimpact the displaced centrally protruding femoral head (Fig. 5-64). This requires inserting a traction screw directly into the greater trochanter in order to provide sufficient lateral traction to disimpact the femoral head. If traction is applied simply to a distal femoral traction pin, reduction is likely to fail since the force vectors need to be directed laterally as well as distally.

After the trochanter screw is inserted using sterile technique, the patient is turned on the opposite side and a pillow or bolster is placed between the thighs to act as a fulcrum. The dislocated femur is adducted over the bolster while the traction screw is pulled laterally to direct the femoral head out of the acetabulum. Often a characteristic pop will be felt just as with any other successful joint reduction. The reduction is considered acceptable if the radiographs demonstrate the femoral head to be returned congruently under the dome of the acetabulum. Slight persistent displacement of the inner acetabular wall or anterior or posterior columns may be accepted since this usually does not affect hip function after the fracture heals. The key to successful closed reduction is restoration of the relationship of the femoral head to the weightbearing dome of the acetabulum (319,320). Precise anatomic reduction of the articular surfaces as emphasized by advocates for open reduction has not proven to be essential for a satisfactory outcome after successful closed treatment (Fig. 5-65). However, posterior subluxation of the femoral head should not be accepted (321,322). Careful CT and other radiographic evaluation may be necessary to rule out persistent posterior displacement. If necessary, stress views may be obtained under fluoroscopy as described by Tornetta (323) to determine the stability of the hip and the posterior acetabulum. Any degree of posterior instability documented clinically or by x-ray requires open reduction and internal fixation to restore posterior stability and congruency to the joint.

Once an adequate reduction is achieved, the patient is transferred to a fracture bed and trochanteric traction is continued using 20 to 30 pounds of weight. In addition, distal femoral

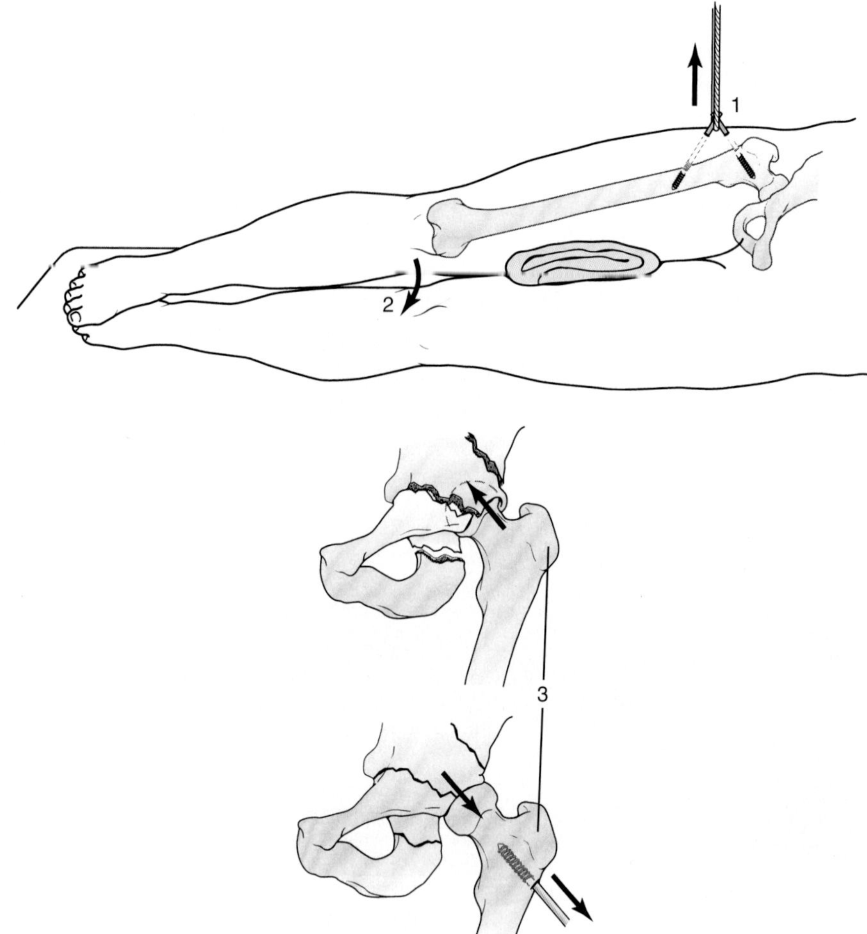

FIGURE 5-64 As with any other dislocation, closed reduction of acetabular fractures should be carried out as soon as possible. With the patient under adequate anesthesia, a trochanteric screw is inserted under sterile technique (*1*). The patient is turned on the opposite side on a pillow. A bolster is placed between the thighs to act as a fulcrum (*2*). The dislocated femur is adducted over the bolster while the traction screw is pulled laterally to lever the femoral head out of the acetabulum (*3*). Often the dislocation will reduce with a popping sensation. If the reduction is successful and confirmed by x-ray, traction is applied to the trochanteric screw as well as to a traction pin inserted in the distal femur. This allows both lateral and longitudinal traction to maintain the femoral head under the dome of the acetabulum. (Modified from Connolly J. *Fractures and dislocations. Closed management.* Philadelphia: WB Saunders, 1995, with permission.)

traction is applied again using 20 to 30 pounds. Adequate continuous traction technique must be maintained until the acetabular fragments begin to consolidate (324).

Many surgeons are reluctant to use lateral trochanteric traction for fear that it increases the risk of infection should surgery become necessary. If the initial attempt at closed reduction is unsuccessful and alignment of the femoral head remains nonconcentric with the acetabular dome, the trochanteric pin should be removed immediately. The patient is then maintained in distal femoral traction until operative reduction can be carried out.

A major objection to closed traction treatment of these fractures is that it mandates continued traction of 6 to 10 weeks in order for the acetabular fragments to heal sufficiently. The healing process cannot be rushed (318). While some traction weight may be removed at 3 to 4 weeks, removing the traction too early will result in loss of reduction and will require reapplication of the traction if an unsatisfactory outcome is to be avoided (Fig. 5-66). The method has numerous advantages and does avoid potential complications of extensive surgery (322,325–329). When reduction by closed methods succeeds, the long-term outcome is as good as operative treatment. Approximately 75% of successful closed reductions of acetabular fractures have satisfactory outcome, while 25% to 30% do poorly. The poor outcomes from closed or open treatment result from the severity of the impact on the articular surface as often as from problems of adequate reduction of the fragmented acetabulum (319,330–335).

SUMMARY

Advantages of Nonoperative Management

The term *nonoperative* is misleading since any closed reduction of a fracture should be considered an operative procedure and approached with appropriate care and planning. Closed reduction, by nonoperative minimally invasive methods, remains the treatment of choice for many fractures today. The objective is to reduce the fracture by manipulation and/or traction, assess the reduction clinically and radiographically, and then maintain alignment by a variety of techniques including casts, fracture

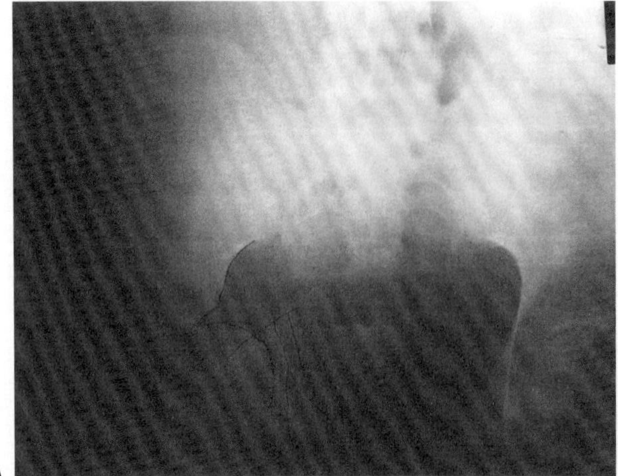

A

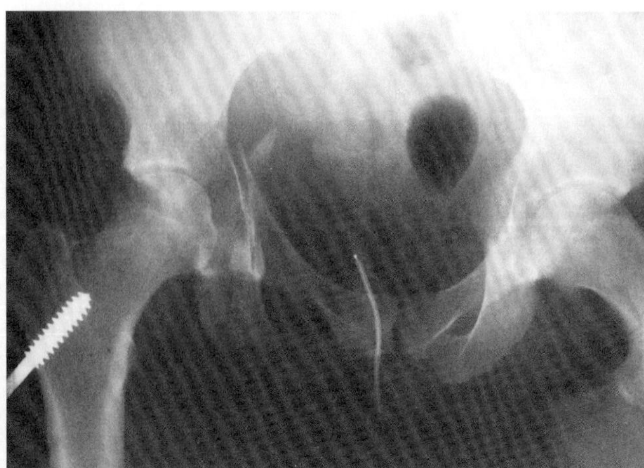

B

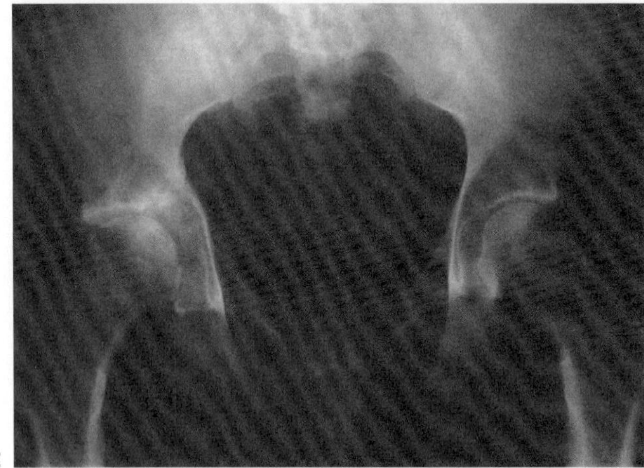

C

FIGURE 5-65 **A.** X-ray of this comminuted fracture of the anterior and posterior acetabular columns shows central protrusion of the femoral head. **B.** The patient was treated by closed reduction with a trochanteric screw and satisfactory repositioning of the femoral head under the acetabular dome was achieved. Subsequently, traction was applied to the trochanteric screw as well as to the distal femur for approximately 6 weeks. **C.** X-ray of the hip at 2 years shows healing of the acetabular fracture and maintenance of a satisfactory joint space with excellent, near-normal motion, and function of the hip joint.

braces, external fixators, or, if necessary, closed intramedullary nailing or percutaneous screw fixation.

Closed reduction, when done well, can avoid infection and the problems of technical errors, which, though infrequent, are real risks of open techniques (34,282,289,290,322,325,327, 321). Closed nonoperative management has generally proven less costly than has operative management of many fractures, if the principles of functional fracture treatment as best described by Sarmiento and others are followed. Emphasis on closed management of fractures is consistent with the growing acceptance of noninvasive or minimally invasive methods of all surgical techniques, not just fracture fixation. Therefore, it is essential that the fracture surgeon understand the mechanics of closed fracture reduction as well as open surgical techniques (34,336).

Disadvantages of Nonoperative Management

With nonoperative techniques, a certain amount of mechanical, analytical, and tactile skills are required and must be learned. Also, there seems to be an unfortunate trend noticed on review of closed malpractice claims (337) that complications after cast treatment of certain fractures, particularly in the tibia, are more likely to lead patients to seek medical-legal recourse than are more significant complications after operative treatment. This may often be based on some arbitrary definitions of an "acceptable" reduction (338), but nevertheless persistent follow-up is essential to ensure against loss of reduction after either nonoperative or operative management.

Nonoperative methods may not be suitable for fractures involving articular surfaces such as the ankle or the knee. Here accurate restoration of articular anatomy is the ideal. Nevertheless, closed reduction by ligamentotaxis with or without percutaneous fixation of periarticular fractures is often preferable to open reduction and attempted rigid fixation of articular fractures that may devascularize small comminuted fracture fragments (235).

Advantages of Operative Treatment

The primary advantage of operative treatment is that well-performed fracture fixation permits anatomic alignment (339)

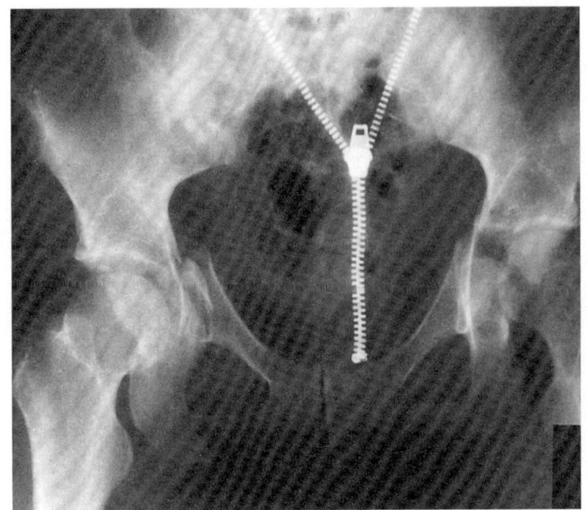
A

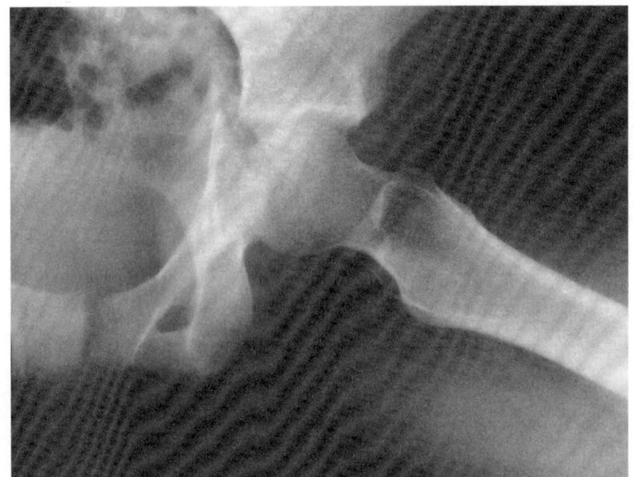
B

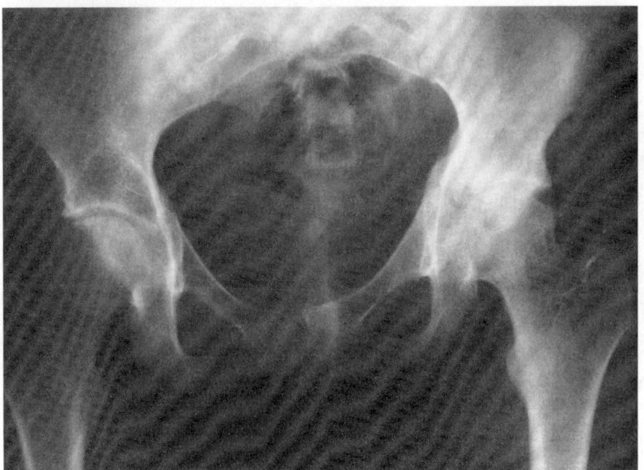
C

FIGURE 5-66 **A.** Anteroposterior x-ray of a patient with bilateral central acetabular fractures treated initially in traction for 3 weeks. The traction was gradually decreased and the patient was allowed out of bed. **B.** Follow-up x-rays when the traction was decreased showed further protrusion of the femoral head into the acetabular fracture on the left. The fracture had involved the anterior and posterior columns, and therefore was more unstable than the fracture of the right hip. The patient was placed back in bilateral traction for an additional 3 weeks. **C.** X-rays of the pelvis at 2½ years show adequate healing of both acetabular fractures with maintenance of the articulation of the femoral head with the acetabular dome bilaterally. The patient had a full range of motion in the right hip and slight limitation of rotation in the left but was asymptomatic with close to normal symmetric relationships between her femoral heads and acetabulor weightbearing domes.

of the fragments, early restoration of joint and muscle function, and rapid mobilization of the patient. The early restoration of mobility for patients with multiple injuries diminishes systemic complications such as phlebitis, pulmonary embolism, and cardiorespiratory problems. The minimally invasive methods of closed reduction and closed nailing or percutaneous screw fixation come close to the ideal of effective fracture immobilization with early patient mobilization. However, this ideal is not always achieved and ineffective fixation is worse than none at all.

Disadvantages of Operative Treatment

A significant disadvantage of operative fixation is the impediment it offers to the effective biologic processes of fracture repair (13,16,336). The reader should recall that the classic Wolff's law of bone formation might be summarized simply as stating that "bone responds to the need for it" (340). The introduction of mechanical fixation of fracture fragments temporarily inhibits or permanently alters signals to the repair processes of bone.

When a fracture is subjected to compression by either a plate or external fixator, callus forms in response to the compressive loading (9,10,341,342). However, the callus is weak when loaded in tension. Thus, a significant number of fractures that have been treated by compression plating or compression fixators have been reported to fail once the plate or the external fixator is removed due to the inability of the seemingly repaired fracture to resist tensile load (10,259–262). This phenomenon has been noted to persist for several years until the callus can be modeled to align itself in the normal longitudinal axis of the bone, and thereby become capable of resisting tension as well as compressive loading.

The management of fractures continues to evolve. Ultimately, our goal should be to maximize closed reduction of fractures and minimize invasive surgery. As we have slowly gained some understanding of the phenomenal processes of skeletal repair, many useful biologic (343–345) and cellular (5,6,11,339,340) methods have become available to aid these repair processes. Consequently, the truly skilled physician who treats fractures must appreciate the biologic cultivation of healing as well as the carpentry of fracture fixation.

ACKNOWLEDGEMENTS

The author deeply appreciates the critique of this revised chapter by Steve Nguyen, MD and other colleagues in the orthopaedic residency program at Orlando Regional Hospital, Florida. Also, the valuable technical assistance of Mrs. Veronica Richardson in revising this chapter is sincerely appreciated.

REFERENCES

1. Manolagas S, Jilka R. Bone marrow, cytokines, and bone remodeling. *N Engl J Med* 1995;332:305–310.
2. Gallagher G. Evolutions: Bone marrow hematopoiesis. *J NIH Res* 1994;6:95–97.
3. Gulati GL. Structure and function of the bone marrow and hematopoiesis. *Hematol Oncol Clin North Am* 1988;2:495–511.
4. Kessinger A. Circulating stem cells—Waxing hematopoietic. *N Engl J Med* 1995;333: 315–316.
5. Caplan A. Mesenchymal stem cells. *J Orthop Res* 1991;9:641–650.
6. Ferrari G, DeAngelis G, Coletta M, et al. Muscle regeneration by bone marrow-derived myogenic progenitors. *Science* 1998;279:1528–1530.
7. Boorstin D. Bergson's creative evolution. In: Boorstin D. *The seekers*. New York: Random House, 1998:245–249.
8. Kenwright J, Goodship A. Controlled mechanical stimulation in the treatment of tibial fractures. *Clin Orthop Rel Res* 1989;241:36–47.
9. Olerud S, Danckwardt-Lilliestrŏm G. Fracture healing in compression osteosynthesis. *Acta Orthop Scand Suppl* 1971;137:1–44.
10. Wirth C, Campbell C, Askew M, et al. The biomechanical effects of compression plates applied to fractures. *J Trauma* 1974;14:563–571.
11. Connolly J. Avoidable causes of non-union. *Clin Orthop Rel Res* 1985;194:226–232.
12. Heppenstall R, Brighton C, Esterhai J, et al. Prognostic factors in nonunion of the tibia: An evaluation of 185 cases treated with constant direct current. *J Trauma* 1984;24: 790–796.
13. McKibben B. The biology of fracture healing in long bones. *J Bone Joint Surg* 1978; 60B:150–162.
14. Rhinelander F, Gracilla R, Phillips R, et al. Microangiography in bone healing. III. Osteotomies with internal fixation. *J Bone Joint Surg* 1967;49:1006.
15. Rhinelander F, Phillips R, Steel W, et al. Microangiography in bone healing. II. Displaced closed fractures. *J Bone Joint Surg* 1968;50A:643–654.
16. Park SH, O'Connor K, McKellop H, et al. The influence of active shear or compressive motion on fracture-healing. *J Bone Joint Surg* 1998;80A:868–877.
17. Puno R, Teynor J, Nagano J, et al. Critical analysis of results of treatment of 201 tibial shaft fractures. *Clin Orthop Rel Res* 1986;212:113–121.
18. Wennberg J, Freeman J, Culp W. Are hospital services rationed in New Haven or over-utilized in Boston. *Lancet* 1987;1:1185–1189.
19. Keller R, Atlas S, Soule D, et al. Relationship between rates and outcomes of operative treatment for lumbar disc herniation and spinal stenosis. *J Bone Joint Surg* 1999;81A: 752–762.
20. Burstein A. Fracture classification systems: Do they work and are they useful? *J Bone Joint Surg* 1993;75:1743.
21. Siebenrock K, Gerber C. The reproducibility of classification of fractures of the proximal end of the humerus. *J Bone Joint Surg* 1993;75A:1751–1755.
22. Sjöden G, Movin T, Güntner M, et al. Poor reproducibility of classification of proximal humeral fractures: additional CT of minor value. *Acta Orthop Scand* 1997;68:239–242.
23. Burkhalter W, Reyes F. Closed treatment of fractures of the hand. *Bull Hosp Joint Dis Orthop Inst* 1984;44:145–162.
24. Carl A, Thomas S. Bilateral sacroiliac joint fracture-dislocation: A case report. *J Trauma* 1990;30:1402–1405.
25. Duwelius P, Connolly J. Closed reduction of tibial plateau fractures. A comparison of functional and roentgenographic end results. *Clin Orthop Rel Res* 1988;220:116–126.
26. Fredrickson B, Yuan H. Nonoperative treatment of the spine: external immobilization. In: Browner B, Jupiter J, Levine A, et al., eds. *Skeletal trauma*, 2nd ed. Philadelphia: WB Saunders, 1992:807–836.
27. Kristensen K, Kiaer T, Blicher J. No arthrosis of the ankle 20 years after malaligned tibial-shaft fracture. *Acta Orthop Scand* 1989;60:208–209.
28. Sarmiento A, Latta L. *Functional fracture bracing: tibia, humerus, and ulna*. Berlin: Springer, 1995.
29. Merchant T, Dietz F. Long-term follow-up after fractures of the tibial and fibular shaft. *J Bone Joint Surg* 1989;71A:599–606.
30. Hägglund G, Hansson L, Norman O. Correction by growth of rotational deformity after femoral fracture in children. *Acta Orthop Scand* 1983;54:858–861.
31. Forrester J, Zederfeldt B, Hayes T, et al. Wolff's law in relation to the healing skin wound. *J Trauma* 1970;10:770–779.
32. Ilizarov G. The tension-stress effect on the genesis and growth of tissues. *Clin Orthop Rel Res* 1989;239:263–271.
33. Claes L, Augat P, Suger G, et al. Influence of size and stability of the osteotomy gap on the success of fracture healing. *J Orthop Res* 1997;15:577–584.
34. Charnley J. *The closed treatment of fractures*, 3rd ed. New York: Churchill Livingstone, 1981.
35. Stewart T. Nonunion of fractures in antiquity, with descriptions of five cases from the new world involving the forearm. *Bull NY Acad Med* 1974;50:875–891.
36. Connolly J, Dehne R. Nonunion of the clavicle and thoracic outlet syndrome. *J Trauma* 1989;29:1127–1133.
37. Shackford S. Taming of the screw: A case report and literature review of limb-threatening complications after plate osteosynthesis of a clavicular nonunion. *J Trauma* 2003; 55:840–843.
38. Bliss S, Weinberger S, Meier M, et al. Clinical problem-solving. The unusual suspect. *N Engl J Med* 2002;347:1876–1881.
39. Kona J, Bosse M, Staeheli JW, et al. Type II distal clavicle fractures: A retrospective review of surgical treatment. *J Orthop Trauma* 1990;4:115–120.
40. Robinson CM, Cairns D. Primary nonoperative treatment of displaced lateral fractures of the clavicle. *J Bone Joint Surg* 2004;86-A:778–782.
41. Ada J, Miller M. Scapular fractures. *Clin Orthop Rel Res* 1991;26:174–180.
42. Nordqvist A, Petersson C. Fracture of the body, neck, or spine of the scapula. A long-term follow-up study. *Clin Orthop Rel Res* 1992;283:139–144.
43. Herscovice D Jr, Fiennes A, Allgŏwer M, et al. The floating shoulder: Ipsilateral clavicle and scapular neck fractures. *J Bone Joint Surg* 1992;74B:362–364.
44. Leung K, Lam T. Open reduction and internal fixation of ipsilateral fractures of the scapular neck and clavicle. *J Bone Joint Surg* 1993;75A:1015–1018.
45. McGinnis M, Denton J. Fractures of the scapula: A retrospective study of 40 fractured scapulae. *J Trauma* 1989;29:1488–1493.
46. Ramos L, Mencía R, Alonso A, et al. Conservative treatment of ipsilateral fractures of the scapula and clavicle. *J Trauma* 1997;42:239–242.
47. Edwards SG, Whittle AP, Wood GW, et al. Nonoperative treatment of ipsilateral fractures of the scapula and clavicle. *J Bone Joint Surg* 2000;82-A:774–780.
48. Court-Brown C, Cattermole H, McQueen M. Impacted valgus fractures of the proximal humerus: The results of non-operative treatment. *J Bone Joint Surg* 2002;84-B:504–508.
49. Horak J, Nilsson B. Epidemiology of fracture of the upper end of the humerus. *Clin Orthop Rel Res* 1975;112:250–253.
50. Kristiansen B, Angermann P, Larsen T. Functional result following fractures of the proximal humerus. A controlled clinical study comparing two periods of immobilization. *Arch Orthop Trauma Surg* 1989;108:339–341.
51. Kumar V, Balasubramaniam P. The role of atmospheric pressure in stabilizing the shoulder. *J Bone Joint Surg* 1985;67B:719–721.
52. Itoi E, Motzkin, Moorey BF, et al. The static rotator cuff does not affect inferior translation of the humerus at the glenohumeral joint. *J Trauma* 1999;47:55–59.
53. Yosipovitch Z, Tikva P, Goldberg I. Inferior subluxation of the humeral head after injury to the shoulder. *J Bone Joint Surg* 1989;71A:751–753.
54. Cofield R. Comminuted fractures of the proximal humerus. *Clin Orthop Rel Res* 1988; 230:49–57.
55. Young T, Wallace W. Conservative treatment of fractures and fracture-dislocations of the upper end of the humerus. *J Bone Joint Surg* 1985;67B:373–377.
56. Ferkel R, Hedley A, Eckhardt J. Anterior fracture-dislocations of the shoulder: Pitfalls in treatment. *J Trauma* 1984;24:363–367.
57. Hersche O, Gerber C. Iatrogenic displacement of fracture-dislocations of the shoulder. *J Bone Joint Surg* 1994;76B:30–33.
58. Bunker T, Anthony P. The pathology of frozen shoulder. *J Bone Joint Surg* 1995;77B: 677–683.
59. Connolly J, Regen E, Evans O. The management of the painful, stiff shoulder. *Clin Orthop Rel Res* 1972;84:97–103.
60. Farragos A, Schmitsch E, McKee M. Complications of intramedullary nailing for fractures of the humeral shaft: A review. *J Orthop Trauma* 1999;13:258–267.
61. Caldwell J. Treatment of fractures of the shaft of the humerus by hanging cast. *Surg Gynecol Obstet* 1940;70:421–425.
62. Sarmiento A, Kinman P, Galvin E, et al. Functional bracing of fractures of the shaft of the humerus. *J Bone Joint Surg* 1977;59A:596–601.
63. Sarmiento A, Latta L. Functional fracture bracing. *J Am Acad Orthop Surg* 1999;7: 66–75.
64. Holdsworth B, Clement D, Rothwell P. Fractures of the radial head-the benefit of aspiration: A prospective controlled trial. *Injury* 1987;18:44–47.
65. Radin E, Riseborough J. Fractures of the radial head. *J Bone Joint Surg* 1966;48A: 1055–1063.
66. Adler J, Shafton G. Radial head fractures: Is excision necessary? *J Trauma* 1963;4: 115–136.
67. Weseley M, Barenfeld P, Eisenstein A. Closed treatment of isolated radial head fractures. *J Trauma* 1983;23:36–39.
68. Khalfayan E, Culp R, Alexander H. Mason type II radial head fractures: operative versus nonoperative treatment. *J Orthop Trauma* 1992;6:283–289.
69. Broberg M, Morrey B. Results of delayed excision of the radial head after fracture. *J Bone Joint Surg* 1986;68:669–674.
70. Gebuhr P, Hŏlmich P, Ørsnes T, et al. Isolated ulnar shaft fractures. Comparison of treatment by a functional brace and long-arm cast. *J Bone Joint Surg* 1992;74B:757–759.
71. Sarmiento A, Kinman P, Murphy R, et al. Treatment of ulnar fractures by functional bracing. *J Bone Joint Surg* 1976;58A:1104–1107.
72. Brakenbury P, Corea J, Blakemore M. Nonunion of isolated fracture of ulnar shaft in adults. *Injury* 1981;12:371–375.
73. Ekelund A, Nilsson O. Early mobilization of isolated ulnar-shaft fractures. *Acta Orthop Scand* 1989;60:261–262.
74. Shively R, Sundaram M. Ununited fractures of the scaphoid in boxers. *Am J Sports Med* 1980;8:440–442.

75. Dias J, Thompson J, Barton N, et al. Suspected scaphoid fractures. The value of radiographs. *J Bone Joint Surg* 1990;72B:98–101.
76. Horri E, Nakamura R, Watanabe K, et al. Scaphoid fracture as a "puncher's fracture." *J Orthop* 1994;8:107–110.
77. Tiel-Van Buul M, Van Beek E, Broekhuizen A, et al. Radiography and scintigraphy of suspected scaphoid fracture. *J Bone Joint Surg* 1993;75B:61–65.
78. Düppe H, Johnell O, Lundborg G, et al. Long term results of fracture of the scaphoid. A follow-up study of more than thirty years. *J Bone Joint Surg* 1994;76A:249–252.
79. Bhandari M, Hanson B. Acute nondisplaced fractures of the scaphoid. *J Orthop Trauma* 2004;18:253–255.
80. Clay N, Dias J, Costigan P, et al. Need the thumb be immobilized in scaphoid fractures? *J Bone Joint Surg* 1991;73B:828–832.
81. Gelberman R, Wolock B, Siegel D. Current concepts review fractures and non-unions of the carpal scaphoid. *J Bone Joint Surg* 1989;71A:1560–1565.
82. Gellman H, Caputo R, Carter V, et al. Comparison of short and long thumb-spica casts for non-displaced fractures of the carpal scaphoid. *J Bone Joint Surg* 1989;71:354–357.
83. Mack G, Bosse M, Gelberman R, et al. The natural history of scaphoid non-union. *J Bone Joint Surg* 1984;66A:504–509.
84. Morgan D, Walters J. A prospective study of 100 consecutive carpal scaphoid fractures. *Aust NZ J Surg* 1984;54:233–241.
85. London P. The broken scaphoid bone. The case against pessimism. *J Bone Joint Surg* 1961;43B:237–243.
86. Reyes F, Latta L. Conservative management of difficult phalangeal fractures. *Clin Orthop Rel Res* 1987;214:23–30.
87. Hunter J, Cowen N. Fifth metacarpal fractures in a compensation clinic population. *J Bone Joint Surg* 1970;52A:1159–1165.
88. Clapper M, O'Brien J, Lyons P. Fractures of the fifth metatarsal. Analysis of a fracture registry. *Clin Orthop Rel Res* 1995;315:238–241.
89. Lawrence S, Botte M. Jones' fractures and related fractures of the proximal fifth metatarsal. *Foot Ankle* 1993;14:358–365.
90. Dameron T Jr. Fractures of the proximal fifth metatarsal: Selecting the best treatment option. *J Am Acad Orthop Surg* 1995;3:110–114.
91. Buckley R, Meek R. Comparison of open versus closed reduction of intraarticular calcaneal fractures: a matched cohort in workmen. *J Orthop Trauma* 1992;6:216–222.
92. Buckley R, Tough S. Displaced intra-articular calcaneal fractures. *J Am Acad Orthop Surg* 2004;12:172–178.
93. Pozo J, Kirwan E, Jackson A. The long-term results of conservative management of severely displaced fractures of the calcaneus. *J Bone Joint Surg* 1984;66B:386–390.
94. Lance E, Carey E Jr, Wade P. Fractures of the os calcis: treatment by early mobilization. *Clin Orthop Rel Res* 1963;30:76–82.
95. Omoto H, Sakurada K, Sugi M, et al. A new method of manual reduction for intra-articular fracture of the calcaneus. *Clin Orthop Rel Res* 1983;177:104–111.
96. Yde J. The Lauge-Hansen classification of malleolar fracture. *Acta Orthop Scand* 1980; 51:181.
97. Rowley D, Norris S, Duckworth T. A prospective trial comparing operative and manipulative treatment of ankle fractures. *J Bone Joint Surg* 1986;68B:610–613.
98. Yablon I, Heller F, Shouse L. The key role of the lateral malleolus in displaced fractures of the ankle. *J Bone Joint Surg* 1977;59A:169–173.
99. Ali M, McLaren C, Rouholamin E, et al. Ankle fractures in the elderly: Nonoperative or operative treatment. *J Orthop Trauma* 1987;1:275–280.
100. Bauer M, Bergstrom B, Hemborg A, et al. Malleolar fractures: Nonoperative versus operative treatment. *Clin Orthop Rel Res* 1985;199:17–27.
101. Bauer M, Jonsson K, Nilsson B. Thirty-year follow-up of ankle fractures. *Acta Orthop Scand* 1985;56:103–106.
102. Cedell C. Is closed treatment of ankle fractures advisable? *Acta Orthop Scand* 1985;56: 101–102.
103. Marti R, Raaymakers E, Nolte P. Malunited ankle fractures. *J Bone Joint Surg* 1990;72B: 709–713.
104. Pankovich A. Fractures of the fibula proximal to the distal tibiofibular syndesmosis. *J Bone Joint Surg* 1978;60A:221–229.
105. Weber B, Simpson L. Corrective lengthening osteotomy of the fibula. *Clin Orthop Rel Res* 1985;199:61–67.
106. Pankovich A. Maisonneuve fracture of the fibula. *J Bone Joint Surg* 1976;58A:337–342.
107. Dickson TB Jr, Kichline PD. Functional management of stress fractures in female athletes using a pneumatic leg brace. *Am J Sports Med* 1987;15:86–89.
108. Sullivan D, Warren F, Pavlov H, et al. Stress fractures in 51 runners. *Clin Orthop Rel Res* 1984;187:188–194.
109. Carter D, Hayes W. Compact bone fatigue damage: A microscopic examination. *Clin Orthop Rel Res* 1977;127:265–274.
110. Hornby R, Evans J, Vardon V. Operative or conservative treatment for trochanteric fractures of the femur. A randomized epidemiological trial in elderly patients. *J Bone Joint Surg* 1989;71B:619–623.
111. Lyon L, Nevins M. Management of hip fractures in nursing home patients: To treat or not to treat? *J Am Geriatr Soc* 1984;32:391–395.
112. Lyon L, Nevins M. Nontreatment of hip fractures in senile patients. *JAMA* 1977;238: 1175–1178.
113. Winter W. Nonoperative treatment of proximal femoral fractures in the demented nonambulatory patient. *Clin Orthop Rel Res* 1987;218:97–103.
114. Fullerton L, Snowdy H. Femoral neck stress fractures. *Am J Sports Med* 1988;16: 365–377.
115. Johansson C, Ekenman I, Törnkvist H, et al. Stress fractures of the femoral neck in athletes. *Am J Sports Med* 1990;18:524–528.
116. Kaltas DS. Stress fractures of the femoral neck in young adults. *J Bone Joint Surg* 1981; 63B:33–37.
117. Raaymakers E, Marti R. Non-operative treatment of impacted femoral neck fractures. *J Bone Joint Surg* 1991;73B:950–954.
118. Aro H, Dahlström S. Conservative management of distraction-type stress fractures of the femoral neck. *J Bone Joint Surg* 1986;68B:65–67.
119. Hansen B, Solgaard S. Impacted fractures of the femoral neck treated by early mobilization and weight-bearing. *Acta Orthop* 1978;49:180–185.
120. Sugano N, Masuhara K, Nakamura N, et al. MRI of early osteonecrosis of the femoral head after transcervical fracture. *J Bone Joint Surg* 1996;78B:253–257.
121. Tooke M, Favero K. Femoral neck fractures in skeletally mature patients, fifty years old or less. *J Bone Joint Surg* 1985;67A:1255–1260.
122. Visuri T, Vara A, Meurman K. Displaced stress fractures of the femoral neck in young male adults: A report of twelve operative cases. *J Trauma* 1988;28:1562–1569.
123. Eastridge B, Burgess A. Pedestrian pelvic fractures: 5-year experience of a major urban trauma center. *J Trauma* 1997;42:695–699.
124. Gilliland M, Ward R, Barton R, et al. Factors affecting mortality in pelvic fractures. *J Trauma* 1982;22:691–693.
125. Rossvoll I, Finsen V. Mortality after pelvic fractures in the elderly. *J Orthop Trauma* 1989;3:115–117.
126. Tile M. Pelvic ring fractures: Should they be fixed? *J Bone Joint Surg* 1988;70B:1–12.
127. Melton L III, Sampson J, Morrey B, et al. Epidemiologic features of pelvic fractures. *Clin Orthop Rel Res* 1981;155:43–47.
128. Mucha P, Farnell M. Analysis of pelvic fracture management. *J Trauma* 1984;24: 379–386.
129. Davidson B, Simmons G, Williamson P, et al. Pelvic fractures associated with open perineal wounds: A survivable injury. *J Trauma* 1993;35:36–40.
130. Gruen G, Leit M, Gruen R, et al. Functional outcome of patients with unstable pelvic ring fractures stabilized with open reduction and internal fixation. *J Trauma* 1995;39: 838–845.
131. Riemer B, Butterfield S, Diamone D, et al. Acute mortality associated with injuries to the pelvic ring: The role of early patient mobilization and external fixation. *J Trauma* 1993;35:671–677.
132. Rothenberger D, Fischer R, Strate R, et al. The mortality associated with pelvic fractures. *Surgery* 1978;84:356–361.
133. Routt Jr ML, Falicov A, et al. Circumferential pelvic antishock sheeting: A temporary resuscitation aid. *J Orthop Trauma* 2002;16:45–48.
134. Lindahl J, Hirvensalo E. Failure of reduction with an external fixator in the management of injuries of the pelvic ring. Long-term evaluation of 110 patients. *J Bone Joint Surg Br* 1999;81:955–962.
135. Henderson R. The long-term results of nonoperatively treated major pelvic disruptions. *J Orthop Trauma* 1989;3:41–47.
136. Kellam J. The role of external fixation in pelvic disruption. *Clin Orthop Rel Res* 1989; 241:66–82.
137. Madsen L, Jensen J, Christensen S. Parturition and pelvic fracture. Follow-up of 34 obstetric patients with a history of pelvic fracture. *Acta Obstet Gynecol Scand* 1983;62: 617–620.
138. Lindsey R, Leggon R, Wright D, et al. Separation of the symphysis pubis in association with childbearing. *J Bone Joint Surg* 1988;70A:289–292.
139. Langloh N, Johnson E, Jackson C. Traumatic sacroiliac disruptions. *J Trauma* 1972; 12:931–935.
140. Semba R, Yasukawa K, Gustilo R. Critical analysis of results of 53 Malgaigne fractures of the pelvis. *J Trauma* 1983;23:535–537.
141. Failinger M, McGanity P. Unstable fractures of the pelvic ring. *J Bone Joint Surg* 1992; 74A:781–791.
142. Kurosaka M, Yoshiya S, Mizuno T, et al. Spontaneous healing of a tear of the anterior cruciate ligament. *J Bone Joint Surg* 1998;80A:1200–1203.
143. Nepola J, Trenhaile S, Miranda M, et al. Vertical shear injuries: Is there a relationship between residual displacement and functional outcome? *J Trauma* 1999;46: 1024–1030.
144. Hwang S, Ahn J. Bilateral fracture-dislocation of the sacroiliac joint: A case report. *J Orthop Trauma* 1991;31:299–300.
145. LaFollette B, Levine M, McNiesh. Bilateral fracture-dislocation of the sacrum. A case report. *J Bone Joint Surg* 1986;68A:1099–1101.
146. Marcus R, Hansen S Jr. Bilateral fracture-dislocation of the sacrum. A case report. *J Bone Joint Surg* 1984;66A:1297–1299.
147. Räf L. Double vertical fractures of the pelvis. *Acta Chir Scand* 1966;131:298–305.
148. Dujardin F, Hossenbaccus M, Duparc F, et al. Long-term functional prognosis of posterior injuries in high-energy pelvic disruption. *J Orthop Trauma* 1998;12:145–151.
149. Miranda M, Riemer B, Butterfield S, et al. Pelvic ring injuries. A long term functional outcome study. *Clin Orthop Rel Res* 1996;329:152–159.
150. Lieberman I, Webb J. Cervical spine injuries in the elderly. *J Bone Joint Surg* 1994;76B: 877–881.
151. Spivak J, Weiss M, Cotler J, et al. Cervical spine injuries in patients 65 and older. *Spine* 1994;19:2302–2306.
152. Slucky A, Eismont F. Treatment of acute injury of the cervical spine. *J Bone Joint Surg* 1994;76A:1882–1896.
153. Beyer C, Cabanela M, Berquist T. Unilateral facet dislocations and fracture-dislocations of the cervical spine. *J Bone Joint Surg* 1991;73B:977–981.
154. Brunette D, Rockswold G. Neurologic recovery following rapid spinal realignment for complete cervical spinal cord injury. *J Trauma* 1987;27:445–447.
155. Cotler H, Miller L, DeLucia F, et al. Closed reduction of cervical spine dislocations. *Clin Orthop Rel Res* 1987;214:185–199.
156. Lee A, MacLean J, Newton D. Rapid traction for reductions of cervical spine dislocations. *J Bone Joint Surg* 1994;76B:352–356.

157. Mirza S, Krengel W, Chapman J, et al. Early versus delayed surgery for acute cervical spinal cord injury. *Clin Orthop Rel Res* 1999;359:104–114.
158. Sabiston C, Wing P, Schweigel J, et al. Closed reduction of dislocations of the lower cervical spine. *J Trauma* 1988;28:832–835.
159. Star A, Jones A, Cotler J, et al. Immediate closed reduction of cervical spine dislocations using traction. *Spine* 1990;15:1068–1072.
160. Bosch A, Stauffer S, Nickel V. Incomplete traumatic quadriplegia. A ten-year review. *JAMA* 1971;216:473–478.
161. Merriam W, Taylor T, Ruff S, et al. A reappraisal of acute traumatic central cord syndromes. *J Bone Joint Surg* 1986;68B:708–713.
162. Scher A. Hyperextension trauma in the elderly: an easily overlooked spinal injury. *J Trauma* 1983;23:1066–1068.
163. Eismont F, Arena M, Green B. Extrusion of an intervertebral disc associated with traumatic subluxation or dislocation of cervical facets. *J Bone Joint Surg* 1991;73A:1555–1560.
164. Fried L. Cervical spinal cord injury during skeletal traction. *JAMA* 1974;229:181–183.
165. Gruenberg M, Rechtine G, Chrin A, et al. Overdistraction of cervical spine injuries with the use of skull traction: A report of two cases. *J Trauma* 1997;42:1152–1156.
166. Ishida Y, Tominaga T. Predictors of neurologic recovery in acute central cervical cord injury with only upper extremity impairment. *Spine* 2002;27:1652–1658.
167. Broom M, Raycroft J. Complications of fractures of the cervical spine in ankylosing spondylitis. *Spine* 1988;13:763–766.
168. Graham B, Van Peteghem P. Fractures of the spine in ankylosing spondylitis. Diagnosis, treatment, and complications. *Spine* 1989;14:803–807.
169. Hunter T, Dubo H. Spinal fractures complicating ankylosing spondylitis. *Arthritis Rheum* 1983;26:751–759.
170. Schwartz M, Fazl M. A conservative philosophy in the management of cervical fractures. *Orthopaedics* 1992;15:303–305.
171. Bucci M, Dauser R, Maynard F, et al. Management of post-traumatic cervical spine instability: operative fusion versus halo vest immobilization. Analysis of 49 cases. *J Trauma* 1988;28:1001–1006.
172. Garfin S, Bottle M, Waters R, et al. Complications in the use of the halo fixation device. *J Bone Joint Surg* 1986;68A:320–325.
173. Johnson R, Owen J, Hart D, et al. Cervical orthoses. A guide to their selection and use. *Clin Orthop Rel Res* 1981;154:134–145.
174. Rockswold G, Bergman T, Ford S. Halo immobilization and surgical fusion: relative indications and effectiveness in the treatment of 140 cervical spine injuries. *J Trauma* 1990;30:893–898.
175. Whitehill R, Richman J, Glaser J. Failure of immobilization of the cervical spine by the halo vest. *J Bone Joint Surg* 1986;68A:326–332.
176. Pepin J, Bourne R, Hawkins R. Odontoid fractures, with special reference to the elderly patient. *Clin Orthop Rel Res* 1985;193:178–183.
177. Schatzker J, Rorabeck C, Waddell J. Non-union of the odontoid process. *Clin Orthop Rel Res* 1975;108:127–137.
178. Polin RS, Szabo T, Bogaev CA, et al. Nonoperative management of types II and III odontoid fractures: the Philadelphia collar versus the halo vest. *Neurosurgery* 1996;38:450–457.
179. Stoney J, O'Brien J, Wilde P. Treatment of type-two odontoid fractures in halothoracic vests. *J Bone Joint Surg* 1998;80B:452–455.
180. Wang G, Mabie K, Whitehill R, et al. The nonsurgical management of odontoid fractures in adults. *Spine* 1984;9:229–230.
181. Hart R, Saterbak A, Clark C. Nonoperative management of dens fracture nonunion in elderly patients without myelopathy. *Spine* 2000;25:1339–1343.
182. Saboe L, Reid D, Davis L, et al. Spine trauma and associated injuries. *J Trauma* 1991;31:43–48.
183. Riggins R, Kraus J. The risk of neurologic damage with fractures of the vertebrae. *J Trauma* 1977;17:126–133.
184. Griffith H, Gleave J, Taylor R. Changing patterns of fracture in the dorsal and lumbar spine. *Br Med J* 1966;1:891–894.
185. Fornasier V, Czitrom A. Collapsed vertebrae. A review of 659 autopsies. *Clin Orthop Relat Res* 1978;131:261–269.
186. Gershon-Cohen J, Rechtman A, Schraer H, et al. Asymptomatic fractures in osteoporotic spines of the aged. *JAMA* 1953;153:625–627.
187. Härmä M, Heliövaara M, Aromaa A, et al. Thoracic spine compression fractures in Finland. *Clin Orthop Rel Res* 1986;205:188–194.
188. Aglietti P, DiMuria G, Taylor T, et al. Conservative treatment of thoracic and lumbar vertebral fractures. *Ital J Orthop Trauma* 1983;9:83–105.
189. Rhyne A III, Banit D, Laxer E, et al. Kyphoplasty: Report of eighty-two thoracolumbar osteoporotic vertebral fractures. *J Orthop Trauma* 2004;18:294–299.
190. Yu SW, Lee PC, Ma CH, et al. Vertebroplasty for the treatment of osteoporotic compression spinal fracture: Comparison of remedial action at different stages of injury. *J Trauma* 2004;56:629–632.
191. Harrington K. Major neurological complications following percutaneous vertebroplasty with polymethylmethacrylate. *J Bone Joint Surg* 2001;83:1070–1073.
192. Bohlman H. Treatment of fractures and dislocations of the thoracic and lumbar spine. *J Bone Joint Surg* 1985;67A:165–169.
193. Bohlman H, Freehafer A, Dejak J. The results of treatment of acute injuries of the upper thoracic spine with paralysis. *J Bone Joint Surg* 1985;67A:360–369.
194. Krompinger W, Fredrickson B, Mino D, et al. Conservative treatment of fractures of the thoracic and lumbar spine. *Orthop Clin North Am* 1986;17:161–170.
195. Berns D, Blaser S, Modic M. Magnetic resonance imaging of the spine. *Clin Orthop Rel Res* 1989;244:78–86.
196. Denis F, Armstrong G, Searls K, et al. Acute thoracolumbar burst fractures in the absence of neurologic deficit. A comparison between operative and nonoperative treatment. *Clin Orthop Rel Res* 1984;189:142–149.
197. McAfee P, Yuan H, Fredrickson B, et al. The value of computed tomography in thoracolumbar fractures. *J Bone Joint Surg* 1983;65A:461–473.
198. Dall B, Stauffer S. Neurologic injury and recovery patterns in burst fractures at the T12 or L1 motion segment. *Clin Orthop Rel Res* 1988;233:171–176.
199. Gertzbein S, Court-Brown C, Marks P, et al. The neurological outcome following surgery for spinal fractures. *Spine* 1988;13:641–643.
200. Gertzbein S, Offierski C. Complete fracture-dislocation of the thoracic spine without spinal cord injury. *J Bone Joint Surg* 1979;61A:449–451.
201. Harryman D. Complete fracture-dislocation of the thoracic spine associated with spontaneous neurologic decompression. *Clin Orthop Rel Res* 1986;207:64–69.
202. McEvoy R, Bradford D. The management of burst fractures of the thoracic and lumbar spine. *Spine* 1985;10:631–637.
203. Simpson A, Williamson D, Golding S, et al. Thoracic spine translocation without cord injury. *J Bone Joint Surg* 1990;72B:80–83.
204. Limb D, Shaw D, Dickson R. Neurological injury in thoracolumbar burst fractures. *J Bone Joint Surg* 1995;77B:774–777.
205. Johnsson R, Herrlin K, Hägglund G, et al. Spinal canal remodeling after thoracolumbar fractures with intraspinal bone fragments. *Acta Orthop Scand* 1977;62:125–127.
206. Black W, Welch H. Advances in diagnostic imaging and overestimations of disease prevalence and the benefits of therapy. *N Engl J Med* 1993;328:1237–1243.
207. Nicoll E. Fractures of the dorso-lumbar spine. *J Bone Joint Surg* 1949;31:376–387.
208. Chan D, Sent N, Kaan K. Nonoperative treatment in burst fractures of the lumbar spine (L2–L5) without neurologic deficits. *Spine* 1993;18:320–325.
209. Knight R, Stornelli D, Chan D, et al. Comparison of operative versus nonoperative treatment of lumbar burst fractures. *Clin Orthop Rel Res* 1993;293:112–121.
210. Young M. Long-term consequences of stable fractures of the thoracic and lumbar vertebral bodies. *J Bone Joint Surg* 1973;55B:295–300.
211. Day B, Kokan P. Compression fractures of the thoracic and lumbar spine from compensable injuries. *Clin Orthop Rel Res* 1977;124:173–176.
212. Hazel W, Jones R, Morrey B, et al. Vertebral fractures without neurological deficit. *J Bone Joint Surg* 1988;70A:1319–1321.
213. Kraemer W, Schemitsch E, Lever J, et al. Functional outcome of thoracolumbar burst fractures without neurological deficit. *J Orthop Trauma* 1996;10:541–544.
214. Weinstein J, Collalto P, Lehmann T. Thoracolumbar "burst" fractures treated conservatively: A long-term follow-up. *Spine* 1988;13:33–38.
215. McAfee P, Bohlman H. Complications following Harrington instrumentation for fractures of the thoracolumbar spine. *J Bone Joint Surg* 1985;67A:672–686.
216. Meyer P Jr, Cotler H, Gireesan G. Operative neurological complications resulting from thoracic and lumbar spine internal fixation. *Clin Orthop Rel Res* 1988;237:125–131.
217. Stauffer S. Current concepts review. Internal fixation of fractures of the thoracolumbar spine. *J Bone Joint Surg* 1984;66A:1136–1138.
218. Gaines R, Humphreys W. A plea for judgment in management of thoracolumbar fractures and fracture-dislocations. *Clin Orthop Rel Res* 1984;189:36–42.
219. Weitzman G. Treatment of stable thoracolumbar spine compression fractures by early ambulation. *Clin Orthop Rel Res* 1971;76:116–122.
220. Weinstein J, Collalto P, Lehmann T. Long-term follow-up of nonoperatively treated thoracolumbar spine fractures. *J Orthop Trauma* 1987;1:152–159.
221. Kupferschmid J, Weaver M, Raves J, et al. Thoracic spine injuries in victims of motorcycle accidents. *J Trauma* 1989;29:593–598.
222. Weber S, Sutherland G. An unusual rotational fracture-dislocation of the thoracic spine without neurologic sequelae internally fixed with a combined anterior and posterior approach. *J Trauma* 1986;26:474–479.
223. Andreychik D, Alander D, Senica K, et al. Burst fractures of the second through fifth lumbar vertebrae. *J Bone Joint Surg* 1996;78A:1156–1165.
224. Mumford J, Weinstein J, Spratt K, et al. Thoracolumbar burst fractures. The clinical efficacy and outcome of nonoperative management. *Spine* 1993;18:955–970.
225. Reid R, Hu R, Davis L, et al. The nonoperative treatment of burst fractures of the thoracolumbar junction. *J Trauma* 1988;28:1188–1193.
226. Vanichkachorn JS, Vaccaro AR. Nonoperative treatment of thoracolumbar fractures. *Orthopaedics* 1997;20:948–955.
227. An H, Simpson M, Ebraheim N, et al. Low lumbar burst fractures: comparison between conservative and surgical treatments. *Orthopaedics* 1992;15:367–373.
228. Bradford D, McBride G. Surgical management of thoracolumbar spine fractures with incomplete neurologic deficits. *Clin Orthop Rel Res* 1987;218:201–215.
229. Wood K, Butterman G, Mehbod A, et al. Operative compared with nonoperative treatment of a thoracolumbar burst fracture without neurological deficit. A prospective, randomized study. *J Bone Joint Surg* 2003;85-A:773–781. Erratum in: *J Bone Joint Surg Am* 2004;86-A:1283.
230. Alms M. Fracture mechanics. *J Bone Joint Surg* 1961;43B:162–166.
231. Brook D, Burstein A, Frankel V. The biomechanics of torsional fractures. *J Bone Joint Surg* 1970;52A:507.
232. Connolly J. Torsional fractures and the third dimension of fracture management. *S Med J* 1980;73:884–891.
233. Sarmiento A, Latta L, Zilioli A, et al. The role of soft tissues in stabilization of tibial fractures. *Clin Orthop Rel Res* 1974;105:116–129.
234. Esposito P, Alexander A, Lichtman D. Delayed overdistraction of a surgically treated thoracolumbar fracture. *Spine* 1985;10:393–396.
235. Bonar S, Marsh JL. Unilateral external fixation for severe pilon fractures. *Foot Ankle* 1993;14:57–64.
236. Clancey G. Percutaneous Kirschner-wire fixation of Colles fractures: a prospective study of thirty cases. *J Bone Joint Surg* 1984;66A:1008–1014.

237. Tornetta P, Weiner L, Bergman M, et al. Pilon fractures: treatment with combined internal and external fixation. *J Orthop Trauma* 1993;7:489–496.
238. Peltier L. A brief history of traction. *J Bone Joint Surg* 1968;50A:1603–1617.
239. Mubarak S, Carroll N. Volkmann's contracture in children: aetiology and prevention. *J Bone Joint Surg* 1979;61B:285–293, 1979.
240. Mustard W, Simmons E. Experimental arterial spasm in the lower extremities produced by traction. *J Bone Joint Surg* 1953;35B:437–441.
241. Atkins R, Duckworth T, Kanis J. Features of algodystrophy after Colles' fracture. *J Bone Joint Surg* 1990;72B:105–110.
242. Hawkins B, Bays P. Catastrophic complication of simple cast treatment: case report. *J Trauma* 1993;34:760–762.
243. Connolly J. *Fractures and dislocations—closed management.* Philadelphia: WB Saunders. 1995:731–745.
244. Connolly J, Csencsitz T. Limb threatening neuropathic complications from ankle fractures in patients with diabetes. *Clin Orthop Rel Res* 1998;348:212–219.
245. Lavalette R, Pope M, Dickstein H. Setting temperatures of plaster casts. *J Bone Joint Surg* 1982;64A:907–911.
246. Kaplan S. Burns following application of plaster splint dressings. Report of two cases. *J Bone Joint Surg* 1981;63A:670–672.
247. Malkin L. Reflex sympathetic dystrophy syndrome following trauma to the foot. *Orthopaedics* 1990;13:851–858.
248. Poplawski Z, Wiley A, Murray J. Post-traumatic dystrophy of the extremities. *J Bone Joint Surg* 1983;65A:642–655.
249. Leach R. New fiber glass casting system. *Clin Orthop Rel Res* 1974;103:109–117.
250. Wytch R, Mitchell C, Ritchie I, et al. New splinting materials. *Prosthet Orthot Int* 1987; II:42–45.
251. Currey J. The mechanical properties of bone. *Clin Orthop Rel Res* 1970;73:210–231.
252. Freeman J, Weaver J, Oden R, et al. Changing patterns in tibial fractures resulting from skiing. *Clin Orthop Rel Res* 1987;216:19–23.
253. Yamada H. *Strength of biological materials.* Baltimore: Williams & Wilkins, 1970.
254. Böstman O. Spiral fractures of the shaft of the tibia. *J Bone Joint Surg* 1986;68B:462–466.
255. Hsien-Chih F, Yun-Wu K, T'ien-Yü S. The integration of modern and traditional chinese medicine in the treatment of fractures. *Chin Med J* 1963;82:493–504, 1963.
256. Shang T, Gu Y, Dong F. Treatment of forearm bone fractures by an integrated method of traditional Chinese and Western medicine. *Clin Orthop Rel Res* 1987;215:56–63.
257. Anderson L. Compression plate fixation and the effect of different types of internal fixation on fracture healing. *J Bone Joint Surg* 1965;47A:191–208.
258. Sarmiento A, Cooper J, Sinclair W. Forearm fractures, early functional bracing: a preliminary report. *J Bone Joint Surg* 1975;57A:297–304.
259. Beaupré G, Csongradi J. Refracture risk after plate removal in the forearm. *J Orthop Trauma* 1996;10:87–92.
260. Langkamer V, Ackroyd C. Internal fixation of forearm fractures in the 1980's: lessons to be learnt. *Injury* 1991;22:97–102.
261. Langkamer V, Ackroyd C. Removal of forearm plates. A review of the complications. *J Bone Joint Surg* 1990;72B:601–604.
262. Rosson J, Shearer J. Refracture after the removal of plates from the forearm. *J Bone Joint Surg* 1991;73B:415–417.
263. Naumark A, Kossoff, Leach R. The disparate diameter: sign of rotational deformity in fractures. *J Can Assoc Radiol* 1983;34:8–11.
264. Matthews L, Kaufer H, Garver D, et al. The effect of supination-pronation of angular malalignment of fractures of both bones of the forearm. *J Bone Joint Surg* 1982;64A: 14–17.
265. Schemitsch E, Richards R. The effect of malunion on functional outcome after plate fixation of fractures of both bones of the forearm in adults. *J Bone Joint Surg* 1992;74A: 1068–1078.
266. Jupiter J. Current concepts review fractures of the distal end of the radius. *J Bone Joint Surg* 1991;73A:461–469.
267. Cooney W III, Dobyns J, Linscheid R. Complications of Colles' fractures. *J Bone Joint Surg* 1980;62A:613–619.
268. Field J, Protheroe D, Atkins R. Algodystrophy after Colles' fracture is associated with secondary tightness of casts. *J Bone Joint Surg* 1994;76:901–905.
269. Edwards G. Intra-articular fractures of the distal part of the radius treated with the small AO external fixator. *J Bone Joint Surg* 1991;73A:1241–1250.
270. Howard P, Stewart H, Hind R, et al. External fixation or plaster for severely displaced comminuted Colles' fractures? *J Bone Joint Surg* 1989;71:68–33.
271. Kongsholm J, Olerud C. Plaster cast versus external fixation for unstable intraarticular Colles' fractures. *Clin Orthop Rel Res* 1989;241:57–65.
272. McQueen M. Redisplaced unstable fractures of the distal radius. *J Bone Joint Surg* 1998; 80B:665–669.
273. Weber S, Szabo R. Severely comminuted distal radial fractures as an unsolved problem: Complications associated with external fixation and pins and plaster techniques. *J Hand Surg* 1986;11A:157–162.
274. James E, Hunter G. The dilemma of painful old os calcis fractures. *Clin Orthop Rel Res* 1983;177:112–115.
275. Crosby L, Fitzgibbons T. Computerized tomography scanning of acute intra-articular fractures of the calcaneus. *J Bone Joint Surg* 1990;72A:852–859.
276. Giachino A, Uhthoff H. Intra-articular fractures of the calcaneus. *J Bone Joint Surg* 1989; 71A:784–786.
277. Stephenson J. Displaced fractures of the os calcis involving the subtalar joint: the key role of the superomedial fragment. *Foot Ankle* 1983;4:91–101.
278. Kitaoka H, Schaap E, Chao E, et al. Displaced intra-articular fractures of the calcaneus treated non-operatively. Clinical results and analysis of motion and ground-reaction and temporal forces. *J Bone Joint Surg* 1994;76A:1531–1540.
279. Mittlmeier T, Morlock M, Hertlein H, et al. Analysis of morphology and gait function after intraarticular calcaneal fracture. *J Orthop Trauma* 1993;7:303–310.
280. Kundel K, Funk E, Brutscher M, et al. Calcaneal fractures: operative versus nonoperative treatment. *J Trauma* 1996;41:839–845.
281. Parmar H, Triffitt P, Gregg P. Intra-articular fractures of the calcaneus treated operatively or conservatively. *J Bone Joint Surg* 1993;75B:932–937.
282. Folk J, Starr A, Early J. Early wound complications of operative treatment of calcaneus fractures: analysis of 190 fractures. *J Orthop Trauma* 1999;13:369–372.
283. Howard JL, Buckley R, McCormack R, et al. Complications following management of displaced intra-articular calcaneal fractures: A prospective randomized trial comparing open reduction internal fixation with nonoperative management. *J Orthop Trauma* 2003:17:241–249.
284. Court-Brown C, Boot D, Kellam J. Fracture dislocation of the calcaneus. *Clin Orthop Rel Res* 1986;213:201–206.
285. Sarmiento A, Gersten L, Sobol P, et al. Tibial shaft fractures treated with functional braces. Experience with 780 fractures. *J Bone Joint Surg* 1989;71B:602–609,
286. Teitz C, Carter D, Frankel V. Problems associated with tibial fractures with intact fibulae. *J Bone Joint Surg* 1980;62:770–775.
287. Haines J, Williams E, Hargadon E, et al. Is conservative treatment of displaced tibial shaft fractures justified? *J Bone Joint Surg* 1984;66:84–88.
288. Oni O, Hui A, Gregg P. The healing of closed tibial shaft fractures. The natural history of union with closed treatment. *J Bone Joint Surg* 1988;70B:787–790.
289. Brown P, Urban J. Early weight-bearing treatment of open fractures of the tibia: an end result of 63 cases. *J Bone Joint Surg* 1969;51A:59–75.
290. Dehne E. Treatment of fractures of the tibial shaft. *Clin Orthop Rel Res* 1969;66: 159–173.
291. Bone L, Sucato D, Stegemann P, et al. Displaced isolated fractures of the tibial shaft treated with either a cast or intramedullary nailing. *J Bone Joint Surg* 1997;79A: 1336–1341.
292. Hooper G, Keddell R, Penny I. Conservative management or closed nailing for tibial shaft fractures. *J Bone Joint Surg* 1991;73B:83–84.
293. Hohl M. *Tibial plateau fractures.* Philadelphia: WB Saunders, 1997:33–59.
294. Sarmiento A, Kinman P, Latta L, et al. Fractures of the proximal tibia and tibial condyles: a clinical and laboratory comparative study. *Clin Orthop Rel Res* 1979;145:136–145.
295. Rasmussen P. Tibial condylar fractures as a cause of degenerative arthritis. *Acta Orthop Scand* 1972;43:566–575.
296. Rasmussen P. Tibial condylar fractures: impairment of knee joint stability as an indication for surgical treatment. *J Bone Joint Surg Am* 1973;55:1331–1350.
297. Lansinger O, Bergman B, Korner L, et al. Tibial condylar fractures. A twenty-year follow-up. *J Bone Joint Surg* 1986;68A:13–19.
298. Lobenhoffer P, Schulze M, Gerich T, et al. Closed reduction/percutaneous fixation of tibial plateau fractures: arthroscopic versus fluoroscopic control of reduction. *J Orthop Trauma* 1999;13:426–431.
299. Koval K, Sanders R, Borrelli J, et al. Indirect reduction and percutaneous screw fixation of displaced tibial plateau fractures. *J Orthop Trauma* 1992;6:340–346.
300. Küntscher G. The Küntscher method of intramedullary fixation. *J Bone Joint Surg* 1958; 40A:17–46.
301. Hardy A. The treatment of femoral fractures by cast-brace application and early ambulation. *J Bone Joint Surg* 1983;65:56–65.
302. Bucholz R, Ross S, Lawrence K. Fatigue fracture of the interlocking nail in the treatment of fractures of the distal part of the femoral shaft. *J Bone Joint Surg* 1987;69A: 1391–1399.
303. Gates D, Alms M, Molina Cruz M. Hinged cast and roller traction for fractured femur. A system of treatment for the third world. *J Bone Joint Surg* 1985;67B:750–756.
304. Mooney V, Connolly J, Johnson K, et al. Fractures of the distal femur. *AAOS Instr Course Lect* 1987;36:427–454.
305. Mooney V, Nickel V, Harcey J, et al. Cast-brace treatment for fractures of the distal part of the femur: a prospective controlled study of 150 patients. *J Bone Joint Surg* 1970;52A:1563–1578.
306. Tile M. Fractures of the acetabulum. *Rockwood and Green's fractures in adults*, vol 2. Philadelphia: Lippincott, 1996:617–619.
307. Phen H, Kumar N, Ireland J. Bilateral central dislocation of the hip following a cerebrovascular accident. *J Bone Joint Surg* 1989;71B:703.
308. Spencer R. Acetabular fractures in older patients. *J Bone Joint Surg* 1989;71B:774–776.
309. Törnkvist H, Schatzker J. Acetabular fractures in the elderly: An easily missed diagnosis. *J Orthop Trauma* 1993;7:233–235.
310. Letournel E. Acetabular fractures: Classification and management. *Clin Orthop Rel Res* 1980;151:81–106.
311. Russell G, Nork S, Routt ML, Perioperative complications associated with operative treatment of acetabular fractures. *J Trauma* 2001;51:1098–1103.
312. Tornetta P III. Displaced acetabular fractures: Indications for operative and nonoperative management. *J Am Acad Orthop Surg* 2001;9:18–28.
313. Rowe C, Lowell J. Prognosis of fractures of the acetabulum. *J Bone Joint Surg* 1961; 43A:30–59.
314. Lowell J. Bursting fractures of the acetabulum, involving the inner wall and superior dome. *AAOS Inst Course Lect* 1973;22:145–158.
315. Eichenholtz S, Stark R. Central acetabular fractures. A review of thirty-five cases. *J Bone Joint Surg* 1964;46A:695–713.
316. Göthlin G, Hindmarsh J. Central dislocation of the hip. The prognosis with conservative management. *Acta Orthop Scand* 1970;41:476–487.
317. Pecorelli F, Della Torre P. Fractures of the acetabulum: conservative treatment and results. *Ital J Orthop Trauma* 1987;13:307–318.
318. Tipton W, D'Ambrosia R, Ryle G. Non-operative management of central fracture dislocations of the hip. *J Bone Joint Surg* 1975;57A:888–893.

319. Heeg M, Oostvogel J, Klasen J. Conservative treatment of acetabular fractures: The role of the weight-bearing dome and anatomic reduction in the ultimate results. *J Trauma* 1987;27:555–559.
320. Heeg M, Otter N, Klasen H. Anterior column fractures of the acetabulum. *J Bone Joint Surg* 1992;74B:554–557.
321. Brumback R, Holt E, McBride M, et al. Acetabular depression fracture accompanying posterior fracture dislocation of the hip. *J Orthop Trauma* 1990;4:42–48.
322. Carnesale P, Stewart M, Barnes S. Acetabular disruption and central fracture-dislocation of the hip. *J Bone Joint Surg* 1975;57A:1054–1059.
323. Tornetta P III. Non-operative management of acetabular fractures. The use of dynamic stress views. *J Bone Joint Surg* 1999;81B:67–70.
324. Johnson J, Barrett A, Anderson C, et al. Roller traction: mobilizing patients with acetabular fractures. *Orthop Nurs* 1995;14:21–24.
325. Daum W, Scarborough M, Gordon W Jr, et al. Heterotopic ossification and other perioperative complications of acetabular fractures. *J Orthop Trauma* 1992;6:427–432.
326. Hull J, Raza S, Stockley I, et al. Surgical management of fractures of the acetabulum: The Sheffield experience 1976–1994. *Injury* 1997;28:35–40.
327. Kaempffe F, Bone L, Border J. Open reduction and internal fixation of acetabular fractures: heterotopic ossification and other complications of treatment. *J Orthop Trauma* 1991;5:439–445.
328. Skie M, Ebraheim N, Podeszwa D, et al. Infection following acetabular and pelvic fractures. *Orthopaedics* 1996;19:68–72.
329. Ylinen P, Santavirta S, Slätis P. Outcome of acetabular fractures: A 7-year follow-up. *J Trauma* 1989;29:19–24.
330. Gruen G, Mears D, Tauxe W. Distinguishing avascular necrosis from segmental impaction of the femoral head following an acetabular fracture: Preliminary report. *J Orthop Trauma* 1988;2:5–9.
331. Heeg M, Klasen H, Visser J. Operative treatment for acetabular fractures. *J Bone Joint Surg* 1990;72B:383–386.
332. Kebaish A, Roy A, Rennie W. Displaced acetabular fractures: Long-term follow-up. *J Trauma* 1991;31:1539–1542.
333. Thompson R, Oegema T, Lewis J, et al. Osteoarthrotic changes after acute transarticular load. *J Bone Joint Surg* 1991;73A:990–1001.
334. Upadhyay S, Moulton A, Srikrishnamurthy K. An analysis of the late effects of traumatic posterior dislocation of the hip without fractures. *J Bone Joint Surg* 1983;65B:150–152.
335. Wright R, Barrett K, Christie M, et al. Acetabular fractures: Long-term follow-up of open reduction and internal fixation. *J Orthop Trauma* 1994;8:397–403.
336. Sarmiento A, Mullis D, Latta L, et al. A quantitative comparative analysis of fracture healing under the influence of compression plating vs. closed weight-bearing treatment. *Clin Orthop Rel Res* 1980;149:232–239.
337. American Academy Orthopaedic Surgeons. Committee on Professional Liability. *Managing orthopaedic malpractice risk.* Chicago: American Academy of Orthopaedic Surgeons, 1996:9–16.
338. Heath C. How Abraham Lincoln dealt with a malpractice suit. *N Engl J Med* 1976;295: 735–736.
339. Perren S. Physical and biological aspects of fracture healing with special reference to internal fixation. *Clin Orthop Rel Res* 1979;138:175–196.
340. Takhano Y, Turner C, Owan I, et al. Elastic anisotropy and collagen orientation of osteonal bone are dependent on the mechanical strain distribution. *J Orthop Res* 1999; 17:59–66.
341. Olerud S, Karlström G. Tibial fractures treated by AO compression osteosynthesis. *Acta Orthop Scand Suppl* 1972;140:1–104.
342. Paavolainen P, Penttinen R, Slätis P, et al. The healing of experimental fractures by compression osteosynthesis: II. Morphometric and chemical analysis. *Acta Orthop Scand* 1979;50:375–383.
343. Croteau S, Rauch F, Silvestri A, Hamdy R. Bone morphogenetic proteins in orthopaedics: from basic science to clinical practice. *Orthopaedics* 1999;22:686–695.
344. Heckman J, Ryaby J, McCabe J, et al. Acceleration of tibial fracture-healing by non-invasive, low intensity pulsed ultrasound. *J Bone Joint Surg* 1994;76A:26–34.
345. Teideman J, Connolly J, Strates B, et al. Treatment of nonunion by percutaneous injection of bone marrow and demineralized bone matrix. *Clin Orthop Rel Res* 1991;268: 294–308.
346. Bruder S, Kurth A, Shea M, et al. Bone regeneration by implantation of purified, culture-expanded human mesenchymal stem cells. *J Bone Joint Surg* 1998;80A:156–162.
347. Connolly J. Clinical use of marrow osteoprogenitor cells to stimulate osteogenesis. *Clin Orthop Rel Res* 1998;355S:S257–S266.

PRINCIPLES OF INTERNAL FIXATION

Christian Krettek and Thomas Gösling

Hans Willenegger recognized the importance of judgment when considering the indications for operative treatment. He promoted excellence of treatment, whether it was operative or nonoperative. When the basic tenets of internal fixation are correctly observed, reliable and predictable outcome is attainable. Weber, defining the foundation for successful application of internal fixation, wrote: "Crucial to the success of these techniques (internal fixation) are (a) an appropriate indication, (b) observance of correct biomechanical principles, and (c) strict aseptic technique" (1). These critical elements form the basis of this chapter.

An improved understanding of the biologic changes associated with internal fixation has led to new philosophies and techniques. Both these new techniques and the conventional techniques of internal fixation are the basis for successful fracture treatment. The basic principles are explained in this chapter.

PREOPERATIVE PLANNING

Meticulous planning is of critical importance and often determines the outcome of the procedure. Successful planning considers not just the operation but the overall treatment concept. The more elective the operation, the more crucial the preoperative planning is. Emergency cases sometimes require immediate surgery and there is less time for planning. The key to preoperative planning is to produce an end result tailored to the needs of the patient. The next step is to analyze which factors will affect treatment. It must then be decided whether internal fixation (IF) is the most appropriate technique of stabilization. The surgeon should ask if the benefits of IF exceed its risks. If IF is chosen as the most appropriate technique to achieve these aims, the question then is whether a one-stage or multistage approach is required. The last step is the actual planning of the IF procedure.

Once the surgeon has defined the optimal end result, the patient's age, general health, profession, and activities must be taken into account. It is important to include the patient in the decision-making process. Aims that are too ambitious may not succeed. For example, below-knee amputation is a disabling procedure, but many patients do better following amputation than after extensive reconstruction (2). In the elderly, early full weight-bearing might be more important than meticulous anatomic reconstruction. Even with a lot of experience, it is often difficult to define the optimal end result for a particular patient.

Not only does soft tissue damage influence the treatment of open fractures, but the treatment of closed fractures as well depends on the degree of soft tissue damage. Closed fractures are usually classified according to Tscherne (see Fig. 52-2) (3). The correct classification of the soft tissue injury in closed fractures is considerably more difficult than in open fractures and requires a lot of experience. The degree of soft tissue injury determines both the timing of the operation and the type of fixation. Even severe closed soft tissue injuries are associated with increased rates of infection, wound healing problems, delayed union, and nonunion (4). Periosteal perfusion is also reduced with closed soft tissue injury (5). IF may represent an additional injury to already-traumatized soft tissues and might be harmful in the early phase; however, fracture instability may lead to further soft tissue damage.

Pathologic fractures due to benign or malignant tumors need special emphasis. The role of surgery often depends on the pathologic diagnosis (see Chap. 20). Special experience in the treatment of bone tumors is necessary and multidisciplinary treatment may be necessary for success. Fracture fixation without knowledge of the pathology can be hazardous, and in any fracture that may be pathologic, appropriate preoperative investigation is essential.

Indications for Internal Fixation

Even in the third millennium, the use of nonoperative treatment is still appropriate for certain types of fractures. The benefits of IF must be balanced against its associated risks. The main advantages of IF are precise restoration of the osseous anatomy and early mobilization with at least partial weight-bearing. The principal disadvantages are the increased risk of infection and the fact that healing may be impaired if this demanding technique is not used properly. Generally speaking, patients are more comfortable after IF than with cast treatment or external fixation.

Displaced intra-articular fractures are best treated by IF, as it is the only fixation method that allows anatomic restoration of the articular surface. Early joint motion is possible, with improvement in the range of movement and the condition of the articular cartilage. Even in the hands of experienced surgeons, displaced fractures of the diaphysis are often unstable after closed reduction and the application of a cast. Comminuted fractures are not suitable for nonoperative treatment. Some fractures, such as displaced fractures of the femoral neck, the femoral head, or the talus, require immediate compression osteosynthesis to reduce the risk of osteonecrosis (6,7). Increasingly, many patients elect to have IF even for nondisplaced fractures, as they may return to their work or sporting activities at an earlier stage. Nevertheless, the decision to operate or not is often based on the surgeon's preference and experience.

Timing of Internal Fixation

The optimal timing for IF is a matter of opinion. In multiply injured patients, clear guidelines exist and are discussed in Chapter 3. Early fixation is also associated with reduced mortality in patients with proximal femoral fractures (8).

The extent of the soft tissue injury may also have a role in the timing of IF. The soft tissue damage associated with diaphyseal fractures is often of less concern because today, definitive immediate stabilization of open long bone fractures with intramedullary (IM) nails is a safe technique and is associated with better results than external fixation (9,10). Closed diaphyseal fractures can also be treated with primary IM nailing regardless of the degree of soft tissue damage (11,12). However, the situation is different in intra-articular fractures associated with significant soft tissue injury, which may require extensive operative treatment. To minimize the risk of infection in these cases, delayed fixation, after recovery of the soft tissues, is recommended. Two-stage or multiple-stage procedures might be necessary before definitive IF is done (13–16). Primary stabilization is usually achieved with a cast or by external fixation. Sometimes logistic problems such as an incomplete diagnosis, surgical inexperience, or inadequate operating facilities or time favor primary provisional stabilization and delayed IF. If primary IF is thought to be of risk to the patient, we use the following protocol for stabilization of complex intra-articular fractures. Immediate CT scan is not required. The surgeon must know which definitive fixation is required later. The patient is brought to the operating room and the stability of the ligaments is checked under anesthesia. An external fixator is applied to restore length and align the fracture as well as possible. The pins of the fixator should be placed appropriately, bearing in mind the need for later definitive IF. Ligamentotaxis is used to reduce the articular component. If closed reduction of the articular fracture is possible, percutaneous lag screw fixation is used. Lag screws should be placed so as not to interfere with later surgery. The patient is returned to the operating room for definitive stabilization when conditions are optimal. In the meantime, a CT scan should be performed. Undertaking the CT scan after primary fixation is advantageous in that the fragments are reduced and the fracture pattern is easier to understand. The position of the lag screws can also be assessed.

Infection Prophylaxis

The use of prophylactic antibiotics has been questioned over many years (17). A study in the early 1960s showed an increased prevalence of infection if antibiotic prophylaxis was used in clean cases (18). Intravenous antibiotic use in routine elective foot and ankle surgery has been shown to be ineffective as prophylaxis for wound infection (19), but today there is evidence that antibiotic prophylaxis reduces the incidence of infection in the treatment of closed fractures. This has been shown in two meta-analyses of randomized controlled trials (20,21). A single-shot application is as effective as multiple doses in preventing local infection. A large single-center randomized controlled trial reached the same conclusion that single-dose prophylaxis with a long-acting broad-spectrum antibiotic substantially reduces the incidence of wound infection and early nosocomial infection after surgery for closed fractures (22). The type of antibiotic may be adapted to the local conditions, but most studies favor second- or third-generation cephalosporins (20–22).

Most surgeons routinely use wound irrigation. This has been proven to be effective in reducing bacterial colonization and the rate of infection (23). Animal studies have shown that antiseptics are more effective than normal saline as an irrigating agent for eradicating germs from a contaminated orthopaedic wound (24). Prophylactic irrigation with antiseptics has been shown to be effective in animal models (25,26). However, the clinical use of antiseptics as prophylaxis remains unproven.

A meta-analysis investigating preoperative hair removal reported no strong evidence against preoperative hair removal, although there is good evidence that shaving should not be used for preoperative depilation. Instead, a depilatory cream or electric clippers, preferably applied immediately before surgery, should be used (27).

Tourniquet

The use of a tourniquet in fracture treatment is somewhat controversial. In the early years of the AO/ASIF, it was suggested that IF should be carried out using a tourniquet because in the absence of bleeding the surgeon might have a clearer view of the anatomic field. A tourniquet also resulted in reduced operating time (28) and reduced intraoperative blood loss (29,30). Animal studies have shown no delay in bone healing (31) if a tourniquet is used.

Nevertheless, the interruption of the blood supply leads to transient local ischemia. This ischemia might be less of a problem in elective musculoskeletal surgery (32). However, in fracture treatment the use of a tourniquet can be associated with postoperative complications. Limb reperfusion after tourniquet ischemia may cause pulmonary microvascular injury. In patients with a femoral fracture as an additional risk factor, the duration of ischemia associated with the use of a tourniquet has been shown to correlate with a longer ventilation time in the ICU (33). Higher incidences of infection have been found (28,34), and a relation with postoperative compartment syndrome has been described (34,35). In reamed nailing a tourniquet may be associated with an increased risk of thermal necrosis (36).

Pressure-related nerve injury might be induced by the application of a tourniquet, especially in the upper arm (37,38). Increased levels of postoperative pain have been reported after tourniquet application (39). The use of an Esmarch bandage to exsanguinate the operative field can lead to pulmonary embolism, especially in trauma patients in whom surgery is delayed (40,41). The actual requirement for a tourniquet in acute fracture treatment must always be considered.

Planning Techniques

The AO/ASIF group recommends preoperative drawings of all planned surgical procedures (42). This planning consists of two components. First, the desired end result is sketched on paper; second, the sequence of surgical procedures required to reach this end result is determined. The more complex the fracture and the fracture fixation techniques, the more important is meticulous preoperative planning.

Preoperative planning facilitates the understanding of a fracture. During the planning phase the surgical process can be repeated as many times as necessary until the surgeon has grasped the full magnitude of the problem and has found the best solution. Trial and error is allowed in the planning but not in the patient! Preoperative planning is especially useful in plate osteosynthesis. The type, shape, and length of the plate can be determined preoperatively. The placement of lag screws also needs detailed planning, which is best done before the skin incision is made. The optimal surgical approach can be chosen, and this prevents unnecessary soft tissue stripping or damage. Preoperative planning reduces the operative time, soft tissue trauma, and degree of disappointment.

The AO/ASIF technique of preoperative planning is based on two orthogonal plane x-rays. The necessary equipment includes tracing paper of good quality or overhead transparencies, colored felt-tipped pens, scissors, a set square or goniometer, an x-ray screen, and a set of relevant implant templates. Before starting the drawings the surgeon must carefully analyze the fracture on both orthogonal x-rays. CT scans are not necessary for the drawing, but they add a lot to the understanding of the morphology of the fracture and the fragments. Each bone fragment that will be included in the reconstruction should be drawn on a single piece of tracing paper to facilitate subsequent reconstruction of the fracture. Each fragment has a near and a far border on the two-dimensional film. The far border must be separately marked, whether by a different color or a dotted line.

There are different techniques to relocate the fragments in the correct position. Direct overlay of the tracing papers is possible with large fragments (Fig. 6-1). In multifragmentary fractures with comminution or defects, the direct overlay technique may be difficult. In these fractures the opposite side can be used as a template. However, this exposes the patient to additional radiation. Care has to be taken to use x-rays of the same size with identical rotation of the beam in relation to the bone. The normal side must be flipped horizontally to be used as a template (Fig. 6-2). The fragments can now be reassembled on the drawn template. Defects can be filled with specially marked bone graft. After reduction the implants used for fixation must be drawn. It is important to plan the exact position of the lag screws to prevent interference with other implants. After the drawing is completed, the main steps of the procedure should be consecutively detailed on the planning sheet. Today preoperative planning can be done with special software. This planning software can be used for corrective as well as acute surgery.

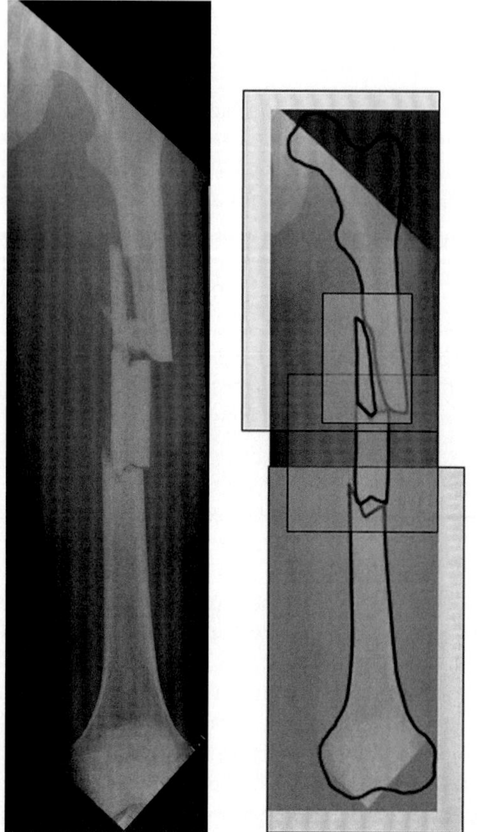

FIGURE 6-1 The direct overlay technique for preoperative planning using an AP view of a segmental femoral fracture as an example. **A.** The proximal fracture has a large butterfly fragment and some minor fragments that will not be reduced or fixed. The distal fracture is transverse. **B.** All fragments that will be reduced or fixed are traced on individual pieces of paper. (*continues*)

REDUCTION

Reduction reverses the process of fracture displacement and is the key to successful IF. After reduction it is essential to hold the reduction until secure fixation of the fracture has been performed. Anatomic reduction was one of the main principles of the AO/ASIF (43). This philosophy has changed somewhat over the past few decades, leading to a differentiation between intra- and extra-articular fractures. Nonanatomic reduction leads to changes in contact pressure of the cartilage in intra-articular fractures, and increased contact pressure predisposes to post-traumatic arthritis. There are no recommendations as to how much intra-articular step-off can be tolerated. The development of osteoarthritis depends not only on the degree of malreduction but also on other factors such as primary cartilage damage, age, whether the fracture is in the upper or lower extremity, the position of the fracture in the joint, and joint stability. Many authors accept a 2-mm intra-articular step-off. Nevertheless, the aim should be an anatomic reduction in intra-articular fractures. In extra-articular fractures the restoration of physiologic alignment and length is of highest priority. Malalignment can cause pain, osteoarthritis, loss of function, implant failure, and nonunion.

Fracture reduction must be performed as carefully as possible. Additional trauma to the soft tissues may result in impaired bone and wound healing and functional recovery in addition to an increased incidence of infection. With each attempted reduction, additional damage to the bone can occur. In the extreme case, a simple fracture can become a complex multifragmentary fracture, making reduction and fixation much more difficult. The use of reduction instruments can be dangerous, especially in osteoporotic bone.

There are two basic reduction techniques: open reduction and closed reduction.

Open Reduction

With open reduction, the fracture is exposed. The exact fit of the fragments can be checked by direct visualization and by palpation of the fracture edges either digitally or with palpation hooks. Interposed soft tissues or bony debris may impede anatomic reduction, and clearance of the fracture is one of the main advantages of open reduction. Usually the periosteum is torn at the fracture; if it lies between the bone ends, it needs to be removed.

Tissue clearance, or debridement, commences with meticulous removal of the periosteum from the fracture. This is done by sharp dissection. At most 1 mm of bone should be denuded of periosteum. Clearance of bony debris is done with a curette or a sharp hook. We also use a brush to clear off the fracture edges. It is advisable to use any spikes or sharp edges of the bone for orientation. In spiral fractures of the lateral malleolus, the distal fragment usually has a posterior bone spike. If this spike is fitted exactly to the corresponding proximal fragment, anatomic reduction is achieved.

Reduction of multiple fragments can be difficult and time-consuming and may have to be done sequentially. Preliminary fixation with Kirschner wires or a reduction forceps may be necessary before the next fragment can be brought into an anatomic position. Detached fragments should not be removed dur-

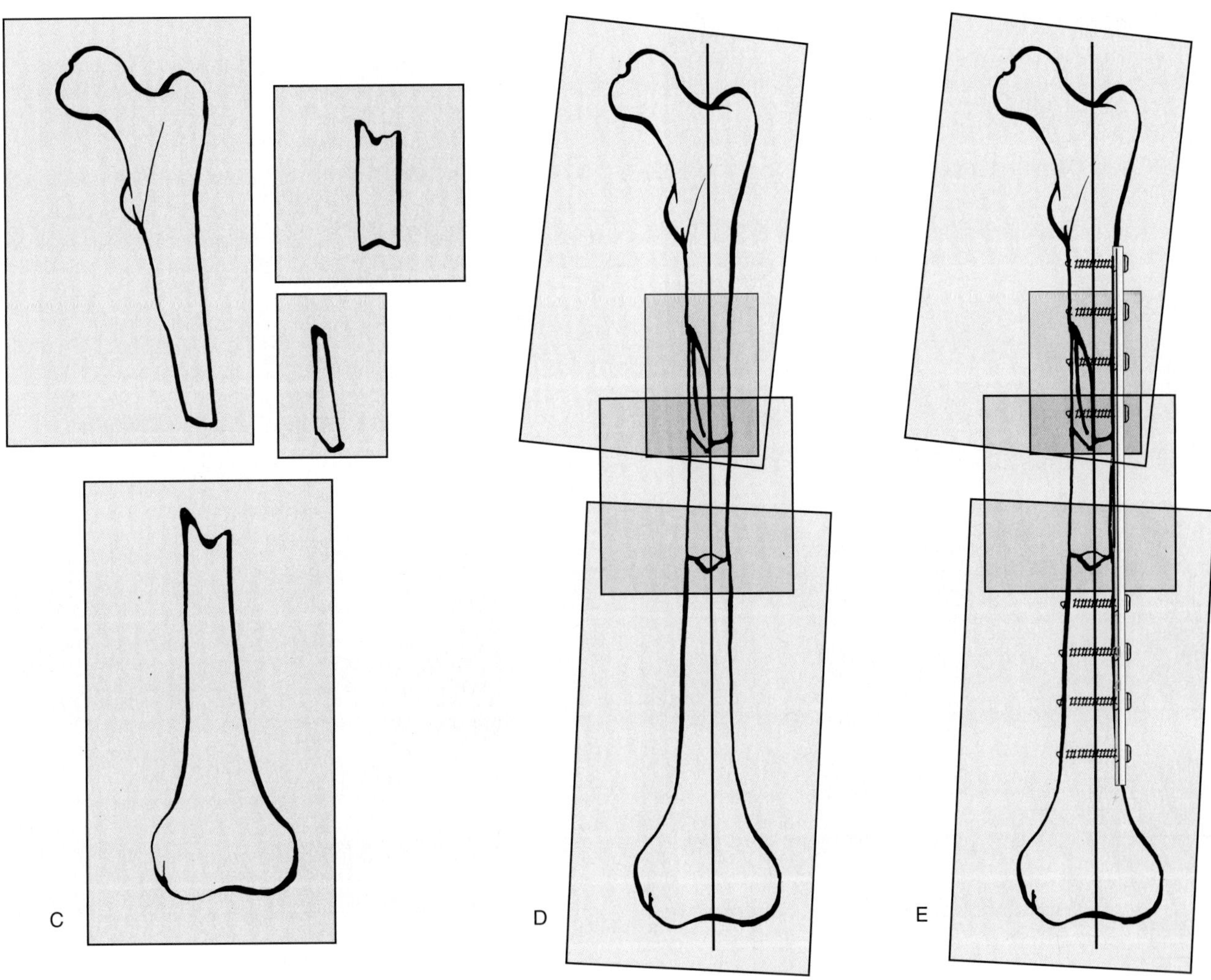

FIGURE 6-1 *(continued)* **C.** In this fracture, four fragments are traced. **D.** A straight line is drawn and the fragments are assembled on the axis. **E.** Percutaneous plating with indirect reduction and bridging plate osteosynthesis is planned. The butterfly fragment is reduced to the proximal main fragment prior to plate positioning. The length of the plate and the number of proximal and distal screws can be determined.

ing the debridement as they can be important to the reconstruction of comminuted fractures.

Closed Reduction

With closed reduction, the fracture remains covered by the surrounding soft tissues. Closed reduction is technically more demanding and cannot be achieved in all fractures. Direct control of reduction may be impeded by the soft tissues, and the surgeon must be familiar with a number of intraoperative reduction techniques (discussed below). The main advantage of closed reduction relates to the biology of the fracture. Secondary damage to the soft tissues with exposure of the fracture can be avoided. The fracture hematoma, with its osteogenic potential, is retained and fracture union is enhanced. The incidence of wound sepsis and deep infection is minimized. However, not all fractures can be reduced closed, and soft tissue interposition, bone debris, and comminution may mean that open reduction has to be undertaken.

Reduction Techniques

Soft Tissue Relaxation

Opposing soft tissue forces can make reduction difficult. In bones with a large surrounding musculature, like the femur, reduction can be particularly difficult to achieve and maintain. Relaxants given by the anesthesiologist can be of use, and appropriate positioning of the patient can also facilitate reduction. Subtrochanteric fractures are difficult to reduce because the proximal fragment is pulled anteriorly and medially by the iliopsoas muscle. This can be counteracted by lifting the upper part of the body. Distal femoral fractures are another example. The

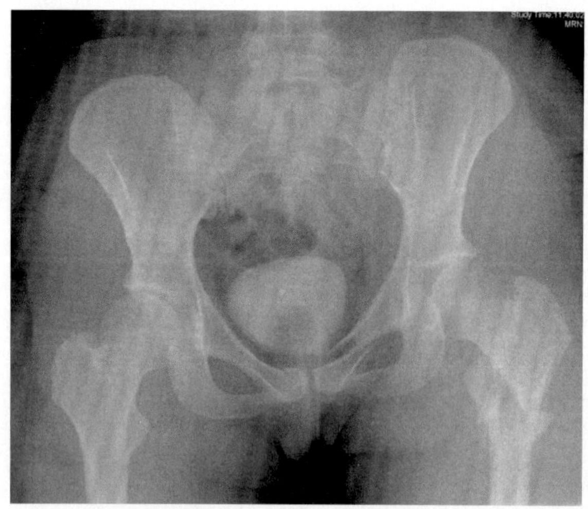

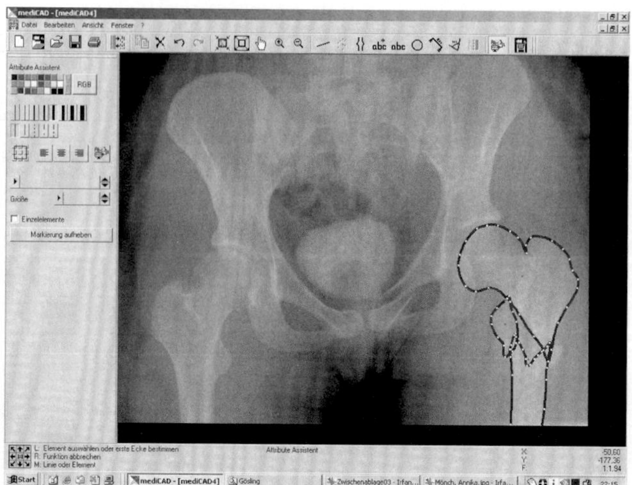

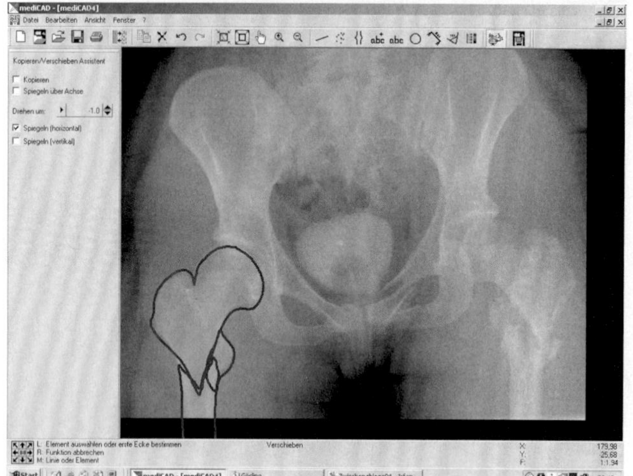

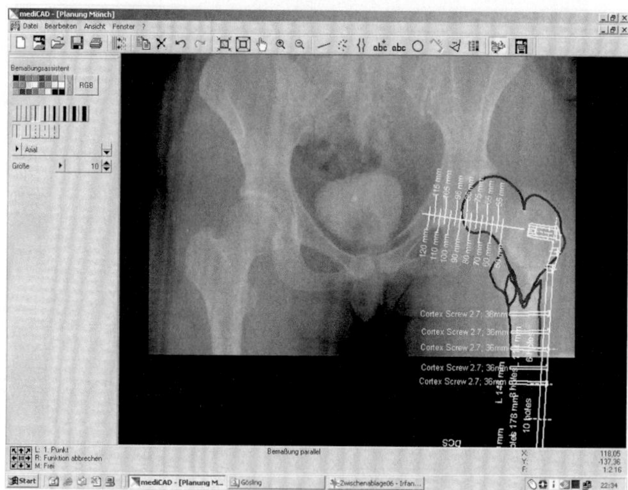

FIGURE 6-2 Overlay technique using the normal side as a template. The planning is done with special software. **A.** A multifragmentary fracture of the proximal femur in an 18-year-old girl. The first step is to upload and to calibrate the digital radiography. **B.** The main fragments are traced manually. **C.** Each fragment is reversed horizontally and matched with the opposite side using an overlay technique. **D.** All fragments are joined to one piece, which is reversed again and shifted to the injured side. The correct dimensions of implant can then be chosen. In this example use of an eight-hole dynamic compression screw with an 85-mm sliding screw and four distal cortical screws is planned.

gastrocnemius muscle pulls the distal fragment into recurvatum (Fig. 6-3). Bending the knee relaxes the muscle and eases reduction. Restoration of the length in femoral shaft fractures can be difficult due to the very strong iliotibial band. With traction along the axis of the shaft, the band tightens and prevents reduction. It is easier to restore the length of the femur in slight valgus alignment, which relaxes the iliotibial band. After the length is restored and both fracture ends are in contact, proper alignment can be restored.

Traction

Traction in the long axis of a bone is one of the most frequently used reduction techniques, especially in diaphyseal fractures associated with shortening. If the forces acting on a fracture are balanced, it may be possible to achieve reduction just with the application of traction. Ligamentotaxis is another method of reducing fractures by traction. With tensioning of the attached ligaments, the articular fragments return to their anatomic position. Ligamentotaxis is widely used for distal tibial and distal radial fractures. Traction can be applied manually, through a fracture table, or by using a distractor or external fixator (44,45).

"Simple Devices"

A number of very simple devices can be used to aid fracture reduction. A towel sling can be used to manipulate a large fragment noninvasively. In combination with an external device, this sling can gradually squeeze the fragment into the right alignment (Fig. 6-4). Simple towel support under a fragment can also

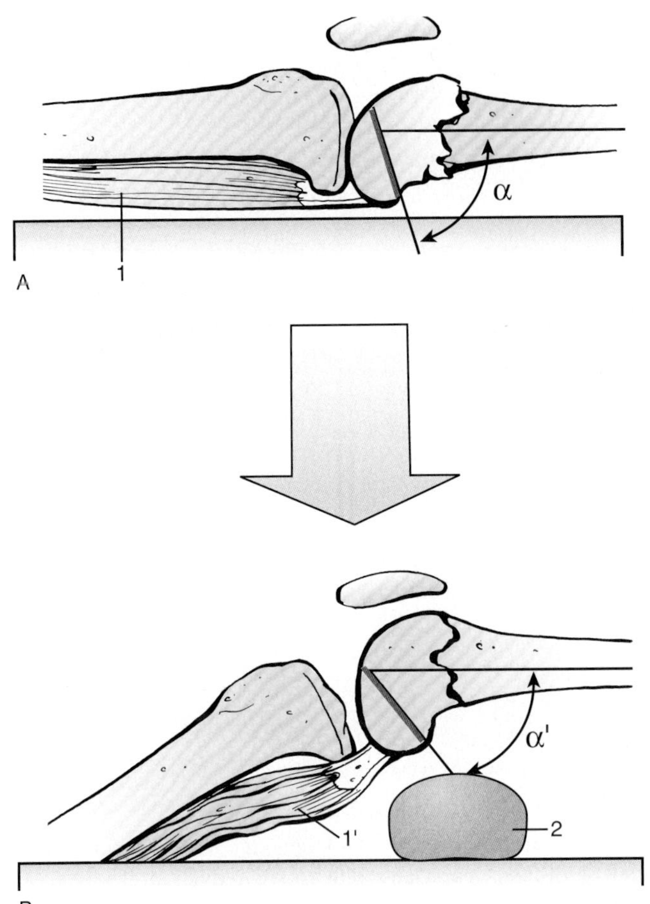

FIGURE 6-3 **A.** A distal femoral fracture has been pulled into recurvatum by gastrocnemius (1). **B.** Knee flexion over a pad (2) relaxes the gastrocnemius and allows fracture reduction. The angle ∝ is therefore altered.

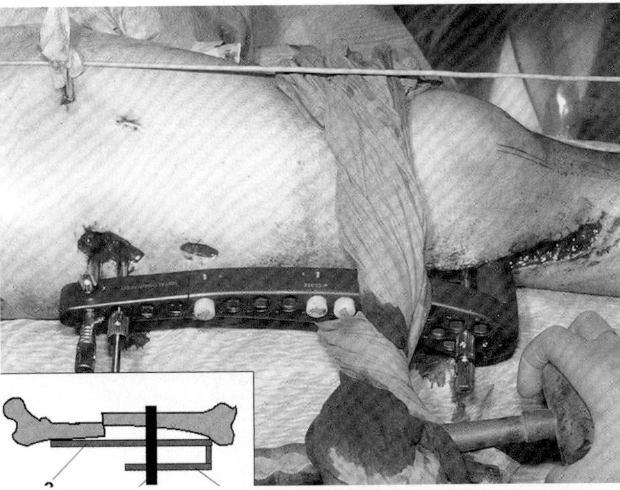

FIGURE 6-4 A distal femoral fracture that is being stabilized treated with the less invasive stabilizing system (LISS). As the towel is tightened, the distal fragment is pulled toward the insertion guide and the LISS plate. Note the cable above the knee, which is used to check the alignment.

align a fracture. A bone hook can manipulate fracture fragments either percutaneously or using an open technique. A hammer may be used to push against a fracture fragment or it can serve as a fulcrum to correct malalignment. An awl, with or without a ball-tip, is useful to push and hold small fragments in position. Cannulated awls allow the minimally invasive insertion of Kirschner wires and subsequent cannulated screw placement (46).

Reduction Forceps

Clamps are used to reduce and maintain fracture reduction. The pointed reduction forcep is probably the most commonly used clamp in fracture treatment. The forcep can be fixed to one single fragment, allowing its manipulation. It can also be used to manipulate two adjacent fragments simultaneously. The reduction forcep is engaged on each fragment. Slight rotational movements and compression of the forcep reduce the fragments. Traction by an assistant or slight pressure on a fragment can be helpful. Locking of the clamp holds the reduction (Fig. 6-5). The forcep should be used gently, as there is a risk of breaking one of the fragments by overenthusiastic manipulation, particularly if the bone is osteoporotic. Forceps or clamps are mainly used for oblique or spiral fractures. In transverse fractures it can be difficult to get a good grip, although a superfi-

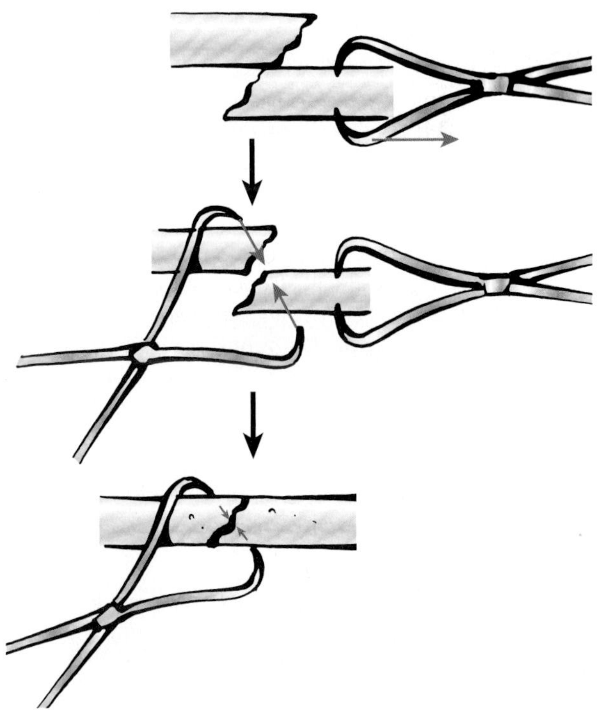

FIGURE 6-5 The technique of using two pointed reduction forceps in an oblique fracture. The first forcep fixes the distal fragment. Traction is then used to restore length. The second forcep is orientated perpendicular to the fracture line and compresses both fracture ends together. Gentle rotation of both clamps allows for an anatomic fit of the fracture edges.

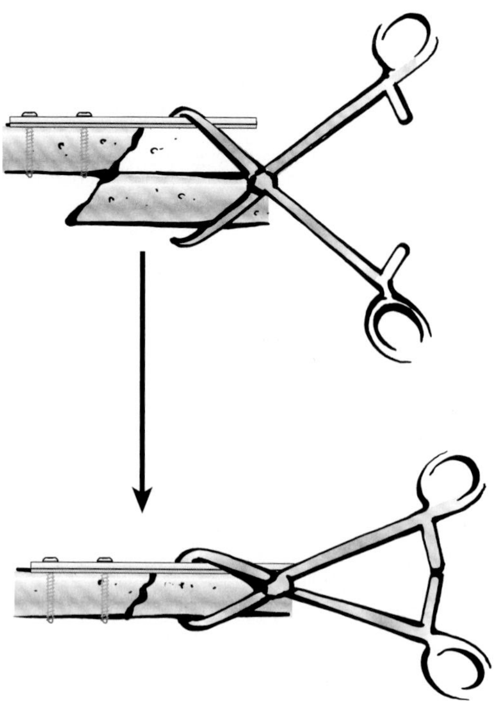

FIGURE 6-6 The serrated jaw can be used to reduce a fragment toward the plate. Traction is used to restore length. Closing of the jaw pushes the fragment toward the plate and holds the fragment in position.

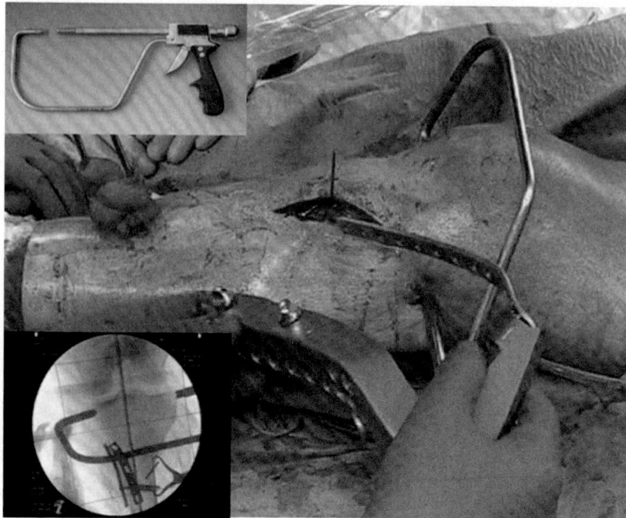

FIGURE 6-7 The collinear clamp. This clamp closes without any rotation. It can be of use in the distal femur and the proximal or distal tibia. The clamp is cannulated, permitting Kirschner wire insertion.

cial drill hole in the cortex can be used to improve fixation. Pointed reduction forceps can be used for open or closed reduction. In closed reduction they can be used percutaneously. Stab incisions should be used to minimize soft tissue damage.

Other useful reduction forceps are the reduction forceps with serrated jaws and the Verbrugge self-centering bone-holding forceps. Both can reduce and hold a plate onto a bone fragment (Fig. 6-6). These forceps are usually used with open reduction techniques. For closed reduction techniques, new instruments have been designed (Fig. 6-7). They allow percutaneous reduction of bone fragments or positioning and retention of plates. A wide range of special forceps are used in particular anatomic regions. Their use is largely dependent on the surgeon's preference.

Intrafocal Manipulation

Kapandji described a technique for Kirschner wire reduction and stabilization of distal radial fractures. The Kirschner wire is inserted percutaneously through the fracture line. Rotating the wire toward the distal mobile fragment results in distraction and volar tilting of the fragment (Fig. 6-8). Drilling the Kirschner wire in the opposite cortex stabilizes the fracture. This technique of reduction is applicable to other locations (47). If the Kirschner wires are too flexible, stronger reduction tools like a chisel can be used. For the reduction of diaphyseal fractures or the iliac wing, the use of a small Hohmann retractor is advised.

Joysticks

The manual manipulation of a fragment covered by soft tissue can be difficult, especially with closed reduction. The use of "joysticks" has been introduced to facilitate the reduction of femoral shaft fractures (48,49). These joysticks allow percutaneous manipulation of the fragments. In the femur, Schanz screws are most effective (Fig. 6-9). The temporarily inserted Schanz screw should be placed close to the fracture. The use of a universal T-handle attached to the screw facilitates the control of the screw and bone. The Schanz screw should not interfere with

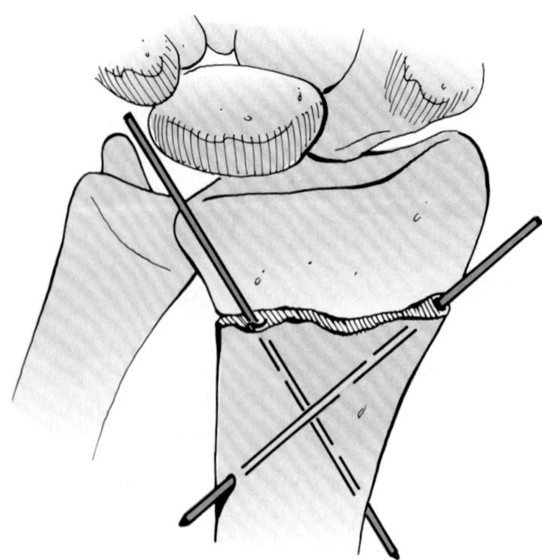

FIGURE 6-8 Kapandjii technique of intrafocal pinning of the distal radius.

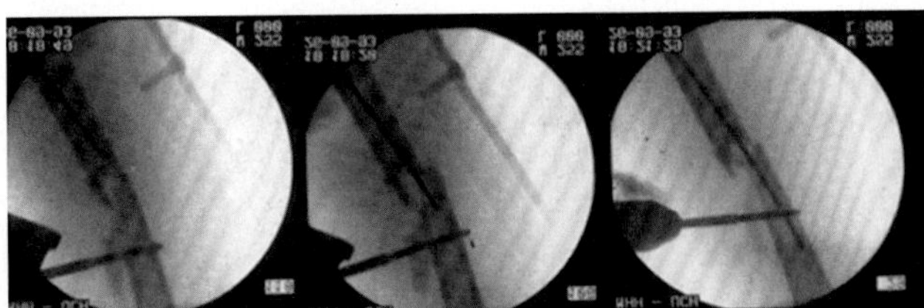

FIGURE 6-9 Sequence of reduction and guide wire insertion in a femoral shaft fracture with a Schanz screw placed in the distal femur. Note that the distal fragment is held in slight valgus to relax the iliotibial band. This valgus position facilitates the passage of the guide wire into the intramedullary canal.

the planned fixation technique. In IM nailing, any screw placed close to the nail insertion point must be intracortical to allow passage of the nail. If Schanz screws are placed in both fragments, the change of their relative positions gives information about the position of the fragments in relation to each other. Manipulation of the Schanz screws will also provide feedback about the position of the fragments. Taking these two points into account, the surgeon can reduce fluoroscopic control and radiation exposure.

Joysticks can be used not only for diaphyseal fractures but also for metaphyseal fractures and even intra-articular fractures. In fractures of the distal femur, the distal radius, or the proximal humerus, joysticks are especially useful for minimally invasive fracture reduction. The size of the joystick depends on the fragment size. Kirschner wires can be used for small fragments. The joysticks can be attached to an external fixator for temporary reduction or for definitive fracture stabilization (Fig. 6-10). Manipulation of intra-articular fragments can be done directly or through a cortical window.

Implants

All implants used for fixation interfere with bone. In some situations the implant can be used not only for fracture stabilization but also for fracture reduction. IM nails are an example of this. They are self-centering in the diaphyses of long bones. An anatomically shaped nail reduces the distal fragment in the sagittal and coronal planes when crossing the fracture, although this does not apply to fractures close to or within the metaphysis, as the widened intramedullary cavity does not permit it. A nail that is not inserted in line with the axis of the bone will produce malalignment. The distal fragment remains centered and lies in line with the nail but not with the proximal fragment.

Plates that exactly fit the anatomy of the broken bone can be used as a reduction tool. This technique is best applied in straight portions of the diaphysis of, for example, the femur, fibula, ulna, or humerus. The plate is fixed with one screw. The nonfixed fragment can be reduced toward the plate using a reduction forceps. This technique can also be used in curved bones or bone fragments, but this is more difficult and needs a lot of experience. If the plate is not contoured in an anatomic shape, malalignment will occur when pulling the fragment toward the plate.

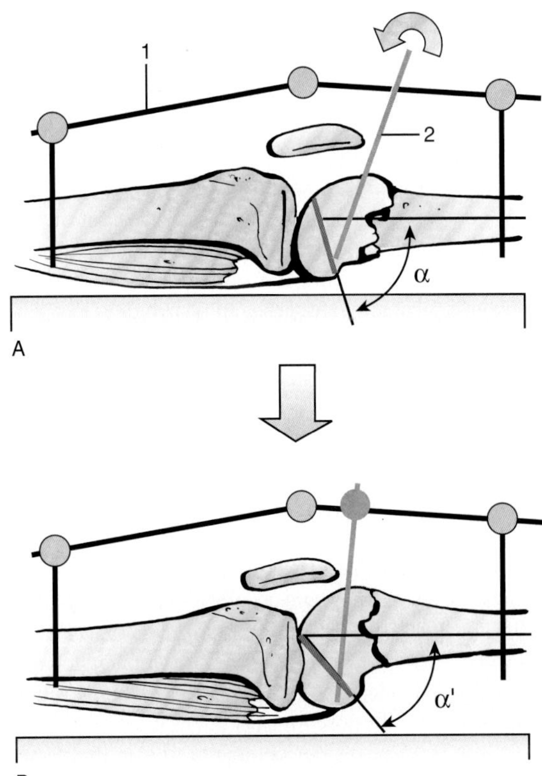

FIGURE 6-10 External femorotibial torsion. **A.** The distal fragment is hyperextended due to the pull of the gastrocnemius muscle. A Schanz screw (2) is inserted as a joystick into the distal fragment. **B.** The joystick is rotated caudally to correct the sagittal malalignment. The Schanz screw is then connected to the external fixator (1). Proper alignment for definitive fracture stabilization is achieved.

Others

Due to difficulties in reduction, multiple inventions are favored by some surgeons in certain situations. The use of a six-axis analysis deformity correction fixator is recommended for selected cases (50). This external fixator can reduce fractures very precisely. The reduction can be done gradually over several days or as a one-stage procedure. The reduction process is often time-consuming, and a lot of experience with the application of ring fixators is essential. The so-called LISS-tractor is a combination of a distractor with a locked screw device. The distractor is integrated into the plate and allows reduction against the plate before final fixation (51).

The AO/ASIF group invented a reduction table for fractures of the lower limb. This table acts as a combination of a fracture table and a distractor. It theoretically permits closed manipulation of the fragments in all six degrees of freedom. However, the device is not very useful. Possibly in the future robots might help to achieve and hold reduction (52)!

Reduction Control

In IF, maintenance of the correct reduction is difficult but essential. With open techniques the reduction can be checked directly by vision or palpation. With less and less invasive surgery being undertaken, other techniques to verify the reduction have become more important, as the incidence of malalignment has increased compared to open techniques (53,54). Intraoperative control is preferred to postoperative control. The threshold to correct malreduction during the primary procedure must be much lower if secondary surgery is to be avoided. Reoperation increases the risk of infection and prolongs rehabilitation time.

Imaging

Radiographic control is most frequently used for the assessment of reduction. It can be used before, during, and after surgery. X-rays in orthogonal planes are the standard imaging technique before and after surgery. During surgery, the use of x-rays can be both difficult and time-consuming. Therefore, if intraoperative x-rays are used, they are usually done at the end of an operation for documentation purposes.

Today fluoroscopy is mainly used for intraoperative imaging. The technique provides real-time visualization of the reduction process. However, fluoroscopy has some disadvantages. The quality of the pictures is poor compared to standard x-rays. It is two-dimensional, and superimposed structures may limit the validity of reduction assessment, particularly in intra-articular fractures. The fluoroscope can show only one plane during fracture reduction, and correct alignment in one plane does not guarantee or predict reduction in the other plane. Imaging of the second plane necessitates turning of the fluoroscope, the patient, or the limb; this risks a loss of reduction. Two orthogonal fluoroscopes may facilitate the control of reduction, but two fluoroscopes are not always available, and they may interfere with the surgical procedure. Another shortcoming of fluoroscopy is the limited field of imaging. Long bones cannot be visualized completely. The surgeon may get a wrong impression about the alignment. Another critical point is the radiation exposure to the patient and the operating staff. For minimally invasive fixation techniques, a duration of radiation exposure of more than 12 minutes has been reported (55,56). The surgeon has to take into account all the shortcomings of fluoroscopy, but today it is the most useful technique for intraoperative imaging.

CT is very valuable in the assessment of intra-articular fractures in different regions of the body (57–60). Steps and gaps are better detected than with conventional x-rays (61). Postoperative CT scans are most sensitive and specific in the detection of malreduction (62,63). It has been shown that a fairly high number of patients need revision surgery after a postoperative CT scan (64). Intraoperative control of reduction is therefore desirable, but usually the use of intraoperative CT scans is limited due to logistical and financial considerations (65,66).

The use of fluoroscopes that can visualize three-dimensional reformatted images looks promising for the intraoperative assessment of reduction. They can be use in a conventional two-dimensional mode or in a three-dimensional mode. With this technique it may be possible to detect and correct reduction anomalies during surgery (Fig. 6-11).

Arthroscopy

Arthroscopy-assisted fracture reduction was introduced in the early 1980s for fractures of the tibial plateau (67). It has been recommended for a number of different locations suitable for arthroscopy (68–71). Arthroscopy offers special advantages if ligaments or menisci are involved. The cartilage surface can be inspected and palpated. Due to the minimally invasive approach, functional results are improved (72). However, when compared to open reduction, the overall alignment may be less good (73). If the joint surface is extremely difficult to visualize despite an open approach, arthroscopic examination can be of use for the assessment of joint congruency. A good example is a calcaneus fracture, where the subtalar joint is difficult to inspect (74). Sometimes it is advisable not to use standard arthroscopy portals. Lateral plateau fractures of the tibia are an ideal indication for arthroscopic-assisted reduction. The lateral meniscus is sometimes disturbed in the assessment of the fracture margins. Therefore, it could be wise to enter the joint by placing the arthroscope below the meniscus.

Intraoperative Axis Control

With closed reduction, the restoration of normal alignment is sometimes difficult (16,75,76). Intraoperatively the assessment of reduction must be made on the small field seen on a fluoroscope. The only method of visualizing the whole extremity during surgery is by using the scout film of a CT scan; however, intraoperative CT scanning is not available in most operating rooms. The knee and ankle joints do not have a functional range of motion in the frontal plane, and malalignment of the lower extremity in the frontal plane may have the most deleterious effect on the patient's functional recovery (77). The so-called cable method is an easy technique for intraoperative assessment of alignment using a fluoroscope (78). The knee is rotated under fluoroscopic control until it is imaged anteroposteriorly. The rotation is held by an assistant. The fluoroscope is moved proximally until the head of the femur is centered. A radiodense cable is placed over the center of the femoral head and held in place. The ankle is imaged using slight rotation of the fluoroscope to give a true anteroposterior mortise view. The cable is tensioned and matched with the middle of the surface of the talar dome. The cable shows the axis of the lower extremity. The fluoroscope is now again centered over the knee. The cable should intersect the tibial joint line in the center. A lateral intersection indicates valgus malalignment and a medial intersection indicates varus malalignment. Another technique uses a Perspex template that contains a nonradiolucent grid. This template is imaged in relation to the bone (79).

Intraoperative Rotation Control

Rotation is particularly difficult to assess in diaphyseal fractures of long bones. In the femur an incidence of malrotation of at

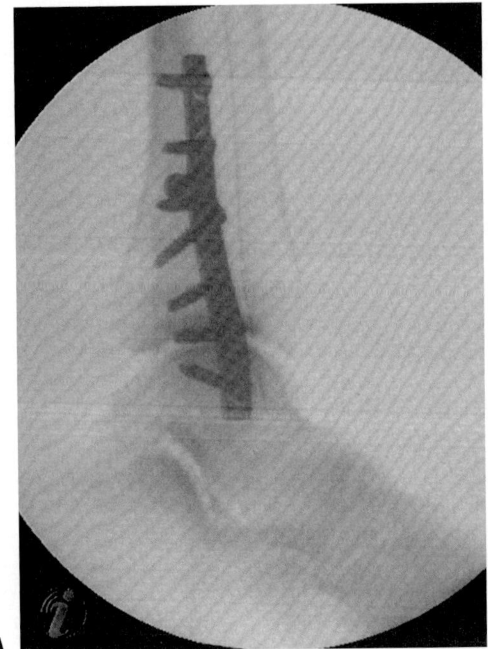
A

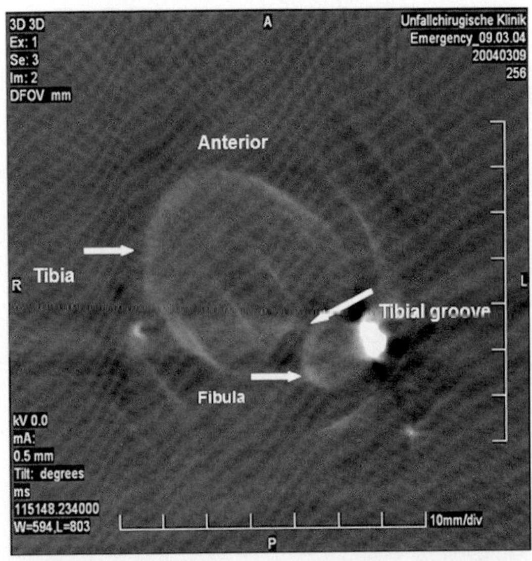

B

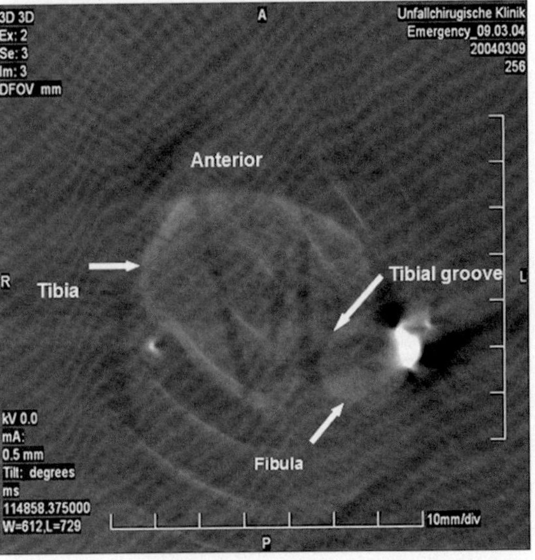

C

FIGURE 6-11 An AO(OTA) type C fracture after open reduction and plate fixation of the fibula without a syndesmosis screw. A syndesmosis screw needs to be inserted secondarily. **A.** Lateral intraoperative fluoroscopy view after closed reduction and screw insertion. **B.** Intraoperative three-dimensional fluoroscopy showed an anterior shift of the distal fibula with consequent incongruency of the tibia and fibula. **C.** After correction of the reduction and screw implantation, a second scan confirmed the correct position of the fibula.

least 10 degrees is reported in more than 40% of patients (80,81). CT is the most reliable method for controlling rotation (82), but the feasibility of using intraoperative CT scanning is limited. Different techniques for intraoperative control exist.

Clinical Rotation Control. Clinical rotation control is not very precise. It can be used to exclude significant rotational differences. To check femoral torsion in the supine position, rotation is done with the hip and knee flexed to 90 degrees. The difference between the sides in maximum internal and external rotation indicates the difference in femoral torsion (Fig. 6-12). Care must be taken not to rotate the pelvis. In the tibia, rotation should be checked with the knee in flexion and the foot dorsiflexed. Internal and external rotation depends on the laxity of the knee and ankle joints. Differences in laxity can alter the correct torsional measurement.

Radiologic Rotation Control. Intraoperative measurement of femoral torsion is difficult. The cortical step sign (Fig. 6-13) and the bone diameter sign provide good hints for the presence of malrotation but are not very sensitive. False-negatives are common, and the absence of these signs does not prove that rotation is correct.

A more precise technique uses the shape of the lesser trochanter on plain x-rays (78). The precise contour of the lesser trochanter depends on the amount of rotation. With increased anteversion, which corresponds to increased internal rotation of the leg, the lesser trochanter enlarges in size. With decreased anteversion, which corresponds to increased external rotation of the leg, the shape of the lesser trochanter decreases until it is covered completely by the shaft. Preoperatively the opposite leg is placed in a reproducible position of rotation. In the original description the patella faces anteriorly (78). Alternatively,

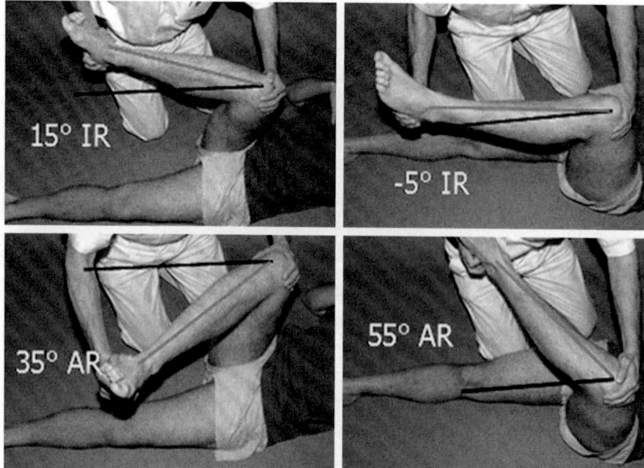

FIGURE 6-12 Clinical measurement of differences in femoral rotation. The measurement is demonstrated with the patient lying on the floor. The same measurement can be done on an operating table in the supine position. To compare the rotation, both femora are placed in maximal internal and external rotation. Care must be taken to stop rotation before the pelvis tilts. This example shows 20 degrees less internal rotation and 20 degrees more external rotation in the left femur. The external rotation difference for the left femur is +20 degrees.

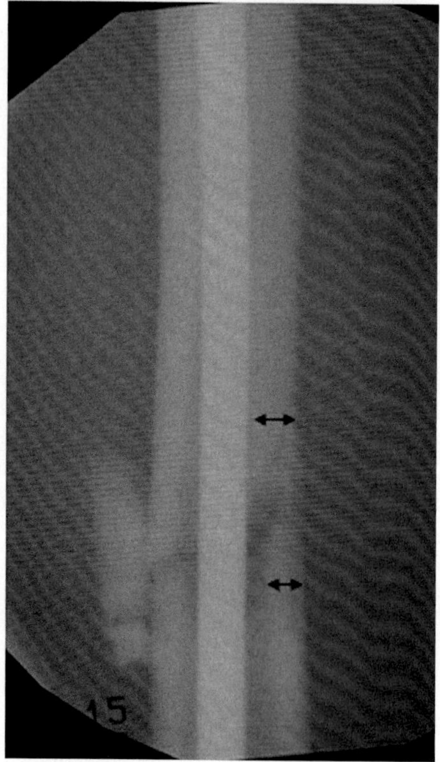

FIGURE 6-13 Same patient as in Figure 6-12, illustrating the cortical step sign. The thickness of the cortex in the proximal fragment is less than in the distal proximal fragment. This suggests malrotation.

the leg can be rotated under fluoroscopic control until the patella is centered upon the femoral condyles. With the leg fixed, the lesser trochanter is imaged and stored in the fluoroscope. To check the rotation, the knee of the operated leg is brought into the same position as described above. The lesser trochanter is imaged and compared to the stored image of the opposite side. Rotation of the proximal fragment is done until both lesser trochanters show the same shape on the anteroposterior view. It is important to center the lesser trochanter exactly on the fluoroscope (Fig. 6-14).

A very precise method for the measurement of tibial torsion with the use of a fluoroscope was described by Clementz (83). The leg is rotated until both condyles match in a lateral view centered on the knee. Holding this position, the fluoroscope is centered on the ankle joint. The fluoroscope is rotated until the anterior and posterior joint surfaces of the medial malleolus match. The amount of rotation of the fluoroscope indicates the degree of tibial torsion.

Computer-Assisted Reduction

Computer-aided orthopaedic surgery (CAOS) is a rapidly progressing technology. It is discussed in detail in Chapter 23. Most applications are for hip and knee replacement. In orthopaedic trauma, both CT-based navigation and fluoroscopy-based navigation are mainly used for screw placement in difficult anatomic regions. Navigated reduction of fractures is under development (84,85). Long bone fractures can be reduced with computer assistance. The fluoroscopic-based navigation system can track the two main fragments. Registration is done with two images in different planes, usually the anteroposterior and lateral planes. The movement of both fragments in both planes is virtually visualized on the navigation system. This technique has two advantages. First, once registration is performed, the surgeon can check the reduction without additional use of the fluoroscope. Second, both planes of the bones are visualized in real time, making reduction much easier. Critical evaluation of the technique is proceeding. CT-based navigation has been introduced for the reduction of pelvic ring fractures with good results (86).

EXTRAMEDULLARY FIXATION TECHNIQUES

Classic Extramedullary Fixation Techniques

Goals

In 1949, Danis stated that there were three requirements for satisfactory internal fixation: the ability to undertake immediate active motion, the complete restoration of the original shape of the bone, and direct union without the formation of visible callus (87). This is achieved with interfragmentary compression using screws, plates, or tension wires. The four principles of the AO-ASIF were anatomic reduction, rigid IF, atraumatic technique for the soft tissue tissues as well as bone, and early pain-free active mobilization during the first 10 postoperative days (88).

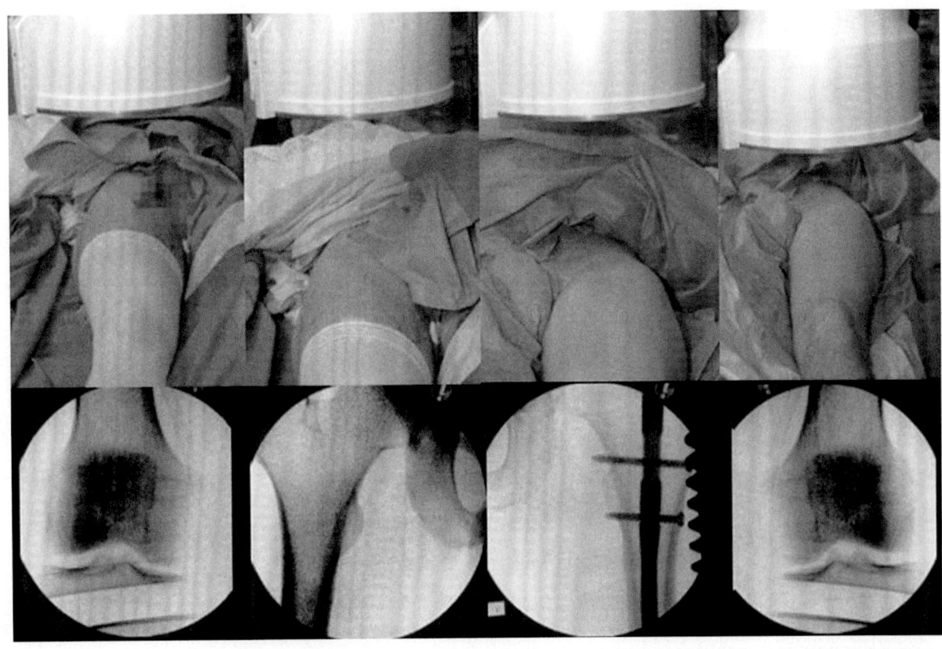

FIGURE 6-14 The intraoperative lesser trochanter method of assessing rotation. The upper row shows the clinical position of the leg. A laser is used to adjust the fluoroscope correctly. The lower row shows the corresponding intensifier image. It is important to have the patella and the lesser trochanter central on the fluoroscope. The measurement starts with the healthy leg (left). With the patella centrally placed, the leg is held manually and the lesser trochanter is imaged. This picture is stored and used as a reference. The same is done on the injured leg. The patella is brought in the same position and the lesser trochanter is imaged. In this example, the lesser trochanter is less visible than on the contralateral side, which indicates less anteversion. Less anteversion corresponds to external rotation of the distal fragment.

Screw Fixation

Screws are the basic component of IF. They are characterized by their material, their dimensions, and their tip and head design. The most commonly used materials are stainless steel and titanium. These materials have different characteristics, and it is important that surgeons understand the differences. When stainless steel bone screws are screwed, they reach a maximum torque. If the screw is tightened further, the screw head will rotate at a constant torque until the screw fails. Titanium screws do not have this constant maximal torque: the torque increases with tightening until failure of the screw occurs. Therefore, surgeons need some experience to tighten titanium screws correctly. Titanium screws also have a significantly lower yield torque where the screws start to permanently deform. The angle to failure is about 50% less for titanium screws than for stainless steel screws. The failure torques are slightly less for titanium (89).

The length of a screw is measured from the outer part of the head to the tip (Fig. 6-15A). The threads are flattened on the side closest to the head and only slightly tilted with respect to the screw axis. This provides a broad pressure-bearing area. Screws can be fully threaded or partially threaded. The nonthreaded portion is called the shaft of the screw. The diameter of the shaft can be less than or equal to the thread diameter. Within the threaded portion, a core diameter (or inner diameter) and a thread diameter (or outer diameter) can be distinguished. The pitch of the screw is the distance between the threads. The lead is the distance through which the screw advances with one 360-degree turn. If the screw is simply threaded, the lead is equal to the pitch; with double threading, the lead is twice the pitch. The mechanics of a screw are directly related to its shape and dimensions.

The surface area of the threads is an important factor that influences pullout strength. The larger the surface area, the greater the pullout strength (90,91). The difference between the thread diameter and the core diameter is called the screw thread depth. The surface area increases with increasing screw thread depth, resulting in higher pullout forces (90,92,93). The core diameter is the most important characteristic determining the bending and fatigue strength of a screw. The ability to increase the surface area at the expense of the core diameter is therefore limited. The forces necessary for screw breakage decrease with a smaller core diameter (93). Furthermore, the core diameter is the principal factor determining fatigue life (94). With finer threads, a smaller pitch increases the pullout strength (90,92). The more threads are engaged within the bone, the greater is the pullout strength (90). The shear strength of the material into which the screw is embedded is another independent variable (90).

To insert screws in bone, a preliminary drill hole is usually made. This drill hole is slightly larger in diameter than the core diameter of the screw. In cortical bone it is usually necessary to tap a thread before the screw can be inserted. The use of tapping is also recommended for hard cancellous bone (93). In porous materials such as normal or soft cancellous bone, the tap enlarges the hole volume by an average of 27%, resulting in a reduced pullout strength (90).

The outer diameter of the tap usually matches the thread diameter of the screw. However, tapping of cancellous bone can be done with a smaller diameter, and this may increase the pullout strength of the screw. Tapping with a pitch different from that of the screw thread must be avoided. This mismatch destroys the surface area of the bone, leading to reduced pullout strength. Measurement of the cortical screw length must be

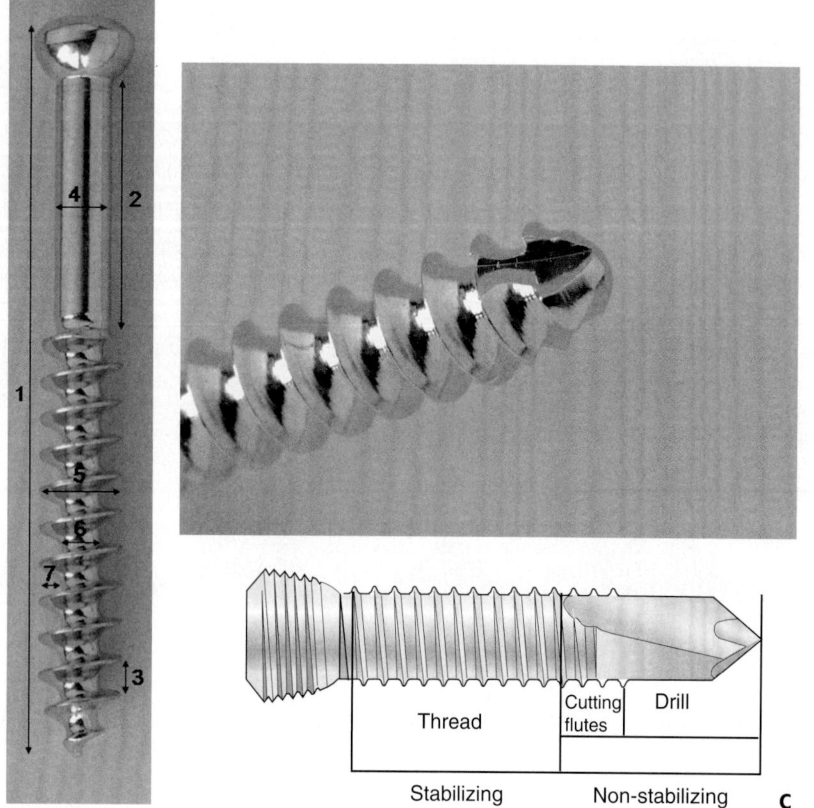

FIGURE 6-15 **A.** Variables that characterize bone screws: *1*, screw length; *2*, shaft length; *3*, pitch; *4*, shaft diameter; *5*, outer diameter; *6*, inner diameter; *7*, thread depth. **B.** An AO 4.5-mm self-tapping screw showing the three cutting flutes. **C.** A self-tapping and self-cutting locking head screw. The drill is located at the tip of the screw, followed by the cutting flutes. The screw threads then stabilize the screw.

done before the drill hole is tapped; otherwise, the depth gauge can damage the bone threads.

Self-tapping screws are beneficial as they reduce operative time and decrease instrumentation use. Self-tapping screws can be divided into thread-forming and thread-cutting screws. Thread-forming screws are suitable for use in soft materials such as cancellous bone. In cortical bone, microfractures of the surrounding bone can be avoided only if the screw diameter is larger than the drill diameter by less than 1% (95). Therefore, thread-cutting is necessary to allow self-tapping screws to be used within cortical bone. The cutting flutes are located at the tip of the screw (see Fig. 6-15B). At least three flutes should be used to facilitate insertion (96). The sharpness of the cutting edges is important (97).

The disadvantage of self-tapping screws concerns their ability to damage the bone threads. Two different mechanisms exist. First, removal and reinsertion of a screw at a different angle causes bending forces. The flutes may cut a new path and damage the initial threads. However, early experimental investigations have shown that with careful reinsertion, there is no weakening of the hold of the screw in bone (98). Second, debris might be caught within the bone threads. With insertion of the screw threads, this debris can cause irregular bone damage. Thus, the cutting-flutes of self-tapping screws have to act as channels for transportation of bone debris. The length of the cutting flutes is usually the same as the threaded part of the tap. Bone debris clearance is dependent on the volume of the cutting flutes. The smaller the volume of the flutes, the more clearing space remains between the flutes (96). For example, the AO 4.5-mm cortex screw produces a bone debris volume of 3 mm^3 within a 5.25-mm-thick cortex (97). Thread-cutting screws have the same pullout strength as non-tapping screws as long as the cutting tip protrudes through the cortex and the same number of screw threads lie within the bone (97). This has to be taken into account when measuring screw length. If the bone is to contain the maximum number of screw threads, the self-tapping tip must penetrate the bone completely. The length of the flutes must be added to the measured screw length (for example, add 2 mm for AO 4.5 cortical screws) (97). The removal of self-tapping screws can be more difficult due to bone growth between the flutes. Turning the screw a little forward loosens the flutes and eases screw removal (97).

Screws are available that are self-drilling as well as self-tapping. The nonthreaded part of the tip, which does not add significantly to pullout strength, is even longer than in self-tapping screws (see Fig. 6-15C). The length of the inserted screw is critical, as the sharp tip will protrude to a greater extent into the soft tissues. These screws are best implanted in a unicortical mode (99), as bicortical placement increases the danger of damaging the threads within the bone. As the tip of the screw hits the second cortex, the threads within the first cortex continue rotating while the screw is not moving forward. This spinning destroys the bony threads within the bone. In fully threaded screws the second cortex contributes only 10% to 20% to the axial screw force. These self-drilling and self-tapping screws produce an even higher amount of bony debris. If these screws are implanted intracortically, the volume of the debris will exceed the clearing space, resulting in a compromised hold.

Most conventional screw heads have a hemispherical undersurface. This shape ensures optimal contact between the screw and the underlying surface. Countersinking a screw results in greater load transfer from the screw to the bone and less soft tissue irritation. Care has to be taken not to penetrate the cortex with the countersink. In bones with a thin cortex, the use of a washer spreads the load over a larger area and prevents cortical breakthrough. Washers have a flat side that is directed to the bone and a countersunk side that provides optimal contact even with an angulated screw. A plate has the same effect as washer. Headless screws allow insertion of the screw underneath the cortex. Specially designed heads can lock within a hole and lead to angular stability between the plate and the screw (see below).

One of the most important facts to bear in mind during insertion of a screw is that tightening is limited to a maximum torque. Above this maximum torque, either the screw or the bone fails. Core diameter and material parameters influence screw failure. Insertion of a screw is characterized by two physical values: the torque that is necessary for insertion of the screw and the resulting axial compression of the screw. Both values are related to each other. Provided that the screw itself does not fail, the relation between the insertion torque and the axial compression is linear while the bone threads are intact. Further tightening results in microfracturing of the bone threads. The increase in axial compression related to increased insertion torque is thereby reduced. Both the axial compression and the insertion torque reach a maximum. Further tightening destroys the bone threads and the axial compression force reduces, sometimes to zero (100,101). Gotzen et al found that microfracturing of the bone occurs above 89% of the maximal axial compression force. They declared this 89% value as the optimal axial compression force and the corresponding torque as the optimal insertion moment (101).

Due to the viscoelasticity of the bone, the maximal axial compression force of the screw falls after removal of the screwdriver. The force decreases rapidly within the first minute and reaches a plateau, called the holding force of the screw. The maximal holding force is reached at the level of microfracturing of the bone thread (101). During insertion the surgeon cannot measure the holding force; the insertion torque is the only indirect indicator. Optimal screw tightening requires experience.

In vivo loosening of correctly placed screws is due to micromotion at the interface between the screw thread and bone (102). This micromotion can be induced by axial pullout forces or by bending moments. In dense bone the resistance of a screw to pullout is high. Screws do not resist bending forces well due to their small core diameter. A 30% increase of the core size increases the bending stiffness by three times (103). Small-diameter screws can have a higher holding force than large-diameter screws (104). The advantage of large-diameter screws lies more in their higher resistance to bending moments than in their resistance to axial pullout. Two facts limit the use of large-diameter screws. First, the holding force of a screw decreases as the outer diameter exceeds 40% of the bone diameter (42). Second, the breaking strength of a bone decreases when the drill hole exceeds 30% of the bone diameter (105).

Types of Bone Screws. The AO/ASIF system differentiates between two basic types of bone screws, cortical and cancellous screws. Cancellous screws have a larger thread depth and a larger pitch than cortical screws. Screws of different sizes exist to meet the requirements of all bones within the body. Screw sizes are named according to the outside diameter of their threaded portion; for example, the 6.5-mm cancellous screw has an outer diameter of 6.5 mm. Cancellous and cortical screws are divided into the subgroups large fragment, small fragment, and mini fragment (Fig. 6-16). These screws have corresponding plates.

Cortical screws are available in diameters from 1.0 to 4.5 mm. A drill hole that is slightly larger than the core diameter is needed. For large fragment screws with a core diameter of 3.0 mm, the drill diameter is 3.2 mm. Cortical screws can be used in both cortical and cancellous bone. The compression force in cortical bone varies between 2,000 and 3,000 N and is much higher than in cancellous bone (106). The compression force depends on the thickness of the cortex. The relationship is linear but not proportional. The maximal compression force is higher for the femoral shaft than for the tibia and the humerus (107). The compression force of a cortical screw depends on the angle of insertion (108), but due to the different relationship between the thickness of the cortex and compression force, the influence of the insertion angle differs. In thin cortices, a perpendicular orientation results in a higher compression force, whereas in thick cortices an angulated orientation results in slightly higher compression. Perpendicular orientation is recommended (108).

Cortical screws are fully threaded. Shaft screws and malleolar screws have the same characteristics as cortical screws, but both screws are partially threaded. Their core diameter and pitch are equal to that of cortical screws. The malleolar screw was specially designed for stabilization of medial malleolus fractures. Tapping is not necessary as it has a trocar cutting tip (97). Due to its large diameter and large screw head, the 4.0-mm cancellous screw is now favored for use in the medial malleolus (97,106). The use of the malleolar screw is now somewhat limited. Removal of these screws can be difficult, as the threads cannot cut their way back out of the healed strong bone around the shaft. Screw breakage can occur on removal (93).

Shaft screws have a shaft diameter equal to the thread diameter. With the increased diameter, the shaft portion is 5 times stiffer and 3.4 times stronger to bending forces (106). Because of this higher resistance to bending forces, shaft screws can be

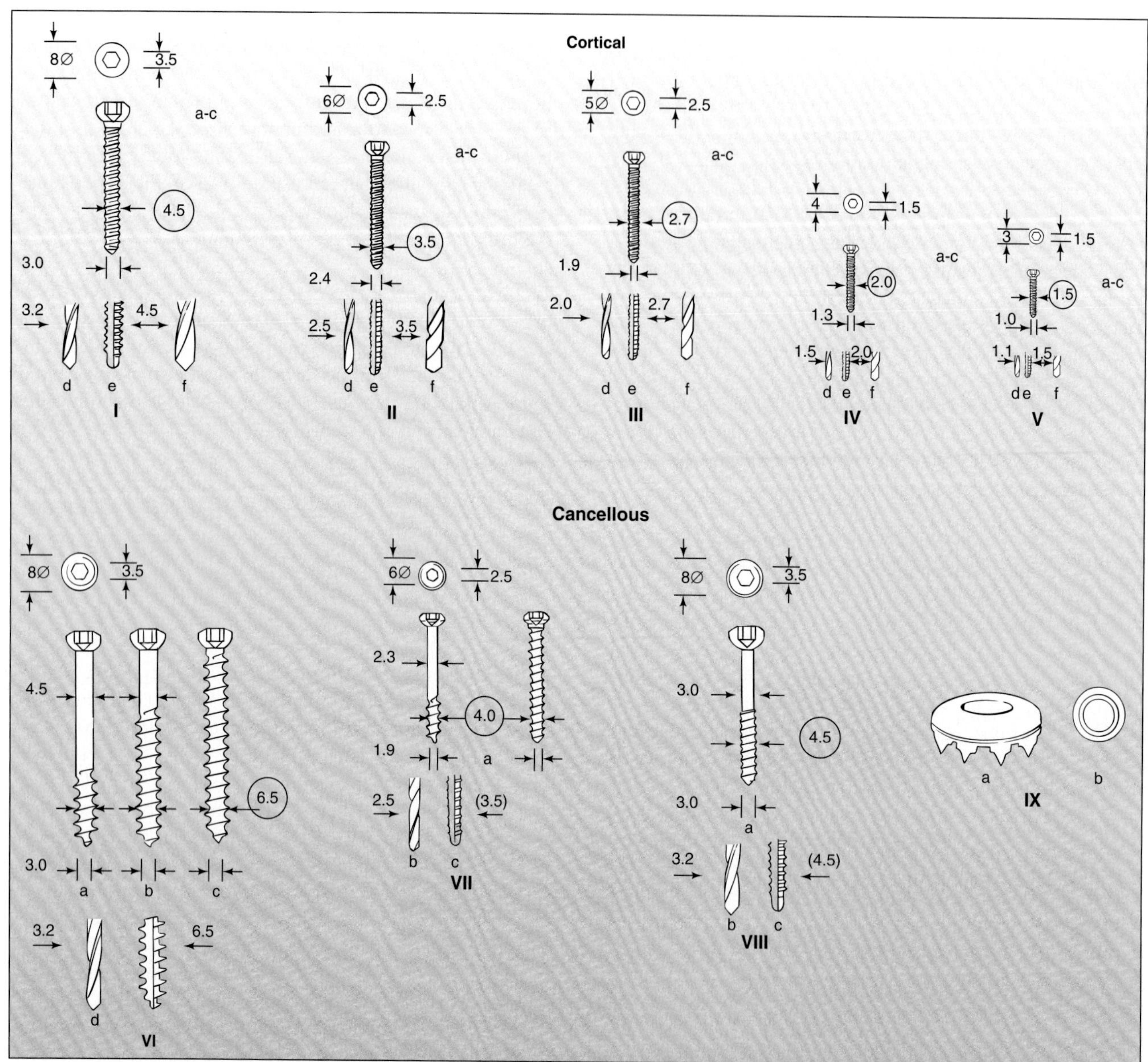

FIGURE 6-16 Solid ASIF screws and their drill bits, taps, and washers. I: 4.5-mm cortex screw: (*a*) 8-mm screw head and 3.5-mm hexagonal recess; (*b*) fully threaded, with 1.75-mm pitch; (*c*) core diameter of 3 mm and outer diameter of 4.5 mm; (*d*) 3.2-mm thread-hole drill bit; (*e*) 4.5-mm tap; (*f*) 4.5-mm glide-hole drill bit. II: 3.5-mm cortex screw: (*a*) 6-mm screw head, with a 2.5-mm hexagonal recess; (*b*) fully threaded, with 1.75-mm pitch; (*c*) 2.4-mm core; (*d*) 2.5-mm thread-hole drill bit; (*e*) 3.5-mm tap; (*f*) 3.5-mm glide-hole drill bit. III: 2.7-mm cortex screw: (*a*) 5-mm head, with 2.5-mm hexagonal recess; (*b*) fully threaded, with 1-mm pitch; (*c*) core diameter of 1.9 mm and outer diameter of 2.7 mm; (*d*) 2-mm thread-hole drill bit; (*e*) 2.7-mm tap; (*f*) 2.7-mm glide-hole drill bit. IV: 2-mm cortex screw: (*a*) 4-mm head, with 1.5-mm hexagonal recess; (*b*) full threaded, with 0.8-mm pitch; (*c*) core diameter of 1.3 mm and outer diameter of 2 mm; (*d*) 1.5-mm thread-hole drill bit; (*e*) 2-mm tap; (*f*) 2-mm glide-hole drill bit. V: 1.5-mm cortex screw: (*a*) 3-mm head, with 1.5-mm hexagonal recess; (*b*) fully threaded, with 0.6-mm pitch; (*c*) core diameter of 1 mm; (*d*) 1.1-mm thread-hole drill bit; (*e*) 1.5-mm tap; (*f*) 1.5-mm glide-hole drill bit. VI: 6.5-mm cancellous screw with 8-mm head having a 3.5-mm hexagonal recess, shaft core of 4.5 mm, and thread core of 3 mm; 3.2-mm drill bit and 6.5-mm tap; (*a*) 16-mm thread length; (*b*) 32-mm thread length; (*c*) fully threaded; (*d*) 3.2-mm drill bit; (*e*) 6.5-mm tap. VII: 4-mm cancellous screw with 6-mm head having 2.5-mm hexagonal recess: (*a*) core diameter is 1.9 mm, pitch 1.75 mm, and requires (*b*) 2.5-mm drill and (*c*) 4.0-mm tap. VIII: 4.5-mm "malleolar" screw with (*a*) 3.0-mm core diameter and self-cutting tip, (*b*) 3.2-mm drill bit and optional (*c*) 4.5-mm tap. IX: Plastic and metal washers.

beneficial to retain interfragmentary compression of a plate that is loaded either by the articulated tension device or by eccentric screw placement. Fully threaded screws can interfere with plate holes if they have to be inserted with a tilt angle. This can compromise the compression force of the screw (109). The insertion of shaft screws necessitates the use of two drill bits, one for the threaded portion (3.2 mm for 4.5-mm screws) and one for the shaft portion (4.5 mm for 4.5-mm screws). The drill for the shaft portion is used first. To center the second drill, a sleeve should be used. With respect to axial pullout, the shaft screw acts a monocortical screw. It is important that the tip of the screw protrudes through the second cortex to achieve a maximum number of threads within the bone.

Cancellous screws have a larger thread depth and a larger pitch than cortical screws. Only large and small fragment cancellous screws are available. Mini-fragment cancellous screws are not required, as the cancellous bone in small-sized bones is dense enough to allow stabilization with cortical screws. Cancellous screws can be fully threaded or partially threaded. The large fragment screws have two predetermined partial thread lengths, 32 mm and 16 mm. The partial thread length of the small fragment screws increases from 5 to 15 mm in proportion to the screw length.

Neutral Screw or Holding Screw. Cortical and cancellous screws can both act as a holding or neutral screw, and the screw threads should match the bone threads. Even with an interfragmentary gap, the fragments are held in the same position. Insertion of the screw has a neutral effect on fragment position. A pilot hole is drilled whose diameter is slightly greater than the core diameter. A drill sleeve should be used to protect the soft tissues. With non–self-tapping screws, the length must be measured before tapping of the bone. If separate tapping is necessary, a sleeve should be used to prevent soft tissue stripping. Finally the screw is inserted.

Lag Screw. Interfragmentary compression with absolutely stable fixation is one of the main principles of conventional IF techniques. One of the strongest and most popular methods of gaining interfragmentary compression is with a lag screw. The interfragmentary compression of a lag screw is about five times higher than the interfragmentary compression of a plate (110). The characteristic of the lag screw is the gliding hole. A lag screw can be fully threaded or partially threaded as long as three criteria are met:

1. The proximal screw thread, whether threaded or not, must not engage bone.
2. The distal screw threads must firmly grip bone.
3. The screw head must firmly abut on the proximal cortex.

Partially threaded screws have the same function as a lag screw as long as the threaded part does not cross the fracture

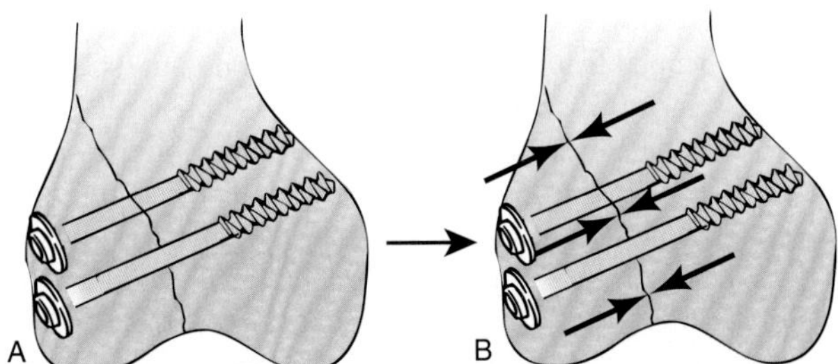

FIGURE 6-17 Lag effect of partially threaded screws. **A.** The threads are located in the distal fragment only. Washers are used to increase the surface area of the screw heads to prevent intrusion of the screw heads into the bone. **B.** With further tightening, the screw heads compress the near fragment toward the far fragment. Compression results within the fracture gap.

line (Fig. 6-17). Threaded screws act as a lag screw when the proximal hole (gliding hole) is drilled with the diameter of the screw thread (Fig. 6-18).

The preparation and insertion of a lag screw is usually done in a standardized manner. The technique is described for the 4.5-mm cortex screw (outer diameter 4.5 mm, core diameter 3.0 mm). The first step is the preparation of the gliding hole. Drilling with the outer diameter of the screw (4.5 mm) is done up to the fracture line. A drill sleeve should be inserted into the proximal cortex. Next, the drilling of the distal grip hole is undertaken. To center the 3.2-mm drill within the extension of the gliding hole, a drill sleeve with an outer diameter of 4.5 mm and an inner diameter of 3.2 mm should be used. As has already been discussed, countersinking of the proximal cortex improves load transfer from the screw head to the bone and reduces soft tissue irritation. If countersinking is desired, it has to be done before measuring the length of the screw. This is best done with a depth gauge. The distal fragment is tapped through the glide hole using the 4.5-mm tap. The length of thread-cutting self-tapping screws must be assessed to ensure that the cutting flutes are beyond the second cortex; otherwise, the holding strength is below that of non–self-tapping screws (97). Fully threaded screws with an overdrilled gliding hole

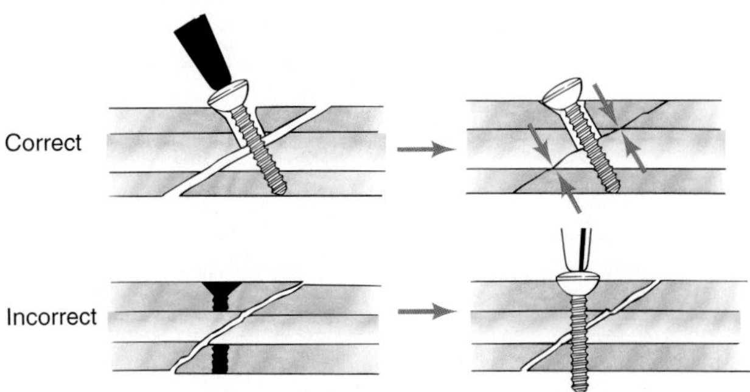

FIGURE 6-18 The use of a fully threaded screw as a lag screw. The proximal fragment is overdrilled and as the screw is tightened, compression is applied to the fracture.

have the advantage of engaging the distal fragment with a maximum number of threads. This leads to a higher holding strength.

The correct insertion angle of a lag screw is important. Maximal interfragmentary compression is achieved if the lag screw is implanted perpendicular to the fracture line (111) (see Fig. 6-18). Mechanical testing has shown that a screw angle of more than 22 degrees from the perpendicular causes the fractures to slide (112). Due to its high interfragmentary compression, the resistance of a single lag screw to a bending moment within the plane of the screw is high. However, one single screw does not neutralize rotation moments within the fracture plane. A second screw, placed either as a neutral or lag screw, enhances stability. With axial loading, a lag screw that is oriented perpendicularly to the axis of the shaft is associated with the least shortening (112). The optimal angle of a lag screw would be a line bisecting the angle between the axis of the bone and the fracture line (42). Tibial spiral fractures can theoretically be treated with pure lag screw fixation (112,113). If the fracture line does not allow an optimal angle of screw insertion, at least one screw should be oriented perpendicular to the axis (43). Short oblique fractures are not suitable for pure lag screw fixation; in these cases, interfragmentary compression is achieved with lag screw fixation. To neutralize torsion moments and axial forces, secondary protection is necessary. This is best done with an additional plate, referred to as a neutralization plate. A combination of rigid fixation and nonrigid fixation, as is seen when a lag screw is used with external fixation, is less successful, as different types of bone healing are combined (114,115).

Double-Threaded Screws. Herbert was the first surgeon to describe the use of a double-threaded screw for compression fixation of scaphoid fractures (116). In place of a head, the screw has a second thread. This second thread has a smaller pitch, leading to a higher lead within the bone. The second thread is fully inserted in the bone, leaving no prominence outside. The different threads induce interfragmentary compression (Fig. 6-19A). These screws are also available in a cannulated form to facilitate insertion. Its design makes the screw very useful in fixing osteochondral fragments.

Plate Fixation

In previous years absolute fracture stability was the principal goal of IF with plates. Absolute stability leads to primary bone healing, and callus formation was seen as a sign of instability, leading to loosening of the fixation. Reduction and fixation was achieved using open techniques, which required extensive surgical approaches and considerable soft tissue dissection. The stability of conventional plate osteosynthesis relies on friction. This friction is induced by compression between the bone and the plate (Fig. 6-20). The lag effect of the screw is the determining factor for the stability. This fixation principle is called "traction." Compression between bone and plate leads to cortical

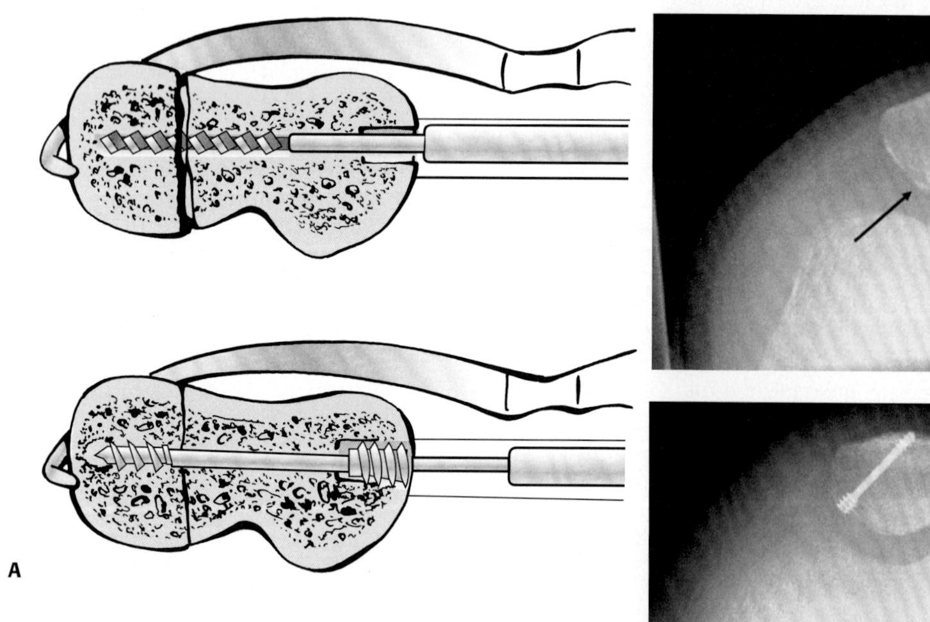

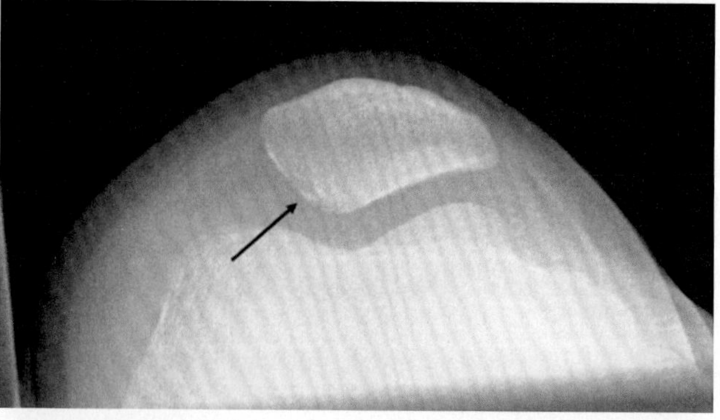

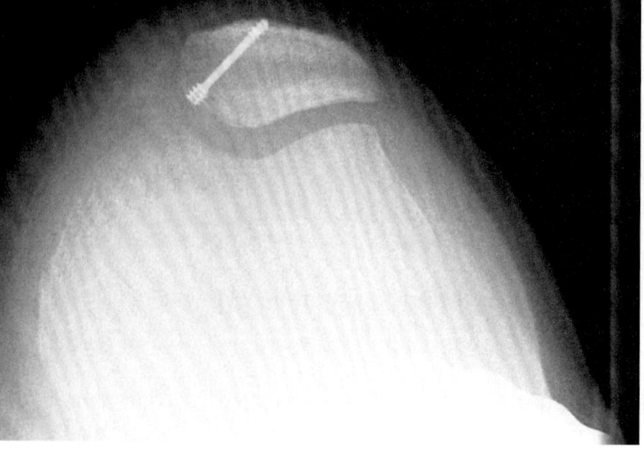

FIGURE 6-19 **A.** The use of a Herbert screw in a scaphoid. The bone is reduced and predrilled (*top*). As the screw is tightened, the fracture is compressed because of the differential pitch size (*bottom*). **B.** Clinical example of the use of a Herbert screw. A young patient had a dislocation of his patella with an osteochondral fragment (*arrow*). **C.** The fragment was loose on arthroscopy and was fixed with a Herbert screw. The proximal thread is buried underneath the cartilage surface.

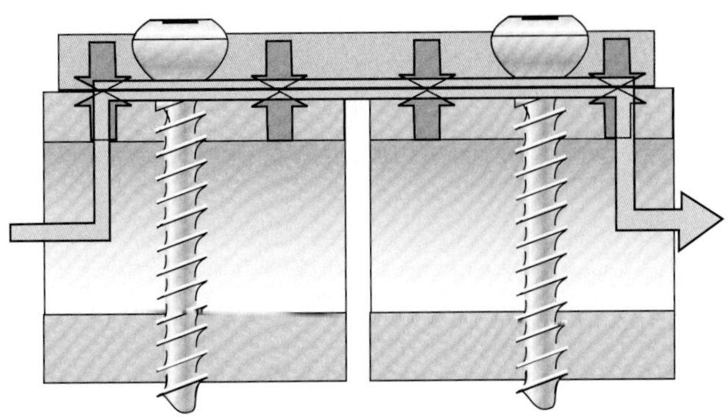

FIGURE 6-20 Conventional plate osteosynthesis relies on compression between the bone and the plate. This compression induces friction. The flux is from the bone through the plate–plate junction and back to the bone.

porosis as a result of impaired periosteal blood supply (117). This phenomenon was referred to as "stress protection." It was thought to delay fracture healing and increase the risk of refracture (118). However, the theory of stress protection of plates has now been abandoned (119–121).

Impaired blood supply not only slows healing but also increases the risk of severe complications such as infection and nonunion. The worst case is an atrophic infected nonunion (122). The compromised blood supply results from both the initial injury to the bone and soft tissues and the additional surgical trauma. A considerable degree of surgical skill and expertise is required to minimize the additional biologic compromise associated with surgery. Nevertheless, osteosynthesis with plates providing rigid fixation is still an important technique of operative fracture treatment.

Plate Design. A considerable number of different types of plates exist. The first plates of the AO/ASIF had a round hole (43). Its spherical shape fitted the spherical shape of the head of the screw. This plate allowed axial compression of the plate by the screws, but due to the shape of the screw hole, the ability to angulate the screws was limited.

Dynamic Compression Plate. The dynamic compression plate (DCP) was introduced in 1969 (123,124). The key to the success of this plate was the design of the screw hole. The holes of the plate are shaped like an inclined, transverse cylinder (Fig. 6-21). Maximal axial compression can be gained if the screw head locks in the transverse part of the hole. This part acts like the standard round hole, but unlike the round hole the screws can be inclined 25 degrees in the longitudinal plane and 7 degrees in the transverse plane. This inclination allows lag screw placement through the plate. Fully threaded lag screws can lose up to 40% compression if their threads wedge within the margin of the screw hole (125). If the screw is inserted close to the

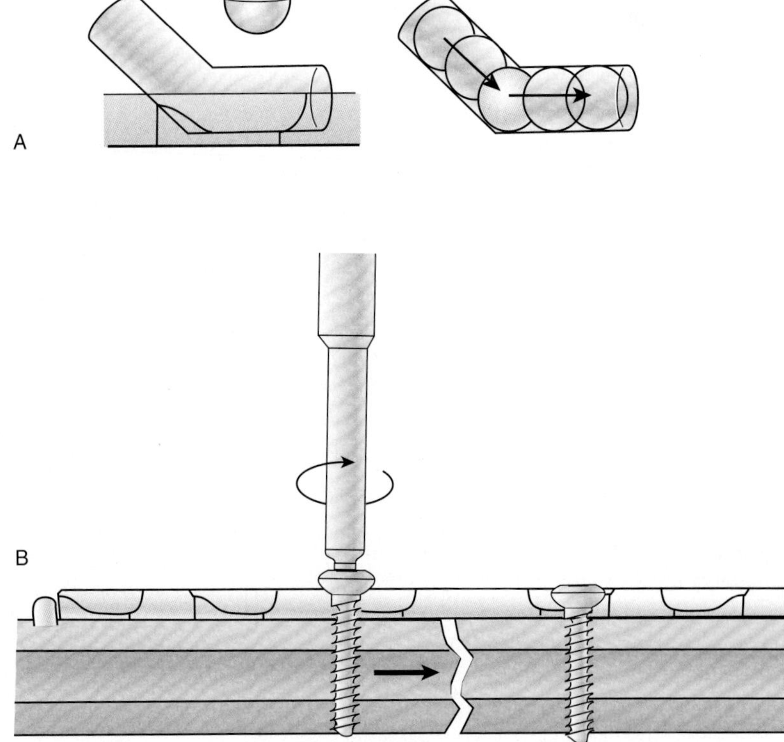

FIGURE 6-21 **A.** The dynamic compression principle. The holes of the plate are shaped like an inclined transverse cylinder. Like a ball, the screw head slides down the cylinder. **B.** In a fixed plate this movement will cause fracture compression.

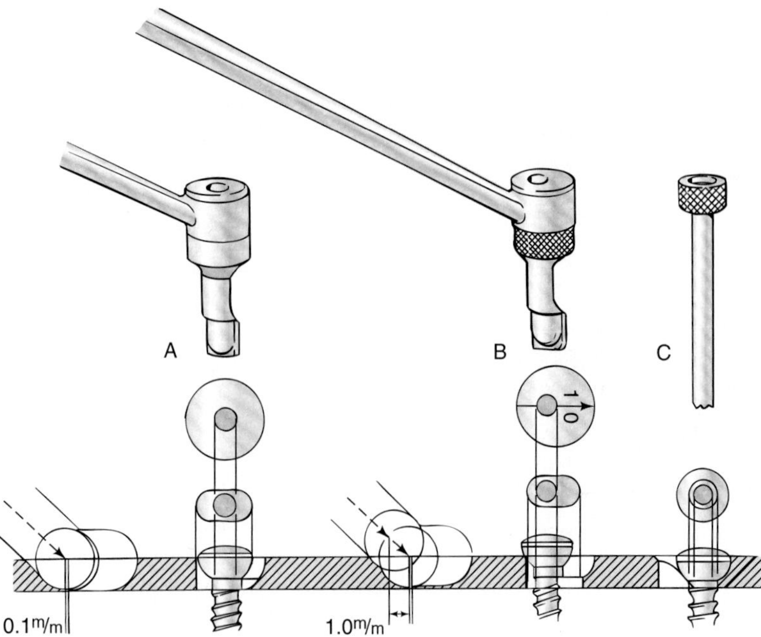

FIGURE 6-22 Drill guides for dynamic compression plates (DCP). **A.** Neutral guide and **(B)** load guide. **C.** The 58-mm drill sleeve, called the coaxial drill sleeve or overdrill sleeve. Drill sleeves for the LC-DCP systems are similar but may be separated from the DCP guides by the presence of notching on their undersurfaces. The neutral guide applies a small displacement force due to the 0.1-mm offset.

inclined part of the hole, the screw head cannot reach maximal compression in the oblique plane, as maximal compression is gained within the transverse part of the hole. Further screw tightening will result in a shift of the plate until the screw head is centered within the transverse part. This shift leads to a second force, which is perpendicular to the axial compression force. If the plate is already fixed to the bone, this shift will result in fracture compression (see Fig. 6-21). One eccentrically placed screw can shift the plate by a maximum of 1 mm. The screw can be inserted in four positions in relation to the hole: extreme load position, load position, neutral position, and buttress position. In the buttress position the screw head is blocked to the border of the hole. Drill guides allow exact positioning of the screw in neutral and load position (Fig. 6-22). The extreme load position and the buttress position are drilled freehand with the usual sleeve. The screw is placed 0.1 mm eccentrically, and therefore 0.1 mm of compression occurs even in the neutral position.

In 1982 a variation of the DCP was introduced, the dynamic compression unit (DCU) (126). In this plate the holes are symmetrical, but an undercut at the periphery of the screw holes allows screw angulation of up to 45 degrees without any impingement on the plate.

LC-DCP (Limited Contact-Dynamic Compression Plate). Compression plating has a deleterious effect on the periosteal blood supply, which may in turn result in significant complications. To minimize these effects, the LC-DCP was invented (109). This plate has a sculpted undersurface that reduces the amount of bone contact by 50% (Fig. 6-23). The newly designed cross-section leads to a more evenly distributed stiffness, and the screw holes do not act as stress risers for implant failure. A special drill guide was designed to ensure accurate screw placement in the load, neutral, or buttress positions. In addition, a universal drill guide permits individual screw positioning. As the outer diameter of the universal drill guide is equal to the outer diameter of the screw, wedging of the threads in the screw hole is prevented.

Tubular Plates. Two different tubular plates exist: the large fragment semitubular plate and the small fragment one-third

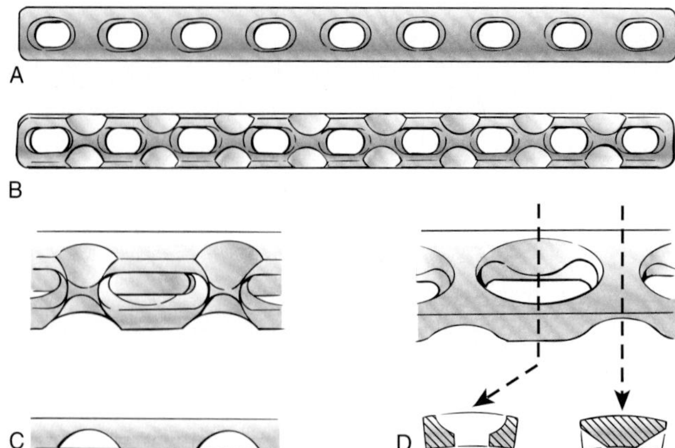

FIGURE 6-23 Titanium limited-contact dynamic compression plate (LC-DCP). **A.** Top view. **B.** Notching on the undersurface. **C.** Revascularization channels. **D.** Double-ramp configuration of the holes (*top*). The two bottom views contrast the geometry of the hole area of the plates with the solid areas.

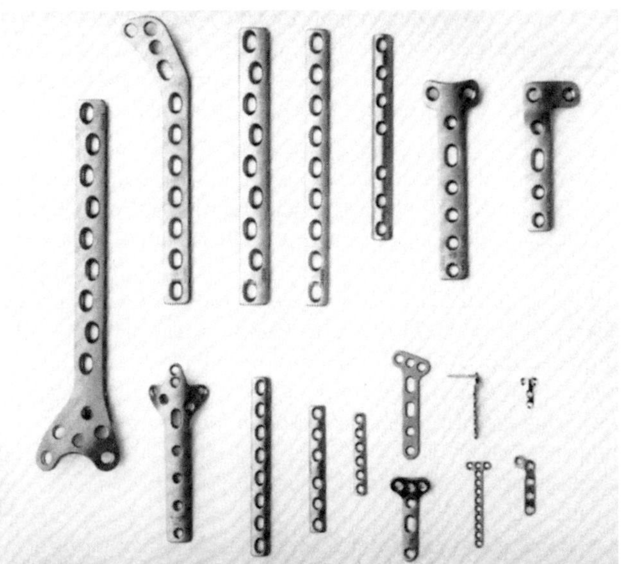

FIGURE 6-24 Titanium ASIF plates include (from *left*) femoral buttress plate; (*top*) tibial buttress plate: 4.5-mm broad LC-DCP: 4.5-mm narrow LC-DCP, semitubular T and L buttress; (*bottom*) cloverleaf: 3.5-mm LC-DCP, one-third tubular, one-fourth tubular, oblique and straight T buttress, and assorted minifragment plates. (Courtesy of Synthes.)

tubular plate (Fig. 6-24). Tubular plates are very thin and can be used in regions where there is little soft tissue cover, such as the distal ulna, olecranon, and lateral malleolus. Due to their thickness these plates do not resist bending moments as well as other plates. The oval hole shape allows eccentric screw placement.

Reconstruction Plates. Contouring of plates into a three-dimensional shape can be difficult, and lateral bending is particularly difficult. Reconstruction plates are characterized by notches between the holes, which facilitate bending. Special bending devices allow contouring in the plane of the plate. These plates have oval holes that allow for compression. Reconstruction plates are very useful for fractures in anatomic regions that require complex three-dimensional contouring, such as the acetabulum. The use of templates that can be molded directly to the bone is advised. Resistance to deformation is lower with these plates.

Precontoured Plates. There are a wide range of precontoured plates that are made to fit the precise shape of a particular anatomic region. They are commonly used in epiphyseal and metaphyseal fractures. Their shape allows multiple screw insertion in different planes in the metaphysis. Different-shaped plates are available for the same anatomic region. Their selection depends mainly on the fracture type, the surgical approach, and the surgeon's preference. Precontoured plates rarely fit the individual anatomy perfectly, and fine contouring is often required. An example of a precontoured plate is shown in Figure 6-25.

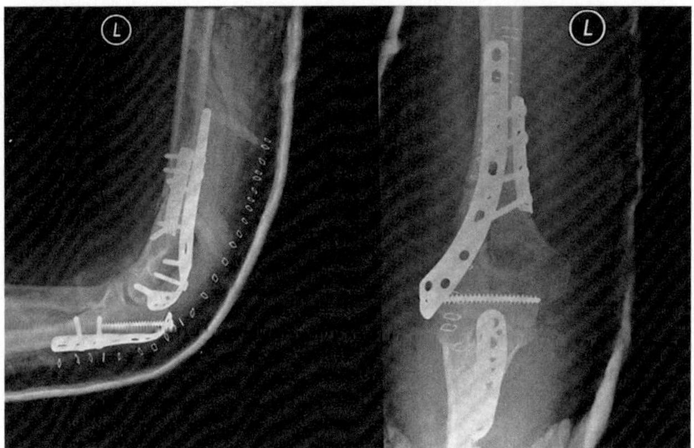

FIGURE 6-25 Distal humeral and olecranon precontoured plates. The olecranon plate has been used to stabilize an olecranon osteotomy. A one-third tubular neutralization plate has also been used.

Blade Plates. The standard blade plates that are widely available are the 130-degree blade plate and the 95-degree blade plate. Conventionally, the 130-degree blade plate was usually used for fractures of the proximal femur and the 95-degree blade plate for fractures of the distal femur. These plates have mixed mechanics. The strong blade affords angular stability when compressive forces are applied to the fracture. The application of blade plates needs meticulous planning. The blade must be correctly placed in all three dimensions; otherwise, malalignment will occur. The use of blade plates requires a lot of experience. Today blade plates are mainly used for corrective osteotomies. In fracture treatment they have been largely replaced by the dynamic hip screw and dynamic condylar screw.

Dynamic Hip Screw and Dynamic Condylar Screw. These plates are derived from blade plates. Their basic mechanical principles are similar. Both screw/plate systems have some advantages over the corresponding blade plates. As they are made of two pieces, the screw can slide within the plate, leading to further compression of the fracture with weight-bearing. The screw is inserted first. In contrast to the blade plate, the position of the plate of the dynamic hip screw and the dynamic condylar screw can be still corrected in the sagittal plane, and only two, instead of three, planes have to be controlled during insertion. Furthermore, minimally invasive plate osteosynthesis is facilitated, as assembly of the screw and the plate can be done after plate insertion. Biomechanical tests show that the dynamic condylar screw is more stable than the equivalent blade plate (127,128). See Chapter 45 for more information on the dynamic hip screw and other sliding hip screw devices.

Principles of Plating. Plate stability depends on the axial force of the screws that compress the plate against the bone. Absolute stability with no screw movement within the screw holes is necessary. Micromovement leads to screw loosening, resulting in decreased fracture compression and loss of stability. Regardless of the type of plate, it is important to impart sufficient compression to the construct. There is a minimum number of screws that need to be inserted into the bone on each side of a fracture to obtain optimal stability. The AO/ASIF recommended six cortices (or three bicortical screws) for the humerus, five cortices for the ulna and radius, seven cortices for the femur, and six cortices for the tibia. In osteoporotic bone this number will need to be increased, with the surgeon often basing the decision about the number of screws on the "compression feeling" achieved during tightening of the screws (42). Angling the screws does not increase plate stability (111).

Most plates can be applied in a number of different ways. The most common types of application are described in this section.

Neutralization Plate. As has already been described, the use of a correctly inserted lag screw will result in significant interfragmentary compression. However, only a few fractures are suitable for fixation using only lag screw fixation. Resistance to bending and torsional moments is often not sufficient, especially if the loads are high. The use of a supplementary plate can neutralize these forces (Fig. 6-26). This neutralization plate does not have any effect on interfragmentary compression, but it protects the lag screw fixation from loosening. The lag screw or screws have to be inserted before the plate, but the lag screw can be inserted through one of the plate holes. This sometimes assists with plate positioning and minimizes soft tissue dissection. Exact contouring of the neutralization plate is necessary.

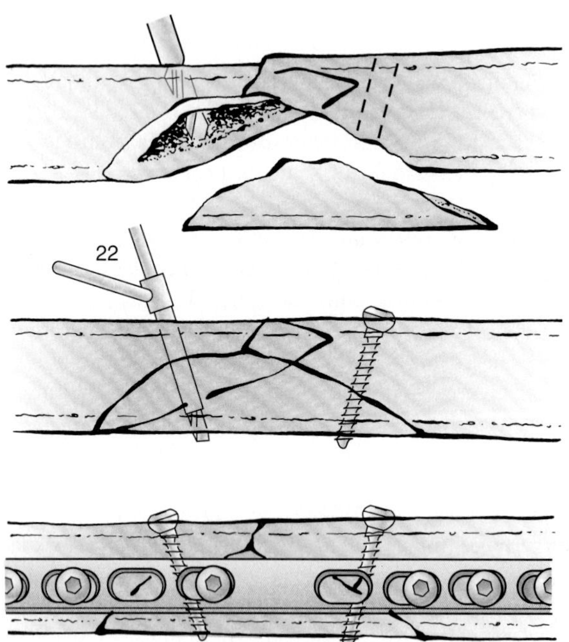

FIGURE 6-26 Technique of neutralization plating. The butterfly fragment is reduced and fixed with two lag screws (one lag screw per main fragment). The lag screws will not withstand the bending forces between the fragments. An additional plate is added that neutralizes the bending forces but does not add any interfragmentary compression.

Buttress Plate. Fractures within the epiphysis or metaphysis are frequently not adequately stabilized by lag screw fixation because of the thin cortex and cancellous nature of the bone. Shear forces and compressive forces must be neutralized by an additional plate. This buttress plate supports the metaphyseal fragment (Fig. 6-27). It works like an avalanche barrier that prevents the snow from sliding downhill. The actual buttress effect is only on the side of the plate. In certain circumstances dual buttress plating may be used, but this is an invasive technique. In plates with DCP holes, the screws must be inserted opposite to the slope to prevent the plate from sliding. Preshaped plates are frequently used as buttress plates, as they conform to the local anatomy. However, exact contouring of the plate is necessary. Some plates have a sliding hole that should be used for the first screw. The sliding hole allows slight corrections of the plate position to obtain the optimal supporting effect.

Antiglide Plate. The antiglide plate is a particular type of buttress plate (129,130). This plate can be used in oblique fractures to prevent sliding of the fragments and subsequent shortening (129). The most basic antiglide plate is the "one-hole antiglide plate." This plate can be either a shortened one-third tubular plate or a washer. The plate with its screw is centered over the spike of an oblique fracture. In this technique drilling is done through the fracture. The antiglide effect leads to compression within the fracture on weight-bearing. An additional lag screw for interfragmentary compression can be used. This screw can be placed either through the plate or outside it.

Compression Plates. Lag screw fixation is one technique used to gain interfragmentary compression. As has already been detailed, lag screw fixation is usually protected by a neutralization plate, which does not contribute to intrafragmentary compression. Plates that cause interfragmentary compression at the fracture are called compression plates. They can be used either in combination with a lag screw or by themselves. The compression gained from the use of a plate is never as high as with lag screw fixation (110). Compression can be generated by using an external tensioning device, bending the plate, using a DCP, or by a combination of all three methods. The principles will be explained with reference to a transverse fracture. Compression with lag screw fixation is not possible in this fracture type, as screws cannot be placed perpendicular to the plane of the fracture.

Prebending. Both the tensioning device and dynamic compression holes lead to eccentric compression of the bone (Fig. 6-28). The cortices close to the plate are under compression, while the opposite cortices are slightly distracted. This distraction is

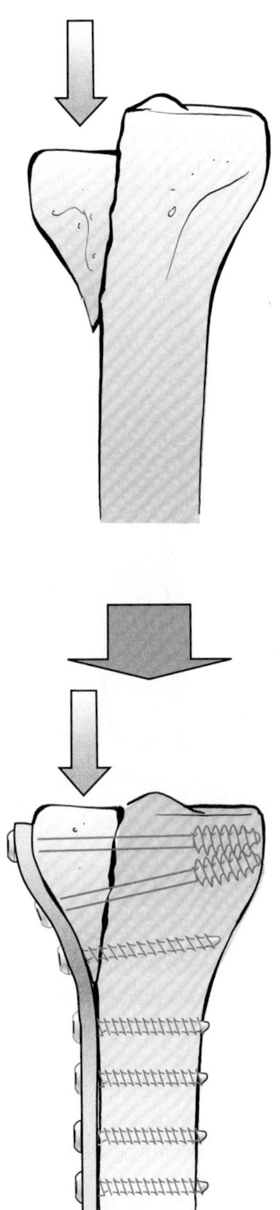

FIGURE 6-27 Function of the buttress plate. The example shows an unstable lateral split fracture of the proximal tibia. The plate buttresses the lateral fragment. It is important to place the screws in eccentric holes close to the fracture.

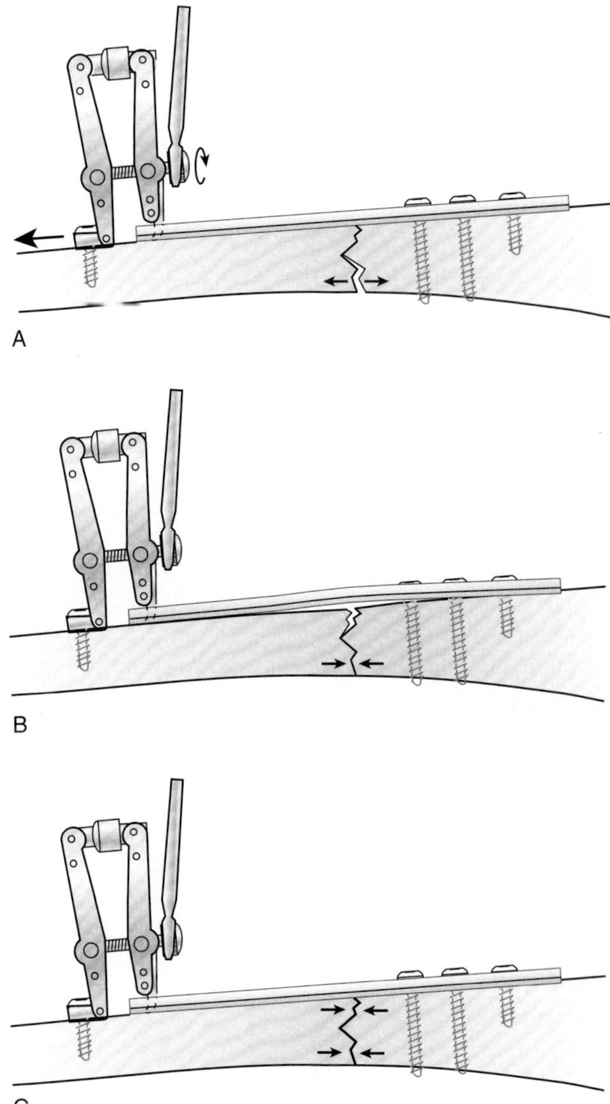

FIGURE 6-28 The use of a prebent plate. **A.** If compression is applied without prebending the plate, there is compression of the cortex under the plate and distraction of the far cortex. **B.** Prebending the plate prevents this. **C.** As tension is applied, the fracture is compressed.

proportional to the applied compression force (131). The resulting gap induces micromovement and disturbed bone healing. An additional lag screw results in more evenly distributed compression and enhances stability (132,133). If the placement of an additional lag screw is not possible, prebending of the plate has to be done. For the 3.5-mm DCP, a prebend of 2 to 4 degrees with 600 N tensioning is recommended (131). Experience is required to gain the optimal interaction between the axial compression force and prebending of the plate. With a prebent plate, compression will result in an even distribution of forces across the fracture site (see Fig. 6-28).

Tensioning Device. After fixation of the plate to the main fragment, the fracture is reduced and held in position with reduction forceps. The articulated tensioning device is opened as much as possible. The hook of the tensioning device is attached to the outer plate hole, which often has a notch that fits the hook of the tensioning device (see Fig. 6-28). The tensioning device is fixed to the "mobile" fragment. Usually unicortical screw fixation is sufficient. In osteoporotic bone, bicortical screw fixation is recommended. The tension device is gradually closed, which results in a shift of the fixed fragment toward the "mobile fragment," with subsequent interfragmentary compression. In oblique fractures the position of the tensioning device is dependent on the fracture morphology. The plate and the tensioning device must be placed in such a way that the fracture spike locks underneath the plate. Otherwise, overriding of the fragment will occur.

Dynamic Compression Hole. As described above, plates like the DCP or LC-DCP generate an axial force with eccentric screw placement. If this axial force is directed toward the fracture, the plate will cause interfragmentary compression less than that associated with the tensioning device (see Fig. 6-21).

Bridge Plating. Bridge plating was originally recommended by the AO/ASIF for comminuted fractures where anatomic restoration was not possible (42,134). The plate was fixed to the main proximal and distal fragments, leaving the fracture untouched (Fig. 6-29). This method of osteosynthesis does not produce rigid fixation, as fracture healing with callus is seen (135). A modification of the bridge plate involves bending the plate in the bridging zone to produce a wave plate (136). This plate was initially used for the treatment of nonunions, as its particular shape allowed surgeons to pack bone graft beneath the wave. The wave shape enabled the surgeon to leave the nonunion untouched and to apply bone grafting underneath the plate (136) (Fig. 6-30).

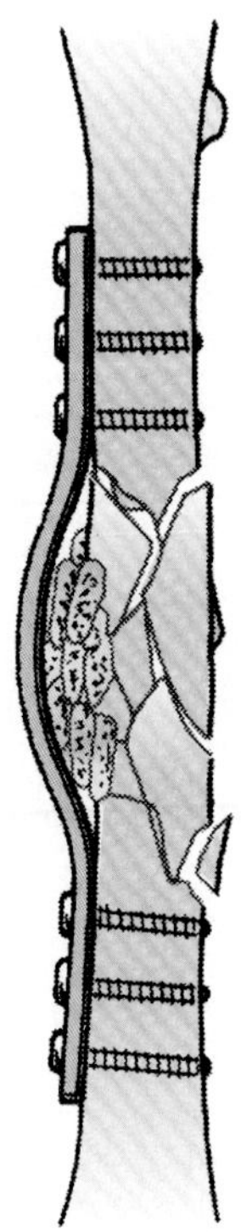

FIGURE 6-30 A wave plate.

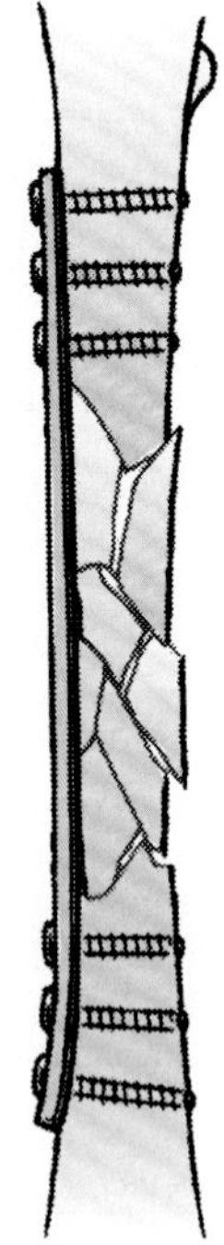

FIGURE 6-29 A bridge plate.

Absolutely stable fixation of bone defects tends to result in bone resorption and nonunion (110,135). To enhance callus formation, plate osteosynthesis must permit micromovement as occurs with IM nailing. This occurs in plate fixation of long defects, as the stiffness of the plate–bone construct is reduced and motion within the fracture gap is achieved during loading. However, even small gaps can be treated with bridge plating, as long as the stiffness of the construct allows micromotion. This results in "elastic" osteosynthesis, which might be considered to be the precursor of minimally invasive plate osteosynthesis (135). In small fracture gaps, the stiffness of the construct is reduced by using a long plate and leaving at least two to four plate holes over the fracture empty.

Cement Augmentation. The incidence of implant failure is higher in pathologic and osteoporotic fractures, often because of poor screw fixation. Müller (137) may have been the first surgeon to use bone cement to increase fixation strength. The mostly commonly used bone cement is polymethylmethacrylate (PMMA). The indications for augmentation with PMMA must be carefully considered, as cement removal and revision osteosynthesis are very difficult. The use of PMMA with internal fixation can be justified when one considers patient outcome in terms of pain relief, mobilization, and restoration of function, in addition to the psychological benefits in patients with limited life expectancy (138).

Biomechanical and clinical studies have shown superior stability with augmented screw fixation (139–143). With cement augmentation the internal fixation has to be performed first. The screws and the plate are then removed and the bone is filled with cement. The screws and plate are reinserted in the same position as the cement hardens.

Cement augmentation is now mainly used in the proximal femur to reduce the incidence of cutout of the screw from the femoral head in the treatment of proximal femoral fractures. Biomechanical studies have shown less implant displacement, especially in very osteoporotic bone (144,145). Recently, clinical and biomechanical tests have examined the use of absorbable calcium phosphate bone cements. These materials are biocompatible, cure at lower temperatures, and have a higher initial stiffness (146,147), but their usefulness has still to be fully determined.

Tension Band Fixation

Eccentric loading of a bone induces compression on the concave side and tension on the convex side. These early concepts of load transfer within bone were developed by Pauwels (148). In a fracture, this eccentric loading leads to bending forces and fracture displacement. An eccentrically placed implant on the convex side can turn distraction forces into compression forces, and compression forces will lead to direct bone healing of the fracture. This is referred to as "tension band plating." To achieve this, the bending moments must be neutralized, the implant must be able to withstand the resulting distraction and compressive forces, and tensioning of the implant must be possible. The cortices on both sides must be intact and exactly reduced. Otherwise, repetitive bending moments may lead to implant failure.

Tension band wiring has the advantage of being less bulky than plating. This is particularly important in fractures in regions such as the patella, olecranon, greater trochanter, and medial malleolus, where the soft tissue cover is thin. In fractures of the patella or olecranon, the tension forces of the muscle are turned into compression forces (Fig. 6-31). Therefore, the compression forces increase with flexion. This principle is called "dynamic tension wiring." In contrast, compression of fractures such as the medial malleolus that are not subjected to muscle pull does not increase with motion. This is called "static tension wiring."

There are a number of different techniques of tension wiring, but the following are essential no matter which technique is used:

1. The wire must withstand the tensile forces.
2. The bone must withstand the compression forces.
3. The opposite cortex must be closed after reduction.

The wire can be fixed around a tendon insertion or through a drill hole in the bone. It can also be looped around the head of a screw or Kirschner wires. The cerclage wire must have some flexibility. Usually wire 1.0 or 1.2 mm in diameter is used. The wire can be looped as a circle or in a figure of eight. It is theoretically advisable to tighten both sides of the wire, or eccentric tension with displacement might occur. Tension wiring is often performed in combination with two Kirschner wires. The application of additional Kirschner wires has some advantages, as the fragments are temporarily fixed by the Kirschner wires and the cerclage wire can be looped around the ends of the wires. Furthermore, the Kirschner wires provide a rotational stability that is not imparted by pure cerclage fixation.

Some technical features are essential for successful tension wiring. The wire fixation must be eccentrically placed on the tensioned side. If a drill hole is used, this hole should be close to the cortex of the tensioned side. The loosening rate of the Kirschner wires is less if they are drilled through the opposite cortex (149). The ends of the Kirschner wires are sometimes prominent, and it is wise to bend the ends of the wires and then bury them.

Minimally Invasive Plate Osteosynthesis (MIPO)

The clinical experience gained from the use of the wave plate (129,150) and bridge plate (134) paved the way for the era of biologic plating (151,152). The emphasis changed from being

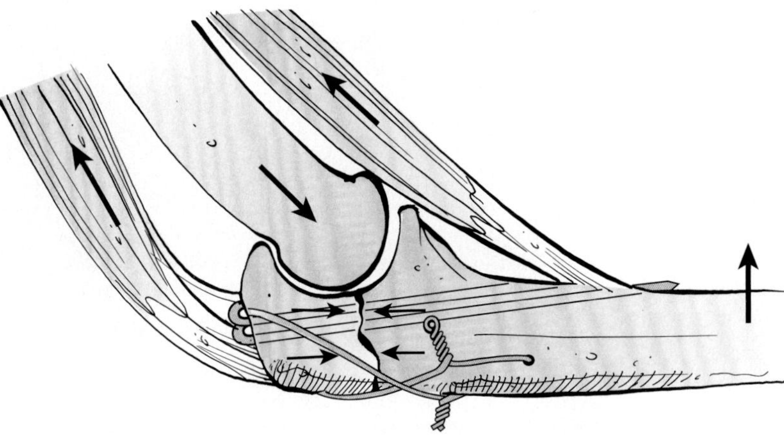

FIGURE 6-31 Tension band fixation of an olecranon fracture.

mainly concerned with the type of implant to protecting the soft tissues by adopting less invasive fixation techniques. These techniques use indirect fracture reduction techniques, and they maintain fracture alignment by plating the fracture without compression. Operative exposure and soft tissue stripping are minimized with preservation of the vasculature and periosteum. The technique of biologic plating aimed to improve rates of fracture union, decrease the use of supplementary bone grafting, and decrease the incidence of complications such as infection or refracture (153).

Philosophy

With the MIPO technique, the fracture site is not exposed and further damage to the soft tissues is prevented or minimized. The philosophy is therefore similar to that of IM nailing. The incision for implant insertion is distant from the fracture, the fracture is reduced closed, and the fixation of the implant to the bone does not interfere with the fracture (Fig. 6-32). The mechanical features of bridge plating cause indirect bone healing.

The MIPO technique can be applied to fractures that do not require anatomic reduction but merely anatomic alignment. These are mainly metaphyseal and diaphyseal fractures. Intra-articular fractures usually require anatomic reduction. If closed reduction cannot be achieved or maintained, an open approach is required. However, to minimize further soft tissue dissection in the metaphysis or diaphysis, a combination of MIPO and open reduction may be undertaken as described for the distal femur (53). With the transarticular approach and retrograde plate osteosynthesis (TARPO) technique, the joint is opened and full exposure is gained (Fig. 6-33). The intra-articular fracture can be reduced and fixed under direct vision. The metaphy-

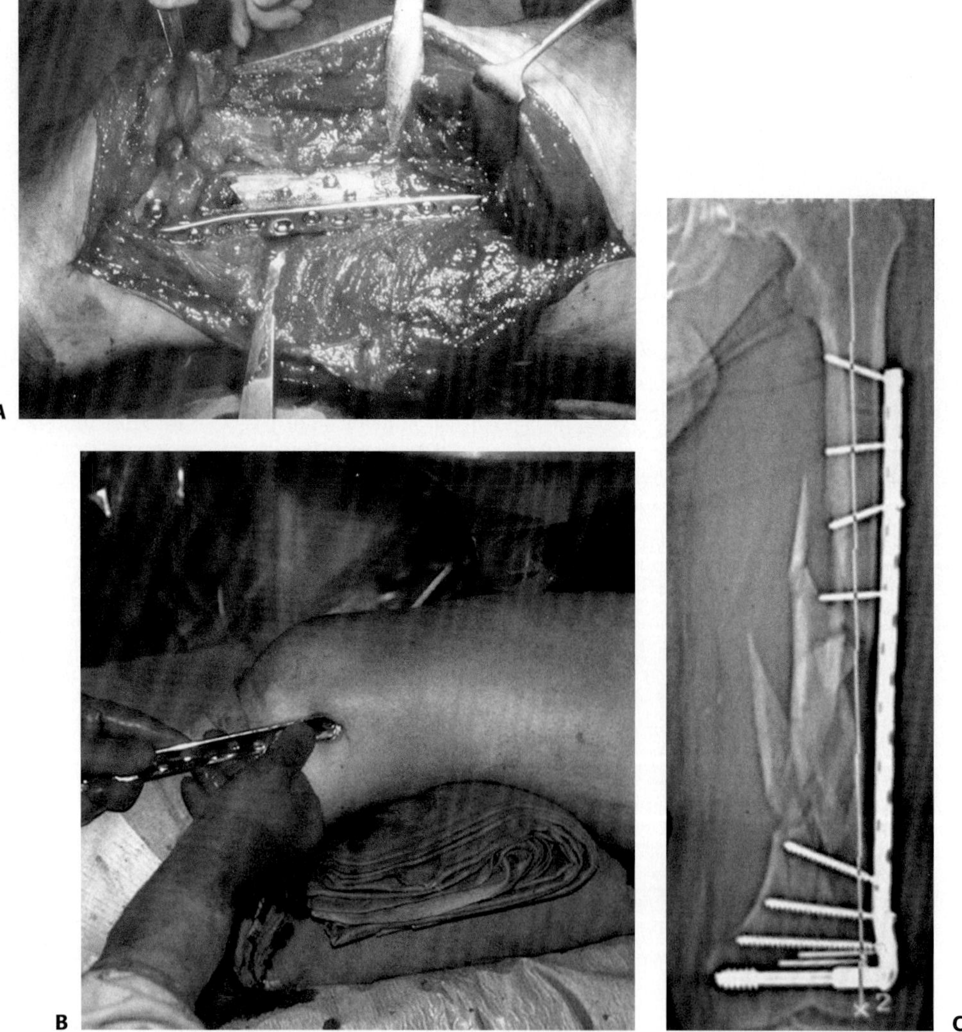

FIGURE 6-32 Minimally invasive surgery used for plate osteosynthesis of the femur. **A.** In the conventional approach, the muscles are detached from the bone. **B.** In a minimally invasive approach, the plate is inserted percutaneously underneath the vastus lateralis muscle. **C.** AP x-ray shows excellent alignment.

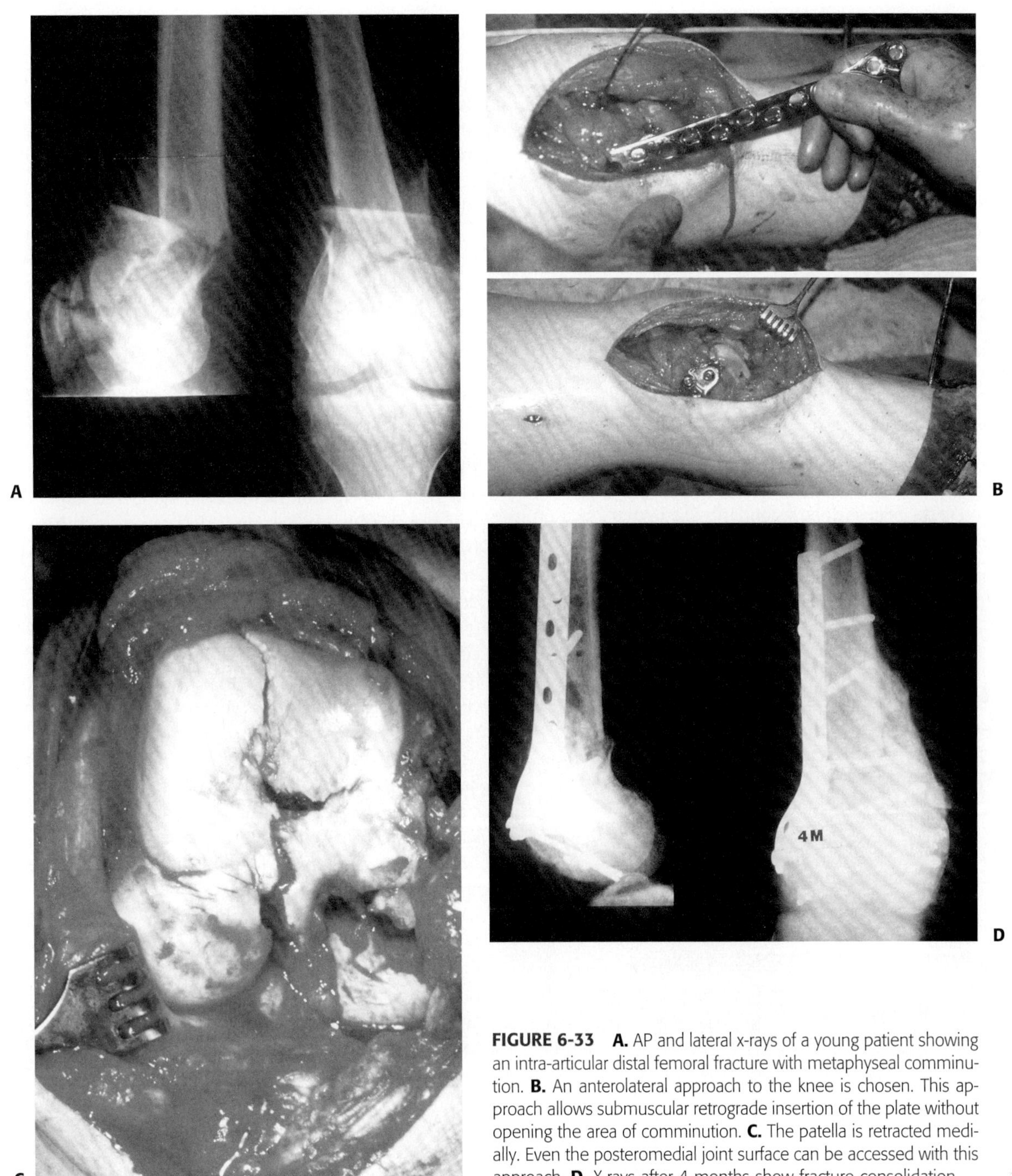

FIGURE 6-33 **A.** AP and lateral x-rays of a young patient showing an intra-articular distal femoral fracture with metaphyseal comminution. **B.** An anterolateral approach to the knee is chosen. This approach allows submuscular retrograde insertion of the plate without opening the area of comminution. **C.** The patella is retracted medially. Even the posteromedial joint surface can be accessed with this approach. **D.** X-rays after 4 months show fracture consolidation.

sis remains untouched. The plate is inserted retrograde through the articular approach.

With the MIPO technique, the incision should be at a safe distance from the fracture site, ideally in an area where the soft tissues are not compromised. A submuscular approach allows for the easy insertion of a plate between the periosteum and the surrounding muscles. Additional soft tissue trauma is minimized. The perforating arteries are preserved and the periosteal vasculature and medullary perfusion is increased compared to conventional plating techniques (154).

Internal Fixators

The concept of internal fixators was devised by a group of Polish surgeons in the 1980s. After carrying out biomechanical studies on plate osteosynthesis, they developed the ZESPOL-system

(155). They based the design of their implants on a number of principles.

1. The screws should be fixed to the plate.
2. Compression between the plate and the bone should be eliminated.
3. The number of screws necessary for stable fixation should be reduced.
4. Plate stability and interfragmentary compression should be preserved.

The system consists of three basic elements (Fig. 6-34):

1. Cancellous or cortical screws with a quadrangular retaining disk and a fine-thread bolt instead of a head.
2. A spherical counternut that fits onto the threaded bolt.
3. A plate with dynamic screw holes.

The counternut locks the screw within the hole of the plate. As with external fixators, the screws have to be inserted first. The fixation to the plate is done secondarily. Temporary fixation of the reduced fracture is necessary until the locked screws provide stability. The plate can be placed close to the bone, subcutaneously, or outside the body. Biomechanical tests showed that axial compression of the ZESPOL system averaged 88% of a conventional compression plate (156). There was an inverse correlation between the compression force and the bone mineral density: in osteoporotic bone the ZESPOL system reached 119% of the axial compression force of a conventional plate.

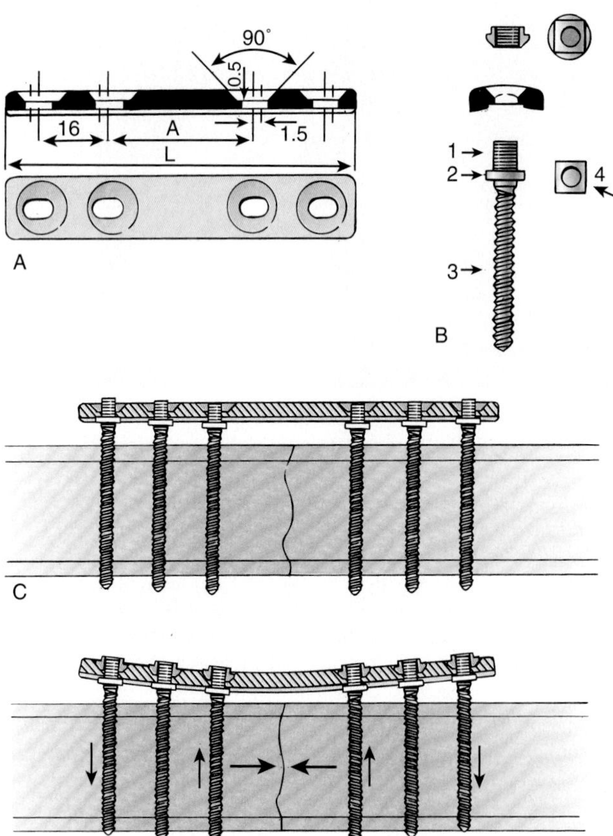

FIGURE 6-34 Zespol plate fixator. **A.** Plate. **B.** Platform screw: (1) tapped pin; (2) screw platform; (3) screw; (4) nut. **C,D.** Screw platforms may be placed variable distances from the bone to create compressive loading with tightening of the nuts.

The Schuhli nut of the AO/ASIF group is based on the same principle (157,158). The counternut is placed beneath the plate and locks the screw head within the plate (Fig. 6-35). The Schuhli nut is compatible with standard AO instrumentation. Axial stiffness is reduced with the use of the Schuhli nut (158), but loss of stiffness under cyclical loading is similar to a conventional plate. With cortical defects, the Schuhli nut improves the stiffness of the construct.

Philosophy

The basic principle of the internal fixator is its angular stability, whereas stability of conventional plate osteosynthesis relies on friction. This friction is caused by compression between the bone and the plate. The lag effect of the screw is the main determinant of stability. In contrast, the principle of fixation of angular stable devices is screw-locking. It does not rely on compression of the screws. Stability is gained by the bone fragments being connected to the fixator through all the screws (Fig. 6-36). The function of the screws of the internal fixator is more akin to that of external fixator pins than to the screws used in conventional plating systems. The internal fixator screws have to neutralize all bending forces. As friction is the main stabilizer in conventional osteosynthesis, these screws are not subjected to high bending forces, and conventional plate osteosynthesis fails when the compression force of the screw decreases and toggling of the screws occurs within the holes. Internal fixators do not impart absolute fracture stability. Elastic deformation of the fixator provides a relatively stable fixation that allows for induction of new bone. Fracture healing takes place by callus formation. As internal fixators do not need compression contact with the bone, precise contouring of the fixator is not necessary. Whereas screw tightening in poorly contoured conventional plates causes fracture malalignment, the internal fixator holds the fragments in position. This feature makes the internal fixator ideal for minimally invasive plate osteosynthesis.

The benefits of angular stability over conventional friction stability are best seen in osteoporotic bone (156,159). Biomechanical tests have shown that the resistance to pullout depends on the loading angle. The lowest stability is seen in screws that are loaded in their long axis, and the highest stability is seen in screws with shear loading perpendicular to the screw (160) (Fig. 6-37). The first corresponds to the conventional screw/plate system and the second to the fixed-angle device. Screws locked in a divergent direction have higher pullout strength than locked parallel screws. This fact is especially important in osteoporotic metaphyseal fractures. The periosteum plays an

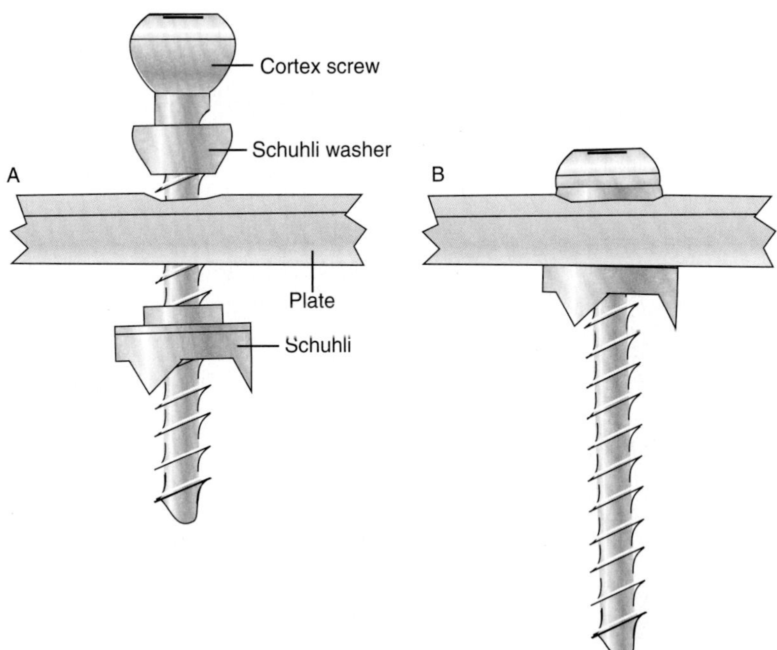

FIGURE 6-35 Principle of the Schuli nut. The standard cortical screw is locked within the plate by the nut underneath the plate.

important role in fracture healing (117,161–163), and as the minimally invasive MIPO technique preserves the periosteum, union tends to be enhanced.

Different Types

Since the introduction of the ZESPOL system and the Schuhli nut, the design of internal fixators has changed, but the basic principle of a locked screw head has remained (99,122,164–168). More recent systems have consisted of a plate and one-piece screws. Two different techniques of securing the screw head in the plate have been evaluated (16,165,168). The first technique uses cold welding of the screw head and the plate. The screw head is made of a titanium alloy, which is harder than the plate. The threaded head can be screwed into the plate hole and locked by cold welding. These screws can be tilted (168). The second technique uses a threaded head that is screwed into a threaded screw hole (Fig. 6-38). The direction of the screw is predicted by the orientation of the threads of the hole. This principle is used by the AO/ASIF for their implants (99,122,167). The locking compression plate (LCP) uses a combi-hole to place either a fixed-angle screw or a conventional compression screw. The shapes of these internal fixators corre-

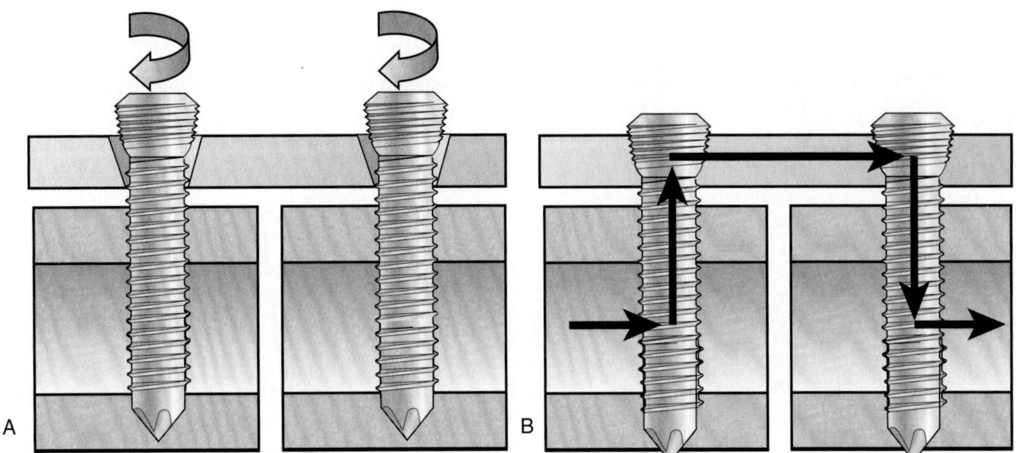

FIGURE 6-36 The mechanical principle of a locked screw plate. **A.** The plate sits slightly off the bone. **B.** Tightening of the screw locks the screw heads within the plate. The plate is not drawn toward the bone, and there is no compression between the bone and the plate. The flux is: bone/screw/plate/screw/bone.

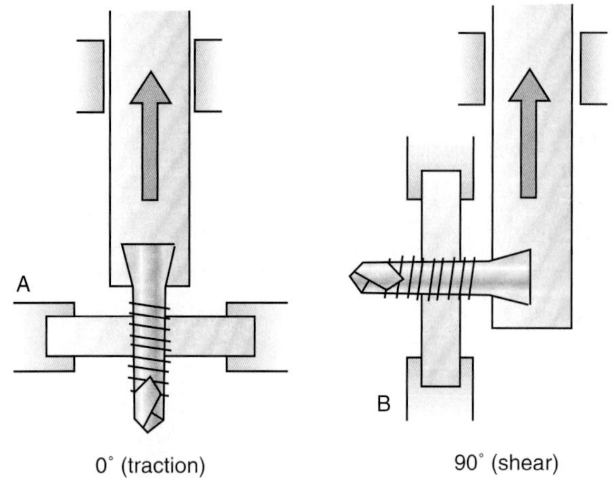

FIGURE 6-37 Different modes of screw loading. **A.** Traction forces: screws of compression plates are loaded in this way. **B.** Shear forces: the bolts/screws of angular stable implants are mainly loaded in this way. (Modified from Seebeck J, Lill C, Morlock MM, Schneider E. Implantatverankerung in osteoporotischem Knochen mittels monokortikaler Schrauben. *Trauma Berufskrankh* 1999;1:411–414.)

spond to the standard AO/ASIF small and large fragment plates (99,165,166).

Basic Principles

The indications for use of an internal fixator are based on many factors, such as fracture location and configuration, the condition of the soft tissues, the presence of other implants, and the experience and preference of the surgeon (166). Internal fixators are ideally used to bridge metaphyseal and diaphyseal multifragmentary fractures using both MIPO and conventional open techniques (16,165,169–174). Biomechanical tests have shown that in the distal femur and femoral diaphysis, internal fixators are associated with less secondary loss of reduction than conventional plates (52,159,175,176) and retrograde femoral nailing (16). Simple transverse or oblique diaphyseal or metaphyseal fractures are still better stabilized by conventional plating techniques (166). Compression osteosynthesis remains the treatment of choice for the fixation of intra-articular fractures.

Lag screw osteosynthesis may be supported by conventional buttress plating in AO type B partial articular fractures. In type C complete articular fractures with comminution of the metaphysis or diaphysis, a combination of articular compression osteosynthesis and metaphyseal bridging with internal fixators may be superior to conventional stabilization techniques. Biomechanical tests have shown that unilateral fracture fixation of bicondylar tibial plateau fractures with an internal fixator is equivalent to conventional bilateral plating (159,177,178). It has also been shown that internal fixators are particularly useful in the treatment of osteoporotic fractures, especially those of the proximal humerus (179), distal humerus (174), distal radius (164), distal femur (Fig. 6-39) (170), and proximal tibia (171).

Periprosthetic fractures are often difficult to treat. These fractures usually occur in patients with poor bone stock. Nailing of these fractures is associated with a stress riser between the nail and the prosthesis, with the risk of a subsequent insufficiency fracture between the nail tip and the prosthesis. Implant overlap leads to higher stability (180). Their use in fractures above a total-knee prosthesis has also been documented (181,182). Unicortical screw placement and their improved stability in osteoporotic bone make internal fixators a useful implant in fractures close to an intramedullary prosthetic stem (Fig. 6-40).

Some basic principles have to be taken into account when using internal fixators. Proper preoperative planning with draw-

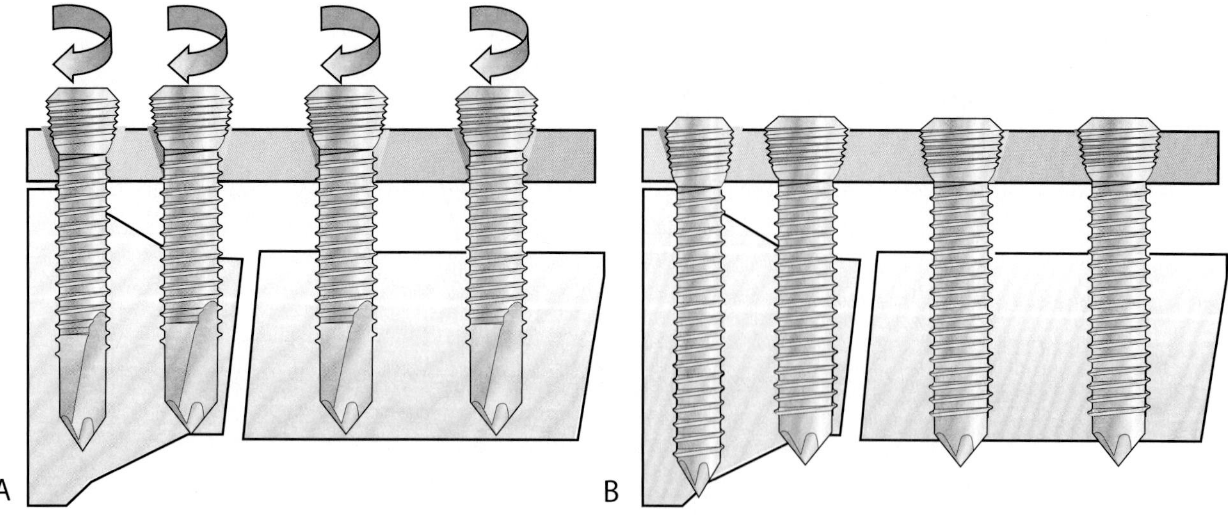

FIGURE 6-38 **A.** The threaded screw head is screwed into the plate. The shape of the plate and the bone may not fit. **B.** Tightening of the screw locks the head within the plate. The position of the bone and plate do not alter. The reduction is maintained.

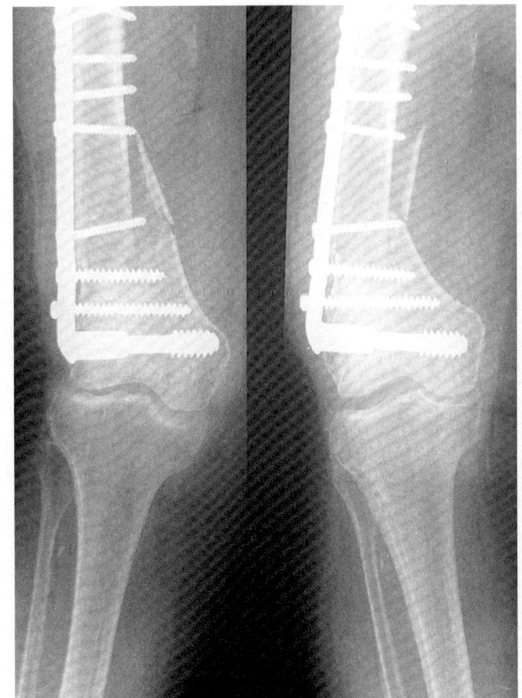

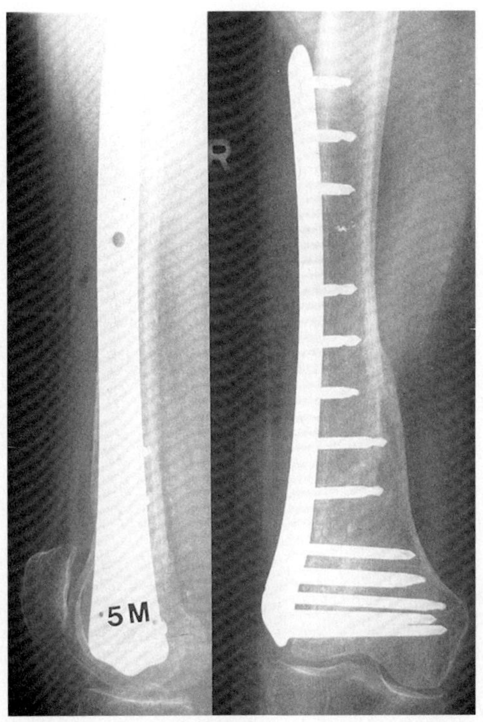

FIGURE 6-39 An 89-year-old osteoporotic woman with a supracondylar femoral fracture. **A.** Initial stabilization was done with a dynamic compression screw. The right-sided x-ray shows instability on varus stress. **B.** The fracture was refixed with a locked screw plate. The patient started immediate weight-bearing. Fracture healing in good alignment was seen 5 months after the operation.

ing of the fracture fixation is helpful. Plate length, screw positions, and screw types should be determined preoperatively. In intra-articular fractures, the joint surface should be reduced and fixed before application of the internal fixator. Precise planning of the position of the interfragmentary screws is essential to prevent any subsequent difficulty in placing the internal fixator. The fracture should be reduced before the internal fixator is applied. Fixation is preferably achieved using an MIPO technique with submuscular plating. With this technique the plate length can be increased without additional soft tissue dissection. The ideal length of the internal fixator can be determined by means of two values, the plate span width and the screw density (114) (Fig. 6-41). The plate span width is the quotient of plate length and overall fracture length. Recommendations by the AO/ASIF group favor a plate span width of more than 2 in comminuted fractures and more than 8 in simple fractures. The plate screw density is the quotient of the number of screws and the number of plate holes. A value between 0.5 and 0.4 is recommended (114). The AO/ASIF guidelines for conventional plate osteosynthesis with regard to a specific number of screws or cortices in each fragment cannot be used for the internal fixator. At least four cortices per main fragment should be used for comminuted fractures and at least three cortices per main fragment for simple fractures (114). Exact contouring of an internal fixator is not necessary. If the internal fixator has to be contoured, the surgeon must avoid bending it at a screw hole. If this is done, adequate locking of the screw head within the hole is not guaranteed. To be sure that no bending will be done within the hole, a threaded drill sleeve or a screw should be inserted before bending. Unicortical locked screws can be used in the diaphysis. In fixators that lock their threaded screws within threaded holes, cold welding with compromised stability can occur if the screws are angulated. Freehand insertion of self-drilling screws can be risky. With locked screws, the surgeon does not have any feedback about the grip of the screw within the bone. Even screws that are placed outside the bone lock firmly within the plate. Predrilling with an aiming device should ensure correct placement of the screw. In osteoporotic bone, bicortical screws should be used.

The outer screws should be inserted first. In curved bones such as the femur, a mismatch of the plate axis and bone axis can occur, which is sometimes difficult to visualize on intraoperative fluoroscopy. Poor placement of the plate may lead to compromised screw fixation within the bone. To ensure correct placement, the incision over the end of the plate should be lengthened to allow digital palpation of the plate and the bone. After the first two screws are inserted, minor degrees of malalignment can be still corrected. The fragments can be pulled onto or pushed away from the plate (Fig. 6-42). This can be done, for example, with the use of a collinear clamp or by inserting a conventional screw. Displaced butterfly fragments can be reduced using the lag effect of a conventional screw. Subsequent

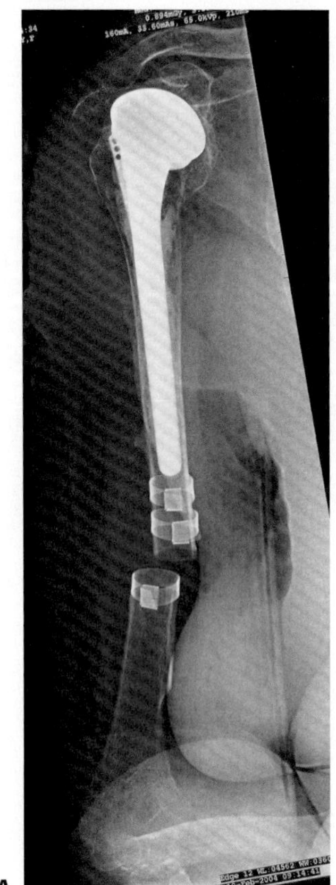

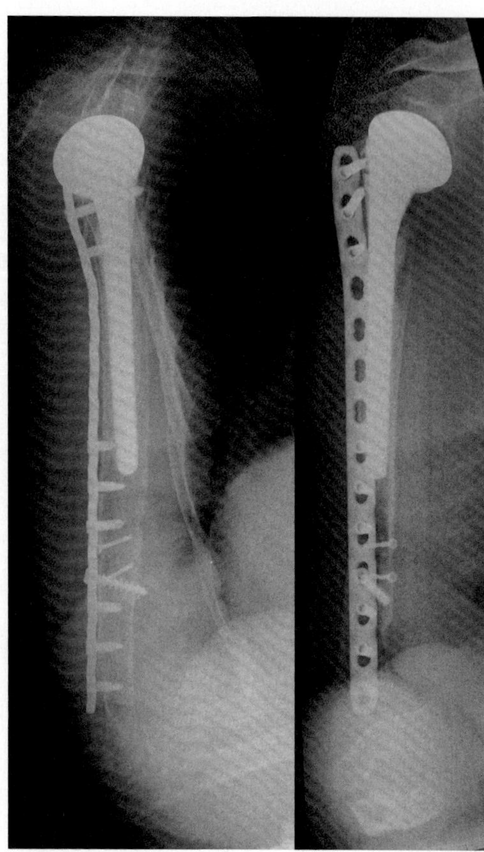

FIGURE 6-40 **A.** A periprosthetic fracture related to a hemiarthroplasty prosthesis. **B.** Treated successfully with a locking compression plate mainly using unicortical screws.

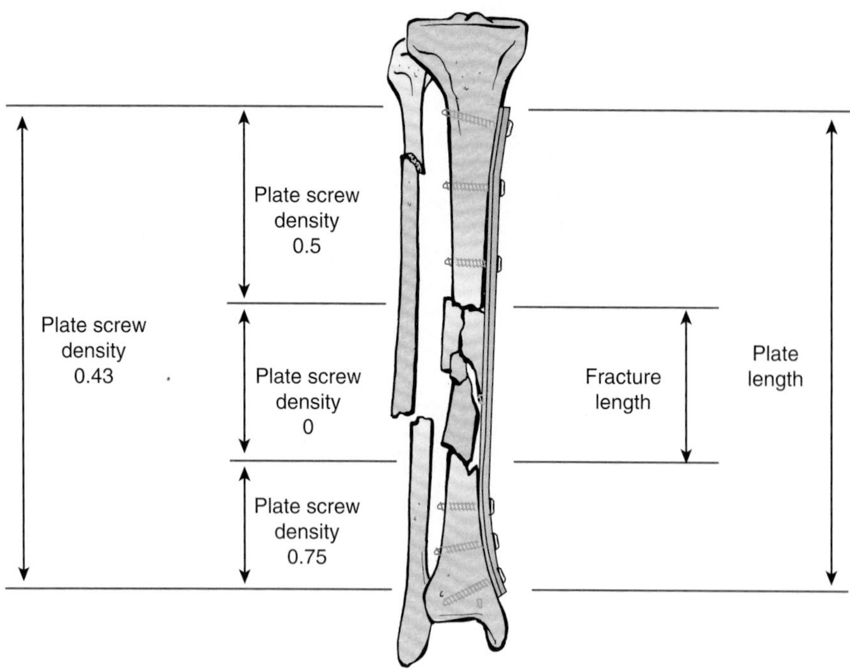

FIGURE 6-41 Plate screw density and fracture/plate quotient according to Gautier. (From Gautier E, Sommer C. Guidelines for the clinical application of the LCP. *Injury* 2003; Suppl2:B63–B76.)

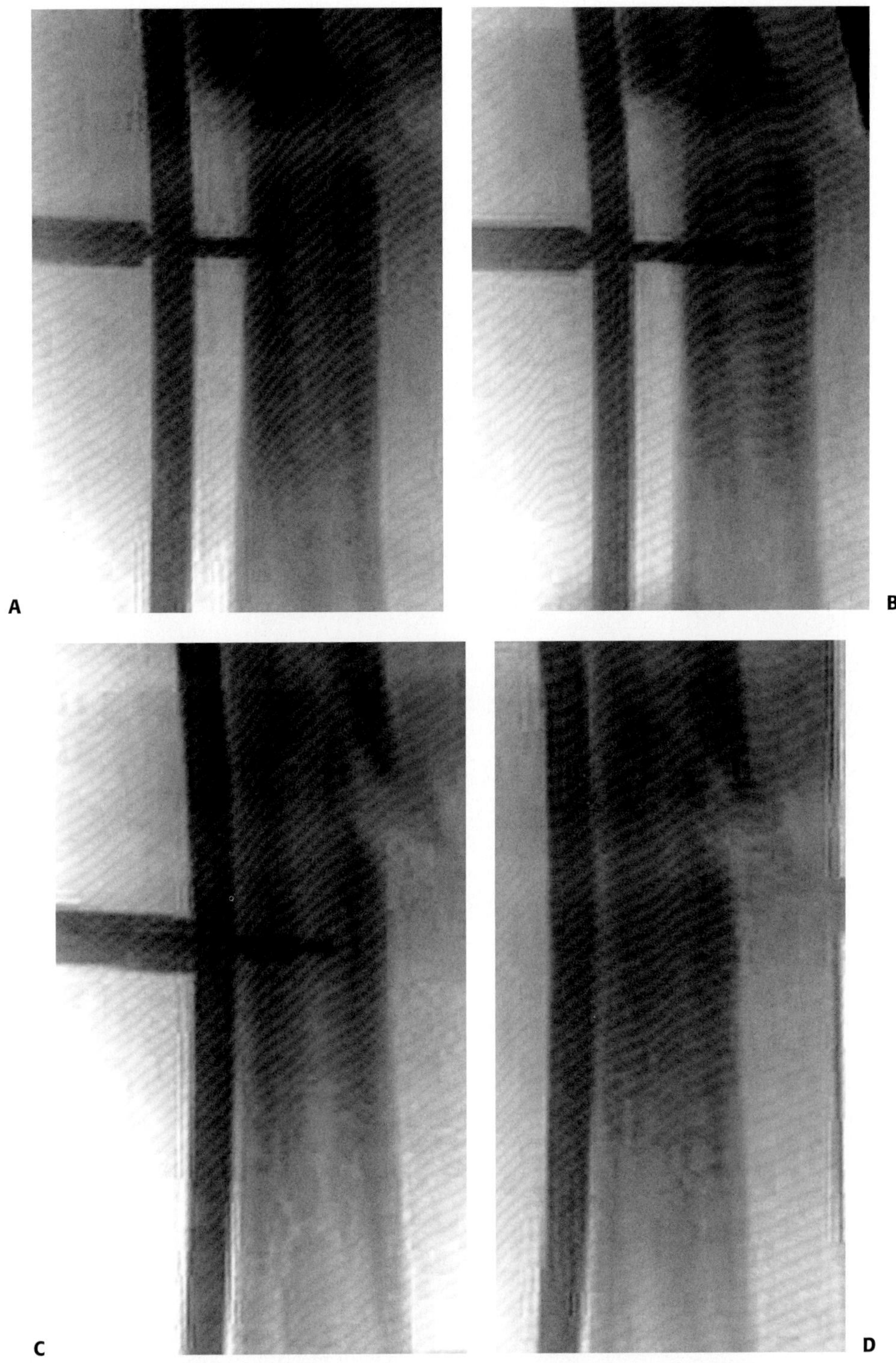

FIGURE 6-42 Intraoperative fluoroscopy shows the function of the so-called whirly-bird. **A.** This reduction device can be used to correct malalignment. **B.** A threaded drill is inserted into near cortex. A counterscrew stabilizes the drill against the aiming guide. **C.** Rotation of the screw results in a relative movement of the drill in relation to the aiming device and plate. **D.** The dislocated fragment can be pulled toward the plate.

removal of the conventional screw is recommended, as the stable fixation of the compression screw and the flexible fixation of the fixator should not be combined (165). In comminuted fractures the screw holes close to the fracture should be used to reduce strain (121). In fractures with a small or no gap, the inner screw holes should be left unfilled to reduce the strain. If the fixation is too stiff, implant failure might occur (165).

INTRAMEDULLARY FIXATION TECHNIQUES

IM fixation techniques permit the placement of an implant in the IM canal of a long bone. Depending on the anatomy, the insertion can be antegrade and retrograde. The entry point depends on the anatomy of the bone but is distant from the fracture site. IM fixation techniques offer the advantages of closed reduction and closed fixation.

History

The first description of IM fixation may have been from Stimson in 1883 (183), who described the insertion of an ivory peg into the medullary canal. Nicolysen, Delbet, and Lambotte all used IM pins for stabilization (184). Hey-Groves used different types of IM devices for the treatment of fractures of the femoral shaft. In 1918 he pointed out the advantages of rapid fixation, preservation of the soft tissues and periosteum, accelerated healing, and abolition of prolonged splintage. His preferred implant was a solid metal rod (185). The Rush brothers described their IM pinning system in 1927.

Probably the most important work in the field of IM fixation was done by the German surgeon Gerhard Küntscher, who perfected the technique of IM nailing. He undertook a considerable number of animal experiments (186) and inserted his first femoral nail in 1939 (187). Following the work of Hey-Groves and the Rush brothers, he recognized the advantages of closed reduction and fixation with respect to fracture healing. However, he also stipulated two further criteria. He stated that the implant must resist loads of several hundred kilograms and that the nail fracture construct must not allow motion, even at high loads. He devised the term "stable osteosynthesis" (188). The principle of fixation was based on compression between the bone and the nail. Therefore, only fractures of the isthmus could be stabilized. To extend the scope of nailing, Küntscher started to ream the IM canal so that compression between the nail and the endosteal surface of the IM canal could be achieved over a greater length (189). Nailing of the tibia was introduced in 1950 by Herzog, who bent the proximal end of the nail (190). Close to his death, Küntscher described the "Detensornagel," which he used for the treatment of comminuted fractures (191). This was the precursor of the interlocking nail, and the idea was carried forward by Klemm and Schellmann (192) from Germany and by Grosse and Kempf (193) from France, who produced the forerunners of the interlocking nails in use today.

Flexible Nails

Flexible nails are actually not nails but pins. Their mechanical characteristics and use are different from IM nails. They are of smaller diameter and are more elastic. They are low-cost implants and have a wide range of indications. Their flexibility allows insertion through a cortical window. There are many different types of flexible nails; the best known are Lottes nails, Rush pins, Ender nails, Morote nails, Nancy nails, Prevot nails, and Bundle nails (194–200). Although many of these devices are called "nails," they do not fulfill the mechanical criteria of a nail.

Mechanics

There are two basic methods of IM pinning. They can act by stabilizing fractures with three- or four-point compression (Fig. 6-43) or by a large number of pins being inserted so that they are jammed into the IM canal (see Fig. 6-43). This is called bundle nailing. Most pins stabilize fractures by three- or four-point compression. These pins are C- or S-shaped. They act like a spring. The equilibrium between the tensioned pin and the bone with its attached soft tissues will hold the alignment.

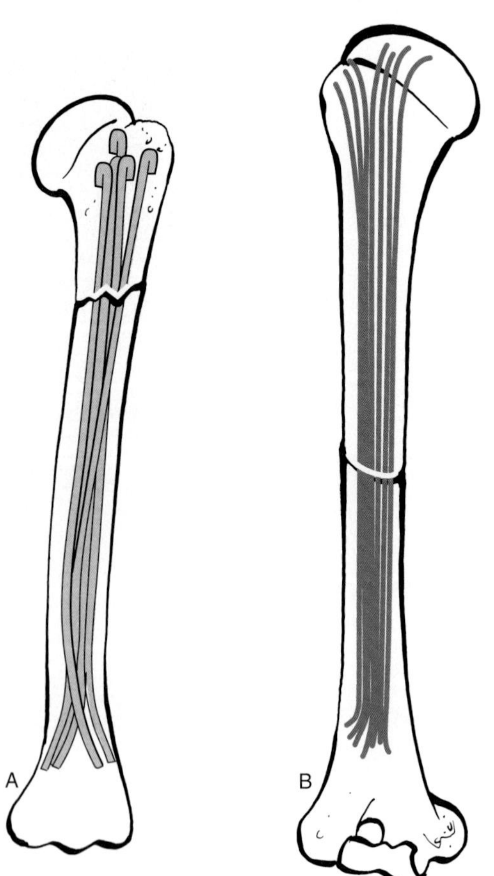

FIGURE 6-43 **A.** Rush pinning of the humerus. Three-point fixation has been used. **B.** Hackethal bundle nailing of the humerus. This method relies on multiple flexible nails being inserted into the diaphysis.

The diameter of the pins depends on the diameter of the IM canal. If possible, two nails with opposite curvature should be implanted. However, some surgeons favor only one rod for mid-shaft fractures (194,201), and bones with a narrow isthmus can only be stabilized with one rod. Most stability is gained if the vertex of the rod is located at the level of the fracture. The stability of the rod depends on its stiffness, which is dependent on its diameter, material, and length. Too stiff a rod does not provide three- or four point compression, and these rods are difficult to insert. The principle of bundle nailing was introduced by Hackethal (202). He inserted many pins into the bone until they jammed within the medullary cavity to provide compression between the nails and the bone.

Both techniques should be seen more as IM splinting than rigid fixation. Bending moments are neutralized, but telescoping and rotational torsion are not prevented with this technique. This applies especially to comminuted fractures, and if used an supplementary external splint may be necessary (200).

Applications

Because of its mechanical properties, flexible pinning in adults tends to be used more in the upper extremity and has been used particularly for fractures of the clavicle (203,204), proximal humerus (205), humeral shaft (206,207), forearm (208), and metacarpals (209). However, even in these fractures an additional external splint may be necessary. In children the main indication for flexible nails is the forearm (210–212), although they are also used for fixation of the femur (196,213,214). Flexible nails have the advantage that they can be inserted through a cortical window at a safe distance from the epiphysis.

Disadvantages

The disadvantages of IM pinning are that additional immobilization is often required (198,200,211) and that the torsional and bending stiffness is much less than that of intact bone and of an IM nail (206,215). Secondary loss of reduction is a problem (216–218), especially in comminuted fractures, which are not sufficiently immobilized by IM three-point stabilization and tend to shorten with loading (216).

Intramedullary Nailing

Since Küntscher's first insertion of a femoral nail for a simple fracture of the femoral diaphysis, there have been a considerable number of modifications of nail design and surgical technique. Different strategies and philosophies of nailing have evolved. The indication for nailing has even been extended to intra-articular fractures.

Mechanics

Elastic deformation is the principle of nail stability. As a nail is hammered into the IM canal, it induces strain, which results in a radially orientated force. This force is proportional to the contact area between the bone and the nail and produces friction that stops the nail from pulling out (Fig. 6-44). Küntscher described this type of stabilization as "elastic locking." To increase the elasticity, the hollow nail has a cloverleaf cross-section with a longitudinal slot. The slot does not significantly reduce the bending stiffness of a nail, but the torsional stiffness is reduced to 15% of its initial value (219,220). Because of this reduced torsional stiffness, slotted nails are much easier to insert. The stabilizing effect of the classic Küntscher nail depends on the elastic locking between the nail and the bone. Due to the shape of the medullary cavity of the femur, only a small part of the bone is in contact compression with the nail. Thus, with the initial technique of IM nailing, only fractures close to the isthmus could be adequately stabilized.

Reaming of the cavity enlarges the diameter of the IM canal. This larger diameter causes two mechanical effects. First, the contact area between the bone and the nail is increased. This widens the scope of fracture stabilization to include most of the diaphysis. The increased contact area leads to increased friction, with a lower incidence of loosening. Second, reaming of the IM canal facilitates the insertion of a nail with a larger diameter, with higher bending and torsional stiffness. Secondary displacement due to bending of the nail is rare if a standard reamed Küntscher nail is used, as the large-diameter implant is the main stabilizer. The weak point is the resistance to axial forces and torsion, as the stability depends on the friction between the bone and the nail. This is a minor problem in simple oblique or transverse fractures, as the contact of the two main fragments provides adequate stability. With comminuted fractures, this is not the case, and the standard Küntscher nail does not prevent shortening in comminuted fractures.

The principle of interlocking nailing is different. These nails have proximal and distal screw holes (Fig. 6-45). The nail is locked to the bone by inserting screws through the bone and the screw holes. The resistance to axial and torsional forces is mainly dependent on the screw–bone interface, and the length of the bone is maintained even if there is a bone defect. The weak points of the construct are the screws themselves and the hold they have in the bone. To improve the screw hold, different techniques have been invented. Vecsei (221) suggested a dowel-bolt for fixation in osteoporotic bone. A similar technique is the so-called modular screw, where the locking screw is inserted into bilaterally placed screws with a high thread depth (Fig. 6-46). The aim of this technique is to increase the surface area within the bone (222). Some nails have a twisted blade instead of the proximal interlocking screw (222,223). In the distal femur, interlocking with a bladelike device has been shown to be 41% stiffer and 20% stronger than with conventional locking bolts (224). The number and orientation of the interlocking screws influence the stability of the nail–bone construct (225,226).

Failure of the interlocking screws leads to significantly higher rates of malunion (227). For small-diameter interlocking screws, failure rates of 12% to 14% have been reported (228,229). Mechanical tests have shown that an increase of interlocking screw diameter significantly increases the fatigue

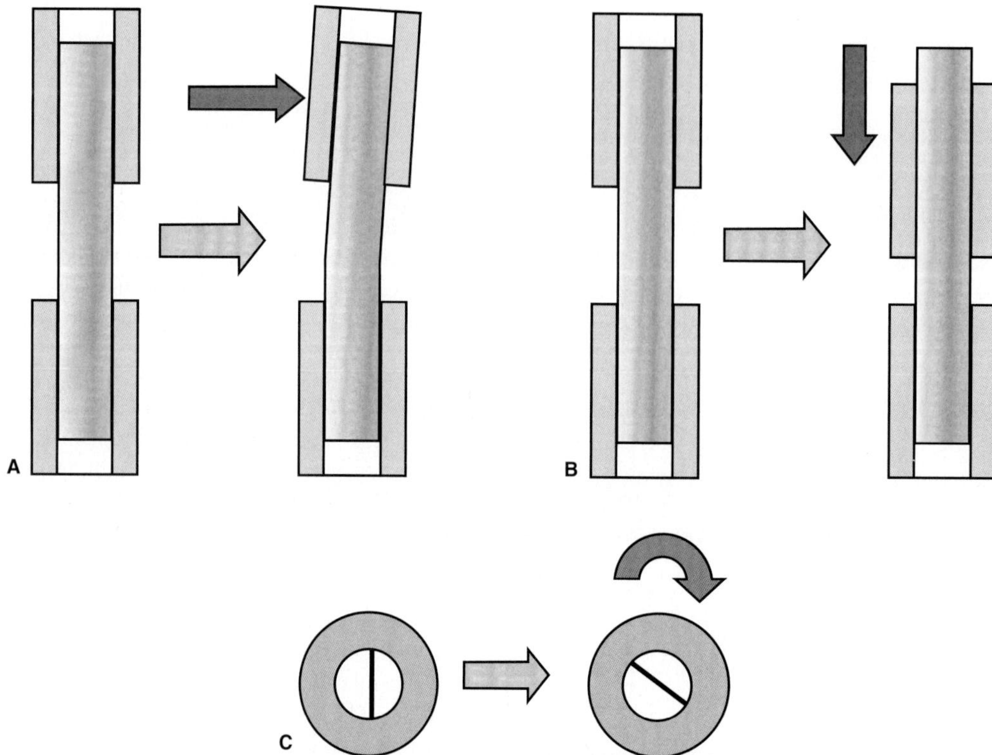

FIGURE 6-44 The basic principle of an IM nail. The nail (*gray color*) can be seen as a rod that is inserted into a tube (*black color*). Ideally the inner diameter of the tube matches the outer diameter of the rod. **A.** Due to the tight fit, the tube is perfectly stabilized against rotation in the frontal or sagittal plane. The positions of the two fragments in relation to the rod do not change. With higher forces, the rod might be bent. **B.** Friction is the main stabilizer against axial shortening. **C.** Friction is the main stabilizer against rotation.

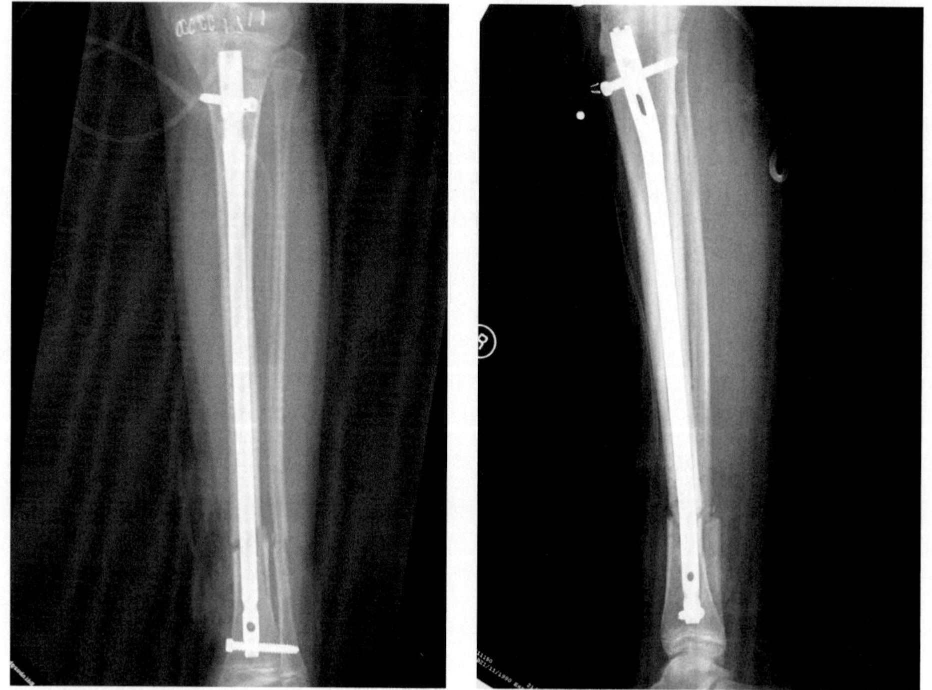

FIGURE 6-45 AP and lateral x-rays of an open tibial fracture treated by locked IM nailing.

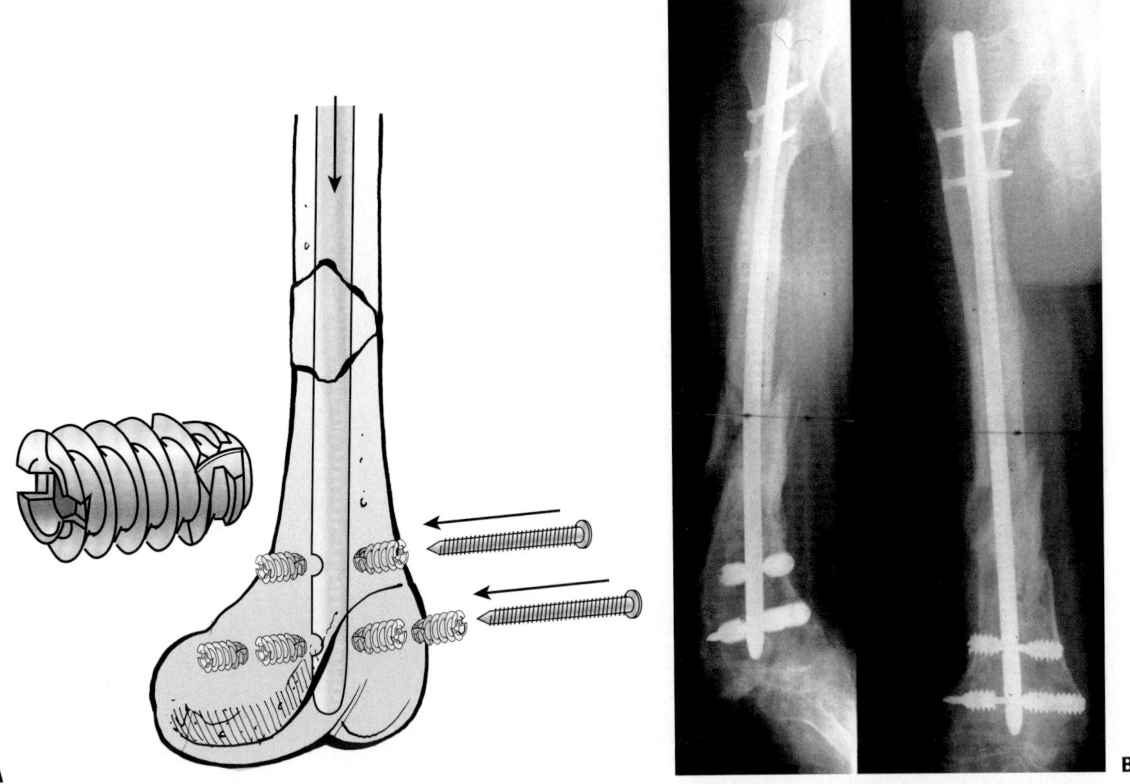

FIGURE 6-46 **A.** The use of the modular screw. The screws are inserted into the osteoporotic bone on both sides of the nail and the locking bolts are inserted through the screws and the locking hole. **B.** A clinical example of the use of the modular screw.

strength. A 20% increase of diameter improved fatigue strength by up to 70% (230).

Inflatable nails have mechanical characteristics similar to that of the classic Küntscher nail. Resistance to axial forces and torsion relies on friction. Unlike the Küntscher nail, the compression force is not generated by elastic deformation during nail insertion. The nail is easily slid in and is then inflated with fluid under high pressure. This pressure generates the compression force that induces friction between the implant and the bone. Biomechanical tests have shown that these nails have significantly less resistance to torsion (231), and clinical studies have shown that the compression effect does not stabilize comminuted fractures (232).

An important mechanical characteristic of IM nails is the working length, which is that portion of the nail that spans the fracture site between areas of fixation in the proximal and distal fragments. In unlocked nails this can vary due to the size of the fracture gap, and in comminuted fractures it can measure several centimeters. In interlocking nails, the working length is the distance between the proximal and distal locking screws. The working length influences nail stiffness in both bending and torsion. In bending, the stiffness is inversely proportional to the square of the working length. In torsion, the stiffness is inversely proportional to the working length (220). Bending stiffness is related to the outer diameter of the nail. Hollow nails, slotted nails, and solid nails do not differ significantly in bending stiffness. Solid nails are, however, significantly stiffer in torsion than hollow and slotted nails (233). Deformation of the nail occurs during insertion. This deformation has been measured by Krettek et al (234,235). In the femur, lateral deformation of up to 20 mm occurs in both solid and slotted nails. Slotted nails show a rotation of 10 degrees (235).

Special Designs for Different Indications. IM nailing is now recommended for wide range of indications in long bone fractures (12,49,225,236–240). The shape of the nail must be adapted to the shape of the medullary cavity. A mismatch may result in malalignment. In the last few years proximal and distal fractures as well as intra-articular fractures have been stabilized by IM nails. Küntscher was the first surgeon to use a Y-shaped nail in the treatment of proximal femoral fractures. Now there are a number of different types of proximal femoral nails (238) (Fig. 6-47). Further information about proximal femoral nails can be found in Chapter 45. Modifications of the configuration and location of locking screws have made standard nails suitable for most indications.

Distraction Nails. Distraction nails offer the opportunity to perform gradual lengthening in a closed fashion (Fig. 6-48). Com-

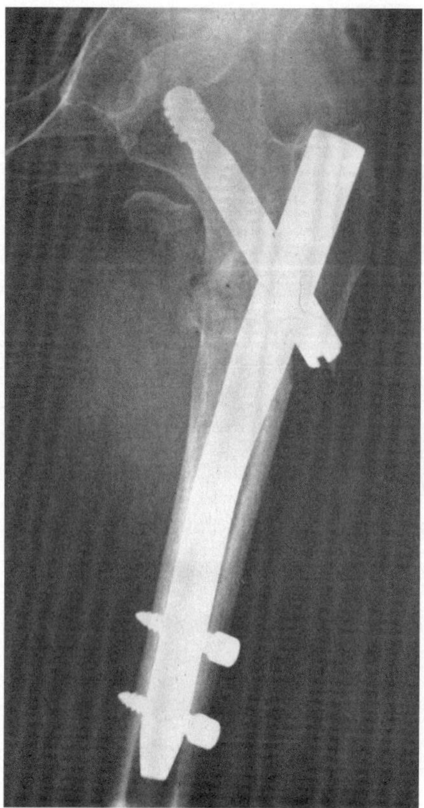

FIGURE 6-47 A proximal femoral IM nail.

pared to distraction osteogenesis by external fixation, this method shows a number of advantages including patient comfort, improved fracture alignment, and a reduced incidence of complications and pain (241–245). These nails are available for lengthening of the tibia and the femur. Two different principles exist. One nail uses a motor with a subcutaneous receiver for gradual lengthening (242). Other nails have a mechanical function with one-way clutches that are activated by alternating rotation. Depending on the device that is used, the amount of rotation that is necessary for elongation differs (243,245). The IM skeletal kinetic distractor (ISKD) activates its clutches by rotations of 3 to 9 degrees. These oscillations are part of the physiologic gait process. A distraction of 1 mm is achieved by 160 rotations of 3 degrees (241,245). Other nails need a rotation of 20 degrees or more for elongation. This may be painful for the patient and might require anesthesia (243).

Pathophysiology of Intramedullary Nailing

IM nailing has both local and systemic effects. These are dependent on the anatomic region, nail design, and surgical technique. In recent years many efforts and resources have been spent to determine whether reaming is beneficial or detrimental to the patient and fracture healing.

Local Changes. Both reamed and unreamed nails cause damage to the endosteal blood supply. Experimental data suggest that reamed nailing deleteriously affects nutrient artery blood flow (246), but the cortical blood supply is significantly reduced after reamed nailing compared with unreamed nailing (247). This applies to both early and late phases. It has been shown that cortical perfusion after reaming is reversible, but it is still significantly reduced after 12 weeks compared to unreamed nailing (248). This reduced perfusion following reaming may be a risk factor for infection, as has been demonstrated in animal experiments (249). Cortical perfusion also depends on the fit of the nail. Tight-fitting nails compromise cortical blood flow to a higher extent than loose-fitting nails (250).

In addition to its effect of bone blood flow, reaming is also associated with the potential risk of heat necrosis. Two series of three cases of osteocutaneous necrosis induced by heat during IM reaming have been reported; all patients in these series had a narrow medullary canal (36,251). In vivo measurements in the tibia have shown significant temperature rises during reaming in canals of 8-mm diameter (252). Blunt reamers and the use of reamers larger in diameter than the medullary canal lead to increased temperature (253). It has been suggested that long bones with very narrow canals should first be reamed manually or an alternative treatment method should be used (251).

These findings have influenced the treatment of fractures associated with severe soft tissue injury in which the extramedullary blood supply is compromised. Some surgeons believe that unreamed nailing is advantageous in the treatment of Gustilo IIIB open fractures (254), citing higher infection rates (9,10). Others have published good results with reamed nailing (255,256). Bhandari et al (257) showed that unreamed nailing was associated with a lower incidence of superficial infection, reoperations, and malunion than external fixation. Clinical studies of both tibial and femoral fractures show that reamed nailing of fractures with low-grade soft tissue injuries significantly reduces the rates of nonunion and implant failure in comparison with unreamed nailing (258–261). In fractures with an intact soft tissue envelope, reaming of the medullary cavity increases significantly the circulation within the surrounding muscles. This increased circulation may improve fracture healing (262).

After reaming of the IM canal, a significant amount of debris collects at the fracture (263). Animal studies have shown that this debris acts like autogenous bone graft (264,265). Reaming does not increase the risk of compartment syndrome (12,258). The peak of compartment pressure is found during insertion of the nail, but the pressure rapidly falls to normal (266,267). Insertion of tight-fitting unreamed nails leads to increased intracompartmental pressure (266). This may be explained by distraction of the fracture gap during insertion of the nail (11).

Systemic. Fat embolism due to IM reaming was described by Küntscher (184). He recommended the avoidance of nailing after trauma in cases of severe injuries or when fat embolism was already present. Fat embolism due to the passage of IM contents into the bloodstream can occur only if the IM pressure associated with instrumentation exceeds the physiologic IM

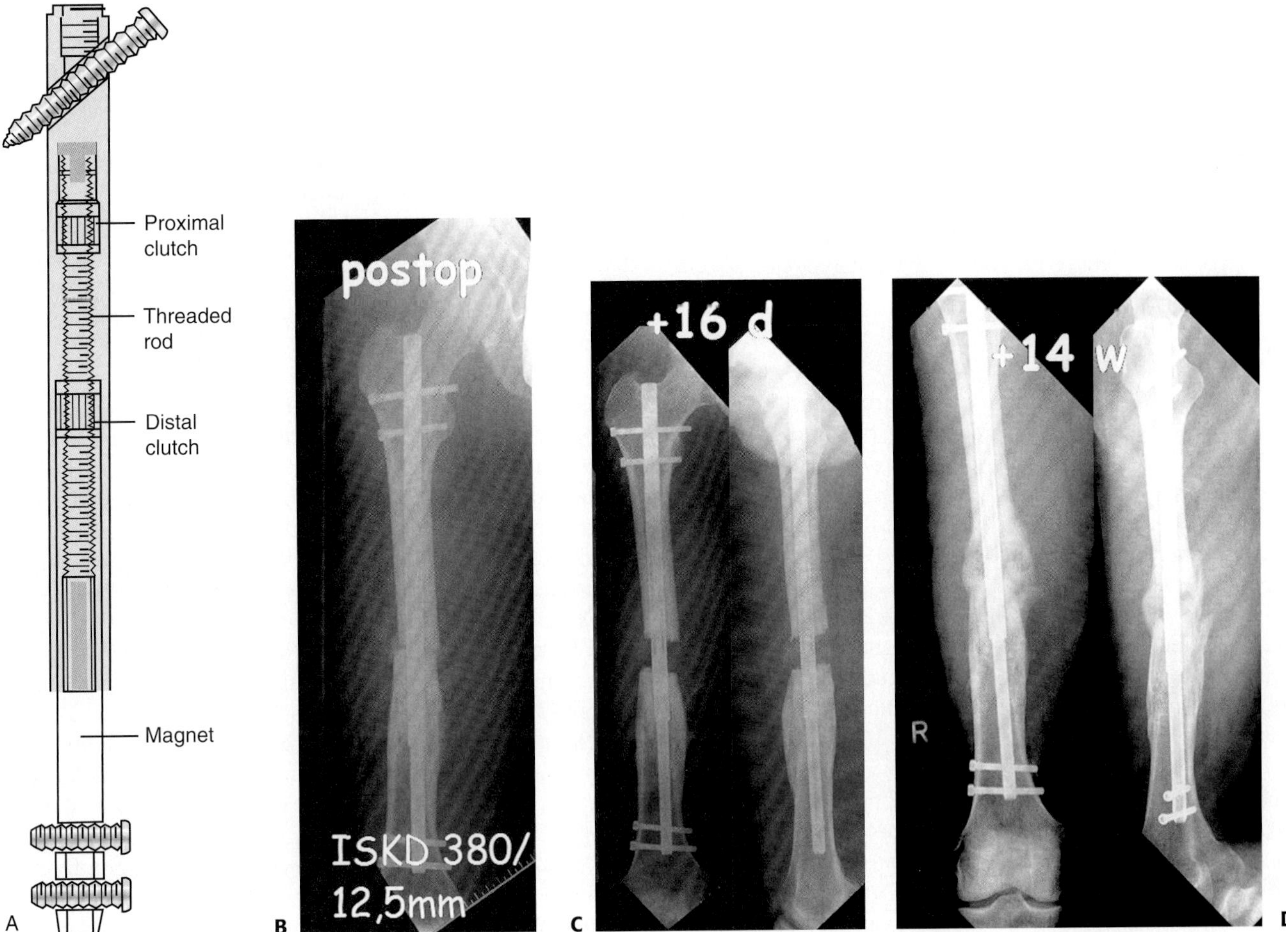

FIGURE 6-48 **A.** The ISKD nail. The nail lengthens over the threaded rod. **B.** Clinical example of distraction in a young male patient with posttraumatic shortening (26 mm). The nail is inserted and the femur is osteotomized. **C.** Amount of distraction 16 days after surgery. **D.** The 26-mm distraction gap has healed after 14 weeks.

pressure and outweighs the effects of the normal blood flow (268). The incidence of fat embolism depends on which bone is involved, with most problems being related to the femur. Reaming of the tibia does not lead to a significant increase of IM pressure (269), and intraoperative echocardiography does not show significant fat embolism in reamed tibial fractures. This phenomenon may be explained by the triangular shape of the tibial IM canal, which may allow some pressure release during reaming or nail insertion (270). In patients with femoral fractures, elevations of pressure between 140 and 830 mm Hg were found after reaming. These pressures vary up to 1,500 mm Hg in animal studies (271). The degree of pressure increase depends on the type of implant, the sharpness of the reamers, the thrust applied during reaming, and the reamer type (272,273). The highest pressure increase occurs during the passage of the first reamer, when the main distal fragment is entered (274). Raised IM pressure causes an elevation of the pulmonary artery pressure, and an increase in intracerebral pressure has also been reported (275).

The release of IM fat causes primary as well secondary systemic effects. Primary effects are directly related to the alteration of blood flow. Following fat embolism a transient increase in pulmonary arterial pressure of about 10 mm Hg occurs (276). However, the mechanical aspects of fat embolism do not explain this increase in pulmonary arterial pressure on their own. Secondary mechanisms such as inflammatory, hemostatic, toxic, and vasoactive reactions modulate the reactions induced by intravenous fat. These may aggravate the mechanical cardiocirculatory reactions (267). Although even the insertion of unreamed nails leads to an increase in IM pressure of about 40 to 70 mm Hg, this is significantly lower than the increase of 420 to 1,500 mm Hg associated with reamed nailing (271).

The following findings are established (268):

- Reamed nailing usually causes a transient alteration in pulmonary arterial pressure. These changes are less sustained after unreamed nailing or plating.
- These changes are more severe if nailing is performed in a nonfractured femur.

- A combination of several preoperative factors aggravates the changes induced by the surgical procedure.
- IM instrumentation induces an acute rise of IM pressure that causes liberation of bone marrow contents into the bloodstream, from where they are transported into the lung. On their way, the thrombi undergo an increase in size, mainly due to adhesion of activated platelets.
- Inside the lung, acute changes cause a transient increase in pulmonary artery pressure and a transient decrease in oxygenation.
- The primary mechanisms are modified and aggravated by a variety of subsequent cascade reactions.

In a randomized clinical study, unreamed nailing was associated with a lower rate of pulmonary complications compared to reamed nailing, but the differences were not statistically significant (277).

The use of a venting hole to reduce the IM pressure increase during reaming is controversial. (278,279). The removal of the medullary contents by suction before inserting the reamers has been shown to be associated with a statistically significant pressure reduction (280). A new development is the use of the rinsing-suction reamer, which in animal studies has been shown to reduce embolism to a negligible amount (281).

General Techniques

Patient Positioning. Poor patient positioning before surgery creates numerous intraoperative problems. No matter which bone is being nailed, the position of the patient must allow unrestricted surgical and radiologic access to the entry point, the fracture, and the areas where interlocking screws will be inserted. Repositioning of the patient is time-consuming and should be avoided, especially in multiply injured patients. There is debate about the need to use fracture tables. Fracture tables were favored for many years for both femoral and tibial nailing (239,269,282,283). Their main advantage is that they help maintain length and alignment. However, prospective randomized studies have shown significantly shorter operative times and less malrotation without the use of a fracture table (284–286). Other disadvantages include pudendal nerve damage with subsequent erectile dysfunction (287,288), contralateral sciatic palsy (289), compartment syndrome of the contralateral leg (290), and pudendal skin necrosis (291). However, there are potential complications associated with nailing without a fracture table, and the decision depends on the experience and preference of the surgeon.

Correct Implant Selection. Selection of the correct diameter and length of the nail is essential before insertion. Inappropriately sized nails may compromise stability, especially in fractures close to or within the metaphysis. Rotational stability increases with the distance between the fracture site and the locking screws (292). If nails or locking screws are too long, they may cause soft tissue irritation and pain. The passage of too wide a nail can have devastating consequences and may explode the diaphysis. This is a greater potential problem with unreamed nailing. The accuracy of templates for preoperative prediction of nail length and diameter has been shown to be poor (293). The preoperative x-rays can be used only if a measuring device is placed at the level of the bone.

Nail length can be precisely measured intraoperatively with a radiolucent ruler under fluoroscopic control. If the injured bone is used to assess length, its length has to be restored under fluoroscopic control and maintained until the measurement is complete. An alternative is to use an IM guide wire to measure nail length, and some guide wires allow fluoroscopic measurement of nail length.

Correct Entry Point. The correct entry point is crucial in IM nailing. For straight nails, the entry point is in line with the axis of the shaft (Fig. 6-49). If correctly placed, stab incisions 2 to 3 cm in length are preferable for the femur and tibia. It has been shown for the tibia that the length of incision correlates with postoperative knee pain (294). An incorrect entry point increases the risk of intraoperative fracture. This applies especially to solid nails, which are more rigid. Iatrogenic fractures are most likely within the neck of the femur (295–297). The mechanics of the femoral neck change depending on the entry point (298).

Malalignment can also be caused by an incorrect entry point, especially in proximal and distal fractures. In midshaft fractures the entry point is not so important, as the nail will "find" its way within the canal. It has been shown that fractures of the proximal tibia tend to go into valgus malalignment if the entry point is too medial and varus malalignment if the entry point is too lateral (299). These experimental data are supported by clinical findings (300). The importance of the correct entry point in preventing malalignment has also been shown in the femur (301).

Anatomic landmarks are not always reliable when determining the exact entry point (302). Whenever a correct entry point is essential, fluoroscopy should be used to determine the exact axis of the bone and the correct insertion point.

Use of Blocking Screws. Nailing of metaphyseal fractures is associated with a higher rate of malalignment than diaphyseal fractures (300,303,304). The technique of blocking or "Poller" screws has been proposed to prevent malalignment in the femur and tibia (305,306). These screws can be used to decrease the functional width of the metaphyseal cavity and to force the nail to pass in a particular direction (Fig. 6-50). The effectiveness of these blocking screws has been proven in clinical studies (306,307).

Blocking screws can be used for alignment, stabilization, and manipulation. The screw is placed perpendicular to the direction in which the implant might displace. In oblique metaphyseal fractures, the blocking screws may help with stabilization because shear forces are transformed into compression forces. They may also help to prevent displacement in renailing procedures, as a second IM nail always tends to follow the previous

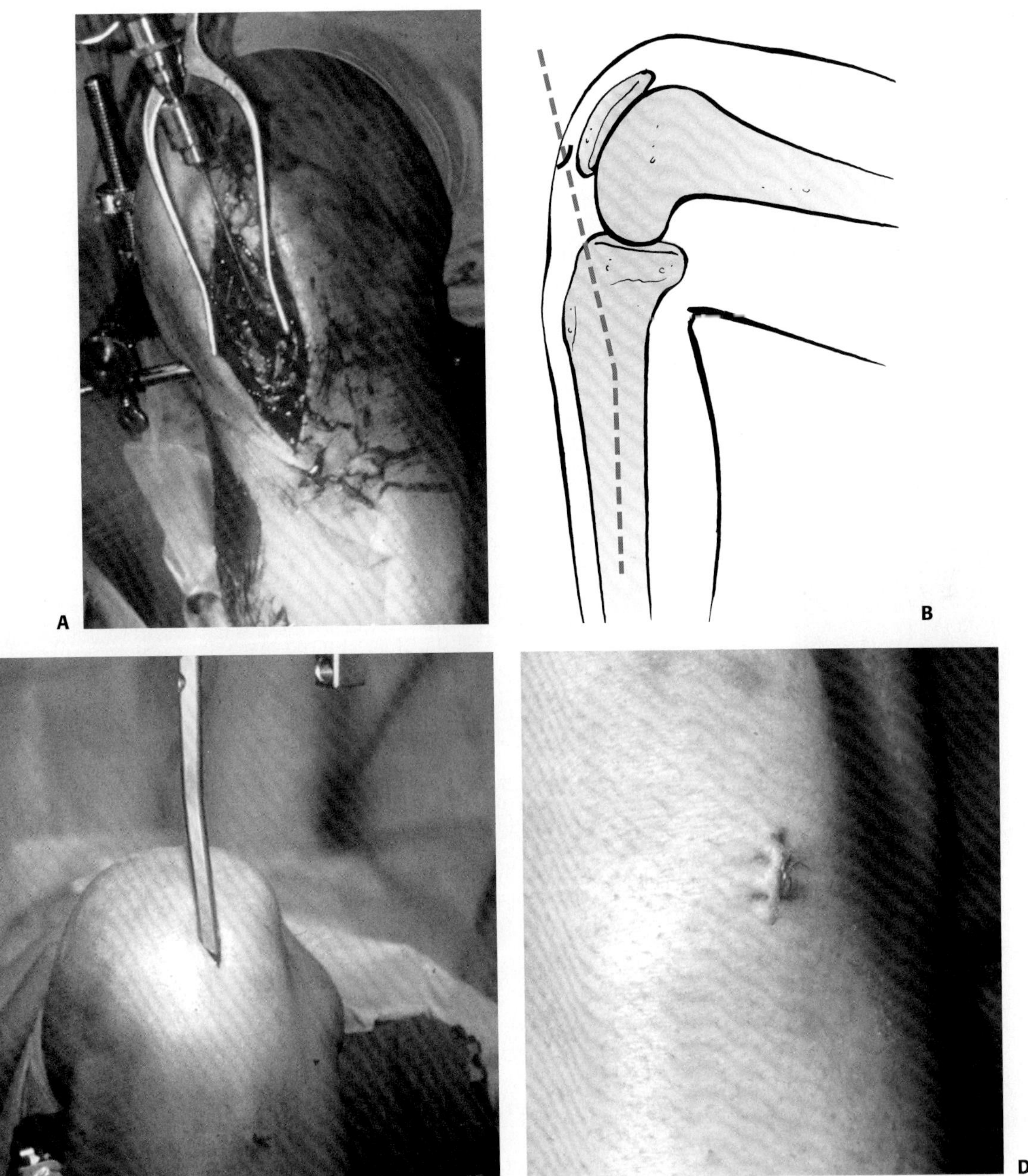

FIGURE 6-49 **A.** An unnecessarily large exposure for the entry point of a tibia nail. **B.** The incision should be in line with the entry point. **C.** With careful planning the incision can be a similar size to the diameter of the nail. **D.** Postoperative picture of the skin incision of the patient in **C.**

track and a blocking screw may prevent this from happening. Similarly, it can be used in situations where the original entry point of the nail was incorrect.

Poller screws can be temporary or definitive, and a drill bit can be used instead of a temporary screw. Their use is not free of risk (Fig. 6-51). As they narrow the medullary cavity, the bone may fracture or preexisting fractures may be extended. The risk is higher if they are used in the diaphysis or in osteoporotic bone.

Locking Techniques. Fracture distraction can occur during nail insertion, this being a particular problem with tight-fitting nails. Distraction causes a rise in compartment pressure (11) and is associated with a higher rate of delayed and nonunion (308). For this reason we recommend that the distal locking screw be placed first. This allows the surgeon to close a distracted fracture by back-slapping the nail. Some nails allow interlocking under compression (309).

Nails can be locked in either dynamic or static modes. Trans-

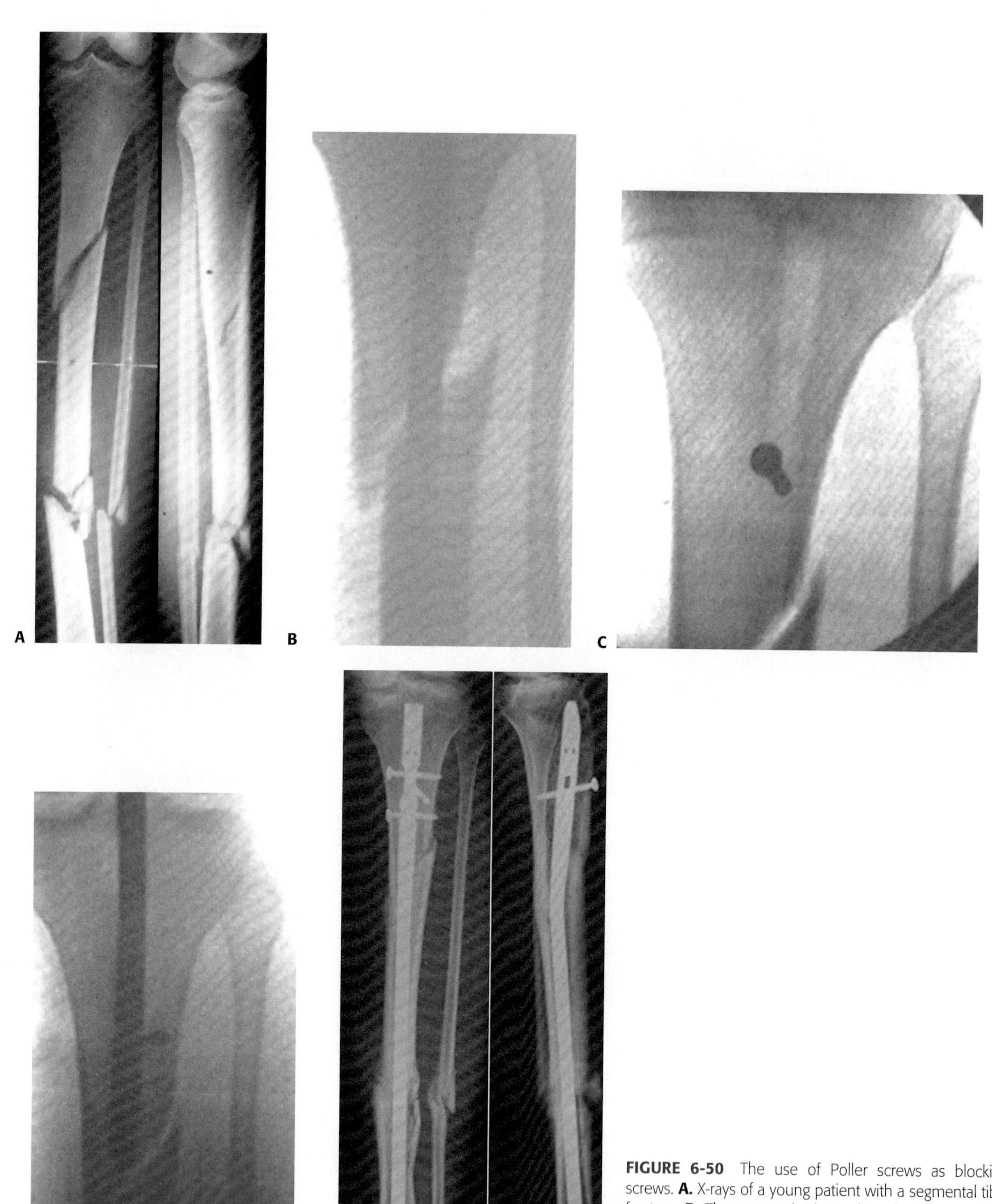

FIGURE 6-50 The use of Poller screws as blocking screws. **A.** X-rays of a young patient with a segmental tibia fracture. **B.** The entry point is too lateral, with a resulting valgus malalignment and medial shift of the proximal fragment. **C.** The nail is removed. A Poller screw is inserted into the wrong canal. **D.** The nail is forced medial to the former canal into a central position. **E.** X-rays after 12 months showed good alignment.

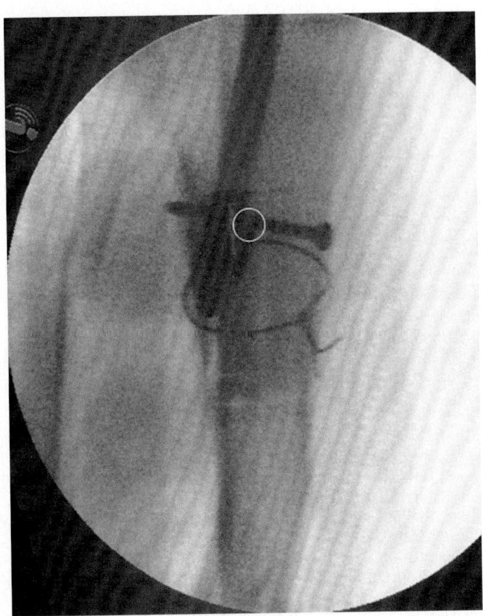

FIGURE 6-51 A serious complication from the use of Poller screws. The AP Poller screw (*white circle*) was positioned to bring the nail into a more medial position. However, the nail slid lateral to the Poller screw and perforated the lateral cortex.

verse, short oblique, and some fractures with butterfly fragments that are axially stable can be dynamically locked. This allows compressive loading of the fracture, which promotes healing (310). In the early days of IM nailing, dynamization was done as a routine procedure 6 to 8 weeks after the initial surgery (192,269) if there was thought to be evidence of delayed union. However, experimental and clinical data have shown that dynamization does not improve union (311,312) and is therefore unnecessary. Although there are some reports that indicate that a single screw is reliable for distal locking of diaphyseal fractures (313,314), we usually lock all distal holes. In a prospective randomized trial of fractures of the tibia, one distal screw failed (59.1%) significantly more often than two distal screws (5%) (315).

Proximal locking is usually easily achieved with an aiming device that can be connected to or is integrated within the insertion guide. Distal locking is much more complicated, as the nail deforms during insertion (234,235), and fluoroscopy-assisted locking is most commonly used. This can be done freehand or with targeting devices. These devices can be mounted onto the fluoroscope (316) or can be used freehand (317). Another alternative is to use a radiolucent drill, which is versatile and easy to use (318). Today radiation-independent targeting devices are also available (319–322). These devices are associated with less radiation exposure compared to the freehand technique. The success rate is similar, but the operative time tends to be longer (320–322). Radiation-independent locking devices are available for the tibia, humerus, and femur. Recently computer-assisted locking has been introduced (323,324). This technique has a high success rate with low radiation exposure, but the locking procedure is prolonged (323).

COATED IMPLANTS

There is a lot of ongoing research concerning the coating of implants. This coating may increase fixation strength, promote healing, or reduce infection. The materials for coating can be inorganic or organic.

Hydroxyapatite (HA)

External fixation studies have provided evidence that HA coating reduces the rate of pin loosening and pin infection (325–327). HA-coated pins also performed well in osteoporotic patients (328). HA coating of standard screws used for internal fixation improves fixation in bone (329). In an experimental study, the extraction torque of HA-coated screws was significantly higher. Furthermore, there was no significant reduction between insertion and extraction torques in the HA-coated group (330). Biomechanical and histomorphologic results suggest the superiority of HA-coated screws in osteopenic cortical bone (331). In proximal femur fractures, coating of the screw head of a dynamic hip screw reduced significantly the rate of cutout (332).

Growth Factors

Animal studies have shown that the local administration of growth factors from coated implants is feasible and significantly accelerates fracture healing (333–336). This application enhances healing in the early phase without altering the normal healing process (337). Local controlled release of growth factors from coated implants does not induce ectopic bone formation (338).

The results clearly demonstrate that the local application of BMP-2 from PDLLA-coated implants is feasible and significantly accelerates fracture healing. Its use may reduce problems in fracture treatment without opening the fracture, implanting further devices, or injection, with its risk of infection or side effects caused by other carriers (334,335).

Antibiotics

The impact of prophylactic antibiotics in reducing postoperative infection is obvious. The concept of inoculating local antibiotics in fractures that are associated with a risk of osteomyelitis is attractive. Gentamicin antibiotic-coated implants have reduced the rate of infection in animal experiments (339,340).

REFERENCES

1. Brunner CF, Weber BG. *Besondere Osteosynthesetechniken*. Berlin: Springer, 1981.
2. Georgiadis GM, Behrens FF, Joyce MJ, et al. Open tibial fractures with severe soft-tissue loss. Limb salvage compared with below-the-knee amputation. *J Bone Joint Surg [Am]* 1993;75:1431–1441.
3. Oestern HJ, Tscherne H. Pathophysiology and classifcation of soft tissue injuries associ-

ated with fractures. In: Tscherne H, Gotzen L, eds. *Fractures with soft tissue injury*. Berlin/Heidelberg/New York: Springer, 1984.

4. Kalicke T, Schlegel U, Printzen G, et al. Influence of a standardized closed soft tissue trauma on resistance to local infection. An experimental study in rats. *J Orthop Res* 2003;21:373–378.
5. Schaser KD, Zhang L, Haas NP, et al. Temporal profile of microvascular disturbances in rat tibial periosteumeum following closed soft tissue trauma. *Langenbecks Arch Surg* 2003;388:323–330.
6. Jain R, Koo M, Kreder HJ, et al. Comparison of early and delayed fixation of subcapital hip fractures in patients sixty years of age or less. *J Bone Joint Surg Am* 2002;84: 1605–1612.
7. Manninger J, Kazar G, Fekete G, et al. Avoidance of avascular necrosis of the femoral head, following fractures of the femoral neck, by early reduction and internal fixation. *Injury* 1985;16:437–448.
8. Elliott J, Beringer T, Kee F, et al. Predicting survival after treatment for fracture of the proximal femur and the effect of delays to surgery. *J Clin Epidemiol* 2003;56:788–795.
9. Schandelmaier P, Krettek C, Rudolf J, et al. Superior results of tibial rodding versus external fixation in grade 3B fractures. *Clin Orthop* 1997;164–172.
10. Tornetta P III, Bergman M, Watnik N, et al. Treatment of grade IIIb open tibial fractures. A prospective randomised comparison of external fixation and non-reamed locked nailing. *J Bone Joint Surg [Br]* 1994;76:13–19.
11. McQueen MM, Gaston P, Court-Brown CM. Acute compartment syndrome. Who is at risk? *J Bone Joint Surg [Br]* 2000;82:200–203.
12. Court-Brown CM. Reamed IM tibial nailing: an overview and analysis of 1106 cases. *J Orthop Trauma* 2004;18:96–101.
13. Sirkin M, Sanders R, DiPasquale T, Herscovici D Jr. A staged protocol for soft tissue management in the treatment of complex pilon fractures. *J Orthop Trauma* 1999;13: 78–84.
14. Patterson MJ, Cole JD. Two-staged delayed open reduction and internal fixation of severe pilon fractures. *J Orthop Trauma* 1999;13:85–91.
15. Blauth M, Bastian L, Krettek C, et al. Surgical options for the treatment of severe tibial pilon fractures: a study of three techniques. *J Orthop Trauma* 2001;15:153–160.
16. Schandelmaier P, Partenheimer A, Koenemann B, et al. Distal femoral fractures and LISS stabilization. *Injury* 2001;32 Suppl. 3:SC55–SC63.
17. Paiement GD, Renaud E, Dagenais G, Gosselin RA. Double-blind randomized prospective study of the efficacy of antibiotic prophylaxis for open reduction and internal fixation of closed ankle fractures. *J Orthop Trauma* 1994;8:64–66.
18. Stevens DB. Postoperative orthopaedic infections. A study of etiological mechanisms. *J Bone Joint Surg [Am]* 1964;46:96–102.
19. Zgonis T, Jolly GP, Garbalosa JC. The efficacy of prophylactic intravenous antibiotics in elective foot and ankle surgery. *J Foot Ankle Surg* 2004;43:97–103.
20. Southwell-Keely JP, Russo RR, March L, et al. Antibiotic prophylaxis in hip fracture surgery: a metaanalysis. *Clin Orthop* 2004;179–184.
21. Gillespie WJ, Walenkamp G. Antibiotic prophylaxis for surgery for proximal femoral and other closed long bone fractures. *Cochrane Database Syst Rev* 2001000244.
22. Boxma H, Broekhuizen T, Patka P, Oosting H. Randomised controlled trial of single-dose antibiotic prophylaxis in surgical treatment of closed fractures: the Dutch Trauma Trial. *Lancet* 1996;347:1133–1137.
23. Badia JM, Torres JM, Tur C, Sitges-Serra A. Saline wound irrigation reduces the postoperative infection rate in guinea pigs. *J Surg Res* 1996;63:457–459.
24. Tarbox BB, Conroy BP, Malicky ES, et al. Benzalkonium chloride. A potential disinfecting irrigation solution for orthopaedic wounds. *Clin Orthop* 1998;255–261.
25. Platt J, Bucknall RA. An experimental evaluation of antiseptic wound irrigation. *J Hosp Infect* 1984;5:181–188.
26. Rosenstein BD, Wilson FC, Funderburk CH. The use of bacitracin irrigation to prevent infection in postoperative skeletal wounds. An experimental study. *J Bone Joint Surg [Am]* 1989;71:427–430.
27. Kjonniksen I, Andersen BM, Sondenaa VG, Segadal L. Preoperative hair removal: a systematic literature review. *AORN J* 2002;75:928–940.
28. Maffulli N, Testa V, Capasso G. Use of a tourniquet in the internal fixation of fractures of the distal part of the fibula. A prospective, randomized trial. *J Bone Joint Surg [Am]* 1993;75:700–703.
29. Jarolem KL, Scott DF, Jaffe WL, et al. A comparison of blood loss and transfusion requirements in total knee arthroplasty with and without arterial tourniquet. *Am J Orthop* 1995;24:906–909.
30. Tetro AM, Rudan JF. The effects of a pneumatic tourniquet on blood loss in total knee arthroplasty. *Can J Surg* 2001;44:33–38.
31. Kase T, Skjeldal S, Nordsletten L, Reikeras O. Healing of tibial fractures is not impaired after acute hindlimb ischemia in rats. *Arch Orthop Trauma Surg* 1998;117:273–276.
32. Simon MA, Mass DP, Zarins CK, et al. The effect of a thigh tourniquet on the incidence of deep venous thrombosis after operations on the fore part of the foot. *J Bone Joint Surg [Am]* 1982;64:188–191.
33. Pollak AN, Battistella F, Pettey J, et al. Reamed femoral nailing in patients with multiple injuries. Adverse effects of tourniquet use. *Clin Orthop* 1997;41–46.
34. Salam AA, Eyres KS, Cleary J, el Sayed HH. The use of a tourniquet when plating tibial fractures. *J Bone Joint Surg [Br]* 1991;73:86–87.
35. Hirvensalo E, Tuominen H, Lapinsuo M, Helio H. Compartment syndrome of the lower limb caused by a tourniquet: a report of two cases. *J Orthop Trauma* 1992;6:469–472.
36. Leunig M, Hertel R. Thermal necrosis after tibial reaming for IM nail fixation. A report of three cases. *J Bone Joint Surg [Br]* 1996;78:584–587.
37. Savvidis E, Parsch K. Prolongierte passagere Paralyse nach pneumatischer Blutsperrenanwendung am Oberarm. *Unfallchirurg* 1999;102:141–144.
38. Hidou M, Huraux C, Viry-Babel F, Laxenaire MC. [Pneumatic tourniquet paralysis. A differential diagnosis after loco-regional anesthesia of the upper limb]. *J Chir (Paris)* 1992;129:213–214.
39. Omeroglu H, Ucaner A, Tabak AY, et al. The effect of using a tourniquet on the intensity of postoperative pain in forearm fractures. A randomized study in 32 surgically treated patients. *Int Orthop* 1998;22:369–373.
40. Darmanis S, Papanikolaou A, Pavlakis D. Fatal intra-operative pulmonary embolism following application of an Esmarch bandage. *Injury* 2002;33:761–764.
41. Lu CW, Chen YS, Wang MJ. Massive pulmonary embolism after application of an Esmarch bandage. *Anesth Analg* 2004;98:1187–1189.
42. Müller ME, Allgöwer M, Schneider E, Willenegger H. *Manual of internal fixarion* Berlin: Springer, 1992.
43. Müller ME, Allgöwer M, Schneider R, Willenegger H. *Manual of internal fixation* Heidelberg: Springer, 1965.
44. Moed BR, Watson JT. Intramedullary nailing of the tibia without a fracture table: the transfixion pin distractor technique. *J Orthop Trauma* 1994;8:195–202.
45. Baumgaertel F, Dahlen C, Stiletto R, Gotzen L. Technique of using the AO-femoral distractor for femoral IM nailing. *J Orthop Trauma* 1994;8:315–321.
46. Neubauer T, Hehli M, Steiner R, Wagner M. [The cannulated osteo-support rod, a new device for the minimally invasive reduction of fractures]. *Unfallchirurg* 2003;106: 649–652.
47. Hilgert RE, Dallek M, Rueger JM. Die minimal-invasive Behandlung massiv dislozierter kindlicher Radiushalsfrakturen durch perkutane Joystick-Reposition und Prevot-Nagelung. *Unfallchirurg* 2002;105:116–119.
48. Georgiadis GM, Burgar AM. Percutaneous skeletal joysticks for closed reduction of femoral shaft fractures during IM nailing. *J Orthop Trauma* 2001;15:570–571.
49. Krettek C, Rudolf J, Schandelmaier P, et al. Unreamed IM nailing of femoral shaft fractures: operative technique and early clinical experience with the standard locking option. *Injury* 1996;27:233–254.
50. Seide K, Wolter D, Kortmann HR. Fracture reduction and deformity correction with the hexapod Ilizarov fixator. *Clin Orthop* 1999;186–195.
51. Babst R, Hehl M, Regazzoni P. LISS Tractor. Kombination des less invasive stabilization systems (LISS) mit dem AO-Distraktor für distale Femur- und proximale Tibiafrakturen. *Unfallchirurg* 2001;104:530–535.
52. Gosling T, Westphal R, Hufner T, et al. Robot-assisted fracture reduction: a preliminary study in the femur shaft. *Med Biol Eng Comput* 2005;43:115–120.
53. Krettek C, Schandelmaier P, Miclau T, et al. Transarticular joint reconstruction and indirect plate osteosynthesis for complex distal supracondylar femoral fractures. *Injury* 1997;28 Suppl. 1:A31–A41.
54. Krettek C, Muller M, Miclau T. Evolution of minimally invasive plate osteosynthesis (MIPO) in the femur. *Injury* 2001;32 Suppl. 3:SC14–SC23.
55. Fuchs M, Schmid A, Eiteljorge T, et al. Exposure of the surgeon to radiation during surgery. *Int.Orthop* 1998;22:153–156.
56. Coetzee JC, van der Merwe EJ. Exposure of surgeons-in-training to radiation during IM fixation of femoral shaft fractures. *S Afr Med J* 1992;81:312–314.
57. Chan PS, Klimkiewicz JJ, Luchetti WT, et al. Impact of CT scan on treatment plan and fracture classification of tibial plateau fractures. *J Orthop Trauma* 1997;2000;11: 484–489.
58. Magid D, Michelson JD, Ney DR, Fishman EK. Adult ankle fractures: comparison of plain films and interactive two- and three-dimensional CT scans. *AJR Am J Roentgenol* 1990;154:1017–1023.
59. Tornetta P III, Gorup J. Axial computed tomography of pilon fractures. *Clin Orthop* 1996;273–276.
60. Dias JJ, Stirling AJ, Finlay DB, Gregg PJ. Computerised axial tomography for tibial plateau fractures. *J Bone Joint Surg [Br]* 1987;69:84–88.
61. Cole RJ, Bindra RR, Evanoff BA, et al. Radiographic evaluation of osseous displacement following intra-articular fractures of the distal radius: reliability of plain radiography versus computed tomography. *J Hand Surg [Am]* 1997;22:792–800.
62. Moed BR, Carr SE, Gruson KI, et al. Computed tomographic assessment of fractures of the posterior wall of the acetabulum after operative treatment. *J Bone Joint Surg [Am]* 2003;85:512–522.
63. Borrell J Jr, Goldfarb C, Catalano L, Evanoff BA. Assessment of articular fragment displacement in acetabular fractures: a comparison of computerized tomography and plain radiographs. *J Orthop Trauma* 2002;16:449–456.
64. Eberl R, Muller EJ, Kaminski A, Muhr G. [The postoperative control CT after a fracture of the acetabulum. A useful quality control measure or an unnecessary exposure to radiation?]. *Unfallchirurg* 2003;106:741–745.
65. Mayr E, Hauser H, Ruter A, Bohndorf K. [Minimally invasive intraoperative CT-guided correction of calcaneal osteosynthesis]. *Unfallchirurg* 1999;102:239–244.
66. Fritz HG, Kuehn D, Haberland N, Kalff R. Anesthesia management for spine surgery using spinal navigation in combination with computed tomography. *Anesth Analg* 2003; 97:863–866.
67. Jennings JE. Arthroscopic management of tibial plateau fractures. *Arthroscopy* 1985;1: 160–168.
68. Kim HS, Jahng JS, Kim SS, et al. Treatment of tibial pilon fractures using ring fixators and arthroscopy. *Clin Orthop* 1997;244–250.
69. Mehta JA, Bain GI, Heptinstall RJ. Anatomical reduction of intra-articular fractures of the distal radius. An arthroscopically-assisted approach. *J Bone Joint Surg [Br]* 2000; 82:79–86.
70. Buchko GM, Johnson DH. Arthroscopy assisted operative management of tibial plateau fractures. *Clin Orthop* 1996;29–36.
71. Holzach P, Matter P, Minter J. Arthroscopically assisted treatment of lateral tibial plateau fractures in skiers: use of a cannulated reduction system. *J Orthop Trauma* 1994;8: 273–281.
72. Ruch DS, Vallee J, Poehling GG, et al. Arthroscopic reduction versus fluoroscopic

reduction in the management of intra-articular distal radius fractures. *Arthroscopy* 2004; 20:225–230.

73. Ohdera T, Tokunaga M, Hiroshima S, et al. Arthroscopic management of tibial plateau fractures: comparison with open reduction method. *Arch Orthop Trauma Surg* 2003; 123:489–493.
74. Gavlik JM, Rammelt S, Zwipp H. The use of subtalar arthroscopy in open reduction and internal fixation of intra-articular calcaneal fractures. *Injury* 2002;33:63–71.
75. Borg T, Larsson S, Lindsjo U. Percutaneous plating of distal tibial fractures. Preliminary results in 21 patients. *Injury* 2004;35:608–614.
76. Krettek C, Schandelmaier P, Miclau T, Tscherne H. Minimally invasive percutaneous plate osteosynthesis (MIPPO) using the DCS in proximal and distal femoral fractures. *Injury* 1997;28 Suppl. 1:A20–A30.
77. Paley D. Consequences of malalignment. In: Paley D, ed. *Principles of deformity correction*. Berlin/Heidelberg/New York: Springer, 2002.
78. Krettek C, Miclau T, Grun O, et al. Intraoperative control of axes, rotation and length in femoral and tibial fractures. Technical note. *Injury* 1998;29 Suppl. 3:C29–C39.
79. Saleh M, Harriman P, Edwards DJ. A radiological method for producing precise limb alignment. *J Bone Joint Surg [Br]* 1991;73:515–516.
80. Prevot N, Charissoux JL, Fiorenza F, et al. Utilisation d'un clou non fendu de Russel-Taylor pour la stabilisation des fractures du femur. A propos de 57 fractures avec 30 etudes tomodensitometriques de la rotation. *Rev Chir Orthop Reparatrice Appar Mot* 1998;84:33–40.
81. Strecker W, Suger G, Kinzl L. Lokale Komplikationen der Marknagelung. *Orthopade* 1996;25:274–291.
82. Hernandez RJ, Tachdjian MO, Poznanski AK, Dias LS. CT determination of femoral torsion. *AJR Am.J Roentgenol* 1981;137:97–101.
83. Clementz BG. Assessment of tibial torsion and rotational deformity with a new fluoroscopic technique. *Clin Orthop* 1989;2000:199–209.
84. Hofstetter R, Slomczykowski M, Krettek C, et al. Computer-assisted fluoroscopy-based reduction of femoral fractures and antetorsion correction. *Comput Aided Surg* 2000;5: 311–325.
85. Schmucki D, Gebhard F, Grutzner PA, et al. Computer aided reduction and imaging. *Injury* 2004;35 Suppl. 1:96–104.
86. Hufner T, Pohlemann T, Tarte S, et al. Computer-assisted fracture reduction of pelvic ring fractures: an in vitro study. *Clin Orthop* 2002;231–239.
87. Danis R. The aims of internal fixation. *Clin Orthop* 1979;138:23–25.
88. Allgower M, Spiegel PG. Internal fixation of fractures: evolution of concepts. *Clin Orthop* 1979;26–29.
89. Disegi JA, Eschbach L. Stainless steel in bone surgery. *Injury* 2000;31 Suppl. 4:2–6.
90. Chapman JR, Harrington RM, Lee KM, et al. Factors affecting the pullout strength of cancellous bone screws. *J Biomech Eng* 1996;118:391–398.
91. Thompson JD, Benjamin JB, Szivek JA. Pullout strengths of cannulated and noncannulated cancellous bone screws. *Clin Orthop* 1997;241–249.
92. DeCoster TA, Heetderks DB, Downey DJ, et al. Optimizing bone screw pullout force. *J Orthop Trauma.* 1990;4:169–174.
93. Perren SM. Force measurements in screw fixation. *J Biomech* 1976;9:669–675.
94. Merk BR, Stern SH, Cordes S, Lautenschlager EP. A fatigue life analysis of small fragment screws. *J Orthop Trauma* 2001;15:494–499.
95. Biliouris TL, Schneider E, Rahn BA, et al. The effect of radial preload on the implant-bone interface: a cadaveric study. *J Orthop Trauma* 1989;3:323–332.
96. Yerby S, Scott CC, Evans NJ, et al. Effect of cutting flute design on cortical bone screw insertion torque and pullout strength. *J Orthop Trauma* 2001;15:216–221.
97. Baumgart FW, Cordey J, Morikawa K, et al. AO/ASIF self-tapping screws (STS). *Injury* 1993;24 Suppl:S1–17.
98. Schatzker J, Sanderson R, Murnaghan JP. The holding power of orthopedic screws in vivo. *Clin Orthop* 1975;115–126.
99. Frigg R. Locking compression plate (LCP). An osteosynthesis plate based on the dynamic compression plate and the point contact fixator (PC-Fix). *Injury* 2001;32 Suppl. 2:63–66.
100. Claes L, Hutzschenreuter P. Das Durchdrehmoment an Zugschrauben mit vorgeschnittenem Kortikalisgewinde. *Z Orthop Ihre Grenzgeb* 1975;2000;113:237–242.
101. Gotzen L, Hutter J, Haas N. Biomechanische Untersuchungen über die. 2000;4,5 mm AO-Corticalisschraube als Zugschraube. Teil 1: Beziehung zwischen Anzugsmoment, Axialkraft und Haltekraft. *Unfallheilkunde* 1980;83:1–7.
102. Ganz R, Perren SM, Ruter A. [Mechanical induction of bone resorption]. *Fortschr Kiefer Gesichtschir* 1975;2000;19:45–48.
103. Perren SM, Frigg R, Hehli M, Tepic S. Lag screw. In: Ruedi TP, Murphy WM, eds. *AO principles of fracture management*. Stuttgart/NewYork: Thieme, 2000.
104. Breuing KH, Gotzen L. Biomechanische Untersuchungen zur Haltekraft der neuen. 2000;3,5–mm-AO-Corticalisschraube. *Hefte Unfallheilkunde* 1986;181:40–46.
105. Burstein AH, Currey J, Frankel VH, et al. Bone strength. The effect of screw holes. *J Bone Joint Surg [Am]* 1972;54:1143–1156.
106. Texhammar R. AO/ASIF instrumentation. In: Texhammar R, Colton C, eds. *AO/ASIF instruments and implants*. Berlin/Heidelberg/New York: Springer, 1993.
107. Hutter J, Gotzen L, Haas N, Kellner W. Biomechanische Untersuchungen über die 4,5 mm AO-Corticalisschraube. *Unfallheilkunde* 1980;83:60–64.
108. Kellner W, Gotzen L, Haas N. Biomechanische Untersuchungen über die. 2000;4,5 mm AO-Corticalisschraube als Zugschraube. Teil. 3: Abhängigkeit der Haltekraft vom Schraubenneigungswinkel. *Unfallheilkunde* 1982;85:413–418.
109. Perren SM. The concept of biological plating using the limited contact-dynamic compression plate (LC-DCP). Scientific background, design and application. *Injury* 1991;22 Suppl. 1:1–41.
110. Perren SM, Buchanan J. Biomechanical aspects of the AO/ASIF technique. In: Texhammar R, Colton C, eds. *AO/ASIF instruments and implants*. Berlin/Heidelberg/NewYork: Springer, 1993.
111. Robert KQ III, Chandler R, Baratta RV, et al. The effect of divergent screw placement on the initial strength of plate-to-bone fixation. *J Trauma* 2003;55:1139–1144.
112. Johner R, Joerger K, Cordey J, Perren SM. Rigidity of pure lag-screw fixation as a function of screw inclination in an in vitro spiral osteotomy. *Clin Orthop* 1983;74–79.
113. Johner R, Wruhs O. Classification of tibial shaft fractures and correlation with results after rigid internal fixation. *Clin Orthop* 1983;7–25.
114. Gautier E, Sommer C. Guidelines for the clinical application of the LCP. *Injury* 2003; 34 Suppl. 2:B63–B76.
115. Krettek C, Haas N, Tscherne H. The role of supplemental lag-screw fixation for open fractures of the tibial shaft treated with external fixation. *J Bone Joint Surg [Am]* 1991; 73:893–897.
116. Herbert TJ, Fisher WE. Management of the fractured scaphoid using a new bone screw. *J Bone Joint Surg [Br]* 1984;66:114–123.
117. Klaue K, Fengels I, Perren SM. Long-term effects of plate osteosynthesis: comparison of four different plates. *Injury* 2000;31 Suppl. 2:S 62.
118. Uhthoff HK, Dubuc FL. Bone structure changes in the dog under rigid internal fixation. *Clin Orthop* 1971;81:165–170.
119. Gautier E, Perren SM. Die Reaktion der Kortikalis nach Verplattung - eine Folge der Belastungsveränderung des Knochens oder Vaskularitätsprobleme. In Wolter D, Zimmer E. *Die Plattenosteosynthese und ihre Konkurrenzverfahren*. Berlin: Springer, 1991.
120. Cordey J, Perren SM, Steinemann SG. Stress protection due to plates: myth or reality? A parametric analysis made using the composite beam theory 11. *Injury* 2000;31 Suppl. 3:C1–13.
121. Gautier E, Perren SM, Cordey J. Strain distribution in plated and unplated sheep tibia: an in vivo experiment. *Injury* 2000;31 Suppl. 3:C37–C44.
122. Perren SM. Evolution and rationale of locked internal fixator technology. Introductory remarks. *Injury* 2001;32 Suppl. 2:B3–B9.
123. Allgower M, Ehrsam R, Ganz R, et al. Clinical experience with a new compression plate DCP. *Acta Orthop Scand Suppl* 1969;125:45–61.
124. Perren SM, Russenberger M, Steinemann S, et al. A dynamic compression plate. *Acta Orthop Scand Suppl* 1969;125:31–41.
125. Klaue K, Frigg R, Perren SM. Die Entlastung der Osteosyntheseplatte durch interfragmentäre Plattenzugschraube. *Helv Chir Acta* 1985;52:19–23.
126. Klaue K. The Dynamic Compression Unit (DCU) for stable internal fixation of bone fractures. MD, Universität Basel, 1982.
127. Jaakkola JI, Lundy DW, Moore T, et al. Supracondylar femur fracture fixation: mechanical comparison of the 95 degrees condylar side plate and screw versus 95 degrees angled blade plate. *Acta Orthop Scand* 2002;73:72–76.
128. Cusick RP, Lucas GL, McQueen DA, Graber CD. Construct stiffness of different fixation methods for supracondylar femoral fractures above total knee prostheses. *Am J Orthop* 2000;29:695–699.
129. Brunner CF, Weber BG. Antigleitplatte. In: Brunner CF, Weber BG, eds. *Besondere Osteosynthesetechniken*. Berlin: Springer, 1981.
130. Winkler B, Weber BG, Simpson LA. The dorsal antiglide plate in the treatment of Danis-Weber type B fractures of the distal fibula. *Clin Orthop* 1990;204–209.
131. Suedkamp NP, Haas N, Krettek C. Biomechanische Untersuchung zur Vorbiegung und Vorspannung an der Kleinfragment-DC-Platte. *Hefte Unfallheilkd* 1986;181:47–52.
132. Gotzen L, Haas N, Strohfeld G. Experimentelle und praktische Grundlagen zur Vorbiegung der schmalen und breiten DC-Platte (DCP). *Unfallheilkunde* 1981;84:121–130.
133. Gotzen L, Haas N, Strohfeld G. Zur Biomechanik der Plattenosteosynthese. Schrage Plattenzugschraube-Plattenvorbiegung. *Unfallheilkunde* 1981;84:439–443.
134. Heitemeyer U, Kemper F, Hierholzer G, Haines J. Severely comminuted femoral shaft fractures: treatment by bridging-plate osteosynthesis. *Arch Orthop Trauma Surg* 1987; 106:327–330.
135. Sturmer KM. Die elastische Plattenosteo-synthese, ihre Biomechanik, Indikation und Technik im Vergleich zur rigiden Osteosynthese. *Unfallchirurg* 1996;99:816–829.
136. Brunner CF, Weber BG. Wellenplatte. In: Brunner CF, Weber BG, eds. *Besondere Osteosynthesetechniken*. Berlin: Springer, 1981.
137. Müller ME. Die Verwendung von Kunstharzen in der Knochenchirurgie. *Arch Orthop Unfallchir* 1964;54:516–522.
138. Habermann ET, Lopez RA. Metastatic disease of bone and treatment of pathological fractures. *Orthop Clin North Am* 1989;20:469–486.
139. Anderson JT, Erickson JM, Thompson RC Jr, Chao EY. Pathologic femoral shaft fractures comparing fixation techniques using cement. *Clin Orthop* 1978;273–278.
140. Benum P. The use of bone cement as an adjunct to internal fixation of supracondylar fractures of osteoporotic femurs. *Acta Orthop Scand* 1977;48:52–56.
141. Cameron HU, Jacob R, Macnab I, Pilliar RM. Use of polymethylmethacrylate to enhance screw fixation in bone. *J Bone Joint Surg [Am]* 1975;57:655–656.
142. Harrington KD. The use of methylmethacrylate as an adjunct in the internal fixation of unstable comminuted intertrochanteric fractures in osteoporotic patients. *J Bone Joint Surg [Am]* 1975;57:744–750.
143. Schatzker J, Horne JG, Sumner-Smith G, et al. Methymethacrylate cement: its curing temperature and effect on articular cartilage. *Can J Surg* 1975;18:172–178.
144. Kramer A, Angst M, Gasser B, Ganz R. [Increasing bone screw anchoring in the femur head by cement administration via the implant: a biomechanical study]. *Z Orthop Ihre Grenzgeb* 2000;138:464–469.
145. Augat P, Rapp S, Claes L. A modified hip screw incorporating injected cement for the fixation of osteoporotic trochanteric fractures. *J Orthop Trauma* 2002;16:311–316.
146. Yetkinler DN, Goodman SB, Reindel ES, et al. Mechanical evaluation of a carbonated apatite cement in the fixation of unstable intertrochanteric fractures. *Acta Orthop Scand* 2002;73:157–164.

147. Goodman SB, Bauer TW, Carter D, et al. Norian SRS cement augmentation in hip fracture treatment. Laboratory and initial clinical results. *Clin Orthop* 1998;42–50.
148. Pauwels F. *Biomechanics of the locomotor apparatus*. Berlin: Springer, 1980.
149. Mullett JH, Shannon F, Noel J, et al. K-wire position in tension band wiring of the olecranon: a comparison of two techniques. *Injury* 2000;31:427–431.
150. Blatter G, Weber BG. Wave plate osteosynthesis as a salvage procedure. *Arch Orthop Trauma Surg* 1990;109:330–333.
151. Gerber C, Mast JW, Ganz R. Biological internal fixation of fractures. *Arch Orthop Trauma Surg* 1990;109:295–303.
152. Ganz R, Mast JW, Weber BG, Perren SM. Clinical aspects of biological plating. *Injury* 1991;22 Suppl. 1:4–5.
153. Miclau T, Martin RE. The evolution of modern plate osteosynthesis. *Injury* 1997;28 Suppl. 1:A3–A6.
154. Farouk O, Krettek C, Miclau T, et al. Minimally invasive plate osteosynthesis and vascularity: preliminary results of a cadaver injection study. *Injury* 1997;28 Suppl. 1: A7–12.
155. Ramotowski W, Granowski R. Das "Zespol"-Osteosynthesesystem: Mechanische Grundlage und klinische Anwendung. *Orthop Praxis* 1984;9:750–758.
156. Hopf T, Osthege S. Die interfragmentäre Kompression des Zespol-Osteosynthese-Systems. Experimentelle biomechanische Untersuchung. *Z Orthop Ihre Grenzgeb* 1987; 125:546–552.
157. Kassab SS, Mast JW, Mayo KA. Patients treated for nonunions with plate and screw fixation and adjunctive locking nuts. *Clin Orthop* 1998;86–92.
158. Kolodziej P, Lee FS, Patel A, et al. Biomechanical evaluation of the schuhli nut. *Clin Orthop* 1998;79–85.
159. Gosling T, Schandelmaier P, Marti A, et al. Less invasive stabilization of complex tibial plateau fractures: a biomechanical evaluation of a unilateral locked screw plate and double plating. *J Orthop Trauma* 2004a;18:546–551.
160. Seebeck J, Lill C, Morlock MM, Schneider E. Implantatverankerung in osteoporotischem Knochen mittels monokortikaler Schrauben. *Trauma Berufskrankh* 1999;1: 411–414.
161. Utvag SE, Grundnes O, Reikeraos O. Effects of periosteumeal stripping on healing of segmental fractures in rats. *J Orthop Trauma* 1996;10:279–284.
162. Utvag SE, Grundnes O, Reikeras O. Early muscle-periosteumeal lesion inhibits fracture healing in rats. *Acta Orthop Scand* 1999;70:62–66.
163. Ozaka A, Tsunoda M, Kinoshita S, Saura R. Role of fracture hematoma and periosteumeum during fracture healing in rats: interaction of fracture hematoma and the periosteumeum in the initial step of the healing process. *J Orthop Sci* 2000;5:64–70.
164. Orbay JL, Fernandez DL. Volar fixation for dorsally displaced fractures of the distal radius: a preliminary report. *J Hand Surg [Am]* 2002;27:205–215.
165. Sommer C, Gautier E, Muller M, et al. First clinical results of the locking compression plate (LCP). *Injury* 2003;34 Suppl. 2:B43–B54.
166. Wagner M. General principles for the clinical use of the LCP. *Injury* 2003;34 Suppl. 2:B31–B42.
167. Frigg R, Appenzeller A, Christensen R, et al. The development of the distal femur less invasive stabilization system (LISS). *Injury* 2001;32 Suppl. 3:SC24–SC31.
168. Wolter D, Schumann U, Seide K. Universeller Titanfixateur interne. Entwicklungsgeschichte, Prinzip, Mechanik, Implantatgestaltung und operativer Einsatz. *Trauma Berufskrankh* 1999;1:307–319.
169. Cole PA, Zlowodzki M, Kregor PJ. Less invasive stabilization system (LISS) for fractures of the proximal tibia: indications, surgical technique and preliminary results of the UMC Clinical Trial 6078. *Injury* 2003;34 Suppl. 1:A16–A29.
170. Schutz M, Muller M, Krettek C, et al. Minimally invasive fracture stabilization of distal femoral fractures with the LISS: a prospective multicenter study. Results of a clinical study with special emphasis on difficult cases. *Injury* 2001;32 Suppl. 3:SC48–SC54.
171. Schutz M, Kaab MJ, Haas N. Stabilization of proximal tibial fractures with the LIS-System: early clinical experience in Berlin. *Injury* 2003;34 Suppl. 1:A30–A35.
172. Stamer DT, Schenk R, Staggers B, et al. Bicondylar tibial plateau fractures treated with a hybrid ring external fixator: a preliminary study. *J Orthop Trauma* 1994;8:455–461.
173. Stannard JP, Wilson TC, Volgas DA, Alonso JE. Fracture stabilization of proximal tibial fractures with the proximal tibial LISS: early experience in Birmingham, Alabama. *Injury* 2003;34 Suppl. 1:A36–A42.
174. Korner J, Lill H, Muller LP, et al. The LCP-concept in the operative treatment of distal humerus fractures: biological, biomechanical and surgical aspects. *Injury* 2003;34 Suppl. 2:B20–B30.
175. Marti A, Fankhauser C, Frenk A, et al. Biomechanical evaluation of the less invasive stabilization system for the internal fixation of distal femur fractures. *J Orthop Trauma* 2001;15:482–487.
176. Koval KJ, Hoehl JJ, Kummer FJ, Simon JA. Distal femoral fixation: a biomechanical comparison of the standard condylar buttress plate, a locked buttress plate, and the 95-degree blade plate. *J Orthop Trauma* 1997;11:521–524.
177. Mueller KL, Karunakar MA, Frankenburg EP, Scott DS. Bicondylar tibial plateau fractures: a biomechanical study. *Clin Orthop* 2003;412:189–195.
178. Goesling T, Frenk A, Appenzeller A, et al. LISS PLT: Design, mechanical and biomechanical characteristics 5991. *Injury* 2003;34:S-A11–S-A15.
179. Lill H, Hepp P, Korner J, et al. Proximal humeral fractures: how stiff should an implant be? A comparative mechanical study with new implants in human specimens. *Arch Orthop Trauma Surg* 2003;123:74–81.
180. Harris T, Ruth JT, Szivek J, Haywood B. The effect of implant overlap on the mechanical properties of the femur. *J Trauma* 2003;54:930–935.
181. Kregor PJ, Hughes JL, Cole PA. Fixation of distal femoral fractures above total knee arthroplasty utilizing the less invasive stabilization system (L.I.S.S.). *Injury* 2001;32 Suppl. 3:SC64–SC75.
182. Althausen PL, Lee MA, Finkemeier CG, et al. Operative stabilization of supracondylar femur fractures above total knee arthroplasty: a comparison of four treatment methods. *J.Arthroplasty* 2003;18:834–839.
183. Stimson LA. *A treatise on fractures*. 1883.
184. Küntscher G. *Praxis der Marknagelung*. Stuttgart, Schattauer, 1962.
185. Hey-Groves EW. Ununited fractures with special reference to gunshot injuries and the use of bone grafting. *J Bone Joint Surg [Br]* 1918;6:203–228.
186. Küntscher G. Die Marknagelung von Knochenbrüchen. Tierexperimenteller Teil. *Klin Wochenschr* 1940;1:6–10.
187. Küntscher G. Die Marknagelung von Knochenbrüchen. *Langenbecks Arch Chir* 1940a; 200:443–455.
188. Küntscher G. Fünfzehn Jahre Marknagel. *Langenbecks Arch Chir* 1955;282:211–227.
189. Küntscher G. Die Technik des Aufweitens der Markhöhle. *Chirurg* 1959;30:28–35.
190. Herzog K. Die Technik der geschlossenen Marknagelung frischer Tibiafrakturen mit dem Rohrschlitznagel. *Chirurg* 1958;29:501–506.
191. Küntscher G. Die Marknagelung des Trümmerbruches. *Langenbecks Arch Chir* 1968; 322:1063–1069.
192. Klemm K, Schellmann WD. Dynamische und statische Verriegelung des Marknagels. *Monatsschr Unfallheilkd Versicher Versorg Verkehrsmed* 1972;75:568–575.
193. Kempf I, Jaeger JH, North J, et al. L'enclouage centro-medullaire du femur et du tibia selon la technique de Kuntscher. Interet du verrouillage du clou. Etude experimentale. *Acta Orthop. Belg* 1976;42 Suppl. 1:29–43.
194. Ender HG. [Treatment of per- and subtrochanteric fractures in old age using elastic nails]. *Hefte Unfallheilkd* 1975;67–71.
195. Levy AS, Levitt LE, Gunther SF, Wetzler MJ. The role of Ender rodding in tibial fractures with an intact fibula. *J Orthop Trauma* 1990;4:75–80.
196. Ligier JN, Metaizeau JP, Prevot J, Lascombes P. Elastic stable IM nailing of femoral shaft fractures in children. *J Bone Joint Surg [Br]* 1988;70:74–77.
197. Lottes JO. Treatment of fractures of the femur with a heavy, large cored, three-flanged medullary nail. *Surgery* 1951;29:868–884.
198. Pankovich AM, Tarabishy IE, Yelda S. Flexible IM nailing of tibial-shaft fractures. *Clin Orthop* 1981;185–195.
199. Waseem M, Paton RW. Percutaneous IM elastic wiring of displaced diaphyseal forearm fractures in children. A modified technique. *Injury* 1999;30:21–24.
200. Wiss DA. Flexible medullary nailing of acute tibial shaft fractures. *Clin Orthop* 1986; 122–132.
201. Rush LV. *Atlas of Rush pin technics*. Berivon: Meridian, 1976.
202. Hackethal KH. [Bundle nailing. A method of marrow nailing of long tubular bones]. *Langenbecks Arch Klin Chir Ver Dtsch Z Chir* 1961;298:1001–1003.
203. Jubel A, Andermahr J, Schiffer G, et al. Elastic stable IM nailing of midclavicular fractures with a titanium nail. *Clin Orthop* 2003;279–285.
204. Enneking TJ, Hartlief MT, Fontijne WP. Rushpin fixation for midshaft clavicular nonunions: good results in 13/14 cases. *Acta Orthop Scand* 1999;70:514–516.
205. Wachtl SW, Marti CB, Hoogewoud HM, et al. Treatment of proximal humerus fracture using multiple IM flexible nails. *Arch Orthop Trauma Surg* 2000;120:171–175.
206. Henley MB, Monroe M, Tencer AF. Biomechanical comparison of methods of fixation of a midshaft osteotomy of the humerus. *J Orthop Trauma* 1991;5:14–20.
207. Neumann HS, Holmenschlager F, Winckler S, Brug E. Bundle nailing of diaphyseal fractures of the humerus. *Acta Orthop Belg* 1995;61 Suppl. 1:159–161.
208. Moerman J, Lenaert A, De Coninck D, et al. Intramedullary fixation of forearm fractures in adults. *Acta Orthop Belg* 1996;62:34–40.
209. Gonzalez MH, Hall RF, Jr. Intramedullary fixation of metacarpal and proximal phalangeal fractures of the hand. *Clin Orthop* 1996;47–54.
210. Lee S, Nicol RO, Stott NS. Intramedullary fixation for pediatric unstable forearm fractures. *Clin Orthop* 2002;245–250.
211. Shoemaker SD, Comstock CP, Mubarak SJ, et al. Intramedullary Kirschner wire fixation of open or unstable forearm fractures in children. *J Pediatr Orthop* 1999;19:329–337.
212. Van der Reis WL, Otsuka NY, Moroz P, Mah J. Intramedullary nailing versus plate fixation for unstable forearm fractures in children. *J Pediatr Orthop* 1998;18:9–13.
213. Carey TP, Galpin RD. Flexible IM nail fixation of pediatric femoral fractures. *Clin Orthop* 1996;110–118.
214. Bar-On E, Sagiv S, Porat S. External fixation or flexible IM nailing for femoral shaft fractures in children. A prospective, randomised study. *J Bone Joint Surg [Br]* 1997;79: 975–978.
215. Carter MD, Gilbert JA, Dahners LE. An evaluation of the bending stiffness of various tibial fixation methods. *Clin Orthop* 1987;289–293.
216. Holbrook JL, Swiontkowski MF, Sanders R. Treatment of open fractures of the tibial shaft: Ender nailing versus external fixation. A randomized, prospective comparison. *J Bone Joint Surg [Am]* 1989;71:1231–1238.
217. Dobozi WR, Larson BJ, Zindrick M, et al. Flexible IM nailing of subtrochanteric fractures of the femur. A multicenter analysis. *Clin Orthop* 1986;68–78.
218. Hoffmann R, Khodadadyan C, Raschke M, et al. [Retrograde IM nailing in proximal fracture of the humerus in the elderly patient. Results of a minimally invasive management concept]. *Zentralbl Chir* 1998;123:1232–1238.
219. Tarr RR, Wiss DA. The mechanics and biology of IM fracture fixation. *Clin Orthop* 1986;10–17.
220. Regoort M, Raaymakers ELFB, Klopper PJ. Mechanical aspects of interlocked nailing. *Hefte zu der Unfallchirurg* 1993;229:41–46.
221. Vecsei V. Der Dübelbolzen: eine Ergänzung zu Verriegelungsnagelung. *Unfallchirurgie* 1980;6:193–198.
222. Krettek C, Schandelmaier P, Tscherne H. Neue Entwicklungen bei der Stabilisierung dia- und metaphysärer Frakturen der langen Röhrenknochen. *Orthopade* 1997;26: 408–421.
223. Grass R, Biewener A, Rammelt S, Zwipp H. [Retrograde locking nail osteosynthesis of

distal femoral fractures with the distal femoral nail (DFN)]. *Unfallchirurg* 2002;2000; 105:298–314.
224. Ito K, Hungerbuhler R, Wahl D, Grass R. Improved IM nail interlocking in osteoporotic bone. *J Orthop Trauma* 2001;15:192–196.
225. Laflamme GY, Heimlich D, Stephen D, et al. Proximal tibial fracture stability with IM nail fixation using oblique interlocking screws. *J Orthop Trauma* 2003;17:496–502.
226. Henley MB, Meier M, Tencer AF. Influences of some design parameters on the biomechanics of the unreamed tibial IM nail. *J Orthop Trauma* 1993;7:311–319.
227. Court-Brown CM, Will E, Christie J, McQueen MM. Reamed or unreamed nailing for closed tibial fractures. A prospective study in Tscherne C1 fractures. *J Bone Joint Surg [Br]* 1996;78:580–583.
228. Whittle AP, Wester W, Russell TA. Fatigue failure in small diameter tibial nails. *Clin Orthop* 1995;119–128.
229. Greitbauer M, Heinz T, Gaebler C, et al. Unreamed nailing of tibial fractures with the solid tibial nail. *Clin Orthop* 1998;105–114.
230. Gaebler C, Stanzl-Tschegg S, Heinze G, et al. Fatigue strength of locking screws and prototypes used in small diameter tibial nails: a biomechanical study. *J Trauma* 1999; 47:379–384.
231. Blum J, Sternstein W, Hessmann MH, et al. Self-locking expandable intramedullary nails offer low rotational stability in biomechanical testing. 2003;
232. Smith WR, Ziran BH, Morgan SJ, et al. Expandable intramedullary nailing for long bone fractures: analysis of results and complications. Presented at Salt Lake City, 2003.
233. Schandelmaier P, Krettek C, Tscherne H. Biomechanical study of nine different tibia locking nails. *J Orthop Trauma* 1996;10:37–44.
234. Krettek C, Mannss J, Konemann B, et al. The deformation of small diameter solid tibial nails with unreamed IM insertion. *J Biomech* 1997;30:391–394.
235. Krettek C, Mannss J, Miclau T, et al. Deformation of femoral nails with IM insertion. *J Orthop Res* 1998;16:572–575.
236. Mittlmeier TW, Stedtfeld HW, Ewert A, et al. Stabilization of proximal humeral fractures with an angular and sliding stable antegrade locking nail (Targon PH). *J Bone Joint Surg [Am]* 2003;85 Suppl. 4:136–146.
237. Rommens PM, Blum J, Runkel M. Retrograde nailing of humeral shaft fractures. *Clin Orthop* 1998;26–39.
238. Schipper IB, Steyerberg EW, Castelein RM, et al. Treatment of unstable trochanteric fractures. Randomised comparison of the gamma nail and the proximal femoral nail. *J Bone Joint Surg [Br]* 2004;86:86–94.
239. Winquist RA, Hansen ST Jr, Clawson DK. Closed IM nailing of femoral fractures. A report of five hundred and twenty cases. *J Bone Joint Surg [Am]* 1984;66:529–539.
240. Seifert J, Stengel D, Matthes G, et al. Retrograde fixation of distal femoral fractures: results using a new nail system. *J Orthop Trauma* 2003;17:488–495.
241. Hankemeier S, Pape HC, Gosling T, et al. Improved comfort in lower limb lengthening with the IM skeletal kinetic distractor. Principles and preliminary clinical experiences. *Arch Orthop Trauma Surg* 2004;124:129–133.
242. Baumgart R, Betz A, Schweiberer L. A fully implantable motorized IM nail for limb lengthening and bone transport. *Clin Orthop* 1997;135–143.
243. Guichet JM, Deromedis B, Donnan LT, et al. Gradual femoral lengthening with the Albizzia IM nail. *J Bone Joint Surg [Am]* 2003;85:838–848.
244. Garcia-Cimbrelo E, Curto de la M, Garcia-Rey E, et al. The IM elongation nail for femoral lengthening. *J Bone Joint Surg [Br]* 2002;84:971–977.
245. Cole JD, Justin D, Kasparis T, et al. The IM skeletal kinetic distractor (ISKD): first clinical results of a new IM nail for lengthening of the femur and tibia. *Injury* 2001; 32 Suppl. 4, SD129–SD139.
246. Brinker MR, Cook SD, Dunlap JN, et al. Early changes in nutrient artery blood flow following tibial nailing with and without reaming: a preliminary study. *J Orthop Trauma* 1999;13:129–133.
247. Klein MP, Rahn BA, Frigg R, et al. Reaming versus non-reaming in medullary nailing: interference with cortical circulation of the canine tibia. *Arch Orthop Trauma Surg* 1990; 109:314–316.
248. Schemitsch EH, Kowalski MJ, Swiontkowski MF, Senft D. Cortical bone blood flow in reamed and unreamed locked IM nailing: a fractured tibia model in sheep. *J Orthop Trauma* 1994;8:373–382.
249. Melcher GA, Metzdorf A, Schlegel U, et al. Influence of reaming versus nonreaming in IM nailing on local infection rate: experimental investigation in rabbits. *J Trauma* 1995;39:1123–1128.
250. Hupel TM, Aksenov SA, Schemitsch EH. Cortical bone blood flow in loose- and tight-fitting locked unreamed IM nailing: a canine segmental tibia fracture model. *J Orthop Trauma* 1998;12:127–135.
251. Ochsner PE, Baumgart F, Kohler G. Heat-induced segmental necrosis after reaming of one humeral and two tibial fractures with a narrow medullary canal. *Injury* 1998;29 Suppl. 2:B1–10.
252. Giannoudis PV, Snowden S, Matthews SJ, et al. Temperature rise during reamed tibial nailing. *Clin Orthop* 2002;255–261.
253. Garcia OG, Mombiela FL, De La Fuente CJ, et al. The influence of the size and condition of the reamers on bone temperature during IM reaming. *J Bone Joint Surg [Am]* 2004; 86:994–999.
254. Gustilo RB, Mendoza RM, Williams DN. Problems in the management of type III (severe) open fractures: a new classification of type III open fractures. *J Trauma* 1984;24: 742–746.
255. Court-Brown CM, McQueen MM, Quaba AA, Christie J. Locked IM nailing of open tibial fractures. *J Bone Joint Surg [Br]* 1991;73:959–964.
256. Keating JF, Blachut PA, O'Brien PJ, Court-Brown CM. Reamed nailing of Gustilo grade-IIIB tibial fractures. *J Bone Joint Surg [Br]* 2000;82:1113–1116.
257. Bhandari M, Guyatt GH, Swiontkowski MF, Schemitsch EH. Treatment of open fractures of the shaft of the tibia. *J Bone Joint Surg [Br]* 2001;83:62–68.
258. Bhandari M, Guyatt GH, Tong D, et al. Reamed versus nonreamed IM nailing of lower extremity long bone fractures: a systematic overview and meta-analysis. *J Orthop Trauma* 2000;14:2–9.
259. Tornetta P III, Tiburzi D. The treatment of femoral shaft fractures using IM interlocked nails with and without IM reaming: a preliminary report. *J Orthop Trauma* 1997;11: 89–92.
260. Canadian Orthopaedic Trauma Society. Nonunion following IM nailing of the femur with and without reaming. Results of a multicenter randomized clinical trial. *J Bone Joint Surg [Am]* 2003;85:2093–2096.
261. Finkemeier CG, Schmidt AH, Kyle RF, et al. A prospective, randomized study of IM nails inserted with and without reaming for the treatment of open and closed fractures of the tibial shaft. *J Orthop Trauma* 2000;14:187–193.
262. Hupel TM, Aksenov SA, Schemitsch EH. Muscle perfusion after IM nailing of the canine tibia. *J Trauma* 1998;45:256–262.
263. Frolke JP, Van de Krol H, Bakker FC, et al. Destination of debris during IM reaming. An experimental study on sheep femurs. *Acta Orthop Belg* 2000;66:337–340.
264. Frölke JP, Bakker FC, Patka P, Haarman HJ. Reaming debris in osteotomized sheep tibiae. *J Trauma* 2001;50:65–69.
265. Hoegel F, Mueller CA, Peter R, et al. Bone debris: dead matter or vital osteoblasts. *J Trauma* 2004;56:363–367.
266. Nassif JM, Gorczyca JT, Cole JK, et al. Effect of acute reamed versus unreamed IM nailing on compartment pressure when treating closed tibial shaft fractures: a randomized prospective study. *J Orthop Trauma* 2000;14:554–558.
267. Tornetta P III, French BG. Compartment pressures during nonreamed tibial nailing without traction. *J Orthop Trauma* 1997;11:24–27.
268. Pape HC, Giannoudis PV, Grimme K, et al. Effects of IM femoral fracture fixation: what is the impact of experimental studies in regards to the clinical knowledge? *Shock* 2002;18:291–300.
269. Brumback RJ. The rationales of interlocking nailing of the femur, tibia, and humerus. *Clin Orthop* 1996;292–320.
270. Wenda K, Runkel M, Degreif J, Ritter G. Pathogenesis and clinical relevance of bone marrow embolism in medullary nailing: demonstrated by intraoperative echocardiography. *Injury* 1993;24 Suppl. 3:S73–S81.
271. Wenda K, Ritter G, Degreif J, Rudigier J. Zur Genese pulmonaler Komplikationen nach Marknagelosteosynthesen. *Unfallchirurg* 1988;91:432–435.
272. Muller C, Frigg R, Pfister U. Effect of flexible drive diameter and reamer design on the increase of pressure in the medullary cavity during reaming. *Injury* 1993;24 Suppl. 3: S40–S47.
273. Muller C, McIff T, Rahn BA, et al. Influence of the compression force on the IM pressure development in reaming of the femoral medullary cavity. *Injury* 1993;24 Suppl. 3: S36–S39.
274. Sturmer KM, Schuchardt W. [New aspects of closed IM nailing and marrow cavity reaming in animal experiments. II. Intramedullary pressure in marrow cavity reaming (author's transl)]. *Unfallheilkunde* 1980;83:346–352.
275. Mousavi M, Kolonja A, Schaden E, et al. Intracranial pressure-alterations during controlled IM reaming of femoral fractures: an animal study. *Injury* 2001;32:679–682.
276. Pape HC, Regel G, Dwenger A, et al. Influences of different methods of IM femoral nailing on lung function in patients with multiple trauma. *J Trauma* 1993;35:709–716.
277. Anwar IA, Battistella FD, Neiman R, et al. Femur fractures and lung complications: a prospective randomized study of reaming. *Clin Orthop* 2004;71–76.
278. Martin R, Leighton RK, Petrie D, et al. Effect of proximal and distal venting during IM nailing. *Clin Orthop* 1996;80–89.
279. Sturmer KM. Measurement of IM pressure in an animal experiment and propositions to reduce the pressure increase. *Injury* 1993;24 Suppl. 3:S7–21.
280. Mueller CA, Rahn BA. Intramedullary pressure increase and increase in cortical temperature during reaming of the femoral medullary cavity: the effect of draining the medullary contents before reaming. *J Trauma* 2003;55:495–503.
281. Joist A, Schult M, Ortmann C, et al. Rinsing-suction reamer attenuates IM pressure increase and fat intravasation in a sheep model. *J Trauma* 2004;57:146–151.
282. Klemm KW, Borner M. Interlocking nailing of complex fractures of the femur and tibia. *Clin Orthop* 1986;89–100.
283. Kempf I, Grosse A, Beck G. Closed locked IM nailing. Its application to comminuted fractures of the femur. *J Bone Joint Surg [Am]* 1985;67:709–720.
284. Wolinsky PR, McCarty EC, Shyr Y, Johnson KD. Length of operative procedures: reamed femoral IM nailing performed with and without a fracture table. *J Orthop Trauma* 1998;12:485–495.
285. McKee MD, Schemitsch EH, Waddell JP, Yoo D. A prospective, randomized clinical trial comparing tibial nailing using fracture table traction versus manual traction. *J Orthop Trauma* 1999;13:463–469.
286. Stephen DJ, Kreder HJ, Schemitsch EH, et al. Femoral IM nailing: comparison of fracture-table and manual traction: a prospective, randomized study. *J Bone Joint Surg [Am]* 2002;84:1514–1521.
287. Amarenco G, Ismael SS, Bayle B, et al. Electrophysiological analysis of pudendal neuropathy following traction. *Muscle Nerve* 2001;24:116–119.
288. Gibson RJ. Erectile dysfunction induced by orthopedic trauma managed with a fracture table. *J Trauma* 2000;48:576.
289. Tait GR, Danton M. Contralateral sciatic nerve palsy following femoral nailing. *J Bone Joint Surg [Br]* 1991;73:689–690.
290. Anglen J, Banovetz J. Compartment syndrome in the well leg resulting from fracture-table positioning. *Clin Orthop* 1994;239–242.
291. Callanan I, Choudhry V, Smith H. Perineal sloughing as a result of pressure necrosis from the traction post during prolonged bilateral femoral nailing. *Injury* 1994;25:472.
292. George CJ, Lindsey RW, Noble PC, et al. Optimal location of a single distal interlocking

screw in IM nailing of distal third femoral shaft fractures. *J Orthop Trauma* 1998;12: 267–272.
293. Krettek C, Blauth M, Miclau T, et al. Accuracy of IM templates in femoral and tibial radiographs. *J Bone Joint Surg [Br]* 1996;78:963–964.
294. Schandelmaier P, Bölderl A, Sailer R, Gösling T. Ability to kneel after tibial nailing: The length of incision matters. *Eur J Trauma* 2002;28[Suppl. 1]:129.
295. Yang KH, Han DY, Park HW, et al. Fracture of the ipsilateral neck of the femur in shaft nailing. The role of CT in diagnosis. *J Bone Joint Surg [Br]* 1998;80:673–678.
296. Apivatthakakul T, Arpornchayanon O. Iatrogenic femoral neck fracture caused by malinsertion of a curved IM nail. *Injury* 2001;32:727–729.
297. Simonian PT, Chapman JR, Selznick HS, et al. Iatrogenic fractures of the femoral neck during closed nailing of the femoral shaft. *J Bone Joint Surg [Br]* 1994;76:293–296.
298. Strand RM, Molster AO, Engesaeter LB, et al. Mechanical effects of different localization of the point of entry in femoral nailing. *Arch Orthop Trauma Surg* 1998;117:35–38.
299. Lembcke O, Ruter A, Beck A. The nail-insertion point in unreamed tibial nailing and its influence on the axial malalignment in proximal tibial fractures. *Arch Orthop Trauma Surg* 2001;121:197–200.
300. Lang GJ, Cohen BE, Bosse MJ, Kellam JF. Proximal third tibial shaft fractures. Should they be nailed? *Clin Orthop* 1995;64–74.
301. Krupp RJ, Malkani AL, Goodin RA, Voor MJ. Optimal entry point for retrograde femoral nailing. *J Orthop Trauma* 2003;17:100–105.
302. Althausen PL, Neiman R, Finkemeier CG, Olson SA. Incision placement for IM tibial nailing: an anatomic study. *J Orthop Trauma* 2002;16:687–690.
303. Freedman EL, Johnson EE. Radiographic analysis of tibial fracture malalignment following IM nailing. *Clin Orthop* 1995;25–33.
304. Ricci WM, Bellabarba C, Lewis R, et al. Angular malalignment after IM nailing of femoral shaft fractures. *J Orthop.Trauma* 2001a;15:90–95.
305. Krettek C, Miclau T, Schandelmaier P, et al. The mechanical effect of blocking screws ("Poller screws") in stabilizing tibia fractures with short proximal or distal fragments after insertion of small-diameter IM nails. *J Orthop Trauma* 1999;13:550–553.
306. Krettek C, Stephan C, Schandelmaier P, et al. The use of Poller screws as blocking screws in stabilising tibial fractures treated with small diameter IM nails. *J Bone Joint Surg [Br]* 1999;81:963–968.
307. Ricci WM, O'Boyle M, Borrelli J, et al. Fractures of the proximal third of the tibial shaft treated with IM nails and blocking screws. *J Orthop Trauma* 2001b;15:264–270.
308. Gaebler C, Berger U, Schandelmaier P, et al. Rates and odds ratios for complications in closed and open tibial fractures treated with unreamed, small diameter tibial nails: a multicenter analysis of 467 cases. *J Orthop Trauma* 2001;15:415–423.
309. Gonschorek O, Hofmann GO, Buhren V. Interlocking compression nailing: a report on 02 applications. *Arch Orthop Trauma Surg* 1998;117:430–437.
310. Georgiadis GM, Minster GJ, Moed BR. Effects of dynamization after interlocking tibial nailing: an experimental study in dogs. *J Orthop Trauma* 1990;4:323–330.
311. Wu CC, Shih CH. Effect of dynamization of a static interlocking nail on fracture healing. *Can J Surg* 1993;36:302–306.
312. Dagrenat D, Moncade N, Cordey J, et al. An experimental study of dynamization following static medullary nailing in comminuted diaphyseal fractures. *Hefte Unfallchirurg* 1993;229:50–58.
313. Hajek PD, Bicknell HR, Jr, Bronson WE, et al. The use of one compared with two distal screws in the treatment of femoral shaft fractures with interlocking IM nailing. A clinical and biomechanical analysis. *J Bone Joint Surg [Am]* 1993;75:519–525.
314. Grover J, Wiss DA. A prospective study of fractures of the femoral shaft treated with a static, IM, interlocking nail comparing one versus two distal screws. *Orthop Clin North Am* 1995;26:139–146.
315. Kneifel T, Buckley R. A comparison of one versus two distal locking screws in tibial fractures treated with unreamed tibial nails: a prospective randomized clinical trial. *Injury* 1996;27:271–273.
316. Kempf I, Grosse A, Taglang G. Das Straβburger Material - der Grosse-Kempf-Nagel. *Hefte Unfallchirurg* 1993;229:75–78.
317. Pennig D, Brug E. [Insertion of distal screws in interlocking nailing using a new free-hand control device]. *Unfallchirurg* 1989;92:331–334.
318. Höntzsch D, Frigg R, Perren SM. Das besondere Instrument: Das Röntgenstrahlendurchlässige Winkelgetriebe der AO (für die distale Verriegelung von Marknägeln). *Operat Orthop Traumatol* 1992;4:286–289.
319. Gugala Z, Nana A, Lindsey RW. Tibial IM nail distal interlocking screw placement: comparison of the free-hand versus distally-based targeting device techniques. *Injury* 2001;32 Suppl. 4:SD21–SD25.
320. Pardiwala D, Prabhu V, Dudhniwala G, Katre R. The AO distal locking aiming device: an evaluation of efficacy and learning curve. *Injury* 2001;32:713–718.
321. Krettek C, Konemann B, Miclau T, et al. A new technique for the distal locking of solid AO unreamed tibial nails. *J Orthop Trauma* 1997;11:446–451.
322. Krettek C, Konemann B, Farouk O, et al. Experimental study of distal interlocking of a solid tibial nail: radiation-independent distal aiming device (DAD) versus freehand technique (FHT). *J Orthop Trauma* 1998a;12:373–378.
323. Suhm N, Jacob AL, Nolte LP, et al. Surgical navigation based on fluoroscopy—clinical application for computer-assisted distal locking of IM implants. *Comput Aided Surg* 2000;5:391–400.
324. Slomczykowski MA, Hofstetter R, Sati M, et al. Novel computer-assisted fluoroscopy system for intraoperative guidance: feasibility study for distal locking of femoral nails. *J Orthop Trauma* 2001;15:122–131.
325. Magyar G, Toksvig-Larsen S, Moroni A. Hydroxyapatite coating of threaded pins enhances fixation. *J Bone Joint Surg [Br]* 1997;79:487–489.
326. Moroni A, Vannini F, Mosca M, Giannini S. State of the art review: techniques to avoid pin loosening and infection in external fixation. *J Orthop Trauma* 2002;16:189–195.
327. Pommer A, Muhr G, David A. Hydroxyapatite-coated Schanz pins in external fixators used for distraction osteogenesis: a randomized, controlled trial. *J Bone Joint Surg [Am]* 2002;84:1162–1166.
328. Moroni A, Faldini C, Marchetti S, et al. Improvement of the bone-pin interface strength in osteoporotic bone with use of hydroxyapatite-coated tapered external-fixation pins. A prospective, randomized clinical study of wrist fractures. *J Bone Joint Surg [Am]* 2001; 83:717–721.
329. Tengvall P, Skoglund B, Askendal A, Aspenberg P. Surface immobilized bisphosphonate improves stainless-steel screw fixation in rats. *Biomaterials* 2004;25:2133–2138.
330. Moroni A, Faldini C, Giannini S, Wippermann B. Plate fixation with hydroxyapatite-coated screws: a comparative loaded study. *Clin Orthop* 2003;262–267.
331. Rocca M, Fini M, Giavaresi G, et al. Osteointegration of hydroxyapatite-coated and uncoated titanium screws in long-term ovariectomized sheep. *Biomaterials* 2002;23: 1017–1023.
332. Moroni A, Faldini C, Pegreffi F, Giannini S. HA-coated screws decrease the incidence of fixation failure in osteoporotic trochanteric fractures. *Clin Orthop* 2004;87–92.
333. Cole BJ, Bostrom MP, Pritchard TL, et al. Use of bone morphogenetic protein 2 on ectopic porous coated implants in the rat. *Clin Orthop* 1997;219–228.
334. Raschke M, Wildemann B, Inden P, et al. Insulin-like growth factor-1 and transforming growth factor-beta1 accelerates osteotomy healing using polylactide-coated implants as a delivery system: a biomechanical and histological study in minipigs. *Bone* 2002; 30:144–151.
335. Schmidmaier G, Wildemann B, Cromme F, et al. Bone morphogenetic protein-2 coating of titanium implants increases biomechanical strength and accelerates bone remodeling in fracture treatment: a biomechanical and histological study in rats. *Bone* 2002;30: 816–822.
336. Schmidmaier G, Wildemann B, Heeger J, et al. Improvement of fracture healing by systemic administration of growth hormone and local application of insulin-like growth factor-1 and transforming growth factor-beta1. *Bone* 2002;31:165–172.
337. Schmidmaier G, Wildemann B, Ostapowicz D, et al. Long-term effects of local growth factor (IGF-I and TGF-beta 1) treatment on fracture healing. A safety study for using growth factors. *J Orthop Res* 2004;22:514–519.
338. Wildemann B, Kandziora F, Krummrey G, et al. Local and controlled release of growth factors (combination of IGF-I and TGF-beta I, and BMP-2 alone) from a polylactide coating of titanium implants does not lead to ectopic bone formation in sheep muscle. *J Control Release* 2004;95:249–256.
339. Lucke M, Schmidmaier G, Sadoni S, et al. Gentamicin coating of metallic implants reduces implant-related osteomyelitis in rats. *Bone* 2003;32:521–531.
340. Price JS, Tencer AF, Arm DM, Bohach GA. Controlled release of antibiotics from coated orthopedic implants. *J Biomed Mater Res* 1996;30:281–286.

PRINCIPLES OF EXTERNAL FIXATION

J. Tracy Watson

HISTORICAL PERSPECTIVE

The history of external fixation dates back to the 19th century, with Malgaigne's description of an ingenious mechanism consisting of a clamp that approximated four transcutaneous metal prongs for use in reducing and maintaining patellar fractures. This was described in 1843, a full 12 years before the introduction of plaster casting techniques (1).

Monolateral External Fixation

The Belgian surgeon Lambotte in 1902 expanded external fixation and was the first to apply a simple unilateral frame in a systematic fashion. He recognized that the metal pins that penetrated bone and protruded through the skin were remarkably well tolerated and could be connected to an external clamp device, which would allow for stabilization of these pins and thus the bone fragments they were attached to (Fig. 7-1) (2). Lambotte's concepts and design evolved and eventually allowed for frame adjustments to occur, including compression and distraction at the fracture site. In Europe, Lambotte's original concepts were expanded significantly, and in 1938 Raul Hoffman devised an external fixator that incorporated a universal ball joint connecting the external ball of the fixator to strong pin-gripping clamps. This universal joint permitted fracture reduc-

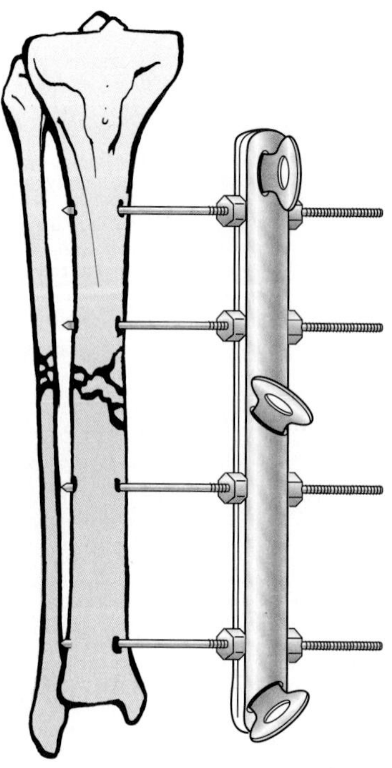

FIGURE 7-1 Lambotte's external fixator, using simple pins and a clamp device.

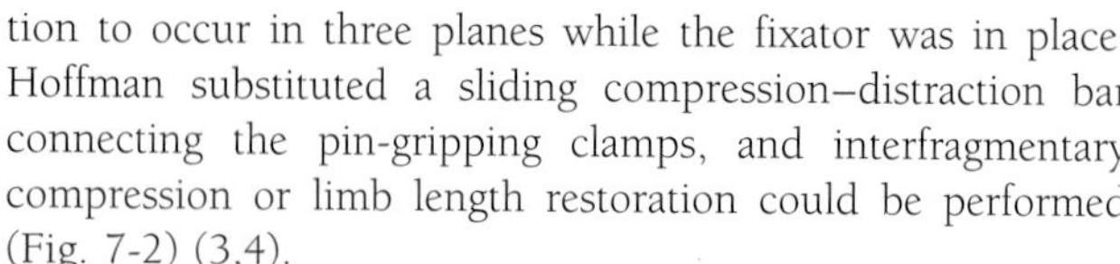

tion to occur in three planes while the fixator was in place. Hoffman substituted a sliding compression–distraction bar connecting the pin-gripping clamps, and interfragmentary compression or limb length restoration could be performed (Fig. 7-2) (3,4).

In the United States, Roger Anderson devised an apparatus for the mechanical reduction of fractures using transcutaneous pins connected to metal clamps. Anderson's early concept called for application of through-and-through transfixion pins. This permitted multiplanar adjustment of the fracture fragments and also allowed compression at the fracture site. After reduction, a cast was applied while the limb was still held by the external device (5). After the cast was applied, the external device was removed and reused on additional patients. Later, Anderson extended this concept and designed an entire external system that connected transcutaneous pins to bars, eliminating the need for a plaster cast (Fig. 7-3) (1).

In 1937 Otto Stader devised a system of fracture management for use in his veterinary practice that permitted stabilization of fractures and also allowed the independent reduction of fracture fragments to occur in three planes (1). The Stader device was refined and enlarged for use in human long bones. In 1942 Lewis and Briedenbach reported their experience with this device for treating fractures of long bones. They were encouraged by the ability to achieve excellent alignment and early

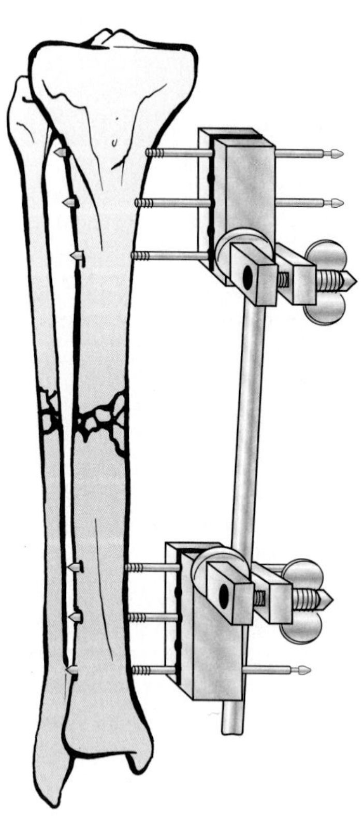

FIGURE 7-2 Hoffman's multi-pin clamp external fixator.

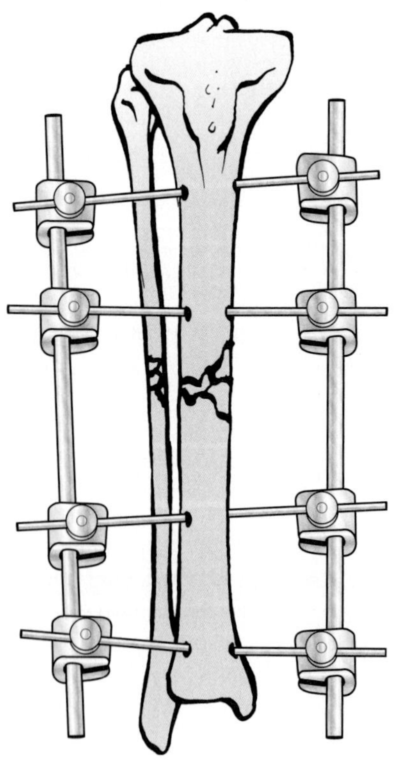

FIGURE 7-3 Anderson device with through-and-through transfixion pins.

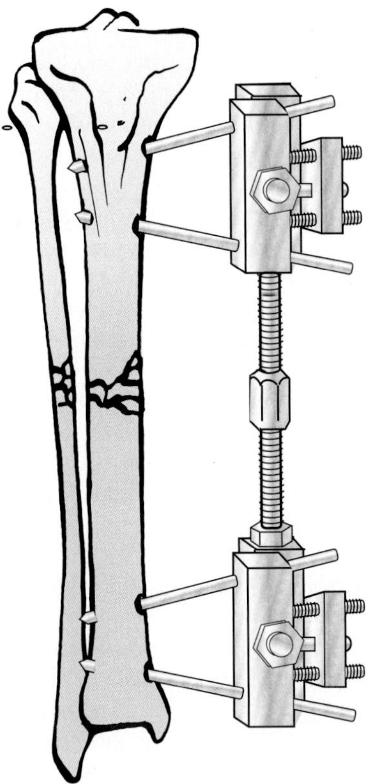

FIGURE 7-4 The Stader device.

ambulation without the need for adjunctive casting (Fig. 7-4) (6).

The use of external fixation techniques by the United States during World War II was documented by Shaar and Kreuz with their use of the Stader splint (7,8). Because of the high incidence of significant complications associated with external fixation, this technique fell into general disfavor because these complications were by and large attributed to the external fixation device and not necessarily to the problems of treating high-energy open fractures. This resulted in a directive issued to military surgeons of the U.S. Armed Forces to discontinue the use of external fixation (1).

After World War II, a study was commissioned by the Committee on Fracture and Trauma Surgery of the American Academy of Orthopaedic Surgeons (AAOS) to investigate the efficacy of and indications for external fixation in clinical fracture management. The study was based on 3,082 questionnaires sent to practicing clinicians who were members of the AAOS, the American Association of Surgery and Trauma, and the Iowa Medical Association. Only 395 replies were analyzed by the committee. Twenty-eight percent of the respondents felt that external skeletal fixation had a definite place in fracture management, while 29.4% felt that external fixation was not inadvisable except in select rare instances (9). Over 43% of respondents had used external fixation at one time but had abandoned it completely at the time of the survey. Based on the results of the survey and concerns that practitioners had with the potential mechanical difficulty associated with these frames, as well as the prospect of converting a closed fracture to an open fracture, the committee concluded that any physicians who contemplated the use of external skeletal fixation required special training under the supervision of a surgeon who had treated at least 200 cases by this method (1). As a consequence, by 1950 the majority of American surgeons were not using this modality. From 1950 to 1970, external fixators were generally unpopular with American orthopaedists, although pins and plaster was still widely used for wrist and tibial fractures.

In Europe, Vidal et al were the first to subject the various assemblies of the external fixator frames to mechanical testing. Vidal used Hoffman's equipment but designed a quadrilateral frame to provide rigid stabilization of complex fracture problems. His biomechanical studies determined that the quadrilateral configuration was quite stable (1,10).

Similarly, Franz Bernie continued with Hoffman's original concept of a unilateral frame using a single connecting bar and half-pins. His extensive clinical experience with a half-pin frame documented the success of this device when treating several large series of fracture problems (11,12).

The European experience in the late 1960s and early 1970s showed that the use of external fixation could not only treat fractures but also could be extended to the treatment of pseudoarthrosis, as well as infections and arthrodesis. The outstanding basic science work on external fixation that was emanating from Europe in the early 1970s, along with the promising clinical results from European centers, stimulated renewed interest in the use of these techniques in North America. This also coincided with the publication of the second edition of the "AO Manual" in 1977 (13). It was at this time that external fixation was recommended for the treatment of acute open fractures. Simultaneously with the recommendations found in the second edition of the "AO Manual," a new tubular monolateral external fixation system was produced. The tubular system of the ASIF gained wide acceptance rapidly because of improved pin design and frame biomechanics, as well as precise indications for their use. These factors contributed to many North American surgeons revisiting and adopting this technique, as well as reporting good clinical results (Fig. 7-5).

Circular External Fixation

External fixation as a modality for fracture treatment continued to remain viable in Russia after World War II. Instead of concentrating on half-pin and monolateral-type configurations, their techniques focused on the use of very thin transfixion wires, which were tensioned to maintain bone segment fixation. By attaching these wires to separate rings, the rings could be individually manipulated to provide for three planes of correction, similar to the concepts pioneered by Hoffman, Bernie, and Vidal. This ability to achieve precise ring positioning resulted in significant flexibility of the device (Fig. 7-6) (14).

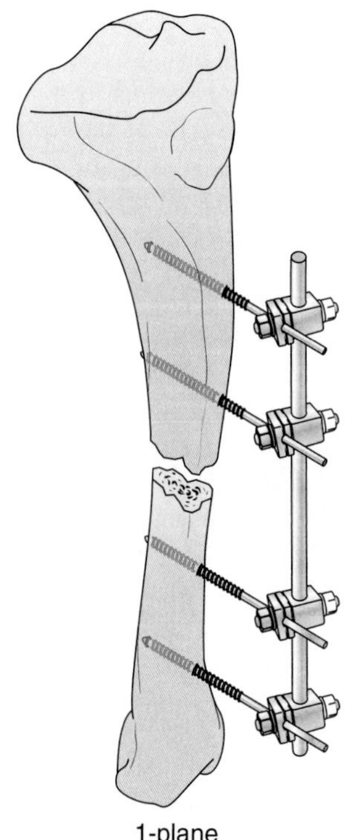

FIGURE 7-5 The "simple monolateral" multicomponent external fixation system that helped renew interest in contemporary external fixation techniques.

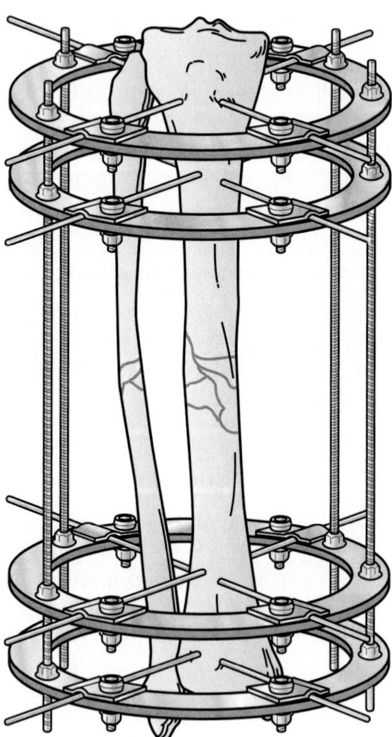

FIGURE 7-6 Ilizarov's circular fixator using small tensioned wires attached to individual rings.

In 1975 Volkoff and Oganesian published a study of a series of patients treated with distraction arthroplasty at the knee and elbow using small transfixion wires attached to ring fixators. Their work went largely unnoticed in North America, even though it was published in the American version of the *Journal of Bone and Joint Surgery* (15).

Dr. David Fisher was exposed to Volkoff's circular apparatus and designed a circular-type fixator. Instead of using thin tensioned wires as with the Russian device, he designed a fixator configuration that allowed for significant pin separation, deviation of pins at various angles, and a semicircular configuration. He determined that fracture site stability could be increased using these circular configuration concepts (1,16).

As the traditional Soviet Ilizarov-type devices were quite cumbersome and complex compared to the more straight forward AO and Hoffman-type fixators, Kroner in 1978 refined and modified the Russian devices by using plastic components and transfixion pins in place of the thin wires used by the Ilizarov technique (17,18).

When the political climate in the Soviet Union changed under different leadership, the possibilities of the Ilizarov method and biology that had previously been unrecognized in the West became more apparent. These techniques were presented at various orthopaedic meetings in Italy and other centers in Western Europe in the late 1970s and early 1980s (1,14,18).

A few select North American surgeons, notably Victor Frankel, James Aronson, Dror Paley, and Stuart Green, were exposed to Ilizarov's work and determined that the methodology applied to difficult contemporary orthopaedic problems had vast potential and began clinical applications in the mid 1980s (14,18). In 1989 Stuart Green, who had significant expertise in treating nonunions and osteomyelitis with external fixation techniques, was entrusted by Ilizarov to translate his original basic science work into English. This was published in *Clinical Orthopaedics and Related Research* in 1989 (18–20).

The North American experience was popularized by a small cadre of American surgeons in the late 1980s. This technique today has become widely accepted for complex problems in traumatology, reconstructive surgery, and limb lengthening. In an effort to simplify and apply these techniques to traumatology, the tensioned ring concept was married to the unilateral fixator and the hybrid external fixator was developed to address periarticular injuries with all the advantages of tensioned wires, while limiting the disadvantages of tethering large musculotendinous units with through-and-through transfixion wire constructs (Fig. 7-7).

Recent advancements in deformity correction have been developed by Charles Taylor and others to correct complex deformities through the use of simple ring constructs using half-pin fixation. The rings are manipulated by a system of adjustable struts, which allow for six-axis correction of bone fragments. The development of this concept, as well as the ability to interface deformity correction with Web-based software, has continued the advancement of contemporary external fixation techniques.

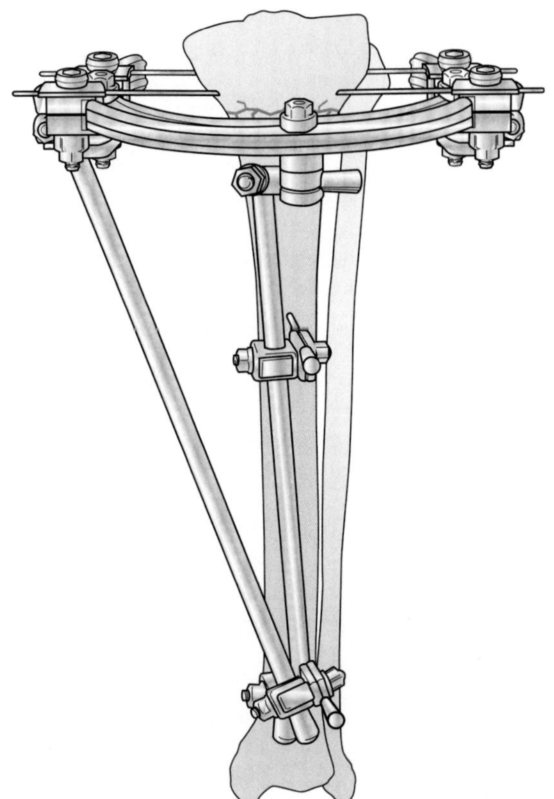

FIGURE 7-7 An early version of a hybrid external fixator that combines periarticular tensioned wires and diaphyseal half-pin configurations.

FRAME TYPES

External fixation systems in current clinical use can be categorized according to the type of bone anchorage used. This is accomplished by using either threaded pins, which are screwed into the bone, or by drilling small-diameter transfixion wires through the bone and then placing the wires under tension to maintain bone fragment position.

The pins or wires are then connected to one another through the use of longitudinal bars or circular rings—thus the distinction between monolateral external fixation (longitudinal connecting bars) and circular external fixation (wires connecting to rings). Circular fixation may use either threaded pins or small tensioned wires to attach the bone to the frame. Monolateral fixation is accomplished using only various-diameter threaded pins, although these may occasionally involve the use of centrally threaded through-and-through transfixion pins.

FRAME BIOMECHANICS

Large Pin Fixation

Large pin fixator constructs are attached to the bone using various sizes of terminally threaded pins. The half-pins have a wide range of diameters, ranging from 2 mm to 6 mm, with all intermediate sizes available. Additionally, there are large-diameter pins with threads in the midportion of the device (i.e., centrally threaded pins) for use in transfixion-type constructs (i.e., Hoffman/Vidal configurations).

The basic indications for large pin external skeletal fixation have specific biomechanical functions, which will be imparted to the fixation construct. The ability to neutralize deforming forces is the most common mechanical principle exploited with external fixation. This is especially true for fresh fractures accompanied by severe soft tissue damage. The acute use of monolateral fixation for the stabilization of fresh fractures is a way of dealing with soft tissue compromise for the immediate posttrauma/postoperative period (21). After resolution of the soft tissue compromise, secondary procedures such as bone grafting or delayed internal fixation are commonly considered. The primary function of fixators used in this way is to provide rigid stability to maintain the fracture and temporary reduction at length to avoid collapse of the fracture construct. However, this type of stabilization is relatively "flexible," and it is nearly impossible to achieve absolute rigidity to achieve primary bone healing using monolateral or less flexible external fixation (see Fig. 7-5).

Monolateral frames can also be used to bring areas of metaphyseal or metadiaphyseal bone into close contact through the use of compression techniques. This may be useful in arthrodesis, osteotomy, or nonunion repair (Fig. 7-8). Similarly, distraction forces can also be applied across pin groups to effect deformity correction, intercalary bone transport, or limb lengthening.

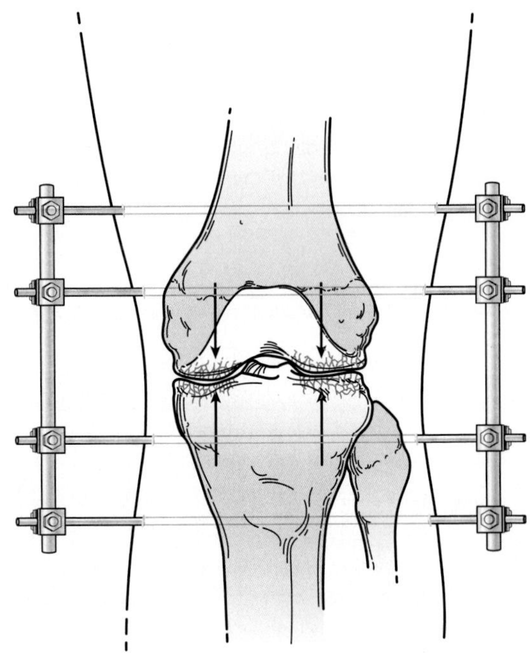

FIGURE 7-8 A simple "compression" monolateral system constructed to achieve arthrodesis of the knee.

Components

No matter what the biomechanical function of the frame type, the most important factor regarding the longevity and performance of the frame is the strength and competency of the pin–bone interface. Pin loosening with subsequent pin sepsis continues to be problematic. There are many biomechanical factors that have been evaluated for the prevention of pin tract problems, and all pin types and designs are based on these concepts (22–27):

1. Pin geometry and thread design
2. The pin–bone interface, biomaterials
3. Pin insertion techniques
4. Pin bone stresses

Pin Design

Both the screw thread design and the type of cutting head have a significant effect on the holding power of screws. Screw diameter is crucial in determining the stiffness of the frame, as well as determining the risk of stress fracture at the pin site entry portal. The bending stiffness of the screw increases as a function of the pins radius raised to the fourth power ($S \approx r^4$). A screw hole greater than 30% of the diameter of the bone results in a 45% reduction in the torsional strength of that bone. In adult bone, a pin diameter of 6 mm is the maximum that can be used to achieve a stable implant without suffering the consequences of stress fracture through the pinhole itself (28–30). In addition to the variable diameter of the pin, the screw thread may also have differing pitch angle and pitch height. The screw design must make allowances for the quality and location of bone to which the screw is applied. Pins that have a small pitch height and low pitch angle are usually applied in regions of dense cortical bone, such as femoral and tibial diaphysis (Fig. 7-9).

As the pitch vertex angle increases and the curvature and the diameter of the thread increase, the area captured by each individual thread is broader, and this pin is more likely to be applied in cancellous bone rather than hard cortical bone. Conical pins have been designed so that the threads taper and increase in diameter from the tip of the pin to the shaft. This allows the pins to increase their purchase theoretically by cutting a new, larger path in the bone. This conical taper also produces a gradual increase in radial preload, and thus the screw–bone contact is optimized (see Fig. 7-9). The micromotion typical of a straight cylindrical screw is avoided (27,31,32).

Insertion Technique

Preloading the implant–bone interface has an effect on pin loosening. Radial preload is a concept that prestresses the pin–bone interface in a circumferential fashion rather than in just one direction (33,34).

Fixator pins are placed with a slight mismatch in the greater thread diameter versus the core diameter of the pilot hole. The small mismatch increases insertion and removal torque, with a decrease in signs of clinical loosening. There is a point at which insertion of pins with a mismatch of greater than 0.4 mm can result in significant microscopic structural damage to the bone surrounding the pin. High degrees of radial preload or a large pilot hole thread diameter mismatch will exceed the elastic limit of cortical bone, with subsequent stress fracture. Thus, the use of oversize pins producing excessive radial preloads is not recommended (25,33,35).

Screw insertion technique also has an effect on the pin–bone interface. The pins typically come in two types, either predrilled or where a drill is used to produce a pilot hole before insertion of the pin. The pilot hole has a root diameter less than or equal to the core diameter of the pin itself (36,37). As a better pilot hole is drilled with a precise cutting tip, the radial preload is also affected, which will also affect the overall pullout strength. The advantages of predrilling using very sharp drills for pilot holes minimizes the risk of thermal necrosis and subsequent bone damage (34). The use of self-tapping cortical pins allows each thread to purchase bone as the pin is slowly advanced (24,38).

There is concern that when using self-drilling pins, the near cortex thread purchase may be stripped as the drill tip of the pin engages the far cortex. As the drill tip on the pin spins to

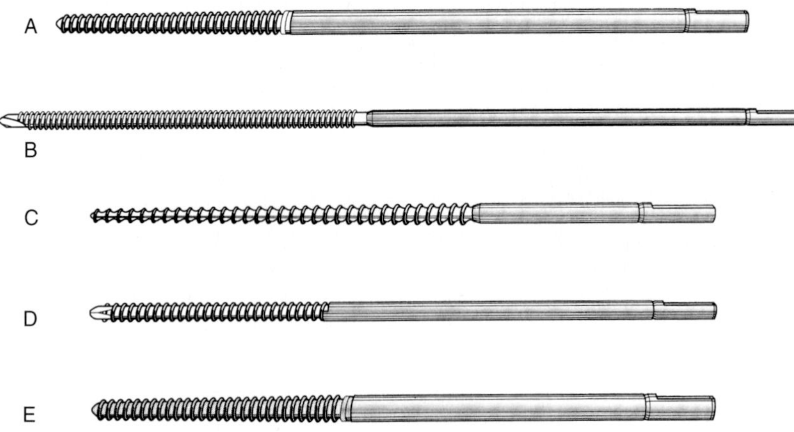

FIGURE 7-9 Various thread designs are used for specific purposes. **A.** The use of tapered pins facilitates subsequent pin removal. **B.** Self-drilling pins with drill-type pin tip. **C.** Pins with a larger thread diameter suitable for cancellous bone insertion. **D.** Pins with small pitch angle and narrow thread diameter are applied in cortical bone. **E.** Hydroxyapatite-coated pins improve the pin–bone interface by encouraging direct bone apposition and ingrowth.

cut the far cortex, the newly purchased bone in the near threads is stripped and the pin stability is compromised (see Fig. 7-9). Some studies indicate a 25% reduction in bone purchase of self-drilling, self-tapping pins compared to that of predrilled pins (39). This is also accompanied by a marked increase in the depth of insertion required to achieve a similar pin purchase or pin "feel" when a self-drilling pin has a long sharp-tipped drilling portion adjacent to the actual threads (40).

Reduction in the length of the drilling portion of the pin means that less of the pin tip needs to project through the far cortex before a firm grip is achieved on the bone. The flutes for tapping the bone run obliquely back down the shaft of the pin. The helical or spiral nature of the flutes steers the bone debris back along the pins and out into the soft tissue. The efficient removal of this bone is mandatory to avoid compacting the cutting flutes and compromising their cutting ability, and increasing the heat of insertion (35). The potential disadvantages of self-drilling pins are, therefore, increased heat of insertion, increased microfracture at both cortices (specifically at the near cortex) with increased bone resorption, and subsequent decreased pullout strength with decreased insertion and extraction torque (31,38). Studies have noted elevated temperatures during insertion with a direct drill technique, where temperatures in excess of 55°C can occur during insertion of self-drilling pins (41). The complication of thermal necrosis with secondary loosening caused by the resorption of nonviable bone is a real concern (Fig. 7-10). Clinically, there does not appear to be any increased incidence of pin tract infection or other pin-associated complications reported with the use of self-drilling pins (37).

Biomaterials

Traditionally, external fixator pins have been composed of stainless steel, offering substantial stiffness (26). Finite element analyses of the near pin–bone interface cortex revealed stress values that were significantly increased by the use of deep threads and by the use of stainless steel as opposed to titanium pins. Titanium has a much a lower modulus of elasticity. Because of the better biocompatibility afforded with titanium and titanium alloys, some investigators prefer the lower pin–bone interface stresses, as well as the better biocompatibility when using titanium, as they feel there is a lower rate of pin sepsis. This may be due to many factors, including an actual bone ingrowth phenomenon seen at the pin–bone interface (31,42,43).

Among the many different techniques to enhance the pin–bone interface fixation, coating the pins with hydroxyapatite (HA) has been shown to be one of the most effective (44–46). Moroni showed that HA-coated tapered pins improved the strength of fixation at the pin–bone interface, which corresponded to a lower rate of pin tract infection (47). The HA coating provides a significant increase in direct bone apposition with a decrease in the fibrous tissue interposition at the pin–bone interface. These advantages provided by HA coating appear to be clinically more relevant when these pins are used in cancellous bone rather than in cortical bone (see Fig. 7-9)

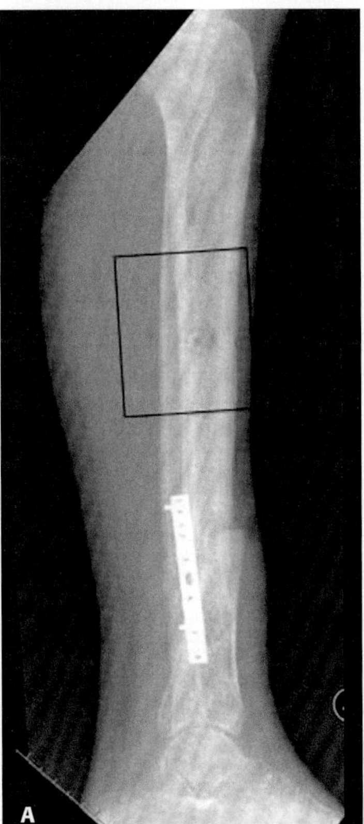

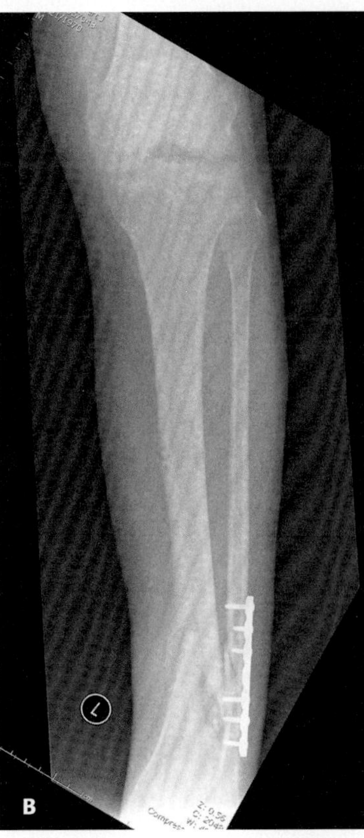

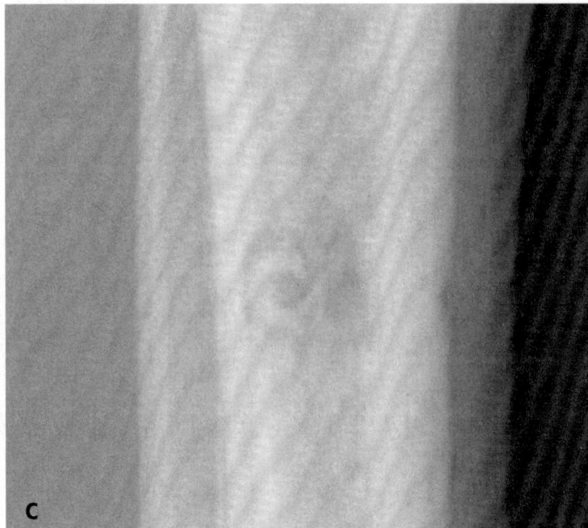

FIGURE 7-10 A,B. Nonunion with varus deformity following failure of hybrid external fixation. Self-drilling pins used in the diaphysis resulted in a ring sequestrum at proximal pin site (*black box*). **C.** Sclerotic bone (dead) at old pin location, with circumferential lucency characteristic of ring sequestrum. This complication required excision of the infected sequestrum.

(45,48). This increase in bone–pin purchase also may make these pins more difficult or painful to remove without anesthesia.

Monolateral Frame Types

Some monolateral frames come with individual separate components, such as separate bars, attachable pin–bar clamps, bar-to-bar clamps, and separate Schanz pins. These "simple monolateral" frames allow for a wide range of flexibility with "build up" or "build down" capabilities. The modular capabilities allow the surgeon to add more pins or bars to the construct to increase the stability of the frame. Similarly, as healing progresses, individual components can be removed to transfer more stresses to the bone. This allows the surgeon to apply a frame specific to the clinical and biomechanical needs of the pathology addressed. A more constrained type of fixator comes preassembled, with a multi-pin clamp at each end of a long rigid tubular body. The telescoping tube allows for axial compression or distraction of this "Monotube" type of fixator.

Simple monolateral fixators have the distinct advantage of allowing individual pins to be placed at different angles and varying obliquities while still connecting to the bar. This is helpful when altering the pin position relative to areas of soft tissue compromise. The advantage of the Monotube type of fixator is its simplicity. Pin placement is predetermined by the multi-pin clamps. Loosening the universal articulations between the body and the clamps allows these frames to be easily manipulated to reduce a fracture. Similarly, compression (dynamization) or distraction can be accomplished by a simple adjustment of the Monotube body (Fig. 7-11).

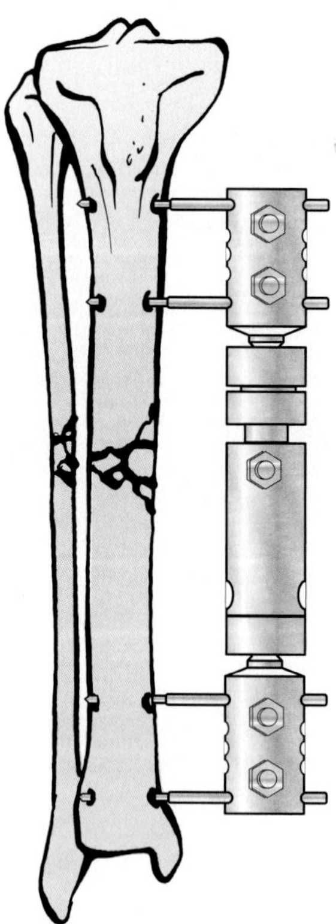

FIGURE 7-11 Large pin "Monotube" fixator. Device has fixed proximal and distal pin clamps and a large telescoping body.

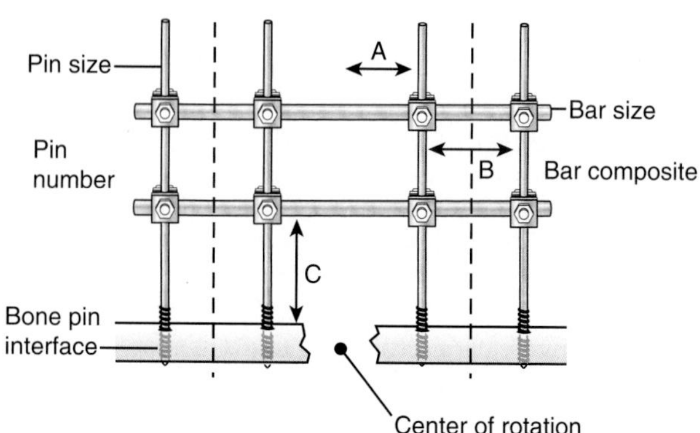

FIGURE 7-12 Factors affecting the stability of monolateral external fixation include pin distance from fracture site, pin separation, bone–bar distance, connecting bar size and composition, pin diameter, pin number, and pin–bone interface. *A*, pin to center of rotation; *B*, pin separation; *C*, bone–bar distance.

Simple Monolateral Fixators

The stability of all monolateral fixators is based on the concept of a simple four-pin frame. Pin number, pin separation, and pin proximity to the fracture site, as well as bone bar distance and the diameter of the pins and connecting bars, all influence the final mechanical stability of the external fixator frame (Fig. 7-12).

Simple four-pin system rigidity can be increased by maximizing pin separation distance on each side of the fracture component as well as increasing the number of pins used. In the case of a four-pin system, using two pins on each limb segment with maximal pin spread and minimizing the bone-connecting bar distance also increases stability (see Fig. 7-12) (49). Behrens used unilateral configurations with stiffness characteristics similar to those of the most rigid one- and two-plane bilateral constructs; these are easily built using the four-pin frame as a basic building block (Fig. 7-13) (50,51). Mechanically most effective

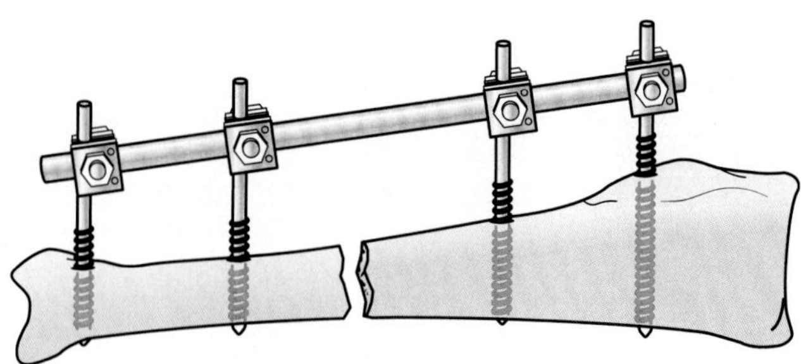

FIGURE 7-13 A simple four-pin external frame is the basic building block for more complex frame configurations.

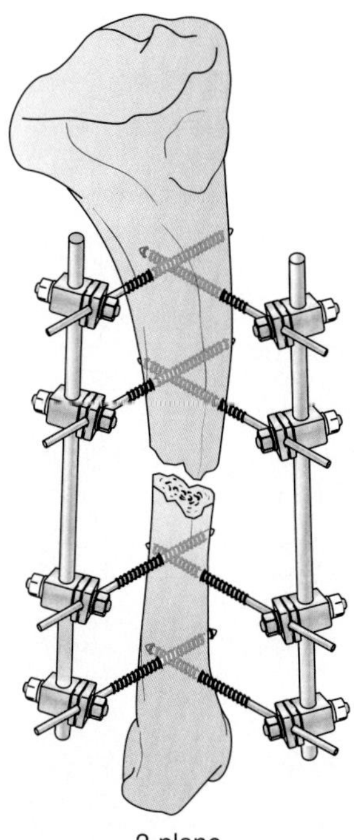

FIGURE 7-14 A delta configuration is composed of two "simple" four-pin frames connected at 90 degrees to each other.

were the delta plane configurations, when two simple four-pin fixators are applied at 90-degree angles to each other and connected (Fig. 7-14). However, single and double stacked bar anterior four-pin frames have the best combination of clinical and mechanical features (Fig. 7-15). The complex delta frames allow for gradual frame build down on a rational basis to slowly transfer more load to the bone. This stepwise frame reduction leads from the most rigid unilateral constructs to frames that allow the most complete force transmission across the fracture site while still providing adequate protection against sagittal bending movements (23,50,51). Studies have shown that a unilateral biplanar delta frame without transfixion pins can be set up with an overall rigidity as good as that of a bilateral transfixion-type device (52).

When the distance from the connecting bar to the bone increases, implant stability decreases. This is clinically significant when dealing with patients with wide areas of soft tissue compromise, which may preclude the ability to place the connecting bar close to the subcutaneous border of the bone. To counteract this, a standard four-pin fixator can be altered to increase the number of pins applied in each fracture segment (see Fig. 7-15) (53).

The materials used to construct the connecting bars have a significant effect on overall frame stability. Kowalski et al showed that carbon fiber bars were approximately 15% stiffer than stainless steel tubes, but that an external fixator with carbon fiber bars achieved 85% of the fixation stiffness achieved with stainless steel tubes (54). They felt that the loss of stiffness of the external fixator construct was likely due to the clamps being less effective in connecting the carbon fiber rods to the pins.

The weakest part of the system is the junction between the fixator body and the clamp or between the fixator clamp and the Schanz pins. Insufficient holding strength on a pin by a clamp may result in a decrease in the overall fixation rigidity, as well as increased motion at the pin–bone interface. Cyclic loading of external fixators has been shown to loosen the tightened screws within the pin clamps. Thus, one needs to be aware of the mechanical yield characteristics of the clamps, bars, and pins throughout treatment (55).

Because of the gradual fatigue of components and loosening of pin-to-bar and bar-to-bar connections, the device should be routinely tightened during treatment (55–57).

Monotube Fixators

Stability of the large Monotube fixators is accomplished in a distinctly different way compared to the simpler monolateral fixators. Most Monotube fixators have a fixed location for their pins mounted in pin clusters. These are connected to the body, and thus the ability to vary pin location is substantially less than with simple monolateral fixators. Because the pin clusters are fixed at either end of the Monotube body, the surgeon cannot maximize pin spread in relation to the fracture site. There is little variability to lower the large Monotube connection bar closer to the bone in an effort to increase stability. These frames are very stable and accomplish their inherent rigidity by having a very large-diameter Monotube connecting body, three to four times the diameter of the simpler monolateral connecting bars. Because of the large body configuration, these devices offer higher bending stiffness, as well as equal torsional stiffness and variable axial stiffness when compared to standard Hoffman-Vidal quadrilateral frames with transfixion pins (see Fig. 7-11) (53,58–61).

These frames have ball joints at either end connecting the large fixator bodies to their respective pin clamp configurations. There has been concern about the ability to achieve stability due to the ball locking mechanism. Chao determined that the ball joint locking cam and fixation screw clamp required periodic tightening during clinical application to prevent loss of frame stiffness under repetitive loading. However, frank clinical failure with these types of ball joint devices has not been demonstrated (58,59,62).

Insufficient holding strength on a pin within a constrained pin clamp may result in the diminution of the overall construct rigidity, as well as pin movement at the pin–bone interface. This is a distinct disadvantage compared to the single-component simple monolateral frames, where each pin has its own pin bone clamp (62). When using Monotube fixators, the use of six pins increased torsional rigidity, but this configuration fails at lower bending loads than the four-pin configuration, reflecting the uneven holding strength of the pin clamp on three pins (62).

The rigidity of a half-pin system is maximal in the plane of

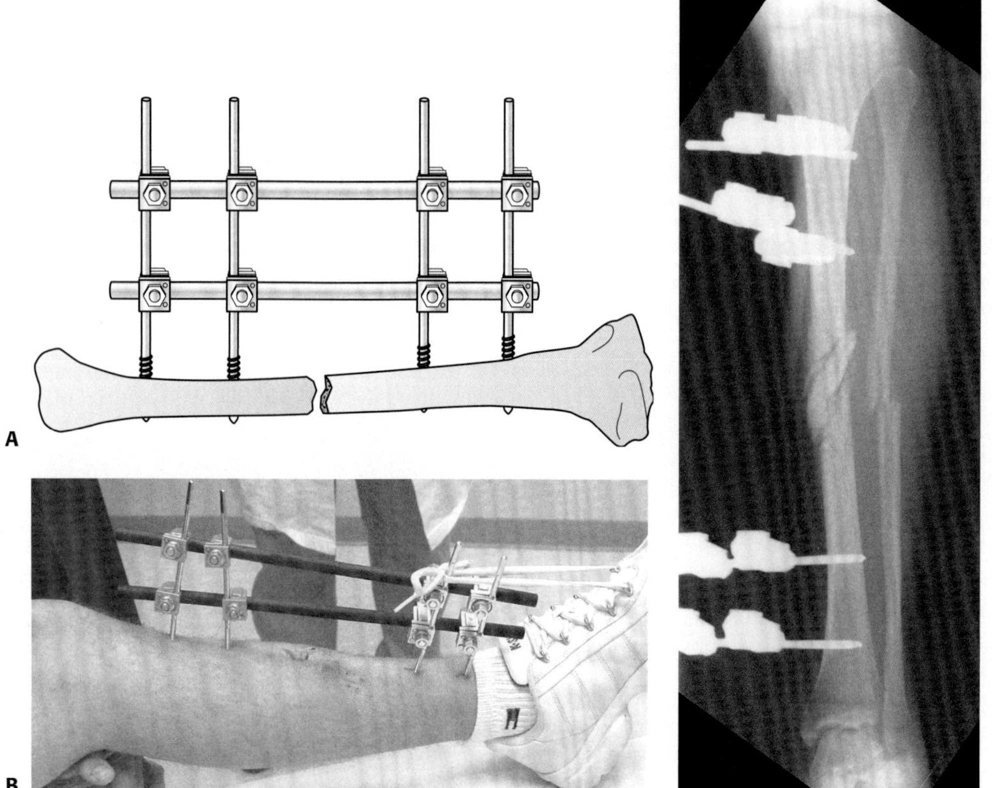

FIGURE 7-15 **A.** The stability of a "simple" four-pin frame can be increased by adding a second connecting bar. A "double-stacked" frame. **B.** The bone–connecting bar distance was increased to avoid soft tissue impingement on the bars. Because of the increased distance to the bone, an additional connecting bar was added to increase the stability of the frame. **C.** Reduction maintained with "simple" four-pin double-stack frame. Early consolidation is noted in this comminuted open fracture.

the pins and is minimal at right angles to this plane. Thus, a simple four-pin frame placed along the anterior border of the tibia will resist the anterior and posterior forces generated with normal stride, while this frame is weakest in mediolateral bending (see Fig. 7-15) (52,63,64). If a fixator could alter the angle of at least one or two pins, this would decrease the overall strength of the construct in the plane of the majority of pins; however, this would be compensated for by increasing the strength of the construct in the plane at right angles (23,50,65).

Shear and Eagan demonstrated that a system in which the pins were placed at 60 degrees to each other offers substantial advantages. With only a 10-degree separation between the pin angles, displacement in response to torsional stress is reduced by 97%. This increase in torsional rigidity occurs until the pin divergence angle reaches about 30 degrees, at which time torsional displacement has all but stopped. The effects on increasing the compressive forces are much less dramatic. A fixator with pins that are placed out of plane to each other (i.e., divergent pin groupings) showed up to a 91% increase in angular and torsion rigidity compared to a traditional monolateral frame, which only allows a linear pin orientation (65). While a rigid frame configuration is not perceived as undesirable, the production of a frame that more closely mimics the biomechanics of normal bone is preferred. An external fixator that allows an offset pin angle of 60 degrees can equalize forces in the sagittal and coronal planes, providing mechanical stimuli much closer to those normally encountered in the sagittal and coronal planes (Fig. 7-16) (65–68).

Steerage Pin Placement

Many investigators are examining alternative pin placements as a way to achieve maximal fracture stability with relative frame simplicity (23,50,52,63–65). This is most problematic when treating highly comminuted fractures or fractures with significant fracture obliquity and increased shear stresses. Standard half-pin application with pins placed perpendicular to the long axis of the bone fails to oppose the shear force vector directly because the pins are placed oblique to the shear force vector, and thus it does not neutralize the cantilever forces induced by this standard pin insertion angle.

Alternatively, when half-pins are placed parallel to the fracture line and thus in direct opposition to the shear force vector, the shear force is actively converted into one of compression, manifesting a dynamic stabilization of the fracture edges (Fig.

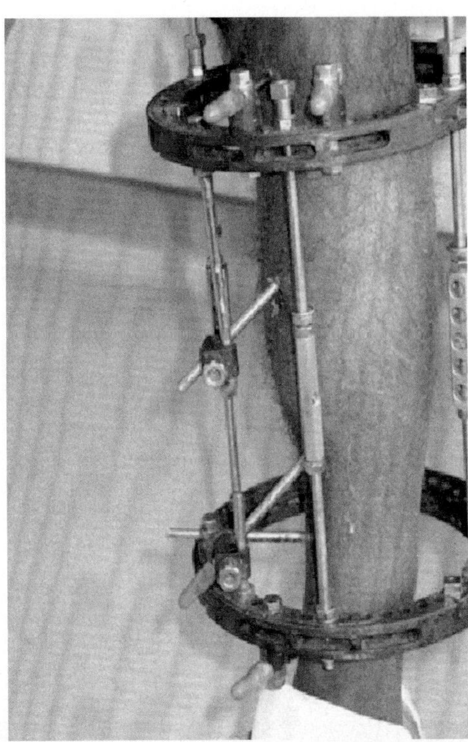

FIGURE 7-16 Frames with nonlinear pin placement neutralize forces similar to the normal forces developed in a tibia. This frame demonstrates pins out of plane to each other in the transverse and sagittal orientations. Six-millimeter HA-coated pins were used, which gives this simple frame very stable mechanics, requiring only three pins on each side of the fracture line.

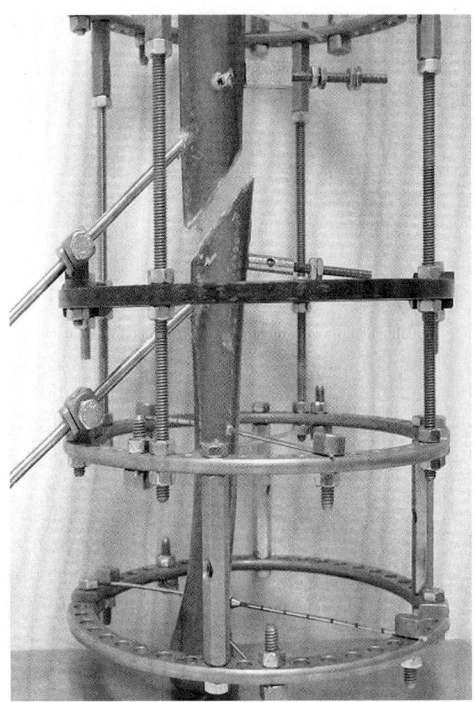

FIGURE 7-17 Steerage pin experimental set-up showing pins placed parallel to the major fracture line, dramatically reducing the shear forces and accentuating compressive forces with axial weight bearing. (Courtesy of David Lowenberg, MD.)

7-17). In this way, compression is dependent on axial load, and the shear phenomenon is almost eliminated. For fracture obliquities of 30 degrees or less, there is inherent stability such that standard modes of fixation can be used without undue concern (69). However, at fracture obliquities greater than 30 degrees, one must respect the inherent shear present with axial loading at the fracture ends. Added steps should therefore be considered to help minimize this shear component, such as the application of the steerage pin concept. At fracture obliquities greater than 60 degrees, shear is a dominating force; even with steerage pins, the forces may be extreme. Frames should be modified to perform strictly as a neutralization device, as interfragmentary compression will be difficult to achieve even with the most complex devices (see Fig. 7-17) (69).

Small Wire Fixation

A major advantage of a monolateral system is that it can be applied in a uniplanar fashion, minimizing the transfixion of soft tissues. The ring-type systems have the disadvantage of transfixion type wires tethering soft tissues as the wires pass from one side of the limb to the other (1,14,18). Because of the smaller wire diameter, the trauma to the soft tissue and bony reaction and intolerance to the wires is minimized. Large pin monolateral fixators rely on stiff pins for frame stability. Upon loading, these pins act as cantilevers and do produce eccentric loading characteristics. Shear forces are regarded to be inhibitory to fracture healing and bone formation, which may be accentuated with certain types of monolateral half-pin stabilization, especially when pins are all in line (70–76). Circular or semicircular fixators allow for multiple planes of fixation, producing frame behavior that largely eliminates the harmful effects of cantilever loading and shear forces while accentuating axial micromotion and dynamization (16,64,67,69,77,78).

Components

Ring fixators are built with longitudinal connecting rods and rings to which the small-diameter tensioned wires are attached. Alternatively, the bone fragments may be attached to the rings by half-pins. The connecting rods may incorporate universal joints, which give these frames their ability to produce gradual multiplanar angular and axial adjustments.

There are several component-related factors that can be manipulated to effect an increase in the stability of the ring fixation construct:

1. Increase wire diameter.
2. Increase wire tension.
3. Increase pin crossing angle to approach 90 degrees.
4. Decrease ring size (distance of ring to bone).

5. Increase number of wires.
6. Use olive wires/drop wires.
7. Close ring position to either side of fracture (pathology) site.
8. Center bone in middle of ring.

Wires

Thin smooth wires of 1.5, 1.8, and 2 mm are the most basic component used in a circular small wire fixator (Fig. 7-18A). Wire strength and stiffness increase as the square of the diameter of the wire ($S \approx d^2$). As these wires are tensioned, they provide increased stability. This occurs by increasing wire stiffness, which simultaneously decreases the axial excursion of the wires during loading. The amount of tension in the wires directly affects the stiffness of the frame. Compression and bending resistance increases as a function of wire tension as tension is gradually increased up to 130 kg. Beyond this threshold, further wire tensioning is difficult to accomplish because commercially available wire-tensioning devices cannot stop the slippage of the wire in the device as the wire is tensioned (see Fig. 7-18B) (14,79,80).

Beaded wires (olive wires) perform many specialized functions. During insertion the beaded portion of the wire is juxtaposed onto the cortex. As the far side of the wire is tensioned, the bead is compressed into the near cortex. This allows olive wires to be inserted to perform interfragmentary compression, which may be useful in fracture applications. These wires act as a source of additional transverse force to help stabilize and correct malunions or nonunions and provide additional support to a limb segment that a smooth wire cannot achieve (14,18).

Wire Tension

During limb lengthening, tension in the wire will inherently be generated from the soft tissue forces achieved through distraction. This may generate tension in the wire as high as 50 kg. If the patient is weight bearing and the limb is loaded, then further wire deflection (tension) occurs. This generates additional tension in the wire. Additional rigidity of the entire construct is also found (the so-called self-stiffening effect of tensioned wires). If the wire was initially tensioned to 130 kg and additional tension is added through lengthening and weight bearing, then the yield point of the wire may be approached,

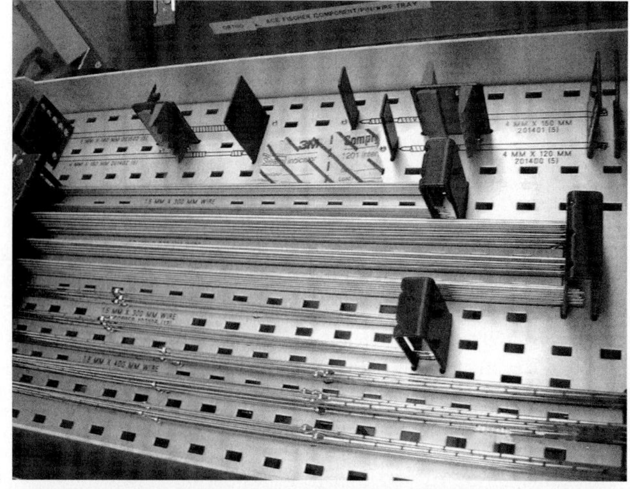
A

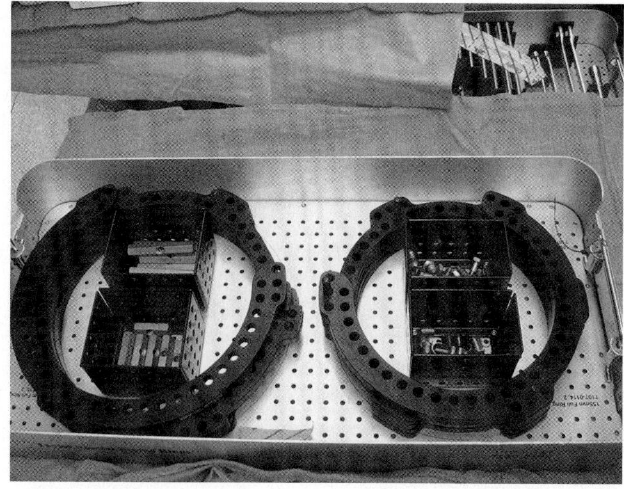
C

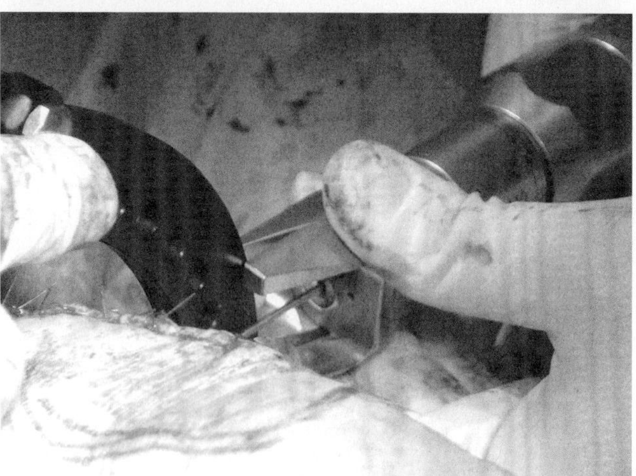
B

FIGURE 7-18 **A.** Smooth and beaded (olive) wires come in the common diameters of 1.5 mm, 1.8 mm, and 2 mm. **B.** A wire tensioning device is used to increase the overall rigidity of the frame construct. **C.** Multiple ring diameters are available to match the diameter of the applied extremity. Too large a ring increases the distance from bone to ring and thus makes the frame less rigid.

with possible wire breakage. A fracture frame is essentially a static fixator where additional wire tension will occur only through weight bearing. Thus, the degree of initial wire tension should take into account the pathology being treated and the treatment forces being generated (14,81–84).

Ring Diameter

The diameter of the ring also affects the stiffness of frame: as the diameter of the ring increases, so does the distance of the ring to the bone. This is similar to the bone–bar distance discussed in the section on half-pin monolateral fixators (see Fig. 7-18C). Because of this increased distance, the frame becomes less stable. Ring diameter and wire tension have a dramatic effect on overall frame stability. As ring diameter increases, the effect of increasing wire tension on gap stiffness and gap displacement is also decreased. Decreasing ring diameter has a greater affect on all variables compared to simply increasing wire tension. Although the effect of wire tension decreases as the ring diameter increases, tensioning wires on frames with larger ring constructs is important because these constructs are inherently less stiff due to longer wires (14,81–85).

Wire Orientation

Wires placed parallel to each other, and parallel to the applied forces, provide little resistance to deformation. The bone can slide along this axis much like a central axle in a wheel. In bending stresses, the frames can be much less rigid due to bowing of the transverse wires and slippage of the bone along these wires. The most stable configuration occurs when two wires intersect as close to 90 degrees as possible. The bending stiffness in the plane of the wire is decreased by a factor of two as the angles between the wires converge from 90 to 45 degrees. Therefore, changing pin orientation to a less acute angle decreases the stiffness in AP bending but has a lesser effect on lateral bending, torsion, and axial compression (82,83,86,87).

Clinically, a wire divergence angle of at least 60 degrees should be attempted (Fig. 7-19). Because this is not always possible due to anatomic constraints of passing transfixion wires, the use of olive wires, or the addition of a wire at a distance off the primary ring (drop wires), significantly improves bending stiffness. The use of two counter-opposed olive wires also improves the shear stiffness (olive wires placed at the same level but from opposite directions, achieving an olive on each side of the bone and thus "locking" in the segment) (18,78,82,83,86,88–90).

Limb Positioning in the Ring

The location of the tibial bone in the limb is actually eccentric to the external soft tissue envelope compared with the humerus or the femur. This is important when placing the rings around the particular extremity. The center of the ring applied may not be located over the actual center of the bone. It may be positioned eccentrically with respect to the ring, affecting the overall stiffness of the frame. If the bone is located off center, this position provides greater stiffness to loading in axial

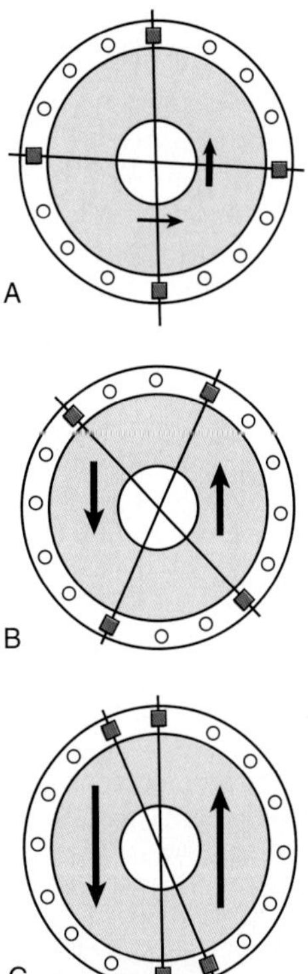

FIGURE 7-19 A. A wire crossing angle of 90 degrees provides the most stable configuration with small mediolateral translations and a rigid frame. **B.** A wire convergence angle of 45 to 60 degrees allows acceptable amounts of translations to occur with satisfactory frame stability. **C.** As the convergence angle decreases, the translation increases dramatically to the point where the bone slides along a single axis. Parallel wires produce a grossly unstable frame configuration.

compression, compared to a construct where the center of the ring is positioned exactly over the center of the bone (14,28,81–83,85–87). Clinically, since most tensioned wire frames are applied to the tibia, this is usually not an issue because the bone is routinely eccentric in the limb as long as the ring is centered on the leg. The eccentric location of the muscular compartments ensures this offset bone position. To place a frame on a tibia with the center/center orientation, a very large ring would be needed; this would vastly increase the ring–bone distance and further decrease the frame stiffness (Fig. 7-20).

A typical four-ring frame consists of eight crossed wires, two wires at each level, and four rings with supporting struts connecting two rings on either side of the fracture (see Fig. 7-6). When this four-ring frame was tested against the standard Hoffman-Vidal quadrilateral transfixion frame, the circular-type frame was noted to be relatively stiff in compression. However, the circular fixators are less rigid than all other monolateral type fixators in all modes of loading, particularly in axial compression (14,81,82,84). However, this may prove to be clinically beneficial to allow for axial micromotion and facilitate secondary bone healing (91). The Ilizarov fixator allowed significantly more axial motion at the fracture site during axial compression

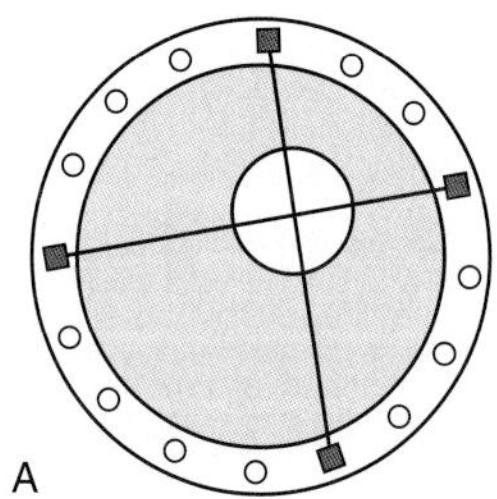

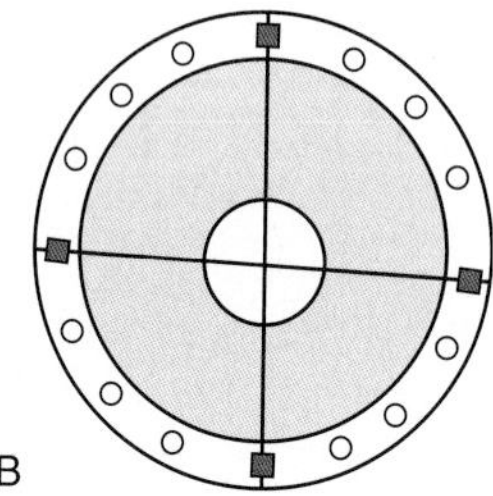

FIGURE 7-20 **A.** Eccentric bone location in the ring, simulating a tibial mounting. **B.** Center/center location of bone in the ring mounting, simulating a femoral or humeral mounting.

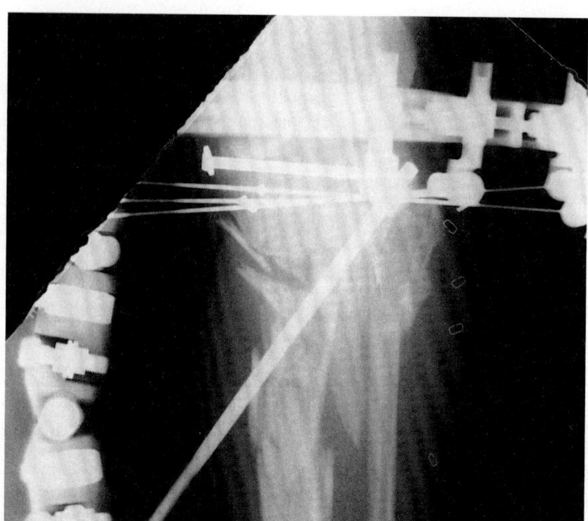

FIGURE 7-21 An early "hybrid" frame showing mechanical instability with a periarticular tensioned wire ring and a monolateral bar connecting only two diaphyseal half-pins.

than the other fixators tested, but the device controlled shear at the fracture site as well as comparative half-pin frames (61,91). The overall stiffness and shear rigidity of the Ilizarov external fixator are similar to those of the half-pin fixators in bending and torsion (18,77,78,86,92–94).

Wire Connecting Bolts

Mechanical slippage between the wire and the fixation bolt is the primary reason for loss of wire tension and thus frame instability. Studies demonstrate that when clamping a wire to the frame, the wire tension is reduced by approximately 7% (95). This may be due to wire deformation by the bolts and as such can reduce wire tension during fixator assembly (96). Slippage can be avoided by adequate torque on the fixation bolt (i.e., greater than 20 Newton meters [Nm]). Material yield accompanied by some wire slippage through the clamps is responsible for the decreased tension at the pin–clamp interface. Although the initial wire tension has an appreciable affect on the wire stiffness, it does not affect the elastic load range of the clamp wire system. To prevent yield of the clamp wire system in clinical practice, the fixator should be assembled with sufficient wires to ensure that the load transmitted to each wire by the patient does not exceed 15 Newtons (57). This is accomplished simply by placing at least two tensioned wires onto each ring present in the frame construct. Adding additional wires will increase frame stiffness in direct proportion to the number of wires in the system. Stiffness of a tensioned wire frame is more dependent on bone preload than on wire number, wire type, or frame design. Preload stiffness can be increased simply by compressing the rings together and achieving bone-on-bone contact (14,28,79,81,83,85,86).

Hybrid Fixators

Because of the complexity involved in the assembly of a full circular ring fixator, hybrid configurations were developed to take advantage of tensioned wires' ability to stabilize complex periarticular fractures. Early designs married a periarticular ring using few tensioned wires to a monolateral bar connected to the shaft using two or three half-pins. Unfortunately these simple frames were shown to be mechanically inferior in their abilities to alleviate cantilever loading, with resultant malunion/nonunion (Fig. 7-21) (89,92,97–99).

Hybrid techniques now should include a ring incorporating multiple levels of fixation in the periarticular fragment. This is accomplished with at least three tensioned wires. If possible, an additional level of periarticular fixation is advantageous using adjunctive half-pins, in addition to the tensioned wires (81,92,100–102).

The use of a single bar connecting the shaft to the periarticular ring places significant stresses on the single connecting clamp and accentuates the harmful off-axis forces generated with weight bearing. Multiple connecting bars or a full circular frame is preferred with a minimum of four half-pins attached to the shaft component (85,94,97–101).

BIOLOGY OF EXTERNAL FIXATION AND DISTRACTION HISTOGENESIS

The fracture repair process proceeds through constant physiologic stages depending on the external forces imparted to the fracture site. Four distinct types of fracture healing have been identified. External fixation facilitates external bridging callus.

External bridging callus is largely under the control of mechanical and other humoral factors and is highly dependent on the integrity of the surrounding soft tissue envelope. The critical cells necessary for healing are derived from the surrounding soft tissues and from the revascularization response that occurs during the inflammatory phase of fracture healing (14,18).

This type of fracture healing has the ability to bridge large gaps and is very tolerant of movement. It results in the development of a large callus with formation of cartilage due to the greater inflammatory response caused by increased micromovement of the fragments (103,104). Migrating mesenchymal cells from the surrounding area reach the fracture ends, where they differentiate into various cell types, primarily cartilage. The cartilage is formed in the well-vascularized granulation tissue due to its ability to repel vessels. These early cartilaginous elements undergo remodeling through endochondral bone formation. This type of indirect bone healing occurs under less rigid interfragmentary stabilization (103,105,106). The rate of this type of healing and the extent of callus in this type of repair can be modulated by mechanical conditions at the fracture site (107). It has been shown that applying cyclic interfragmentary micromotion for short periods of time influences the repair process and leads to a larger area of callus formation compared to fractures that are rigidly fixed (61,70,71,75,91,103,105,106, 108–112). Alternatively, efforts to reduce micromotion by increasing frame stiffness can cause a significant reduction in the rate of healing (57,64,74,113).

Larger interfragmentary movements lead to more fibrocartilage, as well as an increase in the number of blood vessels (108,114). However, as the amount of fibrocartilage increases, the ability for remodeling and bone formation is simultaneously decreased. There appears to be some threshold at which the degree of micromotion becomes inhibitory to this overall remodeling process and thus hypertrophic nonunion can result. However, fractures requiring external fixation in general are usually more complex, which may result in a higher rate of nonunion. Healing problems encountered in these severe injuries may reflect the severity of the local soft tissue and periosteal injury and should not be attributed solely to the inherent features of the external fixation device. Bony healing is not complete until remodeling of the fracture has been achieved. At this stage, the visible fracture lines in the callus decrease and subsequently disappear (14,18,115).

Dynamization

Dynamization converts a static fixator, which seeks to neutralize all forces including axial motion, and allows the passage of forces across the fracture site to occur. As the elasticity of the callus decreases, bone stiffness and strength increase and larger loads can be supported. Thus, the advantages of axial dynamization help to restore cortical contact and produce a stable fracture pattern with inherent mechanical support. Aro described a uniform distribution of callus following dynamization and described this as "secondary contact healing" (71,72). By increasing cortical contact, dynamization attempts to decrease the translational shear forces (70–72). These forces are accepted by most to be the leading factor in producing a predominance of fibrous tissue at the fracture site, with resultant delayed or nonunion (23,66,73,85).

Active dynamization of the fracture occurs with weight bearing or with loading when there is progressive closure of the fracture gap. This usually occurs by making adjustments in the pin bar clamps with simple monolateral fixators or in releasing the body on a Monotube-type fixator. Dynamization also decreases the pin bone stresses and prolongs the lifetime of the frame (14,61,103,116).

There is a race between the gradually increasing load carrying capacity of the healing bone and failure of the pin–bone interface. In unstable fractures, very high stresses can occur at the pin–bone interface, which may create localized yielding failure. In half-pin frames these high stresses are generated primarily at the entry cortex, and stress-related pin–bone failures of half-pins occur mainly in this location (29).

The relative motion of the bone ends at the fracture site is a very important parameter in the healing of the fracture, but the threshold at which this motion becomes deleterious is unknown. Micromotion is the fundamental mechanical force seen within the fracture construct. These factors are imparted to the periosteal callus, and many investigators are studying the quality, magnitude, and timing of micromotion application (18,117). Quantitating micromotion parameters will aid in making frames less rigid and easier to apply.

Limited Open Reduction/Internal Fixation with External Fixation

Inherent in the use of external fixation is the desire to perform limited internal fixation in combination with an external fixator. While this is very useful in metaphyseal bone and has been shown to work well in periarticular fractures, its use in diaphyseal regions must be questioned.

The use of interfragmentary screws seeks to achieve direct bone healing through the use of constant compression. Primary cortical healing occurs only when mechanical immobilization is absolute and bony apposition is perfect. It is very intolerant of movement and is not dependent on external soft tissues. This type of healing is very slow and has no ability to cross gaps, as opposed to external bridging callus (103,111). In many ways, it represents bone healing through gradual remodeling. Primary cortical healing is characterized by sequential cutting cones of osteoclast across the fracture line, with subsequent reestablishment of new osteons. The vasculature develops from a budding process sprouting from the intramedullary blood vessels, which are very fragile and intolerant of motion. The external fixator, on the other hand, does not entirely eliminate extraneous forces, but seeks to limit the degree of micromotion while still allowing movement to occur along a number of vectors (13,18,61, 103,108,111,114). Therefore, because the bone is rigidly fixed with lag screws, very poor bridging callus develops. Because external fixators do not produce absolute rigidity, insufficient cortical healing occurs, demonstrating the worst of both biologic entities (75). This technique has been abandoned in diaphyseal regions because of the increased incidence of pseudoarthrosis (118).

Distraction Osteogenesis

Distraction osteogenesis is the mechanical induction of new bone that occurs between bony surfaces that are gradually pulled apart. Ilizarov described this as "the tension stress effect" (14,18–20). Osteogenesis in the gap of a distracted bone takes place by the formation of a physis-like structure. New bone forms in parallel columns extending in both directions from a central growth region known as the *interzone* (Fig. 7-22). Recruitment of the tissue-forming cells for the interzone originates in the periosteum (14,18,79,119). Under the influence of tension stress, fibroblast-like cells found in the middle of the growth zone have an elongated shape and are oriented along the tension stress vector during distraction. Surrounding the fibroblast-like cells are collagen fibers aligned parallel to the direction of the tension vector. The fibroblastic cells transform into osteoblasts, which deposit osteoid tissue on these collagen fibers. They further differentiate to become osteocytes within the bone matrix laid down on the longitudinal collagen bundles. These cells will become incorporated into their own HA matrix as the collagen bundles are consolidated into bone. This tissue gradually blends into the newly formed bone trabeculae in the regions furthest away from the central interzone. Thus, newly formed bone grows both proximally and distally away from the middle of the distraction zone during elongation. These columns of bone will eventually cross the fibrous interzone to bridge the osteogenic surfaces after distraction (see Fig. 7-22) (14,18–20).

With stable fixation, osteogenesis in the distraction zone proceeds by direct intermembranous ossification, omitting the cartilaginous phase characteristic of endochondral ossification. Distraction osteogenesis also provides a significant neovascularization effect. The fibroblast precursors are concentrated around sinusoidal capillaries. The growth of these newly formed capillaries under the influence of tension stress proceeds very rapidly and in some instances overgrows development of bony distraction, resulting in enfolding of this tremendous capillary response. This dense network of newly formed blood cells has a longitudinal orientation connecting to the surrounding soft tissue vessels by numerous arteries that perforate the regenerate bone. Thus, the regenerate distraction gap is very vascular, with large vascular channels that surround each longitudinal column of distracted collagen. Neovascularization extends from each bone end surface toward the central fibrous interzone. This intense formation of new blood vessels under the influence of tension stress occurs not only in bone but also in the soft tissues. These vessels contain a thin lining of endothelial cells very simi-

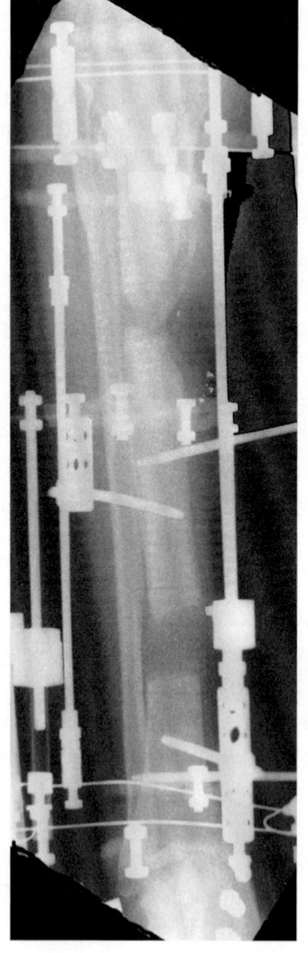
A

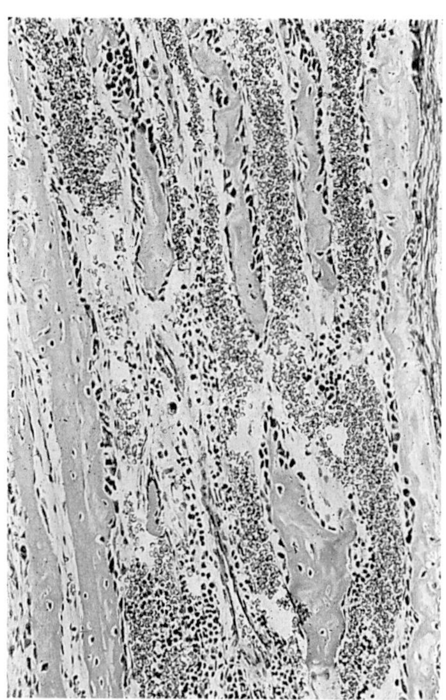
B

FIGURE 7-22 **A.** Interzone (*box*) is the central growth region involved in the genesis of new bone formation during distraction. **B.** Collagen fibrils line up along the vector of distraction. Osteoblasts line the collagen bundles, forming new bone. There are large vascular channels surrounding each collagen bundle.

lar to the neovascular response that occurs in a centripetal fashion during routine fracture healing (see Fig. 7-22).

The rate and rhythm of distraction are crucial in achieving viable tissue after distraction histogenesis. Histologic and biochemical studies have determined that a distraction rate of 0.5 mm/day or less leads to premature consolidation of the lengthening bone, while a distraction rate of 2 mm or greater often results in undesirable changes within the distracted tissues. Faster rates of distraction will disrupt the small vascular channels and areas of cysts can occur, inhibiting mineralization (14,18–20,79,119).

For osteogenesis to proceed more rapidly, optimal preservation of the periosteal tissues, bone marrow, and surrounding soft tissue blood supply at the time of osteotomy is mandatory (14,18,120). The new bone or soft tissues are formed parallel to the tension vector even when the vector is perpendicular to the limb's overall mechanical axis.

Ilizarov recommended that the number of actual distractions (rhythm of distraction) should be at least four, achieving a total of 1 mm of total distraction (rate of distraction) in four divided doses. His work has also shown that constant distraction over a 24-hour period produces a significant increase in the regenerate quality as compared to other variables (14,18–20).

When motion is present at the fracture site, bone resorption always occurs. The greater the interfragmentary motion at the site of the fracture, the greater the resorption of the fragment and the slower the consolidation. The healing process depends on arterial revascularization, and if the fracture fragments are excessively mobile, the local blood supply is traumatized by the moving bone ends (75,108,114). Instability that introduces translational shear across the distraction gap will result in an atrophic fibrous nonunion with mixed cartilage and incomplete vascular channels interspersed within the longitudinal collagen columns. In these areas of mechanical instability, intramembranous ossification is irregular, with islands of endochondral ossification; if local vascularity is insufficient, mineralization will be inhibited, leaving necrotic fibrous areas or vascular cysts.

Circular frames can limit the magnitude of abnormal forces when they are placed in compression (14,79,91,92). This stabilizes the small blood vessels and allows for neutralization of the forces that are destructive to the neovascular region (79,119). This allows endochondral bone remodeling to proceed. Compression osteosynthesis with constant compression on the bone does not suppress the reparative process and does not cause damage or resorption of the bone tissues. Under conditions of both compression and distraction in the presence of stable fixation, bone is actively formed by cellular elements of the endosteum, bone marrow, and periosteum. The osteogenic activity of connective tissue is stimulated by tension stress when the tissue is stabilized. Soon after the end of distraction, the connective tissue is replaced by bone. Therefore, compression (i.e., active compression) or dynamization can facilitate healing of delayed unions or nonunions in this mechanical environment. An increase in axial loading is accompanied by enhanced blood supply, which activates osteogenesis (14,18–20,114). Many authors have demonstrated the positive benefit that axial loading combined with muscular activity has on new bone formation (103–106).

Ilizarov noted that all tissues respond to a slow application of prolonged tension with metaplasia and differentiation into the corresponding tissue type. Bone responds best, followed by muscle, ligament, and tendons in that order. Neurovascular structures respond with gradual new vessels and some degree of nerve and vessel lengthening, but they respond very slowly and are intolerant of acute distraction forces (14,18–20).

As such, this phenomenon of histogenesis can occur indirectly via traction on living tissue, as well as with tension stress simulated by nonviable implants (i.e., the implantation of soft tissue expandable prostheses) (Fig. 7-23) (121).

Muscle growth results from the tension stress effect by increasing the number of myofibrils in preexisting muscle. Muscle also responds by the formation of new muscle tissue through the increased numbers of muscle satellite cells, the appearance of myoblasts and their fusion into myotubes, as well as differentiation of the sarcoplasmic components of the existing muscle fibers into new muscle tissue. Within the newly formed muscle fibers, active formation of myofibrils and sarcomeres also occurs (14,18–20).

Smooth muscle tissue and blood vessels walls are also stimulated by tension stress. Smooth muscle activity and proliferation are accompanied by an increase in the extent and number of intercellular contacts between myocytes and by the formation of new elastic structures. These morphologic changes in the ultrastructure of arterial smooth wall muscle cells resemble the changes seen in the walls of arteries elongated during active prenatal and early postnatal growth (14,18–20).

A similar response also occurs in the connective tissue of fascia, tendons, and dermis. The number of fibroblasts is increased during distraction and an increase in the density of intracellular junctions is multiplied, which is characteristic of fibroblasts in the developing connective tissue of embryos, fetuses, and newborn animals. The adventitial blood vessels in the epineurium and perineurium of major nerve trunks also undergo similar changes (14,18–20).

Distraction, accomplished through the use of a ring fixator or a stable Monotube device, initiates the histogenesis of bone, muscle, nerves, and skin (see Fig. 7-23) (14,18–20,79,119). This facilitates the treatment of complex orthopaedic diseases, including pathologic conditions such as osteomyelitis and fibrous dysplasia. Other conditions that have been historically refractory to standard treatments, such as congenital pseudoarthrosis and severe hemimelias, can also be addressed (18,122–129).

Bone transport methodologies can replace large skeletal defects with normal healthy bone structure that is well vascularized and relatively impervious to stress fractures. The ability to correct significant angular, translational, and axial deformities simultaneously through relatively percutaneous techniques, as well as the fact that these corrections are performed in an ambu-

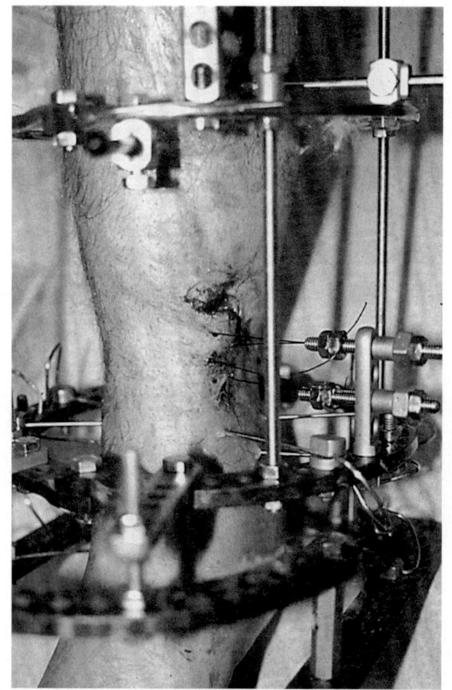

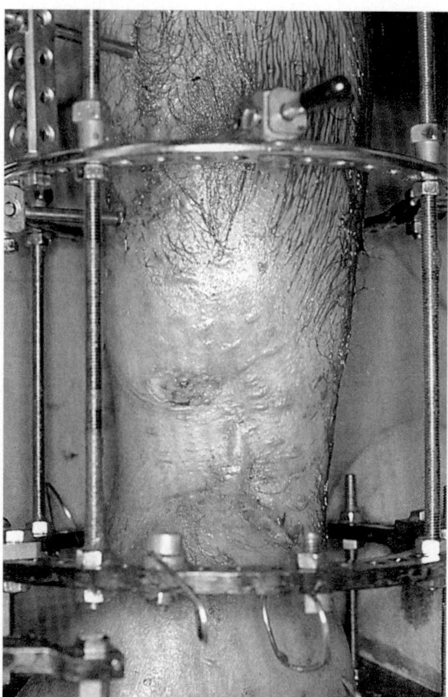

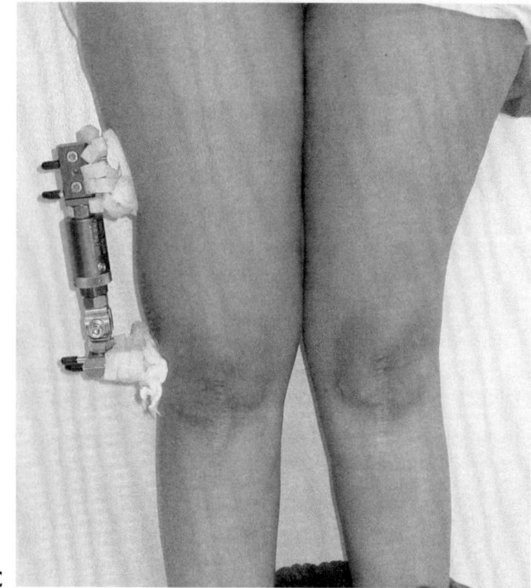

FIGURE 7-23 A,B. Skin and soft tissue defect in concert with an open tibia fracture is closed by gradual distraction using a ring fixator with traction wires attached to skin. **C.** Monotube device used to correct valgus deformity of the right knee (compare with left knee). This is accomplished via gradual distraction across a distal femoral corticotomy.

latory outpatient setting, adds to the attractiveness of this method (Fig. 7-24) (17,18,88,93,130–136).

CONTEMPORARY EXTERNAL FIXATOR APPLICATIONS

Traditionally, external fixation was primarily used in trauma applications. This included the treatment of open fractures and closed fractures with high-grade soft tissue injury or compartment syndrome. For patients with multiple long bone fractures, external fixation has been used as a method for temporary if not definitive stabilization.

Following the introduction of circular and hybrid techniques, indications have been expanded to include the definitive treatment of complex periarticular injuries, which include high-energy tibial plateau and distal tibial pilon fractures.

Given the mechanical and biologic advantages of external fixation, its use in reconstructive orthopaedics has gained wider acceptance. External fixation is currently used for limb lengthening, osteotomy, and deformity correction, as well as bone transport for the reconstruction of bone defects.

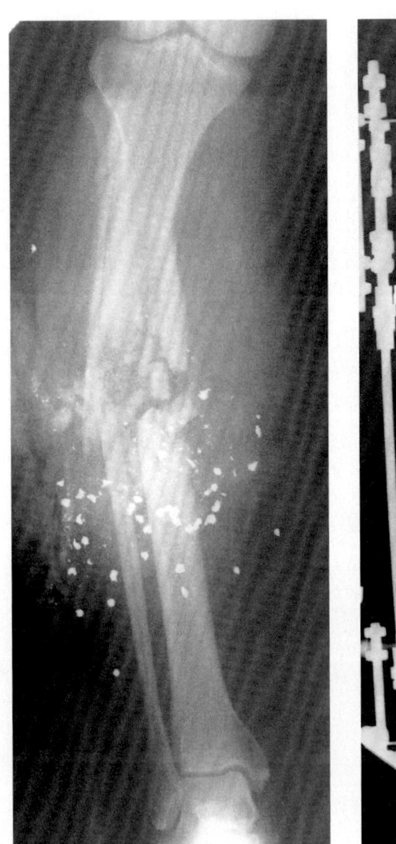
A

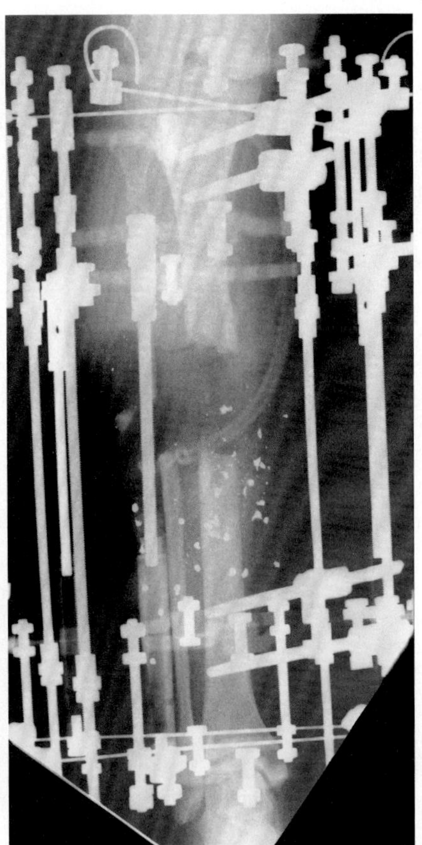
B

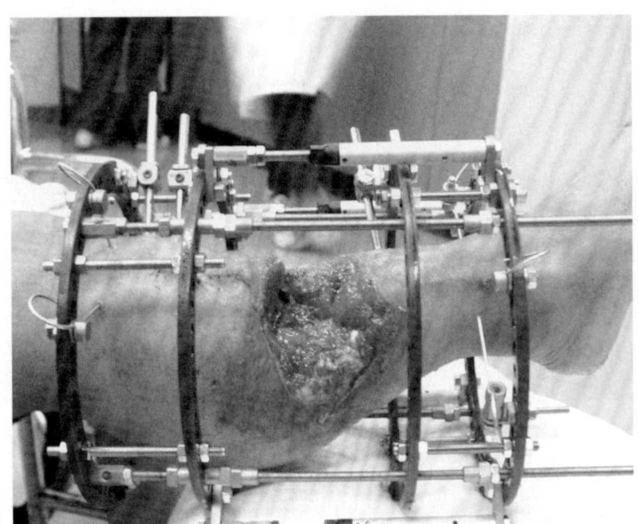
C

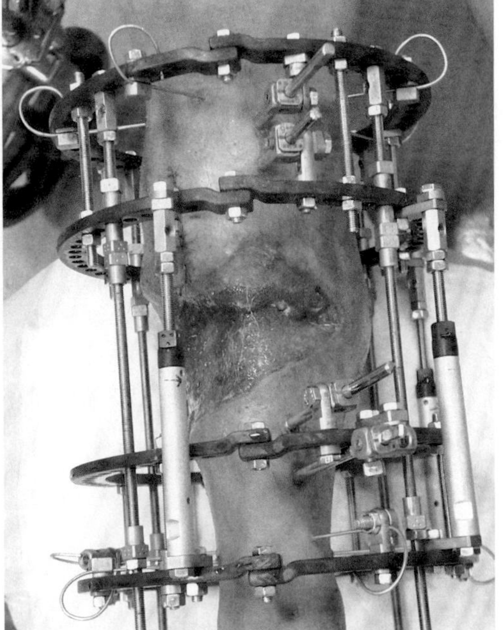
D

FIGURE 7-24 **A,B.** Severe bone and soft tissue loss stabilized with a ring fixator. **C,D.** Gradual distraction (compression) across the defect gradually closes down the defect via soft tissue transport. *(continues)*

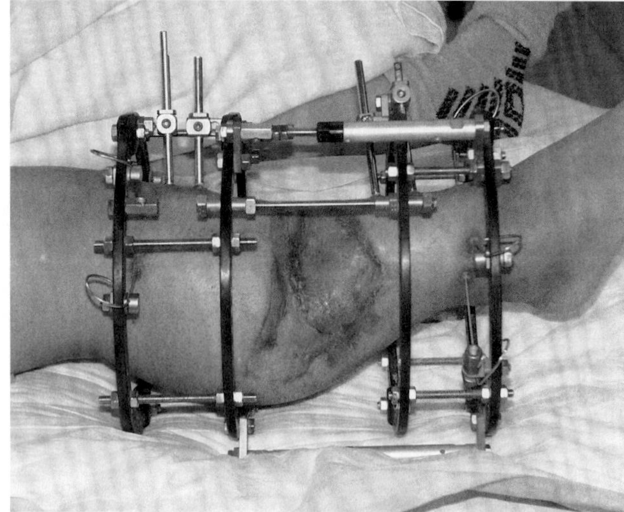

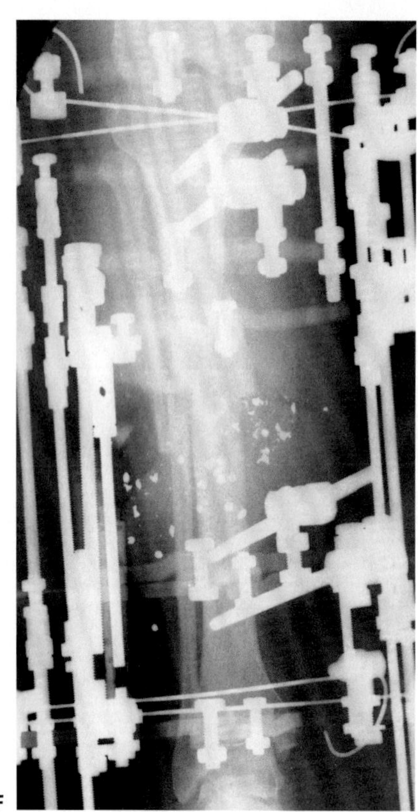

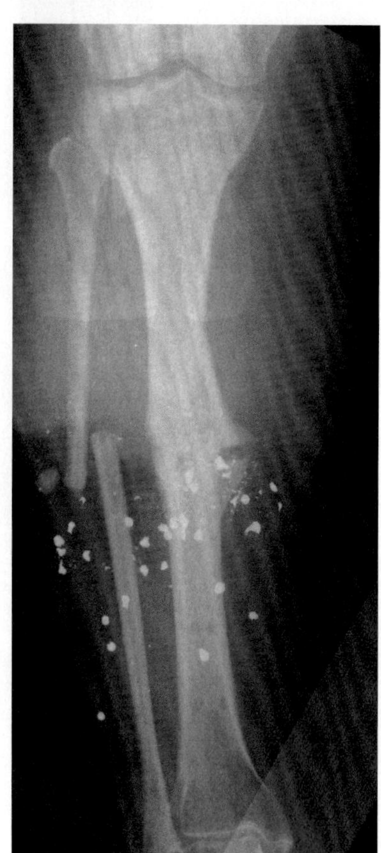

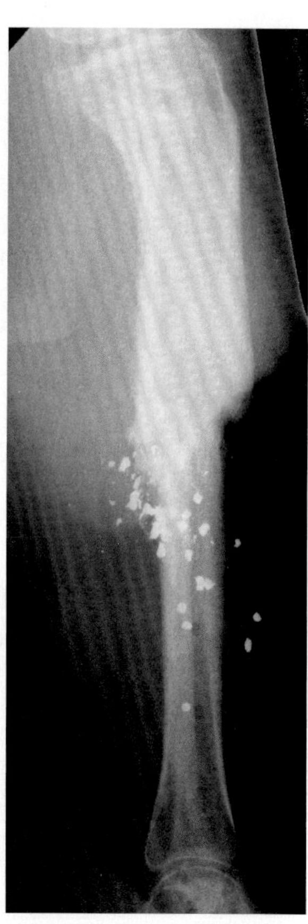

FIGURE 7-24 *(continued)* **E,F.** Skin grafting was performed over reconstructed soft tissues once docking of the bone ends had been completed. **G,H.** Healed tibia later underwent limb lengthening.

The concept of temporary spanning fixation for complex articular injuries has become widely accepted. The ability to achieve an initial reduction via ligamentotaxis substantially decreases the amount of injury-related swelling and edema by reducing large fracture gaps. It is important to achieve an early ligamentotaxis reduction, as a delay for more than a few days will result in an inability to disimpact displaced metaphyseal fragments. When definitive stabilization is attempted, reduction is more difficult by indirect means and may require larger or more extensile types of incisions (137–140).

Many types of temporary "traveling traction" have been described. Most commonly used are the knee- or ankle-bridging constructs. This may be a simple quadrilateral frame, constructed by applying medial and lateral radiolucent external bars to proximal and distal threaded transfixion pins placed across the respective joint. Manual distraction is carried out and a ligamentotaxis reduction achieved. A simple anterior monolateral frame can be used to maintain similar reduction across the knee joint for temporizing the management of knee dislocations, complex distal femoral fractures, and tibial plateau fractures (Fig. 7-25) (137–142).

A simple monolateral frame can be configured in a triangular-type construct about the distal tibial and ankle region in an effort to achieve relative stability. With temporary fixation in place, the patient then can have other procedures or tests performed while effective distraction is maintained and the soft tissues are put to rest (Fig. 7-26).

These techniques are valuable in a polytrauma patient when rapid stabilization is necessary. Simple monolateral or Monotube fixators can be placed very rapidly across long bone injuries, providing adequate stabilization to facilitate the management and resuscitation of the polytrauma patient (143,144).

For periarticular fractures, the decision to convert to definitive stabilization is usually based on the adequacy of soft tissues. A latency period of at least 10 to 14 days is generally required to allow the soft tissues to recover to the extent where contemporary internal fixation techniques can be undertaken safely. Many series have found excellent results with a staged approach consisting of early fracture stabilization using spanning external fixation. This is followed by careful preoperative planning based

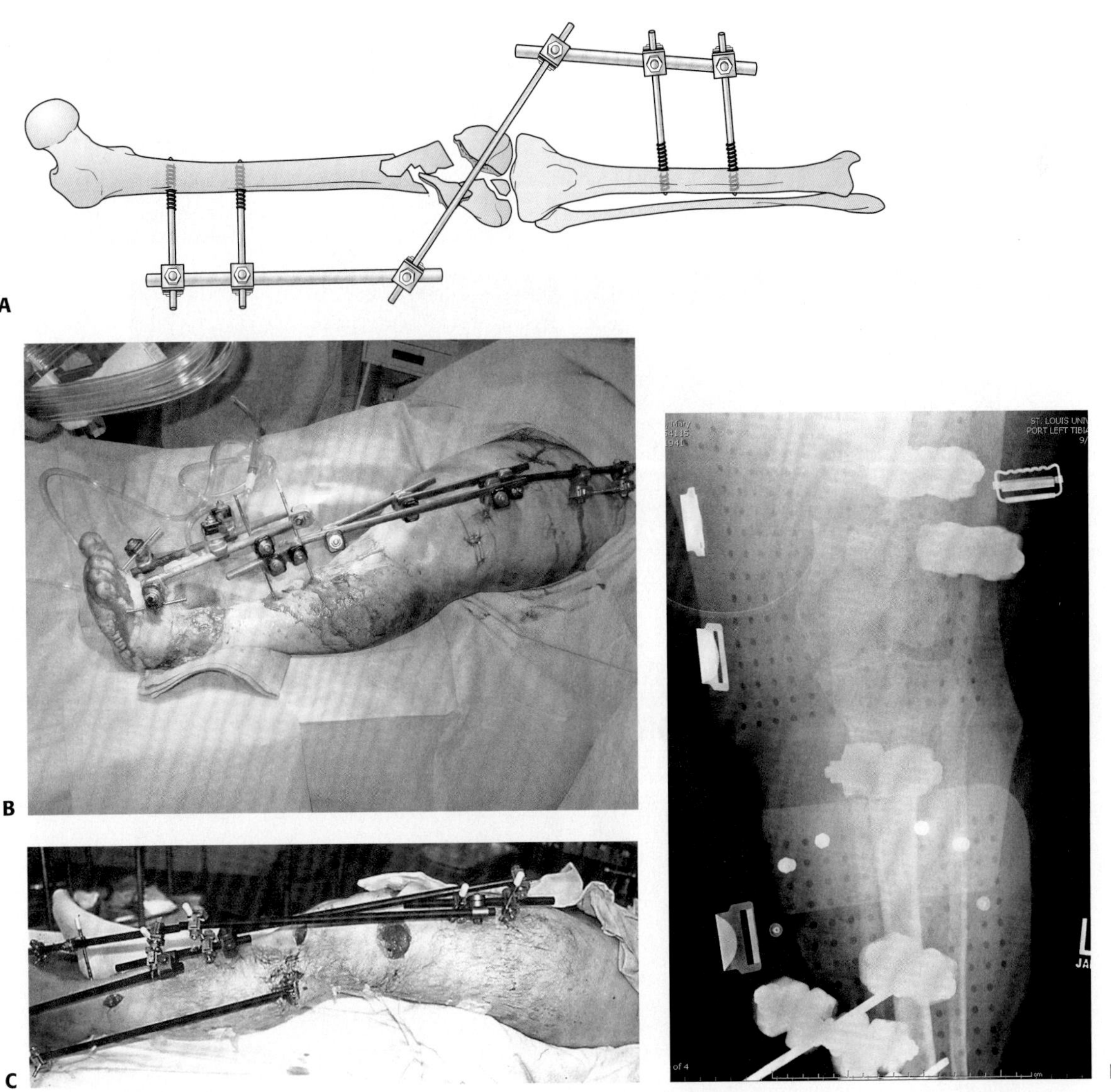

FIGURE 7-25 A. Monolateral components used to temporarily stabilize complex injuries around the knee. **B**. Temporary knee- and ankle-spanning frame placed in a polytrauma patient. **C,D.** Severe crush injuries including a distal femoral and proximal tibial fracture and degloving injury to the foot stabilized with a knee-spanning frame.

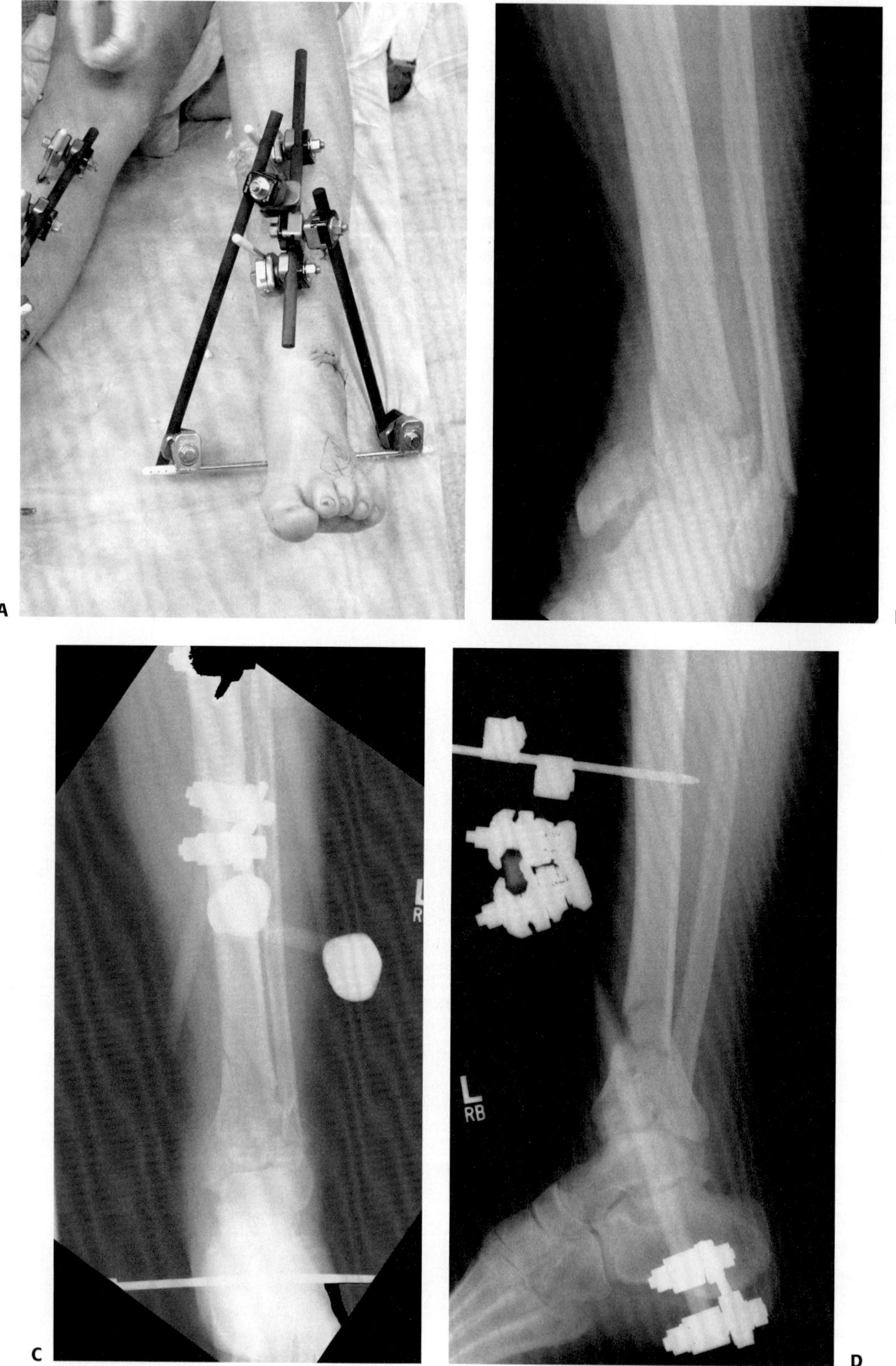

FIGURE 7-26 **A.** Open pilon fracture stabilized with triangular ankle-spanning configuration. **B–D.** The ligamentotaxis reduction achieved with the simple frame facilitates the definitive reconstructive procedures once soft tissue recovery has occurred.

on traction CT scans and the judicious clinical evaluation of the soft tissue injury before definitive internal fixation (137–139,145,146).

With the temporary stabilization of long bone fractures, definitive conversion to intramedullary nailing has had variable success, especially in the tibia. Most authors would suggest early (within the first 2 to 3 weeks of frame application) conversion to intramedullary nailing to avoid colonization of the medullary canal by the external fixator pins. It has been shown that the longer the external fixator remains in place, the greater the risk of complications after conversion to intramedullary devices, especially if the pins are removed and the nail is exchanged at the same operative setting (Fig. 7-27) (125,147).

Stabilization of unstable pelvic fractures has been achieved by the rapid application of simple external fixation for use in the immediate resuscitative period. The application of an external frame affords significant reduction in the volume of the true pelvis, as well as stabilizing the movement of large bony cancellous surfaces along the posterior aspect of the pelvic ring. The ability to provide stabilization and decrease the pelvic volume allows the surgeon to control hemorrhage and has helped to contribute to the low mortality seen with these injuries (148,149).

Anterior pelvic external fixator constructs provide excellent adequate fixation; however, anterior frame application, specifically the supra-acetabular pin application, may be difficult in an obese patient (150). At times the application of an anterior frame may be complicated, cumbersome, and time-consuming,

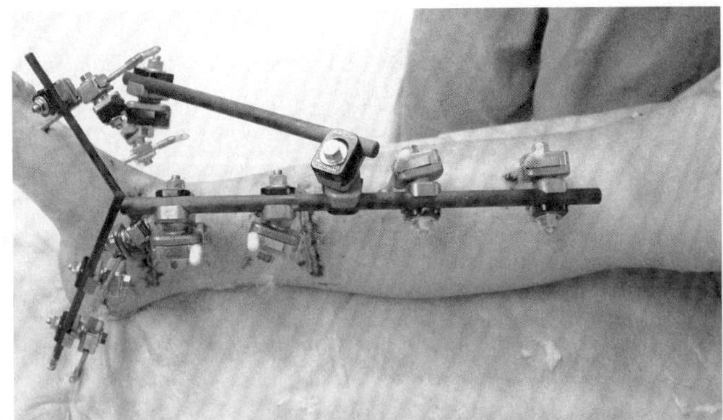

A

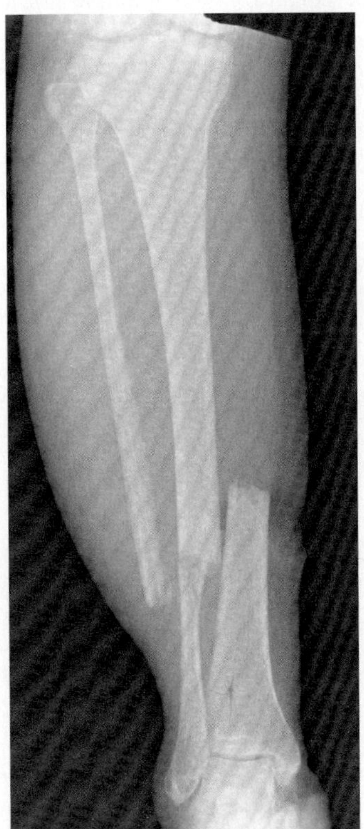

B

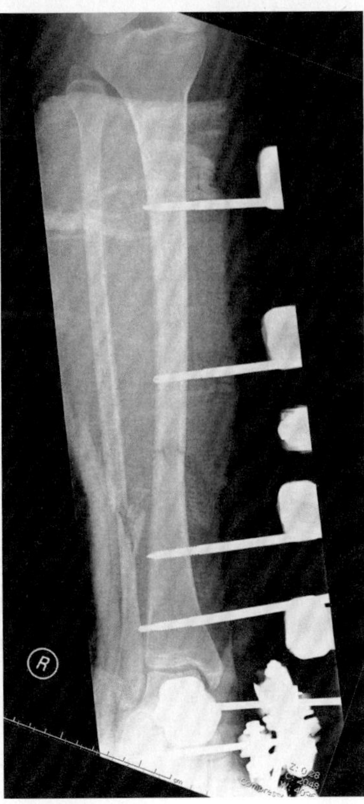

C

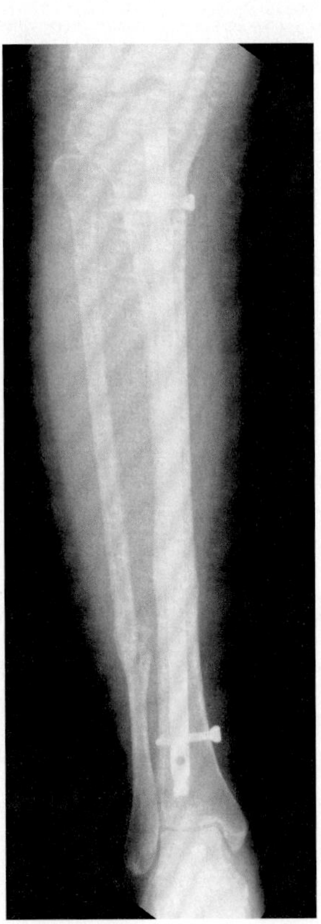

D

FIGURE 7-27 **A.** Open tibial shaft with complex foot injury is temporarily stabilized with a spanning monolateral fixator. **B–D.** An anatomic reduction was achieved and maintained with the frame. Once soft tissues had recovered and the patient's condition had stabilized, the frame was converted to an intramedullary nail at 10 days after the injury.

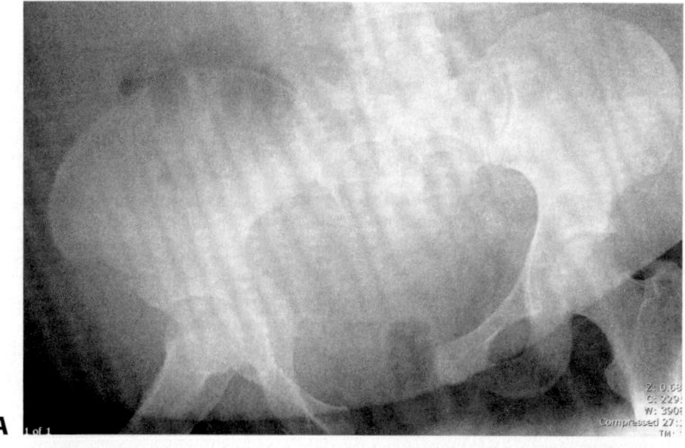

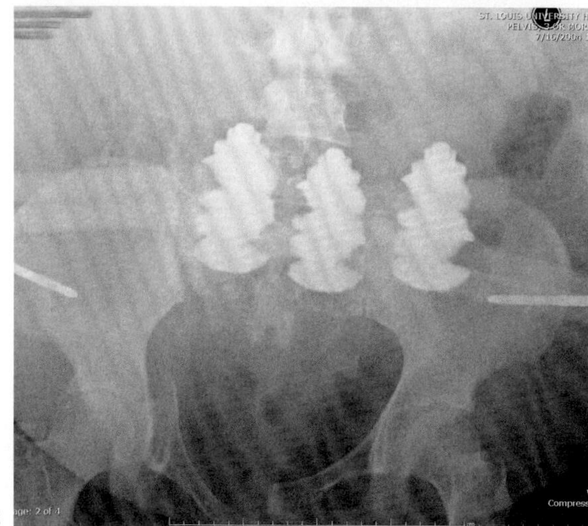

FIGURE 7-28 **A.** Pelvic injury with anterior and posterior disruption and hemodynamic instability. Note large pannus prohibiting supra-acetabular pin placement. **B.** Simple anterior frame applied to help in the resuscitation of the patient and provide temporary pelvic stabilization.

and it may be contraindicated as an emergency application. For this reason, a modification of pelvic external fixation, the so-called C-clamp, is used to provide posterior stability temporarily in patients with massive pelvic ring injuries and massive hemorrhage. Pelvic frames are most useful in fractures that are vertically stable (151). Rotationally unstable fractures such as anterior–posterior compression and lateral compression injuries are best suited for an anterior pelvic frame (Fig. 7-28) (148).

DEFINITIVE FRACTURE MANAGEMENT

The choice of external fixator type depends on the location and complexity of the fracture, as well as the type of wound present when dealing with open injuries. The less stable the fracture pattern, the more complex a frame needs to be applied to control motion at the bone ends. If possible, weight bearing should be a consideration. If periarticular extension or involvement is present, the ability to bridge the joint with the frame provides satisfactory stability for both hard and soft tissues. It is important that the frame be constructed and applied to allow for multiple débridements and subsequent soft tissue reconstruction. This demands that the pins are placed outside the zone of injury to avoid potential pin site contamination with the operative field.

Ring fixators have a definite advantage for extra-articular injuries in that they allow for immediate weight bearing and can gradually correct deformity and malalignment, as well as achieve active compression or distraction at the fracture site.

Monolateral Applications

The major indication for the use of monolateral frames for fracture management is in the distal radius and in the tibial shaft. This is followed closely by temporary application of trauma frames for complex femoral and humeral shaft injuries. Much less common is the use of monolateral frames for forearm injuries.

Specific fixators have been designed for use in the distal radius, which involves applying two pins in the metacarpals and spanning the joint with a specific type of multiaxial body or simple connecting rods. Two pins are then placed in the distal aspect of the radius proximal to the fracture line. Through these devices it is possible to translate the hand in radial, ulnar, and dorsal palmar directions. Following the restoration of palmar tilt by these complex ligamentotaxis maneuvers, wrist position can be adjusted into neutral or extension to help avoid finger stiffness and carpal tunnel syndrome without compromising fracture reduction (152). For unstable fractures, augmentation of the fixator construct with multiple dorsal and radial percutaneous pins corrects the dorsal tilt and maintains the reduction in fractures that are difficult to maintain with distraction ligamentotaxis alone (Fig. 7-29) (32,153,154).

The use of dynamic external fixation devices across the wrist has had mixed results. The concept behind this was to achieve

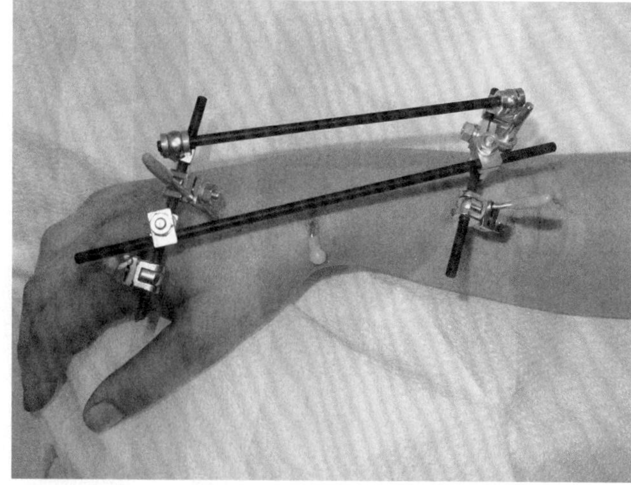

FIGURE 7-29 Mini-fixator used in combination with percutaneous pins to maintain reduction of a distal radius fracture.

a ligamentotaxis reduction as well as to initiate early range of motion by uncoupling the device (155). Early designs had a high degree of unsatisfactory results. External fixation devices function best when maintaining radial length alone. This is best accomplished with frames that do not span the wrist joint but just cross the fracture, leaving the wrist free (156).

The use of external fixation for the management of acute femur fractures is primarily limited to fractures with significant soft tissue or neurovascular compromise or to severely injured patients who cannot tolerate more extensive surgery. Commonly, femoral applications include the use of at least four pins placed along the anterolateral aspect of the femoral shaft. These simple monolateral frames have been shown to provide adequate stabilization for most complex femoral fracture patterns (Fig. 7-30) (157,158). Compared to tibial applications, a femoral frame requires the pins to traverse a greater distance through soft tissues, making accurate pin placement problematic. Fixator constructs with independent pins placed out of plane relative

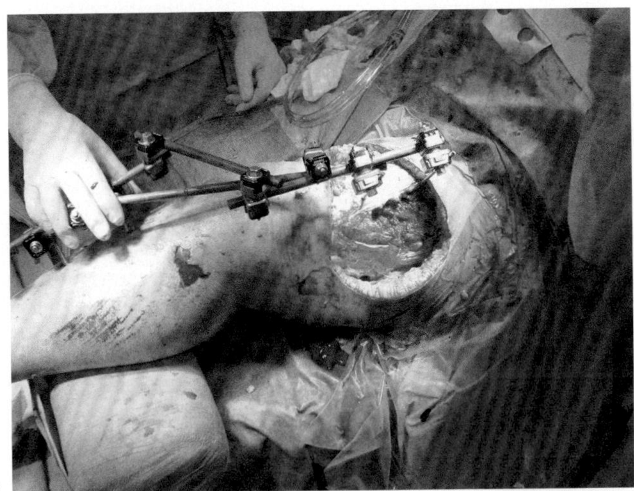

A

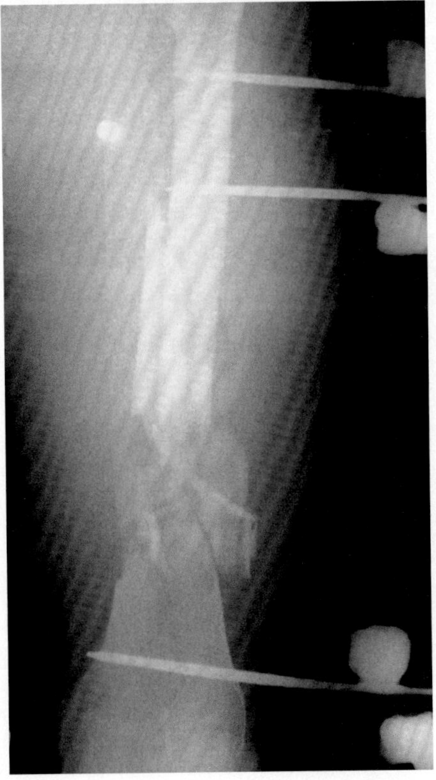

B

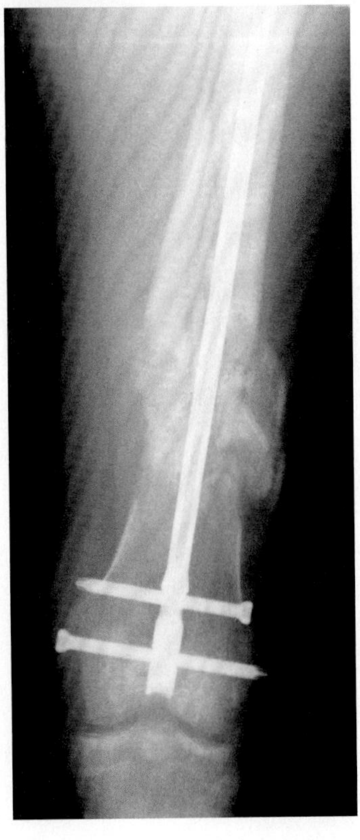

C

FIGURE 7-30 Severe soft tissue injury prevents acute intramedullary nailing of the femoral shaft. Fracture stability required spanning across the knee to maintain reduction. Secondary conversion to an intramedullary nail occurred at 12 days after the injury.

to one another allow for safer pin insertion and show increased stability over Monotube or simple monolateral frames, where pins are placed in a straight line (159,160).

External fixation is an infrequent treatment option for the management of acute humeral shaft fractures. Unlike the tibia, in which fixator half-pins can be placed perpendicular to the subcutaneous medial tibial face, external fixation in the humerus often involves transfixion of crucial musculotendinous units. Side effects of these frames may include pin tract sequelae and an inhibition of shoulder and elbow motion. Therefore, external fixation as a routine treatment method has not been universally embraced. The most frequent indication is the stabilization of severely contaminated open fractures or gunshot wounds that occur in association with vascular disruption. External fixation together with radical débridement has reduced the incidence of chronic infection and improved the prognosis for the vascular repair. Secondary surgical procedures for soft tissue and bony reconstruction are facilitated (13,21,67).

Tibial Fractures

Open tibial diaphyseal fractures are primarily candidates for closed intramedullary nailing, but there are occasions when external fixation is indicated. External fixation is favored when there is significant contamination and severe soft tissue injury or when the fracture configuration extends into the metaphyseal–diaphyseal junction or the joint itself, making intramedullary nailing problematic.

Monolateral external fixation allows for rapid closed reduction, which also helps to limit the operative time and blood loss. It is useful in patients with multiple injuries or if prolonged anesthesia is contraindicated. A simple single- or double-bar unilateral system allows for independent pin placement, while the larger Monotube frames facilitate rapid application with fixed pin couples (23,50).

Contemporary simple monolateral fixators have clamps that allow independent adjustments at each pin–bar interface, allowing wide variability in pin placement; this helps to avoid areas of soft tissue compromise. Because of this feature, simple four-pin placement may be random on either side of the fracture. In general, the most proximal and most distal pins are first inserted as far away from the fracture line as possible and the connecting rod is attached. The rod is positioned close to the bone to increase the strength of the system. The intermediate pins can then be inserted using the multiaxial pin fixation clamps as templates with drill sleeves as guides. Upon placement of these two additional pins, the reduction can then be achieved with minimal difficulty.

Alternatively, the proximal two pins can be connected by a solitary bar and the distal two pins connected by a solitary bar. Both proximal and distal bars are then used as reduction tools to manipulate the fracture into alignment. Once reduction has been achieved, an additional bar-to-bar construct between the two fixed pin couples is connected.

Use of the large Monotube fixators facilitates rapid placement of these devices, with the fixed pin couple acting as a pin template. Two pins are placed through the fixator pin couple proximal to the fracture and two pins are placed through the pin couple distal to the fracture. Care must be taken to allow adequate length of the Monotube frame before final reduction and tightening of the body (Fig. 7-31).

Most Monotube bodies have a very large diameter, which limits the amount of shearing and torsional and bending movements of the fixation construct. Axial compression is achieved by releasing the telescoping mechanism. Dynamic weight bearing is initiated at an early stage once the fracture is deemed stable. In fractures that are highly comminuted, weight bearing is delayed until visible callus is achieved and sufficient stability has been maintained. The telescopic body allows dynamic movement in an axial direction, which is a stimulus for early periosteal healing (70–72).

Because external fixators offer the ability to compress actively across fracture fragments, fracture gaps secondary to comminution and minimal bone loss can be closed directly by this maneuver. Fracture gaps secondary to malalignment can be corrected sequentially as bone union takes place. This can be accomplished with most circular and select monolateral fixators with three-dimensional adjustability (i.e., the large Monotube fixators) (71,72,92).

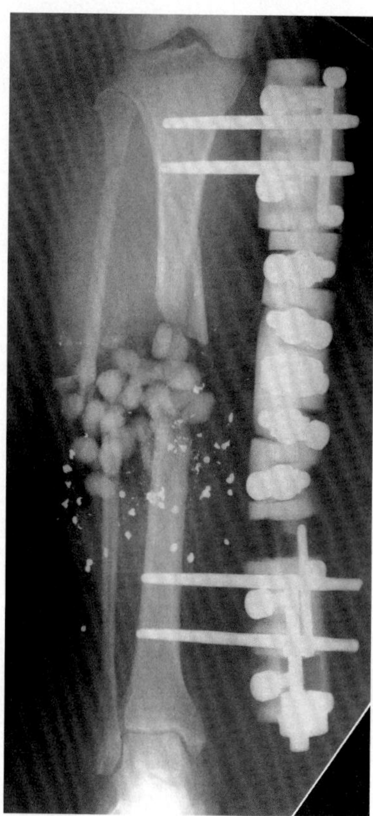

FIGURE 7-31 Monotube fixator allows rapid reduction and stabilization of complex tibia fractures. Antibiotic beads are being used to manage the dead space prior to flap coverage and subsequent grafting procedures.

Closed tibial fractures treated with external fixation heal on an average in 4 to 5 months. In an effort to accelerate this rate, most proponents of external tibial fixation feel that early dynamization or gradual frame disassembly should be performed in an effort to effect load transfer to the fracture and promote secondary callus formation. Research and clinical studies have been inconclusive on the advantages of passive dynamization. However, dynamization does seem to facilitate fracture healing if it is used within the first 6 to 8 weeks after the fracture. Kenwright showed significant improvement in the time to union with active dynamization (103,105,106).

If major bone defect exists at the fracture site, dynamization may result in permanent shortening. If a discrepancy of more than 1.5 to 2 cm will result, then dynamization is not indicated. Most external fixators have bone transport capabilities as an option to regain limb length and skeletal continuity (161).

Often patients with tibia fractures with severe soft tissue injury have concomitant foot injuries as well. These patients require multiple reconstructive procedures and are often initially treated with external fixation techniques such as a bridging frame. It is advantageous to extend these frames down onto the hindfoot and forefoot to avoid the common complication of equinus deformity. This can develop over time, specifically in patients with a wide zone of injury, which can cause the posterior compartment and other tissues to contract (see Fig. 7-27A).

Small Wire External Fixation

Diaphyseal long bone injuries are best managed using half-pin techniques. This is easily accomplished when the fracture occurs in the midportion of the long bone, allowing adequate regions of diaphyseal bone above and below the fracture to be stabilized by half-pins, which achieve solid bicortical pin purchase.

However, as many high-energy fractures involve the metaphyseal regions, transfixion techniques using small tensioned wires are ideally suited to this region. They demonstrate better mechanical stability and longevity compared to traditional half-pin techniques. The use of small tensioned wire circular frames or hybrid frames can be useful for patients with severe tibial metaphyseal injuries that occur in concert with other conditions such as soft tissue compromise, compartment syndrome, or multiple injuries.

Because of the tension exerted on the small periarticular wires, this approach may avoid the need to span the ankle or the knee joint to maintain the reduction. The small tensioned wires may be used in concert with limited open reduction if necessary. Olive wires can be used to achieve and maintain "tension-compression fixation" across small metaphyseal fragments, similar to the effect achieved with small lag screws. Therefore, the combination of smooth and olive wires can be used to neutralize deforming forces across the fracture lines and also help to achieve and maintain compression across the fracture lines (Fig. 7-32) (14,18).

Clinical trials with this methodology have yielded functional results comparable to traditional open techniques while significantly reducing the complications associated with high-energy injuries.

In contrast to other hybrid techniques, a completely circular frame offers more adjustability and will not incur detrimental

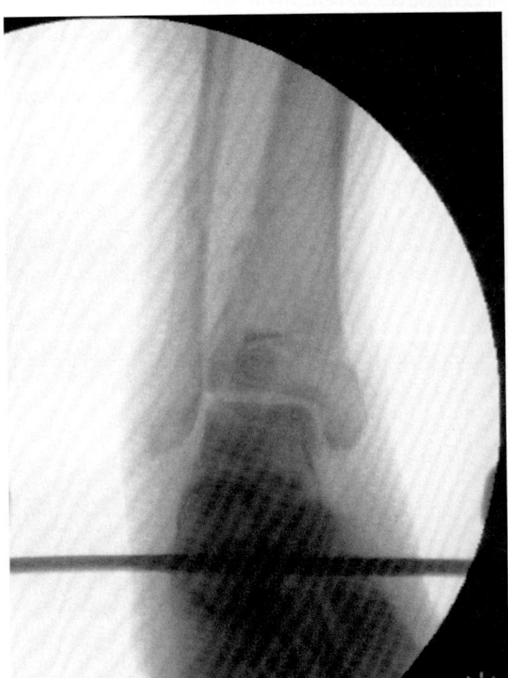
A

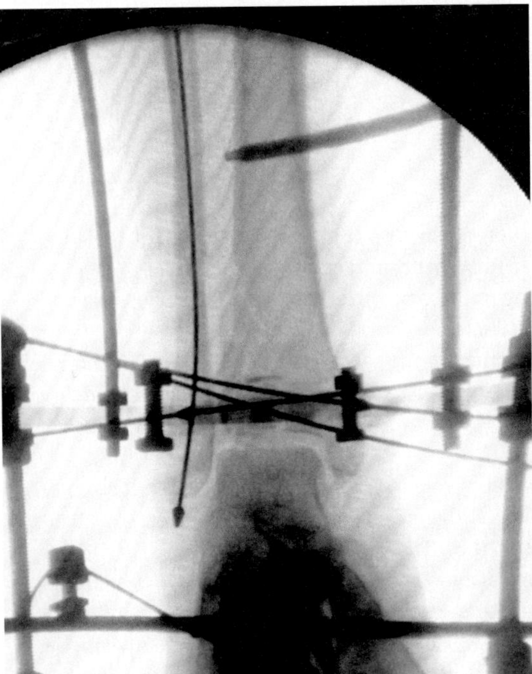
B

FIGURE 7-32 Ring construct using tensioned smooth and olive wires to stabilize small periarticular fracture fragments.

mechanical forces such as cantilever bending. These detrimental forces are commonly generated with traditional hybrid techniques if performed incorrectly. The "hybrid" has evolved to include a traditional monolateral diaphyseal bar attached to a solitary circular periarticular ring. Full ring stabilization is preferable to monolateral shaft stabilization because of the cantilever loading accentuated with this construct. Specifically in the proximal tibia, this type of frame configuration functions similar to a diving board, producing tremendous loads at the metaphyseal–diaphyseal junction, with associated development of nonunion or malunion (90,100,101,140–142,145). If monolateral adaptations are to be used, at least three divergent connecting bars should be attached to the periarticular ring (101). The bars should be oriented to achieve at least 270 degrees of separation to alleviate cantilever loading. An additional disadvantage of this standard "hybrid" construct is the inability to easily dynamize the fixator (89,94,97,98).

Surgical application of a circular hybrid periarticular fixator can be performed with the patient on either a fracture or radiolucent table with calcaneal pin or distal tibial pin traction. Alternatively, femoral distractors or temporary spanning external fixators can be used to obtain preliminary ligamentotaxis and reduction. Additional closed reduction of the condylar and metaphyseal components is achieved by the use of large percutaneously placed reduction forceps. Percutaneous Kirschner wires can also function as joysticks in aiding manipulation of metaphyseal fragments. After reduction of the metaphyseal fragments, olive wires or percutaneous small fragment screws can be used to achieve interfragmentary compression. If necessary, limited incisions are used to elevate the depressed articular fragments as well as bone graft the subchondral defects. At least three periarticular wires are necessary to stabilize these injuries. Most authors using small wire techniques recommend that as many wires as can be inserted safely should be used for maximal stability (101,139,141,142,162,163). Biomechanical data support the use of tensioned wire fixation to stabilize complex fractures of the proximal tibia. The stability achieved with a four-wire fixation construct is comparable to that of dual plating for bicondylar tibial plateau fractures (90,100,141).

When using transfixion wires, care should be taken to avoid the proximal tibial capsular reflection, as well as distal ankle joint to avoid tethering the capsule (164–166). This maintains the wires in an extra-articular location and avoids secondary contamination of the joints, which can result in knee or ankle sepsis (Fig. 7-33).

The treatment of these injuries has also included the use of Monotube ankle bridging and simple monolateral external fixator designs (167,168). These are applied to achieve a distraction reduction across their respective joints, followed by limited open reduction and internal fixation. The advantage of using Monotube constructs for either plateau or pilon fractures is that articular fixation is achieved and maintained without the use of small tensioned wires, and thus the potential for articular contamination is avoided (Fig. 7-34) (63,169).

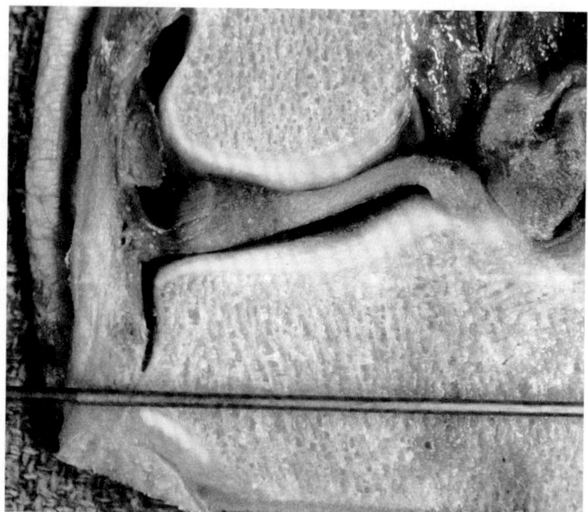

FIGURE 7-33 Anatomic specimen showing the capsular reflections around the knee joint. Care must be taken to avoid capsular penetration when placing periarticular wires around the knee. (Courtesy of Spence Reid, MD.)

Bone Transport

Treatment of acute bone loss after severe tibial shaft fractures continues to be a complex reconstructive problem. Many procedures have been devised to reconstitute bone stock, obtain fracture union, and provide a stable functional limb. Cancellous grafting, whether placed directly into the defect or through a posterolateral approach, has been the most common methodology; however, often this technique requires numerous grafting procedures (130,170). Fibular bypass, tibial fibular synostosis, and ipsilateral direct fibular transfer, as well as free vascularized fibular transfer, have been used to reconstruct these large defects

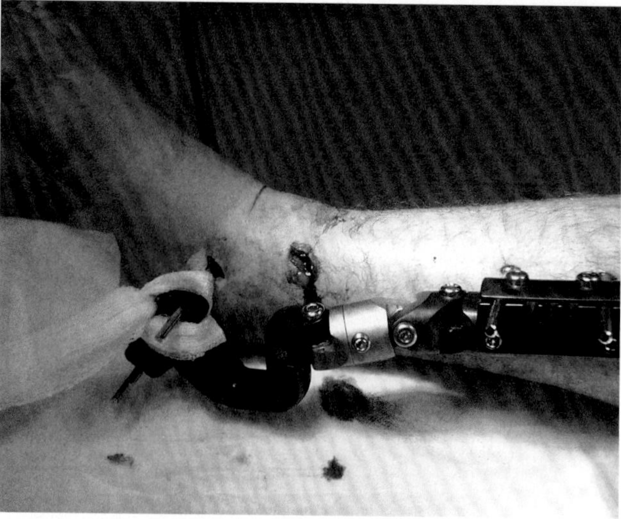

FIGURE 7-34 Monotube ankle-bridging fixator used to provide distraction in combination with limited internal fixation for pilon fractures.

(130,171,172). Internal bone transport has been developed as a primary method of bony reconstruction in acute tibial fractures with bone loss. This technique is indicated for reconstruction of defects greater than 4 cm (14,17,18,88,93,119, 130,132,135,136).

Bone transport can be carried out with a modified Monotube monolateral fixator that has an intercalary sliding mechanism to transport the bone segment. Likewise, ring fixators can also be configured to perform successful intercalary bone transport.

The basic transport frame using a ring fixator consists of four or five rings. A stable proximal and distal ring block is placed at the level of the knee and ankle joints. A transport ring is placed in the midportion of the tibia. Orientation of the frame on the limb is crucial to ensure that the proposed docking site is aligned and will provide sufficient cortical contact for union to occur. Likewise, appropriate alignment using a Monotube construct is also critical to ensure docking site alignment. The intercalary transport component is attached to bone using either transfixion wires or half-pin techniques. An antibiotic cement spacer may be placed in the defect. This block provides additional stability to the frame–bone construct and acts to maintain the transport space. The block remains in place until the next débridement, free flap procedure, or delayed primary closure of the wound (Fig. 7-35).

At the time of definitive wound coverage, the antibiotic block spacer is removed and a solitary string of antibiotic cement beads is placed in the defect. The beads provide and maintain a "potential space" or fibrous tunnel through which the transport segment will travel. This space allows relatively unencumbered movement of the transport segment underneath the flap. If no flap is needed, the wound is closed primarily and the antibiotic beads are still used to maintain the potential space and prevent invagination of the intact soft tissue envelope into the transport pathway (see Fig. 7-35) (17,18,88,93,135,136).

Transport is delayed for at least 3 weeks after free flap coverage. If no flap is used, corticotomy and transport can be undertaken immediately at the time of wound closure. This 3-week delay allows for healing of the flap over the bony defect, as well as early neovascularization of the zone of injury. The delay also allows the free flap anastomosis site to become fully epithelialized so that it can withstand the inevitable tension forces that it is subjected to during the bone transport process (14,18). The transport Schanz pins should be located in the inferior portion of the transport segment, so that they will "pull" the

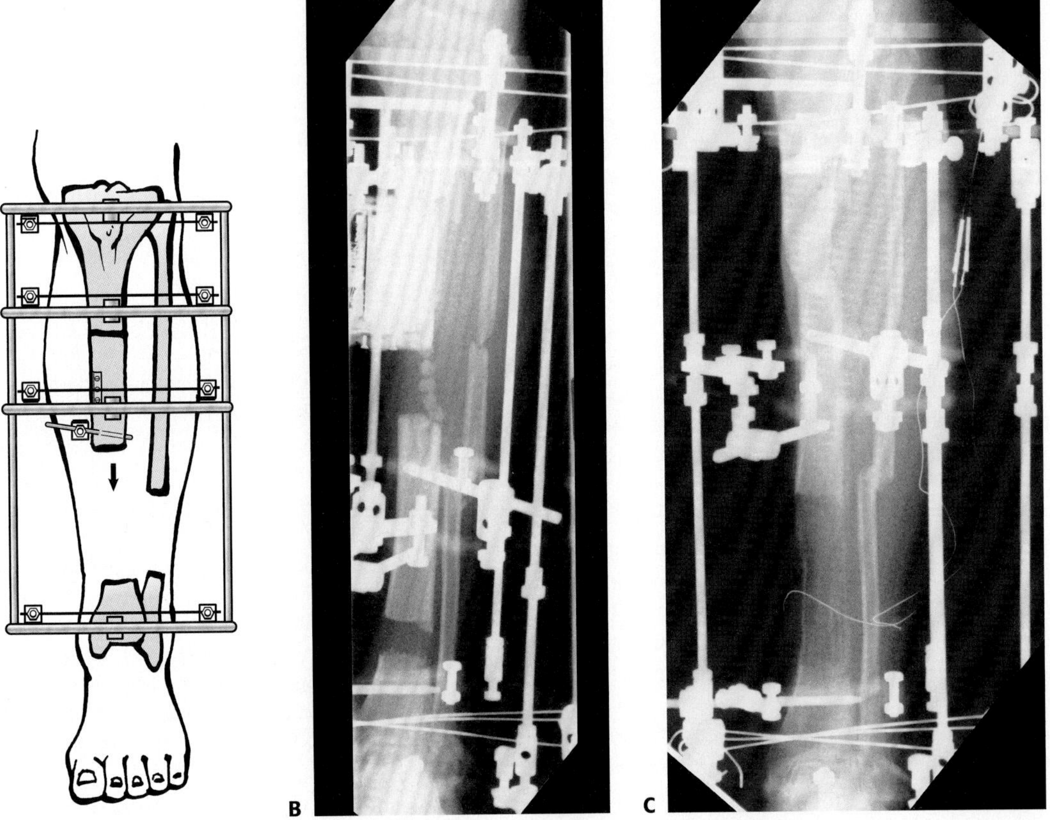

FIGURE 7-35 **A.** A typical four-ring transport frame, attaching the rings to the bone with either transfixion wires or half-pins. **B,C.** Antibiotic beads maintain the potential space in the transport tract. As docking approaches, the beads are removed and autografting to the docking site is carried out.

bone into docking position rather than "push" the transport segment. This would be the case if the pins were located more proximal in the transport segment. This construct results in an unstable situation where the transport segment will tend to deviate during transport (14,17,18,88,136).

After fixation of the transport segment, a proximal or distal corticotomy is performed. Because of the wide zone of injury that often occurs after open tibial fractures, it is better to perform the corticotomy away from any region of soft tissue compromise. A latency period of 7 to 10 days is allowed before the initiation of transport. Distraction begins slowly, at 0.25 to 0.5 mm/day. A slower distraction rate is recommended initially because of the wide variability in injury patterns and vascularity of the limb. In more extensive fractures with a wide zone of injury, transport should be undertaken very slowly and the regenerate bone visualized by approximately 2 to 3 weeks after corticotomy. The distraction rate can then be adjusted, depending on the quality of the regenerative bone. Transport in the acute fracture proceeds at a much slower rate, 0.5 to 0.75 mm per day, as opposed to the standard rate of 1 mm a day typical for standard limb lengthening.

To decrease the transport distance, the limb can be shortened acutely at the time of frame application (130). This shortening aids in soft tissue coverage by decreasing tension and gaps in the soft tissues. In some cases, this approach may allow wounds to be closed by delayed primary closure, secondary intention, or simple skin grafting. Using this technique, extensive free flap coverage may be avoided. However, acute shortening greater than 4 cm is not recommended due to distortion of the neurovascular elements, which results in the development of edema and inability of the musculotendinous units to function properly (see Fig. 7-24) (136). Bone transport continues until the antibiotic beads have been compressed to the width of one bead. At this time, the patient is returned to surgery and the docking site exposed. The beads are removed and the bone ends freshened to achieve punctate bleeding surfaces. A high-speed bur can be used to fashion congruent surfaces on the ends of the proposed docking segments. This ensures maximal cortical contact and increases stability at the docking site. Autogenous iliac crest bone graft is placed directly into the docking site at this time, and distal transport is resumed within 24 hours of the procedure (88,130,136,150).

The docking site is impacted and gradually compressed 0.25 mm every 48 hours until the docking site is radiographically healed. Numerous authors have found that grafting the atrophic docking site aids in the speed of union, with a subsequent decrease in the overall time the patient must remain in the fixator (14,88,130,136,150).

Bone transport is a reliable technique, but it is very time-consuming and requires extreme patient compliance. The principles of transport include a stable external fixation system above and below the defect. The primary importance is the ability to develop a biologically sound wound at the transport location.

Hexapod Fixators

As external fixation devices and techniques have become more sophisticated, the ability to simultaneously correct a complex deformity with a simple device has become more attractive. The Taylor Spatial Frame was designed to allow simultaneous correction in six axes (coronal angulation, translation, sagittal angulation and translation, rotation, and shortening). To achieve this with conventional frames, a complex customized frame mounting would be required. Additionally, the mounting of these traditional frames would be fairly difficult because the rings need to be placed parallel to the respective reference joints, as well as perpendicular to the long axis of the limb. In cases of deformity or fracture, this can be very problematic. "Hexapod"-type frames allow the rings to be positioned in any orientation within their respective limb segment (i.e., above the fracture site). It is not necessary that the rings be parallel to joints or perpendicular to the long axis of the bones. This demanding technique has been vastly simplified using this six-axis hexapod concept (173).

The hexapod is a ring fixator of Ilizarov-type design with a configuration consisting of six distractors and 12 ball joints, allowing for six degrees of freedom of bone fragment displacement. By adjusting the simple distractors, gradual three-dimensional corrections or acute reductions are possible without the need for complicated frame mechanisms (173).

As a fixation device, it is unique in that its optimal use depends on the use of computer software. Once the rings are mounted, the deformity parameters are calculated with respect to angulation and translation in both the AP and lateral planes. Additional information about rotational and axial malalignment is also computed. These deformity parameters are then placed into the software program along with the frame mounting parameters. The frame mounting parameters include data points such as the distance of the frame from the deformity or fracture site location. The overall length of the six struts is also a variable entered into the software calculations. The program then calculates the final strut lengths necessary to achieve a corrected limb alignment. In addition, daily strut adjustments can be calculated to effect correction over a specific time period. The final alignment can be further adjusted using the same software, applying similar deformity and strut parameters.

In the acute application, this frame allows emergent placement of a relatively simple frame. The frame can be attached using either transfixion wires or a minimum of three half-pins on either side of the fracture. An approximate reduction can be achieved grossly at the time of surgery, and the final reduction can be completed over a short period of time using the software program and gradual adjustment of the six struts. The hexapod frames and Internet software offer the advantage of very accurate and precise control of multiple deformities without significant soft tissue dissection. A relatively straightforward and simple external device is applied to effect these corrections. Many early studies have documented the excellent correction achieved for complex deformities, as well as the versatility of this device for immediate fracture management (Fig. 7-36) (173–175).

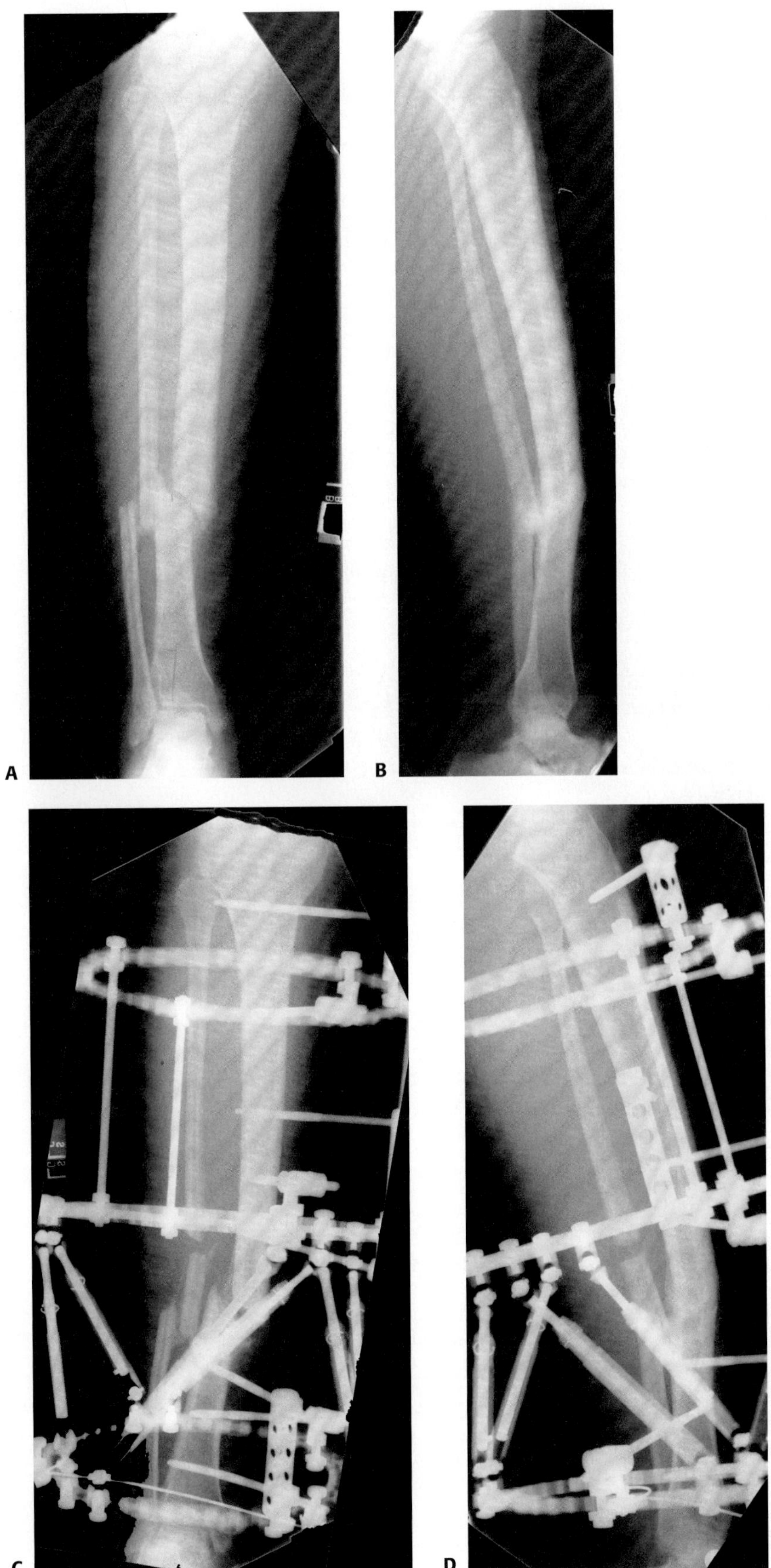

FIGURE 7-36 A,B. Complex tibial nonunion with malrotation, angulation, translation, and leg length discrepancy. **C,D.** Taylor Spatial Frame applied to limb using primarily half-pin attachments. Patient self-adjustment of the six oblique struts will gradually correct all deformity parameters. *(continues)*

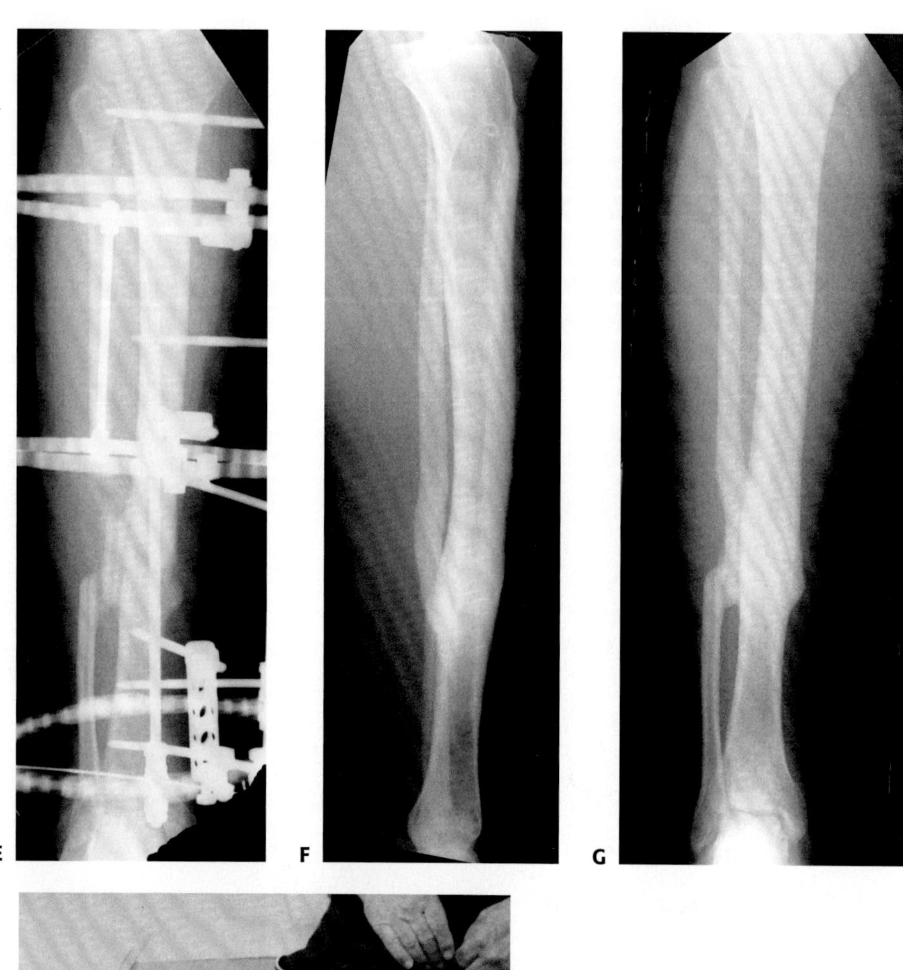

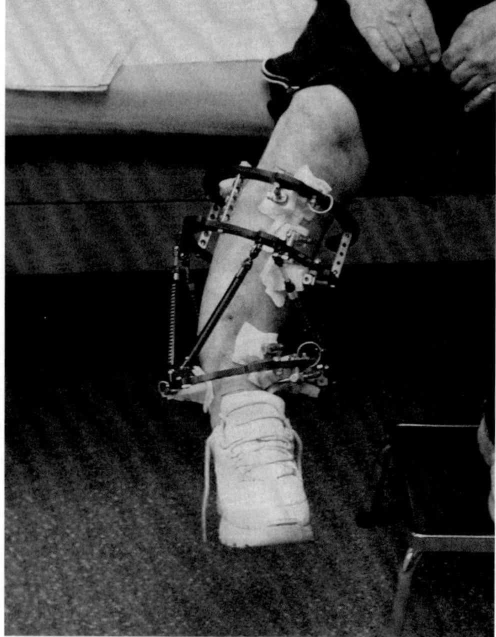

FIGURE 7-36 (*continued*) **E–G.** Complete realignment and consolidation via gradual distraction osteogenesis; no grafting was required to achieve these results. **H.** Clinical view of Taylor Spatial Frame applied to a severe varus combined deformity.

FRAME MANAGEMENT

Often during treatment using external fixators, secondary procedures are required, such as soft tissue coverage procedures or delayed bone grafting. Most external fixator frames can easily be modified or placed out of the zone of injury. Most surgeons find it problematic to drape the fixator out of the operative field and maintain this unusually small area as sterile throughout an entire procedure. The benefits of including an external frame into the operative field include the ability to maintain reduction during secondary conversion procedures, decreasing the time, material cost, and frustration in trying to drape a fixator safely out of the operative field. By using a standardized protocol that includes cleansing the external fixator frame, followed by an alcohol wash, sequential povidone–iodine preparation, paint, and spray with air drying, followed by draping the extremity and fixator directly into the operative field, additional surgery can be safely performed without an increased rate of postoperative wound infection (1,176). It is possible to perform free flaps and other soft tissue procedures directly around the external fixator pins as long as the pins do not communicate directly with the operative site.

Pin Insertion Technique

The integrity of the pin–bone interface is the critical link in the stability of the external fixation system. External fixation pins placed in cancellous metaphyseal bone frequently loosen over time, resulting in fixation failure and an increased risk for infection. The fixation pin in cortical/diaphyseal regions can remain intact and infection-free for extended periods of time. Thus, each pin in the fixation construct should be continually evaluated for these potential problems to avoid an unstable fixator.

The correct insertion technique involves incising the skin directly at the site of pin insertion. Following a generous incision, dissection is carried directly down to bone and the periosteum is incised where anatomically feasible. A small Penfield-type elevator is used to gently reflect the periosteum off the bone at the site of insertion. Extraneous soft tissue tethering and necrosis are avoided by minimizing soft tissue at the site of insertion. A trocar and drill sleeve is advanced directly to bone, minimizing the amount of soft tissue entrapment that might be encountered during predrilling. A sleeve should also be used if a self-drilling pin is selected (Fig. 7-37). Following predrilling, an appropriate depth of pin is advanced to achieve

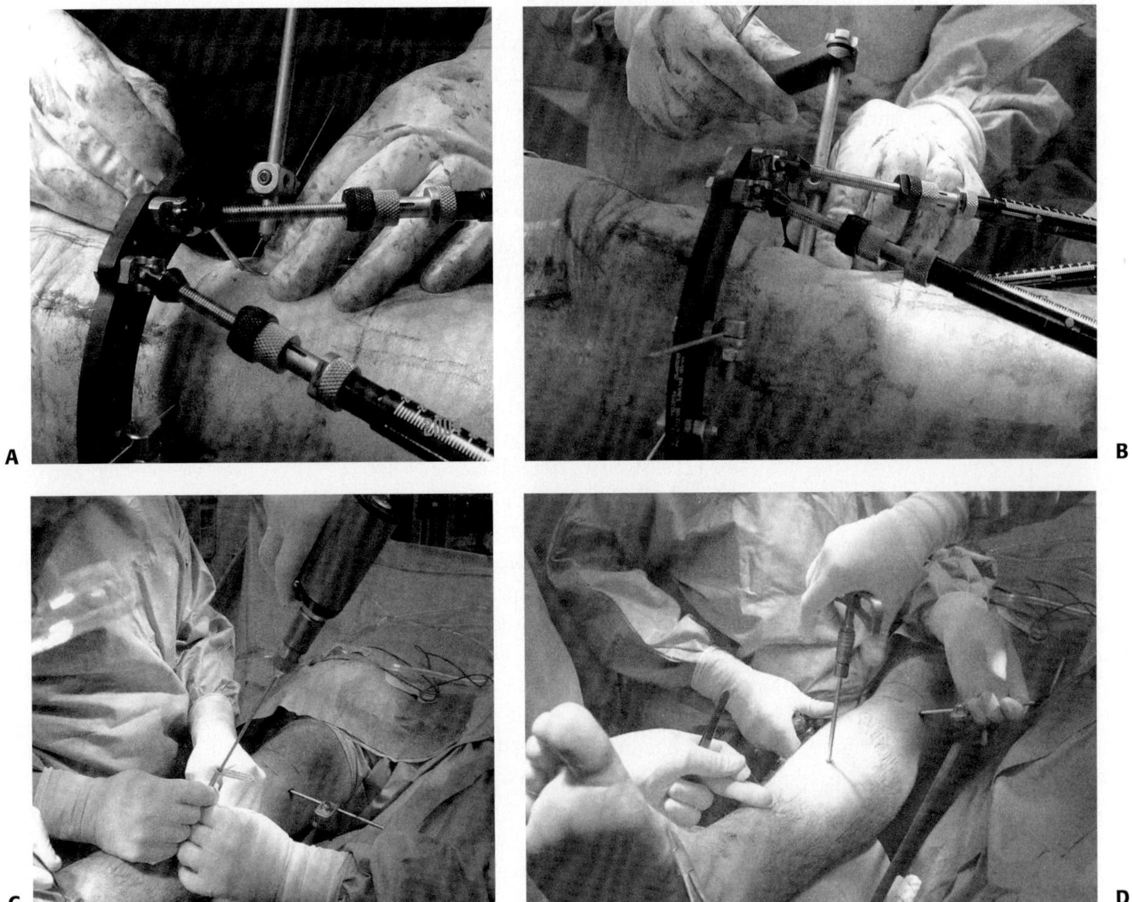

FIGURE 7-37 A trocar/sleeve assembly is used to protect the soft tissues. A drill is used to make the pilot hole, followed by hand insertion of the pin.

bicortical purchase; any soft tissue tethering should be released with a small scalpel (1,14).

Pin Care

The universal standard for pin care has yet to be identified. Pin site recommendations are based more often on clinical preference rather than strict research findings. The pin care protocol should be based on the pathophysiologic processes involved in the development of pin site infection (1). Correct pin site insertion technique removes most of the factors that cause pin site infection and subsequent pin loosening (1,177). If appropriate insertion technique is used, the pin sites will completely heal around each individual pin, much like a pierced earring insertion site heals. Once healed, only showering, without any other pin cleaning procedures, is necessary (178). The occasional removal of a serous crust around the pins using dilute hydrogen peroxide and saline may be necessary (1,14,51,179).

In general, recommendations include using normal saline as the cleansing agent in concert with dilute hydrogen peroxide (1,179). One should avoid ointments for postcleansing care, as these tend to inhibit the normal skin flora and alter the normal skin bacteria, and thus can lead to superinfection or pin site colonization (180). It is important to remove the buildup of crusted material, which will tend to stiffen the pin–skin interface and increase shear forces at the pin–bone interface. This leads to the development of additional necrotic tissues and fluid buildup around the pin (181). Immediate postoperative compressive dressing should be applied to the pin sites to stabilize the pin–skin interface and thus minimize pin–skin motion, which can lead to additional necrotic debris. By "training" the skin, the pin site remains stable (14,18). This allows the skin to heal around the pin undisturbed. Compressive dressings can be removed within 10 days to 2 weeks, once the pin sites are healed (Fig. 7-38A). If pin drainage does develop, then providing pin care three times per day should be undertaken. This may also involve rewrapping and compressing the offending pin site in an effort to minimize the abnormal pin–skin motion (18).

Frame Removal

Definitive treatment with an external fixator demands close scrutiny of the x-rays to ensure that the fracture or distraction site has completely healed before frame removal. Numerous authors have described various techniques, including CT scans, ultrasound, and bone densitometry, to determine the adequacy of fracture healing (14,18,79,119). In general, the patient should be fully weight bearing with minimal pain at the fracture site. The frame should be fully dynamized such that the load is being borne by the patient's limb rather than by the external fixator. For distraction osteogenesis, the x-rays are visualized in the AP and lateral planes. It is necessary to see three out of four neocortices in the regenerate zone reconstituted to ensure that the bone is mechanically stable and able to tolerate frame removal (14,17,81,88,119). Late deformity following frame removal is very common and usually is the result of incomplete healing of the distraction regenerate (14,18). In general, for an adult, the consolidation time (time following the cessation of distraction) is at least 1.5 to 2 times the total distraction time (time from surgery to achieving desired length or transport docking). Consolidation of the anterior cortex of the tibia is always delayed compared to the anterior, lateral, and posterior cortices. The subcutaneous border of the anterior tibia has the least amount of soft tissue coverage and thus blood supply, contributing to this delay. However, mechanical stability requires only three of the four reconstituted cortices.

With standard external fixation techniques, similar precautions should be followed to avoid refracture or nonunion. Four oblique views should be obtained to determine the adequacy of fracture healing before frame removal.

Ease of frame removal in an outpatient or office setting varies depending on the type of fixator pins used. Stainless steel pins are usually easily removed; however, newer pin designs, including titanium pins, as well as HA-coated pins are more problematic. With the biologic ingrowth nature of these biomaterials, pin removal is often difficult, requiring sufficient force to loosen the intact pin–bone interface. This may inflict a significant amount of pain, which may preclude this procedure from occurring in an office setting (43,48). In patients whose treatment time has been prolonged, often a large overgrowth of heterotopic pin keratosis has built up around the pin sites. This can leave an unsightly painful scar if not removed, and therefore it should be excised at the time of pin removal (see Fig. 7-38C).

Frame Reuse

In this era of cost containment for health care, the practice of recycling external fixator components makes sense. Dirschl and Smith reported on a single center's experience with a reuse program. Components in good repair were returned to the operating room stock for reuse, whereas those showing signs of wear were discarded. No component was used more than three times. The medical center charged patients a "loaner fee" equal to the hospital's cost for the inspection, processing, and recycling of fixator components. The mean hospital cost for a fixator decreased 34% as a result of the program. There were no differences in the rates of reoperation or complications before and after institution of the reuse program. No patient had mechanical failure of a new or reused fixator component (182).

Many investigators have evaluated the mechanical properties of recycled fixator components (182–184). A through examination of clinically removed frames, including static mechanical testing, has shown no reduction in performance or catastrophic mechanical failure of recycled parts that showed no visual signs of wear. The potential cost savings, combined with the documented safety of recycled components, makes reuse of these devices attractive.

August 2000 marked a significant change for hospitals or companies that perform in-house reprocessing of single-use medical devices (external fixator components). The U.S. Food

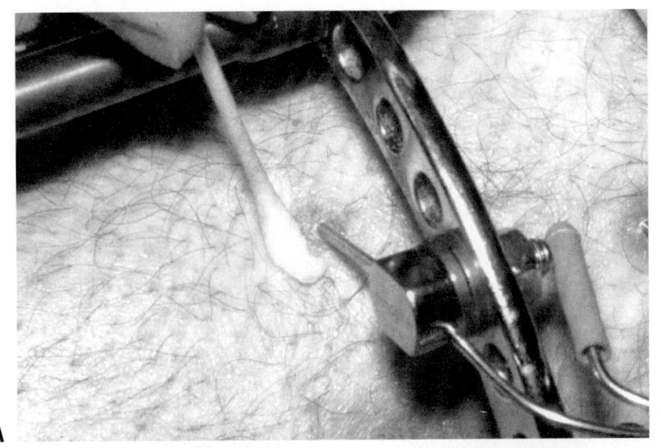
A

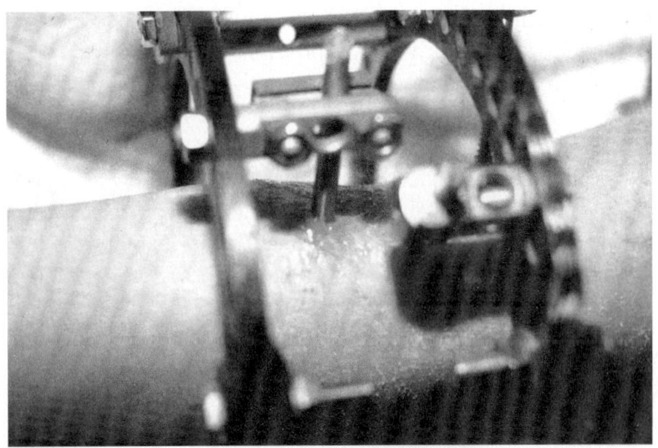
B

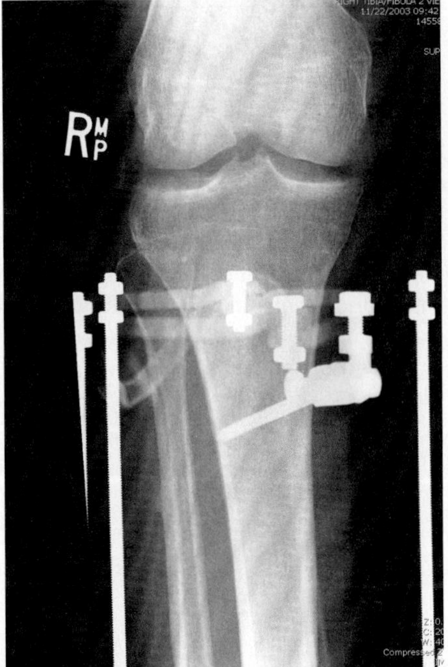

C

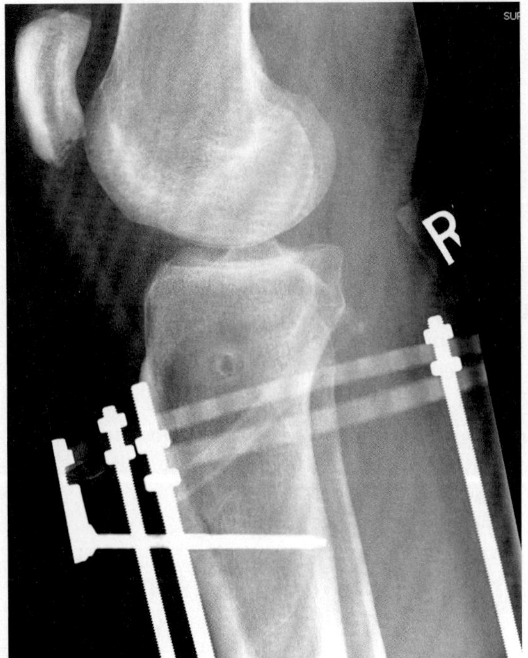

D

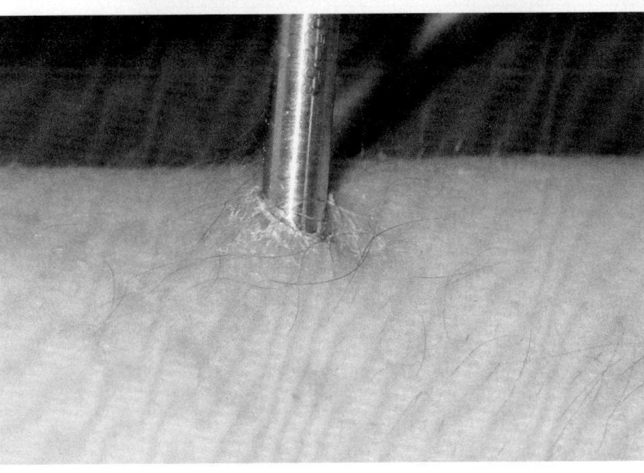
E

FIGURE 7-38 **A.** Healed pin tracts require minimal care other than mild soap and water. **B.** Grade 4 pin tract infection with surrounding erythema and drainage. X-rays of this region must be examined for radiographic signs suggestive of pin loosening. **C,D.** Radiographic evidence of pin sepsis and loosening includes pin sequestrum (*white arrow*) and cortical lucencies (*black circle*). **E.** Long-term pins develop painful hypertrophic keratosis surrounding the pin sites that should be excised at the time of pin removal.

and Drug Administration (FDA) announced new guidelines for hospitals as well as third-party reprocessing companies that now holds them to the same rigorous premarket submission requirements as manufacturers. For every device a hospital wants to reprocess, it must submit information to the FDA that demonstrates the safety and effectiveness of that device following reprocessing. This means that hospitals now face tough choices, with a wide range of factors to consider, such as cost, liability, quality assurance, and device tracking. In the months since the FDA announcement, many hospitals have determined that they lack the resources to meet the arduous premarket submission requirements (510k approval). Hospitals that performed their own reprocessing have been forced to decide whether to continue to recycle at great expense, stop using reprocessed devices altogether, or outsource to a third-party reprocessor. Many have decided to outsource the service.

Reprocessing, whether in-house or by a third-party company, can result in cost savings over the purchase price of new medical devices. Data currently suggest that this does not compromise a hospital's standard of care or patient outcomes, and it may help broaden access to health care in a community by making the best use of a hospital's limited dollars.

Pin Complications

Wire and pin site complications include pin site inflammation, chronic infection, loosening, and metal fatigue failure. Most authors agree that infection rates from external fixation pins have steadily decreased as pin technology has improved but are still very far from zero (185). The rates of frank pin tract infection have been chronicled as anecdotal observations mentioned offhand in many studies regarding external fixation. The major problem in all external fixator studies has been the definition of an infected pin site. Histologic examination of the tissues surrounding the inflamed pin site might lead to the conclusion that almost every pin tract is "infected." The most common wire and pin site complications are now graded by the classification described by Dahl et al (Table 7-1) (186):

- The *Grade 0* pin site appears normal other than marginal erythema and requires only weekly pin care (see Fig. 7-38A).
- *Grade 1* infection shows marginal inflammation, but no drainage is apparent. Treatment requires more frequent pin care consisting of daily cleansing with mild soap or half-strength peroxide and saline solution.
- *Grade 2* pin tract infection consists of an inflamed pin site with serous-type discharge.
- *Grade 3* pin tract infection consists of an inflamed pin site with purulent discharge. Both grade 2 and grade 3 pin tract infections require antibiotics and continued daily pin care.
- *Grade 4* pin tract infection consists of serous or seropurulent drainage in concert with redness, inflammation, and x-rays showing osteolysis of both the near and far cortices. Once osteolysis is visible, showing bicortical involvement, the offending pin should be removed immediately. Local soft tissue débridement of the pin tract with peroxide or other astringent irrigant should be performed. Formal surgical management is unnecessary as long as there are no obvious radiodensities noted on the plain x-rays at the side of osteolysis (see Fig. 7-38).
- *Grade 5* pin tract inflammation consists of inflamed purulent

TABLE 7-1 DAHL Pin Site Classification

Grade	Inflammation	Drainage	X-Ray Findings	Treatment
0	None or marginal	None	None	Weekly care
1	Marginal inflammation	None	None	Frequent pin care with mild soap or half-strength peroxide
2	Inflamed	Serous	None	Same as for grade 1 plus oral antibiotics
3	Inflamed	Purulent	None	Same as grade 2 treatment
4	Inflamed with induration	Seropurulent	Osteolysis at near and far cortices	Pin removal, local wound care
5	Inflamed with induration, tenderness, surrounding erythema	Gross purulent drainage	Sequestrum and medullary abscess	Formal surgical débridement with culture-specific antibiotics

drainage, osteolysis, as well as sequestrum noted around these abscesses within the medullary canal. Deep-seated infection is present. This requires formal irrigation and débridement procedures with delivery of culture-specific antibiotics. In an effort to avoid collapse of the external fixation construct and the establishment of biomechanical frame instability, pin exchange should be carried out in conjunction with the pin removal process.

Premature Consolidation

In patients undergoing distraction osteogenesis, the problem of premature consolidation is most commonly diagnosed as a failure of the corticotomy site to open and lengthen after initiation of distraction. In most instances, the problem is actually an incomplete osteotomy rather than premature healing of the osteotomy site (14,18,136). When this occurs in the tibia, it is a failure to completely osteotomize the posterior lateral cortex. This complication occurs primarily with surgeons inexperienced in performing percutaneous corticotomy techniques. Most experienced surgeons will perform the corticotomy and then manually distract the corticotomy site acutely for 1 to 2 mm under fluoroscopic control to ensure that the corticotomy is complete and can manually be distracted. Using the fixator pins above and below the corticotomy as joysticks, the limb segments can be counter-rotated one against the other under fluoroscopy to ensure that a complete osteotomy has occurred (14,18,136).

Premature consolidation occurs most commonly in the pediatric population, where distraction must begin much sooner compared to adults. It is usually due to a prolonged latency period, allowing significant callus formation to bridge across the corticotomy site. This is seen clinically when examining the frame and seeing excessive deflection of the wires or half-pins, with a concomitant lack of a distraction gap on x-ray. If this is recognized early in the treatment phase, continued slow distraction can be carried out until the premature area of consolidation ruptures (14,18). The patient should be warned that he or she may feel or hear an audible ache, snap, or pop in the limb, with sudden pain and concomitant swelling. Should this occur, the patient should immediately reverse the distraction and compress the region until the pain has subsided. If the patient continues to distract after the premature consolidation zone fractures, significant diastasis in the distraction gap will be created, causing rupture of the neovascular channels. This may result in the formation of cysts, with incomplete regenerate formation and possible regenerate failure (14,18–20,79,81,132).

Should the slow distraction fail to achieve disruption of the premature consolidation, the patient should be returned to the operating room, where closed manipulation can sometimes be successful in achieving complete corticotomy. Should this fail, a repeat corticotomy should be carried out.

The most common causes of incomplete regenerate healing are disruption of the periosteum and soft tissues during corticotomy, too rapid a distraction, and frame instability (18–20,79,81).

The rate and rhythm of distraction should be modulated in accordance with the radiographic visualization of the regenerate bone, including the formation of the interzone and longitudinal orientation of trabecular bone. Any evidence of disruption or nonlinear orientation of the trabecular bone should be a clear sign that frame instability has occurred. Each pin, wire, and ring connection should be checked, and if necessary additional pins or wires should be added to ensure adequate frame stability. This will help to avoid formation of intercalary cartilaginous elements.

Regenerate refracture or late deformity after removal of the apparatus usually presents as a gradual deviation of the limb. This often occurs as a result of the patient and treating surgeon becoming "frame weary," which results in premature frame removal before complete healing of the regenerate or fracture (14,18). One should always error on the conservative side and leave the frame on for an extended period to ensure that the fracture has healed.

Refracture through a docking site is unusual and is usually the result of incomplete healing. What is more common is fracturing through an osteoporotic stress fracture or through a previous pin or wire hole site.

When late deformity or regenerate collapse occurs, this usually leads to an unsatisfactory outcome unless collapse is detected early and the frame reapplied. Untreated, the resulting malunion requires secondary osteotomy procedures.

Pin and wire site fracture, as well as docking site or fracture site refracture, can usually be treated with a cast if detected early, before significant malalignment occurs. However, in complex cases, frame reapplication is required.

Contractures

Muscle contractures usually result from excessive joint distraction. This can occur over an extended period of time, such as with the use of an ankle-bridging Monotube fixator, or temporary traveling traction spanning the knee or ankle (187). A common complication when using lower extremity external fixators is the development of equinus contractures of the foot and ankle. To prevent this, prophylaxis should be encouraged by spanning the tibial frame down onto the forefoot in a neutral position.

Contractures result when the resting muscle length becomes relatively short compared to that of the newly lengthened bone. Thus, tibial lengthening or bone transport can cause flexion contractures at the knee and equinus contractures of the ankle. Measures should be taken to prevent severe muscle contractures when dealing with correction of leg length discrepancy (14,18). This also occurs during the correction of malunions or nonunions where, following the deformity correction, relative length is restored. Preventive measures include avoiding transfixion of tendons and maximizing muscle excursion before placing transfixion wires or half-pins. Physical therapy throughout the course of treatment is helpful, as is splinting and maintaining a plantigrade foot in neutral and the knee in full extension when the patient is at rest.

CONCLUSION

Advances in biomechanics and biomaterials continue to result in improvements in pin and frame technology. External fixation frames can now remain in place for prolonged periods without degradation in the pin–bone interface. Simplified frame mountings have extended the indications for use of these devices beyond acute fracture management to the reconstruction of complex posttraumatic conditions. Cutting-edge technologies such as Web-based software interfacing with digital x-rays, combined with uncomplicated frame adjustments, can now produce anatomic restoration of limbs that previously could not be achieved with external devices. External fixation continues to provide a powerful means to treat a variety of challenging conditions as the ultimate noninvasive tool.

REFERENCES

1. Green SA. *Complications of External Skeletal Fixation: Causes Prevention, and Treatment.* Springfield, IL: Charles C Thomas, 1981.
2. Lambotte A. The operative treatment of fractures: report of fractures committee. *Br Med J* 1912;2:1530.
3. Hoffmann R. Closed osteosynthesis with special references to war surgery. *Acta Chir Scand* 1942;86:255–261.
4. Hoffman R. Osteotaxis: *Transcutaneous Osteosynthesis by Means of Screws and Ball and Socket Joints.* Paris: Gead, 1953.
5. Anderson R. An automatic method of treatment for fractures of the tibia and the fibula. *Surg Gynecol Obstet* 1936;62:865–869.
6. Lewis KM, Breidenbach L, Stader O. The Stader reduction splint for treating fractures of the shafts of the long bones. *Ann Surg* 1942;116:623–631.
7. Shaar CM, Kreuz FP. *Manual of Fractures. Treatment by External Skeletal Fixation.* Philadelphia: WB Saunders, 1943.
8. Shaar CM, Kreuz FP, Jones DT. End results of treatment of fresh fractures by the use of the Stader apparatus. *J Bone Joint Surg* 1944;26:471–474.
9. Johnson HF, Stovall SL. External fixation of fractures. *J Bone Joint Surg [Am]* 1950;32:466–471.
10. Vidal J. External fixation. *Clin Orthop* 1983;180:7–14.
11. Burny F, Bourgois R. [Biomechanical study of the Hoffman external fixation device]. *Acta Orthop Belg* 1972;38(3):265–279.
12. Burny F. Elastic external fixation of fractures of the long bones. *Arch Putti Chir Organi Mov* 1986;36:323–329.
13. Hierholzer G, Ruedi T, Allgower M, et al, eds. *Manual on the AO/ASIF Tubular External Fixator.* Berlin: Springer-Verlag, 1985.
14. A.S.A.M.I. Group, Maiocchi AB, Aronson J, eds. *Operative Principles of Ilizarov: Fracture Treatment, Nonunion, Osteomyelitis, Lengthening, Deformity Correction.* Baltimore: Williams & Wilkins, 1991.
15. Volkov MV, Oganesian OV. Restoration of function in the knee and elbow with a hinge-distractor apparatus. *J Bone Joint Surg [Am]* 1975;57(5):591–600.
16. Fischer DA. Skeletal stabilization with a multiplane external fixation device. Design rationale and preliminary clinical experience. *Clin Orthop* 1983;(180):50–62.
17. Green SA. Skeletal defects: a comparison of bone grafting and bone transport for skeletal defects. *Clin Orthop* 1994;310:111–117.
18. Ilizarov GA. *Transosseous Osteosynthesis. Theoretical and Clinical Aspects of the Regeneration and Growth of Tissue* (Green S, ed). Berlin: Springer Verlag, 1992.
19. Ilizarov GA. The tension-stress effect on the genesis and growth of tissues: Part II. The influence of the rate and frequency of distraction. *Clin Orthop* 1989;(239):263–285.
20. Ilizarov GA. The tension-stress effect on the genesis and growth of tissues. Part I. The influence of stability of fixation and soft-tissue preservation. *Clin Orthop* 1989;(238):249–281.
21. Etter C, Burri C, Claes L, et al. Treatment by external fixation of open fractures associated with severe soft tissue damage of the leg. Biomechanical principles and clinical experience. *Clin Orthop* 1983;(178):80–88.
22. Aro HT, Markel MD, Chao EY. Cortical bone reactions at the interface of external fixation half-pins under different loading conditions. *J Trauma* 1993;35(5):776–785.
23. Behrens F. General theory and principles of external fixation. *Clin Orthop* 1989;241:15–23.
24. Degernes LA, Roe SC, Abrams CF Jr. Holding power of different pin designs and pin insertion methods in avian cortical bone. *Vet Surg* 1998;27(4):301–306.
25. Karnezis IA, Miles AW, Cunningham JL, et al. Axial preload in external fixator half-pins: a preliminary mechanical study of an experimental bone anchorage system. *Clin Biomech* 1999;14(1):69–73.
26. Kasman RA, Chao EY. Fatigue performance of external fixator pins. *J Orthop Res* 1984;2(4):377–384.
27. Lavini FM, Brivio LR, Leso P. Biomechanical factors in designing screws for the Orthofix system. *Clin Orthop* 1994;(308):63–67.
28. Capper M, Soutis C, Oni OO. Pin-hole shear stresses generated by conical and standard external fixation pins. *Biomaterials* 1993;14(11):876–878.
29. Pettine KA, Chao EY, Kelly PJ. Analysis of the external fixator pin-bone interface. *Clin Orthop* 1993;(293):18–27.
30. Seligson D, Donald GD, Stanwyck TS, et al. Consideration of pin diameter and insertion technique for external fixation in diaphyseal bone. *Acta Orthop Belg* 1984;50(4):441–450.
31. Moroni A, Vannini F, Mosca M, et al. State of the art review: techniques to avoid pin loosening and infection in external fixation. *J Orthop Trauma* 2002;16(3):189–195.
32. Nakata RY, Chand Y, Matiko JD, et al. External fixators for wrist fractures: a biomechanical and clinical study. *J Hand Surg [Am]* 1985;10(6 Pt 1):845–851.
33. Biliouris TL, Schneider E, Rahn BA, et al. The effect of radial preload on the implant-bone interface: a cadaveric study. *J Orthop Trauma* 1989;3(4):323–332.
34. Doyle J, Hayes P, Fenlon G. Experimental analysis of effects of pin pretensioning on external fixator rigidity. *Arch Orthop Trauma Surg* 1988;107(6):377–380.
35. Gantous A, Phillips JH. The effects of varying pilot hole size on the holding power of miniscrews and microscrews. *Plast Reconstr Surg* 1995;95(7):1165–1169.
36. Hutchinson DT, Bachus KN, Higgenbotham T. External fixation of the distal radius: to predrill or not to predrill. *J Hand Surg [Am]* 2000;25(6):1064–1068.
37. Seitz WH Jr, Froimson AI, Brooks DB, et al. External fixator pin insertion techniques: biomechanical analysis and clinical relevance. *J Hand Surg [Am]* 1991;16(3):560–563.
38. Clary EM, Roe SC. In vitro biomechanical and histological assessment of pilot hole diameter for positive-profile external skeletal fixation pins in canine tibiae. *Vet Surg* 1996;25(6):453–462.
39. Andrianne Y, Wagenknecht M, Donkerwolcke M, et al. External fixation pin: an in vitro general investigation. *Orthopedics* 1987;10(11):1507–1516.
40. Marti JM, Roe SC. Biomechanical comparison of the trocar tip point and the hollow ground tip point for smooth external skeletal fixation pins. *Vet Surg* 1998;27(5):423–428.
41. Matthews LS, Green CA, Goldstein SA. The thermal effects of skeletal fixation-pin insertion in bone. *J Bone Joint Surg [Am]* 1984;66:1077–1083.
42. Moroni A, Caja VL, Maltarello MC, et al. Biomechanical, scanning electron microscopy, and microhardness analyses of the bone-pin interface in hydroxyapatite coated versus uncoated pins. *J Orthop Trauma* 1997;11(3):154–161.
43. Moroni A, Faldini C, Marchetti S, et al. Improvement of the bone-pin interface strength in osteoporotic bone with use of hydroxyapatite-coated tapered external-fixation pins. A prospective, randomized clinical study of wrist fractures. *J Bone Joint Surg [Am]* 2001;83(5):717–721.
44. Augat P, Claes L, Hanselmann KF, et al. Increase of stability in external fracture fixation by hydroxyapatite-coated bone screws. *J Appl Biomater* 1995;6(2):99–104.
45. Caja VL, Piza G, Navarro A. Hydroxyapatite coating of external fixation pins to decrease axial deformity during tibial lengthening for short stature. *J Bone Joint Surg [Am]* 2003;85(8):1527–1531.
46. Magyar G, Toksvig-Larsen S, Moroni A. Hydroxyapatite coating of threaded pins enhances fixation. *J Bone Joint Surg [Br]* 1997;79(3):487–489.
47. Moroni A, Heikkila J, Magyar G, et al. Fixation strength and pin tract infection of hydroxyapatite-coated tapered pins. *Clin Orthop* 2001;(388):209–217.
48. Moroni A, Faldini C, Pegreffi F, et al. Fixation strength of tapered versus bicylindrical hydroxyapatite-coated external fixation pins: an animal study. *J Biomed Mater Res* 2002;63(1):61–64.
49. Oni OO, Capper M, Soutis C. A finite element analysis of the effect of pin distribution on the rigidity of a unilateral external fixation system. *Injury* 1993;24(8):525–527.
50. Behrens F, Johnson W. Unilateral external fixation. Methods to increase and reduce frame stiffness. *Clin Orthop* 1989;(241):48–56.
51. Bereton V. Pin-site care and the rate of local infection. *J Wound Care* 1998;7(1):42–44.
52. Tencer AF, Claudi B, Pearce S, et al. Development of a variable stiffness external fixation system for stabilization of segmental defects of the tibia. *J Orthop Res* 1984;1(4):395–404.
53. Briggs BT, Chao EY. The mechanical performance of the standard Hoffmann-Vidal external fixation apparatus. *J Bone Joint Surg [Am]* 1982;64(4):566–573.
54. Kowalski M, Schemitsch EH, Harrington RM, et al. Comparative biomechanical evaluation of different external fixation sidebars: stainless-steel tubes versus carbon fiber rods. *J Orthop Trauma* 1996;10(7):470–475.
55. Drijber FL, Finlay JB. Universal joint slippage as a cause of Hoffmann half-frame external fixator failure. *J Biomed Eng* 1992;14(6):509–515. (Erratum in: *J Biomed Eng* 1993;15(2):174.)
56. Harer T, Hontzsch D, Stohr E, et al. [How much are external fixator nuts tightened in general practice?] *Aktuelle Traumatol* 1993;23(4):212–213.
57. Wosar MA, Marcellin-Little DJ, Roe SC. Influence of bolt tightening torque, wire size, and component reuse on wire fixation in circular external fixation. *Vet Surg* 2002;31(6):571–576.
58. Chao EY, Hein TJ. Mechanical performance of the standard Orthofix external fixator. *Orthopedics* 1988;11(7):1057–1069.
59. Hein TJ, Chao EY. Biomechanical analysis of the Orthofix axial external fixator. *Biomed Sci Instrum* 1987;23:39–42.
60. Jaskulka RA, Egkher E, Wielke B. Comparison of the mechanical performance of three types of unilateral, dynamizable external fixators. An experimental study. *Arch Orthop Trauma Surg* 1994;113(5):271–275.
61. Juan JA, Prat J, Vera P, et al. Biomechanical consequences of callus development in Hoffmann, Wagner, Orthofix and Ilizarov external fixators. *J Biomech* 1992;25(9):995–1006.
62. Aro HT, Hein TJ, Chao EY. Mechanical performance of pin clamps in external fixators. *Clin Orthop* 1989;(248):246–253.
63. Thordarson DB, Markolf KL, Cracchiolo A 3rd. External fixation in arthrodesis of the

ankle. A biomechanical study comparing a unilateral frame with a modified transfixion frame. *J Bone Joint Surg [Am]* 1994;76(10):1541–1544.

64. Williams EA, Rand JA, An KN, et al. The early healing of tibial osteotomies stabilized by one-plane or two-plane external fixation. *J Bone Joint Surg [Am]* 1987;69(3):355–365.
65. Shearer J, Egan J. Computerized analysis of pin geometry. In: Coombs R, Green SA, Sarmiento A, eds. *External Fixation and Functional Bracing*. London: Orthotext, 1989: 129–135.
66. Chao EY, Kasman RA, An KN. Rigidity and stress analyses of external fracture fixation devices: a theoretical approach. *J Biomech* 1982;15(12):971–983.
67. Oni OO, Capper M, Soutis C. External fixation of upper limb fractures: the effect of pin offset on fixator stability. *Biomaterials* 1995;16(3):263–264.
68. Schuind FA, Burny F, Chao EY. Biomechanical properties and design considerations in upper extremity external fixation. *Hand Clin* 1993;9(4):543–553.
69. Lowenberg DW, Abruzzo FM, Herzka A, et al. The correlation of shearing force with fracture line migration for progressive fracture obliquities stabilized by external fixation in the tibial model. Proceedings of the 1st Annual A S A M I International, 1998.
70. Arazi M, Yalcin H, Tarakcioglu N, et al. The effects of dynamization and destabilization of the external fixator on fracture healing: a comparative biomechanical study in dogs. *Orthopedics* 2002;25(5):521–524.
71. Aro HT, Chao EY. Bone-healing patterns affected by loading, fracture fragment stability, fracture type, and fracture site compression. *Clin Orthop* 1993;(293):8–17.
72. Aro HT, Kelly PJ, Lewallen DG, et al. The effects of physiologic dynamic compression on bone healing under external fixation. *Clin Orthop* 1990;(256):260–273.
73. Augat P, Burger J, Schorlemmer S, et al. Shear movement at the fracture site delays healing in a diaphyseal fracture model. *J Orthop Res* 2003;21(6):1011–1017.
74. Chao EY, Aro HT, Lewallen DG, et al. The effect of rigidity on fracture healing in external fixation. *Clin Orthop*. 1989;(241):24–35.
75. Park SH, O'Connor K, McKellop H, et al. The influence of active shear or compressive motion on fracture-healing. *J Bone Joint Surg [Am]* 1998;80(6):868–878.
76. Wu JJ, Shyr HS, Chao EY, et al. Comparison of osteotomy healing under external fixation devices with different stiffness characteristics. *J Bone Joint Surg [Am]* 1984; 66(8):1258–1264.
77. McCoy MT, Chao EY, Kasman RA. Comparison of mechanical performance in four types of external fixators. *Clin Orthop* 1983;(180):23–33.
78. Podolsky A, Chao EY. Mechanical performance of Ilizarov circular external fixators in comparison with other external fixators. *Clin Orthop* 1993;(293):61–70.
79. Aronson J, Harrison B, Boyd CM, et al. Mechanical induction of osteogenesis: the importance of pin rigidity. *J Pediatr Orthop* 1988;8(4):396–401.
80. Roberts CS, Antoci V, Antoci V Jr, et al. The accuracy of fine wire tensioners: a comparison of five tensioners used in hybrid and ring external fixation. *J Orthop Trauma* 2004; 18(3):158–162.
81. Aronson J, Harp JH Jr. Mechanical considerations in using tensioned wires in a transosseous external fixation system. *Clin Orthop* 1992;(280):23–29.
82. Calhoun JH, Li F, Ledbetter BR, et al. Biomechanics of the Ilizarov fixator for fracture fixation. *Clin Orthop* 1992;(280):15–22.
83. Calhoun JL, Li F, Bauford WL, et al. Rigidity of half-pins for the Ilizarov external fixator. *Bull Hosp Jt Dis* 1992;52(1):21–26.
84. Cross AR, Lewis DD, Murphy ST, et al. Effects of ring diameter and wire tension on the axial biomechanics of four-ring circular external skeletal fixator constructs. *Am J Vet Res* 2001;62(7):1025–1030.
85. Caja VL, Larsson S, Kim W, et al. Mechanical performance of the Monticelli-Spinelli external fixation system. *Clin Orthop* 1994;(309):257–266.
86. Fleming B, Paley D, Kristiansen T, et al. A biomechanical analysis of the Ilizarov external fixator. *Clin Orthop* 1989;(241):95–105.
87. Orbay GL, Frankel VH, Kummer FJ. The effect of wire configuration on the stability of the Ilizarov external fixator. *Clin Orthop* 1992;(279):299–302.
88. Green SA, Jackson JM, Wall DM, et al. Management of segmental defects by the Ilizarov intercalary bone transport method. *Clin Orthop* 1992;280:136–142.
89. Watson JT, Karges DE, Cramer KE, et al. Analysis of failure of hybrid external fixation techniques for the treatment of distal tibial pilon fractures. Abstract Proceedings, 16th Annual Meeting of the Orthopaedic Trauma Association, San Antonio, TX, Oct. 12–14, 1999.
90. Watson JT, Ripple S, Hoshaw SJ, et al. Hybrid external fixation for tibial plateau fractures: clinical and biomechanical correlation. *Orthop Clin North Am* 2002;33(1): 199–209.
91. Duda GN, Sollmann M, Sporrer S, et al. Interfragmentary motion in tibial osteotomies stabilized with ring fixators. *Clin Orthop* 2002;(396):163–172.
92. Khalily C, Voor MJ, Seligson D. Fracture site motion with Ilizarov and "hybrid" external fixation. *J Orthop Trauma* 1998;12(1):21–26.
93. Saleh M, Rees A. Bifocal surgery for deformity and bone loss after lower-limb fractures. Comparison of bone-transport and compression-distraction methods. *J Bone Joint Surg [Br]* 1995;77(3):429–434.
94. Windhagen H, Glockner R, Bail H, et al. Stiffness characteristics of composite hybrid external fixators. *Clin Orthop* 2002;(405):267–276.
95. Watson MA, Matthias KJ, Maffulli N, et al. Yielding of the clamped-wire system in the Ilizarov external fixator. *Proc Inst Mech Eng [H]* 2003;217(5):367–374.
96. Watson MA, Mathias KJ, Maffulli N, et al. The effect of clamping a tensioned wire: implications for the Ilizarov external fixation system. *Proc Inst Mech Eng [H]* 2003; 217(2):91–98.
97. Pugh KJ, Wolinsky PR, Dawson JM, et al. The biomechanics of hybrid external fixation. *J Orthop Trauma* 1999;13(1):20–26.
98. Pugh KJ, Wolinsky PR, Pienkowski D, et al. Comparative biomechanics of hybrid external fixation. *J Orthop Trauma* 1999;13(6):418–425.
99. Roberts CS, Dodds JC, Perry K, et al. Hybrid external fixation of the proximal tibia: strategies to improve frame stability. *J Orthop Trauma* 2003;17(6):415–420.
100. Ali AM, Saleh M, Bolongaro S, et al. The strength of different fixation techniques for bicondylar tibial plateau fractures: a biomechanical study. *Clin Biomech* 2003;18(9): 864–870.
101. Ali AM, Yang L, Hashmi M, et al. Bicondylar tibial plateau fractures managed with the Sheffield Hybrid Fixator. Biomechanical study and operative technique. *Injury* 2001; 32 Suppl 4:SD86–91.
102. Bronson DG, Samchukov ML, Birch JG. Stabilization of a short juxta-articular bone segment with a circular external fixator. *J Pediatr Orthop B* 2002;11(2):143–149.
103. Kenwright J, Gardner T. Mechanical influences on tibial fracture healing. *Clin Orthop* 1998;(355 Suppl):S179–190.
104. Larsson S, Kim W, Caja VL, et al. Effect of early axial dynamization on tibial bone healing: a study in dogs. *Clin Orthop* 2001;(388):240–251.
105. Kenwright J, Goodship AE. Controlled mechanical stimulation in the treatment of tibial fractures. *Clin Orthop* 1989;(241):36–47.
106. Kenwright J, Richardson JB, Cunningham JL, et al. Axial movement and tibial fractures. A controlled randomised trial of treatment. *J Bone Joint Surg [Br]* 1991;73(4):654–659.
107. Lewallen DG, Chao EY, Kasman RA, et al. Comparison of the effects of compression plates and external fixators on early bone-healing. *J Bone Joint Surg [Am]* 1984;66(7): 1084–1091.
108. Claes L, Eckert-Hubner K, Augat P. The effect of mechanical stability on local vascularization and tissue differentiation in callus healing. *J Orthop Res* 2002;20(5):1099–1105.
109. Goodship AE, Cunningham JL, Kenwright J. Strain rate and timing of stimulation in mechanical modulation of fracture healing. *Clin Orthop* 1998;(355 Suppl):S105–115.
110. Goodship AE, Watkins PE, Rigby HS, et al. The role of fixator frame stiffness in the control of fracture healing. An experimental study. *J Biomech* 1993;26(9):1027–1035.
111. Hart MB, Wu JJ, Chao EY, et al. External skeletal fixation of canine tibial osteotomies. Compression compared with no compression. *J Bone Joint Surg [Am]* 1985;67(4): 598–605.
112. Pettila MH, Sarna S, Paavolainen P, et al. Short-term external support promotes healing in semirigidly fixed fractures. *Clin Orthop* 1997;(343):157–163.
113. Augat P, Merk J, Wolf S, et al. Mechanical stimulation by external application of cyclic tensile strains does not effectively enhance bone healing. *J Orthop Trauma* 2001;15(1): 54–60.
114. Wallace AL, Draper ER, Strachan RK, et al. The vascular response to fracture micromovement. *Clin Orthop* 1994;(301):281–290.
115. Wang ZG, Peng CL, Zheng XL, et al. Force measurement on fracture site with external fixation. *Med Biol Eng Comput* 1997;35(3):289–290.
116. Matsushita T, Nakamura K, Ohnishi I, et al. Sliding performance of unilateral external fixators for tibia. *Med Eng Phys* 1998;20(1):66–69.
117. Cunningham JL, Evans M, Harris JD, et al. The measurement of stiffness of fractures treated with external fixation. *Eng Med* 1987;16(4):229–232.
118. Spiegel PG, VanderSchilden JL. Minimal internal and external fixation in the treatment of open tibia fractures. *Clin Orthop* 1983;(178):96–102.
119. Aronson J, Johnson E, Harp JH. Local bone transportation for treatment of intercalary defects by the Ilizarov technique. Biomechanical and clinical considerations. *Clin Orthop* 1989;(243):71–79.
120. Yasui N, Nakase T, Kawabata H, et al. A technique of percutaneous multidrilling osteotomy for limb lengthening and deformity correction. *J Orthop Sci* 2000;5(2):104–107.
121. Lerner A, Ullmann Y, Stein H, et al. Using the Ilizarov external fixation device for skin expansion. *Ann Plast Surg* 2000;45(5):535–537.
122. Dahl MT. The gradual correction of forearm deformities in multiple hereditary exostoses. *Hand Clin* 1993;9(4):707–718.
123. De la Huerta F. Correction of the neglected clubfoot by the Ilizarov method. *Clin Orthop* 1994;(301):89–93.
124. Kashiwagi N, Suzuki S, Seto Y, et al. Bilateral humeral lengthening in achondroplasia. *Clin Orthop* 2001;(391):251–257.
125. Menon DK, Dougall TW, Pool RD, et al. Augmentative Ilizarov external fixation after failure of diaphyseal union with intramedullary nailing. *J Orthop Trauma* 2002;16(7): 491–497.
126. Noonan KJ, Price CT. Pearls and pitfalls of deformity correction and limb lengthening via monolateral external fixation. *Iowa Orthop J* 1996;16:58–69.
127. Rozbruch SR, DiPaola M, Blyakher A. Fibula lengthening using a modified Ilizarov method. *Orthopedics* 2002;25(11):1241–1244.
128. Stanitski DF, Dahl M, Louie K, et al. Management of late-onset tibia vara in the obese patient by using circular external fixation. *J Pediatr Orthop* 1997;17(5):691–694.
129. Tetsworth KD, Paley D. Accuracy of correction of complex lower-extremity deformities by the Ilizarov method. *Clin Orthop* 1994;(301):102–110.
130. Cierny G, Zorn KE. Segmental tibial defects. Comparing conventional and Ilizarov methodologies. *Clin Orthop* 1994;301:118–123.
131. Manzotti A, Pullen C, Deromedis B, et al. Knee arthrodesis after infected total knee arthroplasty using the Ilizarov method. *Clin Orthop* 2001;(389):143–149.
132. Paley D, Catagni MA, Argnani F, et al. Ilizarov treatment of tibial nonunions with bone loss. *Clin Orthop* 1989;(241):146–165.
133. Sakurakichi K, Tsuchiya H, Uehara K, et al. Ankle arthrodesis combined with tibial lengthening using the Ilizarov apparatus. *J Orthop Sci* 2003;8(1):20–25.
134. Tsuchiya H, Uehara K, Abdel-Wanis ME, et al. Deformity correction followed by lengthening with the Ilizarov method. *Clin Orthop* 2002;(402):176–183.
135. Watson JT, Anders M, Moed BR. Bone loss in tibial shaft fractures: management strategies. *Clin Orthop* 1995;316:1–17.
136. Watson JT. Bone transport. *Techniques in Orthopaedics* 1996;11:2:132–143.
137. Patterson MJ, Cole JD. Two-staged delayed open reduction and internal fixation of severe pilon fractures. *J Orthop Trauma* 1999;13:85–91.

138. Sirkin M, Sanders R, DiPasquale T, et al. A staged protocol for soft tissue management in the treatment of complex pilon fractures. *J Orthop Trauma* 1999;13:78–84.
139. Watson JT, Moed BR, Karges DE, et al. Pilon fractures: treatment protocol based on severity of soft tissue injury. *Clin Orthop* 2000;375:78–90.
140. Watson JT. High-energy fractures of the tibial plateau. *Orthop Clin North Am* 1994;25: 723–752.
141. Watson JT. Hybrid external fixation for tibial plateau fractures. *Am J Knee Surg* 2001; 14(2):135–140.
142. Watson JT. Tibial pilon fractures. *Techniques in Orthopaedics* 1996;11:2:150–159.
143. Haidukewych GJ. Temporary external fixation for the management of complex intra- and periarticular fractures of the lower extremity. *J Orthop Trauma* 2002;16(9): 678–685.
144. Taeger G, Ruchholtz S, Zettl R, et al. Primary external fixation with consecutive procedural modification in polytrauma. *Unfallchirurg* 2002;105(4):315–321.
145. Ali AM, Burton M, Hashmi M, et al. Outcome of complex fractures of the tibial plateau treated with a beam-loading ring fixation system. *J Bone Joint Surg [Br]* 2003;85(5): 691–699.
146. Leung F, Kwok HY, Pun TS, et al. Limited open reduction and Ilizarov external fixation in the treatment of distal tibial fractures. *Injury* 2004;35(3):278–283.
147. Jackson M, Topliss CJ, Atkins RM. Fine wire frame-assisted intramedullary nailing of the tibia. *J Orthop Trauma* 2003;17(3):222–224.
148. Dahners LE, Jacobs RR, McKenzie EB, et al. Biomechanical studies of an anterior pelvic external fixation frame intended for control of vertical shear fractures. *South Med J* 1986;79(7):815–817.
149. Kellam JF. The role of external fixation in pelvic disruptions. *Clin Orthop* 1989;(241): 66–82.
150. Haidukewych GJ, Kumar S, Prpa B. Placement of half-pins for supra-acetabular external fixation: an anatomic study. *Clin Orthop* 2003;(411):269–273.
151. Mears DC, Rubash HE. External and internal fixation of the pelvic ring. *AAOS Instr Course Lect* 1984;33:144–158.
152. Agee JM. External fixation. Technical advances based upon multiplanar ligamentotaxis. *Orthop Clin North Am* 1993;24(2):265–274.
153. Dodds SD, Cornelissen S, Jossan S, et al. A biomechanical comparison of fragment-specific fixation and augmented external fixation for intra-articular distal radius fractures. *J Hand Surg [Am]* 2002;27(6):953–964.
154. Markiewitz AD, Gellman H. Five-pin external fixation and early range of motion for distal radius fractures. *Orthop Clin North Am* 2001;32(2):329–335.
155. Goslings JC, DaSilva MF, Viegas SF, et al. Kinematics of the wrist with a new dynamic external fixation device. *Clin Orthop* 2001;(386):226–234.
156. Flinkkila T, Ristiniemi J, Hyvonen P, et al. Nonbridging external fixation in the treatment of unstable fractures of the distal forearm. *Arch Orthop Trauma Surg* 2003;123(7): 349–352.
157. Blasier RD, Aronson J, Tursky EA. External fixation of pediatric femur fractures. *J Pediatr Orthop* 1997;17(3):342–346.
158. El Hayek T, Daher AA, Meouchy W, et al. External fixators in the treatment of fractures in children. *J Pediatr Orthop B* 2004;13(2):103–109.
159. Bosse MJ, Holmes C, Vossoughi J, et al. Comparison of the Howmedica and Synthes military external fixation frames. *J Orthop Trauma* 1994;8(2):119–126.
160. Dougherty PJ, Vickaryous B, Conley E, et al. A comparison of two military temporary femoral external fixators. *Clin Orthop* 2003(412):176–183.
161. Thakur AJ, Patankar J. Open tibial fractures. Treatment by uniplanar external fixation and early bone grafting. *J Bone Joint Surg [Br]* 1991;73(3):448–451.
162. Endres T, Grass R, Biewener A, et al. [Advantages of minimally invasive reposition, retention, and hybrid Ilizarov fixation for tibial pilon fractures with particular emphasis on C2/C3 fractures]. *Unfallchirurg* 2004;107(4):273–284.
163. Yildiz C, Atesalp AS, Demiralp B, et al. High-velocity gunshot wounds of the tibial plafond managed with Ilizarov external fixation: a report of 13 cases. *J Orthop Trauma* 2003;17(6):421–429.
164. Geller J, Tornetta P 3rd, Tiburzi D, et al. Tension wire position for hybrid external fixation of the proximal tibia. *J Orthop Trauma* 2000;14(7):502–504.
165. Vives MJ, Abidi NA, Ishikawa SN, et al. Soft tissue injuries with the use of safe corridors for transfixion wire placement during external fixation of distal tibia fractures: an anatomic study. *J Orthop Trauma* 2001;15(8):555–559.
166. Vora AM, Haddad SL, Kadakia A, et al. Extracapsular placement of distal tibial transfixation wires. *J Bone Joint Surg [Am]* 2004;86(5):988–993.
167. Bottlang M, Marsh JL, Brown TD. Articulated external fixation of the ankle: minimizing motion resistance by accurate axis alignment. *J Biomech* 1999;32(1):63–70.
168. Fitzpatrick DC, Foels WS, Pedersen DR, et al. An articulated ankle external fixation system that can be aligned with the ankle axis. *Iowa Orthop J* 1995;15:197–203.
169. Sommers MB, Fitzpatrick DC, Kahn KM, et al. Hinged external fixation of the knee: intrinsic factors influencing passive joint motion. *J Orthop Trauma* 2004;18(3): 163–169.
170. Christian EP, Bosse MJ, Robb G. Reconstruction of large diaphyseal defects, without free fibular transfer, in grade IIIB tibial fractures. *J Bone Joint Surg [Am]* 1989;71:994–1002.
171. Edwards CC. Staged reconstruction of complex open tibial fractures using Hoffmann external fixation: clinical decisions and dilemmas. *Clin Orthop* 1983;178:130–161.
172. Enneking WF, Eady JL, Burchardt H. Autogenous cortical bone grafts in the reconstruction of segmental skeletal defects. *J Bone Joint Surg [Am]* 1980;62(7):1039–1058.
173. Seide K, Wolter D, Kortmann HR. Fracture reduction and deformity correction with the hexapod Ilizarov fixator. *Clin Orthop* 1999;363:186–195.
174. Feldman DS, Madan SS, Koval KJ, et al. Correction of tibia vara with six-axis deformity analysis and the Taylor Spatial Frame. *J Pediatr Orthop* 2003;23(3):387–391.
175. Sluga M, Pfeiffer M, Kotz R, et al. Lower limb deformities in children: two-stage correction using the Taylor spatial frame. *J Pediatr Orthop B* 2003;12(2):123–128.
176. Watson JT, Occhietti M, Parmar V. Rate of postoperative wound infections in patients with pre-existing external fixators treated with secondary open procedures. Abstract Proceedings, 15th Annual Meeting of the Orthopaedic Trauma Association, Charlotte, NC, Oct. 22–24, 1999.
177. Parameswaran AD, Roberts CS, Seligson D, et al. Pin tract infection with contemporary external fixation: how much of a problem? *J Orthop Trauma* 2003;17(7):503–507.
178. W-Dahl A, Toksvig-Larsen S, Lindstrand A. No difference between daily and weekly pin site care: a randomized study of 50 patients with external fixation. *Acta Orthop Scand* 2003;74(6):704–708.
179. Gordon JE, Kelly-Hahn J, Carpenter CJ, et al. Pin site care during external fixation in children: results of nihilistic approach. *J Pediatr Orthop* 2000;20(2):163.
180. Marotta JS, Coupe KJ, Milner R, et al. Long-term bactericidal properties of a gentamicin-coated antimicrobial external fixation pin sleeve. *J Bone Joint Surg [Am]* 2003;85,Suppl 4:129–131.
181. Clasper JC, Cannon LB, Stapley SA, et al. Fluid accumulation and the rapid spread of bacteria in the pathogenesis of external fixator pin track infection. *Injury*. 2001;32(5): 377–381.
182. Dirschl DR, Smith IJ. Reuse of external skeletal fixator components: effects on costs and complications. *J Trauma* 1998;44(5):855–858.
183. Dirschl DR, Obremskey WT. Mechanical strength and wear of used EBI external fixators. *Orthopedics* 2002;25(10):1059–1062.
184. Kummer FJ, Frankel VH, Catagni MA. Reuse of Ilizarov frame components: a potential cost savings? *Contemp Orthop* 1992;25(2):125–128.
185. DeJong ES, DeBerardino TM, Brooks DE, et al. Antimicrobial efficacy of external fixator pins coated with a lipid stabilized hydroxyapatite/chlorhexidine complex to prevent pin tract infection in a goat model. *J Trauma* 2001;50(6):1008–1014.
186. Dahl MT, Gulli B, Berg T. Complications of limb lengthening a learning curve. *Clin Orthop* 1994;301:10–18.
187. Simpson AH, Cunningham JL, Kenwright J. The forces which develop in the tissues during leg lengthening. A clinical study. *J Bone Joint Surg [Br]* 1996;78(6):979–983.

BONE AND JOINT HEALING

Joseph A. Buckwalter, Thomas A. Einhorn, and J. L. Marsh

Over the last two decades orthopaedic surgeons have dramatically advanced their ability to restore the structure and function of damaged bones and joints. Using new methods of internal fixation, external fixation, and rehabilitation they now successfully treat even the most severe fractures and many severe joint injuries. New biologic approaches to promoting tissue repair and regeneration will further improve treatment of these injuries (1). Yet, ultimately the results of any treatment of musculoskeletal injuries depends on the skill of the surgeon in taking advantage of the natural healing potential of the tissues that form the skeleton. Surgeons can treat bone and joint injuries without extensive knowledge of these tissues, but they are better able to select the optimal treatment if they have this knowledge. Furthermore, they can treat, and in some instances prevent, complications of musculoskeletal injuries or problems of failed or inadequate healing more effectively when they are as skilled in applying knowledge of tissue healing as they are in the use of surgical techniques.

BONE TISSUE

The mechanical properties of bone are readily apparent. Its tensile strength nearly equals that of cast iron, but it is three times lighter and ten times more flexible. Yet, bone is not a homogenous inert material like iron, or the plastics and metals that form most orthopaedic implants. Its matrix consists of organic and inorganic components and is covered on its internal and external surfaces by cells and cell processes (2). An elaborate system of lacunae, canals, or tunnels containing cells and cell processes, blood vessels, lymphatics, and nerves permeate the matrix, and a variety of specialized cell populations responsible for maintaining the tissue lie within the matrix lacunae and on the bone surfaces (2). In most people bone appears to remain unchanged for decades, but this appearance is deceptive, it is constantly changing in response to mechanical and hormonal signals (3).

Mature bones consist of a central fatty or hematopoietic marrow supported and surrounded by bone tissue and periosteum. Although the three component tissues of bone differ in composition, structure, and function they are not independent. Marrow can serve as a source of bone cells, marrow blood vessels form a critical part of the bone circulatory system and disorders, or mechanical disruption of the marrow can affect the activities of bone and periosteal cells.

Bone consists of mesenchymal cells embedded within an abundant extracellular matrix (2,3). The matrix contains mineral that gives the tissue great strength and stiffness in compression and bending. The organic component of the bone matrix, primarily type I collagen, contributes to bone strength, but also gives bone the plasticity that allows substantial deformation without fracture. Bone matrix also contains a variety of cytokines, including growth factors that stimulate bone formation (2,3). These growth factors appear to have important roles in normal bone metabolism and in fracture healing. The periosteum, consisting of two layers—an outer fibrous layer and an inner more cellular and vascular cambium layer—covers the external bone surfaces and participates in healing of many types of fractures. The thicker, more cellular periosteum of infants and children has a more extensive vascular supply than that of adults. Perhaps because of these differences, the periosteum of children is more active in healing many fractures.

Two types of bone can be distinguished by their mechanical and biological properties: *woven or immature bone* and *lamellar or mature bone* (2). Woven bone forms the embryonic skeleton and is replaced by lamellar bone during development and growth (3). Woven bone also forms the initial fracture repair tissue and is replaced by lamellar bone as the fracture remodels. Compared with lamellar bone, woven bone has a more rapid rate of deposition and resorption, an irregular woven pattern of matrix collagen fibrils consistent with its name, approximately four times the number of osteocytes per unit volume, and an irregular pattern of matrix mineralization. The frequent patchwork formation of woven bone and the spotty pattern of mineralization creates an irregular radiographic appearance that distinguishes the woven bone found in fracture callus from lamellar bone. Because of its lack of collagen fibril orientation, irregular mineralization, and relatively high cell and water concentration, woven bone is less stiff and more easily deformed than lamellar bone.

JOINT TISSUES

All synovial joints share the same basic structure: congruent articulating cartilaginous surfaces supported by subchondral and metaphyseal bone, joint capsules and ligaments that link the bones supporting the articular surfaces and synovial membranes that cover the inner surfaces of the joint except for articular cartilage. Some joints also have dense fibrous tissue menisci that lie between the cartilaginous surfaces and attach to the joint capsule.

Articular cartilage consists of sparsely distributed chondrocytes surrounded by an elaborate, highly organized macromolecular framework filled with water (4). Three classes of molecules (collagens, proteoglycans, and noncollagenous proteins) form the macromolecular framework. Type II collagen fibrils give the cartilage its form and tensile strength, and a variety of quantitatively minor collagens help organize and maintain the meshwork of type II collagen fibrils. The interaction of proteoglycans with water gives the tissue its stiffness to compression and its resiliency and contributes to its durability. The noncollagenous proteins are less well understood than the proteoglycans and collagens, but they appear to help organize and stabilize the matrix, attach chondrocytes to the matrix macromolecules, and possibly help stabilize the chondrocyte phenotype. Unlike the other primary musculoskeletal tissues, cartilage lacks a blood supply, a nerve supply, and a lymphatic supply.

BONE AND JOINT INJURIES

Acute injuries of bones and joints result from applications of forces to the skeleton that exceed the strength of the tissues. Disruptions of bone tissue are called *fractures*. Visible disruptions of articular cartilage also generally are referred to as fractures when they involve both the articular cartilage and subchondral bone, that is, *osteochondral or intra-articular fractures*, and when they involve only the cartilage, that is, *chondral fractures*.

BONE FRACTURE HEALING

Inflammation and Repair

A bone fracture initiates a sequence of inflammation, repair, and remodeling that can restore the injured bone to its original state (5). Inflammation begins immediately after injury and is followed rapidly by repair (6). After repair has replaced the lost and damaged cells and matrix, a prolonged remodeling phase begins. The energy requirements of fracture healing increase rapidly during inflammation and reach a peak during repair, when the cells in the fracture callus are proliferating and synthesizing large volumes of new matrix. These energy requirements remain high until cell density and cell activity begin to decline as remodeling starts (7).

An injury that fractures bone not only damages the cells, blood vessels, and bone matrix (Fig. 8-1), but also the surrounding soft tissues, including the periosteum and muscle. A hematoma accumulates within the medullary canal, between the frac-

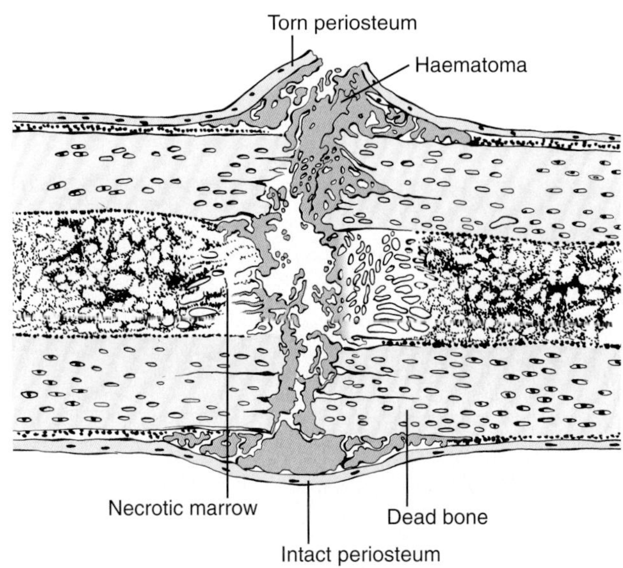

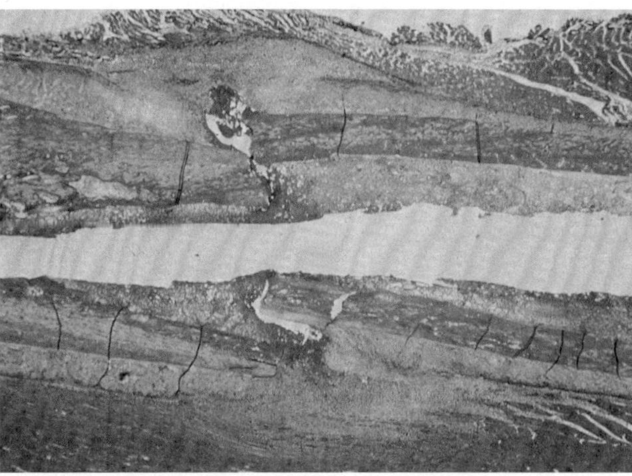

FIGURE 8-1 Initial events following fracture of a long bone diaphysis. **A.** Drawing showing that the periosteum is torn opposite the point of impact, and may remain intact on the other side. A hematoma accumulates beneath the periosteum and between the fracture ends. There is necrotic marrow and cortical bone close to the fracture line. **B.** A photomicrograph of a fractured rat femur three days after injury showing the proliferation of the periosteal repair tissue.

ture ends and beneath elevated periosteum. The damage to the bone blood vessels deprives osteocytes of their nutrition, and they die as far back as the junction of collateral channels, leaving the immediate ends of the fracture without living cells (see Fig. 8-2). Severely damaged periosteum and marrow, as well as other surrounding soft tissues, may also contribute necrotic material to the fracture site.

Inflammatory mediators released from platelets and from dead and injured cells cause blood vessels to dilate and exude plasma leading to the acute edema seen in the region of a fresh fracture. Inflammatory cells migrate to the region, including polymorphonuclear leukocytes followed by macrophages and lymphocytes. These cells also release cytokines that stimulate angiogenesis (8). As the inflammatory response subsides, necrotic tissue and exudate are resorbed, and fibroblasts and chondrocytes appear and start producing a new matrix, the fracture callus (Figs. 8-2 and 8-3).

The factors that stimulate fracture repair probably include the chemotactic factors and growth factors released during inflammation at the fracture site and bone matrix proteins, including growth factors exposed by disruption of the bone tissue (9). Although the inflammation caused by a fracture follows the same sequence for almost every fracture, the amount and composition of repair tissue and the rate of repair may differ depending on whether the fracture occurs through primarily cancellous bone in the epiphyses, metaphyses or vertebral bodies, or through primarily cortical bone in tubular bone diaphyses, the extent of soft tissue disruption surrounding the fracture and other factors that are discussed under the section Variables that Influence Fracture Healing.

The mechanical stability of the fracture site also influences the repair process. The summaries of fracture repair and remodeling that follow immediately below first describe healing of closed fractures that are not rigidly stabilized, that is, fractures where repair proceeds in the presence of motion at the fracture site (Fig. 8-4). A closed clavicle fracture not treated by internal fixation provides an example of repair and remodeling of an unstable fracture. The second summary describes healing of stable fractures, that is, fractures where repair proceeds at a rigidly stable fracture site with the fracture surfaces held in contact. Transverse diaphyseal fractures of the radius and ulna treated by open anatomic reduction and rigid internal fixation provide examples of the repair and remodeling of stable fractures.

Repair and Remodeling of Unstable Fractures

Disruption of blood vessels in the bone, marrow, periosteum, and surrounding tissue at the time of injury results in the extravasation of blood at the fracture site and the formation of a hematoma. Organization of this hematoma is usually recognized as the first step in fracture repair (Fig. 8-2). Experimental work indicates that loss of the hematoma impairs or slows fracture healing (10,11) suggesting that the hematoma and an intact surrounding periosteal soft tissue envelope that contains the hematoma may facilitate the initial stages of repair. Open fractures or treatment of fractures by open reduction disrupts organization of the hematoma, and thereby may slow the repair process. The reasons why a hematoma may affect fracture healing remain uncertain. Presumably, the intact fracture hematoma

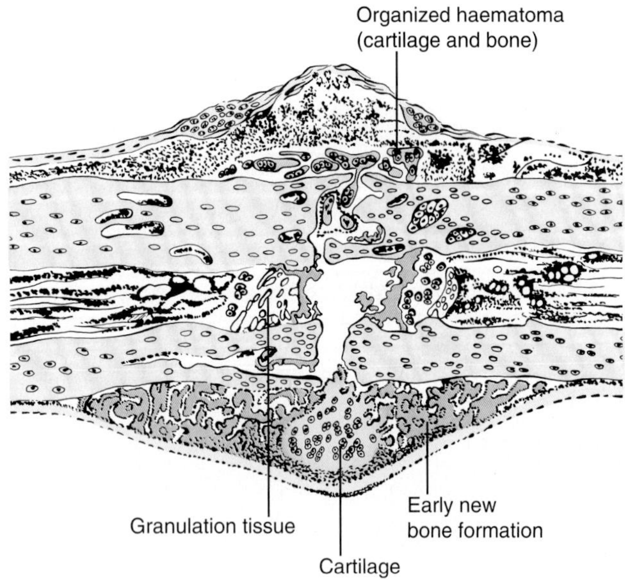

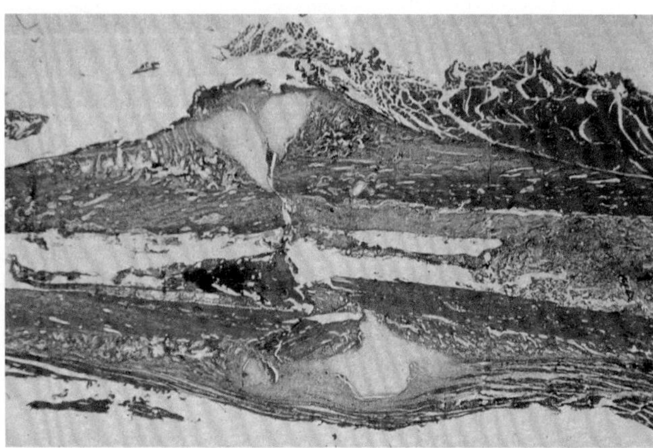

FIGURE 8-2 Early repair of a diaphyseal fracture of a long bone. **A.** Drawing showing organization of the hematoma, early woven bone formation in the subperiosteal regions, and cartilage formation in other areas. Periosteal cells contribute to healing this type of injury. If the fracture is rigidly immobilized or if it occurs primarily through cancellous bone and the cancellous surfaces lie in close apposition, there will be little evidence of fracture callus. **B.** Photomicrograph of a fractured rat femur nine days after injury showing cartilage and bone formation in the subperiosteal regions. (Reprinted from Einhorn TA. The cell and molecular biology of fracture healing. *Clin Orthop Relat Res* 1998;Oct[335 Suppl]:S7–S21.)

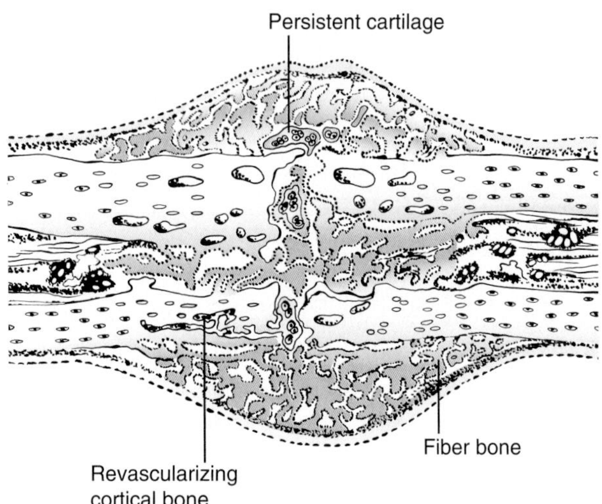

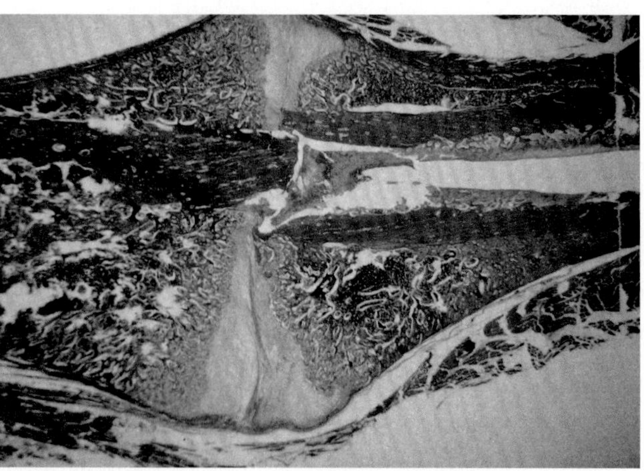

FIGURE 8-3 Progressive fracture healing by fracture callus. **A.** Drawing showing woven or fiber bone bridging the fracture gap and uniting the fracture fragments. Cartilage remains in the regions most distant from ingrowing capillary buds. In many instances, the capillaries are surrounded by new bone. Vessels revascularize the cortical bone at the fracture site. **B.** Photomicrograph of a fractured rat femur 21 days after injury showing fracture callus united the fracture fragments. (Reprinted from Einhorn TA. The cell and molecular biology of fracture healing. *Clin Orthop Relat Res* 1998;Oct[335 Suppl]:S7–S21.)

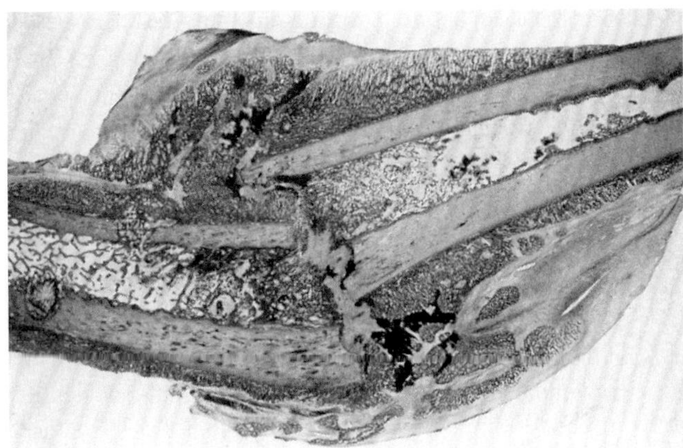

FIGURE 8-4 Light micrograph showing healing of a diaphyseal fracture under conditions of loading and motion. This femur fracture occurred in a pig that continued to use the limb for three weeks. Even though the fracture was not stabilized, it is healing. A large fracture callus consisting primarily of woven bone surrounds and unites the two fracture fragments. As the callus matures it progressively stabilizes the fracture. Notice that the fracture callus contains areas of mineralized and unmineralized cartilage.

provides a fibrin scaffold that facilitates migration of repair cells. In addition, growth factors and other proteins released by platelets and cells in the fracture hematoma mediate the critical initial events in fracture repair including cell migration, proliferation, and synthesis of a repair tissue matrix (8,9).

Although the volume of the vascular bed of an extremity increases shortly after fracture, presumably because of vasodilation, vascular proliferation also occurs in the region of the fracture. It appears that, under ordinary circumstances, the periosteal vessels contribute the majority of capillary buds early in normal bone healing, with the nutrient medullary artery becoming more important later in the process. Fibroblastic growth factors may be important mediators of the angiogenesis in fracture healing, but the exact stimuli responsible for vascular invasion and endothelial cell proliferation have not been defined. When the surgeon interferes with the blood supply to the fracture site, either by stripping the periosteum excessively or by destroying the medullary system through the use of intramedullary nails, repair must proceed with vessels derived from the surviving system.

The bone ends at the fracture site, deprived of their blood supply, become necrotic and are resorbed. In some fractures this may create a radiographically apparent gap at the fracture site several weeks or more after the fracture. The cells responsible for this function, the osteoclasts, come from a different cell line than the cells responsible for bone formation (2,3). They are derived from circulating monocytes in the blood and monocytic precursor cells from the bone marrow, whereas the osteoblasts develop from the undifferentiated mesenchymal cells that migrate into the fracture site.

Pluripotential mesenchymal cells, probably of common origin, form the fibrous tissue, cartilage, and eventually bone at the fracture site. Some of these cells originate in the injured tissues, while others migrate to the injury site with the blood vessels. Cells from the cambium layer of the periosteum form the earliest bone (Fig. 8-1A). Periosteal cells have an especially prominent role in healing childrens' fractures because the periosteum is thicker and more cellular in younger individuals. With increasing age, the periosteum becomes thinner and its contribution to fracture healing becomes less apparent. Osteoblasts from the endosteal surface also participate in bone formation, but surviving osteocytes do not appear to form repair tissue. The majority of cells responsible for osteogenesis during fracture healing appear in the fracture site with the granulation tissue that replaces the hematoma.

The mesenchymal cells at the fracture site proliferate, differentiate, and produce the *fracture callus* consisting of fibrous tissue, cartilage, and woven bone (Fig. 8-3). The fracture callus fills and surrounds the fracture site, and in the early stages of healing can be divided into the hard or bony callus and the softer fibrous and cartilaginous callus. The bone formed initially at the periphery of the callus by intramembranous bone formation is the *hard callus.* The *soft callus* forms in the central regions with low oxygen tension and consists primarily of cartilage and fibrous tissue. Bone gradually replaces the cartilage through the process of endochondral ossification, enlarging the hard callus and increasing the stability of the fracture fragments (Fig. 8-4). This process continues until new bone bridges the fracture site, reestablishing continuity between the cortical bone ends.

The biochemical composition of the fracture callus matrix changes as repair progresses (Fig. 8-5). The cells replace the fibrin clot with a loose fibrous matrix containing glycosaminoglycans, proteoglycans, and types I and III collagen. In many regions they convert this tissue to more dense fibrocartilage or hyaline-like cartilage. With formation of hyaline-like cartilage, type II collagen, cartilage-specific proteoglycan and link protein content increase. Newly formed woven bone remodels to lamellar bone, and with remodeling the content of collagen and other proteins returns to normal levels.

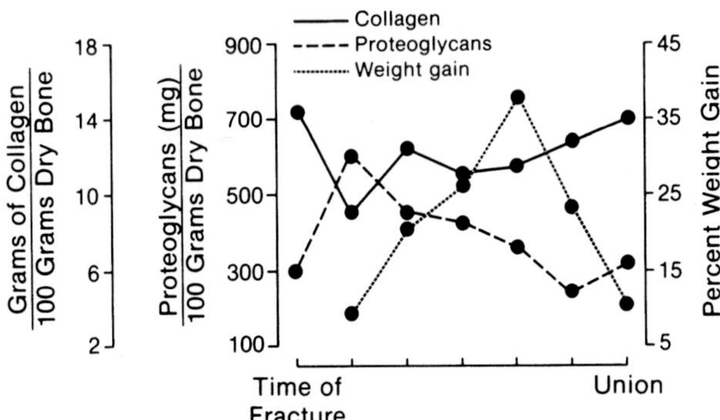

FIGURE 8-5 A schematic representation of the changing composition and mass of fracture callus. Collagen formation precedes significant accumulation of mineral. After an initial rise, proteoglycan concentration falls gradually as fracture healing progresses. The total mass of the fracture callus increases during repair and then decreases during remodeling.

Analysis of fracture repair demonstrates a close correlation between the activation of genes for blood vessel, cartilage, and bone-specific proteins in the cells and the development of granulation tissue, cartilage, and bone (12), demonstrating that fracture repair depends on regulation of gene expression in the repair cells. The simultaneous occurrence of chondrogenesis, endochondral ossification, and intramembranous bone formation in different regions of the fracture callus suggests (Fig. 8-4) that local mediators and small variations in the microenvironment, including mechanical stresses, determine what genes will be expressed and therefore the type of tissue the repair cells form. Local mediators that may influence repair cell function include growth factors released from cells and platelets and oxygen tension. Acidic fibroblast growth factor (FGF), basic FGF, and transforming growth factor beta (TGF-β) may stimulate chondrocyte proliferation and cartilage formation, osteoblast proliferation, and bone synthesis. TGF-β released from platelets immediately after injury may initiate formation of fracture callus. TGF-β synthesis is also associated with cartilage hypertrophy and calcification at the endochondral ossification front.

As mineralization of fracture callus proceeds, the bone ends gradually become enveloped in a fusiform mass of callus containing increasing amounts of woven bone. The increasing mineral content is closely associated with increasing stiffness of the fracture callus (13). Stability of the fracture fragments progressively increases because of the internal and external callus formation, and eventually *clinical union* occurs—that is, the fracture site becomes stable and pain-free. *Radiographic union* occurs when plain radiographs show bone trabeculae or cortical bone crossing the fracture site, and often occurs later than clinical union. However, even at this stage healing is not complete. The immature fracture callus is weaker than normal bone, and it only gains full strength during remodeling.

During the final stages of repair, remodeling of the repair tissue begins with replacement of woven bone by lamellar bone and resorption of unneeded callus. Radioisotope studies show increased activity in fracture sites long after the patient has full restoration of function and plain radiographs show bone union, demonstrating that fracture remodeling continues for years after clinical and radiographic union. Remodeling of fracture repair tissue after all woven bone has been replaced presumably consists of osteoclastic resorption of superfluous or poorly placed trabeculae and formation of new struts of bone along lines of stress.

Although fracture callus remodeling results from an elaborate sequence of cellular and matrix changes, the important functional result for the patient is an increase in mechanical stability. The progressive increase in fracture stability can be described as consisting of four stages (14).

Stage I: A healing bone subjected to torsional testing fails through the original fracture site with a low-stiffness pattern.

Stage II: The bone still fails through the fracture site, but the characteristics of failure indicate a high-stiffness, hard-tissue pattern.

Stage III: The bone fails partly through the original fracture site and partly through the previously intact bone with a high-stiffness, hard-tissue pattern.

Stage IV: Failure does not occur through the fracture site, indicating that new tissue at the fracture site duplicates the mechanical properties of the uninjured tissue.

Despite successful fracture healing, the bone density of the involved limb may be decreased for years (15,16). In one study patients with healed tibial fractures had decreased bone density in the involved limb decades after the injury (16). The clinical significance of these observations remain unclear, but they suggest that fractures, and possibly the decreased loading of a limb after fracture, may cause long lasting changes in the tissues.

Repair and Remodeling of Stabilized Fractures (Primary Bone Healing)

As described above, when motion occurs within certain limits at a fracture site, fracture callus progressively stabilizes the bone fragments and remodeling of the fracture callus eventually produces lamellar bone. However, when the fracture surfaces are rigidly held in contact, fracture healing can occur without grossly visible callus in either cancellous or cortical bone. Some surgeons refer to this type of fracture healing as *primary bone healing*, indicating that it occurs without the formation and replacement of visible fracture callus.

In most fractures that are rigidly stabilized with the bone ends directly apposed there are regions of the fracture line where the bone ends are in contact and other areas where there are small gaps. Where there is contact between bone ends, lamellar bone can form directly across the fracture line by extension of osteons. A cluster of osteoclasts cuts across the fracture line, osteoblasts following the osteoclasts deposit new bone, and blood vessels follow the osteoblasts. The new bone matrix, enclosed osteocytes, and blood vessels form new haversian systems. Where gaps exist that prevent direct extension of osteons across the fracture site, osteoblasts fill the defects with woven bone. After the gap fills with woven bone, haversian remodeling begins, reestablishing normal cortical bone structure. Cutting cones consisting of osteoclasts followed by osteoblasts and blood vessels traverse the woven bone in the fracture gap, depositing lamellar bone and reestablishing the cortical bone blood supply across the fracture site without grossly visible fracture callus. If a segment of cortical bone is necrotic, gap healing by direct extension of osteons still can occur, but at a slower rate, and areas of necrotic cortical bone remain unremodeled for a prolonged period.

Many impacted epiphyseal, metaphyseal, and vertebral body fractures where cancellous and in some regions cortical bone surfaces interlock have sufficient stability to permit primary bone healing at sites where bone surfaces make direct contact. The same type of cancellous bone healing can occur at osteotomies through metaphyseal bone, rigidly stabilized intra-articular fractures and surgical arthrodesis treated with rigid stabilization. Most diaphyseal osteotomies, acute diaphyseal fractures of long bones, and unstable metaphyseal fractures require use of devices that compress and rigidly stabilize the fracture site to allow primary healing.

Failure of Fracture Healing

Despite optimal treatment, some fractures heal slowly or fail to heal (17). It is difficult to set the time when a given fracture should be united, but when healing progresses more slowly than average, the slow progress is referred to as *delayed union*. Watson-Jones (18) described a condition he called *slow union*, where the fracture line remains clearly visible radiographically, but there is no undue separation of the fragments, no cavitation of the surfaces, no calcification, and no sclerosis. This indolent fracture healing may be related to the severity of the injury, poor blood supply, the age and nutritional status of the patient, or other factors. It is not an ununited fracture, but rather a variation of normal healing. Failure of bone healing, or *nonunion*, results from an arrest of the healing process. A nonunion that occurs despite the formation of a large volume of callus around the fracture site is commonly referred to as a *hypertrophic nonunion* (Fig. 8-6), in contrast to an *atrophic nonunion* (Fig. 8-7) where little or no callus forms and bone resorption occurs at the fracture site. In some nonunions, cartilagenous tissue forms over the fracture surfaces and the cavity between the surfaces fills with a clear fluid resembling normal joint or bursal fluid creating a *pseudarthrosis*, or false joint. Pseudarthroses may or may not be painful, but they almost uniformly remain unstable indefinitely. In other nonunions the gap between the bone ends fills with fibrous or fibrocartilagenous tissue. Occasionally dense fibrous and cartilagenous tissue firmly stabilizes a fracture creating a *fibrous union*. Although fibrous unions may be painless and unite the fracture fragments, they fail to restore the normal strength of the bone.

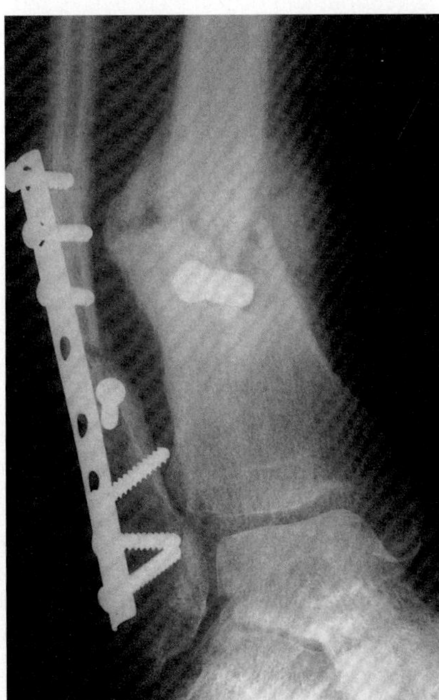

FIGURE 8-6 Hypertrophic delayed union of a distal tibial fracture 5 months after injury. Note the abundant callus but incomplete bridging of the fracture gap.

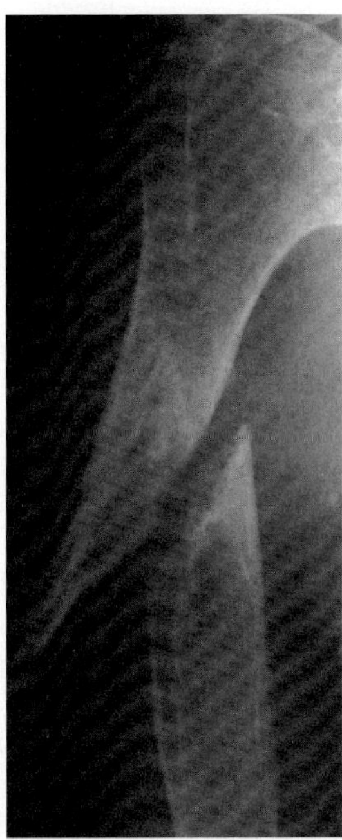

FIGURE 8-7 Atrophic nonunion of a humeral shaft fracture 18 months after fracture. Note the absence of callus.

Variables that Influence Fracture Healing

Occasionally delayed unions or nonunions occur without apparent cause, but in many instances injury, patient, and treatment variables that adversely influenced fracture healing can be identified. These variables include

- Severe soft tissue damage associated with open and high energy closed fractures
- Infection
- Segmental fractures
- Pathologic fractures
- Fractures with soft tissue interposition
- Poor local blood supply
- Systemic diseases
- Malnutrition
- Corticosteroid use
- Iatrogenic interference with healing

Many other variables have been reported to retard bone healing (6). Some of them exert an adverse influence that can be measured in experimental studies, but may not cause clinically significant impairment of fracture healing. Others, like distraction of a fracture site or interposition of soft tissues in a fracture site have not been examined systematically in experimental studies, but clinical experience shows that they can impair fracture healing.

Injury Variables

Open Fractures. Severe open fractures cause soft tissue disruption, fracture displacement, and, in some instances, significant bone loss. Extensive tearing or crushing of the soft tissue disrupts the blood supply to the fracture site, leaving substantial volumes of necrotic bone and soft tissue, impeding or preventing formation of a fracture hematoma and delaying formation of repair tissue. Exposed bone and soft tissue become desiccated, increasing the volume of necrotic tissue and the risk of infection. Early use of vascularized soft tissue flaps to cover bone exposed by severe open fractures can prevent desiccation and facilitate healing of these injuries. In addition to the problems created by the soft tissue damage, open fractures may become infected. Management of this complication usually requires debriding infected bone and soft tissue along with antibiotic treatment. Although infection compromises bone healing, infected fractures can unite if they are stabilized and the infection suppressed. This may leave the patient with chronic osteomyelitis, but in most instances bone union with a chronic infection is a better result than a nonunion.

Severity of Injury. Severe fractures may be open or closed. They may be associated with large soft tissue wounds, loss of soft tissue, displacement and comminution of the bone fragments, loss of bone, and decreased blood supply to the fracture site. Comminution of bone fragments generally indicates that there is also extensive soft tissue injury. However, some patients with osteopenic bone may suffer comminuted fractures from low energy injuries that cause minimal soft tissue injury. Displacement of the fracture fragments and severe trauma to the soft tissues retard fracture healing, probably because the extensive tissue damage increases the volume of necrotic tissue, impedes the migration of mesenchymal cells and vascular invasion, decreases the number of viable mesenchymal cells, and disrupts the local blood supply. Less severe injuries leave an intact soft tissue envelope that contains the fracture hematoma, provides a ready source of mesenchymal cells, a soft tissue tube that directs the repair efforts of these cells, and an internal splint that contributes to immobilization of the fragments.

Intra-articular Fractures. Because they extend into joint surfaces and because joint motion or loading may cause movement of the fracture fragments, intra-articular fractures can present challenging treatment problems. Most intra-articular fractures heal, but if the alignment and congruity of the joint surface is not restored, the joint may be unstable, and in some instances, especially if the fracture is not rigidly stabilized, healing may be delayed or nonunion may occur. However, prolonged immobilization of a joint with an intra-articular fracture frequently causes joint stiffness. For these reasons, surgeons usually attempt to reduce and securely fix unstable intra-articular fractures. This approach ideally restores joint alignment and congruity and allows at least some joint motion while the fracture heals. Unfortunately, restoring joint alignment, congruity and stability in patients with severe intra-articular fractures may require extensive surgical exposure that further compromises the blood supply to the fracture site. Even after reduction and adequate initial stabilization, intra-articular fractures may displace due to high transarticular forces, failure of the stabilization or collapse of the subchondral cancellous bone. This late loss of reduction occurs most frequently after comminuted fractures of the proximal and distal tibia and distal radius.

Segmental Fractures. A segmental fracture of a long bone impairs or disrupts the intramedullary blood supply to the middle fragment. If there is severe soft tissue trauma, the periosteal blood supply to the middle fragment may also be compromised. Possibly because of this, the probability of delayed union or nonunion, proximally or distally, may be increased. These problems occur most frequently in segmental fractures of the tibia, especially at the distal fracture site (19,20). In contrast, segmental fractures of the femur less commonly develop nonunions, presumably because of the better soft tissue coverage and resulting better blood supply. When internal fixation of a segmental fracture is performed, the soft tissue attachments of the middle fragment should be preserved whenever possible.

Soft Tissue Interposition. Interposition of soft tissue including muscle, fascia, tendon, and occasionally nerves and vessels between fracture fragments will compromise fracture healing. The presence of soft tissue interposition should be suspected when the bone fragments cannot be brought into apposition or alignment during attempted closed reduction. If this occurs, an open reduction may be necessary to extricate the interposed tissue and achieve an acceptable position of the fracture fragments.

Damage to Blood Supply. Lack of an adequate vascular supply can significantly delay or prevent fracture healing. Insufficient blood supply for fracture healing may result from a severe soft tissue and bone injury or from the normally limited blood supply to some bones or bone regions. For example, the vulnerable blood supplies of the femoral head, scaphoid, and talar body may predispose these bones to delayed union or nonunion, even in the absence of severe soft tissue damage or fracture displacement. Extensive surgical dissection may also compromise the vascular supply to a fracture site, especially in regions of the skeleton with a vulnerable blood supply or in fractures with associated severe soft tissue injuries, or in regions with minimal surrounding soft tissue, for example, the distal tibia.

Patient Variables

Age. Patient age significantly influences the rate of fracture healing. Infants have the most rapid rate of fracture healing.

The rate of healing declines with increasing age up to skeletal maturity, but following completion of skeletal growth the rate of fracture healing does not appear to decline significantly with increasing age nor does the risk of nonunions significantly increase. One possible reason for the greater healing potential of children may be increased availability of cells that produce repair tissue: younger cells may differentiate more rapidly from the mesenchymal pool and the pool of undifferentiated mesenchymal cells may be larger in children. In addition, the rapid bone remodeling that accompanies growth allows correction of a greater degree of deformity in children.

Nutrition. The cell migration, proliferation, and matrix synthesis necessary to heal a fracture requires substantial energy. Furthermore, to synthesize large volumes of collagens, proteoglycans, and other matrix macromolecules the cells need a steady supply of the components of these molecules: proteins and carbohydrates. As a result, the metabolic state of the patient can alter the outcome of injury, and in severely malnourished patients injuries that would heal rapidly in well-nourished individuals may fail to heal. Although few surgeons in economically developed countries see many severely malnourished patients, they may see relatively large numbers of patients with milder forms of protein-calorie malnutrition and other dietary deficiencies. Jensen and associates (21) found a 42.4% incidence of clinical or subclinical malnutrition in patients undergoing orthopaedic surgical procedures. A study of 490 patients with hip fractures found that 87 of these patients (18%) suffered from malnutrition and that the malnourished patients stayed in the hospital longer, were less likely to recover their pre-fracture level of activity, and were more likely to die within one year of their hip fracture (22).

Because trauma and major surgery can cause malnutrition and thereby decrease immunocompetence (21), surgeons must pay careful attention to nutrition and metabolic balance in patients with multiple injuries (23). Even in well-nourished patients, the nutritional demands of healing multiple injuries can exceed intake (21). Leung and colleagues (7) reported that the adenosine triphosphate (ATP) content of a 2-week rabbit fracture callus was a thousand times greater than the ATP content of normal bone. Others have suggested that a single long-bone fracture can temporarily increase metabolic requirements 20% to 25%, and that multiple injuries and infection can increase metabolic requirements by more than 50% (21,24). Failure to meet these increased nutritional needs may increase mortality and surgical complications including infection, wound dehiscence, impaired healing, and slower rehabilitation. An experimental study of fracture healing demonstrated that fracture callus does not achieve normal strength in states of dietary deficiency, and that a dietary deficiency of protein reduces fracture callus strength and energy storage capacity (25). For these reasons, optimal treatment of injured patients requires assessment of their nutritional status and treatment, which may include nutritional support.

Systemic Hormones. A variety of hormones can influence fracture healing (6). Corticosteroids may compromise fracture healing (26) possibly by inhibiting differentiation of osteoblasts from mesenchymal cells (27) and by decreasing synthesis of bone organic matrix components (26) necessary for repair. Prolonged corticosteroid administration may also decrease bone density and increase the probability of hip, distal radius, rib and vertebral fractures (28). The role of growth hormone in fracture healing remains uncertain. Some experimental work suggests that growth hormone deficiency adversely affects fracture healing and that growth hormone replacement can improve healing (29,30). Other investigations indicate that excess growth hormone may have little or no effect (31,32) and that normal alterations in the level of circulating growth hormone have little effect on fracture healing. Thyroid hormone, calcitonin, insulin, and anabolic steroids have been reported in experimental situations to enhance the rate of fracture healing (6). Diabetes, hypervitaminosis D, and rickets have been shown to retard fracture healing in experimental situations. However, clinical experience shows that fractures heal in patients with hormonal disturbances, although union may be slower than normal.

Nicotine and Other Agents. In addition to hormones a variety of other agents may adversely affect fracture healing. Clinical experience suggests that cigarette smoking inhibits fracture healing, and a study of tibial osteotomy healing in rabbits showed that animals exposed to nicotine healed fractures more slowly and had a higher percentage of nonunions (33). The mechanism of the nicotine effect on bone healing remains unknown, but a study of bone graft incorporation in rabbits showed that nicotine inhibited vascularization of autogenous cancellous bone grafts (34). Agents used to treat malignancies may also inhibit bone healing (35).

Tissue Variables

Form of Bone (Cancellous or Cortical). Healing of cancellous and cortical fractures differs, probably because of the differences in surface area, cellularity, and vascularity. Apposed cancellous bone surfaces usually unite rapidly, possibly because the large surface area of cancellous bone per unit volume creates many points of bone contact rich in cells and blood supply and because osteoblasts will form new bone directly on existing trabeculae. Because woven bone forms across points of cancellous bone contact, stable fractures located primarily in cancellous regions, especially impacted fractures where the trabeculae of the fracture fragments have been forced together so that they interdigitate, form little or no visible external callus and rarely fail to heal. Where fractured cancellous bone surfaces are not impacted, new bone spreads from the points of contact to fill gaps. When a gap is excessively large, two bone-forming fronts grow from the fracture fragments and eventually meet, but if excessive motion occurs, external callus (including cartilage) may develop. In contrast, cortical bone has a much smaller surface area per unit volume and generally a less extensive internal blood supply, and regions of necrotic cortical bone must be removed before new bone can form.

Bone Necrosis. Normally, healing proceeds from both sides of a fracture, but if one fracture fragment has lost its blood supply, healing depends entirely on in-growth of capillaries from the living side or surrounding soft tissues. If one fracture fragment is avascular the fracture can heal, but the rate is slower and the incidence of healing is lower than if both fragments have a normal blood supply (17). If both fragments are avascular, the chances for union decrease further. Traumatic or surgical disruption of blood vessels, infection, prolonged use of corticosteroids, and radiation treatment can cause bone necrosis. Irradiated bone, even when it is not obviously necrotic, often heals at a slower rate than normal bone (36,37). Nonunion may occur in radiated bones (38), probably because of radiation-induced cell death, thrombosis of vessels, and fibrosis of the marrow. These changes may reduce the population of cells that can participate in repair, increase the volume of necrotic tissue, and interfere with the ingrowth of capillaries and migration of fibroblasts into the fracture site.

Bone Disease. Pathologic fractures occur through diseased bone and therefore require less force than that necessary to break normal bone. Commonly recognized causes of pathologic fractures include osteoporosis, osteomalacia, primary malignant bone tumors, metastatic bone tumors, benign bone tumors, bone cysts, osteogenesis imperfecta, fibrous dysplasia, Paget disease, hyperparathyroidism, and infections. Fractures through bone involved with primary or secondary malignancies usually will not heal if the neoplasm is not treated. Subperiosteal new bone and fracture callus may form, but the mass of malignant cells impairs or prevents fracture healing, particularly if the malignant cells continue to destroy bone. Fractures through infected bone present a similar problem. Thus, healing fractures through malignancies or infections usually requires treatment of the underlying local disease or removal of the involved bone. Depending on the extent of bone involvement and the aggressiveness of the lesion, fractures through bones with nonmalignant conditions like simple bone cysts and Paget disease will heal. The most prevalent bone disease, osteoporosis, does not impair fracture healing, but where there is diminished surface contact of apposing cortical or cancellous bone surfaces due to decreased bone mass the time required to restore normal bone mechanical strength may be increased. Furthermore, decreased bone mass reduces the strength and stability of the interface between the bone and screws used for internal fixation. This may lead to failure of internal fixation and subsequent delayed healing or nonunion.

Infection. Infection can slow or prevent bone healing. For fracture healing to proceed at the maximum rate, the local cells must be devoted primarily to healing the fracture. If infection occurs following fracture or if the fracture occurs as a result of the infection, many cells must be diverted to attempt to wall off and eliminate the infection and energy consumption increases. Furthermore, infection may cause necrosis of normal tissue, edema, and thrombosis of blood vessels, thereby retarding or preventing healing. Surgical debridement of infected fractures may cause further tissue damage.

Treatment Variables

Apposition of Fracture Fragments. Decreasing the fracture gap decreases the volume of repair tissue needed to heal a fracture. Restoring fracture fragment apposition is especially important if the surrounding soft tissues have been disrupted or when soft tissues lie between the fracture fragments. When a significant portion of the periosteum and other soft tissue components remain intact or can be rapidly restored, lack of bone fragment apposition may not impair healing.

Loading and Micromotion. The optimal conditions for fracture healing include loading of the repair tissue (39). Based on the available evidence it appears that loading a fracture site stimulates bone formation while decreased loading slows fracture healing (39). In addition, experimental work and clinical experience shows that early or even almost immediate controlled loading and limb movement, including induced micromotion at long bone fracture sites, may promote fracture healing (39). However, the optimal timing, intensity, and pattern of loading for specific fractures have not been defined and probably vary not only among fractures, but among patients.

Fracture Stabilization. Fracture stabilization by traction, cast immobilization, external fixation, and internal fixation can facilitate fracture healing by preventing repeated disruption of repair tissue. Some fractures (e.g., displaced femoral neck and scaphoid fractures) rarely heal if they are not rigidly stabilized. Fracture stability appears to be particularly important for healing when there is extensive associated soft tissue injury, when the blood supply to the fracture site is marginal, and when the fracture occurs within a synovial joint. Excessive motion secondary to ineffective stabilization, repeated manipulation or excessive loading and motion retards fracture healing and may cause nonunion. In these injuries it is probable that the repeated excessive motion disrupts the initial fracture hematoma or granulation tissue, delaying or preventing formation of fracture callus. If excessive motion continues, a cleft forms between the fracture ends, and a pseudarthrosis develops.

Despite the importance of stability for healing of some fractures, motion does not impair healing of other fractures. During the early part of repair, motion occurs at most fractures except for those treated by rigid internal fixation. Fractures with intact surrounding soft tissues that provide some stability in a well-vascularized region of bone may heal rapidly even though palpable motion of the fracture site persists for weeks after injury. For example, closed rib, clavicle, many humeral diaphyseal, and metacarpal and metatarsal fractures heal even though the fracture fragments remain mobile until fracture callus stabilizes them.

Unlike traction, cast immobilization and at least some forms of external fixation, and internal fixation of fractures with metallic implants can produce rigid stabilization of fractures. Although rigid stabilization of a fracture makes possible primary bone repair without cartilage or connective tissue intermediates, it does not accelerate fracture healing. Rigid fixation of fractures makes it possible to restore and maintain anatomic apposition of fracture fragments. This approach has proven especially beneficial in the treatment of intra-articular fractures, diaphyseal fractures of the radius and ulna and other selected diaphyseal and metaphyseal fractures.

Although rigid internal stabilization of fractures with metallic implants has multiple advantages, it also has potential disadvantages. Rigid fixation can alter fracture remodeling and decrease bone density because the stiffness of most implants differs from that of bone. For example, steel is more than ten times as stiff as bone. When a fractured bone, rigidly fixed with a stiff implant, is loaded, the bone is shielded from normal stresses by the more rigid implant. Regional loss of bone mass may occur which increases the probability of re-fracture following removal of the plate (40), although re-fractures following removal of plates may also be due to the presence of screw holes that act as stress risers.

Treatment that Interferes with Healing

Most fractures will heal when treated by a variety of methods. Furthermore, the healing potential of many fractures, especially those in children, can overcome less than optimal treatment, but some surgical and nonsurgical interventions interfere with healing and may cause delayed union or nonunion. Surgical exposure of a fracture site can interfere with healing. The fracture hematoma is disrupted, the blood supply to the fracture site and the surrounding soft tissues may be damaged and opening a closed fracture may lead to infection. Inadequate immobilization of some fractures (for example, scaphoid and femoral neck fractures), distraction of fracture fragments by internal or external fixation devices or traction, repeated manipulations, or excessive early motion of a fracture may interfere with healing.

SYNOVIAL JOINT HEALING

Because cartilage lacks blood vessels, it cannot respond to cell damage with inflammation. However, injuries that disrupt subchondral bone as well as the overlying cartilage initiate the fracture healing process, and the repair tissue from bone will fill an articular cartilage defect. Cartilage healing then follows the sequence of inflammation, repair, and remodeling like that seen in bone or dense fibrous tissue (6,41–43). Unlike these tissues, the repair tissue that fills cartilage defects from subchondral bone initially differentiates toward articular cartilage rather than toward dense fibrous tissue or bone.

In addition to direct mechanical injury, articular cartilage can sustain damage by disruption of the synovial membrane leading to exposure of the articular cartilage. Because of these special features, acute traumatic injuries to synovial joints can be separated into the following categories: disruption of the soft tissues of the synovial joint without direct mechanical cartilage injury, and mechanical injury of articular cartilage.

Healing Following Disruption of Synovial Joint Soft Tissues

Exposure of cartilage to air by traumatic or surgical disruption of the joint capsule and synovial membrane can alter cartilage matrix composition by stimulating degradation of proteoglycans or suppressing synthesis of proteoglycans (42). A decrease in matrix proteoglycan concentration decreases cartilage stiffness and may make the tissue more vulnerable to damage from impact loading. Prompt restoration of the synovial environment by closure of the synovial membrane will allow chondrocytes to repair the damage to the macromolecular framework of the matrix, and the tissue may regain its normal composition and function. However, prolonged exposure of the articular surface to air can desiccate the tissue and kill chondrocytes (44).

It is not clear what duration of exposure causes irreversible damage. The available evidence, based on animal experiments, suggests that damage to the matrix macromolecular framework occurs with any disruption of the synovial membrane (42), but clinical experience suggests that permanent or progressive damage in human joints rarely occurs following temporary disruption of the synovial cavity. Furthermore, cartilage can be restored to its normal condition if the loss of matrix proteoglycans does not exceed the amount the cells can replenish, if a sufficient number of chondrocytes remain viable, and if the collagenous meshwork of the matrix remains intact (45).

Exposure injury to cartilage can be minimized by decreasing the period of time that the cartilage is unprotected by synovium or other soft tissues. If cartilage must remain unprotected, keeping the surface moist with a physiologic solution may be helpful. Because cartilage that has sustained exposure injury may be temporarily more vulnerable to mechanical injury, it seems advisable to minimize immediate impact loading of cartilage that has experienced this type of injury.

Healing Following Damage to the Articular Surface

Acute traumatic injury to articular cartilage may occur through several mechanisms. Osteochondral fractures mechanically disrupt cartilage and bone tissue at the fracture site, but in addition, osteochondral fractures may be associated with blunt trauma limited to cartilage, abrasions of the articular surface, or chondral fractures (41,42,46). Alternatively, blunt trauma to a synovial joint may occur without an associated bone or cartilage fracture. Therefore, acute articular cartilage injuries can be separated into those caused by blunt trauma that does not disrupt or fracture tissue and those caused by blunt trauma or other mechanisms that mechanically disrupt or fracture the tissue. Injuries that fracture or disrupt cartilage can be further divided into those limited to articular cartilage and those affecting both cartilage and subchondral bone.

Blunt Trauma Without Tissue Disruption

Although the effects of acute blunt trauma on articular cartilage have not been extensively studied clinically or experimentally, blunt trauma to joints occurs frequently as an isolated injury or in association with a fracture or dislocation. Among the reasons for the limited number of studies are the lack of clearly defined clinically significant consequences of blunt trauma to cartilage, the ability of cartilage to withstand large acute loads without apparent immediate damage, lack of a clinically detectable injury and repair response in cartilage following blunt trauma, and difficulty in defining the relationship between the intensity of blunt trauma and the extent of cartilage injury (46). Despite these limitations, current information suggests that acute blunt trauma to articular cartilage may damage it even when there is no grossly apparent tissue disruption and these injuries may lead to later degeneration of the articular surface.

Physiologic levels of impact loading have not been demonstrated to produce cartilage injury, and clinical experience suggests that acute impact loading considerably greater than physiologic loading but less than that necessary to produce detectable fractures rarely causes significant articular cartilage injury. However, acute impact loading less than that necessary to produce visible tissue disruption may cause cartilage swelling and increased cartilage collagen fibril diameter and alter the relationships between collagen fibrils and proteoglycans (46). This observation suggests that blunt trauma, under at least some conditions, may disrupt the macromolecular framework of the cartilage matrix and possibly injure cells without producing detectable fracture of the cartilage or bone. Presumably this tissue damage would make cartilage more vulnerable to subsequent injury and progressive deterioration if the cells could not rapidly restore the matrix. This type of injury may help explain the development of articular cartilage degeneration following joint dislocations or other types of acute joint trauma that do not cause visible damage to the articular surface.

Trauma that Disrupts Cartilage

Injuries Limited to Articular Cartilage. Lacerations, traumatically induced splits of articular cartilage perpendicular to the surface, or chondral fractures kill chondrocytes at the site of the injury and disrupt the matrix. Viable chondrocytes near the injury may proliferate, form clusters of new cells, and synthesize new matrix (42). They do not migrate to the site of the injury, and the matrix they synthesize does not fill the defect. A hematoma does not form, and inflammatory cells and fibroblasts do not migrate to the site of injury. This minimal response may be due to the inability of chondrocytes to respond effectively to injury, the inability of undifferentiated mesenchymal cells to invade the tissue defect, and the lack of a clot that attracts cells and gives them a temporary matrix to adhere to and replace with more permanent tissue. Although the response of chondrocytes to injury will not heal a clinically significant cartilage defect, most traumatic defects limited to small areas of articular cartilage do not progress.

Lacerations, fractures, or abrasions of the articular surface tangential or parallel to the surface presumably follow a similar course. Cells directly adjacent to the injury site may die and others may show signs of increased proliferative or synthetic activity. A thin acellular layer of nonfibrillar material may form over an injured surface, but there is no evidence that the cell activity stimulated by the injury restores the articular cartilage to its original state.

Osteochondral Injury. An articular cartilage injury that also damages subchondral bone stimulates bone fracture healing including inflammation, repair, and remodeling (47–49). Blood from ruptured bone blood vessels fills the injury site with a hematoma that extends from the bony injury into the chondral defect. The clot may fill a small chondral defect, generally one less than several millimeters wide, but it usually does not completely fill larger defects. Inflammatory cells migrate through the clot followed by fibroblasts that begin to synthesize a collagenous matrix. In the bone defect and the chondral defect some of the mesenchymal cells assume a rounded shape and begin to synthesize a matrix that closely resembles the matrix of articular cartilage.

Within weeks of injury the repair tissue forming in the chondral portion of the defect and the tissue forming in the bony portion of the defect begin to differ. Tissue in the chondral defect has a higher proportion of repair cells and matrix that resemble hyaline cartilage (Fig. 8-8), while the repair tissue in the bone defect has started to form new bone. Within 6 weeks of injury repair tissue in the two locations is distinguished by the new bone formed in the bone defect, the absence of bone in the chondral defect, and the higher proportion of hyaline cartilage repair tissue in the chondral defect.

While the initial repair of an osteochondral injury usually follows a predictable course, subsequent changes in the cartilage repair tissue vary considerably among similar defects. In some chondral defects the production of a cartilaginous matrix continues and the cells may retain the appearance and some of the functions of chondrocytes, including production of type II collagen and proteoglycans. They rarely if ever restore the matrix to the original state but they may succeed in producing a form of fibrocartilaginous scar that maintains the integrity of the articular surface and provides clinically satisfactory joint function for years. Unfortunately, in many other injuries the cartilage repair tissue deteriorates rather than remodeling. It becomes progressively more fibrillar, and the cells lose the appearance of chondrocytes and appear to become more fibroblastic. The fibrous matrix may begin to fibrillate and fragment, eventually leaving exposed bone (Fig. 8-8). The reasons why healing of some osteochondral injuries results in formation of fibrocartilage that may provide at least temporary joint function, while others fail to repair, have not been well defined.

Variables that Influence Cartilage Healing

Injury Variables

The volume and surface area of cartilage injury and the degrees of disruption of joint congruity and stability can influence joint

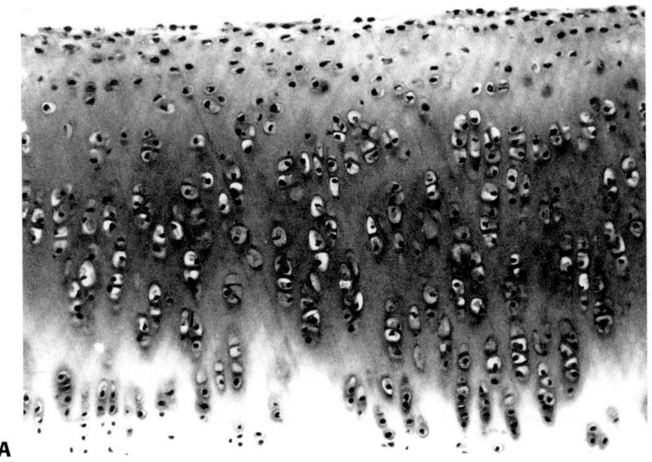

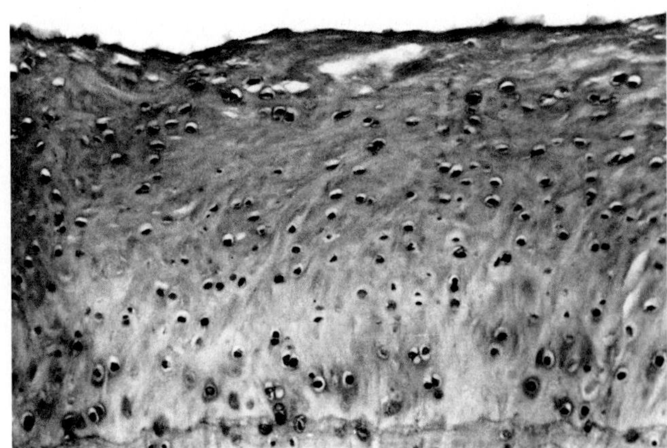

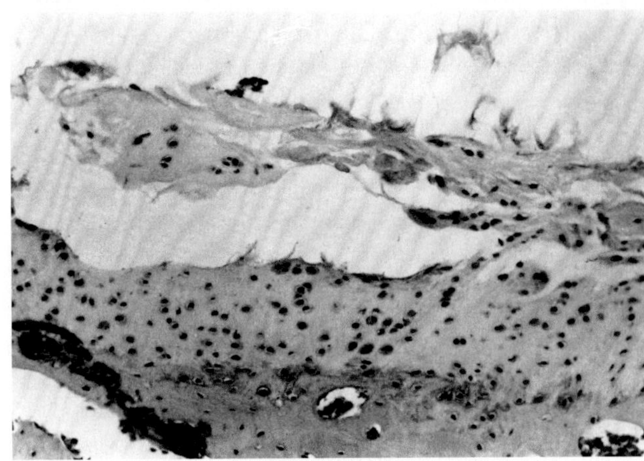

FIGURE 8-8 **A.** Normal rabbit articular cartilage showing the homogenous extracellular matrix. The chondrocytes near the articular surface are relatively small and flattened, whereas those in the middle and deeper zones of the articular cartilage have a more spherical shape. **B.** Well-formed fibrocartilaginous repair cartilage. Notice that the extracellular matrix is more fibrillar and the chondrocytes do not show the same organization as normal articular cartilage. Nonetheless, this repair cartilage does fill the defect in the articular surface. In most instances after osteochondral injury, this type of tissue forms within 6 to 8 weeks. **C.** Photomicrograph showing fibrillation and fragmentation of fibrocartilaginous repair tissue. Because fibrocartilaginous repair tissue lacks the mechanical properties of normal articular cartilage, it often degenerates over time. (Reprinted from Buckwalter JA, Mow VC. Cartilage repair and osteoarthritis. In: Moskowitz RW, Howell DS, Goldberg VM, et al., eds. *Osteoarthritis diagnosis and medical/surgical management*, 2nd ed. Philadelphia: WB Saunders, 1992:86–87, with permission.)

healing (42,43). Furthermore, clinical experience suggests that high intensity joint trauma may cause articular cartilage damage that is not detectable by current imaging methods. The involvement of subchondral bone and joint capsule make treatment more difficult and can adversely influence cartilage healing. Although it is generally accepted that more severe joint injuries are more likely to lead to progressive joint degeneration and osteoarthritis, the relationships between specific injury variables including intensity of force applied to the joint surface, degree of articular surface comminution and incongruity, and the degree of joint instability and the risk of osteoarthritis have not been defined.

Patient Variables

As in other tissues, patient age may influence the healing potential of cartilage injuries (47,50–54). That is, infants or young children have greater potential to heal and remodel chondral and osteochondral injuries than older individuals, although this has not been thoroughly investigated. Other patient variables such as weight, activity level, and systemic disease may be clinically important, but their influence has not been demonstrated.

Treatment Variables

Apposition. Because experimental work indicates that smaller defects in articular cartilage tend to heal more successfully (42,55), it seems reasonable to expect that treatments that decrease the volume and surface area of a chondral defect, such as open reduction and internal fixation of osteochondral fractures, will increase the probability of successful cartilage repair. Experimental work indicates that 1 mm or smaller defects tend to heal more successfully than larger defects (42,55) and eliminating the gap between fragments of articular fractures results in better anatomic restoration of an articular surface. Therefore, decreasing the width of an osteochondral fracture gap should increase the probability of a clinically successful result. However, depending on the location of the chondral injury within the joint and the presence or absence of other injuries to the joint, some separations of osteochondral fractures or loss of segments of the articular surface may not produce clinically significant disturbances of synovial joint function or rapid cartilage deterioration (49).

The clinical results of intra-articular fractures show that articular surfaces can sustain limited traumatic loss of cartilage without immediate disturbance of joint function and possibly without long-term consequences. However, the extent of tolerable loss of the articular surface has not been defined and may vary among joints (49).

Loading and Motion. Prolonged immobilization of a joint following osteochondral fractures can lead to significant adhesions as well as deterioration of uninjured cartilage, resulting in poor synovial joint function. Early motion during the repair and remodeling phases of healing decreases or prevents adhesions and immobilization-induced deterioration of uninjured cartilage. However, loading and motion must be used carefully following injury, because these measures alone will not predictably restore normal articular cartilage structure and composition in clinically significant defects, and excessive loading and motion may damage chondral repair tissue and displace fracture fragments.

Restoration of Joint Congruity. Significant traumatically induced joint incongruity causes mechanical joint dysfunction including instability, locking, catching, and restricted range of motion, and may be associated with progressive deterioration of articular cartilage. It is not clear how much of the long-term cartilage deterioration following injuries that cause joint incongruity is secondary to the traumatic cartilage damage at the time of injury and how much is related to the long-term effects of incongruity. However, in most injuries restoration of acceptable joint congruity avoids immediate problems with mechanical joint dysfunction and may delay or decrease the severity and rate of cartilage deterioration.

Unfortunately, the degree of joint incongruity that can be tolerated without causing long-term joint deterioration has not been well defined. A study of contact stress aberrations following imprecise reduction of experimental human cadaver tibial plateau fractures showed that generally peak local cartilage pressure increased with increasing joint incongruity (fracture fragment step-off), but the results varied among joints (56). In most specimens, cartilage pressure did not increase significantly until the fragment step-off exceeded 1.5 mm. When the step-off was increased to 3 mm, the peak cartilage pressure averaged 75% greater than normal. The authors estimated that the long-term pressure "tolerance level" of cartilage may be much higher, probably about twice the normal level, indicating that simple incongruities of several millimeters should not cause immediate or long-term problems. However, they also found that in some specimens even minor incongruities, as little as 0.25 mm, caused apparently deleterious peak local pressure elevations, suggesting that results may vary even among individuals with the same degree of articular incongruity. Experimental study of intra-articular fractures stabilized with a step-off shows that the articular surface remodels thereby decreasing the original incongruity (57). The long-term results of traumatically induced articular incongruity may also depend on the age of the patient. Skeletally immature individuals may have a greater capacity to remodel incongruities, and age-related alterations in articular cartilage (50) may decrease its capacity to repair injuries or withstand alterations in loading caused by joint incongruity.

Stabilization. Mechanical stabilization of an osteochondral injury in an acceptable position increases the likelihood of satisfactory healing by preventing disruption of the repair tissue and restoring articular cartilage congruity. An equally important benefit of stabilizing osteochondral fractures is that it allows early controlled loading and motion.

CONCLUSION

The primary tissues that form bones and joints—bone and articular cartilage—differ in their composition, structure, and capacity for healing. Bone fractures initiate a response that begins with inflammation (the cellular and vascular response to injury), proceeds through repair (the replacement of damaged or lost cells and matrices with new cells and matrices), and ends with remodeling (removal, replacement, and reorganization of the repair tissue, usually along the lines of mechanical stress). Injury to articular cartilage does not trigger an inflammatory response, but the cells respond to injury with an effort at cell proliferation and synthesis of new matrix. This effort rarely, if ever, restores a normal articular surface. When injuries extend through articular cartilage into bone, the repair tissue that forms in the bone extends into the region of the chondral injury and produces a fibrocartilagenous tissue that in some instances restores a functional articular surface.

The principles of treating acute bone and joint injuries include preventing further tissue damage, avoiding treatments that compromise the natural healing process, and creating the optimal mechanical and biological conditions for healing. This may include removing necrotic tissue, preventing infection, rapidly restoring blood and nerve supply when necessary, and in some circumstances providing apposition, alignment, and stabilization of injured tissue. One of the most important recent advances in the treatment of bone and joint injuries has been the recognition that early controlled loading and motion of the repair and remodeling tissues improves healing of many injuries. However, as with all treatments, this intervention must be used with care, since uncontrolled or excessive loading and motion can adversely affect or even prevent healing. At the tissue level the effect of the mechanical environment on repair and the function of the repair tissue cells are not well understood, and at the clinical level the optimal protocols for loading and motion of musculoskeletal tissue injuries have not been well defined. Although future improvements in treatment of musculoskeletal tissue injuries, including controlled motion and loading of repair and remodeling tissue, use of ultrasound and electrical fields and surgical restoration of apposition and mechanical stability of injured tissue, undoubtedly will advance the practice of orthopaedics, it is not likely that they will restore the original state of the tissue for patients with the most severe musculoskeletal tissue injuries. In particular, large segmental losses of bone and many articular cartilage injuries present especially difficult treatment problems. Future developments that may help improve healing of these injuries include creation and implantation of synthetic matrices and use of growth factors and implanted mesenchymal cells to guide and promote regeneration of bone and articular cartilage.

REFERENCES

1. Buckwalter JA. Can tissue engineering help orthopaedic patients? Clinical needs and criteria for success. In: Sandell LJ, Grodzinsky AJ, eds. *Tissue engineering in musculoskeletal clinical practice*. Rosemont, IL: American Academy of Orthopaedic Surgeons, 2004:3–16.
2. Buckwalter JA, Glimcher MJ, Cooper RR, et al. Bone biology. Part I. Structure, blood supply, cells, matrix and mineralization. *J Bone Joint Surg* 1995;77A:1256–1275.
3. Buckwalter JA, Glimcher MM, Cooper RR, et al. Bone biology II. Formation, form, modeling and remodeling. *J Bone Joint Surg* 1995;77A:1276–1289.
4. Buckwalter JA, Mankin HJ. Articular cartilage I. Tissue design and chondrocyte-matrix interactions. *J Bone Joint Surg* 1997;79A:600–611.
5. Einhorn TA. The cell and molecular biology of fracture healing. *Clin Orthop Relat Res* 1998;Oct(335 Suppl):S7–S21.
6. Buckwalter JA, Einhorn TA, Bolander ME, et al. Healing of musculoskeletal tissues. In: Rockwood CA, Green D, eds. *Fractures*. Philadelphia: Lippincott, 1996:261–304.
7. Leung KS, Sher AH, Lam TSW, et al. Energy metabolism in fracture healing. *J Bone Joint Surg* 1989;71B:567–660.
8. Mark H, Penington A, Nannmark U, et al. Microvascular invasion during endochondral ossification in experimental fractures in rats. *Bone* 2004;35:535–542.
9. Wildemann B, Schmidmaier G, Brenner N, et al. Quantification, localization, and expression of IGF-I and TGF-beta1 during growth factor-stimulated fracture healing. *Calcif Tissue Int* 2004;74:388–397.
10. Grundnes O, Reikeras O. The importance of the hematoma for fracture healing in rats. *Acta Orthop Scand* 1993;64:340–342.
11. Grundnes O, Reikeras O. The role of the hematoma and periosteal sealing for fracture healing in rats. *Acta Orthop Scand* 1993;64:47–49.
12. Sandberg MJ, Aro HT, Vuorio EL. Gene expression during bone repair. *Clin Orthop Relat Res* 1993;289:292–312.
13. Aro HT, Wippermann BW, Hodgson SF, et al. Prediction of properties of fracture callus by measurement of mineral density using micro-bone densitometry. *J Bone Joint Surg* 1989;71A:1020–1030.
14. White AA, Panjabi MM, Southwick WO. The four biomechanical stages of fracture repair. *J Bone Joint Surg* 1977;59A:188–192.
15. Wiel HE, Lips P, Nauta J, et al. Loss of bone in the proximal part of the femur following unstable fractures of the leg. *J Bone Joint Surg* 1994;76A:230–236.
16. Karlsson MK, Nilsson BE, Obrant KJ. Bone mineral loss after lower extremity trauma: 62 cases followed for 15–38 years. *Acta Orthop Scand* 1993;64:362–364.
17. Marsh JL, Buckwalter JA, Evarts CM. Nonunion, delayed union, malunion and avascular necrosis. In: Epps CH, ed. *Complications in orthopaedic surgery*. Philadelphia: Lippincott, 1994:183–211.
18. Watson-Jones R. *Fractures and joint injuries*, Vol. 2. 4th ed. Edinburgh, UK: Livingstone, 1955.
19. Rommens PM, Coosemans W, Broos PL. The difficult healing of segmental fractures of the tibial shaft. *Arch Orthop Traum Surg* 1989;108:238–242.
20. Woll TS, Duwelius PJ. The segmental tibia fracture. Clin Orthop Relat Res 1992;281: 204–207,
21. Jensen JE, Jensen TG, Smith TK, et al. Nutrition in orthopaedic surgery. *J Bone Joint Surg* 1982;64A:1263–1272.
22. Koval KJ, Maurer SG, Su ET, et al. The effects of nutrional status on outcome after hip fracture. *J Orthop Trauma* 1999;13:164–169.
23. Michelsen CG, Askanazi J. Current concepts review: the metabolic response to injury: mechanism and clinical implantations. *J Bone Joint Surg* 1986;68A:782–787.
24. Cuthbertson DP. Further observations of the disturbance of metabolism caused by injury, with particular reference to the dietary requirements of fracture cases. *Br J Surg* 1936; 23:505–520.
25. Einhorn TA, Bonnarens F, Burstein AH. The contributions of dietary protein and mineral to the healing of experimental fractures. A biomechanical study. *J Bone Joint Surg* 1986; 68A:1389–1395.
26. Cruess RL, Sakai T. Effect of cortisone upon synthesis rates of some components of rat bone matrix. *Clin Orthop Relat Res* 1972;86:253–259.
27. Simmons DJ, Kunvin AS. Autoradiographic and biochemical investigations of the effect of cortisone on the bones of the rat. *Clin Orthop Relat Res* 1967;55:201–215.
28. Adinoff AD, Hollister JR. Steroid induced fractures and bone loss in patients with asthma. *N Engl J Med* 1983;309:265–268.
29. Bak B, Jorgensen PH, Andreassen TT. The stimulating effect of growth hormone on fracture healing is dependent on onset and duration of administration. *Clin Orthop Relat Res* 1991;264:295–301.
30. Nielson HM, Bak B, Jorgensen PH, et al. Growth hormone promotes healing of tibial fractures in the rat. *Acta Orthop Scand* 1991;62:244–247.
31. Northmore-Ball MD, Wood MR, Meggitt BF. A biomechanical study of the effects of growth hormone in experimental fracture healing. *J Bone Joint Surg* 1980;62B:391–396.
32. Carpenter JE, Hipp JA, Gerhart TN, et al. Failure of growth hormone to alter the biomechanics of fracture-healing in a rabbit model. *J Bone Joint Surg* 1992;74A:359–367.
33. Raikin SM, Landsman JC, Alexander VA, et al. Effect of nicotine on the rate and strength of long bone fracture healing. *Clin Orthop Relat Res* 1998;Aug(353):231–237.
34. Riebel GD, Boden SD, Whitesides TE, et al. The effect of nicotine on incorporation of cancellous bone graft in an animal model. *Spine* 1995;20:2198–2202.
35. Morcuende JA, Gomez P, Stack J, et al. Effect of chemotherapy on segmental bone healing enhanced by rhBMP-2. *Iowa Orthop J* 2001;21:36–42.
36. Widmann RF, Pelker RR, Friedlander GE, et al. Effects of prefracture irradiation on the biomechanical parameters of fracture healing. *J Orthop Res* 1993;11:422–428.
37. Pelker RR, Friedlander GE. Fracture healing: radiation induced alterations. *Clin Orthop Relat Res* 1997;Aug(341):341:267–282.
38. Goodman AH, Sherman MS. Postirradiation fractures of the femoral neck. *J Bone Joint Surg* 1963;45A:723–730.
39. Buckwalter JA, Grodzinsky AJ. Loading of healing bone, fibrous tissue, and muscle: implications for orthopaedic practice. *J Am Acad Orthop Surg* 1999;7:291–299.
40. Hidaka S, Gustilo RB. Refracture of bones of the forearm after plate removal. *J Bone Joint Surg* 1984;66A:1241–1243.
41. Buckwalter JA, Rosenberg LC, Coutts, R. et al. Articular cartilage: injury and repair. In: Woo SL, Buckwalter JA, eds. *Injury and repair of the musculoskeletal soft tissues*. Park Ridge, IL: American Academy of Orthopaedic Surgeons, 1988:465–482.
42. Buckwalter JA, Rosenberg LA, Hunziker EB. Articular cartilage: Composition, structure, response to injury, and methods of facilitation repair. In: Ewing JW, ed. *Articular cartilage and knee joint function: basic science and arthroscopy*. New York: Raven Press, 1990:19–56.
43. Buckwalter JA. Articular cartilage injuries. *Clin Orthop Relat Res* 2002;Sep(402):21–37.
44. Mitchell N, Shepard N. The deleterious effects of drying on articular cartilage. *J Bone Joint Surg* 1989;71A:89–95.
45. Speer KP, Callaghan JJ, Seaber AV, et al. The effects of exposure of articular cartilage to air. A histochemical and ultrastructural investigation. *J Bone Joint Surg* 1990;72A: 1442–1450.
46. Buckwalter JA. Mechanical injuries of articular cartilage. In: Finerman G, ed. *Biology and biomechanics of the traumatized synovial joint*. Park Ridge IL, American Academy of Orthopaedic Surgeons, 1992:83–96.
47. Buckwalter JA, Brown TD. Joint injury, repair, and remodeling: roles in post-traumatic osteoarthritis. *Clin Orthop Relat Res* 2004;Jun(423):7–16.
48. Buckwalter JA, Martin JA, Olmstead M, et al. Osteochondral repair of primate knee femoral and patellar articular surfaces: implications for preventing post-traumatic osteoarthritis. *Iowa Orthop J* 2003;23:66–74.
49. Marsh JL, Buckwalter J, Gelberman R, et al. Articular fractures: does an anatomic reduction really change the result? *J Bone Joint Surg Am* 2002;84-A:1259–1271.
50. Buckwalter JA, Woo SL-Y, Goldberg VM, et al. Soft tissue aging and musculoskeletal function. *J Bone Joint Surg* 1993;75A:1533–1548.
51. Martin JA, Klingelhutz AJ, Moussavi-Harami F, et al. Effects of oxidative damage and telomerase activity on human articular cartilage chondrocyte senescence. *J Gerontol A Biol Sci Med Sci* 2004;59:324–337.
52. Martin JA, Buckwalter JA. The role of chondrocyte senescence in the pathogenesis of osteoarthritis and in limiting cartilage repair. *J Bone Joint Surg Am* 2003;85-A(suppl 2): 106–110.
53. Martin JA, Buckwalter JA. Telomere erosion and senescence in human articular cartilage chondrocytes. *J Gerontol A Biol Sci Med Sci* 2001;56:B172–179.
54. Martin JA, Ellerbroek SM, Buckwalter JA. Age-related decline in chondrocyte response to insulin-like growth factor-I: the role of growth factor binding proteins. *J Orthop Res* 1997;15:491–498.
55. Convery FR, Akeson WH, Keown GH. The repair of large osteochondral defects: an experimental study in horses. *Clin Orthop Relat Res* 1972;82:253–262.
56. Brown TD, Anderson DD, Nepola JV, et al. Contact stress aberrations following imprecise reduction of simple tibial plateau fractures. *J Orthop Res* 1988;6:851–862.
57. Llinas A, McKellop HA, Marshall GJ, et al. Healing and remodeling of articular incongruities in a rabbit fracture model. *J Bone Joint Surg* 1993;75:1508–1523.

BONE GRAFTING AND ENHANCEMENT OF FRACTURE REPAIR

Sanjeev Kakar, Eleftherios Tsiridis, and Thomas A. Einhorn

CLINICAL NEED

Fracture healing is a well-orchestrated biological process resulting in optimal skeletal repair. Despite this, it is estimated that between 5% and 10% of the fractures occurring annually in the United States exhibit some degree of impaired healing (1). In many instances, the cause is unknown and may be related to inadequate reduction, instability (2), the systemic state of the patient (3,4) or the nature of the traumatic insult itself (5,6). In addition, there are certain areas within the appendicular skeleton that have a predilection to impaired healing due to aspects of the local biomechanical environment or anatomy of the blood supply. Examples include the subtrochanteric region of the femur where, until the introduction of locked intramedullary nailing, control of the mechanical environment was challenging, and the scaphoid where the repair process is influenced by the anatomy of arterial blood flow (7). Despite most fractures healing uneventfully, clinical scenarios arise in which enhancement of fracture repair would be beneficial to ensure rapid restoration of skeletal function.

BONE GRAFTING

Each year, more than 2.2 million bone grafts are performed worldwide, with 450,000 being performed in the United States (8). The indications for grafting include the treatment of delayed unions, failed joint replacements, spinal and long bone arthrodeses, limb salvage reconstructions for malignant bone tumors and complex spine reconstructions for instability and deformity. Approximately 11% of bone grafts are performed in the craniofacial bones.

Autogenous bone graft is still considered the implant of choice for most applications as it naturally provides the basic components required to stimulate skeletal repair. These include osteoinductive growth factors, an osteoconductive extracellular matrix and osteogenic stem cells present in bone marrow elements. *Osteoinduction* refers to the process by which pluripotent mesenchymal stem cells are recruited from the surrounding host tissues and differentiate into bone forming osteoprogenitor cells. This is mediated by graft-derived growth factors such as bone morphogenetic proteins and other peptide signaling molecules (9,10). An *osteoconductive* material is one that acts as a scaffold, supporting ingrowth of capillaries, perivascular tissue and osteoprogenitor cells from the recipient bed. This occurs in an ordered sequence determined by the three dimensional structure of the graft, the local blood supply and the biomechanical forces exerted on the graft and surrounding tissues (10). *Osteogenesis* refers to the process of bone formation. In terms of bone grafting, an osteogenic material is one which contains living cells capable of differentiating into bone.

Despite the effectiveness of autogenous bone graft, several shortcomings exist including donor site morbidity, nerve or arterial injury, and infection rates of between 8% and 10% associated with graft harvesting (11–14). These limitations have prompted the use of an alternate graft material like allogeneic bone. However, despite its ready availability, the risk of disease transmission, diminished biologic and mechanical properties in comparison to autogenous bone, and increased cost have limited its use (15). For these reasons, development of effective bone graft substitutes and strategies for tissue engineering of bone have led to a new field of study for the future of fracture management.

Autologous Bone

Autologous bone graft (also known as autograft, autogenous graft) refers to bone harvested from and implanted into the same individual and includes cancellous bone, cortical bone (nonvascularized and vascularized grafts) and bone marrow. Although much has been written about its use in skeletal reconstruction, relatively little attention has been paid to its application in the healing of fresh fractures.

Bone graft incorporation follows a similar sequence of events to those which occur during fracture repair. Once implanted into the host, hematoma forms around the graft, releasing bioactive molecules such as growth factors and pro-inflammatory cytokines (16). Mediators such as interleukin-1 (IL-1), IL-6, and tumor necrosis factor-alpha (TNFα) are secreted and are chemotactic for hematopoietic cells including neutrophils, macrophages, and osteoclasts. These cells invade the graft, thereby initiating the resorptive phase of incorporation. Peptide signaling molecules such as platelet-derived growth factor (PDGF) and transforming browth factor-beta (TGF-β) facilitate the repair process by acting on mesenchymal cell recruitment and differentiation (17,18).

Once the inflammatory process subsides, formation of a callus occurs. A fibrovascular stroma develops in which host-derived blood vessels and osteogenic precursor cells migrate toward the graft. These pluripotential mesenchymal cells differentiate into osteoblasts and synthesize osteoid. At the same time, the graft undergoes partial necrosis and osteoclasts continue to remove dead bone with release of additional biochemical mediators of repair from its extracellular matrix. Osteoblasts and endosteal lining cells on the surface of the graft may survive the transplantation and contribute to the healing, although the magnitude of this response is not clearly understood. Most likely, the main contribution of the graft is as an osteoinductive and osteoconductive substrate. It provides the necessary physical and chemical properties to support the attachment, spreading, division, and differentiation of normal osteoblastic or osteoblast-like cells to form bone. The remodeling process marks the last stage of graft incorporation with woven bone slowly being transformed into mechanically robust lamellar bone through the coordinated activities of osteoblasts and osteoclasts.

In addition to the biologic events surrounding graft organization, several other local factors have been shown to have an effect on this process (19). The quality of the tissues at the host site, including their vascularity, is particularly important in influencing the rate and extent of graft union. An avascular bed or one that is deficient in endothelial or connective tissue cell precursors, will be less able to respond to the osteoinductive and osteoconductive signals emanating from the graft. This may occur in patients who have undergone previous radiation therapy or who are exposed to a therapeutic or nontherapeutic agent such as glucocorticoid or nicotine, which impairs cell function. Moreover, if mechanical instability exists at the implantation site, granulation and fibrous tissue will develop at the graft–host interface thereby preventing bony union (19).

Autologous Cancellous Bone Graft

The host response to cancellous bone grafts differs from that to cortical bone in terms of its rate and completeness of repair. Cancellous bone, with its large surface area covered by quiescent lining cells or active osteoblasts, has the potential to induce more new bone than cortical bone (20). Bone formation and resorption occur concomitantly. Osteoblasts secrete osteoid onto the surface of necrotic bone, while osteoclasts gradually

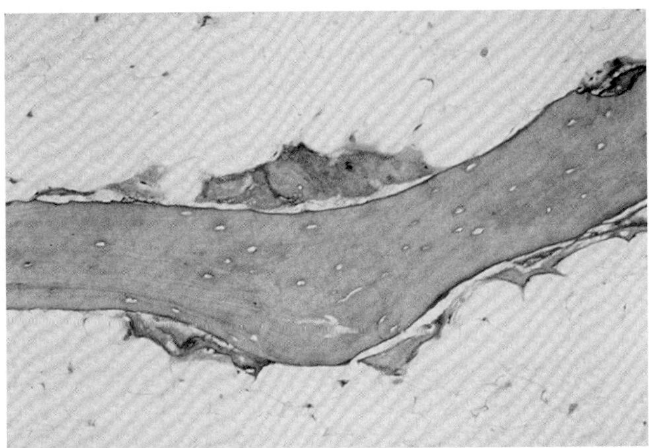

FIGURE 9-1 Low-power photomicrograph showing creeping substitution. Newly formed woven bone, containing osteoblasts with basophilic-staining nuclei, is laid down on dead lamellar bone identified by the presence of empty osteocytic lacunae (× 25; hematoxylin and eosin stain).

resorb the dead trabeculae. This process of *creeping substitution* (21) is characteristic of the late phase of autogenous cancellous bone grafting (Fig. 9-1). Therefore, although a cancellous graft does not provide much, if any, immediate structural support, it incorporates quickly and is completely replaced by host bone and marrow after 1 year (Table 9-1).

Cancellous bone graft is usually harvested in fragments from sites such as the iliac crest, distal radius, greater trochanter and proximal tibial and distal femoral metaphyses (22,23). It is an excellent choice for the treatment of conditions that do not require structural integrity from the graft (24-26).

Autologous Cortical Bone Graft

Cortical bone grafts are usually harvested from the ribs, fibula or shell of the ilium and can be transplanted with or without their vascular pedicle. They are mostly osteoconductive with little or no osteoinductive properties (Table 9-1). The thickness of the matrix of cortical bone limits the diffusion of nutrients to support the survival of any useful fraction of osteocytes after transplantation, thereby limiting its osteogenic properties (27).

Cortical autografts proceed through a similar sequence of incorporation as seen with cancellous grafts. However, because of the density of cortical bone, the rate of revascularization is substantially slower (28–30). This is more commonly seen with nonvascularized grafts where vascular penetration is primarily the result of peripheral osteoclastic resorption and vascular invasion of Volkmann and haversian canals (31).

Vascularized cortical grafts function relatively independently of the host bed (27) as they are implanted with their own functional blood supply. The three main sources for free vascularized bone grafts are the fibula, iliac crest, and rib. The fibula may be isolated on its peroneal vessels, the iliac crest graft uses the deep circumflex iliac artery and vein, while the rib uses the posterior intercostal artery and vein. Once the vessels are successfully anastomosed, greater than 90% of the osteocytes survive the transplantation procedure. Consequently, graft–host union occurs much more rapidly without substantial bone resorption and remodeling as is seen with nonvascularized grafts (32). This lack of resorption and revascularization results in the vascularized grafts providing superior strength during the first 6 weeks after implantation (27). As with cancellous bone, these grafts still require internal or external fixation to provide mechanical stability while they incorporate into the host bed.

TABLE 9-1 Properties of Types of Autologous Bone Grafts

Property	Cancellous	Nonvascularized Cortical	Vascularized Cortical
Osteoconduction	+++	+	+
Osteoinduction	++[a]	+/−	+/−
Osteoprogenitor cells	+++	−	++
Immediate strength	−	+++	+++
Strength at 6 mo	++	++, +++	+++
Strength at 1 yr	+++	+++	+++

[a] Although cancellous bone is widely believed to be osteoinductive, there is no evidence to critically demonstrate that inductive proteins and cytokines are active in autologous cancellous bone graft.
Reprinted with permission from Finkemeier CG. Bone grafting and bone graft substitutes. *J Bone Joint Surg Am* 2002;84:454–464.

Nonvascularized autologous cortical bone grafts can be used to treat segmental bone defects of up to 6 cm in length which require immediate structural support (26). There are no definitive reports regarding the use of nonvascularized grafts for defects of between 6 and 12 cm in length. For defects greater than 12 cm, vascularized grafts are recommended (33). The harvesting of these large grafts, however, is not without problems. Tang et al (34) examined donor site morbidity in 39 patients with avascular necrosis of the femoral head treated by curettage and transplantation of free ipsilateral fibular grafts. Subjective complaints were common and included weakness in 37% of cases. Twenty-nine percent of patients demonstrated weakness in great toe flexion with 43% experiencing difficulty with toe extension.

Autologous Bone Marrow

Bone marrow contains osteogenic precursor cells (35–36) and may become a prime material in the future for use in tissue engineering of bone (37). In the treatment of bony defects, Connolly and Shindell (38) first reported its clinical use in the management of tibial nonunions. Injecting freshly harvested bone marrow into the defects resulted in clinical and radiographic union by 6 months. Others have described similar successes (39,40). Garg and colleagues (40) percutaneously administered autogenous bone marrow to stimulate healing in 20 ununited long bone fractures. Patients were kept nonweight bearing for 6 weeks after surgery, after which they mobilized with protected weight bearing until union was reached. Seventeen out of 20 fractures demonstrated clinical and radiographic union by 5 months. These clinical reports provide encouraging data in support of the use of bone marrow in fracture treatment. However, randomized controlled trials have not been conducted and these will be required to demonstrate true clinical efficacy.

One of the major setbacks associated with bone marrow use is its limited number of osteoprogenitor stem cells. Muschler et al (41) noted that the mean prevalence of colony forming units expressing alkaline phosphatase (CFU-APs), a marker of osteoblast progenitors, is 55 per million nucleated cells. These values undergo a significant age-related decline for both men and women ($p = 0.002$). Muschler and co-workers (42) also noted that the volume of aspirate used for grafting procedures can also affect the number of CFU-APs. As the aspirate volume increases, so does the number of CFU-APs. Contamination of the sample by peripheral blood, however, also grows as the aspiration volume increases. The investigators noted that an increase in the aspiration volume from 1 to 4 mL causes approximately a 50% decrease in the final concentration of CFU-APs. On the basis of these data, the authors recommended that the volume of aspiration from any one site should not be greater than 2 mL. In addition, four 1 mL aspirates will provide almost twice the number of CFU-APs as would one 4 mL aspirate.

As the success of bone marrow grafting depends on the transfer of sufficient numbers of osteoprogenitor cells, investigators have tried to increase the concentrations of these cells. Takigami et al (43) described a technique involving the use of a cell retention system that selectively retains osteoblastic stem cells and progenitors within an implantable graft material. Bone marrow aspirates from the posterior superior iliac spine are taken in 2 mL aliquots and flowed through a customized allograft matrix using the selective cell retention processing system. The resulting graft–bone marrow composite can then be used as an adjunct to stimulate bone formation. In a series of four patients, the authors used this technique to treat tibial, clavicular, and femoral neck nonunions. Results demonstrated stimulation of bony repair thereby providing surgeons with an alternative to iliac crest autograft, which eliminates pain, blood loss and other surgical complications associated with autogenous bone graft harvesting. This was a limited case series and randomized controlled clinical studies are required to demonstrate selective cell retention technology's efficacy on a larger basis.

Allogeneic Bone

The use of allograft bone accounts for approximately one third of bone grafts performed in the United States (44). It is an attractive alternate to autogenous bone as it avoids donor site morbidity and its relative abundance permits it to be tailored to fit the defect size. Despite its use in other areas of orthopaedics such as in spinal surgery (45) or in joint arthroplasty (46), considerably less is known about its use in the repair of fresh fractures or nonunions. This may be in part related to the risk of blood borne disease transmission (47) and suboptimal clinical results compared to autograft (48). These findings may be attributed to its storage and sterilization procedures such as freeze-drying or freezing that are used to lower disease transmission. Freeze-drying or lyophilization involves removal of water and vacuum packing of the tissue. Although this reduces the immunogenecity (49), Pelker et al (50) demonstrated that it also reduces the mechanical integrity of the graft, thereby reducing its load bearing properties. In addition, freeze-drying reduces the allograft osteoinductive potential by inducing the death of its osteogenic cells. Freezing allografts to temperatures of −60°C or below lowers their immunogenecity by diminishing the degradation of enzymes without altering the biomechanical properties.

Allogeneic bone is available in many preparations including morselized and cancellous chips, corticocancellous and cortical grafts, osteochondral segments, and demineralized bone matrix (26). In general, the processes involved in allograft incorporation are similar to those seen with nonvascularized autografts, except that they occur much more slowly and when large grafts are used, incorporation as opposed to resorption and replacement results (51). This is in part related to the lack of viable donor cells that contribute to healing and the immune response that occurs during the inflammatory process of allograft incorporation. This lack of biological activity results in limited revascularization, creeping substitution and remodeling of the graft (52,53). Studies have shown that this lack of vascularization may account for the high incidence of fractures seen with these grafts, which has been reported to occur in between 16% and 50% of grafts (54,55).

Histologically, mononuclear cells invade the graft and surround newly developing blood vessels. These become occluded leading to rapid necrosis of the graft. Necrotic graft bone remains in the host tissue much longer compared to autografts and may be seen for many years after implantation depending upon the size of the graft and its anatomic location (10,30). Osteoinduction and osteoconduction are markedly delayed with osteogenesis occurring 4 to 6 weeks after implantation.

The biological nature of the recipient host bed is a critical factor in facilitating allograft incorporation. A well-vascularized bed aids in the incorporation of the allograft through a combination of revascularization, osteoconduction, and remodeling (56).

Cortical allografts are harvested from a number of sites including the pelvis, ribs, and fibula. They are available as whole bone segments for limb salvage procedures or may be cut longitudinally to yield struts that can be used to fill bone defects or reconstitute cortical bone after periprosthetic fractures (57). In addition to conferring mechanical stability, they may enhance fracture healing and increase bone stock. Their modulus of elasticity is similar to that of host bone resulting in less stress shielding than with other more rigid forms of internal fixation.

The relative inertness of cortical allografts limits their potential to achieve graft–host union. To improve this, autograft harvested from the iliac crest can be placed at the allograft–host bone interface. The autograft provides osteogenic cells and osteoinductive proteins. This technique was described by Wang and Weng (58) in the treatment of distal femoral nonunions. Thirteen patients with femoral nonunions were treated with open reduction and internal fixation with deep-frozen cortical allograft struts. Seven unicortical, five bicortical and one tricortical allografts, with an average length of 10 cm, were used. Autogenous bone grafts were inserted into the defect between the allograft and host femur. All nonunions united at an average of 5 months with an improvement in knee function.

Demineralized Bone Matrix

Demineralized bone matrix (DBM) is produced by acid extraction of allograft bone (59). It contains type I collagen, noncollagenous proteins and osteoinductive growth factors but provides little structural support (60). The bioavailability of the growth factors contained in DBM results in its greater osteoinductive potential than conventional allografts (47). These properties can be affected by different storage, processing, and sterilization procedures. Donor to donor variability in DBM's osteoinductive capacity exists, resulting in the American Association of Tissue Banks and the Food and Drug Administration (FDA) requiring that each batch of DBM be obtained from a single human donor (61).

Implantation of DBM is followed by hematoma formation and an inflammatory process characterized by polymorphonuclear cell migration into the implant within 18 hours. Mesenchymal cells differentiate into cartilage-producing chondrocytes by day 5. The cartilage becomes mineralized and is then invaded by new blood vessels by 10 to 12 days. The accompanying perivascular cells differentiate into osteoblasts leading to new bone formation. Remodeling then occurs with all implanted DBM being eventually resorbed and replaced by host bone (10).

Tiedeman et al (62) reported a case series on the use of DBM in conjunction with bone marrow in the treatment of 48 patients with bony disorders such as comminuted fractures with associated bone loss. Of these 48 patients, 39 were available to follow up and review. Thirty of 39 patients demonstrated bony union. Patients with fracture nonunion represented the most recalcitrant group clinically, with union being achieved in only 61% of these cases. Because no control patients were included in the study, the efficacy of the DBM/bone-marrow composite could not be determined.

Numerous DBM formulations exist based upon refinements of the manufacturing techniques. They are available as a freeze-dried powder, granules, gel, putty, or strips. All have osteoinductive effects in animal studies but no randomized controlled trials have been performed in patients. However, because these materials were originally developed as reprocessed human tissues, clearance for marketing was achieved without the need for randomized controlled trials comparing their efficacy to autologous bone. For this reason, it is unclear how well any of these products perform as bone graft substitutes. Because currently marketed formulations of these products include carrier substances such as glycerol, the FDA now plans to regulate DBM products as class II medical devices. Currently marketed DBM products will most likely be reclassified using the 510K pathway requiring demonstration of substantial equivalence to a predicate device but still not requiring demonstration of efficacy comparable to that achieved with autologous bone graft.

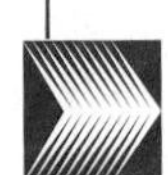

AUTHORS' PREFERRED TREATMENT

We prefer the use of autologous cancellous bone for the augmentation of fractures associated with bone loss, nonunions, and small bone defects requiring grafting (for example, a metaphyseal or mid-diaphyseal cyst that has undergone curettage). Diaphyseal defects up to 12 cm in length can be treated with nonvascularized cortical autografts. For defects more than 12 centimeters, vascularized cortical autografts are recommended. We do not think that there is sufficient information, nor have their been enough studies providing good evidence, to support the use of freshly harvested autologous bone marrow in traumatic or reconstructive orthopaedic surgery. Because the number of osteoprogenitor cells in any human bone marrow aspirate is very small, it is unclear if this complement of cells can support an osteogenic response. However, if surgeons do attempt to use freshly harvested autologous bone marrow, we recommend multiple aspirations of no more than 2 mL each as this will more likely optimize the concentration of osteoprogenitor cells within the aspirates. We have no experience with so-called selective retention methods designed to increase the concentration of osteoprogenitor cells from bone marrow. To our knowledge, the clinical evidence supporting this technology is limited.

There is not much information on the use of allogeneic bone to enhance the healing of fresh fractures or nonunions. We suggest that allogeneic cancellous bone chips be used to augment the healing of fresh fractures associated with bone loss, or nonunions when used in conjunction with autologous bone in order to make up a sufficient volume of graft material. Incorporation of allogeneic strut grafts may also be enhanced by the use of cancellous bone at the junction with the host bone.

Human demineralized bone matrix is a form of allogeneic graft material. Although widely available and known to contain bone morphogenetic protein (BMP), we do not think there is sufficient evidence demonstrating its efficacy in the treatment of fresh fractures or nonunions, or the reconstruction of bone defects. Some authors have used demineralized bone matrix as a delivery vehicle for bone graft substitutes while others have suggested its use in conjunction with autologous cancellous bone to increase the volume of graft material. These reports exist as preclinical animal studies or as anecdotal descriptions. For this reason, we are unable to recommend its use for specific applications at this time.

BONE GRAFT SUBSTITUTES

An ideal bone graft substitute should provide three elements: scaffolding for osteoconduction, growth factors for osteoinduction, and progenitor cells for osteogenesis (63). The currently available materials including calcium phosphate ceramics, calcium sulfate, bioactive glass, biodegradable polymers (64), recombinant human BMPs (OP-1 and BMP-2), and autologous bone marrow cells, each fulfill only one of these criteria. However, there is great interest in improving these materials as the availability of an effective bone graft substitute would solve some of the current limitations associated with the use of autologous bone.

Calcium Phosphate Ceramics

Calcium phosphate ceramics are osteoconductive materials produced by a sintering process in which mineral salts are heated to over 1000°C. Sintering reduces the amount of carbonated apatite, an unstable and weakly soluble form of hydroxyapatite. An ideal osteoconductive scaffold should have the appropriate three-dimensional structure to allow for osteointegration and invasion by cells and blood vessels. It should also be biocompatible and biodegradable with biomechanical properties similar to those of the surrounding bone. Many of the ceramics used as bone grafts enable osteoconduction to occur (65,66). Despite this, their brittleness and poor tensile strength limit their use as bone graft materials.

The first clinical use of calcium phosphate ceramics for the repair of bony defects was reported by Albee in 1920 (67). Since then, several animal studies have reported favorable results. Despite these early experiments, it was not until the 1970s that calcium phosphates, and in particular hydroxyapatite (HA), were synthesized, characterized and used clinically (68–70).

Hydroxyapatite

From a functional perspective, calcium phosphate ceramics can be divided into slow and rapid resorbing ceramics (47). Hydroxyapatite is a slow resorbing compound derived from marine coral (71). A simple hydrothermal treatment process converts it into the more mechanically stable hydroxyapatite form with pore diameters of between 200 and 500 μm, a structure very similar to human trabecular bone (Fig. 9-2).

Interpore (Interpore International, Irvine, CA) is a corraline hydroxyapatite and was the first calcium-phosphate–based bone graft substitute approved by the FDA (Fig. 9-2B). Bucholz et al (73) investigated its use to treat tibial plateau fractures. Forty patients with metaphyseal defects needing operative reduction were randomized into a control group treated with autogenous bone graft or a group treated with Interpore hydroxyapatite. Indications for surgery included valgus instability of the knee secondary to a lateral tibial plateau fracture, varus instability due to a medial plateau injury, articular incongruency of 10 mm or greater, and translation of the major condylar fragment of more than 5 mm. After insertion of the graft, cortical fracture fragments were reduced and a standard AO interfragmentary screw and plate fixation device was used to stabilize the reduction. After an average of 15.4 months for the autograft and 34.5 months for the Interpore-treated groups, radiological and functional knee joint assessments revealed no differences between the two groups. No evidence of ceramic resorption was found in the radiographic follow-up 3 years following implantation, highlighting the potential use of HA as a bone filler.

Tricalcium Phosphate

Tricalcium phosphate (TCP) is a fast resorbing ceramic that undergoes partial conversion to HA once implanted into the body. The HA is resorbed more slowly and will remain in place for years.

Reports have demonstrated the efficacy of TCP as a bone graft substitute. McAndrew et al (70) investigated the suitability of TCP to treat bony defects in a case series of 43 patients with 33 fractures and 13 nonunions. Patients were followed for an average of 1 year. Healing was demonstrated in 90% of the fracture patients and 85% of those with nonunions. Radiographic analysis showed complete resorption of TCP between 6 and 24 months after implantation.

Calcium Phosphate/Collagen Composites

Collagen is the most abundant protein in the extracellular matrix of bone and promotes mineral deposition by providing

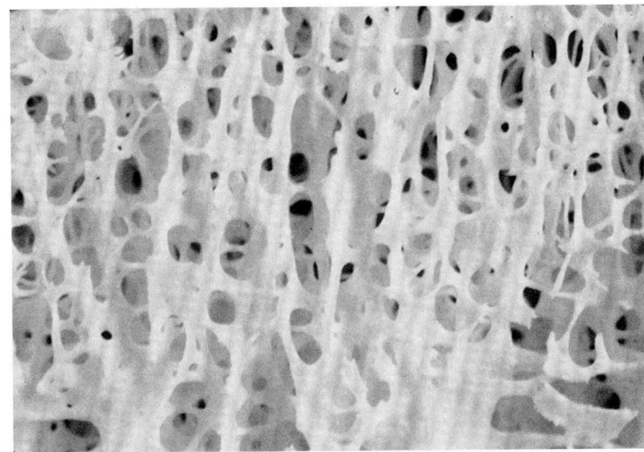
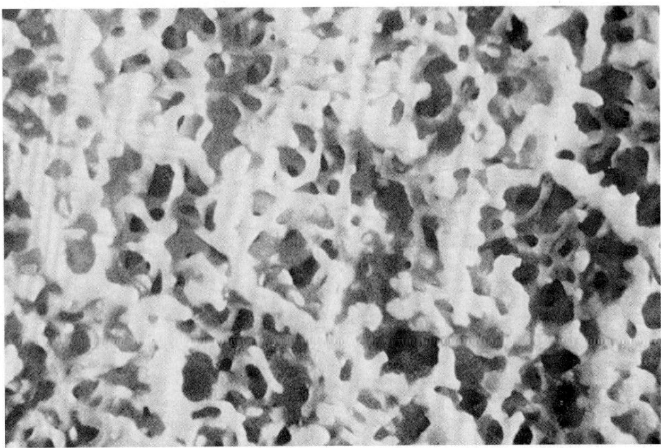

FIGURE 9-2 **A.** High power photograph of cancellous bone demonstrating its interporous structure. (Reprinted with permission from Lee CA, Einhorn TA. The bone organ system. Form and function. In: Marcus R, Feldman D, Kelsey J, eds. *Osteoporosis*, 2nd ed, vol 1. New York: Academic Press, 2001:3–20.) **B.** High power photograph of Interpore, a coralline hydroxyapatite. Note the structural characteristics similar to normal trabecular bone.

binding sites for matrix proteins. Types I and III collagen have been combined with HA, TCP, and autologous bone marrow to form a graft material devoid of structural support but able to function as an effective bone graft substitute or bone graft expander to augment fracture healing. This was demonstrated by Chapman et al (74) who conducted a multicenter prospective, randomized controlled study comparing autogenous bone graft and a composite of bovine collagen, calcium phosphate and autogenous bone marrow (Collagraft, Zimmer, Inc., Warsaw, IN) in the treatment of acute long bone fractures. Two hundred and forty-nine fractures were grafted and followed for a minmum of 2 years. The authors observed no significant differences between the two treatment groups in terms of union rates, functional outcomes and impairments of activities of daily living. The prevalence of complications was similar in the two groups except for higher infection rates in patients receiving autogenous bone grafts. Antibodies to the bovine collagen developed in 12% of patients in the Collagraft-treated group but no specific allergic problems were identified. Similar results using this material have been reported by others (75).

Calcium Sulphate

Calcium sulphate or plaster of paris was first used as a bone filler in the early 1900s (76). It acts as an osteoconductive material which completely resorbs as newly formed bone remodels and restores anatomic features and structural properties.

Moed et al (77) investigated its ability as a bone graft substitute in a prospective nonrandomized clinical study for the treatment of acetabular fractures with intra-articular comminution, marginal impaction, or both. Thirty-one patients (32 fractures) were treated with calcium sulphate pellets. Radiographic analysis demonstrated that the majority of fractures healed successfully with most of the pellets being replaced by bone.

Two groups of investigators reported the use of calcium sulfate as a material which augments or extends the use of autologous bone graft. In a prospective nonrandomized multicenter study, Kelly et al (78) treated 109 patients with bone defects with calcium sulphate pellets alone or mixed with bone marrow aspirate, demineralized bone, or autograft. After 6 months, radiographic results for all patients showed that 99% of the pellets were resorbed and 88% of the defects were filled with trabeculated bone. Borrelli et al (79) treated 26 patients with persistent long bone nonunions or osseous defects after an open fracture, with a mixture of autogenous iliac crest bone graft and medical grade calcium sulphate. Twenty-two patients achieved healing after primary surgery, while a further two demonstrated union after a second procedure. Persistent nonunions were seen in two patients. Despite these encouraging reports, there have been no randomized, controlled trials to study the efficacy of calcium sulfate in the treatment of skeletal injuries.

Calcium Phosphate Cements

Calcium phosphate cements (CPC) can be used to fill bony defects in conjunction with the treatment of acute fractures. This involves the combination of inorganic calcium and phosphate to form an injectable paste which can be delivered into the fracture site. Under physiological conditions, the material begins to harden within minutes, forming a mineral known as dahllite. By 12 hours, dahllite formation is nearly complete, providing the cement with an ultimate compressive strength of 55 MPA. Studies in animals have shown that it is remodeled in vivo and, in some cases, is completely resorbed and replaced by host bone (80).

Sanchez-Sotelo et al (81) conducted a prospective, randomized controlled study examining the use of a commercially available calcium phosphate paste, Norian SRS (Norian Corporation, Cupertino, CA), in the treatment of distal radius fractures. One hundred and ten patients, who were between 50 and 85 years of age, and who had sustained either an AO type A3 or C2 distal radius fracture were enrolled. Patients were prospectively randomized to receive either closed reduction with a short arm cast for 6 weeks or closed reduction and stabilization with Norian SRS for 2 weeks. They were followed for a 12-month period and assessed by radiography, range of motion, and grip strength. The results showed improved functional and radiographic outcomes in the patients treated with Norian SRS. In a subsequent randomized, controlled study, Cassidy et al (82) compared the use of Norian SRS and closed reduction versus closed reduction and application of a cast or external fixator in 323 patients with intra- or extra-articular fractures of the distal radius. Significant clinical differences were seen at 6 to 8 weeks postoperatively, with better grip strength, wrist and digit range of motion, hand function, and less swelling in the patients treated with Norian SRS. By 1 year, these differences had normalized.

In light of the promising results seen with distal radius fractures, Norian SRS has been used to treat other bony injuries. Schildhauer et al (83) reported its use in the treatment of complex calcaneal fractures. Thirty-six joint depression fractures were treated with Norian SRS after standard open reduction and internal fixation. Patients were allowed to weight bear fully as early as 3 weeks postoperatively. Results demonstrated no statistical difference in clinical outcome scores in patients who bore full weight before or after 6 weeks postoperatively suggesting that this cement may permit early full weight bearing after treatment of this fracture.

Lobenhoffer and co-workers (84) used Norian SRS in the treatment of 26 tibial plateau fractures (OTA types B2, B3, and C3) followed for a mean period of 19.7 months. Successive radiographs were taken and clinical parameters were measured using Lysholm and Tegner knee scores. Twenty-two fractures healed without any displacement or complications (two cases required early wound revision secondary to sterile drainage and two cases developed partial loss of fracture reduction between 4 and 8 weeks postoperatively requiring revision surgery). The high mechanical strength of the cement allowed earlier weight bearing after a mean postoperative period of 4.5 weeks. Similar results supporting the use of Norian SRS for filling metaphyseal defects in the treatment of displaced tibial plateau fractures have been reported by others (85) (Fig. 9-3).

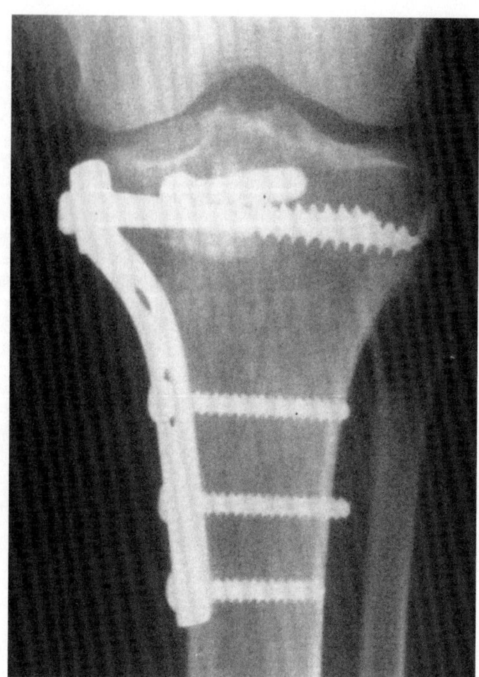

FIGURE 9-3 Radiograph demonstrating the use of Norian SRS for filling metaphyseal defects in the treatment of a displaced tibial plateau fracture. (Reprinted with permission from Bucholz RW, Carlton A, Holmes R. Interporous hydroxyapatite as a bone graft substitute in tibial plateau fractures. *Clin Orthop Relat Res* 1989;240:53–62.)

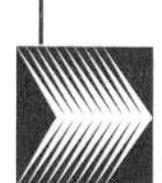

AUTHORS' PREFERRED TREATMENT

Calcium-based bone graft substitutes (tricalcium phosphate, calcium sulfate, calcium phosphate/collagen composites, hydroxyapatite, etc.) are best used as bone void fillers when it is possible to implant them such that they are surrounded by host bone on all sides. It is preferable to use them in parts of the skeleton where tensile strains are low or nonexistent. Calcium sulfate, which is much more rapidly resorbed than the other calcium-based materials, must be used in parts of the skeleton where compressive strength is required for only short periods of time. These materials should not be used to bridge segmental diaphyseal defects or as onlay grafts where the majority of the surface is exposed to soft tissues.

Calcium phosphate-based cement (Norian SRS) has been tested in several randomized controlled clinical trials. Based on these data, its uses to shorten the time in a cast during treatment of distal radius fractures, or to shorten the time to weight bearing in the augmentation of tibial plateau and calcaneal fractures are supported by clinical evidence and are viable treatment options for these indications. It may be useful in other applications such as acetabular fractures and fractures of the hip but sufficient evidence is not yet available for its use in these settings.

ENHANCEMENT OF FRACTURE HEALING WITH GROWTH FACTORS AND RELATED MOLECULES

Growth factors are proteins secreted by cells and function as signaling molecules. They comprise a family of molecules that have autocrine, paracrine, or endocrine effects on appropriate target cells. In addition to promoting cell differentiation, they have direct effects on cell adhesion, proliferation, and migration by modulating the synthesis of proteins, other growth factors and receptors (86).

Bone Morphogenetic Proteins

Since the discovery of the osteoinductive properties of BMP (87), attention has focused on the role of these proteins in embryological development and bone repair in the postnatal skeleton (86,88,89). BMPs are a group of noncollagenous glycoproteins that belong to the TGF-β superfamily. They are synthesized locally and predominantly exert their effects by autocrine and paracrine mechanisms. Fifteen different human BMPs have been identified and their genes cloned (90). For clinical applications, the most extensively studied among these are BMP-2 and BMP-7 (osteogenic protein 1, or OP-1).

The importance of BMPs in bone repair has been the subject of much investigation. Cho et al (88) characterized the temporal expression of BMPs during murine fracture healing, defining specific periods when individual BMPs may exert important roles in normal skeletal repair. BMP-2 showed maximal expression on day one after fracture, suggesting its role as an early response gene in the cascade of healing events. BMPs-3, 4, 7, and 8 exhibited a restricted period of expression from day 14 through day 21, when the resorption of calcified cartilage and osteoblastic recruitment were most active. BMPs-5 and 6 were constitutively expressed from day 3 to day 21.

To determine if BMPs are likely to play a key role during fracture healing in patients, Kloen et al (91) demonstrated the presence of BMPs and their various receptors in human fracture callus. Tissue was obtained from the fracture site of malunions in five patients undergoing revision fracture treatment. Immunohistochemical analysis was performed, and the results demonstrated consistent positive staining for all BMPs and receptors, with immunoreactivity most intense for BMPs-3 and 7. These findings demonstrate that components of the BMP signaling cascade are expressed in human fracture callus and suggest that modulation of the repair process may be possible.

Over the past 20 years, investigators have tested the use of purified or recombinant BMPs in the treatment of several musculoskeletal conditions. While these studies have reported encouraging results, only two randomized, controlled studies have been reported in the treatment of fractures.

In a large prospective, randomized, controlled, partially blinded, multicenter study, Friedlaender et al (92) assessed the efficacy of rhBMP-7 (OP-1) versus iliac crest bone graft in the treatment of 122 patients with 124 tibial nonunions. All nonunions were at least 9 months old and had shown no progress towards healing for the 3 months prior to patient enrollment. Patients were randomized to receive either standard treatment with reduction and fixation with an intramedullary nail and autologous bone graft, or reduction and fixation with an intramedullary nail and implantation of rhBMP-7 (OP-1) on a type I collagen carrier. Results showed that 9 months after surgery, 81% of the 63 patients treated with BMP-7 and 85% of 61 patients treated with autologous bone grafting had achieved clinical union. Radiographic assessments suggested healing in 75% and 84% of these patients, respectively. As these results showed equivalent efficacy between OP-1 and autogenous bone graft, the authors concluded that OP-1 was a safe and effective alternative to bone graft in the treatment of tibial nonunions (Fig. 9-4).

More recently, the BMP-2 Evaluation in Surgery for Tibial Trauma (BESTT) Study Group reported on a large prospective, randomized, controlled multicenter trial evaluating the effects of rhBMP-2 in the treatment of open tibial fractures (93). Four hundred and fifty patients with these injuries were randomized to receive either initial irrigation and debridement followed by treatment with intramedullary (IM) nail fixation alone or IM fixation plus an implant containing either 0.75 mg/kg or 1.5 mg/kg of rhBMP-2 at the time of definitive treatment. The implant was placed over the fracture site at the time of wound closure. After 1 year, there were fewer secondary interventions (returns to the operating room for additional treatment) in the group treated with 1.5 mg/kg rhBMP-2. In addition, those patients treated with 1.5 mg/kg rhBMP-2 had accelerated times to union, improved wound healing, and reduced infection rates (Fig. 9-5).

Despite these promising results, the outcomes in human studies are not as impressive as those seen in animals where greater bone formation and healing has been noted. Diefenderfer et al (94) noted that one of the reasons may be a differential response of human bone marrow stromal cells to BMPs. Bone marrow cells isolated from patients undergoing hip replacement were cultured and grown to confluence with or without dexamethasone, and treated with BMPs. The results demonstrated no significant osteogenic response to BMPs-2, 4, or 7 as determined by alkaline phosphatase induction, unless cells were pretreated with dexamethasone. Moreover, even when cells were pretreated, the alkaline phosphatase response to BMPs was only about 50% of that measured in murine bone marrow cell cultures. The authors concluded that the ability of human bone marrow cells to respond to BMPs may differ substantially from that which exists in lower mammalian species.

Other Peptide Signaling Molecules

Several growth factors, as decribed below, stimulate the activity of chondroprogenitor and osteoprogenitor cells but do not induce cartilage or bone formation from undifferentiated cells. Current interest to understand the role of these molecules in the treatment of fractures is based on the observations that these molecules are expressed during normal fracture healing. Although each has been tested in experimental settings, these factors are not currently available for treatment of patients.

Transforming Growth Factor Beta

Transforming growth factor beta (TGF-β) influences a number of cell processes including the stimulation of mesenchymal stem

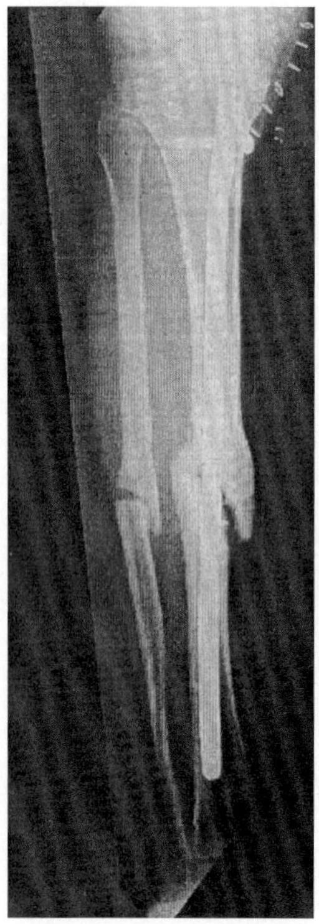
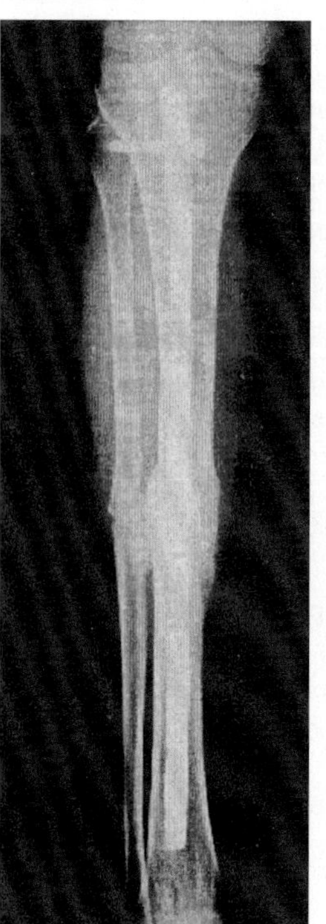
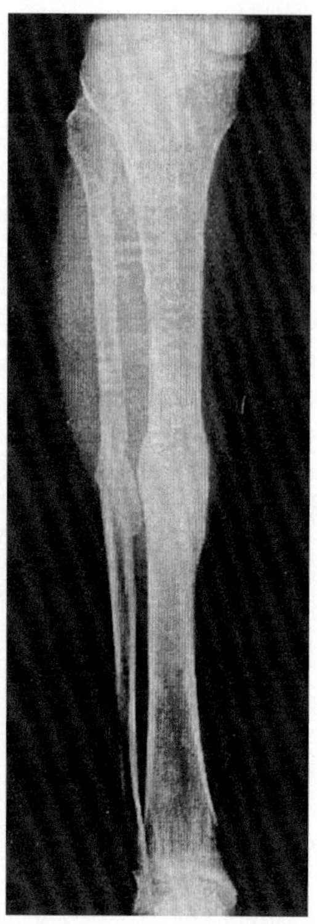

FIGURE 9-4 Sequential radiographs of a tibial nonunion treated with OP-1 immediately postoperatively, 9 months, and 24 months later. Note the bridging callus and subsequent tibial union. [Reprinted with permission from Friedlaender GE, Perry CR, Cole JD, et al. Osteogenic protein 1 (bone morphogenetic protein 7) in the treatment of tibial nonunions. *J Bone Joint Surg Am* 2001;83:S151–S158.]

cell (MSC) growth and differentiation, enhancement of collagen and other extracellular matrix (ECM) protein synthesis. It also functions as a chemotactic factor for fibroblast and macrophage recruitment (95).

Lind et al (96) tested two doses of TGF-β in rabbits in which tibial defects had undergone unilateral plate fixation. After 6 weeks of healing, mechanical testing showed improved bending stiffness only in the group treated with the low dose, and no improvement in the group treated with the high dose. Critchlow et al (97) performed a study of tibial defect healing in rabbits to test the hypothesis that the anabolic effects of TGF-β on bony repair are dependent on the mechanical stability at the fracture site. The results showed that under stable mechanical conditions, a low dose of TGF-β-2 had an insignificant effect on callus development, whereas the higher dose led to a larger callus.

From these studies, TGF-β appears to have some efficacy in

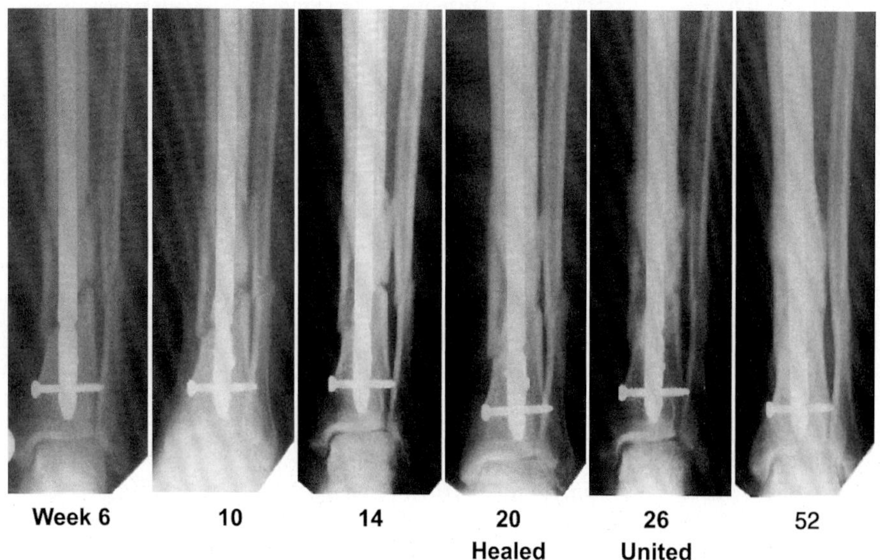

FIGURE 9-5 Radiographs of a patient who had sustained an open fracture of the left tibia (Gustilo-Anderson type IIIB) and was treated with an unreamed intramedullary nail and a 1.50 mg/mL rhBMP-2 implant. The fracture was considered to be clinically healed by 20 weeks, and radiographically healed by 26 weeks. (Reprinted with permission from Govender S, Csimma C, Genant HK, et al. Recombinant human bone morphogenetic protein 2 for treatment of open tibial fractures. A prospective, controlled, randomized study of four hundred and fifty patients. *J Bone Joint Surg Am* 2002;84:2123–2134.)

augmenting fracture healing, however, the effects are highly dose-dependent and not especially robust. To our knowledge, there are no studies underway or planned to test the use of TGF-β in human fracture healing.

Fibroblast Growth Factor

Fibroblast growth factors (FGF) are a group of structurally related compounds that share between 30% to 50% sequence homology. Acidic FGF (aFGF, FGF1) and basic FGF (bFGF, FGF2) are the most well studied members of this family with bFGF considered to be the more potent. It stimulates angiogenesis, endothelial cell migration and is mitogenic for fibroblasts, chondrocytes, and osteoblasts (98,99).

During fracture repair, FGFs differ in their temporal and spatial expression (100). In the early stages, FGF1 and -2 are localized to the proliferating periosteum. This expression is then limited to osteoblasts during intramembranous bone formation and in the chondrocytes and osteoblasts during endochondral bone formation. In light of their active involvement during fracture repair, investigators have studied the potential therapeutic roles of FGF in bone formation. Nakamura and associates (101) studied these effects by injecting bFGF into mid-diaphyseal transverse tibial fractures in dogs. Controls were injected with carrier molecules. Results showed that bFGF enlarged the callus area at four weeks and increased the callus bone mineral content at 8 weeks. Subsequent to the reporting of these findings in animals, at least one biotechnology company initiated preliminary studies in humans in order to set the stage for a multicenter randomized, controlled trial in patients with closed tibia fractures. Those preliminary results have not been reported and the multicenter clinical trial has not been conducted. At this time, the status of the development of FGFs for enhancement of fracture healing in patients is unknown.

Platelet-derived Growth Factor

Platelet-derived growth factor (PDGF) is synthesized by numerous cell types including platelets, macrophages, and endothelial cells. It consists of two polypeptide chains that share 60% amino acid sequence homology (102). PDGFs possess strong mitogenic properties and stimulate the proliferation of osteoblasts (103,104). This is particularly important in fracture healing where they exhibit differential spatial and temporal expression (105). Nash et al (106) examined the efficacy of PDGF on bone formation using a rabbit tibial osteotomy model. Each osteotomy was injected with either collagen or collagen containing 80 μg of PDGF. Results showed an increase in callus formation and a more advanced stage of endosteal and periosteal osteogenic differentiation in the PDGF-treated group compared to the controls. However, there was no improvement in the mechanical properties of the calluses in the group treated with PDGF. Despite these unimpressive results from a single study, there is still interest in the potential role of PDGF in the treatment of fractures and further studies are underway to test its efficacy in experimental models.

Prostaglandin Agonists

Prostaglandins (PG) comprise a group of unsaturated long chain fatty acids. They are synthesized from arachidonic acid by the cyclo-oxygenase enzymes and are known to have profound osteogenic effects when implanted into skeletal sites (107) or systemically infused (108).

In a study of rabbit tibial fractures, Dekel et al (109) demonstrated that PGE_2 caused a dose-dependent stimulation of callus formation and an increase in total bone mineral content. Its effects were also shown to be greatest during the latter stages of fracture healing, suggesting that the primary effect may be to stimulate osteoblasts and osteoprogenitor cells as opposed to undifferentiated Mesenchymal stem cells.

One of the major limitations of PG use in humans is its side effects. These include diarrhea, lethargy, and flushing and are mitigated by the binding of PG to all four of its receptors (EP1, EP2, EP3, EP4). Li and co-workers (107) investigated the effects of CP-533,536, a newly discovered nonprostanoid PGE2 agonist, selective for the EP2 receptor on fracture repair. This receptor primarily regulates bone anabolic activity. Using models of both rat and canine fracture healing, CP-533,536 in a poly-(D, L-lactide-co-glycolide) matrix was delivered to fracture sites in a dose-dependent fashion. Each dose increased callus size, density, and strength compared to the controls. Histologically, extensive endochondral and intramembranous ossification was noted. These data suggest that an EP2-receptor agonist may have a therapeutic role to augment the fracture repair process. Clinical trials are currently underway to investigate this application.

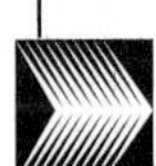

AUTHORS' PREFERRED TREATMENT

We recommend the use of osteogenic protein-1 (OP-1; BMP-7) for the treatment of recalcitrant nonunions of long bones. We recommend the use of BMP-2 for the treatment of open tibia fractures. The other factors and agonists discussed in this section are not yet available and therefore it is not possible to recommend their use at this time.

SYSTEMIC ENHANCEMENT OF FRACTURE HEALING

Parathyroid Hormone

Parathyroid hormone is an important regulator of calcium and phosphate metabolism that acts by enhancing gastrointestinal calcium absorption, increasing calcium and phosphate reabsorption from the kidneys, and participating in the regulation of 1,25 dihydroxyvitamin D synthesis (110). Although the effects of PTH are usually associated with bone resorption, the response of osteoclasts to PTH is more likely mediated via osteoblastic activity as receptors for PTH are found on osteoblast membranes (110). Investigators have shown that while continuous exposure to PTH leads to an increase in osteoclast numbers and activity, intermittent exposure stimulates osteoblasts and results in increased bone formation in rats and humans (111,112).

Clinical trials using PTH (1-34) have shown an increase in bone mass in osteoporotic men and an increase in bone mineral density and a reduction of vertebral and other osteoporotic related fractures in postmenopausal women (113,114). Neer et al (113) assessed the efficacy of PTH (1-34) for improving bone mineral density in a clinical trial involving 1673 postmenopausal women, with prior nontraumatic vertebral fractures. Results demonstrated that PTH increased bone mineral density and reduced the risk of fracture.

Based on this anabolic effect of PTH on the skeleton, several animal studies have been conducted examining PTH effects on the repair of bone. All have demonstrated an enhancement of fracture healing at high doses (115,116). Recently, Alkhiary et al (117) investigated the effect of recombinant PTH on fracture healing in 270 rats that underwent standard, closed femoral fractures and received doses of PTH that are similar to those shown to be effective in the treatment of osteoporosis in postmenopausal women. Using biomechanical tests, histomorphometry and quantitative microcomputed tomography, results demonstrated that daily systemic administration of both a 5 μg/kg/day and 30 μg/kg/day dose enhanced fracture healing by increasing bone mineral density, bone mineral content, and total osseous tissue volume. These findings have supported the initiation of clinical trials to study the role of systemic administration of PTH (1-34) in fracture patients.

Growth Hormone and Insulin-like Growth Factor 1

Growth hormone (GH) and insulin-like growth factors (IGF) play an important role in skeletal development and remodeling. Growth hormone is currently used clinically to treat patients with short stature (118) as it stimulates endochondral ossification, periosteal bone formation, and linear growth. It mediates these effects through the IGF system including the ligands, receptors, IGF binding proteins (IGFBP), IGFBP proteases and activators, and inhibitors of IGFBP proteases (119).

Two IGFs have been identified, IGF-1 (somatomedin C) and IGF-2. Although IGF-2 is the most abundant growth factor in bone, IGF-1 has the greater potency for promoting growth and has been localized in healing fractures of humans (120,121). IGF-1 and IGF-2 promote bone matrix formation (type I collagen and noncollagenous matrix proteins) by fully differentiated osteoblasts (122) and stimulate the proliferation of osteoprogenitor cells once human marrow stromal cells differentiate towards the osteoblast lineage.

Several studies have reported moderate enhancement of skeletal repair using either GH (121,123) or IGF-1 (124). Most recently, Kolbeck et al (125) showed that GH significantly improves the mechanical properties of fracture callus in minipigs. Although it is still unclear if this effect is a direct result of GH or IGF, the potential role of GH as a systemic enhancer of skeletal repair is of great interest.

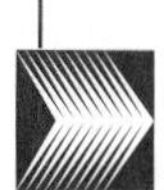

AUTHORS' PREFERRED TREATMENT

Several interesting randomized, controlled clinical trials are currently underway for the use of systemic agents in the enhancement of skeletal repair. At this time, no recommendations can be made as these studies have not yet been completed. The senior author (TAE) has used parathyroid hormone as an adjunct to the repair of fractures in postmenopausal women who would otherwise fulfill the requirements for its use based on their osteoporotic condition. These patients healed their fractures successfully but the association of that healing with the use of parathyroid hormone cannot be firmly established.

PHYSICAL ENHANCEMENT OF SKELETAL REPAIR

The mechanical environment has a direct impact on fracture healing. Direct mechanical perturbation as well as biophysical modalities such as electrical and ultrasound stimulation, have been shown to affect fracture healing. In order to enhance fracture repair by these mechanical measures it is necessary to develop a fundamental understanding of the ways in which the mechanical environment impacts cellular and molecular signaling.

Mechanical Stimulation

The fracture repair process can be modulated by mechanical forces. By controlling the weight bearing status of a limb, the resultant load at the fracture site will influence the stress environment. Sarmiento and associates (126) found that early weight bearing accelerates the fracture healing process. Standardized femoral fractures were produced in rats and stabilized by nonrigid intramedullary fixation. The animals were either allowed to bear weight at an early stage or were kept nonweight bearing by cast immobilization. Histological, radiological, and mechanical differences were present by the second week after fracture. These differences became progressively greater during the next three weeks. The authors attributed these findings to early mobilization facilitating the maturation of callus tissue produced by endochondral ossification.

The degree of stability at the fracture site has a direct impact on the repair process (127). Using a standardized, bilateral tibial canine osteotomy model, compression plating of the fracture was compared with the less stable external fixation performed on the opposite side. At 120 days after injury, bone formation was biomechanically less mature on the external fixator side. These tibiae had significantly less intracortical new-bone formation and more bone porosity when compared with the tibiae that had been treated with compression plates. Endosteal new-bone formation was greater on the plated side. Since the in vitro stiffness of the external fixator was less in all modes tested (compression, distraction, torsion, and anteroposterior bending) except lateral bending, the authors concluded that the rigidity of the fixation may be an important factor in early remodeling of a healing osteotomy.

Several investigators have attempted to modulate fracture healing by altering the mechanical strain environment. In a prospective, randomized clinical trial, Kenwright et al (128) compared the effects of controlled axial micromotion on tibial diaphyseal fracture healing in patients who were treated with external fixation and stratified according to fracture severity and extent of soft tissue injury. A specially designed pneumatic pump was attached to the unilateral frame of one group of patients and delivered a cyclical axial displacement of 1.0 mm at 0.5 Hz for 20 to 30 minutes a day. Fracture healing was assessed clinically, radiologically, and by measurement of the mechanical stiffness of the fracture. Both clinical and mechanical healing were enhanced in the group subjected to micromovement, compared to those treated with frames without micromotion. The differences in healing times were statistically significant and independently related to the treatment method. There was no difference in complication rates between treatment groups.

Distraction Osteogenesis

Limb lengthening was first described by Codivilla in 1905 (129) for the treatment of limb length discrepancies. It was not until the work of Ilizarov (130,131) 50 years later that the technique of distraction osteogenesis gained popularity as a method for enhancing bone regeneration.

Distraction osteogenesis generates new tissue through the application of tensile forces to developing callus via a controlled osteotomy (132,133). It is characterized by three separate stages: (a) the latency phase that immediately follows osteotomy; (b) the active or distraction phase which permits active separation of bony segments; and (c) the consolidation phase where active distraction has ended and healing of the callus begins (134–136). The period of time for each stage varies depending upon the anatomic site and the size of the osseous defect needing repair.

In order to delineate the molecular mechanisms by which distraction osteogenesis promotes new bone formation, Pacicca et al (137) studied the expression of angiogenic factors during this process. They demonstrated the expression of several of these molecules localizing to the leading edge of the distraction gap, where nascent osteogensis was occurring. Expression of these factors was greatest during the active phase of distraction.

Several investigators have utilized the technique of distraction osteogenesis to stimulate new bone formation in the clinical setting. Kocaoglu et al (138) treated 16 patients with hypertrophic nonunions with the Ilizarov distraction method. All patients had at least 1 cm shortening, three patients had a deformity in one plane, and the remainder had a deformity in two planes. All nonunions healed at an average follow-up of 38.1 months, with correction of all preoperative length inequalities and limb angulation to normal anatomic alignment (Fig. 9-6). Sen et al (139) reported on the efficacy of distraction in the management of patients with grade III open tibia fractures. Twenty-four patients who had open tibia fractures with bone (mean bone defect of 5 cm) and soft tissue (mean 2.5 × 3.5 cm) loss and a Mangled Extremity Severe Score of 6 and below were selected and treated with compression-distraction osteogenesis using the Ilizarov-type circular external fixator. After an average of 30 months follow-up, bone assessment results were excellent in 21 and good in three patients. Functional assessment scores were excellent in 19, good in four, and fair in one patient. These findings demonstrate that distraction osteogenesis is a safe, reliable and successful method for the treatment of acute open tibia fractures with bone and soft-tissue loss.

Electrical Stimulation

Fukada and Yasuda (140) first reported the occurrence of piezoelectric potentials in mechanically loaded dry bone in 1957. Since then, many investigators have studied the influence of electrical stimulation on bone formation and growth. In 1971, Freidenberg et al (141) reported the healing of a nonunion after the use of direct current. Within 5 years, over 119 articles had been published highlighting the use of electrical stimulation on bone growth and repair (142).

Currently available devices for electrical stimulation can be categorized as one of three types: constant direct-current (DC) stimulation with the use of percutaneous or implanted electrodes (invasive), capacitive coupling (noninvasive), or time varying inductive coupling produced by a magnetic field (noninvasive). In DC stimulation, stainless steel cathodes are placed in the tissues and electrically induced osteogenesis exhibits a dose response curve in relation to the amount of current that is delivered. Currents below a certain threshold result in no bone formation while those above a certain level lead to cellular necrosis (143). With electromagnetic stimulation, an alternating current produced by externally applied coils leads to a time varying magnetic field that, in turn, induces a time varying electrical field in bone. In capacitative coupling, an electrical field is induced in bone by an external capacitor—that is, two charged metal plates are placed on either side of a limb and are attached to a voltage source (144).

In terms of its applicability to orthopaedics, electrical stimulation has primarily been used in the treatment of nonunions. Brighton and co-workers (144) reported on the treatment of 178 nonunions in 175 patients with DC. Solid bone union was seen in 84% of patients. Patients with a history of osteomyelitis had a healing rate of nearly 75%. The presence of previously

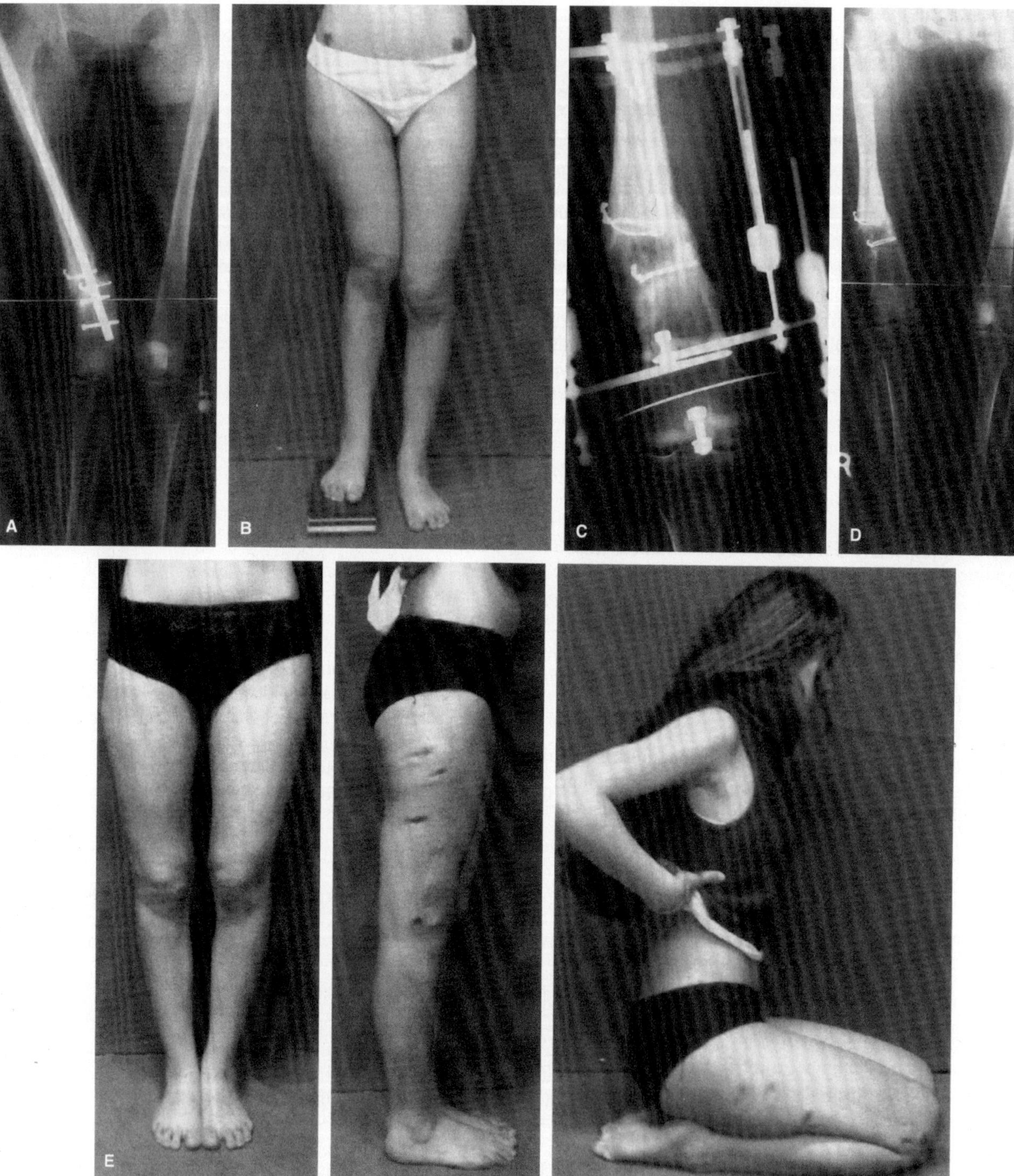

FIGURE 9-6 Radiographs of a 23-year-old woman with a hypertrophic nonunion of the distal femur, with a history of a previous open reduction and internal fixation and a 13-month period of nonunion. **A.** Preoperative anteroposterior radiograph. **B.** Preoperative photograph demonstrating leg length discrepancy. **C.** Callus formation during distraction osteogenesis using an Ilizarov fixator. **D.** Postoperative anteroposterior radiograph 3 months after frame removal. **E.** Postoperative photographs showing correction of leg length discrepancy and knee flexion. (Reprinted with permission from Kocaoglu M, Eralp L, Sen C, et al. Management of stiff hypertrophic nonunions by distraction osteogenesis: a report of 16 cases. *J Orthop Trauma* 2003;17:543–548.)

inserted metallic fixation devices did not affect the healing rate. When this study was expanded to include other centers, an additional 58 out of 89 nonunions achieved similar results. Review of the nonunions treated unsuccessfully with constant direct current suggested that inadequate electricity, the presence of a synovial pseudarthrosis or infection, and dislodgment of the electrodes were the causes of failure with this procedure. Complications of DC were minor and no deep infections resulting from this procedure in patients without previous osteomyelitis were noted. The authors concluded that given proper electrical parameters and proper cast immobilization, a rate of bone union comparable to that seen with bone-graft surgery was achieved.

Similar results were reported by Scott and King (145) in a prospective, double-blind trial using capacitive coupling in patients with established nonunions. In a population of 21 patients, 10 were actively managed and 11 were treated with a placebo unit. Results showed healing in 60% of the patients who had received electrical stimulation. None of the patients managed with the placebo unit demonstrated any bone formation.

Bassett et al (146) reported on the use of pulsed electromagnetic fields (PEMF) in the treatment of ununited tibial diaphyseal fractures. One hundred and twenty-five patients with 127 nonunions underwent long-leg plaster cast immobilization. Patients were treated with nonweight bearing ambulation and a total of 10 hours of PEMF stimulation daily. The authors reported an overall fracture healing rate of 87%, with success being independent of the age or sex, number of previous surgeries, presence of infection, or metal fixation (Fig. 9-7).

Despite the promising results seen in patients with nonunions, the application of this technology to the treatment of fresh fractures has not been clearly defined. Although some studies have shown that pulsed electromagnetic fields favorably influences fracture healing in experimental animals (143), other studies have failed to demonstrate this effect (147). At present, there is a paucity of published clinical studies showing that electrical stimulation enhances the healing of fresh fractures.

An important question concerning the use of electrical stimulation for fractures is whether it is possible to accelerate repair when healing has been slow or when there is early evidence that a nonunion may be developing. Sharrard (148) conducted a double-blind, multicenter trial of the use of pulsed electromagnetic fields in patients who had developed delayed union of tibial fractures. Forty-five tibial fractures that had not united for more than 16 weeks but less than 32 weeks were treated with immobilization in a plaster cast which incorporated the coils of an electromagnetic stimulation unit. The unit was activated for 20 of these fractures and was not turned on for 25. Radiographs showed evidence of union of nine of the fractures that had had active electromagnetic stimulation and in only three of the fractures in the control group ($p = 0.02$).

Ultrasound Stimulation

Low-intensity pulsed ultrasound (LIPUS) has been shown to promote fracture repair and increase the mechanical strength of fracture callus in both animal (149,150) and clinical studies (151,152). In a prospective, randomized double-blind trial, Heckman et al (151) examined the use of US as an adjunct to conventional treatment with a cast in 67 patients with closed or open grade I tibial shaft fractures. Thirty-three fractures were treated with the active device and 34 with the placebo. Using clinical and radiographic criteria, the authors noted that there

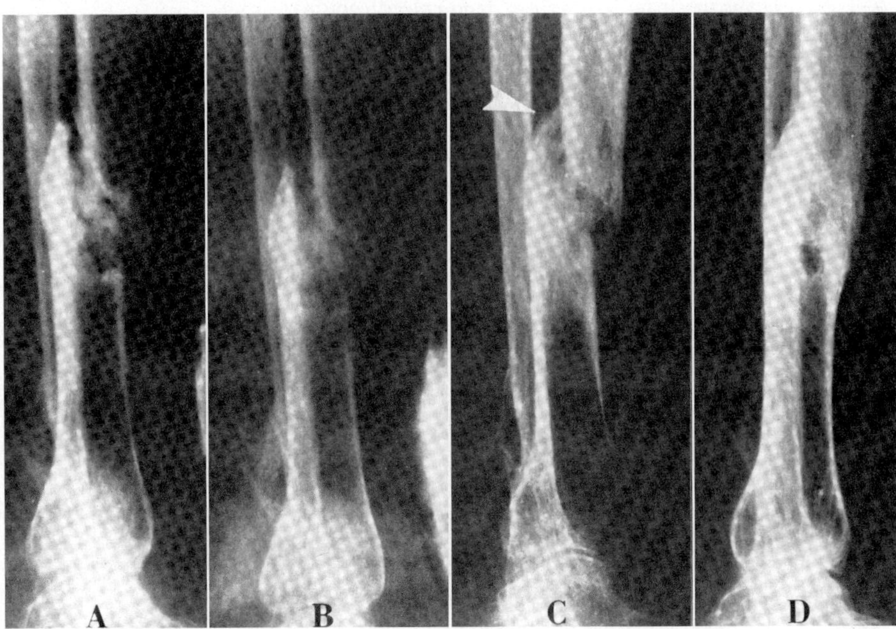

FIGURE 9-7 Sequential radiographs of a 42-year-old woman with tibial nonunion. Note gradual trabecular bone formation and restoration of a medullary cavity in the tibia in response to pulsed electromagnetic fields over a 16-month period. (Reprinted with kind permission from Bassett CAL, Mitchell SN, Gaston SR. Treatment of ununited tibial diaphyseal fractures with pulsing electromagnetic fields. *J Bone Joint Surg Am* 1981; 63:511–523.)

was a statistically significant decrease in the time to union (86 ± 5.8 days in the US treatment group compared with 114 ± 10.4 days in the control group) and in the time to overall healing (96 ± 4.9 days in the US treatment group vs. 154 ± 13.7 days in the controls). There were no issues with patient compliance in the treatment group and no serious complications reported with its use.

In a subsequent multicenter, prospective, randomized double-blind study, Kristiansen and co-workers (152) evaluated the efficacy of LIPUS in the treatment of dorsally angulated distal radius fractures that had been treated with manipulation and a cast. Results demonstrated that time to union was significantly shorter for the fractures that were treated with US compared to the controls (61 ± 3 days compared to 98 ± 5 days). The authors further noted that treatment with US was associated with a significantly smaller loss of reduction (20 ± 6% vs. 43 ± 8%) as determined by the degree of volar angulation as well as with a significant decrease in the mean time until the loss of reduction ceased (12 ± 4 days compared to 25 ± 4 days).

In a study by Cook et al (153), the ability of low intensity US to accelerate the healing of tibial and distal radius fractures in smokers was evaluated. In this patient group, the usual healing time for tibial fractures were 175 ± 27 days and for distal radius fractures were 98 ± 30 days. The investigators were able to show a statistically significant reduction in healing times with the use of US with 103 ± 8.3 days reported in the tibial fracture group and 48 ± 5.1 days in the patients with distal radius fractures. Treatment with US also substantially reduced the incidence of delayed unions in tibias in smokers and nonsmokers. These results are important because they suggest that US can override some of the detrimental effects that smoking has upon fracture healing.

In contrast to the above findings, Emami et al (154) noted that ultrasound did not appear to have a stimulatory role on tibial fracture repair. In a prospective, randomized, double-blinded controlled study, patients with fresh tibial fractures who were treated with a reamed and statically locked intramedullary nail were divided into an ultrasound group and placebo group. They all used an ultrasound device 20 minutes daily for 75 days without knowing whether it was active or inactive. Standardized radiographs were taken every third week until healing and at 6 and 12 months. Results showed that low-intensity ultrasound treatment did not shorten the healing time.

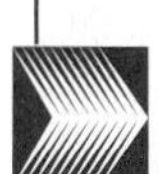

AUTHORS' PREFERRED TREATMENT

The use of controlled micromotion to enhance fracture healing, as described by Goodship and Kenright (155), has not been widely used. Before recommending such treatment, we would encourage surgeons to contact these authors to gain information on how best to employ that technology. The use of appropriately applied distraction osteogenesis for the treatment of nonunions is recommended for surgeons who are experienced with the use of small-pin, ring fixation.

Although not our preferred treatment for nonunions of long bones, we do recognize the data that supports the use of electrical stimulation for these cases. Direct current, capacitive coupling, and pulse electromagnetic fields have all been demonstrated, in randomized controlled trials, to enhance the healing of nonunions. Pulsed electromagnetic fields can also be used for the treatment of delayed unions. There is no evidence that electrical stimulation of any type enhances the healing of fresh fractures.

Ultrasound stimulation can be used for the treatment of fresh closed fractures of the distal radius and tibia when treated in a cast. We also recommend this treatment as an adjunct to the management of closed fractures of long bones in patients who smoke. Because it has not been shown to be successful, we do not recommend the use of ultrasound in the treatment of fractures that have undergone an operation in which fixation devices have been implanted.

CONCLUSIONS AND FUTURE DIRECTIONS

Most fractures heal uneventfully with patients returning to their previous levels of functioning. Unfortunately, however, there is a certain number of cases where difficulties in fracture repair occur and for which alternatives are needed. With improved understanding of the intracellular and extracellular pathways involved in bone healing, our ability to successfully augment this repair process continuously evolves.

Through the advent of tissue engineering, the ability to repair or regenerate the musculoskeletal system is developing rapidly and expanding in its applications. To date, strategies have met with limited success within the clinical setting. With ongoing research to enhance the osteogenic potential of cell concentrates, develop better delivery systems and gene therapy applications for growth factors and osteoinductive substances, this technology will add to current treatment modalities and greatly enhance the management of musculoskeletal injuries and diseases in the future.

REFERENCES

1. Einhorn TA. Current concepts review: Enhancement of fracture healing. *J Bone Joint Surg Am* 1995;77A(6):940–956.
2. Claes L, Augat P, Suger G, et al. Influence of size and stability of the osteotomy gap on success of fracture healing. *J Orthop Res* 1997;15:577–584.
3. Einhorn TA, Bonnarens F, Burnstein AH. The contributions of dietary protein and mineral to the healing of experimental fractures: A biomechanical study. *J Bone Joint Surg Am* 1986;68:1389–1395.
4. Macey LR, Kana SM, Jingushi S, et al. Defects of early fracture healing in experimental diabetes. *J Bone Joint Surg Am* 1989;71:722–733.
5. Nicoll EA. Fractures of the tibial shaft: A survey of 705 cases. *J Bone Joint Surg Br* 1964; 46:373–387.
6. Uhthoff HK, Rahn BA. Healing patterns of metaphyseal fractures. *Clin Orthop Relat Res* 1981;160:295–303.
7. Buckwalter JA, Einhorn TA, Bolander ME, et al. Healing of the musculoskeletal tissues. In: Rockwood, CA Jr, Green DP, Bucholz RW, et al., eds. *Rockwood and Green's fractures in adults*, vol 1. Philadelphia: JB Lippincott, 1996:261–304.
8. Lewandrowski K, Gresser JD, Wise DL, et al. Bioresorbable bone graft substitutes of different osteoconductivities: a histologic evaluation of osteointegration of poly(propyl-

ene glycol-co-fumaric acid-based cement implants in rats. *Biomaterials* 2000;21: 757–764.
9. Urist MR. Bone transplants and implants. In: Urist MR, ed. *Fundamental and clinical bone physiology*. Philadelphia: JB Lippincott, 1980:331–368.
10. Stevenson S. Biology of bone grafts. *Orthop Clin North Am* 1999;39:543–552.
11. Younger EM, Chapman MW. Morbidity at bone graft donor sites. *J Orthop Trauma* 1989;3:192–195.
12. Banwart JC, Asher MA, Hassanein RS. Iliac crest bone graft harvest donor site morbidity: a statistical evaluation. *Spine* 1995;20:1055–1060.
13. Fowler BL, Dall BE, Rowe DE. Complications associated with harvesting autogenous iliac bone graft. *Am J Orthop* 1995;24:895–903.
14. Goulet JA, Senunas LE, DeSilva GL, et al. Autogenous iliac crest bone graft: Complications and functional assessment. *Clin Orthop Relat Res* 1997;339:76–81.
15. Parikh SN. Bone graft substitutes: past, present and future. *J Postgrad Med* 2002;48: 142–148.
16. Bolander MF. Regulation of fracture repair by growth factors. *Proc Soc Exp Biol Med* 1992;200:165–170.
17. Cotran RS, Kumar V, Robbins SL. Healing repair. In: Cotran RS, Kumar V, Robbins SL, eds. *Pathologic basis of disease*. Philadelphia: Saunders, 1989.
18. Joyce ME, Jingushi S, Bolander ME. Transforming growth factor beta in the regulation of fracture repair. *Orthop Clin North Am* 1990;21:199–209.
19. Bauer TW, Muschler GF. Bone graft materials. An overview of the basic science. *Clin Orthop Relat Res* 2000;371:10–27.
20. Friedlaender GE. Current concepts review: Bone grafts. *J Bone Joint Surg Am* 1987;69: 786–790.
21. Goldberg VM, Stevenson S, Shaffer JW. Biology of autografts and allografts. In: Friedlaender GE, Goldberg VM, eds. *Bone and clinical applications*. Park Ridge, IL: American Academy of Orthopaedic Surgeons, 1991:3–12.
22. O'Keefe RM Jr, Riemer BL, Butterfield SL. Harvesting of autogenous cancellous bone graft from the proximal tibial metaphysic. A review of 230 cases. *J Orthop Trauma* 1991;5:469–474.
23. Krause JO, Perry CR. Distal femur as a donor site of autogenous cancellous bone graft. *J Orthop Trauma* 1995;9:145–151.
24. Enneking WF, Eady JL, Burchardt, H. Autogenous cortical bone grafts in the reconstruction of segmental skeletal defects. *J Bone Joint Surg Am* 1980;62A:1039–1058.
25. Moore JR, Weiland AJ, Daniel RK. Use of free vascularized bone grafts in the treatment of bone tumors. *Clin Orthop Relat Res* 1983;175:37–44.
26. Finkemeier CG. Bone grafting and bone graft substitutes. *J Bone Joint Surg Am* 2002; 84A:454–464.
27. Dell PC, Burchardt H, Glowczewskie FP Jr. A roentgenographic, biomechanical and histological evaluation of vascularized and non-vascularized segmental fibula canine autografts. *J Bone Joint Surg Am* 1985;67:105–112.
28. Ray RD. Vascularization of bone graft and implants. *Clin Orthop Relat Res* 1972;87: 43–48.
29. Burchardt H. The biology of bone graft repair. *Clin Orthop Relat Res*1983;42:28–42.
30. Goldberg VM, Stevenson S. The biology of bone grafts. *Semin Arthroplasty* 1996;7:12.
31. Enneking WF, Burchardt H, Puhl JJ, et al. Physical and biological repair in dog cortical bone transplants. *J Bone Joint Surg Am* 1975;57:237–252.
32. Goldberg VM, Shaffer JW, Field G, et al. Biology of vascularized bone grafts. *Orthop Clin North Am* 1987;18:2:179–185.
33. Gazdag AR, Lane JM, Glaser D, et al. Alternatives to autogenous bone graft: efficacy and indications. *J Am Acad Orthop Surg* 1995;3:1–8.
34. Tang CL, Mahoney JL, McKee MD, et al. Donor site morbidity following vascularized fibular grafting. *Microsurgery* 1998;18:383–386.
35. Beresford JN. Osteogenic stem cells and the stromal system of bone and marrow. *Clin Orthop Relat Res* 1989;240:270–280.
36. Connolly JF, Guse R, Tiedeman J, et al. Autologous marrow injection as a substitute for operative grafting of tibial nonunions. *Clin Orthop Relat Res* 1991;266:259–270.
37. Muschler GF, Nakamoto C, Griffith LG. Engineering principles of clinical cell-based tissue engineering. *J Bone Joint Surg Am* 2004;86A:1541–1558.
38. Connolly JF, Shindell R. Percutaneous marrow injection for an ununited tibia. *Nebr Med J* 1986;71:105–107.
39. Healey JH, Zimmerman PA, McDonnell JM, et al. Percutaneous bone marrow grafting of delayed union and nonunion in cancer patients. *Clin Orthop Relat Res* 1990;256: 280–285.
40. Garg NJ, Gaur S, Sharma S. Percutaneous autogenous bone marrow grafting in 20 cases of ununited fracture. *Acta Orthop Scand* 1993;64:671–672.
41. Muschler GF, Nitto H, Boehm CA, et al. Age- and gender-related changes in the cellularity of human bone marrow and the prevalence of osteoblastic progenitors. *J Orthop Res* 2001;19:117–125.
42. Muschler GF, Boehm C, Easley K. Aspiration to obtain osteoblast progenitor cells from human bone marrow: the influence of aspiration volume. *J Bone Joint Surg Am* 1997; 79:1699–1709.
43. Takigami H, Matsukura Y, Muschler GF. Osteoprogenitor cell enriched bone grafts prepared using selective cell retention technology: clinical application in four patients. Raynham, MA: DePuy AcroMed, Inc., 2003.
44. Boyce T, Edwards J, Scarborough N. Allograft bone: the influence of processing on safety and performance. *Orthop Clin North Am* 1999;30:571–581.
45. Dodd CAF, Fergusson CM, Freedman L, et al. Allograft versus autograft bone in scoliosis surgery. *J Bone Joint Surg Br* 1988;70:431–434.
46. Moucha CS, Einhorn TA. Enhancement of skeletal repair. In: Browner BD, Jupiter JB, Levine AM, et al., eds. *Skeletal trauma. Basic science, management and reconstruction*, 3rd ed. Philadelphia: Saunders, 2003:639.
47. Fleming JE Jr, Cornell CN, Muschler GF. Bone cells and matrices in orthopaedic tissue engineering. *Orthop Clin North Am* 2000;31:357–374.
48. Betz RR. Limitations of autograft and allograft: new synthetic solutions. *Orthopaedics* 2002;25(5 Suppl):561–570.
49. Friedlaender GE. Immune responses to ostechondral allografts: current knowledge and future directions. *Clin Orthop Relat Res* 1983;174:58–68.
50. Pelker RR, Friedlaender GE, Markham TC, et al. Effects of freezing and freeze drying on the biomechanical properties of rat bone. *J Orthop Res* 1984;1:405–411.
51. Goldberg VM, Stevenson S. Natural history of autografts and allografts. *Clin Orthop Relat Res* 1987;225:7–16.
52. Burchardt H. Biology of bone transplantation. *Orthop Clin North Am* 1987;18:187–196.
53. Stevenson S, Li XQ, Martin B. The fate of cancellous and cortical bone after transplantation of fresh and frozen tissue antigen matched and mismatched osteochondral allografts in dogs. *J Bone Joint Surg Am* 1991;73A:1143–1156.
54. Enneking WF, Mindell ER. Observations on massive retrieved human allografts. *J Bone Joint Surg Am* 1991;73A:1123–1142.
55. Thompson RC Jr, Pickvance EA, Garry D. Fractures in large-segment allografts. *J Bone Joint Surg Am* 1993;75A:1663–1773.
56. Kerry RM, Masri BA, Garbuz DS, et al. The biology of bone grafting. *Instr Course Lect* 1999;48:645–652.
57. Haddad FS, Duncan CP. Cortical onlay allograft struts in the treatment of periprosthetic femoral fractures. *Instr Course Lect* 2003;52:291–300.
58. Wang JW, Weng LH. Treatment of distal femoral nonunion with internal fixation, cortical allograft struts, and autogenous bone grafting. *J Bone Joint Surg Am* 2003;85A: 436–440.
59. Urist MR, Silverman BF, Buring K, et al. The bone induction principle. *Clin Orthop Relat Res* 1967;53:243–283.
60. Ludwig SC, Boden SD. Osteoinductive bone graft substitutes for spinal fusion: a basic science summary. *Orthop Clin North Am* 1999;30:635–645.
61. *AATB information alert*. McLean, VA: American Association of Tissue Banks, 1993.
62. Tiedeman JJ, Garvin KL, Kile TA, et al. The role of a composite, demineralized bone matrix and bone marrow in the treatment of osseous defects. *Orthopaedics* 1995;18: 1153–1158.
63. Vaccaro AR. The role of the osteoconductive scaffold in synthetic bone graft. *Orthopedics* 2002;25(5 Suppl):S571–S578.
64. Lewandrowski K, Gresser JD, Wise DL, et al. Bioresorbable bone graft substitutes of different osteoconductivities: a histologic evaluation of osteointegration of poly(propylene glycol-co-fumaric acid)-based cement implants in rats. *Biomaterials* 2000;21: 757–764.
65. Ellies LG, Nelson DG, Featherstone JD. Crystallographic structure and surface morphology of sintered carbonated apatites. *J Biomed Mater Res* 1988;22:541–553.
66. Vaes G. Cellular biology and biochemical mechanism of bone resorption: A review of recent developments on the formation, activation and mode of action of osteoclasts. *Clin Orthop Relat Res* 1988;231:239–271.
67. Albee FH. Studies in bone growth: Triple CaP as a stimulus to osteogenesis. *Ann Surg* 1920;71:32–36.
68. Jarcho M, Kay J, Gumaer K, et al. Tissue: cellular and subcellular events at a bone-ceramic hydroxyapatite interface. *J Bioengineering* 1977;1:79–92.
69. Roy D, Linnehan S. Hydroxyapatite formed from coral skeletal carbonate by hydrothermal exchange. *Nature* 1974;247:220–222.
70. McAndrew MP, Gorman PW, Lange TA. Tricalcium phosphate as a bone graft substitute in trauma: preliminary report. *J Orthop Trauma* 1988;2:333–339.
71. Chiroff RT, White EW, Weber KN, et al. Tissue ingrowth of replamine form implants. *J Biomed Mater Res* 1975;9:29–45.
72. Lee CA, Einhorn TA. The bone organ system. Form and function. In: Marcus R, Feldman D, Kelsey J, eds. *Osteoporosis*, 2nd ed, vol 1. New York: Academic Press, 2001: 3–20.
73. Bucholz RW, Carlton A, Holmes R. Interporous hydroxyapatite as a bone graft substitute in tibial plateau fractures. *Clin Orthop Relat Res* 1989;240:53–62.
74. Chapman MW, Bucholz R, Cornell C. Treatment of acute fractures with a collagen calcium phosphate graft material. *J Bone Joint Surg Am* 1997;79:495–502.
75. Cornell CN. Initial clinical experience with the use of Collagraft as a bone graft substitute. *Tech Orthop* 1992;7:55.
76. Dreesman H. Ueber Knochenplombierung. *Bietr Klin Chir* 1892;9:804–810.
77. Moed BR, Willson Carr SE, Craig JG, et al. Calcium sulfate used as bone graft substitute in acetabular fracture fixation. *Clin Orthop Relat Res* 2003;410:303–309.
78. Kelly CM, Wilkins RM, Gitelis S, et al. The use of a surgical grade calcium sulfate as a bone graft substitute: results of a multicenter trial. *Clin Orthop Relat Res* 2001;382: 42–50.
79. Borrelli J Jr, Prickett WD, Ricci WM. Treatment of nonunions and osseous defects with bone graft and calcium sulfate. *Clin Orthop Relat Res* 2003;411:245–254.
80. Constantz BR, Ison IC, Fulmer MT, et al. Skeletal repair by in situ formation of the mineral phase of bone. *Science* 1995;267:1796–1799.
81. Sanchez-Sotelo J, Munuera L, Madero R. Treatment of fractures of the distal radius with a remodellable bone cement. A prospective, randomized study using Norian SRS. *J Bone Joint Surg Br* 2000;82:856–863.
82. Cassidy C, Jupiter JB, Cohen M, et al. Norian SRS cement compared with conventional fixation in distal radius fractures. *J Bone Joint Surg Am* 2003;85:2127–2137.
83. Schildhauer TA, Bauer TW, Josten C, et al. Open reduction and augmentation of internal fixation with an injectable skeletal cement for the treatment of complex calcaneal fractures. *J Orthop Trauma* 2000;14:309–317.
84. Lobenhoffer P, Gerich T, Witte F, et al. Use of an injectable calcium phosphate bone cement in the treatment of tibial plateau fractures: a prospective study of twenty six cases with twenty month mean follow up. *J Orthop Trauma* 2002;16:143–149.

85. Horstmann WG, Verheyen CC, Leemans R. An injectable calcium phosphate cement as a bone graft substitute in the treatment of displaced lateral tibial plateau fractures. *Injury* 2003;34:141–144.
86. Johnson EE, Urist MR, Finerman GA. Repair of segmental defects of the tibia with cancellous bone grafts augmented with human bone morphogenetic protein. A preliminary report. *Clin Orthop Relat Res* 1988;236:249–257.
87. Urist MR. Bone: formation by autoinduction. *Science* 1965;150:893–899.
88. Cho TJ, Gerstenfeld LC, Einhorn TA. Differential temporal expression of members of the transforming growth factor β superfamily during murine fracture healing. *J Bone Miner Res* 2002;17:513–520.
89. Ripamonti U, Duneas N. Tissue morphogenesis and regeneration by bone morphogenetic proteins. *Plast Reconstr Surg* 1998;101:227–239.
90. Croteau S, Rauch F, Silvestri A, et al. Bone morphogenetic proteins in orthopaedics: from basic science to clinical practice. *Orthopaedics* 1999;22:7:686–695.
91. Kloen P, Di Paola M, Borens O, et al. BMP signaling components are expressed in human fracture callus. *Bone* 2003;33:362–371.
92. Friedlaender GE, Perry CR, Cole JD, et al. Osteogenic protein 1 (bone morphogenetic protein 7) in the treatment of tibial nonunions. *J Bone Joint Surg Am* 2001;83: S151–S158.
93. Govender S, Csimma C, Genant HK, et al. Recombinant human bone morphogenetic protein 2 for treatment of open tibial fractures. A prospective, controlled, randomized study of four hundred and fifty patients. *J Bone Joint Surg Am* 2002;84:2123–2134.
94. Diefenderfer DL, Osyczka AM, Garino JP, et al. Regulation of BMP induced transcription in cultured human bone marrow stromal cells. *J Bone Joint Surg Am* 2003;85(Suppl 3): 19–28.
95. Khan SN, Bostrom MP, Lane JM. Bone growth factors. *Orthop Clinic* 2000;31:375–388.
96. Lind M, Schumacker B, Soballe K, et al. Transforming growth factor β enhances fracture healing in rabbit tibiae. *Acta Orthop Scand* 1993;64:553–556.
97. Critchlow MA, Bland YS, Ashhurst DE. The effect of exogenous transforming growth factor β2 on healing fractures in the rabbit. *Bone* 1995;16:521–527.
98. Ingber DE, Folkman J. Mechanochemical switching between growth and differentiation during fibroblast growth factor stimulated angiogenesis in vitro: role of extracellular matrix. *J Cell Biol* 1989;109:317–330.
99. Hurley MM, Abreu C, Harrison JR, et al. Basic fibroblast growth factor inhibits type 1 collagen gene expression in osteoblastic MC3T3E1 cells. *J Bio Chem* 1993;268: 5588–5593.
100. Rundle CH, Miyakoshi N, Ramirez E, et al. Expression of the fibroblast growth factor receptor genes in fracture repair. *Clin Orthop Relat Res* 2002;403:253–263.
101. Nakamura T, et al. Recombinant human basic fibroblast growth factor accelerates fracture healing by enhancing callus remodeling in experimental dog tibial fracture. *J Bone Miner Res* 1998;13:942.
102. Solheim E. Growth factors in bone. *Int Orthop* 1998;22:410–416.
103. Canalis E, McCarthy TL, Centrella M. Effects of platelet derived growth factor on bone formation in vitro. *J Cell Physiol* 1989;140:530–537.
104. Canalis E. Effect of platelet-derived growth factor on DNA and protein synthesis in cultured rat calvaria. *Metabolism* 1981;30:970–975.
105. Andrew JG, Hoyland JA, Freemont AJ, et al. Platelet-derived growth factor expression in normally healing human fractures. *Bone* 1995;16:455–460.
106. Nash TJ, Howlett CR, Martin C, et al. Effect of platelet-derived growth factor on tibial osteotomies in rabbits. *Bone* 1994;15:203–208.
107. Li M, Ke HZ, Qi H, et al. A novel, nonprostanoid EP2 receptor selective prostaglandin E2 agonist stimulates local bone formation and enhances fracture healing. *J Bone Min Res* 2003;18:2033–2042.
108. Ueda K, Saito A, Nakano H, et al. Cortical hyperostosis following long-term administration of prostaglandin E1 in infants with cyanotic congenital heart disease. *J Pediatr* 1980;97:834–836.
109. Dekel S, Lenthall G, Francis MJ. Release of prostaglandins from bone and muscle after tibial fracture. An experimental study in rabbits. *J Bone Joint Surg Br* 1981;63:185–189.
110. Juppner H, Kronenberg HM. Parathyroid hormone. In: Favus MJ, ed. *Primer on the metabolic bone diseases and disorders of mineral metabolism*, 5th ed. Washington, DC: American Society of Bone and Mineral Research, 2003:117–124.
111. Podbesek R, Edouard C, Meunier PJ, et al. Effects of two treatment regimes with synthetic human parathyroid hormone fragment on bone formation and the tissue balance of trabecular bone in greyhounds. *Endocrinology* 1983;112:1000–1006.
112. Hock JM, Gera IJ. Effects of continuous and intermittent administration and inhibition of resorption on the anabolic response of bone to parathyroid hormone. *J Bone Miner Res* 1992;7:65–72.
113. Neer RM, Arnaud CD, Zanchetta JR, et al. Effect of parathyroid hormone (1-34) on fractures and bone mineral density in postmenopausal women with osteoporosis. *N Engl J Med* 2001;344:1434–1441.
114. Dempster DW, Cosman F, Kurland ES, et al. Effects of daily treatment with parathyroid hormone on bone microarchitecture and turnover in patients with osteoporosis: a paired biopsy study. *J Bone Miner Res* 2001;16:1846–1853.
115. Andreassen TT, Ejersted C, Oxlund H. Intermittent parathyroid hormone (1-34) treatment increases callus formation and mechanical strength of healing rat fractures. *J Bone Miner Res* 1999;14:960–968.
116. Holzer G, Majeska RJ, Lundy MW, et al. Parathyroid hormone enhances fracture healing. A preliminary report. *Clin Orthop Relat Res* 1999;366:258–263.
117. Alkhiary YM, Gerstenfeld LC, Krall E, et al. Enhancement of experimental fracture healing by systemic administration of recombinant human parathyroid hormone (PTH 1-34). *J Bone Joint Surg Am* (in print).
118. Ohlsson C, Bengtsson BA, Isaksson OG, et al. Growth hormone and bone. *Endocr Rev* 1998;19:55–79.
119. Kasukawa Y, Miyakoshi N, Mohan S. The anabolic effects of GH/IGF system on bone. *Curr Pharm Des* 2004;10:2577–2592.
120. Andrew JG, Hoyland J, Freemont AJ, et al. Insulinlike growth factor gene expression in human fracture callus. *Calcif Tissue Int* 1993;53:97–102.
121. Bak B, Jorgensen PH, Andreassen TT. Dose response of growth hormone on fracture healing in the rat. *Acta Orthop Scand* 1990;61:54–57.
122. Conover CA. Insulin-like growth factors and the skeleton. In: Canalis E, ed. *Skeletal growth factors*. Philadelphia: Lippincott Williams & Wilkins, 2000.
123. Andreassen TT, Oxlund H. Local anabolic effects of growth hormone on intact bone and healing fractures in rats. *Calcified Tiss Inter* 2003;73:258–264.
124. Thaller SR, Dart A, Tesluk H. The effects of insulin-like growth factor-1 on critical-size calvarial defects in Sprague-Dawley rats. *Ann Plast Surg* 1993;31:429–433.
125. Kolbeck S, Bail H, Schmidmaier G, et al. Homologous growth hormone accelerates bone healing–a biomechanical and histological study. *Bone* 2003;33:628–637.
126. Sarmiento A, Schaeffer JF, Beckerman L, et al. Fracture healing in rat femora as affected by functional weight-bearing. *J Bone Joint Surg Am* 1977;59:369–375.
127. Lewallen DG, Chao EY, Kasman RA, et al. Comparison of the effects of compression plates and external fixators on early bone-healing. *J Bone Joint Surg Am* 1984;66: 1084–1091.
128. Kenwright J, Richardson JB, Cunningham JL, et al. Axial movement and tibial fractures. A controlled randomised trial of treatment. *J Bone Joint Surg Br* 1991:73:654–659.
129. Codivilla A. On the means of lengthening in the lower limbs, the muscles and tissues which are shortened through deformity. *Am J Orthop Surg* 1905;2:353.
130. Ilizarov GA, Khelimskii AM, Saks RG. Characteristics of systemic growth regulation of the limbs under the effects of various factors influencing their growth and length [Russian]. *Ortop Travmatol Protez* 1978;8:37–41.
131. Ilizarov GA, Pereslitskikh PF, Barabash AP. Closed directed longitudino-oblique or spinal osteoclasia of the long tubular bones (experimental study) [Russian]. *Ortop Travmatol Protez* 1978;11:20–23.
132. Meyer U, Meyer T, Wiesmann HP, et al. Mechanical tension in distraction osteogenesis regulates chondrocyte differentiation. *Int J Oral Maxillofac Surg* 2001;30:522–530.
133. Lewinson D, Maor G, Rozen N, et al. Expression of vascular antigens by bone cells during bone regeneration in a membranous bone distraction system. *Histochem Cell Biol* 2001;116:381–388.
134. Sato M, Ochi T, Nakase T, et al. Mechanical tension stress induces expression of bone morphogenetic protein (BMP)-2 and BMP 4, but not BMP6, BMP7 and GDF5 mRNA during distraction osteogenesis. *J Bone Min Res* 1999;14:1084–1095.
135. Tay BK, Le AX, Gould SE, et al. Histochemical and molecular analysis of distraction osteogenesis in a mouse model. *J Orthop Res* 1998;16:636–642.
136. Isefuko S, Joyner CJ, Simpson HRW. A murine model of distraction osteogenesis. *Bone* 2000;27:661–665.
137. Pacicca DM, Patel N, Lee C, et al. Expression of angiogenic factors during distraction osteogenesis. *Bone* 2003;33:889–898.
138. Kocaoglu M, Eralp L, Sen C, et al. Management of stiff hypertrophic nonunions by distraction osteogenesis: a report of 16 cases. *J Orthop Trauma* 2003;17:543–548.
139. Sen C, Kocaoglu M, Eralp L, et al. Bifocal compression-distraction in the acute treatment of grade III open tibia fractures with bone and soft-tissue loss: a report of 24 cases. *J Orthop Trauma* 2004;18:150–157.
140. Fukada E, Yasuda I. On the piezoelectric effect of bone. *J Phys Soc Japan* 1957;12: 1158.
141. Friedenberg ZB, Harlow MC, Brighton CT. Healing of nonunion of the medial malleolus by means of direct current: a case report. *J Trauma* 1971;11:883–885.
142. Brighton CT. Current concepts review. The treatment of nonunions with electricity. *J Bone Joint Surg Am* 1981;63:847–851.
143. Friedenberg ZB, Andrews ET, Smolenski BI, et al. Bone reaction to varying amounts of direct current. *Surg Gynecol Obstet* 1970;131:894–891.
144. Brighton CT, Black J, Friedenberg ZB, et al. A multicenter study of the treatment of non-union with constant direct current. *J Bone Joint Surg Am* 1981;63:2–13.
145. Scott G, King JB. A prospective, double-blind trial of electrical capacitive coupling in the treatment of non-union of long bones. *J Bone Joint Surg Am* 1994;76:820–826.
146. Bassett CAL, Mitchell SN, Gaston SR. Treatment of ununited tibial diaphyseal fractures with pulsing electromagnetic fields. *J Bone Joint Surg Am* 1981;63:511–523.
147. Akai M, Yabuki T, Tateishi T, et al. Mechanical properties of the electrically stimulated callus. An experiment with constant direct current in rabbit fibulae. *Clin Orthop Relat Res* 1984;188:293–302.
148. Sharrard WJW. A double blind trial of pulsed electromagnetic fields for delayed union of tibial fractures. *J Bone Joint Surg Br* 1990;72:347–355.
149. Pilla AA, Mont MA, Nasser PR, et al. Non-invasive low-intensity pulsed ultrasound accelerates bone healing in the rabbit. *J Orthop Trauma* 1990;4:246–253.
150. Yang KH, Parvizi J, Wang SJ, et al. Exposure to low-intensity ultrasound increases aggrecan gene expression in a rat femur fracture model. *J Orthop Res* 1996;14:802–809.
151. Heckman JD, Ryaby JP, McCabe J, et al. Acceleration of tibial fracture-healing by non-invasive, low-intensity pulsed ultrasound. *J Bone Joint Surg Am* 1994;76:26–34.
152. Kristiansen TK, Ryaby JP, McCabe J, et al. Accelerated healing of distal radial fractures with the use of specific, low-intensity ultrasound. A multicenter, prospective, randomized, double-blind, placebo-controlled study. *J Bone Joint Surg Am* 1997;79:961–973.
153. Cook SD, Ryaby JP, McCabe J, et al. Acceleration of tibia and distal radius fracture healing in patients who smoke. *Clin Orthop Relat Res* 1997;337:198–207.
154. Emami A, Petren-Mallmin M, Larsson S. No effect of low-intensity ultrasound on healing time of intramedullary fixed tibial fractures. *J Orthop Trauma* 1999;13:252–257.
155. Goodship AE, Kenwright J. The influence of induced micromovement upon the healing of experimental tibial fractures. *J Bone Joint Surg Br* 1985;674:650–655.

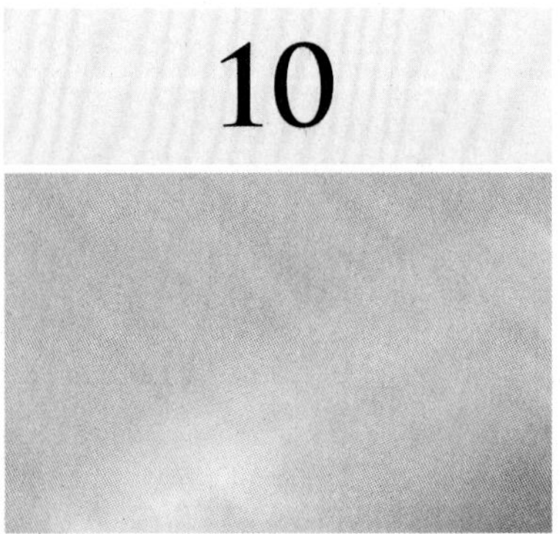

OUTCOME STUDIES IN TRAUMA

Mohit Bhandari

The "outcomes" movement in orthopaedic surgery involves careful attention to the design, statistical analysis, and critical appraisal of clinical research. The delineation between "outcomes" research and "evidence-based medicine" is vague. Since the term evidence-based medicine was coined first at McMaster University, orthopaedic surgeons and researchers have adopted their own style of critical appraisal often coined as "evidence-based orthopaedics (EBO)" using a clear delineation of relevant clinical questions, a thorough search of the literature relating to the questions, a critical appraisal of available evidence and its applicability to the clinical situation, and a balanced application of the conclusions to the clinical problem (1–3).

The balanced application of the evidence (the clinical decision making) is the central point of practicing evidence-based orthopaedics and involves, according to evidence-based medicine principles, integration of our clinical expertise and judgment with patients' perceptions and societal values, and with the best available research evidence (4,5).

Evidence-based orthopaedics involves a hierarchy of evidence, from meta-analyses of high quality randomized trials showing definitive results directly applicable to an individual patient, to relying on physiologic rationale or previous experience with a small number of similar patients. The hallmark of the evidence-based surgeon is that, for particular clinical decisions, he or she knows the strength of the evidence, and therefore the degree of uncertainty.

In the process of adopting evidence-based orthopaedic strategies, surgeons must avoid common misconceptions about evidence-based orthopaedics. Critics mistakenly have suggested that evidence can be derived only from the results of randomized trials, or that statistical significance automatically means clinical relevance. This is not true. This chapter provides a balanced evaluation of all study designs with recommendations to their appropriate use in orthopaedic clinical research.

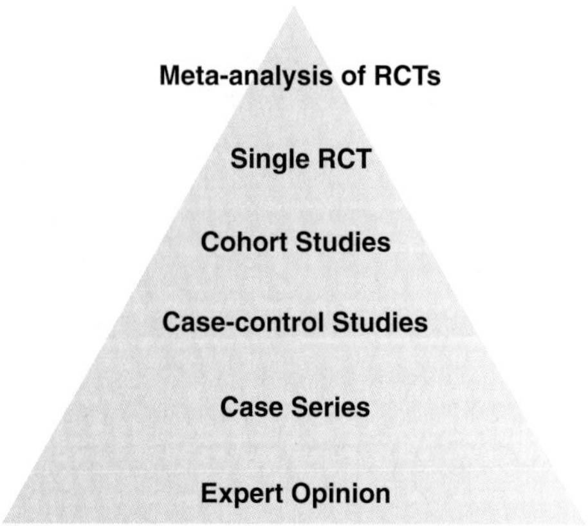

HIERARCHY OF EVIDENCE

Among various study designs, there exists a hierarchy of evidence with randomized controlled trials at the top, controlled observational studies in the middle, and uncontrolled studies and opinion at the bottom (Fig. 10-1) (1,5–7). Sackett et al have proposed a grading system that categorizes the hierarchy of research designs as levels of evidence. Each level (from 1 to 5) is associated with a corresponding grade of recommendation: (i) grade A—consistent level 1 studies; (ii) grade B—consistent level 2 or level 3 studies; (iii) grade C—level 4 studies; and (iv) grade D—level 5 evidence (1,5–7).

Understanding the association between study design and level of evidence is important. The *Journal of Bone and Joint Surgery* (*JBJS*), as of January 2003, has published the level of evidence associated with each published scientific article to provide readers with a gauge of the validity of the study results. Based on a review of several existing evidence ratings, the *JBJS* uses five levels for each of the four different study types (therapeutic, prognostic, diagnostic, and economic or decision modeling studies) (Table 10-1) (8). Level 1 studies may be deemed appropriate for the application to patient care, whereas level 4 studies will be interpreted with caution. For example, readers should be more confident about the results of a high quality multicenter randomized trial of arthroplasty versus internal fixation in patients with hip fracture on revision rates and mortality (level 1 studies) than two separate case series evaluating either arthroplasty or internal fixation on the same outcomes (level 4 studies).

FIGURE 10-1 The hierarchy of evidence with high quality randomized trials at the top and expert opinion at the bottom.

Bhandari et al have evaluated the inter-observer agreement among reviewers with varying levels of epidemiology training in categorizing clinical studies published in the *JBJS* into levels of evidence (9). Among 51 included articles the majority were studies of therapy (68.6%) constituting level 4 evidence (56.9%). Overall, agreement among reviewers for the study type, level of evidence and subcategory within each level was substantial (range in ICC: 0.61–0.75). Epidemiology trained reviewers demonstrated greater agreement (range in ICC: 0.99–1.0) across all aspects of the classification system when compared with nonepidemiology trained reviewers (range in ICC: 0.60–0.75). The findings suggested that epidemiology and nonepidemiology trained reviewers can apply the levels of evidence guide to published studies with acceptable inter-observer agreement. Although reliable, it remains unknown whether this system is valid (9).

The hierarchy of evidence bases its classification on the validity of the study design. Thus, those designs that limit bias to the greatest extent find themselves at the top of the pyramid and those inherently biased designs are at the bottom (Fig. 10-1). Application of the levels of evidence also requires a fundamental understanding of various study designs.

STUDY DESIGNS

The types of study designs used in clinical research can be classified broadly according to whether the study focuses on

TABLE 10-1 Levels of Evidence

	Types of Studies			
	Therapeutic Studies—Investigating the Results of Treatment	Prognostic Studies Investigating the Outcome of Disease	Diagnostic Studies—Investigating a Diagnostic Test	Economic and Decision Analyses—Developing an Economic or Decision Model
Level I	1. Randomized trial (a) Statistically significant difference (b) No statistically significant difference but narrow confidence intervals 2. Systematic Review[2] of level I RCTs (and studies were homogenous)	1. Prospective study[1] 2. Systematic review[2] of level I studies	1. Testing of previously developed diagnostic criteria on consecutive patients (with universally applied reference gold standard) 2. Systematic review[2] of level I studies	1. Clinically sensible costs and alternatives; values obtained from many studies; with multiway sensitivity analyses 2. Systematic review[2] of level I studies
Level II	1. Prospective cohort study[3] 2. Poor quality RCT (e.g., < 80% follow-up) 3. Systematic review[2] (a) Level II studies (b) Nonhomogeneous level 1 studies	1. Retrospective[4] study 2. Untreated controls from an RCT 3. Systematic review[2] of level II studies	1. Development of diagnostic criteria on consecutive patients (with universally applied reference gold standard) 2. Systematic review[2] of level II studies	1. Clinically sensible costs and alternatives; values obtained from limited studies; with multiway sensitivity analyses 2. Systematic review[2] of level II studies
Level III	1. Case control study[5] 2. Retrospective[4] cohort study 3. Systematic review[2] of level III studies		1. Study of nonconsecutive patients (without consistently applied reference gold standard) 2. Systematic review[2] of level III studies	1. Analyses based on limited alternatives and costs; and poor estimates 2. Systematic review[2] of level III studies
Level IV	Case Series (no, or historical, control group)	Case series	1. Case-control study 2. Poor reference standard	Analyses with no sensitivity analyses
Level V	Expert opinion	Expert opinion	Expert opinion	Expert opinion

RCT, randomized controlled trial.

describing the distributions or characteristics of a disease or elucidating its determinants (Fig. 10-2) (7). *Descriptive studies* describe the distribution of a disease, particularly what type of people have the disease, in what locations, and when. Cross sectional studies, case reports, and case series represent types of descriptive studies. *Analytic studies* focus on determinants of a disease by testing a hypothesis with the ultimate goal of judging whether a particular exposure causes or prevents disease. Analytic design strategies are broken into two types: observational studies, such as case-control and cohort studies, and experimental studies, also called clinical trials. The difference between the two types of analytic studies is the role the investigator plays in each of the studies. In the observational study, the investigator simply observes the natural course of events. In the trial, the investigator assigns the intervention or treatment.

Bhandari and Tornetta (6) review each type of study to highlight methodological issues inherent in their design (Table 10-2).

Meta-Analysis (Level 1 Evidence; Grade A Recommendation)

Although not considered to be a primary study design, meta-analysis, deserves mention because it is frequently used in the surgical literature. A meta-analysis is a systematic review that combines the results of multiple studies (of small sample size) to answer a focused clinical question. By its title as a review, meta-analyses are retrospective in nature. The main advantage of meta-analysis is the ability to increase the "total sample size" of the study by combining the results of many smaller studies. When well-designed studies are available on a particular ques-

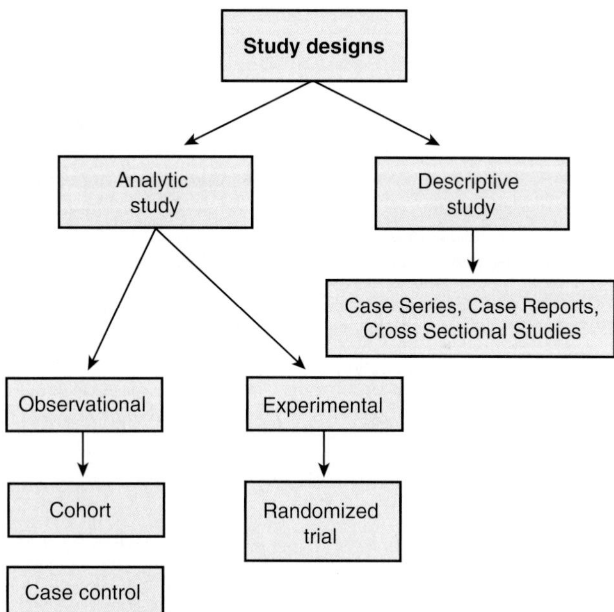

FIGURE 10-2 Categorization of study designs.

tion of interest, a meta-analysis can provide important information to guide clinical practice. Consider the following example. Several small randomized trials have attempted to resolve the issue of whether operative repair of acute Achilles tendon ruptures in younger patients reduces the risk of re-rupture compared with conservative treatment. Of five randomized trials (ranging in sample size from 27 to 111 patients), four found nonsignificant differences in re-rupture rates. These studies were under-powered. Using meta-analytic techniques, the results of these small studies were combined (N = 336 patients) to produce a summary estimate of 3.6% surgery versus 10.6% conservative (relative risk = 0.41, 95% confidence interval, 0.17–0.99, $p = 0.05$) of adequate study power (>80%) to help guide patient care (10).

Another benefit of meta-analysis is the increased impact over traditional reviews (e.g., narrative or nonsystematic reviews). Rigorous systematic reviews received over 2 times the number of mean citations compared with other systematic or narrative reviews (13.8 vs. 6.0, $p = 0.008$) (11).

Authors of meta-analyses can be limited to summarizing the outcomes available, and not necessarily the outcomes of interest. There is often a trade off between pooling data from many studies on common and sometimes less relevant outcomes (e.g., nonunion) versus fewer studies reporting less common outcomes of interest (e.g., avascular necrosis). Thus, the definition eligibility criteria for the studies to be included are an important step in the conduct of a meta-analysis.

While meta-analysis can be a powerful tool, its value is diminished when poor quality studies (e.g., case series) are included in the pooling. Pooled analyses of nonrandomized studies are prone to bias and have limited validity. Surgeons should be aware of these limitations when extrapolating such data to their particular clinical settings.

Randomized Trial (Level 1 Evidence; Grade A Recommendation)

When considering a single study, the randomized trial is the single most important design to limit bias in clinical research (12). While it may seem elementary to explain the term "randomization," most surgeons are unfamiliar with the rationale for random allocation of patients in a trial. Orthopaedic treatment studies attempt to determine the impact of an intervention on events such as nonunions, infections, or mortality—occurrences that we call the trial's target outcomes or target events. Patient age, their underlying severity of fracture, the presence of comorbid conditions, health habits, and a host of other factors typically determine the frequency with which a trial's target outcome occurs (prognostic factors). Randomization gives a patient entering a clinical trial an equal probability (or chance) of being allocated to alternative treatments. Patients can be randomized to alternative treatments by random number tables or computerized randomization systems. Randomization is the only method for controlling for known and unknown prognostic factors between two comparison groups. For instance, in a study comparing plates and intramedullary nails for the treatment of tibial shaft fractures in patients with concomitant head injury, investigators reported imbalance in acetabular fractures between treatment groups. Readers will agree that differences in patient function or mortality may not be attributed to treatment groups, but rather differences in the proportion of patients with acetabular fractures. Realizing this imbalance due to lack of randomization, the investigators employed a less attractive strategy to deal with the imbalance—statistical adjustment for differences between groups. By controlling for the difference in the number of acetabular fractures between groups, the effect of plates versus nails in patients was determined.

Equally important is the concept of "concealment" (not to be confused with blinding) (12). Concealed randomization ensures that surgeons are unable to predict the treatment to which their next patient will be allocated. The safest manner in which to limit this occurrence is a remote 24-hour telephone randomization service. Historically, treatment allocations in surgical trials have been placed within envelopes; while seemingly concealed, envelopes are prone to tampering.

While it is believed that surgical trials cannot be double-blinded due to the relative impossibility of blinding surgeons, Devereaux and colleagues have recently challenged the "classic" definition of double-blinding (13). In a survey of 91 internists and researchers, 17 unique definitions of "double-blinding" were obtained. Moreover, randomized trials in five high profile medical journals (*New England Journal of Medicine*, *Lancet*, *British Medical Journal*, *Annals of Internal Medicine*, and *JAMA*) revealed considerable variability in the reporting of blinding terminology. Common sources of blinding in a randomized trial include: physicians, patients, outcome assessors, and data analysts. Cur-

TABLE 10-2 Study Designs and Common Errors

Study Design	Summary	Common Errors
Meta-Analysis	High quality studies addressing a focused clinical question are critically reviewed and their results statistically combined	Major differences between pooled studies (heterogeneity) Poor quality studies pooled = less valid results
Randomized Trial	Patients are randomized to receive alternative treatments (e.g., cast vs intramedullary nail for tibial shaft fracture) Outcomes (e.g., infection rates) are measured prospectively	Type II (beta) errors—insufficient sample size Type I (alpha) error—overuse of statistical tests and multiple outcomes Lack of blinding Lack of concealed randomization
Prospective Cohort (with Comparison Group)	Patients who receive two different treatments are followed forward in time. Choice of treatment is not randomly assigned (e.g., surgeon preference, patient preference) Comparison group is identified and followed at the same time as the treatment group (i.e., concurrent comparison group) Outcomes (e.g., infection rates) are measured prospectively	Type II (beta) errors—insufficient sample size Type I (alpha) error—overuse of statistical tests and multiple outcomes Lack of adjustment for differences in characteristics between treatment and comparison groups
Prospective Case Series (Without Comparison Group)	Patients who receive a particular treatment are followed fo ward in time (e.g., intramedullary nailing of tibial fractures) No concurrent comparison group is used	Lack of independent or blinded assessment of outcomes Lack of follow-up
Case-Control Study	Patients with an outcome of interest (e.g., infection) are compared backwards in time (retrospective) to similar patients without the outcome of interest (e.g., no infection) Risk factors for a particular outcome can be determined between cases and controls	Type II (beta) errors—insufficient sample size Type I (alpha) error—overuse of statistical tests and multiple outcomes Problems in ascertainment of cases and controls
Retrospective Case Series (with Comparison Group)	Patients with a particular treatment are identified backward in time (i.e., retrospectively). Comparison patients are also identified retrospectively	Type II (beta) errors—insufficent sample size Type I (alpha) error—overuse of statistical tests and multiple outcomes Incomplete reporting in patient charts

rent recommendations for reporting randomized trials include explicit statements about who was blinded in the study rather than using the term "double blinded." Surgical trials can always blind the data analyst, almost always blind the outcome assessor, occasionally blind the patient, and never blind the surgeon. In a review of orthopaedic trials, outcome assessors were blinded only 44% of the time and data analysts were never blinded. However, at least two-thirds of surgical trials could have achieved double-blinding by blinding the outcome assessors, patients, or data analysts (14).

The principle of attributing all patients to the group to which they were randomized results is an *intention-to-treat* principle (Fig. 10-3) (12). This strategy preserves the value of randomization: prognostic factors that we know about, and those we do not know about will be, on average, equally distributed in the two groups, and the effect we see will be just that due to the treatment assigned. When reviewing a report of a randomized trial one should look for evidence that the investigators analyzed

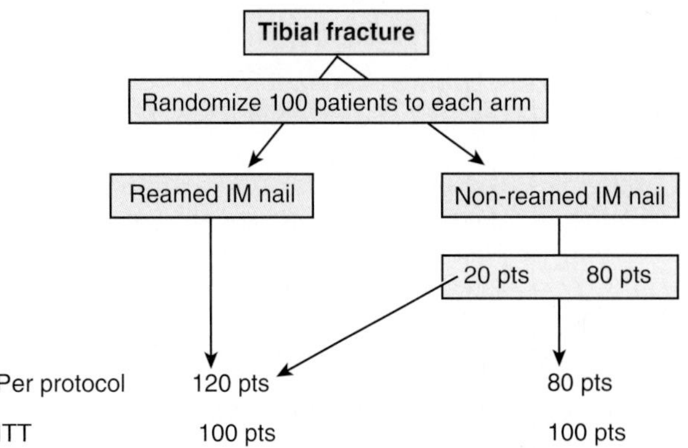

FIGURE 10-3 The intention-to-treat principle: a per protocol analysis analyzes patient outcomes to the treatment they "actually received," whereas intention-to-treat analysis evaluates outcomes based on the treatment to which patients were originally randomized.

all patients in the groups to which they were randomized. Some suggest that an intention to treat approach is too conservative and more susceptible to type II error due to increased biologic variability. Their argument is that an *intention-to-treat* analysis is less likely to show a positive treatment effect, especially for those studies that randomized patients who had little or no chance of benefiting from the intervention.

An alternative approach, referred to as a *per protocol* analysis, reports outcomes on the treatments patients had actually received regardless of the number of crossovers from one treatment to another. This approach is often used to determine whether imbalances in baseline factors actually affect the final result. It may be particularly important when patients who are randomized to one treatment (e.g., reamed or unreamed tibial nail) but never receive either treatment. For example, in a trial of reamed versus unreamed tibial nailing, a patient randomized to a reamed tibial nail who ultimately receives an external fixator due to an intra-operative surgical decision, will be excluded from in *per protocol* analysis; however, recall that this same patient would be included in the reamed tibial nail group in an intention-to-treat analysis.

The overall quality of a randomized trial can be evaluated with a simple checklist (Table 10-3). This checklist provides guides to the assessment of the methodological rigor a trial.

Observational Study (Cohort, Case Series) (Level 2 Evidence; Grade B Recommendation)

Studies in which randomization is not employed can be referred to as nonrandomized, or *observational,* study designs. The role of nonrandomized (observational) comparative studies in evaluating treatments is an area of continued debate: deliberate choice of the treatment for each patient implies that observed outcomes may be caused by differences among people being given the two treatments, rather than the treatments alone (15). Unrecognized confounding factors can interfere with attempts to correct for

TABLE 10-3 Petsky Checklist for Assessing Quality of Reporting

Randomization	1 Yes	1 Partly	0 No
Were the patients assigned randomly?	2 Yes		0 No
Randomization adequately described?	1 Yes		0 No
Was treatment group concealed to investigator?			
Total/4			
Description of outcome measurement adequate?	1 Yes	1 Partly	0 No
Outcome measurements objective?	2 Yes		0 No
Were the assessors blind to treatment?	1 Yes		0 No
Total/4			
Were inclusion/exclusion criteria well defined?	2 Yes	1 Partly	0 No
Number of patients excluded and reason?	2 Yes	1 Partly	0 No
Total/4			
Was the therapy fully described for the treatment group?	2 Yes	1 Partly	0 No
Was the therapy fully described for the controls?	2 Yes	1 Partly	0 No
Total/4			
Statistics	1 Yes	1 Partly	0 No
Was the test stated and was there a *P* value?	2 Yes		0 No
Was the statistical analysis appropriate?	1 Yes		0 No
If the trial was negative, were confidence intervals of post hoc power calculations performed?	1 Yes		0 No
Sample size calculation before the study?			
Total/4 (if positive trial) Total/5 (negative trial)			
Total Score: 20 points (if positive trial)			
21 points (if negative trial)			

identified differences between groups. There has been considerable debate about whether the results of nonrandomized studies are consistent with the results of randomized controlled trials (16–19). Nonrandomized studies, or observational studies, have been reported to overestimate or underestimate treatment effects (16,17).

One example of the pitfalls of nonrandomized studies was reported in a study comparing study designs that addressed the general topic of comparison of arthroplasty and internal fixation for hip fracture (20). Mortality data was available in 13 nonrandomized studies (N = 3108 patients) and in 12 randomized studies (N = 1767 patients). Nonrandomized studies overestimated the risk of mortality by 40% when compared with the results of randomized trials (relative risk 1.44 versus 1.04, respectively) (Fig. 10-4). If we believe the data from the nonrandomized trials, then no surgeon would offer a patient a hemiarthroplasty for a displaced hip fracture given the significant risk of mortality. However, in practice, arthroplasty is generally favored over internal fixation in the treatment of displaced femoral neck fractures. Thus, surgeons believe the randomized trials that report no significant differences in mortality and significant reductions in revisions with arthroplasty.

Important contradictory examples of observational and randomized controlled trial (RCT) results can be found in the surgical literature. An observational study of extracranial to intracranial bypass surgery suggested a "dramatic improvement in the symptomatology of virtually all patients" undergoing the procedure. However, a subsequent large RCT demonstrated a 14% relative increase in the risk of fatal and nonfatal stroke in patients undergoing this procedure compared to medical management (21). These considerations have supported a hierarchy of evidence, with randomized controlled trials at the top, controlled observational studies in the middle, and uncontrolled studies and opinion at the bottom. However, these findings have not been supported in two articles in the *New England Journal of Medicine* that identified nonsignificant differences in results between randomized controlled trials and observational studies (18,19).

Although randomized trials, when available, represent the most valid evidence information, nonrandomized studies can provide invaluable data to generate hypotheses for future studies.

Prospective Observational Study (Level 2 Evidence; Grade B Recommendation)

A prospective observational study identifies a group of patients at a similar point in time and follows them forward in time. Outcomes are determined prior to the start of the study and evaluated at regular time intervals until the conclusion of the study. A comparison group (controls) may also be identified concurrently and followed for the same time period.

While comparison groups are helpful when comparing outcomes of two surgical alternatives, a prospective evaluation of

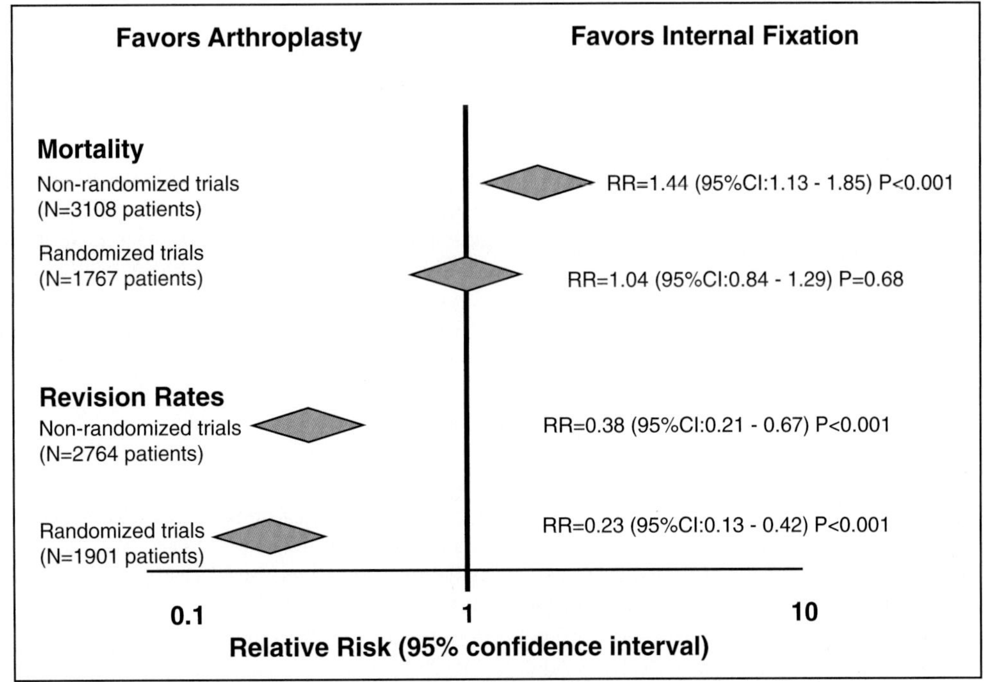

FIGURE 10-4 Estimates from randomized trials tend to provide a more conservative estimate of a treatment effect when compared to nonrandomized studies. Nonrandomized studies over-estimate the benefit of internal fixation regarding mortality by 40%.

a single group of patients with complex injuries can provide information on the frequency of success (radiographic and functional outcomes) and expected complications. This information is most useful when the data collected remains consistent over time, data collected includes important baseline patient characteristics and patient outcomes, and efforts are made to ensure patients are followed over time. Joel Matta's acetabular fracture database is one striking example of a carefully designed single surgeon, prospective database that has consistently collected data on patients over 20 years. With over 1000 patients with acetabular fractures included in this database, the current limits of technique, results, and complications can be reported to serve as a benchmark for future studies. In addition, these types of studies can assist surgeons in discussing the expected risk and outcomes of surgery with their patients during the informed consent process.

Case-Control Study (Level 3 Evidence; Grade B Recommendation)

If the outcome of interest is rare (e.g., mortality or infection), conducting a prospective cohort study may be cost prohibitive. A case-control study is a useful strategy in such circumstances (7). Cases with the outcome of interest are identified retrospectively from a group of patients (e.g., databases) and matched (e.g., by age, gender, severity of injury) with control patients who do not have the outcome of interest. Both groups can be compared for differences in "risk" factors (15). One control may be matched for each case that is identified (1:1 matching). Alternatively, multiple controls may be matched to each case (3:1 or 4:1 matching). The validity of results from case-control studies depend on the accuracy of reporting of the outcomes of interest. For example, investigators conducted a study to determine risk factors for hip fracture among elderly women (22). To accomplish this, they identified 159 women with their first hip fracture and 159 controls (1:1 matching) matched for gender, age, and residence. Risk factors such as perceived safety of the residence, psychotropic drug use, and tendency to fall were also included. Comparison of these factors between the hip fracture and control groups revealed an increased risk of perceived safety (odds ratio = 5.8), psychotropic drug use (odds ratio = 2.6), and tendency to fall (odds ratio = 2.3) among patients who sustained a fracture compared to those who did not.

Retrospective Case Series (Level 4 Evidence; Grade C Recommendation)

The retrospective study design, while less costly and less time consuming, is often limited by bias in the ascertainment of cases and the evaluation of outcomes. Comparison groups can be identified during the same time period as the treatment group (concurrent controls). However, controls from a different period of time can also be used (historical controls). Patient follow-up may be conducted passively (via patient records) or actively (patient follow-up appointment and examination). When patient charts have formed the basis for the outcome evaluation, readers should be convinced that the outcomes were objective measures accurately obtained from patient records. For example, in hospital mortality data is an objective outcome that is likely to have been well documented in patient's charts; however, patient satisfaction or functional outcome is subjective and far less likely to have been recorded with any standardization or consistency.

A case series can provide initial useful information about the safety and complication profile of a new surgical technique or implant. This information is most valid when eligibility criteria for patient inclusion are clearly defined, consecutive patients are screened for eligibility, surgery, and peri-operative care is consistent, outcomes are objective and independently assessed, and follow-up is complete. Unfortunately, the validity of the results can be compromised by inadequate and incomplete reporting of patient characteristics and outcomes in patient charts.

UNDERSTANDING STATISTICS IN TRAUMA OUTCOME STUDIES

Hypothesis Testing

The essential paradigm for statistical inference in the medical literature has been of hypothesis testing. The investigator starts with what is called a *null hypothesis* that the statistical test is designed to consider and, possibly, disprove. Typically, in the null hypothesis, there is no difference between treatments being compared. In a randomized trial in which investigators compare an experimental treatment with a placebo control, one can state the null hypothesis as follows: the true difference in effect on the outcome of interest between the experimental and control treatments is zero. We start with the assumption that the treatments are equally effective and we adhere to this position unless data make it untenable.

In this hypothesis-testing framework, the statistical analysis addresses the question of whether the observed data are consistent with the null hypothesis. The logic of the approach is as follows: even if the treatment truly has no positive or negative impact on the outcome (that is, the effect size is zero), the results observed will seldom show exact equivalence; that is, no difference at all will be observed between the experimental and control groups. As the results diverge farther and farther from the finding of "no difference," the null hypothesis that there is no difference between treatment effects becomes less and less credible. If the difference between results of the treatment and control groups becomes large enough, clinicians must abandon belief in the null hypothesis. We will further develop the underlying logic by describing the role of chance in clinical research.

Let us conduct a hypothetical experiment in which the suspected coin is tossed 10 times and on all 10 occasions, the result is heads (4). How likely is this to have occurred if the coin was indeed unbiased? Most people would conclude that it is highly unlikely that chance could explain this extreme result. We would therefore be ready to reject the hypothesis that the coin is unbiased (the null hypothesis) and conclude that the coin is biased. Statistical methods allow us to be more precise by ascertaining just how unlikely the result is to have occurred simply as a result of chance if the null hypothesis is true. The law of multiplicative probabilities for independent events (where one event in no way influences the other) tells us that the probability of 10 consecutive heads can be found by multiplying the probability of a single head (1/2) 10 times over; that is, 1/2 · 1/2 · 1/2, and so on (4). The probability of getting 10 consecutive heads is then slightly less than 1 in 1000. In a journal article, one would likely see this probability expressed as a *p* value, such as $p < 0.001$.

What Is the *p* Value?

What is the precise meaning of this *p* value? Statistical convention calls results that fall beyond this boundary (that is, *p* value <0.05) *statistically significant*. The meaning of statistically significant, therefore, is "sufficiently unlikely to be due to chance alone that we are ready to reject the null hypothesis." In other words, the *p* value is defined as the probability, under the assumption of no difference (null hypothesis), of obtaining a result equal to or more extreme than what was actually observed.

The 95% Confidence Interval

Investigators usually (though arbitrarily) use the 95% confidence interval (CI). One can consider the 95% CI as defining the range that includes the true difference 95% of the time (12). In other words, if the investigators repeated their study 100 times, it would be expected that the point estimate of their result would lie within the confidence interval 95 of those 100 times. The true point estimate will lie beyond these extremes only 5% of the time, a property of the confidence interval that relates closely to the conventional level of statistical significance of $p < 0.05$.

Measures of Central Tendency and Spread

Investigators will often provide a general summary of data from a clinical or experimental study. A number of measures can be used. These include measures of central tendency (mean, median, and mode) and measures of spread (standard deviation, range). The sample mean is equal to the sum of the measurements divided by the number of observations. The median of a set of measurements is the number that falls in the middle. The mode, however, is the most frequently occurring number in a set of measurements. Continuous variables (such as blood pressure or body weight) can be summarized with a mean if the data is normally distributed. If the data is not normally distributed, then the median may be a better summary statistic. Categorical variables (pain grade: 0, 1, 2, 3, 4, 5) can be summarized with a median.

Along with measures of central tendency, investigators will often include a measure of spread. The standard deviation is derived from the square root of the sample variance. The variance is calculated as the average of the squares of the deviations of the measurements about their mean. The range of a dataset reflects the smallest value and largest value.

Measures of Treatment Effect (Dichotomous Variables)

Information comparing the outcomes (dichotomous—mortality, re-operation) of two procedures can be presented to patients as an odds ratio, a relative risk, a relative risk reduction, an absolute risk reduction, and the number needed to treat (Table 10-4). Both reduction in relative risk and reduction in abso-

TABLE 10-4 Presentation of Results

	Infection	No Infection
Treatment Group	10 A	90 B
Control Group	50 C	50 D

Treatment Event Rate (TER): A(A + B = 10)100 = 10%

The incidence of infection in the treatment group

Control Event Rate (CER): C(C + D = 50)100 = 50%

The incidence of infection in the control group

Relative Risk (RR): TER/CER = 10/50 = 0.2

The relative risk of infection in the treatment group relative to the control group

Relative Risk Reduction (RRR): 1 – RR = 1 – 0.2 = 0.8 or 80%

Treatment reduces the risk of infection by 80% compared to controls

Absolute Risk Reduction (ARR): CER – TER = 50% – 10% = 40%

The actual numerical difference in infection rates between treatment and controls

Number Needed to Treat (NNT): 1/ARR = 1/0.40 = 2.5

For every 2.5 patients who received the treatment, one infection can be prevented

Odds Ratio (OR): AD/BC = (10)(50)/(90)(50)
= 500/4500 = 0.11

The odds of infection in treatment compared to controls is 0.11

luterisk have been reported to have the strongest influences on patient decision-making (23).

Common Statistical Tests

Common statistical tests include those that examine differences between two or more means, differences between proportions, and associations between two or more variables (Table 10-5) (24).

Comparing Two Independent Means

When we wish to test the null hypothesis that the means of two independent samples of normally distributed continuous data are the same, the appropriate test statistic is called *t*, hence the *t*-test. The author of the original article describing the distribution of the *t*-statistic used the pseudonym *Student* leading to the common attribution Student's *t*-test. When the data is non-normally distributed, a nonparametric test such as the Mann-Whitney U or Wilcoxon rank sum test can be used. If the means are paired, such as left and right knees, a paired *t*-test is most appropriate. The nonparametric correlate of this test is the Wilcoxon signed rank test.

Comparing Multiple Independent Means

When three or more different means have to be compared (e.g., hospital stay among three tibial fracture treatment groups—plate fixation, intramedullary nail, and external fixation), single factor analysis of variance is a test of choice. If the test yields statistical significance, investigators can conduct post-hoc comparison tests (usually a series of pairwise comparisons using *t*-tests) to determine where the differences lie. It should be recalled that the *p* value (alpha level) should be adjusted for multiple post-hoc tests. One rather conservative method is the Bonferroni correction factor that simply divides the alpha level ($p = 0.05$) by the number of tests performed.

Comparing Two Proportions

A common situation in the orthopaedic literature is that two proportions are compared. For example, these may be the proportion of patients in each of two treatment groups who experience an infection. The chi-square (χ^2) test is a simple method of determining whether the proportions are really different. When samples are small the χ^2 test becomes rather approximate because the data is discrete but the χ^2 distribution from which the *p* value is calculated is continuous. A Yates' correction is a device which is sometimes used to account for this, but when cell counts in the contingency table become very low (say, less than five) the χ^2 test becomes unreliable and a Fisher's exact test is the test of choice.

Determining Association Between One or More Variables Against One Continuous Variable

When two variables have been shown to be associated, it may be logical to try to use one variable to predict the other. The variable to be predicted is called the dependent variable, and that to be used for prediction is the independent variable. For such a linear relationship, the equation $y = a + bx$ is defined as the regression equation. *a* is a constant and *b* the regression coefficient. Fitting the regression equation, generally using a software package, is the process of calculating values for *a* and *b* which allow the regression line represented by this equation to best fit the observed data. The *P* value reflects the result of a hypothesis test that *x* and *y* are in fact unrelated, or in this case that *b* is equal to zero.

Correlation

The strength of the relationship between two variables (e.g., age vs hospital stay in patients with ankle fractures) can be summarized in a single number, the *correlation coefficient*. The correlation coefficient, which is denoted by the letter *r*, can range from -1.0 (representing the strongest possible negative

TABLE 10-5 Common Statistical Tests

Samples	Data Type and Distribution	Categorical	Ordered Categorical or Continuous and Non-Normal	Continuous and Normal
Two samples	Different individuals	χ^2 test Fisher's exact test	Mann-Whitney U test Wilcoxon rank sum test	Unpaired *t*-test
	Related or matched samples	McNemar's test	Wilcoxon signed rank test	Paired *t*-test
Three or more samples	Different individuals	χ^2 test Fisher's exact test	Kruskal-Wallis statistic	ANOVA
	Related samples	Cochran Q-test	Friedman statistic	Repeated measures ANOVA

Consult a statistician when planning an analysis or planning a study.
(Table adapted from Griffin D, Audige L. Common statistical methods in orthopaedic clinical studies. *Clin Orthop Relat Res* 2003;413:70–79.)

relationship, in which the person who scores the highest on variable scores the lowest on the other variable) to 1.0 (representing the strongest possible positive relationship, in which the person who is older also has the longest hospital stay). A correlation coefficient of zero denotes no relationship between the two variables.

COMMON ERRORS IN THE DESIGN OF ORTHOPAEDIC STUDIES

Any study that compares two or more treatments (e.g., comparative study: randomized trial, observational study with control group, case-control) can be subject to errors in hypothesis testing. For example, when investigators conduct studies to determine whether two treatments have different outcomes, there are four potential outcomes (Fig. 10-5) (1).

- A true positive result (i.e., the study correctly identifies a true difference between treatments)
- A true negative result (i.e., the study correctly identifies no difference between treatment)
- A false negative result—type II (beta) error (i.e., the study incorrectly concludes no difference between treatments when a difference really exists)
- A false positive result—type I (alpha) error (i.e., the study incorrectly concludes a difference between treatments when no difference exists)

Type II Error (Beta Error)

It is perceived that trials of surgical therapies may be sufficiently undersized to have a meaningful impact on clinical practice. Such trials of small sample size are subject to beta (β) errors (type II errors): the probability of concluding that no difference between treatment groups exists, when, in fact, there is a difference (Fig. 10-6). Typically, investigators will accept a beta error rate of 20% ($\beta = 0.20$), which corresponds with a study power of 80%. Most investigators agree that beta error rates greater than 20% (study power less than 80%) are subject to unacceptably high risks of false-negative results.

		Difference	No difference
Results of the study	Difference	Correct conclusion (1-β)	False positive (α error or Type I error)
	No difference	False negative (β error or Type II error)	Correct conclusion (1-α)

FIGURE 10-5 Errors in hypothesis testing: type I and type II errors are presented along with the power of a study ($1 - \beta$).

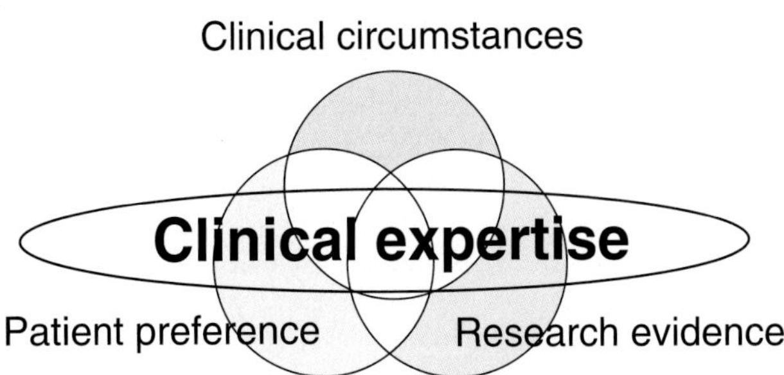

FIGURE 10-6 The current conceptual framework for evidence-based practice encompassing research findings, patients values and preferences, clinical circumstances, and expertise.

In an effort to quantify the extent to which orthopaedic trauma trials were underpowered, Lochner et al reviewed 117 randomized trials in trauma for type II error rates (25). The mean overall study power was 24.65% (range 2%–99%). The potential type II error rate for primary outcomes was 91%. For example, one study demonstrated "no difference" between reamed and nonreamed tibial intramedullary nailing; however, this study was underpowered for this conclusion (study power = 32%). Thus, these conclusions should be interpreted with caution.

Type I Error (Alpha Error)

Most surgeons are less familiar with the concept of concluding that the results of a particular study are true, when, in fact, they are really due to chance (or random sampling error). This erroneous false-positive conclusion is designated as a type I or alpha (α) error (Fig. 10-6) (26). By convention, most studies in orthopaedics adopt an α error rate of 0.05. Thus, investigators can expect a false-positive error about 5% of the time. Ideally, type I error rate is based on one comparison between alternative treatment groups usually designated as the primary outcome measure. In situations where no primary outcome variable has been determined, there is a risk of conducting multiple tests of significance on multiple outcomes measures. This form of data dredging by investigators risks spurious false-positive findings. Several techniques are available to adjust for multiple comparisons, such as the Bonferroni correction.

Most readers are intuitively skeptical when 1 in a list of 20 outcomes measured by an investigator is significant ($p < 0.05$) between two treatment groups. This situation typically occurs when investigators are not sure what they are looking for and therefore test several hypotheses hoping that one may be true. Statistical aspects of the multiple testing issue are straightforward. If n independent associations are examined for statistical significance, the probability that at least one of them will be found statistically significant is $1 - (1 - \alpha)^n$ if all n of the individual null hypotheses are true. Therefore, it is argued that studies that generate a large number of measures of association have markedly greater probability of generating some false-positive results because of random error than does the stated alpha level for individual comparisons.

Bhandari and colleagues conducted a review of recently published randomized trials (within the last 2 years) to determine the risk of type I errors among surgical trials that did not explicitly state a primary outcome (26). One study examining outcomes in two different uncemented total knee arthroplasty designs evaluated 21 different outcome measures and found 13 outcomes were significantly different between groups. As there was no clear statement about a designated primary outcome measure, the risk of a false-positive result was 66% (26).

Misuse of Subgroup Analyses in Orthopaedic Outcome Studies

Subgroup analysis can be defined as treatment outcome comparisons for patients subdivided by baseline characteristics (27,28). For instance, in a study of operative versus nonoperative management of calcaneal fractures, investigators may report no difference in the overall outcome (patient function) but subsequently conduct a series of comparisons across different patient subgroups (gender, disability status, or comorbidities). Subgroup analyses are frequently post-hoc analyses that risk false-positive results (type I error) in which ineffective (or even harmful) treatments may be deemed beneficial in a subgroup. Conducting multiple statistical tests risks spurious false-positive findings. Alternatively, false-negative results may occur because negative subgroup analyses are often underpowered.

Bhandari et al identified important errors in surgical randomized controlled trials related to subgroup analyses. The majority of authors did not report whether subgroup analyses were planned a priori and these analyses often formed the basis of the RCT conclusions. Inferences from such RCTs may be misleading and their application to clinical practice unwarranted (27,28).

In a review of 72 randomized trials (published in orthopaedic and other surgical subspecialties) 27 (38%) RCTs reported a total of 54 subgroup analyses with a minimum of 1 and a maximum of 32 subgroup analyses per study (29). The majority of subgroup analyses 49 (91%) were performed post-hoc and not stated to be pre-planned at the outset of the study nor included in the hypothesis. The majority of investigators inappropriately used tests of significance when comparing outcomes between subgroups of patients (41 subgroup analyses, 76%), however, only 3 of the analyses were performed using statistical test for interaction. Investigators reported differences between subgroups in 31 (57%) of the analyses, all of which were featured in the summary or conclusion of the published paper.

Subgroup analyses should be undertaken and interpreted with caution. The validity of a subgroup analysis can be improved by defining a few important (and biologically plausible) subgroups prior to conducting a study and conducting statistical tests of interaction. When faced with a subgroup analysis in a published scientific paper, readers should ask the following questions: Is the subgroup difference suggested by comparisons within rather than between studies? Did the hypothesis precede rather than follow the analysis? Was the subgroup effect one of a small number of hypothesized effects tested? Is the magnitude of the effect large? Was the effect statistically significant? Is the effect consistent across studies? Is there indirect evidence that supports the hypothesized subgroup effect?

Study Power and Sample Size Calculations

The power of a study is the probability of concluding a difference between two treatments when one actually exists. Power ($1 - \beta$) is simply the complement of the type II error (β). Thus, if we accept a 20% chance of an incorrect study conclusion ($\beta = 0.20$), we are also accepting that we will come to the correct conclusion 80% of the time. Study power can be used before the start of a clinical trial to assist with sample size determination, or following the completion of a study to determine if the negative findings were true (or due to chance).

The power of a statistical test is typically a function of the magnitude of the treatment effect, the designated type I error rate (α), and the sample size (N). When designing a trial, investigators can decide on the desired study power ($1 - \beta$) and calculate the necessary sample to achieve this goal (24).

Comparing Two Continuous Variables

A continuous variable is one with a scale (e.g., blood pressure, functional outcome score, time to healing). For example, in planning a trial of alternate strategies for the treatment of humeral shaft fractures, an investigator may identify a systematic review of the literature which reports that time to fracture healing with treatment A is 110 ± 45 days, while time to healing with treatment B (control group) can be expected to be up to 130 ± 40 days. The expected treatment difference is 20 days and the effect size (mean difference/standard deviation) is 0.5 (20/40). Effect sizes can be categorized as small (0.10), medium (0.30), and large (0.50). The anticipated sample size for this continuous outcome measure is determined by a standard equation.

This study will require approximately 63 patients in total to have sufficient power to identify a difference of 20 days between treatments, if it occurs. An investigator may then audit his or her center's last year and decide if enough patients will present to the center to meet the sample size requirements. Table 10-6 provides additional scenarios and the sample size requirements for varying differences in healing times between treatment and control groups. As the difference between treatments diminishes, the sample size requirements increase (Table 10-6).

Let's consider another study that aims to compare functional outcome scores in patients with ankle fractures treated operatively versus nonoperatively. Previous studies using the functional outcome score have reported standard deviations for op-

TABLE 10-6 Sample Size Requirements for Continuous Outcome (Time to Fracture Healing)

Time to Healing (Control Group)	Time to Healing (Treatment Group)	% Reduction in Time to Healing	Number of Patients Needed Per Group
150 Days	120	20%	16
150 Days	135	10%	63
150 Days	143	5%	289

TABLE 10-7 Sample Size Requirements for Difference Baseline Risks of Pulmonary Embolus

PE Rate Control Group	PE Rate Treatment Group	% Reduction in PE Risk	Number of Patients Needed Per Group
10%	8%	20%	3,213
1%	0.8%	20%	35,001
0.1%	0.08%	20%	352,881

erative and nonoperative cases of 12 points, respectively. Based on previous studies, we want to be able to detect a difference of 5 points on this functional outcome score between treatments.

From equation (1) in the appendix, our proposed study will require 90 patients per treatment arm to have adequate study power [$n_1 = n_2 = 2(12^2)\,(1.96 + 0.84)^2 / 5^2 = 90$].

Reworking the above equation, the study power can be calculated for any given sample size by transforming the above formula and calculating the z-score:

$$z_{1-\beta} = (n_1(\Delta^2)/2(\sigma^2))^{1/2} - z_{1-\alpha/2}$$

The actual study power that corresponds to the calculated z-score can be looked up in readily available statistical literature (6) or on the internet (keyword: z-table) (7,8). From the above example the z-score will be [$0.84 = (90(5^2)/2(12^2))^{1/2} - 1.96$] for a sample size of 90 patients. The corresponding study power for a z-score of 0.84 is 80%.

Comparing Two Dichotomous Variables (When the Outcome Measure Is Dichotomous [Proportion])

A dichotomous variable is typically one that has one of two options (e.g., infection or not, nonunion or not, alive or dead). Let's assume that this same investigator chooses nonunion as the primary outcome instead of time to union. Based on the previous literature, he or she believes that treatment A will result in a 95% union rate and treatment B (control group) will result in a 90% union rate. Now, 869 patients are required for the study to identify a 5% difference in nonunion rates between treatments. An investigator may realize that this number is sufficiently large to prohibit him or her from conducting this trial at one center and may elect to gain support at multiple sites for this trial. For example, in a proposed trial using pulmonary embolus risk as the primary outcome, the number of patients required may be prohibitive (Table 10-7).

Returning to our example of ankle fractures, let us now assume that we wish to change our outcome measure to differences in secondary surgical procedures between operative and nonoperatively treated ankle fractures. We consider a clinically important difference to be 5%. Based on the previous literature, we estimate that the secondary surgical rates in operative and nonoperative treated ankles will be 5% and 10%, respectively. The number of patients required for our study can now be calculated from equation (2) presented in the appendix. Thus, we need 433 patients per treatment arm to have adequate study power for our proposed trial.

$$n_1 = n_2 = [(2 \times 0.075 \times 0.925)^{1/2} \times 1.96 + (0.05 \times 0.95 + 0.1 \times 0.9)^{1/2} \times 0.84]^2 / 0.05^2 = 433$$

Reworking the above equation, the study power can be calculated for any given sample size by transforming the above formula and calculating the z-score:

$$z_{1-\beta} = ((n\,(\Delta^2))^{1/2} - (2p_m q_m)^{1/2}\, z_{1-\alpha/2}) / (p_1 q_1 + p_2 q_2)^{1/2}$$

From the above example the z-core will be $0.84 = ((433 \times 0.05^2)^{1/2} - (2 \times 0.075 \times 0.925)^{1/2} \times 1.96) / (0.05 \times 0.95 + 0.1 \times 0.9)^{1/2}$ for a sample size of 433 patients. The corresponding study power for a z-score of 0.84 is 80%.

MEASURING PATIENT HEALTH AND FUNCTION

The basis of the "outcomes movement" in trauma is a move toward identifying patient relevancy and clinically important measures to evaluate the success (or failure) of surgical interventions. Common to any outcome measure that gains widespread use should be its reliability and validity. Reliability refers to the extent to which an instrument yields the same results in repeated applications in a population with stable health. In other words, reliability represents the extent to which the instrument is free of random error. Validity is an estimation of the extent to which an instrument measures what it was intended to measure. The process of validating an instrument involves accumulating evidence that indicates the degree to which the measure represents what it was intended to represent. Some of these methods include face, content, and construct validity (30,31).

What Is Health-Related Quality of Life?

The World Health Organization defines health as "a state of complete physical, mental, and social well-being." Thus, when measuring health in a clinical or research setting, questioning patient's well-being within each of these domains is necessary to comprehensively represent the concept of health. Instruments that measure aspects of this broad concept of health are often referred to as health-related quality of life (HRQOL) measures. These measures encompass a broad spectrum of items including those associated with activities of daily life, such as work, recreation, household management, and relationships with family, friends, and social groups. HRQOL considers not only the ability to function within these roles but also the degree of satisfaction derived from performing them.

A generic instrument is one that measures general health status inclusive of physical symptoms, function, and emotional dimensions of health. A disadvantage of generic instruments, however, is that they may not be sensitive enough to be able to detect small but important changes (24).

Disease-specific measures, on the other hand, are tailored to inquire about the specific physical, mental, and social aspects of health affected by the disease in question allowing them to detect small important changes (30). Therefore, to provide the most comprehensive evaluation of treatment effects, no matter the disease or intervention, investigators often include both a disease-specific and generic health measure. In fact, many granting agencies and ethics boards insist that a generic instrument be included in the design of proposed clinical studies.

Often the combination of objective end points in a surgical study (i.e., quality of fracture reduction) and validated measures of patient function and quality of life is an ideal combination. While an intra-articular step off in a tibial plafond fracture may be viewed as a less than satisfactory radiograph outcome, there may be no detectable effect on patient function or quality of life (32).

Another factor to consider is the outcome measure's ability to discriminate between patients across a spectrum of the injury in question. Questionnaires may sometimes exhibit ceiling and floor effects. Ceiling effects occur when the instrument is too easy and all respondents score the highest possible score. Alternatively, floor effects can occur if the instrument is very difficult or tapping into rare issues associated with the disease. Most patients will score the lowest possible score. Miranda et al in a study of 80 patients with pelvic fractures found that the severity of pelvic fracture did not alter Short Form-36 and Iowa pelvic scores (33).

Despite increasing severity of the pelvic injury, functional outcomes remained equally poor. This was likely related to the associated soft tissue injuries that created a "floor effect," limiting the ability to discriminate between the orthopaedic injuries.

Common Outcome Instruments Used in Trauma

Beaton and Schemitsch have reported commonly used measures of outcome in orthopaedics (Table 10-8) (31). These include both generic and disease-specific instruments.

EQ-5D/EuroQOL

The EQ-5D, formally described as the EuroQOL, is a five-item scale designed to allow people to describe their health state across five dimensions (15). There are three response categories which combine for a total of 243 possible health states. The preference weight allows a single numeric score from slightly less than zero (theoretically worse than death) to 1 (best health state). EQ-5D scores are used in economic appraisals (such as cost utility analyses) in the construction of quality-adjusted life years for the calculation of cost per quality of life year gained and its comparison across interventions (www.euroqol.org and www.eur.nl/bmg/imta/eq-net/EQ5d.htm).

SF-36

The Short Form-36 (SF-36) is a generic measure of health status. It is probably one of the most widely used measures. The SF-36 has 35 items that fit into one of eight subscales. One additional item is not used in the scores. In 1994 the developers, led by John Ware, produced two summary scores for the SF-36: the physical component score (more heavily weights dimensions of pain, physical function, and role of function physical) and the mental component score (more weight given to mental health, vitality, etc.). The two physical component scores are standardized, so the general population (based on a U.S. sample) will score 50 on average, with a standard deviation of 10. The subscale scores, often presented as a profile graph, are scored on a scale of 0–100 where 100 is a good health state.

S-MFA

The short MFA (S-MFA) is a 46-item questionnaire that is a shortened version of Swionkowski's full Musculoskeletal Functional Assessment. The S-MFA has two main scores—the function index (items 1–34) and the bothersome index (items 35–46). The functional index is subdivided into four subscales (daily activities, emotional status, arm and hand function, and mobility). The S-MFA has been tested in patients with musculoskeletal disorders, as this is the target population. The psychometric properties are high, suggesting that it can be used for monitoring individual patients. The S-MFA was designed to describe the various levels of function in people with musculoskeletal disorders, as well as monitor change over time. It is available free of charge at the website (http://www.ortho.umn.edu/research/clinicaloutcomes.htm).

DASH

The DASH, short for Disabilities of the Arm, Shoulder and Hand, is a 30-item questionnaire designed to measure physical function and disability in any or all disorders of the upper limb. It is therefore designed to be sensitive to disability and change

TABLE 10-8 Commonly Used Outcome Measures*

Type	Measure	Domains/Scales	Number Items	Response Categories	Target Population	Measurement Properties: Internal Consistency	Test–Retest Reliability	Construct Validity	Responsiveness	Comments
Utility	EQ-5D	Mobility Self care Usual activities Anxiety/depression pain	1 1 1 1 1 Total = 5	3	All	N/A	*	**	*	Describes health state which is transcribed into utility using UK data. Indirect measure of utility.
Generic	SF-36 version 2	Physical function Bodily pain Role function—physical Role function—emotional Mental health Vitality Social functioning General health	10 2 4 3 5 4 2 5 Total = 35 + 1 item	3–6	All	**	*	**	**	Version 2 now in use Uses improved scaling for role functioning, and clearer wording Reliability is lower than desired for individual level of interpretation, fine for group
Region	S-MFA	Daily activities Emotional status Arm/hand function Mobility Above combined for functional index[a] Bothersome index	10 7 8 9 34 12	5 point	Musculoskeletal	**	**	**	**	Normative data now available[b] Only measure designed for any musculoskeletal problem
	DASH	Physical function, symptoms (one scale)	30	5	All upper limb musculoskeletal disorders	**	**	*	**	Normative data now available[b] Manual available
	TESS	Physical function in surgical oncology	30	5	Lower limb sarcoma	**	**	*	**	Developed in oncology, however, used in hip fractures

(Continued)

TABLE 10-8 Continued

Type	Measure	Domains/ Scales	Number Items	Response Categories	Target Population	Measurement Properties: Internal Consistency	Test–Retest Reliability	Construct Validity	Respon- siveness	Comments
Specific	WOMAC	Physical function Pain Stiffness	17 5 2	5 or visual analog scale	Osteoarthritis of knee, hip	**	**	**	**	Adopted as key outcome for evaluating knee arthroplasty
	Roland and Morris	Physical function due to low back pain	24	2 (yes/no)	Low back pain	*	**	**	**	Excellent review and comparison with Oswestry in Roland & Fairbanks
	Oswestry	Pain, personal care, lifting, walking, sitting, standing, sleeping, sex life, social life, traveling.	1 each	6 points	Low back pain	**	**	**	**	Excellent review and comparison with Roland in Roland & Fairbanks
	Simple Shoulder Test (SST)	Function-8 Pain Sleep Position	8 1 1 2	2 (yes diffi-cult y/no)	Shoulder disorders	*	**	**	**	Developers suggest reporting % with difficulty in each item, not a summative score. Some psychometrics done using sum of items
	Neck Disability Index	Pain, personal care, lifting, reading, headaches, con-centration, work, driving, sleeping, recreation	1 each	6 point	Whiplash disorders	*	*	*	*	Neck pain has few instruments that have been evaluated for psychometrics. This is most tested
Patient Specific	—	—	—	—	—	—	—	—	—	No patient-specific measure found in literature reviewed

* One or two articles found *in support* of this attribute.

** Multiple articles supporting this attribute.

a From Beaton DE, Schemitsch E. Measures of health-related quality of life and physical function. *Clin Orthop Relat Res* 2003;413 : 90–105.

in disability in the hand as well as in the shoulder. In one study it was directly compared to a shoulder and a wrist measure, and had similar levels of construct validity, responsiveness, and reliability. Another study showed slightly lower properties in the DASH as compared to a wrist specific measure in patients with wrist fracture. Like the S-MFA, the measurement properties of the DASH are quite high (internal consistency 0.96, test–retest 0.95, good validity, and responsiveness) suggesting it could also be used in individual patients in a clinical setting. The DASH is available free of charge on the Internet. It has its own website, but is also available through the American Academy of Orthopaedic Surgeons website. The DASH is one of the questionnaires in the AAOS outcome battery. Several translations are available (www.dash.iwh.on.ca).

WOMAC Osteoarthritis Index

The Western Ontario McMaster (WOMAC) Osteoarthritis Index is a 24-item scale divided into three dimensions: function, pain, and stiffness. The most commonly used response scale is a five-point Likert scale, however, there is a visual analogue scale version. It has been widely used and tested in the field of osteoarthritis and rheumatoid arthritis summarized in a review of its psychometric properties by McConnell et al in 2001 (34). The WOMAC is the most commonly used and endorsed patient-based outcome after hip or knee arthroplasty.

UTILIZING OUTCOME STUDIES IN DECISION MAKING (EVIDENCE-BASED ORTHOPAEDICS)

What Is Evidence-Based Orthopaedics?

The term *evidence-based medicine* (EBM) first appeared in autumn 1990 in a document for applicants to the internal medicine residency program at McMaster University that described EBM as an attitude of enlightened skepticism toward the application of diagnostic, therapeutic, and prognostic technologies. As outlined in the text *Clinical Epidemiology* (1) and first described in the literature in the *ACP Journal Club* in 1991 (2), the EBM approach to practicing medicine relies on an awareness of the evidence on which a clinician's practice is based and the strength of inference permitted by that evidence. The most sophisticated practice of EBM requires, in turn,

- A clear delineation of relevant clinical questions
- A thorough search of the literature relating to the questions
- A critical appraisal of available evidence and its applicability to the clinical situation
- A balanced application of the conclusions to the clinical problem

The balanced application of the evidence (i.e., clinical decision making) is the central point of practicing evidence-based medicine and involves, according to EBM principles, integration of our clinical expertise and judgment with patients' preferences and societal values, as well as with the best available research evidence (Fig. 10-6). The EBM working group at McMaster University has proposed a working model for evidence-based clinical practice that encompasses current research evidence, patient preferences, clinical circumstances, and clinical expertise. EBM is commonly misunderstood as removing clinical expertise as a factor in patient decision making—not so. The common thread that weaves the relationships between patients, circumstances, and research is the experience and skill of the surgeon.

Finding Current Evidence in Trauma

To be effective EBM practitioners, surgeons must acquire the necessary skills to find the "best" evidence available to answer clinically important questions. Reading a few articles published in common orthopaedic journals each month is insufficient preparation for answering the questions that emerge in daily practice. There are at least 100 orthopaedic journals indexed by Medline (4). For surgeons whose principal interest is orthopaedic traumatology, the list is even larger. Given their large clinical demands, surgeons' evidence searches must be time-efficient. Evidence summaries (such as those published in the *Journal of Orthopaedic Trauma*) and systematic reviews (comprehensive literature reviews) are useful resources for surgeons (Table 10-9). The most efficient way to find them is by electronic searching of databases and/or the Internet. With time at a premium, it is important to know where to look and how to develop a search strategy, or filter, to identify the evidence most efficiently and effectively.

User's Guide to Evaluate an Orthopaedic Intervention

Most surgical interventions have inherent benefits and associated risks. Before implementing a new therapy, we should ascertain the benefits and risks of the therapy, and assure ourselves that the resources consumed in the intervention will not be exorbitant. A simple three-step approach can be used when reading an article from the orthopaedic literature (Table 10-10). We recommend you ask whether the study can provide valid results (internal validity), review the results, and consider how the results can be applied to your patient care (generalizability). Lack of randomization, no concealment of treatment allocation, lack of blinding, and incomplete follow-up are serious threats to the validity of a published randomized trial. The User's Guide focuses the assessment on assuring that investigators have considered these issues in the conduct of their study.

Incorporating Evidence-Based Orthopaedics into Daily Trauma Practice

Evidence-based medicine (EBM) is becoming an accepted educational paradigm in medical education at a variety of levels. An analysis of the literature related to journal clubs in residency programs in specialties other than orthopaedic surgery reveals

TABLE 10-9 Finding Current Evidence: Resources

Publications
Evidence-Based Medicine
Using the Medical Literature
Journal of American Medical Association User's Guides
Canadian Medical Association Journal User's Guides
Journal of Bone and Joint Surgery User's Guides
Canadian Journal of Surgery User's Guides

Databases
Best Evidence
Cochrane Library and Cochrane Randomized Trials Register (www.update-software.com/cochrane)
Database of Abstracts of Reviews of Effectiveness (DARE)
Internet Database of Evidence-based Abstracts and Articles (IDEA)
Medline/PubMED (www.ncbi.nlm.nih.gov/entrez/query.fcgi)
EMBASE (European equivalent of Medline)
Clinical Evidence (www.clinicalevidence.org)
SUMsearch (www.sumsearch.uthscsa.edu)
TRIP database (www.tripdatabase.com)

Electronic Publications
American College of Physicians (ACP) Journal Club (www.acpjc.org)
Bandolier: Evidence-based healthcare

Evidence-Based Medicine
National Guideline Clearinghouse (agency of health care policy and research—AHCPR) (www.guidelines.gov)

Internet Resources
Healthweb: Evidence-based Health Care (www.healthweb.org)
Evidence-based medicine from McMaster University (www.hiru.hirunet.mcmaster.ca)
Center for Evidence-Based Medicine (www.cebm.net)
Critically Appraised Topics (CAT) databank (www.cebm.net/toolbox.asp)
New York Academy of Medicine EBM Resource Center (www.ebmny.org)
University of Alberta EBM (www.cebm.med.ualberta.ca/ebm/ebm.htm)

Trauma Links
Edinburgh Orthopaedic Trauma Unit (www.trauma.co.uk/traumalinks.htm)

TABLE 10-10 User's Guide to Orthopaedic Randomized Trials

Validity
Did experimental and control groups begin the study with a similar prognosis?
Were patients randomized?
Was randomization concealed?
Were patients analyzed in the groups to which they were randomized?
Were patients in the treatment and control groups similar with respect to known prognostic factors?
Did experimental and control groups retain a similar prognosis after the study started?
Blinding
Did investigators avoid effects of patient awareness of allocation—were patients blinded?
Were aspects of care that affect prognosis similar in the two groups—were clinicians blinded?
Was outcome assessed in a uniform way in experimental and control groups—were those assessing outcome blinded?
Was follow-up complete?

Results
How large was the treatment effect?
How precise was the estimate of the treatment effect?

Applicability
Can the results be applied to my patient?
Were all patient-important outcomes considered?
Are the likely treatment benefits worth the potential harms and costs?

that the three most common goals were to teach critical appraisal skills (67%), to have an impact on clinical practice (59%), and to keep up with the current literature (56%) (35). The implementation of the structured article review checklist has been found to increase resident satisfaction and improves the perceived educational value of the journal club without increasing resident workload or decreasing attendance at the conference.

Structured review instruments have been applied in a number of orthopaedic training programs; assessments of the outcomes and effectiveness of this format for journal club are ongoing. One example of one structured review instrument for use in orthopaedic training programs is provided in Figure 10-7.

THE FUTURE OF OUTCOME STUDIES IN ORTHOPAEDIC TRAUMA

Over the past 50 years, there has been a vast proliferation of randomized trials. While the strength of evidence is most persuasive in large, randomized trials with small confidence intervals around their treatment effect, this is not always feasible for many clinical problems in orthopaedics. Indeed, only 3% (72 of 2,498 studies) of studies published in orthopaedics reflect randomized trial methodology (14). The design, conduct, and analysis of orthopaedic research has gained widespread appreciation in surgery, particularly orthopaedic surgery. Still, only 14% of the *Journal of Bone and Joint Surgery*'s original contributions represent level I evidence (9). When randomization is not feasible or unethical, prospective observational studies represent the best evidence. Approximately 1 in 5 scientific articles published in *JBJS* represent this level II evidence (9).

Item	Points	Score
1. Study Design		
Randomized Trial or Meta-Analysis (MA) of Randomized Trial	12	
Prospective Observational Study with a Comparison group or MA	10	
Retrospective Observational Study with a Comparison group or MA	8	
Prospective Observational Study with no Comparison group or MA	6	
Retrospective Observational Study with no Comparison group or MA	4	
Cross-Sectional (Single point in time)/Survey	2	
Not Reported/Unable to Discern	0	/12
2. Eligibility Criteria		
Eligibility criteria defined	3	
Eligibility criteria partially defined	2	
Eligibility criteria not reported	0	/3
Ineligible or excluded patients reported	3	
Ineligible or excluded patients partially reported	2	
Ineligible patients or excluded not reported	0	/3
3. Similarity of Comparison Groups at beginning of study		
Groups similar due to randomization	8	
Groups similar by matching cases to controls or p values shown	6	
Groups not similar but statistical tests utilized to correct for imbalances	4	
Authors report groups similar but with no supporting information	2	
Groups not similar , Single Group Only or Not Reported	0	/8
4. Similarity of Comparison Groups at completion of study (omit, if MA)		
Groups remained similar (no crossovers occurred)	4	
Groups dissimilar (crossovers occurred)	2	
Single Group Only or Unsure / Not Reported/Not applicable	0	/4
5. Outcomes assessment		
Main outcomes are objective (ie. don't require major judgement-mortality)	3	
Main outcomes are not objective	1	/3
Outcome assessors independent or blinded	3	
Outcome assessors not independent or not blinded	0	
Unsure	0	/3
6. Follow Up		
90% or greater follow up achieved (prospective, active)	6	
80-89% follow up (prospective, active)	4	
70-79% follow up (prospective, active)	2	
Less than 70% follow up achieved	1	
Not reported or Unsure or Not applicable or Passive Follow Up	0	/6
7. Sample Size		
Pre-study sample size or Power calculation reported	4	
Post-study power calculation reported	2	
Pre-study sample size or Power calculation not reported	0	/4
8. Statistical Tests		
p-Value and Confidence interval(s) Reported	4	
p-Value or Confidence intervals(s) Reported	2	
No statistics reported	0	/4
Total Score		**/50**
If meta-analysis		/46

FIGURE 10-7 A checklist to assess the quality of surgical therapies.

Future studies can provide high quality data on which to base practice if we conduct RCTs whenever feasible, ensure adequate sample size, involve biostatisticians and methodologists, collect data meticulously, and accurately report our results using sensible outcomes and measures of treatment effect. Limiting type II errors (beta errors) will need multicenter initiatives. These larger trials have the advantage of increased generalizability of the results and the potential for large scale and efficient recruitment (1000 patients or more). Single center trials that may have taken a decade to recruit enough patients can now be completed in a few years with collaborative research trials. The obvious drawback with multicenter initiatives is the relative complexity of the design and the cost. It is reasonable to expect that a trial of over 1000 patients will cost over $3 to $4 million to conduct.

CONCLUSION

The purpose of the "outcomes movement" and "evidence-based medicine" is to provide healthcare practitioners and decision makers (physicians, nurses, administrators, regulators) with tools that allow them to gather, access, interpret, and summarize the evidence required to inform their decisions and to explicitly integrate this evidence with the values of patients. In this sense, evidenced-based medicine is not an end in itself, but rather a set of principles and tools that help clinicians distinguish ignorance of evidence from real scientific uncertainty, distinguish evidence from unsubstantiated opinions, and ultimately provide better patient care.

APPENDIX: SAMPLE SIZE CALCULATIONS

1. Continuous Variables

The number of patients required per treatment arm to obtain 80% study power ($\beta = 0.20$) at a 0.05 alpha level of significance is as follows:

$$n_1 = n_2 = 2(\sigma^2)(z_{1-\alpha/2} + z_{1-\beta})^2 / \Delta^2 \qquad (1)$$

where

n_1 = sample size of group one

n_2 = sample size of group two

Δ = difference of outcome parameter between groups (5 points)

σ = sample standard deviations (12)

$z_{1-\alpha/2} = z_{0.975} = 1.96$ (for $\alpha = 0.05$)

$z_{1-\beta} = z_{0.80} = 0.84$ (for $\beta = 0.2$)

2. Dichotomous Variables

The number of patients required per treatment arm to obtain 80% study power ($\beta = 0.20$) at a 0.05 alpha level of significance is as follows:

$$n_1 = n_2 = [(2p_m q_m)^{1/2} z_{1-\alpha/2} + (p_1 q_1 + p_2 q_2)^{1/2} z_{1-\beta}]^2 / \Delta^2 \qquad (2)$$

where

n_1 = sample size of group one

n_2 = sample size of group two

p_1, p_2 = sample probabilities (5% and 10%)

$q_1, q_2 = 1 - p_1, 1 - p_2$ (95% and 90%)

$p_m = (p_1 + p_2)/2$ (7.5%)

$q_m = 1 - p_m$ (92.5%)

Δ = difference $= p_2 - p_1$ (5%)

$z_{1-\alpha/2} = z_{0.975} = 1.96$ (for $\alpha = 0.05$)

$z_{1-\beta} = z_{0.80} = 0.84$ (for $\beta = 0.2$)

REFERENCES

1. Sackett DL, Haynes RB, Guyatt GH, et al. *Clinical epidemiology: A basic science for clinical medicine.* Boston: Little Brown, 1991.
2. Guyatt GH. Evidence-based medicine. *Am Coll Phys J Club* 1991;114:A16.
3. Sackett DL, Richardson WS, Rosenberg WM, et al. *Evidence-based medicine: How to practice and teach EBM.* New York: Churchill Livingstone, 1997.
4. American Medical Association. In: Guyatt GH, Rennie D, eds. *User's guides to the medical literature: A manual for evidence-based clinical practice*, 2nd ed. Chicago: American Medical Association Press, 2001.
5. Bhandari M, Zlowodzki M, Cole PA. From eminence-based practice to evidence-based practice: A paradigm shift. *Minn Med* 2004;4:51–54.
6. Bhandari M, Tornetta P. Issues in the hierarchy of study design, hypothesis testing, and presentation of results. *Tech Orthop* 2004:19:57–65.
7. Brighton B, Bhandari M, Tornetta P III, et al. Hierarchy of evidence: From case reports to randomized controlled trials. *Clin Orthop Relat Res* 2003;413:19–24.
8. Wright JG, Swiontkowski MF, Heckman JD. Introducing levels of evidence to the journal. *J Bone Joint Surg Am* 2003;85A:1–3.
9. Bhandari M, Swiontkowski MF, Einhorn TA, et al. Interobserver agreement in the application of levels of evidence to scientific papers in the American volume of the Journal of Bone and Joint Surgery. *J Bone Joint Surg Am* 2004;86A:1717–1720.
10. Bhandari M, Guyatt GH, Siddiqui F, et al. Operative versus non-operative treatment of achilles tendon rupture—a systematic overview and meta-analysis. *Clin Orthop Relat Res* 2002;400:190–200.
11. Bhandari M, Montori VM, Devereaux PJ, et al. for the Hedges Team. Doubling the impact: Publication of systematic review articles in orthopaedic journals. *J Bone Joint Surg Am* 2004;86:1012–1016.
12. Bhandari M, Guyatt GH, Swiontkowski MF. User's guide to the orthopaedic literature: How to use an article about a surgical therapy. *J Bone Joint Surg* 2001;83A:916–926.
13. Devereaux PJ, Manns BJ, Ghali W, et al. In the dark: physician interpretations and textbook definitions of blinding terminology in randomized controlled trials. *JAMA* 2001;285:2000–2003.
14. Bhandari M, Richards R, Schemitsch EH. The quality of randomized trials in Journal of Bone and Joint Surgery from 1988–2000. *J Bone Joint Surg Am* 2002;84A:388–396.
15. Bhandari M, Guyatt GH, Swiontkowski MF. User's guide to the orthopaedic literature: How to use an article about a prognosis. *J Bone Joint Surg* 2001;83A:1555–1564.
16. Ioannidis JP, Haidich AB, Pappa M, et al. Comparison of evidence of treatment effects in randomized and nonrandomized studies. *JAMA* 2001;286:821–830.
17. Kunz R, Oxman AD. The unpredictability paradox: review of empirical comparisons of randomised and non-randomised clinical trials. *BMJ* 1998;317:1185–1190.
18. Concato J, Shah N, Horwitz RI. Randomized, controlled trials, observational studies, and the hierarchy of research designs. *N Engl J Med* 2000;342:1887–1894.
19. Benson K, Hartz AJ. A comparison of observational studies and randomized, controlled trials. *N Engl J Med* 2000;342:1878–1886.
20. Bhandari M, Tornetta P III, Ellis T, et al. Hierarchy of evidence: Differences in results between non-randomized studies and randomized trials in patients with femoral neck fractures. *Arch Orthop Trauma Surg* 2004;124:10–16.
21. The EC/IC Bypass Study Group. Failure of extracranial–intracranial arterial bypass to reduce the risk of ischemic stroke: Results of an international randomized trial. *N Engl J Med* 1985;313:1191–1200.
22. Haentjens P, Autier P, Boonen S. Clinical risk factors for hip fracture in elderly women: A case-control study. *J Orthop Trauma* 2002;6:379–385.
23. Bhandari M, Tornetta P. Communicating the risks of surgery to patients. *Eur J Trauma* (In press).

24. Griffin D, Audige L. Common statistical methods in orthopaedic clinical studies. *Clin Orthop Relat Res* 2003;413:70–79.
25. Lochner H, Bhandari M, Tornetta P. Type II error rates (beta errrors) in randomized trials in orthopaedic trauma. *J Bone Joint Surg* 2002;83A:1650–1655.
26. Bhandari M, Whang W, Kuo JC, et al. The risk of false-positive results in orthopaedic surgical trials. *Clin Orthop Relat Res* 2003;(413):63–69.
27. Pocock S, Assman S, Enos L, et al. Subgroup analysis, covariate adjustment and baseline comparisons in clinical trial reporting: current practice and problems. *Stats Med* 2002; 21:2917–2930.
28. Yusuf S, Wittes J, Probstfield J, et al. Analysis and interpretation of treatment effects in subgroups of patients in randomized clinical trials. *JAMA* 1991;266:93–98.
29. Bhandari M, Devereaux PJ, Li P, et al. The misuse of baseline comparison tests and subgroup analyses in surgical randomized controlled trials. *Arch Orthop Trauma Surg* (In press).
30. Jackowski D, Guyatt G. A guide to health measurement. *Clin Orthop Relat Res* 2003; 413:80–89.
31. Beaton DE, Schemitsch E. Measures of health-related quality of life and physical function. *Clin Orthop Relat Res* 2003;413:90–105.
32. Marsh JL, Weigel DP, Dirschl DR. Tibial plafond fractures. How do these ankles function over time? *J Bone Joint Surg Am* 2003;85A:287–295.
33. Miranda MA, Riemer BL, Butterfield SL, et al. Pelvic ring injuries. A long term functional outcome study. *Clin Orthop Relat Res* 1996;(329):152–159.
34. McConnell S, Kolopack P, Davis AM. The Western Ontario and McMaster Universities Osteoarthritis Index (WOMAC): A review of its utility and measurement properties. *Arthritis Rheum* 2001;45:453–461.
35. Dirschl DR, Tornetta P 3rd, Bhandari M. Designing, conducting, and evaluating journal clubs in orthopaedic surgery. *Clin Orthop Relat Res* 2003;413:146–157.

IMAGING CONSIDERATIONS IN ORTHOPAEDIC TRAUMA

Andrew H. Schmidt and Kerry M. Kallas

GENERAL CONSIDERATIONS

Medical imaging in the setting of acute trauma contributes greatly to the initial diagnosis and subsequent management of many orthopaedic injuries. In many instances, patients are able to provide details of the injury, and imaging studies often confirm or exclude diagnoses already suggested by the clinical history, mechanism of trauma, and physical examination findings. Imaging also plays a significant role in treating multitrauma patients who may arrive obtunded or unconscious and are therefore unable to localize symptoms or cooperate during the physical examination. Multitrauma patients may also have coexisting neurologic and visceral injury, and orthopaedic imaging may be performed in conjunction with or delayed by associated imaging studies and surgical triage for these injuries.

A wide variety of imaging examinations are available in clinical practice today, and use of a particular modality may be influenced by multiple factors, such as availability, image resolution, invasiveness, cost-effectiveness, patient risk, and requirements for special handling of the trauma patient. Many imaging studies are routinely ordered for specific indications and need no justification; for example, conventional radiographs are used to evaluate for acute bony trauma of the extremities. Particularly with regard to more advanced imaging techniques, however, clinicians must often consider these tradeoffs in deciding whether to pursue additional imaging.

Availability

Although there is widespread availability of conventional radiography in both clinical and hospital settings, there is more variable access to advanced imaging modalities, particularly in rural communities and after hours. Although data are lacking, it has been previously estimated that only 10% of hospitals offer full radiology coverage to emergency departments 24 hours per day (1). Many emergency departments do have continuous access to computed tomography (CT) scanners, but access to more advanced imaging modalities, such as ultrasound (US), nuclear medicine (NM), and magnetic resonance imaging (MRI), varies significantly among hospitals and communities, and may be on an "on-call" basis or not available at all after hours.

Image Resolution

The choice of a particular imaging examination may, in part, be influenced by spatial resolution and contrast resolution. The ability of an imaging modality to resolve small objects of high subject contrast (e.g., bone-muscle interface) as distinct entities is referred to as *spatial resolution*, which is typically measured in line pairs per millimeter (lp/mm); higher values of lp/mm indicate greater resolution. For comparison, the limiting spatial resolution of the human eye is approximately 30 lp/mm. Resolution may also be expressed in millimeters, whereby smaller values represent greater spatial resolution. Table 11-1 lists representative values of limiting spatial resolution for common imaging modalities. Conventional radiographs have considerably better spatial resolution than cross-sectional imaging techniques, although overlapping bony structures often complicate evaluation of osseous anatomy. CT has better spatial resolution than MRI, and is more commonly performed for evaluating finer bony abnormalities, such as avulsion fractures and calcification within tumor matrix.

Contrast resolution refers to the ability to resolve two tissues of similar subject contrast. Conventional radiographs typically have poor soft tissue contrast resolution, whereas CT, and in particular MRI, have much better contrast resolution, in part related to their tomographic nature. For example, on conventional radiographs, subcutaneous fat may be discerned from the underlying muscle groups, although the intermuscular fascial planes cannot be visualized. CT and MRI better demonstrate the subcutaneous fat and intermuscular fascial planes, although MRI shows superior soft tissue contrast resolution compared with CT.

Invasiveness

Most medical imaging procedures are noninvasive, or may require minimally invasive procedures, such as placement of in-

TABLE 11-1 The Limiting Spatial Resolutions of Various Medical Imaging Modalities: The Resolution Levels Achieved in Typical Clinical Usage of the Modality

	Resolution		
Modality	lp/mm	mm	Comments
Screen Film Radiography	6	0.08	Limited by focal spot and detector resolution
Digital Radiography	3	0.17	Limited by size of detector elements
Fluoroscopy	4	0.125	Limited by detector and focal spot
CT	1	0.4	About $^1/_2$-mm pixels
NM–Planar Imaging	<0.1	7	Spatial resolution degrades substantially with distance from detector
SPECT	<0.1	7	Spatial resolution worst toward the center of cross-sectional image slice
PET	0.1	5	Better spatial resolution than other nuclear medicine imaging modalities
MRI	0.5	1.0	Resolution can be improved at higher magnetic fields
US	1.7	0.3 (5 MHz)	Limited by wavelength of sound

SPECT, single photon emission computed tomography; PET, positron emission tomography.
Modified and reprinted with permission from Brushberg JT, Seibert JA, Leidholt EM Jr, et al. *The Essential Physics of Medical Imaging*, 2nd ed. Philadelphia: Lippincott Williams & Wilkins, 2002.

travenous access for contrast administration. Some imaging techniques are more invasive, however, such as peripheral angiography for vascular assessment in the trauma patient, and not only carry more inherent risk to the patient, but also require greater resources and coordination on an emergent basis. When used appropriately, the diagnostic and therapeutic advantages of these procedures can contribute substantially to the patient's management.

Cost-Effectiveness

With increasing pressures on cost containment, studies have been performed to address the cost-effectiveness of algorithms incorporating conventional radiography in diagnosis and follow-up of musculoskeletal trauma (2). Significant costs may be incurred at receiving hospitals as a result of repeating radiographic work-ups for patients who have been transferred from referring facilities along with their original radiographs (3). Several recent studies have shown the benefits of "rules" in deciding when to order radiographs for knee and ankle trauma, resulting in fewer radiographs ordered and reduced cost without increased incidence of missed fractures (2,4–11). Additional studies have also shown the ability to reduce postoperative and follow-up radiographs in treatment of ankle fractures (12,13). Similar studies have addressed the cost-effectiveness of routine pelvic radiography in the setting of blunt trauma, although with mixed results (14,15). Study of pediatric torus fractures has shown that postcasting radiographs are unnecessary and follow-up radiographs do not change fracture management, with the implication of significant cost saving as a result of decreased radiography (16).

Studies have also shown that advanced imaging also contributes to decreased treatment costs in the setting of acute trauma. Multiple studies have shown the cost-effectiveness of MRI in evaluating wrist trauma and suspected scaphoid fractures, in cases where initial conventional radiography was normal (17,18). MRI proved superior to follow-up radiography for diagnosis of occult fractures, resulting in a change in management in up to 89% of cases (19). Cost was found to be similar or reduced in all studies comparing early MRI with more traditional algorithms of casting and radiographic follow-up (17,20). One study showed cost benefits associated with earlier rather than later MRI scanning (19). Similar studies have shown the cost-effectiveness of early limited MRI in the diagnosis and management of occult hip fractures (21).

Patient Risk

As a rule, imaging procedures used in evaluating orthopaedic trauma contribute very little increased risk to the patient; however, handling trauma patients requires special attention. Many trauma patients have potential spine injuries, necessitating the use of spinal precautions and special radiographic views during imaging procedures. Likewise, fractured limbs may be very painful when moved, and there may be changes in fracture reduction or redislocation of an injured joint during manipulation of an extremity for radiographs. Due to pain and disorientation, patients may be unable to lie still during imaging examinations, and may require analgesia and sedation. Sometimes, mechanical ventilation and multiple lines as well as catheters must be managed. Life-support equipment and external fixation devices may also be incompatible with or limit the usefulness of certain examinations, such as conventional radiography and MRI.

Risks associated with ionizing radiation in soft tissues are small, but cumulative, although the information obtained by these imaging studies greatly outweighs these risks. Administering intravenous contrast carries a small risk of adverse events, which may be categorized as mild, moderate, severe, and end organ (22). With traditional high-osmolality ionic contrast media, most adverse reactions are mild to moderate and occur in 5% to 12% of all patients. This incidence is significantly decreased with use of the newer low-osmolality nonionic contrast agents. The occurrence of severe contrast reactions is approximately 1 to 2 per 1,000 patients receiving high-osmolality contrast agents, whereas this number decreases to approximately 1 to 2 per 10,000 patients receiving low-osmolality contrast media (23). Examples of end-organ adverse events include thrombophlebitis related to the injection site, nephrotoxicity, pulseless electrical activity, seizures, and pulmonary edema (22). Peripheral angiography carries a low risk of complications, including bleeding and further vascular injury, although these problems may be minimized with experience and careful technique.

SPECIFIC IMAGING MODALITIES

Radiography

Technical Considerations

Conventional Radiography. Conventional radiography (screen film radiography, plain film radiography) involves the use of x-rays, which are high-energy electromagnetic radiation with wavelengths smaller than ultraviolet light, but longer than gamma rays. X-rays are produced using an x-ray tube, whereby electrons are emitted from a heated tungsten filament and accelerated across a voltage potential to strike a tungsten target. The flow of electrons from filament to the target results in a tube current, and its interaction with the tungsten target generates a spectrum of x-rays and heat. Before leaving the x-ray tube, the x-rays are filtered and collimated into a useable beam. Factors that are set by the technologist to vary the quality and/or quantity of the x-ray beam include the voltage potential (measured in peak kilovoltage [kVp]), tube current (milliamperes [mA]), and exposure time (seconds). The output of the x-ray tube is expressed in mA, calculated by multiplying the tube current (mA) by the exposure time(s). These factors are frequently recorded on radiographs (mainly portable radiographs) for use with future examinations.

After leaving the x-ray tube, the x-ray beam is directed through the patient and onto a screen/film cassette. The x-ray beam is attenuated as it passes through the patient, primarily by two processes, including the photoelectric effect and Compton scatter. Before reaching the screen/film cassette, the transmitted radiation may be further collimated using a lead grid to remove the scatted radiation. Scatter increases with increasing patient thickness and larger fields of view, and is a significant source of image degradation. Scatter may be negligible with extremities, in part related to their smaller size and greater proximity to the cassette; hence, grids may not be required.

Screen/film cassettes are used to capture the transmitted radiation and create the latent image. Intensifying screens absorb x-ray photons, and subsequently emit a greater number of light photons, which are then absorbed by the film. The film consists of a base, which is covered on one or both sides by an emulsion containing silver grains. Absorbed light photons result in liberation of free electrons within the emulsion, which subsequently reduce the silver atoms. When the film is developed, the reduced silver atoms are amplified and appear black on the film. Most screen/film cassettes use a dual-screen and dual-emulsion combination. In order to improve bone detail, a single-screen, single emulsion system may be used.

Portable Radiography. Portable radiography is frequently used to evaluate acute trauma patients, and its use may be complicated by several factors not encountered in the radiology department's controlled environment. Trauma patients frequently are immobile and require special handling precautions, which may make it difficult to obtain routine anteroposterior (AP) and lateral projections. Appropriate placement and alignment of the screen/film cassette may be especially challenging, and if placed behind a backboard or beneath the patient's cart, it may introduce artifacts into the radiograph and obscure anatomy of interest. Objects outside of the patient's body related to his or her resuscitation, including endotracheal tubes, nasogastric tubes, chest tubes, and intravenous access, frequently project onto the radiograph. Casts, splints, and other external fixation devices may also project onto extremity radiographs and limit visualization of underlying bony detail.

Technical factors, such as levels of kVp and mA, also need modification with portable radiography. Portable examinations are often performed with higher kVp settings, which provide for a wider margin of error in selecting other technical factors. Higher kVp values will result in greater scattered radiation, however, and may necessitate the use of a grid with the screen/film cassette. Precise alignment of the grid and cassette to the central beam of the portable x-ray tube is also more difficult because each of the components are not fixed in space, and malalignment results in significant obscuration of the image and degradation in image quality.

Conventional Tomography. Tomography is a specialized application of conventional radiography, where the objective is to image a specific plane of tissue within the body. This is accomplished by a specialized radiography system whereby the patient is kept stationary while the x-ray tube and film cassette move about the patient, usually in a linear fashion, but in opposite directions. Structures within the focal plane of interest are imaged in the same relative location on the film during tube and cassette translations, whereas images of structures located in front or behind the desired plane are blurred out by spreading their images over the entire film. The disadvantages of tomography include long examination times and potential for significant radiation exposure to the patient with larger numbers of images. Moreover, tomography has largely been replaced by more advanced cross-sectional techniques, such as CT and MRI. The use of these advanced technologies has led to a decline in availability of tomography equipment in most imaging departments and a corresponding decrease in technologist experience in performing such examinations.

Digital Radiography. Digital methods of acquiring radiographs have been developed, although several different digital technologies are in use and continue to be refined. In all digital radiography systems, the creation of x-rays and attenuation of the x-ray beam as it passes through the patient remain similar to conventional radiography systems. What differentiates digital radiography systems is the type of image receptor that interacts with the attenuated x-ray beam to create a medical image.

Computed radiography (CR) was first introduced in the late 1970s and has gained wide popularity in radiology departments within the last decade. With CR, the screen/film cassette is replaced by a cassette containing a photostimulatable phosphor deposited onto a substrate. When this type of phosphor interacts with x-rays, electrons are trapped at higher energy levels within the phosphor. The amount of electron trapping is proportional to the incident x-rays and results in the creation of a latent image, which can later be read using a specialized CR cassette reader. The reader scans the phosphor plate using a laser, which releases the electrons from their higher energy states, and results in emission of light as they drop down to lower energy states. The emitted light is captured by a photomultiplier tube, which converts the light into an electrical signal, which is subsequently digitized and stored. This process is done on a point-by-point basis throughout the entire phosphor plate to create a digital image.

Relatively recent advances in flat panel detectors have led to a new digital imaging technology that has been referred to as direct capture radiography, or alternatively, indirect and direct digital radiography (DR). Each of these systems uses flat panel detectors that incorporate a large array of individual detector elements; each one corresponds to a pixel in the final image. In indirect DR, the detector elements are sensitive to light; hence an x-ray intensifying screen is used to convert the incident x-rays into light, which is then captured by the individual detector elements and stored as a net negative charge. In direct DR, the individual detector elements are coated with a photoconductive material (selenium is commonly used). Upon exposure to x-rays, electrons are liberated from the photoconductor and are captured by the underlying detector elements, resulting in a net negative charge within each detector element. With both systems, the negative charges within the array of detector elements are read out electronically, digitized, and stored to create the final image.

Currently, the spatial resolution of conventional radiography is greater than for DR systems. CR and DR, however, offer significant advantages over conventional radiography, including the ability to manipulate digital images and alter image contrast, decreased radiation dose to the patient and radiologic personnel, and greater ease of storage and transmission of radiographs both within and beyond the imaging department. DR systems are expensive to implement, as they require replacement of the entire radiography suite. CR systems are much more economical to implement, as they only require replacement of the screen/film cassettes and purchase of a CR reader. Both digital systems, however, offer ongoing cost savings as a result of decreased numbers of retakes and reduction in film costs. Although digital radiography is likely the future of radiography, it currently does not match conventional radiography for fracture assessment in terms of spatial resolution (Table 11-1).

Applications

Conventional radiography remains the primary diagnostic modality for assessing fractures and dislocations. Orthogonal views, occasionally supplemented by additional specific projections, are sufficient to identify and manage most fractures. In addition to delineating the fracture pattern, conventional radiographs are useful for assessing limb length and alignment and are the primary means by which fracture healing is monitored. In many cases, more subtle indications of injury apparent on conventional radiographs can suggest the need for further diagnostic imaging or intervention. Examples of such cases would be the identification of a posterior fat pad sign in a pediatric elbow, indicating an occult elbow injury, a joint effusion, or the finding of a fat-fluid level in the knee joint capsule indicating osteochondral fracture. Surrounding soft tissues may also be evaluated for and show additional evidence of trauma, including swelling, foreign bodies, and gas. Although conventional radiographs are universally used for assessing fracture healing, one recent report noted that there is very poor interobserver agreement regarding the determination of fracture healing after internal fixation (24).

Orthopedic surgeons' immediate interpretation of conventional radiographs of simple fractures has been shown to be timely, accurate, inexpensive, and contributes to patient care, whereas formal interpretation of the same studies by a radiologist typically occurs after care is rendered, may be inaccurate, adds expense, and does not contribute to patient management (25).

The use of conventional radiography is so fundamental to fracture care that further discussion is unnecessary. Numerous specific examples are found throughout this text.

Fluoroscopy

Technical Considerations

Conventional Fluoroscopy. Fluoroscopy involves the use of low-dose x-rays to image patient anatomy at high temporal resolutions, that is, in real time. Typical components of a fluoroscopy system include an x-ray tube, filters, and a collimator, similar to that used in conventional radiography. The x-ray tube is energized continuously using a low exposure rate, and the x-ray beam is directed through the patient onto an image intensifier. The image intensifier is responsible for converting the attenuated x-ray beam into a visible light image, which is frequently coupled to a closed-circuit television camera to produce a "live" image on a video monitor. An optical coupling system, using high-resolution lenses and mirrors, may also be used to direct the light image to recording devices, such as video recorders and photospot cameras.

The components of the image intensifier are housed in a glass vacuum tube and include a large input phosphor, a photocathode, a series of electrostatic lenses, an anode, and a smaller output phosphor. Incident x-rays are directed onto the input phosphor and are converted into light photons, similar to a radiographic intensifying screen. The light photons are channeled by the phosphor to the adjacent photocathode as a result of the linear crystalline structure of the phosphor matrix. The photocathode is composed of a thin metal layer, containing cesium and antimony, applied to the posterior surface of the input phosphor, which interacts with the light photons and results in emission of electrons. The electrons are then accelerated from the photocathode to the anode by an applied voltage approximating 25,000 V. During the acceleration process, the electrons emitted across the entire cross-sectional area of the photocathode are kept in relative alignment by a series of electrostatic lenses, such that the spatial information they contain is preserved. The electrons are subsequently focused onto the output phosphor, which results in light emission and creation of an image.

Fluoroscopy systems vary in configuration, from permanently installed biplane angiography suites to mobile C-arm designs. Mini C-arm units have become increasingly popular for outpatient clinics. Image intensifiers are produced in different sizes, and measurements refer to the size of the input phosphor. Typical diameters range from 4 to 16 inches (10 to 40 cm) and various sizes may be better suited or standardized to specific applications. Many fluoroscopy systems offer additional magnification modes, which use a smaller area of the input phosphor to create the magnified image. The theoretical resolution of an image intensifier is approximately 4 to 5 lp/mm, with somewhat better resolution obtained in magnification modes (Table 11-1). This is achievable only when the images are output to film. The image intensifier output is usually coupled to a video monitor for real-time viewing, which results in degradation of the resolution achievable by the image intensifier. Resolution of such closed-circuit television systems is typically 1 to 2 lp/mm.

Digital Fluoroscopy. Advances in digital technology have led to the development of digital fluoroscopy systems, which are now common in clinical practice. The output of the image intensifier may be coupled to a high-resolution video camera with subsequently digitized output, or directed onto a charge-coupled device (CCD). A CCD is a small plate containing a large array of photosensitive elements, each of which corresponds to a single pixel in the final digital image. Each element stores charge in proportion to the amount of absorbed light, which is then read out electronically and digitized to produce a pixel value. The matrix of pixel values is then used to create the final digital image. The resolution of a CCD depends on the size of each of its array elements; CCDs with a 1024 matrix may achieve a resolution of 10 lp/mm. The digital nature of the image lends itself to computer postprocessing, including digital subtraction techniques, which improves image contrast. More recent advances in flat panel detector technology using thin film transistor (TFT) arrays may allow replacement of the image intensifier and video camera by TFT panels, resulting in even greater improvement in image contrast.

Applications

Intraoperative Imaging. Intraoperative radiography and fluoroscopy are almost universally used during the operative care of fractures. Imaging techniques are needed during surgery to verify the reduction of fractures, identify the starting portals for intramedullary nails, target cannulated or interlocking screws, and verify implant position (Fig. 11-1). Fluoroscopic assessment of tibial plateau fracture reduction leads to results as good as or better than those obtained with arthroscopic-assisted reduction (26). Norris et al used intraoperative fluoroscopy during the repair of acetabular fractures and found it as effective as postoperative radiographs to assess fracture reduction and comparable to postoperative CT to evaluate for intra-articular extension of hardware (27). Recent advances in "minimally invasive" fracture fixation rely even more on the interpretation of fluoroscopic images (28) (Fig. 11-2).

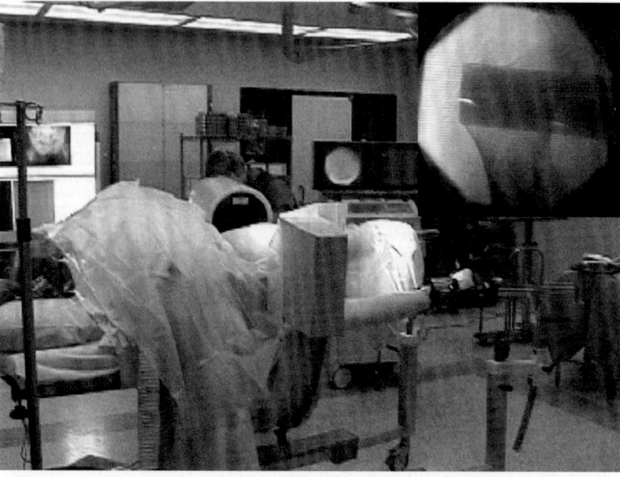

FIGURE 11-2 This intraoperative photograph of a patient in the lateral position for femoral nailing on a fracture table demonstrates the use of fluoroscopy to evaluate fracture reduction and later, to guide implant positioning. The corresponding fluoroscopic image is seen in the upper right corner of the photo.

Despite the benefits of intraoperative fluoroscopy, most surgeons insist on obtaining conventional radiographs at the completion of surgery. Although this practice requires further radiation exposure and adds time and expense, it is important for both clinical and medicolegal documentation. Fluoroscopic images have limited field-of-view, and may not demonstrate the full extend of hardware fixation (as in the case of an intramedullary nail) or overall limb alignment as well as conventional ra-

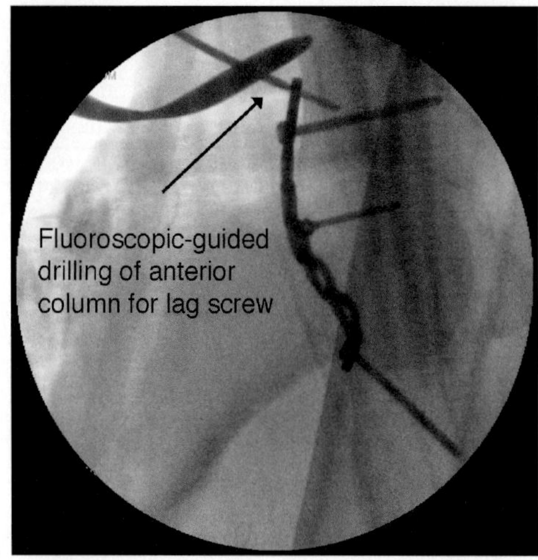

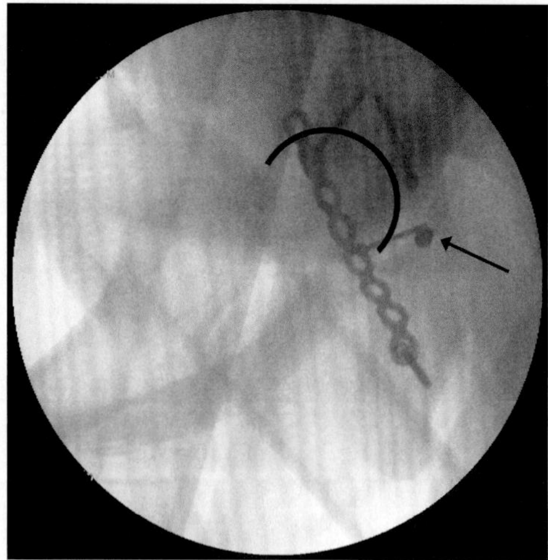

FIGURE 11-1 **A.** Intraoperative fluoroscopic anteroposterior view of the pelvis used to evaluate fracture reduction and guide placement of fixation hardware. Here, intraoperative fluoroscopy is used to target drilling of a lag screw across the anterior column component of an associated transverse and posterior wall fracture repaired from a posterior approach. **B.** Intraoperative imaging is also useful for ensuring that hardware is not within the joint does not extend into the joint space. Multiple views are taken with the C-arm in different positions until the screw of interest is seen "head-on." With this view, it can then be determined whether the screw penetrates the joint surface. The screw can then be compared with the joint space in profile to evaluate for intra-articular extension. In this case, the screw (*arrow*) is clearly outside of the joint.

diographs. Finally, it may be difficult to compare intraoperative fluoroscopic images to later conventional radiographs, so the immediate postoperative radiograph represents an important baseline reference for future comparisons.

Several studies have examined the amount of ionizing radiation that operating room personnel are exposed to during the care of fractures when fluoroscopy is used (29–31). Fortunately, with modern fluoroscopic systems, measurable radiation exposure is limited to the surgeon's hands (30,31), although he or she needs to limit excessive use of the fluoroscope during surgical procedures.

A recent advance in intraoperative fluoroscopy is the ability to generate a cross-sectional, computer-reconstructed axial image in real-time. C-arms that are adapted for this purpose incorporate a motor that rotates the x-ray tube and image intensifier around the patient while taking hundreds of images. Immediate computer processing generates a reconstructed cross-sectional image that is similar to an axial CT image. The ability to obtain immediate cross-sectional images during surgery is a tremendous advance for the repair of intra-articular fractures and in situations when hardware placement requires precision, such as pedicle screws or iliosacral screws.

Surgical Navigation. Although computer-assisted surgical navigation techniques may be performed with cross-sectional imaging data obtained from preoperative CT, fluoroscopy is commonly used for surgical navigation because of its flexibility, convenience, low radiation exposure, and low cost. Although the field of surgical navigation is in its infancy, computer-assisted surgical navigation has already been applied to cervical and thoracic spine fracture fixation (32), placement of percutaneous iliosacral (Fig. 11-3) and anterior column screws in the pelvis (33,34), and intramedullary nailing (35,36).

Fluoroscopic surgical navigation requires a specialized computer-based system, which tracks the position of a hand-held tool in space. It is necessary to "register" the patient's bone

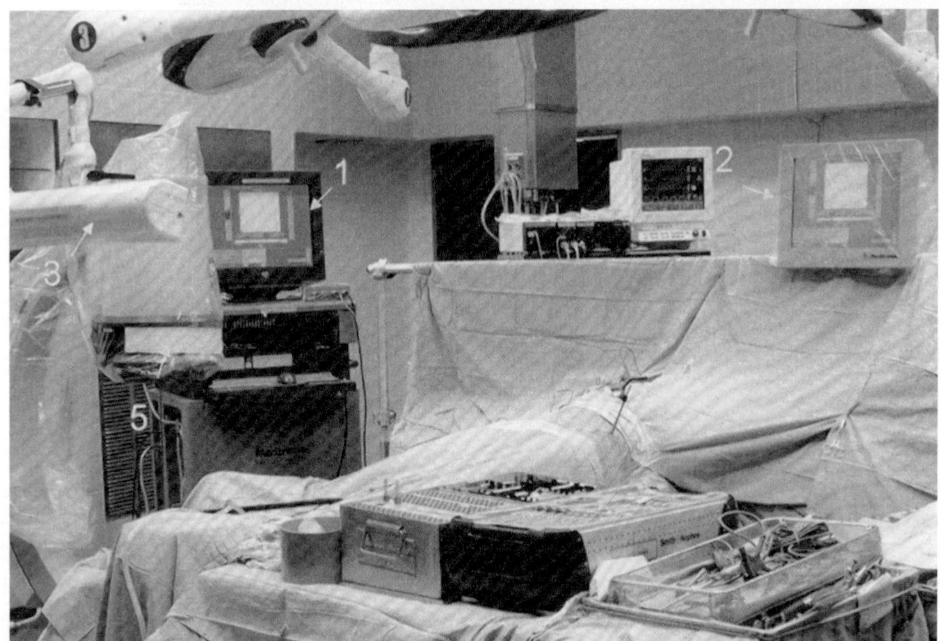

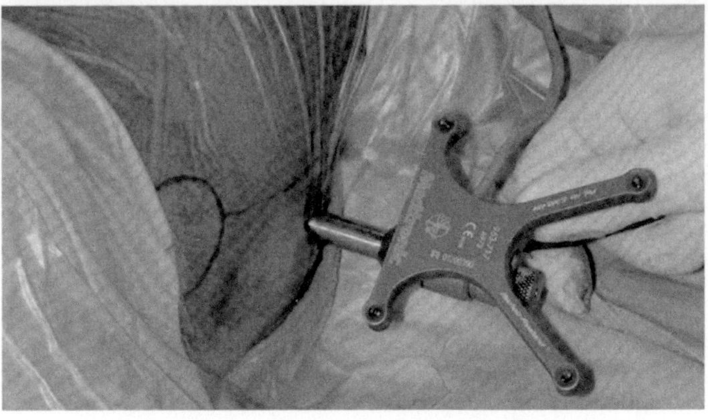

A

FIGURE 11-3 A. Photograph of the intraoperative set-up for computer-assisted fluoroscopic surgical navigation during pelvic surgery. The computer screen (1), surgeon "touch screen" (2), infrared camera (3), reference array (4), and C-arm attachment (5) are visible. (*continues*)

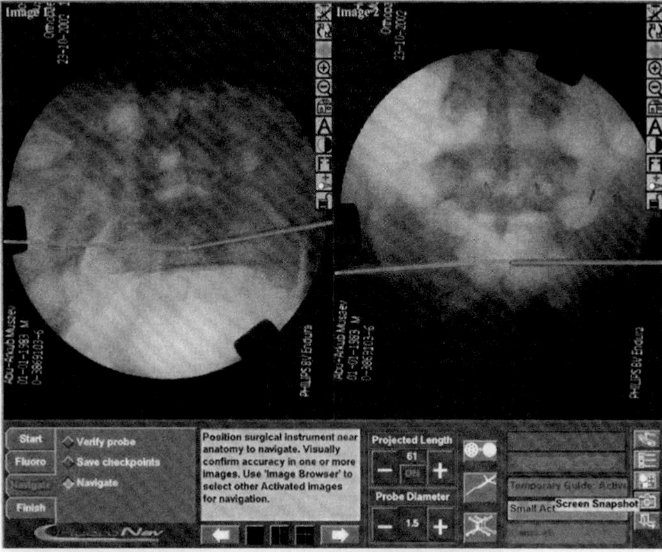

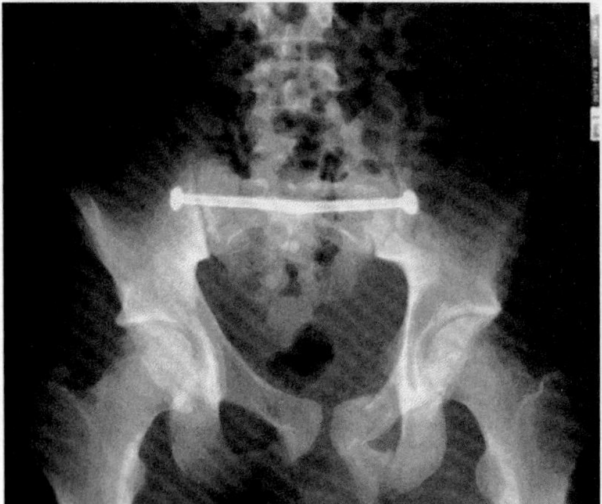

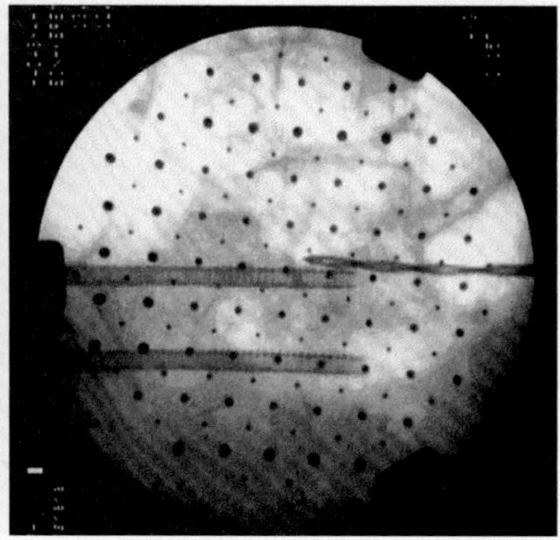

B

FIGURE 11-3 (*continued*) **B.** Fluoroscopic images in two different planes (shown simultaneously) demonstrating placement of iliosacral screws (top). Only two fluoroscopic images are acquired in the desired planes prior to beginning the procedure. The position of the guide pins and drills is visualized in both images (and both planes) in real time. As can be seen, the insertion of the second screw does not require further fluoroscopy. The postoperative pelvic radiograph shows accurate screw placement (lower left). Placement of the guidewire for a third iliosacral screw is verified with conventional fluoroscopy (lower right). All three sacroiliac screws were inserted, using the same preliminary fluoroscopic views, without further exposure to radiation. (Reprinted with permission from Mosheiff R, Khoury A, Weil Y, et al. First generation computerized fluoroscopic navigation in percutaneous pelvic surgery. *J Orthop Trauma* 2004;18(2):106–111.)

within the computer based on preoperative CT data or the use of a generic dataset. Fluoroscopic views need be taken only once; thereafter, all movements of the tool are recorded against the registered bone image and may be displayed in different planes simultaneously, superimposed on the static images by the computer system. This dramatically reduces the need for repeated intraoperative imaging, decreasing the time of surgery and the radiation exposure of the patient and surgical team (Fig. 11-3). Intraoperative changes in the patient's position or in the dimensions of the registered bone (such as might occur during fracture reduction) decrease the accuracy of image registration, however. Surgical navigation has been used for hip fractures, placement of iliosacral screws, and for performing the interlocking of intramedullary nails distally. Although this technology has been proven to be feasible, the clinical importance has not been convincingly shown. Collinge et al compared the safety and efficiency of standard multiplanar fluoroscopy to virtual fluoroscopy for use in the percutaneous insertion of iliosacral screws in 29 cadaver specimens (37). Interestingly, both methods were equally accurate; one screw was incorrectly inserted in each group, and both groups contained examples of screws with minor deviations in trajectory. Although the actual time for screw insertion was less with virtual fluoroscopy (3.5 minutes vs. 7.1 minutes), this was offset by the increased time needed to set up and calibrate the image-guided system (37).

Computed Tomography

Technical Considerations

CT has had the greatest clinical impact of any of the radiographic imaging modalities, such that its inventors (Godfrey Houndsfield and Allan Cormack) received the Nobel Prize for Medicine in 1979. Since its inception in the early 1970s, advances in technology and computer science have guided the development of several new generations of CT scanners, each capable of greater throughput and improved resolution. Although a more detailed review of the history of CT scanners is beyond the scope of this section, a brief description of current concepts in CT scanner technology is presented.

Helical (spiral) CT scanners were developed in the late 1980s and are so named because of the helical path the x-ray beam takes through the patient. The development of "slip ring" technology allowed the gantry (x-ray tube and detectors) to rotate continuously around the patient, whereas with previous-generation scanners, gantry rotation was constrained by electrical cables, which needed to be unwound in between slice acquisitions. With nonhelical scanners, table position was incrementally advanced in between slice acquisitions; with slip ring technology, the table position is advanced continuously while the gantry rotates, resulting in a helical x-ray beam path.

The first dual slice helical scanner was demonstrated in 1992, with 4- and 16-slice models appearing in 1998 and 2001. On the whole, multislice scanners are similar to single-slice helical scanners in many respects. Instead of a single row of detectors, however, multiple rows of detectors are present within the gantry and are designed to allow acquisition of multiple slices at the same time. More recently, the first 64-slice CT scanner has become clinically available, and it is anticipated that this trend will continue with development of even higher-multislice scanners.

With these new technologies, scanning algorithms needed to be modified, which resulted in new terminology and imaging parameters to adjust. For single-slice helical scanners (and older-generation scanners as well), slice thickness is determined by x-ray beam collimation, whereas, for multislice scanners, it is determined by detector width. For single-slice scanners, pitch is defined as the ratio of table movement (mm) per 360 degree rotation to slice thickness (mm). A pitch of 1.0 is comparable to older-generation scanners where the table movement increment was the same as the slice thickness. A pitch of less than 1.0 results in overlapping of the x-ray beam and higher patient radiation dose; a pitch greater than 1.0 results in increased coverage through the patient and decreased radiation dose. In practice, pitch is generally limited to 1.5 to 2.0, although protocols vary. For multislice scanners, the definition of pitch changes to incorporate the detector array width rather than the single slice width and is referred to as *detector pitch*.

The data sets from single-slice and multislice scanners are both helical in nature, and individual slices must be interpolated from the data set. Minimum slice thickness is set by the original x-ray beam collimation (single-slice scanners) or detector width (multislice scanners). Any number of slices may be reconstructed at any position along the long axis of the patient, and in any thickness equal to or greater than the minimal slice thickness. This allows reconstruction of overcontiguous slices (with typically 50% overlap), which increases the sensitivity for detecting small lesions that may otherwise be averaged between adjacent slices, resulting in twice as many images (although with no increase in scan time or additional radiation dose to the patient).

Multiplanar reconstructions (MPR) and three dimensional (3D) reconstructions are also routinely performed with both single-slice and multislice helical scanners. This, in part, is related to the fact that today's CT examinations routinely produce hundreds of images, and MPR and 3D reformatting assist in interpreting these data. Advances in detector technology have allowed slice thickness to decrease to approximately 0.5 mm, allowing acquisition of isotropic voxels. A voxel is the 3D equivalent of a pixel, and represents the volume of tissue represented by a single pixel; isotropic voxels have uniform thickness in all directions. Acquisition of images with isotropic voxels results in multiplanar (nonaxial) reconstructions that have in-plane resolutions equal to that of the original axial image. The use of overcontiguous images is useful in 3D reconstructions to eliminate stair-step artifact.

Orthopaedic hardware results in metallic streak artifact on CT images, which frequently obscures surrounding bone and soft tissue detail. Streak artifact increases with the amount of metal present. Although metal artifact reduction techniques have been developed and significantly improve image quality, at the present time, streak artifact cannot be completely eliminated.

Overall, the advantages of multislice helical scanners include faster scan times and patient throughput, reduced motion artifacts, reduced intravenous contrast requirements, improved lesion detection, and improved multiplanar and 3D reconstructions. Disadvantages include the potential for decreased resolution along the long axis of the patient (related to increased pitch) and a large number of images, resulting in increased reconstruction time and storage requirements.

Applications

Complex Fractures. CT remains the imaging modality of choice for evaluating complex fractures as well as ruling out injury to the spine. In addition to high-resolution axial images, multiplanar reconstructions are commonly performed (Fig. 11-4). Such information provides critical data about the displacement of fracture fragments, including assessment of intra-articular displacement, articular surface depression, and bone loss. Three dimensional reconstructions using surface rendering techniques are often less helpful in fracture management as compared with multiplanar reconstructions. With 3D imaging techniques, fracture planes are frequently obscured by overlying fracture fragments and underestimate the true degree of comminution; however, they may be helpful in evaluating angulation and displacement of fracture fragments, in addition to depression of articular surfaces. With previous-generation CT scanners, evaluation of fracture planes parallel to the scan plane was suboptimal due to volume averaging of the fracture plane with adjacent intact bone. With newer helical scanners, image data are obtained as a volume rather than as individual slices, and multiplanar reconstructions typically have resolution equal to the axial images. For this reason, detection of transversely oriented fracture planes is significantly enhanced. Typical indications for CT include fractures of the proximal humerus, scapula, spine, pelvis, tibial plateau, tibial plafond, and calcaneus, and midfoot.

In the spine, helical CT has become the imaging modality of choice. Despite its greater initial expense, CT has been shown to have sensitivity and specificity of 96%; both greater than conventional plain radiography (38). Grogan et al present a

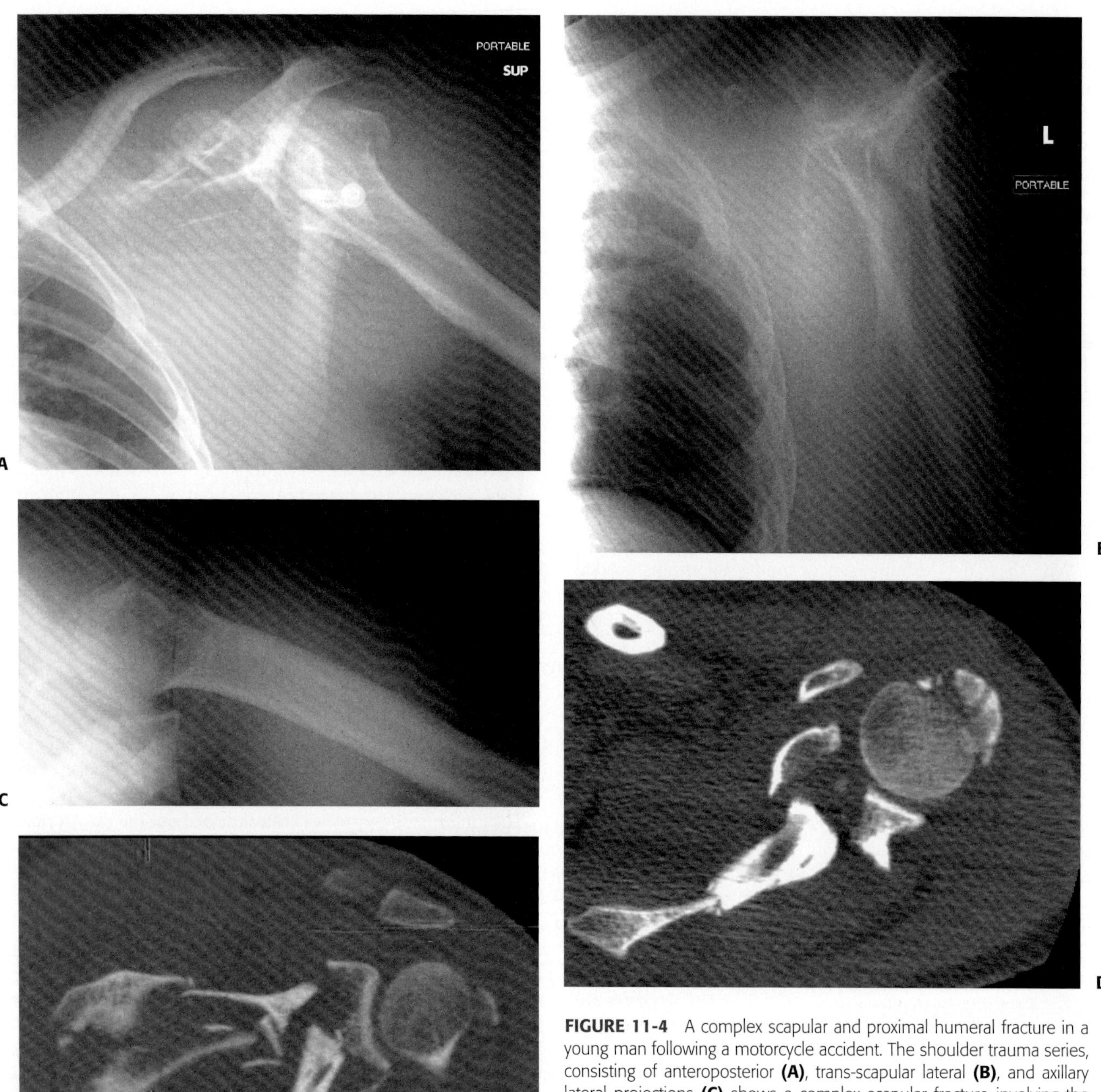

FIGURE 11-4 A complex scapular and proximal humeral fracture in a young man following a motorcycle accident. The shoulder trauma series, consisting of anteroposterior **(A)**, trans-scapular lateral **(B)**, and axillary lateral projections **(C)** shows a complex scapular fracture involving the glenoid fossa, coracoid process, and scapular body as well as fracture of the greater tuberosity of the humerus. Axial CT **(D)** confirms the intra-articular extension of the fracture and better defines the greater tuberosity fracture. Coronal oblique and sagittal oblique reconstructions provide a better additional assessment of the direction and degree of displacement in the cranial-caudal plane of the fracture fragments **(E–F)**. Three-dimensional reconstructions provide anatomic detail about the fracture in any projection **(G–K)**. With 3D reconstruction, specific anatomic structures can be isolated and viewed from any "virtual" angle. Part G illustrates a 3D reconstruction of the injured shoulder viewed from a lateral projection. Note how the humeral head obscures detail about the glenoid fossa fracture. When the humeral head is "removed" (part H) one can better appreciate the pattern of involvement of the glenoid fossa. Finally, the scapula itself can be isolated and viewed from multiple angles, as shown in parts I through K. (*continues*)

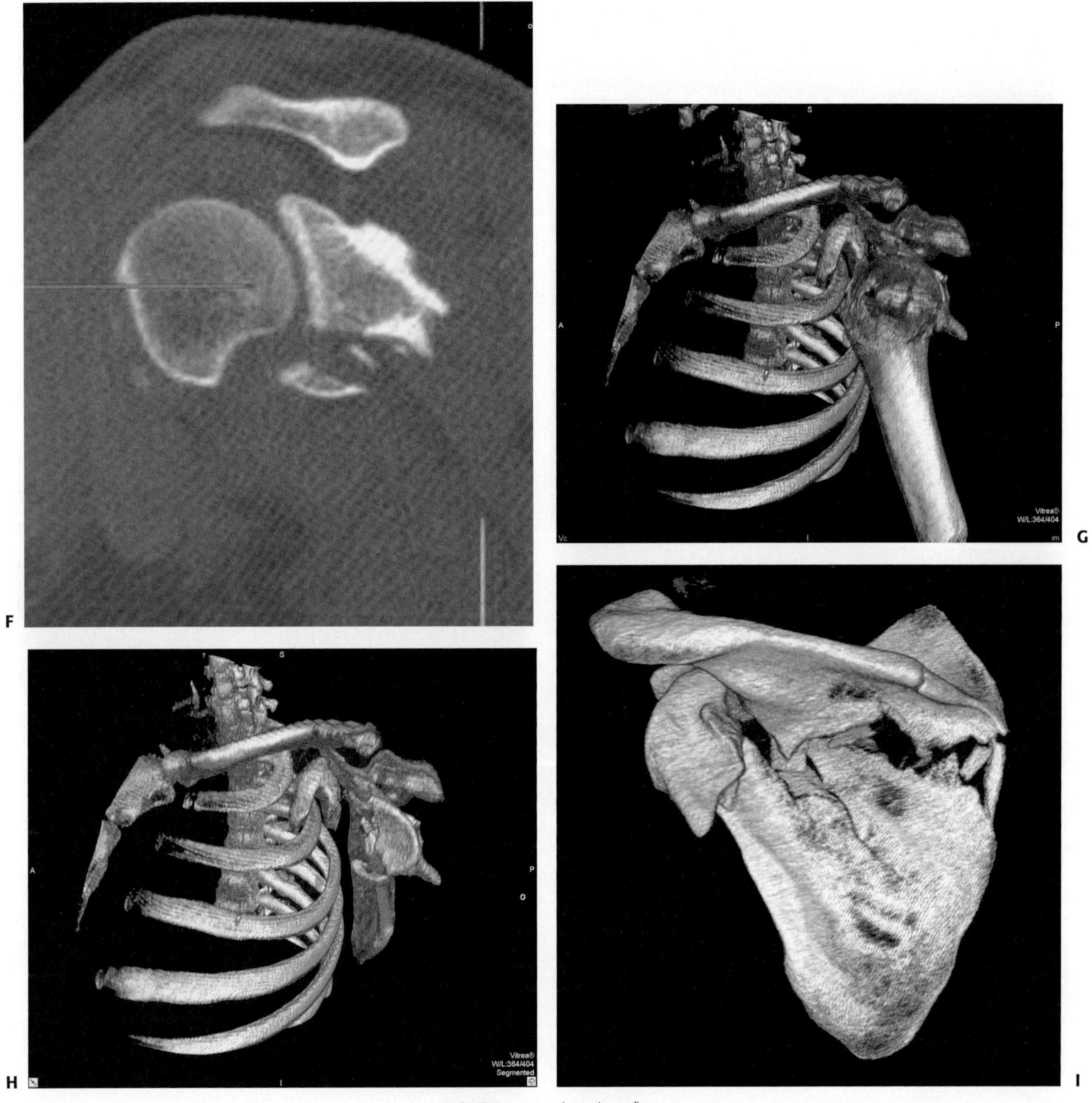

FIGURE 11-4 *(continued)*

decision analysis emphasizing cost minimization, and conclude that helical CT is the preferred initial screening test for detecting cervical spine injury in moderate- to high-risk trauma patients (39). In the upper extremity, CT is commonly performed to evaluate fractures of the proximal humerus and scapula. Multiplanar reconstructions of complex scapular fractures assist in surgical planning (Fig. 11-4). For proximal humeral fractures, simple axial images provide important information about the glenohumeral relationship, demonstrate glenoid rim fractures, and reveal whether the tuberosities of the humerus are fractured. Despite the valuable information that CT provides (with or without multiplanar reconstructions), several studies have shown that the interobserver assessment of proximal humeral and scapular neck fractures was not improved with the addition of CT (40). For distal radial fractures that mandate surgical reconstruction, CT is more accurate than conventional radiogra-

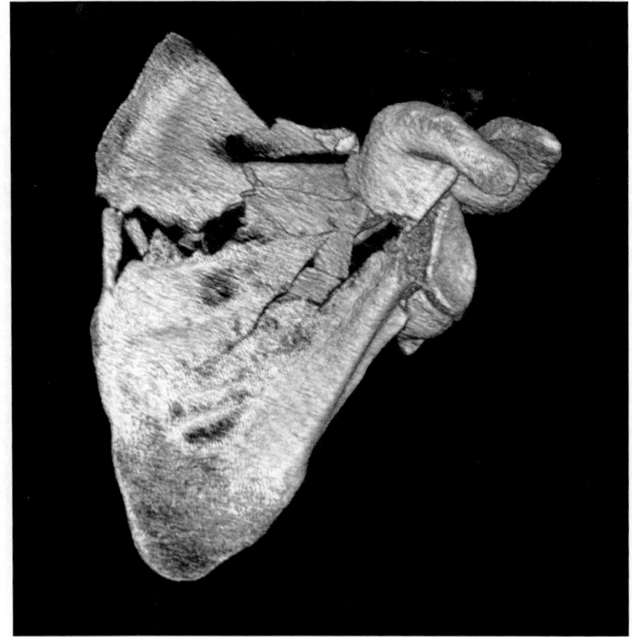
J

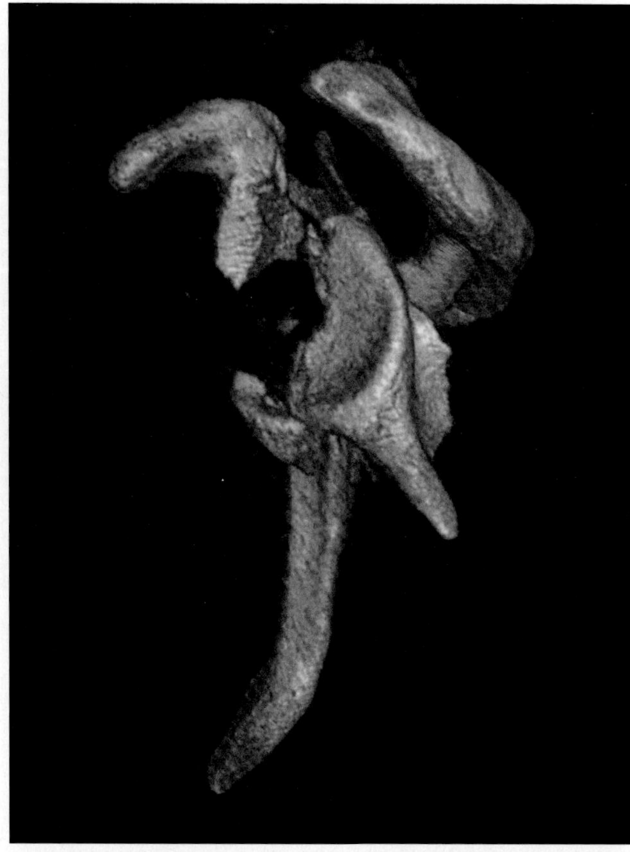
K

FIGURE 11-4 (*continued*)

phy in demonstrating involvement of the distal radioulnar joint, the extent of articular surface depression, and the amount of comminution (40,41).

CT is also routinely used in evaluating pelvic fractures. For the assessment of acetabular fractures, CT is better than conventional plain radiography at identifying intra-articular step-offs and gaps and is considered an essential part of the preoperative evaluation (42). CT demonstrates intra-articular debris in a significant number of patients after hip dislocation (43), and CT should be performed in any patient whose conventional plain radiographs show an incongruent reduction. Because small intra-articular bodies may not be visible on radiographs, one should consider obtaining CT images in all patients who suffer a hip dislocation, even when conventional plain radiographs appear to be normal.

The impact of CT on tibial plateau fracture management is well described (Fig. 11-5) (44). In one study, when using just conventional radiographs for formulating a treatment plan, the mean interobserver kappa coefficient was 0.58, which increased to 0.71 after adding CT. The mean intraobserver kappa coefficient for fracture classification using radiographs was 0.70, which increased to 0.80 with addition of CT. The mean intraobserver kappa coefficient for treatment plan based on radiographs alone was 0.62, which increased to 0.82 after adding CT. With the addition of CT, the fracture classification was changed in 12% of cases, whereas the treatment plan was altered 26% of the time (44). In another study, Wicky et al compared helical CT with 3D reconstructions to conventional radiography in patients with tibial plateau fractures and found that, for the purpose of classification, fractures were underestimated in 43% of cases by radiographs (45). Among a smaller subset of patients in which operative plans were formulated with and without CT, the same investigators found that addition of helical CT 3D reconstructions led to modifications in the surgical plan in more than half the cases (45).

Tornetta and Gorup evaluated the use of preoperative CT in the management of tibial pilon fractures (46). Twenty-two patients were studied with both conventional radiographs and CT. The fracture pattern, number of fragments, degree of comminution, presence of articular impaction, and location of the major fracture line were recorded. CT revealed more fragments in 12 patients, increased impaction in 6 patients, and more severe comminution in 11 patients. The operative plan was changed in 14 (64%) patients, and additional information was gained in 18 (82%) patients (46).

CT is valuable for assessing fractures of the hindfoot. CT reveals bone debris in the subtalar joint of patients with lateral process fractures of the talus (47). In children with Tillaux fractures of the anterolateral distal tibia, CT is better than conventional radiographs in detecting displacement of more than 2 mm, which is considered an indication for surgery (Fig. 11-6) (48). Helical CT is valuable for the preoperative planning of

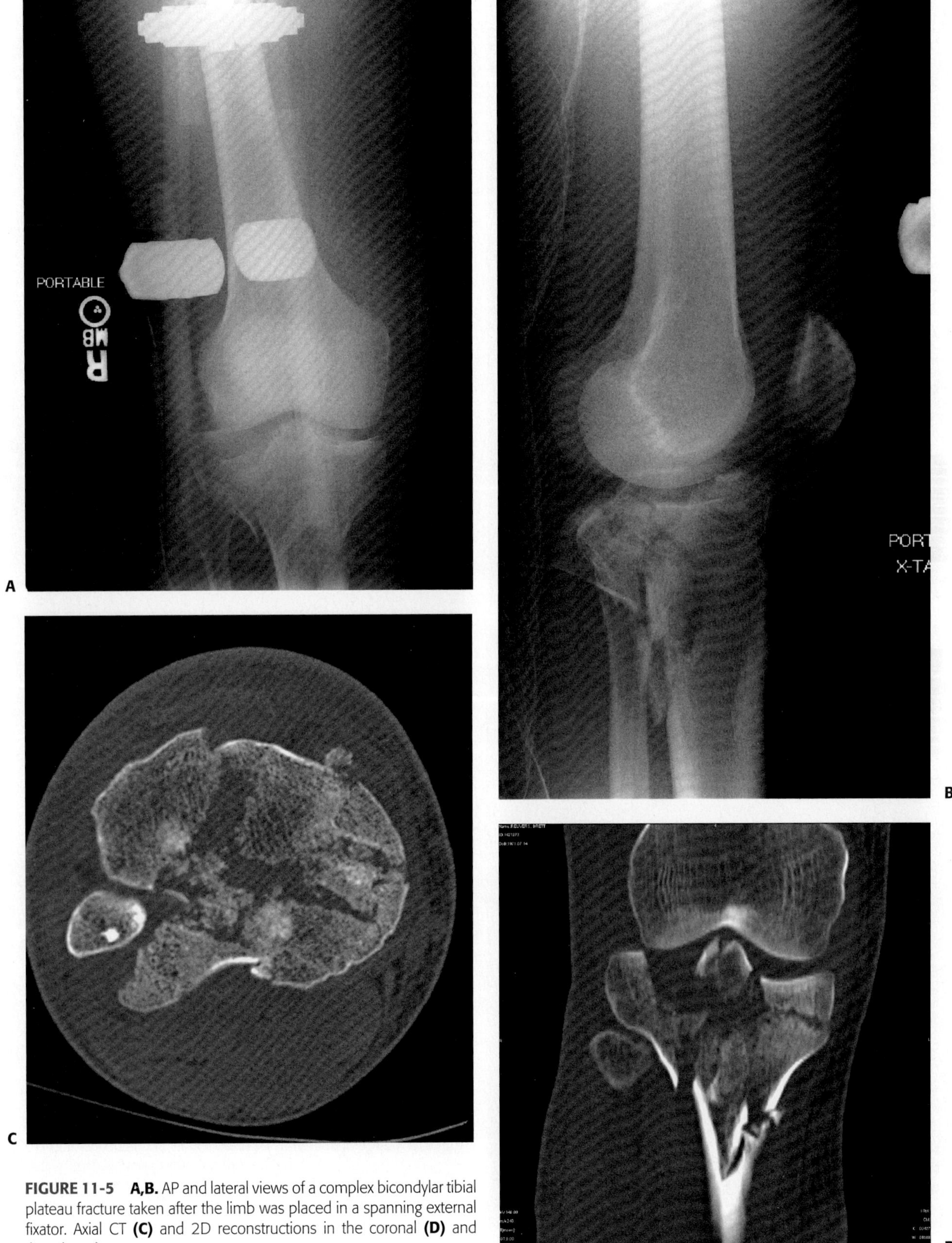

FIGURE 11-5 **A,B.** AP and lateral views of a complex bicondylar tibial plateau fracture taken after the limb was placed in a spanning external fixator. Axial CT **(C)** and 2D reconstructions in the coronal **(D)** and (*continues*)

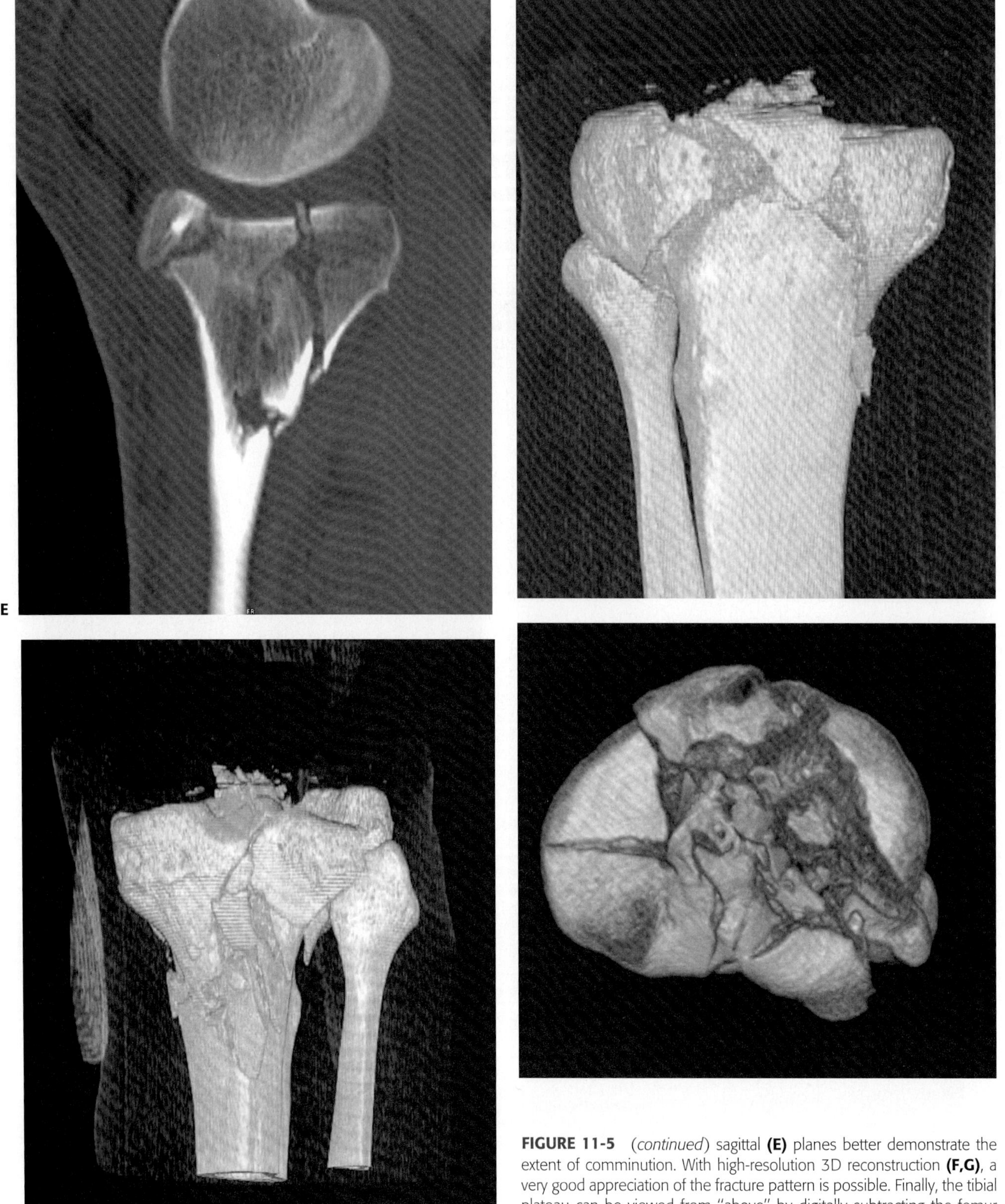

FIGURE 11-5 (*continued*) sagittal **(E)** planes better demonstrate the extent of comminution. With high-resolution 3D reconstruction **(F,G)**, a very good appreciation of the fracture pattern is possible. Finally, the tibial plateau can be viewed from "above" by digitally subtracting the femur and patella and rotating the image **(H)**. For complex fractures such as this, advanced CT imaging is unparalleled.

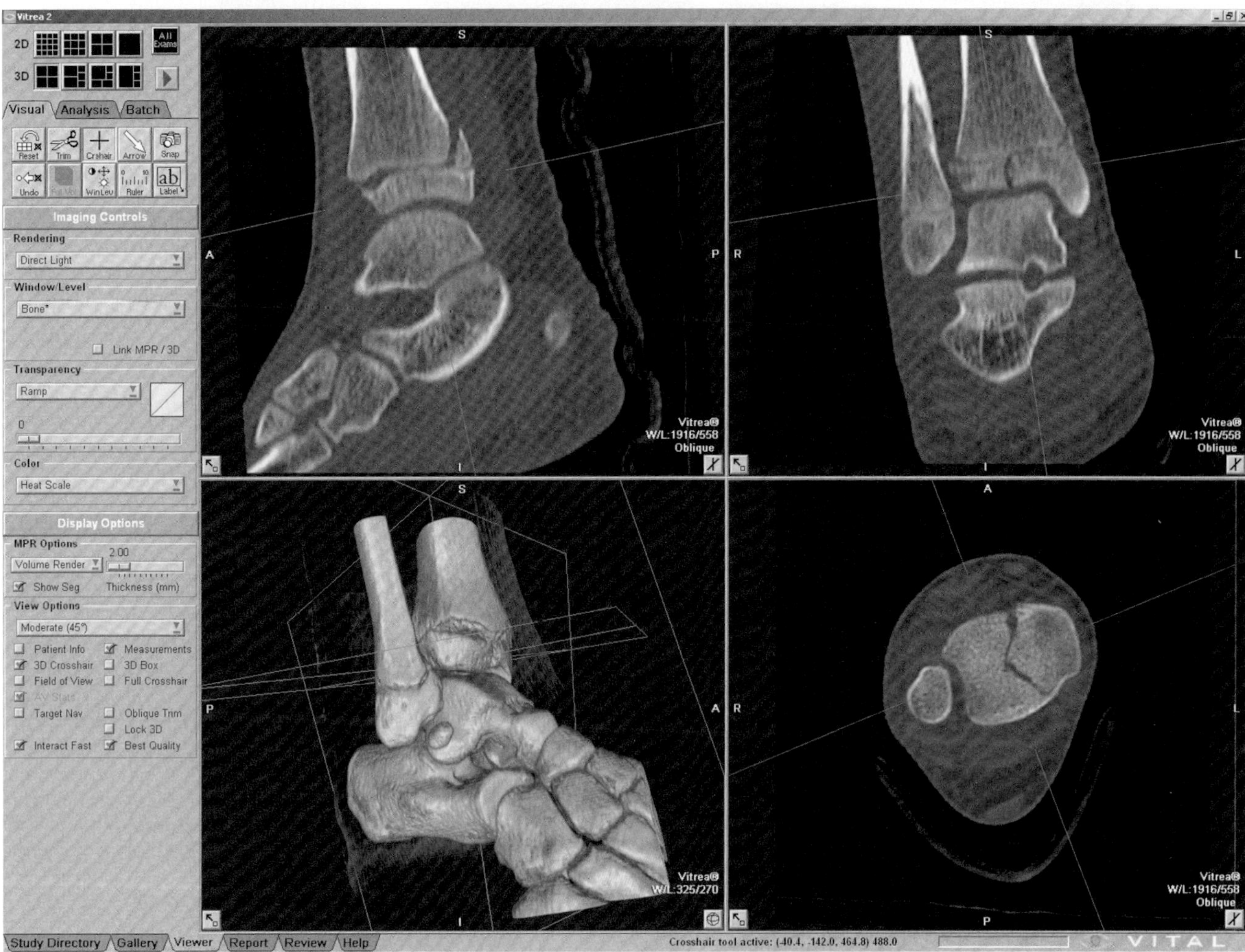

FIGURE 11-6 A triplane fracture as viewed on a digital workstation. Users can visualize axial and reconstructed coronal and sagittal images simultaneously.

calcaneal fractures (49). Axial images of the calcaneus best show hindfoot deformity, whereas multiplanar reconstructions (including 3D imaging with dislocation of the joint) best reveal intra-articular involvement (49).

Postoperative Evaluation of Fracture Reduction. CT is also useful for postoperative assessment of complex fractures. Moed et al compared the functional outcome of 67 patients with posterior wall acetabular fractures with the findings on postoperative CT (50). In this study, postoperative CT more accurately revealed the degree of residual fracture displacement compared with conventional radiographs, and the accuracy of surgical reduction seen on postoperative CT was highly predictive of the clinical outcome (50). Kurozumi et al correlated postoperative radiographs and CT to functional outcomes in 67 patients with intra-articular calcaneal fractures and found that better reduction of the calcaneocuboid joint and posterior facet of the subtalar joint correlated with improved outcome (51).

Healing of Fractures. Conventional radiographs are often limited in demonstrating persistent fracture lines, and such nonunions are more readily demonstrated on CT (Fig. 11-7). CT has also replaced conventional tomography in most centers for the identification of fracture nonunions. Multiplanar CT reconstructions may be needed if the fracture pattern is complex. Assessing partially united fractures can also be difficult, even with CT.

A more interesting role for CT is evaluation of early fracture healing. CT reveals external callus formation earlier than conventional radiographs and allows for more complete and detailed visualization of fracture healing, which may be obscured by overlying casts and/or fixation hardware on radiographs (52). Lynch et al have developed a means of measuring changes in CT density at fracture sites by quantifying the formation of mineralized tissue within fracture gaps, while ignoring loss of bone mineral due to disuse osteoporosis (53). In a preliminary study of seven patients with distal radial fractures, this technique demonstrated increased CT density 2 weeks postfracture

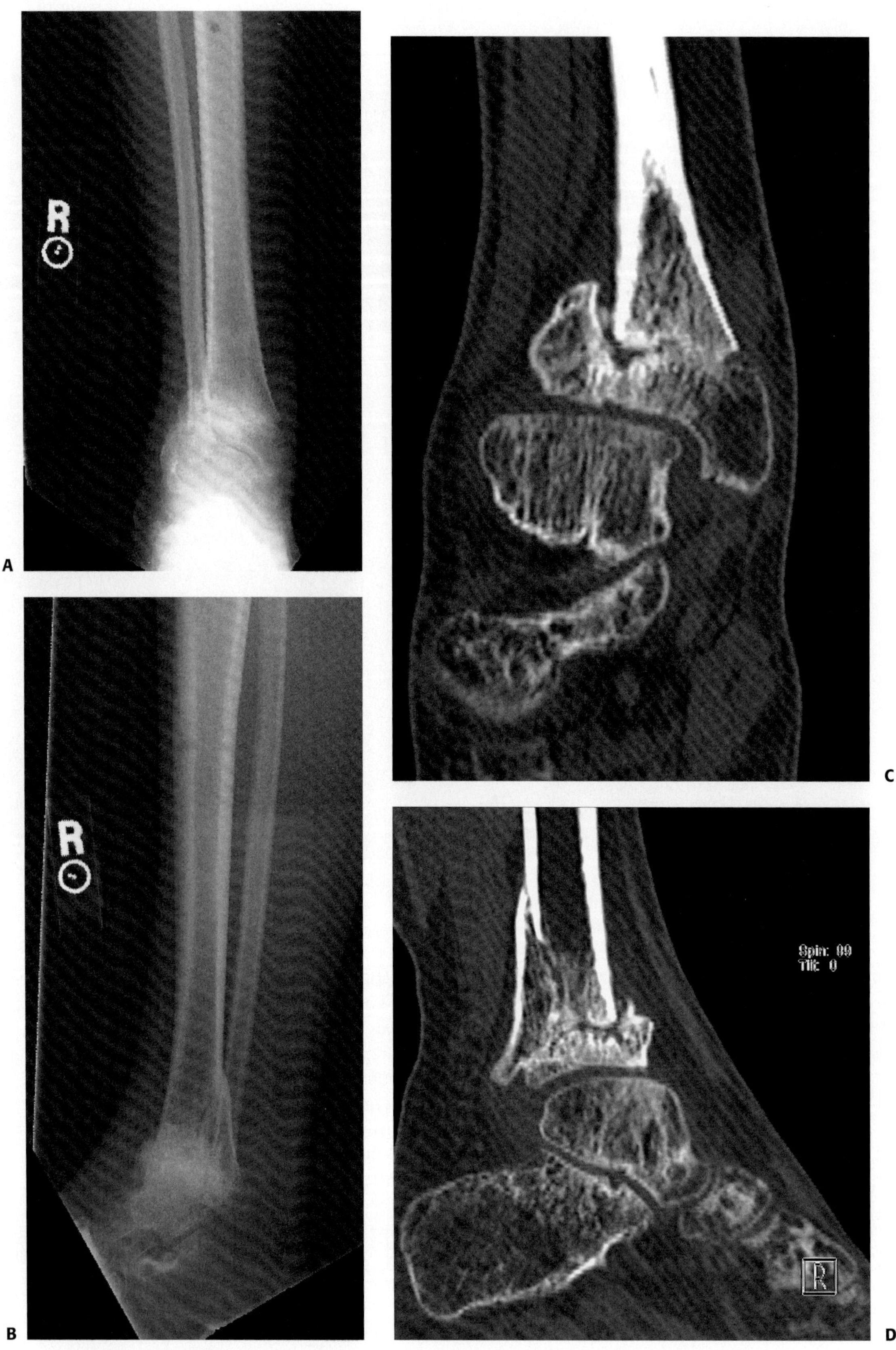

FIGURE 11-7 **A,B.** AP and lateral radiographs of a patient who had external fixation of a distal tibia fracture with progressive deformity. A CT of the nonunion with 2D reconstructions in the coronal and sagittal planes provides unambiguous evidence of fracture nonunion **(C,D)**.

that correlated with the visual appearance of sclerosis and blurring of the fracture line on conventional radiographs (53). It is not yet known whether such information will be predictive of fracture healing complications.

Magnetic Resonance Imaging

Technical Considerations

MRI does not use ionizing radiation. Rather, MRI uses radiofrequency waves, in the presence of a strong magnetic field, to interact with the patient's hydrogen atoms (protons) in order to create images of superb soft tissue contrast. Although the physics of MRI is complex and too detailed to review in this section, the more practical aspects of MRI relevant to the evaluation of orthopaedic imaging will be discussed.

Present-day MRI scanners may be classified according to field strength. The basic unit of measurement of magnetic field strength is the Gauss (G); the earth's magnetic field measures approximately 0.5 G. Field strengths for MRI are much greater and are measured in Tesla (T), which is defined as 10,000 G. Low-field-strength scanners are typically 0.2 to 0.3 T and are commonly used in outpatient settings as "extremity" scanners. High-field-strength scanners are generally those over 1.0 T, with 1.5 T scanners dominating the market and representing more than 90% of installed scanners worldwide. More recently, 3.0 T scanners have become clinically available and should grow in popularity as they become more economical. Advantages to higher-field-strength scanners include increased capability, increased resolution and image quality, and decreased scan time.

Radiofrequency (RF) coils are an important element of any MRI system. RF coils are used to transmit RF waves into the patient, as well as receive RF signals ("echoes") from the patient during the course of the examination. A standard "body" coil is incorporated into scanners as a default coil from which to both send and receive RF signals. The body coil is located within the housing of the magnet, and as a result, is located some distance from the patient. This distance factor decreases the strength of the RF signal received from the patient, although this is not a problem for imaging larger body parts such as the abdomen and pelvis. For smaller body parts, such as extremities in orthopaedic imaging, specialized RF coils are available and are widely used to increase the quality of MRI studies. These coils are usually "receive only" coils, meaning the body coil transmits the RF pulse; some specialty coils, however, incorporate both transmit and receive functions. These smaller coils are placed around or over the body part to be scanned, which decreases the distance from the patient's anatomy to the coil and results in greater signal return from the underlying tissue. This increases the signal-to-noise ratio (SNR) of the resulting images and produces images of greater contrast resolution and higher image quality returning echoes, which may be used to improve image quality, increase spatial resolution, or decrease scan time.

Advances in RF coil technology have led to a wide variety of RF coil designs available today. Volume coils encircle the anatomy of interest and provide increased signal homogeneity. Surface coils are placed over the anatomy of interest and significantly improve near-field signal strength returning from the underlying anatomy. Quadrature and phased-array coil designs incorporate multiple coil elements with electronic coupling to increase signal strength and SNR. Specialized coils are available for orthopaedic imaging and include dedicated phased-array shoulder and wrist coils (shoulder, knee, wrist, small extremities), quadrature extremity (knee, ankle, forefoot) coils, and various sizes of flexible surface coils.

MR images are generated using a series of pulse sequences. The term *pulse sequence* refers to sequence of radiofrequency pulses that are applied in concert with a series of magnetic gradients. These pulses are applied in a particular order and with a particular timing scheme, with the RF coils listening for the resulting "echoes" at specific time intervals. Pulse sequences determine the type of image contrast produced. During each pulse sequence, magnetic gradients are applied to the main magnetic field in order to achieve spatial localization. A magnetic gradient along the long axis of the bore of the magnet (and patient) is used for slice selection, whereas gradients along the transverse plane are responsible for frequency and phase encoding, which result in localization within the transverse plane. Most MRI examinations are particularly loud as a result of rapidly switching the gradients on and off, which necessitates use of earplugs or headphones during the test study. Inherent in all pulse sequences are specifications for parameters such as geometry (imaging plane, field of view, number of slices), resolution (number of frequency and phase encoding steps, slice thickness), and image contrast (repetition time [TR], echo delay time [TE]). A collection of multiple pulse sequences used for a particular examination is often referred to as a *protocol*.

Common sequences used in orthopaedic imaging include spin echo (SE) and gradient-echo (gradient recalled echo [GRE]) imaging. Spin-echo sequences are most frequently used in conjunction with a fast imaging technique, termed *fast* spin-echo (FSE) or *turbo* spin-echo (TSE) imaging, depending on the manufacturer. Spin-echo sequences provide T1-weighted (T1W), proton density (PD), and T2-weighted (T2W) image contrast based on selection of the parameters TR and TE. T1W images tend to depict anatomy well and are sensitive, but not specific, for pathology. T2W images are fluid-sensitive images and tend to depict pathology well. PD images are neither T1W nor T2W, and contrast is derived from differences in proton density within the tissues. PD images are commonly used in orthopaedic imaging, as they result in high SNR images and depict anatomy and pathology well. PD images are often acquired in conjunction with T2W images during the same pulse sequence; in this case, the PD image is referred to as the *first echo*, and the T2W image is called the *second echo*. This combination may also be referred to as a *double echo* (DE, 2E) sequence.

One consequence of FSE/TSE techniques is that fat, like fluid, is relatively bright on PD and T2W sequences. Fat suppression (FS) techniques are necessary to evaluate for edema or fluid with fat-containing tissues, such as bone marrow. Two techniques are commonly used: short TI inversion recovery (STIR) and chemical saturation ("fat-sat," spectral saturation, frequency-selective presaturation). STIR is a distinctive spin-echo pulse sequence that results in suppression of a particular tissue based on the choice of an additional parameter, TI. A relatively short TI value of 150 ms results in suppression of fat-containing tissues. This sequence tends to be relatively low in SNR, and as a consequence, is often performed at lower resolution. The sequence is less affected by variations in magnetic field homogeneity, however, and results in fairly uniform fat suppression throughout the image. Chemical saturation is a frequency-selective RF pulse, which is applied before the normal RF pulse, and effectively eliminates the signal from fat-containing tissues. This may be applied to any of the spin-echo sequences (T1W, PD, T2W); T1W FS sequences are typically used after contrast (gadolinium) enhancement, whereas PD FS and T2W FS sequences are used in evaluating a variety of tissues, including bone marrow and articular cartilage. Chemical saturation is often used in conjunction with lower-resolution fast spin-echo sequences, as the technique decreases SNR as a result of eliminating fat signal, resulting in "grainier" images at higher resolutions. Chemical saturation is also sensitive to inhomogeneities in the external magnetic field, which may result in non-uniform fat suppression across the field of view. This is particularly a problem with extremities positioned off-center with the bore of the magnet, such as the elbow, where the magnetic field is not as uniform compared to isocenter. When uniformity of fat suppression is a problem, STIR images may be substituted. STIR images are not sensitive to gadolinium and cannot be used to evaluate gadolinium-contrast enhancement, and hence are less useful for MR arthrography or intravenous contrast studies.

Developing orthopaedic imaging protocols is a challenging task that involves balancing tradeoffs in signal (SNR), spatial resolution, contrast resolution, and image acquisition time. Low SNR images tend to be "noisy" or "grainy" and unpleasant to view. Higher-resolution techniques result in both lower SNR and longer acquisition times, and may not be practical for all patients; for this reason, lower resolution techniques may be required. Many patients are unable to tolerate long scan times because of pain and limitations on movement during the examination, and, motion artifact may become a problem. MR artifacts (wrap around, motion artifact, pulsation artifact, metallic artifact) represent additional sources of image degradation, and can be difficult at times to eliminate. Newer pulse sequences are available on high-field MR scanners to reduce artifacts associated with orthopaedic implants. When difficulties arise during an MRI examination, pulse sequences often need to be modified in order to obtain the information needed from the examination.

Applications

MRI is frequently performed in evaluating both osseous and soft tissue injury after trauma. MR angiography is a well-established technique for noninvasive evaluation of the arterial system, although it may be impractical for evaluating the multitrauma patient. Evaluation of vascular trauma is accomplished much more rapidly with conventional angiography, which also allows for interventional procedures (e.g., embolization of arterial bleeding). A more controversial application is MR venography (MRV) to detect deep venous thrombosis of the proximal thigh and pelvic veins.

Faster imaging protocols make the use of MRI much more feasible in the acutely injured patient (54), but the practicality of using MRI in trauma patients may be limited by difficulties associated with transporting patients to the MRI suite, as well as MRI incompatibilities with various life-support equipment and patient implants. MRI scan times are also much longer than with CT and other imaging modalities, and may not be tolerated by potentially unstable patients or those in considerable pain.

Osseous Injury. Bone marrow edema (bone bruise, bone marrow contusion) is frequently identified on MRI after trauma. Histologically, these imaging findings correlate with cancellous bone microfractures as well as edema and hemorrhage within the fatty marrow (55). The long-term sequelae of these radiographically occult lesions have not been well defined. Roemer and Bohndorf evaluated 176 consecutive patients with acute knee injuries and found that nearly three-fourths had bone marrow abnormalities (56). The majority of lesions (69%) involved the lateral compartment of the knee; 29% were medial, and 2% were patellofemoral. Many of the lesions resembled edema of the subchondral bone, without other osseous or cartilage injury, while nearly one-fourth represented subchondral impaction fractures and one-third comprised osteochondral or chondral lesions. Forty-nine of these patients had repeat MR studies conducted at least 2 years after their injury. In these patients, only seven of 49 (14%) had persistent signal changes within the marrow space. The extent of signal abnormality was less than originally seen, and none of the patients developed degenerative changes, regardless of the injury type that was initially present. No cases of posttraumatic osteonecrosis were found. Therefore, one must be careful to avoid interpreting marrow signal abnormalities alone on MR imaging as evidence of a true fracture, as this may lead to overtreatment. This distinction is especially problematic in the assessment of hip pain after a fall, where trochanteric bone marrow edema might be interpreted as a fracture, leading to a decision to perform internal fixation.

MRI may be used in the evaluating radiographically occult fractures. Fracture lines are distinctly visualized on PD or T2W images as linear, lower-signal intensity abnormalities silhouetted by higher-signal intensity marrow fat. Fracture lines can also be seen on STIR and PD/T2W FS images, which also show the degree of surrounding reactive marrow edema. Care is needed in interpreting T1W images; however, images as fracture lines may be obscured by surrounding marrow edema, both of which are hypointense in signal intensity on T1W images (57).

MRI has become the imaging modality of choice for identifying occult fractures for which correct early diagnosis is essential, such as femoral neck fractures (Fig. 11-8) (21) and scaphoid fractures (17,19,20,58). Choice of imaging study can result in significant delays in diagnosis and treatment of hip fractures. In one study, 25 patients with hip pain were evaluated for occult fracture with conventional radiographs, scintigraphy, CT, or a combination of studies (59). A final diagnosis was determined

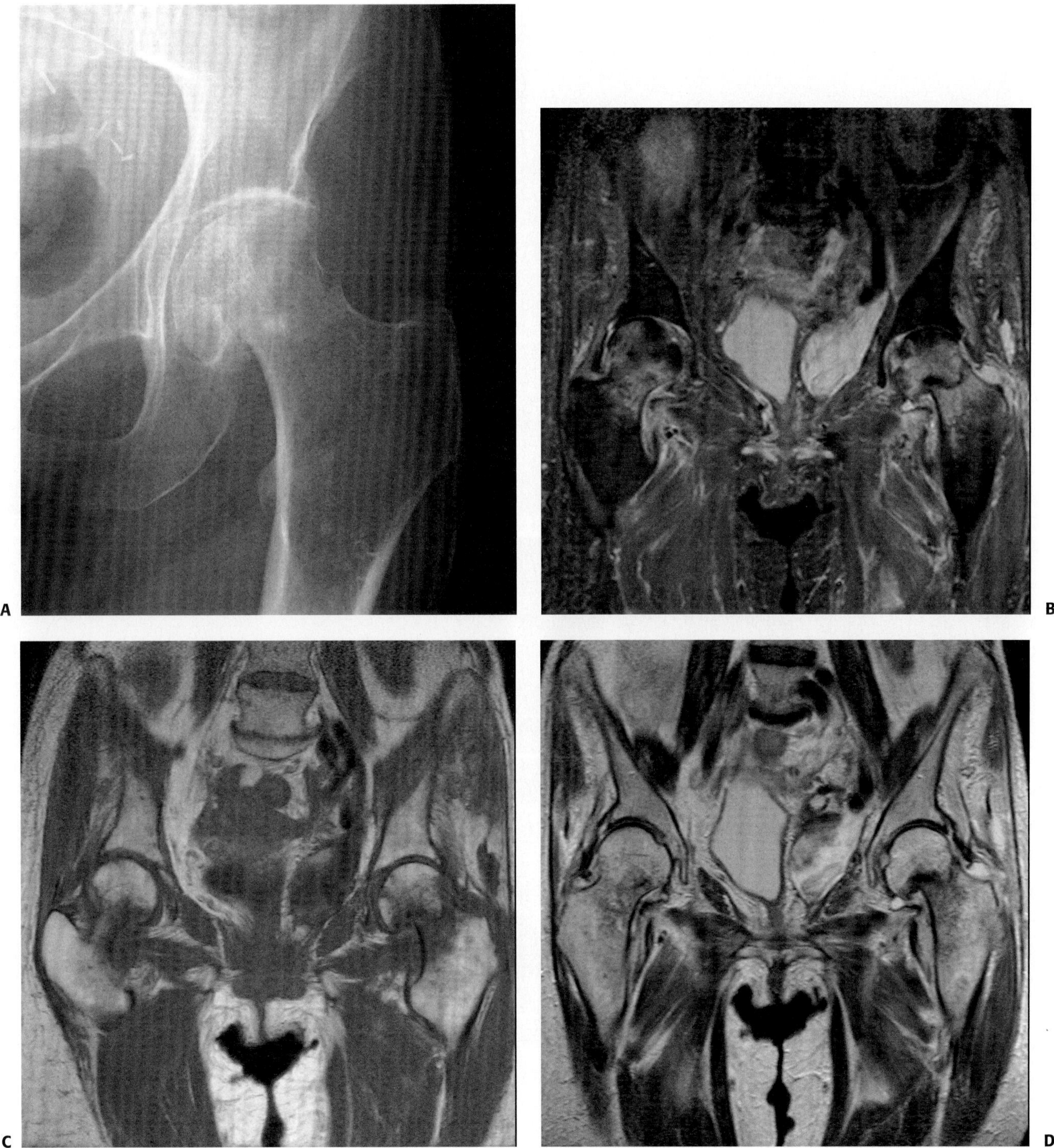

FIGURE 11-8 A. Conventional plain AP radiograph of a patient's hip demonstrates a femoral neck fracture. Although the fracture can be seen on routine radiographs, the patient was at risk for osteonecrosis because of corticosteroid use related to a kidney transplant. Some apparent changes are seen in the bone density of the femoral head. MRI of the pelvis and hip joints confirms the presence of an acute left hip fracture without and demonstrated that there was no osteonecrosis. Incidentally noted is a small developing fracture with surrounding stress reaction in the right femoral neck medially: **(B)** STIR, **(C)** T1-weighted, and **(D)** T2-weighted images. (*continues*)

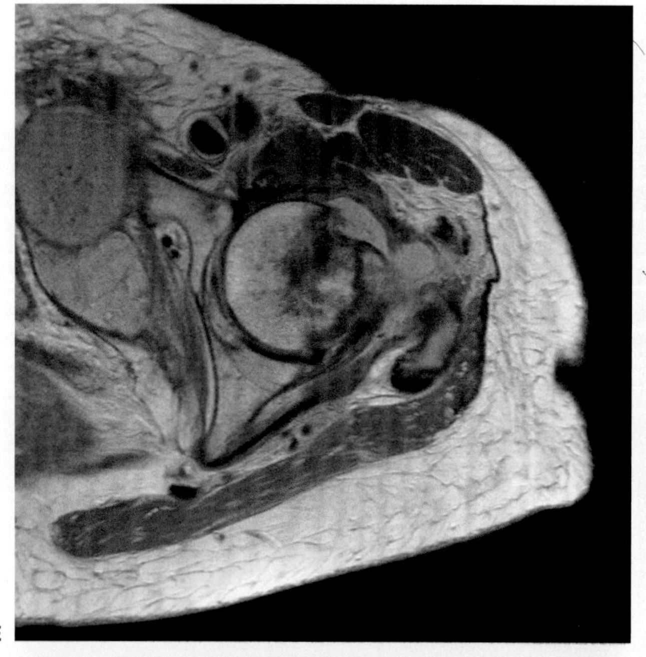
E

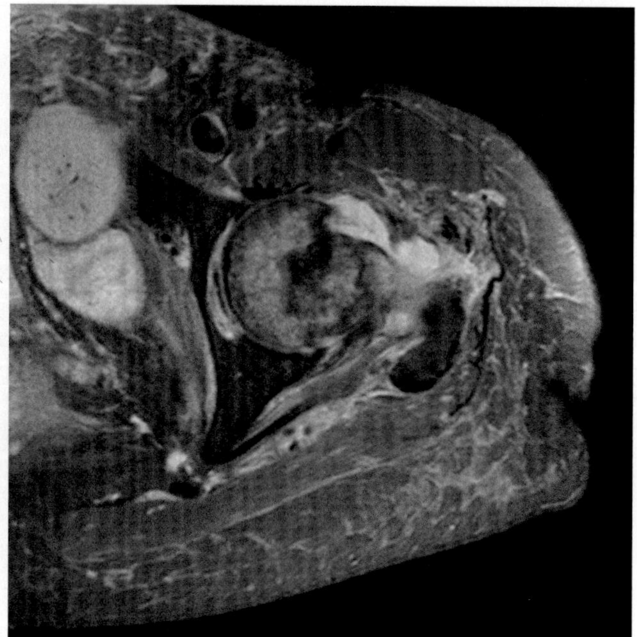
F

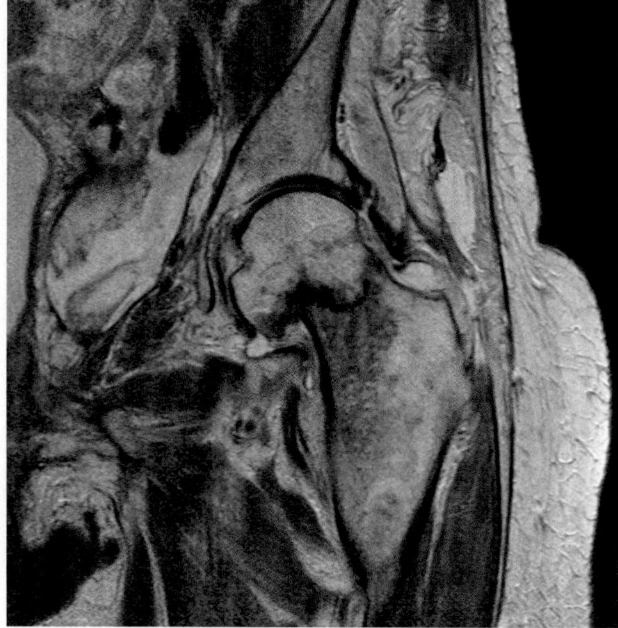
G

FIGURE 11-8 (*continued*) Higher-resolution images of the left hip fracture demonstrating mild impaction at the fracture site without significant angulation. **E.** Axial proton density, **(F)** axial fat-supressed proton density, and **(G)** coronal T2-weighted images. Note inferior pole of kidney transplant in the lower left pelvis with surrounding complex fluid collection.

from repeat radiographs in 10 patients and by scintigraphy in 15 patients. The time to final diagnosis averaged 9.6 days when the diagnosis was made by radiographs, and averaged 5.3 days when the diagnosis was made by scintigraphy. Immediate MRI can dramatically decrease the number of examinations performed and time to diagnosis, resulting in decreased costs of care and possibly reduced complications (60). Rubin et al compared scintigraphy and MRI for the evaluation of clinically suspected, but radiographically occult, hip fractures. Mean time to diagnosis with scintigraphy was greater than 2 days, whereas mean time to diagnosis by MRI was less than 1 day. Patients with hip fractures diagnosed with scintigraphy had a delay to surgery of at least 1 day compared with MRI, and scintigraphy resulted in higher patient costs due to delay in diagnosis (60). MRI has been found to be an excellent aid in diagnosing occult hip fractures, and may reduce subsequent cost and morbidity as a result of definite treatment (61). In many cases, the fracture pattern can be better delineated, which may be of therapeutic importance. Clinicians may be more apt to rely on MRI alone than on NM studies; in one report, clinicians always requested additional imaging for cases in which the bone scan was positive (62). MRI may also identify additional comorbid conditions such as pre-existing osteonecrosis or metastatic disease (61).

Although CT with multiplanar reformatting remains the modality of choice for imaging complex fractures, recent studies indicate that MRI may be valuable in the assessing such injuries as well. In one such study, the impact of MRI on the treatment of tibial plateau fractures was assessed (63). Patients presenting with tibial plateau fracture were assessed with conventional radiographs, CT, and MRI. Three sets of images were prepared for each injury: radiographs alone, radiographs with CT, and radiographs with MRI. Three surgeons were asked to determine the fracture classification and suggest a treatment plan based upon each set of images. The investigators found that the best interobserver variability for both fracture classification and fracture management was seen with the combination of conventional radiographs and MRI. The Schatzker classification of tibial plateau fractures based on conventional radiographs changed an average of 6% with the addition of the CT and 21% with the addition of MRI. MRI changed the treatment plan in 23% of cases. Holt et al studied 21 consecutive patients with tibial plateau fractures who were evaluated with both conventional radiography and MRI before treatment (64). MRI was more accurate in determining fracture classification, in revealing occult fracture lines, and in measuring the displacement and depression of fragments. The MRI findings resulted in a change in the classification of 10 fractures (48%) and a change in the management of four patients (19%). MRI also allowed diagnosis of associated intra-articular and periarticular soft tissue injuries preoperatively.

The role of CT is well recognized in the assessment of spinal trauma, but MRI is increasingly being used to evaluate for associated injuries such as herniated disks with cervical spine injuries and possible spinal cord injury associated with thoracolumbar spine fracture/dislocations. Green and Saifuddin have shown that 77% of patients with spine injury have a secondary injury level identified by whole spine MRI (65). Most commonly, these secondary injuries were bone marrow contusions, but 34% of patients had noncontiguous compression or burst fractures diagnosed by MRI.

Soft Tissue Injury. Because of its superb soft tissue contrast resolution and good spatial resolution, MRI provides an accurate means to assess soft tissue injury. MRI of the shoulder and knee is commonly ordered for evaluation of tendons, ligaments, and cartilage after trauma, frequently related to athletic injuries. Common indications for shoulder MRI following trauma include evaluation of the rotator cuff tendons for tearing, the superior glenoid labrum for superior labral anterior-posterior (SLAP) tears, and the anteroinferior labral-ligamentous complex after glenohumeral joint dislocation (66–68). Standard indications for knee MRI following trauma include evaluation of the cruciate and posterolateral corner ligaments for sprain or disruption, the menisci for tears, and the articular cartilage for osteochondral injury (69–71). Lonner et al compared MRI findings to examination under anesthesia in 10 patients with acute knee dislocations who had later surgical intervention, at which time the pathology was defined (72). Although the investigators considered MRI to be useful for defining the presence of ligamentous injuries in knee dislocations, the clinical examination under anesthesia was more accurate in this series when correlated with findings at surgery (72).

MR arthrography is a potentially valuable technique for assessing intra-articular derangement in many joints. Common indications include distinguishing partial- from full-thickness rotator cuff tears and evaluation of labral-ligamentous pathology in the shoulder, evaluation of the collateral ligaments in the elbow and the intercarpal ligaments in the wrist, demonstrating labral tears in the hip, evaluation of postoperative menisci in the knee, assessing stability of osteochondral lesions, and delineation of intra-articular bodies (73). Direct MR arthrography is performed by intra-articular injection of a dilute gadolinium solution, resulting in distention of the joint capsule and improved delineation of intra-articular structures. Indirect MR arthrography is performed using intravenous injection of gadolinium, with a delay before scanning during which mild exercise may be performed. The indirect technique is based on recognition that the intravenous gadolinium diffuses from the highly vascular synovium into the joint space. The indirect technique does not produce controlled joint distension, however, and is best applied in smaller joints such as the elbow, wrist, ankle, and shoulder (74).

Orthopaedic Hardware. Orthopaedic hardware presents a challenge in MR imaging, as metal distorts the magnetic field and results in large areas of signal void, which frequently obscures adjacent anatomy. New pulse sequence designs are available on high-field MR scanners to reduce artifact associated with orthopaedic implants. Applications for these sequences include evaluation of painful joint replacements, particularly knee and hip prostheses (75–77) and osteonecrosis of the femoral head after pinning femoral neck fractures (Fig. 11-9).

MR Venography. MRI is capable of identifying venous thromboembolism, although the clinical utility of MR venography (MRV) remains somewhat controversial (78,79). In one study, the ability of preoperative contrast venography and MRV to detect deep venous thrombosis (DVT) in the thigh and pelvis was compared in 45 consecutive patients with a displaced acetabular fracture (78). The imaging studies were performed an average of 7 days after injury. Twenty-four asymptomatic thrombi were found with MRV in 15 (33%) of the patients. Ten (42%) of the 24 thrombi were also seen with contrast venography; nine of them were in the thigh. The remaining 14 thrombi (58%) identified on MRV could not be visualized with contrast venography because they were located either in the deep pelvic veins or in the opposite extremity. Thrombus in the internal iliac vein was identified only with MRV. In this study, the findings on MRV resulted in a change in the therapeutic management in 10 (22%) of the 45 patients.

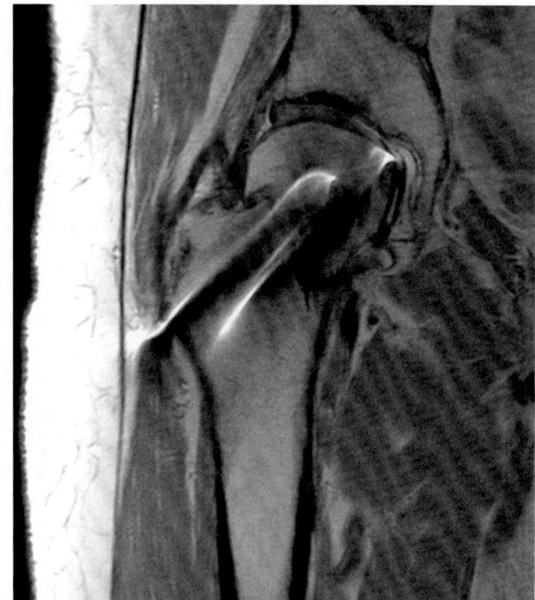

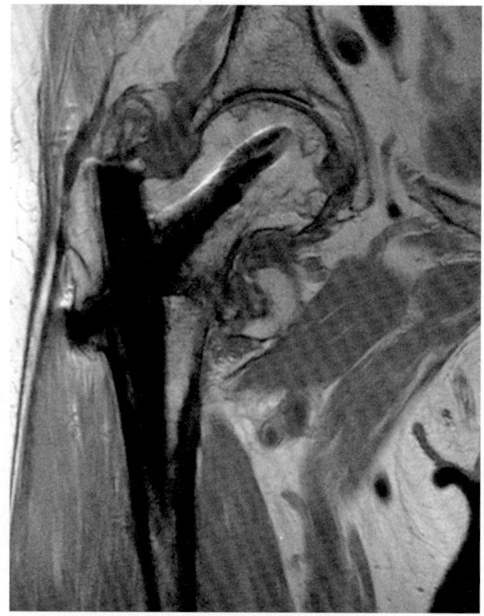

FIGURE 11-9 Metal artifact reduction sequences. **A.** Femoral neck fractures status postpinning with four screws demonstrates nonunion. MRI using metal artifact reduction sequences shows no evidence of avascular necrosis of the femoral head. **B.** An additional case of nonunion of an intertrochanteric fracture which demonstrates avascular necrosis of the femoral head without subchondral fracture or collapse. The intramedullary rod and screw are titanium, which results in fewer artifacts than stainless steel or other alloys.

Nevertheless, MRV was not found to be clinically useful in another series reported by Stover et al (79). In this study, 30 patients with pelvic or acetabular fractures underwent MRV and CT venography to screen for the presence of pelvic venous thrombosis preoperatively. Pelvic DVT was detected by CT venography in two patients (7%) and by MRV in four patients (13%). Invasive selective pelvic venography was performed on the five subjects who tested positive on one or both screening tests; just one CT venography case was validated. The false-positive rate for CT venography was 50%, and the false-positive rate for MRV was 100%.

Arthrography

Technical Considerations

Conventional Arthrography. Arthrography involves distension of a joint capsule using positive or negative contrast agents. Water-soluble, iodinated contrast media is typically used to provide positive contrast, whereas air has been historically used to produce negative contrast. Double-contrast examinations may also be performed using both agents simultaneously, although these techniques are largely of historical interest, as advances in cross-sectional imaging have supplanted double-contrast arthrography techniques.

Injection technique involves placement of a needle into the joint capsule, usually under fluoroscopic or CT guidance. Typically, a 22-gauge needle is used for larger joints, including the shoulder, hip, and knee, and a 25-gauge needle is used for smaller joints, such as the elbow, wrist, ankle, and smaller joints of the hands and feet. The anatomic approach varies according to each joint; for example, a lateral approach into the radiocapitellar joint space is frequently used for the elbow, and anterior approaches are typically used for the shoulder, hip, and tibiotalar joint. Table 11-2 lists technical considerations for arthrography of selected joints. After needle placement, small amounts of contrast are injected until the intra-articular location of the needle tip is confirmed. Contrast is then injected with subsequent distention of the joint capsule, the amount also varies by joint.

Frequently, the injection is performed under fluoroscopy, and sequential spot films are obtained before and during the injection to evaluate the flow of contrast. Pathology is inferred by abnormal communication of contrast with extracapsular structures. Passive and active range of motion are often required to demonstrate pathology, as abnormalities may only be shown after contrast is allowed to work its way through defects in the capsule and into the surrounding soft tissues. Contrast extravasation through capsular abnormalities can be fairly rapid, and may occur during passive or active range of motion. Extravasation may also occur during periods when the fluoroscope is not energized. In addition, the fluoroscope only provides two-dimensional views of bony anatomy, and it is extremely limited in its evaluation of surrounding soft tissues. Consequently, localizing the site of extravasation during conventional arthrography can be quite challenging. Care is also needed to avoid overdistension of the joint capsule, as extravasation through the

TABLE 11-2 Arthrographic Techniques of Selected Joints

Joint	Injection Approach	Needle Size	Volume of Contrast[72]
Shoulder	Anterior glenohumeral joint space	22-gauge 3 1/2 inch spinal needle	15 mL
Elbow	Lateral radiocapitellar joint space	25-gauge 1 1/2 inch needle	10 mL
Wrist	Dorsal radioscaphoid joint space	25-gauge 1 1/2 inch needle	4 mL
Hip	Anterior femoral head/neck junction	22-gauge 3 1/2 inch needle	15 mL
Knee	Medial or lateral patellofemoral joint space	22-gauge 1 1/2 inch needle	40 mL
Ankle	Anterior tibiotalar joint space	22-gauge 3 1/2 inch spinal needle	10 to 12 mL

capsule can occur, leading to subsequent decompression of intra-articular contrast and possible false-positive interpretations.

Complications of arthrography are uncommon, but may include bleeding and infection at the injection site, in addition to allergic reactions related to iodinated contrast media. A small number of patients experience postprocedural pain, possibly related to a mild synovial inflammatory response to the contrast media. Although patients are generally apprehensive about the procedure, they generally tolerate the procedure with less discomfort than expected (80).

Digital Subtraction Arthrography. With the advent of digital imaging, digital subtraction techniques have been developed for fluoroscopy. Typically, a preliminary scout film serves as a "mask," which is subsequently subtracted from images following contrast injection. This significantly improves contrast resolution of the fluoroscopic spot films and enables visualization of contrast that would otherwise be inapparent when adjacent to similar high-density objects, such as joint prostheses. Digital subtraction arthrography (DSA) also allows sequential injection and evaluation of adjacent joint compartments, as a new mask is obtained after injection of the first compartment, which is subsequently subtracted from images acquired during injection of the second compartment. DSA techniques are sensitive to patient motion, however, which produces misregistration artifact as a result of misalignment of the mask and subsequent images. DSA also requires specialized equipment, which may not be available outside of radiology departments.

CT and MR Arthrography. Cross-sectional techniques, such as CT and MRI, have largely replaced conventional arthrography for evaluating internal derangement, but these imaging modalities may be combined with arthrography using appropriate contrast agents for each modality (73,81). For CT arthrography, an arthrogram is first performed using a contrast solution containing saline and water soluble, iodinated contrast media, typically in a 1:1 dilution. Thin-section CT is then performed through the joint, and images in orthogonal planes are reconstructed. For MR arthrography, a very dilute gadolinium solution (typically 1:200 dilution) is injected into the joint, and MR imaging is subsequently performed. In addition to routine sequences, fat suppressed T1-weighted images are used to visualize the injected contrast. With both imaging modalities, evaluation is aided not only by silhouetting intra-articular structures by relatively bright contrast, but also by distension of the joint capsule. This results in separation of intra-articular ligaments and capsular structures and allows more precise evaluation of complex anatomy (Fig. 11-10). Bony and soft tissue abnormalities are directly visualized with these cross-sectional techniques, as compared to conventional arthrography, whereby pathology is inferred based on the appearance of the contrast collection in relation to the bony landmarks.

Applications

Prior to advanced cross-sectional imaging techniques, arthrography was traditionally used for assessing periarticular soft tissue injuries associated with trauma. Today, there are more limited indications for arthrography, although it is frequently performed in combination with CT and MRI to increase the sensitivity and specificity for internal derangement.

Arthrography may be substituted in patients with contraindications to MR imaging, such as pacemakers or intracranial aneurysm clips. CT arthrography is preferred, however, as advances in CT scanner technology have led to marked improvements in resolution and scan time, resulting in high spatial resolution images and multiplanar reconstructions of intra-articular structures.

Upper Extremity. In the upper extremity, shoulder arthrography may be performed to evaluate for full-thickness rotator cuff tears. Extravasation of contrast into the subacromial/subdeltoid

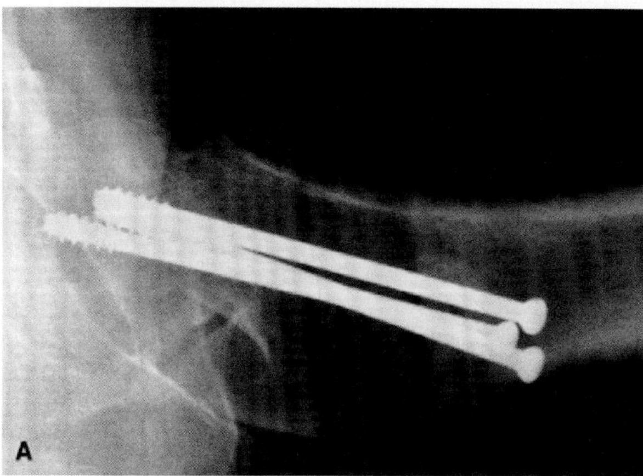

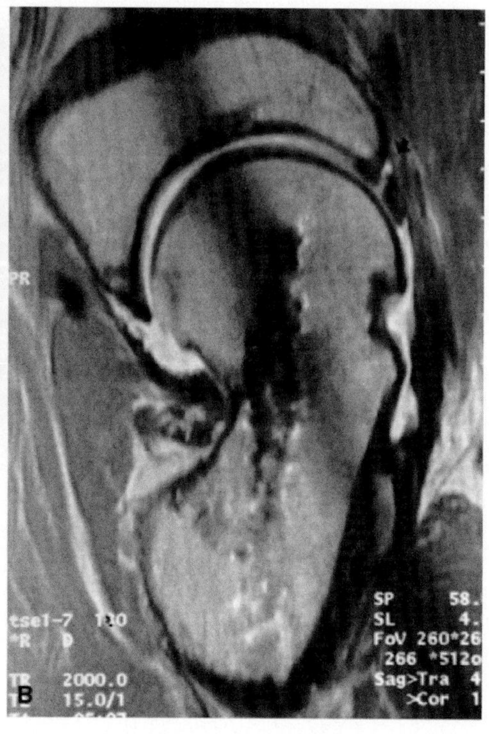

FIGURE 11-10 **A.** Lateral radiograph of the proximal femur after fixation of a femoral neck fracture, showing malunion with retroversion of the femoral neck. **B.** The patient had persistent hip pain, and MR arthrography revealed a tear of the anterior acetabular labrum. Note angular deformity at the site of fracture malunion and residual micrometallic artifact related to insertion of prior screws. (Reprinted with permission from Eijer H, Myers SR, Ganz R. Anterior femoroacetabular impingement after femoral neck fractures. *J Orthop Trauma* 2001;15(7):475–481.)

bursa is diagnostic of a full-thickness tear. Even with careful fluoroscopic observation during the injection process, it is frequently impossible to delineate the site or extent of the tear, as contrast may accumulate in the bursa without visualization of an obvious tract through the torn tendon. Occasionally, no extravasation is seen after completing the injection; however, after passively and/or actively exercising the shoulder, subsequent fluoroscopy reveals contrast flooding the bursa as a result of contrast working itself through a full-thickness tear. Special care is needed in interpreting arthrography of the postoperative rotator cuff, as intact cuff repairs may continue to leak contrast into the bursa.

The value of three-compartment arthrography has been documented in the setting of acute wrist trauma (82,83), as has the value of digital subtraction techniques in wrist arthrography (84,85).

Arthrography has historically been applied to the evaluation of ulnar collateral ligament injuries of the thumb (gamekeeper's thumb). Recent literature has shown MR arthrography to be more accurate in detecting ulnar collateral ligament (UCL) injuries and in evaluating displacement of the torn ligament (86).

Lower Extremity. In the lower extremity, arthrography alone is rarely performed for trauma, but may be combined with CT or MRI for evaluating osteochondral abnormalities (Fig. 11-9) (87). A recent study comparing CT arthrography with MR arthrography suggests that CT arthrography may be more accurate in evaluating cartilage lesions of the ankle joint (88).

Arthrography may also be useful in the evaluation of pain after treating calcaneal fractures with intra-articular extension (89). Matsui et al performed posterior subtalar joint arthrography at a mean of 6 months postinjury in 22 patients; 15 had undergone surgical repair and 7 had been treated nonoperatively. The patients were separated into four groups based on arthrographic findings: normal, narrow, irregular, and ankylosis. Clinical follow-up performed at a mean of 23 months postinjury correlated very well with the earlier arthrographic findings, suggesting that subtalar arthrosis is responsible for much of the symptoms that develop after calcaneal fracture (89).

Pediatric Injuries. Arthrography is valuable in assessing pediatric physeal injuries (especially the elbow) (90–94) that are not visible on conventional radiographs. It is also used intraoperatively to assist with the reduction of pediatric radial head fractures (95).

Dynamic Imaging. Arthrography remains the investigation of choice when dynamic imaging is necessary. In the German literature, Klein et al compared MRI with arthrography and CT arthrography for the diagnosis of wrist pain in 346 patients (96). Imaging findings were correlated with surgical findings in 78 of these patients and with the clinical course in the remainder. Because of its ability to perform functional imaging, arthrography was the best method for evaluating scapholunate ligament tears and defects of the ulnolunate and ulnotriquetral ligaments.

Ultrasonography

Technical Considerations

Conventional Ultrasonography. Ultrasonography (US) refers to the spectrum of sound waves with frequencies greater than 20 kHz (20,000 Hz), which are beyond the audible range of the human ear. Typical frequencies used in medical diagnostic US range from 2.0 to 12 MHz, although frequencies of 20 MHz and higher are in clinical use for more specialized applications involving very small regions of anatomy. Lower frequencies within this range (2 to 5 MHz) allow deeper penetration of the US beam for evaluation of thicker body parts, although at lower spatial resolutions. Higher-frequency US beams (10 to 12 MHz) provide greater spatial resolution and are frequently used in evaluating superficial anatomy, such as tendons.

US beams are generated by transducers, which make use of piezoelectric materials to convert electrical energy into mechanical energy (sound waves). Today's transducer designs are complex and may incorporate hundreds of individual piezoelectric elements, each of which is energized in turn or in combination, such that the individual sound waves combine into an US beam. The US beam propagates into the underlying tissues and is partially reflected back at tissue boundaries due to differences in acoustic impedance between tissues. Acoustic impedance is defined as the product of tissue density and the speed of sound, both of which vary among tissues. Small differences in acoustic impedance will produce smaller reflections of sound waves, whereas large differences in acoustic impedances will result in larger reflections. The reflected echoes travel back to the transducer, where the transducer elements convert the sound waves into electrical signals, which are then used to create the US image.

An US image is composed of an array of pixels, each corresponding to a tissue element at a particular depth and location. Echoes returning from underlying soft tissue elements are generated from reflections of the US beam at tissue interfaces of different acoustic impedance. In addition, smaller cellular elements within tissues can also act as individual "scatterers." Each of these scatterers reflects a small portion of the US beam in all directions. A portion of these scattered echoes are reflected back toward the transducer and are displayed in the image as background "echogenicity" that is characteristic for that tissue. Echoes returning from superficial soft tissues have shorter round trip distances to travel back to the transducer and are detected earlier than those for deeper soft tissues. For this reason, the depth of a tissue element can be calculated using the return time of its corresponding echo. The amplitude of the returning echo determines the brightness, or echogenicity, of a tissue element. As the US beam travels deeper within the soft tissues, it progressively loses energy and subsequent echoes from deeper tissue elements are smaller in amplitude. A correction factor, termed *time gain compensation*, is applied to deeper soft tissues to account for this drop off in echo amplitude. Thus, differences in echogenicity in the resulting US image will be less dependent on tissue depth and more related to differences in acoustic impedance and scattering.

During a single cycle, the transducer sends a short burst of US waves (the US pulse) into the underlying tissues, and then listens for the returning echoes. The time spent sending out the US pulse is a tiny fraction of the listening time, typically about 0.5% of the total cycle time. The pulse repetition frequency determines how many pulses are sent into the underlying tissue over time, and typically ranges between 2,000 and 4,000 cycles/second (2 to 4 kHz). During routine scanning, the transducer is constantly steering and refocusing the US beam within the underlying tissue in order to generate echoes that will correspond to each pixel in the US image. The two dimensional (2D) US image that is generated is typically referred to as *B-mode* ("brightness" mode) *imaging*. The designs of current transducers are quite complex and rely on advanced electronics and scanning algorithms, but have resulted in greater spatial resolution and more advanced feature sets, including 3D and Doppler imaging.

Echogenicity is a term used to describe the relative brightness of echoes returning from tissues or tissue interfaces. Tissues may be described as *hypoechoic* or *hyperechoic* with regard to a reference tissue, in addition to *isoechoic* if two distinct soft tissues share the same level of echogenicity. The descriptor *anechoic* refers to a tissue or medium that produces no reflected echoes and is black on the corresponding US image. Water is the best example of an anechoic medium, as all of the sound waves are transmitted through the medium without any reflections. In such situations, the energy within the US beam will be greater as it reaches the tissues on the far side of the medium and the distal tissues will appear brighter; this is referred to as *increased through transmission*. Conversely, any tissue or medium that blocks transmission of all sound waves will appear highly echogenic at its proximal interface with the US beam and will exhibit "distal acoustic shadowing," whereby the more distal tissues appear black, resembling a shadow. Cortical bone and air are examples where the large differences in acoustic impedance result in marked attenuation of the US beam, producing distal acoustic shadowing.

US examinations are highly operator dependent, and the quality of the examination can be influenced by the sonographer's training, experience performing certain examinations, and understanding of normal anatomy and disease states. US is a real-time examination, and although images that represent the underlying anatomy are saved, these 2D images cannot provide the depth of understanding that real-time visualization provides. For this reason, it may be necessary for the interpreting physician to be present or to image the patient in order to interpret complex examinations.

Doppler US. Doppler US is used to evaluate moving tissues, such as blood flow within vessels. Velocity measurements and directions of flow may be ascertained based on frequency shifts of the returning echoes. When the US beam is reflected from a tissue moving toward the transducer, the returning echoes undergo a slight increase in frequency. Similarly, when interacting with a tissue moving away from the transducer, the US beam will be reflected such that the returning echoes will incur a slight decrease in their frequency. These frequency shifts are used to calculate the speed of the moving tissue, whereas the direction of frequency shift (positive vs. negative) is used to determine the direction of motion relative to the transducer.

Various modes of Doppler operation are available on today's scanners and are frequently used for vascular evaluation. Duplex Doppler imaging combines 2D B-mode imaging with pulsed Doppler imaging; the 2D B-mode image provides an anatomical map to identify vessels for subsequent Doppler interrogation. Color Doppler combines B-mode grayscale imaging with color flow superimposed over vessels, as determined by Doppler imaging. Shades of red and blue are assigned to the vessels based on their velocities and directions and represent flow toward and away from the transducer, respectively. Power Doppler imaging is a signal-processing algorithm that uses the total amplitude of the Doppler signal to generate maps of flow, which are then superimposed on B-mode grayscale images. The corresponding images demonstrate greater sensitivity to slow flow, although no directional information is available.

Applications

Ultrasonography is a simple, noninvasive, relatively inexpensive imaging modality that is now widely available in most hospitals and in many clinics. Diagnostic ultrasonography has an established role in the immediate diagnosis of trauma patients according to the Advanced Trauma Life Support protocol, where it is used in the so-called Focused Abdominal Sonography for Trauma examination for intra-abdominal injury. Ultrasonography also has applications in evaluation of fractures, fracture healing, soft tissue trauma, and venous thromboembolism.

Fractures. Ultrasonography has potential in the assessment of fractures, and may be under-used in this regard. US compares favorably to conventional radiography in the assessment of occult scaphoid fracture in patients with wrist pain (97). Durston et al used US to assess the reduction of pediatric forearm fractures in the emergency department, thereby avoiding multiple trips to the radiology suite while gaining much more rapid assessment of the quality of fracture reduction (98). In some centers, US is used to rule out intra-articular elbow fractures (99). Assessing pediatric elbow injuries is notoriously difficult because of the complex joint anatomy and the multiplicity of its ossification centers, many of which are relatively unossified in childhood. US has proven to be valuable in evaluating lateral condylar fractures, in that it is able to assess the extent of the fracture line through the unossified capitellum and trochlea, in order to distinguish unstable intra-articular fractures from their stable extra-articular counterparts (100).

US may also be clinically useful in evaluating fractures in settings where conventional radiography may not be readily available, such as in military or aerospace settings (101). Dulchavsky et al prospectively evaluated 158 injured extremities by US (102). Nonphysician cast technicians, who had received limited training and were blinded to the patient's radiographic diagnoses, performed the US evaluations. Examinations only required an average of 4 minutes and accurately diagnosed injury in 94% of patients with no false-positive results. Injuries that were diagnosed by US included fractures in the upper arm, forearm, femur, tibia/fibula, hand, and foot.

Fracture Healing. US is a useful method to monitor fracture healing. Moed et al performed sonographic evaluation of patients 6 and 12 weeks after unreamed tibial nailing and found that persistent nail visualization indicated poor callus formation and predicted later healing complications (103). Color Doppler sonography has been shown to demonstrate progressive vascularization of fracture callus and predict delayed callus formation in another study of patients with tibial fractures (104).

Soft Tissue Trauma. Ultrasonography is also well suited for diagnosing musculoskeletal soft tissue injuries and is of proven value in the assessment of many tendon injuries, such as those of the tendoachilles and rotator cuff (105–107). US has been used to assess muscle injury, depicted as a tear or hematoma and subsequent complications such as fibrosis, cystic lesions, or heterotopic ossification (108). US is valuable in localizing foreign bodies within soft tissues; an advantage over conventional radiography is that foreign objects do not need to be radiopaque in order to visualize them (109).

Venous Thromboembolism. US has come to play a very important role in managing venous thromboembolism in trauma patients (110). All trauma patients are at risk for developing deep vein thrombosis (DVT), and venous ultrasonography has become the most widely used imaging modality for DVT diagnosis. In fact, the Intersocietal Commission for the Accreditation of Vascular Laboratories now mandates Duplex Doppler US as the primary instrument for peripheral venous testing (111). Venous scanning performed by skilled operators is the most practical and cost-effective method for assessing DVT of the proximal and distal lower extremity veins. Several US modalities are used to evaluate DVT, including B-mode for real-time visualization of compression of larger veins.

Duplex Doppler for evaluating waveforms and velocities and Color Doppler for depicting patency of veins is particularly useful in the calf and iliac veins (110). The diagnostic accuracy of US is well documented, and the sensitivity and specificity of venous ultrasonography (including all types) for the diagnosis of symptomatic proximal DVT is 97% and 94%, respectively (110). The high specificity of venous ultrasonography is sufficient to initiate treatment of DVT without further confirmation, and the high sensitivity for proximal DVT makes it possible to withhold treatment if the examination is negative (110). When US examinations cannot be performed (uncooperative patient, presence of bandages, casts), an alternative diagnostic procedure, such as contrast venography, may be needed. More advanced imaging modalities, such as CT or MR venography are also available. US is less accurate in the diagnosis of proximal

DVT involving the pelvis; MR venography has been suggested as a more accurate modality for detecting intrapelvic DVT (78).

Nuclear Medicine Imaging

Technical Considerations

Nuclear scintigraphy involves intravenous injection of a radiopharmaceutical with subsequent imaging using a gamma scintillation camera. The radiopharmaceutical is typically composed of two moieties: a radionuclide and a pharmaceutical compound. The pharmaceutical is responsible for localization of the molecule in the body, and the radionuclide allows imaging of the pharmaceutical distribution.

Radionuclides are radioactive isotopes that undergo spontaneous decay, which results in the emission of photons. Photons that are generated in the nucleus of the atom are gamma rays, whereas photons generated by electron transitions within their orbital shells are x-rays. Either may be used for imaging, although the particular choice of a radionuclide predetermines the types and energies of photons that are emitted. In many nuclear medicine (NM) imaging applications, Technetium (^{99m}Tc) is commonly used as the radionuclide due to its favorable imaging properties (140 keV gamma energy), clinically suitable half-life (6 hours), availability (^{99}Mo/^{99m}Tc generator) and ease in labeling of pharmaceuticals. Other radionuclides used in orthopaedic imaging include Gallium (^{67}Ga) and Indium (^{111}In), and are discussed later in this section.

Pharmaceuticals are metabolically active molecules that are designed to localize to target tissues once injected intravenously. There are many different mechanisms of localization, but for orthopaedic imaging, regional blood flow is important for all administered radiopharmaceuticals. Specific radiopharmaceuticals for orthopaedic imaging and their method of localization are discussed later in this section.

Gamma scintillation cameras are specialized detectors that capture photons within a large flat crystal, commonly made of sodium iodide activated with thallium. Photons interact with the scintillation crystal and are converted to visible light, which is then captured by photomultiplier tubes (PMT) coupled to the crystal. The PMT converts the light photon into an electrical signal, which is subsequently amplified and electronically processed. This process results in a single "count" in the final NM image corresponding to a single radioactive decay in the patient.

NM images are formed by placing the gamma scintillation camera over the anatomy of interest and accumulating counts for a specific amount of time, or for a minimum number of counts, typically on the order of hundreds of thousands of counts. Imaging is often performed after a delay to allow localization and/or uptake of the radiopharmaceutical within the target tissues. Delayed imaging demonstrates characteristic patterns of distribution throughout the body for a particular radiopharmaceutical, in addition to abnormal accumulation or absence of activity corresponding to disease states. Consequently, nuclear imaging studies are based on visualization of metabolic function, rather than anatomy. Anatomic features are frequently visualized on NM images, although spatial resolution is typically quite poor compared with other imaging modalities (Table 11-1).

During routine acquisition of NM images, the gamma scintillation camera is left stationary in a single projection, resulting in a planar image. Single photon emission computed tomography (SPECT) is an extension of planar imaging, whereby the gamma camera rotates around the patient, stopping at predefined intervals, to acquire multiple static planar images. Using techniques similar to those in CT, these planar data sets are then processed by computers. Images are typically created in orthogonal tomographic planes (axial, coronal, sagittal), in addition to 3D volumes. Although the main advantage of SPECT over planar images is the improved image contrast resolution as a result of eliminating radioactivity from overlapping anatomy, spatial resolution is similar or slightly decreased compared to planar imaging (Table 11-1).

As nuclear scintigraphy is more of a functional, rather than anatomic, examination, indwelling orthopaedic hardware significantly affects image quality may introduce image artifacts. Hardware can shield the gamma camera from photons arising behind the hardware, resulting in a photopenic defect. Knowledge of indwelling hardware and their characteristic photopenic appearances alleviates misinterpretation of these defects. Multiple projections are also frequently performed during a single examination, which allows evaluation of the activity on multiple sides of the hardware.

Nuclear medicine studies relevant to trauma and orthopaedics are described in the sections to follow.

Skeletal Scintigraphy. Skeletal scintigraphy, commonly referred to as a *bone scan*, is the most commonly performed NM study with respect to the skeletal system. The radiopharmaceutical used is typically a ^{99m}Tc-labelled diphosphonate, which localizes to bone based on chemiadsorption of the phosphorus compound to the mineral phase of bone, particularly at sites of increased osteoblastic activity. Regional blood flow is also important for tracer distribution, as areas of increased regional blood flow deliver greater tracer to the adjacent skeleton, and result in greater uptake. The term *bone scan* typically refers to images obtained after a 2- to 4-hour delay, in order to allow localization of the diphosphonate compound. Three-phase bone scans incorporate additional dynamic and immediate imaging phases. A radionuclide angiogram (first phase) is obtained during transit of radiopharmaceutical through the arterial system. Immediate static images are then obtained for an additional 5 minutes (second phase), and represent "blood pool" or "tissue phase" images. Both of these earlier imaging phases are used to evaluate for regional hyperemia, as evidenced by both increased blood flow and increased surrounding soft tissue uptake.

Normal bone scan images show a characteristic appearance of the skeleton, with slightly greater uptake in the axial skeleton (spine, pelvis) than the extremities. In skeletally immature individuals, there is normal avid uptake in the growth plates, resulting in symmetrically increased bands of activity occurring adjacent to joints and apophyses. Many diseases are characterized by both increased osteoblastic and osteoclastic activity within the bone, in addition to regional hyperemia, and result in greater tracer uptake (hot lesions) than normal bone. These abnormalities may be solitary or multiple, focal, or diffuse in nature. Some pathologic processes, particularly permeative processes (small round cell tumors) or those that elicit little surrounding bone reaction, result in regions of decreased tracer uptake, or "cold" lesions. These lesions may be difficult to detect on routine bone scans. Bone scans are highly sensitive for disease processes, although specificity is poor. A normal bone scan may rule out underlying skeletal abnormality, but a positive bone scan necessitates further workup of the underlying abnormality.

Marrow Imaging. Marrow imaging is performed using ^{99m}Tc-labeled sulfur colloid. The sulfur colloid is composed of particles measuring between 0.1 and 2.0 μm, which are taken up by the reticuloendothelial cells within the liver (85%), spleen (10%), and bone marrow (5%). Uptake is rapid (the half-life lasts for 2 to 3 minutes) and imaging is performed after a 20-minute delay. Current indications for marrow imaging are limited, but include evaluation of osteomyelitis in conjunction with ^{111}In-labeled white blood cell imaging.

Gallium Imaging. Gallium-67 citrate is a radiopharmaceutical that was originally developed as a bone-imaging agent, but was later found to be useful in imaging infection and inflammation. After intravenous injection, gallium binds to transferrin and circulates in the bloodstream. At sites of inflammation or infection, increased regional blood flow and increased vascular permeability result in greater accumulation of gallium. In addition, neutrophils release large amounts of lactoferrin as a part of their inflammatory response; gallium has a higher binding affinity for lactoferrin than transferrin and localizes at the site of inflammation. Gallium is a relatively poor imaging agent, as its photons are not optimum for imaging with present-day gamma cameras, and total body clearance is slow with considerable background activity. Imaging is typically performed at 48 hours, which contributes to delays in diagnosis.

Gallium scans are often interpreted with bone scans for evaluation of osteomyelitis. Gallium activity that is greater than, or in different distribution than, corresponding activity on the bone scan is diagnostic for osteomyelitis.

White Blood Cell Imaging. There are several approaches for using labeled white blood cells (WBC) for diagnosing infection and/or inflammatory processes. Of these, ^{111}Indium oxine- and ^{99m}Tc-labeled hexamethylpropyleneamine (HMPAO) labeled WBC are discussed briefly.

Indium-111 is complexed with oxine, which results in a lipid soluble complex that readily crosses the cell membranes. Approximately 50 mL of blood must be withdrawn and the leukocytes need to be separated from the plasma and red cells. Labeling is accomplished by incubating the leukocytes with the ^{111}Indium oxine complex for 30 minutes. The leukocytes are then resuspended in plasma and reinjected into the patient within a total of 2 to 4 hours. Imaging is typically performed at 24 hours to allow for leukocyte localization and clearance from the blood pool.

^{99m}Tc HMPAO is a cerebral perfusion agent that also crosses cell membranes and may be used to label white blood cells, preferentially granulocytes. Approximately 50 to 75 mL of blood is withdrawn and incubated with the radiopharmaceutical; however, the labeling process is performed in plasma, and cell separation is not needed. The labeled cells are then reinjected, and imaging is performed at 4 hours for the peripheral skeleton.

Labeled WBC studies should be interpreted in combination with sulfur colloid marrow studies for evaluation of osteomyelitis, including infected joint replacements. When used alone, labeled white cell studies may result in false-positive results, as labeled WBCs normally distribute to the bone marrow, in addition to the liver and spleen, after reinjection. The sulfur colloid marrow study is used to map out areas of normal residual marrow activity. Congruent activity is seen within the bone marrow on both examinations. Osteomyelitis results in replacement of marrow activity on the sulfur colloid study, resulting in a photopenic defect, whereas there is significantly increased activity on the corresponding labeled white blood cell study.

Applications

Nuclear medicine imaging is frequently used for further evaluation when conventional radiographs are normal, or to evaluate the significance of abnormalities seen on radiographs. Although typically highly sensitive for disease processes, its poor specificity makes it necessary to correlate the findings with additional clinical history, laboratory evaluation, or imaging examinations. Applications of NM to orthopaedic trauma include evaluation of fractures, osteomyelitis, and osteonecrosis.

Fractures. Bone scans are highly sensitive for acute fractures. Matin et al demonstrated positive scans in 80% of fractures at 24 hours, and in 95% by 72 hours (112). Advanced age and debilitation contributed to nonvisualization of fractures beyond this time frame. The minimum time to return to normal was 5 months, and 90% of fractures returned to normal by 2 years. Due to its poor specificity, scintigraphy can lead to false-positive diagnoses of fracture. Garcia-Morales et al reported five cases of false-positive scans for hip fracture due to collar osteophytes; subsequent MR imaging in these patients was negative (113).

Radiographically negative stress fractures and insufficiency fractures are also well delineated on bone scintigraphy as focal areas of increased radiotracer uptake. Characteristic sites of stress fractures depend on the activity that produced them, although there is considerable overlap. Some fracture patterns show characteristic appearances on scintigraphy. For example, in elderly patients with chronic low back or hip pain, sacral insufficiency fractures reveal a classic "H" pattern of uptake, known as the "Honda" sign (114). Not uncommonly, several focal areas of increased tracer uptake are seen in the skeleton, which presumably represent a combination of acute and more chronic findings. In these cases, three-phase scintigraphy can provide additional information regarding hyperemia and may help to differentiate acute from chronic injuries. Typically, hyperemia resolves within 4 to 8 weeks after initial injury, with the blood flow, then the blood pool, images normalizing.

Scintigraphy may be useful in the early identification of fracture healing complications. Barros et al performed scintigraphy at 6, 12, and 24 weeks with 25 mCi of MDP-Tc99m in 40 patients with tibial shaft fractures that were treated nonsurgically (115). Using the normal leg as a control, an activity index (the ratio of the uptake counts of the injured leg to the normal leg) was calculated. All fractures in this series healed within 20 weeks and the activity ratio index progressively decreased at the three evaluations (115). The investigators speculate that a persistently increased activity index would indicate future development of healing complications, such as delayed union or nonunion, although they did not have any such healing complications in their series (115).

Bone scintigraphy may also be used in evaluating a child with nonaccidental trauma. In a study from Australia, studies of 30 children who were the victims of suspected child abuse and who had both skeletal surveys and bone scintigraphy were retrospectively reviewed (116). Excluding rib fractures, there were 64 bony injuries, of which 33% were seen on both imaging modalities, 44% were seen on skeletal survey only, and 25% of the injuries were seen on bone scans alone. Metaphyseal lesions typical of child abuse were found in 20 cases (31%) on skeletal survey; only 35% of these were identified on bone scan. The investigators felt that both skeletal survey and bone scintigraphy should be performed in cases of suspected child abuse.

Infection. Osteomyelitis may result from hematogenous spread of microorganisms to bone, direct extension from areas of adjacent soft tissue infection, or as a result of open fractures and/or surgery. Persistent pain or delayed healing after surgery can be difficult to evaluate with regard to infection, as conventional radiographs may only show more advanced destructive changes and MR imaging may be very difficult to interpret in light of recent surgery.

Radionuclide imaging has evolved over time with respect to imaging orthopaedic infections. In addition to three-phase bone scans, dual Gallium/bone scintigraphy and labeled WBC studies including combination leukocyte/bone and leukocyte/marrow studies, are valuable in diagnosing both acute and chronic osteomyelitis as well as infected joint replacements. No one study is equally applicable to all clinical situations, however (117).

Although three-phase bone scans have excellent accuracy for detecting osteomyelitis in normal underlying bone, the specificity of this test is markedly reduced in the presence of underlying bone disease.

Dual Gallium (^{67}Ga)/bone scintigraphy has been used to evaluate osteomyelitis. Gallium scintigraphy demonstrates greater accuracy (86%) in diagnosing spinal osteomyelitis compared with ^{111}In-labeled WBC (66%) (118). A recent evaluation of imaging techniques in spinal osteomyelitis and surrounding soft tissue infections has recommended SPECT ^{67}Ga as the radionuclide study of choice when MRI is unavailable or as an adjunct in patients with possible spinal infection in whom the diagnosis remains uncertain (119). Gallium is also better suited for imaging of chronic osteomyelitis when compared with ^{99m}Tc HMPAO-labeled WBCs, which are better for imaging acute infections (120).

^{99m}Tc HMPAO-labeled WBC scintigraphy exhibits high sensitivity (97.7%) and specificity (96.8%) for acute osteomyelitis, although its sensitivity for chronic osteomyelitis is slightly decreased (121). ^{99m}Tc HMPAO-labeled WBC scintigraphy is preferred for evaluating children because of the smaller radiation dose to the spleen and less blood is needed for labeling (122). ^{99m}Tc HMPAO-labeled WBC scintigraphy is superior to ^{99m}Tc bone scintigraphy for children younger than 6 months old due to the poor sensitivity of bone scintigraphy at this age (120). ^{111}In-labeled WBC scintigraphy is preferred in evaluating chronic osteomyelitis, as dual ^{111}In WBC/^{99m}Tc SC studies result in improved accuracy for diagnosis of osteomyelitis in regions containing active bone marrow (120,122). In more complex regions with overlapping bone and soft tissues, such as the skull and hips, simultaneous ^{111}In WBC/^{99m}Tc bone SPECT imaging has been recommended (122).

Dual ^{111}In WBC/^{99m}Tc bone scans have been used to evaluate for osteomyelitis at sites of delayed union or nonunion (123). The sensitivity, specificity, positive and negative predictive values, and accuracy of this approach were 86%, 84%, 69%, 94%, and 82% respectively.

Osteonecrosis. Because scintigraphy is able to demonstrate the vascularity of bone, it is often used to try to assess the risk of osteonecrosis after an injury. Although largely supplanted by MRI, bone scanning can be used to identify osteonecrosis of the femoral head before it is apparent on conventional radiographs (Fig. 11-11) (124). Studies by Drane and Rudd and Mortensson et al have shown that bone scintigraphy cannot predict the risk of osteonecrosis after femoral neck fracture (125,126). Subsequent work has suggested that SPECT imaging may be more accurate in assessing vascularity of the femoral head in fractures of the femoral neck (127).

Angiography

Technical Considerations

Conventional Angiography. Techniques in conventional angiography are well established and involve cannulation of a vessel, commonly a major artery, for subsequent diagnostic and therapeutic interventions. Typically, the right common femoral artery is accessed, although less common access sites include the left common femoral artery, the axillary and brachial arteries, and translumbar aortic approaches, the selection of which depend on the clinical situation and goal of angiography. The Seldinger technique, the standard procedure for cannulating the common femoral artery, involves placing an 18-gauge needle into the

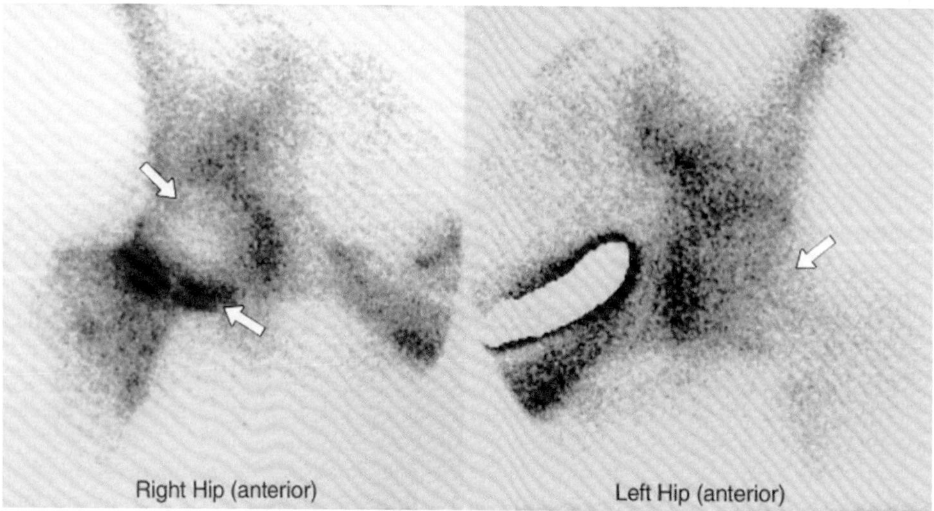

FIGURE 11-11 Pinhole bone scintigraphy (AP views) showing a photon-deficient area centrally in the right femoral head and increased uptake in the femoral neck and subcapital area compared with normal left hip findings. (Reprinted with permission from Yoon TR, Rowe SM, Song EK, et al. Unusual osteonecrosis of the femoral head misdiagnosed as a stress fracture. *J Orthop Trauma* 2004;18(1):43–47.)

artery at the level of the midfemoral head under fluoroscopic guidance. A double wall puncture is preferred, whereby the needle is advanced through both the anterior and posterior arterial walls until contact is made with the femoral head. The needle tip is pulled back slowly until it is within the arterial lumen and pulsatile flow is observed from the needle hub. A guidewire is then passed through the needle and into the vessel lumen, and the needle is then exchanged over the guidewire for a catheter or sheath. Selective catheterization of individual vessels involves advancing the guidewire into the arterial tree, with subsequent advancement of the catheter over the guidewire.

Diagnostic angiography is performed by positioning the catheter tip proximal within the artery of interest and rapidly injecting nonionic iodinated contrast medium, the rate and volume of which is proportional to the size of and flow within the vessel lumen. Rapid fluoroscopic spot filming is timed to coincide with contrast opacification of the arterial tree and documents progressive filling and washout of the vessels. Venous return may also be demonstrated with appropriate delays in filming. Abnormal findings associated with vascular trauma include transection, laceration, dissection, arteriovenous fistula, pseudoaneurysm, mural hematoma, intimal tears, and vasospasm.

Digital subtraction angiography (DSA) is a commonly employed technique, whereby a preliminary fluoroscopic spot film (the "mask") is taken prior to contrast injection, and is subsequently subtracted from dynamic images obtained during contrast injection. The background tissues (bones, soft tissues) are removed from the dynamic arterial images, resulting in greater image contrast resolution. The concentration of iodinated contrast may be reduced using this technique, resulting in a lower total volume of injected contrast medium. Disadvantages of this technique include lower spatial resolution and misregistration artifact, which occurs as a result of patient motion after the mask image has been performed and results in misalignment of the mask during subtraction.

Therapeutic interventions may be performed during angiography, and for trauma patients, most commonly include embolization of bleeding arterial vessels in association with both visceral and bony fractures. Superselective catheterization of the bleeding vessel is first performed, with subsequent occlusion of the vessel using agents administered through the catheter. Temporary and permanent embolic agents are available, and their use is directed by the clinical situation and therapeutic goal. Temporary agents include autologous blood clots and Gelfoam pledgets, whereas permanent agents include micro- and macrocoils, detachable balloons, polyvinyl alcohol, as well as various tissue adhesives and glues. Pre- and postembolization angiograms are performed not only to document occlusion of the bleeding vessel, but also to evaluate for collateral flow around the occluded vessel.

Complications of angiography include puncture site complications (e.g., groin hematoma, arteriovenous fistula, pseudoaneurysm), contrast complications (e.g., anaphylactoid reactions, renal failure), catheter-related complications (e.g., vessel wall dissection, thromboembolism), and therapy-related complications (e.g., tissue necrosis distal to embolization). Complications may be reduced with experience and careful technique by the angiographer.

Computed Tomography Angiography. CTA is a newer and rapidly developing application of multislice helical CT technology. Intravenous nonionic iodinated contrast medium is injected, usually through an antecubital vein, using a volume of 120 to 150 mL at a rate of approximately 3 to 4 mL/second. Scanning is performed after an appropriate delay to ensure passage of contrast through the lungs and heart and into the arterial tree, so that imaging occurs during peak intravascular enhancement throughout the arterial segment of interest. Technical factors such as beam collimation and pitch are adjusted in order to ensure adequate coverage and acceptable scanning times, while preserving high resolution of the study. Images are typically reconstructed from the helical dataset at 1.0-mm slice thicknesses with a 50% overlap. Because a typical CTA study generates hundreds to thousands of images, evaluation of the data is performed using 3D workstations, whereby the images may be viewed using cine modes, multiplanar reconstructions, and interactive real-time volume-rendering techniques. In addition to arterial injury, concomitant complex fractures are also well evaluated on the same study.

Applications

Vascular Trauma. Angiography is an important diagnostic and therapeutic modality in trauma patients with hemodynamic instability due to severe abdominal and pelvic trauma, or extremity injuries with vascular damage (Fig. 11-12). Patients with severe pelvic fractures commonly bleed from fractured bone surfaces and injury to the soft tissues of the pelvic floor. Occasionally, severe venous or arterial injury is present and leads to ongoing hemorrhage and hemodynamic instability. Although management of a hemodynamically unstable patient with a pelvic fracture remains controversial, many experts suggest emergent angiography in these situations (128). The yield in terms of identifiable arterial injury is low; however, when vascular injury is present, embolization using interventional techniques can be life saving. When possible, pelvic angiography can be performed concomitantly with external fixation of the pelvis in patients with severe "open-book" injuries of the pelvic ring (Fig. 11-11).

One traditional indication for angiography has been in the assessment of popliteal artery injury in the patient with definite or suspected knee dislocation. Recently, several studies have clarified the role of angiography in such patients, showing that urgent angiography is not needed unless there are deficits in distal pulses, ideally quantified by determination of the ankle-brachial index (129,130).

MANAGEMENT OF IMAGING DATA

Advances in digital imaging modalities have necessarily been paralleled by advances in distributing, viewing, and storing imaging data. In many instances, the traditional light box has been replaced by digital workstations, the file room has been upgraded with digital archives, and the transport of films has been replaced by digital transmission of images across networks to remote workstations. Many of these changes have evolved in response to the increasing size of digital imaging studies, in addition to the need to use and distribute this information more efficiently within the health care environment. All of these changes have relied on continued improvements in computer networks, workstations, storage devices, and display media, in addition to implementation of standards, to support the evolving digital imaging infrastructure. Although a thorough discussion of digital image management is beyond the scope of this section, a brief review of some of the more common concepts and standards will be presented.

Distribution of Imaging Information

Distribution of medical images is influenced by several factors, including size and volume of imaging studies, computer network infrastructure, and clinical needs by interpreting and referring physicians. Current trends in digital imaging technology have resulted in greater image resolution and greater numbers of images, both of which substantially contribute to increasing sizes of imaging studies. For example, a typical 256 × 256 matrix image, using 2 bytes of storage for each pixel, requires approximately 125 KB of storage per image, whereas a 512 × 512 matrix image requires approximately 500 KB, or four times as much as its lower-resolution counterpart. CT and MRI studies routinely contain 100 to 200 images, resulting in storage requirements of 12 MB to 100 MB per study.

Mediums for distribution include printed films, CD-ROMs, and networks for remote viewing or processing on workstations (Fig. 11-6). Although many imaging departments are transitioning to filmless environments, sheet films are commonly printed and may be necessary outside of the imaging department, such as in private clinics and offices, in addition to the operating room. In particular, hardcopy CT scans and specific radiographic views must remain available to the orthopaedic trauma surgeon to use in the operating room when dealing with complex injuries such as intra-articular fractures and pelvic ring or acetabular fractures. CD-ROM products are increasing in popularity, although computer access is necessary and a greater level of sophistication is needed to use these products. Many imaging devices are connected to networks for transmitting image data to remote locations for image viewing and storage, to which the term "teleradiology" applies. There is a wide variety of network configurations, with descriptors such as local or wide area networks (LAN, WAN), intranets and the Internet. Speed of transmission across networks depends on the various types of communication links within the network (modem, ISDN, DSL, cable modem, T1, T3, fiberoptic cable), as well as the level of network traffic. Data compression is used to decrease the size of imaging studies prior to electronic transmission, and compression schemes are categorized as "lossless" (no loss of original data, typically 3:1 compression) or "lossy" (some loss of data in original image, typically 15:1 or greater compression). Use of the Internet to transmit imaging studies is growing, although patient confidentiality and security issues have received considerable attention.

Imaging studies sent to interpreting physicians are com-

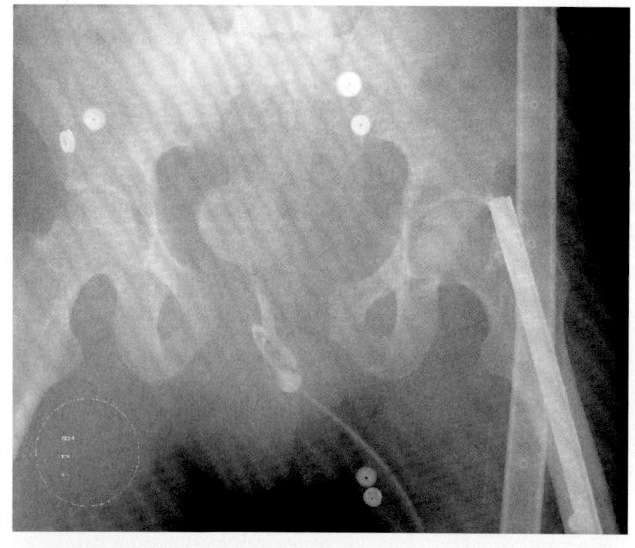

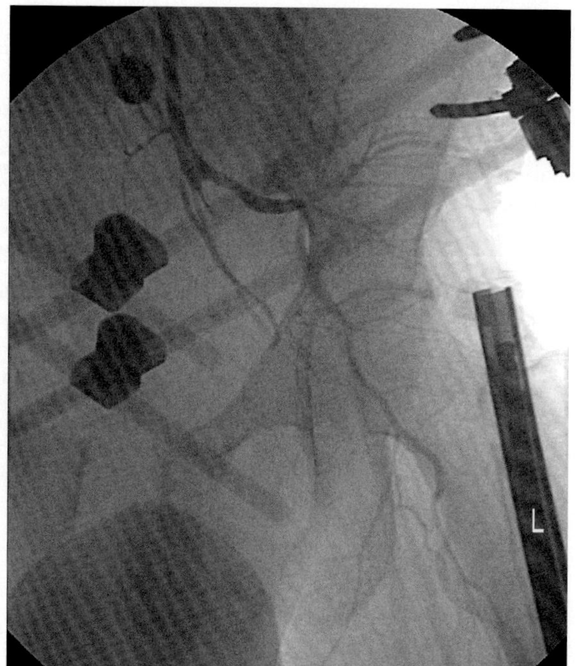

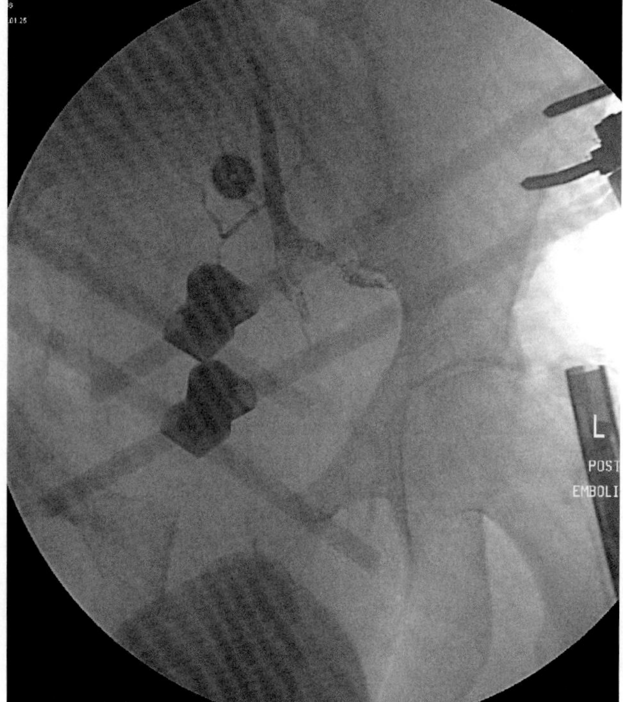

FIGURE 11-12 Pelvic angiography in a hemodynamically unstable trauma patient with a pelvic ring injury. **A.** The AP pelvic radiograph shows wide diastasis of the pubic symphysis. After emergent application of an anterior pelvic external fixator, the patient underwent selective embolization of both right and left internal iliac arteries. **B.** Spot film of the left internal iliac artery demonstrates dissection and nonfilling of multiple medial branches. Contrast fills the left internal iliac artery and its branches before embolization. **C.** Postembolization spot film demonstrates no flow of contrast distal to the embolization coils.

monly viewed on workstations, which are able to display images at full resolution using specific formats ("hanging protocols") and provide advanced capabilities for image processing (Fig. 11-6). Such workstations allow 3D images to be manipulated and reviewed in real-time; some can save movie files of the 3D image onto a disk. Of course, such capabilities are of limited value if they are not available to the orthopaedic trauma surgeon in a timely manner. Current, high-end workstations are expensive and are usually not available outside of the radiology department; normally, less sophisticated viewing stations provide basic access to images outside of the imaging department. In certain environments, use of hardcopy images will remain necessary. Examples of this situation include the operating room, where multiple images of different imaging modalities need to be viewed together by a surgeon in sterile operating garb, and in the clinic where the viewing of multiple studies in chronological order is necessary to observe fracture healing or changes in fracture alignment.

Picture Archive and Communications Systems

A picture archive and communications system (PACS) represents a network of mechanisms used to acquire, view, and store digital images, and at its most basic level includes devices used to acquire digital images (e.g., CT and MRI scanners), workstations whereby images may be viewed and manipulated for diagnostic interpretations, and archives where digital images are stored for later retrieval. PACS may also include viewing stations for departments outside of the radiology department (e.g., emergency room, intensive care unit), and may be contained within their own LAN or exist as a part of a larger WAN. PACS may also communicate with Radiology Information Systems and Hospital Information Systems in order to share and/or modify patient information.

There are many advantages of PACS, including prompt access to clinical images, postprocessing of image data (window levels, multiplanar and 3D reconstructions, measurement and annotations tools), the ability of more than one user to simultaneously view the same images, and reduced filming costs and lost films. On the other hand, significant disadvantages include initial and recurring expenses related to installing and maintaining PACS, massive storage requirements for image archival, and the necessity of support personnel to maintain the network and its components.

Digital Imaging and Communications in Medicine Standards

In 1983, the American College of Radiology (ACR) and the National Electrical Manufacturers Association (NEMA) formed a joint committee to develop a standard by which users could retrieve images and associated information from digital imaging equipment in a form that would be compatible across all manufacturers. Two years later, the first version of the ACR-NEMA standard was published, and in 1988, an updated second version was published, which corrected errors and inconsistencies and added new data elements. The first two versions relied on point-to-point connections between equipment, and by 1988, the growing implementation of networks and PACS necessitated a complete rewriting of the standard, which is currently known as Digital Imaging and Communications in Medicine (DICOM) Version 3.0.

The DICOM standard sets forth a uniform set of rules for communication of medical images and associated information, which are complex, but practical and adaptable. The standard is flexible enough to accommodate a variety of images and image information across a broad range of medical imaging platforms. Conformance with the standard is voluntary, and manufacturers of medical imaging equipment or software who support the standard must provide conformance statements describing their particular implementation of the standard. This does not guarantee that two DICOM-compliant devices will communicate properly with one another; rather, the conformance statement serves as a guide to rule out obvious incompatibilities between equipment.

Digital Imaging and Teleradiology in Orthopaedics

Digital Imaging

Digital imaging is the future of radiology and has definite advantages and disadvantages in the management of musculoskeletal injuries. At present, digital radiography remains inferior to conventional radiography in terms of image spatial resolution (Table 11-1). Work is progressing in digital detector technology that may eventually provide spatial resolution equal to or exceeding that of conventional radiography. In a recent review, Wade et al noted the many potential advantages of digital imaging: reduction of foot traffic between clinics, wards, and the radiology department; increased availability of investigations; increase in the speed of availability; the virtual elimination of missing studies; less radiation exposure; fewer wasted films, and reduction in retrieval times (131). Miller et al describe the medical application of total-body digital radiography for screening trauma patients, using a C-arm–based system initially developed in South Africa to detect theft by diamond miners (132). Full implementation of digital radiography and PACS can be expensive, subject to the nuisances of technological failure, and requires technical support skills that may not be universally available. Traditional printed images will continue to have a role in the operating room, in the clinic, and in other venues where access to the PACS system is not available or appropriate.

Teleradiology

Teleradiology can impact the practice of fracture management in many ways. Teleradiology allows emergency room physicians and/or house staff to send digital images of radiographs or clinical photos to off-site attending orthopaedic staff. There is potential application for community-based orthopaedists to obtain second opinions about fracture management from specialists at tertiary care centers. Traditionally, such consultation required the referring orthopaedic surgeon to obtain, duplicate, and mail hard copies of radiographs to the consulting surgeon, who has then had to communicate his/her opinion to the referring surgeon by telephone. Using teleradiology, the transmission of patient information, imaging studies, and the consultant's evaluation can all be accomplished with greater convenience and less cost.

Ricci and Borrelli demonstrated that teleradiology improved clinical decision-making in the management of acute fractures (133). A series of 123 consecutive fractures was studied; in all cases, a junior orthopaedic resident performed the initial orthopaedic evaluation. All radiographs were digitized and electronically sent to the attending orthopaedist. Treatment plans were formulated and documented at three different times: after verbal communication of the patient's history and injuries, after the digitized radiographs were viewed, and after the original hard-copy radiographs were viewed. The investigators recognized two different types of changes that were made to the initial plan of management: acute treatment changes, and changes in the definitive management of the fracture. Overall, the viewing of digitized radiographs resulted in a change of management in 21% of the fractures. No further changes in management were decided upon after review of the original radiographs. The investigators concluded that the routine use of digitized radiographs improves fracture management (133).

REFERENCES

1. Smith R. Giving emergency radiology its due. Decisions in Imaging Economics, August 2001. Available at http://www.imagingeconomics.com/library/200108-08.asp. Accessed October 15, 2004.
2. Anis AH, Stiell IG, Stewart DG, et al. Cost-effectiveness analysis of the Ottawa Ankle Rules. *Ann Emerg Med* 1995;26:422–428.
3. Thomas SH, Orf J, Peterson C, et al. Frequency and costs of laboratory and radiograph repetition in trauma patients undergoing interfacility transfer. *Am J Emerg Med* 2000; 18:156–158.
4. Bachmann LM, Haberzeth S, Steurer J, et al. The accuracy of the Ottawa knee rule to rule out knee fractures: a systematic review. *Ann Intern Med* 2004;140:121–124.
5. Bulloch B, Neto G, Plint A, et al. Validation of the Ottawa Knee Rule in children: a multicenter study. *Ann Emerg Med* 2003;42:48–55.
6. Emparanza JI, Aginaga JR. Validation of the Ottawa Knee Rules. *Ann Emerg Med* 2001; 38:364–368.
7. Ketelslegers E, Collard X, Vande Berg B, et al. Validation of the Ottawa knee rules in an emergency teaching centre. *Eur Radiol* 2002;12:1218–1220.
8. Leddy JJ, Kesari A, Smolinski RJ. Implementation of the Ottawa ankle rule in a university sports medicine center. *Med Sci Sports Exerc* 2002;34:57–62.
9. Leddy JJ, Smolinski RJ, Lawrence J, et al. Prospective evaluation of the Ottawa Ankle Rules in a university sports medicine center. With a modification to increase specificity for identifying malleolar fractures. *Am J Sports Med* 1998;26:158–165.
10. Nichol G, Stiell IG, Wells GA, et al. An economic analysis of the Ottawa knee rule. *Ann Emerg Med* 1999;34:438–447.
11. Stiell I, Wells G, Laupacis A, et al. Multicentre trial to introduce the Ottawa ankle rules for use of radiography in acute ankle injuries. Multicentre Ankle Rule Study Group. *Br Med J* 1995;311(7005):594–597.
12. Harish S, Vince AS, Patel AD. Routine radiography following ankle fracture fixation: a case for limiting its use. *Injury* 1999;30:699–701.
13. Michelson JD, Ahn U, Magid D. Economic analysis of roentgenogram use in the closed treatment of stable ankle fractures. *J Trauma* 1995;39:1119–1122.
14. Duane TM, Cole FJ Jr, Weireter LJ Jr, et al. Blunt trauma and the role of routine pelvic radiographs. *Am Surg* 2001;67:849–852.
15. Kaneriya PP, Schweitzer ME, Spettell C, et al. The cost-effectiveness of routine pelvic radiography in the evaluation of blunt trauma patients. *Skeletal Radiol* 1999;28: 271–273.
16. Farbman KS, Vinci RJ, Cranley WR, et al. The role of serial radiographs in the management of pediatric torus fractures. *Arch Pediatr Adolesc Med* 1999;153:923–925.
17. Dorsay TA, Major NM, Helms CA. Cost-effectiveness of immediate MR imaging versus traditional follow-up for revealing radiographically occult scaphoid fractures. *Am J Roentgenol* 2001;177:1257–1263.
18. Mack MG, Keim S, Balzer JO, et al. Clinical impact of MRI in acute wrist fractures. *Eur Radiol* 2003;13:612–617.
19. Raby N. Magnetic resonance imaging of suspected scaphoid fractures using a low field dedicated extremity MR system. *Clin Radiol* 2001;56:316–320.
20. Saxena P, McDonald R, Gull S, et al. Diagnostic scanning for suspected scaphoid fractures: an economic evaluation based on cost-minimisation models. *Injury* 2003;34: 503–511.
21. Lim KB, Eng AK, Chng SM, et al. Limited magnetic resonance imaging (MRI) and the occult hip fracture. *Ann Acad Med Singapore* 2002;31(5):607–610.
22. American College of Radiology Committee on Drugs and Contrast Media. Manual on Contrast Media, Version 5.0. Reston, Va: American College of Radiology, 2004;7–10.
23. American College of Radiology Committee on Drugs and Contrast Media. Manual on Contrast Media, Version 5.0. Reston, Va: American College of Radiology, 2004;13.
24. Davis BJ, Roberts PJ, Moorcroft CI, et al. Reliability of radiographs in defining union of internally fixed fractures. *Injury* 2004;35:557–561.
25. Bosse MJ, Brumback RJ, Hash C. Medical cost containment: analysis of dual orthopedic/ radiology interpretation of X-rays in the trauma patient. *J Trauma* 1995;38(2):220–222.
26. Lobenhoffer P, Schulze M, Gerich T, et al. Closed reduction/percutaneous fixation of tibial plateau fractures: arthroscopic versus fluoroscopic control of reduction. *J Orthop Trauma* 1999;13(6):426–431.
27. Norris BL, Hahn DH, Bosse MJ, et al. Intraoperative fluoroscopy to evaluate fracture reduction and hardware placement during acetabular surgery. *J Orthop Trauma* 1999; 13(6):414–417.
28. Krettek C, Miclau T, Grun O, et al. Intraoperative control of axes, rotation and length in femoral and tibial fractures. Technical note. *Injury* 1998;29(Suppl 3):C29–39.
29. Theocharopoulos N, Damilakis J, Perisinakis K, et al. Image-guided reconstruction of femoral fractures: is the staff progeny safe? *Clin Orthop Relat Res* 2005;430:182–188.
30. Blattert TR, Fill UA, Kunz E, et al. Skill dependence of radiation exposure for the orthopaedic surgeon during interlocking nailing of long-bone shaft fractures: a clinical study. *Arch Orthop Trauma Surg* 2004;124(10):659–664.
31. Jones DG, Stoddart J. Radiation use in the orthopaedic theatre: a prospective audit. *Aust N Z J Surg* 1998;68:782–784.
32. Arand M, Hartwig E, Kinzl L, et al. Spinal navigation in cervical fractures–a preliminary clinical study on Judet-osteosynthesis of the axis. *Comput Aided Surg* 2001;6:170–175.
33. Crowl AC, Kahler DM. Closed reduction and percutaneous fixation of anterior column acetabular fractures. *Comput Aided Surg* 2002;7:169–178.
34. Grutzner PA, Rose E, Vock B, et al. Computer-assistierte perkutane Verschraubung des hinteren Beckenrings. Erste Erfahrungen mit einem Bildwandler basierten optoelektronischen Navigationssystem [Computer-assisted screw osteosynthesis of the posterior pelvic ring. Initial experiences with an image reconstruction based optoelectronic navigation system]. *Unfallchirurg* 2002;105:254–260.
35. Kahler DM. Virtual fluoroscopy: a tool for decreasing radiation exposure during femoral intramedullary nailing. *Stud Health Technol Inform* 2001;81:225–228.
36. Suhm N, Jacob AL, Nolte LP, et al. Surgical navigation based on fluoroscopy–clinical application for computer-assisted distal locking of intramedullary implants. *Comput Aided Surg* 2000;5:391–400.
37. Collinge CA, Coons D, Tornetta P, et al. standard multiplanar fluoroscopy versus a fluoroscopically-based navigation system for the percutaneous insertion of iliosacral screws: a cadaver model. *J Orthop Trauma* 2005;19:254–258.
38. Grogan EL, Morris JA Jr, Dittus RS, et al. Cervical spine evaluation in urban trauma centers: lowering institutional costs and complications through helical CT scan. *J Am Coll Surg* 2005;200:160–165.
39. McAdams TR, Blevins FT, Martin TP, et al. The role of plain films and computed tomography in the evaluation of scapular neck fractures. *J Orthop Trauma* 2002;16: 7–11.
40. Cole RJ, Bindra RR, Evanoff BA, et al. Radiographic evaluation of osseous displacement following intra-articular fractures of the distal radius: reliability of plain radiography versus computed tomography. *J Hand Surg Am* 1997;22:792–800.
41. Pruitt DL, Gilula LA, Manske PR, et al. Computed tomography scanning with image reconstruction in evaluation of distal radius fractures. *J Hand Surg Am* 1994;19: 720–727.
42. Borrelli J Jr, Goldfarb C, Catalano L, et al. Assessment of articular fragment displacement in acetabular fractures: a comparison of computerized tomography and plain radiographs. *J Orthop Trauma* 2002;16:449–456.
43. Hougaard K, Lindequist S, Nielsen LB. Computerised tomography after posterior dislocation of the hip. *J Bone Joint Surg Br* 1987;69:556–557.
44. Chan PS, Klimkiewicz JJ, Luchetti WT, et al. Impact of CT scan on treatment plan and fracture classification of tibial plateau fractures. *J Orthop Trauma* 1997;11:484–489.
45. Wicky S, Blaser PF, Blanc CH, et al. Comparison between standard radiography and spiral CT with 3D reconstruction in the evaluation, classification and management of tibial plateau fractures. *Eur Radiol* 2000;10:1227–1232.
46. Tornetta P, Gorup J. Axial computed tomography of pilon fractures. *Clin Orthop* 1996; 323:273–276.
47. Ebraheim NA, Skie MC, Podeszwa DA, et al. Evaluation of process fractures of the talus using computed tomography. *J Orthop Trauma* 1994;8:332–337.
48. Horn BD, Crisci K, Krug M, et al. Radiologic evaluation of juvenile Tillaux fractures of the distal tibia. *J Pediatr Orthop* 2001;21:162–164.
49. Freund M, Thomsen M, Hohendorf B, et al. Optimized preoperative planning of calcaneal fractures using spiral computed tomography. *Eur Radiol* 1999;9:901–906.
50. Moed BR, Carr SE, Gruson KI, et al. Computed tomographic assessment of fractures of the posterior wall of the acetabulum after operative treatment. *J Bone Joint Surg Am* 2003;85:512–522.
51. Kurozumi T, Jinno Y, Sato T, et al. Open reduction for intra-articular calcaneal fractures: evaluation using computed tomography. *Foot Ankle Int* 2003;24:942–948.
52. Grigoryan M, Lynch JA, Fierlinger AL, et al. Quantitative and qualitative assessment of closed fracture healing using computed tomography and conventional radiography. *Acad Radiol* 2003;10:1267–1273.
53. Lynch JA, Grigoryan M, Fierlinger A, et al. Measurement of changes in trabecular bone at fracture sites using X-ray CT and automated image registration and processing. *J Orthop Res* 2004;22:362–367.
54. Eustace S, Adams J, Assaf A. Emergency MR imaging of orthopaedic trauma. Current and future directions. *Radiol Clin North Am* 1999;37:975–994.
55. Rangger C, Kathrein A, Freund MC, et al. Bone bruise of the knee: histology and cryosections in 5 cases. *Acta Orthop Scand* 1998;69:291–294.
56. Roemer FW, Bohndorf K. Long-term osseous sequelae after acute trauma of the knee joint evaluated by MRI. *Skeletal Radiol* 2002;31:615–623.
57. Grangier C, Garcia J, Howarth NR, et al. Role of MRI in the diagnosis of insufficiency fractures of the sacrum and acetabular roof. *Skeletal Radiol* 1997;26:517–524.
58. Kukla C, Gaebler C, Breitenseher MJ, et al. Occult fractures of the scaphoid. The diagnostic usefulness and indirect economic repercussions of radiography versus magnetic resonance scanning. *J Hand Surg Br* 1997;22:810–813.
59. Pool FJ, Crabbe JP. Occult femoral neck fractures in the elderly: optimisation of investigation. *N Z Med J* 1996;109:235–237.
60. Rubin SJ, Marquardt JD, Gottlieb RH, et al. Magnetic resonance imaging: a cost-effective alternative to bone scintigraphy in the evaluation of patients with suspected hip fractures. *Skeletal Radiol* 1998;27:199–204.
61. Haramati N, Staron RB, Barax C, et al. Magnetic resonance imaging of occult fractures of the proximal femur. *Skeletal Radiol* 1994;23:19–22.

62. Deutsch AL, Mink JH, Waxman AD. Occult fractures of the proximal femur: MR imaging. *Radiology* 1989;170:113–116.
63. Yacoubian SV, Nevins RT, Sallis JG, et al. Impact of MRI on treatment plan and fracture classification of tibial plateau fractures. *J Orthop Trauma* 2002;16:632–637.
64. Holt MD, Williams LA, Dent CM. MRI in the management of tibial plateau fractures. *Injury* 1995;26:595–599.
65. Green RAR, Saifuddin A. Whole spine MRI in the assessment of acute vertebral body trauma. *Skeletal Radiol* 2004;33:129–135.
66. Bencardino JT, Garcia AI, Palmer WE. Magnetic resonance imaging of the shoulder: rotator cuff. *Top Magn Reson Imaging* 2003;14:51–67.
67. Tirman PF, Smith ED, Stoller DW, et al. Shoulder imaging in athletes. *Semin Musculoskelet Radiol* 2004;8:29–40.
68. Connell DA, Potter HG. Magnetic resonance evaluation of the labral capsular ligamentous complex: a pictorial review. *Australas Radiol* 1999;43:419–426.
69. White LM, Miniaci A. Cruciate and posterolateral corner injuries in the athlete: clinical and magnetic resonance imaging features. *Semin Musculoskelet Radiol* 2004; 8:111–131.
70. Fritz RC. MR imaging of meniscal and cruciate ligament injuries. *Magn Reson Imaging Clin N Am* 2003;11:283–293.
71. Winalski CS, Gupta KB. Magnetic resonance imaging of focal articular cartilage lesions. *Top Magn Reson Imaging* 2003;14:131–144.
72. Lonner JH, Dupuy DE, Siliski JM. Comparison of magnetic resonance imaging with operative findings in acute traumatic dislocations of the adult knee. *J Orthop Trauma* 2000;14:183–186
73. Steinbach LS, Palmer WE, Schweitzer ME. Special focus session. MR arthrography. *Radiographics* 2002;22:1223–1246.
74. Bergin D, Schweitzer ME. Indirect magnetic resonance arthrography. *Skeletal Radiol* 2003;32:551–558.
75. Sofka CM, Potter HG. MR imaging of joint arthroplasty. *Semin Musculoskelet Radiol* 2002 Mar;6(1):79–85.
76. Sofka CM, Potter HG, Figgie M, et al. Magnetic resonance imaging of total knee arthroplasty. *Clin Orthop Relat Res* 2003 Jan;(406):129–135.
77. Potter HG, Nestor BJ, Sofka CM, et al. Magnetic resonance imaging after total hip arthroplasty: evaluation of periprosthetic soft tissue. *J Bone Joint Surg Am* 2004 Sep; 86–A(9):1947–1954.
78. Montgomery KD, Potter HG, Helfet DL. Magnetic resonance venography to evaluate the deep venous system of the pelvis in patients who have an acetabular fracture. *J Bone Joint Surg Am* 1995;77:1639–1649.
79. Stover MD, Morgan SJ, Bosse MJ, et al. Prospective comparison of contrast-enhanced computed tomography versus magnetic resonance venography in the detection of occult deep pelvic vein thrombosis in patients with pelvic and acetabular fractures. *J Orthop Trauma* 2002;16:613–621.
80. Robbins MI, Anzilotti KF, Katz LD, et al. Patient perception of magnetic resonance arthrography. *Skeletal Radiol* 2000;29:265–269.
81. Farber JM. CT arthrography and postoperative musculoskeletal imaging with multichannel computed tomography. *Semin Musculoskelet Radiol* 2004;8:157–166.
82. Grechenig W, Fellinger M, Seibert FJ, et al. Die arthrography des handgelenks beim frischen trauma [Arthrography of the wrist joint in acute trauma] *Unfallchirurg* 1996; 99:260–266.
83. Grechenig W, Peicha G, Fellinger M, et al. Wrist arthrography after acute trauma to the distal radius: diagnostic accuracy, technique, and sources of diagnostic errors. *Invest Radiol* 1998;33:273–278.
84. Delcoigne L, Durant H, Kunnen M, et al. Digital subtraction in multi-compartment arthrography of the wrist. *J Belge Radiol* 1993;76:7–10.
85. Yin Y, Wilson AJ, Gilula LA. Three-compartment wrist arthrography: direct comparison of digital subtraction with nonsubtraction images. *Radiology* 1995;197:287–290.
86. Ahn JM, Sartoris DJ, Kang HS, et al. Gamekeeper thumb: comparison of MR arthrography with conventional arthrography and MR imaging in cadavers. *Radiology* 1998; 206(3)(Mar):737–744.
87. Loredo R, Sanders TG. Imaging of osteochondral injuries. *Clin Sports Med* 2001;20: 249–278.
88. Schmid MR, Pfirrmann CW, Hodler J, et al. Cartilage lesions in the ankle joint: comparison of MR arthrography and CT arthrography. *Skelet Radiol* 2003;259–265.
89. Matsui Y, Myoui A, Nakahara H, et al. Prognostic significance of posterior subtalar joint arthrography following fractures of the calcaneus. *Arch Orthop Trauma Surg* 1995; 114:257–259.
90. Blane CE, Kling TF Jr, Andrews JC, et al. Arthrography in the posttraumatic elbow in children. *Am J Roentgenol* 1984;143:17–21.
91. Akbarnia BA, Silberstein MJ, Rende RJ, et al. Arthrography in the diagnosis of fractures of the distal end of the humerus in infants. *J Bone Joint Surg Am* 1986;68:599–602.
92. Drvaric DM, Rooks MD. Anterior sleeve fracture of the capitellum. *J Orthop Trauma* 1990;4:188–192.
93. Marzo JM, d'Amato C, Strong M, et al. Usefulness and accuracy of arthrography in management of lateral humeral condyle fractures in children. *J Pediatr Orthop* 1990; 10:317–321.
94. Leet AI, Young C, Hoffer MM. Medial condyle fractures of the humerus in children. *J Pediatr Orthop* 2002;22:2–7.
95. Javed A, Guichet JM. Arthrography for reduction of a fracture of the radial neck in a child with a non-ossified radial epiphysis. *J Bone Joint Surg Br* 2001;83:542–543.
96. Klein HM, Vrsalovic V, Balas R, et al. Bildgebende Diagnostik des Handgelenkes: MRT und Arthrographie/Arthro-CT [Imaging diagnostics of the wrist: MRI and Arthrography/Arthro-CT]. *Rofo Fortschr Geb Rontgenstr Neuen Bildgeb Verfahr* 2002; 174:177–182.
97. Herneth AM, Siegmeth A, Bader TR, et al. Scaphoid fractures: evaluation with high-spatial-resolution US initial results. *Radiology* 2001;220:231–235.
98. Durston W, Swartzentruber R. Ultrasound guided reduction of pediatric forearm fractures in the ED. *Am J Emerg Med* 2000;18:72–77.
99. Kessler T, Winkler H, Weiss C, et al. Sonographie des Ellenbogengelenks bei der Radiuskopfchenfraktur [Ultrasound diagnosis of the elbow joint in fracture of the head of the radius]. *Orthopade* 2002;31:268–270.
100. Vocke-Hell AK, Schmid A. Sonographic differentiation of stable and unstable lateral condyle fractures of the humerus in children. *J Pediatr Orthop B* 2001;10:138–141.
101. Kirkpatrick AW, Brown R, Diebel LN, et al. Rapid diagnosis of an ulnar fracture with portable hand-held ultrasound. *Mil Med* 2003;168:312–313.
102. Dulchavsky SA, Henry SE, Moed BR, et al. Advanced ultrasonic diagnosis of extremity trauma: the FASTER examination. *J Trauma* 2002;53:28–32.
103. Moed BR, Subramanian S, van Holsbeeck M, et al. Ultrasound for the early diagnosis of tibial fracture healing after static interlocked nailing without reaming: clinical results. *J Orthop Trauma* 1998;12:206–213.
104. Caruso G, Lagalla R, Derchi L, et al. Monitoring of fracture calluses with color Doppler sonography. *J Clin Ultrasound* 2000;28:20–27.
105. Bleakney RR, Tallon C, Wong JK, et al. Long-term ultrasonographic features of the Achilles tendon after rupture. *Clin J Sport Med* 2002;12:273–278.
106. Churchill RS, Fehringer EV, Dubinsky TJ, et al. Rotator cuff ultrasonography: diagnostic capabilities. *J Am Acad Orthop Surg* 2004;12:6–11.
107. Roberts CS, Beck DJ, Heinsen J, et al. Review article: diagnostic ultrasonography: applications in orthopaedic surgery. *Clin Orthop* 2002;401:248–264.
108. Peetrons P. Ultrasound of muscles. *Eur Radiol* 2002;12:35–43.
109. Levy AD, Harcke HT. Handheld ultrasound device for detection of non-opaque and semi-opaque foreign bodies in soft tissues. *J Clin Ultrasound* 2003;31:183–188.
110. Zierler BK. Ultrasonography and diagnosis of venous thromboembolism. *Circulation* 2004;109(12 Suppl 1):I9–I14.
111. Intersocietal Accreditation Commission. ICAVL: Essentials and standards for accreditation in noninvasive vascular testing. Part II. Vascular laboratory operations–Peripheral venous testing; 2000: 1–8. Available at: www.intersocietal.org/intersocietal.htm. Accessed June 15, 2004.
112. Matin P. The appearance of bone scans following fractures, including immediate and long-term studies. *J Nucl Med* 1979;20:1227–1231.
113. Garcia-Morales F, Seo GS, Chengazi V, et al. Collar osteophytes: a cause of false-positive findings in bone scans for hip fractures. *Am J Roentgenol* 2003;181:191–194.
114. Peh WC, Khong PL, Yin Y, et al. Imaging of pelvic insufficiency fractures. *Radiographics* 1996;16:335–348.
115. Barros JW, Barbieri CH, Fernandes CD. Scintigraphic evaluation of tibial shaft fracture healing. *Injury* 2000;31:51–54.
116. Mandelstam SA, Cook D, Fitzgerald M, et al. Complementary use of radiological skeletal survey and bone scintigraphy in detection of bony injuries in suspected child abuse. *Arch Dis Child* 2003;88:387–390.
117. Palestro CJ, Torres MA. Radionuclide imaging in orthopedic infections. *Semin Nucl Med* 1997;27:334–345.
118. Palestro CJ. The current role of gallium imaging in infection. *Semin Nucl Med* 1994; 24(2)(Apr):28–41.
119. Love C, Patel M, Lonner BS, et al. Diagnosing spinal osteomyelitis: a comparison of bone and Ga-67 scintigraphy and magnetic resonance imaging. *Clin Nucl Med* 2000; 25:963–977.
120. Peters AM. The utility of [99mTc]HMPAO-leukocytes for imaging infection. *Semin Nucl Med* 1994;24(2)(Apr):110–127.
121. Wolf G, Aigner RM, Schwarz T. Diagnosis of bone infection using 99m Tc-HMPAO labeled leukocytes. *Nucl Med Commun* 2001;22(11)(Nov):1201–1206.
122. Seabold JE, Nepola JV. Imaging techniques for evaluation of postoperative orthopaedic infections. *Q J Nucl Med* 1999;43:21–28.
123. Nepola JV, Seabold JE, Marsh JL, et al. Diagnosis of infection in ununited fractures. Combined imaging with indium-111-labeled leukocytes and technetium-99m methylene diphosphonate *J Bone Joint Surg Am* 1993;75(12)(Dec):1816–1822.
124. Bonnarens F, Hernandez A, D'Ambrosia R. Bone scintigraphic changes in osteonecrosis of the femoral head. *Orthop Clin North Am* 1985;16:697–703.
125. Drane WE, Rudd TG. Femoral head viability following hip fracture. Prognostic role of radionuclide bone imaging. *Clin Nucl Med* 1985;10:141–146.
126. Mortensson W, Rosenborg M, Gretzer H. The role of bone scintigraphy in predicting femoral head collapse following cervical fractures in children. *Acta Radiol* 1990;31: 291–292.
127. Calder SJ, McCaskie AW, Belton IP, et al. Single-photon-emission computerised tomography compared with planar bone scan to assess femoral head vascularity. *J Bone Joint Surg Br* 1995;77:637–639.
128. Dondelinger RF, Trotteur G, Ghaye B, et al. Traumatic injuries: radiological hemostatic intervention at admission. *Eur Radiol* 2002;12:979–993.
129. Klineberg EO, Crites BM, Flinn WR, et al. The role of arteriography in assessing popliteal artery injury in knee dislocations. *J Trauma* 2004;56:786–790.
130. Stannard JP, Sheils TM, Lopez-Ben RR, et al. Vascular injuries in knee dislocations: the role of physical examination in determining the need for arteriography. *J Bone Joint Surg Am* 2004;86:910–915.
131. Wade FA, Oliver CW, McBride K. Digital imaging in trauma and orthopaedic surgery. Is it worth it? *J Bone Joint Surg Br* 2000;82:791–794.
132. Miller LA, Mirvis SE, Harris L, Haan J. Total-body digital radiography for trauma screening: initial experience. *Appl Radiol* 2004;33:8–14.
133. Ricci WM, Borrelli J. Teleradiology in orthopaedic surgery: impact on clinical decision making for acute fracture management. *J Orthop Trauma* 2002;16:1–6.

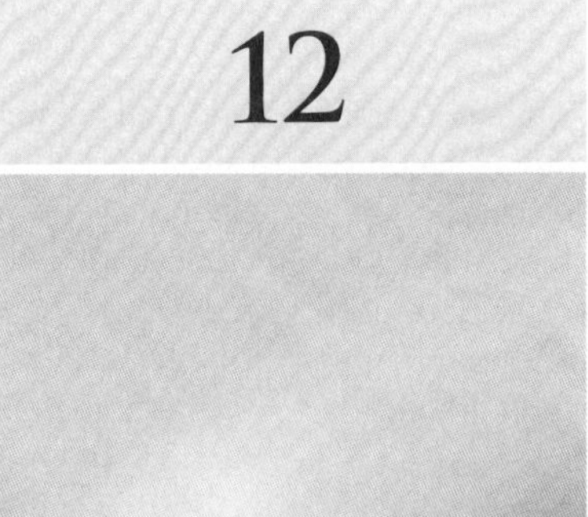

INITIAL MANAGEMENT OF OPEN FRACTURES

Steven A. Olson and Mark D. Willis

An open fracture is one in which a break in the skin allows for direct communication of the fracture site or fracture hematoma with the elements external to the usual protection of the skin. The term "compound fracture" was previously used to describe this injury; however, as it is archaic and nonspecific, it is not used in this chapter. Fractures that are exposed to the environment through breaks in the skin are subsequently referred to as open fractures throughout this text.

Open fractures occur under a wide spectrum of conditions with specific consequences. Bacteria from the environment may contaminate the area of injury, and the quantity of gross contamination may differ with the environment (1,2). The magnitude of force required to produce the fracture is variable as well. Soft-tissue disruption may be minimal with a simple "inside-out" breach of the bone through the skin. Alternatively, high-energy forces delivered during a motor vehicle accident may devitalize the bone and invest soft tissues extensively. This creates an environment more susceptible to infection by any contaminating bacteria (3), limits options for stabilization (4,5), and denies the bone the usual contributions of healing (6). Lastly, in certain cases, diagnosis of the open injury may be difficult as the wound may appear remote to the site of fracture. Missed open injuries can be met with the unfortunate consequence of osteomyelitis or an infected nonunion. Subsequently, when a wound occurs in the same limb segment as a fracture, the fracture must be considered open until proven otherwise. Given these variables, classification and treatment are directed by surgical staging following adequate exploration and debridement.

The prognosis in open fractures is determined primarily by the amount of devitalized soft tissue and the level and type of bacterial contamination. The interplay of these two factors, rather than the fracture pattern alone, is the primary determinant of the outcome (7–9). Outcome subsequently hinges on viable soft-tissue coverage, neurovascular integrity, prevention of infection, and healing of the fracture. This chapter presents concepts and strategies for the early management of open fractures from emergency department to operating room with the intent of maximal limb function as a result. Discussions regarding vascular reconstruction, management of compartment syndrome, and limb salvage versus amputation are found in other chapters. In addition, this chapter focuses the reader on the initial management of open fractures in general. Management schemes relevant to the specific body segments are elaborated upon elsewhere in this text.

HISTORICAL PERSPECTIVE

Hippocrates, it is said, considered war the most appropriate training ground for surgeons. His greatest contribution in this regard lay in his recognition that surgeons can only facilitate healing—they cannot impose it. He recognized the need to accept certain consequences of injury, such as swelling, as essential and admonished against occlusive dressings before such swelling had occurred. He opposed frequent meddling with wounds, except to extrude purulent material, so long as the wound demonstrated progress in repairing itself. He further advocated "iron" (the knife) in treating wounds that did not progress. His principal misconception is generally regarded as his aphorism that held that diseases not curable by steel (knife) are curable by fire (cautery) (10).

Galen and his followers also recognized purulence and admired it, considering it essential to the repair process. Frequent manipulations of a wound and a continuous search for treatments that might be applied to enhance purulence were viewed as desirable in driving the wound to heal. Subsequently, most other schools represented one or the other of these viewpoints as a base for their particular methods of treatment (10).

Brunschwig and Botello, in the 15th and 16th centuries, advocated the removal of nonvital tissue from wounds that did not progress properly. The practice of applying hot oil to cauterize wounds was common in 1538, when Ambroise Paré (1510–1590), a French army surgeon, ran out of hot oil during the siege of Turin. He had only "a digestive made of yolk of egg, oyle of Roses, and Turpentine" and was surprised to find that his patients "dressed with a digestive only" were alive and nearly pain-free the next morning. Paré also advised that "the wound must forthwith be enlarged . . . so that there may be free passage for both the puss or matter . . . obtained therein." The significance of Paré's discoveries were largely unrecognized during his day (11). It remained for Desault, in the 18th century, to reestablish the making of a deep incision to explore a wound, remove dead tissue, and provide drainage. It was he who adopted the term *debridement.* His pupil, Larrey, extended the principle and included the issue of timing. The sooner debridement is done after wounding, he contended, the better the result.

After Mathysen's development of plaster-of-Paris bandages, the principle of occlusive dressings was reintroduced, only to lapse again because of untoward effects from misapplication (10). Lister's introduction of carbolic acid dressings seemed the ultimate item in the galenic search for a magic medication that would persuade wounds to heal. Seized with alacrity, it too proved disappointing, likely because the principles of debridement were too soon forgotten or abandoned—an episode destined to be repeated many times thereafter.

The imperative of debridement of missile wounds was reestablished more firmly during World War I, with the work of Sir Robert Jones caring for allied forces. Thereafter, Trueta brought together the combination of debridement and an occlusive dressing that also served as a splint (the plaster cast) in the treatment of wounded extremities during the Spanish Civil War. Trueta reported only 6 deaths in 1,073 patients treated this way. By contrast with previous experience, his vast number of examples demonstrated the virtues of this method when properly applied (11).

World War II began just after the start of the sulfa era. Sulfa agents supplanted antiseptic solutions, but like them, they were applied directly to injured tissues. Antibiotics were available during the Korean War. The policy of rapid evacuation, wound debridement, and delayed closure was adopted in both the Korean and Vietnam conflicts. This approach remains the standard practice for war wounds today. This practice has profoundly influenced the treatment of open fractures occurring in a civilian setting as well (11). Current recommendations for acute management of open fractures mirror the military model:

1. Provide airway management and urgent resuscitation.
2. Immobilize the injured extremity and apply sterile dressing to the wound.
3. Administer early intravenous antibiotics.
4. Perform urgent operative wound debridement and irrigation, leave the wound open, and stabilize unstable skeletal injuries.
5. Perform repeated debridements, as needed.
6. Delay wound closure/coverage.

The value of close adherence to these principals, particularly aggressive irrigation and debridement with delayed primary closure of wounds and restraint from early internal fixation, is reflected in the recent report of no infections related to open fractures incurred during Operation Enduring Freedom in Afghanistan (12). Alternatively, ongoing investigations continue to examine the rigorous application of these principles. Specifically, one such study, under the direction of the Orthopaedic Trauma Association Open Fracture Study Group, is currently designed to evaluate the effects of primary closure, as compared to delayed closure, of intermediate type, open fractures. The results of these projects will further enhance the management of open fracture wounds and may redefine current clinical practice, i.e., need for recurrent surgical procedures and anesthesia, avoidance of hospital acquired infection in open wounds, and decreased duration of hospitalization.

PRINCIPLES OF MANAGEMENT

Diagnosis

The diagnosis of an open fracture is straightforward in most cases. An injured patient usually has a bleeding deep laceration overlying or near a fracture of the underlying bone. In some cases, the fractured bone may be overtly exposed because of severe soft-tissue loss, eliminating any doubt that an open fracture is present. However, not all open fractures are obvious, and their timely and proper diagnosis and treatment depend on a careful examination of the patient, delineating salient features from the patient's history, a critical reading of x-rays, and good clinical judgment.

Before detailed evaluation of an open fracture takes place, the patient should be stabilized and potential life-threatening injuries must be evaluated and treated according to the Advanced Trauma Life Support principles developed by the American College of Surgeons (13). Maintaining patient's airway, breathing, and circulation are paramount in the initial treatment. Compressive bandages on open, actively bleeding wounds should be applied early. Once the patient is stable, a thorough and systematic search for associated injuries is performed. A cervical collar is placed until a lateral cervical spine (C-spine) x-ray can be obtained. Chest and pelvis x-rays are taken to evaluate for potential sources of hemorrhage or pulmonary dysfunction. As soon as possible, a careful examination of the extremities follows to diagnose fractures and dislocations (13).

The examining physician must document, as best as is possible, the neurologic function and vascular function of each extremity. The surgeon should note the state of circulation to the limb as indicated by capillary blush, the filling of veins, and the status of peripheral pulses. The limb should be examined meticulously for peripheral nerve function. Initial sensory examination by pressure and light touch gives a gross evaluation of limb sensation, but examination for two-point discrimination is often necessary to detect more subtle losses, particularly in the upper extremity. Examination for motor function is difficult in the injured limb owing to pain and splinting secondary to muscle spasm. The normal side should be compared with the abnormal side, and results recorded accurately. This is vital because partial nerve palsy caused by the injury can often be overlooked with an inadequate examination or inexact recording of the findings. Formal motor strength assessment is not practical in the setting of acute injury. The examiner should carefully document an accurate description of which motor groups the patient is able to move. It is helpful to note whether the movement is voluntary or spontaneous (1,2).

After documenting the neurovascular function of the injured limbs, any detected fractures and/or dislocations should be properly aligned or reduced and adequately splinted. Many limbs that have associated signs of vascular insufficiency (cool to touch, diminished or absent pulse, dusky or pale appearance, poor capillary refill) before reduction recover once the vessels have been "unkinked" by realigning the limb. If the limb continues to show signs of vascular insufficiency, an arterial injury should be considered and ruled out.

The location and dimensions of any wounds should be recorded. The skin around the wound(s), including the entire circumference of the extremity, should be examined. Often, significant wounds on the posterior side of the body are initially overlooked. Accordingly, the patient's back and buttocks are evaluated as well. Patients with pelvic or abdominal injuries should have an examination of their perineum. A pelvic fracture in the presence of a vaginal laceration makes it an open fracture. Although bleeding can be from menstruation, it is also a sign of vaginal laceration. Therefore, vaginal examination with a speculum should be done to rule out an occult open pelvic fracture, which occurs in approximately 3.5% of pelvic injuries (14). Appropriate examination of these areas precludes missed diagnoses and provides the opportunity to aggressively treat these occult injuries concurrent to any obvious injuries of the extremities.

Small puncture wounds and deep abrasions on extremities with fractures should be considered to communicate with the fracture until proven otherwise. The presence of crepitance (subcutaneous emphysema from trapped air due to open wounds or gas gangrene) and fluctuance from soft tissue stripping and internal degloving are signs of extensive soft tissue damage that may involve the entire limb (2). In this setting, a small puncture wound or laceration that appears remote from the fracture may indeed communicate with the fracture. Such powerful disruption of the skin, soft tissues, and underlying bone is the culmination of the transfer of energy transmitted to the limb during the injury.

Mechanism of Injury and Related Factors

According to the equation $KE = 0.5\ m\ V^2$, the kinetic energy (KE) is directly proportional to the mass and the square of the velocity of an object at the time of impact with the limb (15). There are a variety of ways in which injuries to the extremities can occur. One of the most severe types of injury is an automobile bumper collision. A 20-mph bumper collision transfers approximately 100,000 foot pounds of energy to the limb that is fixed in position at the time of impact (15) (Table 12-1), which is capable of exceeding the strength and resiliency of bone and the surrounding soft tissues.

Severely injured patients may not be able to give any more than the basic details surrounding the injury, so family members, friends, witnesses, or paramedics should be questioned about the surrounding events to obtain as much useful information as possible (13). The location where the injury occurred is essential to delineate. People exposed to feces or dirt, such as may occur in a farm setting, alert the surgeons to the possibility of clostridial infection and the need for additional antibiotics (penicillin) and more aggressive surgical debridement. Patients with open fractures injured in automobile collisions are at much less risk for development of a clostridial infection. Open fractures that occur in unusual environments, such as a barnyards or gardens, streams or lakes, will likely be contaminated by unusual organisms, such as soil anaerobes and *Aeromonas hydrophilia,* respectively. Injuries caused by lawnmowers and other motorized garden equipment are high-energy injuries with severe contamination (16–19).

The patient's tetanus immunity must be determined (13). Patients who have been immunized within the last 5 years before the injury do not need a booster. Those who were immunized more than 5 years before the injury should receive a tetanus booster. Patients who have never been immunized, or cannot remember the time of their last immunization, should receive a tetanus immunization booster as well as tetanus immune globulin (13).

The surgeon must also inquire about medical illnesses, such as diabetes mellitus, peripheral vascular disease, liver disease, and any immune deficiency syndromes. Any previous injuries and their treatments, especially those involving the acutely injured extremities, should be elicited. Finally, a history of smoking or chronic use of steroids is important to determine because these factors have important negative implications for wound healing. A surgeon deciding whether to salvage a severely injured limb or perform early amputation should have an understanding of all factors, including comorbidities, that affect the success of a complex limb reconstruction.

Radiographic Findings

Radiographic evaluation of the injured extremity is essential for diagnosis and planning of appropriate treatment strategies. Anteroposterior and lateral radiographs are the minimum to properly assess a fracture. Radiographs should be obtained of the joint above and below the site of a fracture in the extremities (13,19). Special radiographic views (e.g., oblique views, inlet/outlet views) may be indicated depending on the injury. Radiographs of the cervical spine and the remainder of the spinal column may be indicated depending on the history of the injury and the patient's symptoms (13).

Radiographs can help verify or diagnose an occult open fracture by showing subcutaneous air or gas in the soft tissues. Air can be sucked into the soft tissues of an extremity as a result of penetrating or blunt trauma because of the occurrence of a

TABLE 12-1 Energy Transmitted by Injury Mechanism

Injury	Energy (ft-lb)
Fall from curb	100
Skiing injury	300–500
High-velocity gunshot wound (single missile)	2,000
20-mph bumper injury (assumes bumper strikes fixed target)	100,000

Data from Chapman MW. Role of bone stability in open fractures. *Instr Course Lect* 1982;31:75–87, with permission.

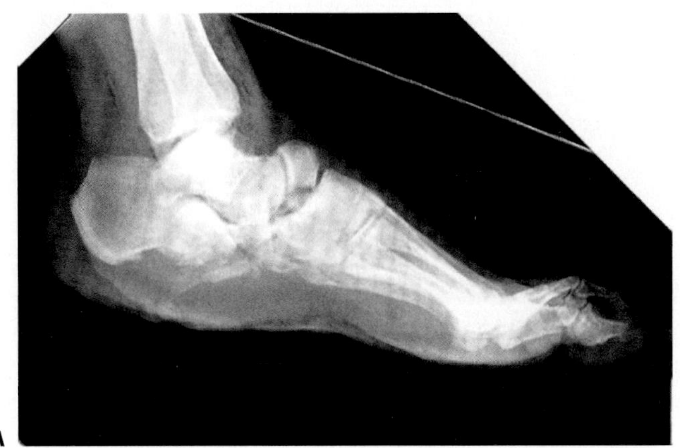

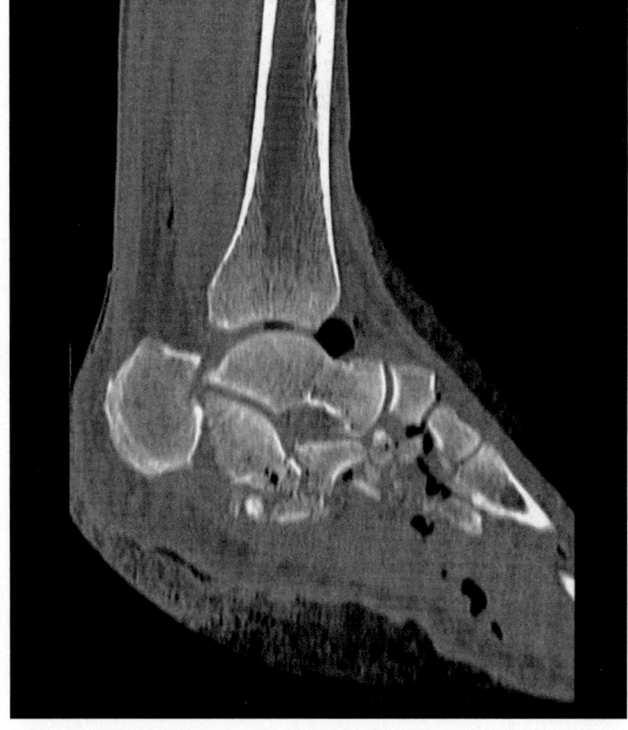

FIGURE 12-1 **A.** Lateral x-ray of a patient with calcaneus fracture. Subcutaneous gas can be seen in and around the foot within the soft tissue envelope. This indicates an open injury has occurred. **B.** Lateral reconstruction of a computerized tomography image of the same injury as shown in Figure 1A. Here the subcutaneous gas can be seen more clearly. Again, this is indicative of an open fracture.

temporary vacuum phenomenon, as energy is dissipated throughout the soft tissues (Fig. 12-1). Gas can also be produced by *Clostridium perfringens* and enteropathogens such as *Escherichia coli* (16). The presence of air or gas in the soft tissues on initial radiographs in the presence of a fracture strongly suggests an open fracture. Additional imaging studies such as a CT scan should be obtained if the patient is stable and there will be no delay in getting the patient to the operating room.

Computed tomography (CT) imaging of extremity injuries should be deferred until the initial management of the open fracture is complete. Indications for additional radiographs may emerge over time. CT scans are useful in pelvic ring and acetabular fractures, as well as other intra-articular fractures. Ideally, CT scans of extremity injuries should be done while the patient is in the scanner for another reason, such as a head or abdominal study, thus making a repeat trip to the scanner unnecessary.

Associated Injuries

Intra-articular penetration can be ruled out by injecting sterile saline with or without methylene blue to distend the joint capsule and watching for fluid extravasation from the open wound (19). Although this test is not 100% sensitive, we have used this technique at our institution for many years and have not had any adverse outcomes. However, we do not use this technique to rule out open fractures because of the potential risk of contaminating a closed fracture hematoma.

The potential for vascular injury should always be considered. The clinician should be alert for "hard signs" of arterial injury, which include (a) absent pulses, (b) active hemorrhage, (c) expanding hematoma, and (d) bruit or thrill. In most institutions, the trauma surgeons or vascular surgeons should be notified of a potential vascular injury. In centers where such physicians are unavailable, an arteriogram should be ordered or an on-table arteriogram performed urgently in the operating suite (2,19).

The presence of nerve injury or deficit is noted on initial physical examination. Deficits persistent after appropriate reduction and splinting are documented. Persistent nerve dysfunction, in certain cases, may warrant exploration and repair.

Once the diagnosis of an open fracture has been made and all other pertinent information regarding the patient's medical history has been obtained, the surgeon is ready to formulate and implement the treatment strategy, the foundation of which is a thorough irrigation and debridement of the open fracture.

Classification

Classification of open fractures is important because it allows comparison of results between surgeons and in scientific publications. The optimal time to classify the open fracture is at the time of debridement of the traumatic wound. However, we present the concepts of classification here to give the reader a reference for further discussions. More important, open fracture classification gives the surgeon guidelines for prognosis and permits us to make some statements about methods of treatment (20,21). In North America and most of the world, the wound classification system of Gustilo and Anderson (18) and the subsequent modification by Gustilo et al (22) is the most widely accepted and quoted. This classification is used throughout this chapter.

There is wide variation in the interpretation and use of the Gustilo-Anderson classification and, in general, there is too much emphasis on wound size. The critical factors in their classification system are (a) the degree of soft-tissue injury and (b) the degree of contamination. A devastating crush injury of the leg necessitating amputation may be associated with only a small skin wound. The size of the skin wound is a poor guide to the classification of the fracture. A very large wound caused by a sharp object, such as a knife, may have minimal associated soft-tissue crush, and therefore may carry a very good prognosis (18,22).

The configuration of the fracture (i.e., the amount of displacement and comminution evident) often points to the amount of energy absorbed by the limb at the time of injury. The fracture configuration is helpful in the classification, but it is secondary to soft-tissue considerations. For these reasons, we have chosen to clarify (rather than modify) the Gustilo-Anderson classification as we use it, in the hope that the reader will find it easier to use and more accurate than descriptions presented elsewhere. Table 12-2 provides a quick reference to these guidelines.

A *type I wound* is caused by a low-energy injury that is usually less than 1 cm long (Fig. 12-2). It is usually caused by the bone piercing from the inside outward rather than by a penetrating injury. Unless the wounding occurs in a highly contaminated environment, the level of bacterial contamination is usually low. A type I classification implies minimal or no muscle damage. As mentioned, a type I wound should not be judged by its size alone because small wounds can be associated with dangerously contaminated wounds (e.g., those occurring in a farmyard) and with high-energy trauma (e.g., crush wounds of the tibia in pedestrians hit by automobiles). The surgeon must take all factors into account when classifying open fractures.

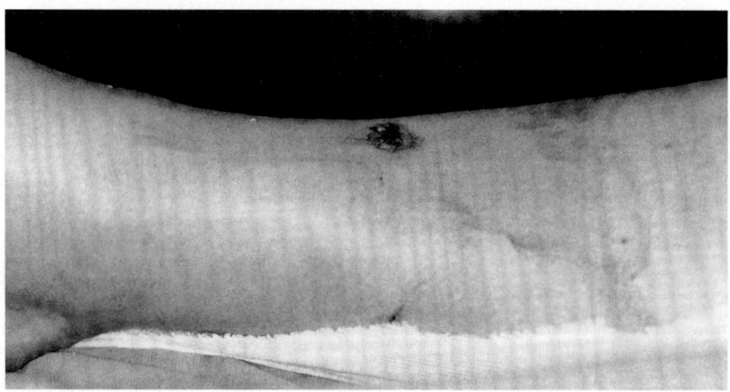

FIGURE 12-2 Type I open tibial fracture.

A *type II wound* is greater than 1 cm in length and has a moderate amount of soft-tissue damage owing to a higher-energy injury (Fig. 12-3). These are usually outside-to-inside injuries. (This is a somewhat broad classification falling between type I and type III wounds.) Some necrotic muscle may be present, but the amount of debridement required is minimal

TABLE 12-2 Classification of Open Fractures

Type	Wound	Level of Contamination	Soft Tissue Injury	Bone Injury
I	<1 cm long	Clean	Minimal	Simple, minimal comminution
II	>1 cm long	Moderate	Moderate, some muscle damage	Moderate comminution
III[a]				
A	Usually >10 cm long	High	Severe with crushing	Usually comminuted; soft tissue coverage of bone possible
B	Usually >10 cm long	High	Very severe loss of coverage; usually requires soft tissue reconstructive surgery	Bone coverage poor; variable, may be moderate to severe comminution
C	Usually >10 cm long	High	Very severe loss of coverage plus vascular injury requiring repair; may require soft tissue reconstructive surgery	Bone coverage poor; variable, may be moderate to severe comminution

[a] Segmental fractures, farmyard injuries, fractures occurring in a highly contaminated environment, shotgun wounds, or high-velocity gunshot wounds automatically result in classification as type III open fracture.

From Chapman MW. The role of intramedullary fixation in open fractures. *Clin Orthop* 1986;212:27.

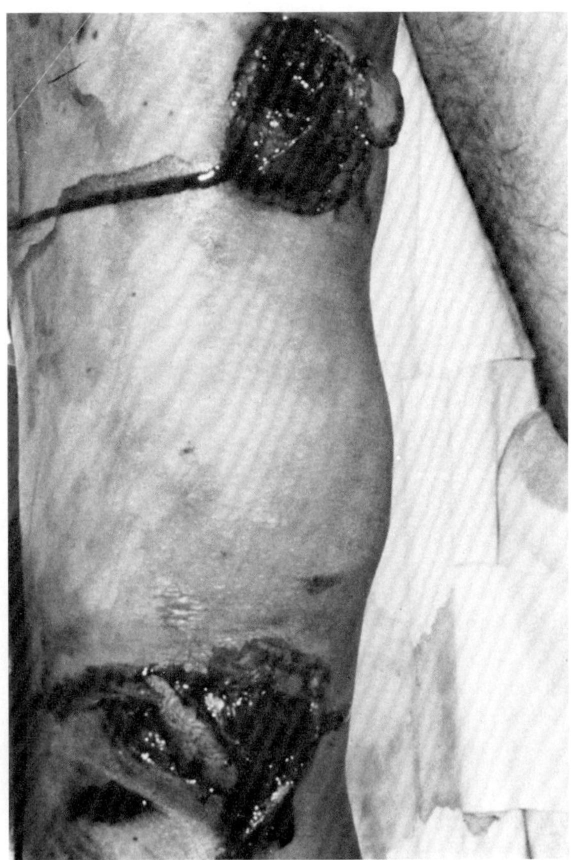

FIGURE 12-3 Type II open tibial fracture.

to moderate, and is usually confined to one compartment. The soft tissue stripped from bone is none to minimal, and wound closure without skin grafts or local flaps should be possible.

A *type III wound* results from a high-energy, outside-to-inside injury and is usually longer than 10 cm with extensive muscle devitalization. In general, the fracture is widely displaced or comminuted, although this is not an essential component (Fig. 12-4). Extensive wound contamination also increases the likelihood of infection and subsequent complications. We include extensive contamination as a reason to classify fractures as type III. Additional factors make an open fracture a type III wound: a close-range shotgun wound, a high-velocity gunshot wound, a segmental fracture with displacement, a fracture with diaphyseal segmental loss, a fracture with an associated major vascular injury requiring repair, a wound occurring in a farmyard or other highly contaminated environment, a fracture caused by the crushing force from a fast-moving vehicle, or an associated compartment syndrome (Table 12-3). The energy of the injury and the degree of soft-tissue devitalization *must* be taken into account when applying this wound classification. Type III wounds can be further classified as follows:

A *type IIIA open fracture* is one in which there is limited stripping of the periosteum and soft tissues from bone, and bone coverage does not present any major problems. The overall soft-tissue envelope about the fracture is usually fairly well preserved. There may be loss of skin, but there is adequate muscle and soft tissue coverage over bone, tendon, and neurovascular bundles.

A *type IIIB open fracture* is one in which there has been extensive stripping of soft tissues and periosteum from bone. Devitali-

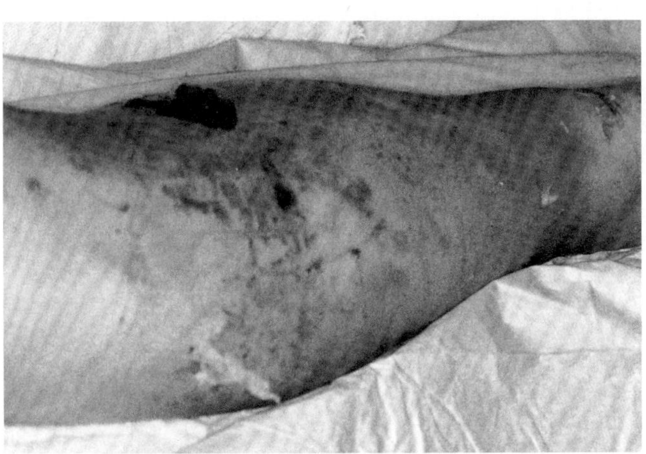

A

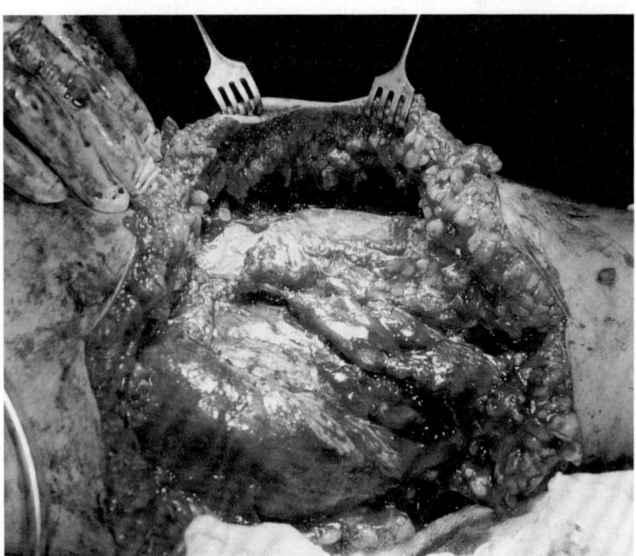

B

FIGURE 12-4 Type III open tibial fracture. **A.** Photograph of the limb of a patient involved in an automobile-versus-pedestrian accident. The soft-tissue defect in the integument is apparent. **B.** Incision of the skin exposes the extent of the underlying degloving and soft-tissue stripping in this injury. This illustrates the concept of zone of injury. The actual zone of the tissue injury extends far proximal and distal to the original traumatic wound.

TABLE 12-3 Factors That Modify Open Fracture Classification Regardless of Initial Skin Defect

Contamination
- A. Exposure to soil
- B. Exposure to water (pools, lakes/streams)
- C. Exposure to fecal material (barnyard)
- D. Exposure to oral flora (bite)
- E. Gross contamination on inspection
- F. Delay in treatment >12 hours

Signs of high-energy mechanisms
- A. Segmental fracture
- B. Bone loss
- C. Compartment syndrome
- D. Crush mechanism
- E. Extensive degloving of subcutaneous fat and skin
- F. Requires flap coverage (any size defect)

zation or loss of soft tissues usually requires a local flap or free tissue transfer, or prolonged use of wound closure adjuncts, such as a wound vacuum for coverage of exposed bone and/or neurovascular bundles.

A *type IIIC open fracture* is one in which there is a major vascular injury requiring repair for salvage of the extremity (Fig. 12-5). A tibia fracture with disruption of the anterior tibial artery but preservation of the posterior tibial artery is not a type IIIC injury. Similarly, an open fracture of the forearm with an intact ulnar or radial artery and well-perfused hand is not a type IIIC injury. Alternatively, open fractures associated with vascular disruption that compromises the viability of the limb and requires repair for reperfusion of the limb are considered type IIIC.

The classification of open fractures according to the Gustilo-Anderson system requires both objective and subjective evaluation of the injured limb (18,22). The classification of an open fracture should be established at the time of operative debridement of the wound. Attempts to classify an open fracture and therefore determine treatment before thorough debridement and assessment of the wound and soft-tissue injury can be misleading.

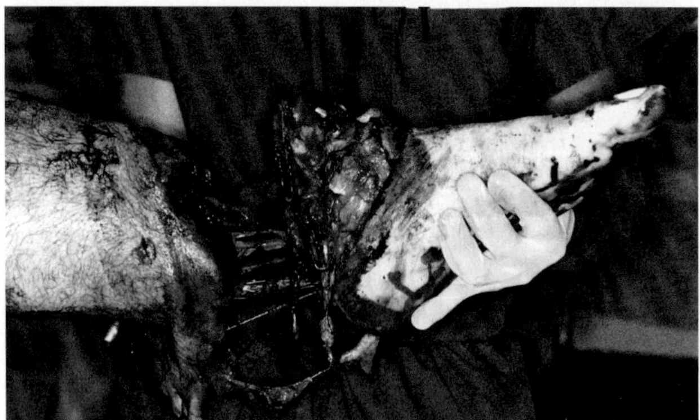

FIGURE 12-5 A type IIIC open tibia fracture. The extent of soft-tissue crush and avulsion in this injury precludes limb salvage. However, if limb salvage were to be performed, vascular repair would be necessary for limb survival.

Brumback and Jones reported on interobserver agreement in the classification of open fractures of the tibia (23). Two hundred forty-five orthopaedic surgeons of varying experience were presented with histories, x-rays, and videos demonstrating physical examination and operative debridement. The participants were asked to classify the fracture according to the Gustilo system. The overall agreement in classification was 60%. The group with least experience (residents and fellows) had an average agreement of 59% (range, 33% to 94%). The most experienced group (trauma fellowship–trained academic surgeons) had an average agreement of 66% (range, 39% to 100%) (23). The authors point out that the classification of open fractures involves an element of subjective judgment with regard to the extent of soft-tissue injury in particular. This is especially so with intermediate types of injury. These observations suggest the reader should critically evaluate the literature when comparing results of open fracture management from different institutions. For example, an article might report that the number of type IIIB open fractures is substantially greater than the number of local flaps and free tissue transfers performed. This observation suggests the use of the Gustilo classification may be skewed to include less severe injuries in the type IIIB category.

Attempts to modify the Gustilo-Anderson system or develop alternative open fracture classification systems have been made. Trafton proposed a classification for open tibia fractures that combined elements of the Gustilo-Anderson and Tscherne (9) classifications into minor, moderate, or major injuries (24). The AO/ASIF group has proposed an open fracture classification to grade soft-tissue injury for use with the AO/ASIF alphanumeric fracture classification system (21). The soft-tissue grade incorporates the degree of injury to the integument (IO for open injuries), muscle tendon injury (MT), and neurovascular injury (NV). Trafton's modified classification offers potential simplicity in classification, whereas the AO/ASIF system offers a detailed and potentially cumbersome system for grading open fractures that may be best suited for research. Neither of these systems has been validated in prospective clinical studies.

The Trauma Department at Hanover, Germany, have developed an open fracture score that considers the AO/ASIF fracture classification; bone loss; loss of soft tissue, skin, and muscle; neurovascular injury and the presence of compartment syndrome; foreign body contamination; final bacteriologic analysis; and time from injury to onset of treatment (Table 12-4) (9,25). This score provides four categories, types I through IV, based on points allocated for each category. This open fracture classification has been reported in a prospective series of open fractures treated in Hanover (9,25).

TABLE 12-4 Hannover Open Fracture Score

	Points
A. Fracture type (AO/OTA fracture classification)	
Type A	1
Type B	2
Type C	4
Bone loss	
<2 cm	1
>2 cm	2
B. Soft tissues	
Skin (wound, contusion, abrasion)	
None	0
<¼ Circumference at level of injury	1
¼ – ½	2
½ – ¾	3
>¾	4
Skin loss	
None	0
<¼ Circumference at level of injury	1
¼ – ½	2
½ – ¾	3
>¾	4
Deep soft tissue injury (e.g., muscles, ligaments, etc.)	
None	0
<¼ Circumference at level of injury	1
¼ – ½	2
½ – 4/4	3
>¾	6
Amputation	
None	0
Subtotal guillotine	20
Subtotal crush	30
C. Ischemia	
None	0
Incomplete (compartment syndrome)	10
Complete <4 h	15
Complete 4–8 h	20
Complete >8 h	25
D. Nerves	
Palmar–plantar sensation	
Yes	0
No	8
Fingers–toes movement	
Yes	0
No	8
E. Contamination	
Foreign bodies/particulate material	
None	0
Single	1
Multiple	2
Massive	10
F. Bacteriology (initial post-debridement culture)	
Aerobe 1 organism	2
Aerobe >1 organism	3
Anaerobe	2
Aerobe and anaerobe	4
G. Onset of treatment (only if soft tissue score >2)	
<6 h	0
6–12 h	1
>12 h	3
Total score	—
Open fracture grade	
Grade 1: 2–3 Points	
Grade 2: 4–19 Points	
Grade 3: 20–69 Points	
Grade 4: >70 Points	

CURRENT TREATMENT

Emergency Department Management

Foreign bodies or obvious debris, such as leaves, stones, or grass, found in open wounds that can be easily removed should be manually removed with sterile forceps. Then, if the patient will be going to surgery within 1 or 2 hours of injury, the wound can be covered with a sterile bandage and the patient transported to the operating room for definitive irrigation and debridement. If the patient will not get to the operating room for several hours or the timing is uncertain, we prefer to irrigate the wound with 1 to 2 L of saline fluid before placing the sterile dressing (2).

Patients with grossly deformed limbs and obviously dislocated joints should not wait for x-rays before receiving a closed reduction and realignment of their injured limbs. Patient should have their open fractures irrigated, covered with sterile dressings, and splinted before going for x-rays.

Some clinicians advocate application of povidone-soaked dressings, but it has been suggested that povidone interferes with osteoblast function, so we use it only when there is extensive wound contamination (26). Patzakis et al (27) advocate a predebridement culture from the wound in the emergency department before administration of antibiotics, or any antiseptics. However, data from our center suggest there is little value in predebridement cultures, so we do not use them (28–30).

Once the sterile dressing is placed, no further wound inspection should be done until the patient is in the operating room. Tscherne et al (9) demonstrated a 4.3% infection rate in open wounds that were covered immediately with a sterile dressing, compared with an 18% infection rate in open wounds left exposed until surgery. To prevent the urge of subsequent physicians to remove the dressings to view the wound, a photograph can be taken and placed in the chart for later review. Serial photographs throughout the treatment of the limb prove to be useful in educating the patient and family, and are often vital in legal proceedings. If photography is not available, then a sketch of the limb and the wound often serves better than paragraphs of written description (31).

In major trauma centers, surgeons from several surgical disciplines are often available for the initial resuscitation and care of the patient. This allows the orthopaedic surgeon to focus on the injuries of the musculoskeletal system. In smaller hospitals, however, the orthopaedic surgeon may be responsible for the complete care of the patient, including resuscitation and maintenance of life until a general surgeon or neurosurgeon can be summoned. In such cases, the measures outlined in Chapter 3 for initial emergent care are critical, permitting the surgeon to proceed with examination of the obviously injured extremity in a methodical and deliberate fashion. In this way, the surgeon can feel comfortable that no other unrecognized injury is likely to emerge suddenly, or that the patient will be further compromised by neglect or oversight. This plea for a deliberate and orderly assessment underscores the fundamental principle that in dealing with the injured, nothing should be taken for granted. To look offers the prospect to know; not to look is to assume.

All open fractures need to be formally treated in the operating room on an urgent basis with meticulous irrigation and thorough but judicious debridement of devitalized soft tissue and devascularized bone fragments (2,19). Because all open fractures are formally debrided, there is little justification for exploration of the wounds in the emergency department. Digital exploration provides little useful information, risks further contamination, and may precipitate profuse bleeding. Local or regional anesthetics administered in the emergency department to alleviate pain or enhance wound exploration are unnecessary, and can hamper subsequent care because they may preclude an accurate neurologic examination on a serial basis, or by subsequent examiners. Obvious foreign bodies are removed with sterile forceps or a sterile gloved hand.

When a small wound in the skin overlies or is in the vicinity of a fracture, immediately the question arises as to whether the wound communicates with the fracture site, thus making it an open fracture. The safest way to answer this question is formal debridement of the wound, tracing it until its deepest extent is established. However, if the wound is treatable in the emergency department and the fracture or joint injury is treatable by closed means, formal debridement, particularly of a very minor wound, in the operating room may not always be necessary. This should be limited to cases with minor wounds, with minimal or no displacement of the associated fracture on x-ray, and minimal signs of soft-tissue trauma (32). The purpose of this limited exploration in the ED setting is to establish whether (a) the wound communicates with the fracture and (b) the underlying tissue is viable in the zone of injury. If there is any question regarding the viability of underlying tissues, the wound should be extended, typically in the operating room. A clinically stable fracture with a small wound and a history of high-risk environment for contamination benefits from operative irrigation and debridement.

Antibiotics

Antibiotics for open fracture wounds should not be considered prophylactic, but therapeutic, because bacteria contaminate these wounds. A recent Cochrane review of antibiotic administration found that the administration of antibiotics in open fractures significantly reduced the rate of infection. Further, the review found there is no ethical reason to perform studies without antibiotic administration (33). Cooney et al (34) found that sepsis was unlikely to occur with fewer than 10^5 bacteria per gram of tissue. Robson et al (35) reported greater than 10^5 organisms per gram of tissue in wounds with a delay in treatment of more than 5 hours. These data support the therapeutic nature of antibiotics in the initial treatment of open fractures. The role of antibiotics is to kill residual organisms and at least inhibit their growth to the point where host protective mechanisms can eradicate them (36,37). Irrigation and debridement and antibiotic administration are by far the most important measures in preventing infection in open fractures, and antibiotics alone certainly cannot be relied on to prevent infection in an inadequately debrided wound (31,38).

The work of Patzakis et al (27) established the basis of our current practice. In a controlled, randomized, prospective study, they compared three groups of open fracture patients: one received immediate administration of cephalothin, one immediate administration of penicillin and streptomycin, and the third group received no antibiotics. The infection rate in the cephalothin group was 2.3%, compared with 9.7% in the penicillin/streptomycin group, and 13.9% in the control group. It is on the basis of this study and subsequent clinical experience that cephalosporins remain the antibiotics of choice for the treatment of open fractures. Early administration of antibiotics during the initial phases of resuscitation decreases the incidence of infection in open fractures. The most common organism producing infection in their series was *Staphylococcus aureus;* most of these infections were resistant to penicillin. Studies have shown that predebridement cultures have no reliable correlation with the eventual infecting organism. The correlation of postdebridement cultures with the eventual infecting organism is moderate at best (29).

An antibiotic with broad-spectrum gram-positive coverage—usually a first-generation cephalosporin derivative—is given in the emergency department for all type I and type II fractures (37,39,40). The addition of an aminoglycoside for gram-negative coverage is recommended for type III injuries (41). Where the strong possibility of significant anaerobic infection is indicated by organic contamination, the addition of penicillin for anaerobic coverage is recommended. Metronidazole is indicated for penicillin allergic individuals or those wounds with severe fecal contamination (Table 12-5). Despite advances in single-agent antibiotic spectrum and delivery, multiagent therapy is still supported in type III open fractures. Patzakis et al (42) conducted a prospective randomized trial of a single broad-spectrum antibiotic (ciprofloxacin) versus multidrug therapy (cefamandole and gentamicin). The rate of infection was no different in type I and II open fractures. In type III open fractures, the infection rates were 31% and 8% ($p < .05$) with single- and multiagent therapy respectively. Subsequently, the use of ciprofloxacin alone may be considered in type I and type II fractures (43–45). However, single-agent therapy with ciprofloxacin alone was not advocated in type III fractures. Fluoroquinolones may be considered as an alternative in patients with known adverse reactions to aminoglycosides or when treating culture-specific, established infections. Authors working in Third World settings have found fluoroquinolones cost-effective treatment for type I and II open fractures (46,47).

Surgical Treatment

Preparation for Surgical Debridement

Preoperative planning determines the order in which multiple fractures are treated, and the teams necessary to treat them (48). The soft-tissue and bone instruments needed should be

TABLE 12-5 Intravenous Antibiotic Therapy for Open Fractures*

	Type I	Type II	Type III	Organic Contamination
Cefazolin 1 g every 8 hours	X	X	X	
Aminoglycoside 3–5 mg/kg/day†			X	
Penicillin 2,000,000 units every 4 hours (or metronidazole 500 mg every 6 hours)				X

* Antibiotic doses for adult patients.
† Varies with renal function of patient.

identified and made available. Open fractures often present unexpected surprises; therefore, a full set of soft-tissue and bone instruments must be immediately available. The surgeon must plan for all contingencies. The full assortment of fixation devices that might be necessary to stabilize the fracture must be available. The optimal position of the patient on the operating table and the need for an orthopaedic fracture table or fluoroscopy must be determined. Occasionally, in a clean type I or II open fracture where primary internal fixation is carried out, immediate cancellous bone grafting may be indicated. If so, a possible bone graft donor site should be selected.

The emergency department splint and dressing are removed. Gentle traction is maintained throughout the surgical preparation to avoid gross deformity at the fracture site and prevent further injury to soft tissues. A tourniquet should be available in the event that tourniquet control of the extremity is needed. A two-phase surgical preparation of the limb may be advisable for severely contaminated wounds. With one preparation set, the entire limb is washed from the fingertips or toes to the tourniquet to eliminate gross contamination. A liter of sterile saline is poured over the wound, and any obvious debris is removed. The second preparation kit is opened and formal surgical preparation of the entire extremity is performed.

Debridement and Irrigation

Debridement (literal translation, *unbridling*) was once used only in the treatment of infected wounds, as an incision to release the purulent contents of the wounds. Gradually, it was realized that removal of necrotic tissue at the time of debridement was beneficial; and finally it was recognized that removal of wound debris and necrotic tissue is best carried out as early as possible after injury.

The objectives of debridement (and irrigation) are as follows:

1. Extension of the traumatized wound to allow identification of the zone of injury.
2. Detection and removal of foreign material, especially organic foreign material.
3. Detection and removal of nonviable tissues.
4. Reduction of bacterial contamination.
5. Creation of a wound that can tolerate the residual bacterial contamination and heal without infection.

The zone of injury is frequently more extensive than suggested by the open wound. Thus, the final fracture classification should be made at the time of debridement. A type I- or II-appearing soft-tissue wound may actually be reclassified to a type III injury, depending on the degree of skeletonization and stripping of soft tissue from the bone proximally or distally (Fig. 12-4). This is strongly suggested by the degree of gross radiologic displacement seen on presentation. It is often necessary to extend type I and II open wounds to expose the complete zone of injury and effect appropriate debridement. This is in contradistinction to the open fracture with a small (<1 cm) wound associated with an undisplaced or minimally displaced, clinically stable fracture. Clinical experience has shown that this variant of open fracture often has a clinical course similar to that of closed fractures regarding both infection and nonunion. This is often seen in open fractures in the upper extremity.

Open fractures of the pelvis are unique in that association with rectal, vaginal, or urologic injury increases the risk of fracture contamination. In effect, these fractures can have external contamination like other open fractures, or they may have internal sources of contamination as well (49). A diverting colostomy is necessary with an open pelvic fracture associated with colonic injury or rectal tear. Severe peroneal laceration may also require fecal diversion.

The tourniquet plays a limited but important role in the management of open fractures. Proper use of a tourniquet in the debridement of open fractures is essential. The surgeon should consider placing the noninflated tourniquet on the limb because it may be necessary to control the severe hemorrhage encountered when a blood clot is removed from an unexpected major arterial injury. Limited inflation of a tourniquet facilitates visualization when dissecting neurovascular structures particularly in the upper extremity. However, the tourniquet should not be inflated unless it is necessary to control bleeding, either for visualization or to limit blood loss, because the anoxia produced by the tourniquet interferes with evaluation of the viability of muscle and may add to preexisting ischemic tissue injury. Transient inflation of the tourniquet for 10 to 20 minutes, followed by release, results in capillary flush. This may be a helpful indicator of soft-tissue viability. A tourniquet should never be inflated while performing intramedullary reaming of any bone. Reaming in this ischemic environment leads to excessive thermal necrosis of the bone. Thus, appropriate use of the tourniquet includes limited indications for inflation during irrigation and debridement. Most of the procedure should be done without tourniquet inflation.

The surgeon should have an established method or plan for wound debridement. We recommend a careful inspection of the initial skin and dermis of the entire wound, followed by inspection of subcutaneous fat, then muscle, and finally bone. In smaller wounds, this may seem redundant. However, in larger, complex wounds, a random approach can lead to an incomplete debridement of nonviable tissue.

Skin and Subcutaneous Fat. An extensile incision is used that provides effective debridement and appropriate visualization of underlying muscle, fascia, and neurovascular structures, as needed, and of the contaminated bone ends. The question of how much of an additional elective incision is required for deep exposure always arises. In wounds caused by high-energy injuries, a useful axiom is that the wound should be equal in length to the diameter of the limb at that level. A better guide is to expose the entire zone of injury. This begins by exploring the traumatic wound and fracture. Proximal and distal extension is continued until healthy tissues are encountered and all areas of periosteal stripping have been identified (2). Although adequate debridement is obviously necessary, the surgeon should not unnecessarily open uninvolved, clean, intact soft-tissue planes. In particular, detaching skin from its underlying fascial attachment should be avoided because the vertical vessels to the skin necessary for the skin's survival will be damaged. Meticulous hemostasis is maintained as debridement progresses because considerable blood can be lost during debridement of even moderate-sized wounds.

Appropriate incisions require good judgment and a willingness to be innovative to avoid the trap of a surgical approach that is not useful or produces further damage, such as distally based flaps that may become necrotic (48,50). Small puncture wounds or holes are excised as well as small, ragged flaps that are not essential to closure (Fig. 12-6). The elliptical wound thus produced is usually easily closed with sutures and can even be left open for spontaneous closure, leaving a simple linear scar. Coring wounds should be avoided because this leaves a round hole that can close only by granulation and scar formation. Many wounds are transverse or oblique to the longitudinal axis of the limb. These can be extended by four means, illustrated in Figure 12-7. In general, crossing the wound results in flaps that are smaller than with the other methods, thus minimizing the risk of flap necrosis while producing the best exposure.

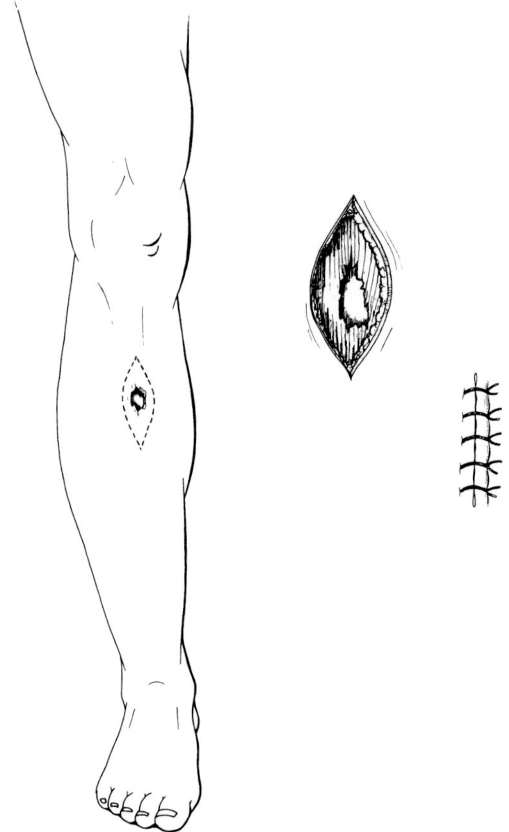

FIGURE 12-6 An elliptical excision of the fracture wound permits proper inspection of the area of injury as well as better closure if the wound is sutured.

The surgeon must be conservative in excision of skin, particularly where it is at a premium (e.g., over the tibia and in the foot and hand). In the hand, for example, particularly in stellate-type lacerations of the digits, excision of skin edges may be contraindicated. Where adequate skin is available, sharp excision of the contaminated and contused skin edge, 1 to 2 mm into good-quality skin with a sharp blade placed at right angles to the skin, removes contaminated and nonviable skin and provides a good wound edge for subsequent closure. This gives the best cosmetic result. The forceps used on skin should always be toothed and should be used with care to avoid further contusion. Frequent changing of the knife blade is necessary to ensure a sharp, well-performed debridement.

A traumatic skin flap that has a base-to-length ratio of more than 1:2, particularly if distally based, frequently has a nonviable tip (51). Some clinicians advocate the injection of an ampule

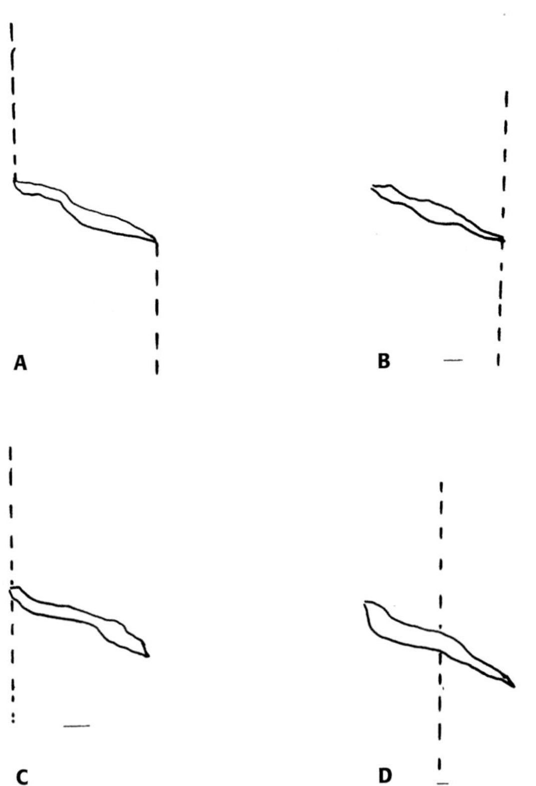

FIGURE 12-7 Methods for extending a traumatic transverse or oblique wound. **A.** The Z-plasty technique produces two large flaps, and risks necrosis of the tips of the flaps. **B,C.** Both of these methods also produce large skin flaps that risk necrosis of the distal portion of the flap. **D.** Incision bisecting the wound results in the smallest flaps. This reduces the risk of flap necrosis and is the preferred incision in most instances.

of fluorescein and visualization of the flap with a Wood's lamp. Obviously, nonviable portions should be excised, but any skin that is marginal should be left; this can always be debrided later, and the major pabulum for infection is not skin but, rather, necrotic muscle. If very large wounds are produced by loss of skin and subsequent coverage is expected to be difficult, it may be possible to harvest skin from the excised flap. A Padgett dermatome works well, set at a 0.010 to 0.012 inch thickness. The graft is run through a 1-to-1.5 or 1-to-3 skin mesher and then widely spread. Often, the graft can be applied immediately to viable muscle and fascia because it does not actually result in closure of the wound and rapidly epithelializes for coverage (51).

Fascia. Any nonviable, damaged, or contaminated fascia should be excised. No marginally viable fascia should be left. We believe limited fasciotomy is indicated in all open fractures secondary to high-energy injuries, and complete fasciotomy of all compartments is often indicated. Frequently, a defect in the fascial layer is present at debridement of an open fracture. Extending this fascial opening to assess the underlying muscle and bone is necessary for an adequate debridement. Therefore, a fasciotomy of the involved myofascial compartment of the open fracture is always indicated as part of the debridement (19).

Muscle. Whereas skin tends to tear or puncture, and fascia to split or shred, muscle, because of its high water content, is subject to hydraulic damage by fluid waves when an injuring object strikes the limb. This is particularly true of high-energy fractures secondary to indirect rapid loading (e.g., a high-velocity skiing injury resulting in comminution of the tibia or femur), in which the bone literally explodes into many fragments. These fragments travel rapidly outward into the muscle and can cause significant muscle damage even when the outer envelope is seemingly undamaged (52). A small bone fragment may pierce the skin, producing what appears to be a very minor type I open fracture, when in fact there may be considerable deep muscle damage. This occurs because the more rapidly bone is loaded before fracture, the more energy is required to fracture it, and the more energy is released from the fracture when it occurs. Because of this absence of direct physical evidence of trauma, it is easy to overlook nonvital muscle because it may not immediately be evident that it has been disturbed or damaged.

In muscle debridement, the approach of "when in doubt, take it out" is the safest. Necrotic muscle is the major pabulum for bacterial growth and poses a great danger in anaerobic infections. Every effort should be made to remove all nonvital muscle tissue, although this always requires careful judgment (2,9,19,53,54). In type I, II, and IIIA open fractures, this may be taken literally, but in types IIIB and IIIC, debridement of an entire muscle or compartment may be necessary to meet this axiom. If the major arterial supply to a severely damaged muscle has been destroyed, the only recourse is total excision. It has been our experience, however, that if even 10% of a muscle belly and its attached tendon can be preserved, significant function is retained. For that reason, there may be an indication for leaving some marginal muscle at the time of initial debridement in severe open fractures, then returning within 24 to 48 hours for redebridement, at which time the muscle will have better declared its viability. The exception to this approach is in wartime or mass casualties, where preservation of life takes precedence over the desire to preserve function (11).

Judgment of the viability of muscle is challenging, and the alliterative quartet provided by Gregory, in the first edition chapter of this textbook, must be addressed by the surgeon: *color, consistency, contractility,* and *capacity to bleed* (Table 12-6). Scully and associates (55), in an attempt to correlate four features with histologic evidence of viability, concluded that consistency and capacity to bleed were the most significant. In our experience, contractility and consistency have been the most reliable because color and capacity to bleed are easily misinterpreted. Remember that the hypoxemia associated with the use of a tourniquet, or in the presence of shock or injury to a major vessel of the involved limb, may make evaluation of these parameters difficult.

Assessment of muscle viability after fasciotomy for compartment syndrome can be difficult. Muscles in the extremities re-

TABLE 12-6 Factors of Muscle Viability

Color	Normally beefy red; rarely, carbon-monoxide exposure can be deceiving
Consistency	Normally firm, not easily disrupted
Capacity to bleed	Can be deceiving because arterioles in necrotic muscle can bleed Typically reliable
Contractility	Responsive to forceps pinch or low cautery setting Typically reliable

ceive their blood supply from small arteries that run in the epimysial layer. Arterioles branch into the central part of the muscle to supply the deeper tissue (56).

Three zones of postischemic muscle changes have been described histologically (57):

1. An inner zone of muscle necrosis in which no swelling occurs.
2. A zone of partial ischemic injury with viable muscle that swells substantially.
3. An outlying zone of normal muscle in which no swelling occurs.

Because of this vascular anatomy, it is possible to have superficial viable muscle and a substantial amount of deeper necrotic muscle, so the surgeon must look beyond the superficial layers during the debridement. This can be accomplished by spreading in the direction of the muscle fibers with a hemostat, permitting the surgeon to assess the character of the deeper muscle tissues without significantly damaging the musculotendinous unit. In addition, whenever there is significant swelling of the muscles with fasciitis, there is a fibrosis of the inner portion of the muscle that can lead to contractures (57).

Tendons. Tendons, unless obviously severely damaged and contaminated, are not a major pabulum for infection, and if essential to function, they should be preserved. Where coverage of tendons by some type of soft tissue is not possible, preservation of the peritenon is essential for tendon survival (19). For that reason, we tend to not debride peritenon but rather copiously irrigate it. If tendon without peritenon must be left exposed in an open wound, a moist dressing must be applied and kept moist until coverage of the tendon can be obtained (see section on definitive wound management). If at all possible, the surgeon should try to swing some muscle, subcutaneous fat, or skin over tendon without peritenon.

Bone. Whereas muscle tissue may mount a defense against invading bacteria, bone tissue is essentially defenseless owing to its relatively poor blood supply. If judgments about muscle viability seem troublesome, judgments about what is to be done with bone fragments are perplexing. In general, small bits of cortical bone that are free of any soft-tissue attachments should be removed. When a large cortical segment is removed in the debridement, the patient is left with a potentially complex reconstruction problem. Bone grafting and bone transport technologies are improving, but the result may still be prolonged disability and increased morbidity for the patient.

The decision to debride segments of the bone can be difficult. When a large bony segment has soft-tissue attachments and is bleeding, it should be retained. The major problem lies with a bone fragment that has only a tenuous soft-tissue attachment or is completely free. It is often tempting to retain it as a perfectly fitting bone graft. In general, completely devascularized bone segments should be debrided. Only in the exceptional circumstance of the open fracture with no significant contamination, such as with an inside-to-out mechanism of injury, should retention of such fragments be considered. Major segments of the articular surface that are dysvascular should be retained regardless of wound type when salvage of the involved joint is to be attempted (19).

The extent of contamination can be difficult to assess. History is often helpful. A history of injury occurring in a highly contaminated environment is suggestive of a significant risk of infection, regardless of the soft-tissue injury. Injuries sustained in environments producing barnyard, soil, or water contamination are especially prone to infectious complications.

Patients presenting with gross contamination in the emergency department should be promptly addressed. Superficial contamination such as leaves, twigs, or clothing should be removed on presentation. It is often helpful to lavage the wound with a liter or more of normal saline to decrease the bacterial count before applying a sterile dressing. Foreign bodies that penetrate into an extremity or body cavity should be approached with caution. Risks of causing further injury or exacerbating hemorrhage by removal of the foreign body are increased in this setting.

At the time of debridement, the wound should be thoroughly inspected for evidence of contamination. The extent of migration of grass, leaves, and the like can be surprising in some wounds. Careful inspection of all degloved areas and skin flaps is necessary to perform a thorough debridement.

Similarly, the fractured ends of long bones should be delivered into the wound for irrigation and debridement. The intramedullary canal should be inspected. Debridement with a curet and irrigation should be used to remove foreign bodies and retained hematoma.

In a series of type III open tibial fractures managed in an external fixator, Edwards et al (58) demonstrated that retention of large dysvascular segments of cortical bone increased the late infection rate by 50% (9% with debridement, and 20% with retention). This suggests that debridement of dysvascular bony segments in severe open fractures leads to a decreased long-term infection rate.

However, in low-energy fractures in which a major cortical bone fragment is essential to an internal fixation construct, when the surgeon is confident that the level of contamination is low and adequate irrigation and debridement has been carried out, the fragment can be retained in the construct (59). This allows for early redebridement if infection intervenes. In addition, retention of a large, segmental fragment of bone may lead to nonunion at one or both ends of the free fragment, and bridging of the nonviable fragment with onlay cancellous bone graft may be advisable at some time during treatment (see section on bone grafting). In the case of free butterfly fragments or segmental pieces in fractures where external fixation will provide the primary stabilization, interfragmentary screw fixation of the free fragment to the adjacent viable bone may be indicated only when no further soft-tissue stripping is necessary, followed by bone grafting across the junction site later (60).

As a general rule, bone debridement initially can be conservative; however, if infection intervenes, early aggressive redebridement of all nonviable bone is important (61–63). It is better to deal with the reconstruction of a large segmental defect than to allow chronic infection to result in chronic osteomyelitis, which may lead to even more bone loss (3). A common judgment error in the management of infected open fractures is the delayed excision of nonviable bone.

Determination of the viability of bone is difficult. Assessment of bone edges for signs of bleeding is the most reliable technique available. Laser Doppler flowmetry has not been definitively tested as a measure of assessing bone viability in the debridement of open fractures (64,65).

As described with tendons, bone without periosteum and not covered by soft tissue quickly desiccates and dies. It is critical, therefore, to preserve any periosteum attached to the bone where bone will not be immediately covered by muscle or subcutaneous fat and skin. It is usually better to thoroughly irrigate periosteum that is attached rather than debride it (see section on wound coverage and coverage).

Joints. Any wound that enters a joint mandates exploration. The wound is debrided as described earlier down to the level of the joint. The traumatic wound itself may permit adequate exploration, or an extensile incision may be necessary. In many joints, however, adequate exploration through the arthrotomy is not possible unless the incision is very large; this is particularly true in the knee and shoulder. Under these circumstances, it may be better to combine debridement of the wound with arthroscopic examination of the joint. If fluid leakage through the wound is a problem, the synovium should be closed and arthroscopic inspection carried out in the usual fashion. It is critical that the entire joint be adequately explored because unexpected foreign bodies or osteochondral fractures are frequently found.

Nerves and Vessels. Nerve injuries amenable to repair should be sutured before delayed primary closure of an open wound. Brisk, small vessel, or arterial bleeders encountered during debridement require immediate ligation or coagulation. Methodical, layer-by-layer hemostasis is important to limit blood loss. General oozing from capillary-sized vessels usually abates with time and compression. Major vessel injuries requiring repair are usually identified before surgery and appropriately planned for but may be encountered unexpectedly during debridement.

Reinstitution of circulation is of primary importance because it is often difficult to know exactly how much time has elapsed from injury to the initiation of vascular repair (66). In our experience, loss of total blood supply to the limb for more than 8 hours nearly always results in amputation. If there has been a significant delay, we prefer to do a very quick irrigation and debridement of the wound to remove only the grossest contamination and then proceed with vascular repair. This is particularly important if the repair must be done through the open fracture wound. There are exceptions, however; for example, if the open fracture wound is anterior to the knee and repair of a popliteal artery requires an independent elective posteromedial exposure, appropriate initial surgical preparation of the limb should be performed using the two-phase method described previously; the traumatic wound is occluded with a barrier drape and exposure is obtained immediately for vascular repair. In the presence of arterial injury necessitating repair, maximal venous outflow is preserved during the debridement (66,67).

In larger vessels, rather than carrying out immediate end-to-end anastomosis or vein grafting, it may be better to insert a temporary shunt. This permits irrigation and debridement and stabilization of the bone before final vascular repair (68). This may be important to establish proper limb length and avoid injury to the vessel during the bone repair.

When vascular repair is necessary, repeat debridement is frequently required and easy visualization of the entire limb to assess circulation is important. For this reason, some clinicians advocate routine internal or external fixation in such situations. Others, notably Connolly (69), have shown that nonoperative immobilization works well, especially in a mass casualty situation.

Fasciotomy

After arterial repair for complete ischemia to the distal limb, massive swelling distal to the site of repair is very common, particularly in the forearm or leg (66–68). Occasionally, collateral circulation provides adequate perfusion to prevent muscle ischemia and subsequent compartment syndrome (70). Because fasciotomy so often becomes necessary, we urge the reader to do it prophylactically in nearly every case. If there is any doubt about its indication, it probably should be done. Moreover, it is better done too early than too late (66,70).

The limb should be carefully examined after the initial procedure for an open fracture. Compartment syndrome can develop insidiously during the initial 24 hours. It is often advisable to measure compartment pressures after the initial procedure to have a baseline for later comparison (71).

Irrigation. There are two adages that apply to open fracture irrigation: "If a little does some good, a lot will do a great deal more," and "The solution to pollution is dilution." The importance of copious irrigation was emphasized by Gustilo and associates (18,39), who recommended that 10 L of normal saline be used for irrigation to decrease the incidence of infection. Whether 10 L should be run through every wound is less important than the fact that irrigation must be thorough and copious. We prefer to use irrigation and debridement simultaneously. Some of the advantages of irrigation are as follows (19,72,73):

1. Initial lavage by flushing away blood and other debris clears the wound for inspection, thus facilitating the removal of foreign material and debridement.
2. Irrigation fluid floats otherwise undetected and often necrotic fronds of fascia, fat, or muscle into the field where they can be seen and excised.
3. Lavage floats contaminated blood clots and loose pieces of tissue and debris from unseen recesses and tissue planes.
4. Lavage of the tissue restores its normal color and facilitates determination of viability.
5. Irrigation reduces the bacterial population.

The ideal method, quantity, and type of irrigation solution used have been investigated vigorously with data that fails to definitively support any particular approach (26,73–79). Available methods of irrigation include pulsatile lavage, water pic, continuous irrigation, and bulb syringe. Each has an advocate. Similarly, the appropriate quantity of irrigation fluid is debatable as well, but based on historical reports of decreased rates of infection, authorities generally advocate at least 9 L of fluid for type III fractures (72). In addition, the benefit of additives has been examined, but the data are confounded by the use of various methods of delivery and the effects of such additives on the host tissues.

Pulsatile lavage offers the advantage of mobilizing particulate matter and freeing such debris from the wound (75). When using pulsatile lavage, Anglen et al (74) demonstrated a 100-fold decrease in the bacterial count of glycocalyx producing *Staphylococcus* compared with bulb syringe irrigation. Alternatively, it has been proposed that microscopic damage to bone architecture produced by high-pressure lavage in in vitro models may alter bone healing in the clinical setting (75,80). Similarly, considerable soft-tissue damage has been demonstrated following high-pressure lavage (81). Bhandari et al (82) demonstrated positive cultures up to 4 cm deep to the surface of highly contaminated wounds in sections of human tibia suggesting bacteria had been driven into the tissue. However, 99% of the surface bacteria were removed (82). Focus has subsequently been placed on the pressure delivered through various systems available.

In an in vitro model, Bhandari et al (75) examined the time-dependent effectiveness of high- and low-pressure systems (75). When implemented within 3 hours of contamination of canine tibiae, low-pressure pulsatile lavage (14 psi at 550 pulsations per minute) was equally effective at removing bacteria with less structural damage to the host when compared with high-pressure pulsatile lavage (70 psi at 1,050 pulsations/minute). However, after 6 hours, low pressure was less effective at removing bacteria. The latter finding was attributed to further adherence of the microorganisms as time allowed for the production of attachment mechanisms. Madden et al (83) noted a similar time-dependent effect in rabbit wounds contaminated by *Staphylococcus aureus* or *Escherichia coli*. In this regard, pulsatile lavage is advocated for dirty wounds to free debris and provide gross decontamination; however, the efficacy of low-pressure, pulsatile lavage after a 6-hour delay is in question. Further studies are required to define the optimal parameters of pressure and pulsations relative to the time of injury.

Bulb syringe lavage and continuous, gravity irrigation through cystoscopy tubing or an equivalent both lack the pressure and pulsatile flow provided by mechanical devices. Advantages include minimizing damage to the bone and surrounding soft tissues (80). Bulb syringe, which has been reported to require up to 200 minutes of irrigation time to process 10 L of fluid, may prove impractical for large open wounds (84). Accordingly, bulb syringe lavage has compared poorly with pulsatile lavage in regards to removing bacteria (74,85). Gravity irrigation provides a means for delivering copious amounts of fluid but has received little attention. In a comparison of pressure lavage (50 psi) versus bulb syringe lavage or gravity irrigation in contaminated rat wounds, pressure lavage was more effective in removing bacteria. This was particularly true in the presence of foreign debris (85). However, in cases where foreign debris is minimal, gravity irrigation should be considered as an effective alternative (72).

"Water pic" devices have been re-introduced as methods of wound irrigation and debridement as well. A continuous stream of water is directed tangentially to the wound surface. Proponents indicate that the device facilitates surface debridement and limits deep, soft tissue involvement (86). The clinical effectiveness in open fracture irrigation has yet to be fully demonstrated. Similarly, irrigation of wounds with hand-held bags of saline under manual compression was recently reported as a fast, and therefore effective, means of delivering large volumes of fluid (10 L in five minutes) (84). However, no outcome data were presented to support this approach.

A number of irrigation additives have been examined concurrent to the focus on method of irrigation delivery. Antiseptics investigated include hydrogen peroxide, povidone-iodine, chlorhexidine, and various alcohol solutions (72). These agents inhibit pathogens by damaging cell walls. Host toxicity through this same mechanism, to include impaired osteoblast function, has been demonstrated as well (26,87). Routine use of these solutions has not been supported as adverse effects including inhibited wound healing and cartilage damage have been reported (88,89).

The benefit of adding antibiotics to irrigation solutions has not been fully demonstrated either. Rosenstein et al (79) noted a decrease in positive cultures following instillation of bacitracin into canine femora inoculated with *Staphylococci*. Alternatively, Conroy demonstrated no difference in positive cultures in rat wounds similarly contaminated and treated with bacitracin irrigation. In a contaminated hardware model, Anglen (74) found no difference in residual bacterial counts when pulsatile irrigation was accomplished with either bacitracin, neomycin, or saline alone (74). However, the addition of soap detergent (Castile soap) to the pulsatile lavage solution decreased the bacterial count 100-fold compared with pulsatile lavage with saline alone. Similar advantages were noted when the surfactant benzalkonium chloride was applied in contaminated rat wounds (77). Although there are no prospective studies comparing the use of antibiotic or surfactant additives in human open fractures, the use of surfactants in heavily contaminated wounds has been proposed as a valuable adjuvant (72). Concerns regarding wound irritation and acceptance of these compounds for clinical use have curtailed the routine application of these agents.

Our current practice in the initial treatment of open fractures is to irrigate type I through IIIA open fractures with a total of 9 L of normal saline with a pulsatile lavage system. As the risk of bacterial adherence is felt to increase with time, this procedure is initiated as soon as possible. For open fractures that are highly contaminated and types IIIB and IIIC, we routinely use an additional 3 L of irrigation. Often, 3 L (one bag) of irrigation is used before debridement, and the remainder is used after a thorough soft tissue debridement is performed.

The patient is frequently returned to the operating room for staged procedures as the soft-tissue injury often continues to evolve. Concerns have been raised that repetitive irrigation may delay fracture healing and promote nonunion as identified by Park et al (90) in a study of bone healing in fractured rabbit tibiae. A dose–response relationship was noted. Those receiving index irrigation alone healed within 10 weeks. Those undergoing repeat irrigation on three occasions had failed to heal by 15 weeks. Less frequent irrigations resulted in further unions by 10 weeks. Adili et al (91) studied the biomechanics of fracture healing in rats following irrigation with pulsatile lavage and bulb syringe. The mechanical strength of the fracture callus was significantly decreased at 3 weeks following pulsatile lavage. However, by 6 weeks, these early effects were no longer noted. The long-term sequelae are unknown. Thus, adequate and aggressive debridements are performed initially to promote early stabilization of the soft tissues and avoid multiple, repetitive procedures at later dates.

SKELETAL STABILIZATION

After initial debridement of the soft-tissue envelope, stabilization is the next priority. Unless the fracture is inherently stable, some form of skeletal stabilization is usually necessary. The goals of skeletal immobilization (4,19) are as follows:

1. Restore length and alignment of long bones.
2. Reduce articular surfaces displaced by fracture.
3. Allow access to the traumatic wound.
4. Facilitate further reconstruction procedures.
5. Allow early use of the limb.
6. Facilitate fracture union and return of function.

Skeletal stabilization options range from traction to plaster immobilization to internal fixation (4,92). In general, the more severe the open fracture, the greater the need for direct skeletal fixation to allow improved access to the traumatic wound. At the outset, reestablishment of good alignment realigns neurovascular structures, which provides optimal circulation to the injured extremity and minimizes the risk of compromising peripheral nerves (19). Restoration of normal length reduces the dead space in which blood can accumulate. Restoration of normal anatomy improves venous and lymphatic return, thereby reducing soft-tissue swelling. At the microscopic level, bone stability helps stabilize soft-tissue planes. This facilitates capillary proliferation and ingrowth to revascularize devitalized bone and soft tissues. Early revascularization of devitalized structures improves local tissue resistance to infection. Stabilization and approximation of soft-tissue planes facilitates diffusion of nutrients and antibodies, as well as white blood cell migration. All of these factors contribute to local wound defense against infection (93,94).

From the standpoint of the whole patient, fracture stability permits muscle rehabilitation and joint motion, which facilitates early return to function. The studies of Salter and associates (95), Mitchell and Shepard (96), and others (97) have shown that rigid internal fixation of osteochondral fractures and early restoration of joint motion are essential to achieve good cartilage healing and prevent joint stiffness and intra-articular adhesions. In multiply injured patients, stabilization of major long bone and axial skeletal fractures permits early mobilization, which facilitates cardiopulmonary care, may prevent thromboembolic phenomena, and has been shown to reduce morbidity and mortality (9,98,99).

As in the treatment of closed fractures, it is difficult to be dogmatic about any one open fracture, and no one technique seems clearly superior to any other in all cases. For the surgeon who deals with open fractures only occasionally or on a temporary basis, the simpler the method, the better. Such a policy creates fewer problems for the first surgeon and provides greater latitude for definitive treatment by the last surgeon. However, the surgeon who treats open fractures on a regular basis must be aware of, and consider the full range of available techniques, and even combine them or, when indicated, improvise (Table 12-7).

Immobilization in Plaster

Plaster-of-Paris casts have limitations in the treatment of open fractures because they may make access to the wound difficult and because they involve a circumferential hard dressing on a limb with the potential for swelling, which can contribute to compartment syndrome. Cast immobilization may be appropriate for type I open injuries in situations where it would normally

TABLE 12-7 Contraindications to Skeletal Fixation

1. Severe osteopenia
2. Severe comminution (i.e., "nonreconstructable")
3. Minimal soft tissue injury with a nondisplaced fracture (i.e., ideal for closed treatment)
4. Severe ongoing local infection
5. Severe systemic compromise precluding anesthesia

be used (e.g., ulnar shaft and nondisplaced tibial fractures) (92,100). These wounds can frequently be left open or closed primarily with one or two sutures after irrigation and debridement. It is usually advisable to apply a splint until the wound has healed and the arm or leg can be placed in a cast. Certain type II open fractures that are minimally displaced, and stable configurations, may be cautiously considered for cast treatment. Wounds that require frequent observation, local dressing changes, and the like are less appropriate for cast management.

A full-length longitudinal cut is always made in the cast with a cast saw after the plaster has dried to produce a univalved cast. Any underlying Webril and stockinette are cut as well. A univalved cast is superior to a bivalved cast in that it can be spread to accommodate the limb without losing adequate fracture immobilization, and it provides more uniform decompression of the limb. A bivalved cast, when spread, provides decompression in only one axis of the limb, results in increased instability, and allows swelling of the skin between the bivalved portions of the cast, which may produce blisters.

There should be an easy way to expose the wound in the cast to inspect it or carry out delayed primary closure. Simply windowing the cast may be unsatisfactory because the window may not be accurately located over the wound. To avoid this, a bubble is made in the cast directly over the wound. This is accomplished by placing a bulky pad of loosely packed cast padding directly over the wound after the dressing and circumferential cast padding have been applied (Fig. 12-8).

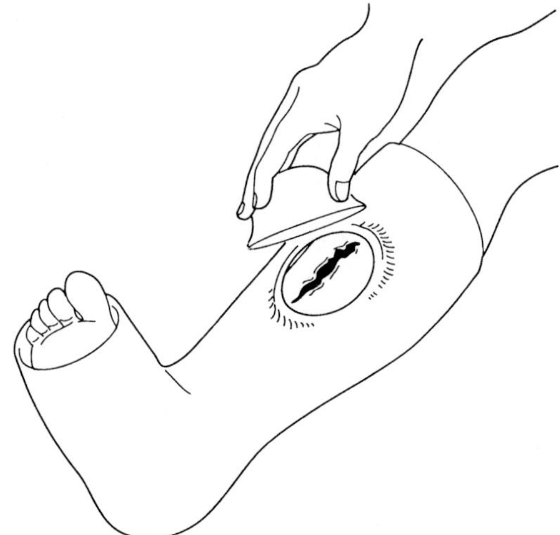

FIGURE 12-8 Bubble in plaster-of-Paris cast can be easily removed for wound care.

Skeletal Traction and Suspension

Balanced skeletal traction, usually as a temporary method, can be used effectively in the femur and occasionally the tibia. Historically, satisfactory results have not been consistently obtained using this modality for definitive management (101). In current practice, the physiologic changes of enforced recumbency, additional expense, and inconsistent final outcomes make the use of skeletal traction for definitive management of open fractures contraindicated in the adult patient (99).

External Skeletal Fixation

In the 1970s and early 1980s, with the emergence of half-pin frames, external fixation finally became the fracture stabilization method of choice for the treatment of most open fractures of long bones (20,58). Many different external fixation devices are now available, each offering unique advantages and features. (See Chapter 7 for a more complete discussion of external fixation methods.) Today, external fixation is most often indicated for type IIIB and IIIC open fractures of the tibia and fibula, and in open fractures of the pelvis (4,49,102,103). More recently, the introduction of ring constructs using highly tensioned wires or half-pin hybrid rings (104,105) has expanded the usefulness of external fixators. Multiple tensioned wires on a ring are useful to stabilize juxta-articular fractures. Limited internal screw fixation with percutaneous cannulated screws facilitates further periarticular reduction. Hybrid fixation frequently incorporates limited internal fixation with variable configurations of external fixation (105). By using the principles of distraction osteogenesis or segmental transport, bone defects can be filled and leg length equalized without needing bone graft (Fig. 12-9) (104).

External fixation devices offer the following advantages (106): (a) they are typically relatively easily and rapidly applied; (b) excellent stability is obtained and reasonably anatomic reduction of major fragments is possible; (c) minimal additional soft-tissue trauma is required for placement, so the risk of wound breakdown and infection is minimized; (d) in most cases, sufficient stability is achieved to allow early joint motion and muscle rehabilitation so the patient is sufficiently mobile that cardiopulmonary care is facilitated in patients with multiple injuries; (e) external fixation offers the option of easily redisplacing the fracture at subsequent debridements; and (f) external fixation may be used as a temporizing frame, restoring the limb

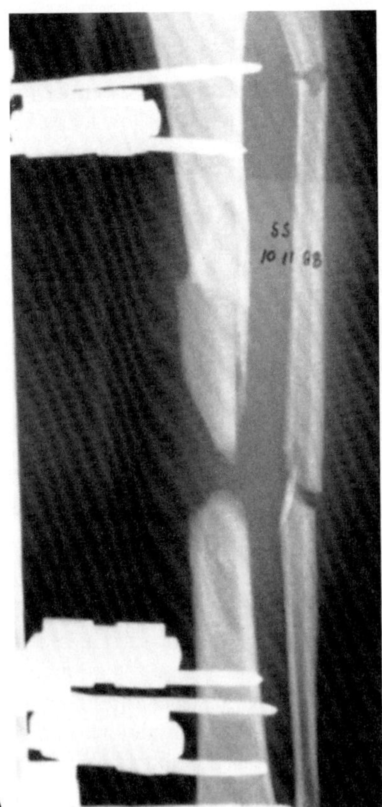

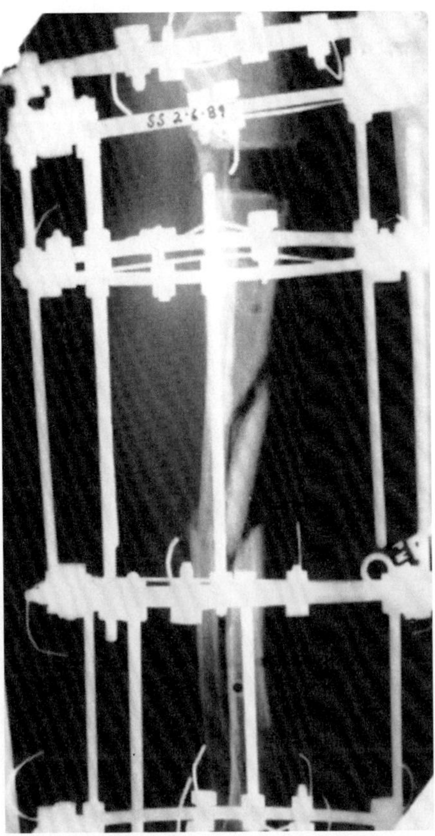

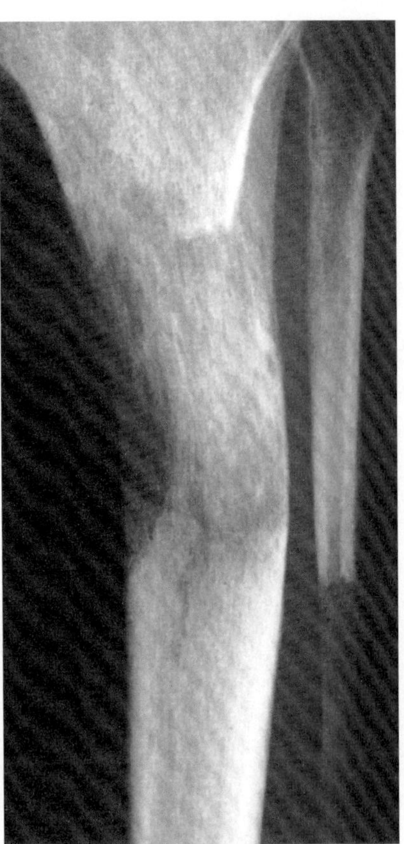

FIGURE 12-9 **A.** Open fracture of the tibia with major segmental bone loss stabilized initially in a uniplanar external fixation. **B.** Appearance after application of a ring fixator and proximal corticectomy for segment transport to close the defect. **C.** Regenerate bone forming in the distraction zone.

to length ("traveling traction") until definitive fixation can be performed.

The disadvantages of external fixators include the following (106): (a) for complex fractures with large wounds, application can be complex and time consuming; (b) the pins may entrap musculotendinous units, restricting functional range of motion and causing patient discomfort; (c) injudiciously placed pins may interfere with soft-tissue reconstructive surgery by preventing the mobilization of flaps; these problems are often worse in the femur and humerus, which are covered by thick muscle envelopes, but can be minimized with the use of half-pin fixators; (d) inappropriate technique of pin insertion may lead to bone necrosis or early loosening of pins, and subsequent pin track infection; loosening is more of a problem in osteopenic bone and cancellous bone; and (e) prolonged use of external fixation devices, particularly non–weight-bearing ones, can lead to delayed union and nonunion of fractures.

Regardless of the external fixator used, there are common points about their application in open fractures, although irrigation and debridement are essential before fixator application. The frame should be applied to obtain as anatomic a reduction as possible. This often requires a provisional reduction be performed before or during fixator application. The pins should be predrilled using a sharp drill bit to avoid bone necrosis. The thick unicortical portion of the tibial crest should be avoided (106) because placing pins there is associated with an increased incidence of pin site necrosis.

In general, pins should be placed through intact soft tissue rather than the traumatic wound. Skin flaps should be loosely approximated before placing the pins to avoid unnecessary tethering of the soft tissues. The less soft tissue between the skin and bone, the less likely pin site problems will occur.

Indications for External Fixation

In fractures in which some type of internal or external fixation is required for stability, internal fixation traditionally is thought to be safest where the risk of infection is the lowest, and external fixation is indicated where the risk of infection is the highest (Table 12-8) (107). However, more recent work suggests that the use of intramedullary nails in open tibial fractures has a similar risk of infection at the traumatic wound site without the risks of pin tract complications (105,108–112). In the upper extremity, the violence of trauma is likely to be less than in the lower extremity and the wounds are usually less severe (113). For this reason, external fixation is used less commonly in the

TABLE 12-8 Relative Indications for Type of Skeletal Fixation in Open Fractures

External fixation
1. Severe contamination—any site

2. Periarticular fractures
   A. Definitive
      1. Distal radius
      2. Elbow dislocation
      3. Selected other sites
   B. Temporizing
      1. Knee
      2. Ankle
      3. Elbow
      4. Wrist
      5. Pelvis

3. Distraction osteogenesis

4. In combination with screw fixation for severe soft tissue injury

Internal fixation
1. Periarticular fractures
   A. Distal/proximal tibia
   B. Distal/proximal femur
   C. Distal/proximal humerus
   D. Proximal ulnar radius
   E. Selected distal radius/ulna
   F. Acetabulum/pelvis

2. Diaphyseal fractures
   A. Femur
   B. Tibia
   C. Humerus
   D. Radius/ulna

upper extremity than the lower extremity for managing open fractures.

In the humerus, external fixation is used for severe type IIIB and IIIC open fractures and in those in which comminution or poor bone quality makes internal fixation impractical or more hazardous. A single-plane, half-pin frame applied laterally works well (106).

One of the best indications for external fixation in the upper extremity is in the management of severe "sideswipe" type III open fractures of the elbow joint that result in major soft-tissue injury, bone loss, and gross instability. A half-pin frame bridging the humerus and the ulna works well. If early motion is desired, a compass-hinge external fixator is useful (114). Most open fractures of the radius and ulna can be safely managed by primary internal fixation with a very low complication rate (113,115). External fixation is most often indicated for unstable, open, comminuted, intra-articular fractures of the distal radius. External fixation from the dorsolateral radius to the second or third metacarpals works well (20,111).

Another indication for external fixation is initial management of open fractures of the pelvis where stability is essential to control hemorrhage, manage the soft tissues, and allow for early mobilization (49). Perineal wounds and ruptured viscera increase the risk of infection in open fractures of the pelvis sufficiently that external fixation is usually the acute management of choice. Fixators work well for controlling the open-book pelvic injury but are inadequate for the stabilization of pelvic ring fractures with vertical instability (54). Bulky and complicated frames have not proven adequate for pelvic ring fractures with vertical instability; therefore, simple frames using two pins in each iliac crest are sufficient for most injuries of the pelvic ring. Those with vertical instability require supplemental skeletal traction or delayed posterior internal fixation (54). Complex open, unstable fractures of the acetabulum, knee, and ankle are well managed initially by external fixators bridging these joints.

In the femur, we now rarely use external fixation in fresh open fractures as definitive treatment. Internal fixation, particularly intramedullary nailing by closed or modified open technique, is possible immediately or on a delayed basis in most cases (52,116–119). We use external fixation as a temporary fixation for diaphyseal fractures of the femur when intramedullary fixation is not possible because of severe physiologic compromise of the patient, or when there is an exceedingly contaminated type III open fracture in which the risk of infection is deemed to be too high. Open fractures of the supracondylar region of the femur are usually secondary to high-velocity trauma. Type IIIA or open supracondylar femur fractures are at increased risk for infection with primary internal fixation (111). In these fractures, initial management with limited internal fixation of the articular component with bridging external fixation of the metaphyseal component is often wise. Subsequent conversion to internal fixation with a bone graft may be possible when the condition of the soft tissues permits (120,121). Similar techniques are used for tibial plateau and pilon fractures with severe soft-tissue injuries. In pilon fractures, a bridging frame with fixation to the calcaneus and the forefoot is advisable to avoid an equinus deformity, and to ensure adequate stabilization (122). In open fractures of the tibia, external fixation remains one of the preferred methods of stabilization (60,123). Reports suggest that nonreamed medullary nails are as effective and have some advantages (105,108–112).

Postoperative Management of External Fixation

There are many protocols for care of external fixation pin sites after insertion. We have found that the primary cause of pin infection is loosening of the pin. The causes for loosening are movement of the skin and soft tissues about the pin, causing soft-tissue necrosis; the introduction of skin bacteria into the interface between the pin and deep soft tissues; and pressure necrosis of soft tissues owing to skin tension from improper skin release and technical errors in pin insertion (106).

The most effective method of skin care we have found is

simple cleansing of the entire external fixation frame, pin tracks, and skin daily with any standard commercial bathing soap to which the patient is not allergic. When the wounds are closed and any incisions around the pin sites have healed, this is easily accomplished during a daily shower by brushing down the frame with a surgical scrub brush and the pins and skin around the pins with a soft toothbrush. An effort must be made to remove all crusts and necrotic debris around the pin tracks. We have found topical antiseptics to be unnecessary, and other ointments and antibiotic solutions are rarely indicated. If any persistent drainage is noted from a pin or persistent discomfort is present, loosening of the pin and infection must be suspected. In such cases, the clamp holding the particular pin is loosened and the pin carefully examined. Frequently, loosening of the pin in the near cortex is found; this can be confirmed by x-ray. Loose pins must never be left in place. These pins are removed and, if necessary, a new pin is placed in a new location. In some cases, this may necessitate removal of the entire frame.

Questions arise regarding conversion of external fixation to internal fixation (120,124–126). The presence of infection in a pin track, whether previous or current, dramatically increases the risk of infection in secondary intramedullary internal fixation. This is generally an issue for external fixators that have been in place for 2 weeks or more. Acute pin track infection is a contraindication to acute conversion to internal fixation. In the absence of pin track infection, the safest measure is first to remove the fixator, temporarily immobilize the limb in a cast or in traction to allow for pin track healing (usually 10 to 14 days), and then proceed to internal fixation. If the fixator has been in place for a short time (<14 days), fixator removal and internal fixation can often be performed during the same anesthetic.

External fixation followed by delayed intramedullary nailing some time after removal of the fixator has resulted in infection rates of 5% to 7% (125–128).

Internal Fixation

The fear of infection has led to the traditionally accepted opinion that immediate internal fixation, or for that matter any internal fixation of open fractures, is contraindicated (107,129). However, this attitude has changed markedly. The prognosis in open fractures has improved dramatically since the two World Wars. Military surgeons, particularly from the Korean and Vietnam wars, have effected a remarkable improvement in the infection rate by using early, meticulous, and aggressive wound debridement and irrigation; immobilizing with plaster casts or traction; and leaving wounds open while using parenteral bactericidal antibiotics (107). These advances have improved the overall prognosis and given surgeons more latitude in the treatment of open fractures (Table 12-8).

Since 1970, reported infection rates in all types of open fractures have ranged from 2.1% to 9.4% (7,58,107,130). Of more importance are the infection rates in each of the fracture types. In 1972, Gustilo and Anderson (18) reported no infections in type I open fractures, an incidence of 3.8% in type II, and 9% in type III. These were fractures treated without internal fixation. Their overall infection rate was 3.2%. In their later series, the infection rate in type I open fractures was unchanged, in type II it was 1.8%, and in type III it was 18.4%, for an overall infection rate of 8.9% (18,39). They attributed this increase in infection rate to an increase in the percentage of severe type III open fractures in their practices. Of note is the 28% infection rate they encountered when type III fractures were internally fixed. Reports of primary internal fixation for open fractures have noted infection rates varying from 6% to 13% with the use of intramedullary fixation (108–110,131). The infection rate in type I open fractures approximates that of clean, elective orthopaedic surgery if a formal, meticulous debridement is carried out, and the traumatic wound is left open.

The indications for immediate internal fixation of open fractures have changed owing to advances in wound care in open fractures, improved antibiotic therapy (and resultant improvement in infection rates), and the technical advances in internal fixation. Gristina and Rovere (132) have shown that the presence of metal, per se, does not promote bacterial growth in vitro. Use of an anti-infective coating of chlorhexidine and chlorhexenol on an intramedullary implant resulted in a lower incidence of infection in an animal model (133). Internal fixation that results in stabilization of the fracture has been shown to have a lower susceptibility to infection than a fracture with gross instability of the fracture site (93,94). Few prospective, paired, randomized studies comparing internal fixation with external fixation for stabilizing open fractures have been reported. The older literature has three such studies (Table 12-9) (100,134,135). These studies showed that external fixation had a lower infection rate and higher rate of union compared with internal fixation. On this basis, the reader would conclude that internal fixation is contraindicated in open fractures. During the same period, however, Lottes and colleagues (136) showed excellent results using closed tibial nailing in the treatment of open fractures of the tibia.

Studies of internal fixation of open fractures published since the 1980s, however, have shown remarkably good results. In these series, the average acute infection rate was 8.9%, with only three cases going on to chronic osteomyelitis—a long-term infection rate of 0.8% (4,129,130). Although bone grafts were required to achieve union in a number of type III open fractures of the tibia, no nonunions occurred. All of the amputations reported occurred early in severe open fractures of the tibia in which an attempt at limb salvage was made, all cases that in the previous decade would have been amputated immediately. It is evident, however, that severe type III open fractures of the tibia remain a problem.

More than a decade ago, Bach and Hansen (137) randomized 59 open tibial shaft fractures (Gustilo type II and type III open fractures) to treatment by application of a plate or external fixator. They found that the prevalence of infection after plate fixation was 35%, compared with 13% after external fixation. Past reports show that reamed interlocking intramedullary nailing

TABLE 12-9 Internal Fixation Versus External Immobilization

Authors	Internal Fixation			External Immobilization		
	No. Cases	% Nonunion	% Infection	No. Cases	% Nonunion	% Infection
Wade and Campbell (100)	51	27	14	58	9	0
Claffey (134)	48	17	35	70	0	0
Gallinaro et al (135)	31	11	17	33	9	3
Totals	130			161		
Average incidence		18	33		9	3

is associated with an increased incidence of infection (19). The advent of minimally invasive techniques of plating that preserve soft tissues have resulted in a resurgence of interest in plate fixation for open fractures in the lower extremity. However, comparative studies of minimally invasive plating and other techniques are not yet available. Keating and colleagues (138) have reported a prospective, randomized trial of reamed versus nonreamed interlocked intramedullary nailing of tibial shaft fractures, and they recorded a 4% incidence of infection in reamed tibial nails and a 2% incidence in nonreamed tibial nails. Schemitsch and colleagues (139,140) reported the effect of reamed versus nonreamed locked tibial nailing on callous blood flow using laser Doppler flowmetry in a sheep model. They reported that the decrease in perfusion after reaming compared with the nonreamed group was an immediate effect of reaming. At 2-, 6-, and 12-week follow-up, there was no difference in callus formation between either group. Lastly, prospective studies comparing nonreamed interlocking tibial nails with external fixation for the treatment of types I, II, IIIA, and IIIB open tibial shaft fractures have reported similar or decreased rates of infection with the use of the nonreamed locked intramedullary nail compared with external fixation (105,110). Table 12-8 lists relative indications for both external fixation and internal fixation in open fractures.

Indications for Immediate Internal Fixation

When considering immediate internal fixation of an open fracture, the surgeon must take into account the "personality" of the fracture, his or her capabilities as a surgeon, the abilities of the operating room team, the adequacy of surgical equipment and implants available, and the particular situation within which the fracture must be treated. For example, will the operating room team be up to the task at 2 o'clock in the morning, and will the patient's general condition permit extensive surgery? Bone quality must be sufficient to hold screws, and the fracture must not be so comminuted that internal fixation is impossible. The surgeon should have a preoperative plan established, and must be skilled with rigid internal fixation methods. Gentleness in the management of the soft tissues is as important as technical ability in fixing the fracture.

Intra-Articular Fractures

Mitchell and Shepard (96) have shown that interfragmentary compression may play a major role in the healing of cartilage in intra-articular fractures. Llinas and colleagues (97) have demonstrated that articular step-offs heal with a different mechanism than full-thickness articular defects. In particular, they found that cartilage and subchondral bone adapt to surface incongruity by modifying their structure. This was most successful when the articular step-off was less than the thickness of the articular cartilage width. They did not find a significant benefit from continuous passive motion. Salter and colleagues (95) have shown that early institution of motion is probably necessary to achieve an optimal result. This requires rigid internal fixation of intra-articular fractures. This is especially true in weight-bearing joints, and clinical experience suggests that intra-articular fractures do best when anatomically reduced and treated with early motion for rehabilitation. These principles are applicable to open as well as closed fractures (20,141). The incidence of extensive soft-tissue injuries associated with open fractures makes this more imperative for open fractures. Intra-articular fractures not requiring internal fixation are those that are nondisplaced and stable, those in patients with limited life expectancies, or those in selected patients with neurologic diseases or paralysis. Severe comminution or underlying bone disease, which makes adequate fixation impossible, is also a contraindication to fixation.

Many open intra-articular fractures have type I wounds. The low infection rate in type I injuries makes it possible immediately to fix these fractures internally with a risk of infection roughly comparable with that of closed fractures if meticulous irrigation and debridement have been done. Because of the increased risk of infection in type II and III open fractures, careful judgment is required. Simple, noncomminuted fractures, such as displaced medial and lateral malleolus fractures, are easily internally fixed with minimum fixation through the open fracture wound. Such a simple procedure adds little to soft-tissue devitalization and accomplishes anatomic reduction and stability that greatly facilitate soft tissue management. Stabilization may even lower the infection rate rather than contribute to it (94,142).

Reports on primary open reduction and internal fixation in type III open articular fractures of the ankle and tibial plateau have shown good results (107,143–146). Early reports of primary open reduction and internal fixation of open distal intra-articular femur fractures have shown good success with type I and type II open fractures, and infection rates in type III fractures ranging from 10% to 45% (111,142). In severe type III open intra-articular fractures, staged surgery or limited internal fixation should be considered. Initially, irrigation and debridement are carried out and the wound is left open. The articular cartilage should be covered by soft tissue. At 3 to 5 days after injury, the patient is returned to the operating room, and if there is no evidence of infection, definitive internal fixation of the fracture can be carried out. After internal fixation, for ultimate safety, the wound can be left open initially and closed 3 to 5 days later. If bone grafting is required, it can be carried out at that time.

Pilon fractures are challenging injuries to treat. Restoration of the articular surface with ligamentotaxis near the anatomic position and reduction of the talus with the use of external fixation to maintain length of the fracture is a safe approach. If the soft-tissue injury is minor to moderate, delayed closure of the wounds with delayed open reduction and internal fixation, as with a closed pilon injury, may be indicated (122). However, if there is a massive injury that requires flap coverage, early internal fixation followed by flap coverage is indicated. After 7 to 21 days, and in the absence of infection, application of a buttress plate or other implants to achieve complete stability can be done more safely. It may be possible at this time to insert cancellous bone grafts. Regardless of the approach used, early motion to restore ankle function is essential (122).

When there is extensive soft-tissue injury or contamination, another approach, at the time of initial debridement, may be indicated. Anatomic reduction and internal fixation can be reserved for the articular fragments alone, with the metaphyseal portion of the fracture managed with external fixation. After successful primary closure, usually 21 or 50 days after injury, acute effects of soft-tissue trauma have resolved and rigid internal fixation of the remainder of the fracture can be undertaken with less risk. This permits early joint mobilization. If the degree of soft-tissue devitalization and contamination causes internal fixation to be delayed longer than 3 weeks after injury, or if the fracture is too comminuted to achieve rigid fixation, it is best to proceed with early joint mobilization in traction or a functional cast-brace.

An optimal end result in intra-articular fractures requires early joint mobilization and muscle rehabilitation. The worst management is to combine the risks of internal fixation with the complications of nonfunctional, external immobilization.

POSTOPERATIVE ANTIBIOTIC USE

The duration of antibiotic administration is controversial (40,147). Older literature suggests continuing intravenous antibiotics until the wound is sealed, using intraoperative cultures for direct antibiotic selection (19,37). More recent work suggests that routine cultures of open fracture wounds at the time of debridement are not cost effective (2,29). Our practice is to take no wound cultures before or after debridement. Antibiotics are given for 48 hours after the initial and any subsequent debridements, as well as after wound closure. This often translates into a patient being on antibiotics for 2 to 4 days following initial presentation and debridement. If signs of infection or drainage occur at any time, the wound is cultured and treatment is based on those cultures (148).

ANTIBIOTIC-IMPREGNATED BEADS

Numerous antibiotics can be incorporated in polymethylmethacrylate (PMMA) without losing their bactericidal activity. They leach out at rates sufficient to produce bactericidal levels in the surrounding fluids and tissues (149). PMMA antibiotic-impregnated beads in type III wounds provide high levels of local antibiotics that are not reached by systemic antibiotics in marginally vascularized soft tissue and bone (150). Commercially manufactured antibiotic beads are becoming available; however, clinical experience is limited (151). At present, antibiotic beads are routinely fabricated by hand intraoperatively. Our preference is to mix 2.4 g of tobramycin or 1 g of vancomycin powder with every 40 g of PMMA bone cement. The mixture is placed into a bead mold to create a series of 6-mm diameter beads strung on multiple-strand stainless-steel wire or nonabsorbable suture. A strand of beads can be packaged individually and sterilized with ethylene oxide gas. When the initial wound is left open, an oxygen-permeable membrane (Op-site) can be applied over the wound (Fig. 12-10). Beads are then removed and replaced as needed at subsequent repeat irrigation and debridements until the wound is closed.

Ostermann et al (152) reported the use of the bead pouch technique as a supplement to parenteral intravenous antibiotics. They compared their results with those obtained in 157 open fractures with systemic antibiotics only, and reported a statistically significant decrease in the infection rate in the group treated with the bead pouch, particularly in type IIIB open fractures. The control fractures had an infection rate of 39%, compared with an infection rate of 7.3% in those treated with a bead pouch. Keating and associates (153) have reported similar results.

Local wound levels of antibiotics produced are higher than those possible using the parenteral route alone. Local tissue levels of tobramycin greater than 400 μg/mL, however, have

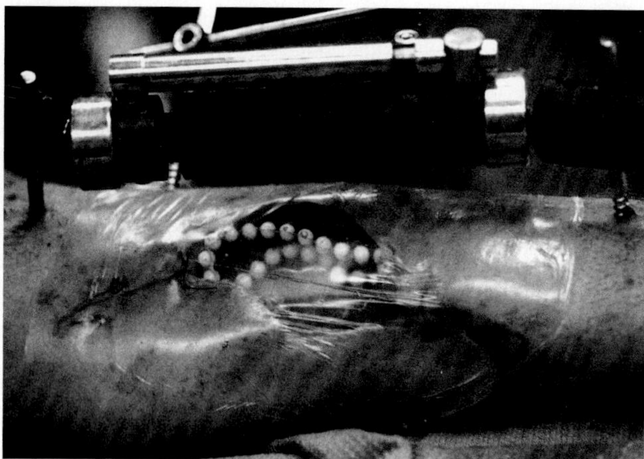

FIGURE 12-10 Photograph illustrating the use of an antibiotic bead pouch. After debridement of the wound, a chain of antibiotic beads is placed into the defect. The defect itself is covered with an oxygen-permeable barrier (Op-site), which allows serum to collect in the defect. The serum bathes the local fracture milieu in a high concentration of antibiotics.

been shown to be toxic to osteoblast cells in tissue culture (154,155). The incidence of delayed union or nonunion associated with the use of the bead pouch technique has not been well studied. Bead pouch treatment for open fractures remains a viable option, but comparative studies with alternative methods of wound treatment are still needed.

Recent advances in the treatment of osteomyelitis with biodegradable antibiotic implants may modify the established approach to local delivery of antibiotics and bone healing in open fractures (156). PMMA beads require eventual removal, and bone grafting is needed to fill any residual, structural defect. Thus, staged procedures are required. Newer osteoconductive materials, such as tobramycin-impregnated calcium sulfate alpha-hemihydrate, provide an opportunity for local antibiotic delivery while concurrently addressing any bone defect (157).

In a recent, prospective study, McKee et al used tobramycin-impregnated calcium sulfate as a local antibiotic delivery devise. Infection was (157) successfully eradicated in 23 of 25 patients with established osteomyelitis. Nine of nine isolated bone defects healed, and union was achieved in 14 of 16 nonunions. Similarly, Beardmore et al (158) examined the outcome of combined demineralized bone matrix and tobramycin-impregnated calcium sulfate in acutely contaminated, goat tibial defects. Intramedullary canal bacterial colony counts were similar in untreated controls and those treated with demineralized bone graft alone. No bacterial growth was noted on culture from tibiae treated with tobramycin-impregnated PMMA or the combined demineralized bone matrix and tobramycin-impregnated calcium sulfate (158). The use of osteoinductive and osteoconductive biodegradable antibiotic implants in human open fractures has not been reported. However, the successful treatment of acutely infected and chronically infected bone defects in the mentioned studies warrants future investigation of these devices in open fractures.

LOCAL NEGATIVE-PRESSURE DRESSINGS

In 1997, Argenta and Morykwas (159) introduced vacuum-assisted wound closure as a means to enhance wound healing through negative pressure dressings. The system consists of a polyurethane foam open cell dressing, which is contoured to the wound and sealed with an occlusive dressing. As negative pressure is applied, effluent from the wound is drawn through a suction tube embedded in the dressing and into a reservoir located in the vacuum device (Fig. 12-11A) (160). Study of this technique in animal wounds demonstrated an increase in local blood flow and an increased rate of granulation tissue formation when compared to moistened saline dressings. Decreased bacterial counts in infected animal wounds receiving negative-pressure therapy further promoted this technique as a revolutionary tool in wound management (161). This method has been successfully employed for wounds encountered by a variety of surgical disciplines (162–164) to include wounds about open fractures and exposed bone (165,166).

Defranzo recently described the successful coverage of wounds involving exposed fractures or bone in 71 of 75 patients. Granulation tissue was noted to form rapidly covering bone and hardware in many cases. Five local fascio- or musculocutaneous flaps were preformed, but no free tissue transfers were required. Vacuum assisted closure was advocated as a "first choice of treatment" in difficult lower extremity wounds (167).

Herscovici (168) has since reported on vacuum-assisted closure of high-energy soft-tissue wounds that would have initially required coverage procedures beyond split thickness skin grafting. Wound sizes varied from 60 to 400 cm^2. Underlying injuries were largely in the lower extremity (18/21) but included elbow, forearm, and acetabular fractures. Twelve wounds (57%) required no further treatment or split thickness skin graft (5/21) alone. Nine (43%) required free tissue transfer; however, the authors suggest that the generation of a favorable wound bed allows for less extensive techniques when obtaining definitive coverage (168).

Negative-pressure dressings have been successfully used in the pediatric population as well. Mooney described the treatment of 27 wounds (11 associated with acute trauma) in patients ranging from 3 days to 18 years of age. Wound closure was obtained with split thickness skin grafting following vacuum-assisted therapy in 15 of 27 cases. Two pedicle flaps for sternal dehiscence and one cross-extremity flap for a leg and foot wound were performed. No vascularized free tissue transfers were required. It was estimated that a minimum of nine patients would have required free tissue transfer had vacuum assisted closure devises not been available (169).

The technique for negative-pressure dressing application begins with basic wound care principles. Devitalized and contaminated materials must be cleared from the wound prior to initial application. Subsequent dressing changes are accomplished in conjunction with operative debridement until the wound is clean and without further necrotic tissue. Once the wound bed

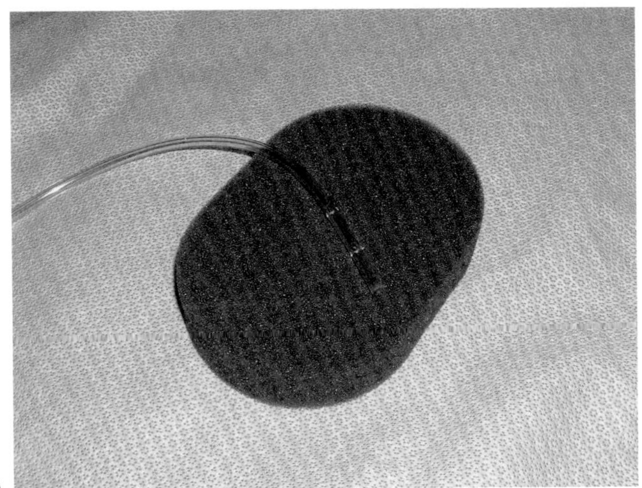

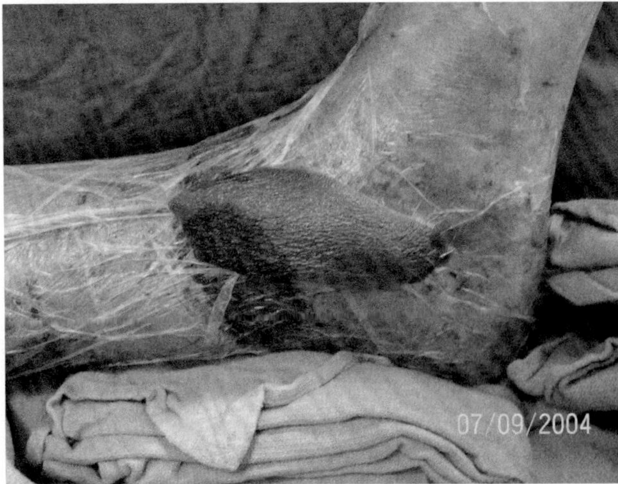

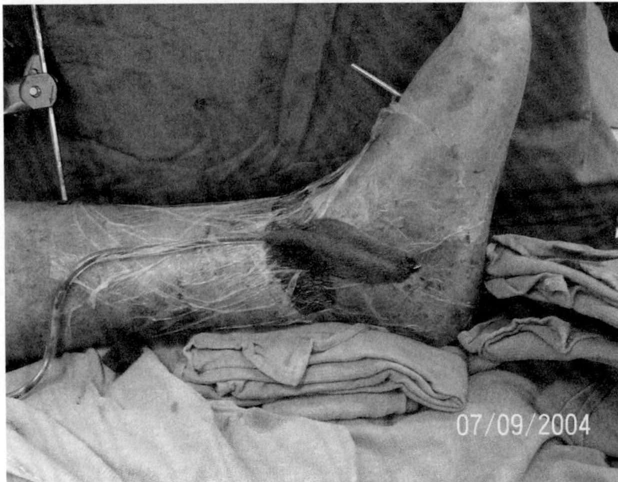

FIGURE 12-11 **A.** Typical reticulated foam sponge and suction tube. **B.** Photograph of medial, pilon fracture wound after debridement and contouring of sponge to fit within confines of wound. **C.** Wound sponge and drainage tube sealed with occlusive drape under suction. Note fixation pins for subsequent, provisional external fixation.

has been surgically prepared, the sponge is cut to fit within the confines of the skin margins (Fig. 12-11B). Direct contact with the entire wound bed is imperative to prevent creation of a dead space or uneven proliferation of granulation tissue (160). Direct contact with the skin is avoided. The suction tube is then inserted into the sponge and the construct sealed into the wound with a clear occlusive dressing (Fig. 12-11C). A mesentery about the suction tube is frequently necessary to prevent air leaks about the interface of the tube with the dressing and skin. The suction tube is then attached to the reservoir, and the vacuum device is activated.

Obtaining airtight seals is sometimes difficult, and technical tricks for application of these devices in difficult regions of anatomy, in conjunction with external fixator devises, or in areas with compromised skin have been described (160,168,170). Exposed tendon or neurovascular structures should be covered with adaptic to prevent interdigitation with the sponge. Skin bridges may be protected with adaptic as well, or a "Y" connector is used to service two sponges with one machine.

Dressing of large wounds may be simplified by tacking sponges in place with staples, particularly if further dressing changes are anticipated under anesthesia. Alternatively, wound sponges can initially be held in place by an occlusive dressing with subsequent introduction of the suction tube through a window in the dressing. The suction tube is then independently secured with a separate adhesive drape, which facilitates creation of a mesentery and airtight seal. A topical skin adhesive can augment this process. In all cases, adequate seals are best obtained when the surrounding skin is effectively blotted dry. When the skin surrounding the wound is abraded or injured, a hydrocolloid type dressing can be placed on the skin, and the occlusive bandage placed onto this dressing. Last, suction from the operative field is a useful means to establish and test the dressing seal should it need to be revised before any break in sterility. Routine wall suction is used to evacuate the dead space in the sponge, which contracts. The suction tube is then clamped. Re-expansion of the sponge implies an air leak that must be identified and revised.

Vacuum devices are routinely operated at 125 mmHg below ambient pressure in accordance with the wound healing experiences demonstrated in animal models. Lower settings (50–75 mmHg) are recommended for extensively weeping wounds or skin grafts (161,171). Intermittent therapy, initially determined to have the most pronounced healing response, is seldom used. Repetitive contraction and expansion of the sponge was poorly tolerated in the clinical setting. Subsequently, continuous therapy has generally been adopted. Wound sponges are typically changed every 48 hours. More frequent changes are recommended in young children as exuberant granulation tissue may rapidly interdigitate with the sponge. Topical lidocaine can be placed on the sponge to facilitate bedside dressing changes once wound stability precludes the need for further operative debridement (160). The duration of therapy is dependant on the size and extent of the wound. Small wounds may heal to completion with negative pressure therapy alone. Larger wounds may require skin grafting once a granulation bed is produced. Alternatively, an extensively exposed fracture site or hardware may mandate flap coverage (159). In these cases, vacuum devises provide self contained, "no touch" wound care between staged, operative debridements while preparing for the tissue transfer.

Negative pressure dressings have caused few complications. Excessive in-growth into the dressing may occur with delayed dressing changes. Maceration of the surrounding skin, local skin irritation from direct contact with the sponge, and shearing of fragile skin during dressing changes are noted infrequently. Caution is exercised when dressing large wounds, particularly in anticoagulated or debilitated patients with extensive edema (low protein levels, heart failure, etc.). Wound effluent can total 1,000 mL per 24 hours. Careful monitoring of fluid status, hemodynamics, and electrolyte status is recommended in conjunction with vigilant monitoring of the system and wound (160).

The decreased frequency of dressing changes relative to traditional wound care contributes to the cost effectiveness of the system. Wound management requires less time of physician and nursing staff as sponges may be left in place for 2 to 4 days. In addition, home therapy systems allow for ambulatory treatment, which facilitates earlier hospital release (172). The cost effectiveness of negative-pressure therapy has been well demonstrated in the setting of chronic pressure ulcers (173). However, in patients with high-energy soft-tissue injuries, Herscovici (168) estimated similar cost between vacuum-assisted closure (average $103/day) when compared to a retrospective, cohort of patients treated with traditional wet-to-dry dressings (average $100/day). The cost effectiveness of vacuum-assisted closure in the acute management of open fractures warrants further examination. This data, in conjunction with the known benefits and complications, will allow for comparison with other adjuvant therapies (i.e., antibiotic beads).

WOUND CLOSURE/COVERAGE

Primary Closure

Primary closure is occasionally indicated. If it is to be done, the following criteria must be met:

1. The original wound must have been fairly clean, and not have occurred in a highly contaminated environment.
2. All necrotic tissue and foreign material have been debrided.
3. Circulation to the limb is essentially normal.
4. Nerve supply to the limb is intact.
5. The patient's general condition is satisfactory and allows careful postoperative assessment.
6. The wound can be closed without tension.
7. Closure will not create a dead space.
8. The patient does not have multisystem injuries.

There is only anecdotal information to support the benefits of routine primary closure of open fractures (174,175). Type I open fracture wounds often meet these criteria; however, the type I wound is usually so small that closure by secondary intention is quite satisfactory. Type III wounds should never be closed primarily. Type II wounds require careful judgment and in general should be left open. Wounds that are more than 8 to 12 hours old at time of initial debridement should not be considered for primary closure. The biggest risk of primary closure is anaerobic infection resulting in gas gangrene. This can occur in very benign-seeming wounds. If the surgeon is inexperienced or in doubt, it seems wise to invoke the axiom, "When in doubt, leave it open," or, even better, "It is never wrong to leave an open fracture open." In rare instances, the soft-tissue injury is so severe that flap coverage is clearly indicated from the initial presentation. This scenario is most common in fractures to the tibia and fibula. Several authors have reported on radical debridement, immediate fracture stabilization, and immediate definitive flap coverage (176–179). Early reports with favorable results are available.

However, in most cases, a flap is not required and an elective portion of the wound made by the surgeon can be closed, leaving the traumatic wound open. It is particularly important to cover primarily tendon without peritenon and bone not covered by periosteum, because desiccation results in the death of these structures. Usually some local muscle or fat can be drawn across these structures, leaving the skin open. The same rationale applies to open joints, where we usually close the capsule over a suction drain and leave the remainder of the wound open.

On the other hand, there seems little question that fractured bones heal most rapidly when they are enclosed by infection-free, pliable, vascularized soft tissues. One of the early objectives of treating an open fracture is to convert it to a closed one. This is probably best accomplished by delayed primary closure.

Delayed Primary Closure

In the healthy adult, the wound-healing process proceeds for the first 5 days or so regardless of whether the wound is closed. As long as closure is achieved before the fifth day, wound strengths at 14 days are comparable with those in wounds closed on the first day. This is why closure before the fifth day is termed *delayed primary closure* (51). There are several advantages to this approach: leaving the wound open minimizes the risk of anaerobic infection, and the delay allows the host to mount local wound defensive mechanisms that permit safer closure than is possible on the first day.

Leaving Wounds Open

Surgeons show a strong tendency to put drains into wounds that have been left open. When draining an established abscess or tissue spaces that tend naturally to reseal themselves (e.g., palmar space, subgluteal space), the reasons for and usefulness of such drains are acknowledged. However, standard mechanical drains (e.g., the Penrose) may irritate the tissues they contact and incite an innocent exudate. The trouble lies in the uncertainty that such an exudate is, in fact, innocent.

Options for management of major soft-tissue wounds include the traditional treatment of packing the wound with gauze dressings inserted to a point just beneath the fascia. The wound should not be packed tightly because this often promotes open "dead space" and prevents adequate drainage. Loosely placed dressings conduct any drainage from the wound to the surface by capillary action. In cases where tendon and bone lack soft-tissue coverage, it may be useful to keep the wound moist by inserting a catheter through which sterile fluid can be dripped, or a bead pouch to prevent tissue desiccation. Negative-pressure dressings can be used as well. Ordinarily, the wound is not exposed on the ward for inspection, but is reexamined at the time of delayed primary closure, 2 to 5 days after injury.

The decision to use a bead pouch or vacuum-assisted closure device is controversial. Both have the advantage of providing a moist, tissue friendly environment for the wound. The bead pouch offers high concentrations of bacterial antibiotics whereas negative-pressure dressings constantly remove effluent from the wound. To date, no comparative trials have been reported for these two methods of wound management. The decision is ultimately based on the treating physician's preference.

Should local symptoms of pain, odor, or obviously excessive drainage appear early on, or should more general signs of fever, leukocytosis, or other problems be noted, early return to the operating room for inspection and repeat irrigation and debridement is warranted. In type III open fractures and those that occurred in a highly contaminated environment, early return to the operating room within 24 to 48 hours may be indicated for wound inspection and repeat irrigation and debridement. This is particularly necessary if the original irrigation and debridement were thought to be marginal.

When wound closure is not possible by approximately the fifth day, particularly when there is residual necrotic tissue in the wound that would benefit from dressing changes, serial dressing changes in the patient's bed may be necessary. This is particularly true if infection intervenes (61). We prefer wet-to-dry dressing changes performed every 12 hours, using either normal saline or half-strength Dakin's solution.

Closure by direct suturing is possible in most cases. Only the minimum amount of suture material is placed deep in the wound. Tension in the closure is avoided because this may produce necrosis of skin edges and deeper soft tissues. If primary closure of the wound without tension is not possible, alternatives are "relaxing" incisions and split-thickness skin grafts. The routine use of suction-irrigation systems is not indicated. Standard suction drainage to eliminate dead space and prevent accumulation of hematoma is used regularly in our practice.

Relaxing Incisions

A linear wound with minimal soft tissue loss may be difficult to close because of underlying swelling. When it is important to obtain full-thickness coverage over bone or other structures, closure can often be effected with a relaxing incision (51,180,181), creating a bipedicular fasciocutaneous flap. Relaxing incisions produce different types of local flaps, the most characteristic being a bipedicular flap. Care must be exercised to place these flaps sufficiently distant from the original wound that the blood supply to the intervening skin is not threatened. This is a particular problem if the skin between the two wounds has been injured. The relaxing incision must be long enough to allow closure of the primary wound without tension. Relaxing incisions are best suited to those areas in which there is some natural mobility of the skin and underlying tissue, such as the thigh and proximal leg, but less so where mobility is limited, as in the lower leg, ankle region, and about the wrist. Local rotational flaps are also helpful in obtaining wound closure (Fig. 12-12). Mechanical devices to aid closure may be useful, but we do not have enough experience with them to advocate their use at this time.

Split-Thickness Skin Grafts

In most cases where the wound bed is composed of viable vascularized soft tissues, a split-thickness skin graft provides the best method of closure (182). This avoids the risk of a bipedicular flap, and is better cosmetically because it leaves only one wound rather than two, because the opened relaxing incision requires split-thickness skin grafting as well. In addition, when edema subsides, the skin graft contracts, and often the resulting wound is much smaller and more cosmetically acceptable. If it is not, late excision and primary closure to produce a cosmetically acceptable wound may be possible.

Split-thickness skin grafts require support from host tissues on which they are deposited and do best when placed directly on viable muscle or well-formed granulation tissue (182). Granulation tissue is not necessary as long as the underlying tissues are well vascularized. Split grafts do not take on bare tendons or on bone not covered by periosteum. Their prospect for survival is somewhat less certain on tissues with a limited blood supply, such as periosteum, fascia, and joint capsule.

Flap Coverage

When soft tissue loss is extensive and closure by primary suture or split-thickness skin graft is not possible, flaps become neces-

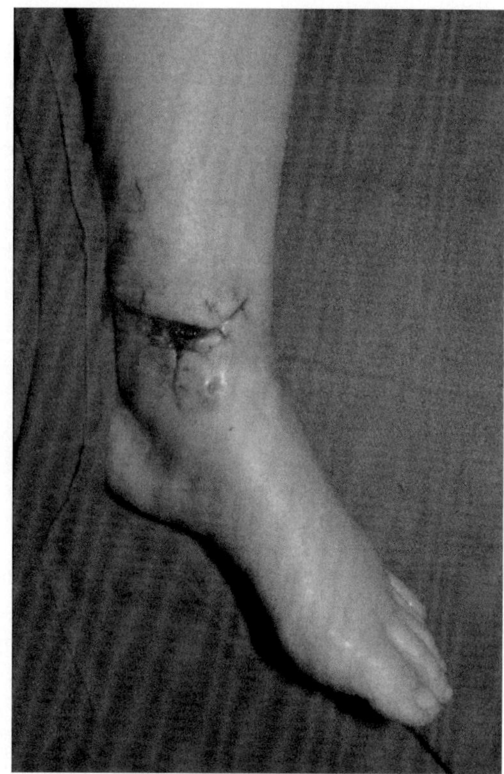

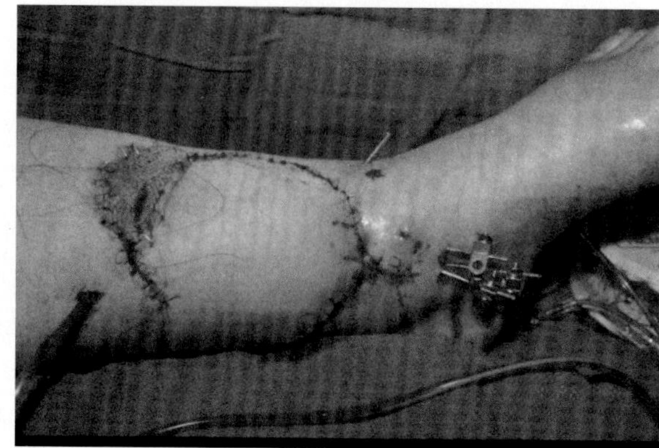

FIGURE 12-12 **A.** AP radiograph of a wound in the distal tibia. This is a transverse wound that has had a longitudinal extension but now has difficulty closing. This can be a common occurrence in patients with poor circulation or severe soft-tissue injury. **B.** The wound is closed after a local rotational flap has been mobilized and inset in this area with a small split-thickness skin graft as well.

sary. The types of flaps available are local fasciocutaneous flaps, local muscle pedicle flaps, remote muscle pedicle flaps, and free microvascularized muscle flaps (6,7,176,180,183,184). This is a very extensive topic in itself and is described in detail in Chapter 16. Suffice it to say that surgeons treating open fractures must be skilled in using all of these flaps or have available a colleague with such skills. Flaps usually are not done at the time of initial irrigation and debridement because it often is very difficult to predict the amount of progressive local tissue necrosis that may occur; a flap placed at this time may, in effect, result in primary closure of the wound (7,51) (Fig. 12-13). Where bone, tendon, and other structures require immediate coverage, we swing a local muscle flap without actually closing the entire wound (180). Otherwise, we believe most flaps are best done at approximately 5 days after injury. Most coverage problems occur in the tibia, and the fracture surgeon should be familiar with the gastrocnemius, soleus, anterior tibial, and flexor hallucis and flexor digitorum local muscle flaps (see Chapter 16) (102).

Biologic Dressings

When closure is not appropriate or cannot be carried out, and arrangements cannot be made for the covering of vulnerable tissues by the transposition of local tissues, biologic dressings of skin or synthetic material may be of value. Homologous human skin, heterologous porcine skin (prepared commercially), and other synthetic dressings may suffice (185). Biobrane has been routinely used to cover fasciotomy sites with good results, and changing these dressings is generally less painful. They seem to be a deterrent to infection, and there is some evidence that existing infection may be suppressed or controlled. Because host granulation tissue invades such grafts, these biologic dressings are frequently followed for indications of adequate wound bed preparation for definitive autogenous grafting. Thus, such grafts need to be changed frequently.

Elevation

Perhaps there is no more critical factor in the control of post-debridement swelling than the simple matter of elevation. Persistent or increased swelling may keep tissues turgid and wound surfaces moist, thereby preventing delayed primary closure. Edematous tissues increase tension on the suture line and may lead to marginal wound necrosis. Other disadvantages of swelling include a possible increase in the prospect of infection, a loss of reduction of fracture should swelling require a cast be split and spread, and probably an increased risk of thrombophlebitis.

Limbs must be elevated in a manner that is comfortable for the patient and guarantees continuous elevation at a level above the heart; however, elevation more than 10 cm above the heart does not enhance lymphatic or venous return but does decrease the arterial input to the limb, which can be hazardous in impending compartment syndrome and in patients with peripheral

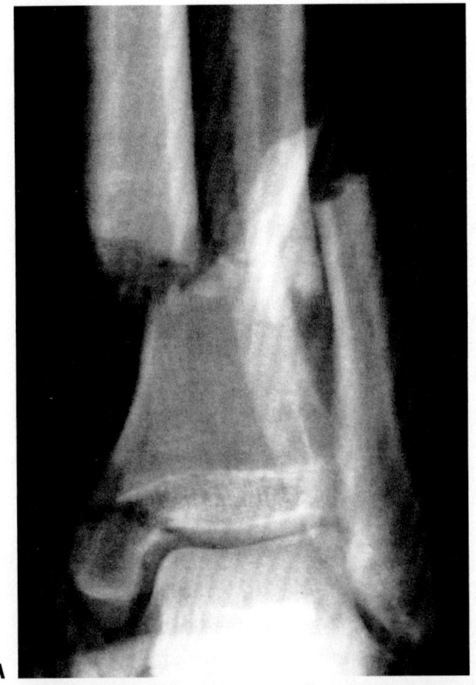

A

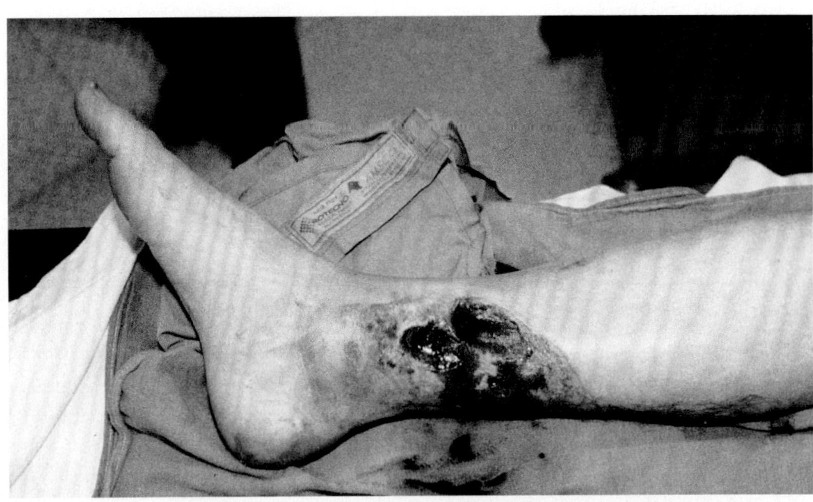

B

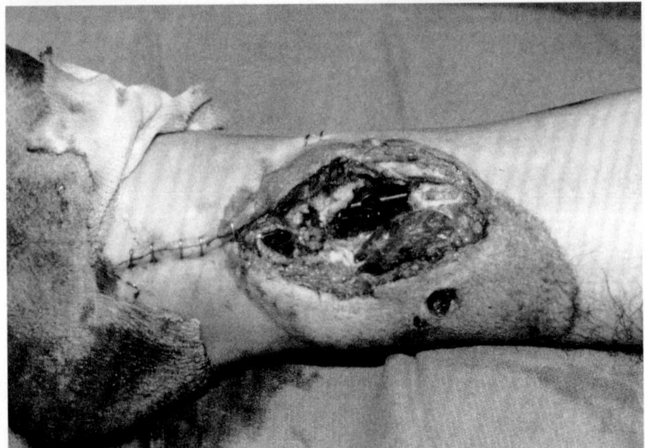

C

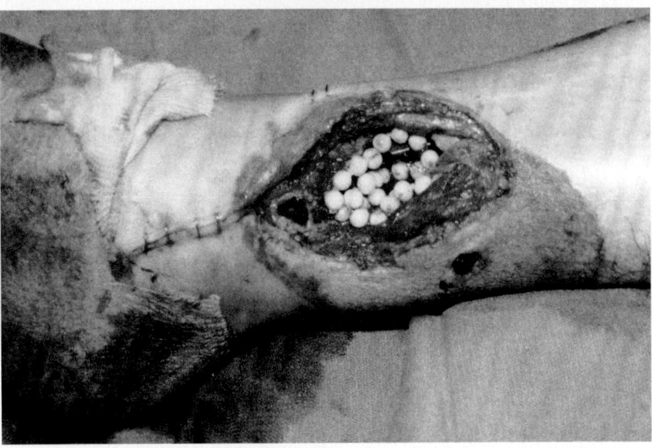

D

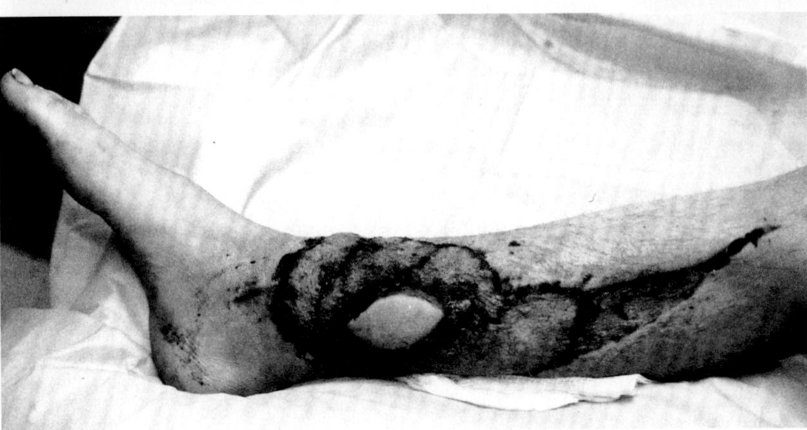

E

FIGURE 12-13 **A.** Anteroposterior x-ray of an open fracture of the tibia and fibula. **B.** Photograph showing the initial traumatic wound, which is based medially. **C.** The fracture is treated with irrigation and debridement of the open wound, plating of the fibular shaft, screw fixation of the medial malleolus, and intramedullary nailing of the distal shaft. This photograph shows the wound after debridement. The intramedullary nail can be seen through bone defect present at the fracture site. **D.** Photograph showing antibiotic beads in place in the fracture defect as an antibiotic bead pouch is being placed. **E.** The soft-tissue defect has been covered with a free vascularized myocutaneous flap.

vascular disease. Under most circumstances, broad slings suspended from the overhead frame serve best.

COMPLICATIONS

The management of open fractures is complex as there are many factors that influence acute treatment in addition to potential complications, which may occur subsequent to initial management. Factors that influence acute treatment include local factors, such as soft-tissue loss, nerve or vessel injury, segmental bone loss, compartment syndrome, and bacterial contamination. Treatment strategies have been presented in this chapter to assist in management of these conditions so as to minimize complications.

Systemic factors may influence treatment as well. Open fractures frequently occur in patients who have sustained multiple injuries or polytrauma to include injury to the head, chest, or abdomen. Such severe injuries invoke a systemic inflammatory response and syndrome (SIRS), which may progress to fulminant and fatal adult respiratory distress syndrome (ARDS) or multisystem organ failure of the lungs, liver, intestines, and kidneys. In models of SIRS, surgery is considered a secondary "hit" or catalyst, which propagates the systemic inflammatory response, and if undertaken injudiciously, may lead to the further systemic insult. In these cases, the orthopaedic surgeon must coordinate care of orthopaedic injuries with the ongoing management of the critically ill patient (186). Antibiotic therapy should be tailored to meet changes in kidney function. Treatment plans for long bone fractures may require modification as reaming for intramedullary nails has been associated with ARDS and subsequent death (187). Recently, the concept of damage control orthopaedics has been promoted. Acute interventions are tailored to minimize the initial surgical insult while providing skeletal stability. These procedures must be balanced with reports of decreased morbidity associated with early definitive fixation of fractures.

Alternatively, a history of diminished immunocompetence must be considered and sought out as this may predispose the patient to poor wound healing and infection. A history of diabetes, immunosuppressive therapy (rheumatologic disease, previous organ transplant, etc.), or immunosuppression acquired by transmittable disease must be identified and investigated (188). Similarly malnutrition, reflected by an absolute lymphocyte count less than 1,500 or albumin less than 3.5 g/dl, may impose additional risks and should be aggressively addressed (189).

Closed head injury occurs in approximately 500,000 persons per year in the United States. Approximately 100,000 will have some form of residual disability. Hypotension during the initial stages of brain injury can lead to further detriment in neurologic outcome (13). Subsequently, plans for operative care, particularly procedures associated with large volume shifts or blood loss, must be coordinated with the treating neurosurgeon and intensive care staff in this patient population. In addition, these patients may not be capable of actively participating in rehabilitative protocols or communicating with attending physicians. Modifications in rehabilitative efforts such as aggressive passive, as opposed to active, motion of affected joints are initiated in anticipation of recovery. Wounds should be closely followed and inspected to look for signs of infection when symptoms cannot be conveyed.

Infection and sepsis are major complications associated with open fractures. A contamination rate of approximately 65% has been reported (27). Infection rates range from 0% to 2% for type I fractures through 10% to 50% for type III fractures (190). Acute infection predisposes the patient to the possibility of acute sepsis and chronic osteomyelitis. Sepsis as the result of an infected open fracture is managed by aggressive irrigation and debridement or possibly amputation when reconstruction appears futile and infection is overwhelming. Several investigators have attempted to look at the relationship between timing of initial operative irrigation and debridement and complications of infection or nonunion (191–194). All authors agree the operative management of an open fracture is an urgent issue, no study has shown a direct relationship between timing of initial operative care and infection. However, there is strong data correlating a delay in antibiotic administration with increased infection rates (33).

Chronic osteomyelitis, which may develop in 5% of cases following open fracture, is similarly managed by repeat debridement of the infective nidus and sequestrum and may require revision of previous reconstructive efforts in certain cases. Sequelae of osteomyelitis include altered structural stability of the bone that affects function (195). Frequently, previously placed hardware must be removed as these metallic surfaces offer a host site for persistent colonization and infection (196). When chronic osteomyelitis requires implant removal prior to fracture union, the patient has an infected nonunion. External fixation constructs are often used to replace internal fixation in attempt to avoid hardware placement within the infected area. Ultimately, the patient must endure the morbidity of repetitive operative procedures and the loss of limb function before resolution of any ongoing infection (197). In severe cases amputation becomes a viable reconstructive option. As such, this complication is aggressively avoided.

In the absence of osteomyelitis, loss of function is occasionally the result of delayed or nonunion. Nonunion rates vary according to the location of the fracture but have been specifically focused upon in the tibia. Nonunion following open tibia fracture may occur in as many as 48% of cases depending on the type of injury and method of treatment (198). Concern for occult infection is always warranted and excluded prior to and concurrent to subsequent intervention. Several authors have identified the presence of an open fracture as a significant risk factor in the development of a nonunion or delayed union (199,200). One recent series of open tibia fractures suggested early administration of bioactive proteins at the time of wound closure decreased the need for secondary interventions for fracture union (201). Further work need to be done in this area. Specific treatment methods regarding delayed union or nonunion are elaborated upon elsewhere in this text. In general, nonunions following open fracture are approached with cautious exclusion of occult infection, delayed reconstruction, and attempts at fixation exclusive of the zone of injury when possible (i.e., external fixation).

Loss of function subsequent to an open fracture is an important complication. Loss of function may result from loss of muscle mass, nerve injury, or unrecognized compartment syndrome. The injury from an open fracture may necessitate the removal of an entire compartment within the extremity. Alternatively, disruption of innervation may further contribute to loss of function within a compartment or limb. In certain cases, particularly within the upper extremity, tendon transfer may be required to obtain satisfactory function. Alternatively, loss of protective sensation due to extensive nerve injury may influence the decision to amputate in the setting of massive trauma. Loss of function due to decreased range of motion is generally addressed with physical therapy or occasionally with arthroscopic or open release. Unrecognized compartment syndrome, however, results in significant morbidity due to contracture, loss of motor function, and variable loss of sensation (202).

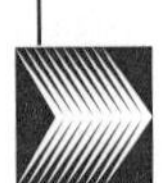

AUTHORS' PREFERRED TREATMENT

The approach to evaluation and treatment of the patient with open fractures follows the discussion outline in this chapter. Several areas of treatment warrant further comment.

Evaluation

Depending upon the practice setting, the orthopedist may find himself/herself in the position of being the primary managing physician of the trauma patient. Physicians practicing in this environment should become very knowledge in the evaluation and management strategies outlined in the "Advanced Trauma Life Support" course as promulgated by the American College of Surgeons. In addition, the orthopedist practicing in the community should become familiar with local and state trauma system guidelines, referral networks for tertiary care, and Emergency Medical Treatment and Active Labor Act (EMTALA) regulations.

Antibiotic therapy should begin early in the process of emergency department evaluation. The initial therapy with gram-positive coverage (i.e., first-generation cephalosporin, or its equivalent) should be given to all patients upon admission once an open fracture is diagnosed. Multidrug therapy for gram-negative and anaerobic organism coverage can be added as the wound, or environmental history of the injury mandates.

Documentation of the initial presentation is increasingly important. With the wide availability of low-cost digital photography, digital images of the injured extremity and wound are now routine in our institution. Physicians using this technology should develop a standardized method for tracking these images so they are available for review in a timely manner by all treating physicians.

Questions of timing of initial radiographic evaluation often arise. Should the x-rays be taken with or without splints? Should radiographs be performed with or without splints? The answer to this question depends upon the systems available in the emergency department in which the physician practices. If radiographs can be taken in the emergency department while the orthopedist can control and align fractures, and still apply splints in a timely manner then performing the radiographs without splints is appropriate. However, if the patient must travel to the Radiology Suite for x-rays to be performed, typically the limb is splinted before obtaining x-rays. There is no justification to delay realignment of the limb or dressing the wound simply to obtain a better x-ray. Details of the fracture pattern can be evaluated with fluoroscopy in the OR, or with other imaging techniques, such as computerized tomography, if needed.

Do complete biplanar images have to be done in the emergency department before traveling to the operating room? Complete imaging is necessary before making the final treatment decision. However, often there is enough information on a single view of the injured limb to determine a basic operative plan. The decision as to complete formal imaging in the emergency department before travel to the OR depends heavily upon the patient's status. Patients in physiologic extremeness, vascular compromise, or with severe contamination of open wounds warrant an abbreviated session of radiology and expedited flow to the operating room. Plain x-rays are often the last studies to be performed after a computerized tomography and angiography, etc. If the patient's physiologic status and wounds are such that definitive fracture stabilization is anticipated at the first operative session, then taking the time to obtain quality biplanar x-rays is recommended. However, if it is anticipated that definitive fixation is not appropriate at the first operating room session, then obtaining a limited series of plain x-rays with plans for intraoperative imaging or delayed formal imaging is a better option in these instances.

Operative Debridement

The question of urgency in proceeding to the operating room for surgical debridement of an open fracture commonly arises. Early aggressive wound debridement and irrigation is universally recommended to decrease the incidence of infection and sepsis. The development of infection is a multifactorial process that involves a number of variables including the extent of soft tissue damage and bacterial contamination, predisposing health conditions of the patient, and the patient's physiologic status upon presentation to name a few. As suspected in such a complex condition developing strong type I evidence of the effect of a single variable, i.e., a time from injury to operative debridement, for a single outcome measure, i.e., infection, is very difficult.

Yet, it is universally accepted among orthopedists that an open fracture in a patient, or especially a family member, is clearly a surgical emergency. It is important to the care of our patients to maintain the relative emergent status of open fractures in our daily practice. It is well known that bacterial contamination will expand in an environment of necrotic tissue. What is unclear is how extensive the tissue necrosis is in a traumatic wound at the time of patient presentation.

Wound debridement is occasionally viewed as an uninteresting part of the operative treatment, to be given to the member of the surgical team with the least experience. However, in reality, wound debridement involves experience and good clinical judgment to be done properly. The key concepts in my experience are:

1. Extend the wound until healthy tissue is found. The extent of injured soft tissue and not the integumentary wound determines the zone of injury for the open fracture.
2. Use a systematic approach to wound debridement once the extent of the zone of injury is determined. In this sense, the older term "wound excision" is appropriate. Excise necrotic tissue layer by layer from skin to bone. This is particularly important in large complex wounds where it is easy to miss areas of contamination without a systematic debridement approach.
3. Use fasciotomy frequently. Of all the tissues in the extremity, retained necrotic muscle poses the greatest threat to the patient in the acute setting. The primary purpose of the debridement is to assess the status of soft tissues, especially muscle. In order to adequately access the muscle the fascia must be opened. A fasciotomy of the involved compartment in which the fracture is open is part of the debridement process.
4. Consider the need for repeat access to damaged tissue. In the setting of a high-energy trauma it is possible to have muscle necrosis that continues to evolve after the initial injury and primary debridement. It is important in this setting to reinspect those areas with potential necrosis. Occasionally definitive skeletal fixation will prevent reinspection of these areas. An example of this is a high-energy tibia fracture with an anterior wound. At the time of initial debridement the deep posterior compartment can be accessed by displacing the fracture. If these posterior tissues appear to be of questionable viability at the end of the primary debridement, consideration should be given to temporizing fixation with an external fixator or splint initially. This allows the fracture to be redisplaced at the time of repeat debridement to access the deep posterior compartment musculature. An IM nail initially will preclude the surgical access. This may necessitate additional incisions if further debridement in this area is necessary.

Skeletal Stabilization

The use of temporary external fixation or spanning external fixator frames is increasingly common. This is due to the recognition that delayed definitive fixation appears beneficial in the setting of the patient with physiologic instability, and many orthopedists practice in multispecialty groups with one or more physicians who perform definitive fracture fixation on a delayed or semielective basis. Regardless of the reason, the basic principles of applying temporary fixation frames are similar.

1. When applying a temporizing external fixator, take the time to use a marking pen to draw potential future surgical incisions that may be used for definitive fixation.
2. Make an effort to align the fracture fragments as anatomically as possible with the use of traction and the spanning external fixator. Maintaining the soft tissues out to length and joints in a reduced position greatly facilitates secondary reconstruction.
3. Temporizing external fixation does not have to be as robust as definitive external fixation. That is, one chance pin per bony segment is often enough to allow for axial traction to realign the bony segments. This may be enough depending upon the fracture pattern and fracture location.
4. Always supplement the temporary external fixation with external splinting. This helps prevent the out of plane displacement that may occur, and provides additional support for the limb. This is particularly important around the foot and ankle where maintaining the foot and ankle in a neutral position prevents late equinus deformity.

Collaborative Planning

Often initial orthopaedic management of open fractures occurs in conjunction with a general surgeon, or other surgical services. Preoperative discussions regarding the choreography of the operation can greatly facilitate the efficiency of the operative procedure for the patient and the surgeon. Issues that can be resolved before the patient enters the operating room include:

1. Choice of operating table. Is a radiolucent table needed?
2. In what order will procedures occur? Who will go first?
3. What equipment is required for the planned procedure?
4. Where will the patient go after the procedure? Is an intensive care unit bed required?
5. What are the anesthetic requirements for the surgical procedure?

Postoperative Dressing

When traumatic wound edges cannot be safely approximated because of tissue loss or extensive contamination the choice of postoperative dressing is not always clear cut. Either an antibiotic bead pouch or negative-pressure dressing such as a wound vacuum may be used. In our experience, both are effective at maintaining a viable wound in most situations after open fractures.

The antibiotic bead pouch technique provides high levels of antibiotic locally in the wound. Maintaining the seal of the bead pouch is often problematic in areas about the foot and ankle. If used here, the skin must be inspected at regular intervals as leaking serum from the bead pouch accumulates in the dependent position under the heel. This can lead to maceration of the skin over the Achilles tendon and skin slough in severe cases. We use the antibiotic bead pouch technique for those wounds that are highly contaminated or occur in an environment that has a likelihood of a high level of bacterial contamination.

Negative-pressure dressings such as a wound vacuum have the advantage of a sealed system with contained drainage. This has resulted in a marked decrease in drainage soaking bed linens of the patient with open fractures. This leads to improved ease of nursing care and potentially to better hygiene for the patient and the wound. We have adopted the use of wound vacuum dressings regularly for open fractures when the tissue bed is clean and without significant contamination. Further investigations are needed to determine the clinical efficacy, as well as the cost effectiveness of these two techniques for postoperative dressings.

Primary wound closure in an open fracture is an increasingly popular topic. The advocates of primary wound closure note that the importance of wound debridement has been widely accepted. As a result of recognition of the importance of adequacy of debridement, primary closure is safe in selected clinical settings. In our practice, primary closure is reserved for patients whose open fractures meet these criteria:

1. A type I or type II open fracture.
2. Viable skin, fascia, and subcutaneous flaps.
3. A thorough debridement can be performed in a timely manner.
4. The skin can be closed without tension.

Those patients who are treated with primary closure of the open fracture wound are followed carefully postoperatively. Any wounds that show signs of increased erythema, increasing pain, or increasing drainage are taken back to the operating room for a second look irrigation and debridement procedure. This technique is best performed by surgeons with extensive experience in the treatment and debridement of open fractures.

REFERENCES

An asterisk denotes a Level 1 evidence-based reference.

1. Olson SA. Open fractures of the tibial shaft. *Instr Course Lect* 1997;46:293–302.
2. Olson SA, Schemitsch EH. Open fractures of the tibial shaft: an update. *Instr Course Lect* 2003;52:623–631.
3. Worlock P. The prevention of infection in open fractures. In: Bunker TD, Colton CL, Webb JK, eds. *Frontiers in fracture management*. Cambridge: Cambridge University Press, 1989.
4. Chapman MW, Mahoney M. The role of internal fixation in the management of open fractures. *Clin Orthop* 1979;138:120–131.
5. Grewe SR, Stephens BO, Perlino C, et al. Influence of internal fixation on wound infections. *J Trauma* 1987;27:1051–1054.
6. Fischer MD, Gustilo RB, Vareka TF. The timing of flap coverage, bone grafting, and intramedullary nailing in patients who have a fracture of the tibial shaft with extensive soft tissue injury. *J Bone Joint Surg Am* 1991;73:1316–1322.
7. Byrd HS, Cierny G III, Tebbetts JB. The management of open tibial fractures with associated soft-tissue loss: external pin fixation with early flap coverage. *Plast Reconstr Surg* 1981;68:73–82.
8. Heier KA, Infante AF, et al. Open fractures of the calcaneus soft-tissue injury determines outcome. *J Bone Joint Surg* 2003;85-A(12):2276–2282.
9. Tscherne H. The management of open fractures. In: *Fractures with soft tissue injuries*. New York: Springer-Verlag, 1984.
10. Wangensteen OH, Wangensteen SD. The rise of surgery from empiric craft to scientific discipline. Minneapolis: University of Minnesota Press, 1978; as cited in Behrens F. Fractures with soft tissue injuries. In: Wangensteen OH, Wangensteen SD, eds. *Skeletal trauma*. Philadelphia: WB Saunders, 1992.
11. Trueta J. *The principles and practice of war surgery with reference to the biological method of the treatment of war wounds and fractures*. St. Louis: CV Mosby, 1943.
12. Lin CPT, David L, Kirk MAJ, et al. Evaluation of orthopaedic injuries in operation enduring freedom. *J Ortho Trauma* 2004;18:300–305.
13. Krantz BE. *Advanced trauma life support for doctors* (ATLS), 6th ed. Chicago: American College of Surgeons, 1997.
14. Neimi TA, Norton LW. Vaginal injuries in patients with pelvic fractures. *J Trauma* 1985;25:547–551.
15. Chapman MW. Role of bone stability in open fractures. *Instr Course Lect* 1982;31: 75–87.
16. Aufranc OC, Jones WN, Bierbaum BE. Gas gangrene complicating fracture of the tibia. *JAMA* 1969;209:2045–2047.
17. Bonatus TJ, Alexander AH. Posttraumatic Aeromonas hydrophilia osteomyelitis. *Orthopedics* 1990;13:118–163.
18. Gustilo RB, Anderson JT. Prevention of infection in the treatment of one thousand and twenty five open fractures of long bones: retrospective and prospective analyses. *J Bone Joint Surg Am* 1976;58:453–458.
19. Olson, SA. Open fractures of the tibial shaft. *J Bone Joint Surg Am* 1996;78:1428–1436.
20. Muller ME, Allgover M, Schneider R, et al. *Manual of internal fixation: techniques recommended by the AO group*. 2nd ed. New York: Springer-Verlag, 1979.
21. Ruedi T, Border JR, Allgower M. Appendix B: classification of soft tissue injuries. In: Allgower M, ed. *Manual of internal fixation*. New York: Springer-Verlag, 1991:151.
22. Gustilo RB, Mendoza RM, Williams DN. Problems in the management of type III (severe) open fractures: a new classification of type III pen fractures. *J Trauma* 1984;24: 742–746.
23. Brumback RJ, Jones AL. Interobserver agreement in the classification of open fractures of the tibia: the results of a survey of 245 orthopaedic surgeons. *J Bone Joint Surg Am* 1994;76:1162–1166.
24. Trafton PG. Tibial shaft fractures. In: Browner BD, Jupiter JB, Levine AM, et al., eds. *Skeletal trauma*. Philadelphia: WB Saunders, 1998:2187–2293.
25. Sudkamp N, Haas N, Flory PJ, et al. Kriterien der Amputation, Rekonstruktion, und Replantation von Extremitaten bei Mehrfachverletzen. *Chirurg* 1989;60:774–781.
26. Kaysinger KK, Nicholson NC, Ramp WK, et al. Toxic effects of wound irrigation solutions on cultured tibiae and osteoblasts. *J Orthop Trauma* 1995;9:303–311.
*27. Patzakis MJ, Harvey JP Jr, Ivler D. The role of antibiotics in the management of open fractures. *J Bone Joint Surg Am* 1974;56:532–541.
28. Carsenti-Etesse H, Donyon F, et al. Epidemiology of bacterial infection during management of open leg fractures. *Eur J Clin Microbiol Infect Dis* 1999;18(5):315–323.
29. Lee J. Efficacy of cultures in the management of open fractures. *Clin Orthop* 1997;339: 71–75.
30. Valenziano CP, Chattar-Cora D, et al. Efficacy of primary wound cultures in long bone open extremity fractures: are they of any value? *Arch Orthop Trauma Surg* 2002;122(5): 259–261.
31. Worlock P, Slack R, Harvey L, et al. The prevention of infection in open fractures: an experimental study of the effect of fracture stability. *Injury* 1994;25:31–38.
32. Yang EC, Eisler J. Treatment of isolated type I open fractures: is emergent operative debridement necessary? *Clin Orthop Relat Res* 2003;(410):289–294.
33. Gosselin RA, Roberts I, Gillespie J. Antibiotics for preventing infection in open limb fractures. *Cochrane Database Syst Rev* 2004;(1):CD003764.
34. Cooney WP III, Fitzgerald RH Jr, Dobyns JH, et al. Quantitative wound cultures in upper extremity trauma. *J Trauma* 1982;22:112–117.
35. Robson MC, Duke WF, Krizek TJ. Rapid bacterial screening in the treatment of civilian wounds. *J Surg Res* 1973;14:426–430.
*36. Braun R, Enzler MA, Rittman WW. A double-blind clinical trial of prophylactic cloxacillin in open fractures. *J Orthop Trauma* 1987;1:12–17.
37. Waterman NG, Howell RS, Babich M. The effects of a prophylactic antibiotic (cephalothin) on the incidence of wound infection. *Arch Surg* 1968;97:365–370.
38. Zalavras CG, Patzakis MJ. Open fractures: evaluation and management. *J Am Acad Orthop Surg* 2003;11(3):212–219.
39. Gustilo RB. Current concepts in the management of open fractures. *Instr Course Lect* 1987;36:359–366.
40. Wilkins J, Patzakis M. Choice and duration of antibiotics in open fractures. *Orthop Clin North Am* 1991;22:433–437.

41. Russell GV Jr, King C, May CG, Pearsall AW 4th. Once daily high-dose gentamicin to prevent infection in open fractures of the tibial shaft: a preliminary investigation. *South Med J* 2001;94(12):1185–1191.
*42. Patzakis MJ, Bains RS, Lee J, et al. Prospective, randomized, double-blind study comparing single-agent antibiotic therapy, ciprofloxacin, to combination antibiotic therapy in open fracture wounds. *J Orthop Trauma* 2000;14:529–533.
43. Alonge TO, Ogunlade SO, Salawu SA, Fashina AN. Microbial isolates in open fractures seen in the accident and emergency unit of a teaching hospital in a developing country. *West Afr J Med* 2002;21(4):302–304.
44. Alonge TO, Salawu SA, Adebisi TA, Fashina AN. The choice of antibiotic in open fractures in a teaching hospital in a developing country. *Int J Clin Pract* 2002;56(5): 353–356.
45. Stevenson J, McNaughton G, Riley J. The use of prophylactic flucloxacillin in treatment of open fractures of the distal phalanx within an accident and emergency department: a double-blind randomized placebo-controlled trial. *J Hand Surg [Br]* 2003;28(5): 388–394.
46. Faisham WI, Nordin S, Aidura M. Bacteriological study and its role in the management of open tibial fracture. *Med J Malaysia* 2001;56(2):201–206.
47. Ikem IC, Oginni LM, Bomgboye EA. Open fractures of the lower limb in Nigeria. *Int Orthop* 2001;25(6):386–388.
48. Mast J, Jakob R, Ganz R. *Planning and reduction technique in fracture surgery*. New York: Springer-Verlag, 1989.
49. Trunkey DD, Chapman MW, Lim RC Jr, et al. Management of pelvic fractures in blunt trauma injury. *J Trauma* 1974;14:912–923.
50. Henry AK. *Extensive exposure*. Edinburgh: E&S Livingstone, 1952.
51. Clifford RP. Skin cover in open tibial fractures. In: Bunker TD, Colton CL, Webb JK, eds. *Frontiers in fracture management*. Cambridge: Cambridge University Press, 1989.
52. Brumback RJ, Ellison PS Jr, Poka A, et al. Intramedullary nailing of open fractures of the femoral shaft. *J Bone Joint Surg Am* 1989;71:1324–1331.
53. Heitmann C, Patzakis MJ, Tetsworth KD, Levin LS. Musculoskeletal sepsis: principles of treatment. *Instr Course Lect* 2003;52:733–743.
54. Tile M, ed. *Fractures of the pelvis and acetabulum*. Baltimore: Williams & Wilkins, 1995.
55. Scully RE, Artz CP, Sako Y. An evaluation of the surgeon's criteria for determining the viability of muscle during debridement. *Arch Surg* 1956;73:1031–1035.
56. Har-Shai Y, Silbermann M, Reis ND, et al. Muscle microcirculatory impairment following acute compartment syndrome in the dog. *Plast Reconstr Surg* 1992;89:283–289.
57. Skjeldal S, Stromsoe K, Alho A, et al. Acute compartment syndrome: for how long can muscle tolerate increased tissue pressure? *Eur J Surg* 1992;158:437–438.
58. Edwards CC, Simons SC, Browner BD, et al. Severe open tibial fractures: results treating 202 injuries with external fixation. *Clin Orthop* 1988;230:98–115.
59. van Winkle BA, Neustein J. Management of open fractures with sterilization of large, contaminated, extruded cortical fragments. *Clin Orthop* 1987;223:275–281.
60. Krettek G, Haas N, Tscherne H. The role of supplemental lag screw fixation for open fractures of the tibial shaft treated with external fixation. *J Bone Joint Surg Am* 1991; 73:893–897.
61. Kindsfater K, Jonassen EA. Osteomyelitis in grade II and III open tibia fractures with late debridement. *J Orthop Trauma* 1995;9:121–127.
62. Orr HW. The treatment of osteomyelitis by drainage and rest. *J Bone Joint Surg* 1927; 9:730–740.
63. Papineau, LJ, Alfageme A, Dalcourt JP, et al. Chronic osteomyelitis: open excision and grafting after saucerization [in French]. *Int Orthop* 1979;3:165–176.
64. Hinsley DE, Hobbs CM, Watkins PE. The role of laser Doppler flowmetry in assessing the viability of bone fragments in an open fracture. *Injury* 2002;33(5):435–438.
65. Swiontkowski MF. Criteria for bone debridement in massive lower limb trauma. *Clin Orthop* 1989;243:41–47.
66. Lange RH, Bach AW, Hansen ST Jr, et al. Open tibial fractures with associated vascular injuries: prognosis for limb salvage. *J Trauma* 1985;25:203–208.
67. Lin CH, Wei FC, Levin LS, et al. The functional outcome of lower extremity fractures with vascular injury. *J Trauma* 1997;43:480–485.
68. Wagner WH, Yellin AE, Weaver FA, et al. Acute treatment of penetrating popliteal artery trauma: the importance of soft tissue injury. *Ann Vasc Surg* 1994;8:557–565.
69. Connolly J. Management of fractures associated with arterial injuries. *Am J Surg* 1970; 120:331.
70. Waikakul S, Sakkarnkosol S, Vandurongwan V. Vascular injuries in compound fractures of the leg with initially adequate circulation. *J Bone Joint Surg Br* 1998;80:254–258.
71. Matsen FA III, Mayo KA, Sheridan GW, et al. Monitoring of intramuscular pressure. *Surgery* 1976;79:702–709.
72. Anglen JO. Wound irrigation in musculoskeletal injury. *J Am Acad Orthop Surg* 2001; 9:219–226.
73. Gross A, Cutright DE, Bhaskar SN. Effectiveness of pulsating water jet lavage in treatment of contaminated, crushed wounds. *Am J Surg* 1972;124:373–377.
74. Anglen J, Apostoles S, Christensen G, et al. The efficacy of various irrigation solutions in removing slime-producing staphylococcus. *J Orthop Trauma* 1994;8:390–396.
75. Bhandari M, Schemitsch EH, Adili A, et al. High and low pressure pulsatile lavage of contaminated tibial fractures: an in vitro study of bacterial adherence and bone damage. *J Orthop Trauma* 1999;13:526–533.
76. Burd T, Christensen GD, Anglen JO, et al. Sequential irrigation with common detergents: a promising new method for decontaminating orthopaedic wounds. *Am J Orthop* 199;28:156–160.
77. Conroy BP, Anglen JO, Simpson WA, et al. Comparison of castile soap, benzalkonium chloride, and bacitracin as irrigation solutions for complex contaminated orthopaedic wounds. *J Orthop Trauma* 1999;13:332–337.
78. Glotzer DJ, Goodman WS, Geronimus LH. Topical antibiotic prophylaxis in contaminated wounds: experimental evaluation. *Arch Surg* 1970;100:589–593.
79. Rosenstein BD, Wilson FC, Thunderburk CH. The use of bacitracin irrigation to prevent infection in postoperative skeletal wounds. *J Bone Joint Surg Am* 1989;71:427–430.
80. Dirschl DR, Duff GP, Dahners LE, et al. High pressure pulsatile lavage irrigation of intraarticular fractures: effects on fracture healing. *J Orthop Trauma* 1998;12:460–463.
81. Boyd JI, Wongworawat MD. High-pressure pulsatile lavage causes soft tissue damage. *Clin Orthop* 2004;427:13–17.
82. Bhandari M, Adili A, Lachowski RJ. High pressure pulsatile lavage of contaminated human tibiae: an in vitro study. *J Orthop Trauma* 1998;12:479–484.
83. Madden J, Edlich RF, Schauerhamer R, et al. Application of principles of fluid dynamics to surgical wound irrigation. *Curr Topics Surg Res* 1971;3:85–93.
84. Karuppasamy K, Hutton MJ, LeF Porteous MJ. A novel system for the irrigation of open fractures. *Injury* 2004;35:980–981.
85. Brown LL, Shelton HT, Bornside GH, et al. Evaluation of wound irrigation by pulsatile jet and conventional methods. *Ann Surg* 1978;187:170–173.
86. Webb LX, Morykwas MJ, Smith TL, et al. High velocity parallel fluid flow for debridement of contaminated wounds in a pig model. Presented at the 16th Annual Meeting of the Orthopaedic Trauma Association, San Antonio, Texas, October 13, 2000.
87. Lineaweaver W, McMorris S, Soucy D, et al. Cellular and bacterial toxicities of topical antimicrobials. *Plast Reconstr Surg* 1985;75:394–396.
88. Menton DN, Brown M. The effects of commercial wound cleansers on cutaneous wound healing in guinea pigs. *Wounds* 1994;6:21–27.
89. van Huyssteen AL, Bracey DJ. Chlorhexidine and chondrolysis in the knee. *J Bone Joint Surg Br* 1999;81:995–996.
90. Park SH, Silva M, Bahk WJ, et al. Effect of repeated irrigation and debridement on fracture healing in an animal model. *J Orthop Res* 2002;20:1197–1204.
91. Adili A, Bhandari M, Schemitsch EH. The biomechanical effect of high-pressure irrigation on diaphyseal fracture healing in vivo. *J Orthop Trauma* 2002;16:413–417.
92. Brown PW, Urban JG. Early weight-bearing treatment of open fractures of the tibia: an end-result study of 63 cases. *J Bone Joint Surg Am* 1969;51:59–75.
93. Curtis MJ, Brown PR, Dick JD, et al. Contaminated fractures of the tibia: a comparison of treatment modalities in animal model. *J Orthop Res* 1995;13:286–295.
94. Rittmann WW, Perren SM. *Cortical bone healing after internal fixation and healing*. New York: Springer-Verlag, 1974.
95. Salter RB, Simmonds DF, Malcolm BW, et al. The biological effect of continuous passive motion on the healing of full-thickness defects in articular cartilage. *J Bone Joint Surg Am* 1980;62:1232–1251.
96. Mitchell N, Shepard N. Healing of articular cartilage in intra-articular fractures in rabbits. *J Bone Joint Surg Am* 1980;62:628–634.
97. Llinas A, McKellop HA, Marshall GJ, et al. Healing and remodeling of articular incongruities in a rabbit fracture model. *J Bone Joint Surg Am* 1993;75:1508–1523.
98. Bone L, McNamira K, Shine B, et al. Mortality in multiple trauma patients with fractures. *J Trauma* 1994;37:262–265.
99. Bone LB, Johnson KD, Weigelt J, et al. Early versus delayed stabilization of femoral fractures: a prospective randomized study. *J Bone Joint Surg Am* 1989;71:336–340.
100. Wade PA, Campbell RD Jr. Open versus closed methods in treating fractures of the leg. *Am J Surg* 1958;95:599–616.
101. Chapman MW. The role of intramedullary fixation in open fractures. *Clin Orthop* 1986; 212:26–34.
102. Small JO, Mollan RA. Management of the soft tissues in open tibial fractures. *Br J Plast Surg* 1992;45:571–577.
103. Trabulsy PP, Kerley SM, Hoffman WY. A prospective study of early soft tissue coverage of grade IIIB tibial fractures. *J Trauma* 1994;36:661–668.
104. Ilazarov GA. *Transosseous osteosynthesis*. Berlin: Springer-Verlag, 1992.
105. Tornetta P III, Bergman M, Watnik N, et al. Treatment of grade 3B open tibial fractures: a prospective randomized comparison of external fixation to non-reamed locked nailing. *J Bone Joint Surg Br* 1994;76:13–19.
106. Green SA. *Complications of external skeletal fixation: causes, prevention and treatment*. Springfield, IL: Charles C Thomas, 1981.
107. Chapman MW. The use of immediate internal fixation in open fractures. *Orthop Clin North Am* 1980;11:579–591.
108. Bonatus T, Olson SA, Lee S, et al. Nonreamed locking intramedullary nailing for open fractures of the tibia. *Clin Orthop* 1997;339:58–64.
109. Helfet DL, Howey T, Dipasquale T, et al. The treatment of open and/or unstable tibia fractures with an unreamed double locked tibial nail. *J Orthop Rev* 1994;[Suppl]:9–17.
110. Henley MB, Chapman JR, Agel J, et al. Treatment of type II, IIIA, and IIIB open fractures of the tibial shaft: a prospective comparison of unreamed interlocking intramedullary nails and half-pin external fixators. *J Orthop Trauma* 1998;12:1–7.
111. Sanders R, Swiontkowski M, Nunley J, et al. The management of fractures with soft-tissue disruptions. *J Bone Joint Surg Am* 1993;75:778–789.
112. Sanders R, Pappas J, Mast J, et al. The salvage of open grade 3B ankle and talus fractures. *J Orthop Trauma* 1992;6:201–208.
113. Moed BR, Kellam JF, Foster RJ, et al. Immediate internal fixation of open fractures of the diaphysis of the forearm. *J Bone Joint Surg Am* 1986;68:1008–1017.
114. Morrey BF. Current concepts in the treatment of fractures of the radial head, the olecranon, and the coronoid. *Instr Course Lect* 1995;44:175–185.
115. Chapman MW, Gordon JE, Zissimos AG. Compression plate fixation of acute fractures of the diaphysis of the radius and ulna. *J Bone Joint Surg Am* 1989;71:159–169.
116. Lhowe GW, Hansen ST. Immediate nailing of open fractures of the femoral shaft. *J Bone Joint Surg Am* 1988;70:812–820.
117. Maurer DJ, Merkow RL, Gustilo RB. Infection after intramedullary nailing of severe open tibial fractures initially treated with external fixation. *J Bone Joint Surg Am* 1989; 71:835–838.
118. Nowotarski PJ, Turen CH, Brumback RJ, Scarboro JM. Conversion of external fixation

to intramedullary nailing for fractures of the shaft of the femur in multiply injured patients. *J Bone Joint Surg* 2000;82–A(6):781–788.
119. O'Brien PJ, Meek RN, Powell JN, et al. Primary intramedullary nailing of open femoral shaft fractures. *J Trauma* 1991;31:113–116.
120. Blachet PA, Meek RN, O'Brien PJ. External fixation and delayed intramedullary nailing of open fractures of the tibial shaft: a sequential protocol. *J Bone Joint Surg Am* 1990; 72:729–735.
121. Marshall PD, Saleh M, Douglas DL. Risk of deep infection with intramedullary following the use of external fixators. *J R Coll Surg Edinb* 1991;36:268–271.
122. Sirkin M, Sanders R, DiPasquale T, et al. A staged protocol for soft tissue management in the treatment of complex pilon fractures. *J Orthop Trauma* 1999;13:78–84.
123. Johnson KD, Bone LB, Scheinberg R. Severe open tibial fractures: a study protocol. *J Orthop Trauma* 1988;2:175–180.
124. Antich-Adrover P, Marti-Garin D, Murias-Alvarez J, et al. External fixation and secondary intramedullary nailing of open tibia fractures: a randomized prospective trial. *J Bone Joint Surg Br* 1997;79:443–447.
125. McGraw JM, Lim EV. Treatment of open tibial-shaft fractures. external fixation and secondary intramedullary nailing. *J Bone Joint Surg Am* 1988;70:900–911.
126. Siebenrock KA, Gerich T, Jakob RP. Sequential intramedullary nailing of open tibial shaft fractures after external fixation. *Arch Orthop Trauma Surg* 1997;116:32–36.
127. Iannocone WM, Taffet R, DeLong WG, et al. Early exchange intramedullary nailing of distal femoral fractures with vascular injury initially stabilized with external fixation. *J Trauma* 1994;37:446–451.
128. Siebenrock KA, Schilling B, Jakob RP. Treatment of complex tibial shaft fractures: arguments for early secondary intramedullary nailing. *Clin Orthop* 1993;290:269–274.
129. Clancey GJ, Hansen ST Jr. Open fractures of the tibia: a review of one hundred and two cases. *J Bone Joint Surg Am* 1978;60:118–122.
130. Ritmann WW, Schibli M, Matter P, et al. Open fractures: long term results in 200 consecutive cases. *Clin Orthop* 1979;138:132–140.
131. Schandelmaier P, Krettek C, Rudolf J, et al. Outcome of tibial shaft fractures with severe soft tissue injury treated by undreamed nailing versus external fixation. *J Trauma* 1995; 39:707–711.
132. Gristina AG, Rovere D. An in vitro study of the effects of metals used in internal fixation on bacterial growth and dissemination. *J Bone Joint Surg Am* 1963;45:1104.
133. Darouiche RO, Farmer J, Chaput C, et al. Anti-infective efficacy of antiseptic-coated intramedullary nails. *J Bone Joint Surg Am* 1998;80:1336–1340.
134. Claffey T. Open fractures of the tibia [Proceedings]. *J Bone Joint Surg Br* 1960;42: 407(abstr).
135. Gallinaro P, Crova M, Denicolai F. Complication in 64 open fractures of the tibia. *Injury* 1974;5:157–160.
136. Lottes JO, Hill LJ, Key JA. Closed reduction, plate fixation and medullary nailing of fractures of both bones of the leg: a comparative end-result study. *J Bone Joint Surg Am* 1952;34:861–877.
137. Bach AW, Hansen ST Jr. Plates versus external fixation in severe open tibial shaft fractures: a randomized trial. *Clin Orthop* 1989;241:89–94.
*138. Keating JF, O'Brien PJ, Blachut PA, et al. Locking intramedullary nailing with and without reaming for open fractures of the tibial shaft: a prospective, randomized study. *J Bone Joint Surg Am* 1997;79:334–341.
139. Schemitsch EH, Kowalski MJ, Swiontkowski MF, et al. Effects of reamed vs. un-reamed locked nailing on callous blood flow and early strength of union in a fracture sheep tibial model. *J Orthop Trauma* 1994;8:373–382.
140. Schemitsch E, Kowalski M, Swiontkowski MF. Soft-tissue blood flow following reamed versus undreamed locked intramedullary nailing: a fractured sheep tibia model. *Ann Plast Surg* 1996;36:70–75.
141. Hawkins LG. Fractures of the neck of the talus. *J Bone Joint Surg Am* 1970;52:991–1002.
142. Yokoyama K, Shindo M, Itoman M, et al. Immediate internal fixation for open fractures of the long bones of the upper and lower extremities. *J Trauma* 1994;37:230–236.
143. Benirschke SK, Agnew SF, Mayo KA, et al. Immediate internal fixation of open complex tibial plateau fractures. *J Orthop Trauma* 1992;6:78–86.
144. Bray TJ, Endicott M, Capra SE. Treatment of open ankle fractures: immediate internal fixation versus closed immobilization and delayed fixation. *Clin Orthop* 1989;240: 47–52.
145. Franklin JL, Johnson KD, Hansen ST. Immediate internal fixation of open ankle fractures. *J Bone Joint Surg Am* 1994;66:1349–1356.
146. Johnson EE, Davlin LB. Open ankle fractures: the indications for immediate open reduction and internal fixation. *Clin Orthop* 1993;292:118–127.
147. Dellinger EP, Caplan ES, Weaver LD, et al. Duration of preventive antibiotic administration for open extremity fractures. *Arch Surg* 1988;123:333–339.
148. Perry CR, Pearson RL, Miller GA. Accuracy of cultures of material from swabbing of the superficial aspect of the wound and needle biopsy in the preoperative assessment of osteomyelitis. *J Bone Joint Surg Am* 1991;73:745–749.
149. Chapman MW, Hadley WK. The effect of polymethylmethacrylate and antibiotic combinations on bacterial viability: an in vitro and preliminary in vivo study. *J Bone Joint Surg Am* 1976;58:76–81.
150. Eckman JB Jr, Henry SL, Mangino PD, et al. Wound and serum levels of tobramycin with the prophylactic use of tobramycin-impregnated polymethylmethacrylate beads in compound fractures. *Clin Orthop* 1988;237:213–215.
151. Buranapanitkit B, Ingviya N, Lim A, et al. In vitro elution of gentamycin from locally implantable beads. *J Musculoskeletal Res* 2000;4:169–176.
152. Ostermann PA, Henry SL, Seligson D. The role of local antibiotic therapy in the management of compound fractures. *Clin Orthop* 1993;295:102–111.
153. Keating JF, Blachut PA, O'Brien PJ, et al. Reamed nailing of open tibial fractures: does the antibiotic bead pouch reduce the deep infection rate? *J Orthop Trauma* 1996;10: 298–303.
154. Edin MI, Miclau T, Lester GE, et al. Effect of cefazolin and vancomycin on osteoblasts in vitro. *Clin Orthop* 1996;333:245–251.
155. Miclau T, Edin ML, Lester GE, et al. Bone toxicity of locally applied aminoglycosides. *J Orthop Trauma* 1995;9:401–406.
156. Zalavras CG, Patzakis MJ, et al. Local antibiotic therapy in the treatment of open fractures and osteomyelitis. *Clin Orthop Relat Res* 2004;(427):86–93.
157. McKee MD, Wild LM, Schemitsch EH, et al. The use of an antibiotic-impregnated, osteoconductive, bioabsorbable bone substitute in the treatment of infected long bone defects: early results of a prospective trial. *J Orthop Trauma* 2002;16:622–627.
158. Beardmore AA, Brooks DE, Wenke JC, et al. Effectiveness of local antibiotic delivery with an osteoinductive and osteoconductive bone-graft substitute. *J Bone Joint Surg Am* 2005;87:107–112.
159. Argenta LC, Morykwas MJ. Vacuum-assisted closure: a new method for wound control and treatment: clinical experience. *Ann Plast Surg* 1997;38:563–577.
160. Webb LX. New techniques in wound management: vacuum-assisted wound closure. *J Am Acad Orthop Surg* 2002;10:303–311.
161. Morykwas MJ, Argenta LC, Shelton-Brown EI, et al. Vacuum-assisted closure: a new method for wound control and treatment: animal studies and basic foundation. *Ann Plast Surg* 1997;38:553–562.
162. Chang KP, Tsai CC, Lin TM, et al. An alternative dressing for skin graft immobilization: negative pressure dressing. *Burns* 2001;27:839–842.
163. Garner GB, Ware DN, Cocanour CS, et al: Vacuum assisted wound closure provides early fascial reapproximation in trauma patients with open abdomens. *Am J Surg* 2001; 182:630–638.
164. Harlen JW. Treatment of open sternal wounds with the vacuum-assisted closure system: a safe, reliable method. *Plast Reconstr Surg* 2002;109:710–712.
165. Fleishmann W, Strecker W, Bombelli M, et al. Vacuum sealing as treatment of soft tissue damage in open fractures. *Unfallchirurg* 1993;96:488–492.
166. Mullner T, Mrkonjic L, Kwasny O, et al. The use of negative pressure to promote the healing of tissue defects: a clinical trial using the vacuum sealing technique. *Br J Plast Surg* 1997;50:194–199.
167. DeFranzo AJ, Argenta LC, Marks MW, et al. The use of vacuum assisted closure therapy for treatment of lower extremity wounds with exposed bone. *Plast Reconstr Surg* 2001; 108:1184–1191.
168. Herscovici D, Sanders RW, Scaduto JM, et al. Vacuum assisted wound closure for the management of patients with high-energy soft tissue injuries. *J Orthop Trauma* 2003; 17:683–686.
169. Mooney JF, Argenta LC, Marks MW, et al. Treatment of soft tissue defects in pediatric patients using the V.A.C. system. *Clin Orthop Rel Res* 2000;376:26–31.
170. Greer SE, Duthie E, Cartolano B, et al. Techniques for applying subatmospheric pressure dressing to wounds in difficult regions of anatomy. *J Wound Ostomy Continence Nurs* 1999;26:250–253.
171. Morykwas MJ, Faler BJ, Pearce DJ, et al. Effects of varying levels of subatmospheric pressure on the rate of granulation tissue formation in experimental wounds in swine. *Ann Plast Surg* 2001;47:547–551.
172. Ballard K, Baxter H. Developments in wound care for difficult to manage wounds. *Br J Nurs* 2000;9:405–412.
173. Philbeck TE, Whittington KT, Millsap MH, et al. The clinical and cost effectiveness of externally applied negative pressure wound therapy in the treatment of wounds in home health Medicare patients. *Ostomy Wound Manage* 1999;45:41–50.
174. DeLong WG Jr, Born CT, Wei SY, et al. Aggressive treatment of 119 open fracture wounds. *J Trauma* 1999;46:1049–1054.
175. Weitz-Marshall AD, Bosse MJ. Timing of closure of open fractures. *J Am Acad Orthop Surg* 2002;10(6):379–384.
176. Godina M. Early microsurgical reconstruction of complex trauma of the extremities. *Plast Reconstr Surg* 1986;78:285–292.
177. Hertel R, Lambert SM, Muller S, et al. On the timing of soft tissue reconstruction for open fractures of the lower leg. *Arch Orthop Trauma Surg* 1999;119:7–12.
178. Sinclair JS, McNally MA, Small JO, et al. Primary free flap cover of open tibial fractures. *Injury* 1997;28:581–587.
179. Yaremchuk MJ, Brumback RJ, Manson PN, et al. Acute and definitive management of traumatic osteocutaneous defects of the lower extremity. *Plast Reconstr Surg* 1987;80: 1–14.
180. Ger R. Then management of open fracture of the tibia with skin loss. *J Trauma* 1970; 10:112–121.
181. Greene TL, Beatty ME. Soft tissue coverage for lower extremity trauma: current practice and techniques. A review. *J Orthop Trauma* 1988;2:158–173.
182. Tanner JC Jr, Vandeput J, Olley JF. The mesh skin graft. *Plast Reconstr Surg* 1964;34: 287–292.
183. Francel TJ, Vander Kolk CA, Hoopes JE, et al. Microvascular soft tissue transplantation for reconstruction of acute tibial fractures: timing of coverage and long-term functional results. *Plast Reconstr Surg* 1992;89:478–487.
184. Lo LJ, Chen YR, Weng CJ, et al. Use of split anterior tibial muscle flap in treating avulsion injury of the leg associated with tibia exposure. *Ann Plast Surg* 1993;31: 112–116.
185. Salisbury RE, Wilmore DW, Silverstein P, et al. Biological dressings for skin graft donor sites. *Arch Surg* 1973;106:705–706.
186. Giannoudis PV. Current concepts of the inflammatory response after major trauma: an update. *Injury* 2003;34:397–404.
187. Giannoudis PV, Abbott C, Stone M, et al. Fatal systemic inflammatory response syndrome following early bilateral femoral nailing. *Intensive Care Med* 1998;24:641–642.
188. Harrison WJ, Lewis CP, Lavy CB. Open fractures of the tibia in HIV positive patients: a prospective controlled single-blind study. *Injury* 2004;35(9):852–856.

189. Schmidt AH, Swiontkowski MF. Pathophysiology of infections after internal fixation of fractures, *J Am Acad Orthop Surg* 2000;8:285–291.
190. Patzakis MJ, Wilkins J. Factors influencing infection rate in open fracture wounds. *Clin Orthop Rel Res* 1989;243:36–40.
191. Harley BJ, Beaupre LA, Jones CA, et al. The effect of time to definitive treatment on the rate of nonunion and infection in open fractures. *J Orthop Trauma* 2002;16(7): 484–490.
192. Khatod M, Botte MJ, Hoyt DB, et al. Outcomes in open tibia fractures: relationship between delay in treatment and infection. *J Trauma* 2003;55(5):949–954.
193. Skaggs DL, Friend L, Alman B, et al. The effect of surgical delay on acute infection following 554 open fractures in children. *J Bone Joint Surg* 2005;87-A(1):8–12.
194. Spencer J, Smith A, Woods D. The effect of time delay on infection in open long-bone fractures: a 5-year prospective audit from a district general hospital. *Ann R Coll Surg Engl* 2004;86(2):108–112.
195. McCarthy EF, Frassica FJ. Infection of bones and joints. In: McCarthy EF, Frassica FJ, eds. *Pathology of bone and joint disorders*. Philadelphia: WB Saunders, 1998.
196. Gristina AG. Biomaterial-centered infection: microbial adhesion versus tissue integration. *Science* 1987;237:1588–1595.
197. Tulner SA, Schaap GR, Strackee SD, et al. Long-term results of multiple-stage treatment for posttraumatic osteomyelitis of the tibia. *J Trauma* 2004;56:633–642.
*198. Bhandari M, Guyatt GH, Swiontkowski MF, et al. Treatment of open fractures of the shaft of the tibia: a systematic overview and meta-analysis. *J Bone Joint Surg Br* 2000; 82:62–68.
199. Bhandari M, Tornetta P, Sprague S, et al. Predictors of reoperation following operative management of fractures of the tibial shaft. *J Orthop Trauma* 2003;17(5):353–361.
200. Muller ME, Allgower M, Schneider R, et al. *Manual of internal fixation: technique recommended by the AO Group*, 2nd ed. New York: Springer-Verlag, 1979.
200. Malik MH, Harwood P, Diggle P, Khan SA. Factors affecting rates of infection and nonunion in intramedullary nailing. *J Bone Joint Surg* 2004;86(4):556–560.
*201. Govender S, Csimma C, Genant HK, et al. Recombinant human bone morphogenetic protein-2 for treatment of open tibial fractures: a prospective, controlled, randomized study of four hundred and fifty patients. *J Bone Joint Surg* 2002;84–A(12):2123–2134.
202. Tsuge K. Management of established Volkmann's contracture. In: Green DP, Hotchkiss RN, Pederson WC, eds. *Green's operative hand surgery*, 4th ed. Philadelphia: Churchill Livingston, 1999.

ACUTE COMPARTMENT SYNDROME

Margaret M. McQueen

Acute compartment syndrome occurs when pressure rises within a confined space in the body, resulting in a critical reduction of the blood flow to the tissues contained within the space. Without urgent decompression, tissue ischemia, necrosis, and functional impairment occur. The acute compartment syndrome should be differentiated from other related conditions.

It is important to be aware of the different definitions associated with a compartment syndrome. Acute compartment syndrome is defined as an elevation of intercompartmental pressure to a level and for a duration that without decompression will cause tissue ischemia and necrosis.

Exertional compartment syndrome is elevation of intercompartmental pressure during exercise, causing ischemia, pain, and, rarely, neurologic symptoms and signs. It is characterized by resolution of symptoms with rest but may proceed to acute compartment syndrome if exercise continues.

Volkmann's ischemic contracture is the end state of neglected acute compartment syndrome, with irreversible muscle necrosis leading to ischemic contractures.

The crush syndrome is the systemic result of muscle necrosis commonly caused by prolonged external compression of an extremity. In crush syndrome, muscle necrosis is established by the time of presentation but intracompartmental pressure may rise as a result of intracompartmental edema, causing a superimposed acute compartment syndrome.

HISTORY

It is now well over a century since the first description of ischemic muscle contractures was published in the medical literature. The first report of the condition was attributed to Hamilton in 1850 by Hildebrand (1) but Hamilton's original description has never been found. The credit for the first full description belongs to Richard Von Volkmann (2), who published a summary of his views in 1881. He stated that paralysis and contractures that appeared after too-tight bandaging of the forearm and hand were ischemic and were caused by prolonged blocking of arterial blood. He recognised that muscle cannot survive longer than 6 hours with complete interruption of its blood flow and that 12 hours or less of too-tight bandaging were enough to result in "dismal permanent crippling." In 1888 Peterson (3) recognized that ischemic contracture could occur in the absence of bandaging but did not postulate a cause.

The first major reports appeared in the English language literature in the early 20th century. At this time it was suggested that swelling after removal of tight bandaging might contribute to the contracture and that the contracture was due to "fibrous-tissue forming elements" or a myositic process (4–6). By the early part of the 20th century, published accounts of the sequence of events in acute compartment syndrome were remarkably similar to those that are known today, with differentiation between acute ischemia caused by major vessel rupture, acute ischemia caused by subfascial tension, the late stage of ischemic contracture, and the separate concept of nerve involvement (7). This paper was the first description of fasciotomy to relieve the pressure. The importance of early fasciotomy was suggested at this time (7,8) and confirmed by prevention of the development of contractures in animal experiments (9).

During the Second World War attention was directed away from these sound conclusions. A belief arose that ischemic contracture was caused by arterial injury and spasm with reflex collateral spasm. Successful results from excision of the damaged artery (10,11) were undoubtedly the result of the fasciotomy carried out as part of the exposure for the surgery. An unfortunate legacy of this belief persists today in the dangerously mistaken view that an acute compartment syndrome cannot exist in the presence of normal peripheral pulses.

The arterial injury theory was challenged by Seddon in 1966 (12). He noted that in all cases of ischemic contracture there was early and gross swelling requiring prompt fasciotomy and that 50% of his cases had palpable peripheral pulses. He was unable to explain muscle infarcts at the same level as the injury on the basis of arterial damage. He recommended early fasciotomy.

In their classic paper McQuillan and Nolan (13) reported on 15 cases complicated by "local ischaemia." They described the vicious circle of increasing tension in an enclosed compartment causing venous obstruction and subsequent reduction in arterial inflow. Their most important conclusion was that delay in performing a fasciotomy was the single cause of failure of treatment.

EPIDEMIOLOGY

Knowledge of the epidemiology of acute compartment syndrome is important in defining the patient at risk for developing acute compartment syndrome. The epidemiology of acute compartment syndrome has been described in a cohort of 164 patients drawn from a defined population in the United Kingdom (14).

The incidence of acute compartment syndrome in a westernized population is 3.1 per 100,000 of the population per annum (14). The annual incidence for males is 7.3 per 100,000 compared to 0.7 per 100,000 for females, a 10-fold increase in risk for males. The age and gender-specific incidences are illustrated in Figure 13-1, showing a type B pattern (see Chapter 4) or the L-shaped pattern described by Buhr and Cooke (15). The mean age for the whole group was 32 years; the median age for males was 30 years and for females 44 years.

The underlying condition causing acute compartment syndrome was most commonly a fracture (69% of cases) (Table 13-1). Similar figures have been reported in children, with 76% of cases caused by fracture, predominantly tibial diaphyseal, distal radius, and forearm (16). The most common fracture associated with acute compartment syndrome in adults is tibial diaphyseal fracture. The prevalence of acute compartment syndrome in tibial diaphyseal fractures is reported as 2.7% to 11% (14,17–22). Differences in prevalence are likely to be due to different diagnostic techniques and selection of patients. The true figure is probably approximately 6% to 8%.

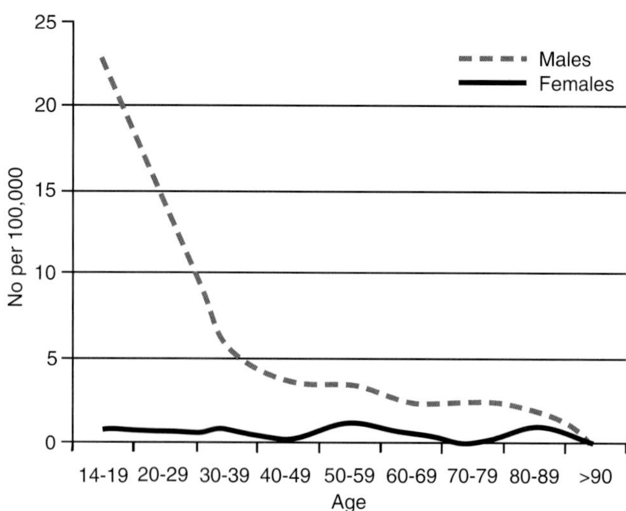

FIGURE 13-1 The annual age- and gender-specific incidence of acute compartment syndrome.

TABLE 13-1 Conditions Associated with Injury Causing Acute Compartment Syndrome Presenting to an Orthopaedic Trauma Unit

Underlying Condition	Percentage of Cases (%)
Tibial diaphyseal fracture	36.0
Soft tissue injury	23.2
Distal radius fracture	9.8
Crush syndrome	7.9
Diaphyseal fracture forearm	7.9
Femoral diaphyseal fracture	3.0
Tibial plateau fracture	3.0
Hand fracture(s)	2.5
Tibial pilon fractures	2.5
Foot fracture(s)	1.8
Ankle fracture	0.6
Elbow fracture dislocation	0.6
Pelvic fracture	0.6
Humeral diaphyseal fracture	0.6

The second most common cause of acute compartment syndrome is soft tissue injury, which added to tibial diaphyseal fracture makes up almost two thirds of the cases. The second most common fracture to be complicated by acute compartment syndrome is the distal radius fracture, which occurs in approximately 0.25% of cases. Forearm diaphyseal fractures are complicated by acute compartment syndrome in 3% of cases. The prevalence of acute compartment syndrome in other anatomic locations is rarely reported. Other less common causes of acute compartment syndrome are listed in Table 13-2 (23–39).

It is now recognized that from adolescence, younger patients are at more risk of compartment syndrome. In tibial diaphyseal fracture the prevalence of acute compartment syndrome is 3 times higher in the under 35-year-old age-group, and in distal radial fractures the prevalence is 35 times less in the older age-group (14). Adolescents have been recognized as having a high rate (8.3%) of compartment syndrome after tibial fracture (17). The only exception to youth being a risk factor in acute compartment syndrome is in cases with soft tissue injury only. These patients have an average age of 36 years and are significantly older than those with a fracture (38).

High-energy injury is generally believed to increase the risks of developing an acute compartment syndrome. However, in tibial diaphyseal fracture complicated by acute compartment syndrome the proportion of high- and low-energy injury shows a slight preponderance of low-energy injury (59%) (14). In the same population there is an equal number of high-energy and low-energy injury in tibial diaphyseal fractures uncomplicated by acute compartment syndrome (39). This suggests acute compartment syndrome may be more prevalent after low-energy injury, possibly because in low-energy injury the compartment boundaries are less likely to be disrupted and an "autodecom-

TABLE 13-2 Causes of Acute Compartment Syndromes

Conditions That Increase Compartment Volume
Fracture
Soft tissue injury
Crush syndrome (including use of the lithotomy position) (23)
Revascularization
Exercise (24)
Fluid infusion (including arthroscopy (25,26)
Arterial puncture (27)
Ruptured ganglia/cysts (28)
Osteotomy (29)
Snake bite (30)
Nephrotic syndrome (31)
Leukemic infiltration (32)
Viral myositis (33)
Acute hematogenous osteomyelitis (34)
Conditions That Reduce Compartment Volume
Burns
Repair of muscle hernia (35)
Medical Comorbidity
Diabetes (36)
Hypothyroidism (37)
Bleeding diathesis/anticoagulants (38)

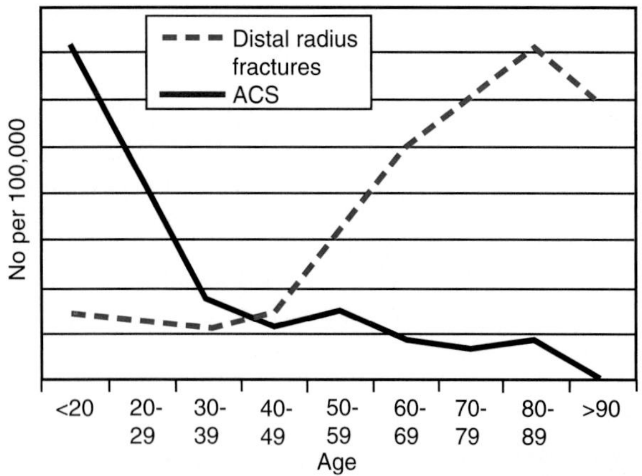

FIGURE 13-2 The annual age-specific incidence of all distal radius fractures compared with the annual age-specific incidence of acute compartment syndrome in distal radial fractures.

pression" effect is avoided. The concept of patients with lower-energy injury being at higher risk is supported by the distribution of severe open fractures in each group. In those complicated by acute compartment syndrome, 20% are Gustilo type III (14); in the whole population of tibial fractures, 60% were type III (39). It is important to note that open tibial diaphyseal fractures remain at risk of acute compartment syndrome, which occurs in around 3% (14), but it would appear that the lower Gustilo types are at more risk, again possibly because of the lack of disruption of the compartment boundaries.

Distal radial and forearm diaphyseal fractures associated with high-energy injury are more likely to be complicated by acute compartment syndrome, probably because of the high preponderance of young males sustaining these types of injury. This is illustrated by a comparison of the age- and gender-related incidence of distal radius fractures complicated by acute compartment syndrome (Fig. 13-2). The likely explanation for the preponderance of young males with acute compartment syndrome is that young men have relatively large muscle volumes, although their compartment size does not change after growth is complete. Thus young men may have less space for swelling of the muscle after injury. Presumably the older person has smaller, hypotrophic muscles, allowing more space for swelling. There may also be a protective effect of hypertension in the older patient.

The second most common type of acute compartment syndrome is that arising in the absence of fractures. The majority of these arise subsequent to soft tissue injury, particularly a crushing injury, but some arise with no preceding history of trauma (38). Patients with acute compartment syndrome without fracture tend to be older and have more medical comorbidities than those with a fracture. They are more evenly distributed between the genders with a male to female ratio of 5:1. The use of anticoagulants seems also to be a risk factor for the development of acute compartment syndrome.

The possible risk factors for the development or late diagnosis of acute compartment syndrome are listed in Table 13-3. As well as demographic risk factors, altered pain perception can delay diagnosis. This can occur if the patient has an altered state of consciousness or with certain types of anesthesia or analgesia (40,41).

PATHOGENESIS

There remains uncertainty about the exact physiologic mechanism of the reduction in blood flow in the acute compartment syndrome, although it is generally accepted that the effect is at the small vessel level, at arteriolar, capillary, or venous levels.

The critical closing pressure theory (42) states that there is a critical closing pressure in the small vessels when the transmural pressure (the difference between intravascular pressure and tissue pressure) drops. Transmural pressure (TM) is balanced by a constricting force (TC) consisting of active and elastic tension derived from smooth muscle action in the vessel walls. The

TABLE 13-3 Risk Factors for Development of or Late Diagnosis of Acute Compartment Syndrome

Demographic	Altered Pain Perception
Youth	Altered conscious level
Male gender	Regional anesthesia
Tibial fracture	Patient-controlled analgesia
High-energy forearm fracture	Children
High-energy femoral diaphyseal fracture	Associated nerve injury
Bleeding diathesis/anticoagulants	

equilibrium between expanding and contracting forces is expressed in a derivation of Laplace's law:

$$TM = TC \div r,$$

where r is the radius of the vessel.

If, as a result of increasing tissue pressure, the transmural pressure drops to a level such that elastic fibers in the vessel wall are no longer stretched and therefore cannot contribute any elastic tension, there will be no further automatic decrease in the radius. TC ÷ r then becomes greater than TM, and active closure of the vessel will occur. This concept has been verified in both animal and human local vascular beds (43–46). Ashton (47) was the first to relate these findings to acute compartment syndrome and concluded that whatever the cause of the raised tissue pressure, blood flow will be decreased and may temporarily cease altogether as a result of a combination of active arteriolar closure and passive capillary compression, depending on vasomotor tone and the height of the total tissue pressure. Critics of this theory (48) doubt the possibility of maintaining arteriolar closure in the presence of ischemia, which is a strong local stimulus for vasodilatation. Ashton (46) noted that flow resumes after 30 to 60 seconds of maintained tissue pressure and attributes this to vessel reopening possibly because of an accumulation of vasodilator metabolites.

A second theory is the arteriovenous (AV) gradient theory (48,49). According to this theory the increases in local tissue pressure reduce the local arteriovenous pressure gradient and thus reduce blood flow. When flow diminishes to less than the metabolic demands of the tissues (not necessarily to zero), then functional abnormalities result.

The relationship between arteriovenous (AV) gradient and the local blood flow (LBF) is summarized in the equation:

$$LBF = Pa - Pv \div R,$$

where Pa is the local arterial pressure, Pv is the local venous pressure and R is the local vascular resistance. Veins are collapsible tubes, and the pressure within them can never be less than the local tissue pressure. If tissue pressure rises as in the acute compartment syndrome, the Pv must rise, also thus reducing the AV gradient (Pa − Pv) and therefore the LBF. At low AV gradients, compensation from local vascular resistance (R) is relatively ineffective (50) and LBF is primarily determined by the AV gradient. Matsen et al (49) presented results on human subjects demonstrating reduction of the AV gradient with elevation of the limb in the presence of raised tissue pressure. This theory has been supported by recent work (51) that demonstrated that with external pressure applied simulating acute compartment syndrome, venous and capillary flow ceased but arterioles were still capable of carrying flow. This disproves the critical closing theory but supports the hypothesis of reduced arteriovenous gradient as the mechanism of reducing blood flow.

A third theory, the microvascular occlusion theory (52), postulates that capillary occlusion is the main mechanism reducing blood flow in acute compartment syndrome. Measurement of capillary pressure in dogs with normal tissue pressures revealed a mean level of 25 mm Hg. Hargens et al (52) suggest that a tissue pressure of similar value is sufficient to reduce capillary blood flow. Resultant muscle ischemia leads to increased capillary membrane permeability to plasma proteins, increasing edema and obstruction of lymphatic vessels by the raised tissue pressure. However, the authors admit that reactive hyperemia and vasodilatation both tend to raise the critical pressure level for microvascular occlusion. This work was done in the presence of normal tissue pressures. However, it has also been pointed out that capillaries are collapsible tubes (48) and that their intravascular pressure ought to rise in the presence of raised tissue pressure. Hargens' theory (52) is supported by more recent work demonstrating reduction of the number of perfused capillaries per unit area with raised tissue pressures (53).

Effects of Raised Tissue Pressure on Muscle

Regardless of the mechanism of vessel closure, reduction in blood flow in the acute compartment syndrome has a profound effect on muscle tissue. Skeletal muscle is the tissue in the extremities most vulnerable to ischemia and is therefore the most important tissue to be considered in acute compartment syndrome. Both the magnitude and duration of pressure elevation have been shown experimentally to be important influences in the extent of muscle damage.

There is now universal agreement that rising tissue pressure leads to a reduction in muscle blood flow. A number of experimental studies have highlighted the importance of perfusion pressure as well as tissue pressure in the reduction of muscle blood flow. Using magnetic resonance measurements of cellular metabolic derangement (pH, tissue oxygenation, and energy stores) and histologic studies, including electronmicroscopy and videomicroscopy studies of capillary blood flow, it has been shown that critical tissue pressure thresholds are 10 to 20 mm Hg below diastolic blood pressure or 25 to 30 mm Hg below mean arterial pressure (53–56). Increased vulnerability in previously traumatized or ischemic muscle has been demonstrated when the critical threshold may occur at tissue pressures more than 30 mm Hg below mean arterial pressure (57).

The ultimate result of reduced blood flow to skeletal muscle is ischemia followed by necrosis, with general agreement that increasing periods of complete ischemia produce increasing irreversible changes (58–60). It has also been shown that muscle necrosis is present in its greatest extent in the central position of the muscle and that external evaluation of the degree of muscle necrosis is unreliable. The duration of muscle ischemia dictates the amount of necrosis, although some muscle fibers are more vulnerable than others to ischemia. For example, the muscles of the anterior compartment of the leg contain type 1 fibers, or red slow-twitch fibers, and the gastrocnemius contains mainly type 2, or white fast-twitch, fibers. Type 1 fibers depend on oxidative metabolism of triglycerides for their energy source and are more vulnerable to oxygen depletion than type 2 fibers, whose metabolism is primarily anaerobic (61). This may explain the particular vulnerability of the anterior compartment to raised intracompartmental pressure.

Effects of Raised Tissue Pressure on Nerve

There is little dispute about the effects of raised tissue pressure on neurologic function. All investigators note a loss of neuromuscular function with raised tissue pressures (62–65) but at varying pressure thresholds and duration. In a study on human neurologic function, Matsen et al (66) found considerable variation of pressure tolerance, which could not be attributed to differences in systemic pressure.

The mechanism of damage to nerve is as yet uncertain and could result from ischemia, ischemia plus compression, toxic effects, or the effects of acidosis.

Effects of Raised Tissue Pressure on Bone

Nonunion is now recognized as a complication of acute compartment syndrome (67–71). It was first suggested by Nario in 1938 (72) that Volkmann's disease caused obliteration of the "musculo-diaphyseal" vessels and caused frequent pseudarthrosis. McQueen (73) observed a reduction in bone blood flow and bone union in rabbit tibiae after an experimentally induced acute compartment syndrome. It is likely that muscle ischemia reduces the capacity for development of the extraosseous blood supply on which long bones depend for healing.

Reperfusion Injury

The reperfusion syndrome is a group of complications following reestablishment of blood flow to ischemic tissues and can occur after fasciotomy and restoration of muscle blood flow in the acute compartment syndrome. Reperfusion is followed by an inflammatory response in the ischemic tissue, which can cause further tissue damage. The trigger for the inflammatory response is probably the breakdown products of muscle (74). Some breakdown products are procoagulants, which activate the intrinsic clotting system. This results in increasing microvascular thrombosis, which in turn increases the extent of muscle damage.

If there is a large amount of muscle involved in the ischemic process, the inflammatory response may become systemic. In acute compartment syndrome this is most likely to occur in the crush syndrome. Procoagulants escape into the systemic circulation and produce systemic coagulopathy, with parallel activation of inflammatory mediators. These then damage vascular endothelium leading to increased permeability and subsequent multiple organ failure. Systemic clotting and the breakdown products of dead and dying cells also lead to activation of white blood cells with the release of additional inflammatory mediators such as histamine, interleukin, oxygen free radicals, thromboxane, and many others (74). This is the basis for the use of agents such as antioxidants, antithromboxanes, antileukotrienes and anti–platelet activating factors, which modify the inflammatory process. Some of these agents have been shown in the laboratory to be capable of reducing muscle injury (75–78).

DIAGNOSIS

Prompt diagnosis of acute compartment syndrome is the key to a successful outcome. Delay in diagnosis has long been recognized as the single cause of failure of the treatment of acute compartment syndrome (13,79–81). Delay in diagnosis may be due to inexperience and lack of awareness of the possibility of acute compartment syndrome, an indefinite and confusing clinical presentation or to anesthetic or analgesic techniques that mask the clinical signs (40,41).

Delay in treatment of the acute compartment syndrome can be catastrophic, leading to serious complications such as permanent sensory and motor deficits, contractures, infection, and, at times, amputation of the limb (22,80). In serious cases there may be systemic injury from the reperfusion syndrome. A clear understanding of the clinical techniques necessary to make an early diagnosis is therefore essential to any physician treating acute compartment syndrome in order to avoid such complications. As well as improving outcome, early recognition and treatment of acute compartment syndrome is associated with decreased indemnity risk in potential malpractice claims (82).

CLINICAL DIAGNOSIS

Pain is considered to be the first symptom of acute compartment syndrome. The pain experienced by the patient is by nature ischemic and usually severe and out of proportion to the clinical situation. Pain may, however, be an unreliable indication of the presence of acute compartment syndrome because it can be very variable in its intensity (83–85), may be absent in acute compartment syndrome associated with nerve injury (86,87), or may be minimal in the deep posterior compartment syndrome (79,85). Pain is present in most cases because of the index injury but cannot be elicited in the unconscious patient. Children may not be able to express the severity of their pain, so restlessness, agitation, and anxiety with increasing analgesic requirements should raise the suspicion of the presence of an acute compartment syndrome (16). Both Shereff (88) and Myerson (89) state that clinical diagnosis of acute compartment syndrome in the foot is so unreliable that other methods should be used.

Pain has been shown to have a sensitivity of only 19% and a specificity of 97% in the diagnosis of acute compartment syndrome, that is, a high proportion of false negative or missed cases but a low proportion of false positive cases (90). There is general agreement, however, that pain, if present, is a relatively early symptom of acute compartment syndrome in the awake, alert patient (90).

Pain with passive stretch of the muscles involved is recognized as a symptom of acute compartment syndrome. Thus pain is increased, for example, in an anterior compartment syndrome when the toes or foot are plantarflexed. This symptom is no more reliable than rest pain because the reasons for unreliability quoted above apply equally to pain on passive stretch. The sensitivity and specificity of pain on passive stretch are similar to those for rest pain (90).

Paresthesias and hypoesthesias may occur in the territory of the nerves traversing the affected compartment and are usually the first sign of nerve ischemia. However, sensory abnormality may be due to concomitant nerve injury (19,87). Ulmer (90) reports a sensitivity of 13% and specificity of 98% for the clinical finding of paresthesias in acute compartment syndrome, a false negative rate that precludes this symptom from being a useful diagnostic tool.

Paralysis of muscle groups affected by the acute compartment syndrome is recognized as being a late sign (90). This sign has equally low sensitivity as others in predicting the presence of acute compartment syndrome, probably because of the difficulty of interpreting the underlying cause of the weakness. This could be inhibition by pain, direct injury to muscle, or associated nerve injury. It is recognized that if a motor deficit develops, full recovery is rare (68,81,91–93). Bradley (93) reported full recovery in only 13% of patients with paralysis as a sign of acute compartment syndrome.

Palpable swelling in the affected compartment can be a further sign of compartment syndrome. However, the degree of swelling is difficult to assess accurately, making this sign subjective. Casts or dressings often obscure compartments at risk and prevent assessment of swelling. Some compartments, such as the deep posterior compartment of the leg, are completely buried under the muscle compartments, obscuring any swelling.

Peripheral pulses and capillary return are always intact in acute compartment syndrome, unless there is major arterial injury or disease or in the very late stages of acute compartment syndrome, when amputation is inevitable. If acute compartment syndrome is suspected and pulses are absent, arteriography is indicated. Conversely, it is dangerous to exclude the diagnosis of acute compartment syndrome because distal pulses are present.

Using a combination of clinical symptoms and signs increases their sensitivity as diagnostic tools (90). However, to achieve a probability of over 90% of acute compartment syndrome being present, three clinical findings must be noted. The third clinical finding is paresis; thus, to achieve an accurate clinical diagnosis of acute compartment syndrome, the condition must be allowed to progress until a late stage. This is clearly unacceptable and has led to a search for earlier, more reliable methods of diagnosis.

COMPARTMENT PRESSURE MONITORING

Following the appreciation that acute compartment syndrome was due to increased tissue pressure within the affected compartment, several techniques were developed to measure intracompartmental pressure (ICP). Raised tissue pressure is the primary event in acute compartment syndrome; thus, changes in ICP will precede the clinical symptoms and signs (20).

Methods of Intracompartmental Pressure Measurement

There are several methods available to measure ICP. One of the first to be used was the needle manometer method (84), using a needle introduced into the compartment and connected to a column filled partly with saline and partly with air. To this column a syringe filled with air is attached, as is a pressure manometer or transducer. The ICP is the pressure that is required to inject air into the tubing and flatten the meniscus between the saline and the air. This method was modified by Matsen et al (94,95) to allow infusion of saline into the compartment. The ICP is the pressure resistance to infusion of saline. These methods, although simple and inexpensive, have some drawbacks. There is a danger of too large a volume being infused, possibly inducing acute compartment syndrome. It is probably the least accurate of the measurement techniques available, with falsely high values having been recorded in comparison with other techniques (96) and falsely low values in cases of very high ICP (97). A needle with only one perforation at its tip can also become easily blocked.

The wick catheter was first described for use in acute compartment syndrome by Mubarak et al (98). This is a modification of the needle technique in which fibrils protrude from the bore of the catheter assembly. This allows a large surface area for measurement and prevents obstruction of the needle; it is ideal for continuous measurement. A disadvantage of this technique is the possibility of a blood clot blocking the tip or air in the column of fluid between the catheter and the transducer, which will dampen the response and give falsely low readings. There is a theoretical risk of retention of wick material in the tissues.

The slit catheter was first described by Rorabeck et al (99). This operates on the same principal as the wick catheter in that it is designed to increase the surface area at the tip of the catheter by means of being cut axially at the end of the catheter (Fig. 13-3). The interstitial pressure is measured through a column of saline attached to a transducer. Patency can be confirmed by

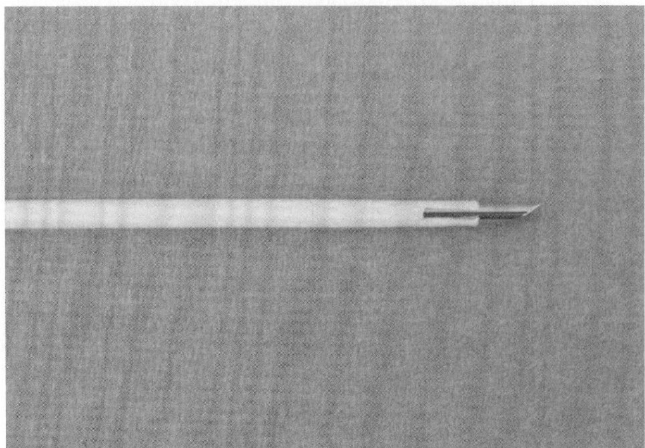

FIGURE 13-3 The tip of a slit catheter. This can be made easily from standard equipment by cutting two slits in the tip of the catheter.

gentle pressure over the catheter tip when an immediate rise in the pressure should be seen. Care must be taken to avoid the presence of air bubbles in the system, because this can, like the wick catheter, result in falsely low readings. The slit catheter is more accurate than the continuous infusion method (96) and is as accurate as the wick catheter (100).

Attempts to improve the reliability of ICP measurement led to the concept of placement of the pressure transducer directly into the compartment by siting it within the lumen of a catheter. The solid state transducer intracompartmental catheter (STIC) was described in 1984 and measurements correlated with conventional pressure monitoring systems (101). This device is now commercially available and is widely used. However, to retain patency of the catheter for continuous monitoring an infusion must be used with its attendant problems. The alternative is intermittent pressure measurement, which is likely to cause significant discomfort to patients and is more labor intensive. Newer systems with the transducer placed at the tip of the catheter do not depend on a column of fluid and therefore avoid the problems of patency (102). However, these systems are more expensive and are a potential problem for resterilization.

All of the methods above measure ICP, which is an indirect way of measuring muscle blood flow and oxygenation. Near infrared spectroscopy measures tissue oxygen saturation noninvasively by means of a probe placed on the skin. This has proven to correlate to tissue pressures experimentally (103), in human volunteers (104), and shows promise but requires further validation in humans subjected to injury (105).

ICP is usually monitored in the anterior compartment because this is most commonly involved in acute compartment syndrome (71) and is easily accessible. There is a risk of missing an acute compartment syndrome in the deep posterior compartments, and some authors recommend measurement of both (106), but measuring two compartments is much more cumbersome. If the anterior compartment alone is monitored, the surgeon must be aware of the small chance of deep posterior acute compartment syndrome and measure the deep posterior compartment pressures if there are unexplained symptoms in the presence of anterior compartment pressures with a safe ΔP. It is important to measure the peak pressure within the limb that usually occurs within 5 cm of the level of the fracture (106). Recommended catheter placement for each of the anatomic areas is summarized in Table 13-4.

TABLE 13-4 Recommended Catheter Placements for Compartmental Pressure Monitoring

Anatomic Area	Catheter Placement
Thigh	Anterior compartment
Leg	Anterior compartment Deep posterior if clinically suspected
Foot	Interosseous compartments Consider calcaneal compartment in hindfoot injuries
Forearm	Flexor compartment
Hand	Interosseous compartment

Threshold for Decompression in Acute Compartment Syndrome

There has been much debate about the critical pressure threshold beyond which decompression of acute compartment syndrome is required. Following appreciation of the nature of acute compartment syndrome being raised pressure, debate centered around the use of tissue pressure alone as indication of the need for decompression. One level believed to be critical was 30 mm Hg of ICP (107,108), because this is a value close to capillary blood pressure. Some authors felt that 40 mm Hg of tissue pressure should be the threshold for decompression (91,94, 101,109), although some recognized a significant individual variation among individuals in their tolerance of raised ICP (49,109). In a series of patients with tibial fractures, a tissue pressure of 50 mm Hg was recommended as a pressure threshold for decompression in normotensive patients (110).

It is now recognized that apparent variation among individuals in their tolerance of raised ICP is due to variations in systemic blood pressure. Whitesides et al (84) were the first to suggest the importance of the difference between the diastolic blood pressure and tissue pressure or ΔP. They stated that there is inadequate perfusion and relative ischemia when the tissue pressure rises to within 10 to 30 mm Hg of the diastolic pressure. There is now good evidence from experimental work to support this concept (55,56) or the similar concept that the difference between mean arterial pressure and tissue pressure should not be less than 30 mm Hg in normal muscle or 40 mm Hg in muscle subject to trauma (54) or antecedent ischemia (57).

This concept was tested in a clinical study designed to test the hypothesis of the differential pressure as a threshold for decompression (20). One hundred and sixteen patients with tibial diaphyseal fractures underwent continuous ICP monitoring both perioperatively and for at least 24 hours postoperatively. The differential pressure between the diastolic blood pressure and the ICP was recorded. Mean pressures over a 12-hour period were calculated to include the duration of elevated pressure in the analysis. Three patients had ΔP of less than 30 mm Hg and underwent fasciotomy. Of the remaining patients, all maintained a ΔP greater than 30 mm Hg despite a number with ICP greater than 40 mm Hg. None of these patients underwent fasciotomy, and none had any sequelae of acute compartment syndrome at final review. The authors concluded that a ΔP of 30 mm Hg is a safe threshold for decompression in acute compartment syndrome. This has recently been validated by the same group (111) who examined the outcome in terms of muscle power and return to function in two groups of patients with tibial fractures. The first group of patients all had an ICP of greater than 30 mm Hg, and the second all had an ICP less than 30 mm Hg. Both groups had maintained a ΔP of greater than 30 mm Hg. There were no differences in the outcomes between the two groups. The concept of the use of ΔP is also supported by Ovre et al (112), who found an unacceptably high rate of fasciotomies (29%) using an ICP of 30 mm Hg as a threshold for decompression.

All of the work quoted above was performed in adults and with reference to leg compartment syndrome. The threshold may differ for children who have a low diastolic pressure and are therefore more likely to have a ΔP less than 30 mm Hg. Mars and Hadley (113) recommend the use of the mean arterial pressure rather than the diastolic pressure to obviate this problem. It has been assumed that these pressure thresholds apply equally to anatomic areas other than the leg, although this has not been formally examined.

The benefit of ICP monitoring in patients at risk of acute compartment syndrome is a significant reduction in the delay to fasciotomy and therefore many fewer patients with sequelae (71). Overtreatment has been cited as a problem with continuous monitoring (114), but this study did not consider the importance of the duration of raised ICP in the diagnosis of acute compartment syndrome. It is important to consider the trend of the ΔP as well as the trend of the ICP. If the ICP is dropping and the ΔP rising, it is safe to observe the patient in anticipation of the ΔP returning within a short time to safe levels. Fasciotomy should not be performed based on a single pressure reading except in extreme cases.

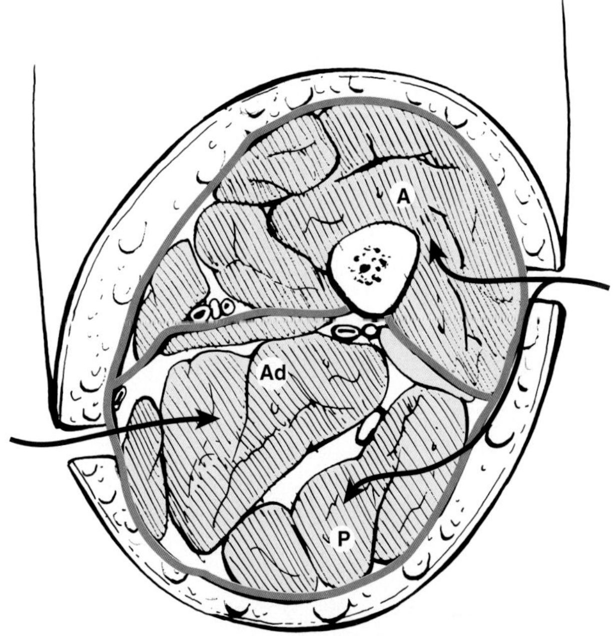

FIGURE 13-4 A cross section of the thigh demonstrating the three compartments and the access to them. *A*, anterior; *P*, posterior; *Ad*, adductor.

SURGICAL AND APPLIED ANATOMY

Thigh

The thigh is divided into three main compartments, which are bounded by the fascia lata and separated by the medial and lateral intermuscular septa (Fig. 13-4). Their contents and the clinical signs of compartment syndrome in each compartment are summarized in Table 13-5. Involvement of the adductor compartment is rare.

Leg

There are four compartments in the leg: anterior, lateral, superficial posterior, and deep posterior (Fig. 13-5).

The anterior compartment is enclosed anteriorly by skin and fascia, laterally by the intermuscular septum, posteriorly by the fibula and interosseous membrane, and medially by the tibia. Its contents and the clinical signs of acute compartment syndrome are listed in Table 13-6.

The lateral compartment is enclosed laterally by skin and fascia, posteriorly by the posterior intermuscular septum, medially by the fibula, and anteriorly by the anterior intermuscular septum. Its contents and the clinical signs of involvement in the acute compartment syndrome are detailed in Table 13-6. The deep peroneal nerve, rarely, may be affected as it passes

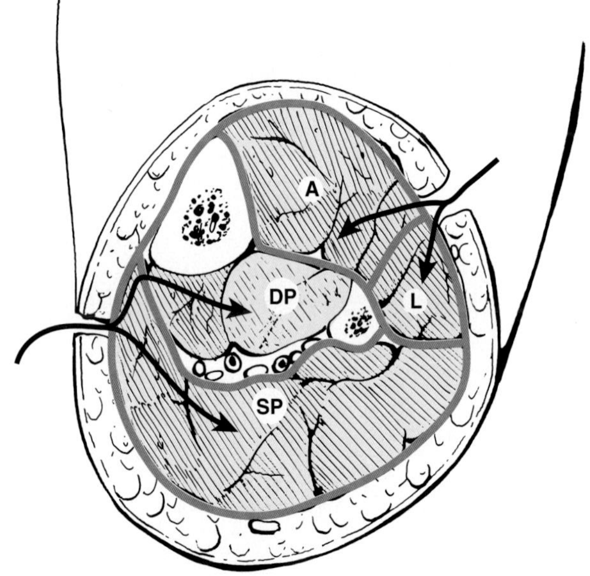

FIGURE 13-5 A cross section of the leg showing the four compartments. The *arrows* show the routes for double-incision four-compartment fasciotomy. *A*, anterior compartment; *L*, lateral compartment; *SP*, superficial posterior compartment; *DP*, deep posterior compartment.

TABLE 13-5 Compartments of the Thigh, Their Contents, and Signs of Acute Compartment Syndrome

Compartment	Contents	Signs
Anterior	Quadriceps muscles Sartorius Femoral nerve	Pain on passive knee flexion Numbness in medial leg/foot Weakness on knee extension
Posterior	Hamstring muscles Sciatic nerve	Pain on passive knee extension Sensory changes rare Weakness on knee flexion
Adductor	Adductor muscles Obturator nerve	Pain passive hip abduction Sensory changes rare Weakness on hip adduction

through the lateral compartment en route to the anterior compartment.

The superficial posterior compartment is bounded anteriorly by the intermuscular septum between the superficial and deep compartments and posteriorly by skin and fascia. Its contents and the clinical signs of acute compartment syndrome are summarized in Table 13-6.

The deep posterior compartment is limited anteriorly by the tibia and interosseous membrane, laterally by the fibula, posteriorly by the intermuscular septum separating it from the superficial posterior compartment, and medially by skin and fascia in the distal part of the leg. Table 13-6 lists the contents of the deep posterior compartment and the likely clinical signs in acute compartment syndrome.

Foot

Until recently most authorities have believed that there are four compartments in the foot: medial, lateral, central, and interosseous (Fig. 13-6). The medial compartment lies on the plantar surface of the hallux, the lateral compartment is on the plantar surface of the fifth metatarsal, and the central compartment lies

TABLE 13-6 Compartments of the Leg, Their Contents, and Clinical Signs of Acute Compartment Syndrome

Compartment	Contents	Signs
Anterior	Tibialis anterior Extensor digitorum longus Extensor hallucis longus Peroneus tertius Deep peroneal (anterior tibial) nerve and vessels	Pain on passive flexion of ankle/toes Numbness of first web space Weakness on ankle/toe flexion
Lateral	Peroneus longus Peroneus brevis Superficial peroneal nerve	Pain on passive foot inversion Numbness of dorsum of foot Weakness of eversion
Superficial posterior	Gastrocnemius Soleus Plantaris Sural nerve	Pain on passive ankle extension Numbness of dorsolateral foot Weakness on plantar flexion
Deep posterior	Tibialis posterior Flexor digitorum longus Flexor hallucis longus Posterior tibial nerve	Pain on passive ankle/toe extension/foot eversion Numbness of sole of foot Weakness on toe/ankle flexion, foot inversion

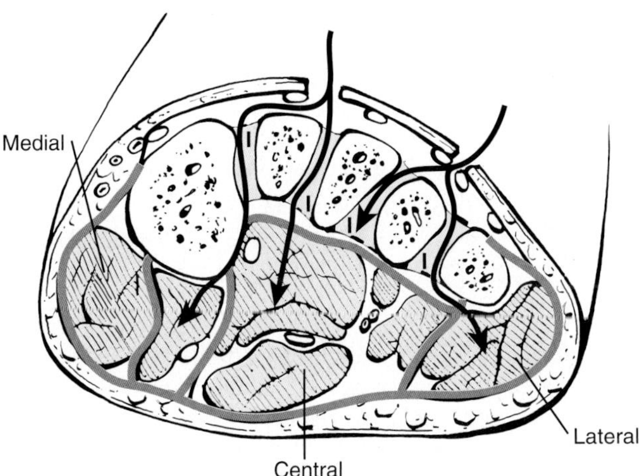

FIGURE 13-6 A cross section of the foot showing access from the dorsum of the foot to the compartments. *I*, interosseous.

on the plantar surface of the foot. The interosseous compartment lies dorsal to the others between the metatarsals. Their contents are shown in Table 13-7.

Manoli and Weber (115) challenged the concept of four compartments using cadaver infusion techniques. They believe that there are nine compartments in the foot, with two central compartments, one superficial containing flexor digitorum brevis and one deep (the calcaneal compartment) (Fig. 13-7) containing quadratus plantae, which communicates with the deep posterior compartment of the leg. They demonstrated that each of the four interosseous muscles and adductor hallucis lie in separate compartments, thus increasing the number of compartments to nine. The clinical importance of these anatomic findings has been challenged after the finding that the barrier between the superficial and calcaneal compartments becomes incompetent at a pressure of 10 mm Hg, much lower than that required to produce an acute compartment syndrome (116). The clinical diagnosis of acute compartment syndrome should be suspected in the presence of severe swelling, but differentiating the affected compartments is extremely difficult.

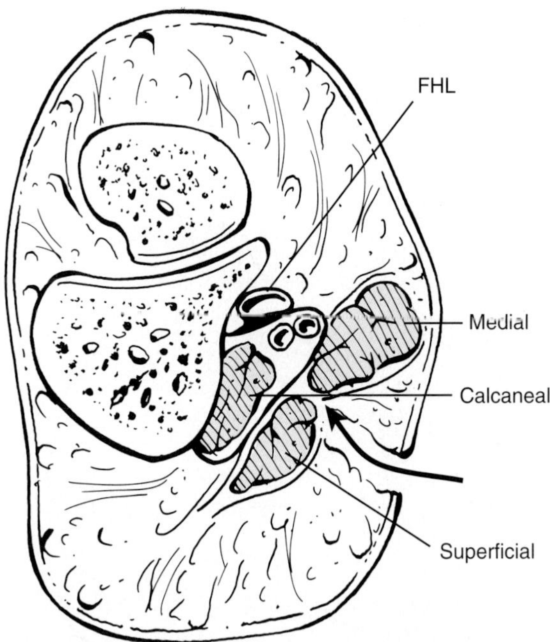

FIGURE 13-7 A section through the hindfoot showing the medial, superficial, and deep central (calcaneal) compartments. The medial approach for release of the calcaneal compartment is shown. *FHL*, flexor hallucis longus.

TABLE 13-7 Compartments of the Foot and Their Contents

Compartment	Contents
Medial	Intrinsic muscles of the great toe
Lateral	Flexor digiti minimi Abductor digiti minimi
Central	
Superficial	Flexor digitorum brevis
Deep (calcaneal)	Quadratus plantae
Adductor hallucis	Adductor hallucis
Interosseous × 4	Interosseous muscles Digital nerves

Arm

There are two compartments in the arm: anterior and posterior (Fig. 13-8). The anterior compartment is bounded by the humerus posteriorly and the lateral and medial intermuscular septa and the brachial fascia anteriorly. Its contents and the clinical signs of acute compartment syndrome are detailed in Table 13-8. In late cases, paralysis of the muscles innervated by the median, ulnar, and radial nerves is seen.

The posterior compartment has the same boundaries as the anterior but lies posterior to the humerus. Its contents and the clinical signs of acute compartment syndrome are listed in Table 13-8.

Forearm

The forearm contains three compartments: volar, dorsal, and "the mobile wad" (Fig. 13-9). The volar compartment has the ulna, radius, and interosseous membrane as its posterior limit and the antebrachial fascia as its anterior limit. Table 13-9 lists the contents and clinical signs of acute compartment syndrome in the volar compartment of the forearm. It has been suggested

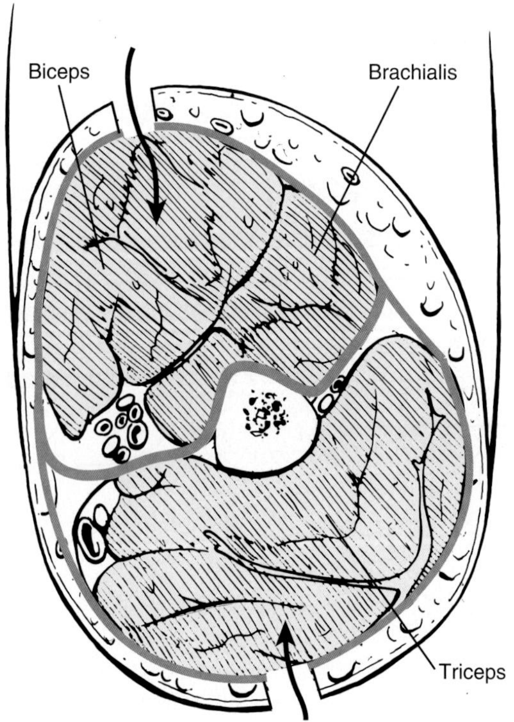

FIGURE 13-8 A cross section of the arm showing the anterior compartment containing biceps and brachialis and the posterior compartment containing triceps.

that the volar compartment of the forearm contains three spaces: the superficial volar, deep volar, and pronator quadratus spaces (117). In practice, however, it is not usually necessary to distinguish between these at fasciotomy (118).

The dorsal compartment of the forearm lies dorsal to the radius, ulna, and interosseous membrane and contains the finger and thumb extensors, abductor pollicis longus, and extensor carpi ulnaris. Its contents and the clinical signs of acute compartment syndrome are summarized in Table 13-9.

Hand

It is generally considered that the hand has 10 muscle compartments: 1 thenar, 1 hypothenar, 1 adductor pollicis, 4 dorsal interosseous, and 3 volar interosseous compartments (Fig. 13-10). The thenar compartment is surrounded by the thenar fascia, the thenar septum, and the first metacarpal. The hypothenar compartment is contained by the hypothenar fascia and septum and the fifth metacarpal. The dorsal interosseous compartments lie between the metacarpals and are bounded by them laterally and the interosseous fascia anteriorly and posteriorly. The volar interosseous compartments lie on the volar aspect of the metacarpals, but it is unlikely that these are functionally separate from the dorsal interosseous compartments because the tissue barrier between the two cannot withstand pressures of more than 15 mm Hg (119). The contents of the hand compartments are detailed in Table 13-10.

Treatment

The single effective treatment for acute compartment syndrome is fasciotomy, which, if delayed, can cause devastating complica-

TABLE 13-8 Compartments of the Arm, Their Contents, and Clinical Signs of Acute Compartment Syndrome

Compartment	Contents	Signs
Anterior	Biceps Brachialis Coracobrachialis Median nerve Ulnar nerve Musculocutaneous nerve Lateral cutaneous nerve Antebrachial nerve Radial nerve (distal third)	Pain on passive elbow extension Numbness with median/ulnar distribution Numbness of volar/lateral distal forearm Weakness on elbow flexion Weakness in median/ulnar motor function
Posterior	Triceps Radial nerve Ulnar nerve (distally)	Pain on passive elbow flexion Numbness with ulnar/radial distribution Weakness on elbow extension Weakness in radial/ulnar motor function

TABLE 13-9 Compartments of the Forearm, Their Contents, and Signs of Acute Compartment Syndrome

Compartment	Contents	Signs
Volar	Flexor carpi radialis longus and brevis Flexor digitorum superficialis and profundus Pronator teres Pronator quadratus Median nerve Ulnar nerve	Pain on passive wrist/finger extension Numbness with median/ulnar distribution Weakness on wrist/finger flexion Weakness in median/ulnar motor function in hand
Dorsal	Extensor digitorum Extensor pollicis longus Abductor pollicis longus Extensor carpi ulnaris	Pain on passive wrist/finger flexion Weakness on wrist/finger flexion
Mobile wad	Brachioradialis Extensor carpi radialis	Pain on passive wrist flexion/elbow extension Weakness on wrist extension/elbow flexion

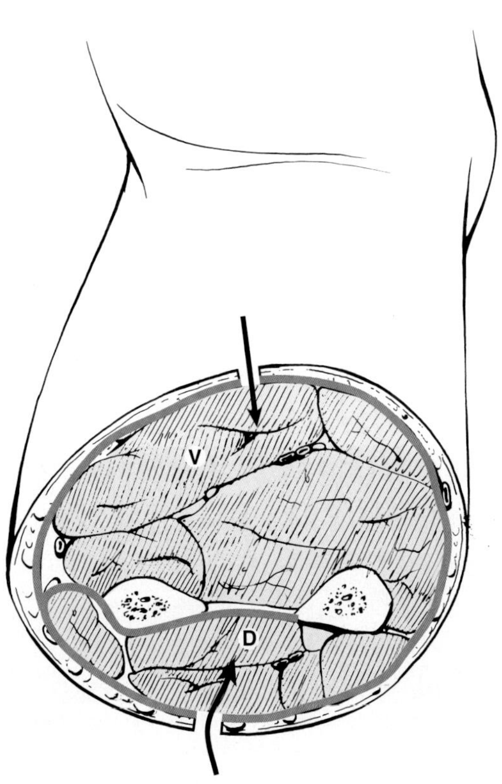

FIGURE 13-9 A cross section of the mid-forearm. The pronator quadratus compartment is not shown as it lies in the distal forearm. *V*, volar; *D*, dorsal.

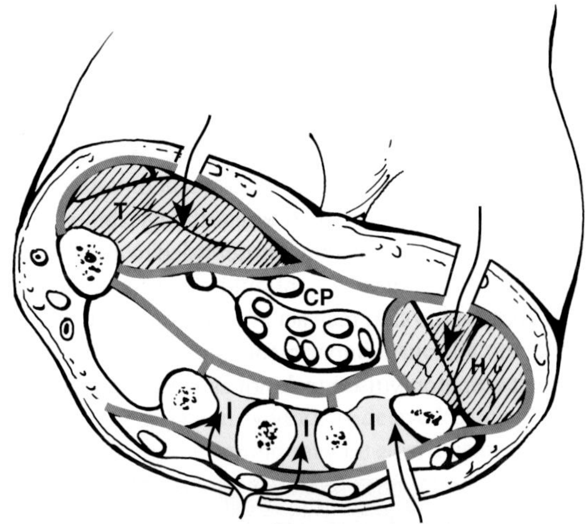

FIGURE 13-10 A cross section of the hand showing the muscle compartments. The adductor pollicis lies more distally. *I*, interosseous; *H*, hypothenar; *T*, thenar; *CP*, central palmar.

tions. However, other preliminary measures should be taken in cases of impending acute compartment syndrome. The process may on occasion be aborted by release of external limiting envelopes such as dressings or plaster casts, including the padding under the cast. Splitting and spreading a cast has been shown to reduce ICP, as has release of dressings (120). The split and spread cast is the only method that can accommodate increasing limb swelling (121). The limb should not be elevated above

ment syndrome treated by fasciotomy (70,81,139,140). In reality, the treatment of the fracture should not be altered by the presence of an acute compartment syndrome, although cast management of a tibial fracture is contraindicated in the presence of acute compartment syndrome. Fasciotomy should be performed before fracture stabilization, to eliminate any unnecessary delay in decompression. Stabilization of the fracture allows easy access to the soft tissues and protects the soft tissues, permitting them to heal.

Reamed intramedullary nailing of the tibia confers excellent stabilization of a diaphyseal fracture and is now probably the treatment of choice in most centers for tibial diaphyseal fracture. Some authors, however, have implicated reaming as a possible cause of acute compartment syndrome (141,142). This was refuted by other studies examining ICP during and after tibial nailing. McQueen et al (143), studying reamed intramedullary nailing, and Tornetta and French (144), studying unreamed intramedullary nailing, agreed that the ICP increased peroperatively and dissipated postoperatively and that nailing did not increase the likelihood of acute compartment syndrome. Nassif et al (145) found no differences in ICP between reamed and unreamed nailing.

Several factors may raise ICP during stabilization of tibial fractures. These include traction, which raises pressure in the deep posterior compartment by approximately 6% per kilogram of weight applied (146). Countertraction using a thigh bar can cause external calf compression if the bar is wrongly positioned and can also decrease arterial flow and venous return, making the leg more vulnerable to ischemia. Elevation of the leg, as in the 90-90 position, decreases the tolerance of the limb to ischemia (66). Thus, excessive traction, poor positioning of the thigh bar, and high elevation of the leg should be avoided in patients at risk for acute compartment syndrome.

COMPLICATIONS OF ACUTE COMPARTMENT SYNDROME

Complications of acute compartment syndrome are unusual if the condition has been treated expeditiously. Delay in diagnosis has been cited as the single reason for failure in the management of acute compartment syndrome (13). Delay to fasciotomy of more than 6 hours is likely to cause significant sequelae (80), including muscle contractures, muscle weakness, sensory loss, infection, and nonunion of fractures (60–71). In severe cases, amputation may be necessary because of infection or lack of function (147).

Late Diagnosis of Acute Compartment Syndrome

There is some debate about the place of decompression when the diagnosis is made late, and muscle necrosis is inevitable, whether it be due to a missed acute compartment syndrome or to the crush syndrome. There seems little to be gained in exploring a closed crush syndrome when complete muscle necrosis is inevitable, except in the circumstances in which there are severe or potentially severe systemic effects when amputation may be necessary. Increased sepsis rates with potentially serious consequences have been reported when these cases have been explored (148). However, if partial muscle necrosis is suspected and compartment monitoring reveals pressures above the threshold for decompression, there may be an indication for fasciotomy to salvage remaining viable muscle. In these circumstances, debridement of necrotic muscle must be thorough to reduce the chances of infection. In rare cases the ICP may be high enough to occlude major vessels. This is a further indication for fasciotomy to salvage the distal part of the limb (148).

It is recommended that if there is no likelihood of any surviving muscle and compartment pressures are low, fasciotomy should be withheld. If there is any possibility of any remaining viable muscle or if compartment pressures are above critical levels, fasciotomy should be performed to preserve any viable muscle. In these circumstances a thorough debridement of necrotic muscle is mandatory.

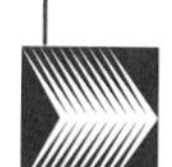

AUTHOR'S PREFERRED TREATMENT

Early diagnosis of acute compartment syndrome is essential, and it is important to be aware of the patients at risk for acute compartment syndrome. Good clinical examination techniques in the alert patient will help to identify the compartments at risk. Compartment monitoring should be used in all at-risk patients, as defined in Table 13-3. In practice this means that all tibial fractures should be monitored, but, if resources to do so are limited, younger patients and male patients should be selected for monitoring. The anterior compartment should be monitored, but in rare cases in which symptoms are present that cannot be explained by the tissue pressures in the anterior compartment, the posterior compartment should also be monitored.

Fasciotomy is performed on the basis of a persistent differential pressure less than 30 mm Hg. If the ΔP is less than 30 mm Hg but the tissue pressure is dropping, as can happen, for example, for a short time after tibial nailing, then the pressure may be observed for a short period in anticipation of the ΔP rising. However, if the ΔP remains less than 30 mm Hg or is decreasing, immediate fasciotomy is indicated. The decision is made primarily on the level of ΔP, with clinical symptoms and signs being used as an adjunct to diagnosis.

I prefer four compartment fasciotomy in the leg because it is simpler and gives an excellent view of all compartments. At this stage, if a fracture is present, it should be stabilized if this has not been done previously. Closure is with a suction-type dressing followed at 48 hours with either direct closure or split skin grafting. There is no indication to prolong closure beyond this unless there is residual muscle necrosis.

FUTURE DIRECTIONS

Acute compartment syndrome remains a potentially devastating complication of fracture. Future development is likely to center around methods of measuring blood flow directly rather than indirectly by ICP measurement. Noninvasive methods of diagnosing acute compartment syndrome are being examined. One such example is near infrared spectroscopy, which measures the amount of oxygenated haemoglobin in muscle tissues transcutaneously (103–105).

Methods of reducing the effects of acute compartment syndrome are also likely to play a part in the future. Some basic science research has already been published on the effects of antioxidants on the outcome of acute compartment syndrome with promising results (78). This work should be extended to human studies in an attempt to reduce the affects of acute compartment syndrome in the clinical situation.

Prevention of acute compartment syndrome is the ultimate goal in its management. Attempts have been made to reduce ICP with the administration of hypertonic fluids intravenously (149), but these have never been successful clinically. However, an experiment on human subjects using tissue ultrafiltration to remove fluid from the compartment has been shown to reduce ICP (150). It remains to be seen whether this technique can be useful clinically.

REFERENCES

1. Hildebrand O. Die Lehre von den ischämischen Muskellahmungen und Kontrakturen. *Z Chir* 1906;108:44–201.
2. Von Volkmann R. Die ischämischen Muskellahmungen und Kontrakturen. *Zentrabl Chir* 1881;51–801.
3. Peterson F. Über ischämische Muskellahmung. *Arch Klin Chir* 1888;37:675–677.
4. Wallis FC. Treatment of paralysis and muscular atrophy after the prolonged use of splints or of an Esmarch's cord. *Practitioner* 1907;67:429–436.
5. Dudgeon LS. Volkmann's contracture. *Lancet* 1902;1:78–85.
6. Rowlands RP. A case of Volkmann's contracture treated by shortening the radius and ulna. *Lancet* 1905;2:1168–1171.
7. Bardenheuer L. Die Anlang und Behandlung der ischaemische Muskellahmungen und Kontrakturen. *Samml Klin Vorträge* 1911;122:437.
8. Murphy JB. Myositis. *JAMA* 1914;63:1249–1255.
9. Jepson PN. Ischaemic contracture: experimental study. *Ann Surg* 1926;84:785–795.
10. Griffiths DL. Volkmann's ischaemic contracture. *Br J Surg* 1940;28:239–260.
11. Foisie PS. Volkmann's ischaemic contracture. *N Engl J Med* 1942;226:671–679.
12. Seddon HJ. Volkmann's ischaemia in the lower limb. *J Bone Joint Surg Br* 1966;48: 627–636.
13. McQuillan WM, Nolan B. Ischaemia complicating injury. *J Bone Joint Surg Br* 1968; 50:482–492.
14. McQueen MM, Gaston P, Court-Brown CM. Acute compartment syndrome: who is at risk? *J Bone Joint Surg Br* 2000;82:200–203.
15. Buhr AJ, Cooke AM. Fracture patterns. *Lancet* 1959;1:531–536.
16. Bae DS, Kadiyala RK, Waters PM. Acute compartment syndrome in children: contemporary diagnosis, treatment and outcome. *J Pediatr Orthop* 2001;21:680–688.
17. Court-Brown CM, Byrnes T, McLaughlin G. Intramedullary nailing of tibial diaphyseal fractures in children with open physes. *Injury* 2003;34:781–785.
18. Blick SS, Brumback PJ, Poka A, et al. Compartment syndrome in open tibial fractures. *J Bone Joint Surg Am* 1986;68:1348–1353.
19. Williams J, Gibbons M, Trindle H, et al. Complications of nailing in closed tibial fractures. *J Orthop Trauma* 1995;9:476–481.
20. McQueen MM, Court-Brown CM. Compartment monitoring in tibial fractures: the pressure threshold for decompression. *J Bone Joint Surg Br* 1996;78:99–104.
21. Finkemeier CG, Schmidt AH, Kyle RF, et al. A prospective randomised study of intramedullary nails inserted with and without reaming for the treatment of open and closed fractures of the tibial shaft. *J Orthop Trauma* 2000;14:187–193.
22. Mullett H, Al-Abed K, Prasad C, et al. Outcome of compartment syndrome following intramedullary nailing of tibial diaphyseal fractures. *Injury* 2001;32:411–413.
23. Mathews PV, Perry JJ, Murray PC. Compartment syndrome of the well leg as a result of the hemi-lithotomy position: a report of two cases and review of literature. *J Orthop Trauma* 2001;15:580–583.
24. McKee MD, Jupiter JB. Acute exercise-induced bilateral anterolateral leg compartment syndrome in a healthy young man. *Am J Orthop* 1995;24:862–864.
25. Seiler JG, Valadie AL, Frederick RW, et al. Perioperative compartment syndrome: a report of four cases. *J Bone Joint Surg Am* 1996;78:600–602.
26. Belanger M, Fadale P. Compartment syndrome of the leg after arthroscopic examination of a tibial plateau fracture: case report and review of the literature. *Arthroscopy* 1997; 13:646–651.
27. Shabat S, Carmel A, Cohen Y, et al. Iatrogenic forearm compartment syndrome in a cardiac intensive care unit induced by brachial artery puncture and acute anticoagulation. *J Interv Cardiol* 2002;15:107–109.
28. Dunlop D, Parker PJ, Keating JF. Ruptured Baker's cyst causing posterior compartment syndrome. *Injury* 1997;28:561–562.
29. Gibson MJ, Barnes MR, Allem MJ, et al. Weakness of foot dorsiflexion and changes in compartment pressures after tibial osteotomy. *J Bone Joint Surg Br* 1986;68:471–475.
30. Vigasio A, Battiston B, De Filippo G, et al. Compartmental syndrome due to viper bite. *Arch Orthop Trauma Surg* 1991;110:175–177.
31. Sweeney HE, O'Brien F. Bilateral anterior tibial compartment syndrome in association with the nephritic syndrome: report of a case. *Arch Intern Med* 1965;116:487–488.
32. Veerandghandam RS, Paz IB, Nadeemanee A. Compartment syndrome of the leg secondary to leukaemic infiltration: a case report and review of the literature. *J Surg Oncol* 1994;55:198–200.
33. Lam R, Lin PH, Alankar S, et al. Acute limb ischaemia secondary to myositis-induced compartment syndrome in a patient with human immunodeficiency virus infection. *J Vasc Surg* 2003;37:1103–1105.
34. Stott NS, Zionts LE, Holtom PD, et al. Acute haematogenous osteomyelitis: an unusual case of compartment syndrome in a child. *Clin Orthop* 1995;317:210–222.
35. Almdahl SM, Due J, Samdal FA. Compartment syndrome with muscle necrosis following repair of hernia of tibialis anterior: case report. *Acta Chir Scand* 1987;153:695–697.
36. Chautems RC, Irmay F, Magnin M, et al. Spontaneous anterior and lateral tibial compartment syndrome in a type 1 diabetic patient: case report. *J Trauma* 1997;43: 140–141.
37. Hsu SI, Thadhani RI, Daniels GH. Acute compartment syndrome in a hypothyroid patient. *Thyroid* 1995;5:305–308.
38. Hope MJ, McQueen MM. Acute compartment syndrome in the absence of fracture. *J Orthop Trauma* 2004;18:220–224.
39. Court-Brown CM, McBirnie J. The epidemiology of tibial fractures. *J Bone Joint Surg Br* 1995;77:417–421.
40. Mubarak SJ, Wilton NCT. Compartment syndromes and epidural analgesia. *J Paediatr Orthop* 1997;17:282–284.
41. Harrington P, Bunola J, Jennings AJ, et al. Acute compartment syndrome masked by intravenous morphine from a patient-controlled analgesia pump. *Injury* 2000;31: 387–389.
42. Burton A. On the physical equilibrium of small blood vessels. *J Biomechanics* 1971;4: 155–158.
43. Nichol J, Girling F, Jerrard W, et al. Fundamental instability of the small blood vessels and critical closing pressures in vascular beds. *Am J Physiol* 1951;164:330–344.
44. Yamada S. Effects of positive tissue pressure on blood flow of the finger. *J Appl Physiol* 1954;6:495–500.
45. Roddie IC, Shepherd JT. Evidence for critical closure of digital resistance vessels with reduced transmural pressure and passive vaso-dilation with increased venous pressure. *J Physiol* 1957;136:498–506.
46. Ashton H. Critical closing pressure in human peripheral vascular beds. *Clin Sci* 1962; 22:79–87.
47. Ashton H. The effect of increased tissue pressure on blood flow. *Clin Orthop* 1975; 113:15–26.
48. Matsen FA. In: *Compartmental Syndromes.* New York: Grune Stratton; 1980.
49. Matsen FA, Wyss CR, Krugmire RB, et al. The effect of limb elevation and dependency on local arteriovenous gradients in normal human limbs with particular reference to limbs with increased tissue pressure. *Clin Orthop* 1980;150:187–195.
50. Henriksen O. Orthostatic changes of blood flow in subcutaneous tissue in patients with arterial insufficiency of the legs. *Scand J Clin Lav Invest* 1974;34:103–109.
51. Vollmar B, Westermann S, Menzer M. Microvascular response to compartment syndrome-like external pressure elevation: an in vivo fluorescence microscopic study in the hamster striated muscle. *J Trauma* 1999;46:91–96.
52. Hargens AR, Akeson WH, Mubarak SJ, et al. Fluid balance within the canine anterolateral compartment and its relationship to compartment syndromes. *J Bone Joint Surg Am* 1978;60:499–505.
53. Hartsock LA, O'Farrell D, Seaber AV, et al. Effect of increased compartment pressure on the microcirculation of skeletal muscle. *Microsurgery* 1998;18:67–71.
54. Heppenstall RB, Sapega AA, Scott R, et al. The compartment syndrome: an experimental and clinical study of muscular energy metabolism using phosphorus nuclear magnetic resonance spectroscopy. *Clin Orthop* 1988;226:138–155.
55. Heckman MM, Whitesides TE, Greve SR, et al. Histologic determination of the ischaemic threshold of muscle in the canine compartment syndrome model. *J Orthop Trauma* 1993;7:199–210.
56. Matava MS, Whitesides TE, Seiler JG, et al. Determination of the compartment pressure threshold of muscle ischaemia in a canine model. *J Trauma* 1994;37:50–58.
57. Bernot M, Gupta R, Dobrasz J, et al. The effect of antecedent ischaemia on the tolerance of skeletal muscle to increased interstitial pressure. *J Orthop Trauma* 1996;10:555–559.
58. Labbe R, Lindsay T, Walker PM. The extent and distribution of skeletal muscle necrosis after graded periods of complete ischaemia. *J Vasc Surg* 1987;6:152–157.
59. Petrasek PF, Homer-Vanmasinkam S, Walker PM. Determinants of ischaemic injury to skeletal muscle. *J Vasc Surg* 1994;19:623–631.

60. Hayes G, Liauw S, Romaschin AD, et al. Separation of reperfusion injury from ischaemia induced necrosis. *Surg Forum* 1988;39:306–308.
61. Lindsay TF, Liauw S, Rouraschin AD, et al. The effect of ischaemia/reperfusion on adenosine nucleotide metabolism and xanthine oxidase production in skeletal muscle. *J Vasc Surg* 1990;12:8–15.
62. Sheridan GW, Matsen FA, Krugmire RB. Further investigations on the pathophysiology of the compartmental syndrome. *Clin Orthop* 1977;123:266–270.
63. Matsen FA, King RV, Krugmire RB, et al. Physiological effects of increased tissue pressure. *Int Orthop* 1979;3:237–244.
64. Hargens AR, Romine JS, Sipe JC, et al. Peripheral nerve conduction block by high muscle compartment pressure. *J Bone Joint Surg Am* 1979;61:192–200.
65. Gelberman RH, Szabo RM, Williamson RV, et al. Tissue pressure threshold for peripheral nerve viability. *Clin Orthop* 1983;178:285–291.
66. Matsen FA, Mayo KA, Krugmire RB, et al. A model compartment syndrome in man with particular reference to the quantification of nerve function. *J Bone Joint Surg Am* 1978;59:648–653.
67. Karlstrom G, Lonnerholm T, Olerud S. Cavus deformity of the foot after fracture of the tibial shaft. *J Bone Joint Surg Am* 1975;57:893–900.
68. Delee JC, Stiehl JB. Open tibia fracture with compartment syndrome. *Clin Orthop* 1981; 160:175–184.
69. Court-Brown CM, McQueen MM. Compartment syndrome delays tibial union. *Acta Orthop Scand* 1987;58:249–252.
70. Turen CH, Burgess AR, Vanco B. Skeletal stabilization for tibial fractures associated with acute compartment syndrome. *Clin Orthop* 1995;315:163–168.
71. McQueen MM, Christie J, Court-Brown CM. Acute compartment syndrome in tibial diaphyseal fractures. *J Bone Joint Surg Br* 1996;78:95–98.
72. Nario CV. La enfermedad de Volkman experimental. *Ann Fac Med Montivideo* 1938; 10:87–128.
73. McQueen MM. *The Effect of Acute Compartment Syndrome on Bone Blood Flow and Bone Union.* MD Thesis 1995, University of Edinburgh.
74. Blaisdell FW. The pathophysiology of skeletal muscle ischaemia and the reperfusion syndrome: a review. *Cardiovasc Surg* 2002;10:620–630.
75. Walker PM, Lindsay TF, Labbe R, et al. Salvage of skeletal muscle with free radical scavengers. *J Vasc Surg* 1987;5:68–75.
76. Adams JG, Dhar A, Shukla SD, et al. Effect of pentoxifylline on tissue injury and platelet-activating factor production during ischaemia–reperfusion injury. *J Vasc Surg* 1995;21:742–748.
77. Kearns SR, Moneley D, Murray P, et al. Oral vitamin C attenuates acute ischaemia–reperfusion injury in skeletal muscle. *J Bone Joint Surg Br* 2001;83:1202–1206.
78. Kearns SR, Daly AF, Sheehan K, et al. Oral vitamin C reduces the injury to skeletal muscle caused by compartment syndrome. *J Bone Joint Surg Br* 2004;86:906–911.
79. Matsen FA, Clawson DK. The deep posterior compartmental syndrome of the leg. *J Bone Joint Surg Am* 1975;57:34–39.
80. Rorabeck CH, Macnab L. Anterior tibial compartment syndrome complicating fractures of the shaft of the tibia. *J Bone Joint Surg Am* 1976;58:549–550.
81. Rorabeck CH. The treatment of compartment syndromes of the leg. *J Bone Joint Surg Br* 1984;66:93–97.
82. Bhattacharyya T, Vrahas M. The medicolegal aspects of compartment syndrome. *J Bone Joint Surg Am* 2004:86:864–868.
83. Eaton RG, Green WT. Volkmann's ischaemia: a volar compartment syndrome of the forearm. *Clin Orthop* 1975;113:58–64.
84. Whitesides TE, Haney TC, Morimoto K, et al. Tissue pressure measurements as a determinant for the need of fasciotomy. *Clin Orthop* 1975;113:43–51.
85. Matsen FA, Krugmire RB. Compartmental syndromes. *Surg Gynaecol Obstet* 1978;147: 943–949.
86. Holden CEA. The pathology and prevention of Volkmann's ischaemic contracture. *J Bone Joint Surg Br* 1979;61:296–300.
87. Wright JG, Bogoch ER, Hastings DE. The 'occult' compartment syndrome. *J Trauma* 1989;29:133–134.
88. Shereff MJ. Compartment syndromes of the foot. *Instr Course Lect* 1990;39:127–132.
89. Myerson MS. Management of compartment syndromes of the foot. *Clin Orthop* 1991; 271:239–248.
90. Ulmer T. The clinical diagnosis of compartment syndrome of the lower leg: are clinical findings predictive of the disorder? *J Orthop Trauma* 2002;16:572–577.
91. Schwartz JT, Brumback RJ, Lakatos R, et al. Acute compartment syndrome of the thigh: a spectrum of injury. *J Bone Joint Surg Am* 1989;71:392–400.
92. Willis RB, Rorabeck CH. Treatment of compartment syndrome in children. *Orthop Clin North Am* 1990;21:401–412.
93. Bradley EL. The anterior tibial compartment syndrome. *Surg Gynaecol Obstet* 1973; 136:289–297.
94. Matsen FA, Mayo KY, Sheridan GW, et al. Monitoring of intramuscular pressure. *Surgery* 1976;79:702–709.
95. Matsen FA, Winquist RA, Krugmire RB. Diagnosis and management of compartmental syndromes. *J Bone Joint Surg Am* 1980;62:286–291.
96. Moed BR, Thorderson PK. Measurement of ICP: a comparison of the slit catheter, side-ported needle and simple needle. *J Bone Joint Surg Am* 1993;75:231–235.
97. Styf JR, Crenshaw A, Hargens AR. Intramuscular pressures during exercise: comparison of measurements with and without infusion. *Acta Orthop Scan* 1989;60:593–596.
98. Mubarak SJ, Hargens AR, Owen CA, et al. The wick catheter technique for measurement of intramuscular pressure. *J Bone Joint Surg Am* 1976;58:1016–1020.
99. Rorabeck CH, Castle GSP, Hardie R, et al. Compartmental pressure measurements: an experimental investigation using the slit catheter. *J Trauma* 1981;21:446–449.
100. Shakespeare DT, Henderson NJ, Clough G. The slit catheter: a comparison with the wick catheter in the measurement of compartment pressure. *Injury* 1982;13:404–408.
101. McDermott AGP, Marble AE, Yabsley RH. Monitoring acute compartment pressures with the STIC catheter. *Clin Orthop* 1984;190:192–198.
102. Willy C, Gerngross H, Sterk J. Measurement of intracompartmental pressure with use of a new electronic transducer-tipped catheter system. *J Bone Joint Surg Am* 1999;81: 158–168.
103. Arbabi S, Brundage SI, Gentilello LM. Near-infrared spectroscopy: a potential method for continuous transcutaneous monitoring for compartmental syndrome in critically injured patients. *J Trauma* 1999;47:829–833.
104. Gentilello LM, Sanzone A, Wang L, et al. Near-infrared spectroscopy versus compartment pressure for the diagnosis of lower extremity compartmental syndrome using electromyelography-determined measurements of neuromuscular function. *J Trauma* 2001;51:1–8.
105. Hope MJ, Simpson H, McQueen MM. Non-invasive acute compartment syndrome monitoring: the influence of haematoma on near-infrared spectroscopy. *Proc AAOS* 2003;4:514.
106. Heckman MM, Whitesides TE, Greive SR, et al. Compartment pressure in association with closed tibial fractures: the relationship between tissue pressure, compartment and the distance from the site of the fracture. *J Bone Joint Surg Am* 1994;76:1285–1292.
107. Mubarak SJ, Owen CA, Hargens AR, et al. Acute compartment syndromes: diagnosis and treatment with the aid of the wick catheter. *J Bone Joint Surg Am* 1978;60: 1091–1095.
108. Hargens AR, Akeson WH, Mubarak SJ, et al. Kappa Delta Award Paper: tissue fluid pressures—from basic research tools to clinical applications. *J Orthop Res* 1989;7: 902–909.
109. Halpern AA, Nagel DA. Compartment syndrome of the forearm: early recognition using tissue pressure measurement. *J Hand Surg* 1979;4:258–263.
110. Halpern AA, Nagel DA. Anterior compartment pressure in patients with tibial fracture. *J Trauma* 1980;20:786–790.
111. White TO, Howell GED, Will EM, et al. Elevated intramuscular compartment pressures do not influence outcome after tibial fracture. *J Trauma* 2003;55:1133–1138.
112. Ovre S, Hvaal K, Holm I, et al. Compartment pressure in nailed tibial fractures: a threshold of 30 mmHg for decompression gives 29% fasciotomies. *Arch Orthop Trauma Surg* 1998;118:29–31.
113. Mars M, Hadley GP. Raised compartmental pressure in children: a basis for management. *Injury* 1998;29:183–185.
114. Janzing HMJ, Broos PLO. Routine monitoring of compartment pressure in patients with tibial fractures: beware of overtreatment! *Injury* 2001;32:415–421.
115. Manoli A, Weber TG. Fasciotomy of the foot: an anatomical study with special reference to release of the calcaneal compartment. *Foot Ankle* 1990;10:267–275.
116. Guyton GP, Shearman CM, Saltzman CL. The compartments of the foot revisited: rethinking the validity of cadaver infusion experiments. *J Bone Joint Surg Br* 2001;83: 245–249.
117. Gerber A, Masquelet AC. Anatomy and intracompartmental pressure measurement technique of the pronator quadratus compartment. *J Hand Surg Am* 2001;26: 1129–1134.
118. Chan PS, Steinberg DR, Pepe MD, et al. The significance of the three volar spaces in forearm compartment syndrome: a clinical and cadaveric correlation. *J Hand Surg Am* 1998;23:1077–1081.
119. Guyton GP, Shearman CM, Saltzman CL. Compartmental divisions of the hand revisited: rethinking the validity of cadaver infusion experiments. *J Bone Joint Surg Br* 2001; 83:241–244.
120. Garfin SR, Mubarak SJ, Evans KL, et al. Quantification of intracompartmental pressure and volume under plaster casts. *J Bone Joint Surg Am* 1981;63:449–453.
121. Younger ASE, Curran P, McQueen MM. Backslabs and plaster casts: which will best accommodate increasing intracompartmental pressures? *Injury* 1990;21:178–181.
122. Gaspard DJ, Kohl RD. Compartmental syndromes in which skin is the limiting boundary. *Clin Orthop* 1975;113:65–68.
123. Mubarak SJ, Owen CA. Double incision fasciotomy of the leg for decompression in compartment syndromes. *J Bone Joint Surg Am* 1977;59:1854–1857.
124. Adkison DP, Bosse MJ, Gaccione DR, et al. Anatomical variations in the course of the superficial peroneal nerve. *J Bone Joint Surg Am* 1991;73:112–114.
125. A report by the British Orthopaedic Association/British Association of Plastic Surgeons working party on the management of open tibial fractures. *Br J Plast Surg* 1997;50: 570–583.
126. Pyne D, Jawad ASM, Padhiar N. Saphenous nerve injury after fasciotomy for compartment syndrome. *Br J Sports Med* 2003;37:541–542.
127. Kelly RP, Whitesides TE. Transfibular route for fasciotomy of the leg. *J Bone Joint Surg Am* 1967;49:1022–1023.
128. Cooper GG. A method of single incision for compartment fasciotomy of the leg. *Eur J Vasc Surg* 1992;6:659–661.
129. Vitale GC, Richardson JD, George SM, et al. Fasciotomy for severe blunt and penetrating trauma of the extremity. *Surg Gynaecol Obstet* 1988;166:397–401.
130. Tarlow SD, Achterman CA, Hayhurst J, et al. Acute compartment syndrome in the thigh complicating fracture of the femur: a report of three cases. *J Bone Joint Surg Am* 1986;68:1439–1443.
131. Myerson M, Manoli A. Compartment syndromes of the foot after calcaneal fractures. *Clin Orthop* 1993;290:142–150.
132. Sanders R. Displaced intra-articular fractures of the calcaneus. *J Bone Joint Surg Am* 2000;82:225–250.
133. Diminick M, Shapiro G, Cornell C. Acute compartment syndrome of the triceps and deltoid. *J Orthop Trauma* 1999;13:225–227.

134. Havig MT, Leversedge FJ, Seiler JG. Forearm compartment pressures: an in vitro analysis of open and endoscopic fasciotomy. *J Hand Surg Am* 1999:24:1289–1297.
135. Janzing H, Broos P. Dermotraction: an effective technique for the closure of fasciotomy—a preliminary report of fifteen patients. *J Orthop Trauma* 2001;15:438–441.
136. Berman SS, Schilling JD, McIntyre KE, et al. Shoelace technique for delayed primary closure of fasciotomies. *Am J Surg* 1994;169:435–436.
137. Fitzgerald AM, Gaston P, Wilson Y, et al. Long term sequelae of fasciotomy wounds. *Br J Plast Surg* 2000;53:690–693.
138. Webb LX. New techniques in wound management: vacuum assisted wound closure. *J Am Acad Orthop Surg* 2002;10:303–311.
139. Gelberman RH. Upper extremity compartment syndromes. In: Mubarak SJ, Hargens AR, eds. *Compartment Syndromes and Volkmann's Contracture.* Philadelphia: WB Saunders; 1981.
140. Gershuni DH, Mubarak SJ, Yani NC, et al. Fracture of the tibia complicated by acute compartment syndrome. *Clin Orthop* 1987;217:221–227.
141. Koval KJ, Clapper MF, Brumback RJ, et al. Complications of reamed intramedullary nailing of the tibia. *J Orthop Trauma* 1991;5:184–189.
142. Moed BR, Strom DE. Compartment syndrome after closed intramedullary nailing of the tibia: a canine model and report of two cases. *J Orthop Trauma* 1991;5:71–77.
143. McQueen MM, Christie J, Court-Brown CM. Compartment pressures after intramedullary nailing of the tibia. *J Bone Joint Surg Br* 1990;72:95–98.
144. Tornetta P, French BG. Compartment pressures during non-reamed tibial nailing without traction. *J Orthop Trauma* 1997;11:24–27.
145. Nassif JM, Gorczyca JT, Cole JK, et al. Effect of acute reamed versus unreamed intramedullary nailing on compartment pressure when treating closed tibial shaft fractures: a randomised prospective study. *J Orthop Trauma* 2000;14:554–558.
146. Shakespeare DT, Henderson NJ. Compartmental pressure changes during calcaneal traction in tibial fractures. *J Bone Joint Surg Br* 1982;64:498–499.
147. Finkelstein JA, Hunter GA, Hu RW. Lower limb compartment syndrome: course after delayed fasciotomy. *J Trauma* 1996;40:342–344.
148. Reis ND, Michaelson M. Crush injury to the lower limbs: treatment of the local injury. *J Bone Joint Surg Am* 1986;68:414–418.
149. Better OS, Zinman C, Reis DN, et al. Hypertonic mannitol ameliorates intracompartmental tamponade in a model compartment syndrome in the dog. *Nephron* 1991;58:344–346.
150. Schmidt AH, Fowler D, Tollefson J, et al. Compartment syndrome ultrafiltration catheters: report of a clinical pilot study of a novel method for management of patients at risk of compartment syndrome. Presented at the Annual Meeting of the Orthopaedic Trauma Association, Hollywood, Florida, 2004.

PENETRATING TRAUMA

Edward A. Perez

Firearms, for better or for worse, are an enduring aspect of American culture. An estimated two thirds of American households possess a firearm (1,2), and more American civilians have been killed by firearms than American soldiers in every war ever fought. Equally as disturbing, fatalities from gunshots in the United States may be as high as 90 times that of any other industrialized nation (1,2,3). The Centers for Disease Control and Prevention reported that between 1993 and 1998 an average of 35,200 fatal injuries and 79,400 nonfatal injuries occurred each year as the result of firearms, and a large urban trauma center reported that gunshot wounds accounted for 24% of orthopaedic admissions and 33% of the average daily orthopaedic census (Fig. 14-1) (4). These alarming numbers were foreseen by Silliphant and Beyer (5), who in 1955 prophetically warned that wound ballistics should "not concern the military surgeon exclusively." This observation is particularly pertinent for orthopaedic surgeons because approximately half of all gunshot injuries are associated with fractures or joint penetration. Although most firearm injuries are caused by low-velocity handguns, with resultant low-energy injuries, a trend toward the use of more damaging, higher-velocity weapons; large-caliber, deforming bullets; and shotguns has been noted (6). Because of the variability of these injuries, treatment concepts continue to evolve, including the extent of debridement, the type and length of antibiotic therapy, and the type of skeletal fixation.

BALLISTICS

Many factors influence the wounding potential of a weapon, including velocity, ammunition, target, and distance. The sci-

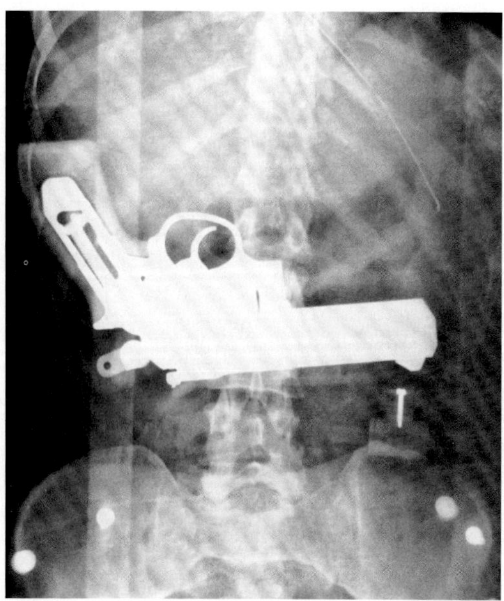

FIGURE 14-1 Handguns are the weapon of choice for urban violence because they are easily carried and concealed. This handgun was discovered during routine x-ray evaluation of a trauma patient.

ence of ballistics studies the behavior of projectiles in flight and their effects on impact. An understanding of the basic principles of ballistics (and firearm-related terminology) will enable the orthopaedic surgeon to more effectively evaluate injuries caused by penetrating trauma (7–9).

Ballistics can be separated into three distinct phases: internal ballistics, external ballistics, and terminal, or wound, ballistics. *Internal* ballistics refers to the characteristics of the projectile within the weapon, whereas *external* ballistics studies the flight of a projectile through the air from the moment it leaves the barrel to the moment it strikes its target. Once a bullet leaves the gun barrel, it starts to decelerate because of impedance from the atmosphere. Projectiles, however, do not behave in a completely stable manner during flight. *Yaw* describes a tilting motion of the projectile as it travels along its flight path. The yaw angle may change dramatically once a bullet contacts its target. *Tumbling* describes the movement of a bullet around its longitudinal axis and usually is insignificant until the target is struck.

Terminal, or *wound*, ballistics describes the effects of the projectile on its target. The amount of kinetic energy transferred to the target tissue is believed to be an important factor in determining wound severity. Kinetic energy is defined (10) as mass multiplied by velocity to the second power:

$$KE = \frac{MV^2}{2}$$

According to this principle, increasing the mass of the bullet or its velocity would increase the wounding potential of a weapon. As an example, a .45-caliber bullet has 5.5 times the amount of kinetic energy as the smaller .25-caliber bullet traveling at the same velocity. The kinetic energy released to the target tissue is equal to the kinetic energy of the missile on exit subtracted from the kinetic energy of the missile on entry (Δ KE = K entry − K exit). Using this formula, a bullet of a given mass and velocity that completely decelerates and becomes lodged in tissue will create a more severe wound than if it had exited the target with little loss of velocity. In general, missiles with greater velocity on impact have a greater change in kinetic energy because of a higher drag within the tissues.

Although important, the transfer of kinetic energy is not the only determinant of wound severity. A large, relatively slow bullet and a smaller, faster bullet may have the same kinetic energy but create different patterns of tissue destruction. The type of tissue struck (adipose, muscle, bone, nerve, artery) and its interaction with the projectile also play key roles.

There are three distinct components of a projectile's effect on tissue: the sonic pressure wave, the permanent cavity, and the temporary cavity (8). A sonic pressure wave precedes the bullet at the time of impact. The velocity of the sonic wave is equivalent to the speed of sound in water (4,800 feet per second), and the wave can produce up to 117 atmospheres of pressure (11). This wave, however, is of extremely brief duration (a few microseconds) and causes no significant tissue disruption. Some investigators believe that the sonic wave may cause neural injury even distant to the site of the missile impact (11), whereas others contend that temporary cavitation may cause the injuries attributed to the sonic wave (8).

The permanent cavity refers to the tissue destroyed by the bullet as it travels within its target (7,8,12). The size of the permanent cavity varies considerably, depending on the type of firearm, the type of ammunition, the distance to the target, and the interaction of the projectile with the target tissues. When the bullet strikes tissue, its flight becomes less stable and its yaw increases. The amount of yaw growth within the tissue is proportional to the degree of yaw at entry (7,8). Tumbling of the bullet within the tissues increases its effective diameter (maximal at 90 degrees of yaw) and as a result increases its wounding capacity. Therefore, it is possible to have a large permanent cavity of tissue destruction underlying a relatively small entrance wound. Tissue destruction also is related to the ratio of a bullet's mass and velocity. A larger, slower bullet causes more tissue crust (permanent cavity) and less radial tissue stretching (temporary cavity) than a smaller, faster bullet. The size of the permanent cavity also depends on the type of ammunition. Bullets that deform and fragment on impact (copper-jacketed, hollow-point) significantly increase tissue destruction.

The temporary cavity is a transient pocket that forms behind the bullet as a result of radial expansion of tissue caused by release of kinetic energy. Pressures created range from 4 atmospheres to subatmospheric (11), and the cavity can be as much as 30 times the size of the projectile (7,8). The effect of temporary cavitation varies with the elasticity of the tissue encountered. Elastic tissue that can easily stretch (lung) sustains less damage than relatively inelastic tissue (liver, bone). Research has shown that a temporary cavity created near a bone can cause it to shatter (13). Bone fragments can become secondary missiles, thus increasing tissue destruction (13). Because the size and effect of temporary cavitation are extremely variable, judgment must be exercised in determining the true amount of tissue damage. It is neither practical nor necessary to excise all tissue affected by the temporary cavity and, in most cases, would do more harm than good. The focus should be on debriding only clearly nonviable tissue and reexploring the wound in 48 hours if necessary.

FIREARMS

Rifles, handguns, and shotguns are three distinct types of firearms. Although it is common practice to categorize these weapons by velocity, the definitions of "high velocity" and "low velocity" are vague. Billings et al (6) defined low velocity as less than 1,000 feet per second (most handguns), medium velocity as 1,000 to 2,000 feet per second (magnum handguns and shotguns), and high velocity as more than 2,000 feet per second (high-powered rifles and military weapons). It is important to keep in mind that not all high-velocity injuries cause significant tissue destruction and that some low-velocity injuries can cause severe destruction. The terms *high-energy* and *low-energy* describe the injury better than missile velocity. High-energy injuries cause severe soft tissue compromise with devitalization of muscles and large permanent cavities, which are associated with higher risks of infection.

Rifles

Rifles usually are considered the most powerful firearm and commonly are used by the military and hunters. Most rifles are capable of firing a projectile at speeds of more than 2,500 feet per second (7,8,14,15). Because wounding potential is related to kinetic energy and kinetic energy is dependent on mass and velocity $\left(KE = \frac{MV^2}{2}\right)$ (1,2,14), it is easy to understand why an M16 rifle propelling a 55-grain bullet at 3,024 feet per second can cause significant bony and soft tissue destruction (16).

Handguns

Handguns are considered the least powerful firearms in common use. A magnum round contains more gunpowder than a standard round, and this increases the velocity and therefore the kinetic energy of the projectile. Magnum loads impart 20 to 60 times more kinetic energy to the bullet than a standard load of the same caliber. A .357 magnum handgun fires a bullet at 1,450 feet per second, approaching the maximal velocity obtainable by a handgun (approximately 1,500 feet per second) (1,13).

Shotguns

Shotguns, a third type of firearm, are popular weapons that are legitimately used worldwide for hunting and sporting activities. The ballistics and wounding capacity of shotguns differ from those of rifles and handguns in several important ways. The severity of shotgun wounds varies widely, ranging from massive tissue destruction at close range to minimal superficial wounding at long range. The type of shot used also affects the wounding potential, because large, heavier shot (buckshot) produces more serious wounds than smaller shot (birdshot) fired from the same distance.

Although a shotgun is capable of inflicting severe injuries (Figs. 14-2 and 14-3), the muzzle velocity does not exceed 2,500 feet per second and shotguns are not considered high velocity firearms (7,8,12,14,17). As an example, the 12-gauge shotgun, which is the most popular in the United States, fires 1⅛ ounces of number 6 shot (the most commonly used ammunition) at a muzzle velocity of 1,255 feet per second. Wound severity is based primarily on the spread and velocity of the pellets or slugs at target impact. The most important determinants of wounding potential are distance to the target and type of ammunition. To cause injury, a projectile must strike the target with sufficient velocity. An impact of 150 feet per second is required to break skin, and an impact velocity of 195 feet per second is necessary to break bone (17).

Wounding potential also is greatly influenced by the type of ammunition used. Buckshot fired at close range can produce some of the most extensive injuries of any civilian firearm. Additionally, buckshot is capable of inflicting significant tissue damage at ranges up to 150 yards. As the distance increases, the buckshot spreads and acts like multiple low-velocity bullets. As an example, each pellet of 00 buckshot, which typically contains nine pellets per shell, behaves similar to an individual .22-caliber bullet when the velocity exceeds 1,000 feet per second (17). A shotgun loaded with birdshot also can cause severe injury

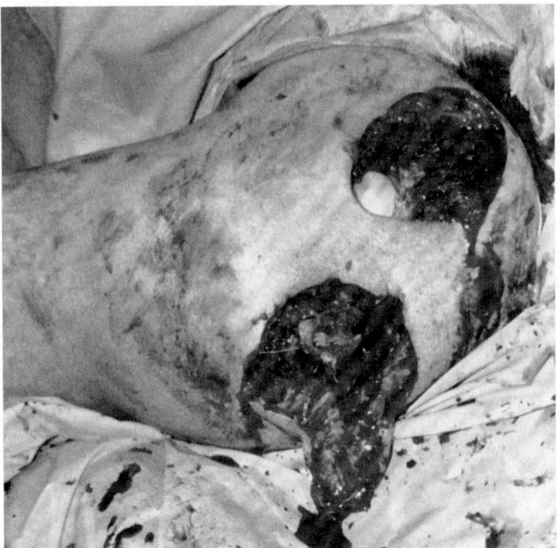

FIGURE 14-2 Perforating wound of the shoulder caused by a close-range shotgun blast.

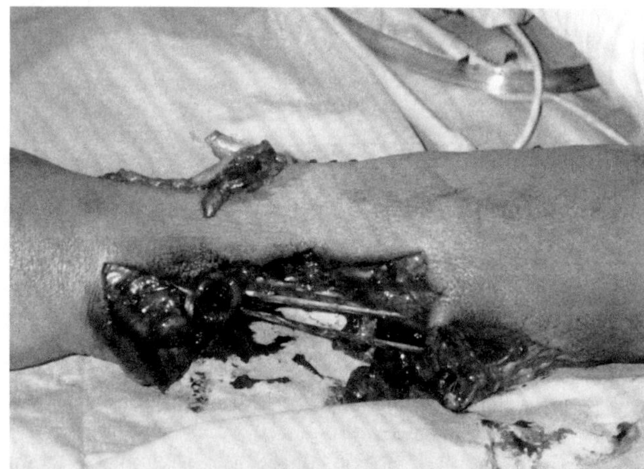
A

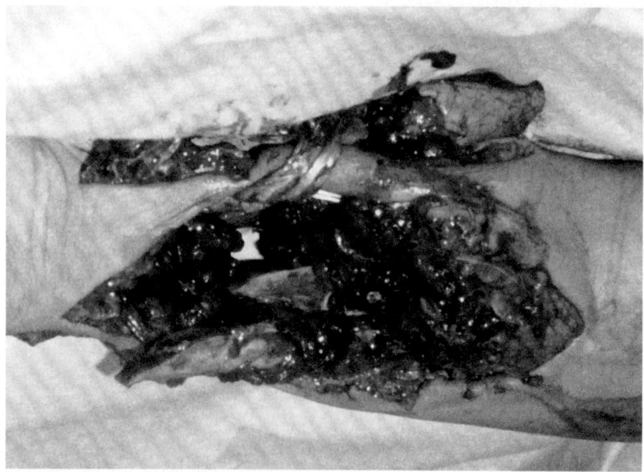
B

FIGURE 14-3 Severe skin, muscle, tendon, bone, and neurovascular damage caused by a close-range shotgun injury. Note the powder marks at the edge of the wound.

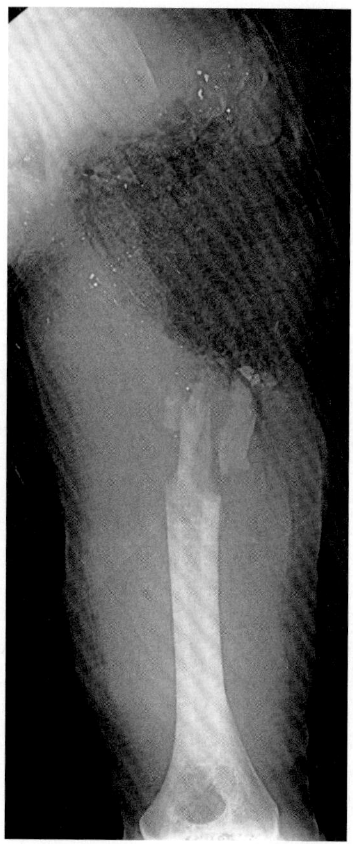

FIGURE 14-4 Severe bony destruction caused by a close-range shotgun blast with birdshot.

at close range (Fig. 14-4), but, unlike buckshot, its wounding potential diminishes rapidly with distance. At a range of more than 7 yards, the pellets behave more like individual BB-gun pellets (18).

MANAGEMENT PRINCIPLES

Initial Evaluation

The first priority in the management of patients with gunshot injuries is the rapid identification and treatment of life-threatening injuries in a systematic process, as outlined by the Advanced Trauma Life Support (ATLS) protocols. Approximately one third of patients with gunshot fractures to the extremities have associated injuries to other organ systems. After the initial survey and the implementation of treatment for life-threatening conditions, a more thorough secondary survey and detailed orthopaedic examination should be performed. The patient should be undressed, and the entire surface of the body, both anteriorly and posteriorly, should be carefully inspected for the presence of wounds. If possible, clothing should be inspected because missing fragments may be found within the wound (Fig. 14-5). The location of the wound (in two dimensions), its size and shape, the apparent amount of soft tissue disruption, and any distinguishing characteristics of the wound and surrounding soft tissue should be documented. One study showed that most clinicians do not accurately describe wounds unless they are prompted to do so (19). A diagram or drawing indicating the exact location of wounds may be helpful (7,19,20). Fackler and Mason (20) cautioned that the average clinician is not adequately trained to differentiate entrance from exit wounds and should not label them as such in the medical record.

A thorough neurovascular examination is extremely important. Any abnormalities necessitate further workup and possible treatment. A high level of suspicion must also be maintained for compartment syndrome in patients with penetrating trauma. The presence of hypotension or shock increases the likelihood of compartment syndrome. Because unconscious patients cannot complain of pain and cannot cooperate with motor and sensory examination, compartmental pressures should be measured if compartment syndrome is suggested by tight, swollen

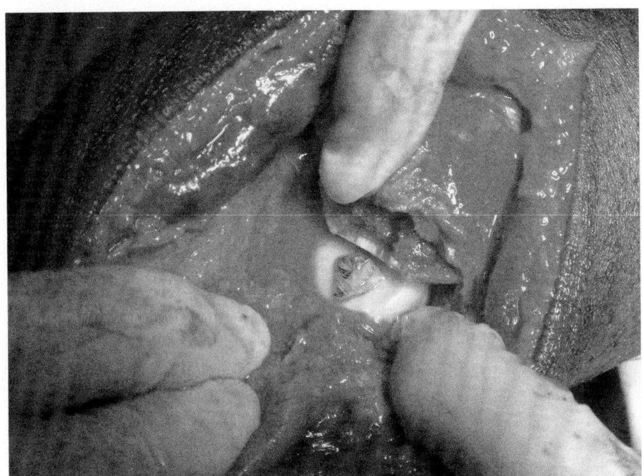

FIGURE 14-5 Pieces of dollar bills carried into the joint by a bullet that penetrated the victim's pockets and knee joint.

limbs in such patients. Timely diagnosis and management are critical to prevent irreversible ischemic damage that threatens the viability of the limb.

X-ray Evaluation

Plain anteroposterior and lateral x-rays should be taken of any extremity or bone thought to be injured. X-rays should include the joints above and below the area of suspected injury. Radiodense markers at the suspected entrance site may aid in evaluation, particularly when multiple wounds are present. In addition to the bony evaluation, the location of any retained projectiles also is identified. A trail of smaller metallic fragments may indicate the path of the bullet. The type of ammunition used and the caliber of the weapon also can sometimes be ascertained from the x-rays. The presence of a large amount of air in the soft tissues, or widespread metallic or bony fragments, may indicate more extensive soft tissue disruption than is appreciable from the size of the entry wound (Fig. 14-6).

Several recognizable patterns of bony injury are caused by penetrating trauma (6,21,22). A low-velocity missile traversing cancellous bone may create a "drill hole." A tangential bullet strike, especially in the metaphyseal area, may cause a unicortical "chip" or "divot" fracture. A higher-velocity weapon, or a direct impact to compact diaphyseal bone, frequently creates a comminuted fracture. Distant fractures may be produced by a torque or fall that occurs after the victim is struck (23).

More specialized imaging studies may be needed to evaluate patients with penetrating musculoskeletal trauma. Arthrography may be necessary to diagnose joint penetration by a projectile when physical examination is equivocal. Computed tomography (CT) should be used for gunshot fractures of the spine and pelvis, to further clarify the nature of the fracture and the precise location of the missile. CT scanning also is helpful in determining whether retained bullet fragments are intra-articular and in planning the treatment of articular injuries.

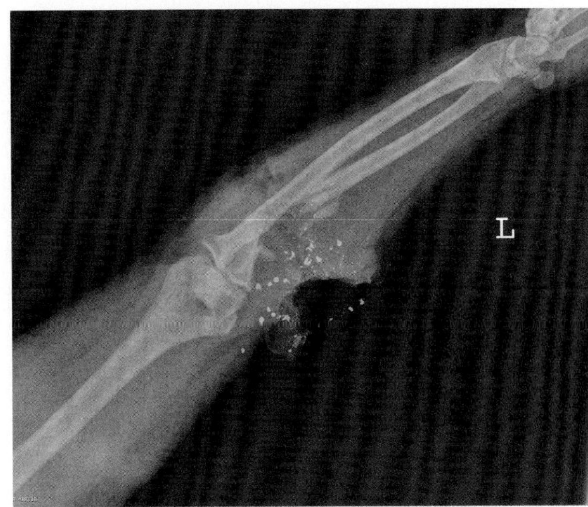

FIGURE 14-6 X-ray findings suggestive of severe soft tissue disruption with wide-spread bony and metallic fragments from gunshot wound of the forearm.

Management of Vascular and Neurologic Injuries

Vascular Injuries

Approximately 10% to 16% of gunshot fractures in the extremities have associated vascular injuries (Fig. 14-7) (24–26). A detailed physical examination is critical to preservation of life

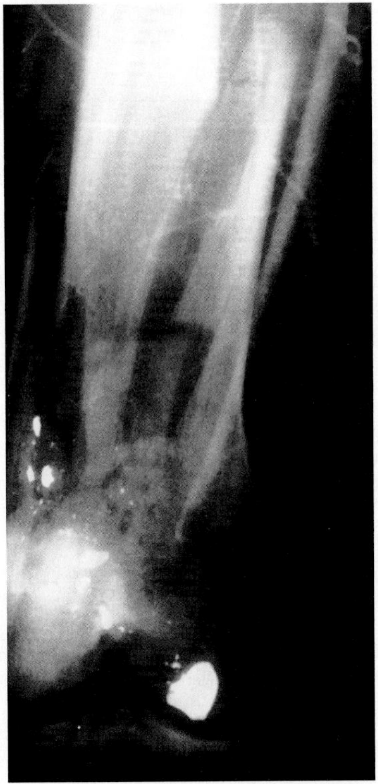

FIGURE 14-7 Arteriogram demonstrating popliteal artery injury in a patient with a gunshot fracture of the distal femur.

and limb. Patients with "hard" signs of arterial injury (absent pulses, expanding or pulsatile hematoma, pulsatile bleeding, bruit or thrill) generally require immediate operative exploration. In such patients, arteriography in the radiography suite needlessly delays treatment. If the location of the injury is unclear, or if a segmental injury may be present, an arteriogram can be done in the operating room. Up to 50% of patients with arterial injury, however, have detectable pulses (24–27). In patients with "soft" signs of arterial injury (neurologic deficit, hypotension without obvious source, large nonexpanding hematoma, bilateral pulse deficit, decreased pulses or those detectable only by Doppler examination), arteriograms can be used to diagnose or exclude arterial injury. Additionally, arteriography has been recommended for proximal injuries that may involve the iliac or axillary arteries, fracture patterns or dislocations that have a high prevalence of associated arterial injuries (knee dislocations), most injuries caused by buckshot, and penetrating injuries in proximity to major vascular structures. Whether to obtain an arteriogram in a patient with a proximity injury but a normal physical examination is a matter of controversy (24–32). Advocates of arteriography cite a 0.3% to 5% prevalence of occult arterial injury in the presence of a normal physical examination. Critics of arteriography in this situation contend that only 1.8% of occult arterial injuries (small intimal flaps, small pseudoaneurysm, arterial spasm) require surgical intervention, and those that do eventually manifest "hard" signs of arterial injury. Patients with no clinical signs of arterial injury, they argue, can be safely observed and monitored with repeated physical examinations. Arteriography itself has a 1% to 4% rate of complications and misses arterial injury in 0.5% to 6% of patients. In some centers, noninvasive vascular studies, such as duplex Doppler ultrasonography, have achieved an accuracy similar to that of arteriography in diagnosing arterial injury.

The algorithm designed by Cornwell (33) is useful in determining the necessity of diagnostic arteriography (Fig. 14-8).

Once the diagnosis of arterial injury has been confirmed, close cooperation is necessary between the general or vascular surgeon and the orthopaedic surgeon (34). The highest priority is placed on the swift restoration of blood flood. This is especially important in patients with prolonged ischemic times. Vein or synthetic grafts often are required. Whether to obtain bony stabilization before or after vascular repair is a matter of debate. Orthopaedic stabilization before vascular repair may unduly prolong ischemic times, whereas an unstable fracture may jeopardize an arterial repair. In ischemic limbs, a temporary vascular shunt can be placed to restore blood flow. Bony stabilization can then be performed, followed by formal vascular repair. Alternatively, the extremity can be first quickly stabilized with a two-pin external fixator, followed by vascular repair, and later definitive orthopaedic management (35). Vascular repair frequently is done before skeletal stabilization. McHenry et al (36) noted no iatrogenic vascular repair injuries, decreased fasciotomy rates, and decreased hospital stay when revascularization (temporary or permanent) was done first. Subsequent orthopaedic intervention must be done carefully to avoid disruption of the vascular anastomosis. In patients with arterial injury whose limbs are still perfused, provisional and sometimes definitive skeletal stabilization often can be safely done before vascular repair. The order of the vascular and orthopaedic interventions usually is left to the discretion of the vascular surgeon. External fixation is most often recommended as the preferred method for initial bony stabilization. This may serve as definitive treatment or may be converted to another method of fixation later. Gunshot femoral fractures with vascular injury can be successfully treated with intramedullary nailing, both immediately and

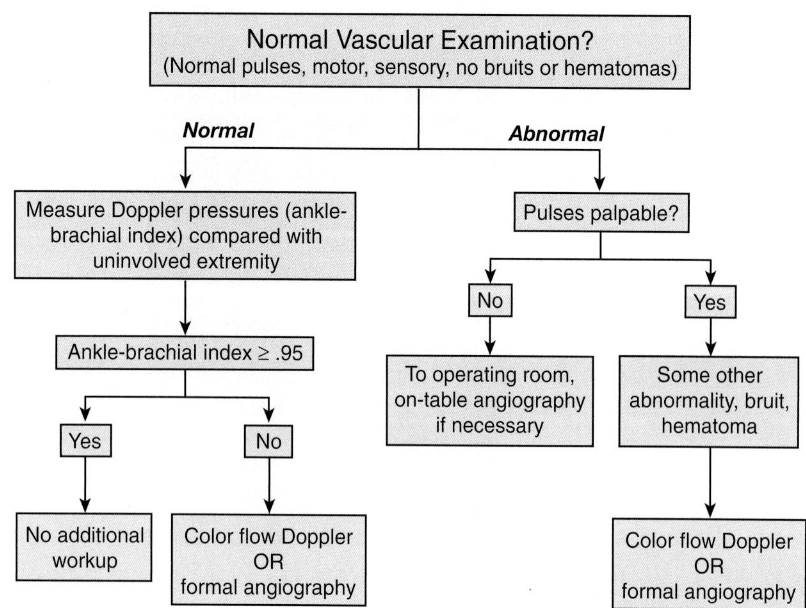

FIGURE 14-8 Algorithm designed by Cornwell (33) for determining the necessity of diagnostic arteriography in patients with gunshot wound to the extremities.

after vascular repair and after short periods of traction or external fixation (37,38).

Nerve Injuries

Nerve injuries accompany approximately 25% or more of gunshot wounds to the extremities (39,40) and are the major determinant in long-term disability. Visser et al (41) noted that nerve injuries often occur concomitantly with vascular injuries, resulting in worse outcomes (39% poor results) than with a vascular injury alone (7% poor results). In two landmark studies of nerve injuries in military conflicts, Sunderland (39) and Omer (42) both noted spontaneous recovery of neurologic deficits in 68% to 69% of patients. Ninety percent of patients with recovery had improved within the first 3 to 9 months. Studies describing nerve injuries inflicted by civilian firearms have reported similar results (7,15,43,44). Because many nerve injuries spontaneously recover, most investigators recommend initial observation. In patients with neurologic deficits and large open wounds, nerves can be explored to determine whether they are in continuity or are severed. The ends of severed nerves are tagged and usually are repaired secondarily when the extent of the nerve injury can be more clearly determined. Patients are followed with clinical examination and may also be evaluated with electromyography and nerve conduction velocity tests to evaluate neurologic recovery. If no recovery is noted within the first 3 to 4 months after injury, nerve exploration should be considered, particularly in proximal injuries. Neurolysis, neuroma resection, end-to-end repair, or nerve grafting can be done as the situation dictates. Omer (42) described significant recovery in only 25% of repaired nerves that had been severed by gunshots.

Management of Soft Tissue Injuries

Low-energy injuries (no evidence of cavitation, myonecrosis, or significant missile debris) usually are caused by low-velocity weapons; rarely a high-velocity through-and-through injury can dissipate energy and lead to a low-energy wound with minimal damage. A low-energy entry wound usually is small, with no significant soft tissue damage. Low-energy soft tissue wounds caused by gunshots do not require extensive debridement. Local wound care (superficial debridement, with or without skin margin excision) is carried out in the emergency department. Wounds are left to heal by secondary intention. Using this approach, we have found the prevalence of infection to be predictably low. Occasionally, a low-velocity penetrating wound to a subcutaneous bone, such as the ulna or tibia, produces bony fragments that protrude from the wound. These loose bone fragments should be removed, and a more formal wound exploration and debridement should be done. Occasionally, low-velocity weapons cause a high-energy injury that may not be immediately noted on examination of the extremity. Long et al (45) classified these injuries as grade 2 in their system (Table 14-1): entrance wound of less than 5 cm but with x-ray evidence of soft tissue destruction (severe comminution, segmental bone destruction, and infiltration of air, bullet, or bone debris in the muscle). Three of seven patients with grade 2 injuries in their series developed infection even with formal debridements. Gugala and Lindsey (43) proposed a classification system based on five parameters: energy, vital structures involved, wound characteristics, fracture, and degree of contamination. The therapeutic usefulness of this extensive classification system has not yet been validated in a clinical setting.

TABLE 14-1 Grading of Gunshot Soft Tissue Wounds

Grade	Wound Size and Appearance	Radiographic Appearance
1	<2 cm, no devitalized muscle	No defect in skin or subcutaneous tissue. Narrow track of metal, bone, air through muscle. Comminution with several large and small fragments.
2	<5 cm, no devitalized muscle	Muscle swelling and a wide area of infiltration with metal, bone, and air. Severe comminution or segmental bone loss.
3	>5 cm or 2 to 5 cm with devitalized muscle	Same as grade 2, plus a defect in the skin and subcutaneous tissue.

Modified from Long WT, Chang W, Brien EW. Grading system for gunshot injuries to the femoral diaphysis in civilians. *Clin Orthop* 2003;408:92–100.

bacteria (bowel perforation), if intra-articular bullet or bone fragments are retained, or if the injury is associated with unstable fractures requiring fixation. Operative debridement of most joints requires arthrotomy, but some joint injuries can be treated arthroscopically (see Fig. 14-10).

It is important to remove intra-articular and intrabursal bullets and bullet fragments to prevent complications from mechanical wear, lead synovitis and arthropathy, and systemic lead toxicity (46–51,53,54). Even bullets lodged in bone but in contact with synovial fluid are at risk for these complications (51). An intra-articular foreign body acts as a mechanical irritant, which can lead to destructive arthritis. Motion of the joint can cause further fragmentation of the bullet and increased absorption of lead by the synovium. This may result in lead arthropathy characterized by reactive synovitis, small mechanical wear particles, periarticular fibrosis, chondrolysis, and severe hypertrophic arthritis. A "ground lead" arthrogram is a characteristic x-ray finding. Lead also can be deposited in cartilage, similar to chondrocalcinosis.

Systemic lead toxicity also can occur in patients with bullets or bullet fragments that remain in contact with synovial fluid or bursal tissue (51). Lead has been shown to be twice as soluble in synovial fluid as it is in serum. Systemic lead toxicity has been diagnosed as early as 2 days and as late as 40 years after intra-articular gunshot wounds (46–49,52). Factors that increase the risk of lead toxicity include bullet or fragment exposure to synovial fluid in a large joint such as the knee or hip, an unjacketed bullet with high lead content, the presence of a large bullet, or fragments or pellets with a large surface area of lead exposed. Symptoms of lead toxicity often are vague and can involve any organ system. Symptoms can include nausea, vomiting, abdominal pain, anorexia, malaise, renal insufficiency, anemia, encephalopathy, seizures, peripheral neuropathy, and, in severe cases, death. Physical findings may include lead lines along the gingival margin. Laboratory findings are variable, but they classically show a microcytic anemia with basophilic stippling. Serum and urine lead levels typically are elevated but may fluctuate. Serum-free erythrocyte protoporphyrin may be elevated as well. Symptoms can fluctuate, and acute crises may occur after metabolic stresses or acute injuries to the lead-containing joint that cause more lead to be released into the system. Lead toxicity is treated with chelation therapy, followed by synovectomy and removal of any remaining intra-articular lead fragments (47). Fragments embedded in bone that are bathed in synovial fluid must be removed as well.

Certain intra-articular injuries deserve special consideration. The hip joint is in close proximity to the abdomen and rectum. Projectiles that penetrate the hip joint may have also traversed the gastrointestinal tract, either before or after joint penetration (Fig. 14-12). This diagnosis frequently is missed and can lead to septic arthritis and cartilage destruction (45,70,81,82). A high index of suspicion, close inspection of the path of the bullet, pelvic x-rays, CT scans, and arthrography can aid in diagnosing this potentially catastrophic injury.

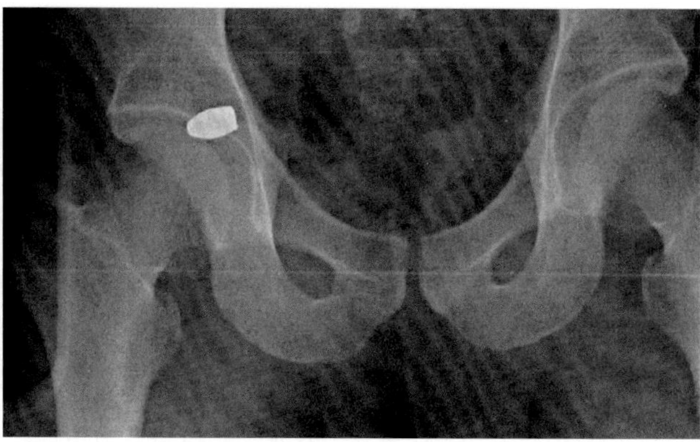

FIGURE 14-12 Bullets in the hip joint pose special risks because of the possibility that they may have traversed the gastrointestinal tract before joint penetration.

Rhee and Martin (55) recommended that all penetrated hips undergo an arthrotomy to remove possible contaminants and debris. Long et al (46) proposed an algorithm for the treatment of gunshot fractures to the hip. Hip injuries caused by low-velocity weapons in which the bullet does not pass through the abdomen or rectum, which have no intra-articular bone or bullet fragments, and that are not associated with unstable fractures can be treated with antibiotics without an arthrotomy. Their protocol includes a 3-day course of intravenous cefazolin and gentamicin. Currently, gunshot wounds that have traversed the hip are treated with an arthrotomy and debridement. Several studies have indicated that gunshot wounds to the pelvis and spine with associated abdominal viscus injury do not require debridement of the fracture bullet path or bullet removal (83–86). Kihtir et al (84) suggested that the rate of infection is related to the treatment of the abdominal injury and not to the debridement of the bullet track, fractures, or bullet removal. However, most authors still recommend debridement for trans-abdominal injuries to the hip joint (45,55,87). Other indications for hip arthrotomy include intra-articular bone or bullet fragments and injuries associated with unstable fractures (Figs. 14-13 and 14-14). Bone and bullet fragments sometimes can be removed arthroscopically by surgeons skilled in this technique. Unstable fractures require operative reduction and fixation.

Some investigators suggest that operative treatment is necessary for all penetrating joint trauma to the knee (Fig. 14-15) (88–90). Berg and Ciullo (91) reported an unexpected amount of joint contamination, including cloth, hair, and skin, found at arthroscopy in three patients with gunshot fractures of the knee (see Fig. 14-5). Tornetta and Hui (79) arthroscopically examined 33 patients with intra-articular gunshot injuries to the knee that were not associated with fractures requiring repair. Overall, five unsuspected chondral injuries and 14 meniscal injuries were identified. Five of seven patients with no x-ray evidence of debris, loose bodies, or intra-articular bullet or bone fragments were found to have either debris or meniscal damage

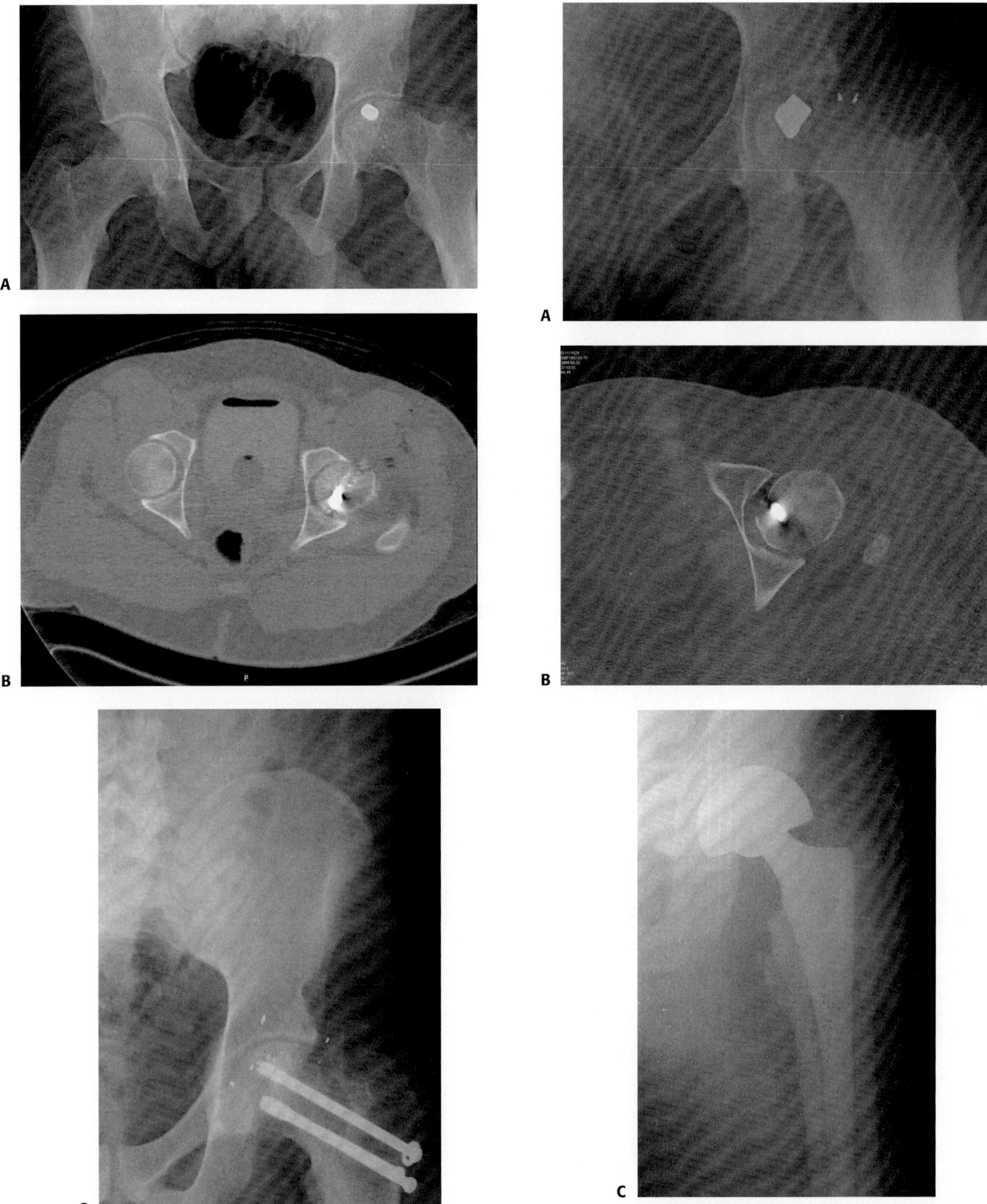

FIGURE 14-13 **A.** Intra-articular bullet in hip joint. **B.** CT shows extent of femoral head fracture. Arthrotomy was required for bullet removal, and the fracture was stabilized with hip screws **(C)**.

FIGURE 14-14 **A,B.** Gunshot injury produced an unstable femoral head fracture, with retained bullet. Open reduction and internal fixation were unsuccessful because of bone loss in the superior portion of the femoral head; hemiarthroplasty was required **(C)**.

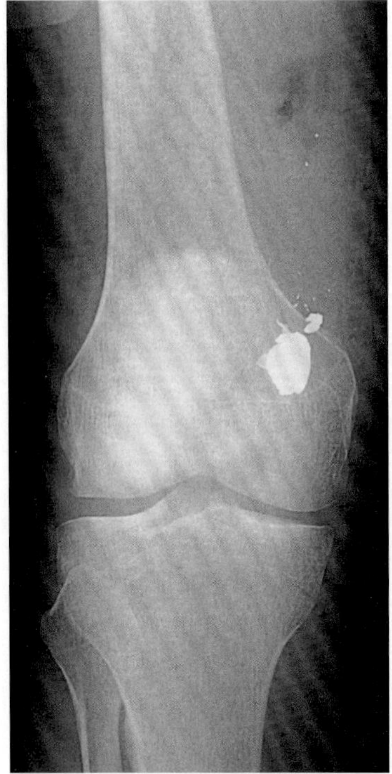

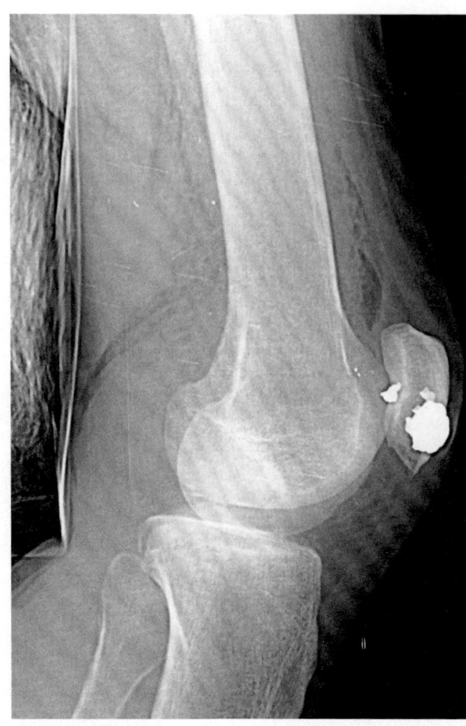

FIGURE 14-15 A,B. Gunshot injury to the knee with a retained intraarticular bullet. Note the knee effusion and intra-articular air in the lateral view **(B)**.

at the time of arthroscopy. Miniarthrotomy was needed in 12 knees to remove loose bodies. Patients received an average of 2 days of antibiotic therapy. No infections occurred. These authors recommended arthroscopic management of all intra-articular injuries caused by low-velocity missiles. We routinely perform an arthroscopic debridement of intra-articular injuries to the knee joint at our institution (Fig. 14-16).

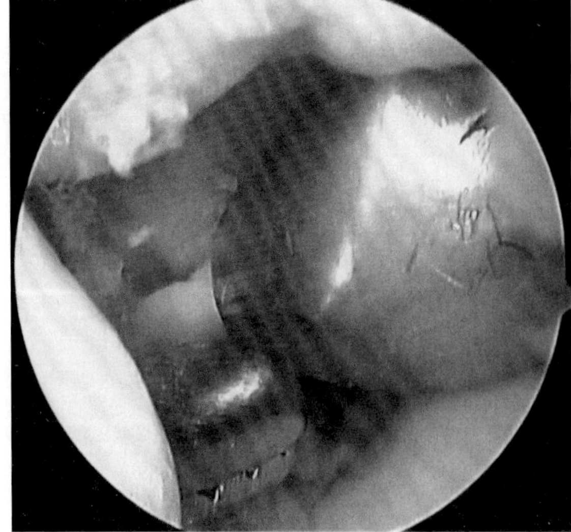

FIGURE 14-16 Arthroscopic bullet removal and debridement are our preferred treatment for intra-articular injuries to the knee joint.

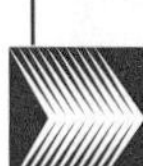

AUTHOR'S PREFERRED TREATMENT

We treat high-energy wounds to the musculoskeletal system with aggressive soft tissue management that includes meticulous operative debridement and irrigation, open wound management, broad-spectrum intravenous antibiotics, and tetanus prophylaxis. Appropriate skeletal fixation is used as indicated by the specific fracture pattern or joint injury and usually is done at the initial debridement if the wound can be adequately cleansed, or the fracture is temporarily stabilized with an external fixator (Fig. 14-17). Debridement and irrigation are repeated every 24 to 48 hours until no further contaminated or devitalized tissue is noted. Delayed soft tissue coverage is done as necessary. Intravenous antibiotics, usually including a first-generation cephalosporin, an aminoglycoside, and penicillin, are given in the emergency department and are continued for 72 hours or longer if wound conditions dictate. Longer periods of antibiotic therapy may be required for patients with severely contaminated wounds and those with wounds in which further development of devitalized tissue is noted at subsequent debridement.

Low-energy injuries causing little soft tissue damage are treated with local debridement and irrigation, and the wounds are left open to heal secondarily. Support exists in the literature for no antibiotic prophylaxis (3,15,44), oral antibiotics (92), single-dose intramuscular cefonicid, (74), and 24 to 72 hours of treatment with intravenous cephalosporin with or without an aminoglycoside (3,44,66) for un-

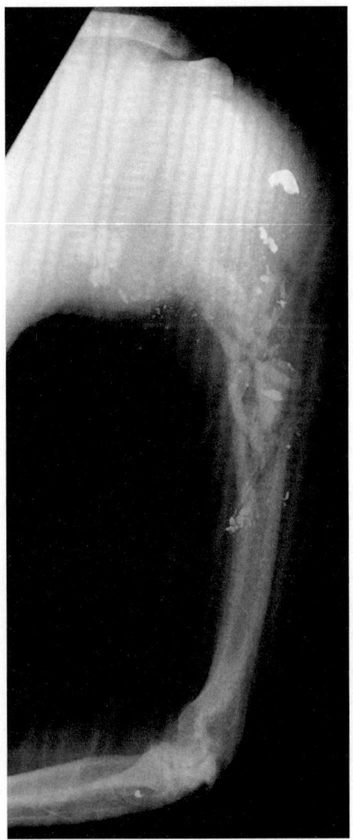

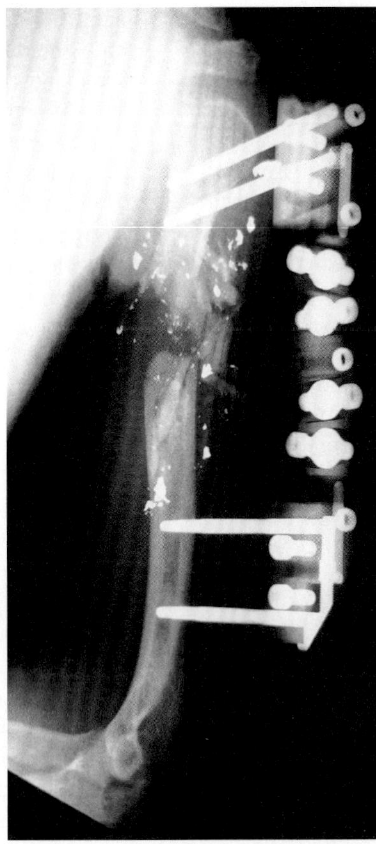

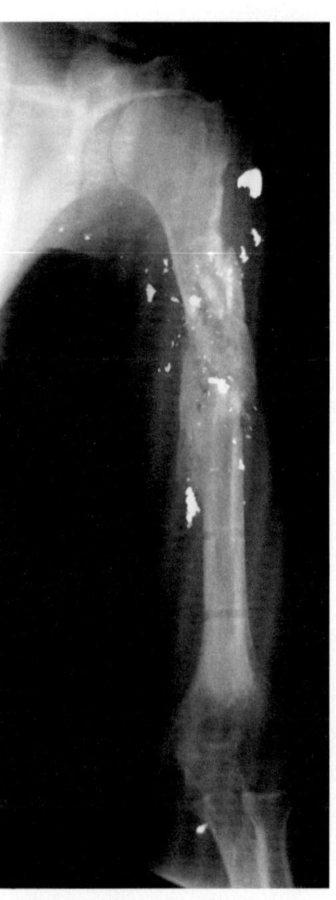

FIGURE 14-17 **A.** Severely comminuted humeral shaft fracture was stabilized with external fixation **(B)**. **C.** Healed fracture after bone grafting and removal of the external fixator.

complicated stable fractures that can be treated on an outpatient basis. At our level 1 trauma center, the most common regimen consists of a single dose of an intravenous cephalosporin in the emergency department, followed by oral cephalexin for 5 days. Fractures are stabilized by appropriate splints or casts as dictated by the location of the fracture. Patients with unstable fractures who are admitted for operative stabilization and patients with wounds or joint injuries for which operative debridement and irrigation are indicated receive an intravenous cephalosporin in the emergency department and for 24 to 48 hours postoperatively. An intravenous aminoglycoside or penicillin is added if contamination is a concern.

Low-energy gunshots to the hip and knee joints that are considered "clean" (the bullet is not retained within the joint, there is no metallic or bony debris in the joint) and require no fracture fixation usually are treated with local debridement and a course of intravenous antibiotics followed by oral antibiotics. An arthrotomy and lavage with intravenous antibiotics are used when there is contamination (clothing or bowel) (see Figs. 14-5 and 14-12), retained bullet or metallic debris in the joint (see Figs. 14-10 and 14-16), bone fragments in the joint, or a fracture pattern that requires fixation (see Figs. 14-13 and 14-14). Arthroscopic debridement and lavage is our preferred method of treatment for the knee and shoulder joints, and formal arthrotomy is used for the hip joint. All high-energy injuries require formal debridement and appropriate antibiotics.

Operative fracture stabilization usually is performed immediately (within 24 hours) if the patient is neurologically and hemodynamically stable. Complex articular injuries or other difficult fractures are splinted, placed in traction, or spanned with an external fixator if conditions are not ideal (surgeon experience, time of day, equipment needs) for definitive skeletal fixation.

UPPER EXTREMITY INJURIES

Gunshot injuries of the upper extremity most commonly involve the forearm, followed in frequency by the humerus and hand. In a series of 66 handgun injuries in children and adolescents (47), 56% of fractures and 54% of soft tissue–only injuries involved the upper extremity. Most gunshot injuries to the upper extremity are low-energy injuries that can be treated as grade I or II open fractures, with the following: minimal debridement of the skin, fascia, muscles; removal of foreign material; fracture stabilization; and appropriate antibiotic therapy (93). Special problems are present with higher energy, more severe injuries.

Stein and Strauss (94) recommended arteriography in all patients with multiple ipsilateral upper extremity gunshot wounds, as well as those with equivocal signs of arterial injury, when the patient's general condition is stable; when physical examination indicates an arterial injury, arteriography is unnecessary, and direct exploration of the involved area should proceed immediately. These authors cited arteriography as being useful for exclusion of arterial injury, evaluation of the site of injury, and planning for surgical treatment of complex wounds. They also emphasized that absence or diminution of the axillary, brachial, radial, and ulnar pulses, combined with other findings, reliably identified arterial injury; apparently normal pulses may be present in 20% of patients with angiographically demonstrable lesions (95,96).

Primary amputation of an injured upper extremity rarely is required. The decision to amputate should be based on the overall clinical assessment that reasonable functional recovery is extremely unlikely (94), as may be the case when combined injury to nerves, bones, soft tissue, and vascular structures is extensive. Close-range shotgun injuries can result in this type of damage. If the patient's life is in immediate jeopardy because of associated injuries, primary extremity amputation may give the best chance for survival.

Proximal Humerus and Shoulder Joint

The primary concerns after low-energy gunshot wounds to the proximal humerus and shoulder joint are the possibility of a pneumothorax and vascular or neurologic injuries. The pleura or major pulmonary vessels can be punctured by a bullet or fracture fragments from the scapula or humerus. In a series of 99 patients with upper extremity vascular injuries caused by low-velocity gunshot wounds, Hardin et al (97) found 21 injuries to the axillary artery and 43 to the brachial artery. Half of those patients with axillary artery lesions had severe functional deficits at final follow-up. Shotgun injuries almost always resulted in permanent functional impairment and often necessitated amputation (see Fig. 14-2). Borman et al (95) also reported that almost one third of their patients with axillary artery and neurologic injuries had serious functional limitations.

Most low-energy gunshot injuries to the shoulder area can be treated nonoperatively (98–100). Nondisplaced and minimally displaced fractures generally can be treated with immobilization, local wound care, and appropriate antibiotics. Indications and techniques for surgery are essentially the same as those for closed proximal humeral fractures (101,102). Displaced fractures of the humeral head and neck can be treated by delayed internal fixation. In injuries with significant destruction of the humeral head hemiarthroplasty may be indicated after healing of the soft tissues. External fixation is useful for fractures associated with large soft tissue defects (Fig. 14-17) (103–107). Gunshot wounds involving the glenohumeral joint should be explored and debrided to remove any foreign bodies. This often can be accomplished arthroscopically (see Fig. 14-10) (108).

Although internal fixation generally is the recommended treatment for "floating shoulder" injuries (ipsilateral fractures of the scapula and clavicle), Edwards et al (109) reported satisfactory results with nonoperative treatment of two such injuries caused by gunshot wounds. One clavicular nonunion resulted from segmental bone loss, but the patient had satisfactory function and required no further treatment.

Humeral Shaft

Low-energy gunshot fractures of the humeral shaft generally can be treated with local wound care, plaster cast, and eventual functional bracing (98). If brachial artery repair is required, stabilization of the fracture is required to protect the vascular repair. Multiple techniques exist, each with its proponents. Compression plating often is the treatment of choice if comminution is not too extensive. Intramedullary nailing is useful for segmental or comminuted humeral fractures, especially in patients with multiple trauma. External fixation is indicated for significant contamination or soft tissue or bone loss (see Fig. 14-17). Other indications for operative treatment of humeral gunshot fractures include multiple trauma necessitating recumbency or the need for crutch-assisted walking, segmental fractures, bilateral humeral fractures, "floating elbow" injuries with ipsilateral forearm fractures, and an inability to maintain a satisfactory reduction by closed means (101).

Balfour and Marrero (98) reported a 2% nonunion rate in 130 patients treated over 15 years with fracture bracing followed by a rehabilitation program. Their contraindications to fracture brace treatment included bedridden patients, patients with vascular injuries, and patients with extremely proximal or distal fractures.

Keller (102) found external fixation to be inferior to functional bracing in 7 gunshot fractures of the humerus, and Joshi et al (100) reported that of 14 gunshot fractures of the humerus, the fracture treated with external fixation resulted in nonunion, as did 1 of 7 treated with fracture bracing; there were no nonunions in the 6 fractures treated with compression plates or intramedullary nails. However, Zinman et al (107) reported external fixation of 26 type III open fractures of the humerus caused by missiles, with excellent results in 14 (61%), good results in 4, fair results in 3, and poor results in 2. All fractures eventually healed. In a series of 38 gunshot fractures of the humeral shaft treated with external fixation, Wisniewski and Radziejowski (106) reported 2 delayed unions and 2 nonunions; superficial pin track infections occurred in 5 patients, 2 of whom had deep wound sepsis and 1 of whom had bone sepsis. These authors attributed a lack of iatrogenic nerve injury to the use of longer skin incisions, blunt muscle dissection, and exposure of the bone for pin insertion in difficult areas.

Wiss and Gellman (110) reported 19 humeral shaft gunshot fractures with associated brachial plexus injuries: 3 treated with plates united, 4 of 6 treated with intramedullary nails developed malunion or nonunion, and 4 of 10 treated with cast bracing developed nonunion.

In a series of 35 open humeral shaft fractures treated at our level 1 trauma center (111), 13 were gunshot injuries. Four of these fractures were treated with splints or braces, 6 were treated with intramedullary nails, 2 with compression plates, and 1 with external fixation. Four patients required brachial artery repair; compression plates were used for fracture stabilization in 2 patients, an intramedullary nail was used in 1 patient, and an external fixator was used in 1 patient. All 13 fractures united. One nailed fracture (type II) that had multiple débridements and split-thickness skin grafting required 7 months for healing, and the fracture (type IIIC) treated with external fixation required iliac crest bone grafting (at 3 months) before healing at 8 months. The proximal locking screw of an intramedullary nail was removed in one patient because of painful impingement.

Elbow

The relatively small soft tissue envelope around the elbow results in gunshot injuries with significant bone destruction as well as neurologic and vascular compromise. These gunshot wounds are among the most difficult to treat. They can cause intra-articular, intercondylar, or supracondylar humeral fractures with major loss of the articular surfaces of the joint, often making joint reconstruction impossible. Because of its position in relation to the skin and underlying bone, the brachial artery is especially vulnerable at the elbow, and arterial injury often is accompanied by nerve injuries, especially to the median nerve. Brachial artery injury can lead to compartment syndrome if repair is delayed, and signs of compartment syndrome (pain and paresthesia) may be absent if nerve injury is also present, leading to delay in diagnosis of increased compartmental pressure.

Displaced fractures with vascular injuries should be stabilized (external or simple internal fixation) before vascular repair, if time permits, to avoid disruption of the repair during fracture reduction and fixation (112). Internal fixation that addresses the specific fracture pattern can be done on a delayed basis if soft tissue coverage is adequate. External fixation across the elbow joint protects an arterial repair, but it often results in loss of elbow motion if it is left in place for longer than 4 to 6 weeks. External fixation also can be used for initial management of fractures with soft tissue or bone loss to maintain alignment and joint space until definitive fixation can be achieved (105).

Forearm

Gunshot wounds of the forearm often are complicated by peripheral nerve injuries, vascular injuries, and the development of compartment syndrome (76,113–120). Fractures in the proximal third of the forearm are most frequently associated with compartment syndrome. Patients should be closely monitored for at least 24 hours after injury, and compartment pressures should be measured if signs of impending compartment syndrome develop.

Although nerve injuries can lead to significant long-term disability, approximately 50% to 70% of nerve injuries resolve spontaneously (113,121). Early dynamic splinting and passive range-of-motion exercises can improve function, and neurolysis or neurorrhaphy can be successful if done 3 to 6 months after injury.

Uncomplicated, nondisplaced gunshot fractures of the forearm without vascular injury generally can be treated with local wound care, appropriate antibiotics, and cast immobilization. Displaced fractures of the radius or ulna or both usually require open reduction with internal fixation (115,119,121). Lenihan et al (121) reported that cast immobilization of displaced fractures of the radius or of both-bone fractures resulted in a high incidence of poor results in their series of 37 low-velocity gunshot extra-articular forearm fractures. The use of a long arm splint until the initial phase of wound healing is completed, followed by delayed primary internal fixation, has been reported to reduce the incidence of malunion and delayed union (110), but this has not been validated in the literature.

Fracture stabilization can be obtained with compression plating (Fig. 14-18), bridge plating, or intramedullary nailing (Fig. 14-19). External fixation can be used for fractures with soft tissue loss or vascular compromise (105). Early cancellous bone grafting may be indicated for comminuted fractures.

Wrist and Hand

Fractures are the most common injuries caused by gunshot injuries to the hand, followed by injuries to nerves, tendons, and arteries (110,122–124). Duncan and Kettelkamp (125) reported that 90% of nerve injuries in 32 low-velocity gunshot hand injuries resolved spontaneously. The primary residual functional impairment of finger function in their patients was related to the location and stability of the fracture. Fractures involving the proximal interphalangeal joints produced the most impairment, followed by fractures of the proximal phalanx. Phillips et al (122) determined that almost half (47%) of the gunshot injuries in their patients (103 injuries) occurred in the metacarpals, followed by the phalanges (32%); injuries to the carpal bones (12%) and the distal radius and ulna (9%) were much less frequent.

Uncomplicated gunshot wounds to the hand can be managed by local wound care, appropriate antibiotics, bulky dressing, splinting, and elevation. The wrist should be splinted in slight extension, the metacarpal joints in 80 to 90 degrees of flexion, and the proximal and distal interphalangeal joints in 10 to 15 degrees of flexion. Splinting of the metacarpal joint in flexion is important to avoid extension contracture of the metacarpal joint, which is difficult to correct. Fingertips should be visible so circulation can be evaluated.

For fracture fixation, I generally follow the principle that fracture treatment is based on location and type of fracture rather than on mechanism. Obviously, the condition of the soft tissue envelope and the comminution of the fracture may dictate the type of fixation used. Low-energy fractures of the proximal humerus and shoulder girdle usually can be treated with local debridement, antibiotics, and immobilization. Low-energy unstable or displaced fractures usually require some form of delayed open reduction with internal fixation, depending on the specific nature of the fracture. Healing of the soft tissue bed must be present before I undertake any reparative or reconstructive procedures in high-energy injuries. For fractures of the humeral shaft that meet the criteria for operative treatment, both locked intramedullary nails and compression plating provide satisfactory results. I usually prefer compression plating for simple fracture patterns, for distal shaft fractures, and after exposure for vascular repair. I choose intramedullary nails for extensively comminuted fractures, segmental fractures, and fractures with poor soft tissue envelopes. External fixation is reserved for fractures that are not suitable for other methods of treatment, such as those with extensive comminution (see Fig. 14-17). Standard open reduction with internal fixation is the technique of choice for fractures involving the distal humerus. Severe articular surface damage or poor soft tissues sometimes necessitate a bridging external fixator. I almost always use a compression plating or bridge plating technique for forearm fractures that require stabilization. Again, extensively comminuted fractures or fractures with poor soft tissue conditions may be treated with intramedullary nails (see Fig. 14-19).

LOWER EXTREMITY FRACTURES

Femoral Shaft

Historically, the management of femoral shaft fractures caused by firearms has been based on the military experience. Traction followed by cast bracing was the most commonly recommended method of stabilization. Over the past few decades, the frequency of low-velocity gunshot fractures in civilians has steadily increased, and treatment principles have evolved. In the late 1970s and early 1980s, conservative treatment was still advocated for gunshot fractures of the femur. In 1982, Ryan et al (129) reported a series of 43 femoral fractures resulting from low-velocity gunshot injuries that were treated with traction and spica casting. All fractures healed with an average of 47 days in traction and 97 days in a spica cast. There were no deep infections. Deformity averaged 5 degrees or less in all but one fracture.

Using their grading system (see Table 14-1) based on 100 femoral gunshot wounds, Long et al (130) reported that no grade 1 injuries developed infections, 42% of grade 2 had deep infections, and 50% of grade 3 injuries had deep infections. They recommended treating grade 1 gunshot injuries as closed fractures, grade 2 injuries as open fractures, and grade 3 injuries as contaminated open fractures.

Although some fractures are stable (metaphyseal drill holes, unicortical chip fractures) and are easily treated nonoperatively, most femoral gunshot fractures are unstable and comminuted, and they may be difficult to align properly in traction. This is especially true of subtrochanteric and supracondylar femoral fractures. Skeletal traction necessitates lengthy hospital stays with associated costs and a prolonged period of functional recovery. Permanent knee stiffness may occur in some patients. Adverse medical consequences of prolonged recumbency, particularly pulmonary complications in multiply injured patients, have been well described in the literature.

The introduction of interlocking intramedullary nails in the mid-1980s dramatically changed the treatment of closed and open femoral shaft fractures, including those caused by gunshots. Closed, locked intramedullary nailing currently is the preferred treatment for most femoral fractures between the femoral condyles and the lesser trochanter (131–136). Reports of femoral fractures caused by firearms that require operative stabilization (129,131,137,138) have cited a high prevalence of Winquist and Hansen grade III or higher comminution (77% to 98% of fractures). These axially and rotationally unstable fractures cannot be adequately treated with flexible or unlocked intramedullary nails. Although plating may be necessary for treatment of proximal femoral fractures that extend into the intertrochanteric region and distal fractures with significant involvement of the femoral condyles, it has little place in the treatment of gunshot fractures of the femoral shaft. Treatment with external fixation often is complicated by pin site infection, knee stiffness, malunion, and nonunion, and it generally is reserved for the most severe open and contaminated fractures, such as shotgun injuries, war wounds, and limbs with questionable viability, often in temporary fashion until definitive intramedullary nailing can be carried out (139).

The changes in philosophy about the optimal timing of nailing of blunt open femoral fractures have extended to gunshot femoral fractures (140–142). It was initially believed that placing isolated femoral fractures in traction, followed by delayed intramedullary nailing at 10 to 14 days when the wound is sealed, would decrease the incidence of infection. In 1991, Wiss et al (143) reported 56 gunshot femoral fractures treated with reamed locked intramedullary nailing. Patients with isolated injuries were placed in traction for 10 to 14 days to allow the soft tissue wounds to heal before nailing. Formal debridement was not done, and all patients received 72 hours of cephalosporins and aminoglycosides. All fractures united, and there were no infections. Complications included one nail failure, two screw failures, two delayed unions, and seven malunions.

Nowotarski and Brumback (144) evaluated 36 low- to mid-velocity gunshot femoral fractures treated with locked intramedullary nailing with 18 hours of injury. All fractures united; however, one delayed union and one nonunion required exchange nailing before healing. No malunions were reported. One infection (2.5%) occurred, which was successfully treated. Patients received an average of 48 hours of cephalosporin antibiotic. Similarly, studies by Brien et al (137) and Wright et al (145) reported satisfactory results with immediate nailing. It appears that immediate reamed locked intramedullary nailing is safe and effective in femoral shaft fractures resulting from low-energy penetrating trauma (Fig. 14-21).

Although reamed intramedullary nailing is the treatment of choice for grades I, II, and IIIA open femoral fractures, the optimal treatment of grade IIIB open fractures is less clear. Grade IIIB open wounds may be associated with close-range shotgun blasts, some high-velocity firearm injuries, and war wounds. Few data are available on the treatment of severe open femoral fractures caused by penetrating trauma. Femoral fractures sustained in the Vietnam War and in earlier wars of the 20th century were predominantly treated with aggressive wound debridement, open wound management, and skeletal traction. In a later report of war injuries (146), external fixation was recommended; osteomyelitis occurred in 8% and pin track infection in 35%.

To avoid the problems associated with prolonged external fixation, staged protocols have been developed, consisting of initial application of an external fixator, followed by early conversion to an intramedullary nail (147–149). Conversion to intramedullary nailing after long periods of external fixation has had unacceptably high rates of infection. Wu and Shih (149) reported a 13.3% infection rate in 15 grade III open femoral fractures initially treated with external fixators that were converted to intramedullary nails at an average of 4 weeks.

A small study by Iannacone et al (147) evaluating the early conversion of external fixation to intramedullary nailing in distal femoral fractures with associated vascular injury is one of the few civilian studies that discusses the treatment of severe penetrating injuries to the femur. Seven fractures were treated with this protocol. The average duration of external fixation was 11 days (range, 3 to 20 days). All external fixators were exchanged for nails in a one-stage procedure. The only infection occurred in a patient with a severe shotgun injury with a soft tissue wound that required coverage with local muscular rotation flaps. The infection resolved after treatment. No vascular complications occurred.

In a larger series of delayed intramedullary nailing of the femur after initial external fixation, Nowotarski et al (148) reported no infections in the four fractures caused by gunshots. Overall their infection rate was 1.7% for their entire series of 54 patients. However, there is no definitive answer on how long an external fixator can be used before conversion to an intramedullary nail with acceptable infection rates. Variables such as initial contamination, time to definitive wound coverage, and presence of pin track infection cloud the picture.

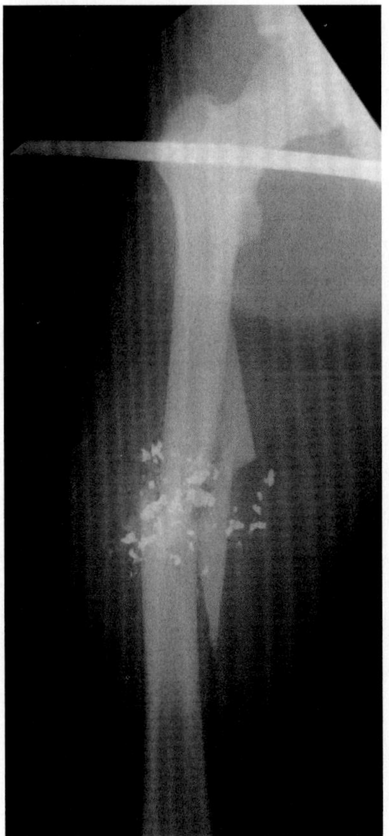
A

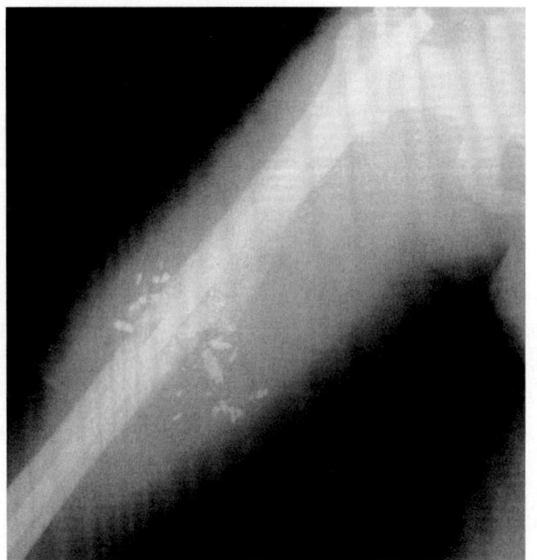
B

FIGURE 14-21 **A.** Comminuted gunshot fracture of the femur. **B.** After treatment with locked intramedullary nailing.

In the most severe injuries, which often include unreconstructable neurologic injury, segmental vascular injury, and skeletal and soft tissue injuries that require complex reconstruction technique, primary amputaton may provide the patient with the best functional result.

Femoral Fractures with Vascular Injury

Arterial injury occurs in a significant percentage of femoral fractures caused by penetrating trauma. Prompt diagnosis and treatment are essential in these limb-threatening injuries (see Fig. 14-7). In four series of low- to mid-velocity gunshot femoral fractures treated by intramedullary nailing (131,143,144,150), the prevalence of associated arterial injury requiring repair ranged from 1.5% to 9%. The true prevalence probably is higher because some femoral fractures with arterial injury were likely treated with other methods.

Historically, the management of penetrating arterial trauma to the extremities has been based on the experience of military surgeons. In World War II, the amputation rate for acute arterial trauma, treated primarily by ligation, was 50%. With the development of techniques of vascular repair, the rate of amputation was reduced to 17.9% in the Korean War and 12.7% in the Vietnam War. Studies of penetrating arterial injuries in civilians report successful limb salvage in up to 94% of patients. Both military and civilian surgeons report a higher rate of amputation when penetrating arterial injuries are associated with fractures. McNamara et al (151) reported 40 patients with humeral, tibial, or femoral fractures with associated vascular injury sustained in the Vietnam War. Twenty-three percent of patients with combined injuries required amputation, compared with only 2.5% of those with vascular injury alone. The failure rate was 60% in fractures associated with popliteal artery injuries.

The orthopaedic management of femoral fractures with associated vascular trauma has changed over the last few decades as well. In the 1960s and 1970s, skeletal traction and other forms of external immobilization were preferred because of more frequent complications with available methods of internal fixation (37,151,152). With the development of improved internal fixation devices, especially locked intramedullary nails, the treatment of femoral fractures with vascular injury in civilians has changed. Several series support the use of internal fixation, both before (38,153), and after vascular repair, for femoral fractures with vascular injury caused by low- to mid-velocity firearms. In four studies of gunshot femoral fractures treated with locked intramedullary nailing (131,143,144,150), nine fractures had associated arterial injuries, most of which were nailed after vascular repair, and no complications were noted.

These results are similar to those obtained at our institution (unpublished data). Between 1986 and 1994, 17 femoral fractures with vascular injury caused by either blunt or penetrating trauma were treated with intramedullary nailing, 13 at the time of vascular repair, 3 after short periods of traction, and 1 after internal fixation. Most of the nailing procedures done on the day of injury were done after vascular repair. All 17 limbs were salvaged, and nailing did not adversely affect any of the vascular repairs. All but a single fracture united, and there was one infection. One patient with a shotgun injury initially treated with external fixation for several weeks developed an infected nonunion.

Nowotarski et al (148) reported a staged approach to treating femoral fractures with vascular injuries. Eight patients with associated vascular injury were included as part of a larger series evaluating the early conversion of external fixation to intramedullary nailing in fractures of the femur. In the eight patients with concomitant vascular injuries, the external fixator was applied before vascular repair. It took an average of 30 minutes to apply the fixator. During conversion of the external fixation to nail placement, the extremity was placed in tibial traction on the fracture table before removal of the external fixator because of movement of the fracture site. There were no infections or vascular complications in the remaining seven patients with associated arterial injuries. Using a similar treatment protocol, Iannacone et al (147,154) evaluated seven distal femoral fractures with vascular injury, including four caused by close-range shotgun blasts. There was one infection in a severe open shotgun injury, and no complications were related to the vascular grafts.

Some investigators recommend external fixation as definitive treatment for femoral fractures with vascular injury (155). Although the prevalence of deep infection is relatively low, pin site infections are common (20%), nonunions may occur in up to 20%, and knee stiffness is a frequent sequela (up to 45%). This method is most appropriate in gunshot fractures associated with severe open wounds resulting from high-velocity weapons or shotguns and in limbs with questionable viability. External fixation is particularly appropriate for war injuries, either as provisional stabilization before evacuation or as definitive treatment in countries lacking advanced orthopaedic equipment and expertise.

Plate fixation has a limited role in the treatment of femoral fractures with vascular injury (156,157). Plates are best suited for extremely proximal fractures involving the intertrochanteric area or extremely distal femoral fractures with intercondylar involvement. In the relatively unusual instance in which a minimally comminuted fracture is exposed during the approach for vascular injuries, plating also can be done through the same incision.

Femoral Fractures with Nerve Injury

The prevalence of nerve palsy associated with gunshot fractures of the femur ranges from 0% to 9%, with an average of about 5% (129,131,137,144). Injuries may be complete or partial, and most commonly involve the peroneal or sciatic nerves. Approximately 50% to 60% of nerve palsies demonstrate complete or significant partial recovery, whereas 40% to 50% exhibit minimal or no recovery. Neurologic recovery can be assessed clinically or by electromyography and nerve conduction velocity studies. If no appreciable recovery is detected after 4 to 6 months, delayed nerve exploration may be considered.

Subtrochanteric and Intertrochanteric Femoral Fractures

Fractures in the subtrochanteric region of the femur have long been recognized as particularly difficult treatment problems. The powerful muscular forces exerted by the flexors and abductors of the hip often cause significant fracture displacement, thus rendering successful nonoperative treatment extremely difficult. High compressive forces are experienced medially, and they increase the stress on implants, particularly if there is medial comminution or bone loss. These problems are compounded in gunshot fractures, which are typically comminuted and have relatively high rates of infection, implant failure, delayed union, and malunion.

Angled-blade plate devices and sliding hip compression screws have been used successfully in subtrochanteric and intertrochanteric fractures of the femur caused by blunt trauma. Complications are frequent, however, when the medial cortical buttress cannot be restored. These devices are best suited for intertrochanteric and high subtrochanteric fractures with minimal comminution. Intramedullary nailing of subtrochanteric fractures (Fig. 14-22) places the nail in a mechanically more advantageous position and allows load sharing by the fractured bone. This technique has reduced some of the complications associated with plate and screw devices.

Wiss et al (143) evaluated 95 subtrochanteric femoral fractures treated with first-generation nails. Three delayed unions, one nonunion, and six malunions were reported. The authors concluded that the biomechanical characteristics of the nail eliminated the necessity for restoration of the medial cortex to achieve stability.

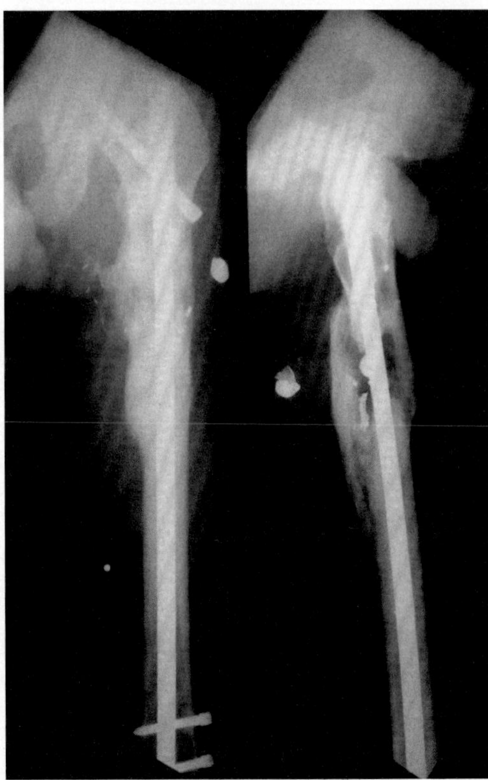

FIGURE 14-22 Low-energy subtrochanteric femoral fracture treated with a second-generation intramedullary nail.

Studies of gunshot femoral fractures by Wiss et al (143), Bergman et al (131), and Nowortarski and Brumback (144) all contained subtrochanteric fractures. Nowortarski and Brumback's series included seven patients treated with second-generation nails. Successful results were obtained in most subtrochanteric fractures in these series.

Distal Femoral Fractures

Supracondylar femoral fractures are difficult injuries to treat because of their proximity to the knee joint, the wide metaphyseal flare, their frequent comminution, and the deforming muscular forces of the quadriceps mechanism and gastrocnemius muscles (Fig. 14-23). Nonoperative treatment by traction and cast bracing was preferred in the 1960s and 1970s (158–160), but internal fixation has produced superior results since the early 1980s because of improvements in implant design. Plate and screw devices developed by the AO group (blade plates, dynamic condylar screws, femoral buttress plates) have been used successfully to treat supracondylar and intercondylar fractures of the femur (161–163). In several large series, infection averaged 0% to 7.7%, nonunion 0% to 7.1%, and malunion 1.7% to 11%, with good and excellent results in 71% to 84% of patients (164,165). These series contained relatively few open injuries and few or no penetrating injuries. The incidence of infection tends to increase when plating techniques are used in open fractures. Current techniques emphasize meticulous soft tissue handling and limited soft tissue stripping.

Locked intramedullary nails inserted in either antegrade or retrograde fashion have been advocated for treatment of supracondylar femoral fractures. Nailing requires little soft tissue disruption. Functional results have been similar to those in fractures treated with plates, and the incidence of infection is generally lower. Tornetta and Tiburzi (150) reported 38 patients with gunshot fractures of the distal femur that were treated with antegrade nailing. The distance from the fracture site to the distal locking screws was less than 5 cm in all patients. All fractures united. There were no deep infections and one superficial infection. Malunion occurred in 3 of 6 patients who underwent the nailing procedure while they were in the lateral position and in 5 of 34 patients who were in the supine position. The authors recommended the supine position for nailing and the use of smooth Steinmann pins as levers to control the distal fragment to reduce the rate of malunion. Antegrade and retrograde nails require approximately 4 cm of intact medial and lateral cortical bone stock in the condyles and are not the preferred treatment for fractures with significant intercondylar comminution.

Patients with severe soft tissue injury may require external fixation, usually spanning the knee joint. Delayed reconstruc-

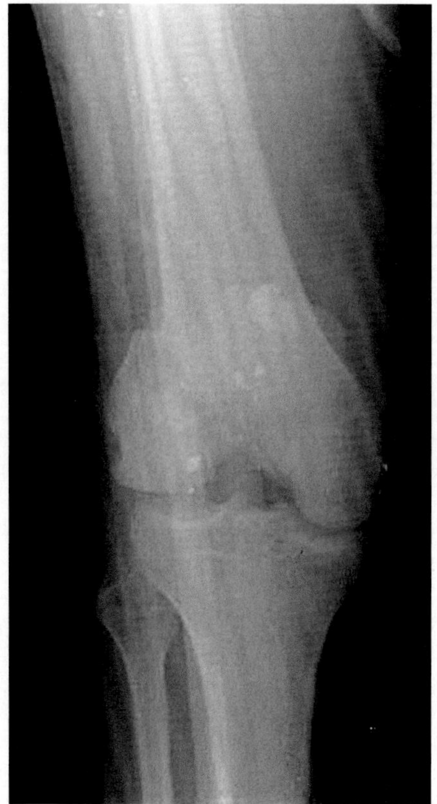

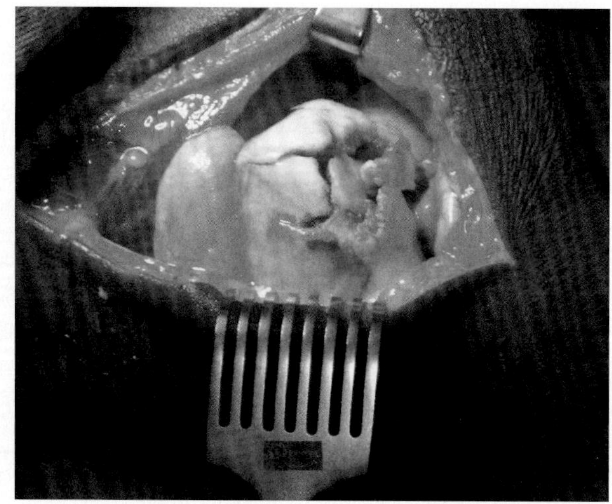

FIGURE 14-23 Gunshot fracture of femoral condyle. Extent of comminution did not appear as severe on x-ray **(A)** as was found intraoperatively **(B)**.

tion can be done after soft tissue healing, or the fixator can remain in place as definitive treatment. In these situations, joint stiffness can be expected. High-energy injuries with severe bone and soft tissue destruction may not be reconstructable and require knee fusion after stabilization of the soft tissues.

Tibial Fractures

Fractures of the tibia caused by penetrating trauma generally can be treated in the same manner as open fractures of the tibia secondary to blunt trauma. Metaphyseal drill-hole fractures, incomplete fractures, and minimally displaced, stable fractures can be treated nonoperatively with casting or functional bracing (Fig. 14-24). Unstable fractures located from 7 cm distal to the knee joint and 4 cm proximal to the ankle joint can be treated with locked intramedullary nailing (see Fig. 14-9). Numerous studies have confirmed the superiority of intramedullary nailing to external fixation in grades I, II, and IIIA open tibial fractures (168–173). Unreamed nailing and external fixation have obtained similar results in grade IIIB open fractures. Although reamed nailing has been presumed to result in an increase in infection in open tibial fractures, reports have refuted this assumption (170). Although some still recommend unreamed nailing in patients with higher-grade open fractures, I prefer minimal reaming to ensure proper nail fit. Plating of open tibial fractures usually is associated with unacceptably high rates of infection. External fixation generally is used for tibial fractures with associated vascular injuries and is preferred for patients with shotgun injuries and severely contaminated wounds. Other indications for external fixation include fractures in unstable patients in whom swift fixation is needed, proximal and distal metaphyseal injuries, and segmental shaft fracture combined with extremely proximal and distal fractures (174–176).

Leffers and Chandler (177) evaluated the treatment of 41 tibial fractures caused by civilian gunshot wounds. Thirty-two fractures were caused by low-velocity firearms, which produced little soft tissue disruption and stable fracture patterns. Most of these patients were successfully treated with casts and functional braces. In this group, there were 2 vascular injuries, 1 compartment syndrome, 3 neurologic deficits, and 2 chronic infections. The 9 patients with intermediate- or high-energy fractures had a much higher percentage of complications. Five were treated with external fixation. There were 5 vascular injuries, 2 compartment syndromes, 4 nerve injuries, 6 chronic infections, and 4 soft tissue healing problems in this subset of 9 patients. The authors recommended surgical debridement, external fixation, and appropriate treatment of vascular injury and compartment syndrome for mid- to high-velocity penetrating injuries of the tibial shaft.

Ten years later, Ferraro and Zinar (178) retrospectively analyzed the treatment of 90 gunshot fractures of the tibia. Fifty-

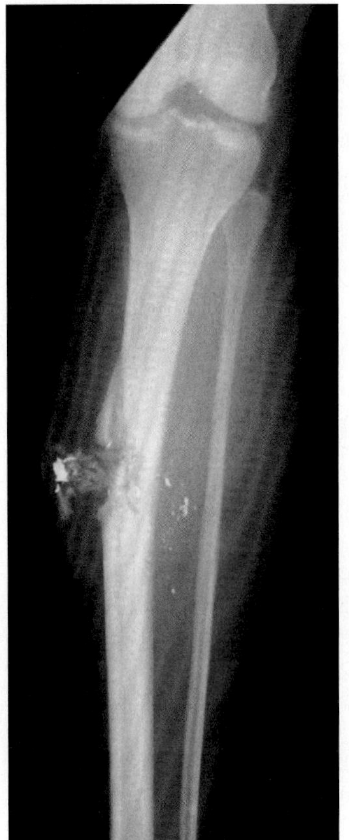

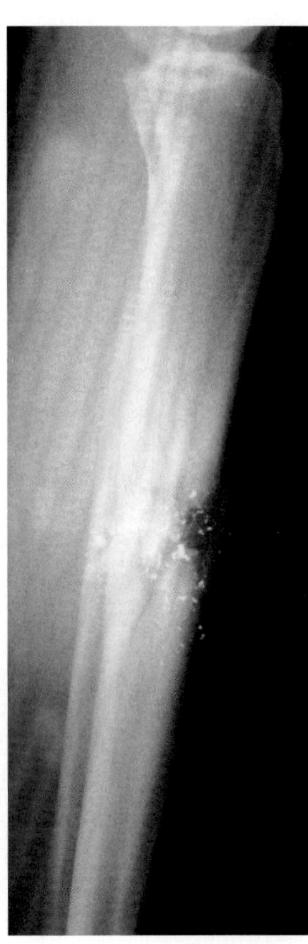

FIGURE 14-24 Stable, unicortical gunshot fractures of the tibia can be treated nonoperatively **(A,B)**.

two fractures were considered stable, and 38 were believed to be unstable based on fracture comminution. All but 2 of the stable fractures were treated in casts and healed within 14 weeks without infection. In the unstable fracture group, 8 were treated in long leg casts and healed in an average of 32 weeks, 16 were treated with external fixation and healed in an average of 27 weeks, and 14 were treated with intramedullary nails and healed in an average of 18 weeks. There were 5 nonunions (3 casts, 1 external fixation of a grade IIIC open injury, and 1 intramedullary nail) and 1 deep infection in the unstable fracture group. The authors recommended intramedullary nailing for unstable fractures when the fracture pattern allows and external fixation for unstable tibial gunshot fractures in which fracture patterns preclude nailing.

Foot Injuries

There are few reports describing the treatment of gunshot wounds to the foot (179–181); however, it is a common injury. It may occur accidentally or as a result of a criminal assault. The foot differs from other areas in the lower extremities in that it has many small joints that may be injured and a thin soft tissue envelope. Gunshot injuries to the foot may damage neurologic or vascular structures, and occasionally fasciotomy is necessary to treat compartment syndrome. Soft tissue coverage with skin grafts or free-tissue flaps may be required for severe injuries. Most fractures can be treated nonoperatively or with percutaneous pin fixation. The infection rate may be higher, regardless of treatment, than that of other gunshot fractures of the extremities, although no definitive studies have shown this to be true. Patients are immobilized in casts or splints for 3 to 6 weeks. Weight bearing is allowed after fracture healing. Early range-of-motion exercises may help to prevent edema, arthrofibrosis, and reflex sympathetic dystrophy. Posttraumatic arthritis may occur after joint injury, and delayed arthrodesis may be required if the foot is painful.

Boucree et al (179) evaluated 101 patients with gunshot injuries to the foot, 81% of whom sustained fractures and 19% had soft tissue injuries only. Ninety-one injuries were low-velocity wounds, 7 resulted from shotguns, and 3 were high-velocity wounds. All patients received intravenous antibiotics, and operative debridement was done in 22 patients with soft tissue wounds larger than 2 cm. Twelve patients developed infections (3 of 3 high-velocity wounds, 3 of 7 shotgun wounds, and 6 of 91 low-velocity wounds).

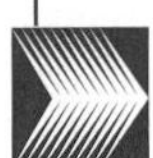

AUTHOR'S PREFERRED TREATMENT

In my institution, almost all low-energy fractures of the femoral shaft, including most intertrochanteric and subtrochanteric fractures, are treated with an intramedullary nailing. I use second-generation nails with femoral head fixation for fractures that include or are proximal to the lesser trochanter. Occasionally, a 95-degree fixed-angle device is used for an intertrochanteric fracture with subtrochanteric extension and displacement of the greater trochanter. Reduction and fixation of the greater trochanter reestablishes the abductor relationship to the femoral shaft. Many high-energy fractures of the femur are initially treated with external fixation until conversion to an intramedullary nail can be safely done, once the soft tissue bed allows.

Extra-articular fractures of the distal femur that have sufficient bone are treated with antegrade or retrograde nailing. Those with a simple split into the joint are treated with retrograde nailing or plate fixation; those with intra-articular comminution usually are fixed with a locked-plate construct.

Close cooperation between the orthopaedist and the general or vascular surgeon is essential when treating femoral fractures with associated vascular injury. In patients whose limbs are ischemic, swift restoration of blood flow is of utmost importance. In these patients, the vascular repair is done before definitive orthopaedic stabilization. A two-pin external fixator can be quickly applied to provide temporary stabilization. Although other investigators have reported using temporary vascular shunts, I have no experience with this technique. In limbs that remain perfused but have vascular injuries that require repair, definitive orthopaedic fixation can be done either before or after vascular repair. At my institution, the decision is left to the vascular surgeon. My colleagues and I prefer antegrade or retrograde locked intramedullary nailing for low-energy gunshot femoral fractures with associated vascular injury between the lesser trochanter and femoral condyles with associated vascular injury. After nailing is done, the vascular status is reassessed, and a completion arteriogram can be obtained. Fasciotomies frequently are required, especially in patients with long ischemic times or concomitant venous injury.

Treatment of gunshot fractures of the tibia follows essentially the same protocol as that for the femur. First is a thorough vascular evaluation with prompt treatment of vascular injuries as necessary. Low-energy injuries with stable fracture patterns are treated with local debridement, tetanus prophylaxis, and appropriate antibiotic treatment. Admittance to the hospital for observation for any soft signs of vascular injury or significant swelling is our policy. If the fracture is unstable, appropriate fracture treatment is carried out: intramedullary nailing of tibial shaft fractures and spanning external fixation of proximal and distal fractures of the tibia that are unsuitable for nailing, usually with staged open reduction and internal fixation when possible. An exception is a low-energy wound to the medial tibia with obvious bone contamination, for which formal debridement is done before intramedullary nailing.

We treat high-energy tibial injuries similar to grade IIIB open fractures. Patients are given cephalosporin and an aminoglycoside (and penicillin if warranted) in the emergency department Initial treatment includes aggressive serial debridements and external fixation. Staged conversion to internal fixation is done if delayed closure or appropriate coverage is attained and the fracture warrants it. We work closely with our plastic surgery colleagues when managing these fractures with severe soft tissue destruction. The decision to amputate relies on judgment and experience and is considered for severe injuries with complex bony, vascular, neurologic, or soft tissue compromise.

Gunshot Wounds to the Spine

Epidemiology

Gunshot wounds to the spine have become more frequent among gunshot injuries treated at major trauma centers, with approximately 50% causing some neurologic deficit (182). Large epidemiologic reviews of gunshot injuries reveal an incidence of 13% to 52% of all spinal cord injuries are caused by firearms, and represent the third most common cause of spinal cord injury (182–186). Victims of gunshot wounds are typically young males, members of minority populations, from lower socioeconomic status, and usually unemployed (185,187,188). Children are not spared from gun violence, and at least one major review (186) demonstrated an equal incidence of spinal cord injury from gunshot wounds and motor vehicle accidents.

The thoracic region is the most common site of injury and carries the worst prognosis for recovery (182,185,189). Gunshot injuries to the spinal cord are more likely to be neurologically complete lesions than are spinal cord injuries caused by blunt trauma (182,185,189), and they are less likely to improve over time (190,191).

The ballistics of wounding are similar to that in other regions of the body (i.e., damage is related to bullet mass, velocity, and deformation on impact), and spinal cord injury can be caused by the bullet directly, by bone fragments, by concussive effects, or by vascular embarrassment. Most civilian injuries are caused from low-velocity handguns and are treated differently from military-type or high-velocity wounds. In general, spinal stability is not compromised with gunshot wounds.

Representing fewer than 1% of spinal cord injuries, stab wounds are uncommon and usually result in a Brown-Séquard syndrome (219). Retained fragments of the wounding instrument may result in continued neurologic compression or delayed infection.

Evaluation

The evaluation of penetrating injuries to the spine begins with the usual ATLS protocol. Rarely is the spinal cord or spinal column injury an emergency, but commonly associated injuries to the brain, neck, thorax, or abdomen can be life-threatening. Classic neurogenic shock does occur, but it is uncommon even with complete injuries, and thorough evaluation for alternative sources of bleeding causing hypotension is essential (193).

It is important to examine the patient's entire body, seeking entrance and exit wounds, because gunshot wounds can be multiple. Special attention should be directed to the patient's posterior neck and both axilla, because these often are overlooked during the physical examination. If a bullet track has crossed the midline of the body, intra-abdominal or intrathoracic injury should be suspected (85,113,114,194–199). While the patient is being examined, routine trauma series x-rays should be obtained. Missile tracks and location and size of wounds should be documented to aid in any future police or legal matters.

All patients must have a detailed neurologic examination with proper documentation of motor and sensory function and reflexes, including the sacral segments. Frequent serial neurologic examinations may be required, especially in patients with mental status changes, intoxication, or distracting injuries.

Conventional x-rays help to localize injury levels, but CT remains the mainstay to identify fracture location and pattern, as well as to locate bullet fragments. Current software algorithms provide remarkable detail, even when metal artifacts are present. Arteriography considerations are the same as for the evaluation of any cervical spine injury, as outlined in Chapter 37.

Spinal stability rarely is affected by gunshot wounds (191,200), and most reported occurrences of instability have been iatrogenic (85,194,201) after decompression and laminectomy. Common stable injury patterns include laminar fractures, body fractures, fracture of one pedicle, fracture of one facet, and disk injuries. Waters et al (202) reported unstable gunshot injuries in the lumbar spine and noted that all patients had fractures of both pedicles or facets. If there is any question of stability, cervical injuries can be evaluated with flexion and extension films once the immediate pain and muscle spasms have resolved (typically 3 to 7 days).

Treatment

Steroids. Current consensus does not support the use of steroids in penetrating injuries to the spine (203,204). Gunshot wounds were specifically excluded from the National Acute Spinal Cord Injury Study in 1990.

Infection. It is a common misconception that bullets are sterilized by being fired from a gun. Even so, spinal infections (osteomyelitis, discitis, and meningitis) from gunshot wounds are rare. Gunshot wounds that do not perforate a hollow viscus (colon, small bowel), pharynx, or trachea must be differentiated from those that do. Simple gunshot wounds can be treated with a few days of intravenous antibiotics, usually a first-generation cephalosporin (182,203). Gunshot injuries that perforate the pharynx, trachea, or hollow viscus require a minimum of 7 days of intravenous antibiotics and preferably 14 days in patients with colonic injuries and those with intra-abdominal complications (85,182,189,194,209). Although antibiotic recommendations vary, a first- or second-generation cephalosporin usually is effective (e.g. cefazolin, cefitin).

Debridement rarely is required, except for high-energy gunshot wounds, and often can lead to significant iatrogenic complications, including instability, epidural abscess, meningitis, wound infections, and persistent cerebrospinal fistula (84,190,191,194,198,201,205–209). The most common infectious complications from gunshot wounds seen at the author's institution are peritonitis, psoas abscesses, and lung abscesses.

Neurologic Injury and Recovery. Gunshot wounds below the level of the conus have a remarkably better prognosis than those occurring above the level of the conus. At the cord level, incomplete lesions fare better than complete lesions (192,202,203,210). One third of patients with complete lesions have nonfunctional improvement, and one third of patients with incomplete lesions regain some useful function (192). For cord-level injuries, cervical and thoracolumbar injuries have a better prognosis than thoracic level injuries.

Late neurologic deterioration rarely occurs, but has been described as long as 15 years after injury (184,211–214), and excision of the retained bullet and reactive tissue should be considered (192,215).

The role of bullet removal has remained controversial, but a few pertinent points can be gleaned from the literature. Data from the Regional Model Spinal Cord Injury Systems suggest that bullet removal is not indicated in cord-level lesions (regardless of whether the lesion is complete or incomplete), but removal promotes neurologic recovery at levels distal to the conus (188). Eismont (182) recommended removal at cervical injury levels to promote recovery of adjacent root function and remove ongoing cord compression. Heary et al (203) reported that outcomes of neurologic incomplete lesions were worse with decompression than without. Prompt bullet removal should be seriously considered for any patient who has neurologic worsening. Delaying laminectomy for 7 to 10 days to allow for clot formation makes dural repair much easier and decreases the risk of persistent cerebrospinal leaks.

Instability. Gunshot wounds rarely result in instability of the spine. The Denis three-column classification system (216) is a useful evaluation tool; however, because of the variety of ways a bullet can pass through the spinal column, a single column injury may result in instability. Common instability patterns include bilateral pedicle fractures or facet fractures. In the cervical spine, extensive comminution of a vertebral body can result in immediate or long-term instability.

Most stable injuries can be treated symptomatically or with a commercial Jewitt brace. More extensive involvement of the vertebral body, pedicles, or facets might require a molded TLSO for better rotational control. If surgical stabilization is required, a posterior approach often is the easiest method. Corpectomy with strut grafting occasionally is required for highly comminuted cervical injuries. Regardless of the treatment, close x-ray follow-up is mandatory to identify progressive kyphotic deformities.

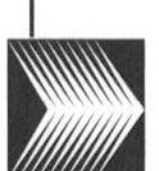

AUTHOR'S PREFERRED TREATMENT

Most patients with gunshot wounds to the spine can be treated conservatively. Each patient is thoroughly evaluated, with emphasis on complete documentation of neurologic status. General surgical involvement is mandatory to identify and treat any intra-abdominal or thoracic injuries. Plain x-rays and CT remain the standards for evaluation of spinal stability, with flexion-extension films obtained as needed. Patients with isolated gunshot injuries are treated with 48 hours of parenteral antibiotic and tetanus prophylaxis as needed. Patients with an injury to the pharynx, trachea, or viscus receive 7 to 14 days of parenteral antibiotics. Steroids are not given. Most patients require no brace or a simple Jewett brace or a hard cervical collar. More unstable injuries often are successfully treated in a molded thoracic lumbosacral orthosis (TLSO). Surgical treatment is infrequent and is reserved for patients demonstrating neurologic decline, retained intracanal bullets at or below the level of the conus or cauda equina, persistent CSF leaks, or spinal instability. When possible, operative intervention is delayed about 7 days to make dural repair easier. Patients with high-velocity gunshot spinal wounds are treated with serial debridement as necessary.

ACKNOWLEDGMENT

The author wishes to acknowledge the contribution of Dr. A. Paige Whittle to this chapter. Much of the information and many of illustrations have come from her, and her contributions are greatly appreciated.

REFERENCES

1. Bartlett CS. Clinical update: gunshot wound ballistics. *Clin Orthop* 2003;408:28–67.
2. Bartlett CS, Helfet DL, Hausman MR, et al. Ballistics and gunshot wounds: effects on musculoskeletal tissues. *J Am Acad Orthop Surg* 2000;8:21–36.
3. Dickey RL, Barnes BC, Kearns RJ, et al. Efficacy of antibiotics in low: velocity gunshot fractures. *J Orthop Trauma* 1989;3:6–10.
4. Brown TD, Michas P, Williams RE, et al. The impact of gunshot wounds on an orthopaedic surgical service in an urban trauma center. *J Orthop Trauma* 1997;11:149–153.
5. Silliphant WM, Beyer J. Wound ballistics. *Mil Med* 1955;117:238-246.
6. Billings JB, Zimmerman MC, Aurori B, et al. Gunshot wounds to the extremities: experience of a level I trauma center. *Orthop Rev* 1991;20:519–524.
7. Fackler ML. Civilian gunshot wounds and ballistics: dispelling the myths. *Emerg Med Clin North Am* 1998;16:17–28.
8. Fackler ML, Bellamy RF, Malinowski JA. The wound profile: illustration of the missile-tissue interaction. *J Trauma* 1988;28:521–529.
9. Rich NM, Metz CW, Hutton JE Jr, et al. Internal versus external fixation of fractures with concomitant vascular injuries in Vietnam. *J Trauma* 1971;11:463–473.
10. Mattox KL, Moore EE, Feliciano DV. *Trauma.* Norwalk, CT: Appleton & Lange, 1988.
11. Harvey E, Korr I, Oster G, et al. Secondary damage in wounding due to pressure changes accompanying the passage of high velocity missiles. *Surgery* 1947;21:218–239
12. Farjo LA, Miclau T. Ballistics and mechanisms of tissue wounding. *Injury* 1997; 28(Suppl 3):S-C12–S-C17.
13. Amato JJ, Syracuse D, Seaver PR Jr, et al. Bone as a secondary missile: an experimental study in the fragmenting of bone by high-velocity missiles. *J Trauma* 1989;29:609–612.
14. DeMuth WE Jr. Bullet velocity as applied to military rifle wounding capacity. *J Trauma* 1969;9:27–31.
15. Ordog GJ, Wasserberger J, Balasubramaniam S, et al. Civilian gunshot wounds: outpatient management. *J Trauma* 1994;36:106–111.
16. Barach E, Tomlanovich M, Nowak R. Ballistics: a pathophysiologic examination of the wounding mechanisms of firearms. II. *J Trauma* 1986;26:374–383.
17. Ordog GJ, Wasserberger J, Balasubramaniam S. Shotgun wound ballistics. *J Trauma* 1988;28:624–631.
18. Deitch EA, Grimes WR. Experience with 112 shotgun wounds to the extremities. *J Trauma* 1984;24:600–603.
19. Ross RT, Hammen PF, Frantz EI, et al. Gunshot wounds: evaluating the adequacy of documentation at a level I trauma center. *J Trauma* 1998;45:151–152.
20. Fackler ML, Mason RT. [Letter.] *J Trauma* 1999;46:741.
21. Rose SC, Fujisaki CL, Moore EE. Incomplete fractures associated with penetrating trauma: etiology, appearance, and natural history. *J Trauma* 1988;28:106–109.
22. Ross RT, Hammen PF, Frantz EI, et al. Gunshot wounds: evaluating the adequacy of documentation at a level I trauma center. *J Trauma* 1998;45:151–152.
23. Hull J, Jones AL, Burgess AR. Extremities: skeleton. In: Ivatury RR, Cayten CG, eds. *The Textbook of Penetrating Trauma.* Philadelphia: Williams & Wilkins; 1966.
24. Alexander JJ, Piotrowski JJ, Graham D, et al. Outcome of complex vascular and orthopedic injuries of the lower extremity. *Am J Surg* 1991;162:111–116.
25. Ashworth EM, Dalsing MC, Glover JL, et al. Lower extremity vascular trauma: a comprehensive aggressive approach. *J Trauma* 1988;28:329–336.
26. Norman J, Gahtan V, Franz M, et al. Occult vascular injuries following gunshot wounds resulting in long bone fractures of the extremities. *Am Surg* 1995;61:146–150.
27. Gahtan V, Bramson R, Norman J. The role of emergent arteriography in penetrating limb trauma. *Am Surg* 1994;60:123–127.
28. Drost TF, Rosemurgy AS, Proctor D, et al. Outcome of treatment of combined orthopedic and arterial trauma to the lower extremity. *J Trauma* 1989;29:1331–1334.
29. Feliciano DV, Herskowitz K, O'Gormon RB, et al. Management of vascular injuries to the lower extremities. *J Trauma* 1988;28:319–328.
30. Flint LM, Richardson JD. Arterial injuries with lower extremity fracture. *Surgery* 1983]: 5–8.
31. Payne WK III, Gabriel RA, Massoud RP. Gunshot wounds to the thigh: evaluation of vascular and subclinical vascular injuries. *Orthop Clin North Am* 1995;26:147–154.
32. Seligson D, Ostermann PAW, Henry SL, et al. The management of open fractures associated with arterial injury requiring vascular repair. *J Trauma* 1994;37:938–940.
33. Cornwell EE III. Current concepts of gunshot wound treatment: a trauma surgeon's perspective. *Clin Orthop* 2003;408:58–64.
34. McCready RA, Procter CD, Hyde FL. Subclavian-axillary vascular trauma. *J Vasc Surg* 1986;3:24–31.
35. Dubravko H, Zarko R, Tomislav T, et al. External fixation in war trauma management of the extremities: experience from the war in Croatia. *J Trauma* 1994;37:831–834.
36. McHenry TP, Holcomb JB, Aoki N, et al. Fractures with major vascular injuries from gunshot wounds: implications of surgical sequence. *J Trauma* 2002;53:717–721.
37. Connolly JF, Wittaker D, Williams E. Femoral and tibial fractures combined with injuries to the femoral or popliteal artery. *J Bone Joint Surg Am* 1971;53:56–68.
38. Starr AJ, Hunt JL, Reinert CM. Treatment of femur fracture with associated vascular injury. *J Trauma* 1996,:17–21.
39. Sunderland S. *Nerves and nerve injury.* New York: Churchill Livingstone; 1972.
40. Woloszyn JT, Uitvlugt GM, Castle ME. Management of civilian gunshot fractures of the extremities. *Clin Orthop* 1988;226:247–251.
41. Visser PA, Hermreck AS, Pierce GE, et al. Prognosis of nerve injuries incurred during acute trauma to peripheral arteries. *Am J Surg* 1980;140:596–599.
42. Omer GE. Injuries to nerves of the upper extremity. *J Bone Joint Surg Am* 1974;56: 1615–1624.
43. Gugala Z, Lindsey RW. Classification of gunshot injuries in civilians. *Clin Orthop* 2003; 408:65–81.
44. Howland WS, Ritchey SJ. Gunshot fractures in civilian practice: an evaluation of the results of limited surgical treatment. *J Bone Joint Surg Am* 1971;53:47–55.
45. Long WT, Brien EW, Boucree JB, et al. Management of civilian gunshot injuries to the hip. *Orthop Clin North Am* 1995;26:123–131.
46. Benzley WC, Rosenthal RE. Lead intoxication 18 months after a gunshot wound. *Clin Orthop* 1984;190:199–203.
47. Bolanos AA, Demizio JP Jr, Vigorita VJ, et al. Lead poisoning from an intra-articular shotgun pellet in the knee treated with arthroscopic extraction and chelation therapy: a case report. *J Bone Joint Surg Am* 1996;78:422–426.
48. Dillman RO, Crumb CK, Lidsky MJ. Lead poisoning from a gunshot wound: report of a case and review of the literature. *Am J Med* 1979;66:509–513.
49. John BE, Boatright D. Lead toxicity from gunshot wound. *South Med J* 1999;92: 223–224.
50. Lees REM, Scott GD, Miles CG. Subacute lead poisoning from retained lead shot. *Can Med Assoc J* 1988;138:130–131.
51. Leonard MH. The solution of lead by synovial fluid. *Clin Orthop* 1969;64:255–261.
52. Linden MA, Manton WI, Stewart RM, et al. Lead poisoning from retained bullets. *Ann Surg* 1982;195:305–313.
53. Meggs WJ, Gerr E, Aly MH, et al. The treatment of lead poisoning from gunshot wounds with succimer (DMSA). *J Toxicol Clin Toxicol* 1994;32:377–386.
54. Switz DM, Elmorshidy ME, Deyerle WM. Bullets, joints, and lead intoxication: a remarkable and instructive case. *Arch Intern Med* 1976;136:939–941.
55. Rhee JM, Martin R. The management of retained bullets in the limbs. *Injury* 1997; 28(Suppl 3):S-C23–S-C28.
56. Janzen DL, Tirman PFJ, Babassa AE, et al. Lead "bursogram" and focal synovitis secondary to a retained intraarticular bullet fragment. *Skeletal Radiol* 1995;24:142–144.
57. Peh WCG, Reinus WR. Lead arthropathy: a cause of delayed onset lead poisoning. *Skeletal Radiol* 1995;24:357–360.
58. Miclau T, Farjo LA. The antibiotic treatment of gunshot wounds. *Injury* 1997;28(Suppl 3):S-C1–S-C5.

59. Simpson BM, Wilson RH, Grant RE. Antibiotic therapy in gunshot wound injuries. *Clin Orthop* 2003;408:82-85.
60. Bender J, Hoekstra S, Levison M. Improving outcome from extremity shotgun injury. *Am Surg* 1993;59:359–364.
61. Tian H, Deng G, Huang M, et al. Quantitative bacteriological study of the wound tract. *J Trauma* 1988;28[Suppl]:215–216.
62. Velmahos GC, Safaoui M, Demetriades D. Management of shotgun wounds: do we need classification systems? *Int Surg* 1999;84:99–104.
63. Weaver LD, Hansrag KK, Idusuyi OB, et al. Gunshot wound injuries. *Orthop Clin North Am* 1995;26:1–7.
64. Thoresby FP, Darlow HM. The mechanics of primary infection of bullets. *Br J Surg* 1967;54:359–361.
65. Wolf AW, Benson DR, Shoji H, et al. Autosterilization in low velocity bullets. *J Trauma* 1978;18:63–65.
66. Hansraj KK, Weaver LD, Todd AO, et al. Efficacy of ceftriaxone versus cefazolin in the prophylactic management of extra-articular cortical violation of bone due to low-velocity gunshot wounds. *Orthop Clin North Am* 1995;26:9–17.
67. Paradies LH, Gregory CF. The early treatment of close-range shotgun wounds to the extremities. *J Bone Joint Surg Am* 1966;48:425–435.
68. Patzakis MJ, Harvey JP, Tyler D. The role of antibiotics in the management of open fractures. *J Bone Joint Surg Am* 1974;56:532–541.
69. Ordog GJ, Sheppard GF, Wasserberger JS, et al. Infection in minor gunshot wounds. *J Trauma* 1993;34:358–365.
70. Brien EW, Brien WW, Long WT, et al. Concomitant injuries of the hip joint and abdomen resulting from gunshot wounds. *Orthopedics* 1992;15:1317–1320.
71. Freeark RJ, Gravier L, Briney W, et al. Gunshot fractures. *Q Bull NW Univ Med School* 1961;35:305–310.
72. Knapp TP, Patzakis MJ, Lee JS, et al. Comparison of intravenous and oral antibiotic therapy in the treatment of fractures caused by low-velocity gunshots. *J Bone Joint Surg Am* 1996;78:1167–1171.
73. Patzakis MJ, Bains RS, Lee J, et al. Prospective, randomized, double-blind study comparing single-agent therapy, ciprofloxacin, to combination antibiotic therapy in open fracture wounds. *J Orthop Trauma* 2000;14:529–533.
74. Geissler WB, Teasedall RD, Tomasin JD, et al. Management of low velocity gunshot-induced fractures. *J Orthop Trauma* 1990;4:39–41.
75. Mellor SG, Cooper GJ, Bowyer GW. Efficacy of delayed administration of benzylpenicillin in the control of infection in penetrating soft-tissue injuries in war. *J Trauma* 1996; 40:5128–5134.
76. Bergman M, Tornetta P, Kerina M, et al. Femur fractures caused by gunshots: treatment by immediate reamed intramedullary nailing. *J Trauma* 1993,:783–785.
77. Ferraro SP Jr, Zinar DM. Management of gunshot fractures of the tibia. *Orthop Clin North Am* 1995°:181–189.
78. Ganocy K, Lindsey RW. The management of civilian intra-articular gunshot wounds: treatment considerations and proposal of a classification system. *Injury* 1998;29(Suppl 1):SA1–SA6.
79. Tornetta P, Hui RC. Intraarticular findings after gunshot wounds through the knee. *J Orthop Trauma* 1997;11:422–424.
80. Ganocy TK II, Lindsey RW. Delayed diagnosis of an intra-articular gunshot injury of the knee: a case report. *J Trauma* 1999;47:158–160.
81. Beceker VV, Brien WW, Patzakis M, et al. Gunshot injuries to the hip and abdomen: the association of joint and intra-abdominal visceral injuries. *J Trauma* 1990;30: 1324–1329.
82. Williams MS, Hutcheson RL, Miller AR. A new technique for removal of intraarticular bullet fragments from the femoral head. *Bull Hosp Joint Dis* 1997;56:107–110.
83. Ivatury RR, Zubowski R, Psarras P, et al. Intra-abdominal abscess after penetrating abdominal trauma. *J Trauma* 1988;28:1238–1243.
84. Kihtir T, Ivatury RR, Simon R, et al. Management of transperitoneal gunshot wounds of the spine. *J Trauma* 1991;31:1579–1583.
85. Kumar A, Wood GW II, Whittle AP. Low-velocity gunshot injuries of the spine with abdominal viscus trauma. *J Orthop Trauma* 1998;7:514–517.
86. Maier RV, Carrico CJ, Heimbach DM. Pyogenic osteomyelitis of axial bones following civilian gunshot wounds. *Am J Surg* 1979;137:378–380.
87. Zura RD, Bosse MJ. Current treatment of gunshot wounds to the hip and pelvis. *Clin Orthop* 2003;408:110–114.
88. Collins DN, Temple D. Open joint injuries: classification and treatment. *Clin Orthop* 1989;243:48–56.
89. Levy AS, Lefkoe TP, Whitelaw GP, et al. Management of penetrating pneumatic nailgun injuries of the knee. *J Orthop Trauma* 1991;5:66–70.
90. McAndrew MP, Johnson KD. Penetrating orthopedic injuries. *Surg Clin North Am* 1991; 71:297–303.
91. Berg EE, Ciullo JV. Arthroscopic débridement after intraarticular low-velocity gunshot wounds. *Arthroscopy* 1993;9:576–579.
92. Dickson K, Watson TS, Haddad C, et al. Outpatient management of low-velocity gunshot-induced fractures. *Orthopedics* 2001;24:951–954.
93. Luce EA, Griffin WO. Shotgun injuries of the upper extremity. *J Trauma* 1978;18: 487–492.
94. Stein JS, Strauss E. Gunshot wounds to the upper extremity: evaluation and management of vascular injuries. *Orthop Clin North Am* 1995;26:29–35.
95. Borman KR, Snyder WH, Weigeit JA. Civilian arterial trauma of the upper extremity: an 11-year experience in 267 patients. *Am J Surg* 1984;148:796–799.
96. McCready RA, Proceter DC, Hyder GL. Subclavian-axillary vascular trauma. *J Vasc Surg* 1986;3:24–31.
97. Hardin WD, O'Connell RC, Adinolfe MF, et al. Traumatic arterial injuries of the upper extremity: determinants of disability. *Am J Surg* 1985;150:266–270.
98. Balfour GW, Marrero CE. Fracture brace for the treatment of humerus shaft fractures caused by gunshot wounds. *Orthop Clin North Am* 1995;26:55–63.
99. Bartlett CS III, Hausman MR, Witschi TH. Gunshot wounds to the shoulder. *Orthop Clin North Am* 1995;26:37–53.
100. Joshi A, Labbe M, Lindsey RW. Humeral fracture secondary to civilian gunshot injury. *Injury* 1998;29(Suppl 1):S-A13–S-A17.
101. Karas EH, Strauss E, Sohail S. Surgical stabilization of humeral shaft fractures due to gunshot wounds. *Orthop Clin North Am* 1995;26:65–73.
102. Keller A. The management of gunshot fractures of the humerus. *Injury* 1995;26:93–96.
103. Reis ND, Zonman C, Besser M, et al. A philosophy of limb salvage in war: use of the fixateur externe. *Mil Med* 1991;156:505–520.
104. Skaggs DL, Hale JM, Buggay S, et al. Use of a hybrid external fixator for a severely comminuted juxta-articular fracture of the distal humerus. *J Orthop Trauma* 1998;12: 439–448.
105. Smith DK, Cooney WP. External fixation of high-energy upper extremity injuries. *J Orthop Trauma* 1990;4:7–18.
106. Wisniewski TF, Radziejowski MJ. Gunshot fractures of the humeral shaft treated with external fixation. *J Orthop Trauma* 1996;10:273–278.
107. Zinman C, Norman D, Hamoud K, et al. External fixation for severe open fractures of the humerus caused by missiles. *J Orthop Trauma* 1997;11:536–539.
108. Tarkin IS, Hatzidakis A, Hoxie SC, et al. Arthroscopic treatment of gunshot wounds to the shoulder. *Arthroscopy* 2003;19:85–89.
109. Edwards SG, Whittle AP, Wood GW II. Nonoperative treatment of ipsilateral fractures of the scapula and clavicle. *J Bone Joint Surg Am* 2000;82:774–780.
110. Wiss DA, Gellman H. Gunshot wounds to the musculoskeletal systems. In: Browner BD, ed. *Skeletal trauma.* Philadelphia: WB Saunders;1992.
111. Heck RK, France JJ, Whittle AP, et al. Treatment of open fractures of the humeral shaft (unpublished data).
112. Trooskin SZ, Sclafani S, Winfield J. The management of vascular injuries of the extremity associated with civilian firearms. *Surg Gynecol Obstet* 1993;176:350.
113. Elstrom JA, Pankovich AM, Egwele R. Extra-articular low-velocity gunshot fractures of the radius and ulna. *J Bone Joint Surg Am* 1978;60:335–341.
114. Fackler ML, Burkhalter WE. Hand and forearm injuries from penetrating projectiles. *J Hand Surg Am* 1992;17:971–975.
115. Foglar C, Ibarra M, Miclau T. Gunshot wounds of the forearm. *Injury* 1997;28(Suppl 3):S-C18–S-C22.
116. Frykberg ER, Dennis JW, Bishop K, et al. The reliability of physical examination in the evaluation of the penetrating extremity trauma for vascular injury: results at one year. *J Trauma* 1991;31:502–505.
117. Hahn M, Strauss E, Yang EC. Gunshot wound to the forearm. *Orthop Clin North Am* 1995;26:85–93.
118. Hammond DC, Gould JS, Hanel DP. Management of acute and chronic vascular injuries to the arm and forearm. *Hand Clin* 1992;8:453–463.
119. Kozin SH, Thoder JJ. The treatment of forearm fractures from penetrating trauma. *Hand Clin* 1999;15:221–231.
120. Moed BR, Fakhouri AJ. Compartment syndrome after low-velocity gunshot wounds to the forearm. *J Orthop Trauma* 1991;5:134–137.
121. Lenihan MR, Brien WW, Gellman H, et al. Fractures of the forearm resulting from low-velocity gunshot wounds. *J Orthop Trauma* 1992;6:32–35.
122. Phillips P III, Hansraj KK, Cox EE II, et al. Gunshot wounds to the hand: the Martin Luther King, Jr. General Hospital experience. *Orthop Clin North Am* 1995;26:95–108.
123. Wilson RH. Gunshots to the hand and upper extremity. *Clin Orthop* 2003;408: 133–144.
124. Wu CD. Low-velocity gunshot fractures of the radius and ulna: case report and review of the literature. *J Trauma* 1995;39:1003–1005.
125. Duncan J, Kettelkamp DB. Low-velocity gunshot wounds of the hand. *Arch Surg* 1974; 109:395–397.
126. Nathan R. The management of penetrating trauma to the hand. *Hand Clin* 1999;15: 193–199.
127. Gonzalez MH, McKay W, Hall RF Jr. Low-velocity gunshot wounds of the metacarpal: treatment by early stable fixation and bone grafting. *J Hand Surg Am* 1993;18:267–270.
128. Cziffer E, Farkas J, Turchanyi B. Management of potentially infected complex hand injuries. *J Hand Surg Am* 1991;16:832–834.
129. Ryan JR, Hensel RT, Salciccioli GG, et al. Fractures of the femur secondary to low-velocity gunshot wounds. *J Trauma* 1981;21:160–162.
130. Long WT, Chang W, Brien EW. Grading system for gunshot injuries to the femoral diaphysis in civilians. *Clin Orthop* 2003;408:92–100.
131. Bergman M, Tronetta P, Kerina M, et al. Femur fractures caused by gunshots: treatment by immediate reamed intramedullary nailing. *J Trauma* 1993;34:783–785.
132. Bone LB, Johnson KD, Weight J, et al. Early versus delayed stabilization of femoral fractures: a prospective, randomized study. *J Bone Joint Surg Am* 1989;71:336–340.
133. Brav E, Jeffress VH. Modified intramedullary nailing in recent gunshot fractures of the femoral shaft. *J Bone Joint Surg Am* 1953;35:141–152.
134. Carr CR, Turnipseed D. Experiences with intramedullary fixation of compound femoral fractures in war wounds. *J Bone Joint Surg Am* 1953;35:153–171.
135. Lhowe DW, Hansen ST. Immediate nailing of open fractures of the femoral shaft. *J Bone Joint Surg Am* 1988;70:812–820.
136. Dicpinigaitis PA, Fay R, Egol KA, et al. Gunshot wounds to the lower extremities. *Am J Orthop* 2002;31:282–203.
137. Brien WW, Kuschner SH, Brien EW, et al. The management of gunshot wounds to the femur. *Orthop Clin North Am* 1995;26:133–138.
138. Tejan J, Lindsey RW. Management of civilian gunshot injuries of the femur: a review of the literature. *Injury* 1998;29(Suppl 1):S-A18–S-A22.
139. Atesalp AS, Yildiz C, Basbozkur M, et al. Treatment of type IIIa open fractures with

Ilizarov fixation and delayed primary closure in high-velocity gunshot wounds. *Mil Med* 2002;167:56–62.

140. Behrman SW, Fabian TC, Kudsk KA, et al. Improved outcome with femur fractures: early versus delayed fixation. *J Trauma* 1990;30:792–797.
141. Healy WL, Brooker AF. Distal femoral fractures: comparisons of open and closed methods of treatment. *Clin Orthop* 1983;174:166–171.
142. Mize RD. Surgical management of complex fractures of the distal femur. *Clin Orthop* 1989;249:77–96.
143. Wiss DA, Brien WW, Becker V Jr. Interlocking nailing for the treatment of femoral fractures due to gunshot wounds. *J Bone Joint Surg Am* 1991;73:598–606.
144. Nowotarski P, Brumback RJ. Immediate interlocking nailing of fractures of the femur caused by low- to mid-velocity gunshots. *J Orthop Trauma* 1994;8:134–141.
145. Wright DG, Levin JS, Esterhai JL, et al. Immediate internal fixation of low-velocity gunshot-related femoral fractures. *J Trauma* 1993;35:678–682.
146. Dubravko H, Zarko R, Tomisalv T, et al. External fixation in war trauma management of the extremities: experience from the war in Croatia. *J Trauma* 1994;37:831–834.
147. Iannacone WM, Bennett FS, Delong WG Jr, et al. Initial experience with treatment of supracondylar femoral fractures using the supracondylar intramedullary nail: a preliminary report. *J Orthop Trauma* 1994;8:322–327.
148. Nowotarski PJ, Turen CH, Brumback RJ, et al. Conversion of external fixation to intramedullary nailing for fractures of the shaft of the femur in multiply injured patients. *J Bone Joint Surg Am* 2000;82:781–788.
149. Wu CC, Shih CH. Treatment of open femoral and tibial shaft fractures: preliminary report on external fixation and secondary intramedullary nailing. *J Formos Med Assoc* 1991;90:1179–1185.
150. Tornetta P III, Tiburzi D. Anterograde interlocked nailing of distal femoral fractures after gunshot wounds. *J Orthop Trauma* 1994;8:220–227.
151. McNamara JJ, Brief DK, Stremple JF, et al. Management of fractures with associated arterial injury in combat casualties. *J Trauma* 1973;13:17–19.
152. Rich NM, Baugh JH, Hughes CW. Acute arterial injuries in Vietnam: 1,000 cases. *J Trauma* 1970;10:359–369.
153. Hafez HM, Woolgar J, Robbs JV. Lower extremity arterial injury: results of 550 cases and review of risk factors associated with limb loss. *J Vasc Surg* 2001;33:1212–1219.
154. Iannacone WM, Taffet R, DeLong WG Jr, et al. Early exchange intramedullary nailing of distal femoral fractures with vascular injury initially stabilized with external fixation. *Injury* 1994;37:446–451.
155. Seligson D, Kristiansen TK. Use of the Wagner apparatus in complicated fractures of the distal femur. *J Trauma* 1978;18:795–799.
156. Back AW, Hansen ST Jr. Plate versus external fixation in severe open tibial shaft fractures: a randomized trial. *Clin Orthop* 1989;241:89–94.
157. Bolhofner BR, Carmen B, Clifford P. The results of open reduction and internal fixation of distal femur fractures using a biologic (indirect) reduction technique. *J Orthop Trauma* 1996;10:373–377.
158. Moore TJ, Watson T, Green SA, et al. Complications of surgically treated supracondylar fractures of the femur. *J Trauma* 1987;27:402–406.
159. Neer CS, Grantham SA, Shelton ML. Supracondylar fracture of the adult femur. *J Bone Joint Surg Am* 1967_:591–613.
160. Stewart MJ, Sisk TD, Wallace SL. Fractures of the distal third of the femur. *J Bone Joint Surg Am* 1966;48:784–807.
161. Merchan ECR, Maestu PR, Blanco RP. Blade-plating of closed displaced supracondylar fractures of the distal femur with the AO system. *J Trauma* 1992;32:174–178.
162. Ostrum RF, Geel C. Indirect reduction and internal fixation of supracondylar femur fractures without bone graft. *J Orthop Trauma* 1995;4:278–284.
163. Sanders R, Regazzoni P, Ruedi TP. Treatment of supracondylar-intercondylar fractures of the femur using the dynamic condylar screw. *J Orthop Trauma* 1994;3:214–222.
164. Danziger MB, Caucci D, Zecher SB, et al. Treatment of intercondylar and supracondylar distal femur fractures using the GSH supracondylar nail. *Am J Orthop* 1995;24: 684–690.
165. Gellman RE, Paiment GD, Green HD, et al. Treatment of supracondylar femoral fractures with a retrograde intramedullary nail. *Clin Orthop* 1996;332:90–96.
166. Giles JB, DeLee JC, Heckman JD, et al. Supracondylar-intercondylar fractures of the femur treated with a supracondylar plate and lag screw. *J Bone Joint Surg Am* 1982;64: 864–870.
167. Leung KS, Shen WY, So WS, et al. Interlocking intramedullary nailing for supracondylar and intercondylar fractures of the distal part of the femur. *J Bone Joint Surg Am* 1991; 73:332–340.
168. Boynton MD, Schmeling GJ. Nonreamed intramedullary nailing of open tibial fractures. *J Am Acad Orthop Surg* 1994;2:107–114.
169. Henley MB, Chapman JR, Agel J, et al. Treatment of type II, IIIA, and IIIB open fractures of the tibial shaft: a prospective comparison of unreamed interlocking intramedullary nails and half-pin external fixators. *J Orthop Trauma* 1998;12:1–7.
170. Keating JF, O'Brien PJ, Blauchut PA, et al. Locking intramedullary nailing with and without reaming for open fractures of the tibial shaft: a prospective, randomized study. *J Bone Joint Surg Am* 1997;79:334–341.
171. Schandelmaier P, Krettek K, Rudolf J, et al. Outcome of tibial shaft fractures with severe soft tissue injury treated by unreamed nailing versus external fixation. *J Trauma* 1995; 39:707–711.
172. Tornetta P III, Bergman M, Watnik N, et al. Treatment of grade IIIB open tibial fractures: a prospective randomized comparison of external fixation and non-reamed locking nailing. *J Bone Joint Surg Br* 1994;76:13–19.
173. Whittle AP, Russell TA, Taylor JC, et al. Treatment of open fractures of the tibial shaft with the use of interlocking nailing without reaming. *J Bone Joint Surg Am* 1992;74: 1162–1171.
174. Brien EW, Long WT, Serocki JH. Management of gunshot wounds to the tibia. *Orthop Clin North Am* 1995;26:165–180.
175. Edwards CC, Simmons SC, Browner BD, et al. Severe open tibial fractures: results treating 202 injuries with external fixation. *Clin Orthop* 1988;230:98–115.
176. Yildiz C, Atesalp AS, Demiralp B, et al. High-velocity gunshot wounds of the tibial plafond managed with Ilizarov external fixation: a report of 13 cases. *J Orthop Trauma* 2003;17:421–419.
177. Leffers D, Chandler RW. Tibial fractures associated with civilian gunshot injuries. *J Trauma* 1985;25:1059–1064.
178. Ferraro SP Jr, Zinar DM. Management of gunshot fractures of the tibia. *Orthop Clin North Am* 1995;26:181–189.
179. Boucree JB Jr, Gabriel RA, Lezine-Hanna JT. Gunshot wounds to the foot. *Orthop Clin North Am* 1995;26:191–197.
180. Durkin RC, Coughlin RR. Management of gunshot wounds of the foot. *Injury* 1998; 28(Suppl 3):S-C6–S-C11.
181. Holmes GB Jr. Gunshot wounds of the foot. *Clin Orthop* 2003;408:861–91.
182. Eismont FJ. Gunshot wounds of the spine. In: Levine AM, Eismont FJ, Garfin SR, et al., eds. *Spine trauma.* Philadelphia: WB Saunders;1998.
183. Benzel EC, Hadden TA, Coleman JE. Civilian gunshot wounds to the spinal cord and cauda equina. *Neurosurgery* 1987;20:281–285.
184. Capen D. Etiology of spinal cord injuries: significant changes over 10 years. Paper presented at the annual meeting of the American Academy of Orthopaedic Surgeons, San Francisco, 1993.
185. Farmer JC, Vaccaro AR, Balderston RA, et al. The changing nature of admissions to a spinal cord injury center: violence on the rise. *J Spinal Disord* 1998;11:400–403.
186. Haffner DL, Hoffer MM, Wiedbusch R. Etiology of children's spinal injuries at Rancho Los Amigos. *Spine* 1993;18:679–684.
187. Smith W, Simmonds JO, Alam ZS, et al. Spinal cord injury caused by gunshot wounds: the cost of rehabilitation. *Clin Orthop* 2003;408:145–151.
188. Waters RL, Sie IH. Spinal cord injuries from gunshot wounds to the spine. *Clin Orthop* 2003;408:120–125.
189. Kitchel SH. Current treatment of gunshot wounds to the spine. *Clin Orthop* 2003;408: 115–119.
190. Velmahos G, Demetriades D. Gunshot wounds of the spine: should retained bullets be removed to prevent infection? *Ann R Coll Surg Engl* 1994;76:85–87.
191. Velmahos G, Demetriades D, Foianini E, et al. A selective approach to the management of gunshot wounds to the back. *Am J Surg* 1997;174:342–346.
192. Waters RL, Hu SS. Penetrating injuries of the spinal cord: stab and gunshot injuries. In: Frymoyer JW, ed. *The Adult Spine: Principles and Practice.* Vol 1. New York: Raven Press; 1991:815–826.
193. Zipnick RI, Scalea TM, Trooskin SZ, et al. Hemodynamic responses to penetrating spinal cord injuries. *J Trauma* 1993;35:578–582.
194. Heiden JS, Weiss MH, Rosenberg AW, et al. Penetrating gunshot wounds of the spine in civilians: review of 38 cases. *J Neurosurg* 1975;42:575–579.
195. Isiklar ZU, Lindsey RE. Gunshot wounds to the spine. *Injury* 1998;29[Suppl 1]: SA7–SA12.
196. Isiklar ZU, Lindsey RW. Low-velocity civilian gunshot wounds of the spine. *Orthopedics* 1997;20:967–972.
197. Payne JE, Berne TV, Kaufman RL, et al. Outcome of treatment of 686 gunshot wounds of the trunk at Los Angeles County-USC Medical Center: implications for the community. *J Trauma* 1993;34:276–281.
198. Waters RL, Adkins RH. The effects of removal of bullet fragments retained in the spinal canal: a collaborative study by the National Spinal Cord Injury Model Systems. *Spine* 1991;16:934–939.
199. Zipnick RI, Scalea TM, Trooskin SZ, et al. Hemodynamic responses to penetrating spinal cord injuries. *J Trauma* 1993;35:578–582.
200. Kupcha PC, An HS, Cotler JM. Gunshot wounds to the cervical spine. *Spine* 1990;15: 1058–1063.
201. Stauffer ES, Wood RW, Kelly EG. Gunshot wounds of the spine: the effects of laminectomy. *J Bone Joint Surg Am* 1979;61:389–392.
202. Waters RL, Adkins RH, Yakura J, et al. Profiles of spinal cord injury and recovery after gunshot injury. *Clin Orthop* 1991;267:14–21.
203. Heary RF, Vaccaro AR, Mesa JJ, et al. Steroids and gunshot wounds to the spine. *Neurosurgery* 1997;41:576–583.
204. Levy ML, Gans W, Wijesinghe HS, et al. Use of methylprednisolone as an adjunct in the management of patients with penetrating spinal cord injury: outcome analysis. *Neurosurgery* 1996;39:1141–1148.
205. Roffi RP, Waters RL, Adkins RH. Gunshot wounds to the spine associated with a perforated viscus. *Spine* 1989;14:808–811.
206. Heary RJ, Vaccaro AR, Mesa JJ, et al. Thoracolumbar infections in penetrating injuries to the spine. *Orthop Clin North Am* 1996;27:69–81.
207. Linn SS, Vaccaro AR, Reisch S, et al. Low-velocity gunshot wounds to the spine with an associated transperitoneal injury. *J Spinal Disord* 1995;8:136–144.
208. Romanick PC, Smith TK, Kopaniky DR, et al. Infection about the spine associated with low-velocity-missile injury to the abdomen. *J Bone Joint Surg Am* 1985;67:1195–1201.
209. Simpson RK Jr, Venger BH, Narayan RK. Treatment of acute penetrating injuries of the spine: a retrospective analysis. *J Trauma* 1989;29:42–46.
210. Robertson DP, Simpson RK. Penetrating injuries restricted to the cauda equina: a retrospective review. *Neurosurgery* 1992;31:265–270.

211. Fung CF, Ng TH. Delayed myelopathy after a stab wound with a retained intraspinal foreign body: case report. *J Trauma* 1992;32:539–541.
212. Jones FD, Woosley RE. Delayed myelopathy secondary to retained intraspinal metallic fragment. *J Neurosurg* 1981;55:979–982.
213. Kuijen JM, Herpers MJ, Beuls EA. Neurogenic claudication, a delayed complication of a retained bullet. *Spine* 1997;22:910–914.
214. Wu WQ. Delayed effects from retained foreign bodies in the spine and spinal cord. *Surg Neurol* 1986;25:214–218.
215. Staniforth P, Watt I. Extradural 'plumboma': a rare case of spinal stenosis. *Br J Radiol* 1982;55:772–774.
216. Denis F. Spinal instability as defined by the three-column spine concept in acute spinal trauma. *Clin Orthop* 1984;189:65–76.

WAR WOUNDS, LIMB SALVAGE, AND TRAUMATIC AMPUTATIONS

Paul J. Dougherty

WEAPONS AND THEIR EFFECTS

Mechanisms of Injury

Weapons of conventional war may be divided into two areas: explosive munitions and small arms. Explosive munitions consist of grenades, mortars, bombs, land mines, and artillery. Small arms consist of handguns, rifles, and machine guns (1,2).

Since World War I, fragments from exploding munitions have accounted for the majority of injuries seen in war (Table 15-1). During more recent operations other than war, land mines and booby traps have accounted for an increased proportion of the wounded. Part of the reason for this increased prevalence is that land mines, once placed, will continue to injure until removed, independent of the course of a conflict. There are vast tracts of minefields that remain in areas of Africa, Asia, and the Balkans (3–6).

Small arms are weapons that fire a bullet from a rifled barrel to a target. The bullet is usually contained in a cartridge consisting of powder, a primer, and a cartridge case all in one unit. They are usually classified by the diameter (size) of the barrel (9 mm, 0.45 in, 7.62 mm). Handguns used by the military are the same as those used by civilian police and others with regards

TABLE 15-1 Casualty Generation by Weapon

	World War I	Bougainville, World War II (US)	Republic of Vietnam (WDMET)
Bullet	28.06	34	30
Mortar	See note[a]	39.5	19
Booby trap/land mine	N/A	1.9	17
Hand grenade	1.21	12.7	11
Artillery	70.4	11	3
Rocket propelled grenade[b]	N/A	N/A	12

Wound Data and Munitions Effectiveness Team, WDMET.
[a] Described as "shell and shrapnel." Would be mostly artillery with some mortars.
[b] Not used in World War I or the Bougainville Campaign.

to size, shape, and caliber. They are usually semi-automatic, which means a bullet is fired every time the trigger is pulled as long as ammunition is in the weapon's magazine (1,2).

Rifles are weapons larger than a handgun and are intended to be fired from the shoulder. Bullets fired from rifles are more aerodynamically shaped and are fired at a faster velocity than those from handguns. The longer barrel, aerodynamic shape, and increased velocity mean the rifle is more accurate over longer ranges (1,2).

Machine guns are intended to fire in the full automatic mode; this occurs when repeated shots are fired as long as the trigger is held down as opposed to the semi-automatic fire described above. Machine guns generally weigh more than rifles and are installed on vehicles and aircraft (1,2).

Modern military rifles are most often the so-called "assault rifles" and have the ability to fire in both full and semi-automatic modes. In an effort to reduce recoil, cartridges used in these weapons are not the full-powered rifle cartridges seen in civilian hunting rifles or military weapons of the first half of the twentieth century (1,2).

Wounds produced by small arms are dependent on several variables. Factors involved with forming gunshot wounds include the size and shape of the projectile, its composition, and the velocity of the projectile. There are two mechanisms of injury to tissue caused by a bullet: the permanent tract and temporary cavity (Fig. 15-1). The permanent tract is tissue that is touched by the bullet. For elastic tissue, such as skeletal muscle, there is a localized area of tissue damage which is proportional to the size of the projectile passing through. A second mechanism, known as temporary cavity, is caused by a transient lateral displacement of tissue which occurs after passage of the projectile. Inelastic tissue, such as liver or bone, may become fractured in this area. Just what the bullet strikes is also important to determine the type of injury seen. The anatomic location and the type of tissue struck (bone versus skeletal muscle, for example) also influence the type of wound seen as well as the clinical

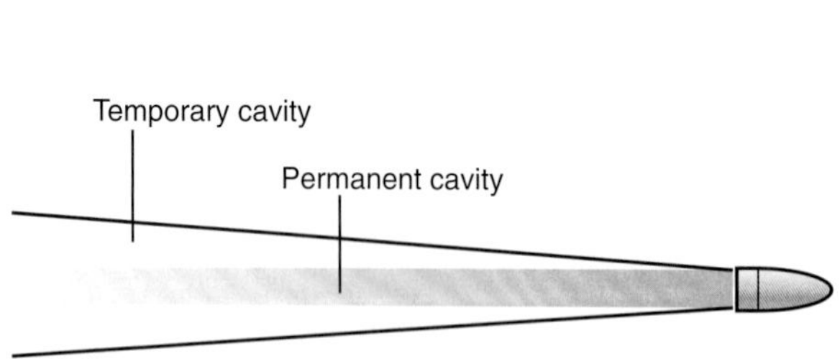

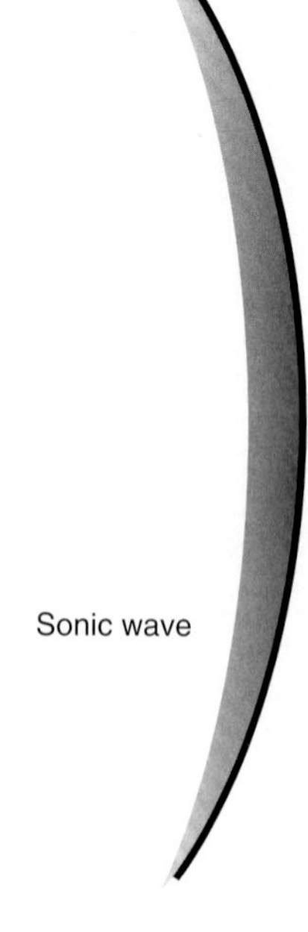

FIGURE 15-1 The two areas of tissue injury: the permanent cavity and the temporary cavity. The permanent cavity is caused by localized areas of cell necrosis proportional to the size of the projectile as it travels through. Temporary cavitization causes a transient lateral displacement of tissue. The shock wave, though measurable, has not been found to cause injury in tissue.

course and outcome. Intermediate targets, such as body armor, may alter the characteristics of a wound seen if the armor is perforated by a bullet (7,8).

Explosive munitions are the most common agents for wounding soldiers on a battlefield. This trend began during World War I (1914–1918) when artillery became more common on the battlefield. This trend continues through today (see Table 15-1). Broad categories of weapons are: bombs, mortars, grenades, artillery, and land mines.

Explosive munitions wound by one or more of three mechanisms: ballistic, blast, or thermal. Ballistic injuries occur from fragments of an exploding munition itself or from material around the explosive device. Blast injuries occur due to a transient blast overpressure caused by the exploding munition. Thermal injuries are caused by a transient increase in local temperature due to the explosion. Blast and thermal injuries occur relatively close to the exploding munition, whereas ballistic injuries also can occur farther from the device (1,2).

Artillery consists of cannon that fire large projectiles for up to several miles. The projectiles may by antivehicle, contain white phosphorous, or be explosive filled. US military artillery cannon range from 105 mm to 8 in (diameter of the cannon barrel). The explosive-filled projectiles are most often used against infantry soldiers. When detonated, they produce fragments of variable shape and size that cause wounds. The fragments produced depend on the casing of the artillery round. More modern artillery casings break up to produce more uniform fragments over a given area. The fragments may range from a few milligrams to several grams in weight. After detonation, fragments may initially travel at several thousand meters per second. This initial velocity rapidly decreases because of the irregular shape of the fragments (1,9).

Grenades are small explosive-filled devices that may be thrown or fired from a special launcher. Grenades may produce smoke for signaling or be designed to disable or destroy tanks or injure soldiers. As with artillery shells, the type of fragments produced is dependent on the composition of the container. Most modern grenades have a notched or pre-fragmented casing that produces fragments of a uniform size when detonated (1,9).

Mortars are weapons that have barrels aimed at a high arc to produce indirect fire. Projectiles fired from mortars may produce smoke, white phosphorus, or explosive fragments. These weapons are smaller and are more limited in range compared with cannon. As with the other weapons described above, fragments produced by the explosive shells vary with the composition of the shell's casing (1,9).

Land mines may be one of two major types: antipersonnel or antivehicle. Antipersonnel land mines are those intended to injure individual soldiers. Antivehicle land mines are intended to destroy or disable vehicles such as tanks (1,9–11). Antipersonnel land mines are classified by the US Army as being: static, bounding, or horizontal spray. Another category, unconventional devices, will be handled separately in this section. Currently there is much concern about land mines throughout the world because of vast tracts that remain in Asia, Africa, and the Balkans. Estimates vary, but somewhere between about 70 and 100 million land mines remain in place, which, until removed, will continue to be a hazard to those living or working in the area (1,9) (Fig. 15-2).

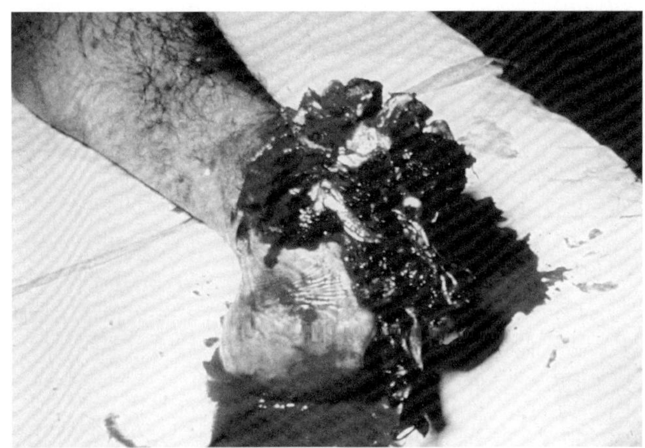

FIGURE 15-2 Land mine injured foot.

Static land mines are those laid on top or buried in soil, which detonate when someone steps on the device. They are the most common type of land mine seen throughout the world. They contain a small amount of explosive (100–200 g) and produce a characteristic pattern of injury.

Russian surgeons obtained considerable experience with land mines during their war in Afghanistan (1979–1988), which prompted them to do both laboratory and clinical investigations on the mechanism of injury. Injuries produced by static land mines are primarily of the lower extremity (Fig. 15-3). There are three areas of injury. First, there is an area of mangling or avulsion (traumatic amputation) that occurs at the midfoot or distal tibia. There is a second area in which the soft tissues are separated from bone along fascial planes in the leg (brisant). This area is a tidewater area in terms of tissue survival; the tissue is compromised but it may heal. The area extends from below the knee to the level of "avulsion" injury of the foot or lower leg. More proximally, injuries may occur from fragments or debris propelled from the land mine but not necessarily from direct effects of the blast itself. The degree of injury is dependent on the size and shape of the individual's limb, the type of footwear and clothing worn, the amount and type of soil overlying the land mine, and the size of the land mine itself (10).

Bounding mines are those land mines which, when tripped, propel a small grenade-like device to about 1 to 2 meters in height. The device then explodes, producing multiple small fragment wounds to those nearby of a similar nature to wounds produced by grenades.

Horizontal spray land mines are those mines which, when tripped, fire fragments in one direction. These land mines may be used to protect a perimeter or during an ambush. The US Army's Claymore mine is such a mine. It fires about 700 steel balls that weigh 10 grains each in one direction. The weapons

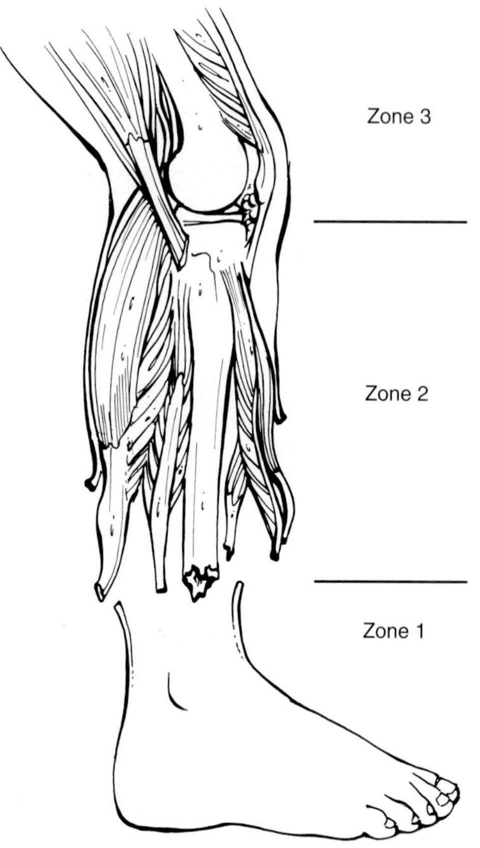

FIGURE 15-3 Russian schema for transtibial amputee.

produce multiple fragment wounds to exposed nearby personnel (1,9) (Fig. 15-4).

Unconventional devices are another category of land mine. These mines are fabricated out of another piece of ordnance, such as a grenade or mortar shell, to detonate when a person either steps on the device or moves a tripwire. These devices may be made out of locally available materials as well. They vary in construction from smaller antipersonnel devices to large explosive devices with several kilograms of explosive to disable or destroy vehicles (1) (Fig. 15-5).

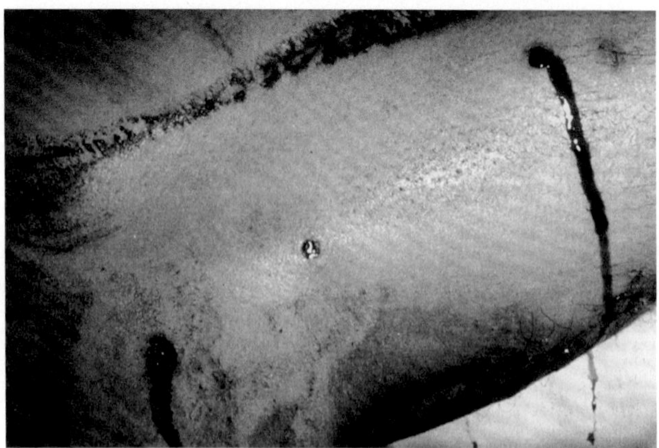

FIGURE 15-4 Limb injury due to Claymore mine. Multiple small punctuate fragment wounds.

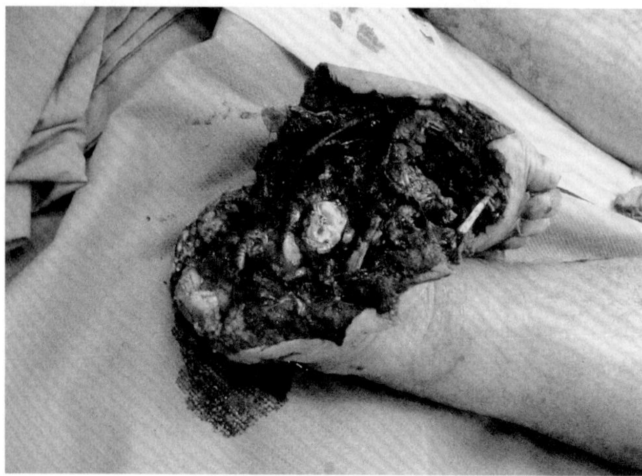

FIGURE 15-5 Land mine amputee.

Bombs are explosive devices that are dropped from aircraft. They may consist of one large explosive device or may carry submunitions distributed more uniformly over a target area. Cluster bombs are an example of the latter device (1,9).

Another type of injury occurs among those who are inside of armored vehicles (11). Most of the world's armies have tanks, infantry fighting vehicles, and armored reconnaissance vehicles within their inventory. Injuries to crewmembers occur both in and around vehicles. Those injured outside of the vehicle have injuries similar to infantrymen. Two types of weapons are used to perforate the armored vehicles envelope to cause injury to the crewmen (antitank land mines may be considered a third type).

First, there is the kinetic energy round. This consists of a hard piece of metal, such as tungsten or depleted uranium, which is fired out of a cannon at a high velocity. The projectiles today are long and narrow and cause a high concentration of pressure over a very small cross-sectional area to defeat the armor plate. If the round penetrates to the crew compartment, injuries may be caused by the penetrating round itself, debris knocked off from the inside of the vehicle itself, or armor debris. Since the penetrating rounds are large, injuries to individuals tend to be catastrophic.

Shaped charges are the other type of weapon seen on the battlefield. They consist of an explosive filled warhead packed around a reverse cone-shaped piece of metal (copper or aluminum). When detonated, the liner collapses and a jet is produced which travels at up to 10,000 feet per second. The jet produces an area of high temperature and pressure over a very small cross-sectional area. When the jet penetrates the armor, it produces two areas of under armor debris. First, there is the jet of the shaped charge. The jet produces catastrophic wounds when it directly hits one of the crewmen. Second, there is an area of under armor debris called spall, which is material knocked off from the inside face of the armored plate itself. Many of today's armored vehicles have liners that do not allow spall debris to form (11).

OVERVIEW OF BATTLE CASUALTIES

The two best epidemiological studies concerning battle casualties consist of data from World War II and the Vietnam War (3–6). A prospective study on battle casualties was conducted during the Bougainville campaign in the Solomon Islands during World War II to assess patient injuries based on the weapon and tactical circumstances. The patients were then followed through their initial surgical care in order to look at outcome. A second study was performed during the Vietnam War to assess 7964 casualties for an 18-month period during the war. The patients in this study (Wound Data and Munitions Effectiveness Team, or WDMET) were evaluated in terms of the tactical situation, the weapons used, the injuries produced, and patient outcome.

Anatomic Distribution of Wounds

The anatomic distribution of wounds among war injured is relatively constant, probably because wounds produced on the battlefield tend to be a random event. Between 60% and 70% of wounded patients admitted to a medical treatment facility have wounds to the extremities, and about 21% of those admitted have fractures. Use of body armor to protect soldiers and airmen was studied in World War II and the Korean War and was found to reduce thoracic and abdominal wounds (12).

Casualty Generation by Weapon and Lethality

The proportion of casualties caused by various weapons from World War I, the Bougainville Campaign in World War II, and the Vietnam War is shown in Table 15-1. The proportion of injuries due to bullets has been relatively constant from conflict to conflict. Recently, fragment producing explosive munitions have accounted for an increasing proportion of casualties seen from the battlefield. This trend is expected to continue (3–6).

The lethality of a weapon is defined as the probability of death given a hit from a particular weapon (Table 15-2). From the Bougainville and WDMET data, the lethality of a bullet wound is about 1/3. Fragments from grenades, mortars, and artillery range from 1/10 to 1/20. Death from tripping a land mine is also about 1/3 (4,6).

TABLE 15-2 Lethality by Weapon

	Bougainville	Vietnam
Weapon		
Bullet	0.32	0.39
Mortar	0.12	0.13
Grenade	0.05	0.13
Artillery	0.11	0.25
Land mine	0.38	0.31

MEDICAL CARE ON THE BATTLEFIELD

Wounded soldiers from the battlefield must be simultaneously treated and moved through the evacuation chain. All major armies throughout the world have made some provisions to care for wounded soldiers. The US military (Army, Navy, and Air Force) have similar echelons of care to treat wounded soldiers (13).

The first treatment of a wounded soldier on the battlefield consists of self-care or buddy care. The first step may be to take cover from hostile fire. Treatment for extremity wounds consists of stopping bleeding, the application of a dressing, and splinting.

The next step is care provided by a medic in which the patient is further evaluated, perhaps with the dressings and splint being adjusted. The medic also has the capability of providing pain relief, antibiotics, and arranging for further evacuation.

A Battalion Aid Station may be the first physician contact that a wounded soldier has. Here the patient is further evaluated, splints and dressings adjusted, and then triaged as to priority for further evacuation and treatment. If the casualty load is light, patients are treated as they arrive. If the casualty load is heavy, patients must be triaged in order to allocate the resources of evacuation and surgical care. Ideally, the triage takes place along the entire evacuation chain. If a patient becomes worse, their priority may increase.

The US Army Medical Company is the next echelon of care in the evacuation scheme. This facility has the capability of providing blood transfusions and has limited x-ray capability. This unit is the first level of care with any bed holding capability. Adjacent to the Medical Company may be the Forward Surgical Team (FST) that provides the first possible surgical support on the battlefield. The purpose of this unit is to provide surgical care of nontransportable patients, in other words those patients whose outcome would be compromised by being evacuated farther for surgical care. Examples of patients who should have surgery at the FST are those with penetrating abdominal wounds who are in shock and those with major traumatic amputations. Because of the mission to treat emergent patients, the FST is staffed with one orthopaedic surgeon and three general surgeons. Having an orthopaedic surgeon is important to make decisions concerning amputations as well as caring for those with multiple injuries. Often those with multiple injuries have major extremity wounds. Because the FST has no bed holding capability, it must be co-located with a medical company to complete its mission. Goals of surgery are to stabilize the patients and prepare them for evacuation. Similar units for the US Navy are the Surgical Company to support the US Marines and the MFST for the US Air Force. While all three are not exactly the same due to the need to meet service specific requirements, they all function at the same level of care.

The US Army's Combat Support Hospital (CSH) is the next echelon of care on the battlefield. The entire unit when assembled has 296 beds which includes intensive care unit capability, six operating rooms, laboratory capability, and is staffed by three orthopaedic surgeons in addition to general surgeons, internists, and emergency room physicians. This hospital is presently deployed as a modular unit in a 40-bed slice with two operating rooms. There are three general surgeons and one orthopaedic surgeon assigned to the hospital in this configuration. This facility is the first surgical echelon for the majority of battlefield patients, including those with orthopaedic injuries. Goals of care at this hospital are to stabilize the patients and to prepare them for evacuation out of the combat zone. Examples of care for patients arriving at the CSH include the treatment of soft tissues, fracture stabilization via casting or external fixator application, or treatment of a partial or complete amputation. The combat support hospital is ideally located near an airfield. The equivalent US Navy hospital is the Fleet Hospital and for the US Air Force the EMEDs Hospital which is a modular system.

Patients may be moved to one of the surgical facilities (FST or CSH) directly from the battlefield depending on the severity of the injury and if the tactical situation permits. In more stationary situations, such as during the Vietnam War, this situation occurred more frequently.

AMPUTATION SURGERY (INCLUDING LIMB SALVAGE)

One of the most visible reminders of the destructiveness of war is the amputee (14–34). Compared to other patient categories, amputees may be characterized as having a higher injury severity, increased morbidity and longer hospitalization than when compared to other battle casualties. Most orthopaedic surgeons have limited experience caring for amputees. As a consequence, it is of paramount importance for military surgeons to study this type of injury and prepare to treat it.

During World Wars I and II, the incidence of amputation was about 3% of all battle casualties (35,36). This figure may be higher during operations other than war (10,20,21). In the series from the Vietnam War, about two-thirds of injuries leading to amputation were caused by land mines or booby traps. This figure is consistent with contemporary reports by the Red Cross surgeons who worked in Afghanistan.

Indications for Surgery

Clear indications for amputation of battlefield casualties include overwhelming sepsis, an unrepairable vascular injury or a partial/complete traumatic amputation (Table 15-3). The anatomic disruption of a posterior tibial nerve in the face of a severe open fracture of the tibia is also an indication. Infection was the leading indication for surgery of American casualties during World War I (37). During World War II, trauma became the main indication for surgery and continues to be so today (15–22,28,30,38,39).

For the majority of battlefield amputees, the decision to amputate is already made for the surgeon. In my review of the indications for surgery of 484 battlefield amputations from the Vietnam War, 89.5% had the amputation for a partial or complete traumatic amputation which necessitated only completion of the amputation via debridement. A further 8.4% had vascular injuries, and 1.9% had an amputation due to infection.

Limb Salvage versus Amputation

A question for every military surgeon should be: could some limbs amputated in previous conflicts be salvaged today? To answer this, we have to decide what advances in trauma care are applicable to battlefield casualties with severely traumatized limbs. Clearly, repair of a vascular injury was attempted on a wide scale during the Korean War, and resulted in a reduction

TABLE 15-3 Indications for Amputation Surgery

	World War I	World War II, European Theater	World War II, Mediterranean Theater	Vietnam, Valley Forge Army General Hospital
Trauma (%)	25.5	64.3	75	89.5
Infection (%)	74.5	14.3	9.5	1.9
Vascular (%)	N/A	21.3	14.5	8.4

in the amputation rate from 50% to 13% in limbs with a vascular injury (40).

The majority of amputations are partial/complete traumatic amputations, requiring only debridement of the residual limb. Late amputations are the result of infection or failed vascular repair. Several authors have analyzed amputations performed late after a patient was transported from Vietnam. Bagg, cited by Burkhalter (41), found that 13 of 200 tibia fractures received at the 106th General Hospital in Japan from Vietnam required an amputation (ten below knee and three above knee).

Schmitt and Armstrong found that open fractures with vascular injury was the cause for nearly half (48%) of the late amputations seen in this facility during the Vietnam War, followed by vascular injuries alone (25%), fractures only (17%), and soft tissue infection (10%) (18).

Recent interest has focused on being able to determine which extremities will require amputation and which will fare best with limb salvage. Since the Vietnam War, the ability to use free flaps to cover bone defects have been used to prevent infection and improve healing. Also, newer designs in external fixation have improved fracture stabilization for severe injuries (42).

Open fractures have been classified since the mid 1970s by the Gustilo and Anderson grading (grade I, II, and III), and later modified to grade IIIA, B, and C depending on severity (43,44). Grade IIIB fractures are open fractures which require local or free flap coverage of the exposed bone. Grade IIIC fractures are those that have a vascular injury that requires repair. Recently, Brumback et al have raised concerns regarding interobserver variability with this classification system (45).

Caudle and Stern (46) reported on 42 IIIB tibial fractures which required a free flap and nine IIIC tibial fractures with a repairable vascular injury. The amputation rate was 17% for the IIIB and 78% for IIIC injuries.

Georgiadis et al (47) evaluated patients with 20 severe tibia fractures that required a free flap for soft tissue coverage. Four required amputation. Average follow-up for 14 patients was 35 months. Concurrently, a further 18 patients with severe tibia fractures had primary amputations. Average follow-up for this group was 44 months. Two of the limb salvage group had a major vascular injury while 15 of the 18 amputees had vascular injuries. Three of the limb salvage patients returned to work, whereas 9 of the 18 amputees returned to work. Average time to full weightbearing was 13 months for the limb salvage and 6 months for the amputation group. Quirke et al (48) evaluated 35 patients with open tibia fractures and major vascular injuries (Gustilo type IIIC). Twenty-one of these patients underwent primary amputation (60%) and a further 14 (40%) underwent vascular repair and fracture stabilization. One underwent late amputation.

Lerner et al (49) studied 109 patients with either a nonunion of the tibia or femur (50), chronic osteomyelitis (39), or lower extremity amputation (20). Comparison was made between these groups to evaluate quality of life parameters using the Psychosocial Adjustment to Illness Scale (PAIS) and Arthritis Impact Measurement Scale (AIMS). A questionnaire was also used to evaluate other demographic factors. Patients with chronic osteomyelitis were more severely affected than the other two groups as measured by the AIMS. Results of the PAIS showed no significant difference between groups.

Attempts to predict when to amputate have resulted in several limb salvage scores. The mangled extremity severity score (MESS) and NISSSA (*n*erve injury, *i*schemia, *s*oft-tissue injury, *s*keletal injury, *s*hock, *a*ge), the Predictive Salvage Index (PSI), and Limb Salvage Index (LSI) have been evaluated in a few studies characterized by small sample sizes and a wide range of injuries (Gustilo IIIB and C) (50–57).

Bosse et al (58–60) have prospectively studied 556 severely injured limbs to assess the clinical utility of the five injury severity scoring systems (MESS, LSI, PSI, NISSSA, and the Hannover Fracture Scale). At 6 months 407 patients retained their limbs. Sixty-three patients had immediate amputations and 86 had delayed amputations. Threshold scores were found to have low sensitivity but relatively high specificity. The use of a limb salvage scores could not be recommended by the authors as a criterion to amputate a limb.

It is unclear as to just what newer techniques developed since the Vietnam War will improve limb survival and function of patients injured on the battlefield. A reasonable scheme for severe open fractures of patients who will undergo a long plane evacuation is to do procedures for saving the limb (stabilize the fracture, vascular repair, wound surgery) and allowing for safe transportation to a site of definitive care. Once in a stable environment, then the patient may undergo more extensive procedures to stabilize the limb, have bone or tissue transfer and undergo rehabilitation. Having definitive stabilization or reconstructive procedures prior to evacuation is not recommended. First, there is not the logistical support to have the necessary equipment for reconstructive procedures at battlefield hospitals. Second, patients undergoing extensive procedures are less able to undergo evacuation without having a complication. Patients in the air evacuation chain are less closely monitored than those in a hospital setting.

Patients who are not moved, such as local civilians, and do receive all of their care near the battlefield should receive the best care possible in this unstable environment. Planning for the long-term care of patients is often not practical. The care team must then assess just what capabilities are present and make the best treatment decision given the available resources.

Traumatic Amputations—Initial Surgical Techniques

Refugee or Civilian Population

Recent experience in treating civilian war casualties by the International Committee of the Red Cross (ICRC) has led to guidelines on the care of amputees in strife torn regions throughout the world. Initial surgical management consists of excision of dead tissue, fashioning flaps, which can be closed later, and placement of the residual limb in a bulky dressing. Inspection of the wound occurs in the operating room a few days later followed by wound closure if the wound condition permits. Patients may be fitted with a prosthesis when the residual limb wound is healed and the edema has subsided. Amputees who have been treated by the ICRC protocol are not evacuated from the facility where the initial amputation was preformed. Often the same surgeons render their entire episode of care at a single facility. This is not a likely scenario in which US military combat casualties will be treated (19,20,23).

A recent report by Simper on the treatment of 111 transtibial amputees in Pakistan recommends a delayed primary closure of the below knee amputation due to war wounds. The environment in which these casualties were injured is significantly different from a conventional battlefield. Patients in this study survived a median evacuation time of 14 hours prior to receiving surgical care, unlike US or Allied soldiers who are evacuated quickly from the battlefield. In this series, delayed primary closure of the residual limbs was performed at a median time of 6.4 days from the initial surgery. Thirteen percent of the amputations failed in this series. Entirely missing from this article is any discussion of fitting prostheses for the patients (19).

Another retrospective report by Atesalp et al compared delayed primary closure to primary closure of the residual limb of 474 patients with transtibial amputations caused by land mine injuries. Of the 392 patients who had primary closure after radical debridement, 11 had revision to a transfemoral level. None of the 82 patients who had delayed primary closure had this complication (22).

Surgeons from the former Soviet Union studied land mine injured patients treated during the war in Afghanistan during the 1980s. The authors concluded that it is difficult to determine at the time of the initial surgery exactly just what tissue will or will not survive. Because of this, they recommended that a "sparing" amputation be performed initially by qualified personnel, that the wound be left open, and for reconstruction to be done at a later time at a specialty center (10).

The treatment of refugees in a theater of operations or in "nation building" efforts remains dependent on the resources which are available to the medical staff. Surgeons treating refugees should not plan procedures that will require extensive long-term care. They should be planned with the patient's host country's current resources in mind, not what is possible at a modern medical center in an industrialized city. In this context, the recommendations by the ICRC (19,22,23) are entirely reasonable and can be used to provide the best care for the most people. Patients in this setting can be cared for by the same surgeon and do not have to undergo evacuation from theater. Fitting of amputees is often problematic, as prostheses are expensive and the rehabilitation requires additional resources.

Patients Who Undergo Evacuation

The open length preserving amputation (formerly called an open circular amputation), is a technique which was relearned by US military surgeons during every conflict of the 20th century (15–18,24–28,30–33,36,38,39). This technique is most applicable to wounded soldiers who must be evacuated after their initial surgery. The amputation should be carried out at the lowest viable level of soft tissue. No consideration for the definitive or final level of amputation should be given. All dead or necrotic tissue should be removed. Often with irregular war wounds an oblique wound is created. Wounds should be left open because it is safer for the patient in the air evacuation system. The limb should be placed in skin traction to prevent bone protrusion and residual limb swelling. The patients should be placed in transportation casts prior to air evacuation. Once a patient is moved to a stable environment, reconstructive procedures and prosthetic fitting may be done. This is the best technique to use because it allows for the safest evacuation of wounded soldiers (see Figs. 15-5 to 15-11).

LaNoue (28) evaluated 230 patients with a transtibial amputation, some of whom had multiple amputations, during the Vietnam War. He found that 41% of the patients had residual limbs that had been closed prior to evacuation and 59% had been left open. Of those closed, 56% failed due to gross infection. He also found that the time to fitting with a permanent prosthesis was also longer, 13 months as opposed to 11 months when the wound was left open.

A formal open length preserving amputation (24,26,28) consists of the following: a circumferential incision is made through the skin and deep fascia at the lowest viable level. This layer is allowed to retract without further dissection. The muscle bundles exposed are then divided circumferentially at the new proximal level of retracted skin edge. The incised muscle bundles will promptly retract proximally, exposing the bone beneath. The soft tissues are then manually retracted proximally to facilitate bone transection at a still higher level. Periosteum should not be stripped. When the amputation is performed properly, the resultant residual limb will have the appearance of a cone with the apex directed proximally. The blood vessels are divided between clamps and are ligated as they are encountered. Named blood vessels are doubly ligated. In addition, a transfixing suture is added to the cuff of large arteries. The artery supplying the sciatic nerve may require separate ligation. Temporary pressure or thromboplastin is applied to the open medullary cavities of large bones to control oozing when necessary. Major nerves are transected 3 to 5 cm above the amputation at the highest possible level without resorting to traction. Major nerves are ligated as they often have a blood vessel associated with them. Cut nerve ends may be injected with a long-acting local anesthetic agent to reduce pain during the postoperative recovery period. Since the amputation has been performed because of irreparable damage to a contaminated, if not grossly septic, extremity, the residual limb should not be closed primarily. The formal open circular amputation is performed at the lowest level of injury. If the zone of injury is oblique then the level of amputation will follow (Fig. 15-6).

Skin Traction

Use of the open length preserving amputation necessitates skin traction to prevent bone protrusion (26,28,30). Skin begins to

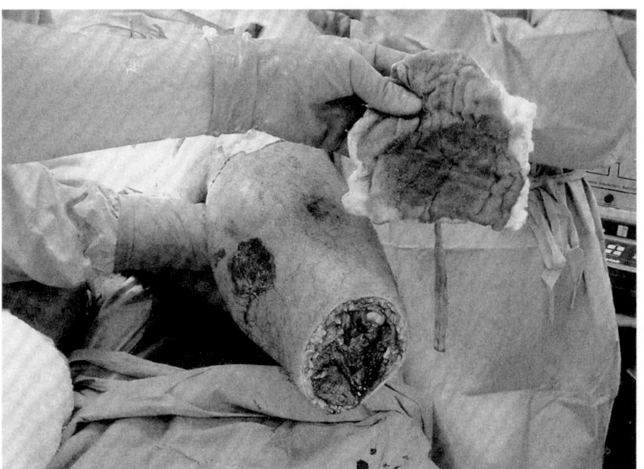

FIGURE 15-6 Transtibial open length preserving amputation. Application of benzoin.

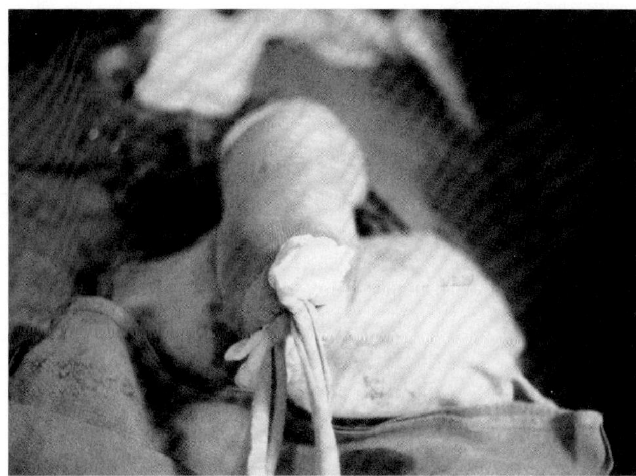

FIGURE 15-8 Stockinette for bed traction.

retract soon after the amputation if traction is not applied to it. The technique is fairly simple. A layer of sterile fine-mesh gauze is placed over the wound, and the recess of the residual limb is dressed loosely with fluffed gauze or other suitable material. A stockinette for skin traction is then applied to the skin above the open residual limb. A liquid adhesive such as benzoin tincture is used to prevent slippage of the stockinette. (Figs. 15-7 and 15-8). The residual limb is wrapped with gentle compression, decreasing proximally, and a few pounds of traction, enough to overcome the elastic recoil of the skin, is applied to the free end of the stockinette. Constrictive dressings proximal to the residual limb should be avoided.

Transportation Casts

Transportation casts are used for patients who will be removed from combat zone hospitals (24,28,30) (Figs. 15-9 to 15-11). They allow for continuous, portable traction to be maintained throughout the evacuation chain as well as support and padding for the soft tissues to make the patient more comfortable. Lower extremity amputees can ambulate on crutches, if the amputation is an isolated injury. Even though they are ambulatory with crutches, a lower extremity amputee should be considered to be a litter patient, however. All constrictive dressings must be loosened to allow for tissue swelling during air craft pressure changes prior to air evacuation. Therefore all casts must be bivalved prior to transport.

Traction attached to the litter or a traction splint, for exam-

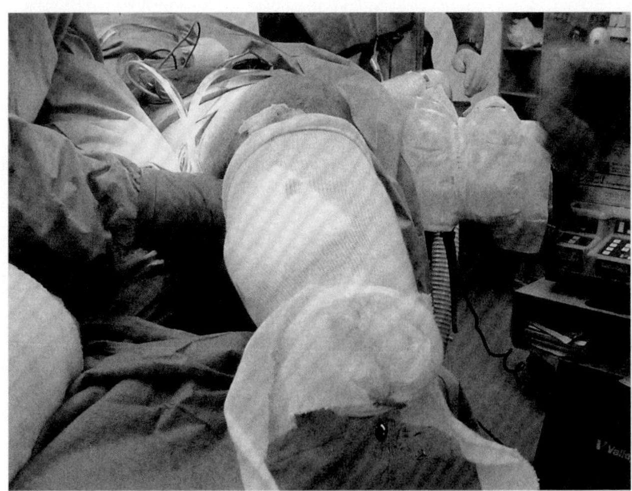

FIGURE 15-7 Application of dressings and stockinette.

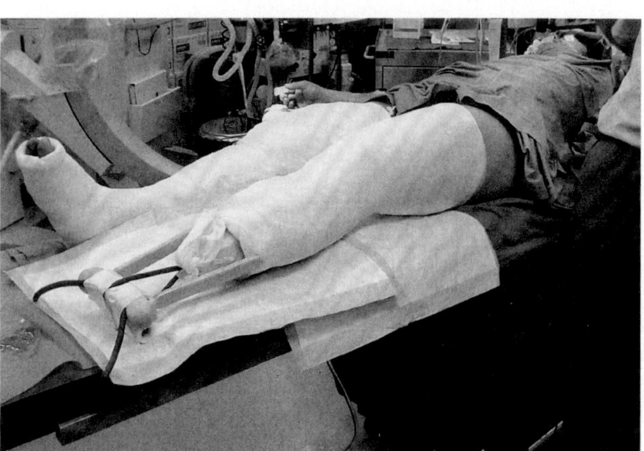

FIGURE 15-9 Transportation cast.

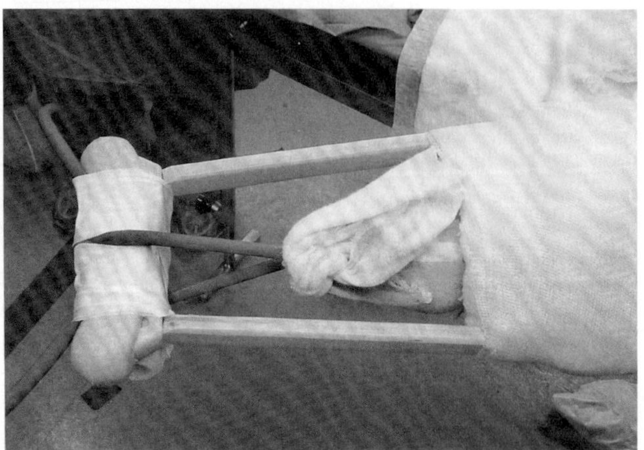

FIGURE 15-10 Outrigger for transportation cast.

ple, does not provide reliable traction that can be maintained throughout the evacuation chain. There is also no soft tissue support provided by these means.

Patients with below knee amputations should be placed in a modified long leg cast. At the time of the last in theater procedure, a cast should be applied after an appropriate dressing has been placed over the wound. It consists of 6-inch wide plaster and 6-inch cotton padding, such as webril. The residual limb end is cleaned, and an adherent such as mastasol is put on the skin. Stockinette is applied over the distal 10 to 15 cm of skin, and the cast applied from the end of the residual limb to the proximal thigh. An outrigger, made of a wire (ladder) splint or crutch is used to maintain traction. For below knee amputees, traction of from 1 to 2 kg should be applied, to overcome the elastic recoil of the skin.

Above knee amputees should be fitted with a hip spica cast. This is best applied at the last surgery in theater. A fracture table can assist the application of the cast. The distal end of the residual limb has stockinette applied as with the below knee amputee after a dressing is placed over the wound. The sacrum and anterior, superior iliac spine are padded with felt. Six-inch cotton padding (webril) is placed from the distal end of the residual limb to the level of the umbilicus. The contralateral thigh is also included. Next, 6-inch plaster is wrapped, beginning with the involved limb first. An outrigger must be incorporated in the distal end to provide traction through the stockinette. The traction should be from 2 to 4 kg, enough to overcome the elastic recoil of the skin. The cotton padding is turned down to the level of the anterior superior iliac spine for the last roll, so that the completed cast leaves the abdomen exposed, which allows for respiratory function in transport.

Below elbow amputees are placed in skin traction by placing a dressing over the wound and applying stockinette in a similar manner to that previously described. A long arm cast is then applied, using 4-inch cotton padding and 4-inch wide plaster. An outrigger, made from a wire splint is applied so that about 2 lb of traction can be maintained on the stockinette.

Above elbow amputees can be placed in traction by applying a dressing to the residual limb end. Stockinette is applied over the end of the residual limb, usually covering all of the residual arm. After padding, a wire splint is fashioned and placed over the distal end of the residual limb. It can then be held in place by plaster. If the wound is proximal, this may not be possible without making a shoulder spica cast.

Military Amputation Specialty Centers

Every major conflict involving the US military during the 20th century saw the development of amputee centers to care for the special needs of those sustaining a limb loss (26–28,30–34,36,61). The centers were started to consolidate the resources of physicians, therapists, nurses, and prosthetists to provide the best care for patients. During World War I the US Army established seven centers to care for 2,635 major amputees (36). During World War II, seven centers were established by the US Army to care for about 16,000 Army amputees (61). The US

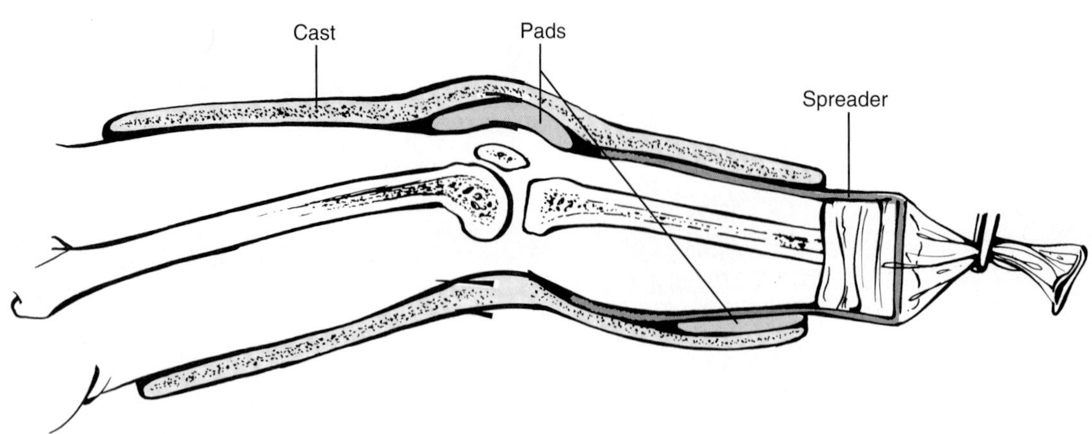

FIGURE 15-11 Cross-sectional drawing of transportation cast for transtibial amputation.

Navy established two centers to care for 1527 amputees seen during that conflict (33,34).

During the Vietnam War, a separate amputee service was started at Valley Forge Army General Hospital for the same reasons amputee centers were established in previous conflicts. This center provided high quality care and research concerning amputees. The lessons learned from the amputation specialty centers are mentioned below.

Definitive Care

A team of surgeons, physiatrists, therapists, and nurses should carefully evaluate patients who are received from overseas. The open residual limb should be evaluated and placed or maintained in skin traction to prevent bone protrusion. Once evaluated, lower extremity amputees should be fitted with a pylon prosthesis as soon as possible, even with the open wounds (Figs. 15-12 and 15-13). This prosthesis should be removable to allow for access to the wound and for skin traction to be applied in bed. Early walking has psychological benefits, improves wound healing, and allows for earlier restoration of proprioception (28,30–32). Wound healing is improved by allowing weightbearing as tolerated and clearing the edema from the residual limb (Fig. 15-14). Upper extremity amputees should also be thoroughly evaluated and placed in a provisional prosthesis to begin activity of daily living training. This training should begin daily under the supervision of occupational therapists (62).

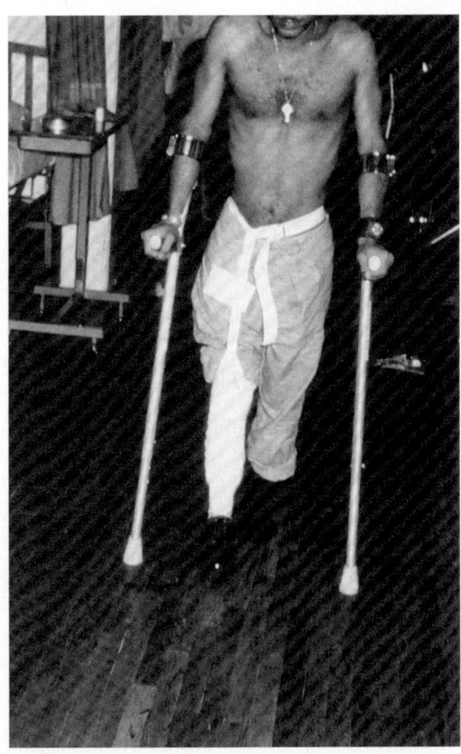

FIGURE 15-12 Walking on pylon, even with open wounds.

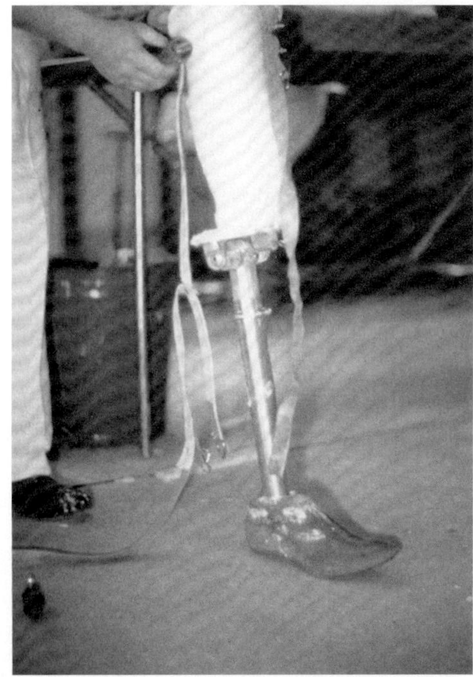

FIGURE 15-13 Close up of pylon.

Most patients will require a second procedure to close the residual limb after the initial open amputation. Consideration will need to be given for the condition of the soft tissues and as to just what level of amputation will provide the best function (28,30).

Refugees and civilians treated at a military hospital or one of the hospitals belonging to a nongovernmental organization such as the ICRC will have their definitive care within the host country. There is often a constraint on resources regarding postoperative care to include prosthetic fitting. In such circum-

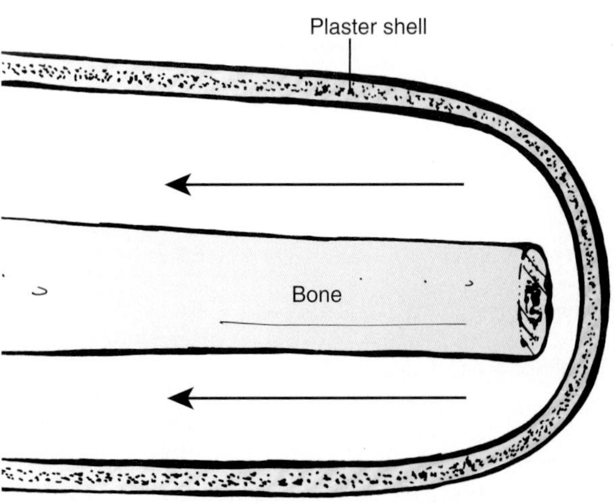

FIGURE 15-14 Pylon with weightbearing.

stances, the surgical team should try and plan for definitive care as soon as possible. If the patient can stay in one place, closure and definitive care may be provided. If the patient must be moved, arrangements for further care should be made as soon as possible. There are a wide variety of situations that surgeons may be exposed to in caring for nonmilitary conflict victims. Because of this, the surgical team needs to assess their own capabilities on a case by case basis in order to provide the best care for patients (19,20).

Levels of Amputation

Upper Extremity Amputations

Upper extremity amputations (Table 15-4) are less frequent in both wartime and civilian settings when compared to lower extremity amputations (15,16,20,28,30,33,34,36,38,39,63). During wartime, the incidence of upper extremity amputees is between 13% and 25%. Rehabilitation should begin as soon as possible for the patients to provide the best possible outcome (62).

Shoulder Disarticulation. Burkhalter reported that 9 of 96 upper extremity amputees had a shoulder disarticulation at Fitzsimmons Army Hospital after the Vietnam War (63). The majority of patients in the series had amputations due to war wounds. This procedure is for nonsalvageable proximal arm injuries or for severe brachial plexopathies.

The surgical technique most often cited was reported by Slocum and others after caring for amputees during World War II (64–66). The patient is placed on the operating room table at a 45 degree angle. An anterior incision is used from the coracoid just medial to the deltoid muscle. As the incision is carried distally, it is then brought circumferentially around the arm and proximally into the axilla. Once through the skin, the cephalic vein is identified and ligated. The deltoid is retracted laterally, and the pectoralis major is incised near its insertion and retracted medially. The axillary artery and vein as well as the thoracoacromial artery are then isolated and ligated before transection. The radial, musculocutaneous, ulnar, and median nerves are isolated, drawn into the field and transected as proximally as possible. Next, the insertions of the coracobrachialis, teres minor and teres major, the deltoid and the origin of the triceps are incised, followed by the subscapularis and the anterior joint capsule. Once the humerus is dissected free the limb may be removed. The deltoid is then sutured inferior to the glenoid to cover the open wound and the skin is closed. There is relatively little fluctuation in the shape of the amputation site after wound healing, therefore the patient may be fitted only with a permanent prosthesis. In one series, three of nine patients with shoulder disarticulations became successful prosthetic wearers (63).

TABLE 15-4 Levels of Amputation

	World War I[a] (36)	World War II (126)	Vietnam (28)
Transhumeral (%)	21.8	6.7	13.9[b]
Transradial (%)	8.4	6.8	
Transfemoral (%)	45.1	35	26.6
Transtibial (%)	12.9	49.8	47.6

[a] Does not include 3.7% knee or 5.2% ankle disarticulations.
[b] Combined transradial and transhumeral.

Transhumeral Amputation. This amputation is performed for severe elbow or arm injuries or for nonsalvageable forearm injuries (63,68) (Fig. 15-15). Other reported indications are infection and brachial plexopathies (69,70). Surgery is done by constructing flaps at the lowest viable level of soft tissue. Very proximal amputations, especially those proximal to the deltoid tuberosity should be fitted with a prosthesis similar to that for a shoulder disarticulation (66,68). Flaps should be made to utilize the available soft tissues and may be irregular in shape. In general, anterior and posterior flaps are made, followed by transection of the muscle more proximally. The brachial artery and vein are isolated and doubly ligated prior to transection. Nerves (radial, ulnar, median, musculocutaneous) are isolated, put on traction and ligated. They are then transected and allowed to retract into the soft tissues to avoid a symptomatic neuroma. Enough muscle should be left to cover the distal end of the bone. The muscle should be sutured to the bone and antagonist muscle groups should be sutured to each other. Skin closure should be done with interrupted sutures. A rigid dressing is placed over the residual limb to reduce swelling. Postoperatively, the patient should begin activities of daily living training. For patients with brachial plexopathies, no advantage has been found in performing a shoulder arthrodesis to stabilize the limb in addition to the amputation. Additional length may be obtained by reflecting a portion of the pectoralis muscle (71). Patients should be fitted with a temporary or practice prosthesis to obtain the best function (63). Functional results in seven patients with transhumeral amputation and subsequent early limb replantation have found that only two of seven had regained useful hand function. The authors felt that tranhumeral replantation may be useful in preserving the elbow with the patient becoming a transradial amputee rather than a transhumeral amputee. The patients in this study all had a discrete transhumeral transection and the distal limb was available for replantation (72). Unfortunately, war wounds are so destructive that they seldom allow for this procedure.

Transradial Amputation. Transradial amputation is most often the direct result of trauma (63). Because function of the transra-

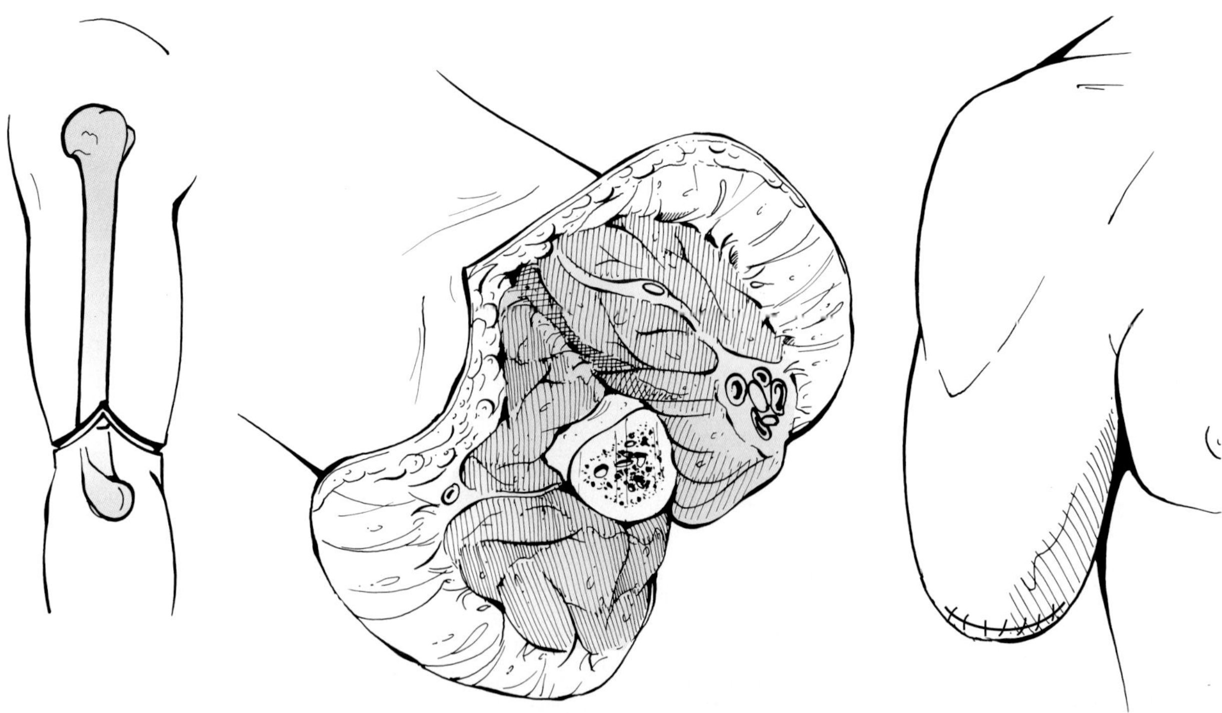

FIGURE 15-15 Transhumeral amputation.

dial amputee is better than that of a transhumeral amputee, every effort should be made to preserve the elbow joint.

A formal transradial amputation is done by creating flaps at the lowest viable level of soft tissue. Because of injury, irregular flaps may be used for soft tissue coverage. The major nerves should be isolated (median, ulnar, radial, lateral antebrachial cutaneous), put under tension, ligated, and then transected and allowed to retract. Major vessels (radial, ulnar) should be isolated and ligated. Muscle groups are then trimmed to provide coverage over the distal bone ends. Myodesis or myoplasty is done to provide muscle coverage over the bone ends and stability (65,73). The skin is then closed with interrupted sutures. A rigid dressing is applied to reduce swelling. A patient should be fitted with a preparatory prosthesis and rehabilitation begun as soon as possible.

Limb length may be added through the use of an Ilizarov fixator (74). Limited data for this procedure exists, making careful application advisable for those using this procedure. Partial thickness skin grafts can be used to cover muscle. A problem with partial thickness skin grafts however is that they are less durable than sensate, full thickness skin. One report lists a reoperation rate of 29% when using them (75).

Krukenberg Amputation. A Krukenberg procedure converts the forearm bones into active, sensate pinchers (76). This procedure is useful for a patient who is blind and has bilateral upper extremity amputations, or has a severe contralateral hand injury. It is also useful in developing nations where prosthetic fitting is limited or not available.

Wrist Disarticulation. A wrist disarticulation is a procedure which may be indicated for a nonsalvageable hand injury. The disadvantage to this procedure is that it provides limited space for the terminal device of the artificial limb and use of a myoelectric prosthesis may be limited by the available space. Advantages are that it preserves forearm rotation and provides an improved area for prosthesis suspension (63,73,77).

The skin flaps created will depend on the extent of injury. Enough skin should be available to form a well contoured residual limb. Myodesis is done to stabilize muscles and provide for function. The triangular fibrocartilage complex must be preserved to allow for stable pronation and supination. Care should be taken to identify the superficial branch of the radial nerve, the dorsal sensory branch of the ulnar nerve, and possibly the medial and lateral antebrachial cutaneous nerves. These should be pulled distally and transected, and allowed to retract away from any bone prominence (77). As with other upper extremity amputees, prosthetic fitting and training should begin as soon as possible. Wright et al found that 8 of 14 patients with a wrist disarticulation were successfully fitted with a prosthesis (67).

Digital Amputation. Amputations of the digits are one of the most common injuries seen in war or peace (77,78). Wartime injuries, as a result of an explosive device, are often not isolated and may include injuries to other parts of the hand and other body regions. Initial surgical procedure(s) should include removal of dead material or foreign debris, leaving wounds open, and performing reconstructive procedures in a stable environment. Microvascular replantation is presently not possible at austere hospitals in strife torn regions due to logistical and personnel constraints (77).

With regard to thumb injuries, all efforts should be made to salvage the digit if at all possible rather than to amputate it, because of its importance with hand function for pinch, grip, and opposition. There are a wide variety of reconstructive procedures, including pollicization and microvascular reconstruction which may be done later in a stable environment. A patient who sustains the loss of a major portion of the thumb should be referred to a center which can perform these procedures as soon as possible (78).

Decisions to salvage the lesser digits are based on the severity of the injury. Injuries proximal to the fingertip at the level of the distal interphalangeal joint should be evaluated in the operating room. At the time of closure, flexor and extensor tendons should be inspected for cleanliness but not sutured together. Digital nerves should be moved away from the suture line to prevent symptomatic neuromas. Closure then should be done to provide the best function (78).

If the amputation is proximal to the insertion of the flexor digitorum sublimus around the level of the proximal interphalangeal joint, there is limited flexion of the digit secondary to the action of the lumbricals working through the extensor tendon. At this level, initial care should be limited to the creation of flaps from locally available tissue. Consideration should also be given to a ray resection. For a severe finger injury, amputation at the metacarpalphalangeal joint versus a ray amputation remains controversial. Better cosmesis is provided by the ray amputation. However, grip strength is decreased when a ray resection is done (78–81).

Fingertip amputations are the most common amputation seen in civilian life. They are common in military life due to training accidents and crush injuries, especially due to heavy hatches on armored vehicles. Treatment is determined by the extent of the initial injury. Soft tissue injuries not involving the nailbed or having exposed bone may be treated with local wound care, particularly in an austere environment. With exposed bone, there are a variety of flaps which may be constructed to cover the digit after bone shortening. Alternatively, rongeuring the bone back until no bone remains exposed is a good option for those taking initial care of patients in a battlefield environment. Cold intolerance and hypersensitivity is reported in 30% to 50% of these patients (82,83).

Lower Extremity Amputations

Hip Disarticulation. A hip disarticulation is a relatively rare procedure (84–89). It is indicated for very proximal (hip) wounds, infection, or uncontrollable hemorrhage. Skin flaps may be made to accommodate the injured tissue. For this procedure, the patient is placed supine on the operating table and a wide preparation is used (85). The surgical field should encompass the back and the anterior surface of the lower abdomen. The field should also extend from midline to midline.

Two main techniques are described: an anterior and posterior flap technique. The posterior flap is performed by making an incision from just medial to the anterior, superior iliac spine distally just anterior to the greater trochanter and posteriorly just distal to the gluteal crease. The second arm of the incision goes from the starting point medially to the pubic tubercle and then posteriorly to the ischial tuberosity and the gluteal crease.

The femoral vessels are isolated, doubly ligated, and then transected. The femoral nerve is also isolated, placed under tension, ligated, then cut and allowed to retract.

The sartorius muscle is then removed from its origin at the anterior superior iliac spine, and followed by transection of the iliopsoas tendon as it insertion. The pectineus muscle and the adductors and gracilis muscle are incised along their origin. The obturator vessels are now exposed. Care is taken not to disrupt the vessels during the dissection to prevent injury and retraction of the vessels within the pelvis.

After abducting the limb, the semimembranosus, semitendinosus and biceps femoris are incised from the ischium. The anterior hip joint capsule is incised and the ligamentum teres is transected.

The patient is then rotated into the lateral position. The skin incision is completed, and the posterior/lateral aspect of the hip is exposed. Incise through the fascia lata and release the abductors close to the trochantes. The gluteus is released from its origin, then the short external rotators (gemelli, pyriformis, and quadratus) are incised as close to the insertion as possible. The sciatic nerve is then isolated, ligated, and cut. It is allowed to retract behind the pyriformis.

Closure is performed by suturing the gemelli and the gluteus medius together, covering the acetabulum. The quadratus femoris and iliopsoas are then approximated. The long posterior medial flap with the gluteus is then brought forward. The gluteal fascia is approximated to the inguinal ligament and the pubic tubercle, completing the muscle closure. Skin closure is then accomplished with interrupted sutures. Care should be taken to provide an even distribution of the excess tissue often seen with the gluteal flap. Drains should be used to prevent hematoma collection, and a bulky dressing should be applied with an elastic spica wrap for the first few days.

A similar technique, using an anterior "racquet"-shaped incision was described by Boyd. This differs in that the posterior gluteal flap is brought forward and sutured to the pectineus and adductor muscle origins (88).

A temporary prosthesis should be fitted as soon as the patient's condition permits and when the patient is ready to participate in physical therapy (89). Once the swelling has subsided, the patient may be considered for prosthetic fitting. Unlike other lower extremity amputations, a period of several months to allow the limb size to stabilize is not necessary.

Transfemoral Amputation. Transfemoral amputations are the second most common major amputation seen in war or peace.

A recent review of battle casualties undergoing this level of amputation found that 29 of 46 (63%) were wounded by land mine injuries, 8 (17.4%) by bullet, 5 (10.9%) by fragments from rocket, grenade mortar, or artillery, and 3 (6.5%) were injured by rocket propelled grenades. Indications for surgery in this study were trauma for 33 of 46 (71.7%), failed vascular repair in 12 of 46 (26.1%), and infection in one patient (90).

For a formal procedure, the patient is placed supine on the operating table (91,92). The surgical prep and drape is done to the hip area and a sterile tourniquet is kept available. With a formal procedure, skin flaps are created for closure of the residual limb. Generally the flaps are anterior and posterior, although because of the injury, the flaps may be medial or lateral or irregular in shape. The muscles are incised more proximally than the skin flaps to allow for myodesis. The bone is transected at the most proximal level, but as much bone length as possible should be preserved to facilitate prosthetic fitting. The major named vessels (femoral profundus and superficial femoral artery) are doubly ligated and then transected. The sciatic nerve is pulled down, ligated, cut, and then allowed to retract to avoid creating a neuroma near the end of the residual limb. Closure is best performed with a myodesis, attaching the adductors to the femur and then the quadriceps to the hamstring muscles. Skin closure is best accomplished by use of interrupted sutures.

Postoperatively, the patient should be placed in a prepatory prosthesis and begin to ambulate with the help of physical therapy when his or her physical condition permits. The final prosthetic fitting should be done when the patient has a stable limb (93,94).

Transtibial Amputation. The transtibial amputation is indicated whenever there is enough soft tissue to cover the residual limb. This is the most common major level of amputation seen in war or peace (14–23,26,28–30,38,39,95). The most common cause of wartime transtibial amputation is a land mine or booby trap. At the site of definitive care, the patient may begin physical therapy and be fitted for a pylon, even with open wounds, until the limb is stable (30,95).

Once the patient is stable and the wounds are clean, a formal transtibial amputation is done. A number of flaps for closure have been described: medial and lateral, anterior and posterior, and long posterior (96,97). A recent Cochrane Review was unable to find superiority of one technique over another (98). Patients with war injuries may have irregular wounds and therefore the flaps used in closure may be irregular in shape. Once the shapes of the flaps have been decided upon, the muscle may be incised to provide for a myodesis. Five nerves (saphenous, tibial, superficial and deep peroneal, and sural) should be identified, isolated, and transected. The three vessels of the leg (tibial, superficial, and deep peroneal) should also be isolated and ligated before their transection. The tibia is transected at the most distal level that still allows for soft tissue coverage. The distal anterior surface is beveled to prevent wear and breakdown of the residual limb in the prosthesis. The fibula is transected 1 to 2 cm proximal to the distal end of the tibia. Myodesis is done to attach the muscle to the tibia through drill holes, with myoplasty to attach the antagonist muscles together to cover the distal end of the tibia. The skin is then closed with interrupted sutures (Figs. 15-16 and 15-17).

Postoperatively, the patient should be placed in a long leg cast with a supracondylar mold and fitted with a pylon and a prosthetic foot. In young, post-traumatic patients, weightbearing may be advanced as tolerated (30,95,97,99).

With those injured in war, the amputation may involve traumatized tissue. The residual limb may be scarred or have retained fragments from the injury itself. Partial thickness skin grafts can be used to cover exposed soft tissue, but they are associated with ulcers and skin breakdown. Because these grafts have decreased sensation, a careful check of the skin should be done as the patient begins prosthetic fitting, and initial fitting with a pylon is usually delayed when skin grafting is used (97).

An Ertl osteomyoplastic amputation may also be performed whereby a bone bridge is created between the tibia and fibula (Fig. 15-18). This bridge is made by creating osteoperiosteal flaps from the tibia and fibula which are then connected, creating a tube which may then fill in and create a bone bridge. Proponents of this procedure feel that it provides a more durable residual limb which is more "end bearing." This technique was used successfully with war amputees from Vietnam at Valley Forge Army General Hospital (30,95,100,101).

Syme's Amputation. Syme's amputations are done for battle casualties with severe foot trauma. The amputation is an ankle disarticulation with preservation of the heel pad (Fig. 15-19). The residual limb is long enough to allow for limited ambulation of a patient without a prosthesis (102–105). Like other amputations, it is two staged. The patient should have forefoot debridement as the initial procedure, leaving the hindfoot intact. LaNoue found that with Vietnam War casualties nearly 90% of those patients who had Syme's amputation prior to evacuation had to be revised (28).

The limb should be prepped and draped to mid calf, and a tourniquet should be applied for surgery (Fig. 15-20). The skin incision is just anterior to the malleoli, going just anterior to the ankle joint on the dorsal side and plantarward as a distal extension of the medial and lateral sides. After the incision is made, the foot is plantarflexed, allowing for more exposure posteriorly. The Achilles tendon is incised from the calcaneus and the soft tissues are sharply removed from the calcaneus and talus, leaving the heel pad on the distal residual limb. The malleoli are then removed, along with the tibial articular surface. The heel flap is then brought forward and sutured to the distal tibia and fibula. To limit dead space and hematoma, a short leg walking cast should be applied and the patient's ambulation training begun if other injuries permit (101–106). When the swelling subsides, the patient may be fitted with a permanent prosthesis.

Partial Foot Amputations. There are several partial foot amputations described for trauma patients (107–109). General indi-

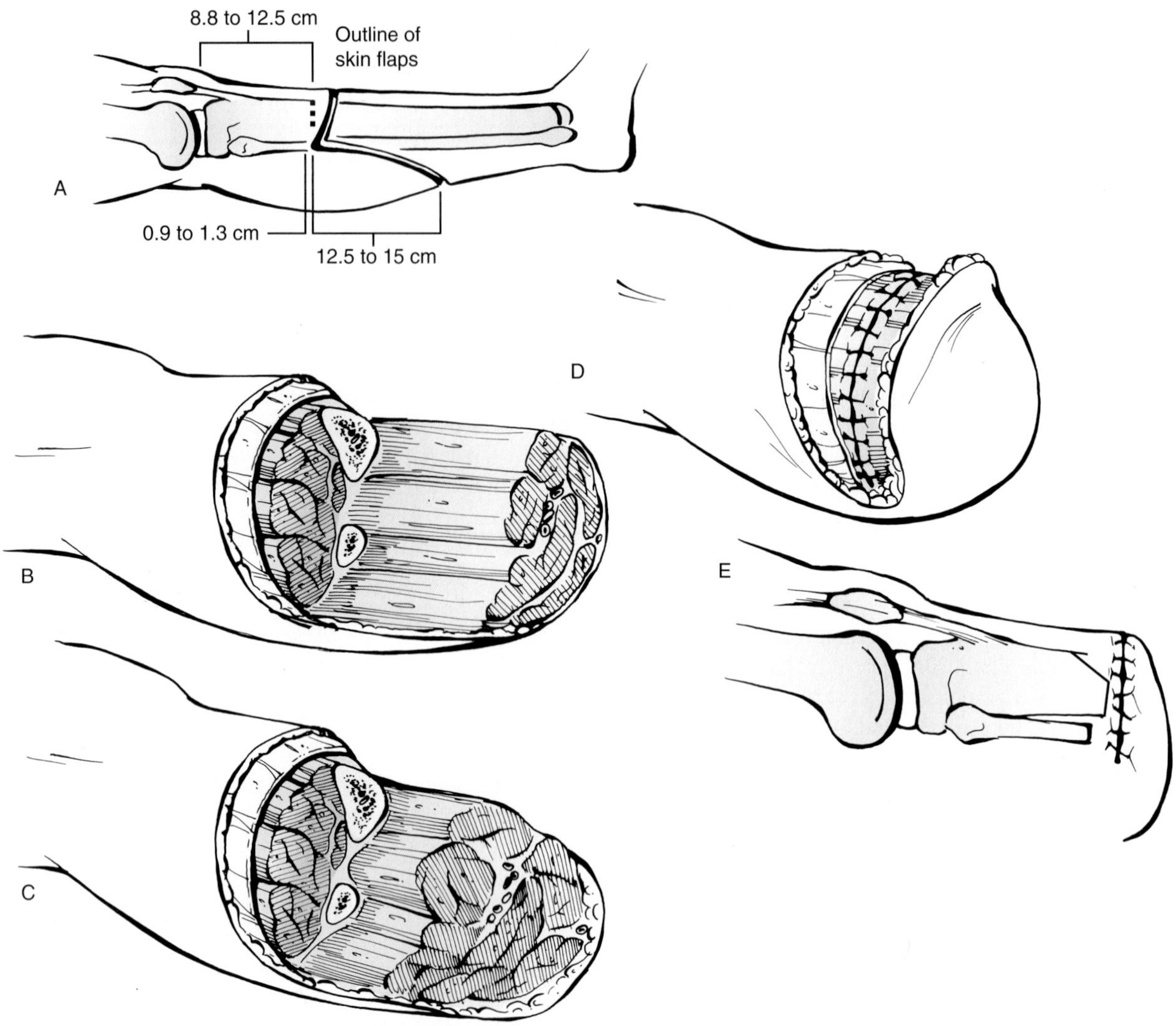

FIGURE 15-16 Transtibial amputation.

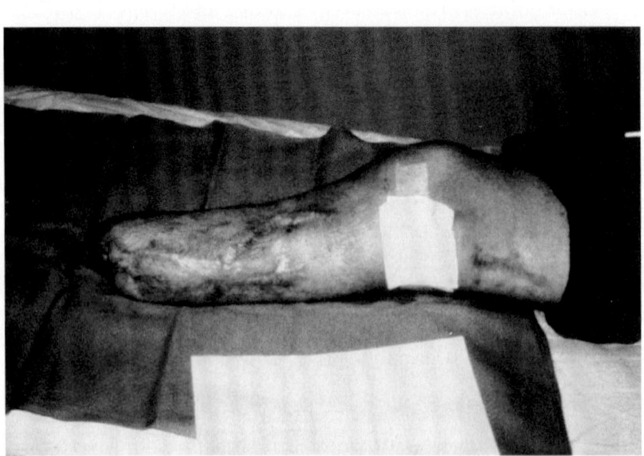

FIGURE 15-17 Closure of traumatic wounds may require irregular flaps.

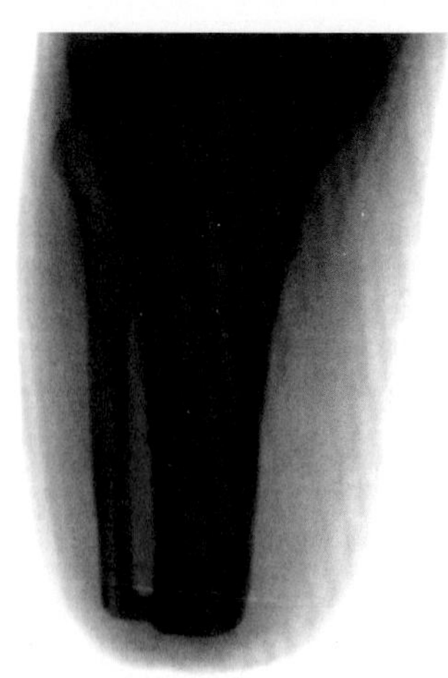

FIGURE 15-18 Ertl osteoperiosteal amputation.

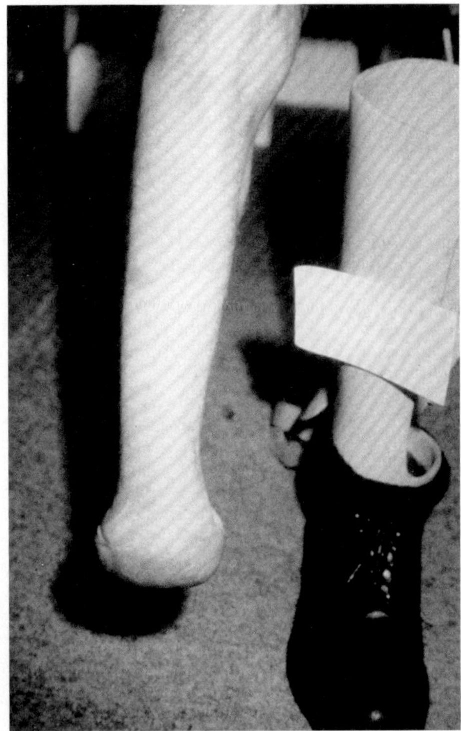

FIGURE 15-19 Symes amputee.

cations include trauma to a limited area of the foot without adequate soft tissue coverage or completion of a partial/complete traumatic amputation. Transmetatarsal amputations may be performed if adequate soft tissue coverage is available, otherwise a more proximal amputation should be performed. A Chopart amputation is at the level of the talonavicular and calcaneocuboid joints, whereas a Lisfranc amputation is through the tarsometatarsal joints. Because an equinus deformity may develop with these amputations, leading to an increase in the distal plantar pressure, their use in trauma patients is limited. This complication may be prevented by transfer of the peroneus brevis tendon to the cuboid and the extensor tendons to the neck of the talus. For late deformity, an Achilles lengthening may be performed. A prosthetic device is required to allow the patient to wear standard shoes. Millstein et al (108) reported good results of patients with partial foot amputations. Worse results were found with those who had skin grafts, those who had a fracture within the residual limb, and those who had more operations. Interestingly, better results were not automatically found with those who had more residual foot length.

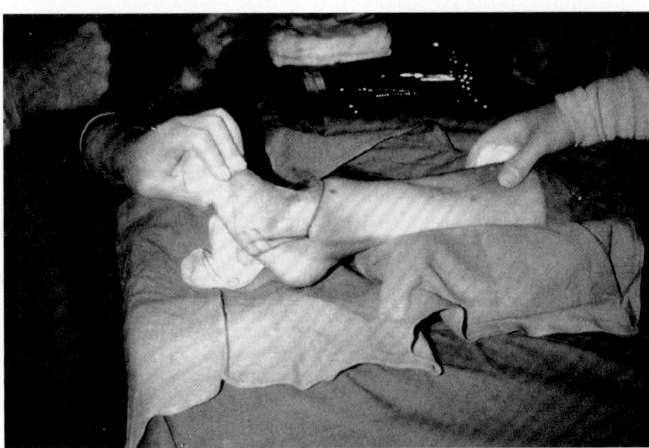

FIGURE 15-20 Symes skin incision.

Postoperative Considerations

Mortality

The overall mortality for those sustaining a traumatic amputation is high. Kellog Speed, later the author of a standard orthopaedic fracture textbook, found that 35 of 121 (29%) major (those proximal to the wrist or ankle) amputees died after admission to his Base Hospital in France in 1918 (110).

Amputee information from the WDMET database of the Vietnam War includes not only those who died in the hospital (died of wounds) but also those who died prior to hospitalization (killed in action). Of 98 major amputees, 35 died before reaching medical care and a further 3 died of wounds after hospitalization. The most common cause of death for this group was hemorrhage. Preventing blood loss of a wounded patient on the battlefield is currently a research interest of the US Army Medical Department (111).

Infection

War wounds are contaminated at the time of injury (112–116). With traumatic amputations, debris is often driven up along fascial planes more proximally, leaving compromised tissue covered with debris. Subsequent colonization, plus the injury itself, places all war wounds at risk for infection. Closure of the residual limb prior to air evacuation has been associated with a high rate of failure. As stated previously, LaNoue (28) found a 52% infection rate with transtibial amputations that were closed prior to evacuation. None of the patients who had their residual limb left open had this complication in his series. Simper (19) found a 13% failure rate of the residual limb in the short term for patients who had a delayed primary closure.

Analysis of data from Israeli battle casualties from the 1973 Yom Kipper War and the 1982 war in Lebanon has shown that the presence of an amputation itself is a high risk for wound infection. Other factors increasing the risk of infection include: multiple operations, polytrauma (injury to other body systems), and open drains (112,113).

Prevention of this complication is dependent upon a number of variables. Patient factors, such as nutritional status and other medical factors may place a patient at risk for having infection or poor wound healing. While this is not usually a problem for healthy soldiers, it is a problem when treating nonmilitary personnel in strife torn regions of the world. Their nutritional status is often poor and the patients may have untreated medical problems. Traumatic amputations are large open wounds that are grossly contaminated. There is an area of compromised tissue in the zone of injury which may or may not survive. This compromised tissue is particularly susceptible to infection. The patient may have other wounds that make the risk of infection higher (19–21,112–116).

Finally, there is the infecting organism itself. Battle wounds are polymicrobial in nature and contain pathogenetic bacteria within hours after wounding. Prevention of wound infection is helped by prompt surgical treatment of the wound—removing the debris, dead tissue, and contaminating organisms (111–116).

Pain

Pain in both the immediate postoperative period and long term is relatively common among amputees (117–121). It is ideal to have pain management services as part of the team caring for amputees to provide treatment in both the immediate postoperative period and for the longer term. In the immediate postoperative period, pain from the incision itself may be complicated by phantom limb pain when the patient has a perception of painful sensation from the missing limb and adequate postoperative pain relief is essential (117–121).

Chronic pain is common in amputees and may contribute to lifestyle limitations with regards to employment or other activities. Phantom limb pain has been reported in 63% to 90% of amputees (119–121).

Residual limb pain may be associated with a neuroma, as described below, or may be due to other reasons such as poor prosthetic fitting, adjacent joint pain, reflex sympathetic dystrophy, or the pain may be referred from another area (119–121). Smith et al (119) reported that there was about a 70% incidence of moderate to severe pain of the residual limb and/or low back. This report also found that low back pain, especially among transfemoral amputees, was more frequent and intense than the residual limb pain.

Nonpainful phantom sensations occur when there is a perception of the amputated limb being present. These may be unpleasant but not necessarily painful sensations. This phenomena has not been as well studied as painful phantom sensations. The incidence of nonpainful phantom sensations was reported to be 80% in one study, and was considered to be moderately or severely bothersome in about 35% of those patients (119–121).

A transected nerve forms a neuroma. It is essential to ensure that the end of the transected nerve is not in an area which is exposed to prosthetic wear. When surgery is done, a nerve should be pulled distally, transected, and then allowed to retract to an area protected by soft tissue. The diagnosis of a symptomatic neuroma may be made when a patient has a localized point of pain, a positive Tinel sign, and the presence of a nodule. If modification of the socket does not bring relief, then excision of the neuroma should be considered (117–121).

Psychological support services should be available at the site of definitive care for all amputees. Between 21% and 52.2% of Vietnam transfemoral and transtibial amputees report the use of psychological support services (90,95). During the initial year after the amputation, clinical depression or post-traumatic stress disorder are the most common diagnoses among military amputees (122,123).

Multiple Amputations

Patients with multiple amputations provide one of the greatest challenges to the amputee care team (124–126). During the Vietnam War, this group comprised 12.8% to 16% of amputees seen at hospitals which had large amputee populations (30,124). In general, the patients require a greater amount of gait training or training for activities of daily living. The care for patients needs to be more individualized than for the patient having a single amputation, and coordination between therapists, physicians, nurses, and prosthetists is paramount.

During the first year postamputation the residual limb may change often in both volume and shape. It is important to follow the patient as volume changes occur and ensure that the prosthesis is changed as well. There may be a need during this period to have frequent temporary socket changes to allow the patient to progress with activities as the shape of the residual limb changes. Often a young amputee will want to be fitted with the permanent prosthesis as soon as possible, even before they have fully healed and have a stable limb. It is important to fit a patient with a permanent prosthesis only when they are ready and the limb is stable. For lower extremity amputees such as at the transtibial or transfemoral level, this is usually between 9 and 18 months.

CONCLUSION

Future conflicts between nations may occur without warning and find US military surgeons treating battle casualties with little or no preparation. It is the goal of military surgeons to be prepared to treat battle casualties and minimize the morbidity and mortality under all circumstances. Preparedness for war not only involves the military surgeon's ability to treat battle casualties but also instructing others in their proper care.

Caring for battle casualties who have sustained amputations is a discontinuous process in military medicine. The documentation of the procedure and care of such casualties can hopefully help future generations of surgeons avoid repeating the mistakes of the past. It is my hope that this review can facilitate the relearning process that is forced on to all orthopedic surgeons who must care for combat casualties. Those who do not learn history are doomed to repeat its mistakes.

Certain principles for the initial management of wartime amputations merit additional emphasis. Initial amputations are performed to save life or limb, with the long-term prosthesis fitting and function as secondary goals. The amputation should be done at the lowest viable level of soft tissue. There are no ideal or standardized levels of amputation in a forward battle treatment facility. For patients who must be evacuated, all residual limbs should be left open, with skin traction applied to prevent skin retraction.

REFERENCES

1. Bellamy RF, Zajtchuk R. The weapons of conventional land warfare. In: Zajtchuk R, ed. *Conventional warfare: ballistic blast and burn injuries*. Washington, DC: Office of the Surgeon General, 1991:1–52.
2. Dougherty PJ, Hetz SP, Fackler ML. Weapons and weapons effects. In: Hetz SP, ed. *Emergency war surgery handbook*, 3rd American ed. Washington DC: Office of the Surgeon General, 2004.
3. Bellamy RF, Zajtchuk R. Assessing the effectiveness of conventional weapons. In: Zajtchuk R, ed. *Conventional warfare: ballistic blast and burn injuries*. Washington, DC: Office of the Surgeon General, 1991:53–82.
4. Bellamy RF. Combat trauma overview. In: *Anesthesia and perioperative care of the combat casualty*. Washington, DC: Office of the Surgeon General, 1995:1–42.
5. Love AG. *The Medical Department of the United States in the World War, Volume XV, Statistics*. Washington, DC: Office of the Surgeon General, 1925:1019.
6. Oughterson AW, Hull HC, Sutherland FA, et al. Study on wound ballistics—Bougainville Campaign. In: Beyer JC, ed. *Wound ballistics*. Washington, DC: Office of the Surgeon General, Department of the Army, 1962:281–436.
7. Fackler ML. Wound ballistics—a review of common misconceptions. *JAMA* 1988;259: 2730–2736.
8. Fackler ML. Missile caused wounds. In: Bowen TF, Bellamy RF, eds. *Emergency war surgery*, 2nd American Revision. Washington, DC: Office of the Surgeon General, Department of the Army, 1988:13–34.
9. Beyer JC, Arima JK, Johnson DW. Enemy ordnance material. In: *Wound ballistics*. Beyer JC, ed. *Wound ballistics*. Washington, DC: Office of the Surgeon General, Department of the Army, 1962:1–90.
10. Necchaev EA, Gritsanov AI, Fomin NF, et al. *Mine blast trauma* (*Experience from the war in Afghanistan*). Stockholm, Sweden: Falths Tryckeri, 1995. Khlunovskaya GP, translator.
11. Dougherty PJ. Armored vehicle crew casualties. *Mil Med* 1990;155:417–420.
12. Herget CM, Coe GB, Beyer JC. Wound ballistics and body armor in Korea. In: Beyer JC, ed. *Wound ballistics*. Washington, DC: Office of the Surgeon General, Department of the Army, 1962:691–767.
13. Bowen TF, Bellamy RF, eds. General considerations of forward surgery. In: *Emergency war surgery*, 2nd American Revision. Washington, DC: Office of the Surgeon General, Department of the Army, 1988:1–9.
14. Aboutanos MB, Baker SP. Wartime civilian casualties: epidemiology and intervention strategies. *J Trauma* 1997;43(4):721–726.
15. Wilbur MC, Willet LV, Buono F. Combat amputees. *Clin Orthop Rel Res* 1970;68: 10–13.
16. McKeever FM. A discussion of controversial points in amputation surgery. *Surg Gynecol Obstet* 1946;82(5):495–511.
17. Seligson D, Baily R. Traumatic amputations. *Clin Orthop* 1976;114:304–306.
18. Schmitt HJ, Armstrong RG. Wounds causing loss of limb. *Surg Gynecol Obstet* 1970; 130(4):682–684.
19. Simper LB. Below-knee amputation in war surgery: a review of 111 amputations with delayed primary closure. *J Trauma* 1993;34:96–98.
20. Korver AJH. Amputees in a hospital of the International Committee or the Red Cross. *Injury* 1993;24:607–609.
21. Korver AJH. Injuries of the lower limbs caused by antipersonnel mines: the experience of the International Committee of the Red Cross. *Injury* 1996;27:477–479.
22. Atesalp AS, Erler K, Gur E, et al. Below-knee amputations as a result of land-mine injuries: comparison of primary closure versus delayed primary closure. *J Trauma* 1999; 47:724–727.
23. Coupland RM. Amputations. In: *War wounds of limbs*. Geneva, Switzerland: Butterworth Heinemann, 1993:61–65.
24. Commander in Chief, Pacific (CINCPAC). *Conference on war surgery*. Tokyo, Japan, 1971:42–47.
25. Kirk NT, McKeever FM. The guillotine amputation. *JAMA* 1944;124(15):1027–1030.
26. Kirk NT. Amputations in war. *JAMA* 1942;120(1):13–16.
27. Kirk NT. *Amputations*. Chicago: WB Conkey, 1924.
28. LaNoue AM. *Care and disposition of amputee war casualties* [student paper]. Ft. Leavenworth, KS: US Army Command & General Staff, April 1971. [See also *Amputee war casualties: errors in initial management*. CME 183 Brooke AMC, 1973.]
29. Traverso LW, Johnson DE, Fleming A, et al. Combat casualties in northern Thailand: emphasis on land mine injuries and levels of amputation. *Mil Med* 1981;146:682–685.
30. Mayfield GW. Vietnam War amputees. In: Burkhalter WE, ed. *Surgery in Vietnam. Orthopedic surgery*. Washington, DC: Office of the Surgeon General and Center for Military History, 1994:131–153.
31. Brown PW. Rehabilitation of the combat-wounded amputee. In: Burkhalter WE, ed. *Surgery in Vietnam. Orthopedic surgery*. Washington, DC: Office of the Surgeon General and Center for Military History, 1994:189–209.
32. Wilson PD. Early weight-bearing in the treatment of amputations of the lower limbs. *J Bone Joint Surg* 1922;4(2):224–247.
33. Kessler HH. Definitive surgical management of amputations. *Naval Med Bull* 1945;44: 1133–1148.
34. Aston MJ. Rehabilitation at the US Naval Hospital, Philadelphia. *Naval Med Bull* 1946; March(Suppl):1–4.
35. Reister FA, ed. *Medical statistics in World War II*. Washington, DC: Office of the Surgeon General, Department of the Army, 1975:112–119.
36. Brackett EG, ed. Amputation service, AEF, care of the amputated in the United States. In: Ireland MW, ed. *The Medical Department of the United States in the World War, Volume XI, Surgery*. Washington, DC: United States Government Printing Office, 1927: 687–748.
37. Callender GR, Coupal JF. Pathology of gas gangrene following war wounds. In: Ireland MW, ed. *The Medical Department of the United States Army in the World War, Volume XII, Pathology of the acute respiratory diseases and of gas gangrene following war wounds*. Washington, DC: United States Government Printing Office, 1929:407–567.
38. Hampton OP, ed. *Orthopaedic surgery in the Mediterranean theater of operations. Surgery in World War II*. Washington, DC: Office of the Surgeon General, 1957:299–331.
39. Cleveland M, ed. Amputations. *Orthopaedic surgery in the European theater of operations*. Washington, DC: Office of the Surgeon General, 1956:155–166.
40. Hughes CW. Arterial repair during the Korean War. *Ann Surg* 1958;147:555–561.
41. Burkhalter WE. Penetrating wounds of the leg with associated fractures of the tibia. In: Burkhalter WE, ed. *Surgery in Vietnam. Orthopedic surgery*. Washington, DC: Office of the Surgeon General and Center of Military History, United States Army, U.S. Government Printing Office, 1994:39–53.
42. Reis ND, Shifrin LZ, Zinman C, et al. A philosophy of limb salvage in war: use of the fixateur externe. *Mil Med* 1991;156:505–520.
43. Gustilo RB, Anderson JT. Prevention of infection in the treatment of one thousand and twenty-five open fractures of long bones. *J Bone Joint Surg* 1976;58A:453–458.
44. Gustilo RB, Mendoza RM, Williams DN. Problems in the management of type III (severe) open fractures. A new classification of type III open fractures. *J Trauma* 1984; 24:742–746.
45. Brumback RJ, Jones AL. Interobserver agreement in the classification of open fractures of the tibia. *J Bone Joint Surg* 1994;76A:1162–1166.
46. Caudle RJ, Stern PJ. Severe open fractures of the tibia. *J Bone Joint Surg* 1987;69A: 801–807.
47. Georgiadis GM, Behrens FF, Joyce MJ, et al. Open tibial fractures with severe soft-tissue loss, limb salvage compared with below knee amputation. *J Bone Joint Surg* 1993; 75A:1431–1441.
48. Quirke TE, Sharma PK, Boss WK, et al. Are type IIIC lower extremity injuries an indication for primary amputation? *J Trauma* 1996;40:992–996.
49. Lerner RT, Esterhai JL, Polomano RC, et al. Quality of life assessment of patient with posttraumatic fracture nonunion, chronic refractory osteomyelitis, and lower-extremity amputation. *Clin Orthop Rel Res* 1993;295:28–36.
50. Gregory RT, Gould RJ, Peclet M, et al. The Mangled Extremity Syndrome (MES): a severity grading system for multisystem injury of the extremity. *J Trauma* 1985;25: 1147–1150.
51. Helfet DL, Howey T, Sanders R, et al. Limb salvage versus amputation: preliminary results of the Mangled Extremity Severity Score. *Clin Orthop Rel Res* 1990;256:80–86.
52. Howe HR, Pooled GV, Hansen KJ, et al. Salvage of lower extremities following combined orthopedic and vascular trauma. A predictive salvage index. *Am Surg* 1987;53: 205–208.
53. McNamara MG, Heckman JD, Corley EG. Severe open fracture of the lower extremity: a retrospective evaluation of the Mangled Extremity Severity Score (MESS). *J Orthop Trauma* 1994;8:81–87.
54. Russell WL, Sailors DM, Whittle TB, et al. Limb salvage versus traumatic amputation. A decision based on a seven-part predictive index. *Ann Surg* 1991;213:473–481.
55. Bonanni F, Rhodes M, Lucke JF. The futility of predictive scoring of mangled lower extremities. *J Trauma* 1993;34:99–104.
56. Durham RM, Mistry BM, Mazuski JE, et al. Outcome and utility of scoring systems in the management of the mangled extremity. *Am J Surg* 1996;172:569–574.
57. Lange RH. Limb reconstruction versus amputation decision making in massive lower extremity trauma. *Clin Orthop Rel Res* 1989;243:92–99.
58. Bosse MJ, MacKenzie EJ, Kellam JF, et al. A prospective evaluation of the clinical utility of the Lower-Extremity Injury Severity Scores. *J Bone Joint Surg* 2001;83A:3–14.
59. Bosse MJ, MacKenzie EJ, Kellam JF, et al. An analysis of outcomes of reconstruction or amputation after leg-threatening injuries. *N Engl J Med* 2002;347:1924–1931.
60. Swiontkowski MF, MacKenzie EJ, Bosse MJ, et al. Factors influencing the decision to amputate or reconstruct after high-energy lower extremity trauma. *J Trauma* 2002;52: 641–649.
61. Peterson LT. The army amputation program. *J Bone Joint Surg* 1944;26:635–638.
62. Pinzur MS, Angelats J, Light TR, et al. Functional outcome following traumatic upper limb amputation and prosthetic limb fitting. *J Hand Surg* 1994;19A:836–839.
63. Burkhalter WE, Mayfield G, Carmona LS. The upper-extremity amputee. *J Bone Joint Surg* 1976;58A:46–51.
64. Slocum DB. *An atlas of amputations*. St. Louis: Mosby Year Book, 1949.
65. Tooms RE. Amputations of the upper extremity. In: Crenshaw AH, ed. *Campbell's operative orthopaedics*, 8th ed. St. Louis: Mosby Year Book, 1992:711–721.
66. McAuliffe JA. Shoulder disarticulation and forequarter amputation. In: Bowker JH, Michael JW, eds. *Atlas in limb prosthetics: surgical, prosthetic, and rehabilitation principles*, 2nd ed. St. Louis: Mosby, 1992:265–275.
67. Wright TW, Hagen AD, Wood MB. Prosthetic usage in major upper extremity amputations. *J Hand Surg* 1995;20A:619–622.
68. McAuliffe JA. Elbow disarticulation and transhumeral amputation. In: Bowker JH, Michael JW, eds. *Atlas in limb prosthetics: surgical, prosthetic, and rehabilitation principles*, 2nd ed. St. Louis: Mosby, 1992:251–253.
69. Zelle BA, Pape HC, Gerich TG, et al. Functional outcome following scapulothoracic dissociation. *J Bone Joint Surg* 2004;86A:2–8.
70. Rorabeck CH. The management of flailed upper extremity in brachial plexus injuries. *J Trauma* 1980;20:49–53.
71. Mazet R. Partial reflection of the pectoralis major muscle. *J Bone Joint Surg* 1953;35A: 681–684.

72. Wood MB, Cooney WP. Above elbow limb replantation: functional results. *J Hand Surg* 1986;11A:682.
73. Ouellette EA. Wrist disarticulation and transradial amputation. In: Bowker JH, Michael JW, eds. *Atlas in limb prosthetics: surgical, prosthetic, and rehabilitation principles*, 2nd ed. St. Louis: Mosby, 1992:429–452.
74. Stricker SJ. Ilizarov lengthening of a posttraumatic below elbow amputation. A case report. *Clin Orthop Rel Res* 1994;306:124–127.
75. Wood MR, Hunter GA, Millstein SG. The value of stump split skin grafting following amputation for trauma in adult upper and lower amputees. *Prosthet Orthot Int* 1987; 11:71–74.
76. Garst RJ. The Krukenberg hand. *J Bone Joint Surg* 1991;73B:385–388.
77. Burkhalter WE, Butler B, Metz W, et al. Experience with delayed primary closure of war wounds of the hand in Viet Nam. *J Bone Joint Surg* 1968;58A:945–954.
78. Louis DS. Amputations. In: Green DP, ed. *Operative hand surgery*, Vol. 1, 2nd ed. New York: Churchill Livingston, 1988:61–119.
79. Peimer CA, Wheeler DR, Barrett A. Hand function following single ray amputation. *J Hand Surg Am* 1999;24:1245–1248.
80. Nuzumalali E, Orhun E, Ozturk K, et al. Results of ray resection and amputation for ring avulsion injury. *J Hand Surg Br* 2003;28:578–581.
81. Melikyan EY, Beg MS, Woodbridge S, et al. Functional results of ray resection. *J Hand Surg* 2003;85A:47–61.
82. Lee LP, Lau PY, Chan CW. A simple and efficient treatment for fingertip injuries. *J Hand Surg Br* 1995;20:63–71.
83. Martin C, Gonzalez del Pino J. Controversies in the treatment of fingertip amputations. Conservative versus surgical reconstruction. *Clin Orthop Rel Res* 1998;353:63–73.
84. Loon HE. The past and present medical significance of hip disarticulation. In: *Selected articles from artificial limbs*. Huntington, NY: RE Kreiger Publishing Company, 1970: 205–222.
85. Tooms RE, Hampton FL. Hip disarticulation and transpelvic amputation. In: Bowker JH, Michael JW, eds. *Atlas in limb prosthetics: surgical, prosthetic, and rehabilitation principles*, 2nd ed. St. Louis: Mosby, 1992:535–538.
86. Wakelin SJ, Oliver CW, Kaufman MH. Hip disarticulation: the evolution of a surgical technique. *Injury* 2004;35:299–308.
87. Lackman RD, Quartararo LG, Farrell ED, et al. Hip disarticulation using the lateral approach: a new technique. *Clin Orthop Rel Res* 2001;392:372–376.
88. Boyd HB. Anatomic disarticulation of the hip. *Surg Gynecol Obstet* 1947;84:346–348.
89. Burgess EM, Romano RL, Zettl JH. The hip disarticulation amputation. In: *The management of lower-extremity amputations*, TR 10-6. Washington, DC: US Government Printing Office, 1969:85–96.
90. Dougherty PJ. Long-term follow-up of unilateral transfemoral amputees from the Vietnam War. *J Trauma* 2003;54:718–723.
91. Gottschalk F. Transfemoral amputation. *Clin Orthop Rel Res* 1999;361:15–22.
92. Gottschalk F. Transfemoral amputation. In: Bowker JH, Michael JW, eds. *Atlas in limb prosthetics: surgical, prosthetic, and rehabilitation principles*, 2nd ed. St. Louis: Mosby, 1992:501–507.
93. Schuhs CM. Prosthetic management. In: Bowker JH, Michael JW, eds. *Atlas in limb prosthetics: surgical, prosthetic, and rehabilitation principles*, 2nd ed. St. Louis: Mosby, 1992:509–533.
94. Burgess EM, Romano RL, Zettl JH. Above knee and knee disarticulation amputations. In: *The management of lower-extremity amputations*, TR 10-6. Washington, DC: US Government Printing Office, 1969:40–73.
95. Dougherty PJ. Transtibial amputees from the Vietnam War. *J Bone Joint Surg* 2001; 83A:383–389.
96. Bowker JH, Goldberg B, Poonekar PD. Transtibial amputation. Surgical procedures and immediate postsurgical management. In: Bowker JH, Michael JW, eds. *Atlas in limb prosthetics: surgical, prosthetic, and rehabilitation principles*, 2nd ed. St. Louis: Mosby, 1992:429–452.
97. Smith DG, Fergason JR. Transtibial amputations. *Clin Orthop Rel Res* 1999;361: 108–115.
98. Tisi PV, Callam MJ. Type of incision for below knee amputation. *Cochrane Database Syst Rev* 2004, accessed April 19, 2005.
99. Burgess EM, Romano RL, Zettl JH. The below-knee amputation. In: *The management of lower-extremity amputations*, TR 10-6. Washington, DC: US Government Printing Office, 1969:13–39.
100. Ertl J. Operationstechik. Uber Amputationsresidual limbfe. *Chirurg* 1949;20:218–224.
101. Deffer PA, Moll JH, LaNoue AM. The Ertl osteoplastic below-knee amputation. (Proceedings) *J Bone Joint Surg* 1971;53A:1028.
102. Wagner FW. The Syme ankle disarticulation. In: Bowker JH, Michael JW, eds. *Atlas in limb prosthetics: surgical, prosthetic, and rehabilitation principles*, 2nd ed. St. Louis: Mosby, 1992:429–452.
103. Alldredge RH, Thompson TC. The technique of the Syme amputation. *J Bone Joint Surg* 1946;28:415–426.
104. Harris RI. Syme's amputation. *J Bone Joint Surg Br* 1956;38:614–632.
105. Pinzur MS. Restoration of walking ability with Syme's ankle disarticulation. *Clin Orthop Rel Res* 1999;361:71–75.
106. Burgess EM, Romano RL, Zettl JH. The Syme amputation. In: *The management of lower-extremity amputations*, TR 10-6. Washington, DC: US Government Printing Office, 1969:74–84.
107. Early JS. Transmetatarsal and midfoot amputations. *Clin Orthop Rel Res* 1999;361: 85–90.
108. Millstein SG, McCowan SA, Hunter GA. Traumatic partial foot amputations in adults. A long-term review. *J Bone Joint Surg Br* 1988;70:251–254.
109. Wagner FW. Partial-foot amputations. In: Bowker JH, Michael JW, eds. *Atlas in limb prosthetics: surgical, prosthetic, and rehabilitation principles*, 2nd ed. St. Louis: Mosby, 1992:389–401.
110. Speed K. Base hospital amputations in war. *JAMA* 1918;17:271–274.
111. Dougherty PJ. Wartime amputations. *Mil Med* 1993;158:755–763.
112. Simchen E, Sacks T. Infection in war wounds: experience during the 1973 October War in Israel. *Ann Surg* 1975;182:754–761.
113. Simchen E, Raz R, Stein H, et al. Risk factors for infection in fracture war wounds (1973 and 1982 wars, Israel). *Mil Med* 1991;156:520–527.
114. Lindberg RB, Wetzler TF, Marshall JD, et al. The bacterial flora of battle wounds at the time of primary debridement. *Ann Surg* 1955;141:369–374.
115. Heggers JP, Barnes ST, Robson MC, et al. Microbial flora of orthopaedic war wounds. *Mil Med* 1969;134:602–603.
116. MacLennan JD. Anaerobic infections in Tripolitania and Tunisia. *Lancet* 1944;246: 203–207.
117. Hoaglund FT, Jergesen HE, Wilson L, et al. Evaluation of problems and needs of veteran lower-limb amputees in the San Francisco Bay area during the period 1977–1980. *J Rehabil R D* 1983;20:57–71.
118. Smith DG, Horn P, Malchow D, et al. Prosthetic history, prosthetic charges and functional outcome of isolated, traumatic below-knee amputee. *J Trauma* 1995;38:44–47.
119. Smith DG, Ehde DM, Legro MW, et al. Phantom limb, residual limb and back pain after lower extremity amputations. *Clin Orthop Rel Res* 1999;361:29–38.
120. Sherman RA, Sherman CJ. A comparison of phantom sensations among amputees whose amputations were of civilian and military origins. *Pain* 1985;21:91–97.
121. Davis RW. Phantom sensation, phantom pain and residual limb pain. *Arch Phys Med Rehabil* 1993;74:79–91.
122. Fitzpatrick MC. The psychologic assessment and psychosocial recovery of the patient with an amputation. *Clin Orthop Rel Res* 1999;361:98–107.
123. Frank JL. The amputee war casualty in a military hospital: observations on psychological management. *Int J Psychiatry Med* 1973;4:1–16.
124. Brown FW. Rehabilitation of bilateral lower-extremity amputees. *J Bone Joint Surg* 1970; 52A:687–700.
125. Dougherty PJ. Long-term follow-up study of bilateral above the knee amputees from the Vietnam War. *J Bone Joint Surg* 1999;81A:1384–1390.
126. McKeever FM. A discussion of controversial points in amputation surgery. *Surg Gynecol Obstet* 1946;82:495–511.

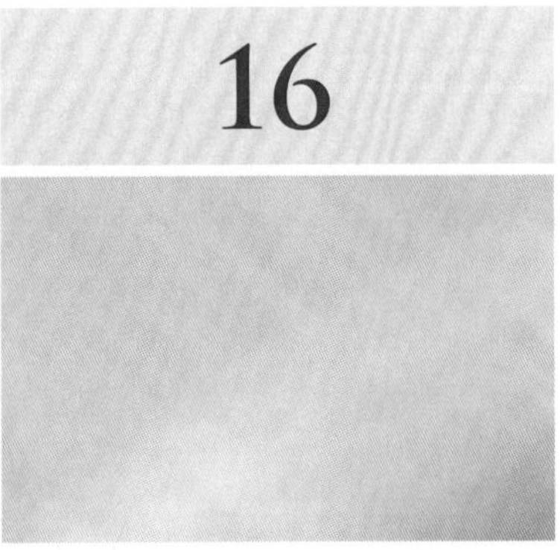

BONE AND SOFT TISSUE RECONSTRUCTION

Lior Heller and L. Scott Levin

Open fractures represent a therapeutic challenge to the orthopaedic surgeon. They are difficult to treat, and the cost of inadequate treatment is high both in financial terms and in continuing patient disability. The etiology of open fractures is varied, and the population affected is heterogeneous. Certain open long bone fractures tend to occur in different age-groups from different causes. Not unexpectedly, young adults tend to be injured in activities such as motorcycling and bicycling or while playing sports. Older patients may sustain fractures after a simple fall. In many cases, open long bone fractures tend to occur in patients who have either other musculoskeletal injuries or injuries to other body systems. This requires that surgeons treating open fractures have adequate training and resources to treat coexisting injuries (1).

HISTORY

The evolution of extremity trauma surgery reflects the development of surgery as a specialty. The management of major extremity trauma has evolved through major stages that include high-level amputations, regional amputation to conserve limb length, wound debridement, vascular repair, flap reconstruction, replantation, and the current concept of acute reconstruction to save limb and preserve function. The problem of open fractures has plagued surgeons since the time of Hippocrates. Drawings from his original writings show crude attempts at external fixation for the purpose of examining and treating wounds (2). Incomplete documents from the ancient Egyptian period reported that comminuted fractures were treated expectantly. Compound fractures were considered a fatal injury because amputation was not a part of the surgical arsenal (3). In the 16th century, Ambroise Pare, considered one of the founding fathers of orthopaedics, warned against the potentially life-threatening condition of gangrene resulting from open fractures, revolutionized amputation surgery by use of the tourniquet, and introduced the development of the hemostatic clamp and vascular ligatures (4). Fortunately, surgical development and refinement has kept pace with people's destructive capacity.

Parallel with the mechanism of limb destruction that has changed during modern wars has been the development of new techniques and concepts for limb salvage such as debridement, vascular reconstruction, soft tissue reconstruction, and the use of microsurgical techniques. Although not all of the problems that confronted trauma surgeons in the past are completely solved, modern methods of open fracture management, skeletal fixation, and soft tissue and bone reconstruction have dramatically improved the potential for limb salvage.

Important advances have taken place in the field of plastic surgery, including the introduction of local flaps and free flaps as efficient methods of closing large post-traumatic soft tissue defects. A better understanding of the anatomy and physiology of free flaps with resultant high rates of success for these autologous tissue transfers and the introduction of distally based fasciocutaneous flaps have improved the surgeon's capability to close almost any soft tissue defects resulting from open fractures (5).

Orthopaedic training and practice has traditionally been dedicated to the care of bone and joint injuries. With the evolution of open methods for fracture fixation and the increasing incidence of high-energy trauma, the need for concomitant soft tissue management in the treatment of open fractures has come to the attention of the orthopaedic traumatologist. The orthopaedic surgeon treating patients with traumatic conditions can no longer isolate care to the diaphysis of long bones or the reconstitution of articular surfaces. Although these goals are vital to the success of overall treatment, the orthopaedist must define a treatment plan for the soft tissues. This treatment plan can be carried out in conjunction with a reconstructive plastic surgeon or by the orthopaedic surgeon alone. The combination of soft tissue management and bone reconstruction permits optimal repair processes to take place in both bone and soft tissue, avoiding the adverse sequelae of failed implants, failed fixation, sepsis, and, ultimately, amputation.

COMPLEX MUSCULOSKELETAL INJURIES

Complex open fractures require effective coordinated care for both bone and soft tissue to achieve successful healing while avoiding infection, but a variety of factors makes this difficult. These factors include compromised vascular supply at the fracture site, marginal soft tissue coverage, and wound contamination. Initial treatment of fractures has improved significantly with the development of antibiotic therapy and aseptic surgical procedures in conjunction with improved stabilization techniques, leading to a significant reduction in the fracture infection rate.

The essential elements of osseous healing of opposed fracture fragments are blood supply and stabilization. Blood supply to bone is derived from nutrient vessels to the long bones, as well as surrounding muscle and fascia. Compromise of a bone's soft tissue envelope or nutrient vasculature places that bone at risk of delayed union, nonunion, or the inability to fight infection if colonized with bacteria following injury.

The role of the soft tissue in fracture healing is not completely elucidated. Different studies suggest that the muscles contiguous to the fracture wound are the immediate source of the blood supply to the fracture (6). Slow healing of certain displaced fractures has been attributed to a paucity of surrounding muscle tissue. Holden (7) tested this concept experimentally and successfully demonstrated the importance of the surrounding muscle in contributing vascular ingrowth to the injured bony cortex. He further showed that when the soft tissue envelope to the muscle was rendered ischemic, revascularization occurred initially in the muscle and secondarily in the skin. The intramedullary circulation did not reconstitute until overlying soft tissue had been revascularized.

OPEN FRACTURES

Historically, treatment of an open fracture in which soft tissue injuries have been neglected, ignored, or mistreated has resulted in therapeutic disasters. It was argued that open reduction with internal fixation of closed or opened fractures did not work. Arguments against internal fixation were that it led to infection, compromised bone healing, and resulted in nonunion.

Two basic principles of the *Arbeitgemeinschaft für Osteosynthesesfragen* (AO) group, established almost 4 decades ago, discuss soft tissue (8). In addition to anatomic reduction and stable internal fixation, careful attention to soft tissue handling, as well as functional rehabilitation of the injured limb, are vital to fracture management. Functional rehabilitation involves the restoration of muscular power and normal biomechanics.

The importance of soft tissue has only recently begun to be recognized. New techniques such as indirect reduction and biologic plating with implants that respect biology and avoid compromising periosteum around bone are being used. Compatible implants such as the limited-contact dynamic compression plate (LC-DCP), point contact plate (PCP), and locking plates with improved metallurgy have been designed to avoid damage to soft tissue created by overvigorous dissection and stripping of the soft tissue envelope (9).

The surrounding soft tissue has been recognized as the vascular envelope nurturing bone back to health, and the importance of its reconstruction early in the post-traumatic course cannot be overemphasized; nor can the importance of anatomy, internervous planes, vascular territories, and atraumatic techniques of dissection (10,11). Rather than relying on brute strength and dissection techniques that result in devascularization of both bone and soft tissue, a keener awareness of delicate soft tissue handling and atraumatic technique by the orthopaedist contributes to the prevention of adverse iatrogenic sequelae following injury. Proper handling of soft tissue includes the use of tools such as skin hooks that permit manipulation of skin and tissue flaps without damage to the soft tissues (Fig. 16-1).

To reconstruct the soft tissue envelope, the surgeon must define what layers are deficient and the size of the deficiency. Subsequently, the surgeon must outline a treatment plan that simultaneously treats bone and soft tissue synergistically.

The soft tissue envelope is composed of several layers, each with a specific function and its own vascular supply. Skin, which consists of epidermis and dermis, is the first soft tissue layer violated in the open fracture, and its disruption defines the open fracture.

The skin has unique properties that enable it to be harvested as a graft. By removing epidermis and partial dermis, a split-thickness skin graft (STSG) can be fabricated; when correctly harvested and applied, this graft can convert an open wound to a closed wound as the graft inosculates and epithelializes. (Inosculation is the process of capillary sprouting that occurs to revascularize a graft such as a skin graft.) These processes reconstitute the outermost layer of the soft tissue envelope. A

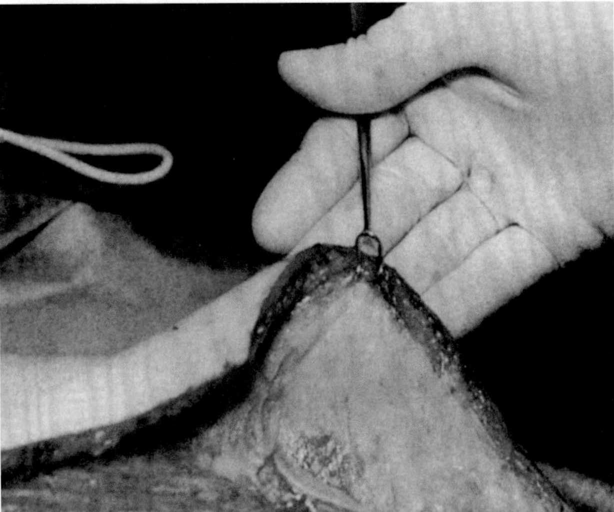

FIGURE 16-1 The skin hook is held between the thumb and index finger and is pulled upward to provide both exposure and traction. The remaining fingers are placed behind the skin to act as a guide to the level of dissection.

skin graft is one of the most basic choices in the reconstructive ladder. The creation of a "sealed" wound defines wound closure, the ultimate goal in soft tissue reconstruction. Wound closure and reconstitution of the epidermal surface may or may not provide long-term stable coverage; however, this is the initial goal when treating open wounds.

The next soft tissue layer, the subcutaneous tissue, is less vascular than the dermal plexus, yet it is important in that it provides a cushion around bony prominences and may be quite specialized, for example, on the plantar surface of the foot.

Fascia is the next deepest layer and surrounds muscle compartments. It contains a rich vascular plexus that can function as the basis for supporting tissue such as skin flaps, which can be transposed or transferred over adjacent, distant, or proximal soft tissue defects.

Muscles are richly vascularized structures that power the locomotor system. They have one of five types of blood supply as outlined by Mathes and Nahai (12) that, in the last 3 decades, have allowed several rungs to be added to the reconstructive ladder. Muscles can be manipulated as transposition flaps, island pedicle flaps, and free-tissue transplantations, so-called free flaps. These microvascular transplants require technically demanding anastomoses of nutrient arteries and veins, as well as the possibility for coaptation of nerves for innervated transfers. Such functional muscle transfers represent the highest rung of the reconstructive ladder and are reserved for specialized situations. Depending on the location and size of soft tissue defects, different muscles may be selected. They can be transplanted with overlying skin if necessary.

The deepest layer of the soft tissue envelope is a richly vascularized layer referred to as the periosteum. This surrounds all long bones and is vital to the response of bone to injury and repair. Recent advances in anatomic dissection and free-tissue transplantation have resulted in use of the periosteum as a free flap to augment conventional methods of bone grafting.

All of the layers of soft tissue just described, including the periosteum, will accept a STSG. Despite contour irregularity, if these layers are healthy and well vascularized, a skin graft can be applied to seal the open wound. This is the first goal in wound management, that is, to reconstitute the epithelial surface of the extremity.

A logical method of reconstruction of the soft tissues must be developed to allow bone to heal and limbs to function normally. The algorithm should be capable of being used by the

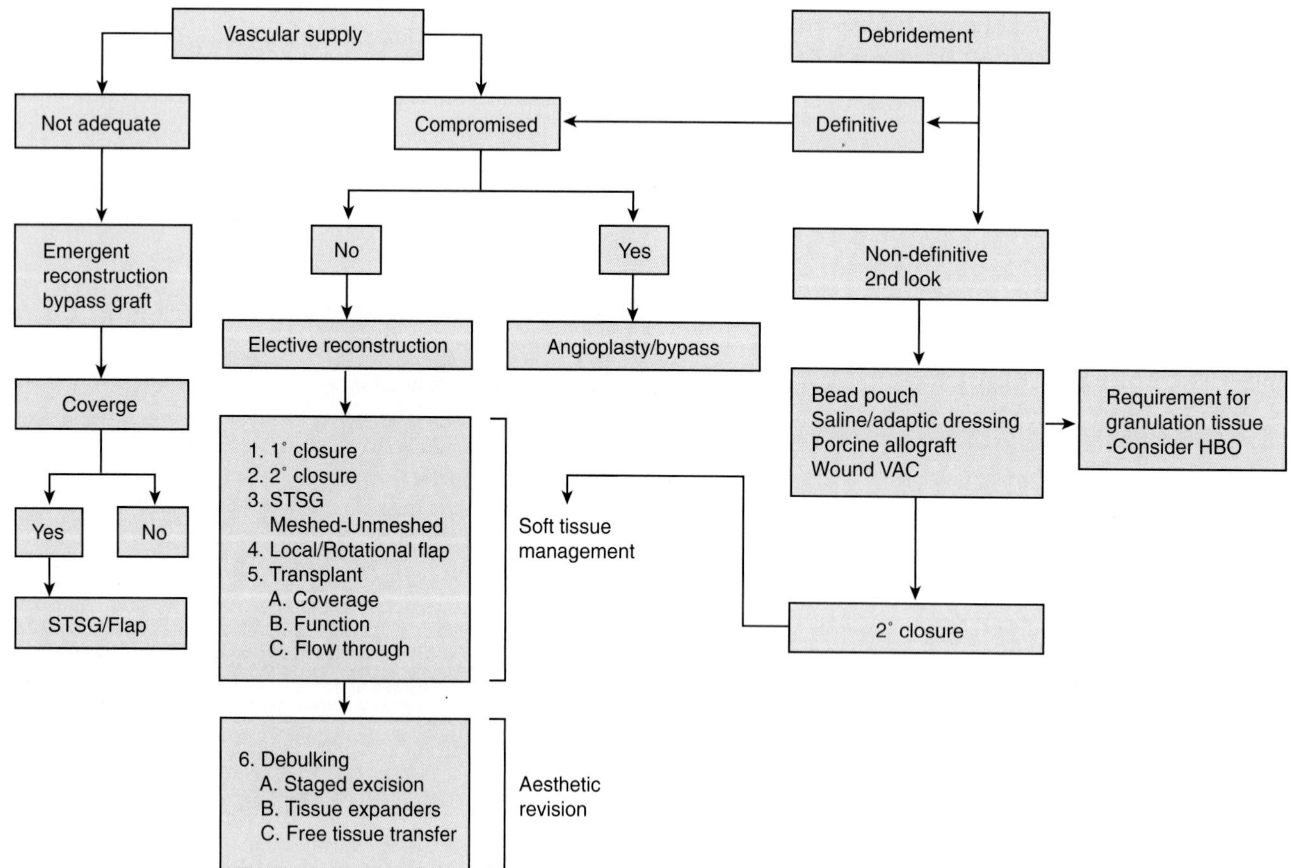

FIGURE 16-2 Reconstructive ladder for soft tissue. (From Levin LS. The reconstructive ladder: an orthoplastic approach. *Orthop Clin North Am* 1993;24:393–409, with permission.)

orthopaedic surgeon in the setting of acute or chronic soft tissue injury with or without fractures. In addition, it should be applicable to chronic conditions, such as osteomyelitis, nonunion, or tumor (13).

In essence, the orthopaedic surgeon must acquire an understanding of the approach used by the plastic surgeon to reconstruct deficiencies in soft tissue. This approach, coupled with knowledge of treatment for bone deficiencies or deformities, serves as an "orthoplastic" philosophy of limb salvage. The reconstructive ladder represents increasingly complex solutions to correspondingly complex problems with the same goal—reconstitution of the soft tissue envelope. The lowest rungs of the ladder are often as important as the top rungs. Understanding the relationship between the needs of the wound and the various techniques offered by the reconstructive ladder is important (Fig. 16-2).

THE RECONSTRUCTIVE LADDER

Patient Evaluation

Evaluation of the patient with soft tissue injury should include determination of the following: the time of injury, mechanism, energy absorption, fracture configuration, systemic injuries, damage to the soft tissue envelope, vascularity of the extremity, sensibility, ultimate salvage of the limb, and underlying medical conditions of the patient (Fig. 16-3). The principles of evaluation of orthopaedic trauma are the same for any basic medical evaluation. These principles apply whether in the outpatient clinic, emergency room, or trauma unit. An evaluation of the perfusion of the traumatized limb is of paramount importance, and, if vascular (arterial) injury is suspected, a vascular surgery consultation should be obtained. Compartment syndrome should be considered and ruled out in any injured extremity,

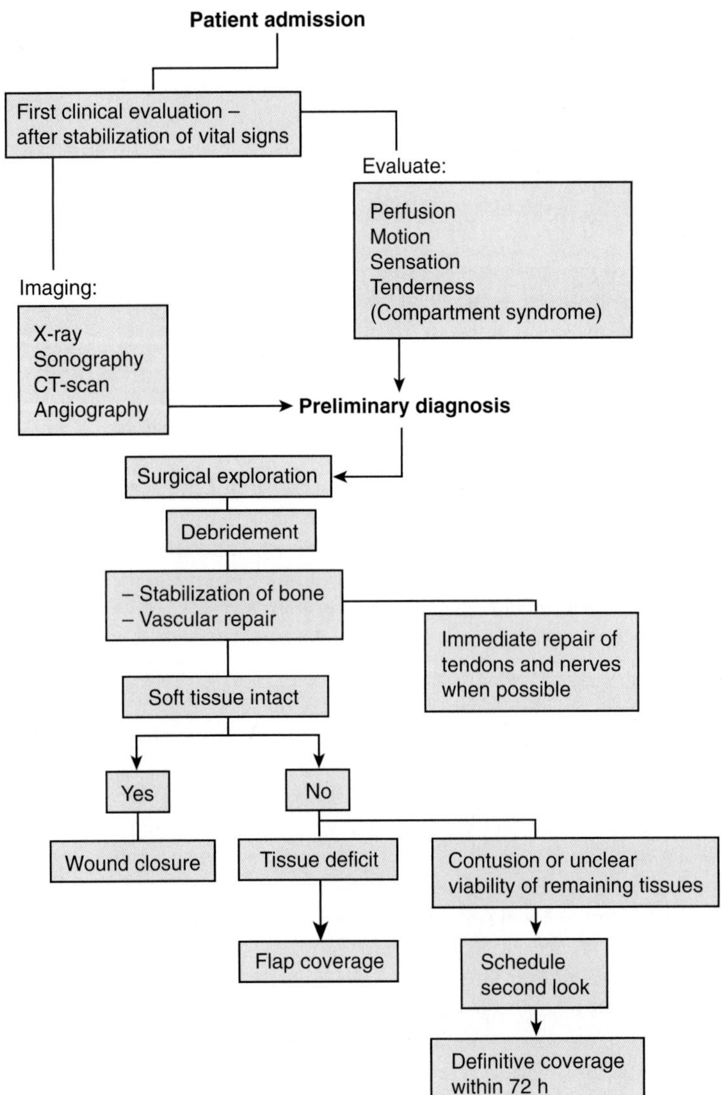

FIGURE 16-3 Patient evaluation, assessment, and management strategy. (From German G, Sherman R, Levin LS. *Decision-making in reconstructive surgery upper-extremity.* New York: Springer-Verlag; 1999, with permission.)

particularly after crush injuries. A general motor examination including the active and passive range of motion, as well as a detailed sensory examination, should be performed. A nerve deficit may be secondary to a spinal cord injury, nerve laceration, compartment syndrome, traction injury, or entrapment between bony fragments. The radiologic evaluation is begun with the standard plain x-ray examination. Computed tomography (CT) is indicated in pelvic fractures, as well as certain joint and spine injuries, and may give valuable information regarding soft tissue damage as well. As a general rule when treating long bone fractures, the joints above and below the fracture should be included in the x-rays.

The wound should be inspected once, and the wound pattern and contamination noted. The next inspection of the wound should then be in the operating room under sterile conditions. Repetitive examination of open wounds in the emergency room has led to higher rates of wound infection and osteomyelitis and should be avoided. In cases of open fractures in polytrauma patients, workup of other injuries may take several hours, not to mention the need for emergent lifesaving visceral surgery that may precede definitive care for open fractures. Prophylactic antibiotics are administered and given on a regular basis until definitive wound debridement and fracture stabilization can be performed.

Classification of Soft Tissue Injury

A classification of the soft tissue injury should allow us to evaluate the results of the treatment, to better inform our patients, and to communicate with our colleagues in a more universal language. It must be reproducible, be easy to remember, and allow prognostication of the injury. The only universally accepted classification of fractures has been a systematic division into "closed" and "open."

Assessment of soft tissue injury is necessary in both open and closed fractures. The degree of soft tissue injury will provide a prognosis and guide fracture management. The different classification schemes can be fairly simple or minutely detailed. The simpler schemes are noncomprehensive and inexact but are the most likely to be used. In 1984, L. Anderson (14) classified open fractures according to the size of the skin wound and to the extent of contamination and necrosis of the wound. As the significance of soft tissue injuries on the influence of bone healing became more apparent, Gustilo and J. T. Anderson (15) devised a three-grade classification in 1976. Type I fractures have a clean wound smaller than 1 cm in size; type II wounds have a laceration bigger than 1 cm and without extensive soft tissue damage; and type III wounds are severe soft tissue lacerations with segmental or severely comminuted fractures in high-energy trauma. Because of problems with the classification of type III injuries, this group was later divided in three subgroups. Type IIIA has a large soft tissue laceration or flaps but allows for adequate soft tissue coverage of bone. Also included in type IIIA are fractures with severe comminution or segmental fractures, regardless of the size of the soft tissue damage. Type IIIB fractures are more severe, with extensive periosteal stripping and soft tissue loss with significant bony exposure and massive contamination. Type IIIC fractures have an arterial injury requiring repair.

A more comprehensive and comparable system, although more difficult to use, is the AO classification (Table 16-1) (16). It incorporates five grades of severity and three categories of tissue. As in the classification of Tscherne and Gotzen (17), a distinction is made between open and closed fractures. The AO classification includes grading the skin, muscle and tendon, and neurovascular structures. A closed fracture involving only skin can be graded in four subgroups. For open fractures, four grades are given. A new feature of this classification is the evaluation for muscle and tendon injuries. Because of the prognostic value, knowledge of the extent of muscle damage and tendon involvement is essential. A common approach in all classification schemes is a determination of the length of laceration of the

TABLE 16-1 Classification and Zones of Injury

AO/ASIF Soft Tissue Injury Classification
Scale
1 Normal (except open fractures)
2–4 Increasing severity of lesion
5 A special situation
Skin lesions (closed fractures)
IC 1 No skin lesion
IC 2 No skin laceration, but contusion
IC 3 Circumferential degloving
IC 4 Extensive, closed degloving
IC 5 Necrosis from contusion
Skin lesions (open fractures)
IO 1 Skin breakage from Inside out
IO 2 Skin breakage <5 cm, edges contused
IO 3 Skin breakage >5 cm, devitalized edges
IO 4 Full thickness contusion, avulsion, soft tissue defect muscle/tendon injury
Muscle tendon injury
MT 1 No muscle injury
MT 2 Circumferential injury, one compartment only
MT 3 Considerable injury, two compartments
MT 4 Muscle defect, tendon laceration, extensive contusion
MT 5 Compartment syndrome/crush injury
Neurovascular injury
NV 1 No neurovascular injury
NV 2 Isolated nerve injury
NV 3 Localized vascular injury
NV 4 Extensive segmental vascular injury
NV 5 Combined neurovascular injury, including subtotal or complete amputation.

skin. As treatment methods have become more comprehensive and more systemic factors are taken into account when treating open fractures, the presence or absence of muscle, nerve, and vascular injury has become more important prognostically. Acute systemic factors, such as shock, associated injuries, or extreme age, have been recognized as important prognostic indicators also. They influence the acute treatment of fractures and the treatment of complications. For example, in osteomyelitis, debilitating factors such as smoking and malnutrition affect the feasibility of reconstruction (18).

Ruedi et al (19) have developed a classification system that characterizes soft tissue injury by addressing several layers of the soft tissue envelope. This classification system determines whether the integument is open or closed. Injuries to muscle, tendon, nerve, and vessels are graded in order of severity. Although this may be more complex than the Gustilo and Anderson (15) classification of open fractures, it is an attempt similar to Tscherne's classification (17) to define in more depth the deficiency and defects of the soft tissues. Factors such as contusion or ecchymosis to skin and muscle must be identified to avoid further damage to these tissues in surgical dissection. Such damage of muscle or fascial territories may make these sites unreliable as replacement tissue.

One of the most important goals in the reconstructive ladder is to provide a physiologic milieu for exposed soft tissue. In the limb with compromised integument and a break in the epithelial surface, underlying subcutaneous tissue, muscle, fascia, bone, and periosteum are exposed, predisposing them to desiccation with inevitable cell death and the risk for infection. To help prevent infection, a sterile, moist bandage should be applied to the wound as soon as possible, bathing the damaged tissues in a physiologic medium such as saline or lactated Ringer's solution.

A biologic dressing is the first rung on the reconstructive ladder. Preventing desiccation of tissue reduces requirements for debridement and preserves simpler options for closure, such as skin grafts.

DEBRIDEMENT

Debridement of damaged tissue is paramount in the treatment of the traumatized limb (Table 16-2 and Fig. 16-4). In most instances, this will result in additional loss of tissue volume, depending on the degree of contamination. The abilities of the reconstructive surgeon, particularly the ability to transplant autogenous tissue such as muscle or skin flaps, have changed the concept of debridement (20,21). Surgeons treating combined injuries must accept the premise that irreversibly damaged or nonviable tissues require replacement, and the zone of injury requires expeditious reconstruction. Marginally viable tissue left behind can subsequently desiccate, infarct, and become infected, further delaying healing. This results in progressive dysfunction related to inflammation, subsequent fibrosis, and pain, which can be avoided if aggressive debridement is undertaken primarily. Critical vascular structures, nerves, and tendons can be cleaned, and prompt coverage may preserve their viability (Fig. 16-5). Debridement may take place in the acute trauma setting or in a chronic wound that has evolved from improper handling of soft tissues initially.

New tools have evolved for debriding wounds, such as ultrasound debridement, which has been used for chronic wounds. The ultrasonic methods have proven to be less painful than the conventional methods of sharp debridement, if used in the

TABLE 16-2 Debridement–Structures

Skin, subcutis	Sharp knife dissection to bleeding dermis. Trim edges 1–2 mm to create clean wound edge. Cut fat back to healthy fat. Punctuate bleeding, minimal hemosiderin staining.
Fascia	May be debrided sharply and should always be removed if not vascularized. Liberal opening/extensive exploration of compartment.
Muscle	Debride to contractile muscle. Color–pink; bleeding from cut myosomes.
Bone	All fragments devoid of significant soft tissue attachments should be removed.
Nerve	Be aware of cutaneous nerves—they may cause painful neuromas. Epineurium can be removed if contaminated (median, radial, and ulnar nerve) with fascicles remaining. If nerve is not vascularized it can remain, provided it does not desiccate, and wound closure is achieved early.
Vessels	Remove any perforated, thrombosed segments. Identify main vascular trunks. If not intact and if there is no flow, segmental vascular debridement: ligate major vessels, clip minor. Identify, mark, and protect major viable vessels that can be used for vascular access during immediate/delayed free tissue transfer.
Pulsatile irrigation	Caveat: avoid implosion of foreign material, hydrodissection of tissue planes and insufflation of tissues.
Deflate tourniquet Decision making on wound closure	Evaluate structures for bleeding.

From German G, Sherman R, Levin LS. *Decision-making in reconstructive surgery upper extremity*. New York: Springer-Verlag; 1999, with permission.

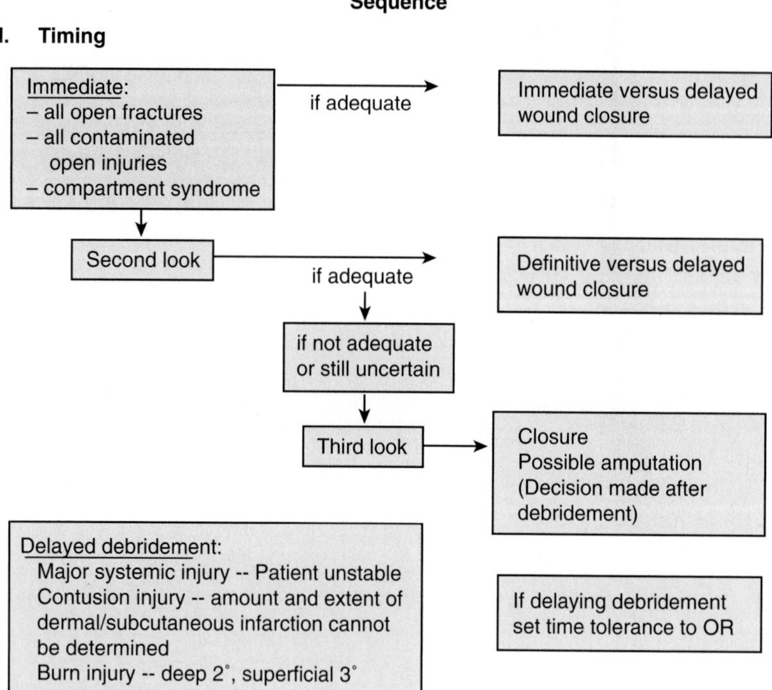

FIGURE 16-4 Debridement. All wounds at some point in time will require debridement to optimize conditions that will allow for wound closure. In cases of open fractures, debridement and stabilization are the most important steps in prophylaxis against sepsis. (From German G, Sherman R, Levin LS. *Decision-making in reconstructive surgery upper-extremity.* New York: Springer-Verlag; 1999, with permission.)

outpatient clinic setting. One advantage of the ultrasound technique is that debridement can be done more precisely in areas where there are patchy areas of granulation tissue that the surgeon would want to preserve.

Other devices such as the Versajet Hydrosurgery System enables the surgeon to hold, cut, and remove damaged tissue and contaminants while simultaneously irrigating the wound. Surgical debridement is accomplished in a single step. The Versajet System uses a high-velocity stream of sterile saline that jets across the hand piece into a suction device that collects fluid and debris from the wound surface (Fig. 16-6). The Versajet requires less irrigant than traditional techniques and confines the irrigant to the wound area. In the acute trauma situation, this obviates the need to change large saline irrigant bags and reservoir waste canisters. This system has multiple power settings depending on the degree of debridement required. One advantage of the hydrosurgery system is that there is less aerosolization of bacteria, which provides less risk to the operating room, staff, and surgeon based on a single wound site. Compared to conventional pulsate irrigation, the Versajet appears to leave significantly less bacteria in the wound.

Debridement of a Fresh Wound

Debridement of the fresh wound (such as the open IIIB or IIIC tibial fractures) is performed in the exsanguinated extremity. This permits the surgeon to carefully observe the appearance of the tissue, detect pockets in the wound, and eliminate all foreign material. In addition, operating under tourniquet prevents unnecessary blood loss during debridement. After debridement is completed, it is simple to identify major bleeders and perform proper hemostasis when the tourniquet is deflated. After release of the tourniquet, the result of debridement can be checked by observing diffuse bleeding throughout the wound.

In the ischemic operative field it is simple to distinguish between healthy and damaged tissue. The basic elements of this judgment are the appearance and consistency of tissues. Healthy tissue in the exsanguinated limb is bright and homogeneous in color. Subcutaneous tissue is yellow, muscles are bright red, and the tendons and fascia have a white and shiny appearance. Damaged tissues are recognized by the presence of foreign bodies, irregular tissue consistency, and irregular distribution of dark red stains, which are hematomas. All nonviable tissue is removed, preferably with a knife. It is not possible to do precise debridement with scissors. Scissors should be used only when dissecting important structures such as nerves, vessels, or tendons.

The edge of the debridement should be in healthy tissue. Avulsed skin and muscles should be removed from the base of the avulsed flap. These tissues are contused, and, in addition, the anatomic pattern of the skin vascularity is not axial as a result

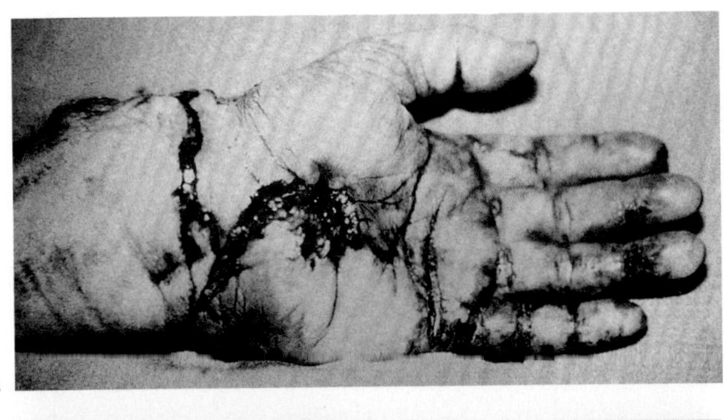
A

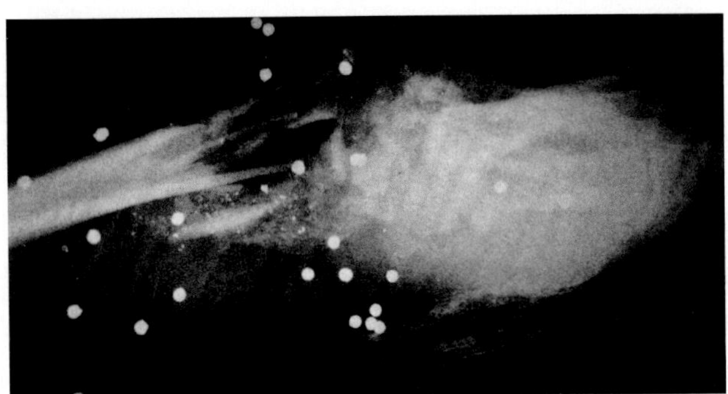
B

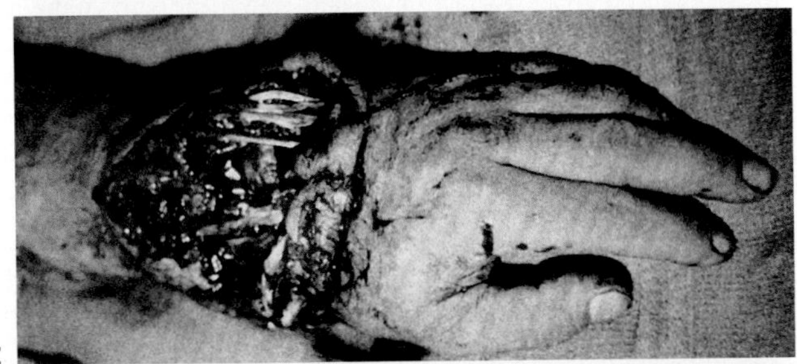
C

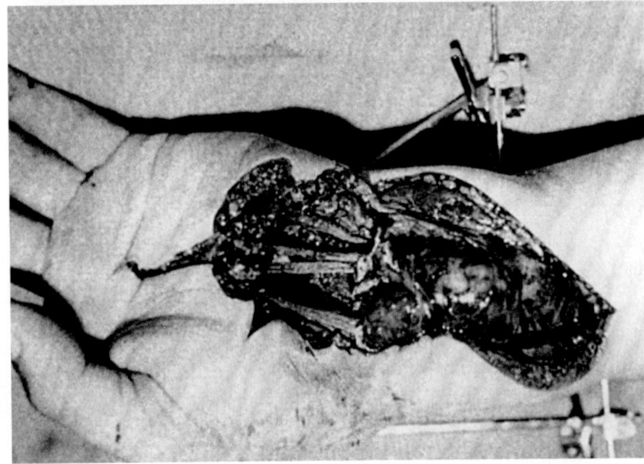
D

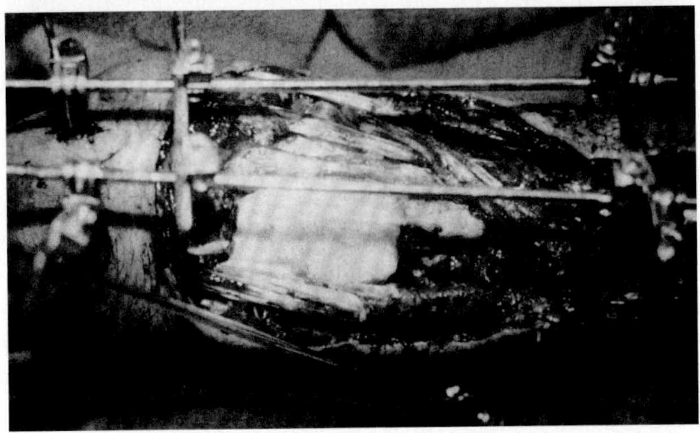
E

FIGURE 16-5 **A.** Gunshot wound to the carpus. **B.** The radiograph portrays significant bone as well as soft tissue destruction. **C,D.** Entrance wound and exit wound shown after debridement and decompression of the carpal tunnel. A through-and-through soft tissue defect is visualized. **E.** The wrist was stabilized with an external fixator, and subsequently a muscle flap was used for coverage and obliteration of the dead space. A tobramycin block was used to preserve space for subsequent wrist arthrodesis with iliac crest bone graft.

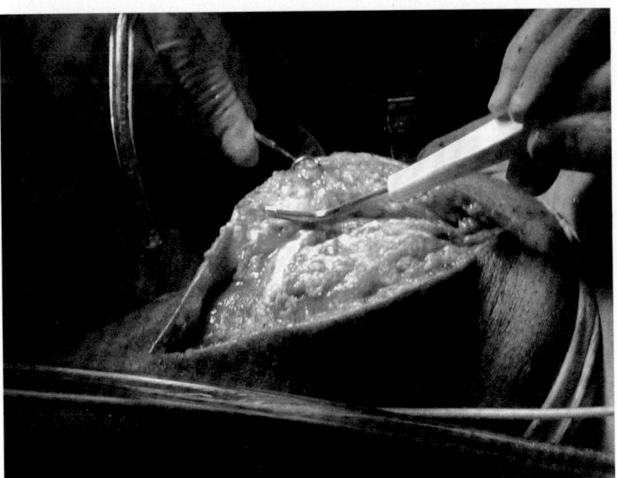

FIGURE 16-6 The Versajet uses fluid-jet technology for soft tissue debridement. The hand piece is shown here in the debridement of a knee wound.

of avulsion of perforators and therefore may be insufficient to maintain viability of such flaps. Denuded tendon, if not frayed, should be cleaned. Disrupted tendons can be sutured or fixed with a suture to surrounding tissue for later reconstruction. Exposed bones are washed with bacitracin solution and mechanically cleansed with bone rongeurs. Free bone fragments usually are removed, and if sections are quite large, they can be stored in the bone bank as bone autografts to be used when soft tissue coverage has been obtained. However, this point is controversial.

Severed vessels are ligated, provided they are not significant to the viability of the injured extremity. If vessels are vital, they are excised to normal-looking margins, and continuity is restored with interposition vein grafts. The nerves are the only structures where debridement is not radical. Those parts that are destroyed without any doubt are removed, and nerve stumps are anchored in the wound so as to avoid retraction and allow later reconstruction with nerve grafts. We prefer that a large cystoclip or hemoclip be applied to the nerve stump so it can be seen on x-ray, and appropriate secondary planning can be done in terms of surgical approach and location of the neuroma stump.

Occasionally, the bed of the wound remains irregular after debridement. With additional incision, it can be made regular in shape, provided that the irregularity is not caused by tissue of functional importance. This maneuver serves to eliminate dead space by permitting the flaps, if they are to be done, close contact with the wound bed, preventing hematoma and subsequent formation of scar.

Chronic Wounds

Debridement of a chronic wound is also done with the limb exsanguinated. Superficial scar is excised completely so that the wound margins are in healthy skin and subcutaneous tissue appears normal. The goal is to treat the chronic wound like a tumor and excise it in its entirety down to normal tissue planes. All scars in the wound should be removed in the same manner as cancer surgeons operate; that is, the knife should always cut through healthy tissues. If functionally important structures are entrapped in the scar, the dissection should commence in the healthy surrounding tissue, passing toward the scar entrapment, where the structures such as nerves or tendons are carefully dissected out.

This portion of the procedure is extremely difficult, and it is necessary to think of the changes in the anatomy due to the injury, previous operations, and the traction exerted by scar tissue. Bone debridement is also very difficult. Although clearly necrotic parts of bone can be recognized, it requires more experience to identify the viable parts of the bone callus and necrotic and inflamed areas in the medullary canal. Studies such as CTs, tomograms, bone scans, and magnetic resonance imaging (MRI) may be helpful in preoperative planning for wound debridement.

Swiontkowski (22) has popularized the use of the laser Doppler to determine bone blood flow in planning for debridement of infected bone. All areas of the bone not covered with periosteum are removed, and those that are exposed are burred under iced saline irrigation to avoid burning bone. If punctuate bleeding is encountered from the cortical bone, the bone is left behind. If not, the bone is removed until the so-called paprika sign popularized by Cierny is identified. This is punctate bleeding from the haversian canals, indicating bone viability. If a sequestrum is in the medullary canal, the anterior part of the bone cortex (such as in the anterior tibia) should be removed to provide a window for access to the medullary canal for placement of muscle flaps, which eliminate dead space and help control infection.

Debridement Technique

The sequence of wound debridement is as follows. The patient is prepped and draped after prescrubbing to remove grime and surface dirt. The tourniquet is inflated after elevating the limb for 5 minutes to exsanguinate it rather than wrapping out with an Esmarch bandage. Next, the wound is superficially washed with bacitracin-impregnated saline solution to remove blood clots or superficial debris. It is advisable to use loupe magnification when debriding. The more complex the wound, the longer the debridement takes. If the wound has been sitting for quite some time and blood is organized in muscle tissues or around fracture ends, half-strength peroxide is used as a first rinse solution to lyse the clot and gain access to the true depths of the wound. The half-strength peroxide will have a tendency to bubble and is washed away with normal saline solution.

Next, a no. 10 or 15 scalpel blade or very sharp scissors is used to excise the skin and dermis, particularly around the edge of the wound, back to normal tissue. Then the subcutaneous layer is inspected and debrided sharply with a no. 15 scalpel to the level of the fascia. All fascia that is stripped, avulsed, or contaminated is then removed. The next layer encountered is muscle; muscle should be resected down to healthy tissue regardless of the amount of muscle removed. Leaving unhealthy necrotic muscle is the surest way to acquire an infection. Periosteum that is elevated from bone should be excised to the level from which it is elevated. Small bone fragments devoid of periosteum or free-floating large segments, although they may be structural, should be removed for fear of colonization, contamination, and infection.

At the conclusion of debridement, the wound is again irrigated; the tourniquet is let down; and then all tissue planes, particularly the muscle, are observed for bleeding as the arterial pressure increases in the limb. Areas that are persistently nonviable, particularly the dermis, skin, and muscle, are excised. Excision then can be done sequentially, watching for punctate bleeding from either the dermis or the muscle. When large flaps have been avulsed, excision is carried out through the skin to the level of bright red blood coming from the dermis on the incision. No attempt should be made to close the wound defect under any undue tension for fear of further ischemic damage to already compromised tissue.

Special Techniques in Debridement

In the chronic bone infection, a motorized burr may be used to debride bone. If the bone is easily removed by the burr, this implies necrosis and nonviability. At the point at which there is punctate bleeding from the haversian canals, indicating good viability of bone, the burring is stopped. Pulsed irrigation systems, while advocated by some, if used too vigorously with too high pressure too close to tissue planes, particularly around tendons, nerves, and vessels, can actually damage tissue and cause swelling. For this reason, we advocate copious but gentle irrigation. A wound that is appropriately debrided sharply down to all healthy tissue requires very little irrigation.

The philosophy of wound debridement should be, again, that of a tumor resection, visualizing all normal tissue planes at the conclusion of debridement. If this is not possible, then a second-look procedure is strongly advised in which the process is started over again, particularly in areas of questionable viability of tissue. This should be done no later than 48 hours, and preferably 24 hours, after the initial debridement. If possible, at least during the first and not later than the second debridement, plans should be under way to obtain wound coverage. This is with closure primarily, delayed closure, skin grafting, or a variety of local or free-tissue transfer procedures discussed elsewhere in this chapter.

Within the reconstructive ladder, options are now available to reconstruct bone as well as soft tissue, and no compromised tissue should be retained. The "wait and see" adage concerning bone devoid of periosteum or muscle that is not bleeding but covering a vital structure should be abandoned. Adequate surgical exposure is critical in the assessment of soft tissue injury, as well as in its treatment. In the patient with a pulseless limb who is brought to the operating room and in whom, despite fluid resuscitation, splinting, and fracture alignment, perfusion does not return to the extremity, arteriography must be performed and vascular repair undertaken.

SELECTION OF RECONSTRUCTION TIME

The optimal time for soft tissue reconstruction in severe open fractures remains controversial. The argument favoring staged procedures is based on the need for a second-look debridement. If there is uncertainty about traumatized and devascularized tissue, a second look is done to allow more adequate resection. The main argument for early reconstruction is to reduce the nosocomial contamination and secondary necrosis of exposed tissues. Late soft tissue reconstruction is associated with a significantly higher infection and flap complication rate when compared with early (within 72 hours) soft tissue coverage (23,24). Godina (25) and other pioneers (26) changed the concept of primary repair and reconstruction of damaged tissue by advancing the phase of reconstruction from a delayed elective procedure to the day of injury. Assuming that an adequate primary debridement is feasible, the outcome should be further improved by immediate soft tissue closure. Immediate reconstruction improves the time to definitive union, decreases the number of operations that are performed, and reduces the infection rate (27).

Patients with IIIB and IIIC open fractures of the lower extremity whose general condition allowed debridement followed by stable internal fixation and immediate soft tissue reconstruction demonstrated a better outcome and a shorter period of convalescence (27). The significantly shorter time to union after immediate reconstruction may be related to the fact that bone infection did not occur. The higher incidence of infection in the delayed group may well be due to the lengthy exposure of the fracture to nosocomial contamination, the secondary damage of exposed tissue, or the necessarily incomplete nature of second-look debridement, particularly in and around a reduced fracture.

PREPARATION OF THE WOUND FOR RECONSTRUCTION

Wound Dressing

The standard protocol for fracture wound management following surgical debridement varies with the severity of the wound. In grades I to IIIA open fracture wounds, the gold standard technique before wound coverage has been packed saline-soaked gauze dressings to eliminate dead space and prevent soft tissue desiccation. The disadvantages of saline-soaked gauze dressings include drying with soft tissue desiccation, nosocomial bacterial contamination, poor dead space management, and, often, significant patient discomfort. Similar benefits are obtained with dressings of gauze soaked in Dakin's solution and half-strength povidone-iodine (Betadine). Dakin's solution is bacteriostatic. Betadine, while bacteriocidal, is controversial because of its soft tissue toxicity. The advantage of all three of these dressing types is that they ensure cleanliness at the time of closure by allowing consistent monitoring of the wound site. In the more severe tibial fractures (grades IIIB and IIIC), aggressive treatment with prophylactic administration of systemic and local antibiotics is recommended.

Fracture wounds with avulsion of the dermal surface but without damage to the underlying muscle may be treated successfully with several techniques. First is emollient coverage. Emollient-type soft tissue coverage may also be indicated to temporize a wound before soft tissue coverage. This may take the form of a hydrogel, such as Vigilion, an antibiotic-impregnated occlusive dressing, such as Scarlet Red, or a simple semipermeable film, such as Bio-occlusive. A copious layer of Neosporin ointment covered by a sterile dressing may also temporize wounds before coverage.

There are four general types of newer wound dressings: semipermeable films (e.g., Opsite, Tegaderm, and Bio-occlusive), hydrogels (e.g., Vigilion), occlusive hydrocolloids (e.g., Duoderm), and synthetic skin substitutes (e.g., Epigard). Application of these new dressings is best when the wound site is surrounded by a border of healthy tissue. Semipermeable films and semiocclusive hydrogels are impermeable to water and bacteria but permeable to oxygen and water vapor. Occlusive hydrocolloids are impermeable to even water vapor and oxygen. For example, Duoderm has an inner adherent surface with an outer impermeable polyurethane foam. Epigard, one of the synthetic skin substitutes, is a nontextile open-matrix polyurethane composed of two layers and backed by a microporous polytetrafluoroethylene film. This matrix allows for new microcirculation to develop in its interstices. However, newer dressings are not without drawbacks, particularly the accumulation of exudate, hematoma, and seroma beneath them (28). In addition to these wound dressings, there is an isolated report on the efficacy of honey as a broad-spectrum antimicrobial found to be effective in controlling *Staphylococcus aureus, Escherichia coli,* and *Pseudomonas aeruginosa,* and *Klebsiella pneumoniae*. Although in need of further clinical verification, honey shows promise for use as a first-line wound dressing agent (29).

Antibiotic Beads

Antibiotic beads have been used effectively to control infection and can be used after the first debridement, until the patient returns to the operating room for a second look at 24 to 48 hours after the initial debridement and fracture stabilization. Advantages of antibiotic beads are that they are able to deliver antibiotics to a compromised wound without systemic effects. The so-called bead pouch, popularized by Henry et al (30), seals the wound, such that transudate from the wound surface is captured, bathing exposed tissues in physiologic fluids that also contain bactericidal levels of antibiotics. Wounds do not desiccate, cell death is avoided, and infection risk is reduced.

The Antibiotic Bead Pouch Technique

One possible solution to the controversy surrounding soft tissue coverage of open tibia fractures lies in local antibiotic delivery achieved via antibiotic-impregnated polymethylmethacrylate (PMMA) (31). The technique of local antibiotic therapy originated with Büchholz in West Germany. It is an application that uses antibiotic-impregnated bone cement to treat infected arthroplasties (29).

Antibiotic-impregnated PMMA beads are strung on steel surgical wire. A chain of medium-sized 6.3-mm PMMA beads is composed of 21 beads each weighing 70 mg and containing a 5.7-mg tobramycin base. The smaller beads are 2 mm in diameter, each weighing 14.5 mg with a 2.2-mm tobramycin base (20 beads per chain). The surgical wire consists of three strands of size 00 surgical wire for the 6.3-mm beads. For the smaller size, four strands of 4-0 steel sutures are used. The custom-made versus commercial fabrication processes differ in that the custom-made beads are polymerized in a mold, whereas the commercial variety is formed in a press with a correspondent increase in temperature and pressure.

The bead pouch technique is most effective in grade III fractures. It is indicated for use in grade I fractures only if primary closure was prevented because of compartment syndrome, marked swelling, or wound edema (31). It is performed in the operating room under sterile conditions. All necrotic, avascular, and contaminated tissue is removed from the fracture site during the initial irrigation and debridement. Wound margins are extended to appropriate widths. Following this, a thorough lavage consisting of bacitracin and normal saline is performed (32). Depending on the severity of the fracture, reduction is accomplished with either an external fixator or a nail.

One or more chains of antibiotic beads are then inserted into the wound surrounding the fracture site. Placement should be such as to fill the soft tissue cavity but leave adequate room for closure. A suction drain (0.32-cm diameter) is placed in the wound. The drain should be positioned so that it exits the hematoma site through normal tissue (32). If possible, the wound should be closed with interrupted sutures. (In wounds with extensive soft tissue damage, closure may not be possible at the time of initial debridement.) Wound coverage is achieved with an adhesive polyethylene wound film, such as Opsite. The semipermeable wound dressing should be stapled to the skin edges, with a second layer wrapped around the entire wound area to prevent leakage of wound secretions. The drain should remain in place for 48 hours. Suction is avoided because it would negate the high bactericidal dosages released by the beads into the wound hematoma. Triple antibiotic coverage of penicillin, cefazolin, and tobramycin is provided parenterally for 5 days (32).

The bead pouch is replaced every 48 to 72 hours in the operating room under sterile conditions. This is done to ensure adequate antibiotic concentrations in the wound environment. Aerobic and anaerobic cultures are taken at each bead change. Final wound closure is achieved through either primary suture closure or, in cases with more extensive soft tissue defects, STSGs or flap coverage.

In more severe fractures the bead pouch provides a solution to much of the debate surrounding delayed or acute soft tissue transfer. The bead pouch delivers high levels of antibiotics locally; therefore, the surgeon can delay definitive coverage until thorough and usually multiple debridements are performed, a clean wound is present, and operative repairs of neurovascular, tendon, and ligamentous structures are done (31). If an acute flap is indicated, the presence of the bead pouch beneath the flap will serve to assuage the fears the surgeon might have of infection occurring beneath the flap.

The bead pouch technique shows significant advantages over saline-soaked, packed gauze dressings in the prevention of desiccation and subsequent soft tissue necrosis. The bead pouch provides an environment in which the bone is enveloped in a warm, moist, protective envelope of soft tissue. This allows for greater infection resistance, increased wound vascularization, and a therapeutic level of antibiotics to be administered at the wound site. This use of antibiotic beads locally is an extremely promising solution to the complications of soft tissue transfer and chronic osteomyelitis.

Hyperbaric Oxygen

Hyperbaric oxygen (HBO) can be used to promote granulation tissue and stimulate angiogenesis in wounds that are compromised, usually on the basis of impaired arterial inflow or compromised venous outflow (33). In addition to exposure to HBO, wound dressings are changed under sterile conditions by chamber personnel, which further improves wound conditions. Patients with gas gangrene associated with fractures require emergent debridement, HBO, antibiotics, and ultimate fracture and soft tissue management (34). Normal tissue oxygen levels are approximately 40 mm Hg. Below 30 mm Hg, normal metabolic activity is significantly impaired (35). In infected wounds and traumatized tissue, oxygen levels frequently fall below 30 mm Hg. HBO enhances oxygen delivery to ischemic and hypoxic wounds, and, even when it causes local vasoconstriction, the overall increase in blood oxygen content results in a net gain so that the net oxygen concentration at the wound increases. It improves neutrophil function, facilitates fibroblast cell division, increases collagen formation, and encourages new capillary budding. The promotion of angiogenesis by HBO is thought to be one of the major factors in promoting the healing of chronic hypoperfused wounds (36).

Vacuum Assisted Closure

Vacuum assisted closure (VAC) is a recently developed tool that exposes a wound to subatmospheric pressure. It has proven to be extremely effective in treating a wide spectrum of wounds, including traumatic wounds and dehisced incisions, with or without exposed hardware (37). The wound cavity is dressed with a cell foam dressing that is connected to an adjustable vacuum source with a negative pressure of −75 to −125 mm Hg. The foam dressing/wound site is sealed with a thin adhesive film, converting the open wound to a controlled closed wound. Pressure is applied continuously or cyclically to the wound. The removal of excess interstitial fluid from the wound periphery results in a decrease in the local interstitial pressure, thus restoring blood flow to compressed or collapsed vessels (38). Along with removal of the chronic fluid, factors that inhibit healing are also removed. An additional mechanism of action of VAC is the mechanical stimulation of cells by tensile forces placed on the tissue as a result of the collapse of the foam dressing by the negative pressure (38).

VAC has become an important part of orthopaedic trauma care. This device decreases edema, increases wound vascularization, fights infection, and promotes granulation tissue (proliferation of capillaries and fibroblasts) (38). The wound VAC is a tool that has several applications in orthopaedic trauma care. It can be used for soft tissue injuries, following initial debridement. If a relatively clean wound can be established, a wound VAC can be applied. This device serves as a barrier dressing and isolates the wound from the hospital environment. Simultaneously, it performs all of the physiologic benefits that have been mentioned. It establishes an environment for granulation to occur. After a second-look procedure it may be used as definitive wound care treatment. Commonly, in large cavitary wounds or wounds with irregular surface topography, the wound VAC can stabilize the wound until definitive treatment can occur. For example, an open tibia fracture that has a large cavitary soft tissue component may benefit from a wound VAC to serve as a barrier dressing from the hospital environment until appropriate soft tissue reconstruction can be performed with either local or, commonly, free-tissue transfer (Fig. 16-7). The advantage of the wound VAC is similar to that of the antibiotic bead pouch

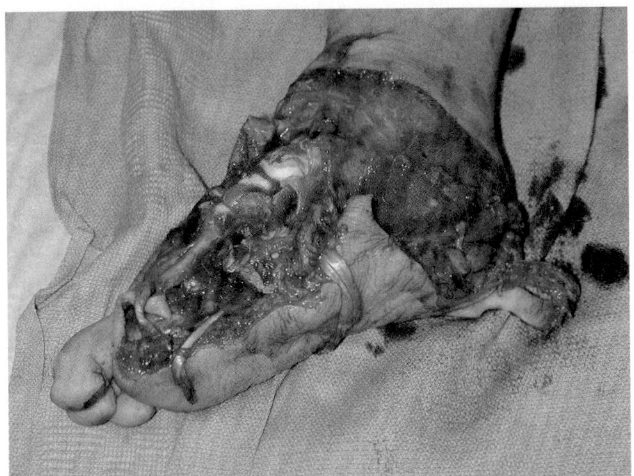

A

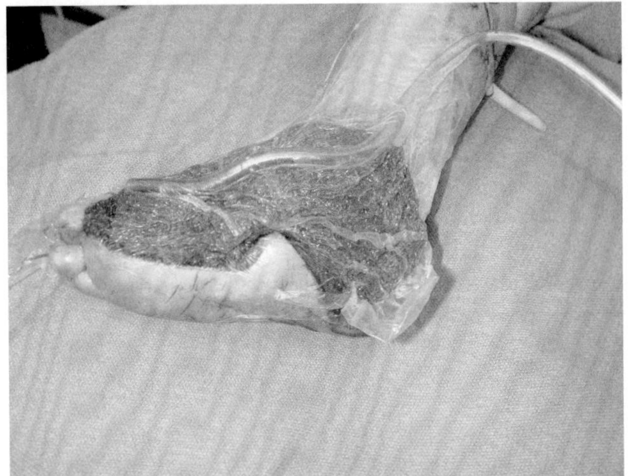

B

C

FIGURE 16-7 **A.** This 4-year-old boy suffered a mutilating injury to both feet when he was run over by a lawnmower. **B.** The wound VAC dressing sponge, tubing, and drape have been applied to the foot following adequate debridement. **C.** The same foot 4 months after debridement, wound VAC treatment, and split-thickness skin grafting.

in that the wound is sealed from the outside world. The advantage of the bead pouch is that there is a high concentration of antibiotics that can be leeched into the tissue. The wound VAC relies more on physiologic rather than pharmaceutical treatment of the wound, in that blood flow can be enhanced and edema can be diminished, making the wound healthier, assuming parenteral antibiotics are given. Another application of the wound VAC has been in the treatment of fasciotomy sites. Traditionally, fasciotomy sites are covered with materials such as saline dressings that require frequent dressing changes on the ward to prevent desiccation. In an era in which hospitals are trying to diminish global costs, particularly in the trauma population, the benefit of the wound VAC is that it can remain on a wound for 2 or 3 days, and sometimes longer, depending on the clinical circumstances. For example, the wound VAC has been a very effective stabilizer of skin grafts that can be used for definitive coverage of open wounds or fasciotomy sites. In these cases the wound VAC stays on for approximately 5 days with a pressure of −75 mm Hg.

Although it is possible to definitively treat certain wounds to completion with a wound VAC, a word of caution should be added regarding the use of this device with exposed hardware such as fixation plates and screws. It is possible that if it is applied long enough, the granulation tissue will grow over exposed plates and screws. The granulation tissue contains bacteria that can colonize the plates and screws, resulting in chronic infection. In addition, when using the wound VAC alone to secure a healed wound, the wound often has a large degree of fibrosis associated with it. Compared with supple soft tissue such as a muscle flap or regional transpositional flap, working through such a scarred bed covered only with a STSG can be difficult, resulting in complications with second procedures such as tendon transfers or bone grafting or even hardware exchange or removal.

Personality of Soft Tissue Injury

The mechanism of injury is also important in determining how soft tissue should be treated and what part of the reconstructive ladder should be applied. A ringer injury, a press injury, and an injury involving heat all carry a poor prognosis. Electrical injuries associated with fracture may appear innocuous but may have significant damage to soft tissue as well as bone. The difficulty in treatment of open fractures is often related to the soft tissues and not to the bone injury.

In any high-energy wound, the zone of injury extends to the soft tissues, similar to the expanding ripples of water where a stone has been thrown. Recognition of this concept is of critical importance in determining the extent of debridement and the need for tissue, preferably imported from a site outside the zone of injury, to reconstruct the soft tissue envelope. The presence of shock, amount of blood loss, and systemic injuries also influence the soft tissue response in the injured limb. The patient with underlying cardiac disease, the elderly patient, the diabetic patient, or the patient with peripheral vascular disease also should be categorized differently from the healthy 20-year-old patient involved in a motor vehicle accident. Patients taking steroids and those who are malnourished or immunocompromised will all have difficulty with wound healing. Smokers not only have difficulty with bone healing but also may have difficulty with perfusion of soft tissue to allow proper healing. These underlying problems must be considered before undertaking reconstruction (39).

Amputation versus Salvage Procedure

In complex extremity injuries, the treating physician must always first determine whether limb salvage is feasible. Before complex and prolonged reconstructions are started on a limb that will ultimately function poorly or not at all, a well-fitted prosthesis should be seen as an excellent option, and early amputation should be considered. Lange (40) and Hansen (41) have delineated a sound algorithm for these difficult wounds.

If neurovascular structures are injured, are they repairable? Is normal plantar sensation obtainable? Does a compartment syndrome exist? Unless it is recognized, muscle ischemia and muscle death will occur, converting potentially viable soft tissue to infarcted muscle and scar. This ultimately increases the need for large block resections and tissue replacement—a higher rung on the reconstructive ladder. Although the evolution of sophisticated microsurgical reconstructive techniques has created the possibility of successful limb salvage in even the most extreme cases, it has become painfully obvious that the technical possibilities are double-edged swords. Hansen (41), in analyzing his vast personal experience with managing open fractures, noted that protracted limb salvage attempts might destroy a patient physically, psychologically, socially, and financially, with adverse consequences for the patient's family as well. In spite of the best attempts, the functional results are often worse than an amputation. Thus, enthusiasm for limb salvage techniques must be tempered by a realistic assessment of the results, not just for the injured part but for the patient as a whole (40). A salvaged limb must function as well as, if not better than, a prosthesis, or heroic attempts at reconstruction are not indicated. Donor-site morbidity should also be considered with free-tissue transfer when approaching a limb reconstruction.

Indicators of a poor prognosis for limb salvage, in order of significance, are (a) massive crush injuries, (b) other high-energy soft tissue injuries, (c) a warm ischemia time longer than 6 hours, (d) severely comminuted or segmental fracture patterns, (e) infrapopliteal arterial injury, (f) prolonged severe hypovolemia shock, and (g) age over 50 years (Fig. 16-8).

The presence or absence of underlying diseases such as diabetes and occupational demands are also important considerations. The same anatomic injury may require a different treatment decision in a 20-year-old laborer than in a 60-year-old diabetic.

Similarly, a given tibial injury may need to be treated differently if there is unreconstructible ipsilateral foot trauma that precludes reasonable limb function even if the leg is salvageable.

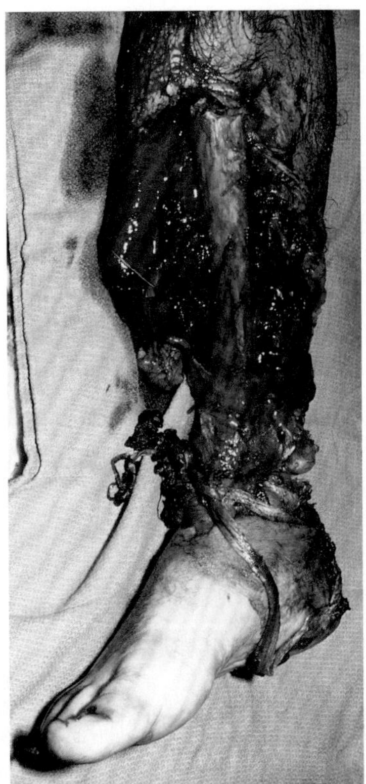

FIGURE 16-8 Grade IIIC fracture. This leg underwent primary amputation because of avulsion of the tibial nerve, ischemia of 9 hours, and significant soft tissue injury.

According to several authors, complete disruption of the tibial nerve (in association with type IIIC tibial fracture) is also a functional liability significant enough to warrant amputation (42–44).

Expedient amputation of a massively traumatized limb, even if it appears salvageable, may also be necessary in the multiply injured patient who cannot tolerate the reconstructive time or metabolic demands of the reconstruction. This is an extremely difficult judgment that is highly individualized and impossible to quantitate.

Type of Fixation

The type of stabilization may also influence the outcome. External fixation has been associated with frequent complications such as pin tract infection and nonunion (45); thus, alternative methods have been considered. At the present time, there is a trend toward immediate and definitive internal fixation, the unreamed nail being the preferred implant for tibial fractures (46,47). Plating seems to be a viable alternative and has a least some theoretical advantages over nailing (48). Worlock et al (49) have shown experimentally a significantly reduced risk of infection with stable plating compared with solid intramedullary nailing.

Indeed, intramedullary nailing or plating is only applicable when the fracture is covered by an adequate soft tissue envelope. If the wound has entered a subacute, colonized phase, internal fixation becomes hazardous (23). Changing to internal fixation after a period of external fixation may be a cause of infection and should therefore be avoided or timed properly (50) (Table 16-3).

TABLE 16-3 Choice of Fracture Fixation

External Fixation	Internal Fixation
Bone comminuted	Intact soft tissue
Severe contamination	Fracture accessible with minimum stripping (in open injuries)
Long delay from injury to OR	Clean wounds
If unable to achieve wound closure in a timely fashion	Internal fixation possible
If second look and debridement is required	Closure possible
If bone or soft tissue is devascularized	Bridge or span plate: can be used with bone graft after wound closure (i.e., flap)
Major soft tissue defects	Intraarticular injuries—absolute indications even in open injuries

From German G, Sherman R, Levin LS. *Decision-making in reconstructive surgery upper-extremity*. New York: Springer-Verlag; 1999, with permission.

TECHNIQUES OF WOUND CLOSURE

After adequate debridement, it may be possible, as in minor hand injuries, to close the wound primarily. This will be done rarely if ever in cases of open fractures because of the danger of contamination or the need for a second-look debridement.

The second rung in the reconstructive ladder is delayed primary closure. This method is considered in cases in which there is uncertainty of the adequacy of the primary debridement and is usually done after the initial edema subsides. Healing by secondary intention refers to epithelialization and wound contraction. This technique may also be applied to abrasions, avoiding the need for skin grafts.

The next level of reconstruction is use of a STSG, either meshed or unmeshed.

Skin Grafting

The skin is composed of dermis and epidermis, which make up approximately 80% to 95% and 5% to 20% of the skin, respectively. The dermis contains sebaceous glands, most of which are appendages of hair follicles (51). Sweat glands and hair follicles are mostly located in the deep dermis. These skin appendages are lined with epithelium, thus allowing for reepithelialization after removal of the epidermis and part of the dermis, as in superficial burns or the harvesting of an STSG.

Although sebaceous glands continue to function after skin grafting, sweat glands (both apocrine and eccrine) undergo temporary loss of nervous control. As a result, newly grafted skin may be dry, requiring moisturizing with common over-the-counter preparations.

Any wound with a full-thickness loss of skin may be considered for skin grafting. Such defects may heal spontaneously but, because of the lack of dermal appendages, do so through the process of contraction and reepithelialization from the wound periphery. When healed, these wounds have skin lacking the normal microanatomy found in native skin. Specifically, there are no rete pegs, epidermal projections into the dermis that anchor the two layers of skin together. Such a wound is relatively unstable in terms of long-term durability. Allowing spontaneous healing of a full-thickness wound is therefore appropriate only for small defects and in certain larger defects, where the contraction process will not distort critical anatomy or cause a functional disturbance such as a joint contracture.

In evaluating a wound for possible skin grafting, the surgeon must assess the adequacy of the wound bed. The process of graft healing will require ingrowth of vessels from the wound, and so relatively avascular tissue provides a poor bed for skin grafting. Exposed bone, tendon, nerve and cartilage, necrotic tissue, and devascularized fat are examples of tissues that provide a poor wound bed. Conversely, well-vascularized tissues such as muscle, periosteum, perichondrium, fascia, healthy fat, epitenon, and dura will all accept skin grafts (Fig. 16-9).

STSGs have less dermis than full-thickness skin grafts (FTSGs), thus allowing more of the natural wound healing process of contraction to occur. They also have less metabolic demand relative to FTSGs and so are more likely to "take" on a vascularly compromised wound. FTSGs are thicker, more durable in the long term, may carry hair follicles allowing future hair growth, allow limited wound contraction, and retain more of their natural donor area pigmentation. In general, FTSGs retain greater sensation than do STSGs.

Because one can expect regeneration of epidermis after harvesting of a STSG, donor sites can be rather large. Despite the spontaneous regeneration noted in these donor sites, there is still a permanent scar, usually noted by subtle textural changes. In certain ethnic groups with a propensity for hypertrophic scarring, however, strict attention must be paid to the location of split-thickness skin harvest. In some Asian or African-American patients, for example, scalp skin may be preferable to thigh skin for this reason. The most common donor sites for STSGs, in order of cosmetic preference, are buttock and thigh, abdomen, back, scalp, chest wall, and arms. Harvesting of a FTSG requires closure of the donor wound, because spontaneous reepithelialization is not possible. As a rule, FTSGs tend to be small and are usually used for reconstruction in the foot or hand.

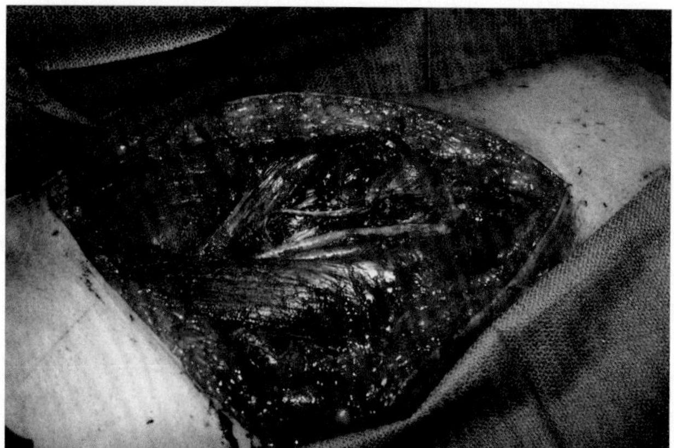

A

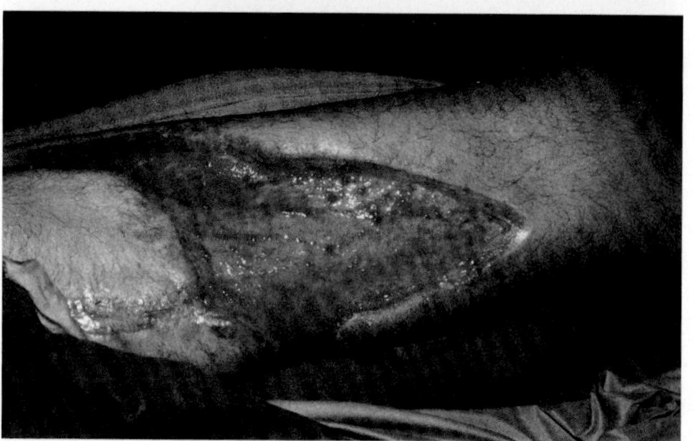

B

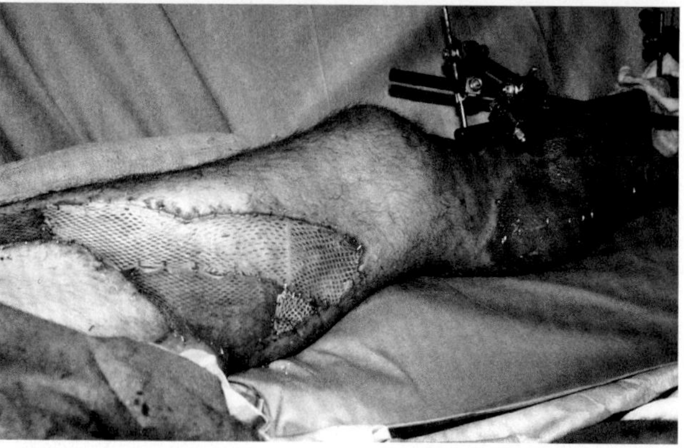

C

FIGURE 16-9 A. Crush injury to the thigh. **B.** The patient was treated with a wound vacuum assisted closure and developed an excellent granulation base. **C.** The wound was closed with mesh split-thickness skin graft.

The healing of skin grafts has been described as a two-step process. Initially, the graft survives by imbibition of wound bed exudate. After approximately 48 hours, new blood vessels begin to sprout from the wound bed and grow up into the graft. Capillaries from the wound bed either connect with graft vessels, a process known as inosculation, or form new vascular channels within the graft, revascularization. During these processes, fibrin and collagen are also assisting in forming a cohesive bond between graft and bed. By the fifth to seventh postgraft day, a skin graft is usually adherent and vascularized, creating a so-called take.

Technique of Skin Grafting

Before skin grafting, the wound must be adequately prepared. All nonviable material must be removed sharply so that the wound bed is left with healthy, preferably bleeding, tissue. A curette is quite useful in this regard. Adequate hemostasis is imperative; however, overuse of the electric cautery creates a charred wound that is unlikely to foster inosculation and revascularization of the graft. Most often after debridement, the wound is elevated and covered with a sponge soaked in normal saline. Usually by the time the graft has been harvested, bleeding from the wound bed has ceased. Topical hemostatic agents such as thrombin may be used to help control the bleeding.

Equipment needed to perform a STSG consists of a dermatome, mesher, mineral oil, suture or staples, and dressings appropriate for both graft and donor site. Dermatomes have evolved from hand-held knives (e.g., Humby knife), to electric and gas-powered devices able to precisely harvest skin of various thicknesses. Most dermatomes require insertion of a disposable blade and have two adjustments that are made by the surgeon. Thickness, measured in thousandths of an inch, is usually set with a dial on the dermatome itself. For most cases, graft thickness is between 12/1000 and 17/1000 of an inch. The clinical setting will dictate an appropriate thickness. One must balance survival (short and long term) of the graft with donor site healing. Therefore, in an elderly patient with "thin" skin a thinner STSG (12/1000 to 13/1000) may be chosen, whereas in a younger patient a thicker STSG (15/1000 to 16/1000) may be preferable. The surgeon must also choose an appropriate width of skin to harvest. This adjustment is made either on the dermatome itself or dependent on an attached cover placed over the blade before harvesting.

The donor site is prepared by first removing any prep solution or other foreign materials from the skin. Mineral oil is applied liberally to both skin and dermatome to aid in gliding. The dermatome is turned on, placed at a 45-degree angle with the skin, and advanced firmly to prevent slippage. As the graft is being harvested, punctate bleeding from a white dermal bed should be seen. If subcutaneous fat is noted, harvesting should be stopped immediately, the graft replaced, and a new donor site chosen with readjustment of the thickness setting on the dermatome. After an adequate amount of skin has been harvested, the dermatome is removed from the skin sharply. The donor area is temporarily covered with a hemostatic agent (local anesthesia with epinephrine or topical thrombin is a popular choice). Donor site dressings will be reviewed later in this discussion.

The skin graft is then meshed for two reasons. First, STSG failure is usually secondary to hematoma formation beneath it, and meshing of the skin will allow drainage postoperatively. Second, when a large amount of graft is needed, meshing will also allow expansion of the graft so that a given piece of skin can cover a larger area. Most popular meshers require placement of the skin on a "card" chosen for the ratio of mesh. Most grafts are meshed at a ratio of 1 to 1.5. Disadvantages of meshing mostly relate to the aesthetics of the healed meshed skin, which retains its meshed appearance in the long term. As a result, grafts to the face and hand, or any other visible location of concern to the patient, are merely "pie-crusted"—multiple holes are placed with a no. 15 scalpel blade to facilitate postoperative drainage.

The STSG is placed carefully on the already prepared graft site and held in place with skin clips applied carefully, first at the periphery. Additional clips are placed in the central portions to encourage adherence. Absorbable or nonabsorbable suture material may be used to affix the graft to the bed, but they offer no advantage in terms of results and take significantly longer to apply. Studies have noted success using fibrin glue (derived from autologous plasma) as an aid in graft adherence (52). The glue was found to improve graft survival, reduce blood loss, and obviate the need for meshing, thus producing a more esthetic result (53).

A myriad of different dressings have been used for the graft site, all with the goal of providing a moist, antimicrobial environment that will facilitate ingrowth of vessels into the graft. A common technique for dressing the graft employs a mixture of acetic acid and glycerin (modified Bunnell's solution) to soak dressings. A layer of nonadherent gauze soaked in this mixture is first placed on the graft. The next layer applied depends on the topography of the graft bed. In a relatively concave bed, there will be a natural tendency for the graft to adhere tightly to the bed and a layer of 4 × 4 gauze soaked in the above mixture followed by a soft, dry, noncompressible gauze wrap is all that is required. In graft beds with hills and valleys, cotton balls soaked in the above mixture and laid carefully in the crevices of the bed will create a custom "moulage" type of dressing that encourages adherence of the graft throughout the bed. Additional 4 × 4 gauze layers and the dry gauze wrap are then placed over this. With small grafts or grafts in areas where a gauze wrap is not logistically possible, a bolster-type bandage may be fashioned with silk or nylon sutures placed at the wound periphery and tied over the dressing to help encourage graft adherence. For grafts placed in a highly mobile area such as the distal extremity, splinting the limb to limit movement may be appropriate as well. Care should be taken to pad the splint so as to prevent any irritation of normal skin under it. After the graft has been properly dressed, the temporary dressing on the donor site is removed. Careful attention must be paid to the donor site, because patients will often complain of more discomfort in this area than at the graft site. A detailed discussion of donor site dressings can be found in a 1991 review (54). In certain patients, any excess STSG should be replaced on the donor site. This will allow rapid (often 3-day) healing of the area of replaced graft.

Treatment of Donor Sites

In general, smaller donor sites should be dressed with semi-occlusive or totally occlusive dressings. This includes clear films (Opsite, Tegaderm) and hydrocolloid dressings (Duoderm). These materials used on a small donor site allow relatively pain-free donor site healing with minimal care, low cost, and low infection rates. When using a clear film, wound exudate (common to any open wound) must be aspirated for the first few days to prevent leakage. A simple way to do this involves prepping the most dependent part of the dressing with alcohol, aspirating tangentially (so as not to prick the skin surface), and then "tire-patching" the dressing with a small IV-size piece of film. In larger donor sites the amount of wound exudate becomes excessive, making these types of dressings impractical. For these wounds semi-open dressings such as Xeroform are preferred. Although slightly more painful, they also allow for donor site healing with minimal care, low cost, and low infection rates.

The technique for a FTSG requires little in the way of instrumentation or equipment. The recipient site is prepared as described above. An appropriate donor site is chosen, and a template is often used to allow harvest of precisely the correct amount of skin. Because of the small size of FTSGs, local anesthesia is commonly employed during their harvesting. FTSGs are almost always used on the face or hands, and thus they are rarely meshed; rather they are "pie-crusted" to facilitate postoperative drainage. The donor site is closed carefully in layers after hemostasis is achieved. After harvest the FTSG is defatted so that only dermis remains on the surface being applied to the wound bed. It is then placed on its recipient bed and held in place with absorbable (e.g., 5-0 chromic) or nonabsorbable (e.g., 5-0 silk or nylon) sutures. Additional sutures can be placed in the midportion. Most FTSGs are dressed with nonadherent gauze, antibiotic ointment (e.g., Bacitracin), and moistened cotton or gauze held in place with a bolster, tie-over dressing.

In addition to autogenous STSGs, certain skin substitutes can be used to provide temporary or even permanent dermal substrates for skin grafting in wounds that otherwise would have required more complex procedures such as flaps. Bioengineered manufactured skin substrates such as Alloderm or Integra have been recent additions to soft tissue treatments that have significant benefits. Alloderm is a dermal collagen matrix that can be placed on an open wound bed that may not be able to take a skin graft. The inoculation of the dermal substrate allows the dermis to regenerate for subsequent skin grafting. Alloderm has been reported for use in diabetic and dysvascular feet as a way to promote healing. It has been the authors' experience that these do not work as well as Integra, which is a bilaminate skin substitute, that has been very effective for wounds that are not suitable for skin grafting but would require higher rungs on the reconstructive ladder for closure, such as a local flap or free flap. Integra is an excellent tool for small wounds or wounds that almost have a dermal substrate but are not yet ready for grafting. Integra can be applied over tendons that are denuded of paratenon, or in cases in which dermis will be required for further reconstruction.

Recently there has been renewed interest in the use of silver. Silver was first used in antiquity, and several products have been developed (e.g., Acticoat) that are silver-impregnated dressings effective against a broad range of bacteria, including aerobic and anaerobic, gram- negative and gram-positive bacteria, yeast, fungi, and viruses. The silver content in these dressings also has anti-inflammatory property that may promote healing as well (Fig. 16-10) (49,55).

When the Integra dressing has been applied to a debrided wound, after 10 to 14 days, the outer laminate (Silastic membrane) is removed, usually revealing a neodermis that is suitable for STSG. Integra, in conjunction with the wound VAC, has been a very effective way to promote a dermal base for skin grafting, obviating the need for more complex procedures such as free-tissue transfer or local regional flaps. Integra is not suitable for placement over large areas of exposed bone cortex, but if a small area required periosteum or dermal substitution, Integra could be used to accomplish this. The treatment requires the cortex to be burred down with a chilled high-speed burr, to achieve punctate bleeding from the haversian system. Integra is then placed over the area with the hope that vascular penetration into the artificial dermis will occur. After 2 weeks, the outer membrane of the Integra can be removed and the neodermis that is created can then be skin grafted. We have successful experience with doing this in cases in which patients were not candidates for free-tissue transfer and with small exposed bone surface areas. The total dimensions should be no greater than 3 cm^2 of exposed bone.

Aftercare and Long-Term Issues

Patients undergoing skin grafting usually do not complain about significant amounts of pain in the grafted area. Mild analgesics such as acetaminophen with codeine will suffice in most cases. The first 3 to 5 days after grafting are the most critical for graft survival, because this is the time when inosculation and revascularization occur. Therefore, it is often prudent with lower extremity grafts to keep patients hospitalized and immobile at strict bed rest with the limb elevated during this period. Many reconstructive surgeons will also place the patient on prophylactic subcutaneous heparin during the time of strict immobilization to prevent deep vein thrombosis. For patients with grafts to either the head and neck or upper extremity, elevation and rest of the affected area as an outpatient is acceptable.

The use of prophylactic antibiotics is controversial, but most reconstructive surgeons will give them at least preoperatively and often for up to 2 to 5 days postoperatively. For a clean wound a first-generation cephalosporin (e.g., Ancef, Kefzol) may be used. In chronic wounds that may have been previously infected, culture-specific antibiotics are appropriate. The dressing on the graft site is usually changed on the fifth to seventh postoperative day or earlier if there are signs or symptoms of infection or hematoma. A FTSG will usually appear quite ecchymotic in the first 7 to 10 days; STSGs may appear paler. In

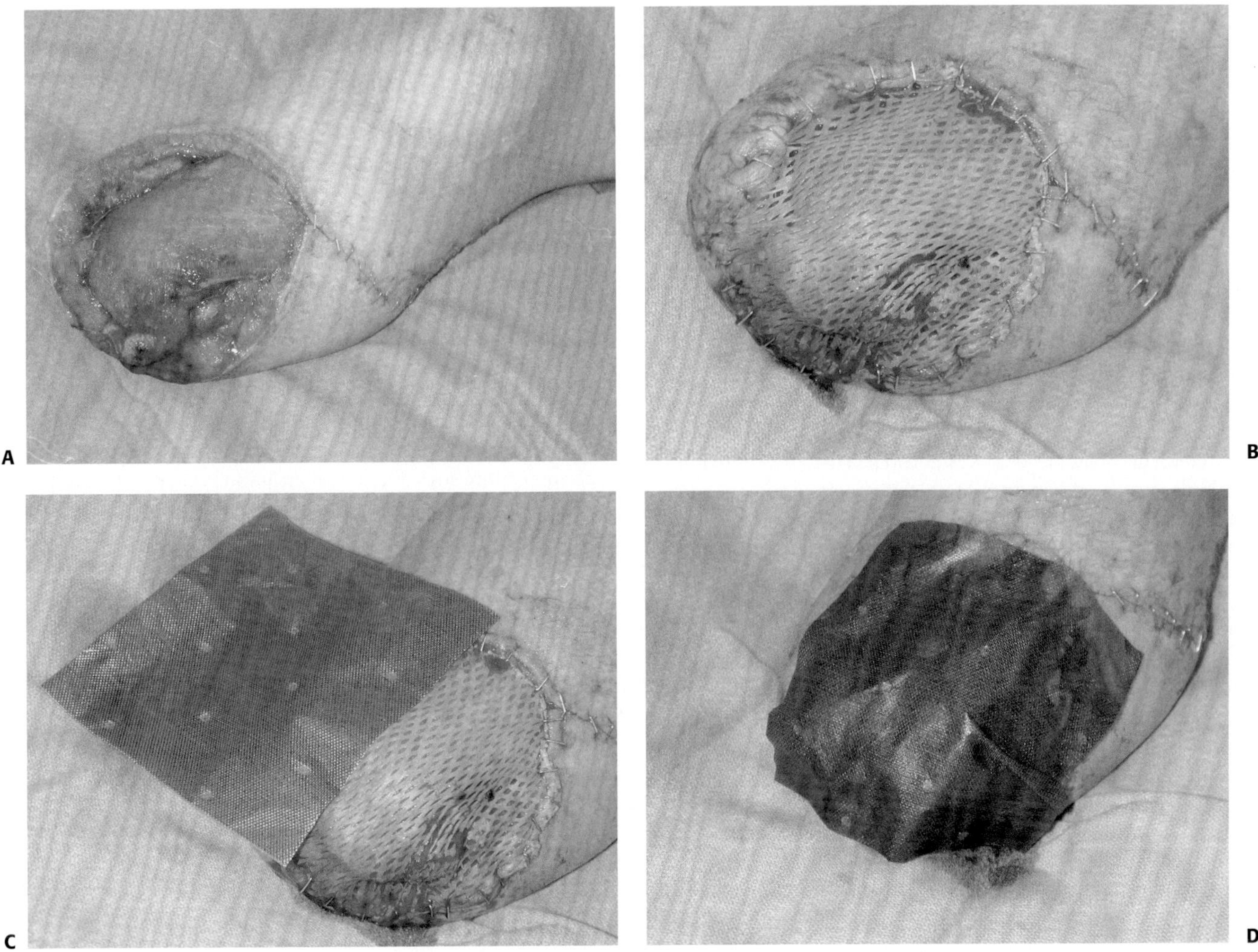

FIGURE 16-10 **A.** This 14-year-old boy was involved in an all-terrain vehicle accident that resulted in a traumatic below-knee amputation. **B.** A split-thickness skin graft has been applied to the wound on the residual limb. **C,D.** The Acticoat silver-impregnated dressing is applied over the skin graft to provide an antimicrobial barrier.

most cases an initial assessment of the take can be made at this point. If the graft is dry, Xeroform gauze and a light bandage are placed over the graft site. For grafts of the head and neck, antibiotic ointment (e.g., Bacitracin) without a bandage may be used. In certain situations the graft may appear moist. In this case, or if there are any signs of infection, the dressing should be changed twice daily, using 0.25% acetic acid–soaked gauze. The graft will often respond favorably to this regimen, effectively saving an otherwise doomed graft.

By the second week, a healthy graft may only need a dressing for protective purposes. The newly healed skin is viable but sensitive, especially to abrasive forces. Newly grafted skin may be dry as a result of the loss of innervation of the sweat glands. Application of an antibiotic ointment in the first 3 weeks, followed by any common skin moisturizer after 3 weeks is helpful. Clips used to secure STSGs should be removed in the first 5 to 10 days to prevent overgrowth of surrounding skin. Sutures used to secure FTSGs should also be removed at this time.

In addition to moisturizing, care should be taken to keep freshly skin grafted areas clean. Sun exposure should be avoided, as with any fresh scar. Patients should be reassured that the initial redness of a STSG donor site will fade over time.

The most common cause of skin graft failure is hematoma beneath the graft, preventing revascularization. Other causes include inadequate immobilization, bacterial contamination, dependency, and incorrect graft orientation (placing the epidermis side down). If a hematoma or infection is identified in the first 3 to 5 days, drainage of the hematoma and local treatment of the infection may be all that is needed for partial or complete graft salvage. As always, attention to detail can help prevent most of the common causes of failure.

FLAPS

A flap is tissue transferred from one anatomic site to another. Vascularity of the transferred tissue is maintained by nutrient vessels within the flap pedicle. The pedicle may either remain attached at its origin or be divided during the transfer and reanastomosed to recipient vessels using microsurgical techniques. Microsurgical transfer of tissue is also known as a free flap (autologous tissue transplantation). Flaps are useful to close defects too large for primary closure and where skin grafts are inadequate. Flaps can contain more than one type of tissue and are named based on the tissues they contain. Examples of compound flaps are fasciocutaneous flaps, which contain skin and underlying fascia, and musculocutaneus flaps, which contain skin, fascia, and muscle. Rotation flaps, such as muscle, skin, and fascia, or a combination, add much-needed vascularized tissue, obliterate dead space, and help to close the wound without tension. When even these options are limited because of wound location or regional donor site deficiencies, free flaps must be considered. The most complex reconstruction employs free-tissue transfer.

Muscle can be transferred into adjacent defects if its native vascular supply is preserved. The utility of any given muscle flap is limited by the size of the muscle and the length of its vascular pedicle and hence the distance it can be transferred. The defect, both functional and cosmetic, created by the muscle transfer must also be considered. Muscle flaps transfer richly vascularized and very immunologically active tissue into wounds that are ischemic or infected (56–58). The bulk of muscle flaps allows contour defects to be resurfaced. Skin can be transferred with the underlying muscle.

Bone can be also used for reconstruction as a free graft or a vascularized graft, alone or together with other tissues such as skin or muscle. Since the development of microvascular techniques, bone grafts from various sites can be transferred with their intact blood supply. Vascularized bone grafts have proved to be advantageous in clinical settings in which nonvascularized bone grafts have been unsatisfactory.

Classification of Muscle Flaps

The classification of muscle type is based on five patterns of muscle circulation (12). A muscle for free-tissue transfer must be able to survive on one vascular pedicle that is dominant and that will support the entire muscle mass. Classification is as follows:

Type 1: one vascular pedicle (extensor digitorum brevis, tensor fascia latae)

Type 2: dominant pedicle and minor pedicles (abductor hallucis longus, gracilis)

Type 3: two dominant pedicles (rectus abdominis, serratus anterior)

Type 4: segmental vascular pedicles (none)

Type 5: one dominant and secondary vascular pedicles (latissimus dorsi, pectoralis major, pectoralis minor)

Unclassified tissue transfers include fillet flaps, as well as combination flaps such as the latissimus dorsi–serratus anterior muscle flap. This is based on one dominant pedicle (thoracodorsal artery).

Pedicle muscle flaps can be local or distal. Gastrocnemius and soleus muscles are examples of local flaps used to cover defects of the leg. A groin flap represents the distal flap group and can cover defects of the dorsum of the hand that need vascularized tissue. Although all muscle transfers can be harvested as the muscle component alone, not all muscles can be harvested with reliable skin overlying it. Examples of muscles with unreliable large skin paddles include the gracilis and pectoralis minor muscles. Including skin with the muscular transfer allows for flap monitoring and provides color and texture match in an extremity that requires muscle for bulk in addition to cutaneous coverage. A musculocutaneous flap is used for a salvage procedure such as to repair an amputation site or a decubitus ulcer with filet flaps from the foot. Here the unique properties of the skin are more durable than a STSG placed over the muscle.

Fasciocutaneous flaps are another option for coverage of defects, especially in cases in which there is no need for bulk. For example, the saphenous fasciocutaneous flap perfused by posteromedial perforators from the saphenous artery may cover defects in the proximal third of the leg. Fascial flaps can be used as pedicled flaps as well as free flaps.

Local Flaps

Gastrocnemius

Use of one head of the gastrocnemius as either a muscle or a musculocutaneous flap has proved to be highly effective in the management of knee and upper leg wounds. The constant dominant proximal vascular pedicle that runs down the length of the muscle makes it one of the most reliable flaps in the body. The muscle can be raised easily, quickly, and safely if attention is paid to the relevant technical and anatomic details. Transposition of the medial head of the gastrocnemius results in little or no functional deficit, provided that the soleus and the lateral head of the gastrocnemius are left intact and functioning.

The gastrocnemius is the most superficial muscle of the posterior calf and consists of two separates heads and extends between the knee and the heel. Each head is considered a separate unit for the purpose of the flap design. The medial head is longer and its muscular fibers extend more inferiorly. Both muscle heads are located superficial to the plantaris and soleus muscles. The distal soleus tendon unites with the gastrocnemius to form a common tendon of insertion. This is a type 1 muscle, and the medial and lateral sural arteries provide independent blood supply to the two muscle heads. These vessels arise from the popliteal artery above the level of the knee joint, and the length of the pedicle is 6 cm. The position of the muscle in the leg can readily be determined by inspection and palpation in most instances. One entire muscle belly or the other is chosen depending on the clinical situation.

The medial head can support a skin flap that extends in width from the medial border of the tibia to the posterior midline of the calf. The point of rotation is the middle popliteal fossa near the origin of the muscle and its blood supply. The skin overlying the muscle and often a "random" extension of the skin and subcutaneous tissue distal to the muscle flap may be included. The lateral gastrocnemius supports a skin flap of smaller dimensions. The skin flap can be extended to within 10 to 15 cm of the lateral malleolus.

The medial gastrocnemius is dissected through a posterior midline incision. The sural nerve and the lesser saphenous vein are two key landmarks that are seen superficial to the muscle belly and preserved. The muscle fascia is split, and the junction of the two heads is incised. Blunt dissection in the plane between the gastrocnemius and the soleus is gently done with the finger. The superficial dissection is then performed, and the muscle is transected distally with a cuff of tendon attached for use in fixation to the wound edge. The tunnel through which the muscle is passed should be of adequate size so as not to constrict the blood supply to the flap. When the flap is elevated as a musculocutaneous flap, the peritenon over the exposed soleus fascia and Achilles tendon should be carefully preserved to provide a suitable bed for the application of a skin graft. In most instances the muscle or musculocutaneous flap will be used as a transposition flap to cover a local defect (59,60). Incising the muscle fascia may improve the contour and increase the length of the muscle available to cover a defect (61). The appearance of the flap may be improved by placing the skin paddle over the distal edge of the muscle and limiting its dimensions to those required by the defect. This flap can be used as an advancement flap to cover upper tibial defects or as a fasciocutaneous flap to cover an amputation stump, and the medial head can be used as a cross leg flap (62,63).

Soleus

The soleus muscle provides several reliable flaps that are frequently the first choice for repair of defects between the knee and the ankle. These defects include exposed bone or open fractures of the long bones or malleoli, exposed internal fixation devices, exposed tendons, stasis ulcer, and unstable scars (64–66).

The value and versatility of the soleus-based flaps result from the following anatomic features: the soleus is the largest, longest muscle beyond the knee, it extends distally on the leg, and its dual neurovascular supply permits splitting of the muscle into two units with musculocutaneous and fasciocutaneous territories. The blood supply is based on the two proximal branches of the posterior tibial artery and venae comitantes and on minor pedicles, which are the four segmental branches of the posterior tibial artery and veins. The distal segmental vascular pedicles permit reversal of soleus segments for distal leg and ankle defects (55), but reversed soleus flaps have been reported to have high failure rates, and their use is reserved for secondary salvage procedures (67). The failure rate may be reduced by transferring only the distal half of the muscle on two distal vascular pedicles and by using only the medial hemisoleus belly (68).

Saphenous Vein Flap

This flap may be used to cover tibial defects either acutely or at a later stage after the fixation of the fractures has been achieved. It also may be used for dense adherent scars over the tibia, as a prelude to secondary bone surgery, or to hasten union in slowly healing of fractures. In addition it has been found to be extremely useful in coverage of the knee joint.

The saphenous vein flap is a unipedicled venous flap based on the saphenous vein in the upper two thirds of the leg (69,70). The flap consists of a rectangular fasciocutaneous island with the vertical axis along the vein. It can be based only on a long patent saphenous vein, and it is preferable not to use this flap when there are adherent, deep scars in the area of the surface markings of the vein. The saphenous venous flap can be designed as a 1:3 proportional rectangle, the vein remaining in the middle along the length of the fasciocutaneous island. The medial extension of the flap usually stops around the area of the subcutaneous portion of the tibia, which is approximately 3 to 5 cm from the long saphenous vein in the upper two thirds of the leg. The flap dimensions are 8 cm in width and 24 cm in length and cover defects by medial, lateral, or posterior transfer of the saphenous venous island (Fig. 16-11).

Free Flaps

Free flaps include isolated transfers, composite tissue transfers, and functioning free muscle transfers. Structural transfers such as vascularized bone grafts or toe transplantation for hand reconstruction are also included in this group of procedures. Specific tissue transfers such as vascular and neural grafts are also an integral part of the microsurgical reconstruction armamentarium. Although such "grafts" do not involve large amounts of tissue, they are considered tissue transplantation and thus included as a free-tissue transfer.

Microsurgery for extremity reconstruction began more than 3 decades ago with the introduction of the operating microscope for anastomosis of blood vessels, described by Jacobson and Suarez (71). Microsurgical repair of digital arteries and digital replantation began in the 1960s (72,73), and microsurgical composite tissue transplantation began in the 1970s. Microsurgeons expanded their efforts from achieving tissue survival to include the improvement of function and appearance in the 1980s. In the 1990s, the emphasis shifted to outcome. Today, composite transplantation or free-tissue transfer routinely not only provides coverage but also facilitates function.

The development of reconstructive microsurgery and the vital role it plays in orthopaedic surgery is credited to the efforts of many investigators who identified new donor sites, expanded indications for free-tissue transfer, and constantly improved microsurgical techniques. The contributions of Mathes and Nahai in summarizing the clinical application for muscle and musculocutaneous flaps should be acknowledged (9,12), as well as the

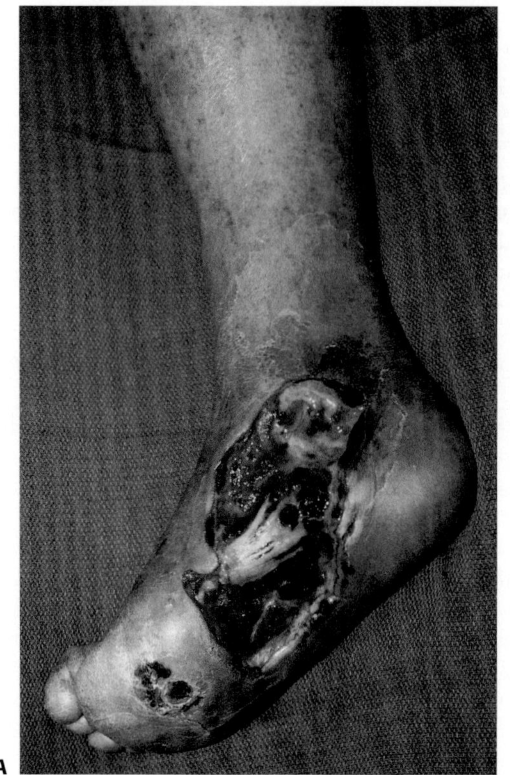

A

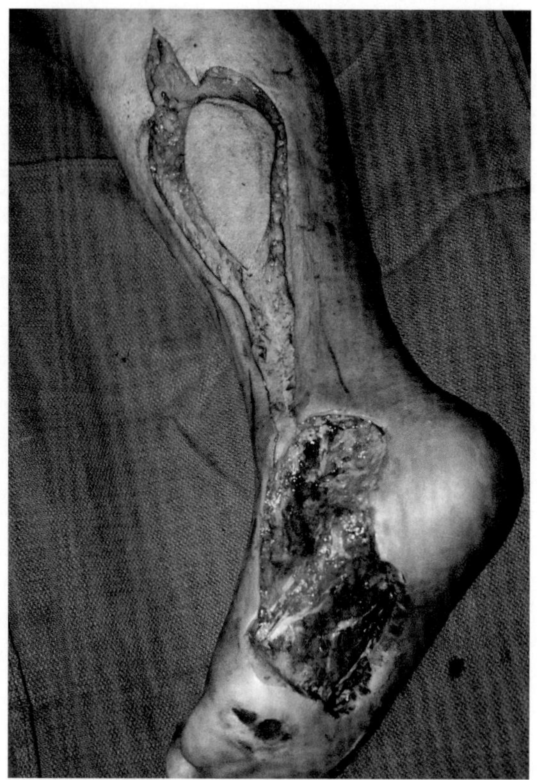

B

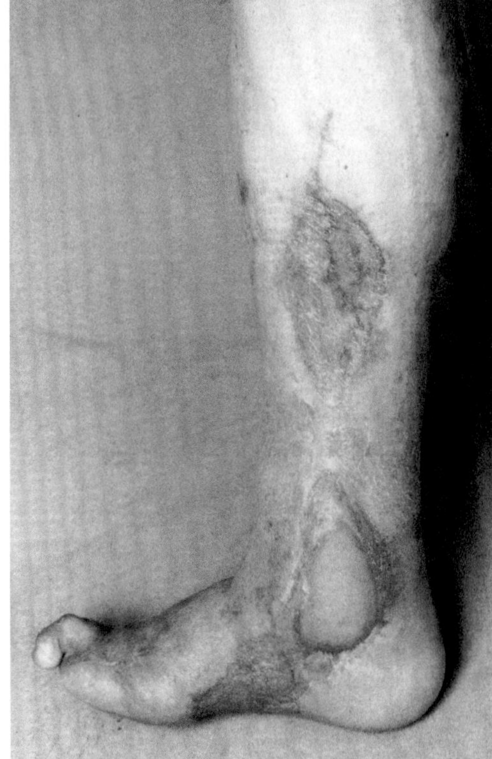

C

FIGURE 16-11 A crush injury to the foot in a patient with diabetes and peripheral vascular disease. He was not a candidate for free-tissue transfer. **A.** Wound before debridement. **B.** Wound after debridement and harvest of saphenous vein flap. **C.** The wound healed with coverage of the exposed medial malleolus. Donor area was covered with split-thickness skin grafts.

pioneering work of Ian Taylor, Harry Buncke, Harold Kleinert, Robert Acland, Bernard O'Brien, and Fu Chan Wei.

Surgeons perform reconstructive procedures in all fields of orthopaedic surgery. For example, the simultaneous management of fractures and associated soft tissue injury, the so-called orthoplastic approach, is now accepted treatment for extremity trauma. It allows for optimal repair processes to take place for bone and soft tissue while avoiding the adverse sequelae of failed fixation, sepsis, and ultimately amputation. Delicate soft tissue handling and an awareness of the blood supply to muscle, fascia, and skin will prevent the orthopaedist from inadvertently damaging tissue, which may result in necrosis and exposure of either bone or implants that require coverage with free flaps. Expeditious repair of soft tissue is important in the care of injured extremities. It facilitates further reconstruction, such as bone grafting or tendon transfers.

A through understanding of free-tissue transfer includes understanding the rationale for tissue transplantation, the timing of the transplant, and the transplant that should be selected. The orthopaedic surgeon should have an understanding of the current techniques of reconstructive microsurgery and should be able to obtain appropriate reconstructive consultation for patients.

Sir Harold Gillies, considered to be one of the fathers of modern reconstructive plastic surgery, used the motto "Replace like with like." The interpretation of this principle with regard to free-tissue transfer is that the reconstructive microsurgeon transplants autogenously vascularized tissue into defects that are the result of trauma, tumor, infection, or congenital defects.

Free-tissue transplantation should be considered for any tissue deficit that cannot be treated by an adjacent tissue rearrangement, skin grafting, or local pedicle flaps. Free-tissue transplantation is selected in instances in which there are "composite deficiencies" such as skin and bone or muscle and skin. Furthermore, free-tissue transplantation may be considered for functional restoration that obviates the need for tendon transfer or nerve grafting, as in brachial plexus injuries, in which free muscle transplantation is performed for functional muscle restoration.

The highest rung on the reconstructive ladder uses free-tissue transfer, possibly in combination with lower rungs of the ladder, such as skin closure, skin grafting, or rotational flaps. An example would be the use of a soleus myoplasty in the middle third of the tibia, as well as requirements for distal third coverage. A free muscle flap such as the latissimus dorsi could be considered in such a case.

INDICATIONS FOR FREE-TISSUE TRANSFER OF THE UPPER EXTREMITY: TRAUMA AND SEPSIS

One of the main advantages of free flaps for hand reconstruction is that they allow early mobilization of the hand following injury. This decreases limb edema and postoperative stiffness. Free flaps allow the possibility of composite tissue reconstruction in one stage, by transferring various combinations of nerve, bone, tendon, skin, and muscle at once. Free flaps can be contoured and cut to precisely fit any defect. Most importantly, the microvascular free tissue transfers have enabled us to adhere more closely to one of the basic principles of any reconstruction effort, as set forth by Gillies, by allowing us to reconstruct these defects with tissue that is most similar to the lost tissue.

Patients who undergo mutilating upper extremity trauma often have the greatest need for free-tissue transfers. Trauma to the hand requires resurfacing using skin, muscle, or free fascial flaps. In the treatment of upper extremity trauma, patients who cannot be treated by conventional techniques such as skin grafting, local flaps, or distant flaps are candidates for free-tissue transfer. It is desirable, when possible, to import tissue rather than use island pedicle flaps that will further compromise upper extremity vascularity. For example, the radial forearm flap, if used for dorsal hand coverage, renders an already-compromised limb more compromised with the use of an island pedicle flap. This requires sacrifice of the radial artery.

For upper extremity sepsis with bone infection involving large intercalary segments either in the humerus or the forearm, the vascularized fibula transplant is an excellent method for reconstruction. Soft tissue sepsis can usually be controlled and treated with local debridement and grafts unless there is massive necrosis requiring coverage, in which case a free skin or muscle flap is selected.

A large selection of free tissue transfers for hand reconstruction is available. One example of the most commonly used flaps in hand reconstruction is the lateral arm flap; this is a fasciocutaneous flap that is a good choice for coverage of either dorsal or palmar defects. It is thin, easy to dissect, and associated with few complications (74).

MICRONEURAL RECONSTRUCTION OF THE UPPER EXTREMITY

Peripheral nerve repair and brachial plexus reconstruction following injuries have evolved parallel to the development of microsurgery. In many cases of peripheral nerve injury, primary repair may not be possible for many reasons, including direct loss of nerve tissue or retraction of nerve stumps following a delay in repair. Primary repair of the gap under tension should always be avoided because it hinders regeneration and reduces blood flow to the repaired nerve (75). Nerve allografting is possible now because of the advances in immunosuppression, although clinical application of peripheral nerve allografting remains under experimental investigation (76).

Different procedures using microsurgical techniques have been described for brachial plexus reconstruction. Some of these techniques include nerve crossing procedures, free muscle transfer, and more recently a combined technique of double free muscle and multiple nerve transfers (77). The transferred muscles, include latissimus dorsi, rectus abdominis, and gracilis. The gracilis muscle is considered to be the best option by many surgeons.

INDICATIONS FOR FREE-TISSUE TRANSFER OF THE LOWER EXTREMITY: TRAUMA AND SEPSIS

In recent years, increasing emphasis has been placed on open reduction and internal fixation in the management of fractures. The importance of proper soft tissue coverage to maintain the vascularity of fragments has also been emphasized. New methods of fractures fixation have evolved, such as indirect reduction and minimal internal fixation, which respect fracture biology and protect soft tissues.

The main indication for salvage of a severely damaged limb is that the limb has potentially intact sensibility. Nerve injuries do not preclude salvage but should be distal enough to permit the return of some function (primarily sensory) within a reasonable amount of time. Conversely, complex lower limb injuries with nerve damage are frequently considered for amputation, because the return to a functional status with a good prosthesis is usually more rapid (78). Advanced age should not be a contraindication to the microvascular limb salvage procedures. Careful preoperative patient evaluation and perioperative monitoring can effectively decrease morbidity and mortality rates to equal those for younger patients (79).

The choice of flap to be used for wound coverage is determined by the size of the wound, the type of tissue deficit, the state of the wound (the colonization, amount of cavitation), the location of the injury, and the length of the pedicle needed. The anastomosis should be done in a "safe zone," where recipient vessels have not been damaged by the initial trauma, either proximal or distal to the zone of injury. The term *zone of injury* refers to the inflammatory response of the soft tissue of the traumatized limb, which extends beyond the gross wound and results in perivascular changes in the blood vessels. These changes include increased friability of the vessels and increased perivascular scar tissue, which can contribute to a higher failure rate, especially in lower limb free-tissue transplantation, presumably because of a higher rate of microvascular thrombosis (80).

Most surgeons avoid the zone of injury by extensive proximal dissection of the recipient vascular pedicle, and some use vein grafts in lower limb reconstruction. Isenberg and Sherman (81) have demonstrated, however, that clinical acceptability of the recipient pedicle (vessel wall pliability and the quality of blood from the transected end of the vessel) was more important than the distance from the wound.

Reconstruction of the traumatized leg can be challenging, because both bony stabilization and soft tissue coverage are required for a successful functional outcome. Free-tissue transfer using microsurgical techniques has allowed surgeons to salvage traumatized extremities in patients who would formerly have required amputation (43,44,82).

OSTEOMYELITIS

Osteomyelitis is now a treatable disease. The Cierny-Mader (13) classification can be used as a guide to treatment. The management of dead space after sequestrectomy relies heavily on the technique of free-tissue transfer. Free muscle flaps provide coverage for the debrided bone and soft tissue, obliterate dead space, improve vascularity, and enhance leukocyte function (83–85).

Advances in skeletal reconstruction and fixation have improved the treatment of patients with osteomyelitis and large (greater than 6 cm) segmental bone defects. In the past, despite successful treatment of osteomyelitis, some patients have required amputation as a result of chronic nonunions. Now, once the bone infection is treated, vascularized bone transplants (86,87), or bone lengthening with the Ilizarov device facilitates reconstruction and provides structural stability for limb function (88).

Local muscles traditionally had been used to treat chronic osteomyelitis, and free flaps have been described more recently for this use. Local gastrocnemius and soleus muscle flaps are still used for coverage of smaller wounds on the upper and middle thirds of the leg, respectively. However, local muscle flaps will not reliably cover defects greater than 25 cm^2 or those on the distal third of the leg, ankle, or foot. For these defects, free-muscle transfers are preferred. The advantages of using the free muscle flaps such as latissimus dorsi (89), serratus anterior (90), and rectus abdominis (91) compared to the local pedicled muscle flaps are that they provide greater bulk (filling larger wounds), have longer pedicles (increasing flexibility in muscle positioning), and carry larger-diameter vessels (facilitating the microanastomoses).

Exposure of plates and screws may occur after open reduction with internal fixation of fractures. This occurs commonly when there is significant tissue edema, creating difficulty in skin closure. It affects the medial pretibial surface of the distal leg more often than the lateral region. Treatment in this situation usually requires free flap coverage (92,93).

TIMING OF FREE-TISSUE TRANSFER

The timing of the wound closure using microsurgical techniques is important. In severe injuries of the lower extremity with associated soft tissue defects, early aggressive wound debridement and soft tissue coverage with a free flap within 5 days was found to reduce postoperative infection, flap failure, nonunion, and chronic osteomyelitis (23,65). Godina (25) emphasized the pathophysiology of high-energy trauma and the importance of radical debridement and early tissue coverage within the first 72 hours.

Lister and Scheker (94) reported the first case of an emergency free flap transfer to the upper extremity in 1988, and they defined the emergency free flap as a "flap transfer performed either at the end of primary debridement or within 24 hours after the injury." Yaremchuk et al (50) recommended that flaps should be transferred between 7 and 14 days after injury and after several debridements. The argument in favor of this approach is that the zone of injury, which often may not be apparent at presentation, can be determined by serial debridements performed in the operating room over several days.

When deciding to perform a primary closure with a free flap, the surgeon should consider two factors: the presence of an exposed vital structure and the risk of infection. An exposed vital structure is defined as "one that will rapidly necrose if not covered by adequate soft tissue" (95). The decision of what constitutes a vital structure depends on circumstances. Tissues such as vessels, nerves, joint surfaces, tendons, and bone denuded of periosteum may lose function and create an environment resulting in infection when left exposed for long periods. In the decision-making process, the surgeon must consider the risk of leaving the vital structure exposed, its functional importance, and the probability of differential recovery of function considering primary or delayed primary coverage.

The risk of infection is the second important factor that should be considered because it may jeopardize the limb, the quality of the functional recovery, or the free flap. As the risk for infection increases, the wisdom of primary closure with a free flap is reduced. Debridement of the wound is the surgeon's most powerful tool to reduce the risk of infection. If radical debridement is not possible, it is not considered safe to do a primary free-flap transfer. Another perspective is that the capability to perform free-tissue transfer allows the surgeon increased freedom to perform radical debridement and may actually reduce the risk of infection (96). Factors such as the mechanism of injury, the elapsed time, and the degree of contamination of the wound should be considered in evaluating the risk of wound infection. In an acute, sharp, noncontaminated injury when closure would be routinely performed if there were no skin loss, there seems to be little reason not to consider an emergency free flap.

Free flaps can be categorized into two different types of transplants: isolated transplants of tissue such as muscle, skin, fascia, bone, or nerve and, more commonly, "composite replacement," which represents a more sophisticated flap. Composite flaps provide more than one function. Examples include myocutaneous, osteocutaneous, or innervated myocutaneous flaps. The type of tissue deficiency and surface requirements will determine the type of flap to be selected.

Tissue transplants are selected with regard to donor site morbidity, recipient site requirements, vascular pedicle length, and anticipated esthetic results. For example, a myocutaneous latissimus dorsi flap would not be transplanted to the dorsum of the foot because of its bulk and the fact that the donor tissue does not match the dorsum of the foot. Other flaps, such as an isolated skin flap (radial forearm flap or lateral arm flap), would be considered a better transplant. Similarly, to fill dead space after sequestrectomy of an infected tibia, a lateral arm flap, which is a small skin flap of approximately 5 by 7 cm, would not be selected because of its lack of bulk and the fact that muscle flaps rather than skin flaps are known to be more effective in the treatment of osteomyelitis. The use of a skin paddle with composite tissue transfers can be done either for contouring or as a monitor for perfusion of the flap.

The next consideration is whether or not dead space needs to be filled. If a flap were used purely for resurfacing, such as on the dorsum of the hand so that secondary tendon reconstruction can be performed, a large bulky flap would not be required. However, if there is significant dead space, a large muscle flap such as a latissimus dorsi flap should be considered. Osseous flaps are also used for structural defects such as intercalary bone defects resulting from trauma, tumor, or infection. If a vascularized bone flap is to be selected, the cross section of the bone defect and the available vascular supply both need to be taken into consideration.

Not all flaps are selected to replace missing tissue. There are instances in which tissue coverage exists but is insufficient in texture or quality. For example, a soft tissue envelope may need to be augmented, for example, when using a scapular flap to cover a knee as a last stage before a total knee replacement. There are free flaps that are performed for purely aesthetic reasons, such as the resurfacing of extremities. This is an unusual use of free-tissue transfer, and it is only done in special cases. A combination of the above factors is what determines free flap selection.

SELECTION OF TISSUE TRANSPLANTATION

Latissimus Dorsi

The latissimus dorsi is a workhorse for extremity coverage. This flap is based on the thoracodorsal artery as the major pedicle and on branches of the intercostals and lumbar arteries as secondary segmental branches. The pedicle length is 8 to 10 cm. The latissimus is innervated by the thoracodorsal nerve, which is a direct branch of the brachial plexus and enters the muscle 10 cm from the apex of the axilla. It is important to identify the anterior border of the muscle preoperatively by having the patient contract the muscle with the hand supported on the hip in a standing position. Marking of the posterior superior iliac spine and scapular tip is helpful. It is also wise to measure 10 cm from the apex of the axilla and place a mark at this site of the pedicle entrance into the muscle.

For harvest, the patient is placed in the lateral decubitus position with an axillary roll. Dissection is most easily accomplished beginning from the anterior border of the muscle, and this method allows early pedicle identification. Elevation of the skin flaps exposes the muscle origins, which are then released from the lumbosacral fascia and iliac crest. The large secondary perforating pedicle must be carefully identified and ligated to avoid troublesome bleeding. After pedicle identification, division of the serratus branch is completed and the entire flap is reflected toward the axilla. Before releasing the muscle peripherally, marking sutures should be placed along the long axis of the muscle every 5 cm if functional transfer is planned in order to allow adequate tension adjustment at the recipient site.

Once the flap is reflected toward the axilla and the arm is abducted, the pedicle may easily be seen entering the muscle. Proximal dissection is performed for the previously determined pedicle length and the muscle insertion is divided. The flap is now ready for transfer. Large suction drains should be left beneath the skin flaps and in the axilla to avoid postoperative hematoma or seroma problems. Some of the problems of this flap are that frequently there is difficulty elevating the flap simultaneously with donor site preparation, particularly if the flap is to be transferred to the upper extremity, and in obese patients the musculocutaneous flap may be excessively thick (Fig. 16-12).

Rectus Abdominis

The rectus can be harvested with the patient in a supine position. This vertically oriented muscle extends between the costal margin and the pubic region and is enclosed by the anterior and posterior rectus sheaths. It is a type 3 muscle (two dominant pedicles) based on the superior epigastric artery and vein and inferior epigastric artery and vein. The pedicle length is 5 to 7 cm superiorly and 8 to 10 cm inferiorly.

Each of the dominant pedicles supplies just over half of the muscle. There is an anastomosis between these vessels that is usually sufficient to support the nondominant half if one of the two pedicles is ligated. Because of the larger size and easier dissection of the inferior epigastric vessel, it is usually used for free-tissue transfer.

The motor innervation is supplied by segmental motor nerves from the seventh through twelfth intercostal nerves that enter the deep surface of the muscle at its middle to lateral aspects. The lateral cutaneous nerves from the seventh through twelfth intercostal nerves provide sensation to the skin territory of the rectus abdominis muscle. The size of the muscle is up to 25×6 cm^2. The skin territory that can be harvested is 21×14 cm^2 and is based on musculocutaneous perforators (96).

Gracilis

The gracilis is a smaller transplant and is useful for defects requiring less bulk than the latissimus or rectus. The gracilis is a type 2 muscle (dominant pedicle and several minor pedicles). It is a thin, flat muscle that lies between the adductor longus and sartorius muscle anteriorly and the semimembranosus posteriorly. The dominant pedicle is the ascending branch of the medial circumflex femoral artery and venae comitantes. The length of the pedicle is 6 cm, and the diameter of the artery is 1.6 mm. The minor pedicles are one or two branches of the superficial femoral artery and venae comitantes. Their length is 2 cm and their diameter is 0.5 mm (97).

Motor innervation is via the anterior branch of the obturator nerve, which is located between the adduction longus and magnus muscles; it usually enters the muscle above the level of the dominant vascular pedicle. The anterior femoral cutaneous nerve (L2-3) provides sensory innervation to the majority of the anterior medial thigh.

This muscle functions as a thigh adductor. The presence of the adductor longus and magnus makes it an expendable muscle.

The size of the muscle is 6×24 cm^2. The skin territory is 16×18 cm^2, but the skin over the distal half of the muscle

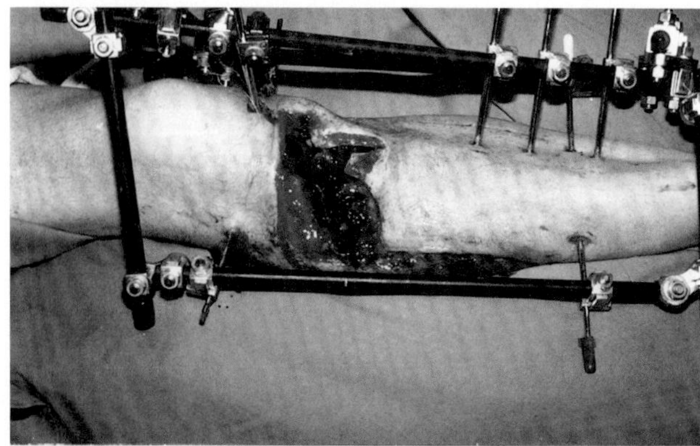

A

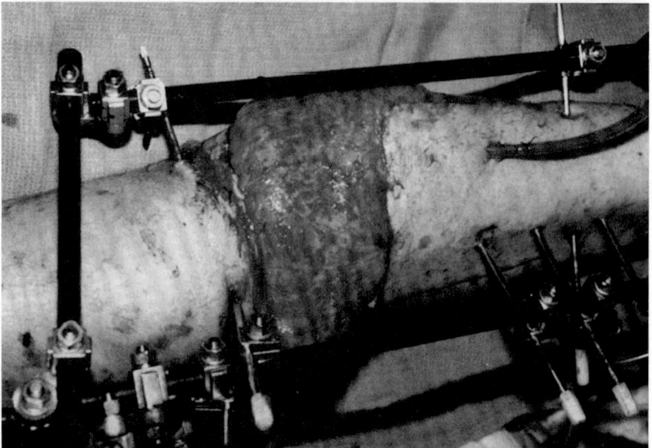

B

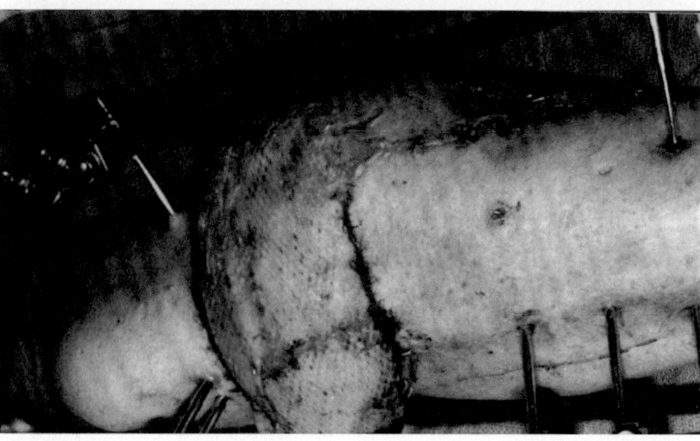

C

FIGURE 16-12 **A.** Proximal tibial fracture. The local tissue was too severely damaged to use a gastrocnemius rotational flap for coverage. **B.** The patient was treated with a latissimus dorsi free flap. **C.** Final result at 2 weeks with skin graft placed over the muscle flap. This case represents the advantages of free-tissue transfer over local flaps in the lower extremity particularly when the local tissue is damaged.

is not reliable when the flap is based on its dominant vascular pedicle with division of the minor vascular pedicles. In obese patients the musculocutaneous flap may be too bulky, necessitating use of a skin graft placed on the muscle.

Fibula

The free fibula transfer has revolutionized the reconstruction of long bone defects. The segment of the fibula that can be harvested varies between 20 to 30 cm. There are two types of vascularization to the fibula provided primarily by the peroneal artery. One source is the nutrient artery, usually unique and branching 6 to 14 cm from the origin of the peroneal artery. The nutrient artery usually enters the bone in its middle third. Periosteal vascularization comes from a series of branches from the peroneal artery and the anterior tibial artery. By isolating the peroneal artery at its origin from the posterior tibial trunk, both medullary and periosteal blood supplies are preserved. The skin on the lateral aspect of the leg gets its blood supply from four to six branches that originate in the peroneal artery.

The harvesting of the fibula is performed under tourniquet, through a lateral approach in a patient who is supine, prone, or in a lateral position. The line of incision runs between the head of the fibula and the lateral malleolus. At the middle of the line a point will indicate the approximate location of the nutrient vessel, and this point should be included in the graft. After incision of the superficial aponeurosis, the dissection is directed straight toward the bone shaft, pushing the peroneal muscles and the musculocutaneous nerve forward and the soleus backward. The bone is reached quickly and the dissection continued above the periosteum of the fibula. Dissection is continued to the interosseous membrane, which is incised to the level of the flexor hallucis longus in the posterior compartment. The graft is then measured and the bone sectioned at both ends, using a Gigli saw, although the peroneal artery has not yet been properly identified. At least 5 cm of fibula should be left intact distally to maintain ankle stability. The bundle is then located and tied at the distal portion of the graft and the dissection continued toward the peroneal-tibial bifurcation. When the recipient is ready, the pedicle is sectioned just below the bifurcation. Inclusion of the skin flap permits postoperative monitoring and simultaneous reconstruction of moderate soft tissue defects. Skin grafting of the donor site is required if the harvested skin flap is wider than 4 cm. For reconstruction of large bony and soft tissue defects, the fibular flap can be used in combination with other soft tissue flaps such as the latissimus dorsi (Fig. 16-13) (98).

Radial Forearm Flap

The radial forearm flap is a thin, well-vascularized fasciocutaneous flap on the ventral aspect of the forearm that was widely

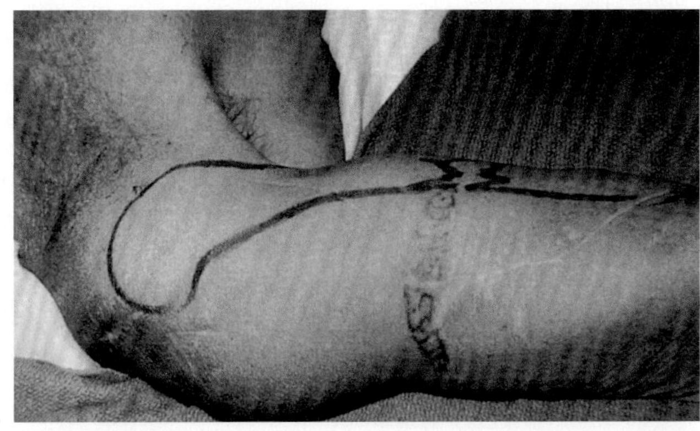
A

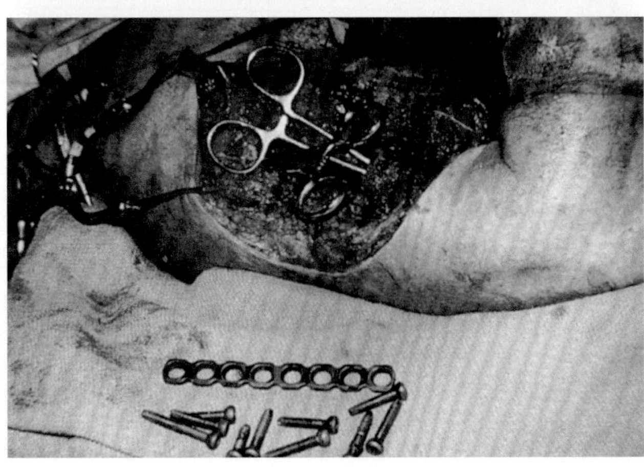
B

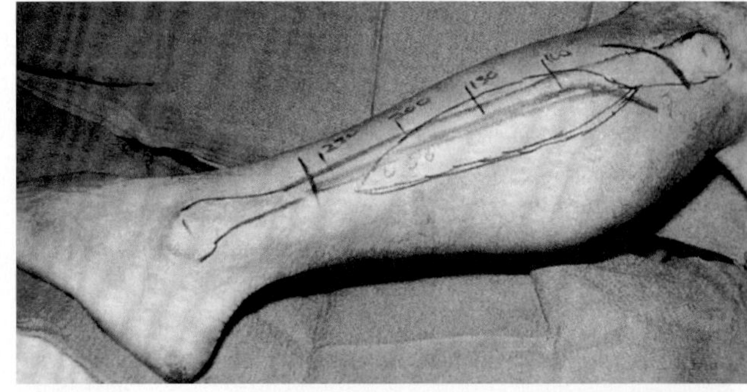
C

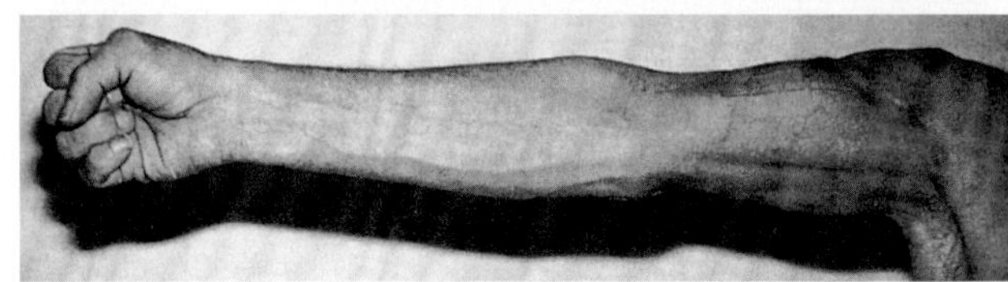
D

FIGURE 16-13 **A.** Humeral nonunion. The patient has undergone five previous attempts to obtain union of the humerus; using a vascularized fibular osteocutaneous flap, union was obtained. **B.** Intraoperative photograph showing both segments of the humeral nonunion, after removal of the hardware. **C.** Preoperative planning of the fibular graft and the skin paddle. **D.** Final appearance.

used in China before it was popularized in the Western literature (34,99). The flap is based on the radial artery, which can achieve a 20-cm pedicle and has a diameter of 2.5 mm. This length of the pedicle facilitates the microsurgical anastomosis out of the zone of injury. The venous drainage is through the venae comitantes of the radial artery, but the flap can include the cephalic vein, the basilic vein, or both.

The flap can contain the lateral antebrachial cutaneous nerve or the medial antebrachial cutaneous nerve and then serve as a neurosensory flap. The size of the flap can be 10×40 cm^2.

A portion of the radius can be included as a vascularized bone graft with this flap (100). The advantages of this flap are a long pedicle and potential sensory innervation. The quality of the bone from the radius is mainly cortical and not of any substantial volume (101). Including the bone in the radial forearm flap may lead to stress fracture of the donor radius. Preliminary tissue expansion will increase the flap dimensions, and, more importantly, it will allow direct closure of the donor defect (102).

Scapular and Parascapular Flap

It is a thin, usually hairless, skin flap from the posterior chest and can be deepithelialized and used as subcutaneous fascial flap, pedicled or free.

The flap is perfused by the cutaneous branches of the circumflex scapular artery and drained by its venae comitantes. The circumflex scapular artery is the main branch of the subscapular artery and the main blood supply to the scapula, the muscles that attach to the scapula and the overlying skin. The length of the pedicle is 5 cm and the diameter of the artery is 2.5 mm. The vascular pattern of this territory makes it possible to raise multiple skin flaps on a single vascular pedicle or to harvest the lateral border of the scapula as an osteocutaneous flap for a complex reconstruction.

The cutaneous territory can be 20×7 cm^2 and can be divided in two components—a horizontal territory (horizontal scapular flap) and a vertical territory (parascapular flap)—based on the branches of the circumflex scapular artery after the vessel courses through the triangular space. Preliminary expansion of the territory of the scapular flap will increase the flap dimensions and permit direct donor site closure. This flap can be combined with other flaps based on subscapular blood supply and may greatly facilitate certain complex reconstructions. These include the latissimus dorsi and serratus anterior flaps, which can supply additional skin, muscle, and bone (rib), if necessary (103–105). The primary indication for the scapular flap is a defect requiring a relatively thin, large cutaneous flap (106). These kinds of defects are often found in the foot (107). The osteoseptocutaneous free scapular flap reconstruction has been described in the lower extremity (108).

Anterolateral Thigh Flap

The anterior lateral thigh flap is currently gaining popularity as the workhorse of the thin flaps. For its harvesting, the patient is placed in the supine position, and a line is drawn from the anterior superior iliac spine to the lateral patella. At this point, using a hand-held Doppler, the descending branch of the lateral circumflex femoral is mapped out, starting at the midpoint of the line. Perforators, which generally cluster within 3 to 4 cm inferolateral to the midpoint, are also mapped using the Doppler. After all perforators are marked, the size of the flap needed should be determined. A template is taken of the area to be reconstructed along with an estimate of the length of pedicle that is needed for reconstruction. The template is then transferred to the anterior thigh to determine size of flap needed. The flap is centered around the perforating vessels. The long axis of the flap should be parallel to the thigh to decrease tension on closure of the donor site. The length of the vascular pedicle can be upward of 15 to 16 cm in length.

Dissection is begun after marking the skin paddle and perforators. The skin is incised down to the fascia overlying the rectus femoris muscle. The medial side of the flap is dissected first. If one is taking this as a fasciocutaneous flap, the fascia is incised and taken off with the skin and subcutaneous tissue. The fascia may be left adherent to the underlying muscles if only skin and subcutaneous tissue is needed.

The dissection is continued medial to lateral until the skin perforators are identified. One can then follow the skin perforators to the main pedicle as a useful landmark. Once the main pedicle is reached, the flap is dissected from its lateral border to the pedicle. At this point, the only remaining attachment to the flap from the patient is the pedicle. The muscles underlying the area of dissection are the rectus femoris and the vastus lateralis muscles. If the flap is based on a septocutaneous perforator, the intermuscular septum between these muscles is where the pedicle descends toward the descending branch of the lateral circumflex femoral vessels. The intermuscular space is then entered, and the pedicle is carefully dissected back to its origin. If the flap is based on a musculocutaneous perforator, the dissection is more tedious. An intramuscular dissection is required. One needs to follow the perforator through the muscle on the anterior surface of the vessel. The branches of the perforator are generally located on the posterior and lateral aspect of the pedicle. Branches are ligated as one proceeds toward the base of the pedicle. A combination of sharp scissor dissection and fine bipolar cautery is used to isolate the pedicle from the surrounding muscle. Some bleeding may occur, but delicate handling of tissue is necessary to avoid damage to terminal vessels that supply the flap's undersurface and spasm of the vessels.

Recipient Vessels

The proper selection of recipient vessels is essential for the success of a free-tissue transfer, especially when the transfer is to the lower extremity. However, a general agreement on which vessels to use has not yet been reached. Conflicting data have been reported on the survival and outcome of the transferred flaps, depending on the vessel used or the location of anastomosis proximal or distal to the zone of injury. For example, the anterior tibial vessels may be preferred for their easy accessibility, whereas the posterior tibial vessels are strongly advocated by others.

Park et al (109) tried to develop an algorithm for recipient vessel selection in free-tissue transfer to the lower extremity. Based on their experience, the most important factors influencing the site of recipient vessel selection were the site of the injury and the vascular status of the lower extremity. The type of flap used, method, and site of microvascular anastomosis were less important factors in determining the recipient vessels.

INFORMED CONSENT AND MEDICAL/ LEGAL ISSUES

Informed consent for free transfer should include an explanation of the principles of microsurgical tissue transplants, as well as the advantages and disadvantages of the procedure. The patient should understand the risk of vascular thrombosis, flap failure loss of limb, and nerve injury. The risks include continued infection, persistent nonunion, and limb losses with or without a successful flap. No guarantees should be given regarding the surgical outcomes. The possibility for salvaging a significantly compromised extremity can be offered using microsurgical techniques either with or without a successful free flap. Limb amputation after free-tissue transfer can be performed for reasons of pain, sepsis, or for persistent bone instability.

POSTOPERATIVE CARE

Postoperative care of free-tissue transfer patients requires that patients be adequately hydrated. Maintenance of proper body temperature and hematocrit is also important. Routine anticoagulation is not utilized.

Flaps are usually monitored for a minimum of 5 days with a laser Doppler in addition to clinical observation. Although the immediate postoperative period of 24 to 48 hours is critical, there have been late occasional failures; thus, laser Doppler monitoring should be continued for 5 days.

Extremities should be elevated at all times to augment venous return. Patients with lower extremity flaps are not allowed to ambulate postoperatively for a minimum of 3 weeks. The inosculation and the healing of the flap to the wound bed, the selection of muscle or skin, and the "take" of the skin graft are factors that go into the timing to determine dependency of the lower extremity. Those patients who have reconstruction around the foot and ankle are most prone to increased venous pressure and resultant edema of the flaps. This edema can result in the dehiscence of the free flap from the surrounding tissue bed. For this reason, these patients are required to keep their limbs elevated and undergo bed to chair transfer for a minimum of 3 weeks. Some experimental data suggest that this period can be shortened. However, it is our experience that this is the amount of time it takes for the flap to mature and develop a sufficient venous return to withstand the hydrostatic pressures associated with standing.

Before proceeding with any other reconstruction such as bone grafting (as in a case of open tibia fracture) or tendon transfers, all wound surfaces must be epithelialized. There must be no edema, cellulitis, granulation tissue, or sinus tracts that could compromise the next stage of reconstruction. For example, in cases of a free muscle flap in the distal third of an open tibia fracture that ultimately requires bone grafting, it is essential that all skin grafts be totally epithelialized to decrease skin colonization of bacteria. It is our preference to remove the external fixator, clean the pin sites, and place the limb in a cast until the pin tracts heal. The flap can be then elevated and an autogenous bone graft safely performed.

MONITORING

Monitoring of a free-tissue transfer is essential to ensure transplant success (Fig. 16-14). Many different monitoring devices and techniques have been used, with varying levels of success. As is true in many situations in medicine, the availability of many solutions to a problem suggests that none is superior or ideal.

Ideal flap monitoring should satisfy several criteria. It should be harmless to the patient or the flap, objective, reproducible, applicable to all types of flaps, and inexpensive. It is important that any monitor be capable of prolonged monitoring and respond rapidly to circulatory changes. Postoperative monitoring techniques can be grouped in four categories: (a) clinical evaluation, (b) direct vessel monitoring, (c) indicators of tissue circulation, and (d) metabolic parameters related to perfusion (110).

Clinical Evaluation

Clinical evaluation remains the gold standard to which all methods of monitoring need to be compared. This involves observation of skin color, temperature, capillary refill, and bleeding characteristics. Clinical observation fulfills many of the criteria of the ideal monitoring system. It is cheap, readily available, and can provide a dynamic picture. The disadvantages are the need for experienced personnel and its use being confined to monitoring surface skin flaps and muscle flaps. Changes are often initially subtle, and by the time they are clinically apparent, salvage of the flap may be impossible because of irreversible tissue damage.

Direct Vessel Monitoring

Direct vessel monitoring can be done by electromagnetic flowmeters. Readings are based on measuring the electric potential induced by blood flow. The ultrasonic Doppler measures sound waves reflected from columns of moving blood cells. Thermocouples measure the temperature difference between preanastomotic and postanastomotic sites on the vascular pedicle using two microthermocouples.

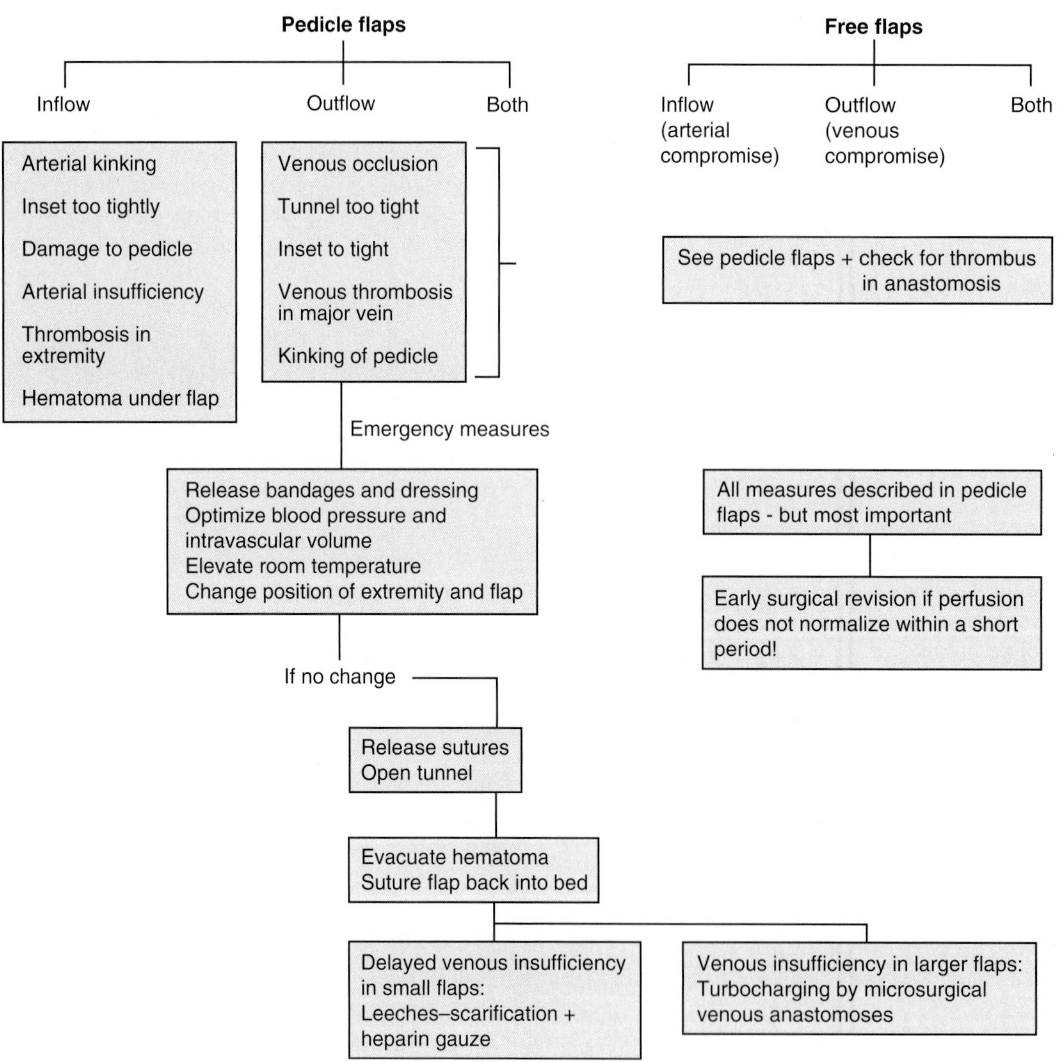

FIGURE 16-14 Monitoring of flaps and impending flap failures. (From German G, Sherman R, Levin LS. *Decision-making in reconstructive surgery upper-extremity*. New York: Springer-Verlag; 1999, with permission.)

Circulation Monitoring

This category of monitoring is based on measuring the change in the temperature of the skin and using it as an indicator of the blood flow in skin. Photoplethysmography is based on the change in the amount of light reflected during change in the local cutaneous blood volume. Laser Doppler flowmetry is based on the same general principles as ultrasound Doppler but measures the frequency shift of light rather than sound waves reflected from moving red blood cells. Pulse oximetry continuously monitors both pulsatility and oxygen saturation, and from these measurements defines blood flow.

Metabolic Monitors

Transcutaneous oxygen monitoring and invasive measurements of PO_2 check the perfusion of tissue transplantations based on metabolic parameters. Levels of tissue oxygen tension have been monitored in flaps and have been shown to reflect the quality of capillary circulation (111).

Monitoring is usually performed in the intensive care unit setting or a step-down setting, depending on the condition of the patient. Absolute values of laser Doppler measurements, patterns, and trends of flow can give valuable information about the dynamic perfusion range of blood flow over time. Low absolute values of perfusion, as well as relative changes from the initial flow, are alarming signs, and immediate clinical evaluation of the flap should be performed. It is our preference to use the laser Doppler to monitor free flaps. The standard practice in our center is to routinely monitor patients in the intensive care unit for the first 24 hours, because this is when the problems most frequently occur following free-tissue transfer.

Based on our experience with laser Doppler monitoring, we suggest classifying the perfusion in one of the following four groups with a corresponding diligence of observation:

1. If the perfusion is within or above the established range, a normal degree of observation is justified.
2. If the observed flow is somewhat low, based on a table of normal blood flow for that flap, a modestly increased level of clinical evaluation is warranted (alert level 1).
3. If the relative flow falls to 50% of the initial flow of that flap and remains at that level for 30 minutes or more, a more aggressive observation of the flap would be indicated (alert level 2).
4. If the absolute flow is lower than 0.4 laser Doppler flow units for 30 minutes, a maximally aggressive clinical observation should occur (alert level 3; "red alert"), and exploration should be strongly considered. This level of flow is typically inconsistent with viability of the flap, regardless of flap type, recipient site, or blood flow history.

In cases of abnormal laser Doppler values, artifact should be ruled out. Falsely low readings can occasionally be the result of a probe becoming slightly detached from the flap. In addition, low readings can be caused by hypovolemia, anemia, and hypothermia (112). Therefore, it is important to closely examine not only the laser Doppler equipment but also the general condition of the patient. Falsely elevated measurements can be caused by vibration, motion of the probe or tissue, location of the probe over a large vessel, or extreme variation in the hematocrit.

Flap Failure and Management (Acute)

The success of free-tissue transfer should be on the order of 95% to 99%. Acute complications occur usually in the first 48 hours and include venous thrombosis, arterial thrombosis, hematoma, hemorrhage, and excessive flap edema. Arterial insufficiency can be recognized by decreased capillary refill, pallor, reduced temperature, and the absence of bleeding after pinprick. This complication can be caused by arterial spasm, vessel plaque, torsion of the pedicle, pressure on the flap, technical error with injury to the pedicle, a flap harvested that is too large for its blood supply, or small vessel disease (due to smoking or diabetes). Management of arterial compromise requires prompt surgical intervention to restore the blood flow (113). Pharmacologic intervention at the time of exploration includes use of vasodilators, calcium channel blockers, and systemic anticoagulants for flap salvage presenting with arterial insufficiency (114). Ultimately, if these pharmacologic agents do not relieve spasm at the level of the arterial inflow, the anastomosis should be redone to rule out intraarterial thrombus.

Venous outflow obstruction can be suspected when the flap has a violaceous color, brisk capillary refill, normal or elevated temperature, and produces dark blood after pinprick. Venous insufficiency can occur as a result of torsion of the pedicle, flap edema, hematoma, or tight closure of the tissue over the pedicle. The venous outflow obstruction can result in extravasation of red blood cells, endothelial breakdown, microvascular collapse, thrombosis in the microcirculation, and, finally, flap death. Given the irreversible nature of the microcirculatory changes in venous congestion that occurs even after short periods of time, the surgeon must recognize venous compromise as early as possible.

These complications can occur alone or in any combination. The clinical observation and the monitoring of the patient (such as with laser Doppler) should alert the surgeon who has to decide between conservative and operative intervention. Conservative treatment may include drainage of the hematoma at the bedside with release of a few sutures to decrease pressure. In cases of venous congestion, leeches may be helpful if insufficient venous outflow cannot be established despite a patent venous anastomosis. The leeches inject a salivary component (hirudin) that inhibits both platelet aggregation and the coagulation cascade. The flap is decongested initially as the leech extracts blood and is further decongested as the bite wound oozes after the leech detaches (113).

The donor site should be given the same attention as the recipient site during the postoperative period. Complications of the donor site include hematoma, seroma, sensory nerve dysfunction, and scar formation.

Treatment of Failure (Late)

Occasionally free flaps, despite early return to the operating room for vascular compromise, do fail. Options for management include the performance of a second free-tissue transfer, noting the technical or physiologic details that led to initial failure. Most of the time, free-tissue transfers that fail are due to technical errors in judgment, whether they be flap harvest, compromise of the pedicle during the harvest, improper microvascular technique during anastomosis, improper insetting resulting in increased tissue tension and edema, or postoperative motion of the extremity resulting in pedicle avulsion. The next decision made by the operating surgeon as to the management of this patient is based on several factors. Obviously, if a patient required a free flap in the first place, a second free flap should be considered. If a decision is made not to redo the flap, it could be left in place using the so-called Crane Principle in which a local flap or free-tissue transfer that progresses to necrosis in part or totally acts as a biologic dressing or eschar over a wound bed. If there is no infection, the eschar can be left on the wound bed with hopes that some healing in the form of granulation can occur underneath it. Ultimately, the eschar is removed and the granulation bed skin grafted, obviating the need for another free-tissue transfer. If wound observation shows that such a bed is not produced, then a second flap must be considered (115).

It is usually our preference not to follow this course, because the flap can become a source of sepsis and further compromise local tissues. Necrotic nonviable flaps should be removed and a temporary wound dressing such as a bead pouch or wound VAC used. Occasionally, when flaps fail in a severely compromised extremity, consideration should be given to amputation in that the morbidity of a second free-tissue transfer and perhaps the resultant extremity state make amputation a more reasonable choice. If a second free flap is considered, obvious errors that led to the original flap compromise need to be recognized. It may be prudent to obtain an arteriogram, evaluate the coagulation profile, and research other issues that might have led to failure.

TEAM APPROACH TO EXTREMITY RECONSTRUCTION

Reconstruction is a coordinated effort between orthopaedic surgeons, vascular surgeons, traumatologists, and plastic surgeons. It is not uncommon in practice for an orthopaedic traumatologist to stabilize a fracture, a vascular surgeon to perform an arterial interposition graft, and, finally, a microsurgeon to do a free-tissue transfer. Communication and careful preoperative planning are important to ensure successful reconstruction. The ability of the reconstructive microsurgeon to deliver the correct tissue at the correct time with the correct composite nature enhances limb salvage.

In instances of bone fracture, the algorithm in Figure 16-15 can be followed with primary hardware placement or external fixator placement, such as an Ilizarov or an AO external fixator. If a bone graft is needed because of missing or devitalized bone, tobramycin beads or silicone spacers can be placed in the bone defect, with subsequent soft tissue coverage. This is then followed by secondary bone grafting with an iliac crest graft, allograft, vascularized graft, intercalary vascularized transplant such as the free fibular graft, or periosteal vascularized flaps (116).

Bone Reconstruction

There are three basic methods to bridge a bony defect in a limb. They are distraction osteogenesis (Ilizarov technique), bone grafting, and free osseous or osteocutaneous flap transfer.

In large bone defects, such as those in the tibia, femur, or humerus, associated with soft tissue, there is a requirement for both bone and soft tissue. For bone defects smaller than 5 cm, conventional bone grafting with corticocancellous grafts can be used to reconstitute the limb. The advent of the Ilizarov device has changed thinking somewhat about intercalary segmental defects, and bone transport can be considered after soft tissue coverage has been obtained (Fig. 16-16).

New evidence suggests that simultaneous Ilizarov and microsurgical tissue transplantation are even higher rungs on the soft tissue reconstructive ladder. In combination with microsurgical transplants, the Ilizarov technique may provide the best reconstructive option by integrating all rungs of the reconstructive ladder. That is, the Ilizarov device can be used to shorten bone acutely and then transport or lengthen bone segments (117). However, the soft tissue requirement of a free-tissue transplant once the limb is shortened can be reduced, changing the selection of muscles or flaps from local flaps to smaller free tissue transplants, such as the gracilis.

Because of the microsurgical capabilities of vascularized tissue transplantation, particularly in the free fibular transfer, such procedures can be used to provide vascularized intercalary segments of bone either following soft tissue envelope reconstruction or simultaneously. In the reconstructive process, the timing of bone grafting is important. When nonvascularized grafts are used, there should be an adequate vascular bed in which to place these grafts. A period of 4 to 6 weeks should be allowed after soft tissue reconstruction of an envelope before conventional grafting is performed.

Ilizarov

The Ilizarov method is a technique for generating both bone and soft tissue through application of tension to the tissue under carefully controlled conditions. This is accomplished by slow distraction (approximately 1 mm/day), divided into small increments (usually every 6 hours) by using an external fixator that is rigid to bending and torsion stress but allows axial micromotion (118,119). The method is used in the treatment of fractures, nonunions, osteomyelitis, deformities, bone loss, and congenital abnormalities. Ilizarov's external fixator is a modular system

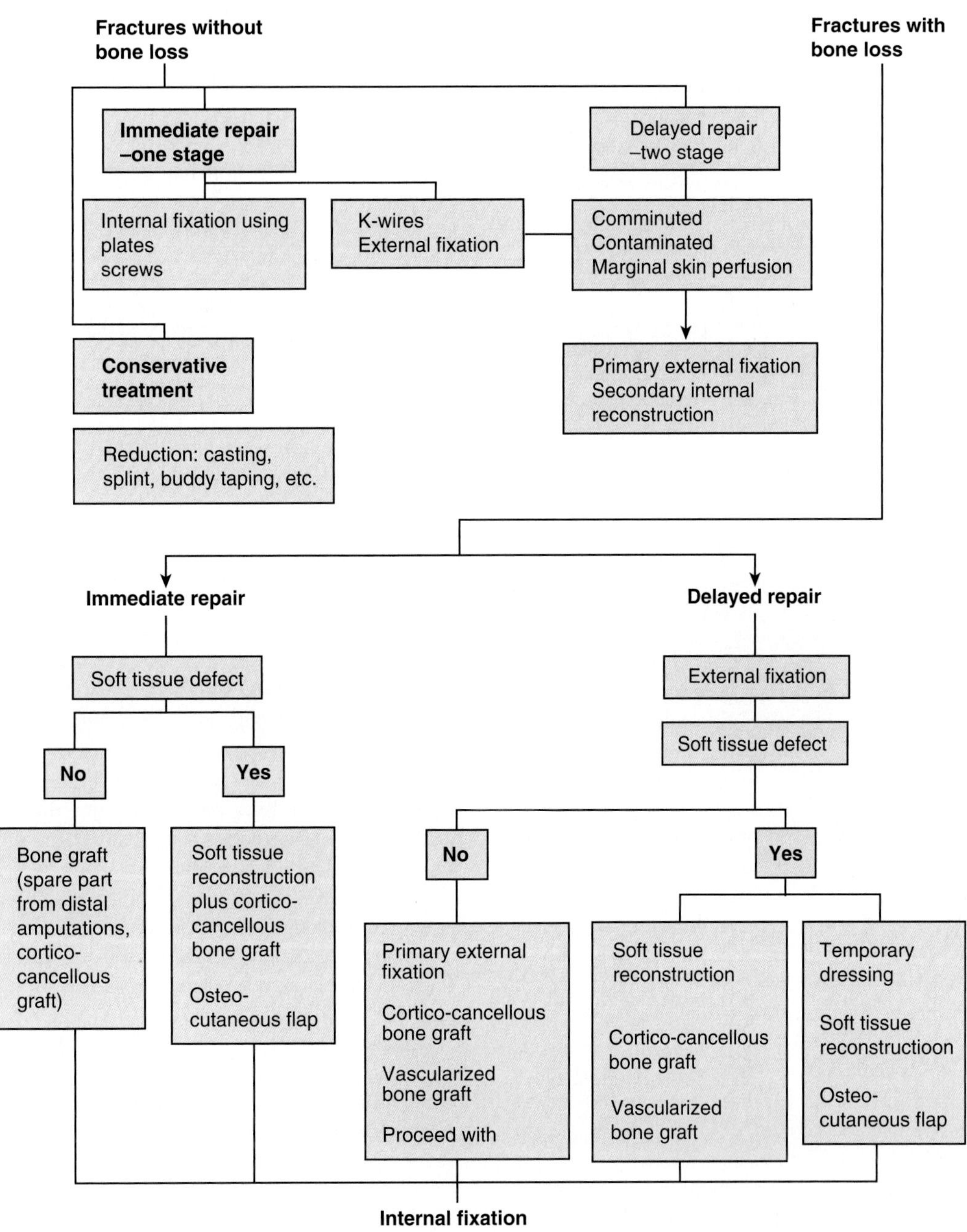

FIGURE 16-15 Fixation devices for fractures. (From German G, Sherman R, Levin LS. *Decision-making in reconstructive surgery upper-extremity*. New York: Springer-Verlag; 1999, with permission.)

of rings with small-diameter stainless steel wires tensioned to between 60 and 130 kg transfixing the extremity (120). The Ilizarov method differs from other techniques for reconstruction of bone and soft tissue in that it is minimally invasive and extremely versatile, it generates tissue (it does not simply stretch it), the fixator permits full weight-bearing and complete function, and it obtains and maintains the reduction of fractures (121).

The Ilizarov fixator and tissue generation method were developed in the western Siberian city of Kurgan. In 1951 Ilizarov discovered that normal tissue could be generated under carefully applied tension; he termed this phenomenon the tension-stress effect (122,123). The tension-stress effect on the bone causes neovascularity, increased metabolic and biosynthetic activity, and orderly cellular proliferation in a similar but not identical manner to normal endochondral ossification at the physis. The tension-stress effect on the bone causes a bipolar fibrous interzone, which matures in an orderly fashion.

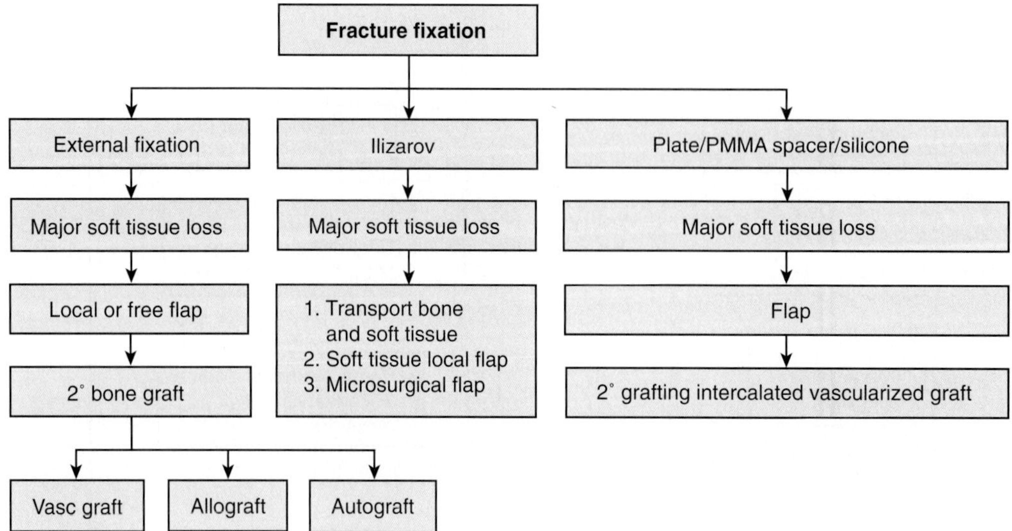

FIGURE 16-16 Segmental bone loss. (From Levin LS. The reconstructive ladder: an orthoplastic approach. *Orthop Clin North Am* 1993;24:393–409, with permission.)

The ability of tissue to grow linearly under conditions of tension applies not only to bone but also to soft tissue. Muscle, nerves, skin, and blood vessels are generated, not stretched, in response to tension; their cellular components proliferate in the direction of the applied tension (117,124).

Fractures associated with defects of bone and soft tissue are ideally treated with the Ilizarov method. Mechanical stability and soft tissue coverage of the fracture can be achieved with this technique (125,126). In cases of bone loss, the bone defect can be filled by two methods: (a) acutely shortening the bone, then gradually lengthening it to restore the original bone length or (b) through bone transport to gradually fill the defect (127,128).

The combined versatility of modern free-tissue transplantation and the Ilizarov method has taken limb salvage to the next level. Four possibilities for combined Ilizarov microsurgery exist. They include the use of Ilizarov as an external fixator for bone stabilization in cases of open fractures. In these cases adequate bone stock is present and will consolidate, usually without bone graft, provided soft tissue coverage is achieved. A need for coverage may occur after the Ilizarov frame is in place and the surgeon recognizes the need for augmentation of the soft tissue envelope. In these cases free-tissue transfer provides coverage only and the frame provides definitive fracture care with options for progressive dynamization by gradual frame disassembly, decreasing rigidity, and increasing load to allow bone healing to occur.

The second combination of Ilizarov and microsurgery is the application of an Ilizarov device after flap placement for correction of evolving deformity such as a malunion. Although the Ilizarov method can treat deformities or malunions without free-tissue transfer, there is a large group of patients who undergo initial stabilization with plates or conventional external fixators. These patients then undergo flap coverage, and, after the soft tissue heals, the bone does not heal or begins to heal with deformity with weight-bearing. If this is recognized early, the Ilizarov can replace the initial external fixator and be used to acutely or gradually align the nascent malunion. If this occurs late, with the bone healed in malalignment, the Ilizarov can be used to realign the limb after osteotomy through the malunion.

In large segmental defects, the Ilizarov can be used to treat the initial fracture by stabilization, followed by callus distraction after the soft tissue is healed.

In cases of bone loss the bone defect can be filled by two methods: (a) acutely shortening the bone, then gradually lengthening it to restore the original bone length or (b) bone transport to gradually fill the defect (127,128). Acute shortening and subsequent lengthening at a site distant from the fracture is indicated in cases requiring nerve or vessel repair. Another advantage of this method is that fracture fragments can be reduced and stabilized under direct vision because these fractures with bone loss always have a soft tissue defect. Free flaps often are used to reconstitute the soft tissue envelope in these cases. The necessary surface area and volume of free flaps are diminished so that the morbidity of the donor site is decreased. For example, in large soft tissue injury with an open tibia fracture, the latissimus dorsi may have been previously selected for coverage. But by acutely shortening the limb and decreasing the soft tissue defect, the gracilis or a slip of the serratus may be harvested. This fulfills the soft tissue requirements but usually involves an easier flap with less morbidity. Disadvantages of this technique are that in cases of treatment of tibial fractures with bone loss, the fibula should be shortened as well, usually through an osteotomy through a separate incision. In addition, blood vessels and nerves may be kinked by the shortening.

Bone transport is another technique used to fill bone and soft tissue defects. This technique maintains the length and alignment of the extremity. The bone defect is filled by first performing a corticotomy at a site proximal, distal or both proximal and distal to the defect. The defect is gradually filled by an "internal lengthening" accomplished by transporting the osteotomized segment toward the defect at a rate of 0.5 to 1 mm/day. There are several advantages of the bone transport method compared with acute shortening. Theoretically, almost no limits exist as to the amount of bone loss that can be filled with this technique. The length and alignment of the extremity are maintained throughout treatment, allowing maximum function and, in the lower extremity, complete ambulation. The soft tissues attached to the transport segment are also transported toward the defect, allowing closure of some soft tissue defects without the use of flaps or grafts (129). Perhaps the most significant disadvantage is that subsequent surgical procedures may be needed as docking occurs, reshaping the ends of the fragments and grafting with autogenous bone. To accelerate bone union, Green et al (128,130) advocate trimming the ends and adding autogenous bone graft.

The Ilizarov technique may be used as a definitive fixation for vascularized bone grafts that are used for bone defects that exceed 6 cm. We prefer to stabilize the osteoseptocutaneous fibular graft in this manner, avoiding the use of internal fixation such as plates or intramedullary nails.

In osteomyelitis, the soft tissue can be managed with free-tissue transfer and the Ilizarov can be used to bridge unstable defects requiring conventional or vascularized bone grafts.

Bone Graft

Bone grafts are classified by their donor origin (autograft vs. allograft), composition (cortical, cancellous, osteochondral), anatomic features (epiphyseal, metaphyseal, diaphyseal), and additional processing (irradiation and demineralization). Each of these features imparts certain properties to a graft that make it suitable or unsuitable for a particular purpose.

Allografts

Allograft tissue is transplanted from one individual to a genetically dissimilar individual of the same species. Allografts can be procured fresh and implanted immediately, which preserves viability of articular chondrocytes; however, other cells such as osteocytes, marrow element, and fibroblasts in the soft tissue attachments probably die. Disadvantages of fresh allograft include size mismatches with the potential recipient and problems of screening for transmittable diseases. Alternatively, allografts can be frozen following procurement. This creates the advantage of storing a spectrum of anatomic sizes and potentially allows a closer anatomic fit for the recipient. Freezing also provides time between procurement and implantation during which screening studies can be performed for infectious agents. Lyophilization of allografts is an expensive preservation technique but makes storage and transportation easier.

Autografts

Fresh, nonvascularized autografts avoid the risk of disease transmission and optimize biologic and immunologic considerations but involve donor site morbidity and have limited utility. Cancellous autograft is primarily used to fill cavitary defects and to supplement osteosynthesis sites. Structural cortical autografts are limited in terms of donor site and include the fibula and iliac crest.

Vascularized Bone Grafts

Pedicled. The advances in surgery, and especially in microsurgery, have made it possible to transfer autogenous bone grafts on vascular pedicles. With the nutrient blood supply preserved, bone cells survive, and healing of the graft to the recipient bone occurs by a mechanism similar to fracture healing rather than by creeping substitution. Thus, graft incorporation is independent of the status of the recipient bed. This is especially significant when the bone defect is located in a scarred or irradiated area that impedes incorporation of conventional autogenous grafts.

Free Vascularized Bone Grafts. Current indications for free vascularized bone grafting are broad. Vascularized bone grafting offers significant advantages in bone defects greater than 6 to 8 cm in length resulting from trauma or infection and requiring extensive sequestrectomy (131,132).

In orthopaedics, indications include refractory nonunion with failure of conventional techniques and congenital pseudarthrosis of the tibia or forearm (133). Future applications may include transfer of a vascularized epiphysis to reconstitute limb growth (134) and transfer of free vascularized allografts (135).

Specialized Free Flaps. Functional composite free flaps, such as the dorsalis pedis with extensor tendons, or innervated transfers, such as the innervated myocutaneous gracilis transplant, represent state-of-the-art reconstruction in which several reconstructive functions are achieved in one procedure.

Other Options

Other options on the reconstructive ladder that need to be considered are emergency free-tissue transfers as outlined by Godina (25). In some severe injuries, an immediate vascularized flap is required to protect exposed structures that, even with temporary wound measures, would be doomed and lead to loss of the extremity. Such instances include exposed vascular grafts or amputation stumps that could be covered by cannibalizing amputated parts. If an injury occurs to an extremity that must be sacrificed, the part can be cannibalized either for vascularized transplanted parts or for conventional parts such as tendon, bone, nerve, or skin grafts.

Heterotopic transplantation as outline by Godina (25) can be considered for parts that would be functional but that cannot be replanted. Simultaneous reconstruction of vascularity and coverage can be obtained with flow-through free flaps, such as the radial forearm flap.

On the highest rung of the reconstructive ladder, to treat compartmental resections resulting from either tumor or unrecognized compartment syndrome (Volkmann's contracture), innervated muscle transfers can be done that not only provide coverage to an extremity but a functioning motor-tendon unit as well. In addition to bone and soft tissue reconstruction, many extremities require nerve grafting. It is crucial to perform nerve grafts in a well-vascularized bed. The choice of vascularized or nonvascularized nerve grafts is still controversial but must be part of the reconstructive algorithm.

RECONSTRUCTIVE ALGORITHM BY REGION

Thus far, discussion in this chapter has focused on patient evaluation, immediate wound care, and the hierarchy of the reconstructive ladder, ranging from simple wound closure to composite tissue transplantation. The remainder of the chapter discusses reconstructive options by region.

Upper Extremity

Although the lower extremity open fracture serves as the prototype for the compound fracture, injuries to the upper extremity are associated with unique properties that influence the selection of techniques for soft tissue reconstruction (136). The upper extremity often sustains mutilating injuries involving skin, muscle, nerve, artery, and tendon without fracture. The reconstructive ladder for such injuries necessitates procedures for wound closure but also requires repair or reconstruction of devitalized tendon, nerve, or missing artery. Reconstruction should address all missing tissues, if feasible, in the first operative procedure. If the surgeon is confident of having achieved an adequate debridement, reconstruction can be performed immediately. A perfect example of this is a replantation injury, in which arteries, nerves, tendons, and damaged soft tissue are treated in a one-stage operation.

In more complex mutilating injuries to the upper extremity, immediate reconstruction is not always possible, and delayed reconstruction of tendons or nerves is necessary. In these instances, soft tissue can be reconstructed with meshed or unmeshed skin graft or, where thicker dermis is needed with less contraction, with full-thickness grafts. Consideration should be given to the esthetic appearance of the limb, more in the upper extremity than in the lower extremity. This may influence whether a split-thickness graft is meshed or unmeshed. The advantage of the meshed split-thickness graft is that the interstices of the graft will allow efflux of edema fluid and blood. Epithelial migration and graft contraction diminish the overall size of the wound when a meshed skin graft is used in comparison with a full-thickness graft.

In patients with tendon devoid of paratenon or with exposed vascular repairs, reconstructive options beyond skin grafting need to be considered. Although fascia or transposition flaps can be used to rotate over exposed tendons, doing so will frequently leave a cosmetic defect or impair venous return from the hand or digits, such as in the cross-finger flap. In the region of the hand, the so-called Chinese flap, the reversed radial forearm flap, the dorsal metacarpal artery flap, and the posterior interosseous artery flap are excellent island pedicle flaps that can be used to reconstitute soft tissue over exposed tendons or bone. The groin flap is another option, but it is associated with the drawback of restricting the extremity, keeping the extremity dependent, and requiring a second-stage release and insetting. In massive defects of the hand in which the groin flap or island pedicle flaps cannot be used, free tissue transplantation should be considered (Table 16-4).

In injuries to the forearm in which there is large tissue loss, the island pedicle flap using the latissimus dorsi as a muscle or myocutaneous flap can be considered. The true practical length of the flap (as an island flap) is to about the midlevel of the forearm, and thus this flap would be more suitable as a free-tissue transplant for areas around the wrist requiring large amounts of tissue. Areas around the elbow and humerus can be treated with skin grafting, a pedicle latissimus flap, or a proximally based radial forearm flap. Innervated transfers are often very effective for restoring function and coverage simultaneously.

Lower Extremity

In the lower extremity with an adequate soft tissue bed, meshed or split-thickness skin grafting can be performed to treat a variety of wounds, including fasciotomy wounds and open wounds with underlying vascularized fascia or muscle. In regions of the lower limb above the knee in ambulatory patients, skin grafting should be considered as the first line of closure, followed by rotational flaps. The island pedicle rectus abdominis muscle can be used in the area around the groin or the trochanter, and the thoracoepigastric flap described by Taylor et al (11) can be considered in the area of the perineum or as far down as the knee. The tensor fascia lata myofasciocutaneous flap can be used without excessive compromise in the ambulatory individual and in open injuries about the posterior pelvis (137); even the superior half of the gluteus maximus muscle can be used without compromising gait (Table 16-5).

For injury to the lower extremity below the knee, the reconstructive ladder beyond skin grafting has expanded in recent years. As a result of the anatomic work by Masquelet and Romana (138), there has been a resurgence of interest in fasciocutaneous and fascial flaps, as well as dermal flaps, that can be used in a variety of clinical circumstances. These include peroneal flaps, the anterior tibial artery flap, the posterior tibial artery

TABLE 16-4 Reconstruction Options for Upper Extremity

	Pedicled Flap		Free Flap	Regional
Palm	Cutaneous	Radial perforator flap Ulnar perforator flap Posterior interosseous flap	Instep island flap (from foot)	
	Fascial	Radial forearm flap Ulnar forearm flap	Temporoparietal fascia flap Serratus flap Lateral arm flap	
Dorsal hand	Cutaneous	Local transposition flaps: Limberg, bilobe, reverse digital island flap Radial perforator flap Ulnar perforator flap Post, interosseous flap		Groin flap
	Fascial	Radial forearm flap Ulnar forearm flap	Lateral arm flap Serratus flap Parascapular flap Anterior thigh flap Gracitis	
Forearm	Muscle Cutaneous and fascial	Radial perforator flap Ulnar perforator flap Radial forearm flap Ulnar forearm flap	Parascapular flap Lateral arm flap	
	Muscle Osteocutaneous	Osteocutaneous posterior interosseus flap Osteocutaneous radial forearm flap Distal pedicle osteocutaneous lateral arm flap Tendocutaneous lateral arm flap	Gracilis Fibula flap Parascapular flap Iliac crest flap	
Shoulder and brachium	Skin	Local transposition flaps Lateral arm flap Parascapular flap Scapula flap	Parascapular flap	
	Muscle	Latissimus dorsi flap Vertical trapezius flap Pectoralis major	Gracilis muscle flap Contralateral latissimus dorsi flap	
	Osteocutaneous	Distal pedicle osteocutaneous lateral arm flap Osteocutaneous radial arm flap	Fibula flap Parascapular flap Iliac crest flap	

flap that functions similar to the radial forearm flap but does not compromise the posterior tibial artery, saphenous and sural flaps, and the peroneal artery flap. The reliability of these flaps is based on an intact vascular plexus. Following extremity trauma, the small fasciocutaneous perforators may be unreliable. In other individuals, such as those with diabetes or peripheral vascular disease, these flaps may also be unreliable but can be considered in the reconstructive ladder.

The classic algorithm for lower extremity coverage involving an open fracture divides the tibia into thirds. In the proximal third, the gastrocnemius muscle flap can be considered for coverage using either the lateral head or the medial head or both. It should be within the reconstructive domain of all orthopaedists to be able to mobilize this flap based on its vascular pedicle (the sural artery and vein) to rotate for coverage of proximal third injuries. However, in some instances, large soft tissue defects exist in the proximal third, and the total volume and surface area coverage of the gastrocnemius muscle is inadequate. In this instance, the surgeon's first consideration should be free tissue transplantation. In the middle third of the tibia, soleus rotational myoplasty has traditionally been performed. More functional impairment to push-off strength occurs when the soleus muscle is used versus the gastrocnemius, and the total surface area in the middle third of the tibia that can effectively be covered is dependent not only on the level of the musculotendinous junction of the soleus but also on the amount of volume

TABLE 16-5 Reconstructive Option for the Lower Extremity

Femur/groin
- STSG
- Tensor fascia lata
- Superior one-half; gluteus maximus
- Thoracoepigastric flap
- Free flap

Leg/Tibia
- Proximal one-third gastrocnemius muscle
- Middle one-third soleus
- Distal one-third: free flap
- Distally based fasciocutaneous flaps

Foot
- STSG
- FTSG
- Abductor hallucis muscle
- Flexor hallucis brevis muscle
- Plantar fascia flap
- Free flap (muscle/skin/innervated?)

FTSG, full-thickness skin graft: STSG, split-thickness skin graft.
From Levin LS. The reconstructive ladder an orthoplastic approach. *Orthop Clin North Am* 1993;24:393–409, with permission.

required. For this reason, with a defect greater than 5 × 8 cm in the middle third of the tibia, the reconstruction option should be directed more toward free-tissue transplantation (Figs. 16-17 and 16-18).

Traditionally, muscle flaps covered with a split-thickness skin graft have been used in the lower extremity, but in large cavitary defects involving compartment resections, composite flaps such as latissimus dorsi, rectus abdominis, or myocutaneous flaps can be considered.

Despite the new possibilities of flaps such as the distally based flexor hallucis longus flap, free-tissue transfer has been reserved for injury to the lower third of the tibia. In injuries with cutaneous loss only, the scapular flap is excellent donor tissue. Other skin flaps include the parascapular, the lateral arm, and the radial forearm. Donor site morbidity and cosmesis are always a consideration in free-tissue transplantation and should be factors in the selection of which flaps to use.

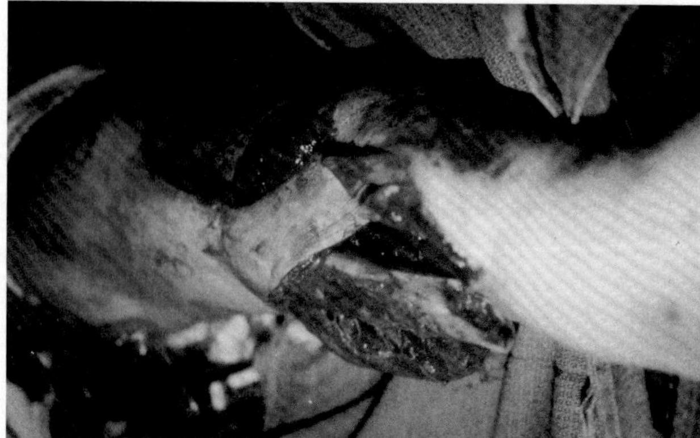
A

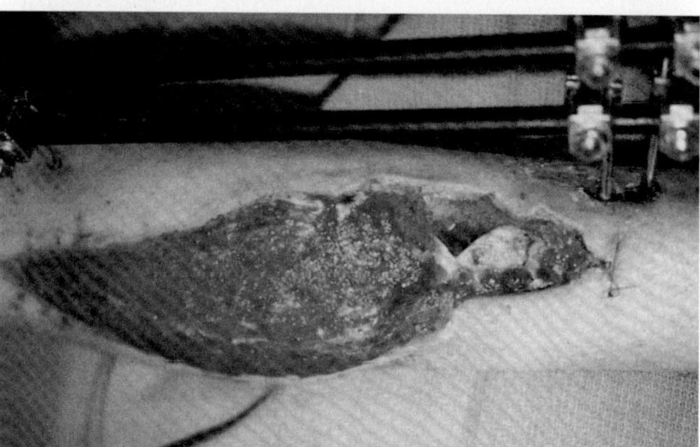
B

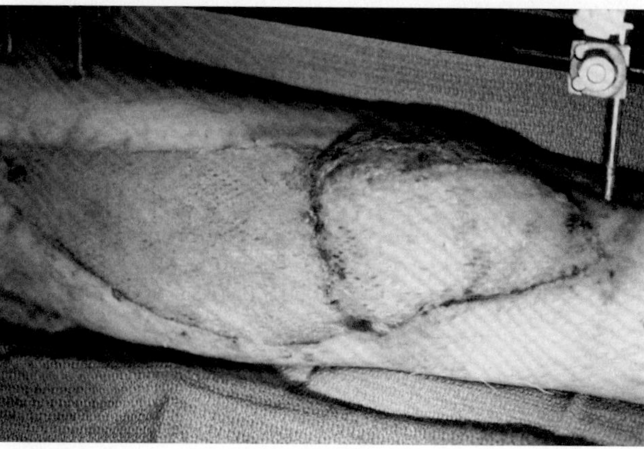
C

FIGURE 16-17 **A.** A IIIB tibia fracture. The patient was treated with a rotational flap that did not provide adequate coverage. **B,C.** The patient needed a free rectus flap for completion of soft tissue coverage. This represents various rungs on the reconstructive ladder used together to complete resurfacing of a traumatized limb.

Foot and Ankle

The soft tissue coverage decision for the foot and ankle can be regionalized. Each anatomic region of the foot has certain characteristics that will influence selection of the free tissue transfer for reconstruction. The foot has special requirements for shoeing and ambulation. The reconstructive ladder for injury to the foot is based on whether there is a fracture, on what part of the foot is exposed, and on whether the area is weight-bearing or non–weight-bearing (Fig. 6-19). The ankle and the dorsum of the foot require thin, pliable soft tissue coverage for exposed tendons that are devoid of paratenon, bones, or joints The weight-bearing surface of the foot (the plantar skin) is unique with respect to its dermal-epidermal characteristics, subcutaneous tissue (in the heel pad), adherent dermal septa to the underlying plantar fascia, and ability to withstand constant pressure

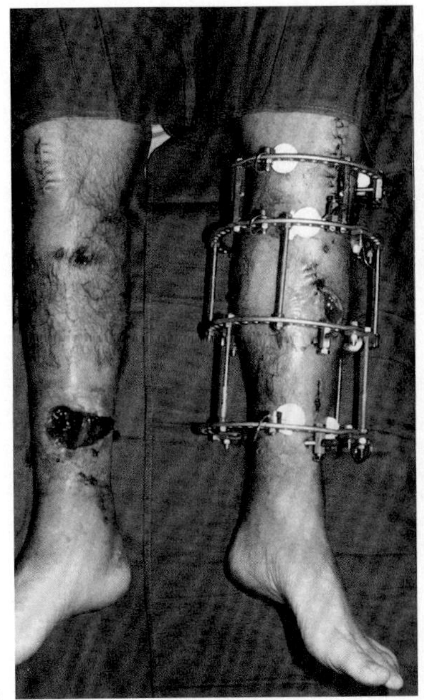
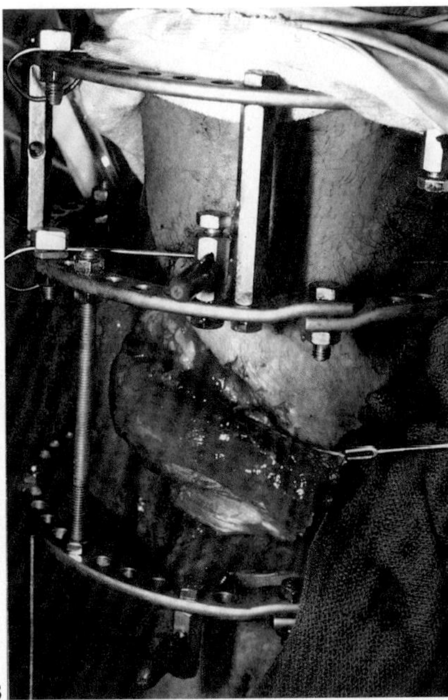
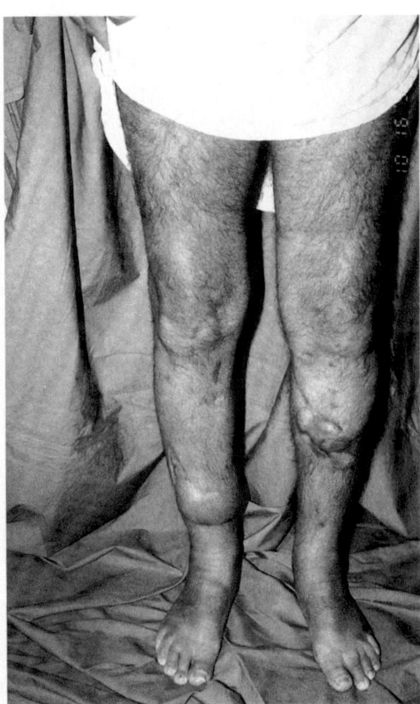

FIGURE 16-18 **A.** Patient with bilateral injuries. On the right leg, the distal third required free muscle transfer in the form of latissimus dorsi muscle flap covered with a split-thickness skin graft. The patient's left leg was stabilized with an Ilizarov fixator. The middle third lesion required a hemisoleus transfer. **B.** The arc of rotation is seen. **C.** Patient standing at 9 months follow-up with both legs healed.

and shear forces. Providing coverage, along with protective sensibility, can be achieved with a free neurosensory flap such as the radial forearm flap (139). Free muscle flaps are used when bulk is necessary to obliterate dead space such as in osteomyelitis, in severe crush injuries with extensive soft tissue loss, and for weight-bearing surfaces (140). However, muscle flaps can often be bulky and, if not contoured properly, may prevent the use of normal shoes.

Plantar Skin Reconstruction

The plantar skin has unique properties. It is thick and heavily keratinized, designed to resist high stress, and anchored to underlying bones and ligaments by thick fibrous connective tissue. The plantar surface acts as a shock-absorbing system for the foot, helping to minimize horizontal and vertical shear forces by its multidirectional fibrous septa (141). The plantar surface of the foot can be divided into three distinct areas with its special requirement to replace like with like.

The forefoot includes the dorsal areas of the metatarsals and toes. The plantar aspect includes the metatarsal heads and the instep. The hindfoot can be divided into the plantar aspect, instep, and lateral aspect of the calcaneus as the major regions requiring reconstruction. The ankle can be divided into the area of the Achilles tendon and the anterior aspect of the tibiotalar joint. In the forefoot, the dorsum and the area over the toes are primarily skin and subcutaneous tissue, making the exposure of tendons and joints more probable with high-energy injury. The plantar forefoot is prone to avulsion because of the vertically oriented septa that bridge from the plantar fascia to the dermal elements of the skin. The heel pad is a very unique structure that contains cushion-like shock absorbing chambers of fat that are not easily replaced.

Around the heel pad, coverage is important to avoid scarring around the tibial nerve and exposure or risk to the posterior tibial tendon. The lateral aspect of the heel in the non–weight-bearing portion is often at risk after internal fixation of calcaneal fractures following an extensive lateral approach. In the ankle, the distal anterior tibia has limited subcutaneous tissue. The skin over the Achilles tendon is also relatively devoid of subcutaneous tissue and frequently requires augmentation after heel cord repair. It is also important to understand the specialized skin, subcutaneous, and fat layers in each region because they will guide reconstruction (Fig. 16-20).

We have classified soft tissue reconstruction of the foot into six categories (A1, A2, B1, B2, C, and D). Each category is associated with unique problems.

Type A: Closed Fractures Treated by Open Reduction with Internal Fixation

Group A1: Inability to Close Skin. In surgical intervention for injuries to the foot, an important factor is soft tissue swelling. Ice, elevation, and a bulky dressing will allow edema to subside, usually within 10 days of the fracture. Although indirect reduction techniques may help, if swelling is not sufficiently decreased, difficulties with wound closure will develop.

Operatively, atraumatic technique, the use of skin hooks

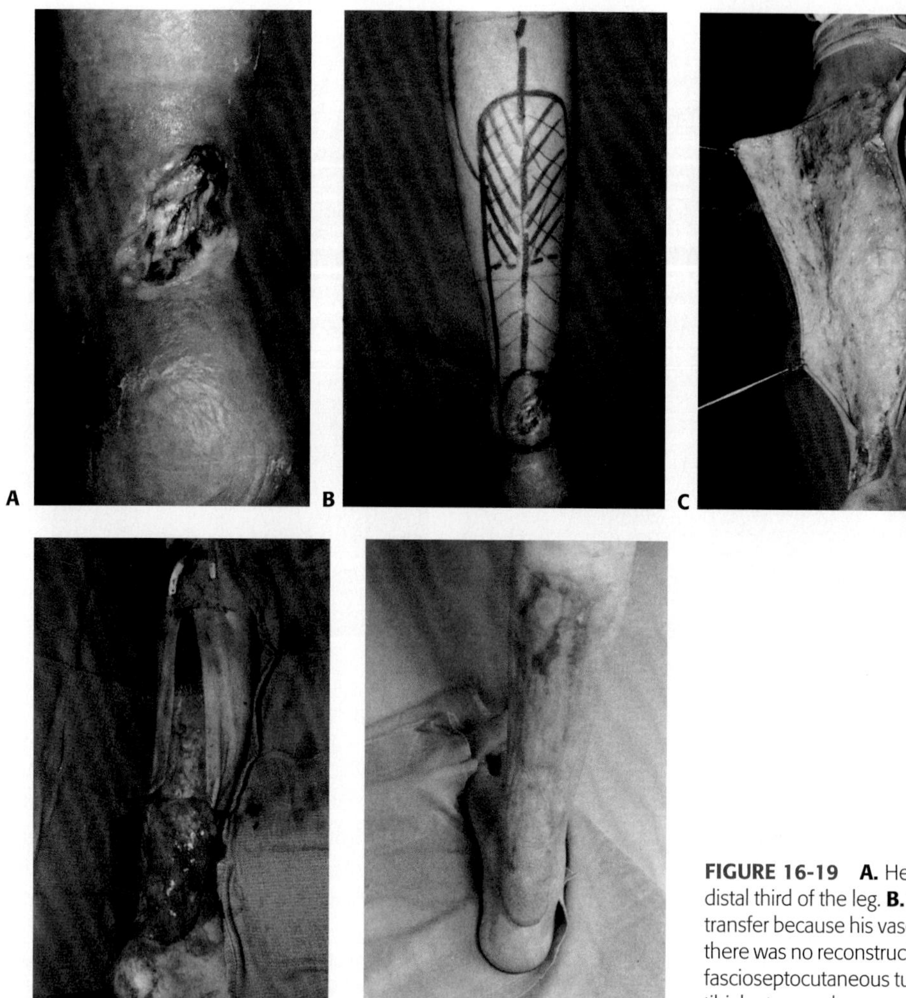

FIGURE 16-19 **A.** Heel cord exposure after soft tissue injury to the distal third of the leg. **B.** The patient was not a candidate for free-tissue transfer because his vascular system was studied with angiography and there was no reconstructable vascular tree to supply donor vessels. **C.** A fascioseptocutaneous turn-down flap was done based on the posterior tibial artery and peroneal perforators. **D.** Intraoperative picture. **E.** Flap turned down.

(rather than self-retaining retractors), loupe magnification, hemostasis during exposure, drains, and postoperative elevation with soft tissue dressings all contribute to permit uncomplicated wound healing. When the wound cannot be closed primarily, porcine allograft, Epigard, or STSG can be applied as temporary coverage. Delayed primary closure may be performed, if possible.

Group A2: Postoperative Wound Breakdown. Postoperatively, wound breakdown may occur. Partial-thickness defects should be managed initially with conservative measures. These include cessation of exercise, daily whirlpools and dressing changes, elevation, and oral antibiotics. This treatment will usually suffice. If plate or bone is visible, however, or if a full-thickness defect has developed, early aggressive, operative soft tissue debridement should be performed.

Subsequent coverage is obtained using local or distal flaps. The decision to use a local flap to cover defects around the foot will depend on (a) the presence of acute infection, (b) the depth of the defect, (c) the presence of an adequate vascular supply, and (d) damage to other areas of the foot that precludes the use of local flaps.

Recently, renewed emphasis has been placed on vascular territories (angiosomes or venosomes) that can be used as local rotation or island flaps. Choices for heel reconstruction include the medial pedis flap, dorsal pedis flap, abductor myocutaneous or fasciocutaneous flap, the peroneal flap, supramalleolar flap, and anterior tibial artery fasciocutaneous flaps (104,116,142,143). Muscle flaps include those from the flexor hallucis brevis or abductor hallucis, which can be rotated to cover small defects about the calcaneus; each of these muscle flaps contains its own vascular supply.

Type B: Requirements for Free Flaps for Foot Reconstruction

Arteriography and, occasionally, venography should be considered before free-tissue transfer. This is especially important in the diabetic and elderly patient in whom proximal lesions may

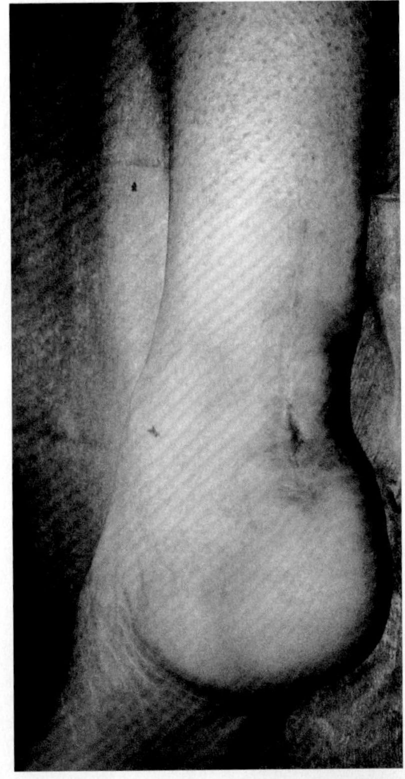

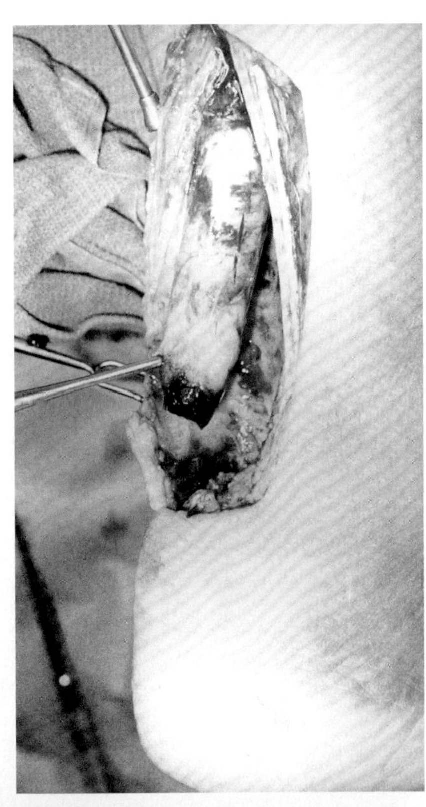

FIGURE 16-20 **A.** Tendon rupture following repair with subsequent chronic granulomatous tendinitis and sinus tract extending to the defect after the heel cord reavulsion. **B.** Intraoperative findings following debridement demonstrating the heel cord. **C.** Fasciocutaneous radial forearm flap in place with palmaris longus tendon used as a vascularized augmentation for heel cord repair. **D.** Immediately after surgery. **E,F.** Follow-up at 9 months showing active dorsiflexion and plantar flexion with stable flap over chronic wound.

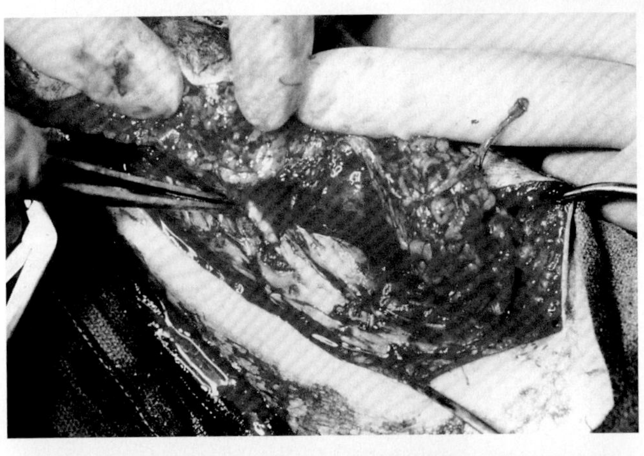

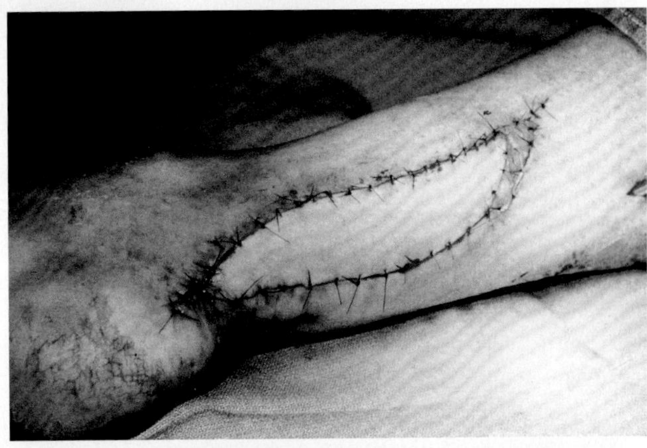

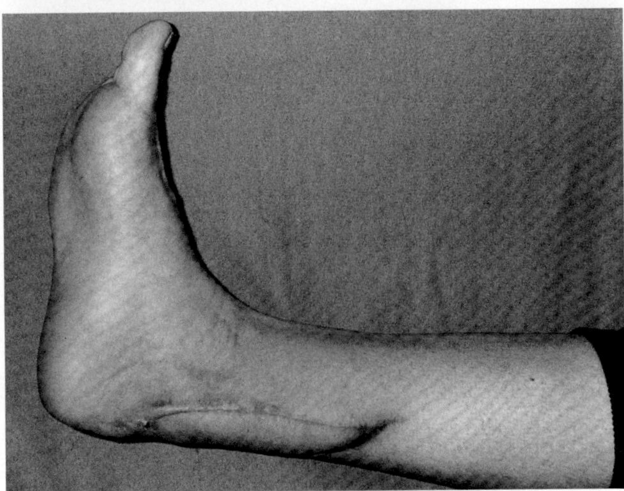

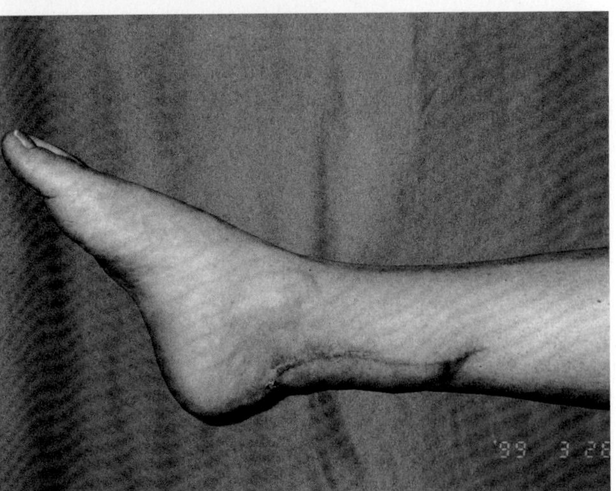

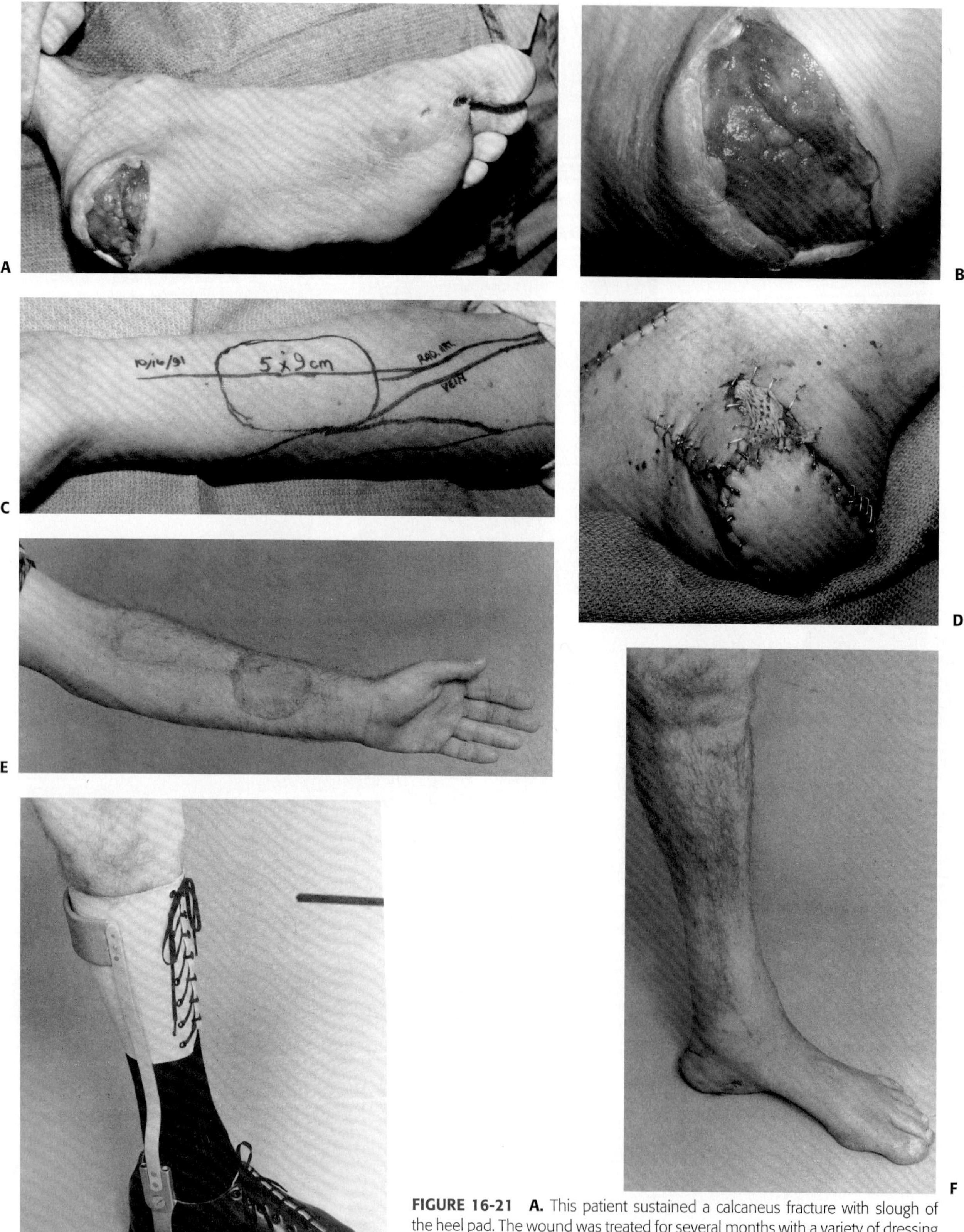

FIGURE 16-21 **A.** This patient sustained a calcaneus fracture with slough of the heel pad. The wound was treated for several months with a variety of dressing changes but did not heal. Calcaneal osteomyelitis was not present. The patient required reconstruction using a radial forearm flap and a vascular graft to provide inflow to the free flap. **B.** Preoperative wound. **C.** Radial forearm flap outlined. **D.** Intraoperative photograph showing heel resurfaced. **E.** Donor forearm at 1 year. **F.** Wound healed at 1 year. **G.** Plantigrade foot standing with ankle-foot orthosis used to unload the heel pad.

preclude inflow in an area of trauma that is already compromised. Flap selection in type B reconstruction is based on need. If cutaneous coverage alone is required, the radial forearm flap provides good coverage (Fig. 16-21).

A long pedicle can be obtained to enable the microsurgeon to perform an anastomosis out of the zone of injury, usually end-to-side on the posterior tibial artery. The lateral arm flap may be selected; however, this often produces significant donor site morbidity. The scapular flap provides cutaneous coverage but tends to be hypermobile after healing. It has less resistance to tangential shear forces if applied to the plantar surface as compared with muscle flaps.

Group B1: Traumatic Large Soft Tissue Loss with Adequate Bone Stock. Good evidence suggests that early coverage of open fractures is the treatment of choice, provided that the wound environment is suitable. The type of soft tissue coverage will depend on, and must be tailored to, the underlying reconstruction.

Group B2: Traumatic Loss of Soft Tissue and Bone. When both a soft tissue and an osseous defect are present, a careful assessment as to appropriate reconstruction must be made. If the injured bone and soft tissue are available and relatively clean, they may be debrided and reattached. If this is not possible, reconstruction would require a free flap, structural bone block iliac crest graft, and internal fixation. Alternatively, an osteocutaneous iliac crest or scapular flap could be used. Careful consideration must be given to a below-knee amputation, because this may ultimately be the fastest and most efficient means of restoring function to the patient (Figs. 16-22 and 16-23).

Type C: Osteomyelitis

Osteomyelitis of the foot usually occurs late and is commonly accompanied by marginal soft tissue overlying implants or bone

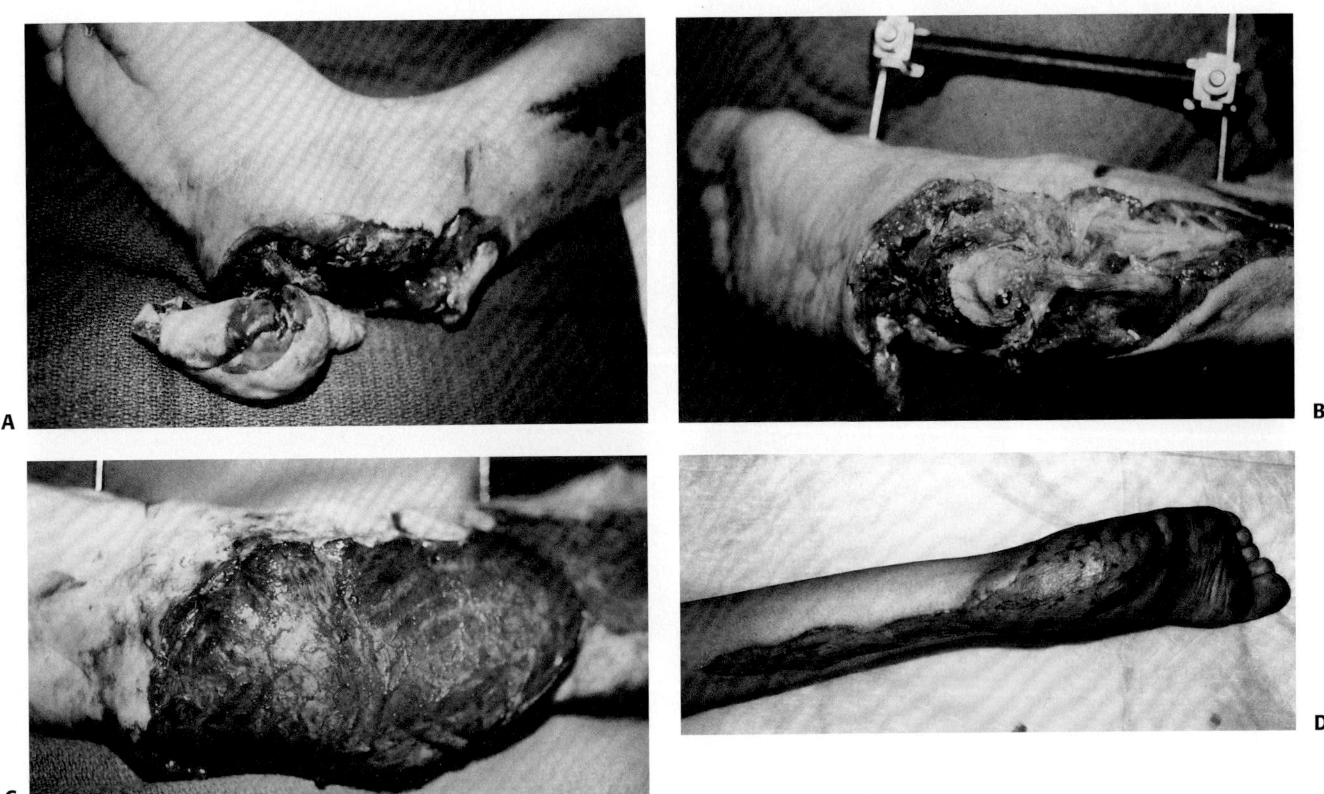

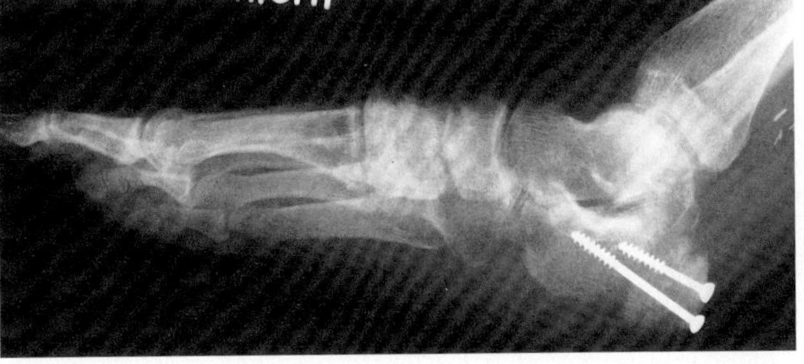

FIGURE 16-22 **A.** Emergency free flap. Patient sustained a lawnmower injury with avulsion of the calcaneal tuberosity and heel skin. **B.** The tuberosity was replaced with an AO 4.5-mm screw, and the heel cord was reattached. An external fixator was placed to keep the foot plantigrade and keep tension off the repair. **C.** An immediate emergency rectus free flap was performed to cover the reconstruction the night of injury. **D,E.** The result of the flap at 6 weeks.

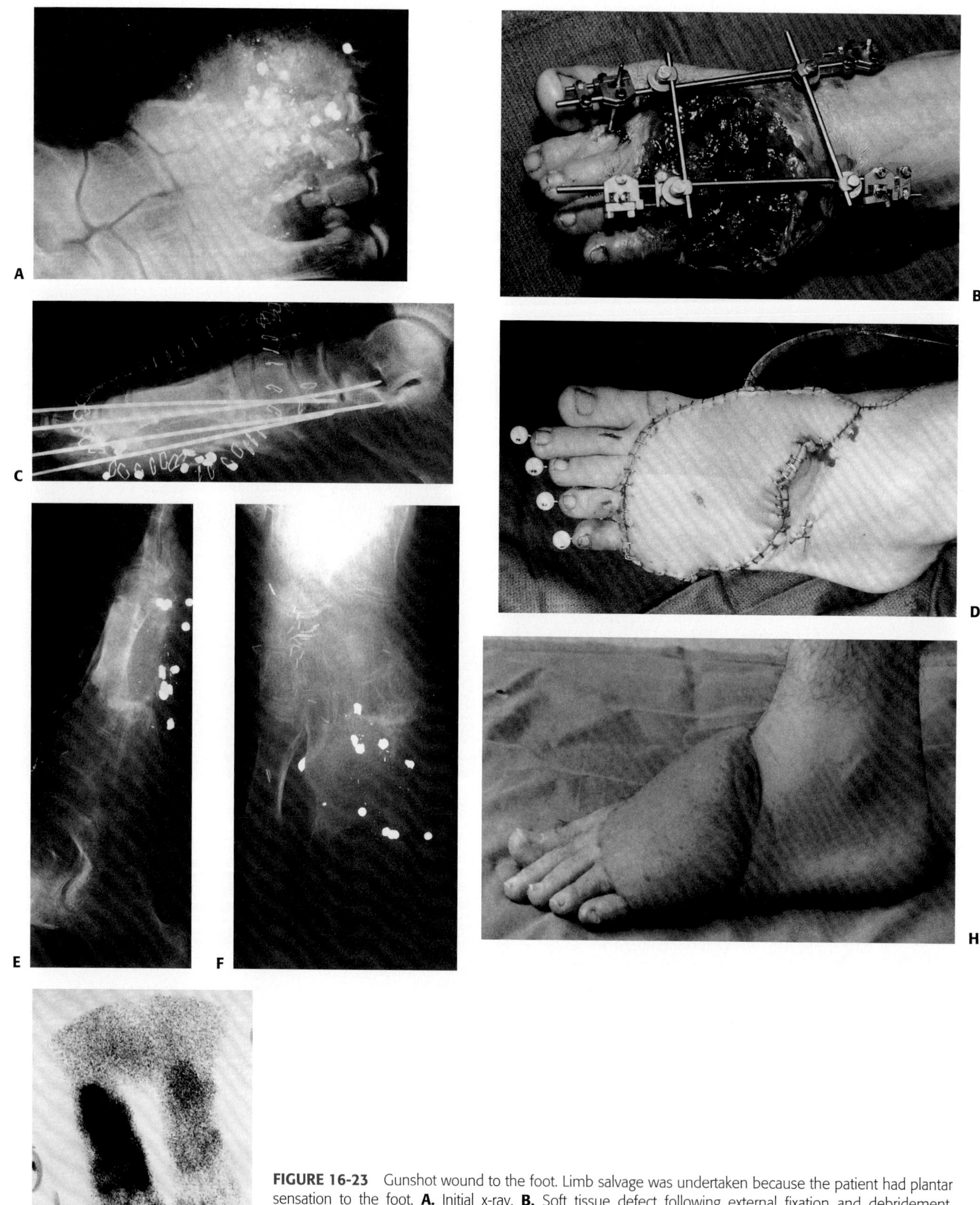

FIGURE 16-23 Gunshot wound to the foot. Limb salvage was undertaken because the patient had plantar sensation to the foot. **A.** Initial x-ray. **B.** Soft tissue defect following external fixation and debridement. **C.** Percutaneous pinning of iliac crest nonvascularized bone graft for intercalary metatarsal reconstruction. **D.** Intraoperative photograph of free scapular flap used to cover bone graft. **E,F.** X-rays at 6 months showing bone graft incorporation. **G.** Bone scan confirming uptake and vascularization of the bone graft. **H.** Final appearance of plantigrade foot at 1 year.

(144). Inflamed, reactive soft tissue cannot be used to close defects if sequestrectomy is performed. Therefore, distant muscle flaps should be strongly considered. Muscle flaps have been shown clinically and experimentally to aid in controlling (not curing) osteomyelitis. Studies by Cierny and Mader (13) have shown in the A host (no systemic illnesses) and B host (systemic illnesses, such as vascular disease, diabetes, history of smoking, or poor nutrition) that osteomyelitis can be controlled using this technique.

Type D: Reconstruction for Unstable Soft Tissue

Problems associated with reconstruction of the heel pad resulting from lack of soft tissue support may require orthotic devices or bracing. These patients often require augmentation of unstable tissue with local or distant flaps. Although the goal of the surgeon is to replace "like with like," according to Gillies, this is virtually impossible in heel pad reconstruction.

Patients receiving noninnervated flaps for soft tissue reconstruction of the heel must be treated in a fashion similar to patients with peripheral neuropathy. Education must be directed toward informing the patient that the foot, although restored and functional, is not normal. The patient must inspect the foot for callosities and irritations. Because of the increased mobility of flaps, particularly skin flaps, a variety of interface problems can occur, either on the flap or at the flap-skin junction. The inability to provide full sensation does not, however, preclude soft tissue reconstruction about the heel in that most patients obtain some degree of proprioceptive feedback and deep sensibility from the underlying muscle, periosteum, and surrounding skin.

AESTHETIC CONSIDERATIONS AFTER LIMB TRAUMA

Limb appearance and function have assumed importance after limb reconstruction. Scar quality and limb contour are important considerations. A favorable scar should be fine-line and situated against a wrinkle, contour junction, or skin line. It should have no contour irregularities or pigmentation abnormalities and not cause distortion or contracture. Scars can be revised or otherwise treated to improve direction, decrease their apparent length, correct distortion of anatomic units, improve surface irregularities, and correct pigment irregularities.

Hypertrophic scars and keloids constitute the unfavorable end of the scar spectrum but must be differentiated to be treated appropriately. Both demonstrate increased collagen deposition (mainly types I and III) during the fibroblastic portion of the proliferative phase of wound healing (5 days to 3 weeks) (145). Keloids are found predominantly in black patients and by definition extend beyond skin wound margins. They may behave quite invasively following the most innocuous skin trauma, for example, a mosquito bite with scratching of the skin. They are familial and exhibit an autosomal dominant pattern of inheritance. Keloids may be located on any part of the body and occur in all age groups except newborns. The hallmarks of this process are greatly increased dermal collagen content, increased collagen synthesis, and decreased collagen degradation (146). Skin levels of the degradative enzyme collagenase are higher in keloids than normal skin, normal scars, or hypertrophic scars and are likely blocked by α_2-macroglobulin. There appears to be a poorly defined immunologic component as well, with greatly increased dermal immunoglobulin (IgG) levels being measured in keloids (147).

Hypertrophic scars are raised and, although initially quite dramatic in color and appearance, tend to gradually regress. They remain within the boundaries of the primary incision or wound and are typified by the hypertrophic burn scar. They are formed at the margins of skin grafts and in deep second- and third-degree burns that are allowed to heal by secondary intention. Among reasons for unfavorable scar formation are location, tension, patient characteristics, and wound closure techniques. The midsternal, deltoid, elbow, knee, and upper breast areas are commonly troublesome, whereas most facial and neck incisions, especially when transverse or in skin lines, heal favorably.

Tension across incisions or wounds is to be avoided whenever possible because it frequently leads to widened, prominent scars. Significant tissue loss from trauma or debridement should raise the possibility of the need for skin grafting, undermining, or flap application. Temporary use of a biologic dressing such as pigskin may allow delayed primary closure of an edematous, overly tight wound such as an extremity fasciotomy wound.

Patient characteristics such as age, race, skin quality, and pigmentation also exert an influence on scar quality. Patient age less than 25 years, heavily pigmented skin, be it Negroid or Caucasian, and thick skin predispose to unfavorable scars. Patients may serve as self-controls in that the quality of previous mature scars is frequently readily apparent and may serve as a guide to scar outcome.

The fundamentals of good wound closure technique remain true and should contribute to a favorable result. Wounds should be free of foreign material and necrotic tissue, closed as soon as possible after wounding, and handled with care. Skin margins should be excised when necrotic and handled with skin hooks or toothed forceps only at the dermal level. Tension should be minimized by judicious undermining if needed or by flaps, skin grafts, or delayed closure. Wound edges require accurate approximation, and closure in layers with eversion using any one of a number of suture techniques. A subcuticular pull-out suture of monofilament may be considered for epidermal approximation. Whether sutures or staples are used is of less importance than having no tension at the epidermal level. Skin tension should be such that staples or sutures may be removed at 6 to 9 days and replaced by Steri-Strips or other tapes. Skin sutures are best tied slightly loosely rather than tightly because postoperative edema almost guarantees skin necrosis with an overly tight closure.

The postoperative treatment of new scars includes early suture removal, massage, avoiding sun exposure, and edema control. Massage reduces wound edema mechanically, may soften wound fibrosis, and helps to desensitize cutaneous reinnervation. Sun exposure after wounding causes scar hyperpigmentation for at least 6 months and should be avoided. Heavy application of sun block may be used if sun avoidance is impossible. Early limb edema control by elevation, limitation of dependency, and judicious use of wraps (for example, Coban) is critical to minimizing wound tension and scar quality. As mentioned above, suture or staple removal as early as possible avoids suture tracts and improves scar quality. Skin sutures should not be used to provide wound edge approximation; dermal sutures serve this function.

Silicone sheet application for up to 12 weeks may provide improvement, at least anecdotally, among those patients with known keloid or hypertrophic scar diathesis or in unfavorable wounds such as ungrafted superficial second-degree burns. In some cases, the improvement even in several-week-old wounds is quite dramatic. This modality is convenient, well tolerated, inexpensive, and painless.

Intralesional corticosteroid injections may also be indicated for patients with a known scar diathesis. An agent such as triamcinolone in a 40 mg/mL concentration with no more than 80 mg given in each 6-week period will frequently blunt the degree of collagen overdeposition seen in these patients. It inhibits the lysylhydroxylase and prolylhydroxylase necessary for collagen synthesis. The effects of steroids are reversible by vitamin A. It also decreases fibroblast migration and increases collagenase activity by decreasing α_2-macroglobulin deposition (148). This wound modulator should be used with caution because it may cause skin atrophy. It is contraindicated in pregnant patients and in patients with peptic ulcer disease.

Options for treatment of the unfavorable scar include revision and dermabrasion. Revision comprises simple excision, breakup of a long scar, and staging. The principles remain constant. Timing of revision is critical and must await scar maturation. Typically, this is 6 to 12 months in adults and up to 24 months in children. The scar's red or pink quality must fade to white. This assumes that the original wound was traumatic or closed under less than ideal circumstances. Scar revision may be performed earlier, weeks to months after injury, if the scar is situated perpendicular to the relaxed skin lines; a primary closure such as this will never be of good quality, regardless of the degree of maturation (149). If a well-planned incision by a careful surgeon in an anatomically favorable area, closed using appropriate techniques, has left an unsatisfactory scar, one should consider whether it is likely to improve with revision.

In revision, the new scar should be situated to fall within existing wrinkle or skin line complexes. A scar immediately adjacent to and parallel to a wrinkle avoids scar retraction and furrowing. Of fundamental importance is that tension be minimized. When undermining is done, the subdermal vascular supply must be preserved.

Dog ears may be excised in a straight-line extension of the original wound. A buried dermal flap technique in which the existing scar is deepithelialized and used for fill helps minimize scar depression. Z-plasty techniques will help to correct scar contracture across joints or in areas where anatomic units are distorted (149). The flaps must be generous for this application; they may be smaller when used to break up a long scar's vertical appearance where no distortion is present. W-plasty techniques may be used to improve scar orientation and appearance when it lies perpendicular to the relaxed skin lines. Local flaps or free flaps may be required when poor scar or soft tissue quality (especially after significant tissue loss or multiple reoperations) contributes to problems with rehabilitation or function. FTSGs, usually taken from the groin, may be used when attempts at revision result in gaping, tight wounds. These may be deepithelialized and overgrafted at a later date for additional thickness. As mentioned above, scar massage, edema control, steroid injection, and silicone sheeting may be useful adjuncts to revision.

In patients with keloids, we have found low-dose radiation to be of benefit in conjunction with scar revision. The keloid is excised immediately within the border of the lesion, closed without tension using subcuticular sutures after dermal approximation, and injected with triamcinolone as described above. The radiation treatment is carried out in 200-rad increments daily for 5 days and is ideally begun on the day of surgery.

Tissue expansion may be very helpful in scar management because it allows revision of large scars in a rapid, two-stage fashion (see below).

Dermabrasion is of value in the treatment of the raised or irregularly contoured scar. It may be used to level high points, but is contraindicated for depressed scars or for those in which the wound edges are "stepped" as a result of poor wound closure technique. The latter wounds should be revised surgically. Dermabrasion may lead to depigmentation, and patients must be warned about this.

Finally, free-tissue transfer may be used. This approach is highly unusual but patients may be inhibited enough psychologically by an unsightly scar that they want to undergo such reconstruction. Careful selection of the flap as well as consideration of donor scar management can result in a satisfactory esthetic result. The use of tissue expanders can help by decreasing donor site morbidity, as well as the need for debulking of flaps, which can result in an improved cosmetic result (150).

STUMP COVERAGE

Despite the success achieved in limb salvage procedures, still a high number of amputations are performed in cases of major trauma and in cases in which the patient is too ill to survive a lengthy operation. The level of amputation itself is an important factor for consideration. In cases of lower limb amputation, below-knee amputation is associated with faster and fuller rehabilitation compared to a through-knee or above-knee amputation. Below-knee amputation decreases the energy required for ambulation, creates a more natural gait, and allows more extensive physical activity (151). The choice of the level of the amputation is dictated by the necessity to cover the stump with appro-

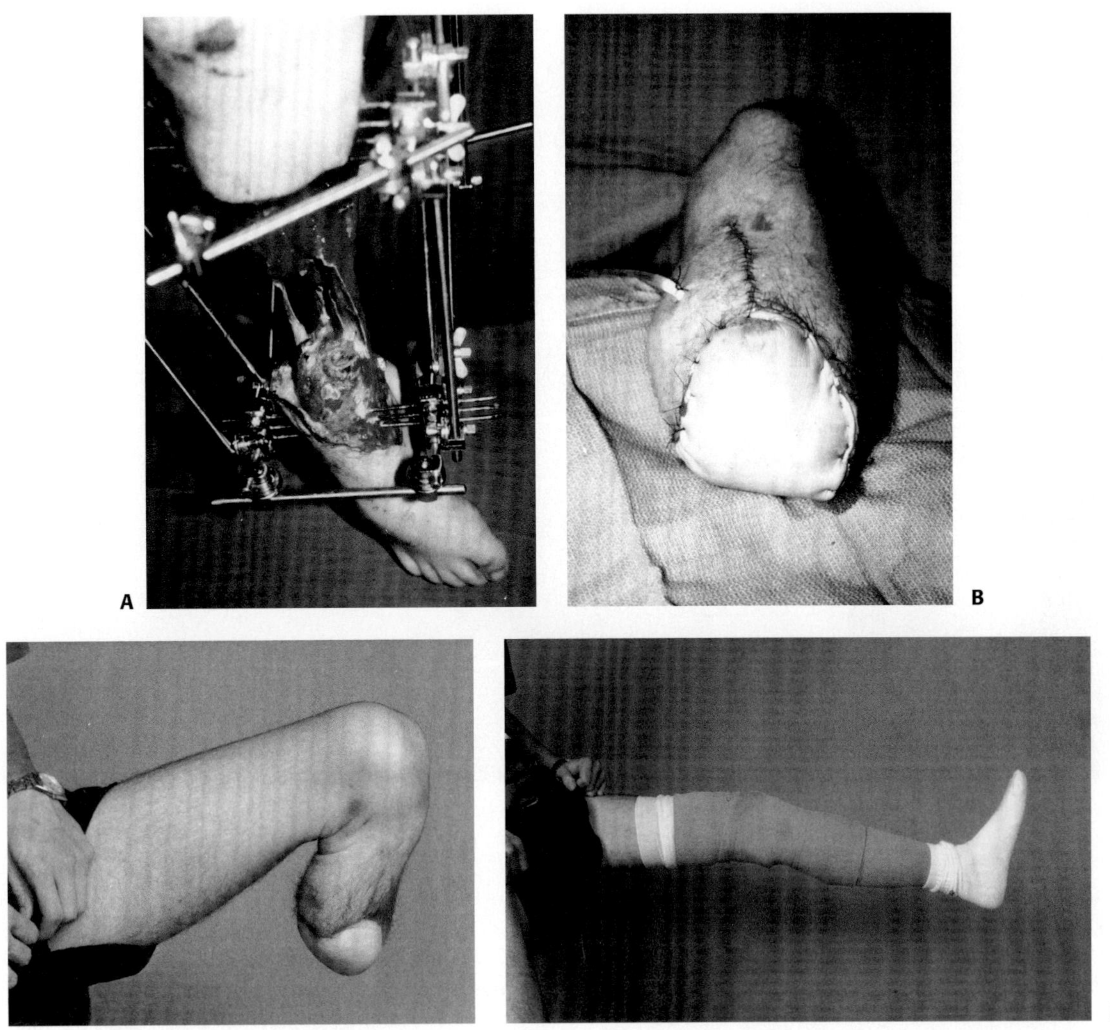

FIGURE 16-24 **A.** Patient with a IIIC fracture with loss of all soft tissue and bone in lower leg. The foot was maintained only by some granulation tissue and the neurovascular bundle that included the posterior tibial nerve. **B.** A plantar filet flap was done as an island pedicle flap to preserve length of the residual limb and provide sensibility for gait training. **C.** Final result with flexion. **D.** Extension wearing prosthesis.

priate soft tissue that is stable enough to withstand the forces acting upon it without ulceration or wound breakdown. STSG of an amputation stump, especially in the lower limb, provides only wound coverage but leaves the need for adequate padding of the amputation stump. In these cases in which a local flap is not available, free flaps should be considered. These flaps can provide coverage of the stump, and, if microneural anastomosis is performed, sensation of the stump can be achieved, providing proprioception within the prosthesis. The amputated part may serve as a donor site (such as a filet foot flap), eliminating donor site morbidity (Fig. 16-24) (152).

TISSUE EXPANSION

Soft tissue expansion enjoys wide use by plastic surgeons around the world and has been used successfully for reconstruction of deformities and for removal of lesions of the extremities (153–156). Soft tissue expansion is best applied in delayed reconstruction, as well as for expansion of free flaps to be used in soft tissue reconstruction of the limbs to lower the morbidity of the donor site (157). This technique requires adequate soft tissue for expansion, and, if only skin is expanded, it should have a thickness and subcutaneous fat that will allow maintenance or restoration of contour at the site of reconstruction (Fig. 16-25).

Sites such as the ankle and the foot can be suitable for expansion but are difficult. There is a high incidence of periexpander infection if the expander is placed next to an open wound in the lower extremity. Judgment will be required in all cases in deciding whether a particular patient is a good candidate for soft tissue expansion.

In the extremities it is preferable to plan a transverse ad-

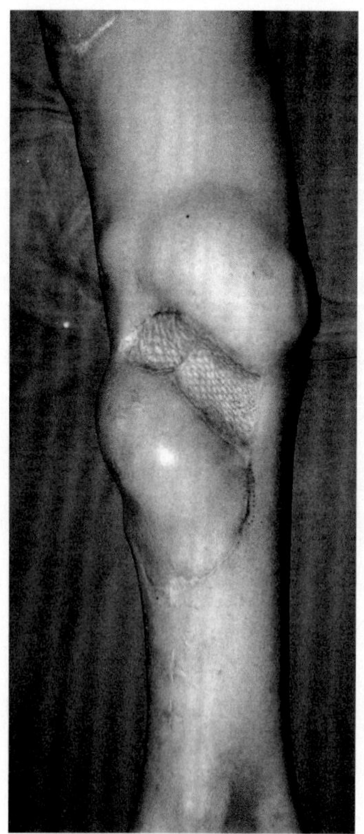

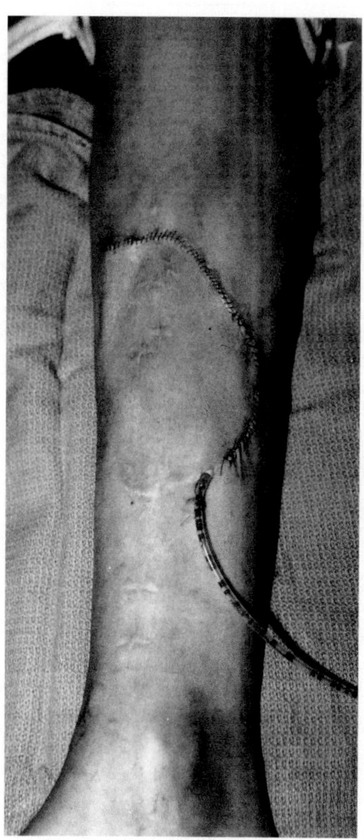

FIGURE 16-25 **A.** Posterior calf deformity after open tibial fracture; tissue expanders under distal and proximal flaps. **B.** Scar excision and primary closure after expander removal.

vancement of tissue instead of an axial advancement (59). The expander should be located just above the muscle fascia. Expansion begins usually 1 to 2 weeks after implantation, is increased once a week, and is continued until the circumference of the extremity has increased by an amount equal to the width of the defect. Complications of soft tissue expansions include infection, dehiscence, seroma, dislocation of the expander, and leakage. One of the most common causes for exposure of an implant is an inadequately dissected pocket. If the pocket is small, the edge of the expander may push against the healing incision and cause a dehiscence.

The advantages of soft tissue expanders are that coverage is with tissue like the tissue that was lost, their use is cost-effective, and the procedure may be conducted on an outpatient basis. Newer techniques such as minimally invasive placement using a balloon dissector and expanders placed through a remote access incision may reduce the delay required for incision healing, minimize complications, and increase the amount of flap gain (158).

FUTURE TECHNOLOGY: PREFABRICATION AND ENDOSCOPIC HARVESTING

Endoscopic Harvesting

The technique of endoscopically assisted flap harvest through small incisions aims to circumvent the disadvantages of the traditional harvesting techniques (157,159). This minimally invasive approach also offers several potential theoretical advantages over traditional harvesting techniques. Magnified visualization of the operative field through the video monitor can help the surgeon achieve better intraoperative hemostasis with less postoperative bleeding. Smaller incisions can potentially result in better wound healing, less nursing care, and less postoperative pain at the donor site. However, these benefits must be weighed against an increased complexity of operating room setup, which leads to increased operative time and cost. Because of lack of tactile sensation and change to two-dimensional video monitor visualization, the endoscopic technique has a steep learning curve. Furthermore, donor site morbidity in the endoscopically assisted technique and the traditional technique must be compared to determine whether this new trend is justified. Recent studies comparing traditional and endoscopic harvesting of the latissimus dorsi revealed no statistically significant differences in the amount of intraoperative bleeding, the incidence of postoperative hematoma, and the incidence of donor site wound infection as assessed by the surgeon. However, a patient questionnaire revealed that, even though it did not reach a statistically significant difference, the endoscopically assisted technique had less pain and allowed earlier and better movement of the upper extremity of the donor site. The patients' attitude and feeling about the scar and overall satisfaction were also higher in the endoscopic group (160).

The search continues for new methods, such as staplers,

that will result in faster and easier methods for microvascular anastomosis. Staplers shorten the operating time and have proved to be safe (161). The vessels suitable for this technique should be chosen carefully, and surgeons using this technique should be also experienced in conventional microsurgery.

It is expected that the time-consuming procedure using interrupted sutures in microvascular surgery will be replaced more and more by the use of running sutures. Furthermore, refinements in laser welding and the development of new glues may take over the role of sutures. The operating microscope itself may also vanish in time. Many microsurgeons prefer to use high-magnification loupes, with which they are able to achieve good results (99,162). Furthermore, advances in video technology now enable the surgeon to view a microsurgical field on a monitor in three dimensions without the necessity to look through the microscope eyepieces (163).

The technique of prefabrication of flaps allows custom flaps to be constructed based on what is required for a specific defect. The exploration of this new frontier may increase the possibility of reconstructive capabilities and decrease the donor morbidity of classical reconstructions (164–166).

Cost and Outcome

The time-consuming and costly nature of microsurgery requires appropriate indications and patient management. To operate in this cost-conscious time, financial as well as functional outcome determinations are critical. Some groups, however, have assembled cost estimates and made initial inroads into outcomes and measurements of cost-effectiveness (167,168).

The versatility and vascularity of free-tissue transfers have made them indispensable tools for reconstructive surgeons. Although free-flap procedures can provide definitive treatment in a single operation, they are expensive and require specialized practitioners. Clearly, a reduction in complications would reduce the cost of these procedures. Currently, efforts are under way to reduce free flap costs at all stages of care by shortening the operating time with the use of new devices, shortening the monitoring time postoperatively, and even exploring in selected patients the possibility of using an outpatient monitoring system (169). In this era of managed care and capitation, expensive procedures are often targeted in cost-containment efforts. Free-flap procedures are costly but they are also effective (170).

REFERENCES

1. Court-Brown CM, Rimmer S, Prakash U, et al. The epidemiology of open long bone fractures. *Injury* 1998;29:529–534.
2. Adams F. *The genuine works of Hippocrates*. New York: Williams Wood; 1891.
3. Aldea PA, Shaw WW. The evolution of the surgical management of severe lower extremity trauma. *Clin Plast Surg* 1986;13:549–569.
4. Kocher MS. Early limb salvage: open tibia fractures of Ambroise Pare (1510–1590) and Percivall Pott (1714–1789). *World J Surg* 1997;21:116–122.
5. Howard M, Court-Brown CM. Epidemiology and management of open fractures of the lower limb. *Br J Hosp Med* 1997;57:582–587.
6. Macnab I, De Haas WG. The role of periosteal blood supply in the healing of fractures of the tibia. *Clin Orthop Rel Res* 1974;105:27–33.
7. Holden C. The role of blood supply to soft tissue in the healing of diaphyseal fractures. *J Bone Joint Surg Am* 1972;54:993.
8. Muhlbauer W, Herndl E, Stock W. The forearm flap. *Plast Reconstr Surg* 1982;70: 336–344.
9. Mathes SJ, Nahai F. *Reconstructive surgery principles, anatomy & techniques*. New York: Churchill Livingstone; 1997.
10. Krettek C, Haas N, Schandelmaier P, et al. [Unreamed tibial nail in tibial shaft fractures with severe soft tissue damage: initial clinical experiences]. *Unfallchirurg* 1991;94: 579–587.
11. Taylor GI, Corlett RJ, Boyd JB. The versatile deep inferior epigastric (inferior rectus abdominis) flap. *Br J Plast Surg* 1984;37:330–350.
12. Mathes SJ, Nahai F. Classification of the vascular anatomy of muscles: experimental and clinical correlation. *Plast Reconstr Surg* 1981;67:177–187.
13. Cierny G 3rd, Mader JT. Approach to adult osteomyelitis. *Orthop Rev* 1987;16: 259–270.
14. Anderson L. Fractures with soft tissue injuries. In: Tscherne H, ed. *Fractures*. Berlin: Springer-Verlag; 1984:4.
15. Gustilo RB, Anderson JT. Prevention of infection in the treatment of one thousand and twenty-five open fractures of long bones: retrospective and prospective analyses. *J Bone Joint Surg Am* 1976;58:453–458.
16. Muller MEAM, Schneider R, et al. *Manual of internal fixation techniques recommended by the AO-ASIF group*. Heidelberg: Springer-Verlag; 1990.
17. Tscherne H, Gotzen GL. *Fractures with soft tissue injuries*. Berlin: Springer-Verlag; 1984: 4–9.
18. Alonso BEAJ. Classification of soft tissue injuries. *Tech Orthop* 1995;10:73–78.
19. Ruedi T, Von Hochstetter A, Schlumpf R. *Surgical approaches for internal fixation*. Heidelberg: Springer-Verlag; 1984.
20. Hansen S. The evolution of musculoskeletal traumatology at Harborview Medical Center. In: Hansen S, Swiontkowski M, eds. *Orthopaedic trauma protocols*. New York: Raven Press; 1993:3–8.
21. Godina M. *A Thesis on the Management of Injuries to the Lower Extremity*. Presernova Druzba Ljuibljana, 1991.
22. Swiontkowski M. Criteria for bone debridement in massive lower limb trauma. *Clin Orthop Rel Res* 1989;243:41–48.
23. Byrd HS, Spicer TE, Cierney GD. Management of open tibial fractures. *Plast Reconstr Surg* 1985;76:719–730.
24. Fischer MD, Gustilo RB, Varecka TF. The timing of flap coverage, bone-grafting, and intramedullary nailing in patients who have a fracture of the tibial shaft with extensive soft tissue injury. *J Bone Joint Surg Am* 1991;73:1316–1322.
25. Godina M. Early microsurgical reconstruction of complex trauma of the extremities. *Plast Reconstr Surg* 1986;78:285–292.
26. Janzekovic Z. Early surgical treatment of the burned surface. *Panminerva Med* 1972; 14:228–232.
27. Hertel R, Lambert SM, Muller S, et al. On the timing of soft tissue reconstruction for open fractures of the lower leg. *Arch Orthop Trauma Surg* 1999;119:7–12.
28. Esterhai JL Jr, Queenan J. Management of soft tissue wounds associated with type III open fractures. *Orthop Clin North Am* 1991;22:427–432.
29. Henry SL, Ostermann PA, Seligson D. The prophylactic use of antibiotic impregnated beads in open fractures. *J Trauma Injury Infect Crit Care* 1990;30:1231–1238.
30. Henry SL, Seligson D, Mangino P, et al. Antibiotic-impregnated beads. I. Bead implantation versus systemic therapy. *Orthop Rev* 1991;20:242–247.
31. Henry SL, Popham GJ, Mangino P, et al. Antibiotic impregnated beads: a production technique. *Contemp Orthop* 1989;19:221–226.
32. Turen CH, DiStasio AJ. Treatment of grade IIIB and grade IIIC open tibial fractures. *Orthop Clin North Am* 1994;25:561–571.
33. Kindwall EP, Gottlieb LJ, Larson DL. Hyperbaric oxygen therapy in plastic surgery: a review article. *Plast Reconstr Surg* 1991;88:898–908.
34. Morykwas MJ, Argenta LC. Nonsurgical modalities to enhance healing and care of soft tissue wounds. *J South Orthop Assoc* 1997;6:279–288.
35. Grim PS, Gottlieb LJ, Boddie A, et al. Hyperbaric oxygen therapy [see comments]. *JAMA* 1990;263:2216–2220.
36. Hunt TK, Zederfeldt B, Goldstick TK. Oxygen and healing. *Am J Surg* 1969;118: 521–525.
37. Argenta LC, Morykwas MJ. Vacuum-assisted closure: a new method for wound control and treatment: clinical experience. *Ann Plast Surg* 1997;38:563–576; discussion 577.
38. Webb LX. New techniques in wound management: vacuum-assisted wound closure. *J Am Acad Orthop Surg* 2002;10:303–311.
39. Levin LS. Personality of soft tissue injury. *Tech Orthop* 1995;10:65–72.
40. Lange RH. Limb reconstruction versus amputation decision making in massive lower extremity trauma. *Clin Orthop* 1989:243:92–99.
41. Hansen ST Jr. The type-IIIC tibial fracture. Salvage or amputation [editorial]. *J Bone Joint Surg Am* 1987;69:799–800.
42. Caudle RJ, Stern PJ. Severe open fractures of the tibia. *J Bone Joint Surg Am* 1987;69: 801–807.
43. Howe HR Jr, Poole GV Jr, Hansen KJ, et al. Salvage of lower extremities following combined orthopedic and vascular trauma: a predictive salvage index. *Am Surg* 1987; 53:205–208.
44. Lange RH, Bach AW, Hansen ST Jr, et al. Open tibial fractures with associated vascular injuries: prognosis for limb salvage. *J Trauma* 1985;25:203–208.
45. Clifford RP, Lyons TJ, Webb JK. Complications of external fixation of open fractures of the tibia. *Injury* 1987;18:174–176.
46. Haas N, Krettek C, Schandelmaier P, et al. A new solid unreamed tibial nail for shaft fractures with severe soft tissue injury. *Injury* 1993;24:49–54.
47. Krettek C, Gluer S, Schandelmaier P, et al. [Intramedullary nailing of open fractures]. *Orthopade* 1996;25:223–233.

48. Clifford RP, Beauchamp CG, Kellam JF, et al. Plate fixation of open fractures of the tibia. *J Bone Joint Surg Br* 1988;70:644–648.
49. Worlock P, Slack R, Harvey L, et al. The prevention of infection in open fractures: an experimental study of the effect of fracture stability. *Injury* 1994;25:31–38.
50. Yaremchuk MJ, Brumback RJ, Manson PN, et al. Acute and definitive management of traumatic osteocutaneous defects of the lower extremity. *Plast Reconstr Surg* 1987;80: 1–14.
51. Rudolph R, Ballantyne DL Jr. Skin grafts. In: McCarthy JG, ed. *Plastic surgery*. Philadelphia: WB Saunders; 1990:221–274.
52. Stuart JD, Morgan RF, Kenney JG. Single-donor fibrin glue for hand burns. *Ann Plast Surg* 1990;24:524–527.
53. Kelton P. Skin grafts. *Sel Read Plast Surg* 1992;7:1–20.
54. Feldman DL. Which dressing for split-thickness skin graft donor sites? [see comments]. *Ann Plast Surg* 1991;27:288–291.
55. McCauley RL, Linares HA, Pelligrini V, et al. *In vitro* toxicity of topical antimicrobial agents to human fibroblasts. *J Surg Res* 1989;46:267–274.
56. Irons GB, Fisher J, Schmitt EHD. Vascularized muscular and musculocutaneous flaps for management of osteomyelitis. *Orthop Clin North Am* 1984;15:473–480.
57. Irons GB Jr, Wood MB. Soft tissue coverage for the treatment of osteomyelitis of the lower part of the leg. *Mayo Clin Proc* 1986;61:382–387.
58. Ruttle PE, Kelly PJ, Arnold PG, et al. Chronic osteomyelitis treated with a muscle flap. *Orthop Clin North Am* 1984;15:451–459.
59. Barfod B, Pers M. Gastrocnemius-plasty for primary closure of compound injuries of the knee. *J Bone Joint Surg Br* 1970;52:124–127.
60. Vasconez LO, Bostwick J III, McCraw J. Coverage of exposed bone by muscle transposition and skin grafting. *Plast Reconstr Surg* 1974;53:526–530.
61. Kroll SS, Marcadis A. Aesthetic considerations of the medial gastrocnemius myocutaneous flap. *Plast Reconstr Surg* 1987;79:67–71.
62. Dibbell DG, Edstrom LE. The gastrocnemius myocutaneous flap. *Clin Plast Surg* 1980; 7:45–50.
63. McCraw JB. Selection of alternative local flaps in the leg and foot. *Clin Plast Surg* 1979; 6:227–246.
64. Byrd HS, Cierny G 3rd, Tebbetts JB. The management of open tibial fractures with associated soft tissue loss: external pin fixation with early flap coverage. *Plast Reconstr Surg* 1981;68:73–82.
65. Ger R. Operative treatment of the avanced stasis ulcer using muscle transposition: a follow-up study. *Am J Surg* 1970;120:376–380.
66. Ger R. Surgical management of ulcerative lesions of the leg. *Curr Probl Surg* 1972: 1–52.
67. Magee WP Jr, Gilbert DA, McInnis WD. Extended muscle and musculocutaneous flaps. *Clin Plast Surg* 1980;7:57–70.
68. Tobin GR. Hemisoleus and reversed hemisoleus flaps. *Plast Reconstr Surg* 1985;76: 87–96.
69. Thatte MR, Thatte RL. Venous flaps. *Plast Reconstr Surg* 1993;91:747–751.
70. Thatte RL, Thatte MR. The saphenous venous flap. *Br J Plast Surg* 1989;42:399–404.
71. Jacobson JH, Suarez SE. Microsurgery and anastomosis of small vessels. *Surg Forum* 1960:243–247.
72. Bunke CM, Schultz WB. Experimental digital amputation and replantation. *Plast Reconstr Surg* 1965;36:62.
73. Kleinert HE, Kasdan ML, Romero JL. Small blood vessels anastomosis for salvaged of severely injured upper extremity. *J Bone Joint Surg Am* 1963;45:788–796.
74. Katsaros J, Schusterman M, Beppu M, et al. The lateral upper arm flap: anatomy and clinical applications. *Ann Plast Surg* 1984;12:489–500.
75. Clark WL, Trumble TE, Swiontkowski MF, et al. Nerve tension and blood flow in a rat model of immediate and delayed repairs. *J Hand Surg Am* 1992;17:677–687.
76. Watchmaker GP, Mackinnon SE. Advances in peripheral nerve repair. *Clin Plast Surg* 1997;24:63–73.
77. Doi K. New reconstructive procedure for brachial plexus injury. *Clin Plast Surg* 1997; 24:75–85.
78. Pederson W. Limb salvage. *Probl Plast Reconstr Surg* 1991;1:125–155.
79. Goldberg JA, Alpert BS, Lineaweaver WC, et al. Microvascular reconstruction of the lower extremity in the elderly. *Clin Plast Surg* 1991;18:459–465.
80. Arnez ZM. Immediate reconstruction of the lower extremity: an update. *Clin Plast Surg* 1991;18:449–457.
81. Isenberg JS, Sherman R. Zone of injury: a valid concept in microvascular reconstruction of the traumatized lower limb? *Ann Plast Surg* 1996;36:270–272.
82. Gustilo RB, Mendoza RM, Williams DN. Problems in the management of type III (severe) open fractures: a new classification of type III open fractures. *J Trauma* 1984;24: 742–746.
83. Eshima I, Mathes SJ, Paty P. Comparison of the intracellular bacterial killing activity of leukocytes in musculocutaneous and random-pattern flaps. *Plast Reconstr Surg* 1990; 86:541–547.
84. Mathes SJ, Alpert BS, Chang N. Use of the muscle flap in chronic osteomyelitis: experimental and clinical correlation. *Plast Reconstr Surg* 1982;69:815–829.
85. Mathes SJ, Feng LJ, Hunt TK. Coverage of the infected wound. *Ann Surg* 1983;198: 420–429.
86. May JW Jr, Jupiter JB, Weiland AJ, et al. Clinical classification of post-traumatic tibial osteomyelitis. *J Bone Joint Surg Am* 1989;71:1422–1428.
87. Peat BG, Liggins DF. Microvascular soft tissue reconstruction for acute tibial fractures: late complications and the role of bone grafting. *Ann Plast Surg* 1990;24:517–520.
88. Anthony JP, Mathes SJ, Alpert BS. The muscle flap in the treatment of chronic lower extremity osteomyelitis: results in patients over 5 years after treatment. *Plast Reconstr Surg* 1991;88:311–318.
89. Bostwick JD, Nahai F, Wallace JG, et al. Sixty latissimus dorsi flaps. *Plast Reconstr Surg* 1979;63:31–41.
90. Harii K, Yamada A, Ishihara K, et al. A free transfer of both latissimus dorsi and serratus anterior flaps with thoracodorsal vessel anastomoses. *Plast Reconstr Surg* 1982;70: 620–629.
91. Bunkis J, Walton RL, Mathes SJ. The rectus abdominis free flap for lower extremity reconstruction. *Ann Plast Surg* 1983;11:373–380.
92. Jones G, Nahai F. Management of complex wounds. *Curr Probl Surg* 1998;35:179–270.
93. Markovich GD, Dorr LD, Klein NE, et al. Muscle flaps in total knee arthroplasty. *Clin Orthop Rel Res* 1995;321:122–130.
94. Lister G, Scheker L. Emergency free flaps to the upper extremity. *J Hand Surg Am* 1988; 13:22–28.
95. Chen S, Tsai YC, Wei FC, et al. Emergency free flaps to the type IIIC tibial fracture. *Ann Plast Surg* 1990;25:223–229.
96. McCabe SJ, Breidenbach WC. The role of emergency free flaps for hand trauma. *Hand Clin* 1999;15:275–288, viii–ix.
97. Giordano PA, Abbes M, Pequignot JP. Gracilis blood supply: anatomical and clinical re-evaluation. *Br J Plast Surg* 1990;43:266–272.
98. Donski PK, Buchler U, Ganz R. Combined osteocutaneous microvascular flap procedure for extensive bone and soft tissue defects in the tibia. *Ann Plast Surg* 1986;16:386–398.
99. Shenaq SM, Klebuc MJ, Vargo D. Free-tissue transfer with the aid of loupe magnification: experience with 251 procedures [see comments]. *Plast Reconstr Surg* 1995;95: 261–269.
100. Cormack GC, Duncan MJ, Lamberty BG. The blood supply of the bone component of the compound osteo-cutaneous radial artery forearm flap: an anatomical study. *Br J Plast Surg* 1986;39:173–175.
101. Swanson E, Boyd JB, Mulholland RS. The radial forearm flap: a biomechanical study of the osteotomized radius. *Plast Reconstr Surg* 1990;85:267–272.
102. Masser MR. The preexpanded radial free flap [see comments]. *Plast Reconstr Surg* 1990; 86:295–301, discussion 302–303.
103. dos Santos LF. The vascular anatomy and dissection of the free scapular flap. *Plast Reconstr Surg* 1984;73:599–604.
104. Reiffel RS, McCarthy JG. Coverage of heel and sole defects: a new subfascial arterialized flap. *Plast Reconstr Surg* 1980;66:250–260.
105. Urbaniak JR, Koman LA, Goldner RD, et al. The vascularized cutaneous scapular flap. *Plast Reconstr Surg* 1982;69:772–778.
106. Barwick WJ, Goodkind DJ, Serafin D. The free scapular flap. *Plast Reconstr Surg* 1982; 69:779–787.
107. Rautio J, Asko-Seljavaara S, Laasonen L, et al. Suitability of the scapular flap for reconstructions of the foot. *Plast Reconstr Surg* 1990;85:922–928.
108. Sekiguchi J, Kobayashi S, Ohmori K. Use of the osteocutaneous free scapular flap on the lower extremities. *Plast Reconstr Surg* 1993;91:103–112.
109. Park S, Han SH, Lee TJ. Algorithm for recipient vessel selection in free tissue transfer to the lower extremity. *Plast Reconstr Surg* 1999;103:1937–1948.
110. Bunke H. *Monitoring in microsurgery: transplantation-replantation*. Philadelphia: Lee & Febiger, 1991.
111. Achauer BM, Black KS, Litke DK. Transcutaneous PO_2 in flaps: a new method of survival prediction. *Plast Reconstr Surg* 1980;65:738–745.
112. Heller L, Levin LS, Klitzman B. Laser Doppler flowmeter monitoring of free tissue transfers: blood flow in normal and complicated cases. *Plast Reconstr Surg* 2001;107: 1739–1745.
113. Utley DS, Koch RJ, Goode RL. The failing flap in facial plastic and reconstructive surgery: role of the medicinal leech. *Laryngoscope* 1998;108:1129–1135.
114. Pang CY, Forrest CR, Morris SF. Pharmacological augmentation of skin flap viability: a hypothesis to mimic the surgical delay phenomenon or a wishful thought. *Ann Plast Surg* 1989;22:293–306.
115. Wheatley MJ, Meltzer TR. The management of unsalvageable free flaps. *J Reconstr Microsurg* 1996;12:227–229.
116. Masquelet AC, Beveridge J, Romana C, et al. The lateral supramalleolar flap. *Plast Reconstr Surg* 1988;81:74–81.
117. Aronson J, Harrison B, Boyd CM, et al. Mechanical induction of osteogenesis: preliminary studies. *Ann Clin Lab Sci* 1988;18:195–203.
118. Fleming B, Paley D, Kristiansen T, et al. A biomechanical analysis of the Ilizarov external fixator. *Clin Orthop* 1989:95–105.
119. Paley D. Biomechanics of the Ilizarov external fixator. In: Bianchi Maiocchi A, Aronson J, eds. *Operative principles of Ilizarov*. Baltimore: Williams & Williams; 1991:33–41.
120. Gugenheim JJ Jr. The Ilizarov method: orthopedic and soft tissue applications. *Clin Plast Surg* 1998;25:567–578.
121. Schwartsman V, Martin SN, Ronquist RA, et al. Tibial fractures: the Ilizarov alternative. *Clin Orthop* 1992;278:207–216.
122. Ilizarov GA. The tension-stress effect on the genesis and growth of tissues. I. The influence of stability of fixation and soft tissue preservation. *Clin Orthop Rel Res* 1989; 238:249–281.
123. Ilizarov GA. The tension-stress effect on the genesis and growth of tissues. II. The influence of the rate and frequency of distraction. *Clin Orthop Rel Res* 1989;239: 263–285.
124. Ippolito E, Peretti G, Bellocci M, et al. Histology and ultrastructure of arteries, veins, and peripheral nerves during limb lengthening. *Clin Orthop* 1994;308:54–62.
125. Dendrinos GK, Kontos S, Lyritsis E. Use of the Ilizarov technique for treatment of non-union of the tibia associated with infection. *J Bone Joint Surg Am* 1995;77:835–846.
126. Feibel RJ, Oliva A, Buncke GM, et al. Soft tissue reconstruction in orthopedic surgery: secondary procedures. *Orthop Clin North Am* 1993;24:537–548.
127. Cierny G 3rd, Zorn KE. Segmental tibial defects: comparing conventional and Ilizarov methodologies. *Clin Orthop* 1994;301:118–123.

128. Green SA, Jackson JM, Wall DM, et al. Management of segmental defects by the Ilizarov intercalary bone transport method. *Clin Orthop Rel Res* 1992;280:136–142.
129. Dendrinos GK, Kontos S, Katsenis D, et al. Treatment of high-energy tibial plateau fractures by the Ilizarov circular fixator. *J Bone Joint Surg Br* 1996;78:710–717.
130. Green SA. Skeletal defects: a comparison of bone grafting and bone transport for segmental skeletal defects. *Clin Orthop Rel Res* 1994;301:111–117.
131. Osterman AL, Bora FW. Free vascularized bone grafting for large-gap nonunion of long bones. *Orthop Clin North Am* 1984;15:131–142.
132. Weiland AJ, Moore JR, Daniel RK. Vascularized bone autografts: experience with 41 cases. *Clin Orthop Rel Res* 1983;174:87–95.
133. Chen CW, Yu ZJ, Wang Y. A new method of treatment of congenital tibial pseudoarthrosis using free vascularised fibular graft: a preliminary report. *Ann Acad Med Singapore* 1979;8:465–473.
134. Nettelblad H, Randolph MA, Weiland AJ. Free microvascular epiphyseal-plate transplantation: an experimental study in dogs. *J Bone Joint Surg Am* 1984;66:1421–1430.
135. Doi K, Akino T, Shigetomi M, et al. Vascularized bone allografts: review of current concepts. *Microsurgery* 1994;15:831–841.
136. Levin LS, Goldner RD, Urbaniak JR, et al. Management of severe musculoskeletal injuries of the upper extremity. *J Orthop Trauma* 1990;4:432–440.
137. Taylor GI, Palmer JH. The vascular territories (angiosomes) of the body: experimental study and clinical applications. *Br J Plast Surg* 1987;40:113–141.
138. Masquelet AC, Romana MC. The medialis pedis flap: a new fasciocutaneous flap. *Plast Reconstr Surg* 1990;85:765–772.
139. Chicarilli ZN, Price GJ. Complete plantar foot coverage with the free neurosensory radial forearm flap. *Plast Reconstr Surg* 1986;78:94–101.
140. May JW Jr, Rohrich RJ. Foot reconstruction using free microvascular muscle flaps with skin grafts. *Clin Plast Surg* 1986;13:681–689.
141. Weinzweig N, Davies BW. Foot and ankle reconstruction using the radial forearm flap: a review of 25 cases. *Plast Reconstr Surg* 1998;102:1999–2005.
142. Harrison DH, Morgan BD. The instep island flap to resurface plantar defects. *Br J Plast Surg* 1981;34:315–318.
143. Hartrampf CR Jr, Scheflan M, Bostwick JD. The flexor digitorum brevis muscle island pedicle flap: a new dimension in heel reconstruction. *Plast Reconstr Surg* 1980;66:264–270.
144. Levin LS, Nunley JA. The management of soft tissue problems associated with calcaneal fractures. *Clin Orthop Rel Res* 1993;290:151–156.
145. Peacock EE Jr, Madden JW, Trier WC. Biologic basis for the treatment of keloids and hypertrophic scars. *South Med J* 1970;63:755–760.
146. Cohen IK, Diegelmann RF, Johnson ML. Effect of corticosteroids on collagen synthesis. *Surgery* 1977;82:15–20.
147. Cohen IK, McCoy BJ, Mohanakumar T, et al. Immunoglobulin, complement, and histocompatibility antigen studies in keloid patients. *Plast Reconstr Surg* 1979;63:689–695.
148. Urioste SS, Arndt KA, Dover JS. Keloids and hypertrophic scars: review and treatment strategies. *Semin Cutan Med Surg* 1999;18:159–171.
149. Borges AF. Timing of scar revision techniques. *Clin Plast Surg* 1990;17:71–76.
150. Chowdary RP, Murphy RX. Delayed debulking of free muscle flaps for aesthetic contouring debulking of free muscle flaps. *Br J Plast Surg* 1992;45:38–41.
151. Arnez ZM, Valdatta L, Sassoon E, et al. Salvage of a below knee amputation stump with a free sensate total sole flap preserving continuity of the posterior tibial nerve. *Br J Plast Surg* 1998;51:470–472.
152. Weinberg MJ, Al-Qattan MM, Mahoney J. "Spare part" forearm free flaps harvested from the amputated limb for coverage of amputation stumps. *J Hand Surg Br* 1997;22:615–619.
153. Antonyshyn O, Gruss JS, Mackinnon SE, et al. Complications of soft tissue expansion. *Br J Plast Surg* 1988;41:239–250.
154. Austad ED. Evolution of the concept of tissue expansion. *Fac Plast Surg* 1988;5:277–279.
155. Manders EK, Oaks TE, Au VK, et al. Soft tissue expansion in the lower extremities. *Plast Reconstr Surg* 1988;81:208–219.
156. Pasyk KA, Argenta LC, Austad ED. Histopathology of human expanded tissue. *Clin Plast Surg* 1987;14:435–445.
157. Miller MJ, Robb GL. Endoscopic technique for free flap harvesting. *Clin Plast Surg* 1995;22:755–773.
158. Kuger K, Levin LS, Klitzman B. Advantages of balloon dissector assisted tissue expander placement: a clinical trial and experimental study. (Submitted.)
159. Fine NA, Orgill DP, Pribaz JJ. Early clinical experience in endoscopic-assisted muscle flap harvest. *Ann Plast Surg* 1994;33:465–469, discussion 469–472.
160. Lin CHWF, Levin LS, Ming CC. Donor-site morbidity comparison between endoscopically assisted and traditional harvest of free latissimus dorsi muscle flap. *Plast Reconstr Surg* 1999;104:1070–1077.
161. Wright JB, Lam K, Buret A, et al. Early healing events in a porcine model of contaminated wounds: effects of nanocrystalline silver on matrix metalloproteinases, cell apoptosis, and healing. *Wound Repair Regen* 2002;10:141–151.
162. Serletti JM, Deuber MA, Guidera PM, et al. Comparison of the operating microscope and loupes for free microvascular tissue transfer [see comments]. *Plast Reconstr Surg* 1995;95:270–276.
163. Franken RJ, Gupta SC, Banis JC Jr, et al. Microsurgery without a microscope: laboratory evaluation of a three-dimensional on-screen microsurgery system. *Microsurgery* 1995;16:746–751.
164. Khouri RK, Koudsi B, Reddi H. Tissue transformation into bone in vivo: a potential practical application. *JAMA* 1991;266:1953–1955.
165. Khouri RK, Upton J, Shaw WW. Principles of flap prefabrication. *Clin Plast Surg* 1992;19:763–771.
166. Morrison WA, Dvir E, Doi K, et al. Prefabrication of thin transferable axial-pattern skin flaps: an experimental study in rabbits [see comments]. *Br J Plast Surg* 1990;43:645–654.
167. Kroll SS, Evans GR, Goldberg D, et al. A comparison of resource costs for head and neck reconstruction with free and pectoralis major flaps. *Plast Reconstr Surg* 1997;99:1282–1286.
168. Laughlin RT, Smith KL, Russell RC, et al. Late functional outcome in patients with tibia fractures covered with free muscle flaps. *J Orthop Trauma* 1993;7:123–129.
169. Kutlu N. Out-patients upper extremity free flaps. *J Reconstr Microsurg* 1998;14:269.
170. Heinz TR, Cowper PA, Levin LS. Microsurgery cost and outcome. *Plast Reconstr Surg* 1999;104:89–96.

SYSTEMIC COMPLICATIONS

David C. Templeman and William A. Marinelli

Complications associated with the management of orthopedic trauma patients are divided into injury specific complications and systemic complications associated with the dysfunction of other organ systems. Injury-specific complications include infection, nonunion, neurologic injuries, and problems that directly relate to a specific musculoskeletal injury. Systemic complications relate to the physiologic changes associated with various injuries such as deep venous thrombosis, pulmonary dysfunction, urinary tract infections, and nutritional compromise. In patients with multiple injuries from blunt trauma, complications of systemic organ dysfunction and multiple system organ failure may occur in association with other severe injuries.

Traditional teachings have focused on the treatment of specific injuries rather than the changes in systemic physiology. In some situations, principles that are appropriate for the care of a specific injury may not be appropriate to the overall care of the multiply injured patient and may even be harmful. A specific example of this concept is fracture stabilization in multiply injured patients with pulmonary contusions. Advances in the understanding and treatment of these systemic associations are developed in this chapter.

The study of the effects of early fracture stabilization began in the 1970s. Early fracture fixation, especially the fixation of femoral fractures, was found to reduce the incidence of pulmonary complications. During this time, the nonoperative management of femoral fractures in patients with multiple injuries was associated with mortality rates between 20% and 30%.

When the concept of early fracture stabilization was applied, it was confirmed that early fracture fixation reduced mortality. Treating patients with femoral traction was associated with higher rates of multiple organ failure compared with early fracture fixation. A comprehensive approach to the patient with multiple injuries became apparent in that the timing of fixation skeletal injuries was critical to the overall care of these patients. This chapter outlines the systemic implications of diagnosing and treating patients with multiple injuries.

MISSED INJURIES

The initial assessment and treatment of multiply injured patients is challenging. Frequently, the management of immediate, life-threatening injuries diverts attention from other injuries, which may then go undetected. These undiagnosed injuries can be a late cause of significant morbidity.

The Advanced Trauma Life Support (ATLS) Course establishes guidelines that set priorities in the initial management of multiply injured patients to help reduce the incidence of missed injuries. Despite the use of protocols, the incidence of missed injuries in multiply injured patients is reported to range from 2% to 50%. Several studies document that the majority of missed injuries involve the extremities, and many of these are fractures (1–3).

ATLS defines two surveys to be used in the assessment of multiply injured patients. The primary survey is designed to rapidly assess a patient for immediate, life-threatening injuries and treat them as they are discovered. The secondary survey is a more thorough examination of all body systems intended to identify all of the injuries the patient has sustained and help plan treatment.

Studies that have examined missed injuries, even with the use of ATLS protocols, have found several associations that clearly place patients at risk for missed injuries.

At-risk patients are those who cannot cooperate because of head injuries or those who are obtunded from drugs or alcohol. In addition, patients whose initial assessment was rushed or compromised because of the need to manage hemodynamic instability are also noted to have a higher incidence of missed injuries. Injuries that are frequently catalogued as missed in these studies are spinal column fractures (including the cervical spine), hand fractures, foot fractures, and neurological injuries (1,2,4).

The tertiary survey, defined as a standardized clinical reassessment within 24 hours of admission is the most effective means to reduce the incidence of missed injuries. In addition, as patients become lucid it is noted that any new complaints during the initial hospitalization be taken seriously. Finally, several studies have documented missed injuries resulting from incomplete communication between the radiologist reviewing films and the treating physician's lack of awareness that an injury was detected by the radiologist (1,3,5).

TRAUMA SCORING SYSTEMS

The initial triage of injured patients to appropriate care centers is improved with the use of the Revised Trauma Score (RTS). The RTS includes the Glasgow Coma Scale, systolic blood pressure, and respiratory rate. Patients with a Glasgow Coma score of less than 13, a systolic blood pressure of less than 90 mmHg, or a respiratory rate of less than 10 or greater than 29 per minute are all criteria for transport to a trauma center. These criteria have been documented to be specific in selecting patients who require the care available at hospitals prepared to manage the severely injured (6).

Injury severity scores (ISS) are a means of quantifying the dose of injury a patient has received. In concept this permits the grouping of comparably injured patients who do not have the same anatomic injuries but have the same severity of injures into groups for the study of delivery systems and methods of care.

The abbreviated injury severity system (AIS) catalogues injuries into six different organ systems. Within each system the injury is graded according to its severity on a scale of 1 (minor) to 5 (critical and life threatening). The scores of the three most severely injured systems are first squared and then added together to arrive at the injury severity score for the patient. Because the ISS only calculates the most severe injury from an organ system—for example, bilateral femoral fractures are scored the same as a single femoral fracture—the system is not as accurate when there are several injuries within a single organ system (6).

The new ISS adds the three highest AIS scores, regardless of anatomic area. In a study of more than 13,000 patients, the NISS was found to be more accurate than the ISS in the prediction of mortality, multiple organ failure, and length of stay. This was particularly true in the patients with blunt trauma and those with orthopaedic injuries.

The ISS correlates with mortality in the elderly, but they die from less severe injuries than younger patients. In a study of high-energy injuries, an ISS of 18 or greater correlated with a mortality rate of 37%. High mortality was associated with the development of acute respiratory distress syndrome (ARDS) and sepsis in these older patients (7,8).

SHOCK

Hypovolemia is the most common cause of shock in the trauma patient. This leads to decreases in the homeostasis of circulation, ventilation, and metabolic functions. Changes in blood pressure and pulse rates are guides to requirements for resuscitation. In young and healthy individuals a 15% blood loss (up to 1,000 mL in a 70-kg male) can occur without little changes in vital signs. With a 30% loss in blood volume (2,500 mL for a 70-kg male), hypotension and tachycardia occur and the patient develops obvious shock (Table 17-1).

Resuscitation is started with crystalloid solutions through large-bore intravenous lines and is monitored by urine output with a goal of 0.5 mL/kg/hr in adults. Central venous catheters and pulmonary catheters are used in severe trauma, chest trauma, and care of elderly adults. With more severe degrees of shock venous constriction occurs, and it becomes necessary to use intravenous cut down of the saphenous or cubital veins. It is estimated that for each liter of blood lost 3 to 4 L of crystalloid solution will be required (9,10).

Only patients with severe exsanguinations require universal donor blood (group O, Rh-negative) because in most centers

TABLE 17-1 Classes of Shock

	Class I	Class II	Class III	Class IV
Blood loss (cc)	<750	750–1,500	1,500–2,000	>2,000
% blood volume	<15%	15%–30%	30%–40%	>40%
Pulse rate (bpm)	<100	>100	>120	>140
Urine output (mL/hr)	>30	20–30	5–15	Negligible

Estimates for a 70-kg male.

cross-matched blood is available within 20 minutes (Table 17-2). Four classes of shock are described that represent the physiologic effects of progressive blood loss. The administration of specific components depends on the results of initial blood samples. Thrombocytopenia is treated at levels of less than 50,000 / μL. Factor-specific deficiencies (hypofibrinogemia, factors V and VIII) are replaced by the use of fresh frozen plasma (6,9,10).

In patients with life-threatening hemorrhage, radiographs of the chest, head, and cervical spine and pelvis when coupled with ultrasound examination of the pelvis will lead to the diagnosis of nearly all cases of massive hemorrhage (10).

Patients that have required large volumes of fluid for resuscitation will frequently develop hypothermia that leads to dysfunctions in coagulation. The warming of these patients is a critical part of their resuscitation and is achieved with the use of warm fluids, warming blankets, and warm inspired air. It is observed that when these patients are hypothermic a vasoconstriction occurs that is followed by vasodilation and relative hypovolemia during the warming period. This results in the need for additional volume replacement; this can be expected while the patient is being warmed (9).

Lactated Ringer's solution is used for initial fluid resuscitation. Large volumes are needed when there is severe blood loss, which may compromise patients with head injuries, in whom hypertonic saline (6.5%) may be more appropriate. Although theoretically beneficial, fluid resuscitation by emergency medial staff before hospitalization has not been shown to reduce mortality rates compared to patients that do not receive prehospital resuscitation. This may be related to delays in transport while obtaining access at the scene of the injury (6,9,10).

DEATH AFTER INJURY

Death after injury from blunt trauma can be divided into three distinct time periods. Immediate death at the accident scene from severe injuries occurs in approximately 45% of patients. The second phase of deaths occurs during the first hours of hospitalization, with only about 10% of trauma deaths occurring at this time. Deaths during the first day are the result of severe head injuries, hemorrhage, or hypoxia; each of these alone or in combination. The third phase of deaths occurs days or weeks after the injury and affects approximately 45% of patients who die as a result of blunt trauma. These late deaths

TABLE 17-2 Guidelines for Fluid Resuscitation

	Rapid Response	Transient Response	No Response
Estimated blood loss	10%–20%	20%–40%	>40%
Need for more crystalloid	Low	High	High
Need for blood	Type and cross match	Type-specific	Emergency release

Adapted from the *Advanced Trauma Life Support for Doctors Student Course Manual*, 6th ed. Chicago: American College of Surgeons; 1997:98.

are due to the effects of head injury, adult respiratory distress syndrome, or multiple system organ failure. Many of these patients have significant musculoskeletal injuries. The development of multiple system organ failure or organ dysfunction after injury is thought to be the result of the systemic inflammatory response to the initial injuries (10–12).

Traditional thought placed little emphasis on the association of musculoskeletal trauma and the development of multiple system organ dysfunction. However, studies of patients that develop multiple system organ failure reveal that these patients have more severe musculoskeletal injuries than patients who did not develop multiple system organ failure. Bone and colleagues demonstrated in a randomized study the beneficial effects of early stabilization of femoral fractures on both morbidity and the length of hospital stay in comparison to patients who did not receive early stabilization of their femoral fractures. Delayed fixation of fractures was also associated with pulmonary compromise (13).

Elderly patients have higher mortality rates with less severe injuries. The reported lethal dose $(LD)_{50}$ ISS for those older than 65 years of age is 20; this is approximately one half of the LD_{50} ISS for those injured who are aged 24 to 44 years (7,8). Tornetta et al have documented the following associations in patients over 60 years of age who die: a lower Glasgow Coma Score compared to that of survivors (11.5 compared to 13.9 points); greater transfusion requirements (10.9 fatalities to 2.9 in survivors); and greater resuscitation requirements (12.4 L in the nonsurvivors contrasted to 4.9 L in the survivors) (8).

ORGAN DYSFUNCTION AND MULTIPLE SYSTEM ORGAN FAILURE IN POLYTRAUMA PATIENTS

Acute Respiratory Failure after Trauma

There are multiple causes of acute respiratory failure in trauma patients. Hypercapnic respiratory failure may develop in patients with significant head trauma secondary to loss of central respiratory drive, patients with high cervical cord injuries, and patients with underlying neuromuscular diseases. Patients with preexisting cardiopulmonary disease may develop respiratory failure with more limited injuries, including patients with obstructive lung disease (e.g., asthma, chronic obstructive pulmonary disease [COPD]), interstitial lung disease (e.g., pulmonary fibrosis), or significant cardiac disease or pulmonary hypertension. ARDS may be a particularly challenging complication of trauma (14,15).

Pulmonary physiology is based on an upright chest, and many individuals assume an upright posture for as many as 16 hours daily. The gradient of capillary hydrostatic pressure is related to the pulmonary vein, with the lung bases having the highest capillary hydrostatic pressure and resulting increase in pulmonary alveolar blood flow but a decrease in alveolar air volume and an increase in alveolar compliance. Pulmonary surfactant is responsible for an increase in compliance and roughly matches alveolar ventilation with alveolar blood flow for efficient systemic oxygenation. The distribution of surfactant means that alveolar oxygenation of capillary blood flow is most efficient with the chest in an upright position (6).

Pulmonary injuries are central to the care of multiply injured patients because they result in a reduction in systemic oxygenation, which affects the function of all organ systems. When patients are supported in the supine position (e.g., fracture immobilization—especially femoral traction), the posterior lung fields are dependent and pulmonary shunting may occur if significant atelectasis develops. This results in a decreased exchange of alveolar oxygen to the pulmonary capillaries. The net effect is a decrease in systemic oxygenation (6,14).

Blunt chest trauma is common to motor vehicle crashes and exists in a spectrum from rib fractures to aortic transections. It is estimated that as many as 1 in 16 people who die at the accident scene exsanguinate as a result of aortic transrections. Many blunt trauma patients sustain pulmonary contusions and hemopneumothoraces. Proper management of their fractures allows these patients to be mobilized, which improves their pulmonary care.

Pulmonary contusions are produced by direct trauma to the lung parenchyma. This causes interstitial hemorrhage, edema, and inflammation. Damaged alveoli are no longer capable of oxygen exchange, and inflammation causes interstitial edema that impedes oxygenation even in the absence of alveolar hemorrhage. Pulmonary contusions are significant as isolated injuries, with mortality rates as high as 20%. Risk factors include age greater than 60 and closed head injuries. The presence or the extent of a lung contusion may not be apparent on initial chest radiographs. Serial chest radiographs 24 hours after admission increased the diagnosis of pulmonary contusion from 42% to 94% in one study of unilateral contusions. Computerized tomography and admission blood gases also fail to estimate the degree of initial damage because pulmonary edema worsens with time after the initial injury. The alveolar injury activates inflammatory cells and results in increased permeability, pulmonary edema, and hypoxia within the first 2 to 4 days after injury. In this period, the performance of other surgeries that increase inflammatory mediators will further pulmonary edema when the inflammatory mediators from remote sites are filtered by the lung (10,12,13,16–18).

The severity of injury is well correlated with levels of inflammatory mediators, immune suppression, and organ dysfunction. After injury the activation of the inflammatory cascade produces a multitude of inflammatory mediators, including the compliment system, cytokines, and macrophages, which act in concert to produce a systemic inflammatory response. Clinically this is manifested as fever, leukocytosis, and pulmonary dysfunction (12,17,18).

Although remote form the lungs, sites of musculoskeletal injuries are rich in inflammatory mediators. Very high levels of inflammatory mediators are present in fracture hematomas. Both the inflammatory mediators and the breakdown of injured tissue to some degree are systemically circulated. Through venous return from the lower extremities, some of these mediators are filtered by the liver and activate hepatic macrophages. These by-products are further circulated through the lungs and induce pulmonary inflammation and edema, which impairs alveolar arterial oxygen exchange. This systemic reduction in oxygenation perpetuates organ system dysfunction (6,10,12,17).

There is ongoing research to identify the specific inflammatory mediators that can be used to predict and measure organ dysfunction and failure. Currently, interleukin-6, neutrophil elastase, erythrocyte sedimentation rate, and platelet count have been correlated with development of organ dysfunction. Interleukin-6 levels are elevated early after injury and are further elevated in certain at-risk patients with early intramedullary nailing and reaming of femoral fractures. Delays in definitive fixation for several days are associated with lower levels of interleukin-6 and a reduction in the incidence of organ dysfunction (12,18–21).

As a result of the above mechanism of tissue necrosis and inflammation, lung dysfunction is frequently observed in patients with severe fractures. Fat embolism syndrome (FES) after fractures is thought to occur from tissue damage caused by marrow embolization of marrow elements, with their subsequent breakdown into toxic free fatty acids within the lung. However, FES develops in only 1% to 5% of patient after fractures. In some animal models, intravascular fat has produced only a negligible inflammatory response. Some of these animal studies indicated that the presence of hypotension combined with intravascular fat was necessary for the development of ARDS. Fat embolism syndrome may present with a wide spectrum of acute lung injury severity, with oxygenation impairment ranging from mild asymptomatic reduction in oxygen saturation to ARDS with severe shunt physiology (13,17,22).

The key pathologic feature of ARDS is diffuse alveolar damage, along with alveolar capillary and epithelial barrier injury, resulting in extravasation of fluid from the pulmonary vasculature into the interstitial and alveolar spaces. This injury results in alveolar edema and collapse, reduction in alveolar volume and total respiratory compliance, and ventilation-perfusion mismatching with shunt physiology (perfusion of unventilated alveoli). When severe, shunt physiology results in marked oxygenation impairment that is relatively refractory to increases in supplemental oxygen. The reduction in alveolar volume and total respiratory compliance is evidenced by elevated airway pressures during positive-pressure ventilation (10,14,17,23).

ARDS may result from direct lung injury from blunt and penetrating trauma to the chest or alveolar injury from either the air–lung or blood–lung interface (Table 17-3). The clinical features, pathophysiology, and management of ARDS have been intensely studied since the initial description of the syndrome in 1967. The mortality of ARDS has reduced from greater than 60% down to 30% to 40% in patients with single organ failure. This reduction in mortality is likely due to the combination of multiple factors, including the adoption of lung protective ventilatory strategies and overall improvement in critical care management. Mechanical ventilation with a lower tidal volume and airway pressure strategy has been demonstrated to reduce ventilator-induced lung injury in animal models and was recently shown to reduce mortality in a large multicenter National Institutes of Health–sponsored prospective randomized trial (14).

TABLE 17-3 Common Causes of ARDS in Trauma Patients

Trauma (blunt or penetrating lung injury)

Air–lung interface
- Aspiration
- Toxic gas or smoke inhalation
- Near-drowning
- Pneumonia

Blood–lung interface
- Sepsis
- Transfusion-related lung injury
- Pancreatitis
- Fat embolism
- Thromboembolism

Neurogenic pulmonary edema from head injury

The understanding of the pathogenesis of ARDS, and its relationship to the early management of multiply injured patients continues to evolve. Current theories relate the development of ARDS and multiple organ failure to the activation of the immune system and the production of inflammatory mediators. Injury stimulates the immune system to produce humoral and cell surface mediators of inflammation and coagulation. Within the immune system there are modulators of inflammation that either promote inflammation as a protective response against inflammation or act to moderate the intensity of the immune response and control the degree of inflammatory response. Imbalances in the regulation of the immune response causing too much inflammation lead to a generalized systemic inflammatory response syndrome (SIRS). SIRS is characterized by endothelial cell damage and interstitial edema, which causes organ dysfunction (10,12,14,17,19).

In contrast, too much suppression of the immune system leads to anergy, or a compensatory response syndrome (CARS), which leads to an increased susceptibility to infection and systemic sepsis. The potential causes of the imbalance in the immune system may be due to either idiosyncratic responses by individuals with genetic predilection or severe injury that overwhelms the immune system (10,12,17).

Systemic Organ Dysfunction

The development of multiple system organ failure frequently occurs in the following sequence. The lung is the usual first target of the SIRS, and ARDS is considered to be the lung's response to inflammation. This is followed by degrees of cardiac, gastrointestinal, renal, hepatic, hematologic, and cerebral failure. Autopsy studies of patients that survive for at least 72 hours almost always show some evidence of multiple system organ dysfunction (6,11,17,24,25).

For the severely injured patient it is postulated that there is an initial state of inflammation caused by the trauma, and that within this state of inflammation there exists a critical balance between the beneficial effects of inflammation and the potential for the immune system to cause tissue damage. This concept is of critical importance in treating this select group of patients as secondary events that could disrupt the balance of the immune system may provoke the onset of multiple system organ dysfunction. These secondary stimuli are referred to as the second hit phenomenon. Suspected secondary stimuli to the immune system include episodes of hypoxia, sepsis, hypovolemia, and blood transfusions. The timing and type of secondary surgery may have a significant impact on furthering the development of immune dysfunction (12,20,26,27).

Central to this theory of first and second hits is the stimulation and release of inflammatory mediators immediately after an injury. There is a direct correlation between the severity of the injury, the levels of inflammatory mediators, and the subsequent development of multiple system organ dysfunction. This is the first hit. The second hit is caused by additional stimulation of the immune system; examples include surgery, infection, and transfusions. One study has documented that preoperative elevations of C-reactive protein and neutrophil elastase or a reduction in platelet counts could be correlated (although not perfectly) with the development of systemic organ dysfunction. These findings may be of critical importance in the timing of major procedures to stabilize fractures. In the future the goal of monitoring inflammatory mediators may be to determine when there is a reduced risk to performing procedures that will increase the inflammatory response (10,11,17, 20,26,28,29).

In one clinical study the measurement of systemic inflammatory mediators was used to judge the recovery of patients from their initial injury. Patients that underwent secondary definitive surgeries 2 to 4 days after injury developed an increased inflammatory response compared to patients who underwent surgery 6 to 8 days after injury. This finding related to patients who underwent surgeries that lasted more than 3 hours. This seems to indicate that there are different inflammatory responses to surgical procedures during different post-traumatic periods (10,20,21,29).

The clinical implications of these studies have been to reorder the priorities and timing of fracture stabilization in select groups of severely injured patients. The recent history of fracture fixation for multiply injured patients established the benefits of intramedullary nailing of femoral fractures within the first 48 hours for patients with two severe injuries. The concept of early definitive fracture fixation has been termed early total care (ETC). However, there appears to be a small subset of patients that may have been adversely affected by ETC, particularly if there was an associated severe pulmonary injury (10,11,17, 20,26,28,29).

Early Total Care

The initial findings that ETC was associated with pulmonary complications were seen after reaming and intramedullary nailing of femoral shaft fractures. Further studies documented that reamed intramedullary nailing (femoral fractures) was a potent stimulator of the immune system. The complications occurred most often in patients with severe hemodynamic shock and severe chest trauma (10,12,20,23,27,30).

These observations led to a change in the initial treatment of these patients directed at initially avoiding profound stimulation of the immune system (reducing the second hit) by stabilizing fractures with less invasive techniques. This concept has been termed damage control orthopedics (DCO) (28,29).

Damage Control Orthopaedics

Conceptually, DCO identifies patients that are at risk for SIRS and organ dysfunction, which includes patients with shock and severe pulmonary injuries and selected patients with severe CNS trauma when it is determined that surgery may lead to hypoxia or hypotension that would extend the primary brain injury. Early temporary fixation of fractures is done with external fixation, which achieves stabilization without profound stimulation of the immune system. The patients are then resuscitated with the benefits of fracture fixation. Delayed definitive fracture fixation is done once the condition of the patient is optimal (Table 17-4) (20,28,29).

The timing of conversion from external fixation to intramedullary nailing of femoral fractures will affect both the potential for the development of organ dysfunction and the possibility of infection from pin tract problems associated with external fixation of femoral fractures. Current studies suggest that a delay of at least 4 days is probably appropriate to allow for a reduction in the inflammatory response to the initial injury. This is based

TABLE 17-4 End Points for Resuscitation

Stable hemodynamic system
Stable oxygen saturation
Lactate level <2 mol/L
No coagulation disturbances
Normal temperature
Urinary output >1 mL/kg/hr
No inotropic support

From Giannoudis PV. Surgical priorities in damage control in polytrauma. *J Bone Joint Surg Br* 2003;85:478–483.

both on observation of the success of resuscitation and an observed decrease of inflammatory mediators in several studies (10,26,28,29).

HEAD INJURIES

The mortality in patients with head injuries is disproportionately higher than other injured patients that do not have head injuries. Many of these patients have ischemic brain injury, which is evident in more than 80% of autopsy studies of those who die from brain injuries (25,31).

The goal in treating injuries of the brain is to avoid extension of the primary brain injury. The primary injury to brain tissue occurs at the time of the initial injury and is worsened by hypoxia, hypotension, increased intracranial pressure, and decreased cranial perfusion. The extension of the initial/primary injury is termed the secondary brain injury (25,31).

This concept of secondary brain injury is observed in patients who die, but are initially lucid after their initial injury. Because hypotension and hypoxia may occur during orthopaedic procedures the timing of fracture fixation in patients with head injuries is both important and controversial.

Cerebral perfusion is a function of the difference between mean arterial blood pressure (MAP) and intracranial pressure (ICP) (expressed as cerebral perfusion pressure [CPP] = MAP − ICP). As ICP increases CPP decreases causing ischemia, with brain death occurring when the oxygen and glucose requirements of the brain are not met. Normal ICP is 10 mm Hg or less, and an ICP of more than 20 mm Hg is considered to require continuous monitoring and treatment.

Aggressive management of intracranial pressure is thought to improve the neurologic outcome. To achieve these goals patients must be resuscitated before proceeding with fracture stabilization. In many situations DCO is beneficial to avoid blood loss or hypotension that is sometimes associated with major orthopedic procedures that in this setting would potentially worsen the patient's head injury (25,28,29,31,32).

Despite this logic, there are few studies that have defined the appropriate timing of fracture surgery in patients with severe head injuries. Two studies that reviewed the literature have differing conclusions. The Eastern Association for the Surgery of Trauma Practice Management Guidelines Work Group concluded that patients with mild, moderate, or severe brain injury who underwent long bone stabilization within 48 hours of injury had similar mortality rates, similar lengths of intensive care stays, similar needs for mechanical ventilation, and similar lengths of hospital stay. Early intramedullary fixation was not found to either enhance or worsen the outcome. The conclusion of this literature review was that timing of long bone stabilization should be individualized to each patient (25,31).

Early stabilization of femoral and tibial fractures in multiply injured patients was studied by Bhandari et al. In this series all patients were treated within 24 hours of injury, which allowed for a comparison of intramedullary nailing and plate fixation of femoral and tibial fractures in patients with head injuries. The severity of the head injury was the most important predictor of death and outcome. This study found that intramedullary nailing did not seem to be contraindicated in patients with lower extremity injuries.

The benefits for the early fixation of patients with head injuries and fractures are theoretically the same as the benefits for other multiply injured patients: decreased respiratory insufficiency, a decrease in soft-tissue damage, and potential reduction in multiple system organ dysfunction and failure. However, as noted, prospective randomized studies of patients with closed head injuries and early as compared to late fracture fixation have not been conducted (25,31).

POSTOPERATIVE FEVER

Normal temperatures range from 35.6°C to 38.2°C with diurnal variations that have a 6 AM nadir and a peak that occurs between 4 and 6 PM. There are two thermal compartments termed the core and shell that have imprecise temperature associations between them. In clinical practice, oral temperatures are most commonly used as the mouth responds quickly to changes in the core temperature and in general is 0.2°C less than the core temperature. Rectal temperatures are commonly used for intubated patients and are usually 0.2°C above the core temperature.

Most textbooks define a temperature greater than 38°C as a fever. Fever is an evolutionary response to multiple stimuli. The function of the immune system is enhanced by fever and enhances antibody production, T cell activation, and cytokine production. In addition the presence of fever seems to inhibit some pathogens, for example *Streptococcus pneumoniae*. There are multiple infectious and noninfectious causes of fever (Tables 17-5 and 17-6).

The evaluation of fever in the postoperative patient can be difficult. The time of the onset of fever after surgery is helpful, whereas the analysis of fever patterns is of less value in determining the cause of the fever. A general guideline to time dependency is fevers occurring in the first 48 hours after surgery are most likely secondary to tissue injury, hematoma, and atelectasis. Ventilator-associated pneumonia usually presents 4 to 5 days after initial intubation. The new onset of fever 5 to 7 days after surgery raises the possibility of a surgical site infection.

The approach to the febrile patient is directed at determining and treating the etiology of the fever. Noninfectious causes of fever need to be considered and treated. The time of onset is a helpful start; early postoperative fevers are evaluated for postoperative atelectasis, with auscultation, incentive spirometry, and a chest radiograph when needed. Later onset fevers require a clinical assessment and, when indicated, obtaining blood cultures and chest radiographs.

NOSOCOMIAL INFECTIONS

Catheter-associated urinary tract infection (CAUTI) is the most common nosocomial infection, constituting over 40% of all ac-

TABLE 17-5 Noninfectious Causes of Fever

Alcohol withdrawal
Postoperative atelectasis
Drug fever
Acute myocardial infarction
Adrenal insufficiency
Acute respiratory distress syndrome
Deep vein thrombosis, pulmonary embolism
Pancreatitis
Hematoma
Injury

quired infections. Infection occurs in as many as 25% of patients who are catheterized for more than 7 days, with the daily risk of 5%. Most CAUTIs are asymptomatic but prompt the use of antibiotic treatment and add $500 to $1000 to acute care costs.

Most microorganisms that cause CAUTIs come from the patient's own perineal and colonic flora or from the hands of health care workers during catheter insertion. In addition to contamination of the catheter at the time of insertion, organisms can ascend from the perineum by capillary action adjacent to the catheter. Most infected catheters become coated by a thick biofilm.

A clean-voided specimen showing more than 10^5 colony-forming units (CFU)/mL is the definition for true infection in the noncatheterized patient; but once organisms are identified in urine from an indwelling catheter, progression to more than 10^5 CFU/mL occurs predictably and rapidly, usually within 72 hours. Most authorities consider concentrations greater than 10^2 CFU/mL in urine collected from the sampling port to indicate a true CAUTI.

The most important risk factor for the development of a CAUTI is catheterization beyond 6 days, with infection in nearly all patients by 30 days. Guidelines for preventing CAUTIs include avoiding unnecessary catheterizations, using alternatives, aseptic insertion techniques, closed drainage systems, dependent drainage, and only necessary manipulation of the drainage system.

Pneumonia is the second most common nosocomial infection, with most infections occurring secondary to aspiration of bacteria colonizing the oropharynx or upper gastrointestinal tract. Because elderly, debilitated patients and postoperative patients are at increased risk, orthopaedic surgeons will encounter these patients in the care of hip fractures and other fractures associated with osteoporosis.

Nosocomial pneumonia is frequently caused by aspiration. Approximately 50% of adults aspirate small volumes during normal sleep. Nearly 100% of intubated patients will aspirate. The development of pneumonia is dependent on the bacterial burden, virulence of colonizing pathogens, and host defense mechanisms.

Factors placing patients at increased risk include a history of smoking, poor dentition, alcoholism, and diabetes.

TABLE 17-6 Infectious Causes of Fever

Pneumonia (ventilator associated)
Intravascular catheter related
Primary gram-negative septicemia
Clostridium difficile colitis
Abdominal sepsis
Candidemia
Complicated wound infection

Risk of Disease Transmission to Health Care Workers

The treatment of trauma patients frequently requires emergent care, which exposes health care workers to large open wounds and places them at risk for blood exposure. In one survey, 87% of surgeons reported a blood skin contact and 39% reported a percutaneous blood exposure in the month before the survey. The diseases of primary concern to health care workers are hepatitis B and C and the human immunodeficiency virus (HIV). The risk of contracting hepatitis is higher than HIV, presumably because of the higher viral titers in the blood of patients with hepatitis in contrast to patients infected with HIV.

Universal precautions are recommended in the care of all trauma patients, and studies indicate that these diseases are more prevalent in trauma patients. Precautions include the use of barriers (gowns, gloves, and facial protection—which should include eye protection) and hand washing after patient contact. Sharp instruments should be disposed in puncture-resistant containers.

It is recommended that all health care workers receive hepatitis B vaccinations. There is currently no effective vaccination nor postexposure prophylaxis for hepatitis C.

Progress continues to be made for the postexposure prophylaxis of HIV, with the use of zidovudine and protease inhibitors.

DEEP VENOUS THROMBOSIS

The landmark study of Geerts et al (33) documented that approximately 60% of patients admitted to a trauma service have evidence of deep venous thrombosis; this study has directed attention to the diagnosis, prophylaxis, and treatment of thromboembolism in injured patients. Deep venous thrombosis represents a spectrum of disease that includes silent thrombi, symptomatic deep venous thrombosis, pulmonary embolism, and death from pulmonary embolism. Two thirds of the patients who die of pulmonary embolism survive less than 20 minutes from the onset of symptoms; a fact that directs efforts toward preventing pulmonary emboli. Because the incidence of death from pulmonary embolism is rare (1% to 2%), there are no randomized prospective studies that establish any form of treatment as being effective in reducing the rate of fatal pulmonary emboli. In contrast, other studies that define asymptomatic thrombi as an end point in treatment are able to document the benefits of many different forms of treatment in reducing the incidence of asymptomatic deep venous thrombosis. Many clinicians are divided in their opinions on the importance of either treatment or prophylaxis because of an incomplete understanding of the natural history of asymptomatic venous thrombosis (33–36).

Venous thromboembolism is multifactorial. The pathophysiology was originally described by Virchow; damage to the vessel wall, venous stasis, and hypercoagulability. All three of these factors are likely to be present in multiply injured patients. Venous stasis is due to immobilization associated with bedrest, damage to the vessel wall can occur at the time of the injury, and hypercoagulability is often present several days after injury. Congenital or acquired thrombophilia also promotes coagulation. Thrombophilia is either inherited or expressed as a genetic mutation. There are clear trends in different ethnic groups; Asians have an extremely low rate of genetic thrombophilia, whereas it is much higher in Northern Europeans. Although biochemical screening tests are not practical or routinely done, a family history for the presence of deep venous thrombosis is a clue to the presence of genetic thrombophilia.

The clinical findings associated with DVT—pain, swelling, and tenderness—are highly unreliable for making the diagnosis. One study indicated that objective testing did not confirm the diagnosis in approximately 70% of patients with the classic signs of DVT. Venography is an accurate method for diagnosis, but is invasive. Noninvasive tests include impedance plethysmography (IPG) and venous Doppler/ultrasonography (D/US). Fibrinogen leg scanning is a radionuclear assay; it is no longer used in the United States because the technique requires the use of a blood product derivative with the risk of disease transmission. Venous ultrasound has largely replaced IPG because it is more accurate and readily available in most institutions. Because venography can be painful, and it is more difficult to perform repetitive tests, it has also been replaced by the use of D/US. The infrequent use of venography over more than the last decade has made this option significantly less available because many radiologists have little or no experience with this modality. However, venography is more accurate in diagnosing calf thrombi and nonocclusive, asymptomatic deep venous thrombi than D/US. The specificity of D/US for deep venous thrombosis of the femoral vein is 95%. The sensitivity and predictive value of D/US for thrombosis of the calf veins is lower (70% and 80%, respectively). In the event of a negative calf ultrasound, one recommended strategy is to repeat US 1 week later to detect the extension of the thrombosis from the calf to the proximal veins (36–38).

However, there is the contention that routine D/US screening performed either once or multiple times is an ineffective approach for managing deep venous thrombosis in trauma patients. In addition to not being cost effective, repetitive screening does not prevent the development or propagation of venous thrombi. The best choice of screening test is also controversial. Although most traumatologists use D/US for the diagnosis of lower extremity thrombi, pelvic thrombi remain difficult to detect, and neither contrast enhanced CT-scans or MRI are documented to be the clear choice of diagnostic test for patients with pelvic or acetabular fractures (36,38).

The clinical symptoms of pulmonary embolism (PE) include transient dyspnea, chest pain, hemoptysis, and, with larger occlusive emboli, symptoms of right-sided heart failure with syncope and hypotension. These symptoms are nonspecific, and the differential diagnosis includes pulmonary infections, musculoskeletal chest wall pain, pericarditis, esophageal spasm, and anxiety (33,37,39).

Because the presenting symptoms are nonspecific, a workup that includes a chest radiograph, electrocardiogram, and an assessment of oxygenation (oximetry or arterial blood gases) are frequently obtained to rule out other cardiorespiratory pathology. Approximately 70% of patients with proven PE will be found to have evidence of venous thrombosis with contrast venography, even when the DVT is clinically silent. Thus, imaging the deep venous system is commonly used as part of the diagnostic strategy in patients with suspected thromboembolic disease. However, lower extremity D/US studies are positive in less than 50% of patients with proven PE. Pulmonary angiography has the gold standard for the diagnosis of PE. A normal pulmonary angiogram excludes the diagnosis and thus is more specific than ventilation-perfusion scans of the lung. A normal perfusion scan also excludes PE. In patients with intermediate probability, lung scans, pulmonary angiogram, or CT angiogram can be used to confirm or exclude PE. Since approximately 1995 the CT pulmonary angiogram has evolved into the most frequently used diagnostic study, with a sensitivity and specificity of at least 90% for identifying central PE (main, lobar, segmental arteries) (38).

Because the risk of recurrence of venous thromboembolism is 5% to 10% per year, some argue for the prevention of the first episode with prophylactic strategies directed at preventing the first thrombotic event. It has been documented that the risk of recurrent venous thromboembolism is higher among men than women (20% vs. 6%). Approaches to prophylaxis for preventing deep venous thrombosis and its complications are divided into mechanical and pharmacologic modalities. Mechanical modalities include graduated stockings, pneumatic compression devices, and vena caval filters. The pharmacologic agents include heparin, low molecular weight heparins, warfarin (Coumadin), and pentasaccharides. The use of these different treatment methods for trauma patients is complex because of the variables of differing musculoskeletal and systemic injuries. The fact that acutely injured patients have active sources of bleeding is a contraindication to the use of pharmacologic prophylaxis until the patient is hemodynamically stable and clinical judgment determines that bleeding has stopped (33,37).

Mechanical prophylaxis includes graduated compression stockings and intermittent compression devices (IPC), which are applied to the foot, the lower leg, or the lower leg and thigh. Although mechanical prophylaxis is not associated with a risk of bleeding, it unfortunately has not been shown to reduce the risk of pulmonary embolism or death. The use of mechanical devices in trauma is hindered by low patient compliance and in many instances the presence of lower extremity fractures that prevent the patients from tolerating the intermittent compression. Despite these drawbacks, mechanical prophylaxis is useful as an adjutant to pharmacologic anticoagulation or in patients who have a high risk of bleeding and cannot receive pharmacologic prophylaxis.

The use of inferior vena cava filters for the prevention of fatal pulmonary embolism in trauma patients is well accepted. Filters are used in patients who have contraindications to anticoagulation or in those who have developed venous thrombosis despite anticoagulation. Common indications for the insertion of vena cava filters include head injuries, multiple long bone fractures, pelvic and acetabular fractures, and patients that have evidence of deep venous thrombosis before a major surgical procedure. Some studies suggest that there is an increased risk for the development of recurrent deep venous thrombosis in patients treated with filters. This suggests that, if possible, anticoagulation therapy should be started, when safe, after the placement of a vena cava filter. The use of retrievable vena cava filters, filters that can be placed and then later removed, has been effective in early use for the prevention of pulmonary embolism in high-risk trauma patients who cannot receive anticoagulation.

In addition to these problems, when a deep venous thrombosis is detected systemic heparinization is often used for treatment. Although not specifically studied in patients after fracture surgery, the use of systemic heparinization within the first week after total hip replacement is associated with a 50% wound complication rate from hematoma formation. Potential and clear contraindications to the use of pharmacologic anticoagulation include associated intracranial bleeding, spinal cord injuries, the observation of splenic injuries, and, in summary, any injury that has a high risk of developing recurrent bleeding with the administration of pharmacologic anticoagulants.

The presence of intracranial injury is a common contraindication to the use of anticoagulation after blunt trauma. Clear protocols for the management of this patient group have not been established, but the danger of using anticoagulation in the presence of intracranial bleeding usually directs treatment to using mechanical devices or repetitive screening to avoid worsening of the intracranial injury. The use of vena caval filters may be beneficial in patients with intracranial injuries, who cannot receive pharmacologic prophylaxis, but are at high risk for thromboembolism. Removable vena caval filters have become available recently and should be considered, particularly in younger patients, especially women of child-bearing age.

Pharmacologic anticoagulation is increasingly used in the management of fracture patients. The mortality rate from pulmonary embolism for patients with hip fractures who do not receive prophylaxis is reported to be 1% to 2%. The use of some form of pharmacologic prophylaxis after fixation of proximal femur fractures is now recommended. However, the indications for the use of anticoagulants for lower extremity fractures distal to the hip is neither established nor well studied. One study that screened patients with fractures distal to the hip reported an 18% incidence of deep venous thrombosis. Factors associated with the development of thrombi included age older than 40, a delay to surgery, and prolonged operative times (33,34,40).

The ideal pharmacologic agent would have qualities of a low complication rate, easy administration, low cost, and excellent bioavailability. Coumadin has been compared with low molecular weight heparin in several prospective and randomized studies of deep venous thrombosis after total hip replacement. These series have documented that low molecular weight heparins reduce the incidence of silent thrombi found on routine screening. This has led many trauma surgeons to the off-label use of low molecular weight heparins in the management of patients after internal fixation of fractures. It is noted that, although this is a current trend, the level of medical evidence in the form of randomized and well-controlled clinical trials for the use of low molecular weight heparins in trauma patients is not established (34,39,41,42).

Given the lack of evidence-based medicine, there is not a clear consensus regarding the differing forms of prophylaxis for venous thromboembolism in patients with major fractures. Despite this, it is important for the treating orthopaedist to consider the patient's risk factors, injuries, surgery, and period of postoperative immobilization. Based on these factors, the physician can develop a strategy for prophylaxis that can be flexible to accommodate the variety of patients and injuries encountered in fracture care.

OUTCOME OF CRITICAL ILLNESS ASSOCIATED WITH ORTHOPEDIC TRAUMA

Historically, outcome studies of critical illness initially focused on short-term mortality (for example, intensive care unit, 28 day, hospital mortality); however, recent investigations have examined important long-term outcomes, including delayed mortality, quality of life (QOL) in survivors, and the social effects on caregivers, including family members. Survival after trauma-related critical illness has significantly improved over the last several decades. Unfortunately, recent studies examining the QOL in survivors after severe and prolonged critical illness, including sepsis and ARDS, have revealed concerning findings, with significant impairments in physical, psychologic, and social functioning. For example, pain is common physical complaint after prolonged critical illness, significantly impairing QOL. In one study of 50 patients from a mixed intensive care unit (ICU) population who proceeded to tracheotomy for prolonged critical illness, 44% of patients reported pain at the highest level of severity (43). Furthermore, many patients survive the acute phase of their critical illness only to suffer prolonged chronic critical illness. These observations have suggested that critical illness should be considered as having at least three components for clinical and research focus: the injury or illness and host characteristics leading to critical illness and ICU admission, the ICU period of critical illness, and subsequent periods of post-ICU care, including hospital ward, intermediate care and rehabilitation, and outpatient care (15). Hopefully, recognizing the physical and psychosocial burdens after critical illness will strengthen our sensitivity to the suffering of patients, families, and caregivers.

ARDS is an unfortunately common complication of trauma and sepsis and may serve as a model of severe and prolonged critical illness. Despite an improvement in mortality over the last 2 decades, survivors of ARDS commonly experience significant impairments in physical, psychologic, and social functioning. Of interest, patients who survive ARDS secondary to sepsis may have greater impairments in QOL than those who survive ARDS secondary to trauma, suggesting the importance of premorbid illness and functional status (44). Although gas exchange is profoundly impaired during the acute phase of ARDS, pulmonary function improves significantly during the first 6 months illness, with only a minority of patients exhibiting moderate to severe impairment. Despite the recovery of pulmonary function, many patients who survive ARDS report significant physical limitations.

Neuromuscular weakness in survivors of prolonged critical illness may be significantly more common than previously appreciated, with one recent study of 109 survivors identifying significant neuromuscular weakness at 12 months after ARDS (45). This study identified generalized weakness with global muscle wasting as the most frequent reason for impairment in a 6-minute walk test; however, foot drop, large joint immobility (heterotropic ossification), and dyspnea were also noted. Earlier studies of septic patients revealed a significant increase in mortality, duration of hospital and rehabilitation care, and overall health care costs in patients with critical illness–acquired neuromuscular weakness. Approximately 50% of ARDS survivors have not returned to work at 1 year after ICU discharge, with weakness and fatigue cited as the most common reasons (45,46). Thus, neuromuscular weakness following critical illness may result in significant and long-lasting impairments in QOL.

Postulated mechanisms for the development of neuromuscular weakness during critical illness include disuse muscle atrophy, inflammation (for example, microvascular thrombosis and ischemia, oxidant injury, apoptosis), corticosteroid-related myopathy, and the use of neuromuscular blockade (47). Effective interventions to enhance neuromuscular function after severe critical illness will ultimately require a greater understanding of the underlying pathophysiology. Studies suggest limiting use of neuromuscular blockade and corticosteroids may be beneficial (47). Furthermore, use of an intensive insulin protocol with tight glucose control has been associated with improved neurophysiologic testing in one study of critically ill surgical patients (48). Pending clinical studies to document efficacy, earlier involvement of physical and occupational therapy and consideration of physical medicine and rehabilitation consultation before hospital discharge seem reasonable.

Neuropsychologic impairment in survivors after critical illness appears to be common and frequently unrecognized. Significant impairments in psychologic and social domains have been identified in survivors of ARDS (44,49,50). Depression appears to be a frequent and disabling complication in survivors of critical illness (49,51). One study identified depression in more than 43% of ARDS survivors on a validated questionnaire administered 6 to 41 months after lung injury (49).

Post-traumatic stress syndrome (PTSD) appears to be related to the frequency of patients' recall of traumatic events in the ICU, with one study revealing 9% incidence of PTSD if one or fewer traumatic events are recalled compared to 41% if two or more traumatic events are recalled (52). In one interesting study examining a mixed ICU patient population, the presence of delusional memories with recall of factual events was associated with the development of PTSD (4). In addition, this study suggested that delusional recall appears to be retained over time but factual recall declines over time.

Cognitive impairment appears to be common after prolonged critical illness, demonstrated in both mixed ICU survivor populations and survivors of ARDS (50,51). In one study of 55 consecutive survivors of ARDS (mean ICU length of stay 29 days) 78% had cognitive impairment at 1 year after ARDS, with one or more of the following: impaired memory, attention, concentration, or decreased mental processing speed (47).

The mechanism by which brain injury during critical illness leads to neuropsychologic impairment is undefined. However, possible mechanisms may be gleaned from observations in septic patients. Reduction in cerebral blood flow, cerebral edema, and disruption in the blood–brain barrier has been identified with septic encephalopathy (53). These observations suggest several potential mechanisms by which systemic inflammation may result in endothelial and neuronal cell injury, including cellular hypoxia, and leukocyte-derived inflammatory mediator and free radical injury.

Effective interventions to reduce the adverse impact of neuropsychologic impairment after critical illness are clearly needed. Pending the results of future research studies, early psychiatric consultation for identification and treatment of depression, anxiety, and PTSD should be considered. Cognitive impairment may be easily missed, and formal neuropsychologic testing may be of significant benefit. For example, neuropsychologic testing may assist in discharge planning, and outpatient assessment may be helpful in evaluating psychosocial functioning and offering occupational guidance. Identification and treatment of sleep disturbance and delirium, commonly present during and after critical illness, may also offer significant benefit. If delusional recall remains associated with the development of PTSD in future studies, interventions to enhance factual recall and reduced delusional recall should be examined. In this regard, sedation and analgesia use during critical illness may alter the recall of ICU experiences in survivors. Although only very preliminary research in this arena is available, the total duration of sedation use may be related to symptoms of depression, and daily interruption of sedation may reduce the development of PTSD (54).

REFERENCES

1. Born CT, Ross SE, Ross SE, et al. Delayed identification of skeletal injury in multisystem trauma: the "missed" fracture. *J Trauma* 1989;29:1643–1646.
2. Brooks A, Holroyd B, Riley B. Missed injury in major trauma patients. *Injury* 2004;35: 407–410.
3. Janjua KJ, Sugrue M, Deane SA. Prospective evaluation of early missed injuries and the role of tertiary trauma survey. *J Trauma* 1998;44:1000–1006; discussion 1006–1007.
4. Jones C, Griffiths RD, Humphris G, et al. Memory, delusions, and the development of acute posttraumatic stress disorder-related symptoms after intensive care. *Crit Care Med* 2001;29:573–580.
5. Hoff WS, Sicoutris CP, Lee SY, et al. Formalized radiology rounds: the final component of the tertiary survey. *J Trauma* 2004;56:291–295.
6. Draaisma JM, Goris JA. Changing patterns of death after injury. In: Border JR, editor. *Blunt Multiple Trauma: Comprehensive Pathophysiology and Care.* New York: Marcel Dekker; 1990.
7. Poole GV, Tinsley M, Tsao AK, et al. Abbreviated injury scale does not reflect the added morbidity of multiple lower extremity fractures. *J Trauma* 1996;40:951–954.
8. Tornetta P III, Mostafavi H, Riina J, et al. Morbidity and mortality in elderly trauma patients. *J Trauma* 1999;46:702–706.
9. Rodriguez JL, Steinberg SM, Bone LB, et al. Resuscitation. In: Border JR, editor. *Blunt Multiple Trauma: Comprehensive Pathophysiology and Care.* New York: Marcel Dekker; 1990.
10. Tscherne H, Regel G. Care of the polytraumatised patient. *J Bone Joint Surg Br* 1996;78: 840–852.
11. Broos PL, Stappaerts KH, Luiten EJ, et al. The importance of early internal fixation in multiply injured patients to prevent late death due to sepsis. *Injury* 1987;18:235–237.
12. Giannoudis PV. Current concepts of the inflammatory response after major trauma: an update. *Injury* 2003;34:397–404.
13. Bone LB, Johnson KD, Weigelt J, et al. Early vs delayed stabilization of femoral fractures: a prospective randomized study. *J Bone Joint Surg Am* 1989;71:336–340.
14. The Acute Respiratory Distress Syndrome Network. Ventilation with lower tidal volumes as compared with traditional tidal volumes for acute lung injury and the acute respiratory distress syndrome. *N Engl J Med* 2000;342:1301–1308.
15. Angus DC, Carlet J. Surviving intensive care: a report from the 2002 Brussels Roundtable. *Intensive Care Med* 2003;29:368–377.
16. Behrman SW, Fabian TC, Kudsk KA, et al. Improved outcome with femur fractures: early vs. delayed fixation. *J Trauma* 1990;30:792–797.
17. Robinson CM. Current concepts of respiratory insufficiency syndromes after fracture. *J Bone Joint Surg Br* 2001;83:781–791.
18. Strecker W, Gebhard F, Perl M, et al. Biochemical characterization of individual injury pattern and injury severity. *Injury* 2003;34:879–887.
19. Michelsen CB, Askanazi J. The metabolic response to injury: mechanisms and clinical implications. *J Bone Joint Surg Am* 1986;68:782–787.
20. Pape HC, Hildebrand F, Pertschy S, et al. Changes in the management of femoral shaft fractures in polytrauma: from early total care to damage control orthopedic surgery. *J Trauma* 2002;53:452–461.
21. Pape HC, van Griensven M, Rice J, et al. Major secondary surgery in blunt trauma patients and perioperative cytokine liberation: determination of the clinical relevance of biochemical markers. *J Trauma* 2001;50:989–1000.
22. Bosse MJ, MacKenzie EJ, Riemer BL, et al. Adult respiratory distress syndrome, pneumonia, and mortality following thoracic injury and a femoral fracture treated either with intramedullary nailing with reaming or with a plate: a comparative study. *J Bone Joint Surg Am* 1997;79:799–809.
23. Anwar IA, Battistella FD, Neiman R, et al. Femur fractures and lung complications: a prospective randomized study of reaming. *Clin Orthop Relat Res* 2004;422:71–76.
24. DeCamp MM, Demling RH. Posttraumatic multisystem organ failure. *JAMA* 1988;260: 530–534.
25. Dunham CM, Bosse MJ, Clancy TV, et al. Practice management guidelines for the optimal timing of long-bone fracture stabilization in polytrauma patients: the east practice management guidelines work group. *J Trauma* 2001;50:958–967.
26. Giannoudis PV. Surgical priorities in damage control in polytrauma. *J Bone Joint Surg Br* 2003;85:478–483.
27. Pape HC, Auf m'Kolk M, Paffrath T, et al. Primary intramedullary femur fixation in multiple trauma patients with associated lung contusion: a cause of posttraumatic ARDS? *J Trauma* 1993;34:540–547.
28. Nowotarski PJ, Turen CH, Brumback RJ, et al. Conversion of external fixation to intramedullary nailing for fractures of the shaft of the femur in multiply injured patients. *J Bone Joint Surg Am* 2000;82:781–788.
29. Scalea TM, Boswell SA, Scott JD, et al. External fixation as a bridge to intramedullary nailing for patients with multiple injuries and with femur fractures: damage control orthopaedics. *J Trauma* 1989;29:1643–1646.
30. Charash WE, Fabian TC, Croce MA. Delayed surgical fixation of femur fractures is a risk factor for pulmonary failure independent of thoracic trauma. *J Trauma* 1994;37: 667–672.
31. McKee MD, Schemitsch EH, Vincent LO, et al. The effect of a femoral fracture on concomitant closed head injury in patients with multiple injuries. *J Trauma* 1997;42: 1041–1045.
32. O'Brien PJ. Fracture fixation in patients having multiple injuries. *Can J Surg* 2003;46: 124–128.
33. Geerts WH, Code KI, Jay RM, et al. A prospective study of venous thromboembolism after major trauma. *N Engl J Med* 1994;331:1601–1606.
34. Fisher CG, Blachut PA, Salvian AJ, et al. Effectiveness of pneumatic leg compression devices for the prevention of thromboembolic disease in orthopaedic trauma patients: a prospective, randomized study of compression alone versus no prophylaxis. *J Orthop Trauma* 1995;9:1–7.
35. Monreal M, Lafoz E, Navarro A, et al. A prospective double-blind trial of a low molecular weight heparin once daily compared with conventional low-dose heparin three times daily to prevent pulmonary embolism and venous thrombosis in patients with hip fracture. *J Trauma* 1989;29:873–875.
36. Oishi CS, Grady-Benson JC, Otis SM, et al. The clinical course of distal deep venous thrombosis after total hip and total knee arthroplasty, as determined with duplex ultrasonography. *J Bone Joint Surg Am* 1994;76:1658–1663.
37. Hirsh J, Hoak J. Management of deep vein thrombosis and pulmonary embolism: a statement for healthcare professionals. *Circulation* 1996;93:2212–2245.
38. Kearon C, Julian JA, Newman TE, et al. Noninvasive diagnosis of deep venous thrombosis. *Ann Intern Med* 1998;128:663–677.
39. Colwell CW Jr, Spiro TE, Trowbridge AA, et al. Use of enoxaparin, a low-molecular-weight heparin, and unfractionated heparin for the prevention of deep venous thrombosis after elective hip replacement: a clinical trial comparing efficacy and safety—Enoxaparin Clinical Trial Group. *J Bone Joint Surg Am* 1994;76:3–14. Erratum in: *J Bone Joint Surg Am* 1994;76:4741.
40. Bergqvist D, Lindblad B, Matzsch T. Low molecular weight heparin for thromboprophylaxis and epidural/spinal anaesthesia: is there a risk? *Acta Anaesthesiol Scand* 1992;36: 605–609.
41. White RH, Romano PS, Zhou H, et al. Incidence and time course of thromboembolic outcomes following total hip or knee arthroplasty. *Arch Intern Med* 1998;158: 1525–1531.
42. Warkentin TE, Levine MN, Hirsh J, et al. Heparin-induced thrombocytopenia in patients treated with low-molecular-weight heparin or unfractionated heparin. *N Engl J Med* 1995;332:1330–1335.
43. Nelson JE, Meier DE, Litke A, et al. The symptom burden of chronic critical illness. *Crit Care Med* 2004;32:1527–1534.
44. Davidson TA, Caldwell ES, Curtis JR, et al. Reduced quality of life in survivors of acute respiratory distress syndrome compared with critically ill control patients. *JAMA* 1999; 281:354–360.
45. Herridge MS, Cheung AM, Tansey CM, et al for the Canadian Critical Care Trials Group. One-year outcomes in survivors of the acute respiratory distress syndrome. *N Engl J Med* 2003;348:683–694.
46. McHugh LG, Milberg JA, Whitcomb ME, et al. Recovery of function in survivors of the acute respiratory distress syndrome. *Am J Respir Crit Care Med* 1994;150:90–94.
47. Deem S, Lee CM, Curtis JR. Update in nonpulmonary critical care: acquired neuromuscular disorders in the intensive care unit. *Am J Respir Crit Care Med* 2003;168:735–739.
48. Van den Berghe G, Wouters P, Weekers F, et al. Intensive insulin therapy in critically ill patients. *N Engl J Med* 2001;345:1359–1367.

49. Weinert CR, Gross CR, Kangas JR, et al. Health-related quality of life after acute lung injury. *Am J Respir Crit Care Med* 1997;156:1120–1128.
50. Hopkins RO, Weaver LK, Pope D, et al. Neuropsychological sequelae and impaired health status in survivors of severe acute respiratory distress syndrome. *Am J Respir Crit Care Med* 1999;160:50–56.
51. Jackson JC, Hart RP, Gordon SM, et al. Six-month neuropsychological outcome of medical intensive care unit patients. *Crit Care Med* 2003;31:1226–1234.
52. Schelling G, Stoll C, Hallar M, et al. Health-related quality of life and posttraumatic stress disorder in survivors of acute respiratory distress syndrome. *Crit Care Med* 1998; 26:651–659.
53. Papadopoulos MC, Davies DC, Moss RF, et al. Pathophysiology of septic encephalopathy: a review. *Crit Care Med* 2000;28:3019–3022.
54. Kress JP, Gehlbach B, Lacy M, et al. The long-term psychological effects of daily sedative interruption on critically ill patients. *Am J Respir Crit Care Med* 2003;168:1457–1461.

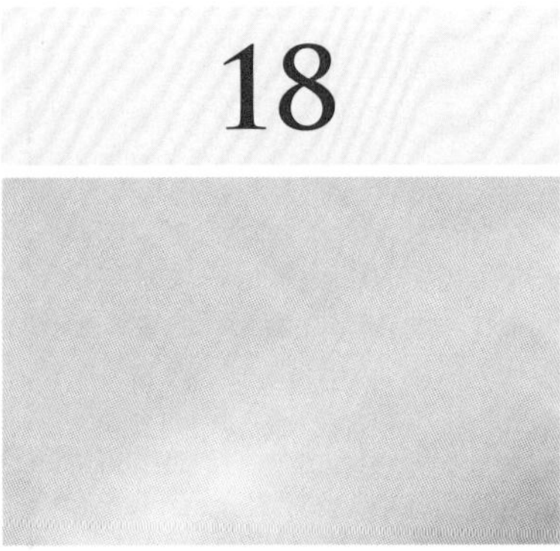

LOCAL COMPLICATIONS

Kirti D. Moholkar and Bruce H. Ziran

A complication is an adverse event that occurs following a procedure (risk of the procedure), treatment (side effect or toxicity), or illness. The most thoughtfully conceived, meticulously prepared and comprehensively planned surgical procedure can also be marred with undesired therapeutic outcomes that can affect the principal illness. With reference to fracture management, *complication* refers to an undesired negative outcome specific to the care of a particular fracture as perceived by the surgeon or by the patient. A complication can also alter the mode and progression of the principal illness, sometimes replacing the severity of the main illness.

Early recognition with prompt appropriate intervention is the best way to avert progression to a potentially disastrous situation. The purpose of this chapter is to provide a framework for reviewing local complications that can result during fracture management. The most common complications of fracture management as listed will be reviewed for etiology, prevention, and subsequent treatment.

1. Complications of cast application
2. Complications of skeletal traction
3. Complications of external fixation
4. Infections in orthopaedics
5. Bleeding complications
6. Vascular injury
7. Neurological injury
8. Complications of bone healing
9. Complex regional pain syndrome
10. Acute pain management

COMPLICATIONS OF CAST APPLICATION

Although recent advances in orthopaedics such as functional bracing and rigid internal fixation have decreased the need for cast immobilization, there is still a group of patients that require formal casting. Plaster of Paris casts are required for immobilizing fractures, correcting deformities, and splinting limbs. Plaster of Paris casts can be a great tool while treating conditions nonoperatively; however, their inadvertent use can result in complications such as macerations, ulcerations, infections, rashes, itching, burns, allergic contact dermatitis, and infections (1–8). One should be particularly cautious in applying casts to patients with loss of protective sensation due to conditions such as diabetes or head injury and in cases of poor skin condition or neurovascular injury (see Fig. 5-31). In these situations, cast application can lead to rapid skin breakdown from pressure necrosis as well as other problems such as Charcot joint changes (9).

Before applying a cast, evidence of neurological injury should be documented. If there is any question of circulatory loss, the cast should not be applied until the circulatory status is clarified and circulation is restored. Infections including gas gangrene, ischemic muscle necrosis from compartment syndrome, and unrecognized vascular injuries can be hidden under a cast and lead to limb loss (4).

Casting Materials

The plaster of Paris bandage consists of a roll of muslin stiffened by starch and soaked with hemihydrates of calcium sulphate. When water is added, the calcium sulphate crystallizes ($CaSO_4 \cdot H_2O + H_2O = CaSO_4 \cdot 2\,H_2O$ + heat). The crystallization of plaster of Paris is an exothermic reaction (3). The setting of this material may be accelerated by increasing the temperature of the water or slowed by cooling the water. As the cast is applied and the plaster of Paris crystallizes, the heat given off can be enough to burn the skin (10) (see Fig. 5-33). This is especially likely if the water used to soak the plaster was too hot. The plaster bandage should be immersed in a water bath that is tepid or at least comfortable to the touch of the person applying it. This is true whether one is applying a circular cast or a longitudinal splint. In fact, thick splints may produce higher exothermic temperatures than casts.

A variety of casting products have become available as a substitute for the classic plaster of Paris cast (11,12). The most widely used is a knitted fiberglass fabric, which is saturated with polyurethane resin. Exposure of this product to water and air initiates a chemical reaction, which causes the tapes to become rigid. Synthetic casting materials present better physical and mechanical properties than the traditional plaster of Paris (11) and are relatively lightweight, strong, radiolucent, and when properly used, resistant to water. The major clinical disadvantage of fiberglass is that it is less malleable and cannot be molded to the limb as well as plaster. In addition, when the fiberglass cast is applied, it accommodates simulated swelling poorly (11).

Swelling

Edema, fluid that persists in the hand or foot, can impede the synchrony of motion between tendons, bones, and joints. An extremity should be elevated and treated in a splint or placed in traction until swelling reduces before placing it in a cast. The cast may be bivalved to accommodate for acute swelling, and then a new cast can be applied once the swelling subsides. Furthermore, the cast needs to be re-examined after acute swelling subsides, because the limb, now smaller, may not be adequately immobilized in the original cast. In this case, a new and better-fitting cast needs to be placed. Swelling distal to the cast is common, and most situations will respond well to limb elevation above the level of the heart. In persistent cases, it is important to either bivalve the cast or to remove and replace the cast.

Complications Associated with Cast Removal

Cast removal requires an oscillating type of saw. The cast saw must be used carefully to avoid lacerating the skin under the cast. It is best to support the cast with the thumb held against the cast in order to avoid pushing the blade through the patient's skin (Fig. 18-1). The use of a cast saw and the noise it produces could make a child apprehensive and agitated, which can be a cause of inadvertent injury (13,14). The use of a cast saw is avoided in children with cardiomyopathy due malignant cardiac arrhythmia triggered by anxiety, which can be fatal (13). Although this method is rarely used, casts can also be removed by wetting and then unwrapping, especially in uncooperative patients and in children.

Inadvertent cast-saw injuries are attributable to inadequately padded casts, improper technique, or blunt saw blades (15). Cast-saw blade temperatures recorded while splitting plaster and fiberglass casts are elevated to a degree that would increase the risk of a second- or third-degree burn (15,16). The saw should not be pulled or pushed parallel to the cast (and skin) surface, instead, multiple gentle thrusts, perpendicular to the cast surface, allow for better proprioceptive feedback and will help avoid skin injury. During removal of fiberglass casts, the saw generates dust that is lower in quantity, but larger in particle size compared to the dust generated when removing plaster of Paris casts. This dust usually consists of glass fibers embedded in cured polyurethane with a minor amount of glass fiber dust. These are not considered to be respirable-sized particles and fall well below the permissible occupational exposure limits for nuisance dusts. Limb swelling after removing the plaster cast can occur, and is called "plaster disease" (17). Supportive elasticized bandages can be provided to reduce such swelling after the removal of plaster casts. Regular exercises and elevation of the limb while the cast is on can reduce such swelling.

Malposition of the Limb

Casts and splints that immobilize limbs in a nonfunctioning position should be avoided, especially for minor injuries. A posterior splint applied for an ankle sprain can leave the foot and ankle in the equinus position, making it impossible for the patient to bear any weight on the limb, promotes edema, and delays recovery from the minor injury (Fig. 18-2). Prolonged lack of function can result in disuse osteoporosis of the foot and subsequent pain with weight bearing (18–20). Casts applied to the upper limb should allow joint motion of the fingers. Similarly, casts on the lower limb should not impinge on or block toe motion.

Pressure Sores

The patient's complaints of a painful cast should never be ignored, and the cast should be changed promptly. Often, this may reveal an area of early skin pressure or irritation that could progress to full-thickness skin loss. Patients who repeatedly request cast changes might be better treated by operative fracture fixation. Although the success of cast treatment depends on proper molding, care should be taken to protect bony prominences such as epicondyles and malleoli, as well as avoiding

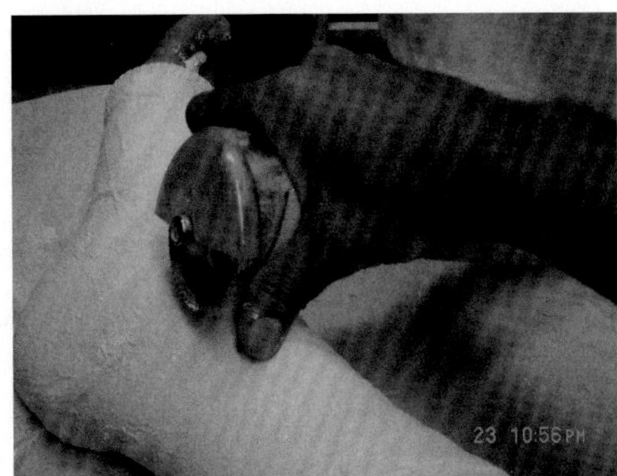

FIGURE 18-1 Safe method to use while cutting the plaster cast with a saw.

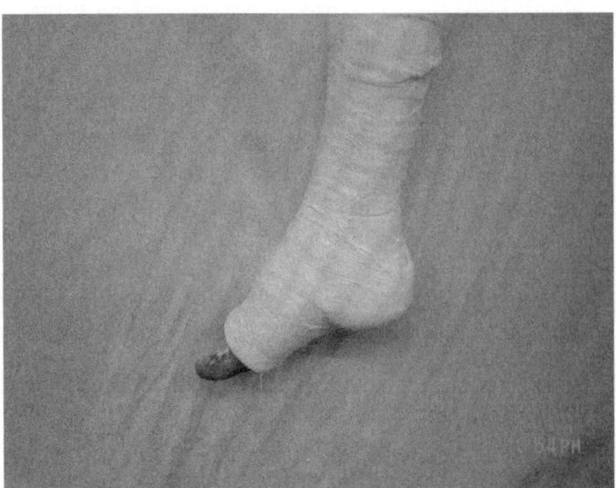

FIGURE 18-2 Cast applied in equinus position.

intrusions into soft areas containing neurovascular structures (cubital and popliteal fossae). Each limb segment requires particular molding methods, and the reader is referred to other classic works on cast techniques, such as Charnley's closed treatment of common fractures (18). Diabetic and vascular ulcers can be treated effectively by means of contact casts. Care should be taken while applying casts to patients with these conditions due to the neurological involvement. These patients are particularly susceptible to thermal, pressure, and friction injury due to contact casts. Regular assessments of the casts and changes should be undertaken.

Allergic Reactions and Contact Dermatitis

Diisocyanates are used in fiberglass casts. Allergic reactions, although temporary, have been reported. Studies have shown that diisocyanates are primarily irritants rather than sensitizers. The skin symptoms of irritation were all mild and temporary (21). These results confirm those of previous studies, which have implicated the quaternary ammonium compound benzalkonium chloride as the allergen responsible for plaster of Paris-induced allergic contact dermatitis (21).

Disuse Atrophy and Muscle Weakness

Muscles that do not function when under cover of plaster will atrophy. Not only can this result in cast loosening, but there may also be functional loss. Motion and isometric exercises should be encouraged. Prolonged non–weight-bearing treatment in a cast can also result in disuse osteopenia, which can complicate recovery. Typically, radiographic features include loss of trabecular pattern, a speckled or mottled appearance of the periarticular surface, and a generalized "washed-out" appearance.

Injury Due to Foreign Objects

Underlying skin injury can result from inserting objects such as fruit seeds, clothes hangers, sticks, pencils, knives, and other objects (22) to relieve skin itching. Explicit instructions and precautions should be given to patients to refrain from such activity. When these types of objects become trapped in the cast, the cast should be changed promptly. In noncommunicative patients, complaints and problems may not be easily solicited, and a change in behavior or disposition should alert the caregiver to potential problems.

Cast Syndrome

Cast syndrome is a rare complication that is seen related to body jacket, shoulder spica, and hip spica. The syndrome occurs due to arteriomesenteric duodenal obstruction, and it is a result of excessive abdomen and chest coverage. The symptoms are severe, and if left untreated, can be potentially lethal. The duodenum passes from right to left across the anterior aspect of the first and second lumbar vertebra. Just above this point, the superior mesenteric artery arises from the abdominal aorta and passes downward with its accompanying veins in the mesentry. There is a potential danger of compression of the third part of the duodenum between the lumbar spine and the aorta posteriorly and the mesentry and vessels anteriorly. This syndrome is precipitated by recumbency and increased lumbar lordosis. Avoiding constrictive body casts that increase lumbar lordosis prevents cast syndrome. Nausea, epigastric fullness, and regurgitation should be carefully evaluated. Because the use of body casts has dropped precipitously, its incidence is low, but should be considered when such a casting method is rendered.

COMPLICATIONS OF TRACTION

There are two types of traction: skin traction and skeletal traction. Traction can be used to reduce and hold fractures, correct deformities, and elevate extremities for managing soft tissue injuries and burns. For hundreds of years, traction has been used to manage fractures and dislocations that are not suitable for treatment by casting or internal fixation (23). With the advancement of orthopaedic technology and techniques, traction is rarely used today.

Skin Traction

The use of skin traction to align a fracture, particularly of the proximal femur, has been common since it was popularized by Buck during the Civil War (24). Skin traction is still used occasionally to stabilize a femur fracture in a child's leg as well as a temporary means of stabilizing adult hip fractures (25,26). Because most of the forces created by skin traction are lost and dissipated in the soft tissue structures, skin traction is rarely used as definitive therapy in adults. Complications can occur as described below.

Application of Skin Traction

Application of skin traction involves using tapes or adhesive materials on the skin, which transmit tensile forces to the limb. Although it provides a more intimate interface and more effective traction, the skin experiences a shear force and is unable to tolerate more than approximately 6 to 10 lbs of traction for a brief length of time. At weights greater than 10 lbs, superficial skin layers may be disrupted and irritated (27). Due to their fragile skin, elderly patients are not good candidates for this type of traction, and deep skin sloughing as well as prolonged hospital stay have been reported as complications (27,28). Prolonged traction tends to pull off the superficial layers of the skin, causing pressure necrosis of the soft tissues. Dermal injury can result in blister formation.

If skin traction is used, injury can be avoided by carefully inspecting the area to be covered by the traction tapes. The skin should be cleaned before applying the adhesive material. A rash, abrasion, or skin wounds are contraindications to skin traction tapes. Hairs on the extremity should be carefully shaved, and tincture benzoin should be applied to the skin after it is cleansed. Even after taking precautionary measures, the skin can still be easily traumatized due to the traction tape's adhesive backing and allergic reaction to the tape and/or the adhesive. The skin under the traction tapes should be inspected regularly for skin breakdown and pressure areas. Bony prominences should be carefully padded to avoid pressure sores. The fibular head, malleoli, femoral condyles, and medial and lateral epicondyle should be padded before applying skin traction. Pressure-related nerve injury due to elastic circumferential wrappings has been reported. Regular attention is needed to assess the peroneal nerve below the knee and ulnar nerve at the elbow for these pressure-related complications. Excessive pain and paresthesias are signs of nerve pressure; circumferential bandages in such circumstances should be immediately removed, and neurological examination should be performed. Increased intracompartmental pressures can also occur (29) due to pressure from within or without. Because circumferential bandaging can result in further increased compartmental pressures and tissue anoxia, patients with skin traction who complain of severe pain should be carefully examined, and elasticized bandages need to be removed.

An alternative to skin traction is a prepackaged sponge-rubber material that can be removed and reapplied (Buck's traction). This option is used most often in the elderly for hip fractures. Although it will not effectively "reduce" the fracture, this method may provide comfort against the involuntary spasm of the hip girdle musculature that can cause fracture motion and pain. Buck's traction is rarely, if ever, used as a definitive method of traction.

Skeletal Traction

If more controlled and powerful traction is desired, or if long-term traction is wanted, skeletal traction is indicated. Kirschner wires and Steinmann's pins are used as fixation devices. It is preferable to use either a large, threaded Steinmann pin (between 1/8 and 1/4 inch) or a fine Kirschner wire that is tensioned for stiffness. Use of the correct traction bow and correct device application is critical to prevent a very painful and troublesome failure of the traction system.

The most commonly used sites for skeletal traction are the proximal tibia, distal tibia, distal femur, os calcis, metacarpals, olecranon, radius, and the ulna (see Fig. 5-27). The pins are placed in metaphyseal bone and strict aseptic precautions should be undertaken to avoid infection. Diaphyseal sites, while providing better bone are usually not feasible, and because most traction pins have a spade tip, there is a risk of thermal injury during placement into hard bone. Sites with possible skin breakdown, infection, hematoma, and fractures should also be avoided.

Infection of the bone or soft tissue around the pin is a common complication of skeletal traction. Traction pin site care is of utmost importance to avoid deep infection and resultant osteomyelitis and ring sequestra. Purulent exudates from pin sites are a sign of infection and should be treated by antibiotics and removal of the device.

Pin tract infection can be minimized or managed by (a) having the pin pass through the least amount of soft tissue possible, (b) minimizing movement of joints adjacent to the traction pin, and (c) routine pin care. As with external fixation pins, the more soft tissue there is around the pin, the greater the risk of pin problems will be. Skin and muscle motion around the pins results in soft tissue irritation that produces a local inflammatory response and increases the risk of bacterial colonization and infection. Stabilizing the soft tissue envelope is the most effective method of preventing irritation.

Placing skeletal traction requires thorough anatomic knowledge of the structures at risk during placement. The first principle is to insert the pins from the side of the limb that contains the most vital structure at risk. In the tibia, care is taken to avoid injuring the superficial peroneal nerve; in the distal femur, it is the adductor hiatus containing the femoral artery; and in the olecranon, it is the ulnar nerve (30).

In osteoporotic bone, there is a distinct risk of the device cutting through the soft bone, especially with greater traction weights. This can occur most in metaphyseal bone. Careful observation and attention to patient complaints of increasing pain are methods to avoid such problems.

Other Complications of Skeletal Traction

Finger stiffness and plantar flexion contractures are common with prolonged use of skeletal traction. Hand physiotherapy should accompany upper limb traction devices. The foot can be kept out of equinus by a plantar support. Routine physiotherapy is important to avoid these problems.

One of the most common complications from skeletal traction is overdistracting the fracture. This has been found to occur particularly in fractures of the distal radius where ligamentotaxis from external fixation can be exerted too vigorously. Overdistraction of the radiocarpal joint can lead to stiffness and even causalgia of the fingers and hand (31). The technique of skeletal traction for cervical spine injuries can also overdistract if the method is applied too vigorously or without careful monitoring of its effect (32,33). Finally, due to the patient's prolonged recumbency, there is an increased risk of thromboembolic events.

COMPLICATIONS OF EXTERNAL FIXATION

External fixation is the oldest of the most commonly used treatment methods for tibial diaphyseal fractures. External fixators date back almost 2,400 years, when Hippocrates described a form of a splint composed of Egyptian leather rings connected by four wooden rods from a cornel tree, which was used to treat a fracture of the tibia (34,35). Technological evolution, better biomechanical knowledge, improved clinical experience, and introduction of newer-generation hybrid fixators have contributed to the increased enthusiasm in the use of external fixation. The most common complications of external fixation are delayed union, pin-tract infection, pin loosening, neurovascular injury, and stiffness of the adjacent joints.

Thermal Injury to the Bone

Thermal injury results from heat generation during the insertion process and may be the cause of ring sequestra. It was thought that inserting pins with power equipment and excessively high rotational velocity might contribute to thermal necrosis. In a human cadaveric study, temperatures in excess of 55°C were observed, and drill speed was found to have an effect on the maximum temperature (36). Pinpoint drill design was a more significant factor, and predrilling was highly effective as a method of minimizing temperature elevation (36). Recent advances in pin design have mostly circumvented this problem. Furthermore, the inevitable wobbling of the manual technique may create a wider opening in the bone that could potentially lead to looseness. Using a power tool with diligent technique will mostly circumvent theoretical problems.

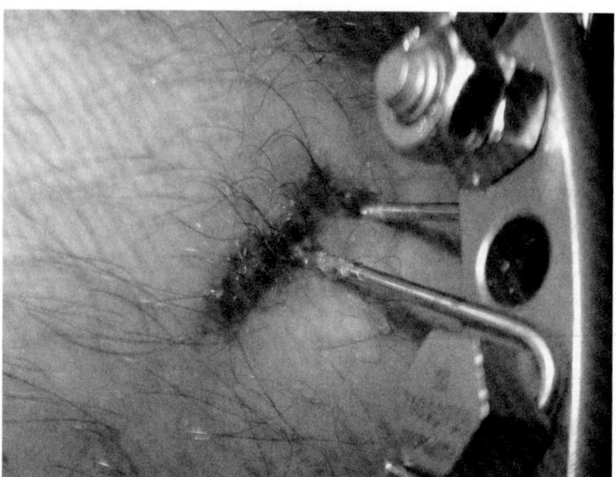

FIGURE 18-3 Pin tract infection.

Pin Loosening

The pin-bone interface is the weakest link in the mechanical stability of external skeletal fixation. Effective precautions should be taken to reduce such stresses and decrease pin loosening. Preloading the pins reduces micromotion and reduces the rate of loosening, but too much radial preload can result in either pressure necrosis or microfractures during placement (37). These stresses at the pin-bone interface can result in bone resorption due to overstrain (38). In addition, rapid failure will occur if the pin is not engaging or through the far cortex. Spade- or trocar-tipped pins should be placed only with predrilling. Current pin designs incorporate a drill tip with flutes that greatly reduce thermal damage to bone and allow simple, rapid, and reliable placement. Care must be exercised to avoid a "transcortical" pin because the flutes of most drill tips do not allow release of cut bone and can result in thermal necrosis. This is because if the flutes are clogged, the tip becomes more similar to a trocar point. Also, newer pin designs with coatings such as hydroxyapatite can result in a better pin-bone interface. There are also designs that use conical pin geometry, which results in a radial preload. While theoretically appealing, conical pin devices have not proven to be better than standard pins, and because of the conical hole created, they cannot be turned back if the pin is inadvertently placed too far. As such, there is little practical need for conical pin designs. Pins with coatings that provide enhanced fixation (hydroxyapatite) have also been introduced, but unless used for definitive and long-term fixation, the increased costs of such devices have not been established.

Pin Tract Infection

Preventing pin tract infections is preferable to treating them (Fig. 18-3). Green stated that the two basic factors that contribute to pin tract infections are tissue necrosis around the pin and excessive pin site tissue motion (39). Pin tract infection has been reported to occur from between 0.5% and 42% (40,41). Pin tract infections can be considered on a spectrum of severity from simple drainage to frank osteomyelitis with resultant ring sequestrum (Fig. 18-4). If cellulitis develops around the pin site, or if a large amount of drainage is occurring, treatment should be started with pin care and an oral cephalosporin. Clinical signs of a deep infection include purulent drainage, swelling, and cellulitis. Chronic osteomyelitis has been reported to occur, but remains infrequent (42). The pathogenesis of infection is complex, but simplistically, biofilm bacteria can colonize the pin and migrate into the limb. While on an inert surface, they avoid host defenses and pharmaceutical intervention. Although colonization itself may not result in failure, the resulting inflammatory response or seeding of the bone around the pin, which may have become necrotic and thus inert also, may result in frank infection.

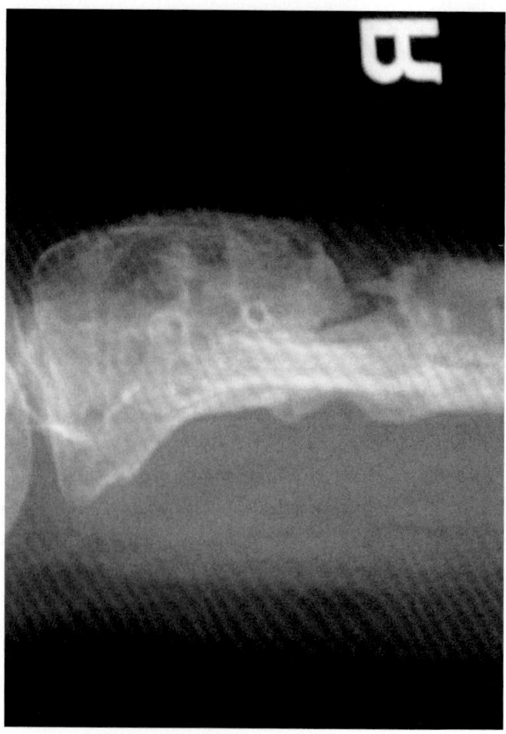

FIGURE 18-4 Ring sequestrum.

Pin tract infections are most common in areas with more soft tissue, such as the humerus and the pelvis. The feet account for only 1% of pin tract infections, and infection is rare in the anteromedial tibia (43–45). In a recent study, patients with fine wire fixation had the lowest incidence of pin tract problems as compared with half-pin fixation, which had a similar risk of pin tract infection (46). Recent studies have shown that the use of hydroxyapatite, silver coating, and polyurethane argentum sleeves on the pins has reduced the incidence of pin tract infections (47–50). Using polyurethane argentum sleeves can significantly reduce pin tract infections, as silver is known to be bactericidal. In one study, the rate of pin-tract infections was reduced to 4.2% (47). In another multicenter, prospective, randomized study, the biomechanical and clinical properties of the bone-pin interface were compared with standard tapered pins and hydroxyapatite-coated tapered pins implanted in patients who underwent femoral and tibial external fixation treatments. The results showed that the hydroxyapatite-coated tapered pins were clinically effective in improving the fixation strength of the bone-pin interface. This improvement corresponded to a lower rate of pin tract-infection.

The frequency (daily or weekly) of pin site care has been recently debated. Although daily pin site care by the patient or a home nurse is recommended (51–53), one study recommended only showering without other physical pin cleaning procedures in children undergoing external fixation procedures (54). Another study found no difference in weekly pin care compared to daily pin care. Excessive use of chemical irritants can actually result in an inflammatory response and can increase the risk of infection. Our current protocol involves daily showering with use of an alcohol pledget to clean the pin, followed by stabilizing the soft tissues around the pin. A gentle compressive dressing covers the skin site and prevents motion that can initiate a local inflammatory response, which can lead to a pin tract infection. Most pin problems can be easily treated with various modalities. The etiology of the problem should be identified. If the problem is due to excessive soft tissue irritation, the soft tissues should be better stabilized with compressive dressings. If there is local skin irritation from chemical treatments, they should be stopped. If there is purulent material and exudate from deep within the wound, packing and antibiotics should be attempted. Prophylactic application of Bactroban ointment and keeping the pins covered is very effective. Allowing the patient to shower and enter into either an antiseptic bath or chlorinated pool is very helpful in stabilizing the skin flora and providing for adequate pin care. It also improves patient morale by promoting personal hygiene. If there is suspicion of a deep pin tract infection, the clamp can be loosened, and if the pin has resistance to turning (e.g., adequate purchase), it can be maintained. If it is frankly loose, it should be promptly taken out. If there is suspicion of osteomyelitis, the pin should be removed, and debridement or curettage of the bone should be performed followed by open packing, in addition to administering intravenous (IV) antibiotics. New pins may need to be placed at different sites if the fracture has not healed.

In cases of bone transport, there will always be some skin irritation as the pins move through the limb, but this is mostly mechanical and resolves with variation of stated treatments. More severe skin problems or skin tenting can be released surgically.

Neurovascular Injury

Nerve and vessel injuries can occur with external fixator placement. Many pins are placed through small incisions without directly visualizing the soft tissue structures deep in the wound. Complications are avoidable with a thorough familiarity of the cross-sectional anatomy and the location of the neurovascular structures (55). The reported incidence of neurovascular complications is 0.6% (55). Meticulous surgical techniques that may reduce complications include using a blunt instrument to dissect the soft tissues and neurovascular structures, allowing the pin or wire to lie directly on bone, and using pin guides to prevent the soft tissue from wrapping around the pins as they turn and advance. The dorsal sensory branch of the radial nerve and the lateral antebrachial nerve (56) in the forearm, the anterior tibial artery, and peroneal nerve at the junction of the third and fourth quarters of the leg and the medial thigh and the saphenous nerve (57) are most often affected and should be protected (58). While treating calcaneal fractures and passing calcaneal pins, the medial calcaneal nerve, which is the most posterior branch of the lateral plantar, and lateral plantar nerves are at significant risk for abutting the pins or being directly injured at the margins of these relatively safe zones (59). Transient radial nerve palsy has been reported to occur in around 5% of cases in a series of 164 humeral fractures (9).

It is fortunate and surprising that vascular injuries are rare. Cadaveric studies show that vessel injury is less likely because the tapered ends of the external fixator pins push the vessels aside. The vascular injuries that occur are largely due to constant pin pressure on the vessel wall (40). Vascular injuries usually occur when the half pins project too far beyond the far cortex. Guides to neurovascular and pin orientation anatomy are available, and the routine use of such educational manuals is strongly recommended (57).

INFECTIONS IN ORTHOPAEDICS

The modern era of infection control in orthopaedic surgery began in 1865 when Lister successfully treated an open fracture with the use of carbolic acid (60). The prophylactic use of antibiotics, in the form of sulfa, was begun during World War II as well as the practice of leaving wounds open (60). Throughout history and even today, some infections remain resistant to our antibiotic compounds, however. Infection will always be a problem for humans and especially in orthopaedics. The incidence has reduced, but the changing microbiology of such infections has increased the patients' morbidity rate. As such, the treatment of orthopaedic infections is not only challenging but varies greatly among surgeons of different backgrounds, philosophies, and experience. We find that a useful way to approach infections is to compare them with a benign tumor. In such cases, the condition rarely is fatal, yet it tends to recur if not adequately treated. In the case of infections, the chemotherapy is antibiotics and tumor surgery principles are very applicable.

Normally, there are millions of bacteria that generally populate skin and body cavities. Table 18-1 shows normal bacterial counts in specific regions of the body. Microorganisms often exist as microbial aggregates in a biofilm slime layer colonizing surfaces within which they are resistant to antagonists. If the right combination of conditions is present along with an inciting event, an infection can be established. Nutrients and free energy are concentrated at the surfaces of the 3D architecture of these bacterial colonies. Colonization of surfaces is not always synonymous with infection. Bacteria such as *Staphylococcus epidermidis*, streptococcal species, and Gram-negative groups are naturally found on skin, oral mucosa, and the intestinal tract. Through evolution, however, bone and cartilage are not teleologically able to support bacterial colonization and are especially susceptible to infection.

TABLE 18-1 Bacteria Commonly Found on the Surfaces of the Human Body

Bacterium	Skin	Conjunctiva	Nose	Pharynx	Mouth
Staphylococcus epidermidis (1)	++	+	++	++	++
*Staphylococcus aureus** (2)	+	+/–	+	+	+
Streptococcus mitis				+	++
Streptococcus salivarius				++	++
*Streptococcus mutans** (3)				+	++
*Enterococcus faecalis** (4)				+/–	+
*Streptococcus pneumoniae** (5)		+/–	+/–	+	+
*Streptococcus pyogenes** (6)	+/–	+/–		+	+
Neisseria sp. (7)		+	+	++	+
*Neisseria meningitidis** (8)			+	++	+
Veillonellae sp.					+
Enterobacteriaceae (Escherichia coli)* (9)		+/–	+/–	+/–	+
Proteus sp.		+/–	+	+	+
*Pseudomonas aeruginosa** (10)				+/–	+/–
*Haemophilus influenzae** (11)		+/–	+	+	+
Bacteroides sp.*					
Bifidobacterium bifidum (12)					
Lactobacillus sp. (13)				+	++
Clostridium sp.* (14)					+/–
Clostridium tetani (15)					

++ = nearly 100 percent, + = common, +/– = rare, * = potential pathogen.

Pathogenesis

When bacteria exist alone or in small clusters that are not colonized, they are in the planktonic state. They are metabolically active and susceptible to the body's host defense systems as well as appropriate antibiotics. Bacterial colonization occurs when bacteria adhere to a surface and begin to undergo a complex and organized process that resists both host and extrinsic efforts at eradication (61). Any inert surface that becomes available to bacteria in a biologic environment can spontaneously acquire a glycoproteinaceous film. In the early stages of colonization, the bacteria can still be killed or contained by host defenses, but there are situations when the bacteria can remain viable: (a) the inoculum is larger than threshold levels, (b) host defense mechanisms are impaired, (c) the tissue on which the bacteria colonize is traumatized (or necrotic), (d) a foreign body is present, and (e) the surface (or tissue) is acellular or inanimate (e.g., dead bone, cartilage, and biomaterials). As a result, colonization alone is not enough for infection, but rather a necessary antecedent.

Bacteria randomly arrive near a bone surface or biomaterial surface by direct contamination, contiguous spreading, or hematogenous seeding. Juxtaposition of the bacteria with a tissue surface or biomaterial is therefore accomplished by van der Waals forces. This interaction allows bacteria to develop "irreversible" cross-links with the surface (adhesin receptor interaction) (62). The surface is anionic and initially repels bacteria (which are also anionic). Adhesion is based on time-dependent specific protein adhesion-receptor interactions, as well as carbohydrate polymer synthesis in addition to charge and physical forces (63). After anchorage to the surface, bacteria begin to create a polysaccharide slime layer, and a "biofilm-enclosed" colony of bacteria forms.

Figure 18-5 documents the activity in a mature biofilm. In this illustration, the pillars of a mature biofilm are visible, distributed on top of a monolayer of surface-associated cells. In addition to fixed cells, there are motile cells that maintain their association with the biofilm for long periods of time, swimming between pillars of biofilm-associated bacteria (64).

The understanding of biofilm bacteria helps explain the recalcitrant nature of orthopaedic infections. The biofilms will only form on inert or nonviable surfaces. The antibiotics need to penetrate this film before gaining access to the bacteria. The definition of a biofilm is best described as a community of sessile bacteria, which are surrounded by a glycocalyx of extracellular matrix. Also, an inert surface such as dead tissue, implants, or debris, provides an area for such bacteria to colonize and form biofilm that will escape the host defense as well as antibiotic treatments. Biofilm (or slime) is formed by bacterial extracapsular exopolysaccharides that bind to surfaces and participate in cell-to-cell aggregation. As orthopaedic implants and materials are increasingly moving toward minimizing the immune response, they are becoming more and more inert. Once colonized on such surfaces, the bacteria are resistant to host defenses and may resist antibiotic action.

Ultimately, the body tries to control the bacterial colonization by increasing the perimeters of action, and as a result, an abscess or involucrum is formed. Alternatively if a sinus develops, there is a method to dispel the detritus and bacteria. Eventually, an equilibrium may come to exist in the form of a chronic infection, which is what many practitioners see in practice. There is usually a history of intermittent symptoms and drainage that responds to an antibiotic. The harmful clinical manifestations of infection are generally due to the release of bacteria into the bloodstream that are metabolically active, the release of toxins, and the release of oxidative enzymes by the host cell. Although they are quite susceptible to the body's host defenses and antibiotics, their numbers and the continued release into the bloodstream, or any weakening of the systemic host, will allow ongoing clinical manifestations. Thus, infection may de-

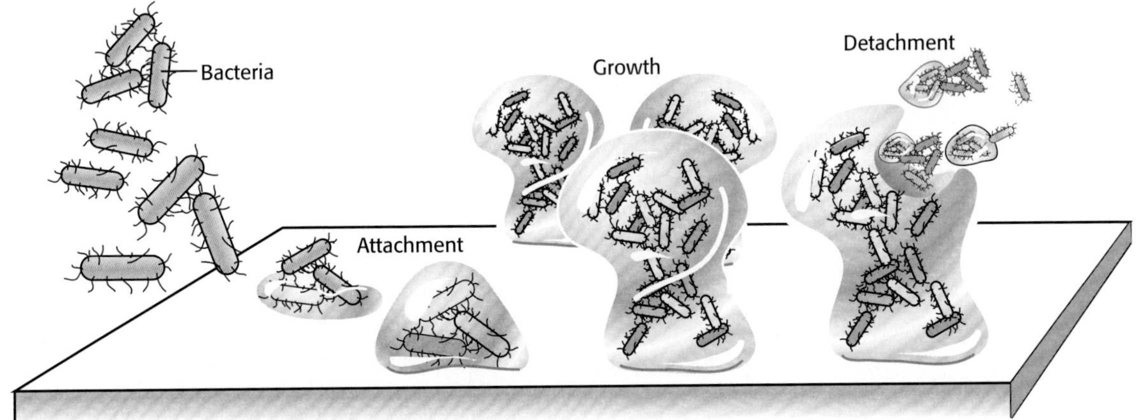

FIGURE 18-5 Illustration of the biofilm bacterial colonization process. First, the bacteria need to find an inert surface (e.g., implant or dead tissue). Implants or dead tissue that have been integrated by the host with some type of surface are not inert and will resist colonization. Then, the colonization process will continue until mature colonies are formed. Once mature, the colonies can change based on environmental signals or signals between colonies.

velop, spread, and persist in this environment. New developments include surface coatings, agents that inhibit colonization or promote dissolution of colonies. Small electric fields, low pH, as well as acidic and negatively charged surfaces seem resistant to biofilms and could become adjunctive treatments. Surface properties on implants or local or systemic drugs may help in the fight.

Adherence to Bone and Biomaterials

Damaged bone acts as a substratum for bacterial colonization. Bone is a relatively acellular composite structure with an organic matrix composed of proline, hydroxyproline, glycine, and alanine (65), which can act as ligands for bacterial adhesion. Devitalized bone devoid of normal periosteum presents a collagen matrix to which bacteria can bind. Moreover, bone sialoprotein has also been suggested as a ligand for bacterial binding to bone (65).

Biomaterials and other foreign bodies are usually inert and susceptible to bacterial colonization because they are inanimate. Regardless of how inert a metal is, it may still modulate molecular events at its surfaces, specifically, receptor-ligand interactions, covalent bonding, and thermodynamic interactions (66,67). The most important feature in a particular metal is its outer surface atomic layer interaction containing glycoproteins and prokaryotic and eukaryotic cells. Stainless steel and cobalt-chromium and titanium alloys are resistant to corrosion through elemental composition, crystalline homogeneity, and the surface oxide passivates. These surface oxides form a reactive interface with bacteria.

Antibiotic Resistance

Following bacterial adherence, the resistance to antibiotics increases (68,69). This resistance property seems to depend on the type of surface to which the organisms are attached. Organisms that adhere to hydrocarbon polymers are extremely resistant to antibiotics. These same organisms, when attached to metals, do not resist antibiotic therapy to the same extent. It has been theorized that bacteria within biofilms have a decreased metabolic rate and undergo phenotypic changes that may influence resistance and virulence (70). It has also been shown that bacteria adherent to surfaces are more resistant to antibiotics their planktonic (free-floating) counterparts. When within the biofilm, antibiotic concentrations of greater than 1,500 times normal are required to penetrate both the biofilm and bacterial cell wall. Even then, most antimicrobials work via interference with cell wall synthesis or reproduction and require metabolically active bacteria to be effective. The bacteria in the biofilm appear dormant, and these characteristics account for the resistant noted clinically.

Acute Posttraumatic Osteomyelitis

Posttraumatic osteomyelitis is a bone infection resulting from trauma that allows pathogenic organisms to enter bone, proliferate in traumatized tissue, and cause a subsequent infection (71). Traumatized soft tissue and bone exposes potential binding sites for bacteria (72). Traumatized tissue also results in compromised blood supply, leading to tissue and bone necrosis, which promotes infection (72). Moreover, the fixation devices that are required in managing fractures serve as additional foci for bacterial colonization (72). In the patient with traumatic injuries, additional factors that contribute to the subsequent development of osteomyelitis are the presence of hypotension, inadequate debridement of the fracture site, malnutrition, alcoholism, and smoking (73,74).

Trauma may lead to interference with the host response to infection. Tissue injury or bacteria triggers (a) activation of the complement cascade that leads to local vasodilation, (b) tissue edema, (c) migration of polymorphonuclear leukocytes to the injury site, and (d) enhanced ability of phagocytes to ingest bacteria (75). Trauma has been reported to delay the inflammatory response to bacteria, to depress cell-mediated immunity, and to impair function of polymorphonuclear leukocytes, including chemotaxis, superoxide production, and microbial killing (75). Cierny and Mader's commonly used system has been shown to have greatest correlation with the patient's general condition rather than the specifics of bone involvement.

Chronic Osteomyelitis

Acute osteomyelitis that is inappropriately treated can become chronic osteomyelitis. General factors that may predispose a patient to this condition include the degree of bone necrosis, nutrition, infecting organism, age, comorbidity, and drug abuse (76). The infecting organism generally varies with the cause of chronic osteomyelitis. Chronic osteomyelitis resulting from acute osteomyelitis is often caused by *Staphylococcus aureus*; however, chronic osteomyelitis occurring after a fracture can be polymicrobial (although in most cases, it is *S. aureus*). IV drug users are commonly found to have *Pseudomonas* or *S. aureus* infections. Gram-negative organisms are now seen in about 50% of all cases of chronic osteomyelitis (76).

The bacterial organisms usually enter the bone directly through interrupted tissue planes as a result of fractures or surgical procedures. Bacteria in bone by themselves are insufficient to produce osteomyelitis. A surgical or traumatic insult sets the stage for the secondary infection (77) creating regions of cortical bone that are no longer perfused adequately. Devitalized bone presents a collagen protein matrix and acellular crystal regions to which bacteria can bind directly (78). The fundamental problem in chronic osteomyelitis and ongoing devascularization of bone is leaving protected pockets of necrotic material to support bacterial growth in relative seclusion from systemic antibiotic therapy. This collection of necrotic tissue, bone, and bacteria is termed the *sequestrum*, and the body's attempt to wall off the offending material with a reactive and inflammatory tissue (either bone or soft-tissue) is called *involucrum*. Note that involucrum can be highly vascular and potentially viable and structural, which should be taken into consideration during surgical debridement.

Classification

Historically, osteomyelitis was classified as either acute or chronic depending on the duration of symptoms. A classification system based on the etiology of the osteomyelitis was developed: type I (hematogenous); type II (osteomyelitis with fracture union); type III (osteomyelitis without fracture union); and type IV (postoperative or posttraumatic osteomyelitis without fracture) (79). In 1984, Weiland et al suggested another classification scheme based on the nature of the bony involvement (80). The categories in this system were the following: type I (open, exposed bone without soft tissue infection); type II (circumferential cortical and endosteal infection); and type III (associated with a segmental defect). In 1989, May et al (70) proposed yet another classification scheme for osteomyelitis, focusing on the tibia. This system was based on the nature of the bone after soft tissue and bony debridement. They proposed the following categories: type I (intact tibia and fibula able to withstand functional loads with no reconstruction needed); type II (intact tibia unable to withstand functional loads requiring bone grafting; type III (<6 cm tibial defect with an intact fibula requiring cancellous bone grant, tibiofibular synostosis, or distraction histogenesis); type IV (<6 cm tibial defect and intact fibula requiring distraction histogenesis, tibiofibular synostosis, or a vascularized bone graft); and type V (>6 cm tibial defect without an intact fibula requiring a possible early amputation).

Perhaps the most widely used system of classification for adult osteomyelitis is that of Cierny and Mader, which identifies the extent of infection as well as the host's condition (81,82) (Fig. 18-6 and Table 18-2). This system is based on four factors: the degree of osseous involvement, the site of involvement, the degree of impairment caused by the disease, and the host's general condition (81). Type I is medullary osteomyelitis (examples of which include hematogenous osteomyelitis and infections of intramedullary rods). Type II is superficial osteomyelitis confined to the bone surface. Type III is localized osteomyelitis involving the full thickness of the cortex but without the loss of axial stability. Type IV is diffuse osteomyelitis involving the circumference of the cortex and loss of axial stability.

TABLE 18-2 Cierny-Mader Staging System for Osteomyelitis

Anatomic Type

Stage 1: Medullary osteomyelitis
Stage 2: Superficial osteomyelitis
Stage 3: Localized osteomyelitis
Stage 4: Diffuse osteomyelitis

Physiologic Class

A host: Healthy

B host:
Bs: Systemic compromise
Bl: Local compromise
Bls: Local and systemic compromise

C host: Treatment worse than the disease

Factors Affecting Immune Surveillance, Metabolism, and Local Vascularity

Systemic factors (Bs): Malnutrition, renal or hepatic failure, diabetes mellitus, chronic hypoxia, immune disease, extremes of age, immunosuppression or immune deficiency

Local factors (Bl): Chronic lymphedema, venous stasis, major vessel compromise, arteritis, extensive scarring, radiation fibrosis, small-vessel disease, neuropathy, tobacco abuse

Reprinted with permission from Cierny G, Mader JT, Pennick H. A clinical staging system of adult osteomyelitis. *Contemp Orthop* 1985;10:17–37.

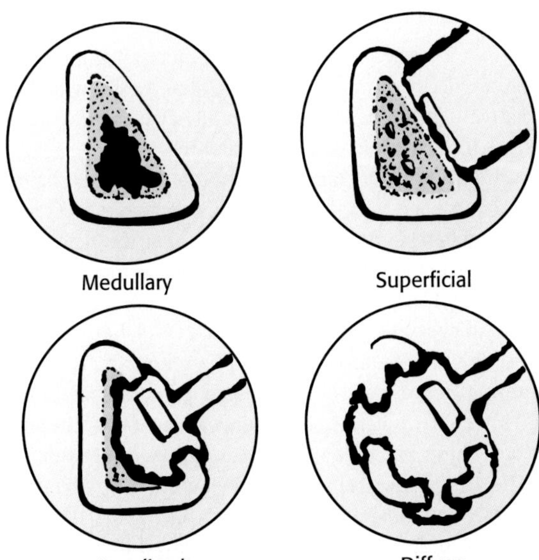

FIGURE 18-6 Cierny and Mader's types of osteomyelitis.

The general condition of the patient is based on factors that affect the response to infection and treatment. Class A patients have normal systemic defenses, metabolic capabilities, and vascular supply to the limb. Class B patients have a local (trauma, prior surgery, local inflammation) or systemic (immunosuppressed, on corticosteroids, peripheral vascular disease) deficiency. Class C patients are those in whom the treatment of the disease (the infection) is worse than the infection itself. In other words, there is greater potential morbidity or mortality from treatment, than from the infection (or noncurative treatment such as suppression) (81). These patients have a poor prognosis for cure. Pairing the four types of osteomyelitis with the three host classes allows for practical treatment strategies. With the use of such a system, Cierny et al proposed a detailed treatment regimen, which defined optimal treatment modalities for each stage and achieved an overall success rate at 2 years equalling

91% for all stages. As one would expect, when broken down by class of host and type of lesion, class A hosts fared the best. In these hosts, success rates of 98% were achieved, even in type IV osteomyelitis. For compromised, class B hosts, success rates were far lower. Depending on anatomic type, success ranged from 79% to 92%.

Organisms in Open Fractures and Trauma

The presence of bacteria in an open wound is not sufficient to cause infection. Approximately 60% to 70% of open fractures are contaminated by bacteria, but a small percentage develop infection, and the risk of subsequent infection is highly correlated with the degree of soft tissue injury (72). With type IIIB open fractures, those in which extensive soft tissue stripping does not allow for adequate coverage over the site, infection can occur in up to 40% of cases (76). Moreover, the bacteria recovered from clinical infections are most likely to be hospital-acquired pathogens such as *S. aureus* or Gram-negative bacilli (including *Pseudomonas aeruginosa*) (83,84). Other bacteria should be considered, depending on the environment, specifically, *Clostridium perfringens* when there is soil contamination, pseudomonas and *Aeromonas hydrophilia* following fresh water injury, and vibrio and *Erysipelothrix* in salt water injury.

Clinical Manifestations

A history of infection or intercurrent illness as well as remote surgery or trauma should raise the clinical suspicion of osteomyelitis. Normal signs of inflammation (rubor, calor, dolor, tumor) may be absent, and the diagnosis of infection when clinical signs are masked can be difficult. Patients can often have a history of infection of another site, such as the lungs, bladder, or skin, especially with a history of trauma. They usually complain of substantial pain in the affected area and may have difficulty with weight bearing. Moreover, reduced activity, malaise, and anorexia may be exhibited. General physical findings include fever, tachycardia, and listlessness. Local findings include swelling and warmth, occasional redness, tenderness to palpation, drainage, and restricted range of motion of adjacent joints.

With a history of trauma, clinical risk factors for infection include a history of open fracture, severe soft tissue injury, a history of substance abuse and smoking, inadequate previous treatment, and an immunocompromised state. Clinical factors affecting treatment that need to be assessed include the time of the infection's onset, the status of the soft tissues, the viability of the bone, the status of fracture healing, implant stability, the host's condition, and the neurovascular examination.

Laboratory Findings

Routine blood cultures are of little help unless the patients have manifestations of systemic disease. Furthermore, blood cultures, which yield coagulase-negative staphylococcus, a common contaminant and common pathogen, must be correlated with other clinical findings before one attributes any clinical significance to them. Laboratory changes that suggest infection include elevations in the white blood cell (WBC) count as well as elevations in the C-reactive protein and erythrocyte sedimentation rate levels. The erythrocyte sedimentation rate may be normal in the first 48 hours, but rises to levels above 100 mm/h, and may remain elevated for weeks (85). Its gradual declination is an indicator of treatment response. Because bacteremia and septicemia are often present, blood cultures should be performed to identify infecting bacteria. Blood cultures are positive in about 50% to 75% of cases (85). Although not a sensitive test for septic arthritis, the detection of antibodies to the teichoic acid cell wall of *S. aureus* has been useful in detecting acute osteomyelitis. The sensitivity approaches 82% in the acute situation and declines to 43% in chronic osteomyelitis (85).

Radiographic Imaging

Radiographically, detectable demineralization may not be seen for at least 10 days (85). When present, it usually signifies trabecular bone destruction. If the infection spreads to the cortex (usually within 3 to 6 weeks), a periosteal reaction may be evident. Unfortunately, radiologic findings in the initial presentation of acute osteomyelitis are often normal. The most common radiographic sign of bone infection is rarefaction, representing diffuse demineralization secondary to inflammatory hyperemia soft tissue swelling with obliteration of tissue planes, trabecular destruction, lysis and cortical permeation, periosteal reactions, and involucrum formation. One study reported that in cases of eventually proven osteomyelitis, 5% of radiograph results were abnormal initially, 33% were abnormal by 1 week, and 90% were abnormal by 4 weeks (86).

Bone Scans

Radionuclide scintigraphy is a very useful diagnostic tool and can be performed with various algorithms. Technetium-99m (^{99m}Tc) is the principal radioisotope employed in most bone scans (87–89). Technetium is formed as a metastable intermediate during the decay of molybdenum-99, has a 6-hour half-life, and is relatively inexpensive, as it is readily available (88). After IV injection, there is rapid distribution of this agent throughout the extracellular fluid. Within several hours, more than half the dose will accumulate in bone, while the remainder is excreted in the urine. There is evidence to suggest that the technetium phosphates bind to both the organic and the inorganic matrix. There is preferential incorporation into metabolically active bone. Bone images are usually acquired 2 to 4 hours after IV injection of the radioisotope. A triple phase bone scan is useful for examining inflammation and related processes. Following the initial injection, dynamic images are captured over the specified region. These are followed by static images at later time points. The first phase represents the blood flow phase, the second phase immediately postinjection represents the bone-pooling phase, and the third phase is a delayed image made at 3 hours when there is decreased soft tissue activity. Classically, osteomyelitis presents as a region of increased blood flow and should appear "hot" on all phases, with focal uptake in the third phase. Other processes such as a healing fracture, a loose prosthesis, and degeneration do not appear hot in the early phase despite a hot appearance in the delayed phase. Reported sensitivities of bone scintigraphy for detecting osteomyelitis vary considerably from 32% to 100%. Reported specificities have ranged from 0% to 100% (90,91).

Gallium-67 citrate binds rapidly to serum proteins, particularly transferrin (92,93). There is uptake in the blood, especially by leukocytes. Gallium has been used in conjunction with ^{99m}Tc to increase the specificity of the bone scan (94,95). Several mechanisms have been postulated to explain the increased activity at sites of inflammation. Enhanced blood flow and increased capillary permeability cause enhanced delivery. Bacteria have high iron requirements and thus avidly take up gallium. Gallium is strongly bound to bacterial siderophores and leukocyte lactoferrins. In regions of inflammation, these proteins are available extracellularly and can bind gallium avidly. Chemotaxis also acts to localize gallium-labeled WBCs at the sites of infection. In a typical study, gallium is injected intravenously, and delayed images are acquired (at 48 to 72 hours). The hallmark of osteomyelitis is focal increased uptake of gallium. Unfortunately, gallium's nonspecific bone uptake can be problematic because any processes causing reactive new bone formation will "light up." In the case of patients with fractures or a prosthesis, osteomyelitis cannot be diagnosed with gallium alone. Most investigators will interpret gallium images along with bone scans. Gallium activity is interpreted as abnormal if it is either incongruous with the bone scan activity or if there is a matching pattern with gallium activity. Reported sensitivities and specificities for the diagnosis of osteomyelitis range from 22% to 100% and 0% to 100%, respectively (88,90,95,96). Despite its lower-than-optimal diagnostic value, gallium still has advantages: (a) it is easily administered, (b) it is the agent of choice in chronic soft tissue infections (less effective in bone infections), and (c) it is a useful agent in following the resolution of an inflammatory process by showing a progressive decline in activity.

Indium-111 (^{111}In-oxine) or ^{99m}Tc-HMPAO-labeled (Ceretec) leukocyte scans are useful as a confirmatory test after a positive Tc-RBC bone scan. The leukocytes migrate to the region of active infection so that the scan can confirm the presence of an active inflammatory reaction. The use of a combined red cell and white cell scan increases both the sensitivity and specificity significantly, and now represents the gold standard of radionuclide testing for infection (97). Due to the variable accuracy of both technetium and gallium scans, most laboratories routinely employ ^{111}In-oxine–labeled leukocytes (93,98–100). Indium WBC preparations require withdrawing approximately 50 mL of autologous whole blood with a leukocyte count of at least 5,000 cells/mm^3. The leukocytes are labeled with 1 mCi of indium oxine and are then reinjected, where they redistribute in the intravascular space. Immediate images thereafter show activity in the lungs, liver, spleen, and blood pool. The half-life is about 7 hours. After 24 hours, only the liver, spleen, and bone marrow show activity. Normal-healing wounds and fully treated infections show no increase in uptake. Leukocytes that migrate to an area of active bone infection will show increased uptake. Most results show improved sensitivity (80% to 100%) and specificity (50% to 100%) for the diagnosis of osteomyelitis (101–105). Indium-labeled WBC scans are generally superior to bone scans and gallium scans in detecting infection. McCarthy et al (106) have reported the diagnostic utility of indium scans in 39 patients with suspected osteomyelitis (confirmed by bone biopsy). Indium scans were 97% sensitive and 82% specific for osteomyelitis. The few false-positive results occurred in patients with overlying soft tissue infections. An accompanying bone scan can help to differentiate bone infection from soft tissue infection. In these situations, the indium scan should be performed before the bone scan to avoid false-positive results (from the remaining technetium uptake). With both tests, the sensitivities and specificities are in excess of 90%.

Until recently, a clinician investigating for the site of infectious foci using nuclear medicine had a choice between ^{67}Ga-citrate imaging and ^{111}In-oxine leukocyte imaging (101), but scientific advances (especially in nuclear medicine) have increased these choices considerably, and continue to increase them. Several techniques in nuclear medicine significantly aid infection diagnosis, including imaging with ^{99m}Tc-hexamethylpropyleneamine oxime (^{99m}Tc-HMPAO) (Ceretec) and ^{99m}Tc-stannous fluoride colloid-labeled leukocytes (104). Each radiopharmaceutical has specific advantages and disadvantages that make it suitable to diagnose different infectious processes (e.g., soft-tissue sepsis, osteomyelitis, abscesses, and infections commonly found in immunocompromised patients) (104,105). ^{99m}Tc-HMPAO scans are being increasingly used, and their kinetics and normal distribution are similar to those of ^{111}In-oxine–labeled leukocytes except for nonspecific activity in urine, kidneys, gall bladder, and the bowel, which results from the elution of secondary ^{99m}Tc-labeled HMPAO complexes.

Labeling the ^{99m}Tc-HMPAO complex is technically identical to ^{111}In-oxine labeling in that it requires separation of leukocytes, but not pure granulocytes, from the whole blood, followed by exposure to the complex. ^{99m}Tc-HMPAO particles are not stable in vivo and elute from cells at a rate of up to 7% per hour. These secondary hydrophilic complexes are released into the blood and excreted through the kidneys and intestine. After labeling, a percentage of leukocytes are damaged, but not killed, by the cell irradiation resulting from internalization of the radionuclide-emitting low-energy electrons (0.4 to 17 keg) (107). Some exceptions are that the ^{99m}Tc-HMPAO label is cheaper and more readily available than the ^{111}In label; that ^{99m}Tc has a much higher photon flux, allowing improved visualization of areas such as the feet; and that ^{99m}Tc-HMPAO localizes in infectious sites more rapidly than does ^{111}In-oxine (102). Producing excellent images of acute soft-tissue sepsis, ^{99m}Tc-HMPAO is the preferred detection agent when sequential imaging at 1 and 4 hours is used. The principal clinical indications for ^{99m}Tc-HMPAO leukocytes include osteomyelitis and soft tissue sepsis. Chronic osteomyelitis, including infected joint prostheses, is better approached with ^{111}In–labeled leukocytes

(107). The use of ^{99m}Tc-HMPAO leukocyte scintigraphy in patients with symptomatic total hip or knee arthroplasty shows improved diagnostic accuracy by means of semiquantitative evaluation (108). ^{99m}Tc-HMPAO can be helpful for children younger than 6 months, as at this age, the sensitivity of ^{99m}Tc-MDP is low (107). ^{99m}Tc-HMPAO is generally more sensitive for the detection of acute osteomyelitis than of chronic osteomyelitis (with a high sensitivity [97.7%] and a specificity of 96.8%) (107). ^{99m}Tc-HMPAO is also able to separate septic from aseptic bone lesions (103).

The combination of ^{99}Tcm-HMPAO leukocytes and ^{99}Tcm-MDP can be recommended as one of the most suitable methods for use in diagnosing bone infection, especially in patients with previous bone disease. In a study involving ^{99m}Tc-HMPAO leucocyte scintigraphy combined with a ^{99m}Tc-MDP bone scintigraphy in the diagnosis of the diabetic foot infection, a sensitivity of 92.6% and specificity of 97.6% was found. Consequently, the HMPAO-Leu/MDP scan is a reliable tool for diagnosing osteomyelitis in the diabetic foot (109).

Marrow scanning is also increasingly used for diagnosing infection. With the use of microcolloid bone marrow scans, more information is available to determine whether there is truly an infection. There is the possibility of leukocyte accumulation with certain inflammatory conditions that could result in a false-positive indium scan. An infection will tend to suppress marrow activity and render the marrow scan cold, while the white cell scan will still be hot. If the white cell scan is hot as is the marrow scan, an infection may not be present. Segura et al looked at technetium-labeled white cell scans (Tc-HMPAO) versus Tc- microcolloid marrow scans in total joints. They found that in 77 patients, the white cell scans had a sensitivity of 96% and a specificity of 30% by itself. When the colloid scan was added, the sensitivity went down to 93%, but the specificity went up to 98%. The addition of a regular red cell scan was not helpful (110). In another study by Palestro et al, an indium white cell scan was compared to technetium sulphur colloid scans to differentiate infection from Charcot arthropathy (111). They found that white cell scans were positive in four out of 20 cases, of which three were infected. In the 16 negative white cell scans, the marrow scan was also negative. In the four positive cases, however, the marrow scan was positive in two cases that were confirmed to be infected. They concluded that white cell scans can be positive in hematopoietically active bones, which can occur in the absence of infection and that marrow scans should be used to confirm the diagnosis.

Indium-Labeled Polyclonal Immunoglobulins

The newer techniques to investigate infection include antigranulocyte antibodies, radiolabeled nonspecific human IgG, interleukins, and antimicrobial peptides (112). The nonspecific polyclonal immunoglobulin (IgG) prepared from human serum gamma globulin and labeled with indium via diethylenetriamine pentaacetic acid (DTPA) chelation, is one of the agents used for detecting osteomyelitis (98,109). Unlike the indium-labeled WBC scans, this agent is easily prepared by simply adding indium chloride to a sterile kit containing a DTPA-IgG complex. The blood half-life is 24 hours, and the primary uptake occurs in the liver. Compared with indium-labeled WBC scans, this technique is easier to perform and has less bone marrow uptake (71). In-IgG scintigraphy is useful for the detection of musculoskeletal infection in patients in whom sterile inflammatory events simulate infectious processes (113).

Magnetic Resonance Imaging

Magnetic resonance imaging (MRI) continues to play an important role in evaluating musculoskeletal infections (114–116). The sensitivity and specificity of MRI for osteomyelitis range from 60% to 100% and 50% to 90%, respectively. It has the spatial resolution necessary to evaluate accurately the extent of the infection in preparation for surgical treatment and localizes any abscess cavities. T1- and T2-weighted imaging is usually sufficient; fat suppression and short T1 inversion recovery (STIR) sequences may be added to better image bone marrow and soft tissue abnormalities. It also has the ability to differentiate between infected bone and involved adjacent soft tissue structures. Images can be acquired in any orientation, and there is no radiation exposure. Gadolinium enhancement should be obtained in the postoperative population to better differentiate postsurgical artifact from infection-related bone marrow edema patterns. Gadolinium may better differentiate abscess formation from diffuse inflammatory changes and noninfectious fluid collections.

Characteristically, active osteomyelitis displays a decreased signal on T1-weighted images and appears bright on T2-weighted images. The process represents the replacement of marrow fat with water from edema, exudate, hyperemia, and ischemia. The MRI signal characteristics that reflect osteomyelitis are intrinsically nonspecific: tumors and fractures can also increase the marrow water content. In patients without prior complications, MRI has been found to be sensitive (but not specific) for osteomyelitis. When a fracture or prior surgery is evident, MRI is less specific in diagnosing infection. Furthermore, in the presence of metallic implants, the artifact makes it difficult to comment on areas near the implant, which may be of primary interest. Certain external fixates are not suitable for MRI and will preclude its use. In these situations, indium-labeled WBC scans are helpful. Although limited, studies show good results in the evaluation of acute osteomyelitis (sensitivities, 92% to 100%; specificities, 89% to 100%) (117). We have found that MRI's best use is helping determine the extent of the infection for operative planning, for example, determining the amount of bone resection that may be needed or identifying occult soft tissue involvement.

Other Modalities

Computed tomography (CT) has assumed a less important role in evaluating osteomyelitis with the widespread use of MRI (118). It remains unsurpassed, however, in the imaging of cortical bone. It is especially useful in delineating the cortical details in chronic osteomyelitis, such as sequestra and foreign bodies (119). It is also useful in evaluating the adequacy of cortical debridement in the staged treatment of chronic osteomyelitis. CT can help differentiate between type III and type IV infections.

The use of fluorine-18 labeled 2-fluoro-2-deoxy-d-glucose positron emission tomography (FDG-PET) scanning enables noninvasive detection and demonstration of the extent of chronic osteomyelitis with 97% accuracy (120). PET is especially accurate in the central skeleton within active bone marrow (118). It is not yet in widespread use, but it remains an adjunctive tool if other methods fail. The overall accuracy of FDG-PET in evaluating infection involving orthopaedic hardware was 96.2% for hip prostheses, 81% for knee prostheses, and 100% in 15 patients with other orthopaedic devices. Among the patients having chronic osteomyelitis, the accuracy is 91% (121). FDG-PET appears to be a sensitive and specific method for detecting infectious foci due to metallic implants in patients with trauma. Sensitivity, specificity, and accuracy were 100%, 93.3%, and 97%, respectively, for all PET data; 100%, 100%, and 100%, respectively, for the central skeleton; and 100%, 87.5%, and 95%, respectively, for the peripheral skeleton (122). 18F-FDG-PET is used to investigate infection in the postoperative spine holds promise to become the standard imaging technique in this difficult patient population, with sensitivity, specificity, and accuracy at 100%, 81%, and 86%, respectively, according to a recent study (123). The accurate differentiation between synovitis, loosening, or infection is often difficult with conventional x-rays, arthrography, or bone scintigraphy. Results suggest that FDG-PET could be a useful tool for differentiating between infected and loose orthopaedic prostheses as well as for detecting only inflammatory tissue such as synovitis (124).

Single photon emission CT (SPECT) provides a qualitative and quantitative look at the volume distribution of biologically significant radiotracers after injection into the human body. SPECT has been used to diagnose spinal prosthetic infection. The overall sensitivity of ^{99m}Tc-HMPAO leukocyte scan with SPECT to detect bone infection was 92%, with a specificity rate of 85% (125).

Because bone scan agents and gallium are usually both positive at fracture sites, they have limited value in detecting infection after a fracture. With no discernible uptake in reactive bone, indium-labeled WBC scans reveal superiority in discovering infection after a fracture. In a prospective study of 20 patients with suspected osteomyelitis superimposed on a delayed union, Esterhai et al (126) reported 100% accuracy of indium-WBC scans. Seabold et al (127) have shown that using indium-WBC scans and bone scans (to differentiate between soft tissue infections) can be 97% specific for osteomyelitis. In chronic or recurrent osteomyelitis, bone scans alone are of less value, as they show increased uptake for up to 2 years after successful treatment and resolution of infection (128). Although gallium scans have historically been shown to be the most optimal method for following the resolution of chronic osteomyelitis, indium-WBC scans appear to be superior. In a prospective study of 50 patients comparing indium-WBC and gallium scans for the detection of osteomyelitis, Merkel et al (129) found that indium-WBC scans were 26% more accurate than gallium scans (83% vs. 57%). All of the clinical data points, from a detailed history of events, a characterization of the host, laboratory studies, clinical examination, as well as adjunctive radiographic studies, are all important in determining the likelihood and extent of infection.

Biopsy

Identifying an organism and determining antibiotic resistance patterns is crucial to a successful outcome in managing osteomyelitis. The procedure can usually be carried out under fluoroscopic guidance. Although sinus tract cultures can be helpful, they should not be the sole guide for antibiotic treatment (126). In a prospective study, Mousa (130) found that 88.7% of sinus tract isolates were identical to operative specimens in 55 patients with chronic bone infection. These results were dependent on aspiration of material by syringe from the depths of an active flowing sinus and immediate inoculation on culture media. Bone biopsy remains the preferred diagnostic procedure in chronic osteomyelitis. Histologic and microbiologic evaluation of percutaneous biopsy samples should be combined in cases of suspected osteomyelitis. The sensitivity of culture in the diagnosis of osteomyelitis could be improved from 42% to 84% by adding histologic evaluation.

Molecular Diagnostics

These procedures are being developed for diagnosing osteomyelitis because some infections remain without an identified pathogen, when using standard techniques. This is particularly true in patients who have been treated with antibiotics shortly before sample collection. These methods target specific macromolecules unique to the infecting pathogens, which are absent in the host cells (131,132). They have the potential to provide rapid results with high accuracy (133). The most commonly used method for diagnosing orthopaedic infections is the polymerase chain reaction (133). Sequences within bacterial 16S ribosomal RNA have served as targets for amplification and detection (133). The polymerase chain reaction has been used to identify very small remnants of bacteria by identifying their nuclear contents. Unfortunately, it cannot easily delineate between nuclear materials from living or dead bacteria, thus increasing the likelihood of false-positive studies. Further investigations are required before these techniques can be widely used, as they lack sufficient sensitivity and specificity, but their use remains promising.

Management and Treatment

The management of osteomyelitis relies on a multidisciplinary approach, combining debridement, soft tissue coverage, and antimicrobial therapy to give the patient the best chance for a cure (134,135). The first step involves identifying (staging the host) and optimizing the host (treating the morbidity of the host and optimizing their physiologic condition, such as nutrition, smoking cessation, diabetes treatment, medical or surgical management of vascular disease). Step two involves classifying the type of osteomyelitis (staging the disease). Next, identifying the organism is required to determine appropriate antimicrobial treatment (the tumor analogy of chemotherapy). Once the extent of disease, the nature of the host and infecting organism are noted, a determination should be made regarding one of several general treatment algorithms. The treatment options available include attempted ablation and cure of the offending infection or in selective cases, such as C hosts, that are not suitable for this line of treatment, some type of suppressive treatment. Attempted ablation and complete cure has numerous issues, and decision making steps will often require the tumor equivalent of a wide resection with "clean" margins. Although a surgically clean bed with extensive resection is desirable, efforts should be made to maintain axial stability when possible. Thus, retention of a well-vascularized but affected involucrum, or a viable segment of bone adjacent to infection, may be feasible. At some point, if adequate resection will result in a reconstruction that is too extensive and unsuitable for the host status, amputation is the best option and should not be considered a failure. In some cases of life- or limb-threatening infection, a "debulking" of the infection may be a suitable first step followed by chronic suppression. In such a circumstance, identifying the infecting bacteria is required to allow use of a specific antibiotic; otherwise, broad-spectrum antibiotics are needed.

In a cohort study of 32 patients who had had an average of 3.2 surgical operations for osteomyelitis, Pape et al (136) found that reaming of the medullary canal was so successful that 84% of patients were able to return to their previous profession and 97% were pain-free. Evidence for treating an infected intramedullary nail has been derived largely from observational data. Pommer et al (137) found that reaming an infected intramedullary canal resulted in eradication of infection in all patients with initially infected intramedullary nails compared with 62% of those with multiple operations before nailing.

Irrigating Solutions

The original intent of pulsatile irrigation was based on early studies on infections that recommended that the bacteria should be "knocked off" any surface. Although such mechanical cleansing may work acutely, mature colonies are not easily eradicated with this method. Furthermore, there is evidence that the velocity of the liquid stream may be deleterious to both bone and soft tissue cells (138). As a result, detergent-type compounds or surfactant solutions have been recently investigated as a way of disrupting the hydrophobic or electrostatic forces that drive the initial stages of bacterial surface adhesion. A sequential surfactant irrigation protocol was developed and shown to be effective in the polymicrobial wound with established infection. Several studies have examined the relative merits of various irrigating solutions in the debridement of infected soft tissue and bone (139–141). Irrigation with saline alone has been shown in animal studies to reduce colony counts by half in contaminated wounds (142); however, conflicting studies have shown no beneficial effect of saline (143,144). The effect of irrigation with various irrigating solutions in removing adherent staphylococci from bone and soft tissues has been reported (145). In vitro studies have shown that although solutions such as Betadine and hydrogen peroxide are effective in eliminating bacteria, they are also toxic to osteoblasts. Detergents (soaps) have been shown to be the only irrigating solutions that remove additional bacteria above the effect of mechanical irrigation alone (145). Moreover, soap solutions have been found to have minimal effects on bone formation and osteoblast numbers in vitro (142). The proposed mechanism of their effect is based on the formation of micelles that overcome the strength of the interaction between the organisms and bone. Castille soap has recently been reported to be useful in this situation (139,141). Evidence-based clinical studies are pending.

Antibiotic Depot Devices and Techniques

Bucholz introduced the concept of local antibiotic therapy in the form of antibiotics soaked in bone cement to treat infected arthroplasties in the 1970s. On the basis of the success noted in reducing arthroplasty infections, interest developed in applying antibiotic- saturated cement as a therapy for osteomyelitis (146). Keating et al reported a 4% infection rate in 53 open tibial fractures with tobramycin-saturated beads (147). Ostermann et al reported a significant difference in infection rates of type IIIB fractures with use of aminoglycoside beads plus parenteral antibiotics (6.9%/112 patients) compared to patients receiving only parenteral antibiotics (40.7%/27 patients) (148).

Use of antibiotic depots allows for high local concentrations of antibiotic with little systemic absorption. Antibiotic release is biphasic, most occurring during the first hours to days post-implantation, and the remaining elution persists for weeks and sometimes for years. Some of the other antibiotics that have been tried with PMMA include clindamycin, which elutes well, but is not available as a pharmaceutical-grade powder; fluoroquinolones in cement powder has not been reported; erythromycin was applied earlier in some studies, but a subsequent study demonstrated inadequate elution of erythromycin from Palacos cement; macrolides and azalides are unavailable; tetracycline and colistin fail to elute from the Palacos cement in clinically meaningful quantities. One problem with PMMA depot systems is that they require removal and in staged treatments of infections, the PMMA spacers can become encased in scar and very difficult to remove. When used acutely for open fractures or short courses, their removal is generally not problematic and has even been described percutaneously. There is an entire issue of *Clinical Orthopedics and Related Research* (No. 295) dedicated to the use of PMMA antibiotic depot methods for trauma to which the reader is referred for more in-depth information (149). There are a number of commercial antibiotic-impregnated PMMA cements available, and they are just becoming accessible in the US. Most of the antibiotic cement use in the US has been off-label by the surgeon, and despite very encouraging results from several studies, their approval has been slow. Tobramycin (Nebcin) can be substituted for gentamicin, as it is available as a pharmaceutical-grade powder, whereas gentamicin is not. Unfortunately, the manufacturing of this antibiotic has ceased, and other formulations are being investigated. Other generic compounds may contain carriers and impurities that alter the handling of the cement composite, and as a result, other alternatives may need to be explored. Vancomycin is a heat-stable, excellent choice for local antibiotic delivery and should be considered when there is a chance of resistant staphylococcal organisms.

There are also newer types of material available for local delivery of antibiotics that are resorbable and do not require removal. Surgical-grade calcium sulfate (Osteoset) has been utilized recently and reported for use in both open fractures and infections. Although the calcium sulfate products have been promoted to also be a bone graft substitute, there are little human data in fractures and infections demonstrating this dual function of depot and graft. Another important consideration is that calcium sulphates and carbonate will absorb or dissolve independent of bone formation, whereas calcium phosphates tend to be replaced with bone very slowly. Furthermore, large volumes of the calcium sulphate can result in an osmotic effect that results in fluid accumulation and the potential for seroma formation and wound drainage. When mixed with fluid and blood, the calcium drainage looks like bloody pus and may prompt extra surgical treatments. Unpublished studies using calcium-based graft material have shown unacceptable complication rates (OTA 2004). Because setting times can reach 30 to 45 minutes, adding tobramycin may be impractical. Consequently, despite a seemingly novel concept, such products should be used with caution and experience.

Gentamicin-soaked hydroxyapatite ceramic beads simulate a bone graft by serving as an osteoconductive matrix, but they are resorbed slowly, and after elution, may behave as a foreign body with potential reinfection. Gentamicin-impregnated polylactide-polyglycolide copolymer implants are biodegradable and may not need removal once implanted. There is little clinical experience with this type of implant, however, and they can elicit an inflammatory response that may mimic acute infection.

Debridement Techniques

If surgical treatment is chosen, the hallmark of treatment is debridement. All nonviable and inert structures should be debrided to remove the infected material and debris without destabilizing the bony structure. The goal is to convert a necrotic, hypoxic, infected wound into a viable wound. The critical judgment for the clinician occurs when there is potentially infected bone that may be partially vascularized and that is critically needed to maintain the bone's structural stability. Sinus tracts present for more than 1 year should be excised and sent for pathologic examination to rule out an occult carcinoma (150). Soft tissue retraction should be minimal, and flaps should not be created. On one hand, leaving behind infection may result in recurrence, but resection and subsequent destabilization would involve extensive surgical reconstruction and its associated risks.

Meticulous debridement is one of the most important initial steps in treating infected bone and soft tissue. The paprika sign has classically determined the limits of debridement, which are characterized by punctuate cortical or cancellous bleeding. Efforts should be made to limit any periosteal stripping that may further devitalize the bone. Reactive new bone surrounding an area of chronic infection is living and usually does not require debridement. The sequestrum needs to be identified and removed, whereas the involucrum may be preserved. Rapid debridement may be achieved with a high-speed bur used with continuous irrigation to limit thermal necrosis. Laser Doppler flowmetry may facilitate an accurate assessment of the bone's microvascular status, thereby identifying it for removal (151). Laser Doppler flowmetry is the only in vivo method of blood flow determination that provides instantaneous determinations of perfusion and is nondestructive.

When the medullary canal is infected, intramedullary reaming is a good method of debridement. In general, one should overream the medullary canal by 2 mm. Lavage can be performed from the entry portal with egress through a vent or previous locking screw holes. Dull reamers and heat generation should be avoided to prevent further cortical necrosis. Intramedullary reaming of the canal as a debridement technique has shown favorable results in treating medullary osteomyelitis. In one series, 25 patients with posttraumatic osteomyelitis (22 of whom were treated with intramedullary reaming) were followed for at least 6 months (146). At a mean postoperative evaluation of 26 months, 21 of the 22 patients were free of any recurrent infection. In a more recent study, 40 patients suffering from chronic osteomyelitis were treated with intramedullary reaming. Only four patients suffered a recurrent infection after intramedullary reaming (152).

If the medullary infection is too proximal (or distal) for a tight reamer fit, a trough must be created to debride the canal directly (saucerization). An oval-shaped trough is biomechanically the most desirable in comparison to other geometries and results in little diminution of the bone's torsional strength (Fig. 18-7). Indications for stabilization are simply those in which the bone's stability is compromised postdebridement or if there is mechanical instability of a preexisting implant. Greater than 30% loss of circumferential cortical contact or any segmental resection requires stabilization.

External Fixation

When a debridement has necessitated a segmental bone resection, applying a circular external fixator can stabilize the bone ends, help improve limb blood flow, and provide a method to regenerate missing bone via distraction osteogenesis (144). In adults, an average of approximately 2 months is required for every centimeter of lengthening. Healing at the docking site is not reliable and may require bone grafting. Pin-site infections,

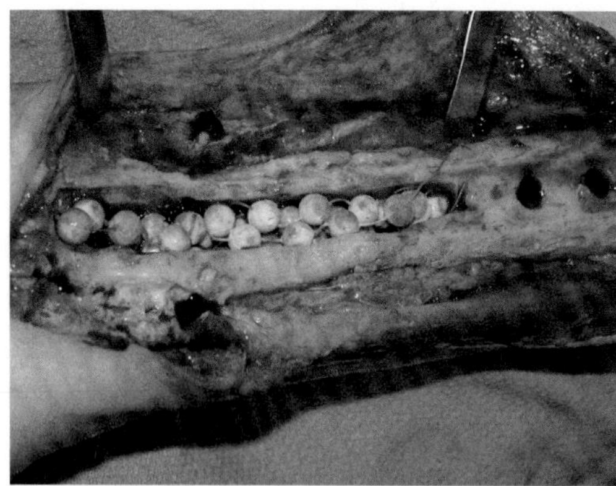

FIGURE 18-7 Photo of trough created in bone after infection with plating. Structural integrity is maintained.

pin loosening, and premature or failed bone consolidation bone can occur, but are less common with increasing experience. Green compared the use of circular external fixators alone with open cancellous bone grafting for intercalary defects in long bones. He found docking-site healing problems in the external fixator group and donor-site morbidity in the bone-graft group (39,42). In a similar study of patients with segmental tibial defects, Cierny and Zorn (153) found that patients treated with the Ilizarov external fixator experienced shorter operating room times, shorter hospital stays, and similar complication rates to those treated with bone grafting and soft tissue coverage procedures. Ueng et al (154) followed 15 patients with femoral diaphyseal infected nonunions managed with a two-stage protocol including antibiotic-impregnated beads, definitive external skeletal fixation, and staged bone grafting, and found no recurrence of osteomyelitis (154). Similarly, Marsh et al (155) found that segmental excision, distraction osteogenesis, and gradual correction of deformity were 100% effective in eliminating infection in a series of patients with osteomyelitis. The promising outcomes with ring fixation support its use in treating bone defects in osteomyelitis. With this method, patient selection is paramount for success. Recently, an external fixation risk index has been proposed for identifying patients who are at an increased risk of a major complication (failure of implant, failure of union) after the application of external fixation (156). Alcohol use, low socioeconomic status, and smoking history were all independent predictors of poor outcomes with external fixation. Moreover, the odds of having an adverse outcome increased nine times when all three factors were present.

Bone Grafting Techniques

Once all nonviable tissue has been removed and when the defect is stable mechanically and biologically viable, consideration must be given to bone grafting. Standard techniques include open cancellous bone grafting, posterolateral bone grafting, or soft tissue transfer before cancellous bone grafting. Esterhai et al (157) found that treatment of chronic osteomyelitis complicating nonunion and segmental defects of the tibia was less successful with open cancellous bone grafting. Healing by secondary intention is best demonstrated by the open cancellous grafting technique as popularized by Papineau and described by Cierny (82). The Papineau technique involves local debridement followed by a period of open management until a healthy granulation tissue covers the wound base, after which fresh autogenous cancellous graft is packed into the defect, followed by frequent dressing changes until the graft becomes incorporated. If needed, split-thickness skin grafting is performed at a later date. This type of management places high metabolic demands on the host because it requires the host to control infection and incorporate bone graft. This treatment method has been superseded by more successful methods and is usually reserved as a last resort in certain cases.

If structural augmentation is required (greater than 30% to 50% volume loss) or if nonunion is present, autogenous cancellous bone grafts are usually indicated. In a noncompromised (A host) patient with a clean wound, these grafts can be placed directly beneath local or transferred muscle at the time of wound closure. Cierny reported a success rate of 93% using this approach and recommended adding a powdered, pathogen-specific antibiotic to the cancellous grafts at the time of insertion (82). Some investigators recommend staged bone grafting in systemically and/or locally compromised (B hosts) patients, in the presence of internal fixation, or when massive grafting is required (greater than 50 mL) (158). In the interim, the osseous dead space can be maintained with antibiotic-saturated PMMA beads.

Segmental defects can be reconstructed using massive cancellous grafting in a staged reconstruction, free bone transfer, or the bone transport techniques of Ilizarov (158,159). The Ilizarov technique offers unique, comprehensive solutions to the problems associated with treating a large, infected bone segment. Using the established techniques of stable external fixation, atraumatic corticotomy, and appropriate delay before distraction, large skeletal defects can be spanned. This reconstructive ability permits radical segmental debridement of infected regions. The defect is slowly replaced with innate bone and behind it, highly vascular regenerate bone forms, which has been shown to increase global blood flow to the entire extremity (159,160). Some investigators suggest that muscle flaps appropriate for the soft tissue defect should be used before initiating transport (160). Ilizarov has shown that this step may not be necessary because the skin and soft tissue will move with the transporting segment and close the soft tissue defect as the bone gap closes (161). Furthermore, during treatment, the patient is encouraged to resume functional use of the limb. Walking, working, sports, and swimming are all possible, but the patient must be compliant and motivated. Many outpatient visits and adjustments are required, and minor pin-tract infections are common.

Acute Postoperative Infection

Frequently, the clinician is faced with a situation wherein there is a recent reconstruction with the presence of metallic implants and other inert biologic tissue (compromised bone or bone graft). In the case of an angry-appearing wound, if there are obvious signs of infection such as erythema, copious drainage, edema, and fever, acute surgical debridement and irrigation is needed. If there is satisfactory fixation and stability of the construct, only nonessential elements such as excess bone graft should be removed. Placing an antibiotic delivery depot (either PMMA or resorbable) with a more aggressive antibiotic regimen may curb the infection until healing has taken place. If this treatment is undertaken, suppression on antibiotics should continue until such time, and when adequate healing has occurred. There should be strong consideration of redebridement, hardware removal, and an intraoperative decision as to whether more antibiotic depot treatment is required. This algorithm is followed with the hypothesis that the original wound was contaminated and was probably colonized with bacteria (with biofilm formation on all inert structures in the wound), and that the debulking and suppression was in an effort to prevent the need to "start over." With our current understanding of biofilm bacteria, it would be unlikely that the wound could be bacteria-free, and more likely that infection would recur. It is for this reason that the threshold of hardware removal and re-debridement is lower than normal. If this approach is not successful, there should be consideration of "starting over," which entails completely removing and debriding inert substances, placing an antibiotic depot system, temporary stabilization with an external fixator or cast, and a staged reconstruction. Unlike the literature in arthroplasty, there is not much scientific literature on success/failure rates in such circumstances for fractures. It should be noted however, that bones can heal in the presence of active infection and unlike arthroplasty, where the implant is considered permanent, the fracture setting allows for implant removal once bone healing has taken place.

More often, the situation is not so obvious, and there may only be slight erythema, possibly some serous drainage, and minimal overt evidence of deep infection. Diagnostic studies such as CT scans and bone scans can offer some information, but are most useful if negative. Most wounds have a potential space that fills with hematoma and can accumulate inflammatory cells, which can lead to erroneous test readings. If the patient has taken nonsteroidal anti-inflammatory drugs (NSAIDs) and is taking anticoagulants, a short interruption of the anticoagulant (if not contraindicated) and continuation of a broad-spectrum antibiotic should be attempted. The antibiotic is used because active wound drainage provides a potential route for secondary bacterial contamination with hospital-acquired organisms. If there is little response to such treatment, then surgical exploration with deep cultures or an aspiration of a fluid collection should be performed. Contact dermatitis must be differentiated from wound infection and suture reaction; both cause erythema around the wound. Contact dermatitis is readily recognized by the characteristic shape of the erythematous area. An erythematous plaque following the shape of a bandage strongly suggests contact dermatitis. The presence of vesicles and pruritus further add clues to the diagnosis.

Dehiscence results when a wound fails to heal. The healing wound has minimal tensile strength, and, although re-epithelialization occurs rapidly, fibroplasia and subsequent collagen production are initiated after a delay of approximately 5 days. The remodeling of collagen gradually increases the tensile strength of the wound. The wound regains 3% to 5% of its original strength at 2 weeks; 15%, at 3 weeks; 35%, at 1 month; and increases to a final strength of 80%, after several months.

Sutures are foreign bodies and can cause an immunologically mediated tissue response, clinically evident as erythema. This reaction must be differentiated from true wound infection and contact dermatitis. Many factors may contribute to suture reactivity. The larger the caliber of the suture is, and longer the sutures stay in, the more reactivity occurs. Synthetic or wire sutures are much less reactive than natural sutures (e.g., silk, cotton, catgut); a monofilament suture is less reactive than a braided suture.

The following is an algorithm for acute infection:

1. Hardware stable + bone not healed = retain hardware, antibiotics until healed, then hardware removal
2. Hardware unstable + bone not healed = remove hardware, antibiotics, temporary stabilization, spacer, and reconstruction when clean
3. Hardware stable + bone healed = remove hardware, debride with effort not to destabilize, control dead space, and antibiotics
4. Hardware stable + bone not healed + systemic effects = remove hardware, temporary stabilization, spacer, antibiotics, and reconstruction when able. Consider amputation if unsuitable host

Principles of Antimicrobial Therapy

Antimicrobial therapy is often prolonged and requires outpatient management. Antibiotics must allow bone penetration and must be nontoxic, convenient to administer, and cost effective. It is recommended that antibiotic should be administered intravenously for at least the first 2 weeks (162). Antibiotic selection should be based on in vitro susceptibilities of the microorganisms causing infection. Table 18-3 outlines the more commonly used regimens for initial osteomyelitis treatment. Regimens should be tailored to meet the patient's specific needs. Because of the increasing complexity of antibiotics available, as well as the side effects and possible complications, the collaborative efforts of a dedicated infectious disease specialist greatly facilitate the treatment process. Early reports suggest that such an arrangement may improve outcomes, although this has not been borne out with level I evidence-based data.

The need for long-term treatment remains debated. There is no consensus on duration of treatment; some physicians propose as few as 2 weeks, and others suggest longer-term therapy. Short-term therapy is based on the premise of an excellent debridement, healthy host tissue, and a healthy host. Those who advocate longer-term treatment point to what we have learned

TABLE 18-3 Initial Antibiotic Regimens for Patients with Posttraumatic Osteomyelitis

Organism Antibiotics	Antibiotic(s) of First Choice	Alternative
Staphylococcus aureus or coagulase-negative (methicillin-sensitive) staphylococci	Oxacillin 2 g IV Q 6 hours or clindamycin phosphate 900 mg IV Q 8 hours	First-generation cephalosporin or vancomycin
S. aureus or coagulase-negative (methicillin-resistant) staphylococci	Vancomycin 1 g IV Q 12 hours plus rifampin	Linezolid, trimethoprim-sulfamethoxazole or minocycline plus rifampin
Varied streptococci (groups A and B β-hemolytic organisms or penicillin-sensitive *Streptococcus pneumoniae*)	Penicillin G, 4 million units IV Q 6 hours	Clindamycin, erythromycin, vancomycin or ceftriaxone
Intermediate penicillin-resistant *S. pneumoniae*	Ceftriaxone 2 g IV Q 24 hours	Erythromycin, clindamycin, or levofloxacin
Penicillin-resistant *S. pneumoniae*	Vancomycin 1 g IV Q 12 hours	Levofloxacin
Enterococcus species	Ampicillin 2 g IV Q 6 hours or vancomycin 1 g IV Q 12 hours	Ampicillin-sulbactam (Unasyn), linezolid
Enteric Gram-negative rods	Fluoroquinolone (e.g., ciprofloxacin 750 mg orally BID)	Third-generation cephalosporin
Serratia species or *Pseudomonas aeruginosa*	Levofloxacin 500 mg IV Q 24 hours, cefepime 2 g IV Q 12 hours plus fluoroquinolone	Ertapenem (Invanz) 1 g IV Q 24 hours
Anaerobes	Clindamycin 900 mg IV Q 8 hours	For Gram-negative anaerobes: amoxicillin-clavulanate (Augmentin) or metronidazole (Flagyl)
Mixed aerobic and anaerobic organisms	Amoxicillin-clavulanate, 875 mg and 125 mg, respectively, orally BID	Ertapenem 1 g IV Q 24 hours

from biofilm technology and recommend such treatment when there are reconstructions involving large volumes of graft and implants (inert materials) (163). The theory behind this idea is that until complete revascularization takes place, the inert material is a potential site for bacteria colonization, either from the bloodstream, or from remnants in the tissue bed. Use of an appropriate suppressive oral agent can help minimize the risk of bacterial seeding of the reconstructive site. As such, proper selection and monitoring of the antibiotics is imperative. The agents to be selected should be the least toxic and least expensive, and should require once or twice daily administration for convenience and compliance. Table 18-4 outlines several oral antibiotics with excellent oral bioavailability (drug that attains similar serum and tissue concentration whether given orally or intravenously) that may be substituted for IV antibiotics whenever possible as long as the microorganism is susceptible to these agents.

There has been an increase of vancomycin-resistant *Enterococcus* especially in the ICU and now emerging vancomycin-resistant *Staphylococci*. Vancomycin should be used only if there is a high rate of infection caused by methicillin-resistant *S. aureus* or methicillin-resistant S. *epidermidis*. For perioperative prophylaxis, a single dose of vancomycin administered immediately before the surgery followed by two to three doses postoperatively should be adequate. Vancomycin should only be used for Type I hypersensitivity to cephalosporins, which includes urticaria, laryngeal edema, and bronchospasm with or without cardiovascular shock. An alternative for cefazolin would be clindamycin.

Suppressive Treatment

When radical surgical debridement procedures cannot be performed (C host), if hardware has been left in place in order to maintain stability (acute infection), or if the patient refuses surgical treatment, eradication of the infection is unlikely. In such cases, suppressive antibiotics may be in order, which consist of long-term oral antibiotic administration. Microbiological

TABLE 18-4 Selected Oral Antimicrobial Agents with Excellent Oral Bioavailability Commonly Used to Treat Patients with Musculoskeletal Infection

Fluoroquinolone
Ciprofloxacin
Levofloxacin
Gatifloxacin
Metronidazole
Linezolid
Rifampin
Trimethoprim-sulfamethoxazole
Azoles
Fluconazole
Itraconazole

diagnosis should be attempted, and the patient must be compliant. Even in this scenario, the duration of suppressive antibiotic therapy is not clearly defined. Generally, a minimum 6-month course is usually administered with hope that the infection will be contained (but not eradicated) by the host mechanism. In some situations, suppressive therapy must be continued lifelong.

Other Considerations

Recently, there has been a plethora of nonautogenous bone graft alternatives. Most often, bone grafting is generally performed after the infected nonunion is treated, so the situation resembles that of an aseptic nonunion. Such treatment and grafts will be discussed further in the section on nonunion treatment.

In situations involving a destroyed articulation, there may be little option other than fusion or amputation. This is generally the accepted norm for trauma surgeons. There is a growing trend, however, and crossover between trauma and reconstruction, wherein the traumatologists are performing arthroplasty. Stemming from some experience in acute geriatric fractures, this treatment method also offers hope of function to young patients without a critical articulation. The hip, knee, and possibly the elbow are three joints that are not well tolerated in the fused state. Accepting a higher (but still low) rate of reinfection and failure, arthroplastic reconstruction may not provide longevity, but may greatly improve the short-term quality of life and function for such patients. This is especially true if consideration is given to long-term suppression until the tissue envelope adequately revascularizes and establishes host defenses. This topic will obviously be an area of further research.

Wound Dressing

In choosing a wound dressing, several characteristics should be considered (144): (a) optimization of wound healing, (b) preventing infection, (c) ability to absorb exudate, (d) biocompatibility, (e) hypoallergenicity, and (f) occlusivity. Generally, there are four types of wound dressings: semi-impermeable films, hydrogels, occlusive hydrocolloids, and synthetic skin substitutes. Several semi-impermeable membranes are available (OpSite, Tegaderm, Bio-Occlusive). The permeability of these dressings to water and oxygen is 2,500 g/m^2 per 24 hours and 7,000 mL/m^2 per 24 hours, respectively (144). The occlusive hydrocolloids (Duoderm) have permeability to water vapor and oxygen of 30 g/m^2 per 24 hours and 150 mL/m^2 per 24 hours, respectively (164). Alvarez has reported that re-epithelialization beneath a hydrocolloid dressing was greatest, followed by a polyurethane film, air exposure, and wet-to-dry dressings. Collagen synthesis was shown to be greater in the wounds exposed to air, followed by the hydrocolloid, polyurethane, and wet-to-dry dressings. In wounds with exposed bone, the dressings should prevent wound and bone desiccation as well as secondary contamination. There is no consensus or scientific study that demonstrates superiority of any one type of dressing.

Soft Tissue Coverage

Soft tissue reconstruction in osteomyelitis is limited to the use of muscle flaps. The timing of flap coverage in infected bone remains controversial. Although satisfactory results in chronic osteomyelitis have been reported with a single-stage procedure, most investigators advocate a two-stage technique. The first step consists of thorough debridement and culture and initiating empiric antibiotic coverage. Definitive soft tissue reconstruction is generally performed in 5 to 7 days. This interval allows time for the final culture results from the initial debridement to be obtained and also allows specific antibiotic therapy directed against all cultured pathogens to be initiated. Macroscopically, muscle flaps are pliable enough to completely fill dead space within the debridement cavity with vascularized tissue. The flaps also serve as a vascular bed for immediate skin grafting.

Because of the markedly increased blood supply of muscle compared with skin, local oxygen tension, delivery of leukocytes, and antibiotic levels have all been shown to increase in the presence of a muscle flap (165). Anthony and Mathes (165) followed 34 consecutive patients with chronic osteomyelitis of the distal lower extremity treated with debridement, a 10- to 14-day course of culture specific antibiotics, and immediate muscle flap coverage, and found a 96% success rate at a minimum 5-year follow-up. Other investigators have reported success rates of 80% to 100% in the use of muscle flaps to cover osteomyelitic wounds (166).

Wound VAC

Recently, a new method of wound treatment has provided a valuable adjunct for patients with complex issues who may not be candidates for soft tissue flaps. Vacuum-assisted closure (VAC) therapy is a system that uses suction to help promote wound healing. Negative pressure is applied across the wound through a medium, which helps distribute the pressure evenly across the wound. The advantages of this negative-pressure system are that the local blood flow increases, the infected material and the colonizing bacteria are removed, tissue edema is reduced, and there is mechanical contraction of the wound. VAC may help wounds that are chronic, acute, due to trauma from injury, and wounds that will not close properly (167). The VAC therapy system consists of a computer-controlled therapy unit, plastic tubing and canister, foam dressing, and a clear adhesive dressing. The foam dressing goes on the wound. One end of the tube will connect to the foam, and the other end connects to the canister. The canister connects to the VAC system. The wound area needs to be sealed with clear adhesive drapes. When the machine is started, the foam dressing will shrink (see Fig. 16-7B). The frequency of changing the dressings varies between 2 to 7 days. If the dressings are changed too frequently, it can hamper granulation tissue formation.

Hyperbaric Oxygen

Hyperbaric oxygen (HBO) therapy, together with advanced antibiotics, debridement, modern orthopaedic devices, and aggressive wound care, has been shown to be of great benefit in reducing the morbidity and mortality of severe and refractory musculoskeletal infections, as well as the cost of the care in managing these hard-to-treat problems (168). In the field of orthopaedics, HBO alone or as adjunctive therapy has proved useful in managing osteomyelitis, nonhealing wounds (diabetic foot ulcers and chronic ulcers from chronic limb ischemia), and acute osteomyelitis in critical locations such as the skull or sternum (169).

The following information explains the mechanisms of action of HBO therapy in treating osteomyelitis. First, HBO enhances oxygen-dependent leukocyte killing through the production of hydrogen peroxide and superoxide, by providing increased oxygen tension in the hypoxic tissue. In earlier animal studies, the oxygen tension of infected bone increased from 23 mm Hg to 104 mm Hg in response to HBO at 2 atm (170). Because the bactericidal activity of leukocytes in vitro is directly related to local oxygen tension, transient reversal of hypoxia might increase the clearance of bacteria (171). Second, optimal tissue oxygen tension enhances osteogenesis (172) and neovascularization (173) to fill the dead space with new bone and soft tissues. HBO has also been shown to enhance osteoclastic activity (174) to remove bony debris. Synergistic effects of HBO on bone healing with bone morphogenic protein (BMP) have also been shown (175). Finally, HBO has also been shown to potentiate the antimicrobial effects of aminoglycosides, and possibly sulpha drugs and vancomycin, in the killing of susceptible bacteria (170).

HBO appears to be clinically effective with supportive literature, although none of the studies are randomized and controlled. Although there are conflicting reports, the majority of the literature supports the adjunctive use of HBO. Unfortunately, it is also expensive and not always well tolerated by the patient. The major effect of HBO is to hyperoxygenate the blood and tissues and thereby increase the diffusion gradient into necrotic tissues. Currently, it is indicated for clostridial infections, crush injuries, necrotizing tissue infections, and refractory osteomyelitis.

COMPLICATIONS OF BONE HEALING

Pathophysiology of Fracture Healing

Bone has a remarkable capacity to heal after complete disruption. The cascade of events that leads to restoring skeletal integrity after an injury may be divided into clinically and histologically identifiable stages. Bone heals in one of two ways, either through endochondral ossification, or via direct osteonal healing. The fracture heals by callus formation in endochondral ossification. In the latter, there is no callus formation, and absolute and rigid stabilization is needed to allow a direct osteonal healing of the fracture site. This is typically the situation with rigid fixation and interfragmentary compression between two bone segments.

The Stages of Fracture Healing

Immediately after a fracture, a series of events occurs involving an overlapping cascade of events, including hematoma formation, inflammation, repair and remodeling (Fig. 18-8).

Hematoma Formation

After an injury to the bone, the gap is filled with blood from the ruptured periosteal and endosteal vessels and the accompanying soft tissue trauma. This blood distends the soft tissues and clots to form a hematoma. Numerous factors are released from the cellular elements present and from those recruited to the area from chemotactic stimuli. The signal-rich environment allows for the inception of a temporal and spatial sequence of events that lead to healing. As the hematoma matures, an inflammatory phase begins to prepare for healing (see Fig. 8-1A).

The Inflammatory Response

Osteocytes deprived of nutrition at the fracture ends die and play a passive role in the repair process. Osteoclasts remove necrotic bone, and the macrophages remove the hematoma. Presence of necrotic material incites an inflammatory response in the inflammatory phase (first few weeks), and numerous biochemical chemotactic substances are released. It clinically corresponds with pain, swelling, erythema and increased local temperature. The clot from the hematoma serves as a source of signaling molecules with the capacity to initiate the cascade of cellular events critical to fracture healing. The inflammatory

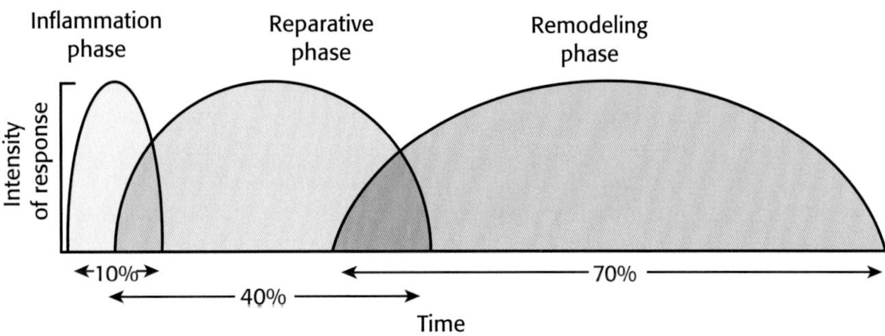

FIGURE 18-8 Stages of fracture healing.

cells secreting cytokines interleukin-1 and 6 regulate the early events in the fracture healing process. The degranulating platelets in the clot may release signaling molecules, such as transforming growth factor-beta (TGF-β) and platelet-derived growth factor, which are important in regulating cellular proliferation and differentiation of committed mesenchymal stem cells. The polypeptide fibroblast growth factor may be responsible for cell migration and matrix synthesis.

The Reparative Phase

As the inflammatory phase abates, the repair process commences (see Fig. 8-2A). The BMPs act on the undifferentiated perivascular mesenchymal cells. BMPs are osteoinductive and induce metaplasia of mesenchymal cells into osteoblasts. TGF-β induces mesenchymal cells to produce type II collagen and proteoglycans. It also induces osteoblasts to produce collagen. Undifferentiated mesenchymal cells move to the site of the injury and have a capacity to be transformed into osteoblasts, chondroblasts, and fibroblasts (176). Polymorphonuclear leukocytes, histiocytes, and mast cells help to remove tissue debris. Vasoactive substances (nitric oxide and endothelial stimulating angiogenesis factor) play a role in increasing tissue vascularity and trigger neoangiogenesis. Reticulin and collagen fibrils that have formed in the hematoma lie scattered within the fibrin scaffold (177). The cell population also includes osteoclasts that begin to clean up dead bone. The granulation tissue that subsequently forms comprises a thick cellular mass, and in appropriate strain environments, endochondral ossification occurs with islands of immature bone and hypertrophic chondrocytes. This thick cellular mass forms the callus (or splint) between the fracture fragments on the periosteal and endosteal surface and helps reduce interfragmentary motion (see Fig. 8-3A). The callus with immature or woven bone becomes densely mineralized and solidifies, thereby reducing further the movement between the fractured bone ends. As this external (bridging) callus forms from the fractured hematoma, the internal (medullary) callus forms more slowly and occurs later. Periosteal callus originates from the osteoprogenitor cells of the inner cambial layer of the periosteum.

The immature (woven) bone is transformed into mature or lamellar bone by continuing osteoblastic and osteoclastic activity. This process takes about 8 to 12 weeks. In some places, this conversion takes place by membranous ossification and in other places, it occurs by endochondral ossification. At this point, external mechanical stimuli can have the greatest affect on fracture healing because mechanical stability is crucial at this stage.

Remodeling

Reshaping the solid bone bridging the fracture site occurs at this stage. It is a continuous process of alternating bone resorption and formation. The muscular forces and weight bearing stresses help in remodeling. Remodeling allows the bone to assume its normal configuration and shape based on the stresses to which it is exposed (Wolff's law). Thicker lamellae are laid down where the stresses are high, excess bone is carved away, slight deformity is corrected, and the medullary cavity is reformed. Fracture healing is said to be complete when repopulation of the marrow space occurs. This process continues for months to years.

Fracture Healing Based on Type of Stabilization

Primary Bone Healing (Direct Bone Healing)

This form of bone healing occurs in anatomically reduced, stably fixed fractures. Healing occurs by direct osteonal penetration and haversian remodeling with no external bridging callus (Fig. 18-9). The haversian remodeling has two main functions: revascularization of necrotic fracture ends and reconstitution of inter-

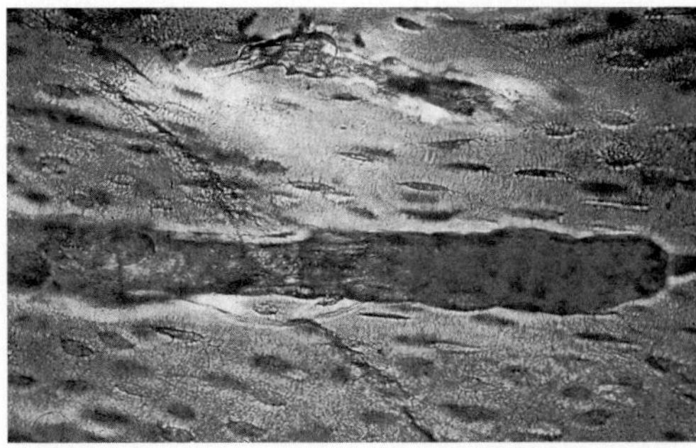

FIGURE 18-9 Histologic example of direct osteonal healing with minimal callous and endochondral processes. The healing crosses the fracture line directly.

cortical union. It has also been referred to as *contact healing* in contact areas and *gap healing* in noncontact areas.

In contact healing, there is no ingrowth of mesodermal cells from the periosteum or endosteum. At approximately 4 weeks after fixation, haversian canals proliferate along the longitudinal axis of the bone. The remodeling osteoclastic cutting cones travel across the fracture site followed by a mantle of osteoblasts. The osteoblasts deposit circumferential bone lamellae behind the cutting cone to produces a haversian system (osteon). Gap healing occurs when a fracture that is perfectly reduced has irregular surfaces that create gaps between the fragments. Under stable conditions, the fracture gap is filled with woven bone, which will then be remodeled. Even with rigid internal fixation, gaps greater than 1 mm are partially filled with fibrous tissue, which is subsequently replaced by bone in a process similar to secondary bone healing. Beyond such distances and when there is enough strain, the healing process occurs with the endochondral method described previously.

Fracture Healing in Cancellous Bone

When there is direct contact between the cancellous bone fragments, healing occurs by creeping substitution. New trabeculae formed by intramembranous ossification are laid down on the original trabeculae to produce bone between the two fragments. There is no terminal death and no bridging callus. Once union is established, remodeling occurs.

Distraction Osteogenesis

Distraction osteogenesis was described by Ilizarov. Bone repair is induced by gradual controlled distraction after an interval of induction, which is usually after 5 to 7 days. Bone formation takes place through a process that is more similar to intramembranous ossification. Although it is not within the scope of this chapter, it is mentioned for the sake of completeness.

Mechanical Basis of Fracture Healing

Shortly after the initial phase of healing, in vascularized areas, and if there is sufficient immobilization, there are strain environments that allow the process of endochondral ossification to proceed. Although there are numerous cellular, piezoelectric, biologic, and mechanical processes occurring, the Perren's interfragmentary strain theory (178) helps explain the mechanical basis of healing. Each tissue type has various strain tolerances, for example, granulation and fibroblastic tissue can elongate up to 100% before failure. Thus, these cells are able to proliferate in strain environments that experience motion. Cartilage and bone, on the other hand, can tolerate much less strain, from 2% to 10% and <2%, respectively.

Perren theorized that the magnitude of interfragmentary strain would determine the subsequent differentiation of the fracture gap tissue. He felt that interfragmentary strains above 100% would lead to nonunion. Strains between 10% and 100% would lead to sustain initial fibrous tissue formation. Strains between 2% and 10% would lead to cartilage formation and an endochondral ossification formation. Strains under 2% would lead to direct bone formation and primary fracture healing.

As granulation tissue forms, and theoretically some type of immobilization exists, such as casting or internal fixation, motion between fragments will decrease. During callus formation (lasting from 1 to 5 months), cells proliferate and differentiate to produce osteoblasts and chondroblasts. The osteoblasts and chondroblasts synthesize the extracellular organic matrices of woven bone and cartilage respectively, and the newly formed bone is mineralized. As these "stiffer" cells proliferate, the construct is further stiffened, which produces strain environments low enough to allow cartilage and bone healing. This concept helps clarify why stabilization methods that allow too much motion may result in higher nonunion rates. It also helps explain why simple transverse fractures may have more difficulty healing than longer fracture segments with some comminution. In the more comminuted fractures, the limb motion is distributed among a greater distance and "per length-unit strain" is less than when the same limb motion is borne by a single transverse fracture gap. In the latter, a seemingly small amount of motion can easily exceed strain limits for bone formation. In such situations, the body may try to reduce motion by forming bone adjacent to the fracture segment, thus increasing its inertial cross-sectional moment, in an attempt to decrease motion in the central most portions of the fracture. The failure of this process is frequently demonstrated as a hypertrophic nonunion.

There is often a "race" between healing and implant failure. Implants rarely fail by catastrophic overload as presented in static tests. Usually, there is a fatigue failure of the "construct," whether between the bone-implant interface, or the implant itself. Understanding the biology of healing and the mechanics of fixation are critical to monitoring healing, as it can be very difficult to accurately determine healing. In the absence of any biologic activity such as atrophic nonunions, construct failure may be delayed. There can also be situations in which the bone erroneously appears to be healing, or healed. In these situations, failure is even more delayed. To understand this phenomenon, the concepts of load sharing and fatigue failure are important to understand. If the load that is borne by the limb during functional activity is partially transmitted through axially stable bone-on-bone contact within the construct, then the implant and bone are considered "load sharing." If there is no bone-on-bone contact and the implant must bear nearly 100% of the load, it is a "load-bearing" construct. In load-bearing situations, the implant and the bone-implant interfaces experience much higher stresses than in the load-sharing construct. Such high stresses can result in earlier construct failure. This is due to a common concept of materials wherein a material or construct can withstand less cyclic loading before failure with increasingly higher stresses. For each implant and construct there is a stress below which an infinite number of cycles can be borne. This is termed the *endurance limit*. Thus, one can see that in load-sharing situations, the stresses experienced by any part of the construct are less than with load-bearing situations, and can delay failure until a later time (cycles). It is for this reason that failure is often delayed in some complex reconstructions that may initially be load-sharing, but because of completely avascular bone segments, complete healing does not occur, and there is eventual and progressive failure. It is also possible, that the construct is such that each element is under its endurance limit, and in this situation, failure can be indefinitely delayed or quite late. These concepts as well as monitoring for evidence of biologic activity (vascularity) are important when making treatment decisions.

Delayed Union

Five million fractures occur annually in the United States. Five to 10% of (250,000 to 500,000) will result in delayed or nonunion with considerable morbidity (179). Delayed union is defined as a fracture that has not healed within its expected healing time. Such slow healing may be due to patient factors, local tissue factors, or due to the fracture geometry and its treatment. Although delayed unions can go on to heal, it is the usual stepping-stone to nonunion. A brisk biologic response without early healing may not technically qualify for a nonunion, but instead a delayed union, and may prompt a change in treatment that results in healing. Histologically, delayed unions differ slightly from the pattern described for spontaneous healing. Callus formation is prominent, and the interfragmentary tissue consists of fibrous tissue or fibrocartilage, which slowly undergoes bony substitution. Inadequate fracture reduction, regardless of its cause, may be a prime reason for delayed union or nonunion.

Nonunion

Failure to show any progressive change in radiographic appearance for at least 3 months after the period of time during which normal fracture union was expected to take place is evidence of nonunion (180). There are several published definitions of nonunion, but none is universally accepted. A nonunion exists when repair is not complete within the period expected for a specific fracture and when cellular activity at the fracture site ceases (176). Nonunion is the cessation of both the periosteal and endosteal healing responses without bridging (181). Fracture nonunion occurs when the reparative cascade of fracture healing phases is interrupted with accompanying failure of radiographic progression.

Generally, as a definition, failure of a fracture to heal in 6 to 8 months constitutes nonunion (182). Nonunion occurs when there is failure of the biology (high-energy injuries with devascularization), failure of the host (nicotine, vascular disease, other comorbidities), failure of mechanics (improper stabilization), or treatment failure (iatrogenic devascularization) (183). If there has been any previous surgery to the limb, there should always be the suspicion of infection as the cause of nonunion.

Classification of Nonunions

As proposed by Weber and Czech, nonunions are first categorized as viable (hypertrophic or vascular nonunion) and nonviable (atrophic or avascular nonunion), based on whether the fracture site is capable of a biologic reaction (184). Hypertrophic nonunion can be further subdivided into elephant foot, horse hoof and oligotrophic nonunion. Paley and Herzenberg classify nonunions according to clinical mobility with the following numbers: (1) stiff (<5 degrees mobility), (2) partially mobile (5 to 20 degrees mobility), or (3) flail (>20° mobility) (185). These categories roughly correlate to the three Weber-Czech categories.

Hypertrophic Nonunions

The hypertrophic nonunion shows that although adequate vascularity exists, there is insufficient mechanical stability (Fig. 18-10). This can result from inadequate surgical technique, improper fixation, or premature motion at the fracture site. Elephant foot nonunions are rich in callus and usually result from early weight bearing and/or insecure fixation in a reduced fracture with viable fragments.

Horse hoof nonunions are mildly hypertrophic and exhibit less callus. These usually result after unstable fracture fixation. Oligotrophic nonunions have little callus but still demonstrate some biologic capacity. They usually occur because of major displacement of a fracture, fragment distraction, and internal fixation without proper apposition of the fragments. Hypertrophic nonunions respond well to treatment and stable fixation by means of plates (186) intramedullary nails (187,188) or external fixation (161). Infection can also mimic a vascular nonunion and should always be considered. Usually, the callus is infected and may be part of the involucrum, and there may be rarefactions and irregularities in the callus, as well as evidence of hardware failure. Laboratory and diagnostic studies should be considered in such situations, as the treatment algorithm is quite different between infected and aseptic nonunions.

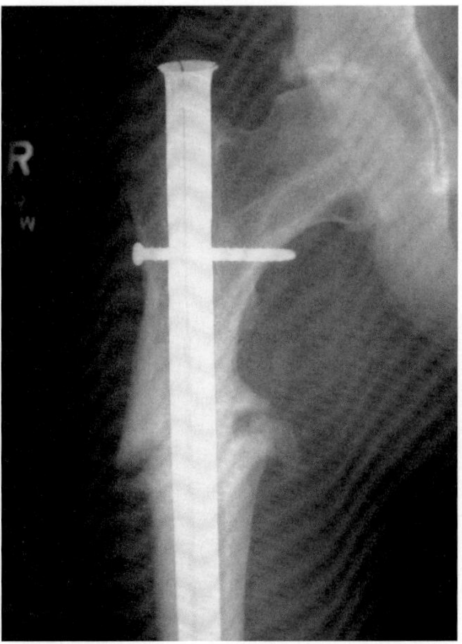

FIGURE 18-10 Hypertrophic nonunion.

Atrophic Nonunions

Atrophic nonunions are characterized by absence of callus, avascular bone ends, and poor healing potential (Fig. 18-11). Atrophic nonunions are subdivided into torsion wedge, comminuted, and defect nonunion. Torsion wedge nonunions are the result of intercalary fragments with poor blood supply. These occur when there are multiple comminuted devascularized fragments. Defect nonunions result due to bone loss with large gaps between the bones. Here, the gap is usually filled with an avascular scar tissue with poor osteogenic potential. Treating these nonunions is difficult due to the common association of fracture gaps, infection, and poor vascularity.

There is a special subgroup of nonunions that contains a fibrous capsule around a freely mobile nonunion. This cavity is filled with a viscous fluid, creating the appearance of a joint, and is referred to as a *pseudoarthrosis*. These are uncommonly seen in modern times.

Infected Nonunions

These nonunions require consideration of the infection (Fig. 18-12). After adequate treatment of the infection, the infected nonunion resembles an aseptic nonunion. Due to the infection and subsequent ablative surgery, they may have less biologic potential, so they behave more like an atrophic nonunion and frequently have segmental defects. An aggressive approach is required to treat infected nonunions due to the common associations of inadequate soft tissue coverage, poor vascularity, and loose fixation devices (189).

Risk Factors for Nonunion

Severity of Local Injury

Fractures associated with more extensive bone or soft tissue trauma have less biologic potential for healing. Because fracture healing requires adequate vascularity and differentiation of mesenchymal cells, a wide "zone of injury" will be a greater risk for both infection and development of atrophic behavior. In simpler fractures, the soft tissue envelope is intact, providing a ready source of mesenchymal cells as well as a better blood supply. Loss of bone substance or gaps between fracture fragments leads to a condition in which the cells' ability to bridge the gap is compromised. This is especially true for bones with less soft tissue surroundings such as the tibia, as compared to the femur, or for bones with less vascular options, such as the femoral neck. When a bone is fractured, the normal nutrient artery and centripetal blood flow is disrupted. In such situations, the blood flow to the bone reverses and depends on the periosteal capillary plexus and muscle envelope. This is why iatrogenic injury to periosteal tissues during surgical stabilization is of utmost importance and should be avoided. Maintenance of any muscle, tendon, or ligament attachments to bone may be crucial to maintaining their biologic healing potential (178,190).

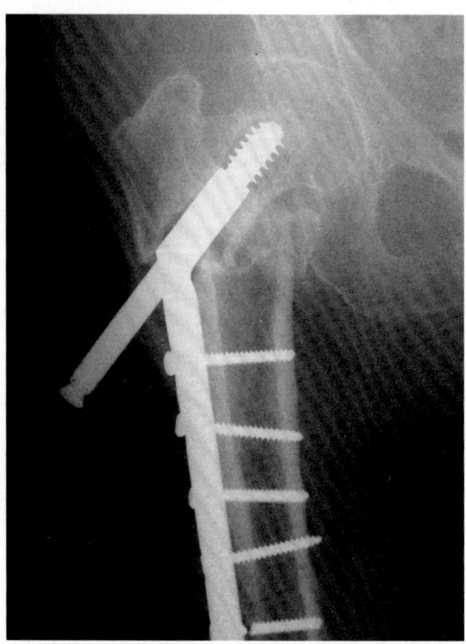

FIGURE 18-12 Infected nonunion.

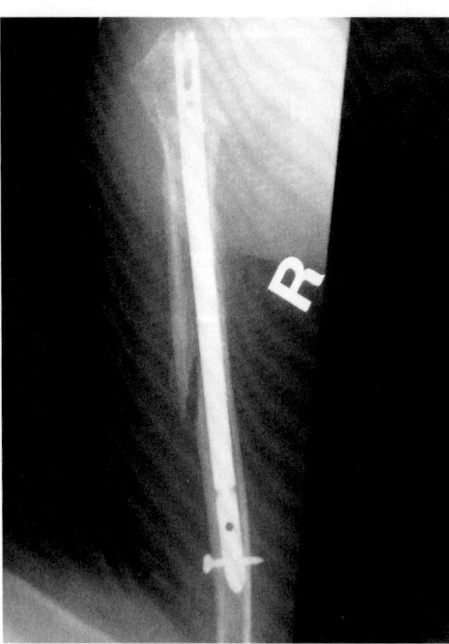

FIGURE 18-11 Atrophic nonunion.

Type of Bone

Cortical and cancellous bones react somewhat differently. Cancellous bone unites very rapidly, and the union occurs at points of direct contact. Repair in cancellous bone is rapid because there are many points of bone contact, which are rich in cells and blood supply. Gaps in cancellous bone are filled by the spread of new bone from the points of contact. Cortical bone unites by two mechanisms, based on the local conditions. If apposition of cortical bone ends occurs with rigid immobilization, end-to-end healing takes place from the cortical surfaces with very little external callus. If on the other hand, there are small fracture gaps or some degree of motion, repair occurs by external callus. Certain bones are known for a predisposition to nonunion due to their tenuous blood supply. The femoral neck, scaphoid, fifth metatarsal, and the talus are some examples.

Excessive Motion

Inadequate immobilization leads to delayed union or nonunion. Repeated manipulation has been shown to retard fracture healing. The initial fibrin scaffolding, which is the first step in fracture repair, is disrupted if immobilization is not adequate and if the bony bridge of external callus fails to form properly. If inadequate immobilization continues throughout the repair process, a nonunion can develop, and if excessive, this can lead to the classic pseudarthrosis. Fixation methods should be appropriate for the injury and the bone. Bone responds poorly to shear and best to compressive forces. As described previously, the local strain environment is crucial for bone healing. This may be the paradoxical reason why some transverse fractures do not heal as reliably as those with more comminution.

Radiation Necrosis

Bone that has been irradiated heals at a slower rate with a higher risk of nonunion. The threshold for osseous radiation injury is believed to be 3,000 cGy, with cell death occurring at 5,000 cGy. Radiation interferes with fracture healing by more than one mechanism. It may cause vascular and cellular damage (176). Radiation causes cell death in the local region, thrombosis of vessels, fibrosis of the marrow, and reduced capillary ingrowth. Through experiments on rats, Green (191) found that radiation suppresses osteoblastic proliferation and neovascularization at the fracture site. In growing bone, radiation decreases chondroblastic mitotic activity, reduces the size of the lacunae, and diminishes osteoid replacement of primary cartilage (191).

Systemic Factors

Age

It is well known that fractures heal very rapidly in young patients and the rapid remodeling that accompanies growth allows correction of a greater degree of deformities. Experimental work (192) using titrated thymidine shows that in young animals, there is more rapid differentiation of cells from the mesenchymal pool, which makes them available for the repair process. Elderly animals heal at a slower rate than younger animals, but in clinical practice in humans, this is difficult to document. In a series of 842 patients examining the incidence of nonunions by location (bone), children were less likely to develop nonunions than adults (193). Nonunions in fractured tibia, in children are extremely rare (194) except in the presence of congenital pseudarthrosis. The thicker periosteum and the better vascularity of the bone are related to the lower incidence of nonunions in children (195). It has also been shown that although the elderly can still heal normally, the numbers of stem cells available for healing decrease with age. This is especially true with autogenous pelvic graft, which already has a paucity of osteogenic cells.

Illness and Malnutrition

Chronic illness and malnutrition have been linked with poorer fracture healing (196). Phosphorus and calcium deficiencies appear to delay callus formation in rats secondary to reduced mineralization (197). Protein dietary deficiency has been shown to reduce callus strength (198). Protein deprivation has shown a profound detrimental effect on fracture healing in an experiment involving rats (199). When compared with controls, malnourished animals had callus composed primarily of fibrous-type tissue and had decreased periosteal and external callus. Based on mechanical testing results, callus from malnourished animals showed reduced strength and stiffness (199).

Anemia

Anemia due to blood loss and iron deficiency can delay bone healing. In a rat model, marked weakness of callus strength was identified at 3, 6, and 8 weeks after fracture in anemic animals (200). The histological differences observed between the anemic and control groups were marked retardation of fracture healing in the anemic group, with the incidence of nonunion reaching 33% compared to 0% in the control group. The likely explanation for the effect of anemia on fracture healing could be altered secondary to tissue oxygenation. Bone cellular metabolism depends on the oxygen tension and circulating wound blood volume (200). Iron could be responsible for delaying bone healing by interfering with the enzyme system responsible for transporting the cytochrome chain involving iron and copper.

Hormones

Corticosteroids are powerful inhibitors of fracture healing (201).They inhibit the differentiation of osteoblasts from mesenchymal cells and decrease the synthesis rates of the major components of bone matrix mandatory for repair. Growth hormone is a potent stimulator of fracture healing. Experimental work has shown that the alterations in the level of circulating growth hormone profoundly influence the fracture-healing rate (201, 202). Sex steroids play an essential role in maintaining bone health throughout life. Osteoblast cells appear to be stimulated by androgens in vitro; however their use in vivo is limited due to their virilizing side effects as well as alterations in lipoprotein profiles. In an experiment to compare fracture healing in a rat femoral defect model, sustained delivery of dihydrotestosterone has been shown to stimulate the osteoblastic activities, which eventually causes an increase in the cortical bone density (203).

In humans, type I diabetes is associated with a decrease in skeletal mass and delayed fracture healing (204,205). Patients with diabetes exhibit reduced bone mineral density as measured by dual x-ray absorptiometry of the lumbar spine and proximal femur (206). In a 12-year prospective study, bone formation was shown to be reduced in diabetic humans, suggesting that they have diminished osteoblastic activity, compared with normal individuals (207). Animal model experiments have suggested that diabetes inhibits cell proliferation during fracture healing due to decreased platelet-derived growth factor levels (208). Diabetic animals fail to regulate osteoblast differentiation, which in turn, leads to decreased bone formation (208).

Smoking

Smoking, and specifically the effect of nicotine, has been shown to be a potent inhibitor of fracture healing. Cigarette smoking is well documented to place the patient at a higher risk of delayed union and nonunion (209). Empirical clinical observation suggests that cigarette smoking has an inhibitory effect on long bone fracture healing. The primary reason for this effect is thought to be both constriction of small blood vessels caused by nicotine and the inhibition of growth of new blood vessels. It has been shown to adversely affect bone mineral density, lumbar disk disease, the rate of hip fractures, and the dynamics of bone and wound healing (210). Smoking is associated with an increased risk of complications in patients with open tibial fractures (209). There is an increased rate of flap failure, delayed union, and nonunion (209). Although scientific and clinical information on smoking and its consequences suggests differing degrees of correlation between smoking and orthopaedic conditions, most available data suggest a real and reproducible relationship (210).

NSAIDs

Prostaglandins are known to play an important role in bone repair and normal bone homeostasis. Prostaglandins are released as part of the inflammatory response. They are synthesized from arachidonic acid by the cyclooxygenase enzymes, COX-1 and COX-2. NSAIDS inhibit COX activity and have become the primary means of alleviating chronic pain associated with rheumatoid and osteoarthritis. They are also widely used as analgesics in treating acute postsurgical and traumatic pain. Although these data raise concerns about the use of COX-2–specific inhibitors as anti-inflammatory or analgesic drugs in patients undergoing orthopaedic procedures, clinical reports have been largely inconclusive concerning the effects of NSAIDs on bone healing. Because animal data suggest that the effects of COX-2 inhibitors are both dose-dependent and reversible, in the absence of scientifically sound clinical evidence, it is suggested that physicians consider short-term administration or use of other drugs in managing these patients (211).

Treatment of Nonunions

Enhancement of Fixation

In situations when excessive motion is present but where there is biologic potential (e.g., hypertrophic nonunions), the treatment consists of enhancing stability. In many situations, compression plating is sufficient. A mild deformity may be corrected with use of a plate, but in cases where the deformity is not as mobile, surgical release (e.g., osteotomy or takedown of nonunion) may be required. It is not always necessary to change implant types. For example, small-caliber nails that are not canal filling have been shown to result in more problems in healing and require a greater number of procedures to obtain healing in open tibia fractures (212). Revision reamed nailing using a larger nail with compression may be adequate. Failed plating may just require revision compression plating. The same is true with external fixation and the common principle would be to apply compression and improve stability of the fixation.

Bone Grafting

In 1879, Macewen demonstrated the use of his pioneering bone grafts in Glasgow (213). In the 1920s and 1930s, Campbell and Phemister popularized the use of autografts for delayed unions and nonunions of fractures (214). Wilson and Charnley used cancellous bone graft strips to treat nonunions (193,215). Autogenous bone was preferred to allograft, as the success rate was 88% for autogenous, compared to 70% for allograft (216).

There are several elements required for the success of bone graft to obtain healing. The graft needs to be osteoconductive, which provides scaffolding upon which new bone can grow. It needs to be osteoinductive, which provides the biologic signals to recruit and influence cellular activity of bone formation. These two components were thought to be the essential elements for healing. Recently, other vital elements have been recognized as also being necessary. In order for bone to form, there needs to be a cell with osteogenic potential. Although autograft is thought to provide such cells, Muschler has shown that with pelvic autograft, only from 1/20,000 to 1/100,000 of the cells are osteogenic cells (217). Furthermore, considering that these cells are living and require vascularity for oxygen and nutrition, these cells may not survive long enough to participate in osteogenesis when implanted into an avascular nonunion site. Thus, there must be some local or systemic recruitment that takes place as well as revascularization. The exact temporal and spatial sequence and elements for healing are still being elucidated.

Dating back to the classic work of Urist, allograft bone that was processed was found to contain proteins from the TGF-β family of proteins that were osteoinductive. Since then, a number of BMPs have been identified and found to have significant potential to heal osseous defects. When processed with allograft bone, demineralized bone matrix has been applied in numerous circumstances instead of autograft bone. BMP-2, 6, and 9 may play an important role in inducing osteoblast differentiation of mesenchymal stem cells (218). Most commercial preparations of BMPs have been found to work quite well in laboratory and animal studies, but they have not been proven as effective in human trials. One problem is that performing well-controlled level I evidence-based trials for such products is hard if not impossible (177). The incidence of nonunions is low compared to other conditions, and controlling for the numerous parameters such as injury, patient, and prior treatments, makes such studies nearly impossible to perform. What remains then, are studies with strict inclusion criteria and cohort or descriptive reports that require more cautious interpretation. Although successful animal testing is necessary, it is not sufficient. As such, animal studies should be interpreted with scrutiny and a "burden of proof" is required, where efficacy in primates, and finally, in controlled clinical trials in humans is needed. There are currently two products with such scientific methodology that have been shown to be effective. Osteogenic Protein-1 (OP-1,

Stryker, Mahwah, NJ), which is a recombinant BMP-7 has been demonstrated to be effective in nonunions and Infuse (Wyeth, NYSE:WYE), which is a recombinant BMP-2 has been effective in acute fractures (218). Other products in uncontrolled clinical evaluations have shown promise, and numerous other products are currently being evaluated and await peer review.

Osseous Transplants

Large-defect nonunions have been successfully treated with osseous cortical implants (219). From what has been shown in the tumor literature (220), cortical grafts do not become fully revascularized or incorporated with host bone, and they seem to form junctional bone welds to host bone. Because the allograft bone does not remodel, it is subject to failure in the active patient. Vascularized cortical autograft has been attempted using fibula and iliac crest. Vascularized fibula transfer is a valuable technique for reconstructing extensive long bone defects in the upper extremity. This vascularized bone is viable bone, in which the osteocytes and osteoblasts survive, and due to the preservation of bone-forming capacity, bone fusion occurs early. The fibula, a tubular bone, is similar to the shape of the forearm and does not overstuff the forearm; hence wound closure is usually not a problem. This procedure has been used for reconstructing the lower extremity, but has been subject to delayed stress fractures due to its size. If used in the lower extremity, a prolonged period of protected weight bearing is needed to allow the bone to remodel and hypertrophy (219). As a result, it has been used more often in upper-extremity situations than in the lower extremity. In the lower extremity, when defects exceed 4 to 6 cm, massive grafting has been challenging, as this is a large cavity and bed of bone to revascularize. In these situations, using distraction osteogenesis as developed by Ilizarov has been more applicable. The methodology of the Ilizarov technique is well described in the literature and has been extensively applied to complex posttraumatic situations (221). With this method, the defect is slowly filled in by creating an osteotomy remote from the injury site, and in a slow and controlled manner, transporting host bone into the defect. The distracting osteotomy site slowly fills with "regenerate" bone that forms in a unique manner and ossifies by intramembranous ossification. The soft tissues, vessels, and nerves all accommodate well to this method, and the patient is allowed and encouraged to participate in functional activity as well as weight bearing. Although the Ilizarov technique requires close and diligent management, it provides a superb method for posttraumatic reconstruction. The bone formed is "autogenous" and the patient is functional during treatment. The method also allows correction of deformity, treatment of infection, and it provides an alternative for hypertrophic nonunions.

Use of Electricity in Treating Nonunions

John Birch, a general surgeon, first used electricity clinically to heal fractures (222). In 1841, Edward Hartshorne first reported the successful use of electricity in treating tibial nonunions (222). Friedberg, in 1971, reported electrical stimulation (222), and many investigators have reported its use in successfully treating nonunions since that time (222–224).

These devices may use direct current (DC), pulsed electromagnetic fields (PEMF), combined magnetic fields (CMF), alternating current, or capacitive coupling to provide electrical stimulation to a fracture site. Electrical fields have been generated in bone invasively by placing electrodes into the healing fracture site, or noninvasively by capacitative or inductive coupling. Electric and electromagnetic fields are, collectively, one form of biophysical technique, which regulates extracellular matrix synthesis and may be useful in clinically stimulating repair of fractures and nonunions (225). These techniques have been used clinically to treat fresh fractures, osteotomies, spinal fusions, as well as delayed and nonunions (226–228).

Capacitative Coupling

Bassett (226) developed this noninvasive technique, which requires accurate placement of two coils around the fracture site. The limb is immobilized in plaster, and the coils are placed on the plaster around the fracture site. Potentials of 1 to 10 V at frequencies of 20 to 200 kHz are applied, which produces electrical fields in the tissue of approximately 1 to 100 mV/cm (225). Capacitative coupling promotes bone healing of fracture nonunions (229). In a study to compare healing rates employing DC, capacitive coupling, or bone graft, the findings suggested that bone graft surgery yielded a poorer union rate when there was a previous bone graft failure, and capacitive coupling had a poorer union rate in the presence of an atrophic nonunion (230).

Direct Electrical Current

Direct electrical current techniques stimulate osteogenesis at the cathode at currents of 5 to 100 mA. Direct current can be provided by semi-invasive or invasive methods. The semi-invasive technique of Friedenberg (222) is composed of (a) a power pack that supplies a current of 20 mA, (b) an anode consisting of a stainless steel grid applied to the skin, and (c) stainless cathode k wires. The tip of the cathode is inserted through the skin into the nonunion using an image intensifier. The overall success rate reported by Heppenstall in 50 forearm nonunions treated with 3 months semi-invasive DC stimulation in the absence of gap or infection was 80% (231). The invasive technique was devised by Patterson (232) and involves a small operation to insert a generator that supplies a constant current of 20 mA. A platinized anode with a titanium cathode is made into a form of helix and placed across the site of nonunion. Zichner reported his experience with invasive use of DC with success in 1981 (233). Implantable DC stimulation is effective in managing established nonunions of the extremities (234).

Inductive Coupling

Electrical fields can be produced in bone by inductive coupling (IC) with an external time varying or pulsed electromagnetic field. This technique uses a single or double current-carrying coil, which is driven by an external field generator and also induces a secondary electrical field in the bone.

PEMF

Exogenous electromagnetic fields are produced to promote fracture healing by either invasive or noninvasive methods. It has been shown that shear stresses on bone liberate electrical potentials on osteocyte membrane, which promote fracture healing. In vitro electromagnetic fields on osteoblasts stimulate secretion of BMP-2 and 4, TGF-β, and IGF–II, which in turn, promote fracture healing. Pulsed electromagnetic stimulation has been shown to be an effective modality, especially for hypertrophic nonunions (230), but it does not address issues of instability, deformity, or leg length inequality.

Heckman et al (235) reported healing in 64% of 149 patients using PEMF, and that the healing rate was higher for the tibia than for the femur or humerus. As understanding of the mechanisms of action expands, specific requirements for field energetics are being defined and the range of treatable conditions is broadened. These conditions include nerve regeneration, wound healing, and diabetes (236). PEMF augments angiogenesis primarily by stimulating endothelial release of FGF-2, inducing paracrine and autocrine changes in the surrounding tissue. These findings suggest a potential role for PEMF in therapeutic angiogenesis (237).

CMF

CMF stimulators use an external coil system with a combination of direct and alternating currents to produce both static and alternating magnetic fields. The CMF units are available in different sizes and coil designs to accommodate various fracture locations. The size and bulk of CMF technology coils may affect patient compliance, but the units are recommended for only 30 minutes of use per day. CMFs, a new type of biophysical stimulus, have been shown to act by stimulating endogenous production of growth factors that regulate the healing process (65).

Pulsed Ultrasound

Ultrasound bone growth stimulation is designed to transmit low-density, pulsed high-frequency acoustic pressure waves to accelerate healing of fresh fractures and to promote healing of delayed unions and nonunions that are refractory to standard treatment (238). Pulsed ultrasound units are also worn externally and consist of a battery power pack and transducer head. The unit may be applied directly to the skin overlying the fracture site, or by windowing a cast if necessary. There is evidence from randomized trials that low-intensity pulsed ultrasound treatment may significantly reduce the time to fracture healing for fractures treated nonoperatively. Treatment with the active ultrasound device also substantially reduced the incidence of tibial delayed unions in smokers and nonsmokers. Using the active ultrasound device accelerates cortical and cancellous bone fracture healing, substantially mitigates the delayed healing effects of smoking, speeds the return to normal activity, and reduces the long-term complication of delayed union (239). There does not appear to be any additional benefit to ultrasound treatment after intramedullary nailing with prior reaming (238). Its use is gaining wider acceptance, and its ease of use is well tolerated by patients.

BLEEDING COMPLICATIONS

Hemorrhage is the most common cause of shock in patients with polytrauma, leading to cellular hypoxia and death (240). This situation can arise in the field of orthopaedics when the injuries involve unstable pelvic injuries and long bone fractures in combination with visceral injuries such as in the liver and spleen. Bilateral fractures of the femora can result in significant blood loss of up to 3 to 4 units per fracture. Hemorrhage associated with unstable pelvic fractures is commonly venous and may be amenable to angiographic embolization, so if facilities are available, this option should be explored. The antishock pelvic clamp can be applied in the emergency departments in suitable situations to reduce the pelvic volume and reduce exsanguinating hemorrhage by tamponade effect. Blood transfusion is common and is required in a multiply injured patient. Early mortality is usually secondary to uncontrolled hemorrhage, whereas late mortality is due to associated injuries and sepsis-induced multiple organ failure (241,242). A large body of experimental and clinical research has greatly expanded our knowledge of cellular mechanisms and clinical outcomes in resuscitating patients with hypovolemic shock (240). Aggressive resuscitation to correct tissue hypoperfusion within 24 hours of injury is associated with improved clinical outcomes (240). Blood substitutes, hypertonic saline, and minimally invasive hemodynamic monitoring techniques have the potential of optimizing fluid resuscitation in patients with polytrauma (240). In patients with multiple injuries who are in an "unstable" or "in extremis" clinical condition, damage-control orthopaedics is the current treatment of choice (241,242). By performing limited surgical interventions, the subsequent reduction in blood loss and transfusion requirements can only be beneficial in these critically ill patients, reducing the risk of developing systemic complications and early mortality (241). Advanced blood banks ensure adequate supply of whole blood and fractionated products in the form of packed red cells, plasma, and platelets. Prevalence of blood-borne diseases necessitates thorough screening as a standard procedure in most blood banks.

Disseminated intravascular coagulation is one of the complications of massive blood transfusion. Massive resuscitations, however, are associated with specific complications such as hypothermia, coagulopathy, and abdominal compartment syndrome (240). Acute disseminated intravascular coagulation is characterized by generalized bleeding, which ranges from petechiae to exsanguinating hemorrhage, or microcirculatory and macrocirculatory thrombosis. This leads to hypoperfusion, infarction, and end-organ damage. In severe cases, patients may develop fever and a shock-like picture with tachycardia, tachypnea, and hypotension. Platelet count should be monitored after 7 to 10 U of red packed cells are transfused. Sepsis and multiple-organ system failure occur days after acute hemorrhagic shock.

A normal hemostatic response to vascular injury involves the initial formation of a platelet plug followed by a fibrin-platelet clot, and it depends on the adequate quantity and function of coagulation factors and platelets. A medication or disease state that affects any step in this coagulation cascade has the potential to cause bleeding. Additionally, inadequate hemostasis during surgery and mechanical factors, such as hypertension and trauma, can cause bleeding complications. An increased risk of severe intraoperative bleeding complications has been shown when warfarin, aspirin, NSAIDs, and antiplatelet agents are used in the context of various types of surgeries, from orthopaedic surgery to ophthalmologic surgery. A few recent studies focusing on cutaneous surgery failed to demonstrate a significant difference in postoperative bleeding complications in patients who continue anticoagulant medications compared with those who discontinue them in the preoperative period. Because of the relative paucity of studies, however, no consensus on how to manage these patients has been achieved.

Postoperative bleeding usually arises within the first 24 hours after surgery. Minor postoperative bleeding from wound edges is not uncommon, and it usually results from excessive activity on the patient's part—from trauma to the wound or from the increase in blood flow, which occurs when the vasoconstrictive effect of epinephrine diminishes.

A hematoma can have deleterious consequences as it exerts pressure on the wound edges; it may lead to ischemia, tissue necrosis, and dehiscence. The collection of blood is also an excellent medium for bacterial growth and places the wound at increased risk of infection. If discovered in the acute postoperative period (within the first few days), the hematoma is still gel-like and may be expressed from the wound through the suture line or by partial takedown of the repair. A large, expanding hematoma requires immediate suture removal to release the tension on the wound. After several days, the hematoma evolves into a more solidified mass, and its removal is more difficult. If discovered at this point, one must assess for wound compromise to determine whether the wound needs to be opened. If the wound does not appear to be compromised, the patient may be treated with a pressure dressing and close follow-up care. Antibiotics should be considered. The natural history of hematomas includes liquefaction, which occurs between 7 to 14 days. At this point, one may be able to aspirate the hematoma with a large-gauge needle. Placing drains for the first 24 hours after surgery may be helpful prophylactically or in managing wounds susceptible to drainage. Long-term drain placement may not be of any benefit and may provide a route for bacterial colonization.

VASCULAR INJURIES

Vascular injuries associated with fractures and dislocations may produce a catastrophic situation if treatment is delayed. The complications of vascular injuries to the extremities can range from infection and thrombosis to gangrene, amputation, and sometimes death. Extremity vascular injury may result from penetrating injuries such as gunshot wounds and knife injuries. Industrial accidents can result in penetrating injuries (e.g., nail guns). Iatrogenic arterial injury is increasingly frequent and may result from any invasive diagnostic or therapeutic procedure (243). Blunt vascular injury can result from motor vehicle accidents, falls, assaults, and crush injuries.

It is especially important that orthopaedic surgeons are trained in evaluating vascular injuries associated with fractures and dislocations, as they may be the first surgeons to evaluate the injury. It is also important to recognize that vascular injuries may occur during treatment of a fracture and/or a dislocation, and it is extremely important that these injuries are recognized and treated appropriately.

Arterial Injuries

There are five specific types of vascular injuries: intimal flaps, disruptions or subintimal hematomas, wall defects, complete transection, and arterial venous fistula. The intimal flaps and subintimal hematomas are usually associated with blunt trauma, but the wall defects, complete transections, and arterial venous fistulas are frequently seen with penetrating wounds. When an arterial vessel is transected, vascular spasm coupled with low systemic blood pressure appears to promote clotting at the injury site and helps to preserve vital organ perfusion better than that which occurs with ongoing uncontrolled hemorrhage. Arterial injuries occurring as a result of sudden forces that produce traction or torsion account for the majority of civilian injuries. These injuries will generally produce an elevated flap of intima or an intramural hematoma. It is important to recognize that flow past these injured areas may be present initially but diminishes as the lumen narrows. It is also possible that an injured artery after initially going into spasm may produce catastrophic hemorrhage after the spasm is relieved. Thrombosis may occur within minutes or hours of an injury or may be a later manifestation, depending on such factors as the degree of underlying atherosclerosis or associated venous injury.

Vascular injuries can be associated with fractures in areas where the vessels are close to the osseous structures or are held in a fixed position by muscles, ligaments, or adjacent bones. The femoral artery is vulnerable to injury along the entire femoral shaft. After it courses through the adductor canal, the popliteal artery and veins traverse the posterior surface of the knee joint capsule and are tethered in position by the tendinous hiatus of the adductor magnus superiorly and the soleus tendon insertion and interosseous membrane inferiorly. It is for this reason that posterior dislocation of the knee and fractures involving the femoral condyles or tibial plateaus carry a high risk of vascular injury, particularly if there is posterior fragment displacement. The collateral geniculate branches are not well protected by soft tissue and frequently are also injured or unable to compensate for sudden interruption of flow through the main channel. Popliteal artery injury is common in high-velocity dislocations. Angiography is indicated in known or suspected peripheral vascular injury when the injury's location is not certain, when multiple injury sites may be present, when the diagnosis requires confirmation, or when transcatheter treatment may be the therapy of choice. If there is any doubt or suspicion, prompt angiography should be considered. Arteriograms can be helpful but should not delay operative treatment of obvious arterial injuries (244).

In Hoover's (245) series of popliteal artery injuries accompanying closed trauma to the knee, 75% went on to amputation despite surgical intervention, and only one patient's foot regained full viability and usefulness. Fortunately, injuries to the popliteal artery, the tibial-peroneal trunk, or the trifurcation occur in less than 3% of all tibial fractures. Posterior dislocations of the knee may result in an injury to the popliteal artery. Two large studies, one by Dennis et al (246) and the other by Kendall et al (247), demonstrated a relatively low incidence of surgical repair of 5.4% to 16.2%. These two studies have reflected a definite lower tendency toward an operative approach to nonocclusive lesions such as an intimal defect or narrowing of the popliteal artery.

A study from a level I trauma center assessing popliteal artery injuries found the amputation rate as high as 19% (248). The single most important factor determining the ultimate fate of the limb with vascular compromise is the duration of limb ischemia. A warm limb ischemic time of less than 6 hours was associated with an amputation rate of 6.7% compared with 33% in limbs with warm ischemic times of more than 6 hours in one recent series (249). Shock is also important in the outcome of the ischemic limb, as hypotension and distal vasoconstriction predispose to early soft tissue necrosis (249). A large study involving 550 patients with 641 lower-limb arterial injuries found that lower-limb arterial injuries carry a high amputation rate. Stab injuries are the least likely to lead to amputation, whereas high-velocity firearm injuries are the most likely to do so.

There is a distinct difference between the upper extremity and lower extremity in regard to collateral circulation. In the upper extremity, the collateral circulation is normally more extensive than in the lower, so that damage to a major upper extremity artery is less likely to lead to gangrene and amputation. It is interesting to note that numerous reports of successful brachial artery ligation have been recorded in the earlier literature, but most investigators today advocate vascular repair whenever possible for injuries that occur at this level. Injuries to numerous other arteries, including the thyrocervical trunk, subscapular, radial, ulnar, obturator, hypogastric, posterior tibial, and dorsalis pedis have been reported sporadically in conjunction with skeletal trauma. Their complications tend to be hemorrhagic rather than ischemic, because parallel patent collateral arteries are usually present. Also, they are frequently recognized and treated early, and therefore the results are often excellent. The nature of the arterial injury is frequently variable and may occur as an immediate or as a late complication of a bone or joint injury.

There are very few vessels that cannot be ligated in extremis, at varying risk to life and limb. Although not routinely recommended, if necessary, the common and external carotid, subclavian, axillary and internal iliac arteries can be ligated with few consequences. Ligation of the internal carotid artery carries a 10% to 20% risk of stroke. Ligation of the external iliac artery, common femoral or superficial femoral artery has a significant risk of critical limb ischemia after ligation. Ischemia is more likely if there is significant soft tissue injury and destruction of supporting collateral circulation. Arteries of the celiac axis can be ligated but ligating the superior or inferior mesenteric artery will almost inevitably lead to gut necrosis in the young trauma patient. Arterial defects may be repaired by lateral arteriorrhaphy, patch angioplasty, direct end-to-end anastomosis, interposition grafts, or arterial bypass. Clear communication should be established between the orthopaedic surgeons and their vascular colleagues in treating peripheral vascular injuries. The vascular interventions can range from operative visualization of normal vascular anatomy for diagnostic purposes to reconstructing entire segments of injured vessels. If the injured vessel is less than 2 cm, primary anastomosis can be performed. The ends of a transected artery usually retract. If the ends can be approximated without tension, a direct end-to-end anastomosis repair can be employed. Mobilization of the two ends may be necessary and aided by division of minor arterial branches. Where approximation of the vessels is not possible, a reversed vein graft, or synthetic graft is used to repair the defect. If there is a concomitant vein injury, it should usually be repaired first, if possible, to avoid low-flow thrombosis of the arterial repair. If the patient's condition and hemodynamic status allow prolonged operative intervention, replacing an injured peripheral arterial segment is best accomplished with autologous vein. Polytetrafluoroethylene can be used in some situations. It has been successfully used in contaminated fields with a low infection rate (250) for both venous and arterial reconstruction. In many trauma centers, conventional angiography and potential transcatheter embolization are used in patients with pelvic trauma who continue to hemorrhage despite external fixation and who already have undergone an abdominal exploration if an associated solid organ injury is known (251). In other trauma centers, angiography may be obtained before external fixation or surgical abdominal exploration if significant hemorrhage is present, even in unstable patients (252). Angiography remains the gold-standard investigation for the further investigation and delineation of vascular injury.

Fasciotomy should be performed if the muscular compartments are considered tight or in cases of delayed repair, but should not be performed routinely (249). Orthopaedic stabilization of fractures using external fixators is appropriate in cases of combined vascular injury and long bone fracture with prolonged duration of ischemia, major soft-tissue loss, or significant wound contamination. Factors associated with amputation are the severity of shock and soft-tissue injury ($p < 0.01$) and tibial artery injury compared with more proximal injury (253).

Arteriovenous fistulas may occur and require proper reconstruction. False aneurysms may also develop during the treatment course of a patient with an arterial injury. Angiographic embolization has been a very valuable method for managing this type of complication. The clinician must be aware of this possibility when a large mass is in an extremity after a significant injury. The presence of a thrill and bruit over the injury site should alert the examiner to consider the existence of arteriovenous fistulas. The simple technique of listening with a stethoscope over a soft tissue mass can identify a bruit, which is frequently present with an arteriovenous fistula. This possibility must be kept in mind with all gunshot-type injuries associated with fractures. Angiography is a reliable diagnostic tool, and should be used in all vitally stable patients. Surgical or nonsurgical closure of arteriovenous fistulas will prevent local and systemic complications that might be irreversible in long-standing fistulas (254).

Venous Injuries

Isolated venous injuries are not commonly associated with skeletal trauma except in the pelvis. In contrast, the combination of venous and arterial disruption after skeletal trauma is common and occurs more frequently than is appreciated. The exact incidence of this occurrence varies, but is directly related to the anatomic relationships of the artery and the vein. Rich et al (249), reviewing a series of 1,000 major arterial injuries occurring in Vietnam, found the overall incidence of concomitant venous injuries was 37.7%; but with popliteal artery injuries, the incidence rose to 58.7%. In general, these injuries are lacerations, often multiple, producing hematomas. One of the side effects of venous injuries is that thrombosis may follow as a delayed event. If this occurs, the hemodynamic and hydrostatic effects may be significant, particularly after attempted arterial repair, because improved arterial inflow may then only contribute to hematoma formation, distal edema, and progressive tissue destruction. It has been shown that venous occlusion in the groin area results in a significant adverse effect on femoral arterial inflow (255). There has been an increased awareness of the detrimental effects of popliteal venous ligation regarding tissue viability of the lower extremity; for this reason, there has been an increased incidence of attempted repair of this structure in the lower extremities (256). This is not to state that the repaired veins remain open, as it has been shown that close to 60% of interpositional grafts and greater than 20% of simple venous direct repairs are temporarily occluded in the postoperative period (257). Despite this finding, it is still felt that venous injuries in the groin or in the popliteal area require repair rather than ligation if the patient is stable and does not have any associated life-threatening problems. Obviously, if the patient has a life-threatening problem, it is appropriate to consider venous ligation in these areas, as since prolonged anesthesia is required for repair.

In patients who present with a cold pulseless extremity, it is vitally important to re-establish the arterial inflow as soon as possible. The guideline that has been useful in managing patients with this type of problem is the general dictum that muscle can survive up until 6 hours of ischemia (258). After that, the chances of survival are dramatically diminished. Re-establishing blood flow may be accomplished either by a temporary intraluminal vascular shunt or by a formal repair.

Amputation

An early or primary amputation may be indicated in a severely damaged extremity, particularly with massive soft tissue loss and significant bone destruction. This is a clinical decision that the attending surgeon will make when the patient is brought to the operating room for initial treatment of the severe injury. Guidelines for managing the mangled extremity have been outlined in other chapters. This type of treatment requires a thorough discussion with the patient and family before any attempted surgical treatment of a severely damaged extremity. It is strongly advised that the possibility of amputation is documented in the surgery consent form that the patient signs. Preoperative and intraoperative photographs are obtained to document the severity of the injury and the fact that an amputation was the treatment of choice. In general, surgeons strongly lean toward attempting to save a limb rather than to consider an amputation. This tendency is dangerous, however, when the patient's life may be at stake if inappropriate salvage techniques are attempted and the patient subsequently experiences complications such as muscle death and breakdown followed by renal shutdown and death. The vast majority of patients requiring amputation have usually sustained significant open injuries either in military combat or in industrial, farm, or vehicular accidents. To achieve a proper amputation, several operations may be required to obtain proper bone length and viable muscle with a useful stump for prosthetic application. Early amputation may also be indicated when there is a failure of orthopaedic, vascular, or peripheral nerve reconstruction. Waddell and Lenczner (259) have shown that most clinical indications for delayed amputation are present within 2 to 10 days after the initial injury. Patients are very resistant to the idea of amputation, which accounts for the majority of cases that are delayed beyond this relatively short time interval. Fortunately, this clinical situation occurs in less than 20% of cases during the management of civilian injuries.

Compartment Syndrome

Compartment syndrome is a painful, limb- and life-threatening condition due to prolonged interruption of blood flow to a limb, and if left untreated, may lead to cellular ischemia and activation of cellular and humoral inflammatory responses. Increased pressure in a tight osteofascial compartment, such as the fascial compartments of the lower limb above capillary and venous pressure, can cause vascular stasis, cellular ischemia, and death. It results when perfusion pressure falls below tissue pressure in a closed anatomic space. Compartment syndrome is not confined to the distal lower extremity and can occur in the thigh, buttock, and forearm. Soft tissue injury and muscle necrosis can be sufficient to produce acute compartment syndrome in the absence of a fracture (260).

Clinically, there is intense, disproportionate pain in the limb, worsened by passive flexion pressures. The classic sign of acute compartment syndrome is pain occurring in an extremity after an injury, especially when the muscle is stretched. Often, the patient complains of severe pain out of proportion to examination and a burning sensation or tightness. The traditional five Ps (pain, paraesthesia, pallor, pulselessness, paralysis) should be observed with caution. Pain and paraesthesia are the reliable signs (261). Patients who are unconscious have spinal cord injury or epidural anesthesia should be monitored cautiously, as the early, reversible signs of compartment syndrome may be lost, and diagnosis relies on a high index of suspicion and measurement of compartment pressure. Intracompartmental pressure monitoring should be considered for an early diagnosis of acute compartment syndrome in uncooperative, polytraumatized patients with tibial shaft fractures (262). In young children, pain in an injured extremity should be interpreted carefully due to inability to gather a detailed history. Compartment syndrome has been reported in children after closed reduction and intramedullary fixation and after elective ulnar-shortening osteotomies (263). High suspicion shall be maintained while monitoring pain in an injured extremity. Extra vigilance with the use of patient-controlled analgesia (PCA) is needed in patients with intramedullary nailing following tibial shaft fractures as the diagnosis could be delayed, leading to lasting sequelae secondary to delayed decompression (264).

Early diagnosis is extremely important because of irreversible tissue injury approximately 6 hours after ischemia onset. Early fasciotomy not only improves patient outcome, but is also associated with decreased indemnity risk (265). The aphorism, "If you think about doing a fasciotomy, you probably should do one" still holds true. Morbidity from fasciotomy is minimal and the procedure should be performed as soon as possible (266). Fasciotomy is associated with a minor risk of wound infection, but limb loss and death result from persisting ischemia, muscle necrosis, and multiorgan failure, not from infected fasciotomy wounds (267). In delayed cases, routine fasciotomy may not be successful (268).

If confirmation of the diagnosis is required, compartment pressure readings may be obtained (269). Many surgeon use 30 mm Hg as a cutoff mark for performing fasciotomy. The wick catheter technique is capable of important clinical applications in diagnosing and treating acute and chronic compartment syndromes (270). Clinically, the side-ported needle or the slit catheter can be used to obtain accurate measurements of compartment pressure. A handheld measuring instrument such as the slit catheter is now an option. Under local anesthesia, the catheter is inserted into the appropriate compartment, and the pressure is recorded. Development of a compartment syndrome depends not only on intracompartment pressure but also on systemic blood pressure. Values that are 10 to 30 mm Hg less than the diastolic blood pressure indicate a possible compartment pressure problem, although the specific pressure limits have been a topic of considerable discussion in the medical literature (271). A difference of less than 30 mm Hg between the diastolic and tissue pressures has been validated clinically, and it is recommended that at this level, serious consideration should be given to decompression of the affected compartments. Use of this pressure threshold with compartment monitoring has been shown to decrease the delay to fasciotomy by 50 % and significantly reduce the late complications of acute compartment syndrome (272).

Compartment pressure measurements should be performed at the level of the fracture as well as at locations proximal and distal to the zone of the fracture to determine the highest tissue pressure's location. In a study on closed tibial fractures, the peak pressure was usually found at the level of the fracture and was always located within 5 cm of the fracture (258,273). Clinical vigilance still forms the mainstay in detecting compartment syndrome (CS), and measured tests are more likely to confirm clinical diagnosis. Further information on compartment syndrome is found in Chapter 13.

Other Modalities

Muscle oxyhemoglobin level measured by using near-infrared wavelength reflection spectroscopy strongly reflects compartment pressure, perfusion pressure, and loss of dorsiflexion twitch. Currently available portable near-infrared devices may provide the benefit of continuous, noninvasive monitoring for CS. Further studies to determine the role of this technology in the detection of compartmental syndrome are warranted (273). MR imaging with a variety of pulse sequences including fat suppression, magnetization transfer imaging, and IV gadopentetate dimeglumine administration can help make the diagnosis of a manifest compartment syndrome in clinically ambiguous cases. It visualizes the affected compartments and allows the surgeon to selectively split the fascial spaces (274). Ultrasound aids in evaluating arterial flow as well as in visualizing any deep venous thrombosis. The pulsed-phase locked loop ultrasonic device may be used as a low-cost, portable and noninvasive alternative to current methods for diagnosing acute compartment syndrome. It measures submicrometer displacements of the fascial walls. These displacements occur due to muscle compartment volume expansion of the lower leg and are related to changes in intramuscular pressure (IMP). In the cadaveric tests, the pulse-phase locked loop detected changes in compartment diameter resulting from IMP changes of 1 mm Hg and from infusions of 0.25 mL saline increments (275).

NERVE INJURIES

Trauma to peripheral nerves is relatively common, and most damage results from blunt trauma and penetrating missiles (276). Fortunately, in the vast majority of cases, the nerve is not divided. Injury to the nerve results in damage to the involved nerve cells, connective tissue elements, and the related lymphatics and blood vessels.

The functional unit of the nerve is a neuron. The neurons are constant after birth, and they cannot be replaced after injury. Injury to a peripheral nerve stimulates an initiation of a sequence of biochemical and morphologic alterations. After injury, the nerve cell body size enlarges for 10 to 20 days. This "hypertrophy" is visible for the course of the regenerative process, and "atrophy" back to normal size occurs once healing is complete. Hemorrhage and edema are apparent immediately at the severed ends. The swelling and tissue constituents form a clot that is evident for 7 to 10 days (277,278).

In either case, within 24 to 72 hours, neurofibrillar degeneration occurs for a minimum of two to three nodes of Ranvier proximal to the point of injury. The myelin sheath loses its layered appearance, macrophage invasion begins to clear and remove degenerated myelin from the damaged nerve tissue, and Schwann cells respond vigorously and proliferate to form dense cords along the axis of the now-digested axoplasm. Mesenchymal cells proliferate in response to the inflammatory process and stimulate collagen deposition at the end of the proximal stump. This, in conjunction with fibrin remnants from the initial hemorrhage, may lead to form a neuroma (277,279). Approximately 2 to 20 days after injury, axoplasmic regeneration may begin. At the site of injury, cellular proliferation of Schwann cells has already commenced. The Schwann cell outgrowth attempts to connect the proximal stump with the Schwann cell elements of the distal nerve stump. The Schwann cell attempts to grow concurrently with the axoplasm, thus providing a framework for axonal growth (277,278). If surgical realignment or nerve stump approximation does not occur, the migration axoplasm may form a neuroma, a meshwork of organized clot elements, mainly fibrin strands, that provides an errant scaffolding framework for axonal migration. As the Schwann cells migrate distally, their pathway is deviated to align with the random fibrin clot at the nerve stump. The regenerating axons follow the Schwann tubules and continue the random growth pattern. Axoplasm migration in this disorganized tissue produces multifilamentous branching that attempts to seek the distal nerve stump (278).

Extraneural connective tissue may also produce ingrowth to the injury site and can distort and block the path of axon migration. In contrast, surgical repair of peripheral nerve injury permits smooth, unbranched axoplasmic migration into the distal stump. It is hypothesized that axoplasmic branching attempts to compensate for the neuroma roadblock to ensure axonal migration into the distal stump (280,281).

Pathophysiology and Classification of Nerve Injury

There is no single classification system that can describe all the variations of nerve injury. In 1943, Seddon introduced a nerve injury classification based on three main types of nerve fiber injury and whether there is continuity of the nerve. The three types are neurapraxia, axonotmesis, and neurotmesis (282).

Neurapraxia

In this case, there is an interruption in conduction of the impulse down the nerve fiber, and recovery takes place without wallerian degeneration. Neurapraxia is the mildest form of nerve injury. It is probably a biochemical lesion caused by concussion or shock-like injuries to the fiber. In the case of the role nerve, neurapraxia is brought about by compression or relatively mild, blunt blows, including some low-velocity missile injuries close to the nerve. There is a temporary loss of function, which is reversible within hours to months of the injury (the average time is 6 to 8 weeks). There is frequently greater involvement of motor than sensory function, and autonomic function is retained.

Axonotmesis

Axonotmesis involves loss of the relative continuity of the axon and myelin, but preservation of the nerve's connective tissue framework (the encapsulating tissue, the epineurium, and perineurium) are preserved. Because axonal continuity is lost, wallerian degeneration occurs. Electromyography performed 2 to 3 weeks later shows fibrillations and denervation potentials in musculature distal to the injury site. There is usually an element of retrograde proximal degeneration of the axon; regeneration to occur, this loss must first be overcome. The regeneration fibers must cross the injury site, and regeneration through the proximal or retrograde area of degeneration may require several weeks. The neural growth then progresses down to the distal site, such as the wrist or hand. Proximal lesions may grow distally as fast as 2 to 3 mm per day, and distal lesions may grow as slowly as 1.5 mm per day.

Neurotmesis

Neurotmesis is the more severe lesion with little potential of recovering and usually occurs on severe contusion, stretch, or complete laceration. The axon and the encapsulating connective tissue lose their continuity. The last (extreme) degree of neurotmesis is transsection, but most neurotmetic injuries do not produce gross loss of nerve continuity, but rather internal disruption of the nerve's architecture sufficient to involve perineurium and endoneurium as well as axons and their covering. Denervation changes recorded by electromyography are the same as those seen with axonotmetic injury. There is a complete loss of motor, sensory, and autonomic function. If the nerve loss has been completely divided, axonal regeneration causes a neuroma to form in the proximal stump.

Nerve Healing and Reconstruction

A peripheral nerve regenerates at a rate of approximately 1 mm per day (283). At the beginning stage of regeneration, the proximal axon stump sprouts buds that comprise the nerve growth cone (284). Axonal regeneration is guided toward the distal end of the nerve by a gradient of diffusible chemical substances by a process called *neurotropism* (284). The axonal buds preferentially move toward neural tissue, but cannot differentiate between sensory or motor fascicles. The distal fascicle's size appears to be the most significant factor in determining the regenerating growth cone's target (284). Misdirected axonal buds may result in mismatched nerve connections. Aberrant motor nerve innervations can cause abnormal movements. Abnormal sensory nerve innervations can cause misperception of the location of touch or pain (285). Motor endplates must be reinnervated within 18 months of trauma for function to be preserved (286). Preventing motor endplate degradation is important to ensure motor functionality after regeneration is complete (287).

Nerve Reconstruction

Sharp lacerations without loss of nerve substance or partial lacerations are fixed by primary nerve repair. Primary repair is direct suturing of the nerve immediately after injury. The repair can be carried out by epineurial repair, in which the separated nerve endings are sutured together using a microsuture (288) (usually 8–0 or 10–0 Ethicon). Pure sensory or motor nerves yield better results when this repair technique is used (284,288). In a crushing nerve injury, group fascicular repair is indicated. In crush nerve injuries or delayed repair, group fascicular repair improves fascicular alignment. Individual fascicle repair is not practiced widely because it is technically difficult (284). During secondary nerve repairs, bones can be shortened to add length to a nerve. Nerve transposition across a flexed joint (e.g., the ulnar nerve in the elbow) is another strategy for gauging nerve length in secondary repairs (284). These techniques can gain as much as an approximate 10% increase in available nerve length (284), but within 3 weeks after injury, a nerve may lose as much as 8% of its length (284). Many surgeons prefer delayed suture to primary suture because this method allows the wound to heal, and it decreases the risk of infection. Neurolysis is performed on intraneural and extraneural scar tissue to release regenerating nerve fibers in the hope of improving functional recovery (287). Nerve grafting is carried out if nerve length is lost. Sural nerve is a standard nerve autograft and is favorable due to the ease in harvesting it and the ratio of axons to the epineurium (284). Results from autograft use are slightly more favorable than allograft use (284). Artificial conduits have not proven to be as successful as conventional nerve autografts (284). Brain-derived neurotrophic factor and collagen tubulization have been used in an attempt to create a reliable artificial conduit for axonal regeneration (289).

Iatrogenic Nerve Injury

Inadvertent nerve damage is one of the most dreaded complications of surgery. Patients should be warned of the possibility of nerve injury during discussion of informed consent. Nerve injury may be transient and reversible or permanent. Thorough knowledge of the anatomy, with special attention to known danger zones, is required to anticipate vital structures as they are approached. Effects of local anesthesia may result in temporary sensory or motor nerve paralysis; these conditions resolve within 1 day. Neurapraxia refers to a deficit caused by inadvertent pressure or tension during surgery and may result in sensory or motor deficits, but generally resolves within months.

Complications of Nerve Injury

Following acute nerve injury, a variety of pain syndromes can develop (290). Painful neuromas and entrapment syndromes can arise at the injury site and can cause extreme local tenderness and pain. The presence of neuroma formation indicates axonotmesis or neurotmesis. The shape and location of the neuroma may provide an estimation of the prognosis. A fusiform neuroma indicates integrity of some fascicles in the area of injury. Location of the neuroma within the nerve trunk may indicate the lesion's severity. Lateral neuromas suggest partial neurotmesis with functional tissue remaining. If the injury does not exceed 50% of the width of the nerve trunk, spontaneous recovery may occur without surgical intervention. If greater than 50% involvement is present, however, resection and neurorrhaphy is indicated. Bulbous and dumbbell-shaped neuromas suggest widespread neurotmesis with poor prognosis for spontaneous recovery. Excision of the neuroma and neurorrhaphy is indicated in these cases (290–292).

In 1872, Mitchell coined the term *phantom limb* to describe the phenomena in which amputees continue to report a sensory awareness of a limb that has been amputated (293). The term *phantom limb pain* is now commonly used to describe pains that are referred to the phantom limb. The idea that pain can be referred to a phantom limb clearly implies that central neural mechanisms are involved. Unlike the peripheral theories of referred pain, there is absolutely no opportunity for phantom limb pain to result from a branching of nerves from an injured region to the area of reference.

It has been reported that as many as 79% of amputees describe their phantom pains as similar to pains felt in the limb before amputation (294). Reports of pain memories in phantom limbs appear to be less common when there has been a discontinuity, or a pain-free interval, between the experience of pain and the amputation. This may explain why relief of preamputation pain by continuous epidural block for 3 days prior to amputation (295), as well as after amputation (296), decreases the incidence of phantom limb pain 6 months later. Furthermore, there appears to be a higher probability that pain will persist in the phantom limb if pain is experienced at or near the time of amputation (294), or if preamputation pain is very intense or of long duration (297).

After a cutaneous injury, both the injured skin and the uninjured skin adjacent to the injury become more sensitive to specific types of sensory stimulation. In particular, the injured skin becomes more sensitive to nonnoxious heating or stroking (thermal and mechanical allodynia), as well as to noxious heating or punctate stimulation (thermal and mechanical hyperalgesia). In contrast to the injured skin, the adjacent uninjured skin appears to become more sensitive to mechanical (but not thermal) stimuli with hyperalgesia to punctate stimulation spreading farther and lasting much longer (13 to 24 hours) than allodynia to stroking (1 to 2 hours) (298).

First described by Martyn (299), referred pain is a condition in which pain is not localized within the injured region, but at an adjacent or distant site. Referred pains often occur following injury of deep tissue such as muscle, joints, or viscera. It has been shown that the distribution of referred pain increases with the intensity (300) and duration (301) of the noxious stimulation from the injured deep tissue.

COMPLEX REGIONAL PAIN SYNDROMES

Historical Review

The earliest description of severe burning pain after peripheral nerve injury is that by the surgeon Ambroise Paré in the 17th century (302). King Charles IX, ill with smallpox, was bled by inducing a lancet wound to the arm. After this therapy, the king suffered from persistent pain, muscle contracture, and an inability to flex or extend his arm. Paré was called on to treat the king, whose symptoms finally disappeared. In 1872, Weir Mitchell (293) described the term *causalgia*—the severe burning pain, allodynia, and autonomic changes in an extremity. Causalgia occurred after nerve injury endured by Civil War soldiers as a result of gunshot wounds. Soon, similar symptoms were being noted in patients after trauma or surgery in nonmilitary patients, many of whom had no obvious nerve injury. In 1900, Paul Sudeck described regional demineralization accompanying posttraumatic pain (303). In 1916, Leriche (304) noticed improvement in causalgia patients after sympathectomy and proposed that causalgia was caused by excessive activity of the sympathetic nervous system (SNS). He also noted that sympathectomy could effect permanent relief. In 1946, Evans introduced the term *reflex sympathetic dystrophy* (305). In 1994, the International Association for the Study of Pain renamed reflex sympathetic dystrophy as *complex regional pain syndrome* (CRPS I) and causalgia as CRPS II to adopt a consensus terminology and to create uniform diagnostic criteria (306).

A number of clinical syndromes appear under CRPS, including reflex sympathetic dystrophy, algodystrophy, Sudeck's atrophy, shoulder-hand syndrome, and causalgia. *Complex* denotes the varied and dynamic nature of the clinical presentation, both within a single individual over time and among individuals with seemingly similar disorders (306). It also indicates the features of inflammation, autonomic, cutaneous, motor, and dystrophic changes that distinguish this from other forms of neuropathic pain. *Regional*, as in the wider distribution of symptoms and findings beyond the area of the original lesion, is a hallmark of these disorders. Such symptoms and signs usually affect the distal part of a limb, but can occasionally involve discrete regions or spread to other body areas. Pain is the sine qua non for the CRPS, particularly pain that is disproportionate to the inciting event. This is not just burning pain, but includes spontaneous pain and thermal or mechanically induced allodynia. As a syndrome, the constellation of symptoms and signs of CRPS represents a series of correlated events that are sufficient to be designated as a distinctive entity, even though it is not known what constitutes each of these events or which are essential, nor the nature of the pathologic changes that ensue.

According to the International Association for the Study of Pain, CRPS I occurs without a known nerve lesion, while CRPS II comprises similar symptoms after an identifiable nerve lesion. Although Diagnostic Criterion I is an "initiating noxious event," usually trauma or surgery, identical clinical problems occur occasionally without evidence of trauma (306). It is likely that these patients have had an internal nonobvious trauma, such as tissue infarction. Criterion II states that there must be "hyperalgesia, continuing pain, or allodynia, with which the pain is disproportionate to any inciting event." Criterion III requires "evidence at some time of edema, changes in skin blood flow, or abnormal sudomotor activity in the region of the pain." Criterion IV requires absence of an alternative explanation for the symptoms. The only additional criterion for CRPS II is the presence of a known nerve injury.

Pathophysiology and Autonomic Dysfunction

The pathogenesis of CRPS has been the subject of much attention (306). Many theories have been proposed to explain this disease, although none has proved conclusive. It is quite possible that the true poorly understood mechanism is a combination of several of the current theories. The autonomic nervous system appears to be involved, although there is no scientific proof of such involvement. It is hypothesized that the fundamental abnormality in type I CRPS is an ongoing nociceptor input that maintains the central state of hyperexcitability for prolonged periods (307,308). Thus, the principle difference between sympathetically maintained pain and sympathetically independent pain appears to be the mechanism of generation and maintenance of the nociceptor input to the spinal cord. In sympathetically maintained pain, the nociceptor input is maintained by an interaction between primary afferents and sympathetic efferents through an alpha-adrenergic mechanism (309). In sympathetically independent pain, however, the maintaining nociceptor input arises from other causes, such as peripheral nerve stimulation (e.g., a neuroma). Consequently, both peripheral and central mechanisms play roles in the syndrome's pathophysiology. In addition, studies involving several animal models of nerve injury have shown an interaction between primary afferents and sympathetic efferents (308,310).

By definition, sympathetically maintained pain is eliminated by an anesthetic blockade of the sympathetic efferents that serve the painful area (308,311).

Central Nervous System Abnormalities

Sympathetic denervation and denervation hypersensitivity cannot completely explain the vasomotor and sudomotor abnormalities. First, in CRPS I, there is no overt nerve lesion (312). Second, in CRPS II, the autonomic symptoms spread beyond the territory of the lesioned nerve. A continuous functional inhibition of vasoconstrictor activity induced by central mechanisms might also lead to secondary end-organ supersensitivity (decentralization supersensitivity) in the absence of structural damage to sympathetic fibers (313).

Inflammation

The role of inflammation and the immune system (314,315) is not clear in the available research. Some of the features of CRPS (e.g., vasomotor abnormalities, swelling, and pain) have been attributed to sympathetic dysfunction and could be explained by inflammation without the requirement for a sympathetic contribution. Particularly in its early phase, it is quite likely that there is an inflammatory component to CRPS I (316,317). Corticosteroids have been shown to be beneficial, which is in keeping with this idea (318). In addition, scintigraphy using radio-labeled immunoglobulins shows extensive plasma extravasation in patients with acute CRPS I (319). Analysis of joint fluid and synovial biopsies in patients with CRPS has shown an increase in protein concentration, synovial hypervascularity, and neutrophil infiltration (320,321). As a result, the weight of evidence does indicate that inflammatory processes are involved in the pathogenesis of early CRPS.

Classification

Pain syndromes resulting from a trivial injury such as a fracture, sprain, or burns are referred to as *CRPS I* (formerly reflex sympathetic dystrophy [RSD]). Reflex sympathetic dystrophy is defined as a pain syndrome in which the pain is accompanied by loss of function and evidence of autonomic dysfunction (322). Syndromes caused by frank nerve damage (caused by crush injuries, gunshot wounds, or laceration injuries) are termed *CRPS II* (formerly *causalgia*). Collectively, these syndromes can be considered on a continuum of SNS dysfunction, as outlined by Vernon (323). Viewed as such, causalgia would be found at one end of the continuum, representing frank nerve damage with little supposed intervertebral dysfunction, with reflex sympathetic dysfunction at the opposite end, representing little nerve damage, but possible intervertebral dysfunction.

Clinical Signs and Symptoms

The signs and symptoms of CRPS compose a triad of pain, vasomotor changes, and trophic changes (summarized in Table 18-5). Symptoms present generally within 3 weeks to 6 months of the initial injury (324). The initial insult is usually a traumatic injury (crush injury, laceration for CRPS II) or significant noxious event (burn, blunt trauma, sprain for CRPS I). Additional triggers that may cause CRPS I can include stroke, shingles, surgery, occupational injury, or medical conditions such as vascular disease, infection, or myocardial infarction (325,326). The initial injury is thought to cause a reactive vasomotor reflex spasm, followed by a loss of vascular tone, which leads to vasodilation and rapid bone resorption (327). Subsequent decreased mobility leads to decreased circulation, which ultimately causes fibrosis and shortening of involved ligaments (20).

TABLE 18-5 Signs and Symptoms of the Complex Regional Pain Syndromes

Category/System	Common Signs and Symptoms
Autonomic	Bilateral temperature difference on palpation Skin discoloration Subcutaneous thickening Peripheral edema
Sensory	Increased sensitivity to pin-prick, light touch, temperature Muscle belly tenderness Hyperalgesia over bony prominences
Motor	Muscle atrophy and weakness Joint stiffness Muscle contractures Mechanical allodynia
Radiologic	Osteopenia revealed by plain films/ nucleotide bone scans

Clinical Course

The clinical course of CRPS is divided into three stages, although the validity of assigning fixed stages of symptom progression has been questioned. Staging is based on both the severity and chronologic development of symptoms. Stage I is the early, mild stage; stage II, moderate; and stage III, severe.

Stage I CRPS

Stage I CRPS is characterized by mild symptoms and begins within days or weeks of the precipitating injury. Sharp, burning pain, swelling, and dysfunction are localized, and although mild in comparison to the later stages of CRPS, the symptoms are more serious than would normally be expected for the injury. This exaggerated response is a key diagnostic factor when dealing with possible cases of CRPS. Allodynia is generally absent during stage I (256), although hyperesthesia is present, and the limb is relatively immobile and sensitive. Stage I (acute) may last up to 3 months.

Stage II CRPS

Stage II is marked by increasing dysfunction and symptom severity and is defined by the increased chronicity of the symptoms. Pain persists and increases in severity, as does sensitivity. Changes to the distal portions of the affected limb reflect the growing autonomic dysfunction. The limb is increasingly moist and cold, edema increases, and the skin becomes mottled. Continued immobilization leads to increasing joint stiffness, and myofascial contractures are possible (323). CRPS at stage II may respond to treatment, but often persists for several months. Stage II (dystrophic) can last 3 to 12 months.

Stage III CRPS

Stage III is the most severe stage, where symptoms that have developed during stage II reach a level of near intolerance. Stage III (atrophic) occurs from 1 year on. Severe aching and throbbing pain is present, and the limb is effectively immobilized and functionally useless. Chronic autonomic dysfunction leads to dystrophic changes to skin, muscle tissue, and bone tissue. Halted growth of nails and hair accompanies dystrophic changes to the skin, muscles become atrophied, and regional osteoporosis is observed on plain films (328) and bone scans (326). At this stage, the symptoms are unresponsive to treatment, and the condition is considered permanent.

Diagnosis

CRPS can range from minor involvement including one or more fingers to involvement of the entire extremity presenting with wide variation of pain and dysfunction. Due to the similarities between CRPS symptoms and those found in many acute traumatic injuries such as sprains or fractures, diagnosing CRPS is difficult. Important information can be gained from physical examination, bone scanning, and specific neural blockade tests that can aid in the diagnosis of CRPS. As with most conditions, several differential diagnoses must be considered.

There are three prerequisites underlying the development of CRPS that are required for diagnosis: a persistent lesion or injury, a predisposing constitution and an abnormal sympathetic reflex arc (329,330).

CRPS I can be seen after a wide range of injuries and operations. The primary etiological factor associated with the expression of CRPS I is trauma (57.4%), surgery (22.9%), and overuse syndromes (19.7%) (329). CRPS I has been associated with diseases such as stroke and diabetes mellitus. Constitutional traits and susceptible personality makes the appearance of these disorders more likely after injury (322,331). Some traits associated with CRPS include anxiety, dependency, insecurity, an overpowering sense of dissatisfaction, and other personality disturbances (322,331).

Initially, other conditions should be ruled out, and thereafter, a presumptive diagnosis can be made on the presence of some or all signs and symptoms. The exact diagnostic criterion remains controversial. Today, diagnosis of CRPS I takes into consideration the criteria established in the consensus report of an ad hoc committee of the American Association for Hand Surgery on the definition of RSD syndrome, as well as the criteria outlined by Kozin (325). Diagnostic criteria include persistent diffuse pain as well as the loss of hand function and autonomic dysfunction. Evidence of autonomic dysfunction can be based on changes in skin and/or soft tissue blood flow, as reflected by an increase or decrease in temperature and sweating. CRPS I can be confirmed if interruption of the sympathetic reflex produces relief of symptoms; however, failure of relief of sympathetic blockade does not rule out the condition. CRPS should not be excluded until after at least three or more blocks have been carried out with no amelioration of the symptoms (329).

Physical Examination

Clinical signs and symptoms reflect the wide spectrum of symptoms that are observed in CRPS patients. Pain can be described as burning, throbbing, shooting, or aching. Physical examination may reveal skin discoloration, edema, and subcutaneous thickening. Palpation may reveal temperature differences between the affected and unaffected limbs. In addition, temperature readings may be taken using thermistors or thermography (332). Sensory dysfunction can be observed during physical examination. Light touch, pinprick, and temperature evaluation can elicit and illustrate morbidity. Deep palpation can show tenderness of muscle groups, and palpation over bony prominences can help evaluate the presence and severity of hyperalgesia. In addition, atrophy of hair, skin, and nails can be seen.

Psychological Factors

Psychological and social factors are readily recognized issues in analyzing the disorder. In patients with either CRPS I or II, there is a significant amount of major psychiatric comorbidity. Major depressive disorder and personality abnormalities are regularly found (327,333).

Radiography

Radiography has played a role in diagnosing this condition since Sudeck described osteoporosis as part of the atrophic phase of RSD; however, there is also controversy regarding the radiographic findings in RSD (334). Radiological evaluation is generally performed on suspected CRPS patients, and plain films may show osteopenia in the affected limb. It has been reported that visible osteopenia may not be detectable until 2 to 4 weeks after the onset of symptoms (335). The osteopenia is greater than would be expected by disuse alone (327). Despite a clear clinical diagnosis of CRPS, up to one-third of patients have normal, plain radiographs (336). In a prospective study of 60 patients with tibial fractures, 18 patients developed reflex sympathetic dystrophy at the time of bone union. The degree of bone loss (osteopenia) was independent of the type of management and of the time to fracture union (337).

Bone Scans

Nucleotide bone scans or scintigraphy has become the preferred diagnostic test to demonstrate dystrophic changes in bone, where increased uptake on the affected side indicates CRPS-induced osteopenia. Scintigraphic patterns of uptake on a three-phase bone scan constitute the best objective, strictly diagnostic test, particularly in the hand. Although several investigators have advocated using the bone scan in this setting (338), one study concluded that scintigraphy should not be considered as the definitive technique for diagnosing RSD (307). In another recent series of 134 patients with RSD, 51 had a bone scan, but only 53% were interpreted as consistent with RSD (307). MacKinnon and Holder have adopted the strictest criteria for diagnosis and consequently have shown the greatest predictive value is a favorable response to treatment (332). For use in the hand, they required a diffuse increase in delayed periarticular tracer uptake in all joints of the affected hand, and have reported positive and negative predictive values of 88% and 99%, respectively (332). Adults with RSD have a characteristic delayed bone scan pattern consisting of diffusely increased uptake with juxta-articular attenuation (339).

A three-phase bone scan was used to investigate 63 patients with arm pain of unexplained etiology; 25% of these patients were identified with definite (or probable) RSD on Kozin's criteria (340). The value of bone scanning as a diagnostic test was evaluated. The 3-hour delayed images revealed a specificity of 92% and a sensitivity of 50%. These values were not improved when data from the blood pool phase were added. Symptoms that lasted less than 6 months or patient age greater than 50 years increased the test's sensitivity (340). In another study by Zyluk and Birkenfeld (341), three-phase bone scans were performed in 65 patients with posttraumatic RSD to evaluate which changes in uptake of the tracer appear before and after treatment. At final imaging, the mean uptake ratios of patients with good, moderate, and poor response to treatment did not differ significantly. This suggests that although three-phase bone scintigraphy may be valuable in making the diagnosis of RSD, it has no worth in monitoring the treatment course of RSD. These equivocal findings have led some investigators to suggest other noninvasive imaging studies. Nazarian et al (342) found that patients with reflex sympathetic dystrophy of the lower extremity had increased power Doppler flow compared with asymptomatic control subjects. A local anesthetic block of the appropriate sympathetic ganglia represents the best practical combined diagnostic and prognostic test in the management of the patient evaluated for suspected CRPS. Successful achievement of a sympathetic blockade, evidenced by Horner's syndrome (miosis, ptosis, anhidrosis) and warming of the affected extremity in conjunction with relief of the chief complaint of pain confirms the diagnosis of CRPS. Although failure of pain relief does not rule out the diagnosis of CRPS, a positive response with relief of symptoms all but confirms the diagnosis, and, more importantly, predicts a favorable response to a series of therapeutic sympathetic blocks.

Modified Sympathetic Blockade Testing

Many of the symptoms and findings discussed previously are common to both CRPS and less serious acute traumatic injuries. Therefore, more sophisticated tests have been developed to aid in the definitive diagnosis of CRPS. The most common test involves injecting a neural blockade and analyzing the response in the affected limb. In such tests, normal saline solution is used as a control, and Novocaine (5% procaine hydrochloride) is used as a pharmacologic neural blocker. The solution is injected into either the stellate ganglion, when the arm is involved, or the lumbar paravertebral ganglia, when the lower limbs are involved. Alternative neural blockade tests include injection of guanethidine, an intravenously administered agent that depletes presynaptic noradrenaline stores, thus producing an initial exaggeration of symptoms, followed by relief in CRPS patients. Also, the phentolamine test may be administered, whereby α-adrenoreceptors are blocked, and relief of symptoms and pain indicates increased peripheral sympathetic activity (343). Each of these latter tests may be modified and used as treatments, as discussed in the information to follow.

Treatment

Physical Medicine and Rehabilitation

Physical medicine and rehabilitation should be the first step in treating CRPS and serves by treating the secondary complications of CRPS, such as decreased joint range of motion and tendon excursion. Improving stiffness and mobility is likely to provide additional general benefits, such as ameliorating depression and offering pain control. A randomized, controlled study showed that physical and, to a lesser extent, occupational therapies reduced pain and improved active mobility in patients with recent-onset CRPS type I (344). Elevation, massage, and contrast baths have also been used (345). Surgical stockings or elastic bandages can be used to minimize edema in an affected extremity. Dynamic splinting and stress-loading programs of traction can improve range of motion (346). If contractures are not prevented or treated with physical therapy, orthopaedic surgery may become necessary.

Physical therapy is emphasized in treating CRPS to maintain and increase joint range of motion and muscle strength. Early intervention with physical therapy is important, as immobilization and mechanical allodynia increase as CRPS progresses, making physical activity and therapy difficult. For patients with CRPS in the leg or foot, assisted walking is useful to maintain motion while limiting pain caused by weight bearing and movement (347). Massage therapy, alternating hot and cold baths, and whirlpool therapy for tactile desensitization have proven to be effective adjuncts to physical therapy (348), and transcutaneous electrical nerve stimulation (TENS) has shown some effectiveness, although there are conflicting reports regarding its usefulness (349).

Acupuncture

There is no evidence to support acupuncture in the treatment of CRPS. One small study did not show any statistical differences between acupuncture and sham groups (350).

TENS

TENS has been found to be effective in 50% to 90% of pediatric patients with CRPS (351). This treatment method is worth attempting, as it is noninvasive and does not have side effects (with the exception of an occasional skin irritation) (351).

Psychiatric Treatment

Due to the discrepancy between CRPS patients' subjective complaints of pain and the limited objective evidence of underlying pathology, psychiatric factors are considered as one of the causes of CRPS. Although many patients with long-term CRPS battle depression and anxiety, these conditions usually are a consequence, rather than a cause, of their pain (352). Some very depressed patients may need more aggressive psychiatric treatment such as electroconvulsive therapy (353).

Alternative Therapies

Alternative approaches for treating CRPS are gaining favor with patients, possibly due to the relative ineffectiveness and unreliability of some medical treatments. Recently, a clinical investigation of the efficacy of qigong, a form of traditional Eastern healing, was undertaken. Patients received either qi emission or qigong instruction, including home exercise, from a qigong master, or a set of similar instructions from a sham master. After the first six to 10 training sessions, 82% of the experimental group showed improvement, versus 45% of controls. By the final training session, 91% of the experimental group experienced analgesia, compared to 36% in the control group. Anxiety was also decreased in each group, although to a significantly higher degree in the treatment group (352). The investigators accounted for factors such as pre-experimental hypnotizability and concluded that qigong is an effective treatment for the pain and psychological effects (depression, anxiety) associated with CRPS.

The success of qigong suggests that there may be a role for nonconventional treatment modalities in the management of CRPS patients. Grunert et al (353) found that a combination of thermal biofeedback, relaxation training, and supportive psychotherapy was effective as a pain reduction strategy for patients with RSD, with 14 of 20 patients returning to work at 1-year follow-up. In addition, there may be a role for spinal manipulative therapy in the relief of sympathetically mediated pain and effects. Muramatsu et al (354) treated 17 patients with CRPS using manipulation therapy and regional anesthesia and found satisfactory results in 88% of patients. They found good results when treating CRPS type I, early-stage disease, and upper-limb involvement.

Pharmacologic Treatment

Patients with CRPS are seen much earlier by the orthopaedist than the pain clinician. In the early stage of the disease, there are more treatment options than in the established case. The other side of the coin could be that these patients would recover anyway; so the results of early treatment are more favorable. Oral steroids have been shown to be effective to reduce pain and edema at 12 weeks in a small, randomized, controlled study where oral prednisolone was administered to patients over a duration of 3 months (355). There is evidence for efficacy of corticosteroids, which decrease inflammation, relieve pain, and minimize ectopic electrical activity after nerve injury (356). In a placebo-controlled study, the frequency of shoulder-hand syndrome in patients with stroke hemiparesis was shown to be reduced after administration of methylprednisone for 4 weeks (357). Patients with CRPS can develop bone resorption in the affected area (358), although this likely is a secondary consequence of reduced mobility and loss of innervation to the bone. For this reason, inhibitors of osteoclast activity (e.g., bisphosphonates or regulators of bone metabolism) have been evaluated as treatments for recent-onset CRPS. The mechanisms by which calcitonin and bisphosphonates control pain in early CRPS are unclear. Bisphosphonates hinder the synthesis of prostaglandin E2, proteolytic enzymes, lactic acid, and proinflammatory cytokines (200); calcitonin inhibits the synthesis of proteolytic enzymes and lactic acid. None of these agents can be administered orally; calcitonin is available as a nasal spray and bisphosphonates usually are administered intravenously. Open-label studies suggest that pamidronate can reduce pain and improve range of motion (359). In a randomized, controlled study, 300 mg of clodronate administered intravenously to patients daily for 10 days resulted in lasting pain relief (360).

Noradrenergic Tricyclic Antidepressants

The tricyclic antidepressants work due to their antihyperalgesic and antidepressant action; their efficacy is well demonstrated in neuropathic pain syndromes such as postherpetic neuralgia and diabetic neuropathy (361). Their antihyperalgesic effects seem to be related to several known actions, including enhancement of noradrenergic descending inhibitory pathways and partial sodium-channel blockade.

Sympathetic Blockade

Sympathetic blockade has been the most popular treatment for CRPS since the 1930s (362). Neural blockade can be regional or local, pharmacologic or surgical. Surgical sympathectomy is a late-stage option in patients for whom pharmacologic blockade has failed. Pharmacologic blockade can be used either locally or regionally. Regional blockade utilizes guanethidine, whereas local anesthetics are used at either the stellate ganglion or the lumbar paravertebral ganglion (308). Guanethidine, reserpine, bretylium, methylprednisolone, and lidocaine have been used individually as neural blockers, with varying success (333,363).

Zyluk (338,341,363) reported the treatment results of 36 patients with upper extremity RSD. Each patient received regional IV blocks of methylprednisolone and lidocaine with post-treatment physiotherapy (finger exercises and whirlpool therapy); 69% of the patients described their outcomes as good, meaning that they had relief of spontaneous pain and no limitations in finger movement. Smoking has been implicated in RSD by increasing the local and systemic effects of the SNS, and cessation of tobacco use is a rational recommendation during treatment (47).

Spinal Cord Stimulators

Spinal cord stimulation is a form of therapy used to treat CRPS I (364). It involves an electrical generator that delivers pulses to a specific spinal cord area. The leads can be implanted by laminectomy or percutaneously and the source of power is supplied by an implanted battery or by an external radiofrequency transmitter.

ACUTE PAIN MANAGEMENT

The cost of pain (from all causes) to US society—in productive time lost, health care expenses, and compensation was estimated to be $61.2 billion per year from 2001 to 2002 (179), and it continues to increase every year. Pain results from physical disorders and also from combinations of physiological, pathological, emotional, psychological, cognitive, environmental, and social factors. Pain sensation is a protective function and occurs whenever tissue is being injured or damaged. Tissue injury and concomitant pain evoke an endocrine-metabolic response, which is characterized by increased catecholamine and cortisol levels. Pain and the associated stress response observed in trauma patients should always be viewed as detrimental, and the rationale for treatment of posttraumatic and postoperative pain must be prioritized if morbidity secondary to trauma is to be minimized. The postoperative management of pain in the trauma patient is facilitated by a multidisciplinary approach that includes consulting a pain management specialist. The pain specialist functions as an integral member of the trauma team to provide the effective and appropriate relief of pain (365).

Pain management may be needed in three phases after injury. The first phase is following injury, which lasts about 0 to 5 hours. During this immediate stage, many patients feel very little pain. The second is the acute phase lasting several days, where pain is a prominent feature (366). The third phase involves managing chronic pain. The chronic stage is characterized by complex behavioral disturbances in conjunction with pain. In this chapter, we describe the management of acute and early postoperative pain. Plans for pain management must consider surgical concerns. Regional anesthesia may mask the pain associated with a developing compartment syndrome (367), and the results can be catastrophic. Likewise, narcotic analgesia may preclude the use of frequent neurological examinations in the patient with an altered mental status due to head injury or drug intoxication. This makes the multidisciplinary postoperative pain management vital and must include input from the various surgical services responsible for the patient. The early management of pain in the trauma patient serves many important functions. Pain control attenuates the physiologic response to stress and reduces the morbidity associated with trauma. Adequate pain relief permits early mobilization, facilitates rehabilitation, and decreases the detrimental effects of prolonged immobilization and may decrease the incidence of chronic pain syndromes (368,369).

Acute pain management has been vastly improved in recent years (370). Trauma patients, particularly complex multiple-trauma individuals, require a highly specialized team to provide optimal care and outcome. The rationale of analgesic management is to reduce pain intensity to tolerable levels and the treatment should not alter the body's physiological responses. Hypovolemia and reduced organ perfusion should be kept in mind, as conventional drugs in normal doses can produce high serum levels causing undesirable side effects. Due to trauma, tissue oxygenation could be hampered, and therapy affecting respiration and oxygenation should be avoided. Medications affecting the state of consciousness should be eschewed, especially in a drugged or head-injured patient. Drugs affecting the intracranial pressure should be used with caution. Depositing local anesthetic agents into the epidural space can cause a considerable increase in intracranial pressure (371). Adequate knowledge of drug interactions and the use of appropriate methods of analgesia can minimize adverse drug effects (372). Drugs should not be administered orally, as gastric emptying could be delayed. The intramuscular (IM) route is not suitable, particularly for the patient with diminished tissue perfusion, because the drug will be poorly absorbed.

Managing Acute Pain

Opioid Analgesics

Narcotic analgesia is commonly used to manage acute pain. Morphine is usually administered intravenously and acts within 15 to 20 minutes. Morphine is usually administered in IV doses of up to 10 mg. Clonidine combined with opioids produces an additive and, in some cases, a synergistic effect at the spinal cord level (373). Clonidine can be used with morphine, fentanyl or sufentanil in treating acute pain (374). Meperidine, 10 to 20 mg administered intravenously provides adequate analgesia in 10 minutes. Meperidine is the most powerful cardiovascular depressant of all narcotics, so it should be used with great caution in the hypovolemic trauma victim and also has potential hazards in the elderly (375). Midazolam has been shown to produce an additive effect with opioids (376). Midazolam binds to a benzodiazepine site on the GABA-A receptor, producing an increase in the amplitude and duration of the GABA-induced synaptic current (377). At the supraspinal level, midazolam has been shown to inhibit the opioid antinociceptive effect (378). Analgesic synergism has been noted with midazolam and with this combination, analgesia can be achieved at lower dosages (359). Clinical studies have focused on the delivery of combined intrathecal midazolam and bupivacaine. Pain scores were not reportedly different and, although there was a reduction in opioid supplementation, the opioid side effects were not reduced (379). Fentanyl and alfentanil are probably the most suitable drugs for the relief of acute pain (380,381). Fentanyl, unlike morphine has an extremely rapid onset *of* action (381). Under close monitoring of airway and ventilation, an initial loading dose of fentanyl, 2 to 4 mg/kg, over a 20-minute period, followed by a 1- to 1.5-mg/kg per hour infusion, can provide rapid and effective pain control. Alfentanil can be given as a 20-mg/kg per infusion. Doses of this magnitude produced depression of the carbon dioxide response curve, but respiratory function returns to normal within 1 hour after discontinuing alfentanil (362,382).

Sublingual and Oral Narcotics

Buprenorphine, a relatively new partial agonist-analgesic with a long duration of action (6 to 8 hours), can be given sublingually. It has obvious advantages for both the patient and the nursing staff and has been shown to produce effective postoperative analgesia (383). A common side effect of this drug is nausea, which may be unresponsive to conventional antiemetics, including naloxone (384). The plasma buprenorphine concentration following a 0.4-mg sublingual dose rises slowly and reaches a peak in about 3 hours (142,174,203,236,252,261 265,280,285,295,383,385). The drug may be given postoperatively on a regular basis every 8 hours for 3 or 4 days if required.

Buccal morphine (13.3 mg) is a relatively new preparation that has been used in Europe. Studies suggest that it produces postoperative analgesia comparable to IM morphine (386). Its use is limited, as the effect of these preparations is not as potent as IV or epidural opiates.

IM Narcotics

Administering narcotic analgesics by the IM route is generally the most common method for providing postoperative analgesia (387). The analgesia may last for too short a duration due to multiple factors, among which are poor prescribing by physicians (poor drug choice, inadequate dose, and inappropriate dosing interval) (388). The clinician should administer the first dose of an appropriately chosen drug, monitor its effect, and then decide on a suitable dose to be given at an appropriate dosing interval, within the tolerable confines of side effects, for at least the first 24 hours. Morphine sulfate (10 to 12 mg) and meperidine (80 to 100 mg) are the narcotic agents most commonly used, but newer agents are now being used more often.

PCA

Further refinements of IV analgesia techniques have led to the use of patient-controlled demand systems (381). These devices consist of an electronic apparatus that administers a preset bolus of the drug when the patient presses a bedside button. All devices include safeguards to prevent the patient from receiving more than a preset number of doses hourly. Most patients maintain their own level of analgesia and do not use the maximal available dose. One of the limiting factors is the expensive apparatus that is required for this type of analgesia.

When prescribing postoperative PCA therapy, the ideal drug should (a) have a rapid onset of analgesic action, (b) be highly efficacious in relieving pain, (c) have an intermediate duration of action, and (d) be associated with no side effects. Although there is no ideal narcotic analgesic, a large number of analgesic drugs can be used for managing postoperative pain with a PCA system, such as. hydromorphone (Dilaudid), fentanyl (Sublimaze), sufentanil (Sufenta), pentazocine (Talwin), butorphanol (Stadol), and nalbuphine (Nubain). Morphine and meperidine remain the most widely used parenteral analgesics (389).

Errors in using the PCA system should be avoided and are preventable by adequate training of the nursing staff and carefully instructing the patients. Opiate-related side effects (e.g., nausea, vomiting, and constipation) are expected to occur in 10% of patients (390).

Local Anesthetics

In the patient with compromised circulatory function, utmost care must be exercised when administering drugs that have further depressant effects on cardiac and/or cerebral function. Routes of administration that produce sympathetic blockade are inappropriate in the hypovolemic patient; this precludes using spinal or epidural analgesia until the blood volume has been restored to normal. When assessment of limb function and pain is important (e.g., compartment syndromes, plaster casts), long-acting peripheral nerve blocks are inappropriate to use. Equally inappropriate is the use of regional anesthesia in trauma victims. Therefore, local anesthetic provides adequate pain relief without interfering with the physiological circulatory and cerebral state of the injured patient. Moreover, other therapeutic measures, including surgery, can often be carried out using only the local anesthetic, which obviates the need for a general anesthetic and avoids potential hazards in a patient with a full stomach. Local anesthetics can be administered by infiltration, peripheral nerve block, and conduction blockade. Peripheral nerve blocks deserve wider use because they usually produce total and long-lasting analgesia, with minimal side effects. Furthermore, they often make the administration of a general anesthetic unnecessary and, in fact, shorten the patient's hospital stay (391). The use of regional anesthesia has been recommended for disaster situations (392).

Nerve Blocks

Infiltration

Orthopaedists and neurosurgeons have been infiltrating wound edges with a long-acting local anesthetic agent such as bupivacaine for some time, and use of the technique has more recently been advocated for producing postoperative analgesia for other incisions (393).

Peripheral Nerve Block

Peripheral nerve blocks can be administered by a single injection or by a continuous catheter technique. With the single-injection technique, a long-acting local anesthetic agent is used, and the block is repeated as required. With the continuous technique, a catheter is inserted adjacent to the nerve(s) and intermittent doses or a continuous infusion of local anesthetic agent can be administered. When continuous infusion is used following an initial bolus dose of bupivacaine, 0.25%, 0.1 to 0.25 mg/kg per hour (approximately 5 mL/hr), it produces adequate analgesia, with plasma bupivacaine levels maintained below toxic range (1.5 to 1.7 mg/mL) (494). In practice, these techniques have been performed primarily to produce anesthesia for surgery and are continued postoperatively to provide analgesia. Thus, analgesia by this method is usually confined to the limbs; the brachial plexus, femoral nerve, and lumbar plexus are blocked most frequently. Occasionally, the trauma patient poses limitations for these blocks—time constraints might not permit the insertion of a preoperative catheter, and the need for surgical assessment of the limb postoperatively could preclude prolonged blockade. In the absence of these conditions, however, peripheral nerve blocks, by providing excellent analgesia, improving the mobilization of the injured limb, and augmenting the blood flow to the extremity not only speed the return to function but also probably lessen the risk of the limb's reflex sympathetic changes.

Trauma patients, particularly complex multiple-trauma individuals, require a highly specialized team to provide optimal care and outcome. The anesthesiologist has the training and expertise to offer regional techniques that are often necessary in the early posttraumatic period. Pain-management physicians should assume active roles in trauma patient therapy because they know the pain to expect from different lesions and the associated morbidity. Monitoring the patient's progress demands daily attention to detail.

Neuraxial Catheters

As previously discussed, epidural catheters may be inserted into the thoracic or lumbar regions of the spine to provide pain relief in the thorax, abdomen, or lower extremities. The benefits of epidural analgesia in the postinjury period include smaller doses of narcotics with less respiratory depression, improved pulmonary toilet, and early mobilization (395). Using smaller doses of narcotics may be especially beneficial in the head-injured patient to decrease pain, prevent further agitation, and facilitate the ongoing assessment of mental status (366). Continuous infusions are frequently used to provide ongoing pain relief. The infusion solely of local anesthetics through the epidural catheter permits the safe IV use of narcotic analgesics for pain relief from other injuries.

Spinal catheters permit intermittent or continuous dosing by infusion and require smaller doses of medications than epidural catheters for effective pain relief.

Peripheral Catheters or Nerve Blocks

Brachial plexus catheters may be inserted to permit intermittent bolus dosing or continuous infusions of medications for managing pain in isolated upper-extremity injuries. This technique also provides a sympathectomy, which is beneficial after vascular repair or replantation and may prevent the development of chronic pain syndromes.

Catheters may be inserted into the femoral nerve sheath or the popliteal fossa to provide lower-extremity analgesia in the postinjury period. Compared with brachial plexus catheters, these techniques offer similar advantages and have a low complication rate (385).

Intercostal Nerve Blocks and Intrapleural Catheters

Intercostal nerve blocks provide excellent relief of the pain associated with multiple rib fractures. The relief is temporary (limited by the administered local anesthetic agent's duration of action), however, and the nerve blocks must be repeated frequently. Intercostal nerve blocks carry the risk of a pneumothorax; therefore, bilateral nerve blocks are avoided in the absence of thoracostomy tubes (366).

The placement of an intrapleural catheter provides excellent pain relief after chest trauma. The catheter allows dosing with either intermittent or continuous infusion methods. If a thoracostomy tube is in place, temporary clamping during bolus dosing is necessary to prevent immediate suctioning of the local anesthetic medication. Increased peak plasma levels of local anesthetics may predispose to local anesthetic toxicity with this technique (366). Another advantage with either of these techniques is the ability to use narcotic analgesic medications to manage pain from other sites.

REFERENCES

1. Connolly JF, Csencsitz TA. Limb threatening neuropathic complications from ankle fractures in patients with diabetes. *Clin Orthop* 1998;(348):212–219.
2. Griffith R, Channon C. The law of negligence and community nursing: a case study. *Br J Community Nurs* 2004;9(6):257–259.
3. Kaplan SS. Burns following application of plaster splint dressings. Report of two cases. *J Bone Joint Surg (Am)* 1981;63(4):670–672.
4. Lavalette R, Pope MH, Dickstein H. Setting temperatures of plaster casts. The influence of technical variables. *J Bone Joint Surg (Am)* 1982;64(6):907–911.
5. Lovell CR, Staniforth P. Contact allergy to benzalkonium chloride in plaster of Paris. *Contact Dermatitis* 1981;7(6):343–344.
6. Marks MI, Guruswamy A, Gross RH. Ringworm resulting from swimming with a polyurethane cast. *J Pediatr Orthop* 1983;3(4):511–512.
7. Newman. C. Cast care with the Goretex cast liner: patient education manual. Flagstaff, Ariz: WL Gore and Associates Inc, 1990.
8. Selesnick H RJ, Ellison PS. Waterproof cast liner: a 5-year prospective study. *Orthop Transactions* 1996;20:256.
9. Burny F, HM, Adrianne Y, et al. A review of 164 cases. External Fixation of the humerus.
10. Leach R. New fiber glass casting system. *Clin Orthop* 1974;103:109–117.
11. Schuind F, Moulart F, Leigeois JM, et al. Orthopaedic Immobilization. *Acta Orthop Belg* 2002;68(5):439–461.
12. Wytch R, Mitchell C, Ritchie IK, et al. New splinting materials. *Prosthet Orthot Int* 1987; 11(1):42–45.
13. Katz K, Fogelman R, Attias J, et al. Anxiety reaction in children during removal of their plaster cast with a saw. *J Bone Joint Surg (Br)* 2001;83(3):388–390.
14. Ansari MZ, Swarup S, Ghani R, et al. Oscillating saw injuries during removal of plaster. *Eur J Emerg Med* 1998;5(1):37–39.
15. Killian JT, White S, Lenning L. Cast-saw burns: comparison of technique versus material versus saws. *J Pediatr Orthop* 1999;19(5):683–687.
16. Dubowitz G, Miller DM. Cast adrift: Gortex cast liners allow greater patient activity. *Wilderness Environ Med* 2003;14(3):167–168.
17. Muller ME, Willenegger H. *Manual of internal fixation*. New York: Springer-Verlag, 1970.
18. Charnley J. *The closed treatment of common fractures*. Edinburgh: Churchill Livingstone, 1961.
19. Malkin LH. Reflex sympathetic dystrophy syndrome following trauma to the foot. *Orthopedics* 1990;13(8):851–858.
20. Poplawski ZJ, Wiley AM, Murray JF. Post-traumatic dystrophy of the extremities. *J Bone Joint Surg (Am)* 1983;65(5):642–655.
21. Wong DA, Watson AB. Allergic contact dermatitis due to benzalkonium chloride in plaster of Paris. *Australas J Dermatol* 2001;42(1):33–35.
22. Terzioglu A, Aslan G, Sarifakioglu N, et al. Pressure sore from a fruit seed under a hip spica cast. *Ann Plast Surg* 2002;48(1):103–104.
23. Peltier LF. A brief history of traction. *J Bone Joint Surg (Am)* 1968;50(8):1603–1617.
24. Rosen JE, Chen FS, Hiebert R, et al. Efficacy of preoperative skin traction in hip fracture patients: a prospective, randomized study. *J Orthop Trauma* 2001;15(2):81–85.
25. Jerre R, Doshe A, Karlsson J. Preoperative skin traction in patients with hip fractures is not useful. *Clin Orthop* 2000;(378):169–173.
26. Parker MJ, Handoll HH. Pre-operative traction for fractures of the proximal femur. *Cochrane Database Syst Rev* 2003(3):CD000168.
27. Shabat S, Gepstein R, Mann G, et al. Deep skin slough following skin traction for hip fractures. *J Tissue Viability* 2002;12(3):108–112.

28. Janzing H, Broos P, Romnens P. Compartment syndrome as complication of skin traction, in children with femoral fractures. *Acta Chir Belg* 1996;96(3):135–137.
29. Mustard WT, Simmons EH. Experimental arterial spasm in the lower extremities produced by traction. *J Bone Joint Surg (Br)* 1953;35-B(3):437–441.
30. Levi N. Is preoperative tibial traction responsible for peroneal nerve palsy in patients with a fractured hip? *Acta Orthop Belg* 1998;64(3):273–276.
31. Esposito PW, Alexander AH, Lichtman DM. Delayed overdistraction of a surgically treated unstable thoracolumbar fracture. A case report. *Spine* 1985;10(4):393–396.
32. Fried LC. Cervical spinal cord injury during skeletal traction. *JAMA* 1974;229(2): 181–183.
33. Gruenberg MF, Rechtine GR, Chrin AM, et al. Overdistraction of cervical spine injuries with the use of skull traction: a report of two cases. *J Trauma* 1997;42(6):1152–1156.
34. Hippocrates. An abridged report on external skeletal fixation. 1939. *Clin Orthop* 1989;(241):3–4.
35. Hippocrates. The works of Hippocrates. Baltimore: Williams and Wilkins, 1939.
36. Matthews LS, Green CA, Goldstein SA. The thermal effects of skeletal fixation-pin insertion in bone. *J Bone Joint Surg (Am)* 1984;66(7):1077–1083.
37. Muller ME, Willenegger H. *Manual der Osteosynthese*. Berlin: Springer-Verlag, 1992.
38. Aro HT, Chao EY. Bone-healing patterns affected by loading, fracture fragment stability, fracture type, and fracture site compression. *Clin Orthop* 1993;(293):8–17.
39. Green SA. Complications of external skeletal fixation. *Clin Orthop* 1983;(180):109–116.
40. Dwyer NS. Preliminary report upon a new fixation device for fractures of long bones. *Injury* 1973;5(2):141–144.
41. Steinfield PH, Cobelli NJ, Sadler AH, et al. Open tibial fractures treated by anterior half-pin frame fixation. *Clin Orthop* 1988;(228):208–214.
42. Green SA, Ripley MJ. Chronic osteomyelitis in pin tracks. *J Bone Joint Surg (Am)* 1984; 66(7):1092–1098.
43. Edwards CC GP, Kenzora JE, Browner BD. Treatment of 50 severe open injuries about the ankle using external fixation. *J Bone Joint Surg Orth Trans* 1982;6:415.
44. Edwards CC, Browner BD, Baugher WH. The use of external fixators in the upper extremity. *J Bone Joint Surg Orthop Trans* 1982;6:403.
45. Rubash HE, Mears DC. External fixation of the pelvis. *Instr Course Lect* 1983;32: 329–348.
46. Parameswaran AD, Roberts CS, Seligson D, et al. Pin tract infection with contemporary external fixation: how much of a problem? *J Orthop Trauma* 2003;17(7):503–507.
47. DeJong ES, DeBerardino TM, Brooks DE, et al. Antimicrobial efficacy of external fixator pins coated with a lipid stabilized hydroxyapatite/chlorhexidine complex to prevent pin tract infection in a goat model. *J Trauma* 2001;50(6):1008–1014.
48. Forster H, Marotta JS, Heseltine K, et al. Bactericidal activity of antimicrobial coated polyurethane sleeves for external fixation pins. *J Orthop Res* 2004;22(3):671–677.
49. Moroni A, Heikkila J, Magyar G, et al. Fixation strength and pin tract infection of hydroxyapatite-coated tapered pins. *Clin Orthop* 2001;(388):209–217.
50. Pommer A, Muhr G, David A. Hydroxyapatite-coated Schanz pins in external fixators used for distraction osteogenesis: a randomized, controlled trial. *J Bone Joint Surg (Am)* 2002;84-A (7):1162–1166.
51. McKenzie LL. In search of a standard for pin site care. *Orthop Nurs* 1999;18(2):73–78.
52. Olson RS. Halo skeletal traction pin site care: toward developing a standard of care. *Rehabil Nurs* 1996;21(5):243–246, 257.
53. Sims M, Saleh M. Protocols for the care of external fixator pin sites. *Prof Nurse* 1996; 11(4):261–264.
54. Dahl W, Toksvig-Larsen S, Lindstrand A. No difference between daily and weekly pin site care: a randomized study of 50 patients with external fixation. *Acta Orthop Scand* 2003; 74(6):704–708.
55. Moskovich R. Proximal tibial transfixion for skeletal traction. An anatomic study of neurovascular structures. *Clin Orthop* 1987;(214):264–268.
56. Hassan DM, Johnston GH. Safety of the limited open technique of bone-transfixing threaded-pin placement for external fixation of distal radial fractures: a cadaver study. *Can J Surg* 1999;42(5):363–365.
57. Vives MJ, Abidi NA, Ishikawa SN, et al. Soft tissue injuries with the use of safe corridors for transfixion wire placement during external fixation of distal tibia fractures: an anatomic study. *J Orthop Trauma* 2001;15(8):555–559.
58. Lim EV, Lavadia WT, Blebea J. Vascular impingement by external fixator pins: a case report. *J Trauma* 1995;38(5):833–835.
59. Casey D, McConnell T, Parekh S, et al. Percutaneous pin placement in the medial calcaneus: is anywhere safe? *J Orthop Trauma* 2002;16(1):26–29.
60. Olson SA, Finkemeier CG, Moehring HD. Open fractures. In: Bucholz RW, Heckman JD, eds. *Rockwood and Green's Fractures in Adults*, vol 1, 5th ed. Philadelphia: Lippincott-Raven, 2001:285–317.
61. Gristina AG, Naylor PT, Myrvik QN. Mechanisms of musculoskeletal sepsis. *Orthop Clin N Am* 1991;22(3):363–371.
62. Dankert J, Hogt A, Feijen J. Bacterial adhesion, colonization and infection. Biomedical polymers. *Crit Rev Biocompat* 1986;2:219–301.
63. Jefferson KK. What drives bacteria to produce a bio film? *FEMS Microbiol Lett* 2004; 236(2):163–173.
64. Watnick P, Kolter R. Biofilm, city of microbes. *J Bacteriol* 2000;182(10):2675–2679.
65. Mann S. Molecular recognition in bio mineralization. *Nature* 1988;332:119–124.
66. Fischer B, Vaudaux P, Magnin M, et al. Novel animal model for studying the molecular mechanisms of bacterial adhesion to bone-implanted metallic devices: role of fibronectin in Staphylococcus aureus adhesion. *J Orthop Res* 1996;14(6):914–920.
67. Gustilo RB, Gruninger RP, Tsukayama DT. Microbial adhesion and the pathogenesis of biomaterial-centered infections. In: *Orthopaedic infection*. Philadelphia: WB Saunders, 1989:3–25.
68. Naylor P JR, Myrvik Q. Antibiotic sensitivity of biomaterial adherent staphylococcus epidermidis. *Orthop Trans* 1988;12:524–525.
69. Nichols WW, Dorrington SM, Slack MP, et al. Inhibition of tobramycin diffusion by binding to alginate. *Antimicrob Agents Chemother* 1988;32(4):518–523.
70. Toguchi A, Siano M, Burkart M, et al. Genetics of swarming motility in Salmonella enterica serovar typhimurium: critical role for lipopolysaccharide. *J Bacteriol* 2000; 182(22):6308–6321.
71. Meadows SE, Zuckerman JD, Koval KJ. Posttraumatic tibial osteomyelitis: diagnosis, classification, and treatment. *Bull Hosp Jt Dis* 1993;52(2):11–16.
72. Tsukayama DT. Pathophysiology of posttraumatic osteomyelitis. *Clin Orthop* 1999; (360):22–29.
73. Evans RP, Nelson CL, Harrison BH. The effect of wound environment on the incidence of acute osteomyelitis. *Clin Orthop* 1993;(286):289–297.
74. Toh CL, Jupiter JB. The infected nonunion of the tibia. *Clin Orthop* 1995;(315): 176–191.
75. Hoch RC, Rodriguez R, Manning T, et al. Effects of accidental trauma on cytokine and endotoxin production. *Crit Care Med* 1993;21(6):839–845.
76. Cunha B, Dee R, Klein N, et al. Bone and Joint infections. In: Dee R, Hurst L, Gruber M, et al, eds. *Principles of orthopaedic practice*, 2nd ed. New York: McGraw-Hill, 1997: 317–344.
77. Morrissy RT, Haynes DW. Acute hematogenous osteomyelitis: a model with trauma as an etiology. J Pediatr Orthop 1989;9(4):447–456.
78. May JW Jr, Jupiter JB, Weiland AJ, et al. Clinical classification of post-traumatic tibial osteomyelitis. *J Bone Joint Surg (Am)* 1989;71(9):1422–1428.
79. Kelly PJ. Infected non-union of the femur and tibia. *Orthop Clin N Am* 1984;15(Jul)(3): 481–490.
80. Weiland AJ, Moore JR, Daniel RK. The efficacy of free tissue transfer in the treatment of osteomyelitis. *J Bone Joint Surg (Am)* 1984;66(Feb)(2):181–193.
81. Cierny G III. Chronic osteomyelitis: results of treatment. *Instr Course Lect* 1990;39: 495–508.
82. Cierny G, Mader JT. The surgical treatment of adult osteomyelitis. In: Evarts CM, ed. *Surgery of the musculoskeletal system*. Vol. 4. New York: Churchill-Livingstone, 1983: 15–35.
83. Haas DW, McAndrew MP. Bacterial osteomyelitis in adults: evolving considerations in diagnosis and treatment. *Am J Med* 1996;101(5):550–561.
84. Mader JT, Calhoun J. Long-bone osteomyelitis diagnosis and management. *Hosp Pract* (Off Ed) 1994;29(10):71–76, 79, 83 passim.
85. Wheat J. Diagnostic strategies in osteomyelitis. *Am J Med* 1985;78(6B):218–224.
86. Ash JM, Gilday DL. The futility of bone scanning in neonatal osteomyelitis: concise communication. *J Nucl Med* 1980;21(5):417–420.
87. Court-Brown CM, Keating JF, McQueen MM. Infection after intramedullary nailing of the tibia. Incidence and protocol for management. *J Bone Joint Surg (Br)* 1992;74(5): 770–774.
88. Datz FL. *Gamuts in nuclear medicine*, 2nd ed. Norwalk, CT: Appleton-Century-Crofts, 1983:82–85.
89. Fink-Bennett D, Balon HR, Irwin R. Sequential technetium-99m sulfur colloid/indium-111 white blood cell imaging in macroglobulinemia of Waldenstrom. *Clin Nucl Med* 1990;15(6):389–91.
90. Schauwecker DS, Braunstein EM, Wheat LJ. Diagnostic imaging of osteomyelitis. *Infect Dis Clin N Am* 1990;4(3):441–463.
91. Wald ER, Mirro R, Gartner JC. Pitfalls on the diagnosis of acute osteomyelitis by bone scan. *Clin Pediatr (Phila)* 1980;19(9):597–601.
92. Borman TR, Johnson RA, Sherman FC. Gallium scintigraphy for diagnosis of septic arthritis and osteomyelitis in children. *J Pediatr Orthop* 1986;6(3):317–325.
93. Rubin RH, Fischman AJ, Needleman M, et al. Radiolabelled, nonspecific, polyclonal human immunoglobulin in the detection of focal inflammation by scintigraphy: comparison with gallium-67 citrate and technetium-99m-labeled albumin. *J Nucl Med* 1989; 30(3):385–389.
94. Esterhai J, Alavi A, Mandell GA, et al. Sequential technetium-99m/gallium-67 scintigraphic evaluation of subclinical osteomyelitis complicating fracture non-union. *J Orthop Res* 1985;3(2):219–225.
95. Hartshorne MF, Graham G, Lancaster J, et al. Gallium-67/technetium-99m methylene diphosphonate ratio imaging: early rabbit osteomyelitis and fracture. *J Nucl Med* 1985; 26(3):272–277.
96. Merkel KD, Brown ML, Fitzgerald RH, Jr. Sequential technetium-99m HMDP-gallium-67 citrate imaging for the evaluation of infection in the painful prosthesis. *J Nucl Med* 1986;27(9):1413–1417.
97. Magnuson JE, Brown ML, Hauser MF, et al. In-111-labeled leukocyte scintigraphy in suspected orthopedic prosthesis infection: comparison with other imaging modalities. *Radiology* 1988;168(1):235–239.
98. Schauwecker DS. Osteomyelitis: diagnosis with In-111-labeled leukocytes. *Radiology* 1989;171(1):141–146.
99. Seabold JE, Flickinger FW, Kao SC, et al. Indium-111-leukocyte/technetium-99m-MDP bone and magnetic resonance imaging: difficulty of diagnosing osteomyelitis in patients with neuropathic osteoarthropathy. *J Nucl Med* 1990;31(5):549–556.
100. Van Nostrand D, Abreu SH, Callaghan JJ, et al. In-111-labeled white blood cell uptake in noninfected closed fracture in humans: prospective study. *Radiology* 1988;167(2): 495–498.
101. Datz F. Infection imaging. *Semin Nucl Med* 1994;24:89–91.
102. Datz FL. Abdominal abscess detection: gallium, 111In-, and 99mTc-labeled leukocytes, and polyclonal and monoclonal antibodies. *Semin Nucl Med* 1996;26(1):51–64.
103. Datz FL, Seabold JE, Brown ML, et al. Procedure guideline for technetium-99m-HMPAO-labeled leukocyte scintigraphy for suspected infection/inflammation. Society of Nuclear Medicine. *J Nucl Med* 1997;38(6):987–990.
104. Hughes DK. 99mTc-HMPAO-, and 99mTc-stannous fluoride colloid-labeled leukocytes and with 67Ga-citrate. *J Nuc Med Tech* 2003;31(4):196–201.

105. Hauet JR, Barge ML, Fajon O, et al. Sternal infection and retrosternal abscess shown on Tc-99m HMPAO-labelled leukocyte scintigraphy. *Clin Nucl Med* 2004;29(3):194–195.
106. McCarthy K, Velchik MG, Alavi A, et al. Indium-111-labeled white blood cells in the detection of osteomyelitis complicated by a pre-existing condition. *J Nucl Med* 1988; 29(6):1015–21.
107. Peters AM. The utility of [99mTc] HMPAO-leukocytes for imaging infection. *Semin Nucl Med* 1994;24(2):110–127.
108. Wolf G, Aigner RM, Schwarz T. Diagnosis of bone infection using 99m Tc-HMPAO labelled leukocytes. *Nucl Med Commun* 2001;22(11):1201–1206.
109. Poirier JY, Garin E, Derrien C, et al. Diagnosis of osteomyelitis in the diabetic foot with a 99mTc-HMPAO leucocyte scintigraphy combined with a 99mTc-MDP bone scintigraphy. *Diabetes Metab* 2002;28(6 Pt 1):485–490.
110. Segura AB, Munoz A, Brulles YR, et al. What is the role of bone scintigraphy in the diagnosis of infected joint prostheses. *Nuc Med Commun* 2004;25(May)(5): 527–532.
111. Palestro CJ, Mehta HH, Patel M, et al. Marrow versus infection in the Charcot joint: indium-111 leukocyte and technetium-99m sulphur colloid scintigraphy. *J Nuc Med* 1998;39(Feb)(2): 346–350.
112. Boerman OC, Rennen H, Oyen WJ, et al. Radiopharmaceuticals to image infection and inflammation. *Semin Nucl Med* 2001;31(4):286–295.
113. Molina-Murphy IL, Palmer EL, Scott JA, et al. Polyclonal, non-specific 111In-IgG scintigraphy in the evaluation of complicated osteomyelitis and septic arthritis. *Q J Nucl Med* 1999;43(1):29–37.
114. Modic MT, Feiglin DH, Piraino DW, et al. Vertebral osteomyelitis: assessment using MR. *Radiology* 1985;157(1):157–166.
115. Quinn SF, Murray W, Clark RA, et al. MR imaging of chronic osteomyelitis. *J Comput Assist Tomogr* 1988;12(1):113–117.
116. Tang JS, Gold RH, Bassett LW, et al. Musculoskeletal infection of the extremities: evaluation with MR imaging. *Radiology* 1988;166(1 Pt 1):205–209.
117. Unger E, Moldofsky P, Gatenby R, et al. Diagnosis of osteomyelitis by MR imaging. *Am J Roentgenol* 1988;150(3):605–610.
118. David R, Barron BJ, Madewell JE. Osteomyelitis, acute and chronic. *Radiol Clin N Am* 1987; 25(6):1171–1201.
119. Tehranzadeh J, Wang F, Mesgarzadeh M. Magnetic resonance imaging of osteomyelitis. *Crit Rev Diagn Imaging* 1992;33(6):495–534.
120. Dich VQ, Nelson JD, Haltalin KC. Osteomyelitis in infants and children. A review of 163 cases. *Am J Dis Child* 1975;129(11):1273–1278.
121. Chacko TK, Zhuang H, Nakhoda KZ, et al. Applications of fluorodeoxyglucose positron emission tomography in the diagnosis of infection. *Nucl Med Commun* 2003;24(6): 615–624.
122. Schiesser M, Stumpe KD, Trentz O, et al. Detection of metallic implant-associated infections with FDG PET in patients with trauma: correlation with microbiologic results. *Radiology* 2003;226(2):391–398.
123. De Winter F, Vogelaers D, Gemmel F, et al. Promising role of 18-F-fluoro-D-deoxyglucose positron emission tomography in clinical infectious diseases. *Eur J Clin Microbiol Infect Dis* 2002;21(4):247–57.
124. Manthey N, Reinhard P, Moog F, et al. The use of [18 F] fluorodeoxyglucose positron emission tomography to differentiate between synovitis, loosening and infection of hip and knee prostheses. *Nucl Med Commun* 2002;23(7):645–653.
125. Weon YC, Yang SO, Choi YY, et al. Use of Tc-99m HMPAO leukocyte scans to evaluate bone infection: incremental value of additional SPECT images. *Clin Nucl Med* 2000; 25(7):519–526.
126. Esterhai JL Jr, Goll SR, McCarthy KE, et al. Indium-111 leukocyte scintigraphic detection of subclinical osteomyelitis complicating delayed and non-union long bone fractures: a prospective study. *J Orthop Res* 1987;5(1):1–6.
127. Seabold JE, Nepola JV, Conrad GR, et al. Detection of osteomyelitis at fracture nonunion sites: comparison of two scintigraphic methods. *Am J Roentgenol* 1989;152(5): 1021–1027.
128. Graham GD, Lundy MM, Frederick RJ, et al. Predicting the cure of osteomyelitis under treatment: concise communication. *J Nucl Med* 1983;24(2):110–113.
129. Merkel KD, Brown ML, Dewanjee MK, et al. Comparison of indium-labeled-leukocyte imaging with sequential technetium-gallium scanning in the diagnosis of low-grade musculoskeletal sepsis. A prospective study. *J Bone Joint Surg (Am)* 1985;67(3): 465–476.
130. Mousa HA. Evaluation of sinus-track cultures in chronic bone infection. *J Bone Joint Surg (Br)* 1997;79(Jul)(4):567–569.
131. Eisenstein BI. The polymerase chain reaction. A new method of using molecular genetics for medical diagnosis. *N Engl J Med* 1990;322(3):178–183.
132. Tompkins LS. The use of molecular methods in infectious diseases. *N Engl J Med* 1992; 327(18):1290–1297.
133. Hoeffel DP, Hinrichs SH, Garvin KL. Molecular diagnostics for the detection of musculoskeletal infection. *Clin Orthop* 1999;(360):37–46.
134. Eckardt JJ, Wirganowicz PZ, Mar T. An aggressive surgical approach to the management of chronic osteomyelitis. *Clin Orthop* 1994;(298):229–239.
135. Marsh JL, Prokuski L, Biermann JS. Chronic infected tibial non-union with bone loss. Conventional techniques versus bone transport. *Clin Orthop* 1994;(301):139–146.
136. Pape HC, Zwipp H, Regel G, et al. Chronic treatment refractory osteomyelitis of long tubular bones—possibilities and risks of intramedullary boring. *Unfallchirurg* 1995; 98(3):139–144.
137. Pommer A, David A, Richter J, et al. Intramedullary boring in infected intramedullary nail osteosyntheses of the tibia and femur. *Unfallchirurg* 1998;101(8):628–633.
138. Anglen JO. Wound irrigation in musculoskeletal injury. *J Am Acad Orthop Surg* 2001; 9:219–226.
139. Anglen JO, Apostoles S, Christensen G, et al. The efficacy of various irrigation solutions in removing slime-producing Staphylococcus. *J Orthop Trauma* 1994;8(5):390–396.
140. Dirschl DR, Wilson FC. Topical antibiotic irrigation in the prophylaxis of operative wound infections in orthopedic surgery. *Orthop Clin N Am* 1991;22(3):419–426.
141. Moussa FW, Gainor BJ, Anglen JO, et al. Disinfecting agents for removing adherent bacteria from orthopaedic hardware. *Clin Orthop* 1996;(329):255–262.
142. Benjamin JB, Volz RG. Efficacy of a topical antibiotic irrigant in decreasing or eliminating bacterial contamination in surgical wounds. *Clin Orthop* 1984(184):114–117.
143. Casten DF, Nach RJ, Spinzia J. An experimental and clinical Study of the effectiveness of antibiotic wound irrigation in preventing infection. *Surg Gynecol Obstet* 1964;118: 783–787.
144. Condie J, Ferguson DJ. Experimental wound infections: contamination versus surgical technique. *Surgery* 1961;50:367–371.
145. Bhandari M, Schemitsch EH, Adili A, et al. High and low pressure pulsatile lavage of contaminated tibial fractures: an in vitro study of bacterial adherence and bone damage. *J Orthop Trauma* 1999;13(8):526–533.
146. Rosenstein BD, Wilson FC, Funderburk CH. The use of bacitracin irrigation to prevent infection in postoperative skeletal wounds. An experimental study. *J Bone Joint Surg (Am)* 1989;71(3):427–430.
147. Keating JF, Blachut PA, O'Brien PJ, et al. Reamed nailing of open tibial fractures: does the antibiotic bead pouch reduce the deep infection rate? *J Orthop Trauma* 1996;10(5): 298–303.
148. Ostermann PA, Henry SL, Seligson D. Value of adjuvant local antibiotic administration in therapy of open fractures. A comparative analysis of 704 consecutive cases. *Langenbecks Arch Chir* 1993;378(1):32–36.
149. Patzakis MJ, Mazur K, Wilkins J, et al. Septopal beads and autogenous bone grafting for bone defects in patients with chronic osteomyelitis. *Clin Orthop Relat Res* 1993; 295:112–118.
150. Sankaran-Kutty M, Corea JR, Ali MS, et al. Squamous cell carcinoma in chronic osteomyelitis. Report of a case and review of the literature. *Clin Orthop Relat Res* 1985; (Sep)(198):264–267.
151. Duwelius PJ, Schmidt AH. Assessment of bone viability in patients with osteomyelitis: preliminary clinical experience with laser Doppler flowmetry. *J Orthop Trauma* 1992; 6(3):327–332.
152. Ochsner PE, Brunazzi MG. Intramedullary reaming and soft tissue procedures in treatment of chronic osteomyelitis of long bones. *Orthopedics* 1994;17(May)(5):433–440.
153. Cierny G III, Zorn KE. Segmental tibial defects. Comparing conventional and Ilizarov methodologies. *Clin Orthop* 1994;(301):118–123.
154. Ueng SW, Wei FC, Shih CH. Management of femoral diaphyseal infected nonunion with antibiotic beads local therapy, external skeletal fixation, and staged bone grafting. *J Trauma* 1999;46(1):97–103.
155. Marsh DR, Shah S, Elliott J, et al. The Ilizarov method in non-union, malunion and infection of fractures. *J Bone Joint Surg (Br)* 1997;79(2):273–279.
156. Smith W SP, Stewart D, et al. The relationship of socioeconomic risk factors and complication rates in external fixation of the tibia. Presented at the 15th Annual Meeting of the Orthopaedic Trauma Association, October 22, 1999.
157. Esterhai JL Jr, Sennett B, Gelb H, et al. Treatment of chronic osteomyelitis complicating non-union and segmental defects of the tibia with open cancellous bone graft, posterolateral bone graft, and soft-tissue transfer. *J Trauma* 1990;30(1):49–54
158. McNally MA, Small JO, Tofighi HG, et al. Two-stage management of chronic osteomyelitis of the long bones. The Belfast technique. *J Bone Joint Surg (Br)* 1993;75(3):375–380.
159. Wood MB, Cooney WP III, Irons GB Jr. Skeletal reconstruction by vascularized bone transfer: indications and results. *Mayo Clin Proc* 1985;60(11):729–734.
160. Fiebel RJ, Oliva A, Jackson RL, et al. Simultaneous free-tissue transfer and Ilizarov distraction osteosynthesis in lower extremity salvage: case report and review of the literature. *J Trauma* 1994;37(2):322–327.
161. Ilizarov GA. The treatment of pseudarthrosis complicated by osteomyelitis and the elimination of purulent cavities. In: *Transosseous osteomyelitis: theoretical and clinical aspects of the regeneration and growth of tissue.* Berlin: Springer-Verlag, 1993:495–547.
162. Tetzlaff TR, McCracken GH Jr, Nelson JD. Oral antibiotic therapy for skeletal infections of children. II. Therapy of osteomyelitis and suppurative arthritis. *J Pediatr* 1978;92(3): 485–490.
163. Ziran BH, Rao N, Hall RA. A dedicated team approach enhances outcomes of osteomyelitis treatment. *Clin Orthop Relat Res* 2003;(Sep)(414):31–36.
164. Esterhai JL Jr, Queenan J. Management of soft tissue wounds associated with type III open fractures. *Orthop Clin N Am* 1991;22(3):427–432.
165. Anthony JP, Mathes SJ. Update on chronic osteomyelitis. *Clin Plast Surg* 1991;18(3): 515–523.
166. Anthony JP, Mathes SJ, Alpert BS. The muscle flap in the treatment of chronic lower extremity osteomyelitis: results in patients over 5 years after treatment. *Plast Reconstr Surg* 1991;88(2):311–318.
167. Argenta LC, Morykwas MJ. Vacuum-assisted closure: a new method for wound control and treatment: clinical experience. *Ann Plast Surg* 1997;38(6):563–576; discussion 577.
168. Wang J, Li F, Calhoun JH, et al. The role and effectiveness of adjunctive hyperbaric oxygen therapy in the management of musculoskeletal disorders. *J Postgrad Med* 2002; 48(3):226–231.
169. Petzold T, Feindt PR, Carl UM, et al. Hyperbaric oxygen therapy in deep sternal wound infection after heart transplantation. *Chest* 1999;115(5):1455–1458.
170. Mader JT, Adams KR, Wallace WR, et al. Hyperbaric oxygen as adjunctive therapy for osteomyelitis. *Infect Dis Clin N Am* 1990;4(3):433–440.
171. Knighton DR, Halliday B, Hunt TK. Oxygen as an antibiotic. The effect of inspired oxygen on infection. *Arch Surg* 1984;119(2):199–204.
172. Sawai T, Niimi A, Takahashi H, et al. Histologic study of the effect of hyperbaric oxygen therapy on autogenous free bone grafts. *J Oral Maxillofac Surg* 1996;54(8):975–981.

173. Sheikh AY, Gibson JJ, Rollins MD, et al. Effect of hyperoxia on vascular endothelial growth factor levels in a wound model. *Arch Surg* 2000;135(11):1293–1297.
174. Barth E, Sullivan T, Berg E. Animal model for evaluating bone repair with and without adjunctive hyperbaric oxygen therapy (HBO): comparing dose schedules. J Invest Surg 1990; 3(4):387–392.
175. Okubo Y, Bessho K, Fujimura K, et al. Effect of hyperbaric oxygenation on bone induced by recombinant human bone morphogenetic protein-2. *Br J Oral Maxillofac Surg* 2001; 39(2):91–5.
176. Buckwater J, Cruess RL. Healing of musculoskeletal tissues. In: Green DP, ed. *Fractures*. Rockwood Calif: Lippincott, 1991:81.
177. Cornell CN. Initial clinical experience with use of Collagraft as bone graft substitute. *Tech Orthop* 1992;7:55–63.
178. Perren SM, Huggler A, Russenberger M, et al. The reaction of cortical bone to compression. *Acta Orthop Scand* 1969;125(Suppl):19–29.
179. Centers for Disease Control and Prevention. Medical expenditures attributable to injuries—United States, 2000. *Morb Mortal Wkly Rep* 2004;53(1):1–4.
180. Heppenstall RB. Fracture Treatment and Healing. Philadelphia: Saunders, 1980.
181. Marsh D. Concepts of fracture union, delayed union, and non-union. *Clin Orthop* 1998; (355 Suppl):S22–S30.
182. Rodriguez-Merchan EC, Gomez-Castresana F. Internal fixation of nonunions. *Clin Orthop* 2004;(419):13–20.
183. Rosacker JA, Jarosvawu K. Both bone fractures of the forearm. *Orthopedics* 1981;4: 1353.
184. Weber B, Czech O. *Pseudarthrosis*. Bern: Hans Huber, 1976.
185. Paley D, Catagni MA, Argnani F, et al. Ilizarov treatment of tibial non-union with bone loss. *Clin Orthop* 1989;(241):146–165.
186. Muller ME, Thomas RJ. Treatment of non-union in fractures of long bones. *Clin Orthop* 1979;138:141–153.
187. Kempf I, Grosse A, Rigaut P. The treatment of noninfected pseudarthrosis of the femur and tibia with locked intramedullary nailing. *Clin Orthop* 1986;212:142–154.
188. Webb LX, Winquist RA, Hansen ST. Intramedullary nailing and reaming for delayed union or nonunion of the femoral shaft. A report of 105 consecutive cases. *Clin Orthop* 1986;(212):133–141.
189. Wray JB. The biochemical characteristics of the fracture hematoma in man. *Surg Gynecol Obstet* 1970;130(5):847–852.
190. Wallace AL, Draper ER, Strachan RK, et al. The effect of devascularisation upon early bone healing in dynamic external fixation. *J Bone Joint Surg (Br)* 1991;73(5):819–825.
191. Green N, French S, Rodriquez G, et al. Radiation-induced delayed union of fractures. *Radiology* 1969;93(3):635–641.
192. Tonna EA, Cronkite EP. The periosteum. Autoradiographic studies on cellular proliferation and transformation utilizing tritiated thymidine. *Clin Orthop* 1963;30:218–233.
193. Boyd H. Observations on non-union of the shafts of long bones, with a statistical analysis of 842 patients. *J Bone Joint Surgery* 1961;3A:159.
194. Blount W. *Fractures in children*. Baltimore: Williams & Wilkins, 1955.
195. Buckwater JA. Bone structure and function. Park Ridge, Illinois: American Academy of Orthopaedic Surgeons. 1987:27. American Academy of Orthopaedics Surgeons exhibit, Atlanta, Feb 9–14, 1984.
196. Blount W. *Fractures in children*. Baltimore: Williams & Wilkins, 1944.
197. Doepfner W. Consequences of calcium and/or phosphorus deficient diets on various parameters of callus formation and on growth rate in young rats. *Br J Pharmacol* 1970; 39(1):188P–189P.
198. Einhorn TA, Bonnarens F, Burstein AH. The contributions of dietary protein and mineral to the healing of experimental fractures. A biomechanical study. *J Bone Joint Surg (Am)* 1986;68(9):1389–1395.
199. Day SM, DeHeer DH. Reversal of the detrimental effects of chronic protein malnutrition on long bone fracture healing. *J Orthop Trauma* 2001;15(1):47–53.
200. Rothman RH, Klemek JS, Toton JJ. The effect of iron deficiency anemia on fracture healing. *Clin Orthop* 1971;77:276–283.
201. Koskinen EV, Ryoppy SA, Lindholm TS. Bone formation by induction under the influence of growth hormone and cortisone. *Isr J Med Sci* 1971;7(3):378–380.
202. Nichols JT, Toto PD, Choukas NC. The proliferative capacity and DNA synthesis of osteoblasts during fracture repair in normal and hypophysectomized rats. *Oral Surg Oral Med Oral Pathol* 1968;25(3):418–426.
203. Benghuzzi H, Tucci M, Tsao A, et al. Stimulation of osteogenesis by means of sustained delivery of various natural androgenic hormones. *Biomed Sci Instrum* 2004;40:99–104.
204. Herskind AM, Christensen K, Norgaard-Andersen K, et al. Diabetes mellitus and healing of closed fractures. *Diabetes Metab* 1992;18(1):63–64.
205. Soejima K, Landing BH. Osteoporosis in juvenile-onset diabetes mellitus: morphometric and comparative studies. *Pediatr Pathol* 1986;6(2–3):289–299.
206. Munoz-Torres M, Jodar E, Escobar-Jimenez F, et al. Bone mineral density measured by dual X-ray absorptiometry in Spanish patients with insulin-dependent diabetes mellitus. *Calcif Tissue Int* 1996;58(5):316–319.
207. Krakauer JC, McKenna MJ, Buderer NF, et al. Bone loss and bone turnover in diabetes. *Diabetes* 1995;44(7):775–782.
208. Lu H, Kraut D, Gerstenfeld LC, Graves DT. Diabetes interferes with the bone formation by affecting the expression of transcription factors that regulate osteoblast differentiation. *Endocrinology* 2003;144(1):346–352.
209. Adams CI, Keating JF, Court-Brown CM. Cigarette smoking and open tibial fractures. *Injury* 2001;32(1):61–65.
210. Porter SE, Hanley EN Jr. The musculoskeletal effects of smoking. *J Am Acad Orthop Surg* 2001;9(1):9–17.
211. Einhorn TA. Cox-2: Where are we in 2003? The role of cyclooxygenase-2 in bone repair. *Arthritis Res Ther* 2003;5(1):5–7.
212. Simon AM, Manigrasso MB, O'Connor JP. Cyclo-oxygenase 2 function is essential for bone fracture healing. *J Bone Miner Res* 2002;17(6):963–976.
213. Wilson J. Cancellous strip bone grafting. *J Bone Joint Surg (Am)* 1957;39:585.
214. Muller ME, Schner R, Willeneger H. *Manuel of forearm fixation*. Berlin: Springer-Verlag, 1979.
215. Charnley J. *The closed treatment of common fractures*. Edinburgh: Churchill Livingstone, 1961:245.
216. Taylor C. Delayed union and Nonunion of fractures in Campbell's operative orthopaedics, 8th ed, Crenshaw A, ed.
217. Friedlaender GE, Perry CR, Cole JD, et al. Osteogenic protein-1 (bone morphogenetic protein-7) in the treatment of tibial nonunions. *J Bone Joint Surg (Am)* 2001;83-A(Suppl 1)(Pt 2):S151–S158.
218. Cheng H, Jiang W, Phillips FM, et al. Osteogenic activity of the fourteen types of human bone morphogenetic proteins (BMPs). *J Bone Joint Surg (Am)* 2003; 85-A(8): 1544 52.
219. Zaretski A, Amir A, Meller I, et al. Free fibula long bone reconstruction in orthopedic oncology: a surgical algorithm for reconstructive options. *Plast Reconstr Surg* 2004; 113(7):1989–2000.
220. Enneking WF, Eady JL, Burchardt H. Autogenous cortical bone grafts in the reconstruction of segmental skeletal defects. *J Bone Joint Surg (Am)* 1980;62(7):1039–1058.
221. Mekhail AO, Abraham E, Gruber B, et al. Bone transport in the management of posttraumatic bone defects in the lower extremity. *J Trauma* 2004;56(2):368–378.
222. Friedenberg ZB, Harlow MC, Brighton CT. Healing of non-union of the medial malleolus by means of direct current: a case report. *J Trauma* 1971;11(10):883–885.
223. Patterson DC, Lewis GN, Cass CA. Treatment of delayed union and non-union with an implanted direct current stimulator. *Clin Orthop* 1980;148: 117–128.
224. Srivastava KP, Saxena AK. Electrical stimulation in delayed union of long bones. *Acta Orthop Scand* 1977;48(6):561–565.
225. Aaron RK, Ciombor DM, Simon BJ. Treatment of nonunions with electric and electromagnetic fields. *Clin Orthop* 2004;(419):21–29.
226. Bassett CA, Pawluk RJ, Pilla AA. Acceleration of fracture repair by electromagnetic fields. A surgically noninvasive method. *Ann N Y Acad Sci* 1974;238:242–262.
227. Goodwin CB, Brighton CT, Guyer RD, et al. A double-blind study of capacitively coupled electrical stimulation as an adjunct to lumbar spinal fusions. *Spine* 1999; 24(13):1349–56; discussion, 1357.
228. Traina G, Massari L, Cadossi R. Electrical stimulation of tibial osteotomies. A double blind study. In: Bersani F, ed. *Electricity and magnetism in biology and medicine*. New York: Kluwer Academic/ Plenum, 1999:137–138.
229. Abeed RI, Naseer M, Abel EW. Capacitively coupled electrical stimulation treatment: results from patients with failed long bone fracture unions. *J Orthop Trauma* 1998; 12(7):510–513.
230. Brighton CT, Shaman P, Heppenstall RB, et al. Tibial non-union treated with direct current, capacitive coupling, or bone graft. *Clin Orthop* 1995(321):223–234.
231. Heppenstall RB, Brighton CT, Esterhai JL Jr, et al. Clinical and roentgenographic evaluation of non-union of the forearm in relation to treatment with D.C. electrical stimulation. *J Trauma* 1983;23(8):740–744.
232. Paterson DC, Hillier TM, Carter RF, et al. Experimental delayed union of the dog tibia and its use in assessing the effect of an electrical bone growth stimulator. *Clin Orthop* 1977;(128):340–350.
233. Zichner L. Repair of nonunions by electrically pulsed current stimulation. *Clin Orthop* 1981(161):115–121.
234. Nelson FR, Brighton CT, Ryaby J, et al. Use of physical forces in bone healing. *J Am Acad Orthop Surg* 2003;11(5):344–354.
235. Heckman JD, Ingram AJ, Loyd RD, et al. Non-union treatment with pulsed electromagnetic fields. *Clin Orthop* 1981(161):58–66.
236. Bassett CA. Beneficial effects of electromagnetic fields. *J Cell Biochem* 1993;51:387–393.
237. Linovitz RJ, Pathria M, Bernhardt M, et al. Combined magnetic fields accelerate and increase spine fusion: a double-blind, randomized, placebo controlled study. *Spine* 2002;27(13):1383–1389; discussion, 1389.
238. Busse JW, Bhandari M, Kulkarni AV, et al. The effect of low-intensity pulsed ultrasound therapy on time to fracture healing: a meta-analysis. *CMAJ* 2002;166(4):437–441.
239. Cook SD, Ryaby JP, McCabe J, et al. Acceleration of tibia and distal radius fracture healing in patients who smoke. *Clin Orthop* 1997;(337):198–207.
240. Shafi S, Kauder DR. Fluid resuscitation and blood replacement in patients with polytrauma. *Clin Orthop* 2004(422):37–42.
241. Giannoudis PV, Pape HC. Damage control orthopaedics in unstable pelvic ring injuries. *Injury* 2004;35(7):671–677.
242. Pryor JP, Reilly PM. Initial care of the patient with blunt polytrauma. *Clin Orthop* 2004; 422:30–36.
243. Giswold ME, Landry GJ, Taylor LM, et al. Iatrogenic arterial injury is an increasingly important cause of arterial trauma. *Am J Surg* 2004;187–185; 590–592.
244. Abou-Sayed H, Berger DL. Blunt lower-extremity trauma and popliteal artery injuries: revisiting the case for selective arteriography. *Arch Surg* 2002;137(5):585–589.
245. Hoover NW. Injuries of the popliteal artery associated with fractures and dislocations. *Surg Clin N Am* 1961;41:1099.
246. Dennis JW, Jagger C, Butcher JL, et al. Reassessing the role of arteriograms in the management of posterior knee dislocations. *J Trauma* 1993;35:692–697.
247. Kendall RW, Taylor DC, Salvian AJ, et al. The role of arteriography in assessing vascular injuries associated with dislocations of the knee. *J Trauma* 1993;35:875–878.
248. Sagraves SG, Conquest AM, Albrecht RJ, et al. Popliteal artery trauma in a rural level I trauma center. *Am Surg* 2003;69(6):485–489; discussion, 490.
249. Rich NM, Baugh JH, Hughes CW. Popliteal artery injuries in Vietnam. *Am J Surg* 1969; 118(4):531–534.
250. Shah DM, Leather RP, Corson JD, et al. Polytetrafluoroethylene grafts in the rapid

reconstruction of acute contaminated peripheral vascular injuries. *Am J Surg* 1984; 148(2):229–233.
251. Panetta T, Sclafani SJ, Goldstein AS, et al. Percutaneous transcatheter embolization for massive bleeding from pelvic fractures. *J Trauma* 1985;25(11):1021–1029.
252. Ben-Menachem Y, Coldwell DM, Young JW, et al. Hemorrhage associated with pelvic fractures: causes, diagnosis, and emergent management. *Am J Roentgenol* 1991;157(5): 1005–1014.
253. Faris IB, Raptis S, Fitridge R. Arterial injury in the lower limb from blunt trauma. *Aust N Z J Surg* 1997;67(1):25–30.
254. Ilijevski N, Radak D, Radevic B, et al. Popliteal traumatic arteriovenous fistulas. *J Trauma* 2002;52(4):739–744.
255. Hobson RW II, Howard EW, Wright CB, et al. Hemodynamics of canine femoral venous ligation: significance in combined arterial and venous injuries. *Surgery* 1973;74(6): 824–829.
256. Pasch AR, Bishara RA, Schuler JJ, et al. Results of venous reconstruction after civilian vascular trauma. *Arch Surg* 1986;121(5):607–611.
257. Meyer J, Walsh J, Schuler J, et al. The early fate of venous repair after civilian vascular trauma. A clinical, hemodynamic, and venographic assessment. *Ann Surg* 1987;206(4): 458–464.
258. Heckman MM, Whitesides TE Jr, Grewe SR, et al. Compartment pressure in association with closed tibial fractures. The relationship between tissue pressure, compartment, and the distance from the site of the fracture. *J Bone Joint Surg (Am)* 1994;76(9): 1285–1292.
259. Waddell JP, Lenczner EM. Arterial injury associated with skeletal trauma. *Injury* 1974; 6(1):28–32.
260. Hope MJ, McQueen MM. Acute compartment syndrome in the absence of fracture. *J Orthop Trauma* 2004;18(4):220–224.
261. Bae DS, Kadiyala RK, Waters PM. Acute compartment syndrome in children: contemporary diagnosis, treatment, and outcome. *J Pediatr Orthop* 2001;21(5):680–688.
262. Ozkayin N, Aktuglu K. Monitoring of uncooperative, polytraumatized patients with tibial shaft fractures for acute compartment syndrome. *Ulus Travma Derg* 2004;10(2): 128–132.
263. Yuan PS, Pring ME, Gaynor TP, et al. Compartment syndrome following intramedullary fixation of pediatric forearm fractures. *J Pediatr Orthop* 2004;24(4):370–375.
264. Richards H, Langston A, Kulkarni R, et al. Does patient controlled analgesia delay the diagnosis of compartment syndrome following intramedullary nailing of the tibia? *Injury* 2004;35(3):296–298.
265. Bhattacharyya T, Vrahas MS. The medical-legal aspects of compartment syndrome. *J Bone Joint Surg (Am)* 2004;86-A(4):864–868.
266. Nerlich M, Dziadzka S, Schmidt U. Compartment syndrome of the lower leg. Long-term results. *Unfallchirurg* 1991;94(5):257–261.
267. Rush DS, Frame SB, Bell RM, et al. Does open fasciotomy contribute to morbidity and mortality after acute lower extremity ischemia and revascularization? *J Vasc Surg* 1989; 10(3):343–350.
268. Finkelstein JA, Hunter GA, Hu RW. Lower limb compartment syndrome: course after delayed fasciotomy. *J Trauma* 1996;40(3):342–344.
269. Whitesides TE, Haney TC, Morimoto K, et al. Tissue pressure measurements as a determinant for the need of fasciotomy. *Clin Orthop* 1975;113:43–451
270. Mubarak SJ, Hargens AR, Owen CA, et al. The wick catheter technique for measurement of intramuscular pressure. A new research and clinical tool. *J Bone Joint Surg* 1976; 58A:1016–1020.
271. Rorabeck CH. Exertional tibialis posterior compartment syndrome. *Clin Orthop Relat Res* 1986;208:61–64.
272. McQueen M. Acute compartment syndrome. *Acta Chir Belg* 1998;98(4):166–170.
273. Garr JL, Gentilello LM, Cole PA, et al. Monitoring for compartmental syndrome using near-infrared spectroscopy: a non-invasive, continuous, transcutaneous monitoring technique. *J Trauma* 1999;46(4):613–616; discussion, 617–618.
274. Rominger MB, Lukosch CJ, Bachmann GF. MR imaging of compartment syndrome of the lower leg: a case control study. *Eur Radiol* 2004;14(8):1432–1439.
275. Lynch JE, Heyman JS, Hargens AR. Ultrasonic device for the noninvasive diagnosis of compartment syndrome. *Physiol Meas* 2004;25(1):N1–N9.
276. Colohan AR, Pitts LH, Rosegay H. Injury to the peripheral nerves. In: Feliciano DV, Moore EE, Mattox KL, eds. *Trauma*, 3rd ed. Stamford, CT: Appleton & Lange, 1996: 853–862.
277. Almquist E, Eeg-Olofsson O. Sensory-nerve-conduction velocity and two-point discrimmination in sutured nerves. *J Bone Joint Surg (Am)* 1970;52(4):791–796.
278. Ducker TB, Kempe LG, Hayes GJ. The metabolic background for peripheral nerve surgery. *J Neurosurg* 1969;30(3):270–280.
279. Blumcke S, Niedorf HR. Axoplasmic alterations in the proximal and distal stumps of transacted nerves. *Act Neuropath* 1966;7:44.
280. Bassett CA, Campbell JB, Husby J. Peripheral nerve and spinal cord regeneration: factors leading to success of a tubulation technique employing millipore. *Exp Neurol* 1959;1: 386–406.
281. Weiss P. Nerve patterns: The mechanics of nerve growth. *Growth* 1941;5:163.
282. Seddon HJ. Nerve injuries. *J Univ Mich Med Center* 1965:31:4.
283. Ristic S, Strauch RJ, Rosenwasser MP. The assessment and treatment of nerve dysfunction after trauma around the elbow. *Clin Orthop* 2000;(370):138–153.
284. Trumble TE. Pathophysiology and repair. Peripheral nerve injury. In: Feliciano DV, Moore EE, Mattox KL, eds. *Trauma*, 4th ed. New York, NY: McGraw-Hill, 2000: 1047–1055.
285. Berkow R. The Merck Manual of Medical Information. West Point, NJ: Merck Research Laboratoris, 1997:30.
286. Schwartz SI. *Principles of surgery*, 7th ed. New York: McGraw Hill, 1999.
287. Greenfield LJ: *Surgery: scientific principles and practice*, 2nd ed. Philadelphia: Lippincott-Raven, 1997:2172–2173.
288. Townsend PL. Microsurgical techniques in reconstructive surgery. In: Farndon J, Keen G, eds. *Operative surgery and management*, 3rd ed. Oxford, UK: Butterworth-Heinemann, 1994:434–435.
289. Utley DS, Lewin SL, Cheng ET, et al. Brain-derived neurotrophic factor and collagen tubulization enhance functional recovery after peripheral nerve transection and repair. *Arch Otolaryngol Head Neck Surg* 1996;122(4):407–413.
290. Clark WK. Surgery for injection injuries of peripheral nerves. *Surg Clin N Am* 1972; 52(5):1325–1328.
291. Kline DG, Nulsen FE. The neuroma in continuity. Its preoperative and operative management. *Surg Clin N Am* 1972;52(5):1189–1209.
292. Swaim SF. Peripheral nerve surgery in the dog. *J Am Vet Med Assoc* 1972;161(8): 905–911.
293. Mitchell S. Injuries of their nerves and their consequences. New York: Dover Publications, 1965.
294. Katz J, Melzack R. Pain 'memories' in phantom limbs: review and clinical observations. *Pain* 1990;43(3):319–336.
295. Bach S, Noreng MF, Tjellden NU. Phantom limb pain in amputees during the first 12 months following limb amputation, after preoperative lumbar epidural blockade. *Pain* 1988;33(3):297–301.
296. Jahangiri M, Jayatunga AP, Bradley JW, et al. Prevention of phantom pain after major lower limb amputation by epidural infusion of diamorphine, clonidine and bupivacaine. *Ann R Coll Surg Engl* 1994;76(5):324–326.
297. Jensen TS, Krebs B, Nielsen J, et al. Non-painful phantom limb phenomena in amputees: incidence, clinical characteristics and temporal course. *Acta Neurol Scand* 1984; 70:407–414.
298. Meyer RA. Peripheral neural mechanisms of nociception. In: Wall PD, Melzack R, eds. *Textbook of pain*. Edinburgh: Livingstone Churchill, 1994:13–44.
299. Martyn S. On the physiological meaning of inframammary pain. *Br Med J* 1864;2: 296–298.
300. Kellgren JH. Observations on referred pain arising from muscle. *Clin Sci* 1938;3: 175–190.
301. McAuliffe G, Goodell H, Wolff H. Experimental studies on headache pain from the nasal and paranasal structures. *Proc Assoc Res Nervous Mental Dis* 1943;23:185–208.
302. Paré A. In: Johnson T, translator. The Collected Works of Ambroise Paré, Book 10. Of the cure of wounds of the nervous parts. Pound Ridge, UK: Milford House, 1934: 400–402.
303. Sudeck P. Die akute (trophoneurotische) Knochenatrophie nach Entzündungen und Traumen der Extremitäten. *Deut Med Wschr* 1902.
304. Leriche R. De la causalgie envisagee comme une nevrite due sympathique etde son traitment par la denudation et l'excision des plexus nerveux peri-arteriels. *Presse Med* 1916;24:178–180.
305. Evans JA. Reflex sympathetic dystrophy. *Surg Gynecol Obstet* 1946;82:36–44.
306. Boas RA. A Workshop Report on RSD (now CRPS). Seattle, IASP Press. Complex regional pain syndromes, 1995.
307. Allen G, Galer BS, Schwartz L. Epidemiology of complex regional pain syndrome: a retrospective chart review of 134 patients. *Pain* 1999; 80(3):539–544.
308. Scadding JW. Development of ongoing activity, mechanosensitivity, and adrenaline sensitivity in severed peripheral nerve axons. *Exp Neurol* 1981;73(2):345–364.
309. Task Force on Taxonomy: Classification of Chronic pain: Description of Chronic Pain Syndromes and Definitions of Pain Terms. Seattle: IASP Press, 1994.
310. Devor M, Janig W. Activation of myelinated afferents ending in a neuroma by stimulation of the sympathetic supply in the rat. *Neurosci Lett* 1981;24(1):43–47.
311. Schurmann M, Gradl G, Wizgal I, et al. Clinical and physiologic evaluation of stellate ganglion blockade for complex regional pain syndrome type I. *Clin J Pain* 2001;17(1): 94–100.
312. Goldstein DS, Tack C, Li ST. Sympathetic innervation and function in reflex sympathetic dystrophy. *Ann Neurol* 2000;48(1):49–59.
313. Blair SJ, Chinthagada M, Hoppenstehdt D, et al. Role of neuropeptides in pathogenesis of reflex sympathetic dystrophy. *Acta Orthop Belg* 1998;64(4):448–451.
314. Jänig WM, Mathias CM. *Neurobiology of the autonomic nervous system*. Oxford: Oxford University Press, 1994.
315. Calder JS, Holten I, McAllister RM. Evidence for immune system involvement in reflex sympathetic dystrophy. *J Hand Surg (Br)* 1998;23(2):147–150.
316. Leitha T, Korpan M, Staudenherz A, et al. Five phase bone scintigraphy supports the pathophysiological concept of a subclinical inflammatory process in reflex sympathetic dystrophy. *Q J Nucl Med* 1996;40(2):188–193.
317. Van der Laan L, Goris RJ. Reflex sympathetic dystrophy. An exaggerated regional inflammatory response? *Hand Clin* 1997;13(3):373–385.
318. Yung Chung O, Bruehl SP. Complex regional pain syndrome. *Curr Treat Options Neurol* 2003;5(6):499–511.
319. Oyen WJ, Arntz IE, Claessens RM, et al. Reflex sympathetic dystrophy of the hand: an excessive inflammatory response? Pain 1993;55(2):151–157.
320. Leis S, Weber M, Isselmann A, et al. Substance-P-induced protein extravasation is bilaterally increased in complex regional pain syndrome. *Exp Neurol* 2003;183(1): 197–204.
321. Leis S, Weber M, Schmelz M, et al. Facilitated neurogenic inflammation in unaffected limbs of patients with complex regional pain syndrome. *Neurosci Lett* 2004;359(3): 163–166.
322. Amadio PC, Mackinnon SE, Merritt WH, et al. Reflex sympathetic dystrophy syndrome: consensus report of an ad hoc committee of the American Association for Hand Surgery on the definition of reflex sympathetic dystrophy syndrome. *Plast Reconstr Surg* 1991; 87(2):371–375.
323. Vernon H. Reflex sympathetic dystrophy and chiropractic. *Adv Chir* 1995:183–194.

324. Levine DZ. Burning pain in an extremity. Breaking the destructive cycle of reflex sympathetic dystrophy. *Postgrad Med* 1991;90(2):175–178, 183–185.
325. Kozin F. Reflex sympathetic dystrophy syndrome: a review. *Clin Exp Rheumatol* 1992; 10(4):401–409.
326. Muneshige H, Toda K, Kimura H, et al. Does a viral infection cause complex regional pain syndrome? *Acupunct Electrother Res* 2003;28(3–4):183–192.
327. Paice E. Reflex sympathetic dystrophy. *Br Med J* 1995;310(6995):1645–1648.
328. Reuben SS, Sklar J. Intravenous regional anesthesia with clonidine in the management of complex regional pain syndrome of the knee. *J Clin Anesth* 2002;14(2):87–91.
329. Soucacos PN, Diznitsas LA, Beris AE, et al. Reflex sympathetic dystrophy of the upper extremity. Clinical features and response to multimodal management. *Hand Clinics* 1997;13:339–354.
330. Soucacos PN, Diznitsas LA, Beris AE, et al. Clinical criteria and treatment of segmental versus upper extremity reflex sympathetic dystrophy. *Acta Orthopaedica Belgica (Acta Orthop Belg)* 1998;64(Sep)(3):314–321.
331. Hardy MA, Merritt WH. Psychological evaluation and pain assessment in patients with reflex sympathetic dystrophy. *J Hand Therapy* 1988;3:154–164.
332. Mackinnon SE, Holder LE. The use of three-phase radionuclide bone scanning in the diagnosis of reflex sympathetic dystrophy. *J Hand Surg (Am)* 1984;9(4):556–563.
333. Monti DA, Herring CL, Schwartzman RJ, et al. Personality assessment of patients with complex regional pain syndrome type I. *Clin J Pain* 1998;14:295–302.
334. Schiepers C, Bormans I, De Roo M. Three-phase bone scan and dynamic vascular scintigraphy in algoneurodystrophy of the upper extremity. *Acta Orthop Belg* 1998; 64(3):322–327.
335. Tietjen R. Reflex sympathetic dystrophy of the knee. *Clin Orthop* 1986;(209):234–243.
336. McDougall IR, Keeling CA. Complications of fractures and their healing. *Semin Nucl Med* 1988;18(2):113–125.
337. Sarangi PP, Ward AJ, Smith EJ, et al. Algodystrophy and osteoporosis after tibial fractures. *J Bone Joint Surg (Br)* 1993;75(3):450–452.
338. Zyluk A. The usefulness of quantitative evaluation of three-phase scintigraphy in the diagnosis of post-traumatic reflex sympathetic dystrophy. *J Hand Surg (Br)* 1999;24(1): 16–21.
339. Goldsmith DP, Vivino FB, Eichenfield AH, et al. Nuclear imaging and clinical features of childhood reflex neurovascular dystrophy: comparison with adults. *Arthritis Rheum* 1989;32(4):480–485.
340. Werner R, Davidoff G, Jackson MD, et al. Factors affecting the sensitivity and specificity of the three-phase technetium bone scan in the diagnosis of reflex sympathetic dystrophy syndrome in the upper extremity. *J Hand Surg (Am)* 1989;14(3):520–523.
341. Zyluk A, Birkenfeld B. Quantitative evaluation of three-phase bone scintigraphy before and after the treatment of post-traumatic reflex sympathetic dystrophy. *Nucl Med Commun* 1999;20(4):327–333.
342. Nazarian LN, Schweitzer ME, Mandel S, et al. Increased soft-tissue blood flow in patients with reflex sympathetic dystrophy of the lower extremity revealed by power Doppler sonography. *Am J Roentgenol* 1998;171(5):1245–1250.
343. Charlton JE. Management of sympathetic pain. *Br Med Bull* 1991;47:601–618.
344. Oerlemans HM, Oostendorp RA, de Boo T, et al. Pain and reduced mobility in complex regional pain syndrome I: outcome of a prospective randomised controlled clinical trial of adjuvant physical therapy versus occupational therapy. *Pain* 1999;83(1):77–83.
345. Bengtson K. Physical modalities for complex regional pain syndrome. *Hand Clin* 1997; 13:443–454.
346. Watson HK, Carlson L. Treatment of reflex sympathetic dystrophy of the hand with an active "stress loading" program. *J Hand Surg (Am)* 1987;12(5 Pt 1):779–785.
347. Lopez RF. Reflex sympathetic dystrophy. Timely diagnosis and treatment can prevent severe contractures. *Postgrad Med* 1997;101(4):185–190.
348. Seale KS. Reflex sympathetic dystrophy of the lower extremity. *Clin Orthop* 1989;(243): 80–85.
349. Abram SE, Lightfoot RW. Treatment of long standing causalgia with prazosin. *Reg Anaesth* 1981;6:79–81.
350. Korpan MI, Dezu Y, Schneider B, et al. Acupuncture in the treatment of posttraumatic pain syndrome. *Acta Orthop Belg* 1999;65(2):197–201.
351. Spacek A, Hoerauf K, Kress HG. Pain management of complex regional pain syndrome (CRPS). *Acta Anaesthesiol Scand* 1998;(Suppl)42:13–15.
352. Wu WH, Bandilla E, Ciccone DS, et al. Effects of qigong on late-stage complex regional pain syndrome. *Altern Ther Health Med* 1999;5(1):45–54.
353. Grunert BK, Devine CA, Sanger JR, et al. Thermal self-regulation for pain control in reflex sympathetic dystrophy syndrome. *J Hand Surg (Am)* 1990;15(4):615–618.
354. Muramatsu K, Kawai S, Akino T, et al. Treatment of chronic regional pain syndrome using manipulation therapy and regional anesthesia. *J Trauma* 1998;44(1):189–192.
355. Christensen K, Jensen EM, Noer I. The reflex dystrophy syndrome response to treatment with systemic corticosteroids. *Acta Chir Scand* 1982;148(8):653–655.
356. Devor M, Govrin-Lippmann R, Raber P. Corticosteroids suppress ectopic neural discharge originating in experimental neuromas. *Pain* 1985;22(2):127–137.
357. Braus DF, Krauss JK, Strobel J. The shoulder-hand syndrome after stroke: a prospective clinical trial. *Ann Neurol* 1994;36(5):728–733.
358. Fraioli F, Fabbri A, Gnessi L, et al. Subarachnoid injection of salmon calcitonin induces analgesia in man. *Eur J Pharmacol* 1982;78(3):381–382.
359. Maillefert JF, Cortet B, Aho S. Pooled results from 2 trials evaluating biphosphonates in reflex sympathetic dystrophy. *J Rheumatol* 1999;26(8):1856–1857.
360. Varenna M, Zucchi F, Ghiringhelli D, et al. Intravenous clodronate in the treatment of reflex sympathetic dystrophy syndrome. A randomized, double blind, placebo controlled study. *J Rheumatol* 2000;27(6):1477–1483.
361. Max MB, Lynch SA, Muir J, et al. Effects of desipramine, amitriptyline, and fluoxetine on pain in diabetic neuropathy. *N Engl J Med* 1992;326(19):1250–1256.
362. Verre M, De Santis F, Glyronakis S, et al. Pharmacological sympathetic block in complex regional pain syndrome. *Clin Ter* 2002;153(6):367–372.
363. Zyluk A. Results of the treatment of posttraumatic reflex sympathetic dystrophy of the upper extremity with regional intravenous blocks of methylprednisolone and lidocaine. *Acta Orthop Belg* 1998;64(4):452–456.
364. Grabow TS, Tella PK, Raja SN. Spinal cord stimulation for complex regional pain syndrome: an evidence-based medicine review of the literature. *Clin J Pain* 2003;19(6): 371–383.
365. Stewart WF, Ricci JA, Chee E, et al. Lost productive time and cost due to common pain conditions in the US workforce. *JAMA* 2003;290(18):2443–2454.
366. Rauck RL. Trauma. In: Raj PP, ed. *Pain medicine*. St. Louis: Mosby, 1996:346–357.
367. Ananthanarayan C, Castro C, McKee N, Sakotic G. Compartment syndrome following intravenous regional anesthesia. *Can J Anaesth* 2000;47(11):1094–1098.
368. Grande CM, Smith CE, Stene JK. Trauma anesthesia. In: Longnecker DE, Tinker JH, Morgan GE, eds. *Principles and practice of anesthesiology*, 2nd ed. St. Louis: Mosby-Year Book, 1998:2138–2164.
369. Rosenberg AD. Perioperative anesthetic management of orthopedic injuries. 1999.
370. Carr DB, Goudas LC. Acute pain. *Lancet* 1999;353(9169):2051–2058.
371. Grocott HP, Mutch WA. Epidural anesthesia and acutely increased intracranial pressure. Lumbar epidural space hydrodynamics in a porcine model. *Anesthesiology* 1996; 85(5):1086–91.
372. Butcher D. Pharmacological techniques for managing acute pain in emergency departments. *Emerg Nurse* 2004;12(1):26–35 (quiz 36).
373. Eisenach JC, De Kock M, Klimscha W. alpha (2)-adrenergic agonists for regional anesthesia. A clinical review of clonidine (1984–1995). *Anesthesiology* 1996;85(3): 655–674.
374. Eisenach JC, Detweiler DJ, Tong C, et al. Cerebrospinal fluid nor epinephrine and acetylcholine concentrations during acute pain. *Anesth Analg* 1996;82(3):621–626.
375. Koppert W, Weigand M, Neumann F, et al. Perioperative intravenous lidocaine has preventive effects on postoperative pain and morphine consumption after major abdominal surgery. *Anesth Analg* 2004;98(4):1050–1055.
376. Wang C, Chakrabarti MK, Whitwam JG. Synergism between the antinociceptive effects of intrathecal midazolam and fentanyl on both A delta and C somatosympathetic reflexes. *Neuropharmacology* 1993;32(3):303–305.
377. Luger TJ, Hayashi T, Lorenz IH, et al. Mechanisms of the influence of midazolam on morphine antinociception at spinal and supraspinal levels in rats. *Eur J Pharmacol* 1994; 271(2–3):421–31.
378. Nishiyama T, Gyermek L, Lee C, et al. Analgesic interaction between intrathecal midazolam and glutamate receptor antagonists on thermal-induced pain in rats. *Anesthesiology* 1999;91(2):531–537.
379. Valentine JM, Lyons G, Bellamy MC. The effect of intrathecal midazolam on postoperative pain. *Eur J Anaesthesiol* 1996;13(6):589–593.
380. Hagelberg N, Aalto S, Kajander J, et al. Alfentanil increases cortical dopamine D2/D3 receptor binding in healthy subjects. *Pain* 2004;109(1–2):86–93.
381. Katz J, Schmid R, Snijdelaar DG, et al. Pre-emptive analgesia using intravenous fentanyl plus low-dose ketamine for radical prostatectomy under general anesthesia does not produce short-term or long-term reductions in pain or analgesic use. *Pain* 2004;110(3): 707–718.
382. Hicks RW, Becker SC, Krenzischeck D, et al. Medication errors in the PACU: a secondary analysis of MEDMARX findings. *J Perianesth Nurs* 2004;19(1):18–28.
383. Aygun S, Kocoglu H, Goksu S, et al. Postoperative patient-controlled analgesia with intravenous tramadol, intravenous fentanyl, epidural tramadol and epidural ropivacaine + fentanyl combination. *Eur J Gynaecol Oncol* 2004;25(4):498–501.
384. Mishra LD, Nath SS, Gairola RL, et al. Buprenorphine-soaked absorbable gelatin sponge: an alternative method for postlaminectomy pain relief. *J Neurosurg Anesthesiol* 2004;16(2):115–21.
385. Ben-David B, Schmalenberger K, Chelly JE. Analgesia after total knee arthroplasty: is continuous sciatic blockade needed in addition to continuous femoral blockade? *Anesth Analg* 2004;98(3):747–749.
386. Coda BA, O'Sullivan B, Donaldson G, et al. Comparative efficacy of patient-controlled administration of morphine, hydromorphone, or sufentanil for the treatment of oral mucositis pain following bone marrow transplantation. *Pain* 1997;72(3):333–346.
387. Wilder-Smith CH, Hill L, Dyer RA, et al. Postoperative sensitization and pain after cesarean delivery and the effects of single in doses of tramadol and diclofenac alone and in combination. *Anesth Analg* 2003;97(2):526–533.
388. Weis OF, Sriwatanakul K, Alloza JL. Attitudes of patients, house staff and nurses towards postoperative analgesic care. *Anesth Analg* 1983;62:70.
389. Adams RJ, Armstrong EP, Erstad BL. Prescribing and self-administration of morphine in Hispanic and non Hispanic Caucasian patients treated with patient-controlled analgesia. *J Pain Palliat Care Pharmacother* 2004;18(2):29–38.
390. Colwell CW Jr. The use of the pain pump and patient-controlled analgesia in joint reconstruction. *Am J Orthop* 2004;33(Suppl 5):10–12.
391. Patel N, Smith CE. Pain management in trauma. *Anesthesiol Clin N Am* 1999;17: 295–309.
392. Raw RM. Regional anaesthesia in mountain rescue. *S Afr Med J* 2004;94(1):8–9.
393. Hadzic A, Arliss J, Kerimoglu B, et al. A comparison of infraclavicular nerve block versus general anesthesia for hand and wrist day-case surgeries. *Anesthesiology* 2004; 101(1):127–132.
394. Kirkpatrick AF, Bednarczyk LR, Hime GW, et al. Bupivacaine blood levels during continuous interscalene block. *Anesthesiology* 1985;62(1):65–67.
395. Charghi R, Backman S, Christou N, et al. Patient controlled i.v. analgesia is an acceptable pain management strategy in morbidly obese patients undergoing gastric bypass surgery. A retrospective comparison with epidural analgesia. *Can J Anaesth* 2003;50(7): 672–678.

OSTEOPOROTIC FRACTURES

Magnus K. Karlsson, Karl J. Obrant, and Per Olof Josefsson

EPIDEMIOLOGY

Osteoporosis was first observed in Egypt in 990 BC and has therefore been known about for many centuries (1). The definition of osteoporosis is a bone mineral density (BMD) of 2.5 standard deviations or more below the young normal mean (2) (Table 19-1). Using this definition a quarter of all post-menopausal American caucasians, a total of 26 million caucasian American women, are osteoporotic (3). The number of fragility fractures, those of the proximal humerus, distal forearm, vertebrae, pelvis, hip, and the tibial condyles have risen exponentially during the same period (Fig. 19-1) (4,5). These fractures show a number of common epidemiological features. The incidence is higher in women than men and increases exponentially with age (Fig. 19-2). The fractures also occur at sites where there is a large proportion of trabecular bone (4–6). The reason for the increase in incidence is not fully understood. The changes in population demographics, particularly the high incidence of elderly in the population as well as changes in BMD and other risk factors have all influenced the incidence of osteoporotic fractures.

One of the commonest risk factors associated with fracture is a fall (7–11). Approximately one third of community dwellers aged 65 years or more and 50% to 60% of residents of nursing and old people's homes fall each year with women falling more than men (11–14). Fractures, dislocations, or serious soft tissue injuries result from about 10% to 15% of the falls in patients living in the community (11,14,15) and from about 15% to 20% of falls in institutionalized patients (14–16). Fractures occur in 3% to 12% of falls in the elderly being more common in women than men (10). Hip fractures occur in <1% of falls (10–17). The annual incidence of hip fractures in those with a tendency to fall is 7% but is 14% amongst frequent fallers. In the United States falls are responsible for the second highest injury-related cost to the economy (18). Unintentional falling is an important cause of mortality in the elderly. Twenty-three percent of injury-related deaths in patients over 65 years of age and 34% in those over 85 years of age occur as a result of a fall (19). It is therefore obvious that a major goal in fracture prevention must be to reduce the frequency of falls (20).

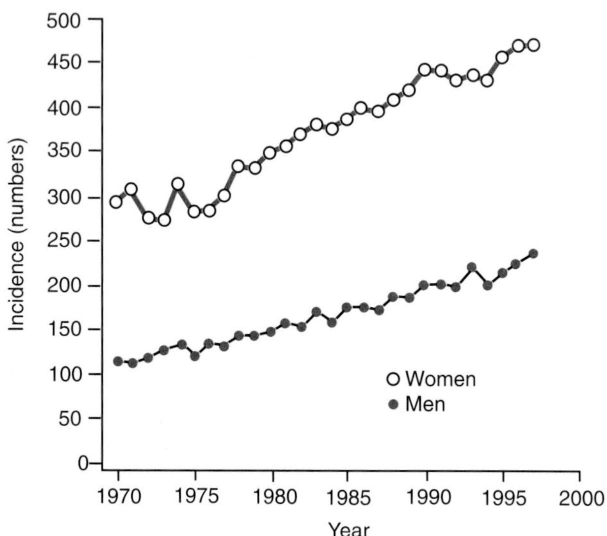

FIGURE 19-1 Age-adjusted incidence (per 100,000-persons) of hip fractures in Finland in women and men aged 50 years or older between 1970 and 1997. (Reprinted with permission from Kannus P, Niemi S, Parkkari J, et al. Hip fractures in Finland between 1970 and 1997 and predictions for the future. *Lancet* 1999;353:802–805.)

TABLE 19-1 World Health Organization Definition of Normal Bone Mineral Density, Osteopenia, Osteoporosis, Established Osteoporosis

Diagnostic Category	Definition	BMD T-Score
Normal bone mass	BMD above 1 standard deviation below the average young adult value	≥−1
Osteopenia	BMD between 1 and 2.5 standard deviations below the average young adult value	−1 to −2.5
Osteoporosis	BMD more than 2.5 standard deviations below the average young adult value	≤−2.5
Severe osteoporosis or established osteoporosis	BMD more than 2.5 standard deviations below the average young adult value and at least one osteoporotic fracture	≤−2.5

World Health Organization. Assessment of fracture risk and its application to screening for postmenopausal osteoporosis. Report of a WHO Study Group. *World Health Organ Tech Rep Ser* 1994;843:1–129.

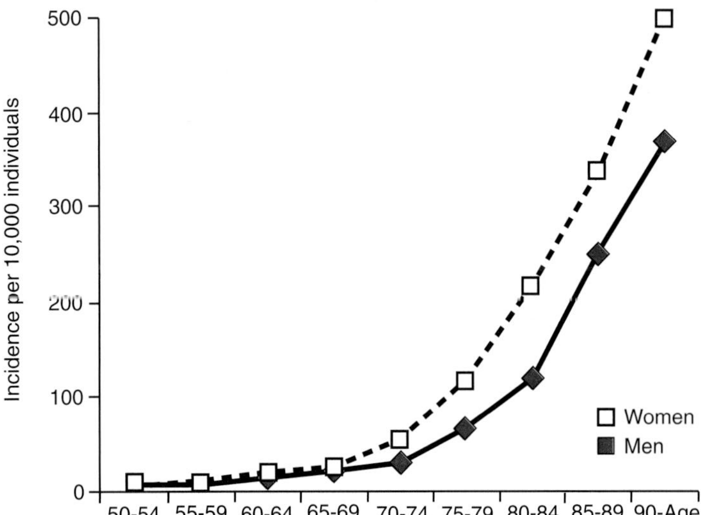

FIGURE 19-2 Incidence of hip fractures per 10,000 inhabitants in Malmö, Sweden 1992–1995. (Rogmark C, Sernbo I, Johnell O, Nilsson JA. A trend-break. *Acta Orthop Scand* 1999;70: 19–22.)

Fragility fractures also impose an enormous cost on society. Hip fracture is a major cause of hospital admission in the elderly and in the U.S. the direct cost of hip fractures was more than $7 billion per year in 1992 (21) and £750 million per year in 1994 in the United Kingdom (22). In addition the cost of nursing home care for patients who had hip fractures in the U.S. in 1992 was estimated to be $1.5 billion (21). The costs and outcome of hip fractures are often closely monitored as this fracture is usually regarded as the most significant osteoporotic fracture. The mortality attributable to osteoporosis is most obviously associated with hip fractures with the highest incidence occurring in the first 6 months after fracture (23). Hip fractures are also associated with up to 20% reduction in expected survival (24) and with the highest mortality in men (25), older patients (26), and in non-Caucasians (26). Additionally many patients become permanently disabled after hip fracture with the proportion who cannot walk rising from 20% to 50% after the fracture (27). A third of patients become totally dependent and require institutional care (28).

The highest incidence of hip fractures has been reported in Caucasians living in North Europe followed by Caucasians living in North America and Asians, with the lowest incidence being recorded in the African-American population (29). The female-to-male ratio is 3:1 in Caucasians, but 1:1 in Chinese and the Bantu (29). The incidence is age-dependent in both men and women rising from 2 per 100,000 person-years among Caucasian women less than 35 years of age to 3032 per 100,000 person-years in women of at least 85 years of age (Fig. 19-2) (30). The incidence of hip fracture has also increased during the last 40 years (4,5) even if recent data suggests either a leveling off or a slight downturn in North America and Europe (Fig. 19-3) (31). In contrast to this the incidence of hip fractures in developing Asian countries has rapidly increased during the last few decades (32) so that by the year 2050 it is estimated that 6.3 million hip fractures will occur globally, more than half of these in Asia (Fig. 19-3) (33).

The prevalence of vertebral fractures also varies in different ethnic groups being higher in Scandinavian, American, and Hong Kong Chinese females than in Eastern European females. The rates in male Hong Kong Chinese and male American Caucasians are lower than in male Europeans (34–36). The female-to-male ratio is 2:1 in Caucasians and the prevalence is age-dependent in both men and women. In North America this rises from <20 per 100,000 person-years in men and women under 45 years of age to 1,200 per 100,000 person-years in both men and women of at least 85 years of age (34). According to Swedish data the incidence of vertebral fracture has increased from 1950 to 1983 (37) but this trend has not been confirmed in Denmark (38) or in Rochester, Minnesota, U.S. (35). Mortality following a vertebral fracture is increased in men and women although it is less than after hip fracture (40). Patients with vertebral fractures also experience a reduction in quality of life usually as a result of back pain. They also have functional limitation, depression, disability, and loss of height (41,42).

PATHOGENESIS OF OSTEOPOROSIS

During the first decades in life there is an increase in skeletal size and BMD accrual (43,44). The BMD at age 20 to 30 years is described as the peak bone mass being the highest BMD that the individual will reach in life. It occurs in different skeletal regions at different ages (44). The factors that determine bone mineral density are poorly understood but studies in twins indicate that 60% to 80% of the BMD is determined by heredity (45). Other important factors are environmental factors such as the level of estrogen, testosterone, and growth hormone in addition to the level of exercise and nutrition as well as any diseases that interfere with normal growth (45,46). It is also likely that both anabolic and catabolic environmental factors have the greatest impact on bone during skeletal growth. For example, the skeletal response to exercise is most pronounced

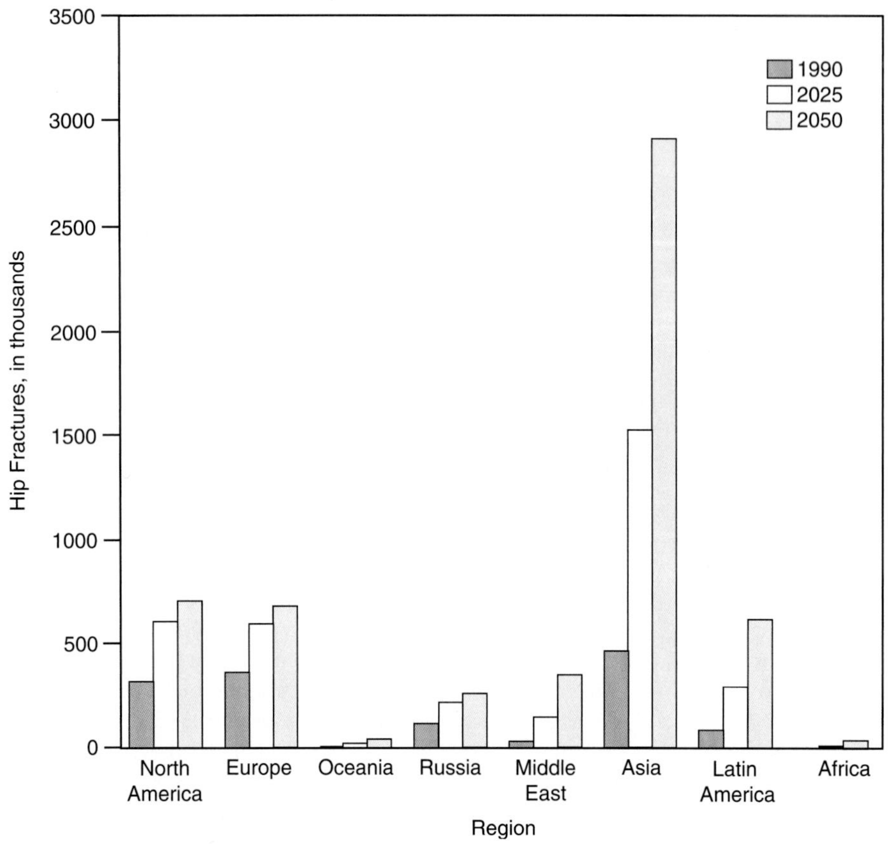

FIGURE 19-3 Estimated numbers of hip fractures in eight geographic regions in 1990, 2025, and 2050. (Reprinted with permission from Cooper C, Campion G, Melton LJ 3rd. Hip fractures in the elderly: a world-wide projection. *Osteoporos Int* 1992;2:285–289.)

during the pre- and early pubertal years, this being the period of fastest growth and the highest accrual of BMD (43,44,47) (Fig. 19-4).

Once peak bone mass is reached the BMD is virtually stable or shows a slight decrease until menopause. At the menopause the levels of estradiol and estrone drop to about 25% and 50% of their pre-menopausal values. At this time they are mainly produced by extra-glandular conversion of androgen precursors in muscles and adipose tissues. As the female sex hormones are probably the most important hormones regulating BMD, an accelerated loss of BMD naturally occurs during the 5 to 10 years after the menopause (48,49). At this time the increase in the number of sites undergoing active remodeling leads to BMD loss (48,49), trabecular perforation (50), and an increased risk of fracture (49). The processes that lead to age-related bone loss are probably multifactorial. With increasing age calcium absorption is impaired, which may lead to secondary hyperparathyroidism and accelerated bone loss. There is also a reduced production of active vitamin D due to thinning of the skin and reduced exposure to sunlight (51). This process is exacerbated by estrogen deficiency in both elderly men and women (51).

Cell cultures have also shown that osteoblasts undergo up to 50 population doublings but that the cells age. In patients with osteoporosis osteoblasts seem to undergo fewer population doublings resulting in an alteration of the relationship between

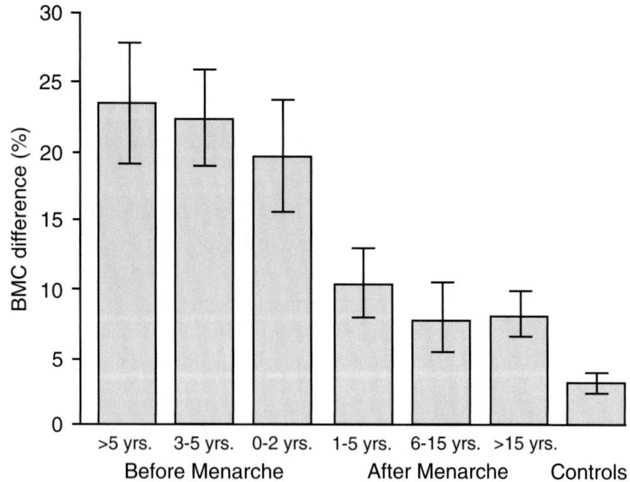

FIGURE 19-4 The mean (95% confidence interval) playing-to-nonplaying arm difference in bone mineral content of humeral shaft in 105 female tennis and squash players and their 50 controls according to biological age at which training was started (i.e., starting age of playing relative to age at menarche). (Reprinted with permission from Kannus P, Haapasalo H, Sankelo M, et al. Effect of starting age of physical activity on bone mass in the dominant arm of tennis and squash players. *Ann Intern Med* 1995; 123:27–31.)

bone formation and bone resorption (52). This may explain the insufficiency of the osteoblasts that has been demonstrated in elderly patients with osteoporosis (51). Thus, the main difference between osteoporotic and nonosteoporotic individuals seems to be mainly related to defective bone formation. Bone turnover in osteoporotic individuals may be elevated, normal, or reduced but the imbalance between resorption and formation always seems to be present although it is more pronounced with increased bone turnover (53). In addition, collagen synthesis and secretion of other osteotropic factors diminishes with age, a fact that could also influence skeletal strength (52).

As there is no demonstrable underlying medical cause for osteoporosis in 80% of women and 50% of men who present with fragility fractures, a diagnosis of primary involutional osteoporosis is often made (54). Riggs and Melton (54) subdivided primary osteoporosis into type I and type II osteoporosis. Type I is directly related to the loss of ovarian function after the menopause and type II is an exaggeration of the normal aging process. A recent study has emphasized the importance of estrogen in bone loss in both men and women and proposed a link between type I and type II osteoporosis (51). However, it is important to realize that involutional osteoporosis is multifactorial, although the roles of each specific factor are still poorly understood. If there is a cause for osteoporosis such as an endocrine, metabolic, gastrointestinal, renal, or hematologic disorder in addition to certain hereditary diseases and drug treatment, the diagnosis is that of secondary osteoporosis (Table 19-2). The higher proportion of secondary osteoporosis in men than women is usually attributed to alcoholism, malignant disease, long-term corticosteroid treatment, and hypogonadism (Table 19-2) (55).

TABLE 19-2 Diseases and Conditions Associated with Secondary Osteoporosis

Hormonal	**Rheumatological**
Hypogonadism	Rheumatoid arthritis and related diseases
Cushing syndrome	Ankylosing spondylitis
Addison disease	
Hyperthyroidism	
Hyperparathyroidism	**Hematological**
Acromegaly	Multiple myeloma and related diseases
Nutritional	Hemochromatosis
Severe malnutrition (e.g., anorexia nervosa)	Hemophilia
	Mastocytosis
	Thalassemia
Malabsorption (e.g., postgastrecomy)	Leukemia and lymphoma
Severe liver disease	
	Other
	Paralysis or total immobilization
Hereditary	Chronic obstructive lung disease
Osteogenesis imperfecta	Diffuse metastatic carcinoma
Ehlers-Danlos syndrome	Hypercalcemia of malignancy
Homocystinuria	
Congenital porphyria	
Hypophosphatasia	

ASSESSMENT OF BONE MINERAL DENSITY

The ability to measure BMD has been one of the most significant advances in the investigation and treatment of osteoporosis as BMD correlates strongly with bone strength. Variation in the level of bone mineral density accounts for 60% to 80% of bone strength, but it is important to realize that bone strength depends not only on the amount of mineral measured by current techniques but also on the structural characteristics of the skeleton such as size, shape, and three-dimensional architecture. Up until now the prediction of bone strength and risk of fracture has mainly been based on densitometric measurements but current research evaluating the macro- and microgeometrical structure of bone will probably improve the prediction of bone strength and the risk of fracture (48,56,57).

Single Photon Absorptiometry and Dual Photon Absorptiometry

The first specific bone scanning method to be developed, the single photon absorptiometry technique (SPA), used a single energy radionuclide. The technique of photon absorptiometry relies on the relationship between bone mineral content and the ease with which photons pass through skeletal tissue (Table 19-3). The denser the skeleton the more photons are absorbed by the bone tissue. This method can only be used in regions with minimal soft tissue, usually the distal radius or the calcaneus, as the scan cannot differentiate between absorption in soft tissue and bone (48–58). Dual photon absorptiometry (DPA), which uses two different photon energies, was developed to separately evaluate the absorption in soft tissue and bone so that skeletal structures surrounded by soft tissues could be evaluated. However, because of low precision relative to the rate of change of BMD dual photon absorptiometry was not suitable for monitoring longitudinal changes (58).

Dual Energy X-Ray Absorptiometry

Dual x-ray absorptiometry (DXA) was introduced in 1987 (59). This method uses x-rays as the photon source avoiding the problems of isotope source decay and replacement. The scan time is reduced to minutes with markedly improved scan image quality and resolution. However, the most important advance was that precision was markedly improved compared to the DPA technique making the technique adequate for longitudinal monitoring of BMD. DXA is currently the most used scanning technique for predicting the risk of fractures, establishing or confirming the diagnosis of osteoporosis, selecting patients for therapy and for monitoring the effective-

TABLE 19-3 Methods for Bone Mineral Measurement

Ionizing Radiation		Nonionizing Radiation
Gamma Radiation	*X-Ray*	
Single photon absorptiometry (SPA)	Radiogrammetry	
Dual photon absorptiometry (DPA)	Single x-ray absorptiometry (SXA)	Ultrasound
Neutron activation analysis (NAA)	Dual x-ray absorptiometry (DXA)	Magnetic resonance tomography (MRT)
Compton scattering technique	Quantitative computed tomography (QCT)	

ness of therapy (Table 19-3) (60). Fan-beam DXA technology offers semiautomatic vertebral morphometry (MXA) for screening vertebral deformities with scanning in the lateral projection (61). Thus far, fan-beam DXA technology has been used in research to screen for the presence of fractures but in the future this technique may be used to improve fracture prediction. When deciding treatment strategies for osteoporosis most clinicians currently use the hip scan, or occasionally the spine scan in younger patients, as the gold standard. Newer and smaller DXA equipment that measures the radius or the calcaneus, is promising because of lower cost and because the machines are portable. However, further studies must be undertaken before these machines can be recommended in general screening programs.

Quantitative Ultrasound

Quantitative ultrasound (QUS) transmits a signal through the bone in the range of 100 kHz up to 2 MHz. It started in 1984 with the introduction of parameter broadband ultrasound attenuation (BUA) (Table 19-3) (62). This parameter evaluated the attenuation in the bone, this being mainly caused by scattering but also by absorption (62). Attenuation seems to reflect not only the amount of mineral in the bone but also the bone structure, elasticity, and strength. Bone microstructure and material properties have both been shown to affect QUS parameters and studies have supported the view that QUS can predict fractures independent of the BMD value estimated by DXA scan (56,63). It has been suggested that BUA is not only influenced by BMD but also by the microarchitecture of bone whereas the speed of sound (SOS) may vary with the elasticity of bone (56,63). Therefore, QUS approaches may provide a better insight into skeletal status as it relates to mechanical strength (Table 19-3) (56,63). The two parameters BUA and SOS are often combined in weighted averages, most commonly presented as "stiffness," quantitative ultrasound index (QUI), or "soundness." However, none of the indices reflects biomechanical stiffness nor do they supply additional information over those provided by BUA and SOS. However, they are practical to use as they summarize BUA and SOS and have a lower precision error. They are probably better suited for monitoring (63,64).

The main use of QUS is in the assessment of fracture risk. The two largest prospective studies with sample sizes of 6500 to 10,000 women showed that QUS measured at the calcaneus can be used to predict future hip fracture risk equally as well as DXA measurements (56,65). Typically the risk of fracture increases by approximately a factor of 2 if a QUS value is reduced by one standard deviation but this varies between devices and QUS parameters as well as between different types of fractures (56,65). The use of QUS in monitoring and diagnosis requires further study.

Quantified Computer Tomography

Quantified computer tomography (QCT) is a powerful technique that measures the density of different tissues (57). Standard CT scanners can be adapted to provide qualitative bone density measurements. QCT is the only densitometric technique that measures the actual volumetric bone density. Other ionizing techniques measure the amount of mineral within the scanned area (57,58). This is done with QCT by selecting a region in the central portion of the vertebral body, or any other specified area, and measuring the true density of trabecular bone. It is also possible to specifically select cortical bone and estimate bone size and shape. In recent years smaller peripheral QCT (pQCT) units have been manufactured capable of measuring BMD in the forearm and leg. The previous problems of high radiation exposure and poor reproducibility compared to DXA have been minimized with the new versions of pQCT software. Although promising this method has thus far been mainly used for research purposes and currently no prospective data exists that evaluates the use of pQCT in fracture prediction. There are a number of other techniques using ionizing and nonionizing sources in the evaluation of BMD but none of these methods are in use in clinical practice (Table 19-3).

ASSESSMENT OF BONE METABOLISM BY BIOCHEMICAL BONE MARKERS

Bone Formation

Bone contains hydroxyapatite crystals, which are present in the matrix, consisting of about 90% type I collagen and 10% noncollagenous proteins including osteocalcin, the dominant noncollagenous protein in bone. The basic structure of collagen is a triple helix consisting of two α-1 and 1 α-2 chains with a high content of glycine, proline, and hydroxyproline. Pro-collagen is formed in the osteoblasts and after secretion to the extracellular space the pro-collagen I extension peptides are split at the amino-terminals (PINP) and carboxy-terminals (PICP) before final fibril formation. These extension peptides are a marker of bone formation and can be measured in blood (66). However type I collagen is present in many tissues, particularly the skin and the relative contribution from these sites to circulating PICP and PINP has not been clarified. In addition during bone formation the osteoblasts secrete noncollagenous small proteins that become incorporated in the matrix. One of these, osteocalcin, or bone GLA protein (BGP), can be measured in blood as a marker of bone formation (66,67). Alkaline phosphatase (ALP) and bone-specific alkaline phosphatase (BALP), an enzyme involved in the mineralization of bone are also used as markers of bone formation (Table 19-4) (66–68).

Bone Resorption

Urinary hydroxyproline (Hyp) was widely used to estimate the degradation of bone collagen and as such was a marker of bone resorption. However, as this marker is present in all types of collagen and the excretion is largely dependent on collagen rich food the clinical interpretation of Hyp is difficult (66). The collagen molecules aggregate to fibrils that are stabilized by covalent cross-links. The pyridinium cross-links comprise pyridinoline (Pyr) and deoxypyridinoline (D-Pyr) which are present in all mature collagen except skin. As D-Pyr is only present in significant amounts in bone it is considered to be more bone-specific than Pyr. The pyridinium cross-links are measured as total pyridinolines, free pyridinolines, and telopeptides, the peptide cross-link fragments at the N-terminal (NTX) and C-terminals (CTX), and in serum as markers of bone resorption (66–69). During bone resorption osteoclasts also secrete tartrate-resistant acid phosphatase isoenzymes (TRACP) and the serum concentration of this enzyme, and in particular TRACP type 5b has been used as a marker of bone resorption (70,71). However, the enzyme is not specific to bone and it is difficult to separate from isoenzymes derived from other tissues such as platelets and erythrocytes. Another collagen degradation product used to estimate bone resorption is C-terminal cross-linking telopeptide of type I collagen which is found both in serum and urine (Table 19-4).

TABLE 19-4 Measurements of Bone Turnover, Evaluating Bone Formation and Resorption, by Bone Metabolic Markers

Markers of Bone Formation
Serum
Osteocalcin (OC)
Bone-specific alkaline phosphatase (BALP)
Total alkaline phosphatase (ALP)
Procollagen I C-terminal extension peptide (PICP)
Procollagen I N-terminal extension peptide (PINP)
Markers of Bone Resorption
Serum
Tartrate-resistant acid phosphatase (TRACP)
Tartrate-resistant acid phosphatase 5b (TRACP 5b)
C-terminal cross-linking telopeptide of type I collagen (CTX)
N-terminal cross-linking telopeptide of type I collagen (NTX)
C-terminal cross-linking telopeptide of type I collagen generated by metalloproteinases (ICTP)
Urine
Deoxypyridinoline (D-Pyr)
Pyridinoline (Pyr)
Hydroxyproline (Hyp)
C-terminal cross-linking telopeptide of type I collagen (CTX)
N-terminal crosslinking telopeptide of type I collagen (NTX)

As most of the bone metabolic markers are affected by underlying factors such as diurnal rhythm, day-to-day variations, seasonal variations, menstrual variations, age, sex, diet, alcohol intake, systemic diseases, medication, and physical activity (72,73), the interpretation of bone markers must be undertaken with care. Markers have proved to be useful in epidemiological and intervention studies in which groups of patients are studied, and in patients with metabolic diseases associated with high bone turnover such as Paget's disease. However, guidelines for classifying and evaluating individual patients with osteoporosis are less well defined. For example, it is not possible to separate a large skeleton with a low turnover from a small skeleton with a high turnover. Nevertheless, some studies have shown that measurement of a single marker of bone turnover or a combination of markers can identify groups of patients with low bone mass. Currently no data consistently prove that such measurements will predict low BMD or a future fracture in an isolated patient (74). Biomechanical markers of bone turnover may also have a role in short-term monitoring of treatment (75). It remains to be proven if measurements of bone markers will add to the predictive values obtained by BMD measurement.

TABLE 19-5 Risk Factors for Osteoporosis, Falls, and Fractures

Risk Factor	Osteoporosis	Fall	Fracture
Low bone mineral density			+
Older age	+	+	+
Female	+	+	+
Primary or secondary amenorrhoea	+		+
Primary or secondary hypogonadism in men	+		+
Premature menopause	+		+
Postmenopausal status	+	+	+
Tallness		+	+
Low body weight	+		+
Long hip axis length			+
Previous fragility fracture	+	+	+
Family history of fracture			+
White or Asian ethnic origin			+
Immobility/low physical activity	+	+	+
Current smoking	+	+	+
High caffeine intake			+
Alcohol abuse	+	+	+
High bone turnover	+		+
Osteomalacia/vitamin D deficiency	+	+	+
Low dietary calcium intake	+		+
Chronic illnesses	+	+	+
Glucocorticoid therapy	+		+
Sedative medications		+	+
Visual impairment		+	+
Cognitive impairment		+	+
Neurologic diseases		+	+
Lower limb disability	+	+	+
Hyperthyroidism	+		+

(Continued)

TABLE 19-5 Continued

Risk Factor	Osteoporosis	Fall	Fracture
Hyperparathyroidism	+		+
Malabsorption	+		+
Celiac disease	+		+
Gastrectomy	+		+
Chronic arthritis	+	+	+
Chronic renal/liver diseases	+		+
Cushing's syndrome	+		+
Malignancies	+		+
Organ transplantations	+		+
Nursing home resident		+	+

RISK FACTORS FOR OSTEOPOROSIS AND FRAGILITY FRACTURES

Risk factors for fragility fractures can be divided into two main types. Those related to trauma such as a tendency to fall and those related to bone strength such as BMD, skeletal architecture, and bone size (Table 19-5) (48,56,76). However, several risk factors such as immobility and aging may operate through both skeletal and extra-skeletal routes. For example, fracture risk increases with age partly due to increased bone loss and partly due to the fact that older patients are at greater risk of fracture than younger patients, independent of their BMD level. Clinically it is important to determine all risk factors as women with multiple risk factors and low BMD are at an especially high risk of fracture (Table 19-5 and Fig. 19-5) (76).

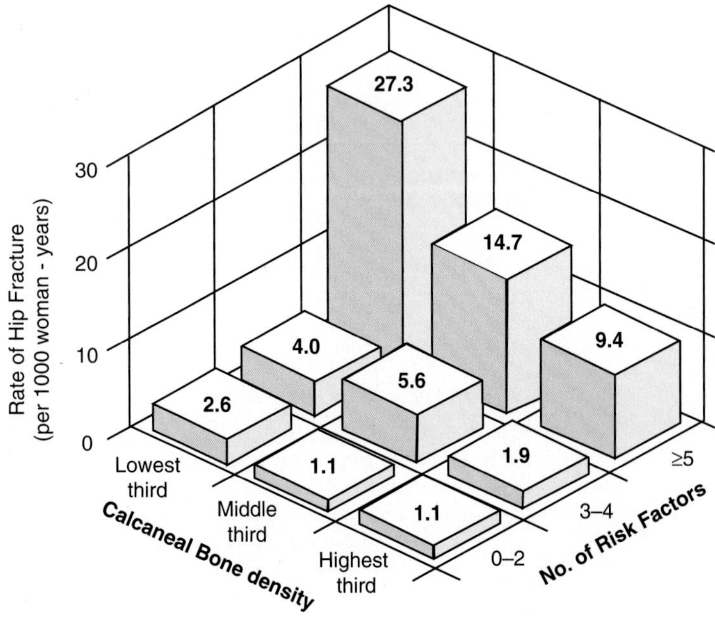

FIGURE 19-5 Annual risk of hip fracture according to the number of risk factors and the age-specific calcaneal bone density. (Reprinted with permission from Cummings SR, Nevitt MC, Browner WS, et al. Risk factors for hip fracture in white women. Study of Osteoporotic Fractures Research Group. *N Engl J Med* 1995;332:767–773.)

Bone Mineral Density

At present BMD is probably the best surrogate measure of the breaking strength of bone. Furthermore the diagnosis of osteoporosis is only defined by BMD measurement using the DXA technique and only in women (Table 19-1) (2). BMD was not originally designed to be used as a criterion for therapeutic intervention but to identify the proportion of the population at increased risk of fracture. Using this criterion 30% of the American post-menopausal female population are now recognized as having osteoporosis (77). The definition of osteopenia (Table 19-1) as a BMD between −1 and −2.5 standard deviations (SD) below the young normal mean was meant to describe a group of individuals at increased risk of developing osteoporosis but still not having a particularly high risk of fracture. The classification of established osteoporosis adds the risk factor of previous fracture to the treatment protocol in an individual patient (2,78). Clinicians must understand that the risk of fracture increases exponentially with decreasing BMD (79). No specific BMD level signifies a "fracture threshold." The definition of the disease osteoporosis is only arbitrarily chosen. A decreased BMD of 1 SD is thought to generally increase the fracture risk by about 1.5 times but it may be up to 2.5 times according to the measured region (Table 19-6) (80,81). One study which followed 8134 non-African American women over 65 years of age found that the age-adjusted relative risk of hip fracture was 1.6 for each 1 SD decrease in BMD in the lumbar spine and 2.6 for each 1 SD decrease in BMD in the femoral neck (Table 19-6) (81). It has also been shown that peripheral measurements of the radius and calcaneus can predict future fractures (78,82).

Data also suggests that the QUS of the calcaneus will independently predict the risk of hip fracture in elderly women as well as a DXA scan (56,65). In the EPIDOS study 5662 elderly women with a mean age of 80.4 years were assessed with calcaneal ultrasound and femoral neck DXA. The relative risk of hip fracture for a 1 SD reduction was 2.0 for ultrasound broadband attenuation, 1.7 for speed of sound (SOS), and 1.9 for femoral BMD measured by the DXA technique (56,65). Prospective validation using studies of peri- and early post-menopausal women are needed before bone ultrasound can be recommended for fracture risk assessment in these groups.

Even if BMD is an excellent screening tool for fracture population screening for osteoporosis is not recommended (83). It is recommended that patients are selected for bone densitometry on the basis of significant risk factors. There are several well-established risk factors related to secondary osteoporosis and further diagnosis by BMD is indicated in these patients even if they are asymptomatic (Table 19-5). Similarly the diagnosis of osteoporosis may be confirmed with bone densitometry in patients with previous low-trauma fractures, radiological evidence of osteopenia, or a vertebral deformity.

Skeletal Geometry

The geometry of the femoral neck probably plays an important part in the risk of sustaining a hip fracture. The length of the femoral neck, the hip axis length (HAL), measured between the external border of the greater trochanter and the inner pelvic rim has been shown to be an independent predictor of hip fracture (84). A new algorithm was developed by Yoshikawa et al (85) and Beck et al (86) using the principles of single plane engineering. This estimates femoral neck mechanical strength from an antero-posterior DXA scan, a so-called hip strength analysis (HSA). A similar geometric approach for the prediction of fractures has also been undertaken from forearm bone scans (48). Preliminary data indicates that the inclusion of geometric analyses in the estimate of risk factors could possibly improve fracture prediction (48,87).

Heredity

Twin and family studies have demonstrated that 60% to 80% of bone mass is determined by genetic factors (45). This is probably true during both growth and aging. Daughters of mothers with osteoporosis have a relatively low BMD compared to age-matched daughters of mothers without osteoporosis (45).

TABLE 19-6 Age-adjusted Relative Increase in Risk of Fractures[a]

Site of Measurement	Forearm Fracture	Hip Fracture	Vertebral Fracture	All Fractures
Distal radius	1.7 (1.4–2.0)	1.8 (1.4–2.2)	1.7 (1.4–2.1)	1.4 (1.3–1.6)
Femoral neck	1.4 (1.4–1.6)	2.6 (2.0–3.5)	1.8 (1.1–2.7)	1.6 (1.4–1.8)
Lumbar spine	1.5 (1.3–1.8)	1.6 (1.2–2.2)	2.3 (1.9–2.8)	1.5 (1.4–1.7)

[a] In women for every 1 standard deviation decrease in bone mineral density (absorptiometry) below the mean value for age (95% confidence interval). From Marshall D, Johnell O, Wedel H. Meta-analysis of how well measures of bone mineral density predict occurrence of osteoporotic fractures. *Br Med J* 1996;312:1254–1259.

The risk of sustaining a hip fracture in women with a maternal history of hip fracture is about twice that of women without such a history, independent of BMD (76). One of the first groups to demonstrate a relationship between genetic polymorphism and bone mass was Kelly et al (88), even though the paper was later withdrawn. Subsequent studies have only implied a minor association between BMD and a vitamin D receptor. However recent studies have indicated the importance of genetic polymorphism in a variety of genes. It is likely that there is an association between a specific polymorphism in the type I collagen (89), transforming growth factor beta (TGF-β) (90), the estrogen receptor (91), and the type I collagen gene (COLIA1) (92) and low BMD and fractures. It is probable that new associations between genetic polymorphism and BMD will be made but as osteoporosis is a polygenic disease it is also probable that no single gene will provide sufficient information to predict the risk of fracture. However a combination of a number of genes, perhaps in conjunction with BMD measurements and other risk factors could facilitate prediction of individuals at high risk of fracture.

History of Previous Fracture

Fractures caused by a fall from a standing height are often related to osteoporosis and it is estimated that osteoporosis plays a role in up to 75% of fractures in people aged 45 years or older (93). Women who have had either vertebral fractures or nonspine fractures also have an increased risk of sustaining new vertebral fractures (78) and women who have had wrist fractures have an increased risk of sustaining new hip fractures (94) independent of the BMD. In the study of osteoporotic fractures (SOF), which included 9516 white women of 65 years or older, it was found that a history of fracture increased the risk of hip fracture by 50% independent of the BMD (76). In addition any type of fracture sustained since the age of 15 years increases the risk of having subsequent fractures by 70% in peri-menopausal women aged 47 to 56 years independent of BMD (95). Because the risk is independent of BMD a history of fractures may indicate an increased tendency to fall, the existence of extra-skeletal risk factors or a defect in bone strength other than a low BMD.

Falls

One third of the elderly population fall annually, the incidence of falls causing injury increasing with age (12). The incidence is higher in the institutionalized elderly compared with elderly patients living at home (13). Frequent falling is also one of the most common risk factors for fractures and virtually the same risk factors for falls also account for fractures (Table 19-5) (7–11). Intrinsic risk factors for falls (10,11,14,16,17) include:

- Old age
- Female gender
- Low body mass
- Medical comorbidities
- Musculoskeletal diseases
- Cognitive impairment
- Gait and balance disorders
- Sensory impairments
- Postural hypotension
- History of previous falls
- Use of certain medications
    - Benzodiazepines
    - Sedative-hypnotic drugs
    - Antidepressants
    - Anti-hypertensive medication
    - Anti-arrhythmic drugs
    - Diuretics
    - Anti-seizure medications

In contrast environmental hazards such as rugs, slippery and uneven floor surfaces, poor lighting, electrical cords, foot stools without handrails, slippery top surfaces, and unsuitable footwear are often classified as extrinsic risk factors (10,11, 14,16,17,96). Extrinsic factors play a progressively smaller role in falls as age advances largely because it is the intrinsic factors that assume a much more important role as chronic illness becomes a more significant problem (97).

Age

Most risk factors associated with fractures become more prevalent with advancing age, the risk of sustaining a hip fracture increasing 1.5 to 2 times every 5 years (81,98). During the peri-menopausal years the risk of fracture is increased in peri-menopausal women as compared with pre-menopausal women independent of BMD (79) indicating that risk factors other than BMD account for the increase (56).

Gender

Females are at greater risk of osteoporotic fractures. Lower peak BMD, faster bone loss, smaller bone size, and the higher prevalence of falls in women may explain this. Mechanical properties of bone are not only dependent on BMD but also on size, geometry, and architecture. Gender differences and the recurrence of fracture may be explained in part by the larger cross-sectional area of bones in men and differences in periosteal bone apposition with aging (48,99).

Weight

Low body weight is associated with low BMD (100) and increased fracture incidence (17). Gaining weight after the age of 25 years provides protection against hip fracture (76), while in contrast, losing weight greatly increases the risk of osteoporotic fractures (101). The Framingham study reported that the relative risk of fracture was found to be 0.63 in individuals 114%

to 123% overweight and 0.33 in individuals more than 138% overweight (102). Obesity may protect the skeleton in several ways. These are increased extra-glandular production of estrone in the fat tissue, improved vitamin D status due to storage of vitamin D in fatty tissues, the provision of a local cushioning effect at the hip when falling, and a denser and stronger skeleton due to increased loading in obese people.

Body Length

Tall individuals seem to have an increased risk of having a hip fracture (76,103). The reason could be that tall individuals fall further thus hitting the ground with greater force (104) or because tall individuals have a longer hip axis length (84).

Calcium Intake

Studies evaluating the relationship between dietary calcium intake and hip fracture risk have given conflicting results (98,105,106). Errors in the measurement of dietary calcium intake and slow changes in BMD may explain this but it appears that increased dietary calcium partially prevents bone loss, although the effect in populations with high calcium is small (107).

Smoking

Studies suggest that current smokers have a low BMD and more fractures than nonsmokers (108). A large meta-analysis supported this view reporting that smoking is a risk factor for osteoporotic fractures, independent of BMD, in post-menopausal women (109). This could be due to the fact that smokers, in comparison with nonsmokers, have an earlier menopause, are slimmer, have a reduced extra-glandular production of estrogens, have an increased metabolic clearance rate of estrogens, and that smoking inhibits the function of osteoclasts.

Caffeine

Studies report that a high caffeine intake in the elderly is associated with an increased fracture risk (76,110). In contrast high caffeine consumption does not appear to be associated with an increased risk of fracture in peri-menopausal women (95,111,112). Thus, the adverse effects of caffeine on bone may be only important in the elderly.

Alcohol

Individuals who abuse alcohol have an increasing risk of sustaining fractures partly due to poor balance, associated illnesses, frequent falls and accidents, but also due to the adverse effect of alcohol on bone metabolism (112). Alcohol exerts a direct toxic effect on bone cells. It affects osteoblast proliferation in vitro and reduces matrix protein synthesis in vivo (113). In contrast moderate alcohol consumption does not appear to be a risk factor for osteoporosis or fracture (100).

Immobility

Osteoclasts are sensitive to mechanical loading and a reduced loading as occurs in immobile patients leads to increased BMD loss (114). Immobility also contributes to decreased muscle strength, this being a major risk factor for falls (100,115,116). Decreased muscle strength may also have a direct negative influence on BMD (100,115,116). Increased hip fracture risk has been reported to be linked with poor quadriceps strength associated with immobility independent of the BMD (15). Several studies have confirmed this showing that mobile women have a lower risk of hip fracture compared to less mobile women (46,76). However, it is not known whether the adverse effect of physical inactivity and immobility are mediated by decreased BMD, coexisting illnesses and increased risk of falls, or all of these factors.

Medical Conditions

Impaired health and chronic illnesses predispose to fractures by impairing BMD, bone quality, and muscle function. They also tend to decrease physical activity and to increase the likelihood of falling. Diseases and conditions that have been found to increase the risk of sustaining fractures (17,76,115,117,118) include:

- Hyperthyroidism
- Decreased visual acuity
- Poor depth perception
- Mental impairment or dementia
- Impaired neuromuscular function (e.g., the inability to rise from a chair without using the arms)
- Hypercortisolism
- Hypogonadism
- Hyperparathyroidism
- Osteomalacia
- Renal and hepatic diseases
- Certain malignancies
- Rheumatoid arthritis
- Paget's disease
- Gastrectomy and organ transplantation

Many of these conditions are considered to be associated with fall-related risk factors rather than BMD-related factors (11,119).

Drug Treatment

A variety of drugs are related to an increased risk of hip fracture independent of the BMD (76). Studies have reported that treatment with corticosteroids, long-acting benzodiazepines, or anticonvulsant drugs (especially phenytoin), gonadotrophin-releasing hormone agonists, tamoxifen, long-term treatment with heparin, cytotoxic drugs, and lithium are associated with an increased risk of hip fracture (76,118). This association remains after adjusting for BMD suggesting that the associated illnesses, impaired health, and increased likelihood of falls affect the risk of fracture (76,118).

How to Use the Risk Factors

Several risk factors can be modified. It is possible to influence BMD and the likelihood of falling (120,121) but prevention requires a multifaceted strategy including environmental changes, the provision of adequate calcium intake, supporting physical activity, improving functional ability, correcting or treating health disorders, and avoiding poly-pharmacy (120,121). In individuals with risk factors other than low BMD these factors should be addressed.

Other risk factors cannot be modified. These risk factors, together with the modifiable risk factors can be used to identify at-risk groups suitable for bone densitometry and amenable to different treatment strategies. In the Study of Osteoporotic Fractures Caucasian women over 60 years were classified according to their calcaneal BMD and the number of clinical risk factors for hip fracture (76). The relationship between BMD and fracture risk was least apparent with few clinical risk factors. Thus women with a higher calcaneal BMD with more than four clinical risk factors had a higher risk of sustaining a hip fracture than women with lower BMDs but few other risk fractures (Fig. 19-5). The highest risk for hip fractures was found in women with the lowest BMDs who had more than four clinical risk factors.

PREVENTION OF OSTEOPOROTIC FRACTURES

Half of all women and one third of all men will sustain a fragility fracture during their lifetime (33). Increased morbidity and mortality and the high costs associated with the rising incidence of osteoporotic fractures makes it imperative to implement prevention strategies in the community (122,123). Hip and vertebral fractures in women are most commonly discussed but other fragility fractures are associated with significant problems as well (124). In addition as the number of fractures in men and children has increased we must also discuss these groups (47,125,126). However, general screening to detect low BMD is not considered to be cost-effective as a modest deficit in BMD is associated with a low absolute risk of sustaining a fracture. The use of drug treatment in these groups would mean a considerable therapeutic investment to save a relatively small number of fractures. Furthermore, studies show that it is only individuals with osteoporosis in whom drugs will reduce the incidence of fractures. It is unclear whether individuals with a more modest deficit in BMD benefit from drug treatment (Table 19-6) (127–137). If the aim of health care is to reduce the fracture rate in the community widely accessible, inexpensive intervention programs with no adverse effects are required.

Nonpharmacological Prevention of Osteoporotic Fractures

Nutrition

Normal skeletal health is dependent on a balanced diet with an adequate intake of calories, minerals, and proteins. Calcium is the most important nutrient for attaining adequate peak bone mass but there is no universal consensus about the daily requirement. The 1994 consensus conference discussing the optimum calcium intake recommended a daily intake of 1200 to 1500 mg for adolescents, 1000 mg for adults up to 65 years of age, and 1500 mg for post-menopausal women not receiving estrogen and for elderly individuals (138). Although the results of most studies indicate a beneficial effect from calcium supplements, especially in individuals with a low intake, the long-term effect of a high dietary calcium on BMD is unclear. Calcium also seems to work as a threshold nutritional element with about 400 mg per day as a limit. Below this, increasing calcium intake seems beneficial and necessary (139). The positive correlation between dietary calcium and BMD has been shown in children (140), adolescents (141), and young women (142) indicating that higher calcium intake results in a higher BMD. It has been calculated that variations in calcium nutrition early in life may account for as much as 5% to 10% difference in peak adult bone mass, which would contribute to more than 50% of the difference in the rates of hip fracture in later life (143).

Calcium absorption is also dependent on the vitamin D level and serum concentrations of 25-hydroxyvitamin D decline with age. The current recommendation is that the daily intake of vitamin D should be about 400 to 800 IU if exposure to sunlight is low especially in the elderly who have decreased ability to activate precursors in the skin, decreased ability to hydroxylase vitamin D in the kidney and liver, reduced dietary intake, and diminished absorption from food. Another problem in frail elderly individuals is achieving an adequate intake of protein, total energy, and a variety of other nutritional components such as phosphorus, magnesium, zinc, copper, iron, fluoride, sodium, vitamins D, A, C, and K—all of which are required for normal bone health.

Physical Activity

Bone tissue seems to be most adaptive to mechanical load during periods of rapid skeletal change as in puberty. Mechanical loading increases BMD but also improves bone structure, geometry, architecture, and possibly material properties such as strength, stiffness, and its energy-absorbing capacity (47,144). The biological purpose of this adaptation is to achieve a skeleton which is more resistant to load but still as light as possible to facilitate mobility (144). Data has unequivocally shown that physical activity may increase BMD, skeletal geometry, and bone strength by up to 30% to 50% (46,47,145) in those individuals in whom training is initiated before puberty (Fig. 19-4) (46,47). The reason for this can be explained by the fact that the adolescent growth spurt is the only time in life when bone is added in substantial amounts to both sides of the bone cortex by endosteal and periosteal apposition (146). The importance of regarding exercise during growth as a prevention strategy for fragility fractures in old age originates from the data that relate exercise to increased peak bone mass and show that 60% to 70% of the variance in BMD at 65 years of age is attributed to achieved peak bone mass (45).

Bone tissue is also able to respond to exercise in adulthood although to a lesser extent than during growth. During adulthood physical activity should be regarded more as bone-preserving rather than bone building as most studies show a 1% to 3% increase in BMD with exercise (147,148). Nevertheless the exercise-induced bone-preserving effect in adulthood may be of great importance in maintaining bone strength and preventing age-related fractures as only a small increase in BMD on group level is associated with a significant reduction in the risk of fracture (81). Furthermore, exercise may cause a reduction in the incidence of fracture through nonskeletal effects (149,150). In the post-menopausal period physical activity may prevent age-related bone loss (151,152). Brisk walking, climbing up and down stairs, dancing, and callisthenics are the most suitable activities for older people since they are easily available and are inexpensive and safe (149). It also appears that exercise should be life long if bone strength is to be maintained as cessation of exercise is followed by a rapid decline of the exercise-achieved BMD (145).

Regular impact loading activities that create high magnitude strains and versatile strain distributions throughout the bone structure best improve bone strength (46,144,145,148,152, 153). Squash, tennis, badminton, aerobics, step exercises, volleyball, basketball, soccer, gymnastics, weight and power training, and similar sports may best fulfill these demands (46,144). In contrast, endurance training such as long distance running, swimming, and cycling has not proved as effective in increasing BMD (46).

The best proof that exercise could be used to prevent fractures would be gained from studies that had the incidence of fracture as their outcome criterion. Unfortunately no such randomized controlled trials exist. Instead we have to rely on prospective and retrospective observational and case control studies. These types of studies consistently show that both past and current physical activity is associated with a reduced risk of hip fracture in women and men, the risk reduction being up to 50% (149,150). Several studies also report a dose-response relationship that further supports the probability of a link. It seems that vigorous activity during youth followed by more moderate activity during adulthood is the best combination to prevent hip fracture as vigorous activity in old age may actually increase the incidence of falls that cause injury (154,155). Studies focusing on physical activity and fractures other than hip fractures are few and present contradictory results. If anything, these studies suggest that lifetime physical activity protects against all types of fractures although it must be appreciated that vigorous activity in the elderly may increase the risk of falls and therefore fractures (149,150,155,156). Activity programs for the elderly must therefore be designed specifically for each individual and be based on the physical abilities of that person. They should be undertaken with caution and after proper training (155). It would seem that promotion of life long physical activities is probably one of the most important goals in public health programs of the new millennium (154,155).

Prevention of Falls

Recent prospective randomized controlled trials have shown that exercise can reduce the risk of falling in elderly and frail individuals (120,159–161). Exercise, including balance training, improves balance and decreases the risk of falling. The greatest effect was seen in those who were most compliant with the program (162–164). In several recent studies Tai Chi has been shown to be an effective intervention reducing falls by almost 50% (120,157). The effectiveness of modifying other risk factors has not been demonstrated in controlled studies. However, it makes sense to modify the home environment to eliminate as many elements as possible that could lead to falls. As previous falls are an independent risk factor for future falls, it is especially important to evaluate each elderly person who has fallen for any risk factors in the home environment. This has been successfully utilized in the PROFET study (Prevention of Falls in the Elderly Trial) in which intervention decreased the risk of falls by 70% in patients who had presented to emergency departments with fall-related injuries (158). The key elements of such programs of risk reduction are:

1. Individual management so that factors relevant to a particular patient are addressed
2. Reduction of environmental hazards
3. Appropriate reduction of medication
4. Education of the individual in behavior strategies
5. Exercise programs to improve strength, balance, and aerobic capacity

Hip Protectors

More than 90% of hip fractures are related to direct impact on the hip (165). Falls directly on the hip increase the odds ratio for a hip fracture by about 20-fold (104). In nursing home patients who fall on their hips the risk of fracture is 25% in women and 33% in men (166). Energy absorption in the soft tissues surrounding the hip has been shown to protect against hip fractures (167,168) and as much as 75% of the energy in a fall can be absorbed (168). This partly explains why being overweight protects against hip fractures (169). Based on these facts various hip padding systems have been developed. There are a number of different types, including an energy shunting type (horseshoe) system (170), a crash helmet type (171,172), an energy absorptive type (173), and an airbag type (174), de-

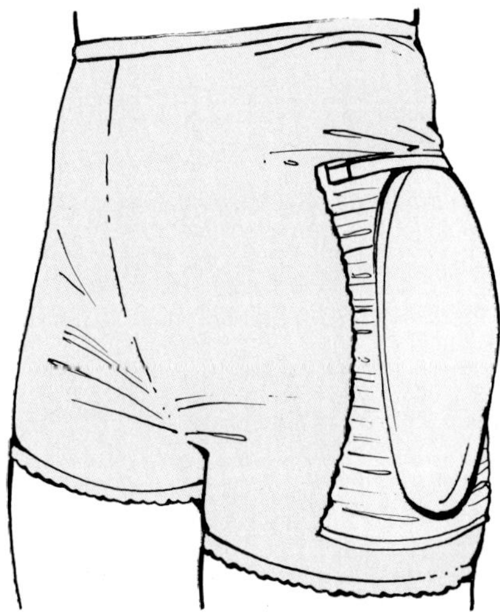

FIGURE 19-6 The hip protector underwear.

signed to reduce the impact of the skeleton in a fall (Fig. 19-6) (104,165,166,175). Randomized controlled trials, including nursing home residents and those frail elderly living at home, have shown a protective effect of 34% by hip protectors when using pooled data (166,175,178). So far no studies have shown that hip protectors have a general protective effect in people living at home. The most significant problem with this type of prevention strategy appears to be compliance. Based on a subgroup analysis in a previously reported nursing home study the compliance in the use of hip protectors was 24% (166) and in a more recent community-based study an initial acceptance rate of 57% decreased to 40% after 2 years (20).

Pharmacological Prevention of Osteoporotic Fractures

Calcium and Vitamin D

Calcium supplements, generally prescribed as 500 to 1000 mg daily, are known to slow the rate of bone loss in the elderly and in individuals with a low calcium intake (140–142). There are also studies that suggest that calcium supplements may reduce the incidence of fractures but usually calcium supplementation is regarded as an adjunctive treatment for osteoporosis (179–181). Calcium supplements are safe, although mild gastrointestinal disturbances such as constipation have been reported. The risk of kidney stones related to increased urinary calcium excretion does not appear to be a problem.

There is evidence that vitamin D is also useful in the treatment of osteoporosis. A French study including 3270 elderly women who lived in old people's homes and who were treated daily for 3 years with 1,200 mg calcium and 800 IU vitamin D showed a 29% reduction in the incidence of hip fracture and a 24% reduction in the incidence of nonvertebral fracture compared with a placebo group (Table 19-7) (132,133). Another study reported a similar trend with a 50% reduction in nonvertebral fractures in patients whose daily diet was supplemented with calcium and vitamin D (107). A British study, including 2686 men and women living in their own homes, reported that calcium and vitamin D treatment over a 5-year period reduced the risk of fracture by 22% and the risk of fractures in the hip, forearm, or spine by 33% (182). This study implied that calcium and vitamin D treatment might decrease fracture risk in nursing home residents who did not have a deficient calcium intake. In contrast a study of 2,578 elderly healthy Dutch women with a high calcium intake who were treated daily with 400 IU vitamin D over 3.5 years showed no effect on the risk of hip fracture (183). A recently published meta-analysis reported that vitamin D treatment alone did not reduce the risk of fractures (184). However, in combination with calcium the risk of hip fractures was reduced by 26% in elderly care home residents. Although in healthy individuals living in their own home there was no reduction in the incidence of hip fracture, the risk of sustaining vertebral fractures was reduced by 54% (184). Similar results were published in another meta-analysis that totaled 8124 individuals (185). Thus, the literature suggests that calcium and vitamin D should be used routinely in elderly individuals living in old people's homes because of a high prevalence of vitamin D deficiency as a result of low intake, low exposure to sunlight, and impaired vitamin D synthesis in the skin. Vitamin D in this dosage is safe and does not require monitoring. When compliance is low, 150,000 to 300,000 IU can be given intramuscularly twice a year. Calcium and vitamin D also reduce cortisone-induced bone loss. Currently there is controversy regarding whether calcium and vitamin D supplementation in healthy elderly people with an adequate intake of dairy products influences the risk of fracture (182,184,185).

Hormone Replacement Therapy

Estrogen reduces bone loss in post-menopausal women by inhibiting bone resorption resulting in, at best, a 5% increase in BMD over 1 to 3 years (49,186). Additional calcium supplementation seems to further enhance the beneficial effects of hormone replacement therapy (HRT) treatment (187). Recent data also suggests that smaller doses of HRT than those often used in early post-menopausal women, in the range of 0.5 to 1 mg of oral 17-estradiol, 25 mg of transdermal 17-estradiol, or 0.3 mg of conjugated equine estrogens have a similar beneficial skeletal effect. Estrogen influences BMD loss for as long as the drug is given (188). When HRT is stopped bone loss mimics bone loss after the menopause (189–191). Fracture data from the Million Women Study, a prospective observational study including 138,737 post-menopausal women followed for 1.9 to 3.9 years supports this finding (192).

There is also data to support the theory that fracture risk is reduced by estrogen treatment. Case-control and cohort studies suggest that HRT decreases the risk of hip fracture by about 30% (102). Two controlled studies of osteoporotic women indicate a 50% reduction in the risk of fractures of the spine (49,193). Another meta-analysis of controlled trials supports this report-

TABLE 19-7 Randomized Controlled Trials with Incidence of Vertebral and Hip Fractures Over 3 Years[a]

	Study (Ref.)	Risk Profile of Patients at Baseline	Sex	Mean Age (yr)	No. Patients	Fracture Incidence		
						Placebo	Drug	Relative Risk (95% CI or p value)
Vertebral Fracture Drug								
HRT	WHI (135)	Healthy postmenopausal women	Female	63	16,608	0.74%	0.48%	0.66 (0.44–0.98)
Raloxifen 60 mg	MORE-1 (136)	No vertebral fracture	Female	65	3,012	5%	2 %	0.50 (0.4–0.8)
Raloxifene 60 mg	MORE-2 (136)	Vertebral fractures	Female	68	1,539	21%	15%	0.70 (0.6–0.9)
Alendronate 5–10 mg	FIT-1 (131)	Vertebral fractures	Female	71	2,027	15%	8%	0.53 (0.41–0.68)
Alendronate 5–0 mg	FIT-2 (130)	No vertebral fractures	Female	68	4,432	3%	2%	0.56 (0.39–0.8)
		Subgroup T-score ≤2.5	Female	–	1,631	4%	2%	0.50 (0.31–0.82)
Alendronate	Orwoll et al (137)	FN T-score ≤2 or ≥1 and a fragility fracture	Male	63	241	7.1%	0.8%	0.11 ($p = 0.02$)
Risedronate 5 mg	VERT-US (128)	Vertebral fractures	Female	69	1,628	16%	11%	0.51 (0.36–0.73)
Risedronate 5 mg	VERT-MN (129)	Vertebral fractures	Female	71	815	29%	18%	0.59 (0.43–0.82)
Calcitonin 200 IU	PROOF (223)	Vertebral fractures	Female	69	557	16%	11%	0.67 (0.47–0.97)
Rh 1–34 PTH 20 μg	Neer et al (226)	Vertebral fractures	Female	69	892	14%	5%	0.35 (0.22–0.55)
Strontium 2 g	Meunier et al (229)	T-score ≤2.5 and vertebral fracture	Female	69	1,649	24.4%	17.7%	0.59 (0.48–0.73)

Hip Fracture Drug								
Calcium 1.2 g/Vit D 800 IU	Chapuy (132)	Living in care home	Female	84	3,270	4.2%	2.4%	0.73 (p = 0.043)
HRT	WHI (135)	Healthy postmenopausal women	Female	63	16,608	0.77%	0.52%	0.66 (0.45–0.98)
Raloxifen 60 and 120 mg	MORE (136)	Osteoporosis (T-score ≤2.5) with or without vertebral fractures	Female	67	7,705	0.7%	0.8%	1.1 (0.6–1.9)
Alendronate 5–10 mg	FIT-1 (131)	Vertebral fractures	Female	71	2,027	2.2%	1.1%	0.49 (0.23–0.99)
Alendronate 5 and 10 mg	FIT-2 (130)	T-score ≤2.5	Female	–	1,631	1.6%	0.72%	0.44 (0.18–0.97)
Risedronate 5 mg	VERT-US (128)	T-score ≤1.6	Female	68	4,432	0.8%	0.65%	0.79 (0.43–1.44)
Risedronate 5 mg	VERT-MN (129)	Vertebral fractures	Female	69	1,628	1.8%	1.4%	N/A
Risedronate 2.5 and 5 mg	HIP (127)	Vertebral fractures	Female	71	815	2.7%	2.2%	N/A
		70–80 yr with osteoporosis	Female	74	5,445	3.2%	1.9%	0.6 (0.4–0.9)
		Subgroup prevalent vertebral fx	Female	–	–	5.7%	2.3%	0.4 (0.2–0.8)
Calcitonin 200 IU	PROOF (223)	>80 yr with or without osteoporosis	Female	83	3,886	5.1%	4.2%	0.8 (0.6–1.2)
Rh 1–34 PTH 20 μg	Neer et al (226)	Vertebral fractures	Female	69	557	1.8%	1.2%	0.5 (0.2–1.6)
		Vertebral fractures	Female	69	892	0.74%	0.0037%	N/A

[a] If not specifically presented otherwise, with % of patients and relative risk (95% confidence interval or p value) in trials done with calcium and vitamin D, hormone replacement therapy (HRT), raloxifen, alendronate, risedronate, nasal calcitonin, 1–34 fragment of recombinant human parathyroid hormone (Rh 1–34 PTH), and strontium ranelate in the treatment of postmenopausal osteoporosis.

Follow-up period when calculating incidence and relative risk: WHI 5.2 years, FIT-2 2.4 years extrapolated to 3 years, PROOF 5 years data extrapolated to 3 years, Chapuy et al 18 months, Trivedi et al 5 years, Neer et al data 21 months.

N/A, not available.

ing a 33% reduction of vertebral fractures with HRT (194). A further study including 22 randomized trials shows a 27% reduction in nonvertebral fractures and specifically a 40% reduction in both hip and wrist fractures (195). The study that finally supported the theory that estrogen in combination with gestagen reduces the risk of fracture was the Women's Health Initiative Study (WHI). This study included 161,809 healthy post-menopausal women including 16,608 involved in fracture evaluation over a 5.2-year period (134,135). After this period the planned 8-year follow-up study was canceled when the adverse negative effects outweighed the positive effects. The study reported that estrogen reduced hip fracture incidence by 34%, vertebral fractures by 34%, fragility fractures by 23%, and all fractures by 24% (Table 19-7) (135). One recently published meta-analysis including more than 20,000 women followed for an average of 4.9 years supported the WHI study results reporting that the general fracture risk was reduced by 28% (196).

The down side of HRT is that it has many serious adverse effects including vaginal bleeding, breast tenderness, deep vein thrombosis and pulmonary embolism, stroke, heart disease, gall bladder disease, and an increased risk of breast, endometrial, and ovarian cancer after long-term use (134,135,197–199). Women who have had a hysterectomy can be given estrogen alone but in others estrogen and a progestagen should be given cyclically or in a combined continuous regime to reduce the risk of endometrial cancer (200). We should also be aware that the WHI study evaluated younger post-menopausal women, not only elderly women with osteoporosis, this being the important group for fracture reduction. Whether estrogen influences steroid-induced bone loss is unclear. In most countries estrogen is not recommended as the primary preventative agent for osteoporosis.

Selective Estrogen Receptor Modulators

In contrast to HRT, which has multiple target organs leading to a number of adverse effects, selective estrogen receptor modulators (SERMs) act as estrogen agonists or antagonists depending on the target tissue. Raloxifene acts as an antagonist of estrogen in the breast and the endometrium but acts as an agonist on bone and lipid metabolism. Raloxifene has been shown to prevent menopausal bone loss, decrease bone turnover to premenopausal levels, and reduce the incidence of fracture. The evaluation of fracture incidence is based on one large randomized controlled trial, the MORE study (Multiple Outcomes of Raloxifene Evaluation), involving 7,705 women with osteoporosis (Table 19-7). This study reported a 30% reduction of vertebral fractures in women who did not have a previous vertebral fracture and a 50% reduction in women who had a previous vertebral fracture (136). No effects were found on nonvertebral fractures (136). Raloxifene also lowers the frequency of breast cancer by 70% (201,202) but increases the incidence of venous thrombosis and pulmonary embolism at a similar rate to HRT (203). The ongoing RUTH study (Raloxifene Use for The Heart trial) will provide more data regarding the effects of raloxifene. As new SERMs are now in phase III trials, it is likely that the number of these drugs available for use will increase in the future.

Tibolone is a synthetic steroid that has been used for the prevention of osteoporosis. It acts on estrogen, progesterone, and androgen receptors either directly or indirectly through metabolites and has different effects from different target tissues. Tibolone prevents bone loss in post-menopausal women (204), but so far there is no data regarding fractures.

Bisphosphonates

Bisphosphonates are stable analogues of pyrophosphates characterized by a phosphorous-carbon-phosphorous bond that strongly binds to the hydroxyapatite crystal with a half-life in bone of several years. The drug inhibits bone resorption by reducing the recruitment and activity of osteoclasts and by increasing their apoptosis (205). Because food, calcium, iron, coffee, tea, and orange juice reduce the absorption of bisphosphonates, the drug should be taken while fasting. There are mild adverse effects including dyspepsia, abdominal pain, and diarrhea in addition to esophagitis that may force a patient to stop the medication (206). This problem is reduced if the drug is taken in one weekly dose compared to daily administration (207). There are also reports that etidronate can induce a mineralization defect in bone after long-term use.

Etidronate was the first bisphosphonate used for treatment of low BMD. A dose of 400 mg per day was given for 2 weeks and then repeated every 3 months. The increase in BMD is reported to be about 4% and results show a reduction of the rate of vertebral fractures after 2 years of treatment (208,209). A longer term study showed no fracture reduction after 3 years of treatment (210). One recently published meta-analysis, including 13 randomized controlled studies of etidronate with more than 1-year follow-up, reported that the risk of sustaining vertebral fractures was reduced by 40% whereas there was no effect on any other fracture (211). Etidronate seems to reduce steroid-induced bone loss but any effect on the fracture incidence is as yet unclear (211).

Alendronate is a bisphosphonate that prevents post-menopausal bone loss (212,213). In 2027 osteoporotic women with at least one previous vertebral fracture, a 5 mg daily dose for 2 years followed by 10 mg daily for a third year was associated with a reduction of about 47% in vertebral, wrist, and hip fractures compared with a placebo (Table 19-7) (131). A 4-year study of the use of alendronate in women with low BMD, but without a preexisting vertebral fracture supported these results in finding a nonsignificant decrease in the frequency of fractures ($p = 0.07$) and a 45% reduction in new vertebral fractures (Table 19-7) (130). When the data from these two studies was pooled and only women with osteoporosis were included, it was found that alendronate did reduce the risk of fracture with 12 to 18 months of treatment (130,131,214). Another placebo controlled study using 10 mg of alendronate daily in 1,908 post-menopausal women with a BMD T-score below −2 SD reported a 47% reduced risk of nonvertebral fracture after 1 year (215). The incidence of radiologically confirmed vertebral fracture was also reduced by 89% in men with 2 years of treatment with alendronate (Table 19-7) (137). A recently published meta-analysis, including 11 randomized controlled trials of the use of alendronate with more than a 1-year follow-up, reported that the risk of sustaining vertebral fractures was reduced by 48% whereas in those who were treated with 10 mg of alendronate daily there was also a 49% risk reduction in sustaining nonvertebral fractures (216). The optimum duration of treatment remains unknown with one study suggesting that there may be no additional benefit after 5 years of treatment (217). Alendronate seems to reduce steroid-induced bone loss but whether there is any effect on fracture incidence has not been fully evaluated as yet.

Risedronate is another bisphosphonate that prevents post-menopausal bone loss (218). A study of 2,400 women who had had previous vertebral fractures and were given 5 mg of risedronate per day showed that this reduced the incidence of new vertebral fractures by 65% after the first year and by 41% over 3 years (Table 19-7) (128). Risedronate treatment over 3 years also reduced the incidence of vertebral fractures by 49% in another study which included 1,226 patients who had at least two previous vertebral fractures (Table 19-7) (129). The overall incidence of nonvertebral fractures in the two studies was reduced by 30% to 40% (128,129). However the data supporting the reduction in the incidence of hip fracture by risedronate is less clear. Risedronate treatment in 5,445 osteoporotic women aged 70 to 79 years showed a 40% reduction in hip fracture ($p = 0.02$) over 3 years reaching 60% in those with a previous vertebral fracture (127). In contrast the same treatment in 3896 women older than 80 years who had clinical risk factors for falls, but without BMD assessment in most cases, had no effect on the rate of hip fractures (127). These data suggest that bisphosphonates may have an anti-fracture effect in individuals with low BMD. A meta-analysis of the effect of risedronate contained five studies that included vertebral fractures and seven studies with nonvertebral fractures. This meta-analysis reported that risedronate reduced the risk of vertebral fractures by 36% and nonvertebral fractures by 27% (219).

There are other bisphosphonates but they require further evaluation with regards to their potential to reduce the incidence of fracture. A dose of 800 mg daily of clodronate seems to reduce the number of vertebral fractures by 46% (220). Tiludronate is used for the treatment of Paget's disease of bone but cannot be recommended for the treatment of osteoporosis because of an absence of data regarding fractures in phase III trials. Orally administered daily pamidronate may be effective in osteoporosis but has a high incidence of upper gastrointestinal symptoms which reduce its value (221). In contrast intravenous infusion of pamidronate is commonly used in malignant bone disease and in Paget's disease of bone with only minor side effects (222), but as no data regarding fractures are available this bisphosphonate cannot be recommended for fracture prevention. Ibandronate and zoledronate are two other bisphosphonates now in clinical trials but without data regarding fractures.

Calcitonin

Calcitonin is produced by the thyroid C cells. It reduces bone absorption by osteoclast inhibition. The treatment can be provided by subcutaneous or intramuscular injection. Side effects include nausea, facial flushes, and diarrhea. This compares unfavorably with the intranasal administration of salmon calcitonin in which 200 IU daily provides treatment that has no such side effects. The PROOF study (Prevent Recurrence Of Osteoporotic Fractures), a 5-year controlled trial of 1,255 post-menopausal women with osteoporosis, reported that 200 IU of intranasal salmon calcitonin per day reduced vertebral fracture risk by 31% while no effects were found on peripheral fractures (Table 19-7) (223). However, this study must be interpreted with care as 60% of individuals were lost to follow-up. Doses of 100 and 400 IU had no effect and no consistent effect on BMD and bone turnover markers were noted (223). A meta-analysis of 30 randomized controlled studies provided evidence that calcitonin reduces the risk of vertebral fractures by 54% (224). Whether calcitonin influences steroid-induced bone loss is as yet unclear.

Parathyroid Hormone

Continuous treatment by parathyroid hormone (PTH) results in increased bone resorption and bone loss. By contrast intermittent PTH treatment in individuals with osteoporosis stimulates bone formation, increases BMD, and reduces the risk of fractures (225,226). In one randomized controlled trial including 1637 post-menopausal women with a previous vertebral fracture 20 μg of subcutaneous recombinant human PTH administered daily for a median of 19 months reduced the incidence of new vertebral fractures by 65% and 40 μg reduced the incidence by 69% (Table 19-7) (226). The reduction in the incidence of nonvertebral fragility fractures was 53% with both doses during the same period while BMD increased by 9% and 13% in the spine and by 3% and 6%, respectively, in the femoral neck with the two doses after 21 months of treatment. Injection with PTH has adverse effects, mainly nausea and headache.

Strontium

Strontium ranelate treatment is also associated with reduced bone resorption and possibly with increased bone formation (227). A rise in BMD and a reduction in vertebral fracture incidence have been suggested in phase II trials (228). One recently published study suggests that strontium reduces fractures (229). This was a randomized study of 1649 post-menopausal women with osteoporosis and at least one previous vertebral fracture. Two grams of strontium ranelate per day, administered for 3 years, increased BMD and reduced the risk of sustaining new vertebral fractures by 49% during the first year and 41% during the entire 3-year period (Table 19-7). In addition there were no more adverse effects in the treatment group than in the placebo group. Since these results are relatively new further information will be required to examine the role of strontium ranelate in the prevention of fragility fractures.

Fluoride

Fluoride is a mineral which is incorporated into the hydroxyapatite crystal of bone. It stimulates osteoblast recruitment and activity and increases BMD in the spine but less so in the hip (230,231). However, controlled trials have failed to show that fluoride reduces fractures. If anything it seems as though the incidence of nonvertebral fractures might increase. Currently fluoride cannot be recommended for the treatment of osteoporosis.

Other Drugs

Several other drugs have been used in the treatment of osteoporosis. Studies report an increase in BMD with their use but none provide adequate data about fractures. Alfacalcidol and calcitriol are vitamin D analogues occasionally used as treatment for osteoporosis. Studies show a small increase in spine BMD, but as there is inadequate data regarding fractures, treatment with these drugs cannot be regarded as having the potential to reduce fractures (232,234). Vitamin K has also been suggested as a treatment for osteoporosis and it has been reported that a low intake of vitamin K is associated with an increased risk of hip fracture (235). Treatment with menatetrenone, a vitamin K2 compound, has shown improved BMD (236), but currently there are no randomized controlled trials with an adequate sample size evaluating the effect of vitamin K. Growth hormone is another drug used in the treatment of osteoporosis as it theoretically could increase muscle strength and BMD. There is, however, no proof that it prevents bone loss and reduces fracture risk in post-menopausal women. Ipriflavone, a synthetic compound belonging to the family of isoflavones, may prevent bone loss but it does not seem to reduce the incidence of fractures in osteoporotic women (237). Finally statins increase BMD in animal studies (238), but further information is required about their effects in humans before it can be recommended for the prevention of fragility fractures.

SPECIFIC SURGICAL CONSIDERATIONS FOR TREATING FRACTURES IN AN OSTEOPOROTIC BONE

If an older patient with osteoporosis sustains a fracture there are several important age-related factors to consider when planning treatment. The functional demands in the elderly are different from young healthy people and long-term immobilization in bed must be avoided. Delaying fracture treatment by more than one day has been reported to increase mortality in the elderly (239,240). Thus, it is probably even more important in the elderly to achieve a stable fracture fixation that will reduce pain and facilitate mobilization. Reduced bone mass, increased bone brittleness, and structural changes such as medullary expansion must be taken into account in the osteoporotic patient when deciding the type of surgical method to be used. It must also be understood that the osteoporotic patient usually has low physical demands and a reduced life expectancy when making a decision regarding treatment. For example long-term complications following arthroplasty will not occur in the majority of elderly patients. Thus, joint replacement surgery is a good option after displaced femoral neck fractures as the stability provided by the implant permits immediate weightbearing and mobilization (241). The major problem in osteoporotic fracture treatment is fixation of the device to the bone as bone failure is much more common than implant breakage. Internal fixation devices such as sliding nail plates, intramedullary nails, and tension band constructs that permit skeletal loading minimize stress at the implant–bone interface. Some osteoporotic fractures are also associated with bone loss. If this occurs it is important to achieve bone contact between the two main fragments even if this results in shortening of the extremity. Good bone contact will improve the chance of healing, reduce the healing period, and also reduce the strains on the fixation device. If plates are used these should be used as tension bands which require cortical contact opposite the plates. In addition long plates, where the spacing of the screws are more important than the number of screws, should be used as they will distribute the forces over a larger area reducing the risk of bone failure (242).

Several types of fragility fractures such as fractures of the humerus, distal radius, and closed fractures of the tibial diaphysis can be mobilized in a sling, cast, or brace (243). Immobilization in casts has the disadvantage of immobilizing the joints adjacent to the fracture often leading to joint stiffness. Furthermore, a cast does not control fracture shortening which is often seen in osteoporotic bone; and if the subcutaneous tissue is very mobile, as it often is in the elderly, cast fixation will not provide adequate fracture fixation. External fixators can be used but the main problem with external fixation in osteoporotic bone is the same as for screw fixation, namely loss of fixation. Loosening of the device is often followed by pin infection and local bone resorption sometimes leading to a secondary fracture at the pin site (244). The introduction of hydroxyapatite coated pins has reduced the complication as fixation is improved compared to using titanium-coated and standard pins (245). Another method of improving fixation and avoiding bone resorption is to anchor the screws with polymethylmethacrylate bone cement. This can be inserted into the bone and allowed to harden before drilling or it can be inserted into the screw holes just before the screws are inserted. The screws can then be tightened after the cement hardens (Fig. 19-7). If this method is used it is important that the cement does not penetrate the fracture so as to interfere with fracture healing.

Metaphyseal fractures in osteoporotic bone are associated with specific fixation problems as the metaphyseal fragment is often very small. To improve fixation and resist bending forces a screw and plate construct with a locked angle between the plate and metaphyseal screw is often used. Recently locked plates have been introduced threaded screw holes in the plates, which create angular stability between the screws and the plates. The LISS system (less invasive stabilization system) and the LCP (locking compression plates) are examples of such plates. The

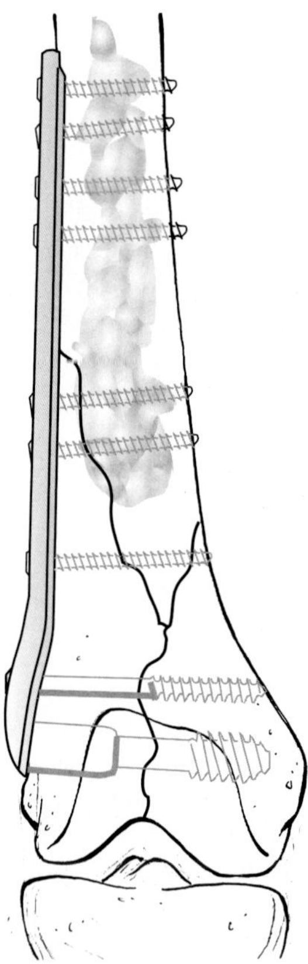

FIGURE 19-7 A displaced diaphyseal femur fracture primarily treated by open reduction and open fixation with an angle plate with augmentation of the screw fixation in the bone by polymethylmethacrylate.

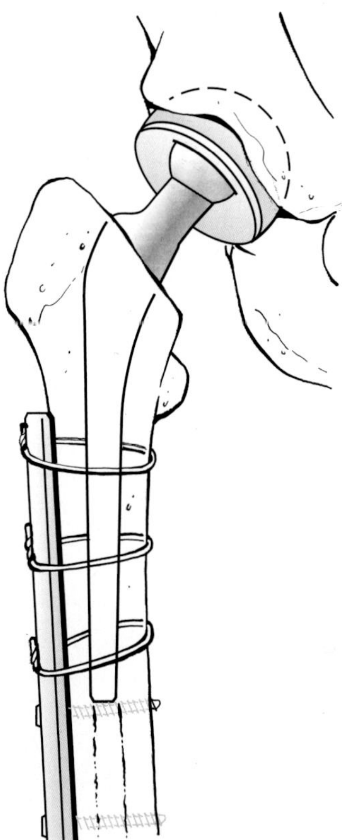

FIGURE 19-9 A periprosthetic femur fracture primarily treated by open reduction and open fixation with a plate with wires for fixation around the femoral shaft.

LCP provides 3 times greater stability than a standard lateral condylar buttress plate and about 2.5 times greater stability than a 95-degree condylar plate in axial loading (246). Biomechanically this is explained by the fact that the LCP also uses multiple screws for metaphyseal fixation (Fig. 19-8). A particular problem that often rules out the use of screws and plates in osteoporotic bone is the periprosthetic fracture. These can be treated with plates using wires for fixation around the femoral shaft (Fig. 19-9).

Intramedullary nailing is a popular treatment for osteoporotic long-bone fractures. It is biomechanically more favorable than plates and screws and will usually permit immediate weightbearing. With the introduction of interlocking nails it is also possible to nail fractures that are close to the metaphyseal regions in long bones. The fixation can be improved by the use of several interlocking screws in different directions or by augmentation of the screws with bone cement. It is also important to realize that as osteoporosis is accompanied by increased diameter of the intramedullary canal (48) wider nails must often be used in older patients. It is possible that even if osteoporosis does not impair fracture healing the diminished bone mass might increase the time taken to restore adequate bone strength. There are experimental studies that show a reduced rate of healing in estrogen-deficient animals (247). As fracture fixation is reduced in osteoporotic bone it would be advantageous to accelerate the healing process. Therefore autogenous cancellous bone graft is often recommended to enhance fracture healing as the osteoconductive bone matrix, osteoinductive growth factors, and mesenchymal stem cells present in this type of graft are thought to stimulate the healing process. However, in patients with osteoporosis the amount of cancellous bone available for grafting is reduced often necessitating the use of allografts, which are biologically inferior to autografts and carry the additional risk of disease transmission. To overcome these problems growth factors are available to induce new bone formation. There are also biodegradable synthetic products such as calcium

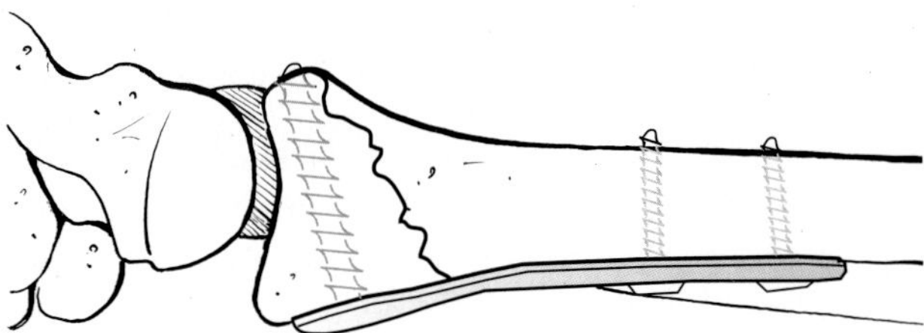

FIGURE 19-8 A metaphyseal distal radius fracture primarily treated by open reduction and open fixation with a locking compression plate (LCP).

phosphate cement which fill defects in osteoporotic bone. These have mainly been used in the treatment of distal radial fractures (248–251). Further studies are required before we can define the role of these products in routine clinical work.

Vertebroplasty and Kyphoplasty

Treatment of vertebral compression fractures has usually been nonoperative, the amount of disability directly relating to the number of fractured vertebrae. Within the last few years vertebroplasty and kyphoplasty have been introduced as new treatment modalities although they have not yet been fully evaluated. In both techniques the crushed vertebrae are filled with material, usually polymethylmethacrylate bone cement in order to avoid further compression. Kyphoplasty also aims to reduce fracture compression before the bone cement is injected. The operative techniques for these procedures have been described elsewhere (252) and will therefore only be reviewed briefly in this chapter.

Vertebroplasty was initially described in 1987 (253). Kyphoplasty has evolved from vertebroplasty in the last few years. Both procedures can usually be undertaken under local anaesthetic. The patient is positioned prone on bolsters in an attempt to reduce the kyphosis and a trochar and cannula is inserted through the pedicle into the posterior or central areas of the vertebral body. Radiopaque bone cement is then injected under fluoroscopic guidance into the vertebral body (Fig. 19-10). Care must be taken not to inject the cement outside the vertebral body and particularly not to inject it into the spinal canal. In kyphoplasty the patient is placed in the same position, but once the cannula has been inserted an inflated balloon is introduced into the vertebral body under manometric control. The objective is to partially or fully reduce the compressed vertebral body. After this has been done the balloon is removed and the operation proceeds as for vertebroplasty (Fig. 19-11). There has been considerable interest in these two techniques but unfortunately little evidence-based information exists as to their success. Despite this the impression is that both procedures are associated with good pain relief. A retrospective study of 500 patients showed that vertebroplasty was associated with significant pain reduction and an improvement in functional status in 50% of the patients 7 months after the procedure. The results were obtained regardless of the number of vertebral fractures that were treated (254). A controlled study has indicated that there is significant relief from symptoms and improvement in function within 24 hours of the procedure (255). However, 6 to 12 months after the procedure there was no evidence of any difference between the groups of patients. The weakness of this study is that the controls comprised the individuals who declined vertebroplasty. Overall, however, it appears that the technique produces short-term pain relief but the long-term results are less clear.

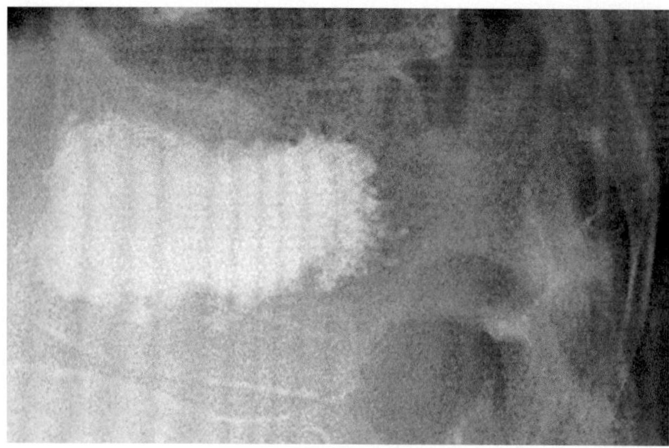

FIGURE 19-10 Vertebroplasty performed in the lumbar spine.

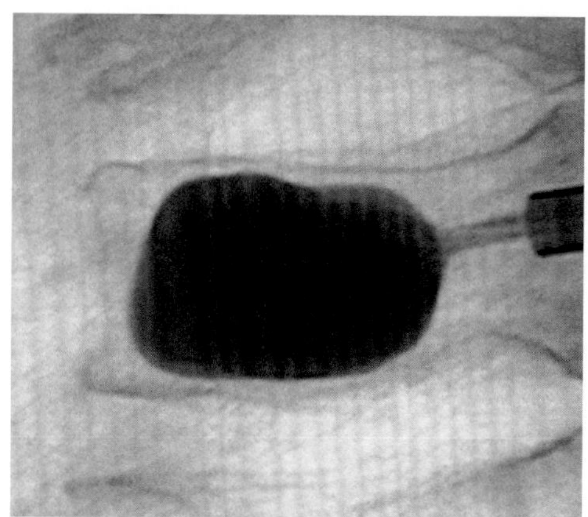

FIGURE 19-11 Kyphoplasty performed in the lumbar spine.

The results of kyphoplasty tend also to be presented in short-term evaluations of the technique. A number of studies report that between 20% to 50% of patients showed no restoration of vertebral body height after the procedure (256,257) while others report mean reduction in the kyphosis of about 10 degrees (257). Most studies indicate good pain relief immediately after the procedure but there is conflicting evidence about long-term results (256,257). A retrospective controlled study comparing kyphoplasty with nonoperated controls showed that the procedure was associated with immediate pain relief and functional improvement compared with the patient's status before surgery and with the controlled group (258). Hospital stay was also longer in the nonoperatively treated group.

Theoretically the technique of kyphoplasty should minimize cement leakage into the surrounding tissue. However, there are as yet no studies that directly compare vertebroplasty and kyphoplasty, although observational studies report an incidence of at least 10% cement leakage in patients treated with kyphoplasty which is similar to the incidence noted after vertebroplasty (256–258). More serious adverse events have been reported. These are extravasation into segmental veins (258), leakage into the spinal canal with associated neurological disturbance, and peri-operative pulmonary edema with myocardial infarction and rib fractures (256,257). There is also the additional potential problem of a surgical procedure altering the biomechanical forces in the spine resulting in new vertebral fractures. One paper has described 12% of patients with new vertebral fractures within 2 years of a vertebroplasty, most being adjacent to the operated vertebrae (259). It is likely however that the complication rate is higher as this study only included symptomatic vertebral fractures and the follow-up was restricted to only 16% of the operated patients.

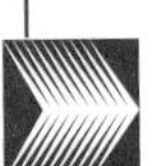

AUTHORS' PREFERRED TREATMENT OF OSTEOPOROSIS AND OSTEOPOROTIC FRACTURES

Prevention Strategies

There are a number of pharmacological and nonpharmacological agents that have been proven to reduce the incidence of osteoporotic fractures. It can no longer be regarded as acceptable clinical practice to avoid investigating or treating patients with osteoporosis who present with low-energy fractures. One fragility fracture indicates further fractures and it should be borne in mind that BMD measurement has a better predictive ability for future fractures than blood pressure has for a future stroke. The evaluation of the patient must include a history of risk factors and in many cases a BMD scan. Prevention strategies may involve both pharmacological and nonpharmacological approaches.

Increased physical activity is the first recommendation we make to virtually all patients with a fragility fracture, independent of age. There is good evidence in the literature that physical activity is beneficial for BMD and reduces the incidence of fracture, especially in post-menopausal women (150,151). We believe that the recommendation to increase physical activity is advantageous not only from the point of view of reducing the risk of future fracture but also for other sound biological reasons. There is good evidence that calcium and vitamin D supplementation can reduce the risk of sustaining a hip fracture in elderly institutionalized patients (133). At the moment there is no evidence that any other nutritional supplement has the same effect. The fact that hip fracture patients are considerably thinner than age-matched individuals without a fracture (260) suggests that increased nutritional intake including calcium, vitamin D, and proteins may also provide protection from future fractures. We therefore recommend a well-balanced diet in patients presenting with a low-energy fracture.

The use of hip protectors in the frail elderly has been shown to reduce the incidence of hip fracture in a number of randomized controlled trials (166,175,178). Currently we recommend hip protectors mainly to institutionalized individuals partly because of the low compliance and lack of data showing benefit to the elderly living in their own homes. Pharmacologic prevention is based on several double-blinded prospective randomized controlled trials showing drug treatment reduces the incidence of fracture. Calcium and vitamin D given together in sufficient dosage have been shown to reduce the incidence of fracture particularly in elderly institutionalized patients (107,133,261). We believe that 500 to 1,000 mg calcium and 400 to 800 IU of vitamin D should be provided to almost all elderly individuals. These doses do not give rise to significant side effects except for occasional gastrointestinal discomfort.

In individuals with osteoporosis who require further treatment we believe that bisphosphonates are usually the drug of choice. Studies indicate that bisphosphonates reduce the risk of fracture compared with no treatment (128,262). Because of the possibility of gastrointestinal disturbances, particularly esophagitis, we prescribe a weekly dose which has been proven to reduce these effects (207). Selected estrogen receptor modulators (SERMs) can also be recommended for fracture prevention as they have been shown to be successful in randomized controlled trials (136). However, the relative effect of bisphosphonates and the fact that they have increased side effects such as thromboembolism (203) mean that SERMs are our second choice for pharmacologic prevention.

Subcutaneous parathyroid hormone (PTH) has been documented to reduce fractures (226,263,264). However, because of its expense, the requirement for daily injections and the incidence of potential side effects we only use this drug in the most severe cases of osteoporosis or in those patients who get severe adverse effects with other drugs. We try to avoid giving PTH to younger patients with osteoporosis because of the lack of long-term data. There is data indicating that estrogen reduces fracture incidence in post-menopausal women (134,135), however, because of the serious side effects that were discussed earlier in this chapter we currently do not use estrogen as a first-line treatment option in osteoporosis.

Surgical Strategies

In general we treat low-energy fractures in the upper and lower limbs slightly differently. Most fractures of the upper limb are treated nonoperatively because of the difficulties of internally fixing these fractures and the lower functional demands in the older osteoporotic patient. Open reduction and internal fixation of proximal humeral fractures in the elderly often give disappointing results and we tend to reserve surgical treatment for severely displaced fractures. Hemi-arthroplasty of the shoulder is not as successful as arthroplasty of the hip joint. We reserve this option for complex fractures such as four-part fractures (265,266).

We usually try to treat displaced distal humeral fractures by open reduction and internal fixation (267) using elbow arthroplasty as a reconstruction procedure for painful nonunions despite the fact that good results of arthroplasty in the management of distal intra-articular fractures have been published (268). Individuals with distal radius fractures that heal in more than 10 degrees of dorsal angulation and/or radial shortening of more than 2 mm have been reported to have a poorer functional outcome than in individuals with more displacement (269). We therefore treat displaced distal radial fractures with external fixation (244,251). However, it is important to assess the functional demands of patients with distal radial fractures and we occasionally treat these patients in a plaster cast without fracture reduction.

In the lower limb we aim to achieve stable fixation to allow immediate weightbearing and early mobilization (239,240). We treat most osteoporotic acetabular fractures nonoperatively with a period of non-weightbearing mobilization although primary arthroplasty is considered for selected patients. Displaced femoral neck fractures are treated with primary joint replacement as randomized controlled studies have shown this technique to be advantageous when compared to pinning (241,270). In patients who have a displaced femoral neck fracture and are more than 70 years of age we use arthroplasty whereas pinning remains our first choice in patients below 70 years of age and in patients with undisplaced fractures (241,270). The standard treatment for trochanteric fractures is a sliding hip screw (271) and in virtually all patients with hip fractures early mobilization and weightbearing is encouraged (271).

We usually treat femoral diaphyseal fractures with closed reduction and antegrade intramedullary nailing whereas unstable distal femoral fractures are usually treated by open reduction and internal fixation. Retrograde nails are sometimes used to bridge long comminuted femoral fractures. We believe that this technique provides a more stable construct either with a blade plate or a dynamic condylar screw (271,273). The LISS plate probably provides a better alternative especially for peri-prosthetic fractures (274).

Fractures of the proximal distal tibia are treated in the same way as in patients who do not have osteoporosis. If a stable fixation is achieved we permit mobilization after 2 to 6 weeks in a cast although full weightbearing is usually not allowed within 8 to 12 weeks (250,275).

We regard vertebroplasty and kyphoplasty as promising new operative treatments for osteoporotic vertebral fractures. However we would caution surgeons that clinical studies must indicate that these new techniques are useful before the treatment can be widely recommended.

TABLE 19-8 10-Year Probability of Fracture (%) According to Age and Risk Relative to the Average Population[a]

Relative Risk	50 yr	60 yr	70 yr	80 yr
Hip fracture (male)				
1	0.84	1.26	3.68	9.53
2	1.68	2.50	7.21	17.89
3	2.58	3.73	10.59	25.26
4	3.33	4.94	13.83	31.75
Hip fracture (female)				
1	0.57	2.40	7.87	18.0
2	1.14	4.75	15.1	32.0
3	1.71	7.04	21.7	42.9
4	2.27	9.27	27.7	51.6
Hip, clinical spine, humeral, Colles fracture (male)				
1	3.3	4.7	7.0	12.6
2	6.5	9.1	13.5	23.1
3	9.6	13.3	19.4	23.9
4	12.6	17.3	24.9	39.3
Hip, clinical spine, humeral, Colles fracture (female)				
1	5.8	9.6	16.1	21.5
2	11.3	18.2	29.4	37.4
3	16.5	26.0	40.0	49.2
4	21.4	33.1	49.5	58.1

[a] In Sweden.

From Kanis JA, Oden A, Johnell O, et al. The burden of osteoporotic fractures: a method for setting intervention thresholds. *Osteoporos Int* 2001;12:417–427.

FUTURE PERSPECTIVE

Few doctors see as many patients with osteoporosis as orthopaedic surgeons. The diagnosis is often made in the orthopaedic wards or in the outpatient clinic after a low-energy fracture has occurred. Orthopaedic surgeons must be careful that they do not just concentrate on the technical aspects of fracture fixation and that they appreciate the considerable consequences of osteoporosis. Identification of subjects at high risk of future fracture constitutes the most rational approach to fracture prevention. We believe that it is the responsibility of the orthopaedic surgeon to arrange for patients who present with low-energy fractures to be properly advised and investigated for osteoporosis. It is also the responsibility of every orthopaedic surgeon to be aware of the different treatment modalities that exist and to appropriately advise the patient.

The investigation and treatment of osteoporosis is not necessarily the province of the orthopaedic surgeon. Referral to an appropriate physician interested in investigation and treatment is however the responsibility of the orthopaedic surgeon. We think it likely that the prediction of the risk of future fractures will determine treatment strategy. Table 19-8 shows the 10-year fracture probability for the common osteoporotic fractures in Sweden according to the population at risk (276). A relative risk of 2 means that the risk of sustaining a fracture has doubled. Similar tables can help us to estimate the risk of fracture from the relative risk estimates that are achieved from bone scans and investigation of risk factors (Fig. 19-5). When a hip fracture alone is considered a 10-year probability of 10% or more provides a cost-effective threshold for treating women (277). As the aim of the assessment of fracture is to target cost-effective treatment interventions—that is, to include those at the highest risk—we can hopefully more easily decide who to treat with similar risk calculations.

REFERENCES

An asterisk denotes a Level I evidence-based reference.

1. Dequeker J, Ortner DJ, Stix AI, et al. Hip fracture and osteoporosis in a XIIth Dynasty female skeleton from Lisht, upper Egypt. *J Bone Miner Res* 1997;12:881–888.
2. World Health Organization. Assessment of fracture risk and its application to screening for postmenopausal osteoporosis. Report of a WHO Study Group. *World Health Organ Tech Rep Ser* 1994;843:1–129.
3. Melton LJ 3rd. How many women have osteoporosis now? *J Bone Miner Res* 1995;10:175–177.
4. Obrant KJ, Bengner U, Johnell O, et al. Increasing age-adjusted risk of fragility fractures: a sign of increasing osteoporosis in successive generations? *Calcif Tissue Int* 1989;44:157–167.
5. Bengner U. Epidemiological changes over 30 years in an urban population. Thesis, Lund University, Lund, Sweden, 1987.
6. Melton LJ, 3rd, Riggs BL. *Osteoporosis: etiology, diagnosis and management*. New York: Raven Press, 1995:225–248.
7. Melton LJ, 3rd, Riggs BL. Risk factors for injury after a fall. *Clin Geriatr Med* 1985;1:525–539.

*8. Tinetti ME, Doucette JT, Claus EB. The contribution of predisposing and situational risk factors to serious fall injuries. *J Am Geriatr Soc* 1995;43:1207–1213.

9. Greenspan SL, Myers ER, Maitland LA, et al. Fall severity and bone mineral density as risk factors for hip fracture in ambulatory elderly. *JAMA* 1994;271:128–133.

*10. Tinetti ME, Doucette J, Claus E, et al. Risk factors for serious injury during falls by older persons in the community. *J Am Geriatr Soc* 1995;43:1214–1221.

*11. Tinetti ME, Speechley M, Ginter SF. Risk factors for falls among elderly persons living in the community. *N Engl J Med* 1988;319:1701–1707.

12. Ryynanen OP, Kivela SL, Honkanen R, et al. Incidence of falling injuries leading to medical treatment in the elderly. *Public Health* 1991;105:373–386.

*13. Luukinen H, Koski K, Honkanen R, et al. Incidence of injury-causing falls among older adults by place of residence: a population-based study. *J Am Geriatr Soc* 1995;43:871–876.

*14. Tinetti ME. Factors associated with serious injury during falls by ambulatory nursing home residents. *J Am Geriatr Soc* 1987;35:644–648.

*15. Nguyen T, Sambrook P, Kelly P, et al. Prediction of osteoporotic fractures by postural instability and bone density. *BMJ* 1993;307:1111–1115.

*16. Tinetti ME, Liu WL, Ginter SF. Mechanical restraint use and fall-related injuries among residents of skilled nursing facilities. *Ann Intern Med* 1992;116:369–374.

*17. Grisso JA, Kelsey JL, Strom BL, et al. Risk factors for falls as a cause of hip fracture in women. The Northeast Hip Fracture Study Group. *N Engl J Med* 1991;324:1326–1331.

18. Rice D, MacKenzie E. Cost of injury in the United States: A report to Congress. San Francisco: University of California, 1989.
19. Fingerhut LA, Warner M. Injury chartbook. In: *Health, United States, 1996–1997*. Hyattsville, MD: U.S. Department of Health and Human Services, Centers for Disease Control and Prevention, National Center for Health Statistics, 1997. DHHS Publication No. (PHS) 97-1232.
20. Hindso K. Behavioral attitude towards hip protectors in elderly orthopedic patients. *Osteoporosis Int* 1998;8:119.
21. Praemer A, Furner S, Rice D. *Musculoskeletal condition in the United States*. Park Ridge, IL: American Academy of Orthopaedic Surgeons, 1992.
22. Advisory Group on Osteoporosis. Report. London: Department of Health, 1994.

*23. Weiss NS, Liff JM, Ure CL, et al. Mortality in women following hip fracture. *J Chronic Dis* 1983;36:879–882.

24. Cummings SR, Kelsey JL, Nevitt MC, et al. Epidemiology of osteoporosis and osteoporotic fractures. *Epidemiol Rev* 1985;7:178–208.
25. Sexson SB, Lehner JT. Factors affecting hip fracture mortality. *J Orthop Trauma* 1987;1:298–305.
26. Kellie SE, Brody JA. Sex-specific and race-specific hip fracture rates. *Am J Public Health* 1990;80:326–328.
27. Holbrook T, Grazier K, Kelsey J, et al. *The frequency of occurrence, impact and cost of selected musculoskeletal conditions in the United States*. Chicago: American Academy of Orthopaedic Surgeons, 1984.

*28. Bonar SK, Tinetti ME, Speechley M, et al. Factors associated with short- versus long-term skilled nursing facility placement among community-living hip fracture patients. *J Am Geriatr Soc* 1990;38:1139–1144.

29. Villa M, Nelson L. Race, ethnicity and osteoporosis. In: Marcus R, Feldman D, Kelsey J, eds. *Osteoporosis*. San Diego: Academic Press, 1996:435–447.
30. Cooper C, Melton LJ 3rd. Epidemiology of osteoporosis. *Trends Endocrinol Metab* 1992;314:224–229.
31. Rogmark C, Sernbo I, Johnell O, et al. Incidence of hip fractures in Malmo, Sweden, 1992–1995. A trend-break. *Acta Orthop Scand* 1999;70:19–22.
32. Melton LJ 3rd, Atkinson EJ, Madhok R. Downturn in hip fracture incidence. *Public Health Rep* 1996;111:146–150, discussion 151.
33. Cooper C, Campion G, Melton LJ 3rd. Hip fractures in the elderly: a world-wide projection. *Osteoporos Int* 1992;2:285–289.
34. O'Neill TW, Felsenberg D, Varlow J, et al. The prevalence of vertebral deformity in European men and women: the European Vertebral Osteoporosis Study. *J Bone Miner Res* 1996;11:1010–1018.
35. Melton LJ 3rd, Lane AW, Cooper C, et al. Prevalence and incidence of vertebral deformities. *Osteoporos Int* 1993;3:113–119.
36. Lau EM, Chan HH, Woo J, et al. Normal ranges for vertebral height ratios and prevalence of vertebral fracture in Hong Kong Chinese: a comparison with American Caucasians. *J Bone Miner Res* 1996;11:1364–1368.
37. Bengner U, Johnell O, Redlund-Johnell I. Changes in incidence and prevalence of vertebral fractures during 30 years. *Calcif Tissue Int* 1988;42:293–296.
38. Hansen M, Overgaard K, A G, Christiansen C. Does the prevalence of vertebral fractures increase? *Osteoporosis 1990*. Copenhagen, 1990:95.
39. Nevitt MC, Cummings SR. Type of fall and risk of hip and wrist fractures: the study of osteoporotic fractures. The Study of Osteoporotic Fractures Research Group. *J Am Geriatr Soc* 1993;41:1226–1234.

*40. Hasserius R, Karlsson MK, Nilsson BE, et al. Prevalent vertebral deformities predict increased mortality and increased fracture rate in both men and women: a 10-year population-based study of 598 individuals from the Swedish cohort in the European Vertebral Osteoporosis Study. *Osteoporos Int* 2003;14:61–68.

41. Ettinger B, Block JE, Smith R, et al. An examination of the association between vertebral deformities, physical disabilities and psychosocial problems. *Maturitas* 1988;10:283–296.

*42. Ettinger B, Black DM, Nevitt MC, et al. Contribution of vertebral deformities to chronic back pain and disability. The Study of Osteoporotic Fractures Research Group. *J Bone Miner Res* 1992;7:449–456.

43. Bailey DA, McKay HA, Mirwald RL, et al. A six-year longitudinal study of the relationship of physical activity to bone mineral accrual in growing children: the university of Saskatchewan bone mineral accrual study. *J Bone Miner Res* 1999;14:1672–1679.
44. Sundberg M. Skeletal growth and effects of physical activity during adolescence. Thesis, Lunds University, Lund, Sweden, 2001.
45. Seeman E, Tsalamandris C, Formica C, et al. Reduced femoral neck bone density in the daughters of women with hip fractures: the role of low peak bone density in the pathogenesis of osteoporosis. *J Bone Miner Res* 1994;9:739–743.
46. Karlsson M, Bass S, Seeman E. The evidence that exercise during growth or adulthood reduces the risk of fragility fractures is weak. *Best Pract Res Clin Rheumatol* 2001;15:429–450.
47. Kannus P, Haapasalo H, Sankelo M, et al. Effect of starting age of physical activity on bone mass in the dominant arm of tennis and squash players. *Ann Intern Med* 1995;123:27–31.
48. Ahlborg HG, Johnell O, Turner CH, et al. Bone loss and bone size after menopause. *N Engl J Med* 2003;349:327–334.

*49. Lindsay R, Hart DM, Forrest C, et al. Prevention of spinal osteoporosis in oophorectomised women. *Lancet* 1980;2:1151–1154.

50. Parfitt AM. Age-related structural changes in trabecular and cortical bone: cellular mechanisms and biomechanical consequences. *Calcif Tissue Int* 1984;36(Suppl 1): S123–S128.
51. Riggs BL, Khosla S, Melton LJ 3rd. A unitary model for involutional osteoporosis: estrogen deficiency causes both type I and type II osteoporosis in postmenopausal women and contributes to bone loss in aging men. *J Bone Miner Res* 1998;13:763–773.
52. Kassem M, Ankersen L, Eriksen EF, et al. Demonstration of cellular aging and senescence in serially passaged long-term cultures of human trabecular osteoblasts. *Osteoporos Int* 1997;7:514–524.
53. Eriksen EF, Hodgson SF, Eastell R, et al. Cancellous bone remodeling in type I (postmenopausal) osteoporosis: quantitative assessment of rates of formation, resorption, and bone loss at tissue and cellular levels. *J Bone Miner Res* 1990;5:311–319.
54. Riggs BL, Melton LJ 3rd. Clinical review 8: Clinical heterogeneity of involutional osteoporosis: implications for preventive therapy. *J Clin Endocrinol Metab* 1990;70: 1229–1232.
55. Toussirot E, Royet O, Wendling D. [Aetiologic features of osteoporosis in male patients aged less than 50 years: study of 28 cases with a comparative series of 30 patients over the age of 50]. *Rev Med Interne* 1998;19:479–485.
56. Bauer DC, Gluer CC, Cauley JA, et al. Broadband ultrasound attenuation predicts fractures strongly and independently of densitometry in older women. A prospective study. Study of Osteoporotic Fractures Research Group. *Arch Intern Med* 1997;157: 629–634.
57. Genant HK, Cann CE, Ettinger B, et al. Quantitative computed tomography of vertebral spongiosa: a sensitive method for detecting early bone loss after oophorectomy. *Ann Intern Med* 1982;97:699–705.
58. Nilsson BE, Johnell O, Petersson C. In vivo bone-mineral measurement. How and why—a review. *Acta Orthop Scand* 1990;61:275–281.
59. Kelly TL, Slovik DM, Schoenfeld DA, et al. Quantitative digital radiography versus dual photon absorptiometry of the lumbar spine. *J Clin Endocrinol Metab* 1988;67:839–844.
60. Mazess RB, Barden HS, Bisek JP, et al. Dual-energy x-ray absorptiometry for total-body and regional bone-mineral and soft-tissue composition. *Am J Clin Nutr* 1990;51: 1106–1112.
61. Steiger P, Cummings SR, Genant HK, et al. Morphometric x-ray absorptiometry of the spine: correlation in vivo with morphometric radiography. Study of Osteoporotic Fractures Research Group. *Osteoporos Int* 1994;4:238–244.
62. Langton CM, Palmer SB, Porter RW. The measurement of broadband ultrasonic attenuation in cancellous bone. *Eng Med* 1984;13:89–91.
63. Gluer CC. Quantitative ultrasound techniques for the assessment of osteoporosis: expert agreement on current status. The International Quantitative Ultrasound Consensus Group. *J Bone Miner Res* 1997;12:1280–1288.
64. Morris FL, Naughton GA, Gibbs JL, et al. Prospective ten-month exercise intervention in premenarcheal girls: positive effects on bone and lean mass. *J Bone Miner Res* 1997; 12:1453–1462.
65. Hans D, Dargent-Molina P, Schott AM, et al. Ultrasonographic heel measurements to predict hip fracture in elderly women: the EPIDOS prospective study. *Lancet* 1996; 348:511–514.
66. Russell RG. The assessment of bone metabolism in vivo using biochemical approaches. *Horm Metab Res* 1997;29:138–144.
67. Masters PW, Jones RG, Purves DA, et al. Commercial assays for serum osteocalcin give clinically discordant results. *Clin Chem* 1994;40:358–363.
68. Woitge HW, Seibel MJ, Ziegler R. Comparison of total and bone-specific alkaline phosphatase in patients with nonskeletal disorder or metabolic bone diseases. *Clin Chem* 1996;42:1796–1804.
69. Kollerup G, Thamsborg G, Bhatia H, et al. Quantitation of urinary hydroxypyridinium cross-links from collagen by high-performance liquid chromatography. *Scand J Clin Lab Invest* 1992;52:657–662.
70. Minkin C. Bone acid phosphatase: tartrate-resistant acid phosphatase as a marker of osteoclast function. *Calcif Tissue Int* 1982;34:285–290.
71. Gerdhem P, Ivaska KK, Alatalo SL, et al. Biochemical markers of bone metabolism and prediction of fracture in elderly women. *J Bone Miner Res* 2004;19:386–393. Epub Dec 22, 2003.
72. Woitge HW, Scheidt-Nave C, Kissling C, et al. Seasonal variation of biochemical indexes of bone turnover: results of a population-based study. *J Clin Endocrinol Metab* 1998; 83:68–75.
73. Greenspan SL, Dresner-Pollak R, Parker RA, et al. Diurnal variation of bone mineral turnover in elderly men and women. *Calcif Tissue Int* 1997;60:419–423.
74. Ravn P, Fledelius C, Rosenquist C, et al. High bone turnover is associated with low bone mass in both pre- and postmenopausal women. *Bone* 1996;19:291–298.
75. Harris ST, Gertz BJ, Genant HK, et al. The effect of short term treatment with alendronate on vertebral density and biochemical markers of bone remodeling in early postmenopausal women. *J Clin Endocrinol Metab* 1993;76:1399–1406.
*76. Cummings SR, Nevitt MC, Browner WS, et al. Risk factors for hip fracture in white women. Study of Osteoporotic Fractures Research Group. *N Engl J Med* 1995;332: 767–773.
77. Looker AC, Wahner HW, Dunn WL, et al. Proximal femur bone mineral levels of US adults. *Osteoporos Int* 1995;5:389–409.
*78. Ross PD, Davis JW, Epstein RS, et al. Pre-existing fractures and bone mass predict vertebral fracture incidence in women. *Ann Intern Med* 1991;114:919–923.
*79. Kroger H, Huopio J, Honkanen R, et al. Prediction of fracture risk using axial bone mineral density in a perimenopausal population: a prospective study. *J Bone Miner Res* 1995;10:302–306.
*80. Marshall D, Johnell O, Wedel H. Meta-analysis of how well measures of bone mineral density predict occurrence of osteoporotic fractures. *BMJ* 1996;312:1254–1259.
*81. Cummings SR, Black DM, Nevitt MC, et al. Bone density at various sites for prediction of hip fractures. The Study of Osteoporotic Fractures Research Group. *Lancet* 1993; 341:72–75.
*82. Hui SL, Slemenda CW, Johnston CC Jr. Baseline measurement of bone mass predicts fracture in white women. *Ann Intern Med* 1989;111:355–361.
83. Who are candidates for prevention and treatment for osteoporosis? *Osteoporos Int* 1997; 7:1–6.
84. Faulkner KG, Cummings SR, Black D, et al. Simple measurement of femoral geometry predicts hip fracture: the study of osteoporotic fractures. *J Bone Miner Res* 1993;8: 1211–1217.
85. Yoshikawa T, Turner CH, Peacock M, et al. Geometric structure of the femoral neck measured using dual-energy x-ray absorptiometry. *J Bone Miner Res* 1994;9: 1053–1064.
86. Beck TJ, Ruff CB, Warden KE, et al. Predicting femoral neck strength from bone mineral data. A structural approach. *Invest Radiol* 1990;25:6–18.
87. Crabtree N, Adams J, Pols H, et al. Age, gender and geographical effects on hip geometry and bone mineral distribution: The EPOS study. *Osteoporos Int* 1997;7:291.
88. Kelly PJ, Morrison N, Sambrook PN, et al. Genetics and osteoporosis: role of the vitamin D receptor gene. *Agents Actions* 1994;42:i–ii.
89. Grant SF, Reid DM, Blake G, et al. Reduced bone density and osteoporosis associated with a polymorphic Sp1 binding site in the collagen type I alpha 1 gene. *Nat Genet* 1996;14:203–205.
90. Langdahl BL, Knudsen JY, Jensen HK, et al. A sequence variation: 713-8delC in the transforming growth factor-beta 1 gene has higher prevalence in osteoporotic women than in normal women and is associated with very low bone mass in osteoporotic women and increased bone turnover in both osteoporotic and normal women. *Bone* 1997;20:289–294.
91. Kobayashi S, Inoue S, Hosoi T, et al. Association of bone mineral density with polymorphism of the estrogen receptor gene. *J Bone Miner Res* 1996;11:306–311.
92. Uitterlinden AG, Burger H, Huang Q, et al. Relation of alleles of the collagen type I alpha1 gene to bone density and the risk of osteoporotic fractures in postmenopausal women. *N Engl J Med* 1998;338:1016–1021.
93. Cooper C, Melton LJ 3rd. Magnitude and impact of osteoporosis and fractures. In: Marcus R, Feldman D, Kelsey J, eds. *Osteoporosis*. San Diego: Academic Press, 1996: 419–434.
*94. Mallmin H, Ljunghall S, Persson I, et al. Fracture of the distal forearm as a forecaster of subsequent hip fracture: a population-based cohort study with 24 years of follow-up. *Calcif Tissue Int* 1993;52:269–272.
*95. Huopio J, Kröger H, Honkanen R, et al. Risk factors for perimenopausal fractures. A prospective population-based study. *Osteoporos Int* 1998;8(Suppl 3):6.
*96. Rizzo JA, Baker DI, McAvay G, et al. The cost-effectiveness of a multifactorial targeted prevention program for falls among community elderly persons. *Med Care* 1996;34: 954–969.
97. Perry BC. Falls among the elderly: a review of the methods and conclusions of epidemiologic studies. *J Am Geriatr Soc* 1982;30:367–371.
*98. Paganini-Hill A, Chao A, Ross RK, et al. Exercise and other factors in the prevention of hip fracture: the Leisure World study. *Epidemiology* 1991;2:16–25.
99. Ruff CB, Hayes WC. Sex differences in age-related remodeling of the femur and tibia. *J Orthop Res* 1988;6:886–896.
100. Kroger H, Tuppurainen M, Honkanen R, et al. Bone mineral density and risk factors for osteoporosis—a population-based study of 1600 perimenopausal women. *Calcif Tissue Int* 1994;55:1–7.
*101. Ensrud KE, Cauley J, Lipschutz R, et al. Weight change and fractures in older women. Study of Osteoporotic Fractures Research Group. *Arch Intern Med* 1997;157:857–863.
102. Kiel DP, Felson DT, Anderson JJ, et al. Hip fracture and the use of estrogens in postmenopausal women. The Framingham Study. *N Engl J Med* 1987;317:1169–1174.
*103. Meyer HE, Tverdal A, Falch JA. Risk factors for hip fracture in middle-aged Norwegian women and men. *Am J Epidemiol* 1993;137:1203–1211.
104. Hayes WC, Myers ER, Morris JN, et al. Impact near the hip dominates fracture risk in elderly nursing home residents who fall. *Calcif Tissue Int* 1993;52:192–198.
105. Johnell O, Gullberg B, Kanis JA, et al. Risk factors for hip fracture in European women: the MEDOS Study. Mediterranean Osteoporosis Study. *J Bone Miner Res* 1995;10: 1802–1815.
*106. Wickham CA, Walsh K, Cooper C, et al. Dietary calcium, physical activity, and risk of hip fracture: a prospective study. *BMJ* 1989;299:889–892.
*107. Dawson-Hughes B, Harris SS, Krall EA, et al. Effect of calcium and vitamin D supplementation on bone density in men and women 65 years of age or older. *N Engl J Med* 1997;337:670–676.
108. Daniell HW. Osteoporosis of the slender smoker. Vertebral compression fractures and loss of metacarpal cortex in relation to postmenopausal cigarette smoking and lack of obesity. *Arch Intern Med* 1976;136:298–304.
109. Law MR, Hackshaw AK. A meta-analysis of cigarette smoking, bone mineral density and risk of hip fracture: recognition of a major effect. *Br Med J* 1997;315:841–846.
*110. Kiel DP, Felson DT, Hannan MT, et al. Caffeine and the risk of hip fracture: the Framingham Study. *Am J Epidemiol* 1990;132:675–684.
*111. Torgerson DJ, Campbell MK, Thomas RE, et al. Prediction of perimenopausal fractures by bone mineral density and other risk factors. *J Bone Miner Res* 1996;11:293–297.
*112. Hernandez-Avila M, Colditz GA, Stampfer MJ, et al. Caffeine, moderate alcohol intake, and risk of fractures of the hip and forearm in middle-aged women. *Am J Clin Nutr* 1991;54:157–163.

113. Nielsen HK, Lundby L, Rasmussen K, et al. Alcohol decreases serum osteocalcin in a dose-dependent way in normal subjects. *Calcif Tissue Int* 1990;46:173–178.
*114. Graafmans WC, Ooms ME, Bezemer PD, et al. Different risk profiles for hip fractures and distal forearm fractures: a prospective study. *Osteoporos Int* 1996;6:427–431.
*115. Graafmans WC, Ooms ME, Hofstee HM, et al. Falls in the elderly: a prospective study of risk factors and risk profiles. *Am J Epidemiol* 1996;143:1129–1136.
*116. Koski K, Luukinen H, Laippala P, et al. Physiological factors and medications as predictors of injurious falls by elderly people: a prospective population-based study. *Age Ageing* 1996;25:29–38.
*117. Dargent-Molina P, Favier F, Grandjean H, et al. Fall-related factors and risk of hip fracture: the EPIDOS prospective study. *Lancet* 1996;348:145–149.
118. Kanis JA, Delmas P, Burckhardt P, et al. Guidelines for diagnosis and management of osteoporosis. The European Foundation for Osteoporosis and Bone Disease. *Osteoporos Int* 1997;7:390–406.
119. Myers AH, Baker SP, Van Natta ML, et al. Risk factors associated with falls and injuries among elderly institutionalized persons. *Am J Epidemiol* 1991;133:1179–1190.
*120. Province MA, Hadley EC, Hornbrook MC, et al. The effects of exercise on falls in elderly patients. A preplanned meta-analysis of the FICSIT Trials. Frailty and Injuries: Cooperative Studies of Intervention Techniques. *JAMA* 1995;273:1341–1347.
*121. Tinetti ME, McAvay G, Claus E. Does multiple risk factor reduction explain the reduction in fall rate in the Yale FICSIT Trial? Frailty and Injuries Cooperative Studies of Intervention Techniques. *Am J Epidemiol* 1996;144:389–399.
*122. Cooper C, Atkinson EJ, Jacobsen SJ, et al. Population-based study of survival after osteoporotic fractures. *Am J Epidemiol* 1993;137:1001–1005.
*123. Poor G, Atkinson EJ, O'Fallon WM, et al. Determinants of reduced survival following hip fractures in men. *Clin Orthop Rel Res* 1995:260–265.
124. Ray NF, Chan JK, Thamer M, et al. Medical expenditures for the treatment of osteoporotic fractures in the United States in 1995: report from the National Osteoporosis Foundation. *J Bone Miner Res* 1997;12:24–35.
125. Seeman E. The dilemma of osteoporosis in men. *Am J Med* 1995;98:76S–88S.
*126. Center JR, Nguyen TV, Schneider D, et al. Mortality after all major types of osteoporotic fractures in men and women: an observational study. *Lancet* 1999;353:878–882.
*127. McClung MR, Geusens P, Miller PD, et al. Effect of risedronate on the risk of hip fracture in elderly women. Hip Intervention Program Study Group. *N Engl J Med* 2001; 344:333–340.
*128. Harris ST, Watts NB, Genant HK, et al. Effects of risedronate treatment on vertebral and nonvertebral fractures in women with postmenopausal osteoporosis: a randomized controlled trial. Vertebral Efficacy With Risedronate Therapy (VERT) Study Group. *JAMA* 1999;282:1344–1352.
*129. Reginster J, Minne HW, Sorensen OH, et al. Randomized trial of the effects of risedronate on vertebral fractures in women with established postmenopausal osteoporosis. Vertebral Efficacy with Risedronate Therapy (VERT) Study Group. *Osteoporos Int* 2000; 11:83–91.
*130. Cummings SR, Black DM, Thompson DE, et al. Effect of alendronate on risk of fracture in women with low bone density but without vertebral fractures: results from the Fracture Intervention Trial. *JAMA* 1998;280:2077–2082.
*131. Black DM, Cummings SR, Karpf DB, et al. Randomised trial of effect of alendronate on risk of fracture in women with existing vertebral fractures. Fracture Intervention Trial Research Group. *Lancet* 1996;348:1535–1541.
*132. Chapuy MC, Arlot ME, Delmas PD, et al. Effect of calcium and cholecalciferol treatment for three years on hip fractures in elderly women. *Br Med J* 1994;308:1081–1082.
*133. Chapuy MC, Arlot ME, Duboeuf F, et al. Vitamin D3 and calcium to prevent hip fractures in the elderly women. *N Engl J Med* 1992;327:1637–1642.
*134. Manson JE, Hsia J, Johnson KC, et al. Estrogen plus progestin and the risk of coronary heart disease. *N Engl J Med* 2003;349:523–534.
*135. Rossouw JE, Anderson GL, Prentice RL, et al. Risks and benefits of estrogen plus progestin in healthy postmenopausal women: principal results from the Women's Health Initiative randomized controlled trial. *JAMA* 2002;288:321–333.
*136. Ettinger B, Black DM, Mitlak BH, et al. Reduction of vertebral fracture risk in postmenopausal women with osteoporosis treated with raloxifene: results from a 3-year randomized clinical trial. Multiple Outcomes of Raloxifene Evaluation (MORE) Investigators. *JAMA* 1999;282:637–645.
*137. Orwoll E, Ettinger M, Weiss S, et al. Alendronate for the treatment of osteoporosis in men. *N Engl J Med* 2000;343:604–610.
138. NIH consensus development panel on optimal calcium intake. *JAMA* 1994;272: 1942–1948.
139. Matkovic V, Heaney RP. Calcium balance during human growth: evidence for threshold behavior. *Am J Clin Nutr* 1992;55:992–996.
140. Lee WT, Leung SS, Ng MY, et al. Bone mineral content of two populations of Chinese children with different calcium intakes. *Bone Miner* 1993;23:195–206.
141. Ilich JZ, Skugor M, Hangartner T, et al. Relation of nutrition, body composition and physical activity to skeletal development: a cross-sectional study in preadolescent females. *J Am Coll Nutr* 1998;17:136–147.
142. Teegarden D, Lyle RM, McCabe GP, et al. Dietary calcium, protein, and phosphorus are related to bone mineral density and content in young women. *Am J Clin Nutr* 1998; 68:749–754.
143. Matkovic V, Kostial K, Simonovic I, et al. Bone status and fracture rates in two regions of Yugoslavia. *Am J Clin Nutr* 1979;32:540–549.
144. Kannus P, Sievanen H, Vuori I. Physical loading, exercise, and bone. *Bone* 1996;18: 1S–3S.
145. Karlsson MK, Linden C, Karlsson C, et al. Exercise during growth and bone mineral density and fractures in old age. *Lancet* 2000;355:469–470.
146. Parfitt AM. The two faces of growth: benefits and risks to bone integrity. *Osteoporos Int* 1994;4:382–398.
*147. Bassey EJ, Ramsdale SJ. Increase in femoral bone density in young women following high-impact exercise. *Osteoporos Int* 1994;4:72–75.
*148. Heinonen A, Kannus P, Sievanen H, et al. Randomised controlled trial of effect of high-impact exercise on selected risk factors for osteoporotic fractures. *Lancet* 1996;348: 1343–1347.
149. Joakimsen RM, Magnus JH, Fonnebo V. Physical activity and predisposition for hip fractures: a review. *Osteoporos Int* 1997;7:503–513.
*150. Gregg EW, Cauley JA, Seeley DG, et al. Physical activity and osteoporotic fracture risk in older women. Study of Osteoporotic Fractures Research Group. *Ann Intern Med* 1998;129:81–88.
*151. Dalsky GP, Stocke KS, Ehsani AA, et al. Weight-bearing exercise training and lumbar bone mineral content in postmenopausal women. *Ann Intern Med* 1988;108:824–828.
*152. Heinonen A, Oja P, Sievanen H, et al. Effect of two training regimens on bone mineral density in healthy perimenopausal women: a randomized controlled trial. *J Bone Miner Res* 1998;13;483–490.
153. Lanyon LE. Using functional loading to influence bone mass and architecture; objectives, mechanisms, and relationship with estrogen of the mechanically adaptive process in bone. *Bone* 1996;18:37S–43S.
154. Jaglal SB, Kreiger N, Darlington G. Past and recent physical activity and risk of hip fracture. *Am J Epidemiol* 1993;138:107–118.
155. Slemenda C. Prevention of hip fractures: risk factor modification. *Am J Med* 1997;103: 65S–71S, discussion 71S–73S.
*156. Mallmin H, Ljunghall S, Persson I, et al. Risk factors for fractures of the distal forearm: a population-based case-control study. *Osteoporos Int* 1994;4:298–304.
*157. Wolf SL, Barnhart HX, Ellison GL, et al. The effect of Tai Chi Quan and computerized balance training on postural stability in older subjects. Atlanta FICSIT Group. Frailty and Injuries: Cooperative Studies on Intervention Techniques. *Phys Ther* 1997;77: 371–381, discussion 382–384.
*158. Close J, Ellis M, Hooper R, et al. Prevention of falls in the elderly trial (PROFET): a randomised controlled trial. *Lancet* 1999;353:93–97.
*159. Campbell AJ, Robertson MC, Gardner MM, et al. Falls prevention over 2 years: a randomized controlled trial in women 80 years and older. *Age Ageing* 1999;28: 513–518.
*160. Gardner MM, Robertson MC, Campbell AJ. Exercise in preventing falls and fall related injuries in older people: a review of randomised controlled trials. *Br J Sports Med* 2000; 34:7–17.
*161. Gillespie LD, Gillespie WJ, Robertson MC, et al. Interventions for preventing falls in elderly people. *Cochrane Database Syst Rev* 2003:CD000340.
*162. Lord SR, Ward JA, Williams P, et al. The effect of a 12-month exercise trial on balance, strength, and falls in older women: a randomized controlled trial. *J Am Geriatr Soc* 1995;43:1198–1206.
*163. Shumway-Cook A, Gruber W, Baldwin M, et al. The effect of multidimensional exercises on balance, mobility, and fall risk in community-dwelling older adults. *Phys Ther* 1997;77:46–57.
*164. Wolfson L, Whipple R, Derby C, et al. Balance and strength training in older adults: intervention gains and Tai Chi maintenance. *J Am Geriatr Soc* 1996;44:498–506.
165. Cummings SR, Nevitt MC. A hypothesis: the causes of hip fractures. *J Gerontol* 1989; 44:M107–111.
*166. Lauritzen JB, Petersen MM, Lund B. Effect of external hip protectors on hip fractures. *Lancet* 1993;341:11–13.
167. Lotz JC, Hayes WC. The use of quantitative computed tomography to estimate risk of fracture of the hip from falls. *J Bone Joint Surg Am* 1990;72:689–700.
168. Lauritzen JB. Estimate of hip fracture threshold adjusted for energy absorption in soft tissue. *J Nucl Med* 1994;21:S48.
169. Lauritzen JB. Body fat distribution and hip fractures. *Acta Orthop Scand* 1992;63:S89.
170. Hayes WC. *Bone fracture prevention garment and method.* Washington, DC: U.S. Patent and Trademark Office, 1992.
171. Lauritzen JB. Impacts in patients with hip fractures and in vitro study of the padding effect: introduction of a hip protector. *Acta Orthop Scand* 1990;61:S239.
172. Parkkari J, Kannus P, Heikkila J, et al. Energy-shunting external hip protector attenuates the peak femoral impact force below the theoretical fracture threshold: an in vitro biomechanical study under falling conditions of the elderly. *J Bone Miner Res* 1995; 10:1437–1442.
173. Sellberg M. The development of a passive protective device for the elderly to prevent hip fractures from accidental falls. *Advances in Bioengineering* 1992;22:505–508.
174. Charpentier P. A hip protector based on airbag technology. *Bone* 1996;18:S117.
*175. Kannus P, Parkkari J, Niemi S, et al. Prevention of hip fracture in elderly people with use of a hip protector. *N Engl J Med* 2000;343:1506–1513.
176. Heikinheimo RJ. To fall but not break—safety pants. *Proceeding of the 13th Triennial Congress of the International Ergonomics Association*, Tampere, Finland, 1997.
*177. Harada A, Mizuno M, Takemura M, et al. Hip fracture prevention trial using hip protectors in Japanese nursing homes. *Osteoporos Int* 2001;12:215–221.
*178. Ekman A, Mallmin H, Michaelsson K, Ljunghall S. External hip protectors to prevent osteoporotic hip fractures. *Lancet* 1997;350:563–564.
*179. Dawson-Hughes B, Dallal GE, Krall EA, et al. A controlled trial of the effect of calcium supplementation on bone density in postmenopausal women. *N Engl J Med* 1990;323: 878–883.
*180. Reid IR, Ames RW, Evans MC, et al. Long-term effects of calcium supplementation on bone loss and fractures in postmenopausal women: a randomized controlled trial. *Am J Med* 1995;98:331–335.
181. Recker RR, Hinders S, Davies KM, et al. Correcting calcium nutritional deficiency prevents spine fractures in elderly women. *J Bone Miner Res* 1996;11:1961–1966.

*182. Trivedi DP, Doll R, Khaw KT. Effect of four monthly oral vitamin D3 (cholecalciferol) supplementation on fractures and mortality in men and women living in the community: randomised double blind controlled trial. *BMJ* 2003;326:469.
*183. Lips P, Graafmans WC, Ooms ME, et al. Vitamin D supplementation and fracture incidence in elderly persons. A randomized, placebo-controlled clinical trial. *Ann Intern Med* 1996;124:400–406.
*184. Gillespie WJ, Avenell A, Henry DA, et al. Vitamin D and vitamin D analogues for preventing fractures associated with involutional and post-menopausal osteoporosis. *Cochrane Database Syst Rev* 2001:CD000227.
*185. Papadimitropoulos E, Wells G, Shea B, et al. Meta-analyses of therapies for postmenopausal osteoporosis. VIII: Meta-analysis of the efficacy of vitamin D treatment in preventing osteoporosis in postmenopausal women. *Endocr Rev* 2002;23:560–569.
*186. PEPI Writing Group Effects of hormone therapy on bone mineral density: results from the postmenopausal estrogen/progestin interventions (PEPI) trial. The Writing Group for the PEPI. *JAMA* 1996;276:1389–1396.
187. Nieves JW, Komar L, Cosman F, et al. Calcium potentiates the effect of estrogen and calcitonin on bone mass: review and analysis. *Am J Clin Nutr* 1998;67:18–24.
188. Ahlborg HG, Johnell O, Karlsson MK. Long term effects of oestrogen therapy on bone loss in postmenopausal women: a 23 year prospective study. *BJOG* 2004;111:335–359.
189. Christiansen C, Christensen MS, Transbol I. Bone mass in postmenopausal women after withdrawal of oestrogen/gestagen replacement therapy. *Lancet* 1981;1:459–461.
190. Felson DT, Zhang Y, Hannan MT, et al. The effect of postmenopausal estrogen therapy on bone density in elderly women. *N Engl J Med* 1993;329:1141–1146.
191. Lindsay R, Hart DM, Fogelman I. Bone mass after withdrawal of oestrogen replacement. *Lancet* 1981;1:729.
192. Banks E, Beral V, Reeves G, et al. Fracture incidence in relation to the pattern of use of hormone therapy in postmenopausal women. *JAMA* 2004;291:2212–2220.
193. Lufkin EG, Wahner HW, O'Fallon WM, et al. Treatment of postmenopausal osteoporosis with transdermal estrogen. *Ann Intern Med* 1992;117:1–9.
*194. Torgerson DJ, Bell-Syer SE. Hormone replacement therapy and prevention of vertebral fractures: a meta-analysis of randomised trials. *BMC Musculoskelet Disord* 2001;2:7.
*195. Torgerson DJ, Bell-Syer SE. Hormone replacement therapy and prevention of nonvertebral fractures: a meta-analysis of randomized trials. *JAMA* 2001;285:2891–2897.
*196. Beral V, Banks E, Reeves G. Evidence from randomised trials on the long-term effects of hormone replacement therapy. *Lancet* 2002;360:942–944.
197. Grodstein F, Stampfer MJ, Goldhaber SZ, et al. Prospective study of exogenous hormones and risk of pulmonary embolism in women. *Lancet* 1996;348:983–987.
198. Bergkvist L, Persson I. Hormone replacement therapy and breast cancer. A review of current knowledge. *Drug Saf* 1996;15:360–370.
199. Colditz GA, Hankinson SE, Hunter DJ, et al. The use of estrogens and progestins and the risk of breast cancer in postmenopausal women. *N Engl J Med* 1995;332: 1589–1593.
200. Beresford SA, Weiss NS, Voigt LF, et al. Risk of endometrial cancer in relation to use of oestrogen combined with cyclic progestagen therapy in postmenopausal women. *Lancet* 1997;349:458–461.
*201. Cummings SR, Eckert S, Krueger KA, et al. The effect of raloxifene on risk of breast cancer in postmenopausal women: results from the MORE randomized trial. Multiple Outcomes of Raloxifene Evaluation. *JAMA* 1999;281:2189–2197.
*202. Cauley JA, Norton L, Lippman ME, et al. Continued breast cancer risk reduction in postmenopausal women treated with raloxifene: 4-year results from the MORE trial. Multiple outcomes of raloxifene evaluation. *Breast Cancer Res Treat* 2001;65:125–134.
*203. Barrett-Connor E, Grady D, Sashegyi A, et al. Raloxifene and cardiovascular events in osteoporotic postmenopausal women: four-year results from the MORE (Multiple Outcomes of Raloxifene Evaluation) randomized trial. *JAMA* 2002;287:847–857.
*204. Bjarnason NH, Bjarnason K, Haarbo J, et al. Tibolone: prevention of bone loss in late postmenopausal women. *J Clin Endocrinol Metab* 1996;81:2419–2422.
205. Fleisch H. *Bisphosphonates in bone disease: from the laboratory to the patient.* San Diego: Academic Press, 2000.
206. de Groen PC, Lubbe DF, Hirsch LJ, et al. Esophagitis associated with the use of alendronate. *N Engl J Med* 1996;335:1016–1021.
*207. Schnitzer T, Bone HG, Crepaldi G, et al. Therapeutic equivalence of alendronate 70 mg once-weekly and alendronate 10 mg daily in the treatment of osteoporosis. Alendronate Once-Weekly Study Group. *Aging (Milano)* 2000;12:1–12.
*208. Storm T, Thamsborg G, Steiniche T, et al. Effect of intermittent cyclical etidronate therapy on bone mass and fracture rate in women with postmenopausal osteoporosis. *N Engl J Med* 1990;322:1265–1271.
*209. Watts NB, Harris ST, Genant HK, et al. Intermittent cyclical etidronate treatment of postmenopausal osteoporosis. *N Engl J Med* 1990;323:73–79.
*210. Harris ST, Watts NB, Jackson RD, et al. Four-year study of intermittent cyclic etidronate treatment of postmenopausal osteoporosis: three years of blinded therapy followed by one year of open therapy. *Am J Med* 1993;95:557–567.
*211. Cranney A, Guyatt G, Krolicki N, et al. A meta-analysis of etidronate for the treatment of postmenopausal osteoporosis. *Osteoporos Int* 2001;12:140–151.
*212. Hosking D, Chilvers CE, Christiansen C, et al. Prevention of bone loss with alendronate in postmenopausal women under 60 years of age. Early Postmenopausal Intervention Cohort Study Group. *N Engl J Med* 1998;338:485–492.
*213. McClung M, Clemmesen B, Daifotis A, et al. Alendronate prevents postmenopausal bone loss in women without osteoporosis. A double-blind, randomized, controlled trial. Alendronate Osteoporosis Prevention Study Group. *Ann Intern Med* 1998;128: 253–261.
*214. Black DM, Thompson DE, Bauer DC, et al. Fracture risk reduction with alendronate in women with osteoporosis: the Fracture Intervention Trial. FIT Research Group. *J Clin Endocrinol Metab* 2000;85:4118–4124.
*215. Pols HA, Felsenberg D, Hanley DA, et al. Multinational, placebo-controlled, randomized trial of the effects of alendronate on bone density and fracture risk in postmenopausal women with low bone mass: results of the FOSIT study. Foxamax International Trial Study Group. *Osteoporos Int* 1999;9:461–468.
*216. Cranney A, Wells G, Willan A, et al. Meta-analyses of therapies for postmenopausal osteoporosis. II. Meta-analysis of alendronate for the treatment of postmenopausal women. *Endocr Rev* 2002;23:508–516.
*217. Tonino RP, Meunier PJ, Emkey R, et al. Skeletal benefits of alendronate: 7-year treatment of postmenopausal osteoporotic women. Phase III Osteoporosis Treatment Study Group. *J Clin Endocrinol Metab* 2000;85:3109–3115.
*218. Mortensen L, Charles P, Bekker PJ, et al. Risedronate increases bone mass in an early postmenopausal population: two years of treatment plus one year of follow-up. *J Clin Endocrinol Metab* 1998;83:396–402.
*219. Cranney A, Tugwell P, Adachi J, et al. Meta-analyses of therapies for postmenopausal osteoporosis. III. Meta-analysis of risedronate for the treatment of postmenopausal osteoporosis. *Endocr Rev* 2002;23:517–523.
*220. McCloskey E, Selby P, de Takats D, et al. Effects of clodronate on vertebral fracture risk in osteoporosis: a 1-year interim analysis. *Bone* 2001;28:310–315.
*221. Lufkin EG, Argueta R, Whitaker MD, et al. Pamidronate: an unrecognized problem in gastrointestinal tolerability. *Osteoporos Int* 1994;4:320–322.
*222. Reid IR, Wattie DJ, Evans MC, et al. Continuous therapy with pamidronate, a potent bisphosphonate, in postmenopausal osteoporosis. *J Clin Endocrinol Metab* 1994;79: 1595–1599.
*223. Chesnut CH 3rd, Silverman S, Andriano K, et al. A randomized trial of nasal spray salmon calcitonin in postmenopausal women with established osteoporosis to prevent recurrence of osteoporotic fractures study. PROOF Study Group. *Am J Med* 2000;109: 267–276.
*224. Cranney A, Tugwell P, Zytaruk N, et al. Meta-analyses of therapies for postmenopausal osteoporosis. VI. Meta-analysis of calcitonin for the treatment of postmenopausal osteoporosis. *Endocr Rev* 2002;23:540–551.
225. Seeman E, Delmas PD. Reconstructing the skeleton with intermittent parathyroid hormone. *Trends Endocrinol Metab* 2001;12:281–283.
*226. Neer RM, Arnaud CD, Zanchetta JR, et al. Effect of parathyroid hormone (1-34) on fractures and bone mineral density in postmenopausal women with osteoporosis. *N Engl J Med* 2001;344:1434–1441.
227. Marie PJ, Hott M, Modrowski D, et al. An uncoupling agent containing strontium prevents bone loss by depressing bone resorption and maintaining bone formation in estrogen-deficient rats. *J Bone Miner Res* 1993;8:607–615.
*228. Meunier PJ, Slosman DO, Delmas PD, et al. Strontium ranelate: dose-dependent effects in established postmenopausal vertebral osteoporosis—a 2-year randomized placebo controlled trial. *J Clin Endocrinol Metab* 2002;87:2060–2066.
*229. Meunier PJ, Roux C, Seeman E, et al. The effects of strontium ranelate on the risk of vertebral fracture in women with postmenopausal osteoporosis. *N Engl J Med* 2004; 350:459–468.
*230. Meunier PJ, Sebert JL, Reginster JY, et al. Fluoride salts are no better at preventing new vertebral fractures than calcium-vitamin D in postmenopausal osteoporosis: the FAVO Study. *Osteoporos Int* 1998;8:4–12.
*231. Riggs BL, Hodgson SF, O'Fallon WM, et al. Effect of fluoride treatment on the fracture rate in postmenopausal women with osteoporosis. *N Engl J Med* 1990;322:802–809.
*232. Orimo H, Shiraki M, Hayashi T, et al. Reduced occurrence of vertebral crush fractures in senile osteoporosis treated with 1 alpha (OH)-vitamin D3. *Bone Miner* 1987;3:47–52.
*233. Gallagher JC, Riggs BL, Recker RR, et al. The effect of calcitriol on patients with postmenopausal osteoporosis with special reference to fracture frequency. *Proc Soc Exp Biol Med* 1989;191:287–292.
*234. Gallagher JC, Goldgar D. Treatment of postmenopausal osteoporosis with high doses of synthetic calcitriol. A randomized controlled study. *Ann Intern Med* 1990;113: 649–655.
235. Feskanich D, Weber P, Willett WC, et al. Vitamin K intake and hip fractures in women: a prospective study. *Am J Clin Nutr* 1999;69:74–79.
236. Orimo H, Shiraki M. Clinical evaluation of menatetrenone in the treatment of involutional osteoporosis. *The IVth International Symposium on Osteoporosis*, Hong Kong, 1993.
*237. Alexandersen P, Toussaint A, Christiansen C, et al. Ipriflavone in the treatment of postmenopausal osteoporosis: a randomized controlled trial. *JAMA* 2001;285: 1482–1488.
238. Mundy G, Garrett R, Harris S, et al. Stimulation of bone formation in vitro and in rodents by statins. *Science* 1999;286:1946–1949.
*239. Casaletto JA, Gatt R. Post-operative mortality related to waiting time for hip fracture surgery. *Injury* 2004;35:114–120.
*240. Dorotka R, Schoechtner H, Buchinger W. The influence of immediate surgical treatment of proximal femoral fractures on mortality and quality of life. Operation within six hours of the fracture versus later than six hours. *J Bone Joint Surg Br* 2003;85:1107–1113.
*241. Rogmark C, Carlsson A, Johnell O, et al. A prospective randomised trial of internal fixation versus arthroplasty for displaced fractures of the neck of the femur. Functional outcome for 450 patients at two years. *J Bone Joint Surg Br* 2002;84:183–188.
242. Tornkvist H, Hearn TC, Schatzker J. The strength of plate fixation in relation to the number and spacing of bone screws. *J Orthop Trauma* 1996;10:204–208.
243. Sarmiento A, Sharpe FE, Ebramzadeh E, et al. Factors influencing the outcome of closed tibial fractures treated with functional bracing. *Clin Orthop Relat Res* 1995:8–24.
244. Ahlborg HG, Josefsson PO. Pin-tract complications in external fixation of fractures of the distal radius. *Acta Orthop Scand* 1999;70:116–168.
245. Moroni A, Toksvig-Larsen S, Maltarello MC, et al. A comparison of hydroxyapatite-coated, titanium-coated, and uncoated tapered external-fixation pins. An in vivo study in sheep. *J Bone Joint Surg Am* 1998;80:547–554.
246. Koval KJ, Hoehl JJ, Kummer FJ, et al. Distal femoral fixation: a biomechanical compari-

son of the standard condylar buttress plate, a locked buttress plate, and the 95-degree blade plate. *J Orthop Trauma* 1997;11:521–524.

247. Walsh WR, Sherman P, Howlett CR, et al. Fracture healing in a rat osteopenia model. *Clin Orthop* 1997:218–227.

*248. Chapman MW, Bucholz R, Cornell C. Treatment of acute fractures with a collagen-calcium phosphate graft material. A randomized clinical trial. *J Bone Joint Surg Am* 1997;79:495–502.

249. Gazdag AR, Lane JM, Glaser D, et al. Alternatives to Autogenous Bone Graft: Efficacy and Indications. *J Am Acad Orthop Surg* 1995;3:1–8.

250. Keating JF. Tibial plateau fractures in the older patient. *Bull Hosp Jt Dis* 1999;58:19–23.

*251. Kopylov P, Runnqvist K, Jonsson K, et al. Norian SRS versus external fixation in redisplaced distal radial fractures. A randomized study in 40 patients. *Acta Orthop Scand* 1999;70:1–5.

252. Rao RD, Singrakhia MD. Painful osteoporotic vertebral fracture. Pathogenesis, evaluation, and roles of vertebroplasty and kyphoplasty in its management. *J Bone Joint Surg Am* 2003;85-A:2010–2022.

253. Galibert P, Deramond H, Rosat P, et al. [Preliminary note on the treatment of vertebral angioma by percutaneous acrylic vertebroplasty]. *Neurochirurgie* 1987;33:166–168.

254. Evans AJ, Jensen ME, Kip KE, et al. Vertebral compression fractures: pain reduction and improvement in functional mobility after percutaneous polymethylmethacrylate vertebroplasty retrospective report of 245 cases. *Radiology* 2003;226:366–372.

255. Diamond TH, Champion B, Clark WA. Management of acute osteoporotic vertebral fractures: a nonrandomized trial comparing percutaneous vertebroplasty with conservative therapy. *Am J Med* 2003;114:257–265.

256. Lieberman IH, Dudeney S, Reinhardt MK, et al. Initial outcome and efficacy of "kyphoplasty" in the treatment of painful osteoporotic vertebral compression fractures. *Spine* 2001;26:1631–1638.

257. Phillips FM, Ho E, Campbell-Hupp M, et al. Early radiographic and clinical results of balloon kyphoplasty for the treatment of osteoporotic vertebral compression fractures. *Spine* 2003;28:2260–2265, discussion 2265–2267.

258. Weisskopf M, Herlein S, Birnbaum K, et al. [Kyphoplasty—a new minimally invasive treatment for repositioning and stabilising vertebral bodies]. *Z Orthop Ihre Grenzgeb* 2003;141:406–411.

259. Uppin AA, Hirsch JA, Centenera LV, et al. Occurrence of new vertebral body fracture after percutaneous vertebroplasty in patients with osteoporosis. *Radiology* 2003;226: 119–124.

260. Karlsson MK, Johnell O, Nilsson BE, et al. Bone mineral mass in hip fracture patients. *Bone* 1993;14:161–165.

261. Grados F, Brazier M, Kamel S, et al. Effects on bone mineral density of calcium and vitamin D supplementation in elderly women with vitamin D deficiency. *Joint Bone Spine* 2003;70:203–208.

262. Black DM, Cummings SR, Stone K, et al. A new approach to defining normal vertebral dimensions. *J Bone Miner Res* 1991;6:883–892.

*263. Body JJ, Gaich GA, Scheele WH, et al. A randomized double-blind trial to compare the efficacy of teriparatide [recombinant human parathyroid hormone (1-34)] with alendronate in postmenopausal women with osteoporosis. *J Clin Endocrinol Metab* 2002; 87:4528–4535.

*264. Black DM, Greenspan SL, Ensrud KE, et al. The effects of parathyroid hormone and alendronate alone or in combination in postmenopausal osteoporosis. *N Engl J Med* 2003;349:1207–1215.

265. Zyto K. Non-operative treatment of comminuted fractures of the proximal humerus in elderly patients. *Injury* 1998;29:349–352.

*266. Robinson CM, Page RS, Hill RM, et al. Primary hemiarthroplasty for treatment of proximal humeral fractures. *J Bone Joint Surg Am* 2003;85-A:1215–1223.

267. Robinson CM, Hill RM, Jacobs N, et al. Adult distal humeral metaphyseal fractures: epidemiology and results of treatment. *J Orthop Trauma* 2003;17:38–47.

268. Frankle MA, Herscovici D, Jr., DiPasquale TG, et al. A comparison of open reduction and internal fixation and primary total elbow arthroplasty in the treatment of intraarticular distal humerus fractures in women older than age 65. *J Orthop Trauma* 2003;17: 473–480.

269. McQueen M, Caspers J. Colles fracture: does the anatomical result affect the final function? *J Bone Joint Surg Br* 1988;70:649–651.

270. Bhandari M, Devereaux PJ, Swiontkowski MF, et al. Internal fixation compared with arthroplasty for displaced fractures of the femoral neck. A meta-analysis. *J Bone Joint Surg Am* 2003;85-A:1673–1681.

271. Adams CI, Robinson CM, Court-Brown CM, et al. Prospective randomized controlled trial of an intramedullary nail versus dynamic screw and plate for intertrochanteric fractures of the femur. *J Orthop Trauma* 2001;15:394–400.

272. Schatzker J. Fractures of the distal femur revisited. *Clin Orthop Rel Res* 1998:43–56.

*273. Armstrong R, Milliren A, Schrantz W, et al. Retrograde interlocked intramedullary nailing of supracondylar distal femur fractures in an average 76-year-old patient population. *Orthopedics* 2003;26:627–629.

274. Althausen PL, Lee MA, Finkemeier CG, et al. Operative stabilization of supracondylar femur fractures above total knee arthroplasty: a comparison of four treatment methods. *J Arthroplasty* 2003;18:834–839.

275. Rasmussen PS. Tibial condylar fractures. Impairment of knee joint stability as an indication for surgical treatment. *J Bone Joint Surg Am* 1973;55:1331–1350.

276. Kanis JA, Oden A, Johnell O, et al. The burden of osteoporotic fractures: a method for setting intervention thresholds. *Osteoporos Int* 2001;12:417–427.

277. Kanis JA, Dawson A, Oden A, et al. Cost-effectiveness of preventing hip fracture in the general female population. *Osteoporos Int* 2001;12:356–361.

278. Kannus P, Niemi S, Parkkari J, et al. Hip fractures in Finland between 1970 and 1997 and predictions for the future. *Lancet* 1999;353:802–805.

279. McQueen MM. Redisplaced unstable fractures of the distal radius: a randomised prospective study of bridging versus non-bridging external fixation. *J Bone Joint Surg Br* 1998;80:665–669.

PATHOLOGIC FRACTURES

Kristy L. Weber

Pathologic fractures occur in bone that is not normal. Weakened bone predisposes the patient to failure during normal activity or after minor trauma. Failure (pathologic fracture) of bone under these circumstances should alert the orthopaedic surgeon to the presence of an underlying condition. Successful management of the patient requires recognition, diagnosis, and treatment of the condition affecting the bone. The management of the fracture may be dramatically altered by the associated pathologic condition, and failure to recognize a condition such as osteoporosis or metastatic bone disease may be detrimental to the patient's life or affected extremity.

When planning the management of patients with a pathologic fracture and systemic skeletal disease, it is best to separate the underlying diseases into correctable and uncorrectable conditions. Correctable diseases include renal osteodystrophy, hyperparathyroidism, osteomalacia, and disuse osteoporosis. Uncorrectable diseases include osteogenesis imperfecta, polyostotic fibrous dysplasia, postmenopausal osteoporosis, Paget's disease, and osteopetrosis. All of these disorders involve bones that are weak and predisposed to fracture or plastic deformation. The fracture callus may not form normally, and healing often occurs slowly. Many of these patients have an increased incidence of fracture, delayed union, and nonunion.

If the underlying process is correctable, appropriate treatment should be initiated. If the underlying process cannot be corrected, the condition of the remainder of the skeleton must be considered when planning treatment of the fracture. A primary goal in the management of patients with any systemic skeletal disease is to prevent disuse osteoporosis, which may lead to additional pathologic fractures.

Osteoporosis is the most common condition associated with pathologic fractures, but the management of patients with this condition may only require minor modifications of conventional fracture care. In contrast, the treatment of patients with metastatic bone disease and actual or impending pathologic fractures necessitates a multidisciplinary approach to care with different principles applied to fracture fixation. This chapter will primarily focus on the evaluation and treatment of patients with metastatic bone disease and pathologic fractures. It will briefly cover the management of fractures in patients with primary benign and malignant bone tumors. In addition, treatment of patients with metabolic abnormalities and decreased bone density unrelated to malignancy will be addressed. The majority of patients with pathologic fractures are treated by general orthopaedic surgeons. It is important that all orthopaedic surgeons have a basic understanding of the principles involved in the care of these patients so that appropriate treatment is initiated.

Currently, an estimated 10 million Americans more than 50 years of age have osteoporosis, whereas another 34 million have osteomalacia and are at risk for developing osteoporosis (1). Approximately 1.5 million people sustain a pathologic fracture related to osteoporosis each year (2). Of senior citizens, 20% who sustain a hip fracture die within 1 year (3). One of every two women more than 50 years of age will have an osteoporosis-related fracture in her lifetime (4). Other skeletal conditions such as Paget's disease affect an estimated one million people in the United States, whereas approximately 20,000 to 50,000 Americans have osteogenesis imperfecta (1).

The American Cancer Society estimates that 1.3 million new cancer cases were diagnosed in 2003, and approximately 50% of these tumors can metastasize to the skeleton (5). With improved medical treatment of many cancers, especially breast, lung, and prostate, patients are living longer. There is an increased prevalence of bone metastasis in this population, which increases the chances that these patients will develop a pathologic fracture. The majority of bone metastases originate from cancers of the breast, lung, and prostate, followed by the thyroid and kidney. The most common sites of metastasis in the skeleton include the spine, pelvis, ribs, skull, and proximal long bones (6).

TABLE 20-1 Evaluation of a Patient with a Lytic Bone Lesion

1. History: thyroid, breast, or prostate nodule
2. Review of systems: gastrointestinal symptoms, weight loss, flank pain, hematuria
3. Physical examination: lymph nodes, thyroid, breast, lungs, abdomen, prostate, testicles, and rectum
4. Plain x-rays: chest, affected bone, humerus, pelvis, femur, spine
5. 99mTc bone scan/FDG-PET scan: total body
6. CT scan: chest, abdomen, pelvis
7. Laboratory: complete blood count, erythrocyte sedimentation rate, calcium, phosphate, urinalysis, prostate-specific antigen, immunoelectrophoresis, and alkaline phosphatase
8. Biopsy: needle vs. open

FDG, Fluorine-18 deoxyglucose; PET, positron emission tomography; CT, computed tomography.

EVALUATION OF THE PATIENT WITH AN IMPENDING OR ACTUAL PATHOLOGIC FRACTURE

Clinical

History

A comprehensive evaluation of a patient with a lytic bone lesion or pathologic fracture is essential (Table 20-1) (6). A thorough history must be obtained to understand the circumstances surrounding the current injury. Certain signs or fracture features should alert the orthopaedic surgeon to the possibility of an associated pathologic process (Table 20-2). The degree of trauma and presence of pain before the injury may provide information about the underlying bone strength. Pain is the most common presenting symptom, ranging from a dull ache to an intense pain exacerbated by weightbearing. Patients must be asked specifically about previously diagnosed or treated cancer; otherwise they may consider themselves cured and not volunteer this information. A history of radiation is important. Standard review of systems and questions about recent weight loss, fevers, night sweats, and fatigue are important. Questions about relevant risk factors such as smoking, dietary habits, and toxic exposures should be asked.

TABLE 20-2 Factors Suggesting a Pathologic Fracture

- Spontaneous fracture
- Fracture after minor trauma
- Pain at the site before the fracture
- Multiple recent fractures
- Unusual fracture pattern ("banana fracture")
- Patient >45 years of age
- History of primary malignancy

Physical Examination

The physical examination should include careful evaluation of the affected skeletal region. Palpation of a mass or fracture and a detailed neurologic examination of the extremities are essential. All extremities and the entire spine should be evaluated for additional lesions or lymphadenopathy, because patients can have multiple sites of involvement with bone metastasis, lymphoma, or osteoporosis. A physical examination should include careful evaluation of all possible primary sites (breast, prostate, thyroid) and a stool guaiac test.

Laboratory Studies

Disturbances in hematologic and/or metabolic parameters can lead to the diagnosis of a primary or secondary disorder associated with a pathologic fracture. In all patients in whom a pathologic process is suspected, a baseline laboratory profile should include a complete blood count with differential, erythrocyte sedimentation rate, serum chemistries, blood urea nitrogen, serum glucose, liver function tests, protein, albumin, calcium, phosphorus, and alkaline phosphatase. Patients with widespread bone metastases exhibit anemia of chronic disease, hypercalcemia, and increased alkaline phosphatase. The hemoglobin is also low in patients with multiple myeloma. A standard urinalysis is necessary to look for microscopic hematuria, which suggests renal cell carcinoma (RCC), and a 24-hour urine collection is necessary for a complete metabolic evaluation. Serum and urine protein electrophoreses are important to exclude multiple myeloma. Thyroid function tests, carcinoembryonic antigen, CA125, and prostate-specific antigen are serum markers for specific tumors. N-telopeptide and C-telopeptide are new biological markers of bone collagen breakdown that can be measured in the serum and urine. These markers are used to confirm increased destruction caused by bone metastasis, measure the overall extent of bone involvement, and assess the response of the bone to bisphosphonates (7,8).

Patients with osteoporosis have normal values for the aforementioned laboratory tests, whereas patients with osteomalacia have low serum calcium and phosphorus, high serum alkaline phosphatase, high urinary phosphorus, and high urinary hydroxyproline values (Table 20-3). Patients with primary hyperparathyroidism have high serum calcium, alkaline phosphatase, and parathyroid hormone with low serum phosphorus. They also have high urinary calcium, phosphorus, and hydroxyproline. Patients with renal osteodystrophy have low serum calcium with high serum phosphorus, alkaline phosphatase, and blood urea nitrogen. When secondary hyperparathyroidism develops in these patients, the serum calcium increases to at or above normal values with elevated parathyroid hormone levels. Urine values are difficult to assess in patients with secondary hyperparathyroidism owing to abnormal glomerular filtration. Patients with Paget's disease have normal values for serum calcium and phosphorus but markedly elevated levels of alkaline phosphatase and urinary hydroxyproline. Prostate-specific antigen is a sensitive measurement of prostate cancer. A value less than 10 ng/mL essentially excludes the presence of bone metastasis (9). Remember that serum calcium is a measurement of unbound calcium in the serum, and, therefore, determination of serum protein is necessary to interpret the calcium level. If the serum protein is lower than normal, the normal range of serum calcium is lowered.

Associated Medical Problems

The clinical problems encountered by patients with metastatic bone disease are substantial. Patients often have marked pain

TABLE 20-3 Disorders Producing Osteopenia

	Laboratory Value			
Disorder	Serum Calcium	Serum Phosphorus	Serum Alkaline Phosphatase	Urine
Osteoporosis	Normal	Normal	Normal	Normal Ca
Osteomalacia	Normal	Normal	Normal	Low Ca
Hyperparathyroidism	Normal to high	Normal to low	Normal	High Ca
Renal osteodystrophy	Low	High	High	
Paget's disease	Normal	Normal	Very high	Hydroxyproline
Myeloma[a]	Normal	Normal	Normal	Protein

[a] Abnormal serum or urine immunoelectrophoresis.

and pathologic fractures that leave them unable to ambulate or perform their activities of daily living. Patients with spinal fractures may develop neurologic deficits that lead to paralysis. Patients with impending or actual extremity fractures may be forced to remain on bedrest for prolonged periods of time, predisposing them to hypercalcemia. Anemia is a common hematologic abnormality in these patients. The most encompassing and tragic concern of patients with pathologic fractures from metastatic disease is the general loss in their quality of life.

Approximately 40% of the 75,000 cases of hypercalcemia diagnosed in the United States each year are related to hypercalcemia of malignancy, most commonly associated with cancers of the lung, breast, kidney, and genitourinary tract (10). The remainder are caused by primary hyperparathyroidism. Rarely, the two causes occur simultaneously. The orthopaedic surgeon managing a patient with metastatic carcinoma to bone must be aware of the risks, symptoms, and management of hypercalcemia because it can be lethal if untreated (Table 20-4).

Hypercalcemia is not usually the presenting sign of malignancy, but it portends a poor prognosis for the patient. As many as 60% of patients with hypercalcemia will survive less than 3 months, and only 20% will be alive at 1 year (11). Often the symptoms are nonspecific, so it is easier to diagnose the problem by measuring the serum calcium. There is not a reliable correlation between the severity of the hypercalcemia and the degree of skeletal involvement. Patients with lung cancer often develop hypercalcemia without obvious bone metastases, whereas hypercalcemia in multiple myeloma or breast carcinoma correlates with the extent of bone metastases (12). Histologic evidence suggests that the presence of metastatic disease in bone is not necessary to see diffuse osteoclastic activity associated with clinical hypercalcemia.

Once the patient with hypercalcemia is identified, a treatment plan must be established that usually involves inpatient care. Vigorous volume repletion is a temporizing measure, so treatment must focus on reducing the degree of bone resorption. This can be accomplished by treating the tumor directly or by using bisphosphonates to reduce osteoclastic activity (13–15). Correction of any electrolyte imbalance or hypercalcemia should ideally be done before surgery.

TABLE 20-4 Signs and Symptoms of Hypercalcemia

Neurologic: headache, confusion, irritability, blurred vision

Gastrointestinal: anorexia, nausea, vomiting, abdominal pain, constipation, weight loss

Musculoskeletal: fatigue, weakness, joint and bone pain, unsteady gait

Urinary: nocturia, polydypsia, polyuria, urinary tract infections

Radiographic Workup

Plain X-Rays

The most important imaging study used to evaluate a patient with a destructive bone lesion or pathologic fracture is a plain x-ray in two planes. The x-rays should be carefully reviewed with attention to specific lesions and overall bone quality. Specifically they should be examined for diagnostic clues such as generalized osteopenia, periosteal reaction, cortical thinning, Looser's lines, and abnormal soft tissue shadows. A series of questions to assist in determining the underlying process was popularized by W. Enneking, MD, and can be reviewed in Table 20-5. The entire affected bone should be imaged to identify all possible lesions, and remember that referred pain to distal sites may be caused by a more proximal lesion.

Osteopenia is the radiographic term used to indicate inadequate bone (osteoporosis) or inadequately mineralized bone (osteomalacia). These two disorders cannot be definitively distinguished on plain x-rays, but there are some suggestive differential clues. Looser's lines (compression-side radiolucent lines), calcification of small vessels, and phalangeal periosteal reaction are features of osteomalacia or hyperparathyroidism. Thin cortices and loss of the normal trabecular pattern without other abnormalities are more suggestive of osteoporosis.

When an osteolytic or osteoblastic lesion is noted in otherwise normal bone, the diagnosis is most likely a tumor. It is important to determine whether the lesion is inactive, active, or aggressive. Small osteolytic lesions surrounded by a rim of reactive bone without endosteal or periosteal reaction are usually inactive or minimally active (benign) primary bone tumors. Lesions that erode the cortex but are contained by periosteum are usually active benign or low-grade malignant bone tumors. Large lesions that destroy the cortex are usually aggressive, malignant lesions that can be primary or metastatic. A permeative or "moth-eaten" pattern of cortical destruction is highly suggestive of malignancy. Most destructive bone lesions in patients more than 45 years of age are the result of metastatic carcinoma followed by multiple myeloma and lymphoma; however, a solitary bone lesion should be fully evaluated to rule out a primary bone tumor such as a chondrosarcoma, malignant fibrous histiocytoma, or osteosarcoma (6).

The radiographic appearance of bone metastasis can be osteolytic, osteoblastic, or mixed. Osteolytic destruction is most common and occurs in metastases from cancers of the lung, thyroid, kidney, and colon (Fig. 20-1). An osteoblastic appearance with sclerosis of the bone is common in metastatic prostate cancer. Metastatic breast cancer often has a mixed osteolytic and osteoblastic appearance in the bone (Fig. 20-2). The radiographic appearance is determined by the balance of bone destruction by osteoclasts and bone production by osteoblasts. Tumor cells secrete factors that interact with host cells in the bone microenvironment and affect the cycle of normal bone turnover (16–20). An isolated avulsion of the lesser trochanter is almost always pathologic, and this specific injury should arouse suspicion of occult metastatic disease and an imminent

TABLE 20-5 Evaluation of Plain X-rays

Question	Option	Interpretation
1. Where is the lesion?	Epiphysis vs metaphysis vs diaphysis Cortex vs medullary canal Long bone (femur, humerus) vs flat bone (pelvis, scapula)	
2. What is the lesion doing to the bone?	Bone destruction (osteolysis) -Total -Diffuse -Minimal	
3. What is the bone doing to the lesion?	Well-defined reactive rim Intact but abundant periosteal reaction Periosteal reaction that cannot keep up with tumor (Codman's triangle)	Benign or slow-growing Aggressive Highly malignant
4. What are the clues to the tissue type within the lesion?	Calcification Ossification Ground glass	Bone infarct/cartilage tumor Osteosarcoma/osteoblastoma Fibrous dysplasia

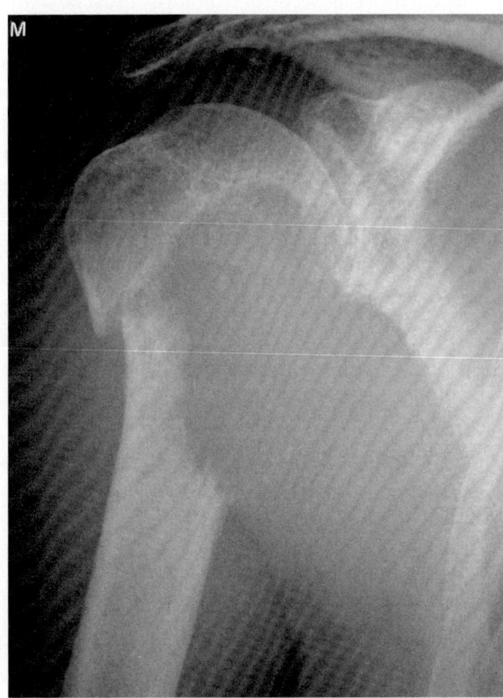

FIGURE 20-1 Anteroposterior x-ray of the right shoulder in a 55-year-old male with metastatic renal cell carcinoma (RCC). He had pain for 6 weeks before sustaining a minor injury to the right shoulder. Note the purely lytic lesion with a pathologic fracture through the surgical neck of the humerus.

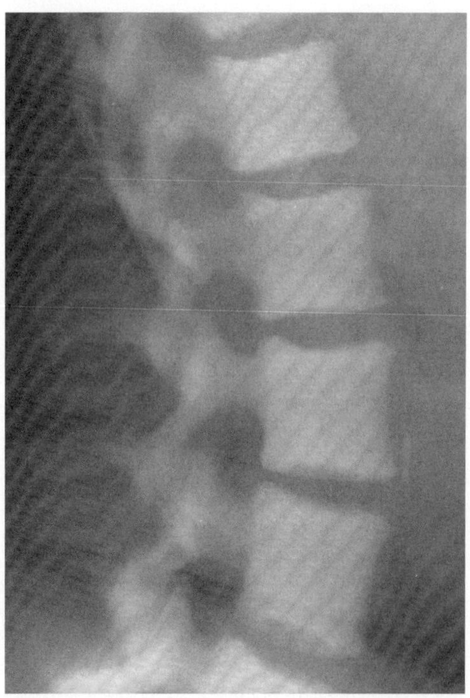

FIGURE 20-2 Lateral x-ray of the lumbar vertebral bodies in a 56-year-old woman with metastatic breast cancer. Note their osteoblastic appearance because of an imbalance in bone production over bone destruction.

femoral neck fracture (21). A cortical lesion in adults is usually a metastasis (22,23).

Nuclear Medicine Studies

When a metastasis is suspected, the remainder of the skeleton should be evaluated for additional bony sites of disease. Technetium bone scintigraphy is helpful in determining the extent of metastatic disease in the skeleton because it detects osteoblastic activity and is quite sensitive (Fig. 20-3). Multiple myeloma is falsely negative on a bone scan as are occasional cases of metastatic RCC because of the decreased osteoblastic response to the tumor. More recently, positron emission tomography (PET) scanning has become the gold standard in metabolic imaging and is now used to screen patients for metastatic disease. Fluorine-18 deoxyglucose provides a way to quantitate glucose metabolism with higher tracer accumulation in more aggressive malignancies. It directly measures the presence of tumor, which makes it superior to scintigraphy (24,25). In a recent study, PET/computed tomography (CT) scanning had higher sensitivity and specificity than PET scanning alone for detection of malignant bone lesions (26).

Three-Dimensional Imaging/Angiography

Magnetic resonance imaging (MRI) is not generally used to evaluate metastatic lesions in the extremities because it is not cost-effective, but it is useful in the evaluation of patients with spinal metastasis to define the relationship of tumor to the underlying neurologic structures. A standard angiogram is still useful when embolizing feeding tumor vessels in vascular lesions such as metastatic RCC or multiple myeloma. If the vascular supply to a lesion needs to be assessed but not embolized, MR or CT angiograms give greater detail than a traditional angiogram.

Further imaging studies are necessary to search for a primary lesion when metastatic carcinoma to the skeleton is suspected and has not been identified with examination of the breast, thyroid, and prostate (27). Recommended radiographic staging studies include a chest x-ray and CT scans of the chest, abdomen, and pelvis. A mammogram should be performed if breast cancer is suspected. If multiple myeloma is considered, a skeletal survey including skull films is recommended. PET scanning is also being used to detect unknown primary lesions.

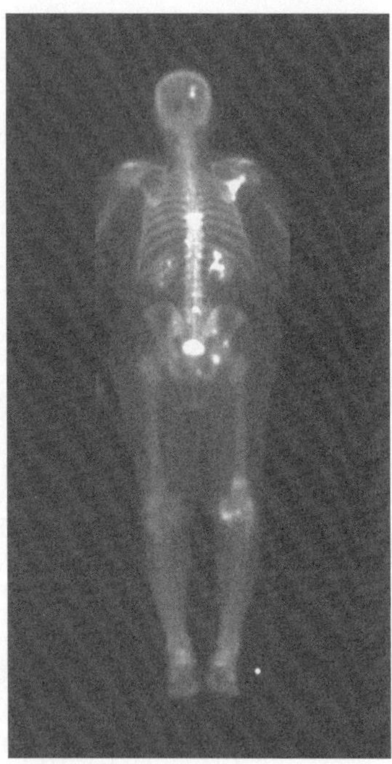

FIGURE 20-3 A technetium bone scan in a patient with widely metastatic adenocarcinoma. There are multiple sites of increased uptake throughout the skeleton. These correspond to areas of increased osteoblastic activity in response to the tumor.

When and How to Biopsy

A thorough history and physical examination with appropriate imaging studies often leads to the correct diagnosis, particularly in the case of widespread metastatic bone disease. However, a solitary bone lesion in a patient with or without a history of cancer should be biopsied to obtain an accurate diagnosis. Presuming a solitary lesion is a bone metastasis in an older patient may lead you to perform the wrong operation, thereby potentially compromising the life and limb of the patient if the lesion is actually a sarcoma.

If a tissue diagnosis is necessary, a biopsy must be performed. There are several ways to biopsy an unknown skeletal lesion, and either a needle or open incisional biopsy is reasonable depending on the availability of expert musculoskeletal radiologists and pathologists (28). A needle biopsy is usually definitive when differentiating a carcinoma from a sarcoma. Immunohistochemical staining may allow determination of the primary site of origin of a carcinoma. When there is a pathologic fracture through a lytic lesion, the biopsy can be complicated because of bleeding and early fracture callus. The fracture should be stabilized initially with traction or a cast to allow preliminary staging studies to be completed. If a needle biopsy is definitive, contamination from an open biopsy is avoided.

If a needle biopsy is nondiagnostic, a careful incisional biopsy should be performed using oncologic principles so as not to preclude subsequent surgical treatment (29). When possible, the tissue should be obtained from a site unaffected by the fracture. The biopsy should be as small as possible, in a longitudinal fashion in line with the extremity, and with excellent hemostasis. Tissues contaminated by a post-biopsy hematoma must be considered contaminated by tumor cells. Cultures should always be sent at the time of biopsy to rule out infection, which can be confused radiographically with a tumor. If a definitive diagnosis of metastatic disease can be made on an intraoperative frozen section, surgical treatment of the pathologic fracture can be performed at the same operative setting. If the frozen section is not diagnostic, it is best to wait for the permanent sections before definitively treating the tumor and fracture.

IMPENDING PATHOLOGIC FRACTURES

As stated earlier in this chapter, the most common pathologic fracture is caused by osteoporosis. In most situations these fractures should be managed in a standard fashion as recommended in the accompanying chapters of this text. Modifications such as the addition of methylmethacrylate or locking plate fixation may be necessary because of the weakened bone (30). Pathologic fractures caused by metastatic bone disease demand special considerations that will be discussed in further detail.

Bone metastases are painful even without an associated fracture. Treatment options for known skeletal metastasis include (a) prophylactic surgical stabilization before radiation therapy or (b) radiation and/or chemotherapy without prophylactic fixation (6,31). The term *impending fracture* is used throughout the literature on metastatic disease, but there are no clear guidelines supported by prospective clinical studies to define this term. Retrospective studies have formed the basis to guide the indications for prophylactic fixation, but they are often limited by the use of plain x-rays, subjective patient information, and an inadequate understanding of the biomechanical factors involved in the bone affected by metastatic carcinoma (32,33). Although experienced orthopaedic surgeons may have an intuitive sense for which lesions are at high risk for fracture, there is considerable controversy about what constitutes an impending fracture and little reliable data to guide treatment.

Classification Systems

Factors necessary for the assessment of fracture risk include the x-ray appearance of the lesion and the patient's symptoms. Fidler assessed preoperative and postoperative pain in patients with impending fractures and found that, among patients with 50% to 75% cortical involvement, all had moderate to severe pain preoperatively and no or only slight pain after prophylactic internal fixation (32). Commonly, a lesion is considered to be at risk for fracture if it is painful, larger than 2.5 cm, and involves more than 50% of the cortex (33). In an attempt to quantify this risk, Mirels developed a scoring system based on the presence or absence of pain, and the size, location, and radiographic appearance of the lesion (34). Each of the four variables is assigned from 1 to 3 points (Table 20-6). Mirels analyzed 78 lesions previously irradiated without prophylactic surgical fixation. Over a 6-month period, 27 lesions (35%) fractured and 51 lesions remained stable. Mean scores of 7 in the nonfracture group and 10 in the fracture group were calculated. The author concluded that lesions scoring 7 or lower can be safely irradiated, whereas lesions scoring 8 or higher require prophylactic internal fixation before irradiation (34).

Subsequently, Hipp and colleagues attempted to quantify the risk of pathologic fracture in patients with metastatic bone disease (35). They defined fracture risk as the load-bearing requirement of the bone divided by its load-bearing capacity. The load-bearing requirement depends on the patient's age, weight, activity level, and ability to protect the site. The load-bearing capacity depends on the amount of bone loss, modulus of the remaining bone, and location of the defect with respect to the type of load applied. A more recent biomechanical study of simulated lytic defects in whale vertebral bodies demonstrated that relative fracture risk in vivo could be predicted by a structural rigidity analysis using cross-sectional imaging data (36). Although this system provides a comprehensive method to determine the risk of pathologic fracture, it is not routinely used in the clinical setting.

Patients treated with prophylactic stabilization of an impending fracture fare better than those treated after a fracture: shorter hospitalization (average 2 days), discharge more likely (40%), more immediate pain relief, faster and less complicated surgery, less blood loss, quicker return to premorbid function, improved

TABLE 20-6 Mirel's Criteria for Risk of Fracture

	Number Assigned		
Variable	1	2	3
Site	Upper extremity	Lower extremity	Peritrochanteric
Pain	Mild	Moderate	Severe
Lesion[a]	Blastic	Mixed	Lytic
Size	$<^1/_3$ diameter of the bone	$^1/_3$–$^2/_3$ diameter of the bone	$>^2/_3$ diameter of the bone

Each patient's situation is assessed by assigning a number (1, 2, or 3) to each aspect of his or her presentation (site, pain, lesion, and size) and then adding the numbers to obtain a total number to indicate the patient's risk for fracture. Mirel's data suggest that those patients whose total number is 7 or less can be observed, but those with a number of 8 or more should have prophylactic internal fixation.

[a] By radiography.

survival, and fewer hardware complications (37,38). Elective stabilization also allows the medical oncologist and surgeon to coordinate operative treatment and systemic chemotherapy. One critical caveat when treating patients with impending pathologic fractures is that fracture risk is greatest during the surgical positioning, preparation, and draping. When patients are anesthetized they cannot protect the affected extremity and must rely on the surgical team to proceed carefully. Low energy fractures will occur after very minor trauma or a twisting movement. If a pathologic fracture occurs, damage to the surrounding soft tissues is minimal compared with traumatic fractures in healthy bone.

The goals of surgical treatment in a patient with an impending pathologic fracture are to alleviate pain, reduce narcotic use, restore skeletal stability, and regain functional independence (6,31). However, the decision to proceed with operative intervention is multifactorial and must be individualized. Factors included in the decision-making are (a) life expectancy of the patient, (b) patient comorbidities, (c) extent of the disease, (d) tumor histology, (e) anticipated future oncologic treatments, and (f) degree of pain. Patients with a life expectancy of less than 6 weeks may not gain significant benefit from major reconstructive surgery. However, an accurate prognosis is not always possible and the decision of whether to proceed with surgery should be discussed with the multidisciplinary team, the patient, and the patient's family.

TREATMENT OPTIONS FOR PATIENTS WITH METASTATIC OR SYSTEMIC DISEASE

General Considerations

Patients with cancer are living longer. More patients are living with bone metastasis. Because of the advances in systemic treatment, pain control, and local modalities including radiation and surgery, the philosophy has changed from one of palliation for immediate demise to aggressive care to improve the quality of remaining life. The local bone lesion can be treated with nonsurgical management (radiation, functional bracing, and bisphosphonates) or surgical stabilization with or without resection. Medical treatment with bisphosphonates has decreased the incidence of pathologic fractures by inhibition of osteoclast-mediated bone destruction (39). Patients with small bone lesions, especially in nonweightbearing bones, are often candidates for radiation therapy rather than surgical stabilization. Surgical intervention is often used for large lytic lesions at risk for fracture or for existing pathologic fractures. Postoperatively, external beam radiation is used as an adjuvant local treatment unless the metastatic lesion is completely resected (6,40).

After treatment for a pathologic fracture, the bone may or may not heal. The factors that influence whether healing will occur include location of the lesion, extent of bony destruction, tumor histology, type of treatment, and length of patient survival. Gainor and Buchert determined the most important factor affecting union was length of patient survival (41). After studying 129 pathologic long bone fractures, they found the overall rate of fracture healing in their study to be 34%; however, it was 74% in the group of patients who survived more than 6 months. Among different tumor histologies, fractures secondary to multiple myeloma were most likely to heal (41).

Surgical Guidelines

Specific surgical guidelines will be outlined in the subsequent sections of this chapter pertaining to different areas of the extremities, pelvis, and spine. Surgical treatment of metastatic bone disease uses the most current internal fixation devices and prosthetic replacements. The ideal reconstruction allows immediate weightbearing and is durable enough to not require revision for the increased lifespan of patients with metastatic bone disease (31). It should be assumed that the fixation device used will be load-bearing because only 30% to 40% of pathologic fractures unite even after radiation treatment (41,42).

Depending on the forces through a particular area of the skeleton, bone quality, and likelihood of tumor progression, standard internal fixation may be contraindicated. An intramedullary device or modular prosthesis provides more definitive stability. Polymethylmethacrylate (PMMA) is often used to increase the strength of the fixation, but it should not be used solely to replace a segment of bone. PMMA improves the bending strength of a fixation construct and the outcome of fixation in both animal and human studies (43,44). It does not affect the use of therapeutic radiation, nor are the properties of the PMMA affected adversely by the radiation (45). Autogenous bone graft is not generally used in the treatment of extremity fractures from metastatic bone disease. Segmental allografts are also rarely indicated because they require a prolonged healing time.

If the patient is expected to die of metastatic cancer, the most expedient reconstruction with the least risk of complication or failure should be used. In the majority of cases, this requires metal and PMMA. When a prosthesis is used to replace a joint affected by a metastatic lesion or pathologic fracture, it should be cemented into the host bone. Ideally, the patient should be allowed to bear weight as tolerated after the surgical procedure. Another rule when treating patients with metastatic disease is to prophylactically stabilize as much of the affected bone as possible. When an intramedullary device is indicated, the entire femur, humerus, or tibia should be treated with a statically locked nail (46–48). For femoral lesions, a reconstruction nail is used to stabilize the femoral neck even if no lesion is present at the time of surgery.

Some carcinomas are relatively resistant to chemotherapy and radiation therapy when they spread to the skeleton. RCC is a notable example. Surgical treatment is often indicated even for small RCC lesions because they tend to progress despite standard medical treatment and external beam radiation (49). Depending on the patient's expected lifespan and location of the lesion, open treatment with thorough curettage of metastatic RCC followed by intramedullary fixation and PMMA will decrease the tumor burden (50). Postoperative radiation is used to prevent growth of the residual microscopic disease (40). When complete resection and joint replacement can be performed for metastatic RCC, the chances of preventing bone destruction from recurrent tumor are increased (51,52).

Metastatic cancers that are hypervascular put the patient at risk for life-threatening intraoperative hemorrhage if precautions are not taken. Metastatic RCC is the most likely lesion to cause excessive blood loss, but metastatic thyroid cancer and multiple myeloma can also be hypervascular. When possible, a tourniquet should be used with these lesions. However, most metastases occur in the proximal extremities, precluding use of a tourniquet. Excessive blood loss can often be avoided if preoperative angiographic embolization is performed by an interventional radiologist within 36 hours of the surgical procedure (53). Patients with metastatic RCC often have only one functioning kidney, so a careful evaluation of their renal status should be performed before injecting nephrotoxic dye for angiography.

Multidisciplinary Team Approach

Patients who present with a pathologic fracture are often medically debilitated and require multidisciplinary care. In addition to an orthopaedic surgeon, the comprehensive team includes a medical oncologist, radiation oncologist, physical/occupational therapist, and psychologist/psychiatrist. Nutrition is of particular concern; serum prealbumin should be measured and improved if it is low. This may require the addition of enteral or parenteral hyperalimentation perioperatively. Patients may have relative bone marrow suppression and will require adequate replacement of blood products. Perioperative antibiotic coverage, prophylaxis for embolic events, aggressive postoperative pulmonary toilet, and early mobilization are all instituted as standard treatment.

Nonoperative Treatment

Bracing

Bracing of an impending or actual pathologic fracture should be performed if the patient is not a surgical candidate. Nonsurgical candidates are those with limited life expectancies, severe comorbidities, small lesions, or radiosensitive tumors (6). The use of a fracture brace works well for lesions in the upper extremity. Patients should limit weightbearing on the affected extremity. A braced lesion may heal with or without radiation therapy. Lesions most amenable to bracing are those in the humeral diaphysis, forearm, and occasionally the tibia. Patients with proximal humeral lesions can be treated with a sling, and those with distal humeral lesions can be immobilized in a posterior elbow splint with or without a hinge. If a patient has multiple lesions requiring the use of all extremities to ambulate, surgical stabilization will provide better support than a brace.

Upper Extremity Fractures

Twenty percent of osseous metastases occur in the upper extremity with approximately 50% occurring in the humerus. Upper extremity metastases can result in significant functional impairment by hindering personal hygiene, independent ambulation, meal management, ability to use external aids, and general activities of daily living (6). When making decisions about treatment of upper extremity metastasis, the benefits to quality of life should outweigh the risks of potential surgery. Contractures of the shoulder and elbow are common with or without surgical treatment, and these joints should be kept moving. Gentle pendulum exercises can maintain motion in the shoulder and, with appropriate precautions against using torsion, are safe for most proximal and mid-humeral impending fractures. Gravity-assisted elbow flexion and extension exercises can also be performed safely by most patients.

Scapula/Clavicle

Metastatic lesions to the clavicle and scapula are generally treated nonoperatively with shoulder immobilization, radiation, and/or medical management. Occasionally a large, destructive metastasis will occur in the inferior body or articular portion (glenoid) of the scapula. As uncontrollable pain dictates, these areas of the scapula can be resected.

Proximal Humerus

Fractures involving the humeral head or neck are treated with a proximal humeral replacement or intramedullary fixation. If substantial bone is available in the proximal humerus, an intramedullary locked device with multiple proximal screws is acceptable and maintains shoulder range of motion (48). Methylmethacrylate may be required to supplement the fixation. When there is extensive destruction of the proximal humerus or a fracture leaving minimal bone for proximal fixation, resection of the lesion and reconstruction with a cemented proximal humeral endoprosthesis is indicated (54). This modular construct replaces a variable amount of proximal humerus and has a long cemented stem to protect the remainder of the bone (Fig. 20-4). In the face of disease progression, it can be modified to a total humeral prosthesis. Involvement of the glenoid is rare, so replacement of this articular surface is generally not necessary. The goal of a proximal humeral replacement is pain relief and local control of the tumor; range of motion and stability are often limited because of poor soft tissue attachments to the construct. A synthetic vascular graft or mesh sutured to the glenoid labrum and around the prosthetic humeral head can offer some stability. Postoperative radiation therapy is used in cases when intralesional treatment is performed.

Humeral Diaphysis

Humeral diaphyseal lesions can be surgically treated with locked intramedullary fixation or an intercalary metal spacer (48,55–58). Locked intramedullary humeral nails span the entire humerus and provide mechanical and rotational stability (Fig. 20-5). As previously mentioned, PMMA improves implant stability and supplements poor bone quality when used with surgical stabilization (43). Intercalary spacers offer a modular reconstructive option after resection of large diaphyseal lesions

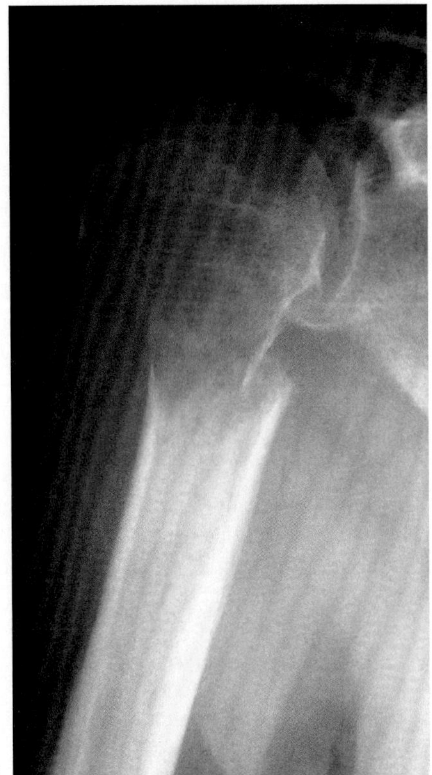

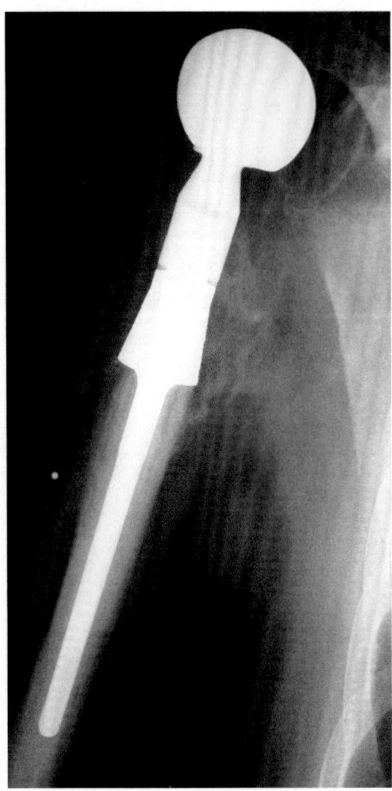

FIGURE 20-4 **A.** Anteroposterior x-ray of the right proximal humerus in a 54-year-old male with multiple myeloma. He has a displaced fracture through the humeral neck with a large lytic lesion filling the proximal humerus. **B.** Postoperative x-ray after resection of the proximal humerus and modular prosthetic replacement. The stem is cemented into the native humerus. Excellent pain control was achieved with this reconstruction.

(55). They are used in segmental defects and cases of failed fixation caused by progressive disease. Intercalary spacers can be used after complete resection of a metastatic lesion in the humeral diaphysis, minimizing blood loss in hypervascular lesions and often alleviating the need for postoperative radiation. Damron et al and Henry et al reported that intercalary spacers provide immediate stable fixation, excellent pain relief, and early return of function (55,59). Plate fixation produces good to excellent functional results in nonpathologic humeral fractures; however, drawbacks for their use in metastatic disease include the need for extensive exposure of the humerus and the inability to protect the entire bone. With disease progression, plate fixation of the humerus is at risk of failure.

Distal Humerus

Distal humeral lesions are treated with flexible intramedullary nails, bicondylar plate fixation or resection with modular distal humeral reconstruction. Flexible nails, inserted in a retrograde manner through small medial and lateral incisions, offer ease of insertion, the ability to span the entire humerus, excellent functional recovery, and preservation of the elbow joint. Curettage of the distal humeral lesion allows an open reduction in the case of a fracture and the opportunity to use PMMA in the lesion to gain rotational stability. Orthogonal plate fixation is similar to nonpathologic fracture care, but, when combined with PMMA, it can provide a stable elbow. This method of fixation does not protect the proximal humerus against a future metastatic lesion or fracture. A distal humeral resection and modular endoprosthetic reconstruction of the elbow is the best option for massive bone loss involving the condyles (60).

Forearm/Hand

Metastases distal to the elbow are unusual, and the most common are from the lung, breast, and kidney (61). Metastatic lesions to the radius and ulna can be treated with flexible rods or rigid plate fixation. Pathologic fractures of the radial head can be treated with resection. Intralesional surgery is preferred for hand metastases with curettage, internal fixation, and cementation. If the lesion is distal or extensive, amputation may be the best option.

Pelvic/Acetabular Fractures

Classification and Treatment

Many bone metastases or pathologic fractures in the bony pelvis do not affect weight-bearing; consequently, they do not require surgical intervention. Lesions of the iliac wing, superior/inferior pubic rami, or sacroiliac region fit into this category. Insufficiency fractures caused by osteoporosis frequently occur in these locations and are managed with protected weightbearing until the pain diminishes (62,63).

Periacetabular lesions, however, affect ambulatory status and often present a difficult surgical problem (64–66). The situation is magnified if there is protrusion of the femoral head through

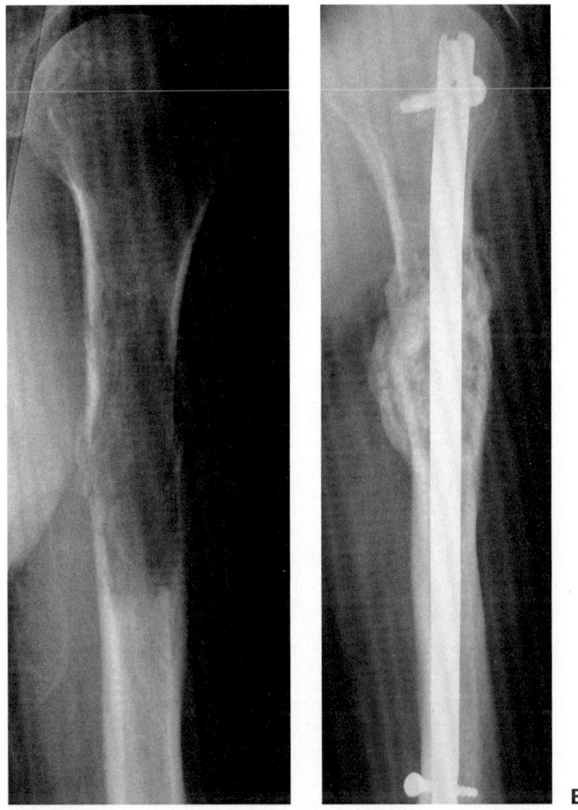

FIGURE 20-5 A. Anteroposterior x-ray of the left humerus in a 58-year-old male with multiple myeloma. This minimally displaced fracture was the presenting feature of his disease. **B.** Postoperative x-ray 6 months after closed intramedullary humeral nail placement. With systemic chemotherapy and external beam radiation to the left humerus, the fracture and lesion have healed.

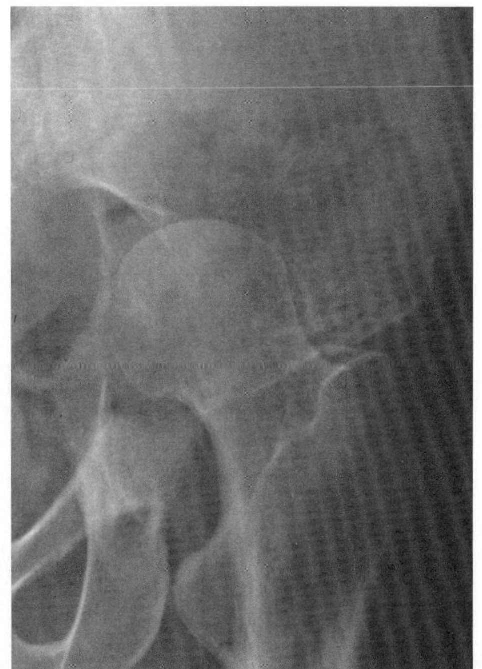

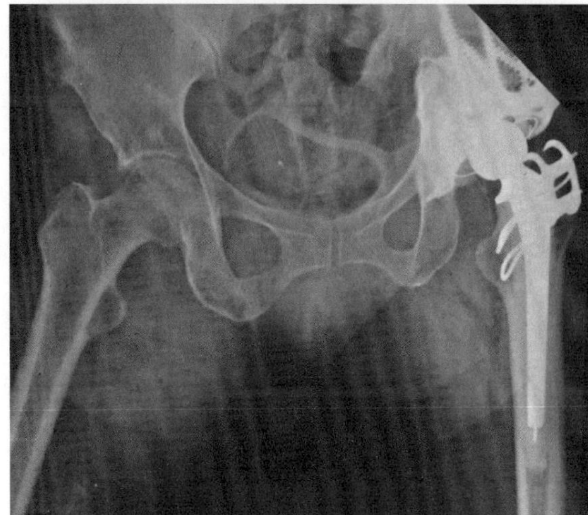

FIGURE 20-6 A. Anteroposterior x-ray of the left hip in a 61-year-old woman with metastatic breast cancer. Note the femoral head protrusion into the pelvis through a pathologic acetabular fracture. It is important to try and identify metastatic lesions before they fracture so that prophylactic fixation can be performed. Note the extensive bone loss in the superior dome and medial wall. This would be categorized as a Class II lesion. **B.** Postoperative x-ray after acetabular reconstruction with an antiprotrusio cage, multiple screws, and polymethylmethacrylate.

a pathologic acetabular fracture (Fig. 20-6). All pathologic fractures or defects in this location should be assessed with CT scans with three-dimensional reconstructions. There are several classification systems for acetabular defects. However, when assessing metastatic disease to the acetabulum, various modifications of the Harrington classification are used. This system classifies the location and extent of the defect and guides the technical considerations of fixation (64). The modification used in my practice describes Class I lesions as minor acetabular defects with maintenance of the lateral cortices and superior and medial walls. A conventional cemented acetabular component provides sufficient support. Class II lesions are major acetabular defects with a deficient medial wall and superior dome. An antiprotrusio device or medial mesh is necessary (Fig. 20-6). Class III lesions are massive defects with deficient lateral cortices and superior dome. There is no substantial peripheral rim for fixation of a metal component; therefore, weightbearing stresses must be transmitted from the acetabular component into bone unaffected by the tumor, usually near the sacroiliac joint. An acetabular cage should be used with long screw fixation into any remaining pubis, ischium, and ilium. The massive bony defect is filled with PMMA to provide immediate stability after long screws and threaded 5/16-inch Steinman pins anchor the construct. A polyethylene cup is then cemented into the acetabular cage in the correct orientation (Fig. 20-7). Class IV lesions involve pelvic discontinuity and can be treated expediently with resection and reconstruction using a saddle prosthesis (67). The

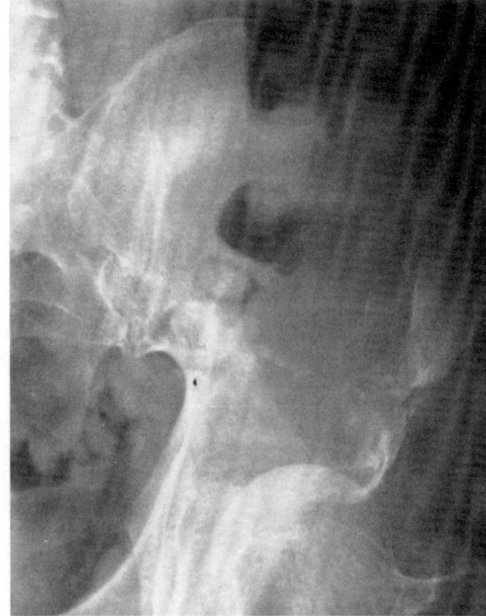

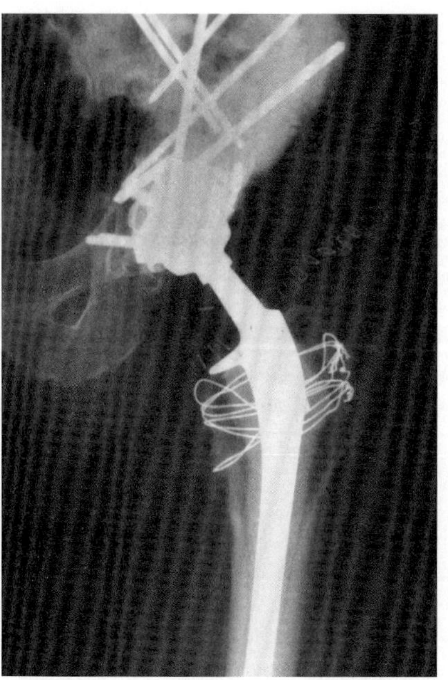

FIGURE 20-7 **A.** Anteroposterior x-ray of the left acetabulum in a 49-year-old woman with metastatic RCC and a Class III acetabular lesion. Note the massive bone destruction of the periacetabular region, precluding peripheral rim fixation. Arterial embolization of the tumor to decrease intraoperative bleeding is recommended. **B.** Postoperative x-ray after reconstruction using a cemented acetabular cage with long Steinman pins transmitting stress into the sacroiliac region.

use of a pelvic prosthesis is more common in Europe (68). With these techniques, satisfactory pain relief and function can be achieved in 70% to 75% of patients. Complications are common and occur in 20% to 30% of cases (64,66,69). Extensive blood loss can be anticipated with massive lytic defects. This demanding surgery is probably best performed by someone with extensive experience treating this type of lesion. The trabecular metal, tantalum, may provide new options for acetabular fixation by allowing early bone ingrowth. It can be used in combination with a cemented acetabular cage (70).

Lower Extremity Fractures

The femur is the most common long bone to be affected by metastases (71). The proximal third is involved in 50% of cases with the intertrochanteric region accounting for 20% of cases. Metastatic disease to the femur is the most painful of all bone metastases, likely because of the high weightbearing stresses through the proximal region. Pathologic fractures of the femur suddenly alter the quality of a patient's life and threaten an individual's level of independence. Without proper surgical attention, the patient with a pathologic fracture of the femur will be confined to bed, a situation that is medically and psychologically devastating.

Painful destructive lesions in the proximal femur should be prophylactically stabilized whenever possible because of the high incidence of subsequent fracture and the comparative ease of the operation. The development of bone metastasis is an ongoing process, so it is important to stabilize as much of the femur as possible (47). Generally, it is recommended that the tip of the chosen fixation device should bypass a given lesion by at least two times the diameter of the femur.

Femoral Neck

Pathologic fractures of the femoral head and neck rarely heal, and the neoplastic process tends to progress (Fig. 20-8) (72). Accordingly, there is a high incidence of failure if traditional fracture fixation devices are used (73). The procedure of choice for patients with metastatic disease to the femoral head or neck is a cemented replacement prosthesis (Fig. 20-9) (72,74). The decision to use a hemiarthroplasty versus a total hip replacement depends on the presence of acetabular involvement. This must be carefully scrutinized because acetabular disease can go unrecognized. All tumor tissue should be curetted from the femoral canal before implanting the prosthesis. When there are adjacent lesions in the subtrochanteric region or proximal diaphysis, a long-stemmed cemented femoral component should be used for prophylactic fixation distally, avoiding a future pathologic fracture through a distal lesion and allowing full weight-bearing postoperatively. When there are no additional lesions in the femur, the length of the cemented femoral stem is controversial. The risk of significant cardiopulmonary problems

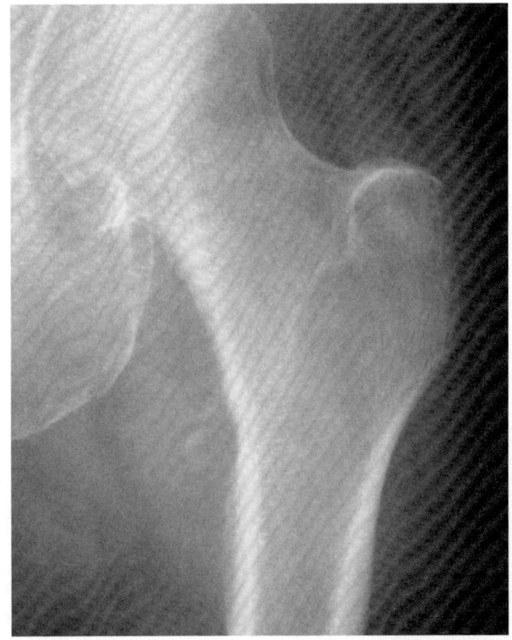

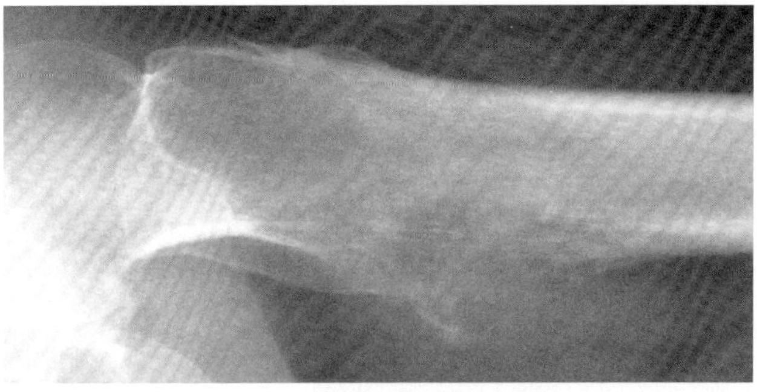

FIGURE 20-8 Anteroposterior **(A)** and lateral **(B)** x-rays of the left hip in a 52-year-old woman with metastatic lung carcinoma. There is an impending fracture caused by a lytic lesion in the medial aspect of the femoral neck.

from monomer embolization after pressurizing the extra cement and long stem within the canal must be weighed against the potential risk of future metastasis distal to the tip of the prosthesis if a shorter stem is used. If long-stemmed femoral components are used, it is important to inject the cement into the canal while it is still in a fairly liquid state (75).

Intertrochanteric Region

Traditional fixation of an intertrochanteric fracture with a screw and side-plate construct has a high rate of failure when used in the setting of metastatic bone disease, even when supplemented with adjuvant PMMA and postoperative radiation. The standard of care is intramedullary fixation or prosthetic replacement (46,47). The choice of fixation in this region of the femur depends on the extent of the lesion and whether it is radiosensitive. If bone with sufficient strength remains in the femoral head and neck, and local control is likely to be achieved with postoperative external beam radiation, an intramedullary reconstruction device is recommended that will allow the patient the highest level of function. A cephalomedullary nail protects the femoral neck and is used for all metastatic lesions or pathologic fractures of the femur when an intramedullary device is indicated. If the destruction is more extensive, a cemented calcar-replacing prosthesis is required. The same issues arise related to the length of the femoral stem as discussed in the previous section.

Subtrochanteric Region

Using traditional fixation for subtrochanteric fractures in patients with metastatic bone disease will usually end in failure. This region of the femur is subjected to forces of up to four to six times body weight. Statically locked intramedullary fixation with or without PMMA will stabilize the area and provide weightbearing support (76). Even impending fractures should be statically locked because the lesion can fracture later causing shortening of the femur. A modular proximal femoral prosthesis is reserved for cases with extensive bone destruction or used as a salvage device for failed internal fixation (Fig. 20-9) (74,77). It can also be used when a wide resection is necessary for a pathologic fracture through a primary bone sarcoma. There is an increased risk of dislocation and abductor mechanism weakness with a megaprosthesis, but this should not prevent its use in patients with radioresistant or locally aggressive tumors. A bipolar head is used to provide more stability if the acetabulum is not involved with metastatic disease. Excellent pain relief and local tumor control can be obtained after tumor resection and reconstruction.

Femoral Diaphysis

Pathologic fractures of the femoral diaphysis are treated most effectively with a statically locked cephalomedullary nail, with or without PMMA (Fig. 20-10) (46,47). Plate fixation, although more rigid, will not protect a large enough segment of bone and is prone to failure with disease progression. Cephalomedullary nail fixation protects the entire bone and is technically simple, especially when performed prophylactically. A trochanteric or piriformis entry point can be used, and the canal is slowly overreamed 1.0 to 1.5 mm to avoid high impaction forces during rod placement (78). Because the device will be loadbearing if the fracture does not unite, the largest possible diameter nail should be used.

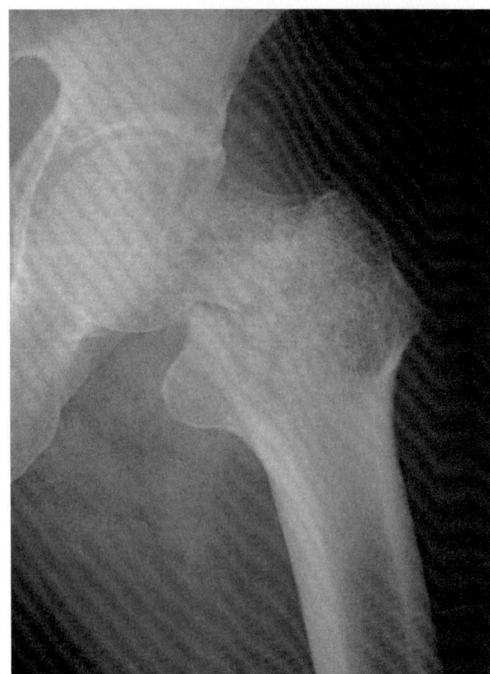

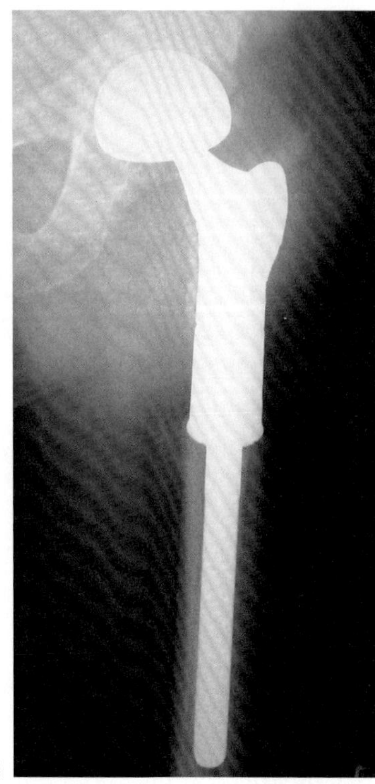

FIGURE 20-9 **A.** Anteroposterior x-ray of the left proximal femur in a 77-year-old man with a dedifferentiated chondrosarcoma. He had 3 months of hip pain before developing a pathologic fracture of the femoral neck through a lesion with a calcified cartilage matrix. An open biopsy confirmed the diagnosis. **B.** Postoperative x-ray after a wide resection of the chondrosarcoma and reconstruction with a proximal femoral replacement. The hip abductors are sutured back to holes in the trochanteric portion of the prosthesis, and the patient is braced postoperatively.

Supracondylar Femur

The choice of fixation for pathologic supracondylar femur fractures depends on the extent of local bone destruction and the presence of additional lesions located in the proximal femur. The distal lesions can be a treatment challenge because of frequent comminution and poor bone stock, especially in older patients. Options include lateral locking plate fixation supplemented with PMMA or a modular distal femoral prosthesis (28). A retrograde nail has the drawback of potentially seeding the knee joint with tumor while failing to provide fixation to the femoral neck region. The locking plate provides stable fixation after curettage and cementation of the metastatic lesion. The modular endoprosthesis is the optimal choice for local control when there is massive destruction of the femoral condyles, because it allows the lesion to be resected en bloc (79).

Tibia

Metastases distal to the knee are uncommon, but, for proximal tibial lesions, similar principles should be used as for lesions in the supracondylar femoral area. A locking plate with PMMA after thorough curettage of the lesion is generally sufficient. Extensive lesions require a modular proximal tibial prosthesis. Tibial diaphyseal lesions and fractures should be managed with a locked intramedullary device. Various techniques can be used for pathologic fractures of the distal tibia, but standard internal fixation methods are generally advised with generous use of PMMA to augment the construct (80). The treatment of foot and ankle lesions must be individualized to maintain maximal function (81).

Spinal Fractures

Between 5% and 10% of patients who die of metastatic carcinoma will have microscopic disease in their spine (82,83). The metastases most commonly involve the vertebral body rather than the posterior elements. The majority of these patients will not have clinically significant spine disease during their lifetime and will not need treatment specific to this location. The lesions are often discovered incidentally on a bone scan during a routine metastatic workup in a patient with known cancer. However, if the disease progresses, it can cause moderate to severe pain persisting for months before the onset of focal neurologic deficits. Occasionally the onset of pain is sudden after a pathologic compression fracture.

When the patient does not have a history of cancer, it must be decided whether a compression fracture is secondary to osteoporosis or a bone metastasis. If the patient has a history of cancer or if the patient's current symptoms, physical examination, laboratory studies, or imaging suggest a primary carcinoma or myeloma, the patient should be evaluated for a compression fracture caused by metastatic disease. It is imperative to consider spinal metastasis in any patient with cancer who experiences back pain. A delay in diagnosis can allow progression and possible neurologic compromise leading to permanent functional deficits. Patients with a suspected malignancy should undergo a biopsy, but others should be treated symptomatically. If a patient treated for an osteoporotic compression fracture does not respond to the treatment, or if there is progressive destruction of bone, a biopsy should also be performed. Percutaneous

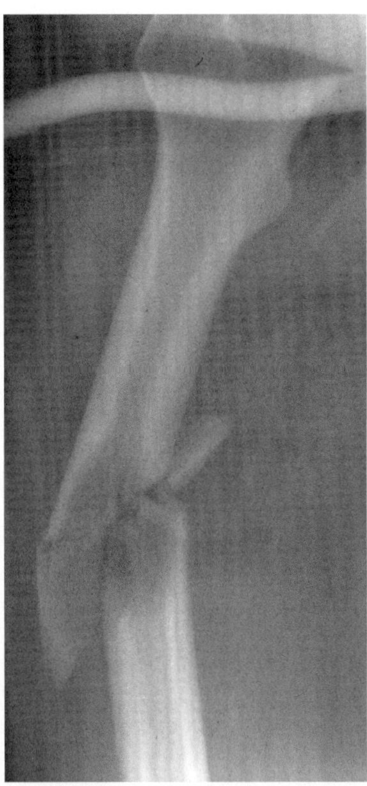

FIGURE 20-10 Anteroposterior x-ray of the right femur in a 33-year-old man with metastatic pheochromocytoma. He had pain for 8 weeks before falling onto the right leg. A purely lytic lesion is noted at the fracture site. He was treated with a femoral cephalomedullary nail to protect the length of the femur from future metastatic lesions.

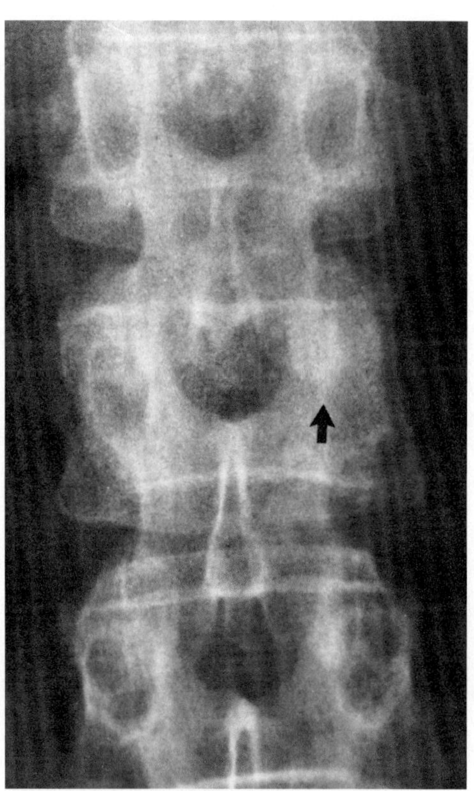

FIGURE 20-11 This anteroposterior x-ray of the lumbar spine in a patient who had back pain shows a subtle finding that is often called the "winking owl." The cortical bone of the pedicles is seen at the upper outer corners of the vertebral bodies as dense, round structures because the view is cross-sectional. When metastatic deposits involve the vertebrae, the cortices of the pedicles are usually thinned and therefore cannot be seen on plain x-rays. This "missing" pedicle (*arrow*) is the closed or "winked" eye and is almost pathognomonic of metastatic disease.

CT-guided needle biopsy of vertebral lesions can be performed with local anesthesia and intravenous sedation.

The classic plain radiographic finding in metastatic involvement of the spine is loss of a pedicle on an anteroposterior view (Fig. 20-11). MRI can be used to differentiate an osteoporotic compression fracture from one caused by a malignant lesion (84). When there is complete replacement of the vertebral segment, multiple vertebral body lesions, pedicle involvement, and an intact intervertebral disk, metastatic disease is most likely (Fig. 20-12). Some patients with myeloma, lymphoma, or leukemia may present with osteopenia of the vertebrae. To determine whether the patient has a hematologic malignancy, a bone marrow aspirate should be considered. Most of these patients will have systemic findings (e.g., weight loss, fatigue, fever). If a metastatic deposit in the spine is identified, the patient is at risk of having additional skeletal deposits.

Treatment options for patients with symptomatic metastatic disease to the spine include nonoperative management with radiation, corticosteroids, and bracing, minimally invasive techniques such as kyphoplasty and vertebroplasty, and surgical treatment with adjuvant radiation (85–90). Several spine scoring systems for the evaluation of patients with vertebral metastasis have been reported, but no system has been universally adopted to guide treatment (91,92).

Generally, the symptoms with a vertebral compression fracture caused by osteoporosis are minor and can be successfully controlled with temporarily decreased activity or bracing. If the patient has asymptomatic vertebral metastases that are not at risk for pathologic fracture, systemic treatment can be used to address the primary and metastatic disease. Regular imaging of the spine should be performed to ensure that further tumor growth is identified quickly. Often, early recognition of a spinal metastasis allows pain relief with nonoperative management. If the patient has pain but no neurologic compromise or risk of impending fracture, radiation treatment is indicated. Radiation is also used on radiation-sensitive tumors such as lymphoma or myeloma even when they present with neurologic compromise. The tumor response is usually sufficiently rapid such that the risk of permanent neurologic loss is no higher than that seen after surgical decompression. When there is minimal or no bone destruction and cord compression is caused by tumor extension, emergency radiation is recommended (93). The pa-

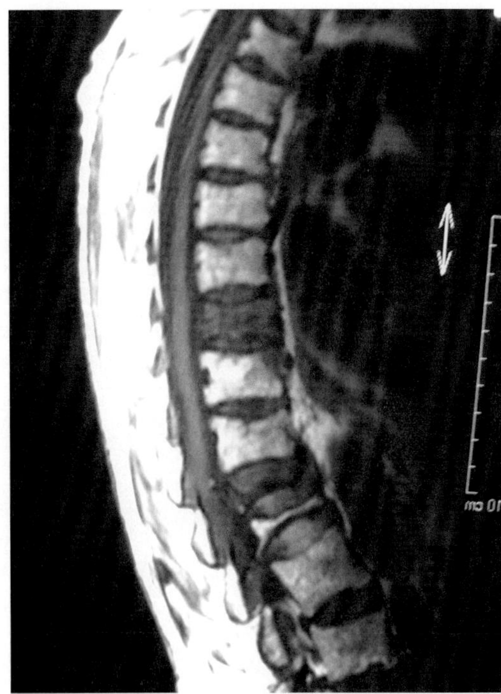

FIGURE 20-12 A sagittal view of a magnetic resonance imaging (MRI) scan in a patient with metastatic disease to the spine. Note the multiple lesions and an area of bone and tumor extension against the spinal cord. The entire vertebral body was involved. This patient had a history of metastatic cancer.

tient should also be treated with a short course of high-dose corticosteroids to reduce the edema surrounding the tumor that contributes to the compression and neurologic damage. Other indications for radiation treatment of vertebral metastases include patients with medical comorbidities precluding surgery, patients with 6 weeks or less to live, and patients with multilevel disease. Radiation should be added preoperatively or postoperatively to improve local disease control when patients are treated with surgery (40).

Indications for surgical treatment of vertebral metastases include progression of disease after radiation, neurologic compromise because of bony impingement or radioresistant tumor within the spinal canal, an impending fracture or spinal instability because of pathologic fracture or progressive deformity. The goals of surgery are to maintain or restore neurologic function and spinal stability (82).

When surgical treatment is necessary to relieve compression of the spinal cord, decompression and stabilization are required. Before surgery, an MRI is used to verify the level of the lesion and rule out the possibility of compression at additional levels. A preoperative angiogram with embolization of feeder vessels should be considered in patients with highly vascular metastasis, such as RCC, to reduce intraoperative blood loss (53). Relief of symptoms can often be accomplished by a posterior decompression and fusion using instrumentation (85). When there is anterior collapse of the vertebrae and anterior compression of the spinal cord resulting in kyphosis, the patient is treated with an anterior decompression and stabilization (87,89,94). When the posterior elements are involved with tumor and the cord is compressed anteriorly, the patient should have an anterior decompression with posterior stabilization and fusion (Fig. 20-13) (90). Internal fixation is indicated to provide immediate stability for all but the most limited decompressions. In recent years, there has been considerable improvement in the available implants to manage structural deficiency of the spine including pedicle screws, cages, and more sophisticated plates and rods. Specific techniques for anterior and posterior decompression and stabilization, including the use of modern instrumentation systems, are described in the literature (90). Surgical implants should ideally be titanium for easier assessment of recurrent disease on an MRI scan. As patients live longer with their metastatic disease, aggressive surgical treatment of their spinal lesions can enhance quality of life. However, the magnitude of the operative procedure should not exceed the patient's chance of surviving the surgery or the surgeon's level of competence.

Kyphoplasty/Vertebroplasty

Minimally invasive treatments for metastatic disease of the spine have been used to control pain in patients who have developed compression fractures (86,88). Vertebroplasty or kyphoplasty

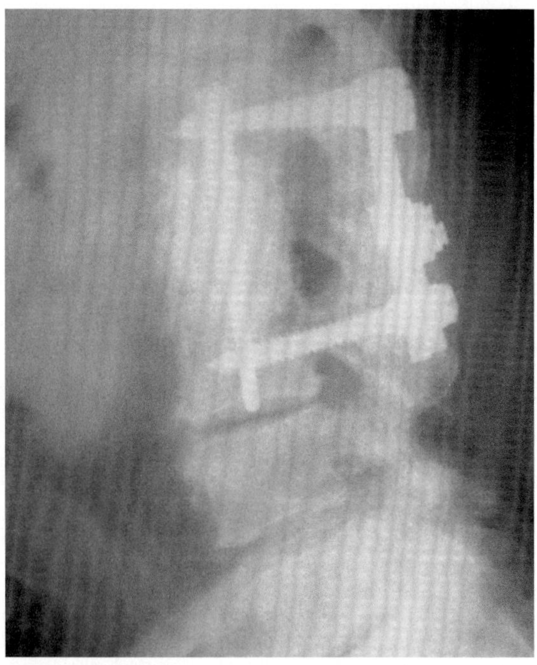

FIGURE 20-13 Lateral x-ray showing spinal instrumentation after treatment of a patient with multiple myeloma who had extension of tumor compressing the spinal cord and neurologic compromise unresponsive to radiation. Anterior and posterior decompression with resection of the involved body and instrumentation was necessary to stabilize the segment. Pedicle screws and PMMA contributed to the construct.

can be used for pathologic vertebral body fractures caused by osteoporosis, metastatic carcinoma, or multiple myeloma. Indications include patients with stable compression fractures who have normal neurologic function but persistent pain. One technique, vertebroplasty, involves percutaneous direct injection of PMMA through the pedicle to maintain vertebral height. More recently, kyphoplasty is a way of regaining vertebral body height by expanding the compression fracture with a balloon before injecting the PMMA (Fig. 20-14). Reported complications include extrusion of cement around the neurologic structures, so this procedure should only be performed after careful consideration of the risks.

Complications

Because patients with pathologic fractures are often older and have multiple associated medical problems, the chance of perioperative complications is increased. These patients have the same risks as those with nonpathologic fractures when they consent to surgical treatment, but some complications are more likely in patients with widespread cancer. Two of the most concerning problems are tumor progression with resultant hardware failure and cardiopulmonary compromise.

Bone metastases that are unresponsive to chemotherapy and radiation will continue to destroy bone so that the existing hardware or prosthesis is load-bearing rather than load-sharing. Using the principles of surgical treatment outlined in this chapter will minimize the risk of hardware failure, but inevitably some constructs will still fail. The salvage of failed reconstructions must be individualized, but modular endoprostheses can frequently be used to salvage failed intramedullary fixation (Fig. 20-15) (77). Again, the patient's lifespan and general health must be favorable before they are indicated for a prolonged procedure.

Cardiopulmonary compromise is a noted risk in patients with bone metastases. First, many of these patients have pulmonary metastases or primary lung tumors that make ventilation more difficult. Some patients will have a surgical procedure for a bone metastases and fail postoperative attempts at extubation, remaining in an intensive care setting for a prolonged time. Second, the placement of long-stemmed cemented femoral prostheses or prophylactic femoral or humeral nails must be done carefully to avoid embolic events. Careful suction of the canal and slow reaming are tips to decrease this complication (75,78).

Role of Adjuvant Radiation and Medical Treatment

External Beam Radiation

External beam radiation is used to treat pain secondary to bone metastases, halt the progression of bony destruction, and allow healing of an impending pathologic fracture. It is a reasonable alternative to surgical treatment for certain lesions. When the

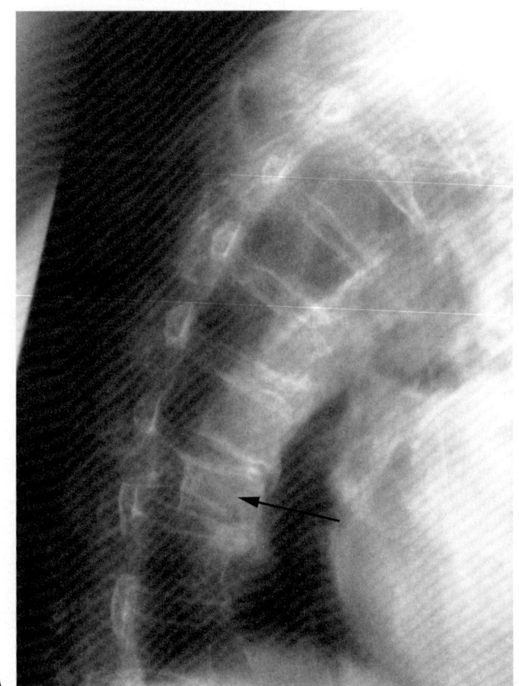
A

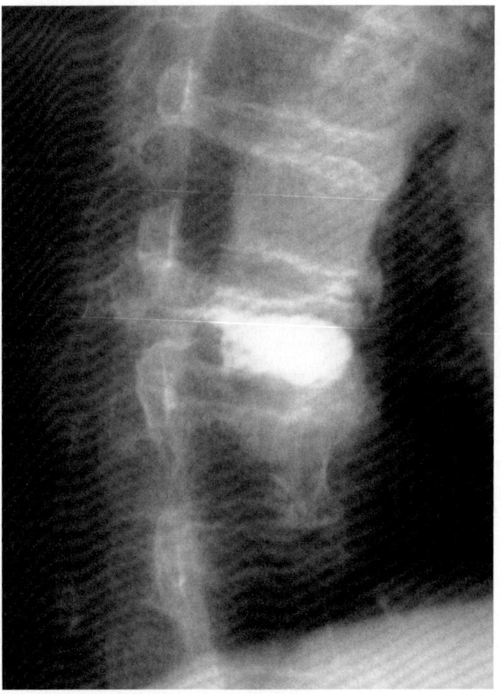
B

FIGURE 20-14 **A.** Lateral x-ray of a patient with senile osteoporosis and a thoracic compression fracture. **B.** Lateral x-ray after treatment with kyphoplasty to regain vertebral height and relieve pain. Note that the methylmethacrylate is relatively well contained. The fracture reduction is minimal, but she had complete pain relief 2 weeks after the procedure.

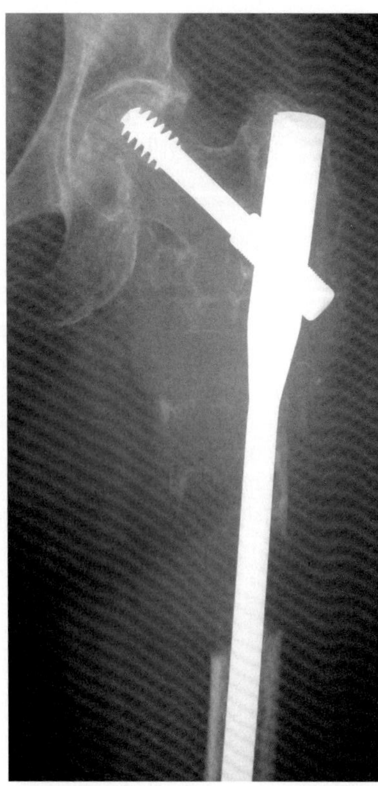

FIGURE 20-15 Anteroposterior x-ray of the left proximal femur in a 68-year-old man previously treated with an intramedullary nail for metastatic RCC of the subtrochanteric region of the femur. Disease progression has caused severe pain and failure of the reconstruction. The patient was treated with resection of the proximal femur and reconstruction with a modular proximal femoral prosthesis.

endpoint is pain relief, local radiation therapy typically results in partial relief in more than 80% of patients with bone metastases and complete pain relief in 50% to 60% of cases (95). Variability in response rates depends on multiple factors including the histology and location of the lesion (96). The onset of symptomatic relief usually occurs in the first 1 to 2 weeks, but maximal relief may take several months. Radiation is used in the postoperative setting to increase local tumor control after surgical stabilization. Retrospective data have shown that postoperative radiation improves limb function and decreases the rate of second orthopedic procedures (40). The majority of patients in this study had the entire prosthesis or internal fixation device included in the treatment field. Radiation can usually begin 2 weeks after the surgical procedure if there are no wound complications.

Systemic Radionucleotides

Systemic therapy for bone metastasis using radioactive bone-seeking agents provides palliation of bone pain. It may be appropriate for widespread bone metastases when more traditional forms of radiation have reached their limit or when standard radiation techniques are not feasible because of surrounding normal tissue tolerances. Strontium-89 and samarium-153 are used clinically and are preferentially taken up at sites of active bone mineral turnover similar to bisphosphonates (97). There is a greater uptake of the radionucleotides in metastatic lesions than in normal bone. Robinson and associates reported clinical response rates of 80% for bone pain improvement in patients with breast cancer, with 20% of patients becoming totally pain free (98).

Bisphosphonates

Bisphosphonates bind preferentially to the bone matrix and inhibit osteoclastic bone resorption (99). They decrease the depth of resorption cavities at osteoclastic binding sites, inhibit osteoclastic function, alter the morphology of the osteoclast ruffled border, and inhibit maturation and recruitment of osteoclasts from the monocyte/macrophage cell line. Bisphosphonates promote osteoclast apoptosis, and some data indicate that they have similar direct effects on tumor cells (13). Intravenous bisphosphonates have been used with success to treat bone pain and hypercalcemia in breast cancer, and they are most commonly used as an adjunct to other systemic therapies (39).

A combined analysis of two studies that evaluated the use of the bisphosphonate pamidronate included 751 patients treated with hormone therapy or chemotherapy for lytic bone metastases from breast cancer (39). Skeletal events in the pamidronate group were 51% versus 64% in the placebo arm, and the time to first event overall was 12.7 months versus 7 months in the placebo group. The time to a new pathologic fracture was substantially prolonged at 25.2 months for the pamidronate-treated patients versus 12.8 months for the placebo-treated patients. The median time to need for radiation had not been reached for the pamidronate group compared with 16 months for the placebo group (39).

Controversies and Future Directions

Two of the main controversies in the management of patients with metastatic bone disease include (a) the ideal length of a cemented femoral stem in patients with metastatic disease about the hip and (b) the specific characteristics that define an impending fracture. These topics were discussed previously.

There is also continued debate as to the surgical treatment of patients with a solitary metastasis. There is literature to suggest that wide resection of a solitary RCC metastasis leads to increased survival (50–52). However, it has not been shown that these data are applicable to metastatic disease from other primary sites. The study recommending resection of solitary RCC metastasis was conducted before widespread use of PET scanning, which allows discovery of smaller foci of active disease. It is likely that many patients presumed to have solitary metastasis would have additional sites of disease if screened with PET imaging. However, a patient with a solitary metastasis from any origin who has been tumor-free for several years should be considered a candidate for a resection. RCC and follicular cell thyroid carcinoma are the two tumors most likely to produce isolated bone metastasis years after therapy for the primary tumor.

Future directions in the surgical treatment of patients with metastatic bone disease of the spine and extremities will likely include more widespread use and applications for trabecular metal. The tantalum acetabular components allow excellent bone ingrowth and are being used more routinely in revision joint arthroplasty to reconstruct large acetabular defects (31,70). No studies are currently available to assess the use of trabecular metal in patients with metastatic disease who have massive bone loss or prior radiation. Further advances in this type of metal fixation may allow improvement in the attachment of soft tissues to megaprostheses after tumor resection.

Interventional radiologists are working more closely with orthopaedic surgeons to manage patients with bone metastases. Radiofrequency ablation is being used more frequently for palliative treatment of painful metastatic lesions. It provides an alternative to external beam radiation or surgery (100). A recent study of patients with pelvic and sacral metastases treated with radiofrequency ablation showed a clinical benefit with significant pain relief in 95% of patients (101,102). Most of these patients had failed to respond to prior treatment or were considered to be poor candidates for narcotic medication or radiation. Another new procedure termed *acetabuloplasty* is similar to vertebroplasty in that PMMA is injected percutaneously into an acetabular defect to provide pain relief and possibly avoid a major surgical reconstruction (31,103).

TREATMENT OPTIONS FOR PATIENTS WITH PATHOLOGIC FRACTURES THROUGH PRIMARY BONE TUMORS

Benign Bone Tumors

Benign bone tumors occur most commonly in children and young adults. Most tumors gradually enlarge until the patient reaches skeletal maturity, and then they resolve or become inactive. Inactive lesions do not require surgical treatment. Active or aggressive benign lesions often require intralesional curettage with or without bone grafting to remove the tumor and allow healing of the underlying bone. A pathologic fracture through a benign bone tumor may change the course of treatment. Because of the age and activity level of patients who have benign bone tumors, pathologic fractures are not uncommon.

In general, the treatment of a pathologic fracture through a benign bone lesion depends on the activity of the underlying lesion. Most can be treated nonoperatively in a cast until the fracture heals. At that time, treatment of the benign tumor can be addressed. Indications for surgical treatment of the fracture include unacceptable deformity in a cast, open fracture, fracture nonunion, or association with active or aggressive lesions such as giant cell tumor or aneurysmal bone cyst (ABC). The treatment of pathologic fractures in the context of specific benign bone tumors is discussed next. The reader is referred to comprehensive musculoskeletal oncology texts to learn more about the diagnosis and treatment of the individual tumors.

Unicameral Bone Cyst

Two thirds of patients with a unicameral bone cyst (UBC) present with a pathologic fracture (104). The majority of these lesions are located in the proximal humerus or proximal femur. A humeral fracture should be allowed to heal in a satisfactory position to see whether the fracture stimulates healing of the cyst (Fig. 20-16). If the cyst has not healed spontaneously after the fracture callus remodels, corticosteroid injection into the cyst is recommended. A displaced fracture through a proximal femoral UBC in a child usually requires open reduction, bone grafting of the cyst, and internal fixation.

Aneurysmal Bone Cyst

An ABC is an active benign lesion that can grow rapidly in the metaphysis of a young patient, simulating a malignancy (104). Despite its occasional aggressive growth pattern, pathologic fractures are uncommon. Approximately 15% to 20% of lesions occur in the posterior elements of the spine and can cause neu-

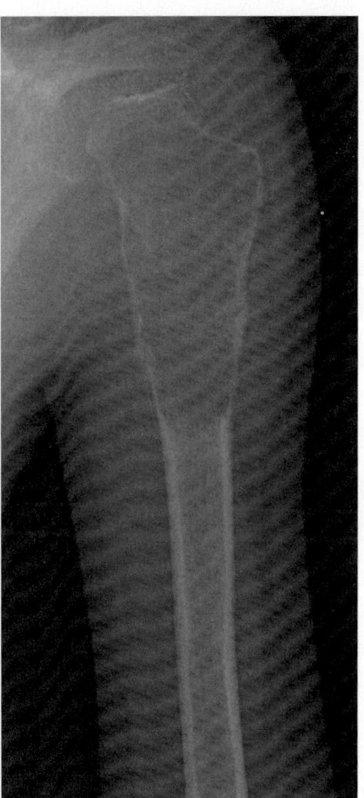

FIGURE 20-16 Anteroposterior x-ray of the left humerus in an 8-year-old boy with a pathologic fracture through a unicameral bone cyst (UBC). There is extensive involvement of the humeral metaphysis. The cyst starts in the proximal metaphysis and will appear to move distally with growth of the humerus. This patient was treated with a sling until the fracture healed and then had intralesional injection of corticosteroids to treat the UBC.

rologic compromise. The standard treatment for an ABC with or without a fracture is intralesional curettage and bone grafting. Depending on the age of the patient and location of the ABC, a pathologic fracture might require internal fixation at the time of curettage.

Eosinophilic Granuloma

An eosinophilic granuloma is a solitary lesion in the spectrum of disease known as Langerhans cell histiocytosis. It is a benign bone tumor, and affected patients present with pain. This tumor can cause collapse of a vertebral body (vertebra plana) and neurologic symptoms. Patients with symptomatic vertebra plana are braced, and eventually the vertebral height is restored (105). For extremity lesions that do not spontaneously resolve, the standard of care is intralesional corticosteroid injection. Open curettage is reserved for selected lesions that fail to respond or are unsuitable for steroid injection because of the size, location, or aggressiveness of the lesion (106). A pathologic fracture should be allowed to heal before performing a needle biopsy and injection so the fracture callus does not confuse the histologic picture.

Nonossifying Fibroma

Nonossifying fibromas are extremely common lytic lesions in young patients. They spontaneously resolve after skeletal maturity. They are asymptomatic, but large lesions can fracture. Common pathologic fracture locations include the distal tibia, distal femur, and proximal tibia (Fig. 20-17). Patients with multiple lesions have a higher risk of fracture. Pathologic fractures can be treated successfully in the majority of cases with closed reduction and cast immobilization (107). If the lesion persists after fracture consolidation, curettage and bone grafting can be performed if necessary. If a fracture is unstable and cannot be reduced in a closed fashion, curettage and bone grafting are combined with internal fixation.

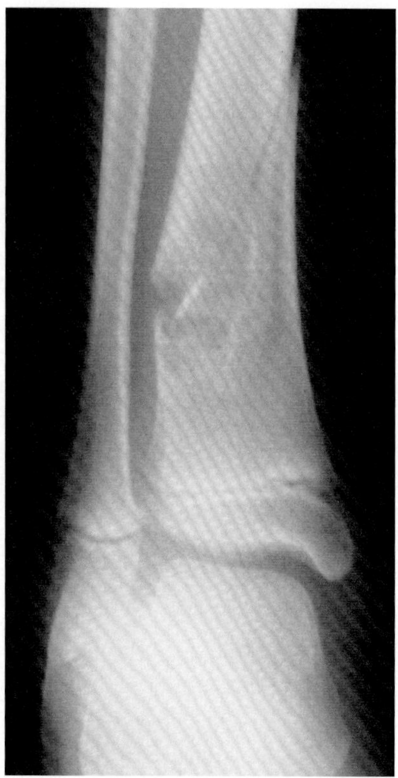

FIGURE 20-17 Anteroposterior x-ray of the distal tibia of a 10-year-old boy. The well-developed reactive rim of bone around the eccentric, metaphyseal, radiolucent lesion is virtually diagnostic of a nonossifying fibroma (NOF). The patient had no symptoms until he slid into second base and caught his foot, twisting his lower leg. He heard a crack and had acute pain. The fracture was treated in a cast and healed, but the NOF remained 2 more years before healing completely.

Enchondroma

Enchondromas are benign cartilage tumors that are asymptomatic unless associated with a pathologic fracture (108). The lesions in long bones rarely fracture. Those most prone to pathologic fractures and pain occur in the small bones of the hand (Fig. 20-18). Some advocate nonsurgical treatment of these lesions, because the fracture occasionally stimulates resolution of the enchondroma. Most agree that surgical intervention, if performed, should be delayed until the fracture has healed (109). Surgical treatment of the enchondroma eliminates the future risk of pathologic fracture and avoids progressive deformity. Whether to bone graft the lesion after curettage remains controversial. Multiple enchondromas with frequent hand fractures and deformities occur in Ollier's disease and Maffucci's syndrome.

Fibrous Dysplasia

Fibrous dysplasia is more consistent with a developmental abnormality than a true neoplasm and occurs in both monostotic and polyostotic forms (110). Most solitary lesions of fibrous dysplasia are asymptomatic, but patients can present with a painful pathologic fracture or bowed extremity. In the polyostotic form, lesions involve multiple areas of a single bone or multiple bones in one extremity, and fractures occur in 85% of these patients. The structural bone strength is decreased in fibrous dysplasia, and sequential fractures can result in progressive deformity producing the classic Shepherd's crook varus appearance of the proximal femur. The fractures are rarely displaced and heal well.

Pathologic fractures or symptomatic lesions in the upper extremity and spine can be treated nonoperatively, whereas lower extremity fractures usually require internal fixation (111). Extensive areas of fibrous dysplasia in high-stress weightbearing areas are treated with prophylactic internal fixation. The lesion should be biopsied at the time of surgery to confirm the diagnosis before proceeding with intramedullary fixation to stabilize long bones. The goal is to strengthen and straighten the bone, not to resect the lesion. Internal fixation does not alter the disease process but provides mechanical support and pain relief. A more recent, but unproven, option is medical treatment with bisphosphonates alone or in combination with surgery (112).

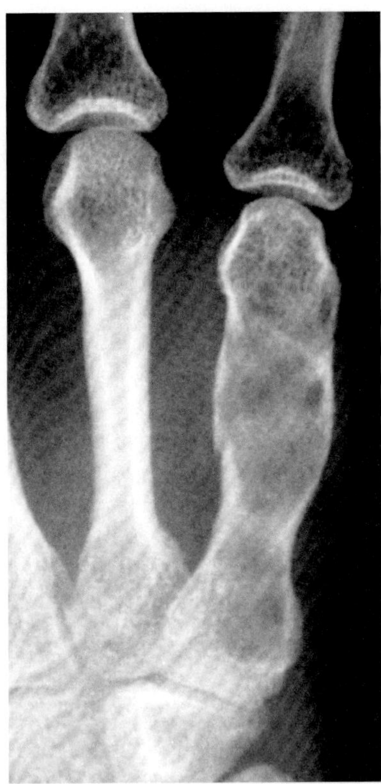

FIGURE 20-18 Anteroposterior x-ray of the hand in a 25-year-old female. She sustained minimal trauma and has a nondisplaced fracture of the fifth metacarpal. She had previously fractured this metacarpal through a known enchondroma. She had closed treatment for the second fracture followed by curettage and allograft bone placement in the enchondroma.

Giant Cell Tumor

Giant cell tumor is an aggressive benign bone tumor that occurs in young adults (113). Ten percent of patients present with a pathologic fracture. In patients whose adjacent joint can be preserved, the giant cell tumor should be treated with thorough curettage and bone grafting or cementation. Internal fixation is usually necessary after a pathologic fracture because there is usually extensive bone loss and deformity. Adjuvant treatment with phenol or cryosurgery should be used with caution in patients when a pathologic fracture exposes adjacent soft tissues. Primary resection and reconstruction is only necessary when the associated joint is destroyed.

Malignant Bone Tumors

Primary malignant bone tumors are treated with a combination of surgery, chemotherapy, and/or radiation. We previously discussed multiple myeloma, a primary malignant bone tumor that has a systemic presentation and occurs in older patients. Pathologic fractures in patients with myeloma, lymphoma, and metastatic carcinoma can be treated with fixation through the tumor because they are systemic diseases treated primarily with chemotherapy and radiation. The overall survival of the patients is not compromised by palliative surgical stabilization. Primary malignant bone tumors such as osteosarcoma, Ewing's sarcoma, and chondrosarcoma are treated much differently than systemic disease. These tumors grow initially in the bone and can metastasize to the lungs. Local control of the primary lesion is usually achieved by complete surgical resection. A pathologic fracture through the lesion theoretically decreases the chance of local control, because tumor cells spread through the hematoma. Amputation becomes a real consideration for patients with a pathologic fracture through these tumors.

Before initiating treatment for a patient with a pathologic fracture through a presumed primary bone sarcoma, the patient should have staging studies and a histologic diagnosis. An appropriate staging workup includes a CT scan of the chest for all patients, and a bone marrow biopsy when Ewing's sarcoma is suspected. The biopsy of a presumed bone sarcoma is especially difficult in the setting of an associated pathologic fracture. The fracture hematoma and healing process alter the histology and may confuse the pathologist. Whenever possible, the biopsy should be performed away from the fracture. When there is an extraosseous soft tissue mass associated with the tumor, an image-guided needle biopsy is usually adequate. When the lesion is intraosseous and fracture callus is present, an open biopsy is preferred.

Internal fixation of a pathologic fracture through a primary sarcoma may compromise the limb and life of the patient. If the patient will be treated with preoperative chemotherapy, cast immobilization of the fracture is preferred. The fracture usually heals during systemic treatment, and a cast avoids potential pin tract infections in neutropenic patients stabilized with an external fixator.

Patients with a pathologic fracture through a primary malignancy of bone require a coordinated multidisciplinary team that includes a medical oncologist, radiation oncologist, musculoskeletal pathologist, radiologist, physical therapist, and orthopaedic oncologist; only with the full complement of care can these patients achieve the best quality of life and maximum overall survival.

Osteosarcoma/Ewing's Sarcoma

These two sarcomas are the most common primary bone tumors in children. Approximately 10% of patients present with a pathologic fracture. Closed treatment of the fracture in a cast is indicated after a needle or open biopsy is performed. When staging is complete, preoperative chemotherapy is used for patients with osteosarcoma or Ewing's sarcoma. After 3 to 4 months of systemic therapy, a decision is made about local control of the primary tumor. For patients with osteosarcoma, surgical resection is indicated. If patients have a clinical and radiographic response to chemotherapy, a limb salvage procedure is generally preferred. Recent articles have shown no difference in overall survival for patients with osteosarcoma and a pathologic fracture that are treated with limb salvage compared with amputation (114,115). Close follow-up is necessary to watch for local recurrence.

Local control in Ewing's sarcoma can be achieved with surgical resection, radiation, or both. In reconstructible sites, most patients are treated with limb salvage surgery to remove all chemotherapy-resistant clones and avoid the risks of radiation in a growing child. However, in patients with a pathologic fracture treated with surgical resection, consideration should be given to adding radiation as a postoperative adjuvant to improve the chance of local control and avoid amputation (116).

Chondrosarcoma

Chondrosarcoma occurs in middle-aged and older adults. The pelvis is a common site, but displaced pathologic fractures are rare in this location. The most common location of a pathologic fracture through a chondrosarcoma is in the proximal femur (Fig. 20-19). A serious mistake is to assume the fracture is secondary to metastatic carcinoma and place an intramedullary rod through the lesion. This act generally precludes any safe limb salvage option for the patient. An older patient with a solitary lytic lesion should be staged appropriately and a biopsy performed to confirm the diagnosis before any surgical treatment.

The treatment of a patient with a chondrosarcoma is in the hands of an orthopaedic oncologist. Chemotherapy and radiation are not effective for this tumor. Therefore, a pathologic fracture greatly compromises the local area, because any stray tumor cells not resected will likely grow into a locally recurrent lesion (117). A displaced fracture through a chondrosarcoma is a reason to consider amputation, especially if wide resection cannot be achieved with a limb salvage procedure.

CONCLUSION

Any process that reduces bone strength predisposes a patient to a pathologic fracture during normal activity or after minimal trauma. It must be recognized as a pathologic fracture if the patient is to be treated properly.

- The most common cause for a pathologic fracture is osteoporosis or osteomalacia.
- Patients with osteoporosis or osteomalacia require evaluation and management of the underlying disorder.
- Patients more than 45 years of age with a pathologic fracture or lytic lesion are much more likely to have metastatic bone disease than a primary bone tumor.
- The prognosis for patients with metastatic bone disease is improving because of early recognition and better adjuvant treatment; therefore, many patients will live more than 2 years.
- Do not immediately assume that a lytic lesion or pathologic fracture is from metastatic disease. A thorough workup and possible biopsy are required.
- Prophylactic fixation for impending fractures from metastatic disease is technically easier for the surgeon and allows a quicker patient recovery.
- The Mirels scoring system is available to guide the treatment of an impending fracture from metastatic bone disease.
- Femoral neck fractures from metastatic bone disease require

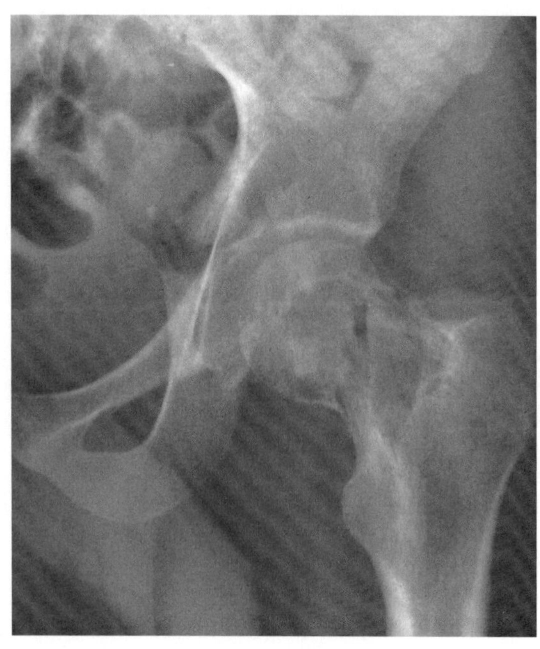
A

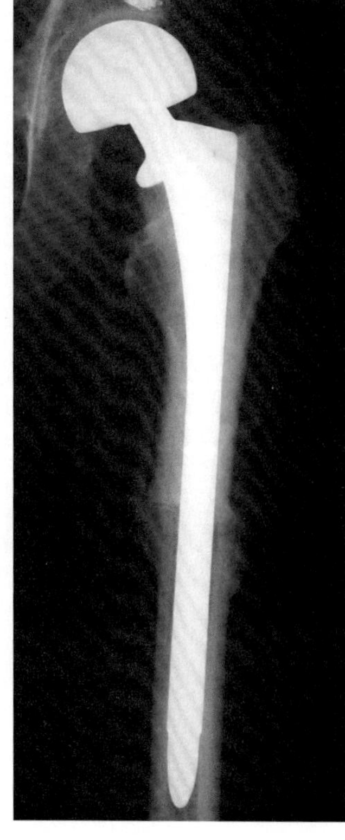
B

FIGURE 20-19 **A.** Anteroposterior x-ray of the left hip in a 24-year-old male with a pathologic fracture of the femoral neck. He had pain for 6 months before sustaining the fracture after minimal trauma. This history in a young healthy patient should raise suspicion of an underlying process in the bone. There is matrix production within the lesion, and an open biopsy revealed a grade 2 chondrosarcoma. **B.** X-ray 18 months after resection of the proximal femur and hip capsule and reconstruction with an allograft-prosthetic composite. The prosthesis is cemented into the allograft and press-fit into the host bone. The patient was free of local recurrence when he died of metastatic disease 2 years later.

a cemented hip prosthesis, because internal fixation has a high rate of failure with disease progression.

- When surgery is required for metastatic disease to the spine, decompression and stabilization with internal fixation are generally necessary.
- Surgical reconstruction for pathologic fractures should be durable enough to allow immediate weightbearing and last throughout the patient's expected lifespan.
- A pathologic fracture through a primary malignant bone tumor is treated much differently than a fracture through a metastatic lesion.
- Treatment of patients with pathologic fractures requires the presence of a multidisciplinary team composed of orthopaedic surgeons, medical oncologists, radiation oncologists, endocrinologists, radiologists, pathologists, pain specialists, nutritionists, physical therapists, and psychologists/psychiatrists.

REFERENCES

1. U.S. Department of Health and Human Services. Bone Heath and Osteoporosis: A Report of the Surgeon General. Rockville, MD: U.S. Department of Health and Human Services, Office of the Surgeon General; 2004.
2. Riggs BL, Melton LJ III. The worldwide problem of osteoporosis: insights afforded by epidemiology. *Bone* 1995;17(5 Suppl):505S–511S.
3. Leibson CL, Tosteson AN, Gabriel SE, et al. Mortality, disability, and nursing home use for persons with and without hip fracture: a population-based study. *J Am Geriatr Soc* 2002;50(10):1644–1650.
4. Cummings SR, Melton LJ. Epidemiology and outcomes of osteoporotic fractures. *Lancet* 2002;359(9319):1761–1767.
5. Jemal A, Tiwari RC, Murray T, et al. Cancer statistics 2004. *Cancer J Clin* 2004;54(1): 8–29.
6. Weber KL, Lewis VO, Randall L, et al. An approach to the management of the patient with metastatic bone disease. *Instr Course Lect* 2004;53:663–676.
7. Coleman RE. The clinical use of bone resorption markers in patients with malignant bone disease. *Cancer* 2002;94(10):2521–2533.
8. Demers LM, Costa L, Lipton A. Biochemical markers and skeletal metastases. *Clin Orthop* 2003;S415:S138–S147.
9. Chybowski FM, Larson-Keller JJ, Bergstralh EJ, et al. Predicting radionucleotide bone scan finding in patients with newly diagnosed untreated prostatic cancer: prostate specific antigen is superior to all other clinical parameters. *J Urol* 1991;145:313–318.
10. Ralston S, Fogelman I, Gardner MD, et al. Hypercalcemia and metastatic bone disease: is there a casual link? *Lancet* 1982;2:903–905.
11. Fisken RA, Heath DA, Somers S, et al. Hypercalcemia in hospital patients. *Lancet* 1981; 1:202–207.
12. Sherry MM, Greco FA, Johnson DH, et al. Metastatic breast cancer confined to the skeletal system: an indolent disease. *Am J Med* 1986;81:381–386.
13. Coleman RE, Purohit OP, Black C, et al. Double-blind, randomized, placebo-controlled, dose-finding study or oral ibandronate in patient with metastatic bone disease. *Ann Oncol* 1999;10:311–316.
14. Gucalp R, Theriault R, Gill I, et al. Treatment of cancer-associated hypercalcemia: double blind comparison of rapid and slow intravenous infusion regimens of pamidronate disodium and saline alone. *Arch Intern Med* 1994;154:1935–1944.
15. Major P, Lortholary A, Hon J, et al. Zoledronic acid is superior to pamidronate in the treatment of hypercalcemia of malignancy: a pooled analysis of two randomized, controlled clinical trials. *J Clin Oncol* 2001;19:558–567.
16. Clohisy DR, Palkert D, Pedurovsky I, et al. Human breast cancer induces osteoclast activation and increases the number of osteoclasts at sites of tumor osteolysis. *J Ortho Res* 1996;14(3):396–402.
17. Guise TA. Molecular mechanisms of osteolytic bone metastases. *Cancer* 2000;88: 2892–2898.
18. Roodman GD. Biology of osteoclast activation in cancer. *J Clin Oncol* 2001;19: 3562–3571.
19. Teitelbaum SL. Bone resorption by osteoclasts. *Science* 2000;289(5484):1504–1508.
20. Weber KL, Gebhardt MC. Specialty update: what's new in musculoskeletal oncology. *J Bone Joint Surg* 2003;85(4):761–767.
21. Bertin KC, Horstman J, Coleman SS. Isolated fractures of the lesser trochanter in adults: an initial manifestation of metastatic malignant disease. *J Bone Joint Surg* 1984;66: 770–773.
22. Coerkamp EG, Kroon HM. Cortical bone metastasis. *Radiology* 1988;169:525–528.
23. Greenspan A, Norman A. Osteolytic cortical destruction: an unusual pattern of skeletal metastases. *Skeletal Radiol* 1988;17:402–406.
24. Ohta M, Tokuda Y, Suzuki Y, et al. Whole body PET for the evaluation for bony metastases in patients with breast cancer: comparison with 99Tcm-MDP bone scintigraphy. *Nucl Med Commun* 2001;22(8):875–879.
25. Peterson JJ, Kransdorf MJ, O'Conner ML. Diagnosis of occult bone metastases: positron emission tomography. *Clin Orthop* 2003;(415 Suppl):S120–S128.
26. Even-Sapir E, Metser U, Flusser G, et al. Assessment of malignant skeletal disease: initial experience with 18F-fluoride PET/CT and comparison between 18F-Fluoride PET and 18F-fluoride PET/CT. *J Nucl Med* 2004;45(2):272–278.
27. Rougraff BT, Kneisl JS, Simon MA. Skeletal metastases of unknown origin: a prospective study of a diagnostic strategy. *J Bone Joint Surg* 1993;75:1276–1281.
28. Weber KL. Specialty update: what's new in musculoskeletal oncology. *J Bone Joint Surg* 2004;86:1104–1109.
29. Mankin HJ, Mankin CJ, Simon MA. The hazards of the biopsy, revisited. Members of the Musculoskeletal Tumor Society. *J Bone Joint Surg* 1996;78:656–663.
30. Bartucci EJ, Gonzalez MH, Cooperman DR, et al. The effect of adjunctive methylmethacrylate on failures of fixation and function in patients with intertrochanteric fractures and osteoporosis. *J Bone Joint Surg* 1985;67:1094–1107.
31. Jacofsky DJ, Papagelopoulos PJ, Sim FH. Advances and challenges in the surgical treatment of metastatic bone disease. *Clin Orthop* 2003;(415 Suppl):S14–S18.
32. Fidler M. Prophylactic internal fixation of secondary neoplastic deposits in long bones. *Br Med J* 1973;1:341–343.
33. Snell W, Beals RL. Femoral metastases and fractures from breast carcinoma. *Surg Gynecol Obstet* 1964:119:22–24.
34. Mirels H. Metastatic disease in long bones: a proposed scoring system for diagnosing impending pathological fractures. *Clin Orthop* 1989;249:256–265.
35. Hipp JA, Springfield DS, Hayes WC. Predicting pathologic fracture risk in the management of metastatic bone defects. *Clin Orthop* 1995;312:120–135.
36. Hong J, Cabe GD, Tedrow JR, et al. Failure of trabecular bone with simulated lytic defects can be predicted non-invasively by structural analysis. *J Orthop Res* 2004;22(3): 479–486.
37. Bunting RW, Boublik M, Blevins FT, et al. Functional outcome of pathologic fracture secondary to malignant diseases in a rehabilitation hospital. *Cancer* 1992;69:98–102.
38. Katzer A, Meenen NM, Grabbe F, et al. Surgery of skeletal metastases. *Arch Orthop Trauma Surg* 2002;122(5):251–258.
39. Lipton A, Theriault RL, Hortobagyi GN, et al. Pamidronate prevents skeletal complications and is effective palliative treatment in women with breast carcinoma and osteolytic bone metastases: long term follow-up of two randomized, placebo-controlled trials. *Cancer* 2000;88:1082–1090.
40. Townsend P, Smalley S, Cozad S. Role of postoperative radiation therapy after stabilization of fractures caused by metastatic disease. *Int J Radiat Oncol Biol Phys* 1995;31:43.
41. Gainor BJ, Buchert P. Fracture healing in metastatic bone disease. *Clin Orthop* 1983; 178:297–302.
42. Brown RK, Pelker RR, Friedlaender GE, et al. Postfracture irradiation effects on the biomechanical and histologic parameters of fracture healing. *J Orthop Res* 1991;9: 876–882.
43. Harrington KD, Sim FH, Enis JE, et al. Methylmethacrylate as an adjunct in internal fixation of pathologic fractures. *J Bone Joint Surg* 1976;58(8):1047–1055.
44. Sim FH, Daugherty TW, Ivins JC. The adjunctive use of methylmethacrylate in fixation of pathological fractures. *J Bone Joint Surg* 1974;56:40–48.
45. Eftekhar NS, Thurston CW. Effect of irradiation on acrylic cement with special reference to fixation of pathological fractures. *J Biomech* 1975;8:53–56.
46. Ward WG, Spang J, Howe D, et al. Femoral recon nails for metastatic disease: indications, technique, and results. *Am J Orthop* 2000;29(9 Suppl):34–42.
47. Weber KL, O'Connor MI. Operative treatment of long bone metastases: focus on the femur. *Clin Orthop* 2003;S276–S278.
48. Yazawa Y, Frassica FJ, Chao EY, et al. Metastatic bone disease: a study of the surgical treatment of 166 pathologic humeral and femoral fractures. *Clin Orthop* 1990;251: 213–219.
49. Russo P. Renal cell carcinoma: presentation, staging, and surgical treatment. *Semin Oncol* 2000;27:160–176.
50. Durr HR, Maier M, Pfahler M, et al. Surgical treatment of osseous metastases in patients with renal cell carcinoma. *Clin Orthop* 1999:367:283–290.
51. Jung ST, Ghert MA, Harrelson JM, et al. Treatment of osseous metastases in patients with renal cell carcinoma. *Clin Orthop* 2003;(409):223–231.
52. Swanson DA. Surgery for metastases of renal cell carcinoma. *Scand J Surg* 2004;93(2): 150–155.
53. Chatziioannou AN, Johnson ME, Penumaticos SG, et al. Preoperative embolization of bone metastases from renal cell carcinoma. *Eur J Radiol* 2000;10:593–596.
54. Kumar D, Grimer RJ, Abudu A, et al. Endoprosthetic replacement of the proximal humerus. Long-term results. *J Bone Joint Surg Br* 2003;85(5):717–722.
55. Damron TA, Sim FH, Shives TC, et al. Intercalary spacers in the treatment of segmentally destructive diaphyseal humeral lesions in disseminated malignancies. *Clin Orthop* 1996;324:233–243.
56. Damron TA, Rock MG, Choudhury SN, et al. Biomechanical analysis of prophylactic fixation for middle third humeral impending pathologic fractures. *Clin Orthop* 1999; 363:240–248.
57. Dijkstra S, Stapert J, Boxma H, et al. Treatment of pathological fractures of the humeral shaft due to bone metastases: a comparison of intramedullary locking nail and plate osteosynthesis with adjunctive bone cement. *Eur J Surg Oncol* 1996;22:621–626.
58. Redmond BJ, Biermann JS, Blasier RB. Interlocking intramedullary nailing of pathological fractures of the shaft of the humerus. *J Bone Joint Surg* 1996;78:891–896.

59. Henry JC, Damron TA, Weiner MM, et al. Biomechanical analysis of humeral diaphyseal segmental defect fixation. *Clin Orthop* 2002;(396):231–239.
60. Weber KL, Lin PP, Yasko AW. Complex segmental elbow reconstruction after tumor resection. *Clin Orthop* 2003;415:31–44.
61. Leeson MC, Makley JT, Carter JR. Metastatic skeletal disease distal to the elbow and knee. *Clin Orthop* 1986;206:94–99.
62. Brahme SK, Cervilla V, Vinct V, et al. Magnetic resonance appearance of sacral insufficiency fractures. *Skeletal Radiol* 1990;19:489–493.
63. Newhouse KE, El-Khoury GY, Buckwalter JA. Occult sacral fractures in osteopenic patients. *J Bone Joint Surg* 1992;74:1472–1477.
64. Harrington KD. The management of acetabular insufficiency secondary to metastatic malignant disease. *J Bone Joint Surg* 1981;63(4):653–664.
65. Kunisada T, Choong PF. Major reconstruction for periacetabular metastasis: early complications and outcome following surgical treatment in 40 hips. *Acta Orthop Scand* 2000;71(6):585–590.
66. Vena VE, Hsu J, Rosier RN, et al. Pelvic reconstruction for severe periacetabular metastatic disease. *Clin Orthop* 1999;(362):171–180.
67. Aboulafia AJ, Buch R, Mathews J, Li W, et al. Reconstruction using the saddle prosthesis following excision of primary and metastatic periacetabular tumors. *Clin Orthop* 1995;(314):203–213.
68. Abudu A, Grimer RJ, Cannon SR, et al. Reconstruction of the hemipelvis after the excision of malignant tumors. Complications and functional outcome of prostheses. *J Bone Joint Surg Br* 1997;79(5):773–779.
69. Marco RA, Sheth DS, Boland PJ, et al. Functional and oncological outcome of acetabular reconstruction for the treatment of metastatic disease. *J Bone Joint Surg* 2000;82(5):642–651.
70. Bobyn JD, Stackpool GJ, Hacking SA, et al. Characteristics of bone ingrowth and interface mechanics of a new porous tantalum biomaterial. *J Bone Joint Surg Br* 1999;81(5):907–914.
71. Ward WG, Spang J, Howe D. Metastatic disease of the femur. Surgical management. *Orthop Clin North Am* 2000;31(4):633–645.
72. Lane JM, Sculco TP, Zolan S. Treatment of pathological fractures of the hip by endoprosthetic replacement. *J Bone Joint Surg* 1980;62(6):954–959.
73. Behr JT, Dobozi WR, Badrinath K. The treatment of pathologic and impending pathologic fractures of the proximal femur in the elderly. *Clin Orthop* 1985;(198):173–178.
74. Papagelopoulos PJ, Galanis EC, Greipp PR, et al. Prosthetic hip replacement for pathologic or impending pathologic fractures in myeloma. *Clin Orthop* 1997;(341):192–205.
75. Churchill DL, Incavo SJ, Uroskie JA, et al. Femoral stem insertion generates high bone cement pressurization. *Clin Orthop* 2001;(393):335–344.
76. Weikert DR, Schwartz HS. Intramedullary nailing for impending pathological subtrochanteric fractures. *J Bone Joint Surg Br* 1991;73(4):668–670.
77. Sim FH, Chao EY. Hip salvage by proximal femoral replacement. *J Bone Joint Surg* 1981;63(8):1228–1239.
78. Barwood SA, Wilson JL, Molnar RR, et al. The incidence of acute cardiorespiratory and vascular dysfunction following intramedullary nail fixation of femoral metastasis. *Acta Orthop Scand* 2000;71(2):147–152.
79. Eckardt JJ, Kabo M, Kelly CM, et al. Endoprosthetic reconstruction for bone metastases. *Clin Orthop* 2003;S254–S262.
80. De Geeter K, Reynders P, Samson I, et al. Metastatic fractures of the tibia. *Acta Orthop Belg* 2001;67(1):54–59.
81. Hattrup SJ, Amadio PC, Sim FH, et al. Metastatic tumors of the foot and ankle. *Foot Ankle* 1988;8(5):243–247.
82. Boland PJ, Lane JM, Sundaresan N. Metastatic disease of the spine. *Clin Orthop* 1982;169:95–102.
83. Suen KC, Lau LL, Yermakov V. Cancer and old age. An autopsy study of 3,535 patients over 65 years old. *Cancer* 1974;33:1164–1168.
84. Yuh WTC, Zacharck CK, Barloon TJ, et al. Vertebral compression fractures: distinction between benign and malignant causes with MR imaging. *Radiology* 1989;172:215–218.
85. Akeyson EW, McCutcheon IE. Single-stage posterior vertebrectomy and replacement combined with posterior instrumentation for spinal metastasis. *J Neurosurg* 1996;85(2):211–220.
86. Dudeney S, Lieberman IH, Reinhardt MK, et al. Kyphoplasty in the treatment of osteolytic vertebral compression fractures as a result of multiple myeloma. *J Clin Oncol* 2002;20(9):2382–2387.
87. Harrington KD. Anterior decompression and stabilization of the spine as a treatment for vertebral collapse and spinal cord compression from metastatic malignancy. *Clin Orthop* 1988;233:177–197.
88. Lieberman I, Reinhardt MK. Vertebroplasty and kyphoplasty for osteolytic vertebral collapse. *Clin Orthop* 2003;(415 Suppl):S176–S186.
89. Liu JK, Apfelbau RI, Chiles BW III, et al. Cervical spinal metastasis: anterior reconstruction and stabilization techniques after tumor resection. *Neurosurg Focus* 2003;15(5):E2.
90. Turgut M, Gul B, Girgin O, et al. Role of surgical treatment in 70 patients with vertebral metastasis causing cord or root compression. *Arch Orthop Trauma Surg* 1997;116:415–419.
91. Tokuhashi Y, Matsuzaki H, Toriyama S. A scoring system for the preoperative evaluation of metastatic spine tumor prognosis. *Spine* 1990;15:1110.
92. Tomita K, Kawahara N. Kobayashi T, et al. Surgical strategy for spinal metastasis. *Spine* 2001;26:298.
93. Rades D, Blach M, Nerreter V, et al. Metastatic spinal cord compression. Influence of time between onset of motoric deficits and start of irradiation on therapeutic effect. *Strahlenther Onkol* 1999;175(8):378–381.
94. Kanayama M, Ng JT, Cunningham BW, et al. Biomechanical analysis of anterior versus circumferential spinal reconstruction for various anatomic stages of tumor lesions. *Spine* 1999;24(5):445–450.
95. Bates T, Yarnold JR, Blitzer P, et al. Bone metastasis consensus statement. *Int J Radiat Oncol Biol Phys* 1992;23:215.
96. Arcangeli G, Micheli A, Arcangeli F, et al. The responsiveness of bone metastases to radiotherapy: the effect of site, histology and radiation dose on pain relief. *Radiother Oncol* 1989;14:95–101.
97. Serafini AN. Therapy of metastatic bone pain. *J Nucl Med* 2001;42:895–906.
98. Robinson RG, Blake GM, Preston DF, et al. Strontium–8: treatment results and kinetics in patients with painful metastatic prostate and breast cancer in bone. *Radiographics* 1989;9:271.
99. Rogers MJ, Gordon S, Benford HL, et al. Cellular and molecular mechanisms of action of bisphosphonates. *Cancer* 2000;88:2961–2978.
100. Gronemeyer DH, Schirp S, Gevargez A. Image-guided radiofrequency ablation of spinal tumors: preliminary experience with an expandable array electrode. *Cancer J* 2002;8(1):33–39.
101. Callstrom MR, Charboneau JW, Goetz MP, et al. Painful metastases involving bone: feasibility of percutaneous CT- and US-guided radio-frequency ablation. *Radiology* 2002;224:87–97.
102. Goetz MP, Callstrom MR, Charboneau JW, et al. Percutaneous image-guided radiofrequency ablation of painful metastases involving bone: a multicenter study. *J Clin Oncol* 2004;22:300–306.
103. Weill A, Kobaiter H, Chiras J. Acetabulum malignancies: technique and impact on pain of percutaneous injection of acrylic surgical cement. *Eur Radiol* 1998;8(1):123–129.
104. Campanacci M, Capanna R, Picci P. Unicameral and aneurysmal bone cysts. *Clin Orthop* 1986;204:25–36.
105. Raab P, Hohmann F, Kuhl J, et al. Vertebral remodeling in eosinophilic granuloma of the spine. A long-term follow-up. *Spine* 1998;23(12):1351–1354.
106. Yasko AW, Fanning CV, Ayala AG, et al. Percutaneous techniques for the diagnosis and treatment of localized Langerhans-cell histiocytosis (eosinophilic granuloma of bone). *J Bone Joint Surg* 1998;80(2):219–228.
107. Easley ME, Kneisl JS. Pathologic fractures through nonossifying fibromas: is prophylactic treatment warranted? *J Pediatr Orthop* 1997;17:808–813.
108. Scarborough M, Moreau G. Benign cartilage tumors. *Orthop Clin N Am* 1996;27:683–589.
109. Tordai P, Lugnegard H. Is the treatment of enchondroma in the hand by simple curettage a rewarding method? *J Hand Surg* 1990;15B:331–334.
110. Stephenson R, London M, Hankin F, et al. Fibrous dysplasia: an analysis of option for treatment. *J Bone Joint Surg* 1987;69-A:400–409.
111. Guille JT, Jumar SJ, MacEwin GD. Fibrous dysplasia of the proximal part of the femur. Long-term results of curettage and bone-grafting and mechanical realignment. *J Bone Joint Surg* 1998;80:648–658.
112. Lane JM, Khan SN, O'Connor WJ, et al. Bisphosphonate therapy in fibrous dysplasia. *Clin Orthop* 2001;382:6–12.
113. Campanacci M, Baldini N, Boriani S, et al. Giant cell tumor of bone. *J Bone Joint Surg* 1987;69:106–114.
114. Bacci G, Ferrari S, Longhi A, et al. Nonmetastatic osteosarcoma of the extremity with pathologic fracture at presentation: local and systemic control by amputation or limb salvage after preoperative chemotherapy. *Acta Orthop Scand* 2003;74(4):449–54.
115. Scully SP, Ghert MA, Zurakowski D, et al. Pathologic fracture in osteosarcoma: prognostic importance and treatment implications. *J Bone Joint Surg* 2002;84-A(1):49–57.
116. Fuchs B, Valenzuela RG, Sim FH. Pathologic fracture as a complication in the treatment of Ewing's sarcoma. *Clin Orthop* 2003;(415):25–30.
117. Bjornsson J, McLeod RA, Unni KK, et al. Primary chondrosarcoma of long bones and limb girdles. *Cancer* 1998;15;83(10):2105–2119.

21

STRESS FRACTURES

David C. Teague

Much has changed in our understanding of stress fractures since Breithaupt's 1855 initial account describing a syndrome of painful swollen feet among marching Prussian soldiers (1). It wasn't until 1956 that the first report of the condition was shown in athletes (2). Originally the domain of military recruits and military physicians, recreational and competitive athletes with stress fractures now commonly present to civilian practitioners. Athletic populations involved in team and individual sports increasingly develop overuse injuries, and stress fractures have been reported in most bones in the body.

Stress fracture incidences evade precise determination in athletic populations due to variability in training programs and lack of standardized reporting (3). Track and field teams have shown incidences from 10% to 31%, with lesser but substantial numbers noted for participants in gymnastics, ballet, figure skating, basketball, crew, soccer, and lacrosse (4,5). United States military recruits develop lower-extremity stress fractures at a gender-dependent rate of up to 4% in men and 7% in women (6–9).

By convention, stress fractures occur in normal bone when the bone is subjected to abnormal or unaccustomed stresses. This condition is distinct from insufficiency fractures, wherein normal stresses applied to abnormal bone produce fracture.

PRINCIPLES OF MANAGEMENT

Pathophysiology of Injury

Various forces exert loads on bone during all physical activities. Ground and joint reaction forces as well as muscle forces stress the bone by applying force across unit areas of bone. These stresses yield local deformation or change in length, termed *strain*. Stress, a measure of the load applied, produces strain or bone deformation in a given direction (10).

According to Wolff's law, normal loads delivered to normal bone produce normal bone remodeling (11). This remodeling response to cyclic loading entails initial osteoclastic bone resorption followed by osteoblastic new bone formation within cortical bone, as well as on the trabeculae of cancellous bone (12,13). The resorption process peaks at 3 weeks, but it takes 3 months to adequately create the new bone to complete the remodeling cycle (14–17). When optimally loaded and enough time is provided for remodeling, bone mass remains static, no stress fracture or injury ensues, and the bone becomes stronger (16–20). Repetitive loading, however, outstrips the bone's ability to create new bone in the resorption tunnels and engenders a resorption-dominated accelerated remodeling process that actually weakens the bone (14,8,20–22). With continued repetitive loading, a positive feedback mechanism develops in which increased mechanical usage stimulates bone turnover, resulting in focally increased remodeling space or porosity and decreased bone mass. This weakened site is more susceptible to further microdamage, which will incite additional resorption. Ultimately, stress fracture can result from continued loading superimposed on the focally decreased bone mass generated by progressively larger resorption sites (23).

Signs and Symptoms

A careful history of load-related pain often points to the likely diagnosis of stress fracture. Most athletes can accurately characterize their symptom progression and relate the gradual onset of vague pain over a period of weeks during training. Symptoms are initially described as mild and present only during the stress or activity (18). The symptoms very often occur during the first few weeks after an increase in training volume or intensity, a change in technique or surface, or an alteration of footwear. Any change in a previously regimented training program may be the inciting historical event (10,22,24). For nonathletes, a recent atypical increase in activity (e.g., a vacation with a great deal more walking than usual or a new aerobic exercise program) may be described (25). If left unchecked, the process may progress to persistent pain after training, pain at rest, and even night pain. Pertinent historical questions relate to potential risk factors. History of previous stress fractures or other painful sites, and the presence of eating disorders, leg length discrepancy, or muscle imbalance should be evaluated. In the female patient, age of menarche and presence of menstrual irregularities must be considered. For athletes, training regimen alterations are usually the root cause of the pain. For runners, the most common training change is a significant increase in the distance run during a brief period of training (26). Furthermore, the potential impact to the patient must be assessed. For example, a scholarship athlete may wish to make different treatment choices than a weekend runner.

The hallmark physical finding is focal bone pain with palpation and stressing, but findings vary depending on the stress fracture's location and the time from injury onset to presentation. When the site is accessible, local swelling may be noted. Percussion of the bone typically produces pain, but passive and active range of motion of adjacent joints does not. The anatomical location of the pain can help in the diagnosis. For example, femoral diaphyseal fractures occur typically in the medial cortex, so lateral thigh pain is not likely to be correlated with a stress fracture (25). Inaccessible sites require indirect physical tests for diagnosis. For example, pain produced by hip extension while standing on the opposite leg may implicate stress fractures of the pars interarticularis (27).

Risk Factors

In general, the predominant risk factor for developing a stress fracture is an increase in training frequency and intensity. Work based on concepts by Grimston and Frost allows analysis of the factors that may lead to the bone's failure to successfully adapt to the mechanical loads to which it is exposed (28–30). Mechanical competence of bone depends on properties such as bone density and geometry, all related to cellular activity. The theoretical mechanosensory system of bone, classically considered as Wolff's law, can be understood as a mechanostat that senses strain, compares it to a given threshold, and initiates an adaptive cellular response. Physiological, mechanical, and pharmacological factors generate mechanostat responses by providing functional stimuli to the bone. Systemic constraints on bone health (e.g., genetics or eating disorders) may impede the bone's ability to respond despite messages from the mechanostat.

In contrast to elderly patients with osteoporosis and bone density measurements predictive of fragility fracture risks, the majority of young active individuals have normal bone density (31). Little work points to any significant connection between bone density and risk of stress fracture in men. Studies of male soldiers and runners typically find no difference in tibial bone density between those with and without stress fractures (32–34). Although not clearly causally related, low bone density may be a risk factor for women (35). A multivariate analysis shows a strong association between low femoral neck bone density and risk of stress fracture in female military recruits (36). An 8% lower bone density at the tibia was identified in a subgroup of female track athletes who developed tibial stress fractures (33). The density measures for these women were still higher than those for similar less-active nonathletes, perhaps suggesting that the bone density athletes require may be greater than that needed by the general population. In summary, bone density measurement does not appear to be a useful screening tool for stress fractures (35).

Smaller bone size appears to predispose to stress fracture (28). In a prospective evaluation of more than 600 military recruits, up to 10% smaller tibial width and cross-sectional area was found among those who developed stress fractures (37). Similar results for male runners are reported (34). Although bone geometry likely impacts stress fracture development, currently no practical imaging system allows this variable to be used as a screening tool.

Activity that produces repetitive loading can lead to stress fracture development. Multiple factors influence the clinical responses to bone loading (28). Most studies support the notion that poor baseline physical fitness predisposes to stress fracture development when there is a significant increase in activity (38–40), but well-conditioned athletes also develop stress fractures, so other factors must be considered. Load magnitude and rate appear to present the most significant stimulation of bone cellular dynamics, so the training regimen of soldiers and athletes often merits scrutiny (28). Training modifications including rest periods (41,42), banning concrete as a training surface (24,43), use of running shoes (24,44), and restricting high-impact activities (42,45,46) can reduce the incidence of stress fractures in military recruits. Surveys of athletes relate changes in training in more than 80% before the onset of a stress fracture.

Increased training volume is related to higher stress fracture risks in ballet dancers and runners (47,48).

The role of flexibility, either too much or not enough, cannot be conclusively documented to contribute to stress fracture development (28). Many investigators have evaluated factors including joint mobility, laxity, and muscle length. Only limited ankle dorsiflexion and increased hip external rotation have been somewhat implicated in stress fracture development (32,49,50). Similarly, the contribution of foot structure to stress fracture risk is controversial (51,52). For example, some studies support an association in male military recruits between high midfoot arch and greater risk of stress fracture (51,53). This correlation does not appear in all studies, however (54). The stress fracture and foot type relationship is likely variable depending on which bone is involved. Leg length discrepancy actually appears to increase the chance of stress fracture for military and athletic individuals, but the risk is not specific to either the shorter or the longer limb (33,47,55).

Impact attenuation during training should alter the functional stimuli transmitted to the bone. Conventionally, the training surface is considered to be a factor in the development of stress fracture. Most physicians advise athletes to avoid training on hard, uneven surfaces, but no clear scientific data support or refute this recommendation (28). Although ground reaction forces decrease with more compliant running surfaces, running or walking on these same surfaces may result in more or earlier muscle fatigue (56,57).

No studies demonstrate a correlation between a host of body size and composition factors and the incidence of stress fractures (28). Height, weight, body mass index, body girth and width, as well as many other variables, have been investigated (33,48,58,59). Even in military recruits who display more variability in body size than typical groups of similar athletes, no consistent associations between stress fractures and body size and composition can be shown (32,39,40,46).

Whereas multiple endogenous hormones affect skeletal homeostasis, sex hormones, primarily in women, appear to have substantial impact on the stress fracture risks. There is no relationship between lowered testosterone levels and stress fractures for male athletes (60). Even when testosterone levels are decreased, they are typically within the range of normal for healthy adult men (61–63). Conversely, female athletes with menstrual irregularities are uniformly found to have an increased risk for developing stress fractures. These women with menstrual disturbances present a relative risk for stress fractures that is two to four times higher than for eumenorrheic athletes (35). Additionally, amenorrheic athletes are at a higher risk of developing multiple stress fractures (64). Lifetime menstrual history similarly yields information regarding the risk of stress fracture, and the historically regular athletes report a risk that is 20% less than those with very irregular menstrual cycles.

The mechanism that produces increased stress fracture risk with menstrual disturbance is unclear and most certainly multifactorial. Nevertheless, the association is unassailable and is frequently found presenting together with eating disorders and osteopenia. This combination, known as the *female athlete triad*, mandates that attention is directed to all facets of the patient's condition (35,65). Eating disorders occur more commonly in female athletes than males (66,67). Even active-duty female soldiers admit to an 8% prevalence of eating disorders (68). Disordered eating patterns appear to increase the risk of stress fractures in ballet dancers and young adult female track athletes (69,70). Without a doubt, extreme weight-control behavior in college athletes doubles the risk of stress fracture (71). Note that low calcium intake does not appear to be an important risk factor in otherwise healthy athletes and military recruits (35).

Stress fractures occur in people of all ages. The peak incidence appears in late adolescence and early adulthood among military recruits, competitive and recreational athletes, and dancers. (8,52,72–75). Age is an important factor in determining the location of stress fractures, but age does not appear to be an important factor in their etiology (72).

Imaging Modalities

The diagnosis of a stress fracture often does not require imaging studies, especially when a careful history and a classic physical examination combine to make the diagnosis with certainty; however, several radiographic modalities are at the disposal of the clinician for definitive documentation and differential evaluations. Plain x-rays, bone scintigraphy, computed tomography (CT), and magnetic resonance imaging (MRI) scans are now the routine examinations that are used to evaluate and diagnose stress fractures.

Plain X-rays

X-rays obtained very early in the stress fracture process typically are not effective in demonstrating an abnormality. Findings rarely appear before 2 to 3 weeks from the onset of symptoms. New periosteal bone formation, the classic radiographic marker of a healing response, often does not appear until 3 months from symptom onset. In some patients, radiographic changes never appear for a number of stress fractures (76). When changes are evident, a number of findings confirm the presence of a stress fracture, rendering this modality poorly sensitive but highly specific. Only 20% of bone scan foci positive for stress fractures correlate with positive plain film findings (77,78). The false-negative rate for x-rays approaches 100% for early grade I bone scan positive lesions, but drops to 24% for grade III lesions, demonstrating that stress fractures have more ability to remodel and respond to the altered stresses later in their course, and the later response is often apparent on plain x-rays.

Findings associated with fractures may include periosteal bone formation, horizontal or oblique linear patterns of sclerosis, endosteal callus, and a frank fracture line. The initial radiographic sign of a progressing stress fracture is the gray cortex, which corresponds to a low-density cortical area affected by increased osteoclastic bone resorption activity (10) (Fig. 21-1). As the process evolves in long bones, the stress fracture undergoes marginal resorption and may yield an ovoid lucency within

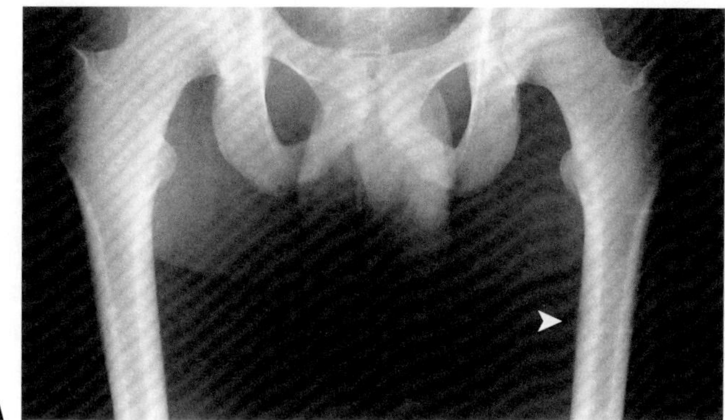

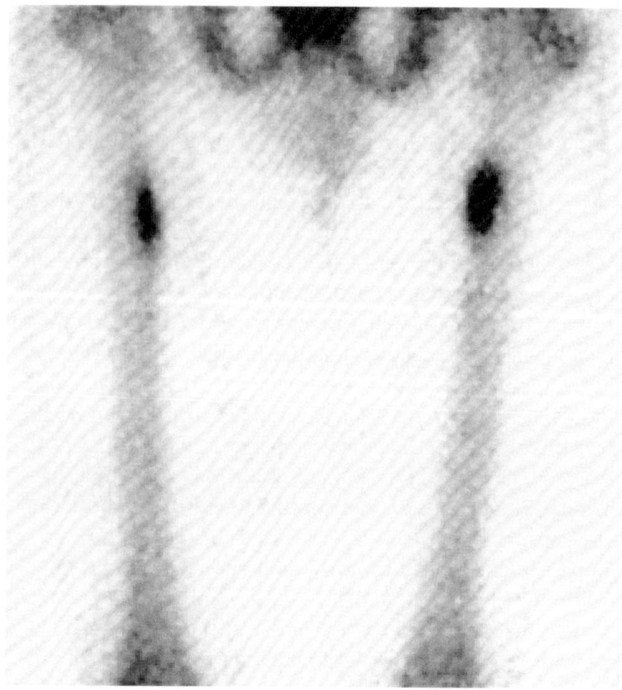

FIGURE 21-1 Imaging studies for a 20-year-old distance runner with bilateral proximal activity-related thigh pain. **A.** Plain film demonstrates the gray cortex on the left femur (arrow) with minimal changes on the right. **B.** Delayed spot image scintigraphic study shows grade 3 increased activity at the left proximal femur, while the right side shows a slightly less intense increased signal.

a thickened area of cortical hyperostosis (27). A late-stage stress fracture in cortical bone appears as a radiolucent line with extension partially or completely across the cortex. Similar-stage stress fractures in cancellous bone demonstrate a fracture lucency oriented perpendicular to the trabeculae. Healing is noted by focal sclerosis in areas of cancellous bone, whereas diaphyseal healing involves both periosteal and endosteal cortical thickening (27). Plain films are most likely to present positive findings in the fibula and metatarsals. Films should be centered over the painful, suspected bone and typically are not helpful in discerning stress injuries to the pars interarticularis. Some investigators contend that plain films are unlikely to yield positive results when investigating possible tibial stress fractures, and others state the femur, pars, and tarsal bones are least likely to yield remarkable findings on initial plain film investigation. (27,76).

Scintigraphy

When x-ray findings are conclusive, additional studies are not required. If multiple sites of stress fracture are possible based on history and physical examination, or if plain films do not support the presumptive diagnosis of stress fracture, three-phase bone scintigraphy has been the study of choice. Bone scan has long been considered the most sensitive test for stress fracture, with sensitivity approaching 100% (10,76), but the sensitivity is not coupled with high specificity, so clinical features must be correlated.

Isotopes are atoms with identical atomic numbers but different atomic weights, and a nuclide is the nucleus of a given isotope. Nuclides or isotopes with differences in numbers of protons and neutrons are unstable and give off particles or electromagnetic radiation in their transition to stability known as *radioactive decay*. These materials are synonymously called *radionuclides* or *radioisotopes*. When used for diagnostic purposes, the materials are termed *radiopharmaceuticals* and *radiotracers* (79).

Technetium-99m methylene diphosphonate (^{99m}Tc MDP) is the usual radioisotope utilized for bone scans. Gamma radiation is emitted, and the whole body dose for a bone scan is about 0.13 to 0.19 rad. The bladder dose, where the radioactivity is concentrated in the urine, is 2.62 to 3.90 rads, hence the need for frequent voiding during and after the scanning period.

^{99m}Tc MDP is available in good supply at low cost, has a 6-hour half-life, and emits gamma energy at an ideal frequency for gamma cameras used in diagnostic imaging (79).

The radioisotope is administered as a bolus intravenously. The mechanism of uptake in bone is not precisely elucidated, but blood flow to the bone is a fundamental requirement. In normal bone, uptake is in proportion to blood flow to the bone. In abnormal situations such as stress fractures that are accompanied by high bone vascularity, factors other than bone blood flow play a larger role in radiotracer uptake. New bone formation proves to be the most important factor in the uptake, whereas bone destruction without new bone formation yields no increase in uptake (27,79).

Bone scintigraphy is performed in three phases, two early and one delayed. The initial images acquired immediately after radiotracer injection are representative of blood perfusion to bone as well as soft tissue and correspond roughly to contrast angiography. The second set of images, obtained approximately

2 to 5 minutes after injection and termed the *blood pool scans*, show radionuclide location in the soft tissues or extravascular space. These images reflect the extent of hyperemia and capillary permeability, and generally correspond to the acuity and severity of the injury. At 2 to 4 hours after injection, the delayed images document radionuclide accumulation in the skeleton and, to a lesser extent, the soft tissue. Over this time, 50% of the diphosphonate tracer is postulated to be adsorbed on the hydroxyapatite matrix of bone, with special affinity for new bone formation sites (76).

Given a correlating history and physical examination, the scintigraphic diagnosis of stress fracture is made by focal increased uptake on the third-phase images. Stress fractures are positive on all three phases, but periostitis develops positive foci only on the delayed images (27,80,81). Other soft tissue injuries are positive only in the first two phases, allowing some differentiation between bony and soft tissue pathology; however, the lack of specificity remains a disadvantage of this modality (27,76). The typical list of conditions producing similar localized uptake includes osteoid osteoma, other bony tumors, osteomyelitis, bony infarct, and bony dysplasias. Due to its improved ability to differentiate many of these conditions, MRI scanning may be the diagnostic method of choice in certain settings.

Radionuclide scans can be positive within hours of a bone injury (27). Acute stress fractures are positive on all three phases. As bony healing proceeds, the initial phase perfusion scan normalizes first. Within the ensuing few weeks, the blood pool second-phase images return to normal. Because bony remodeling continues for an extended time period, focal uptake on the delayed images resolves last. Uptake gradually diminishes in intensity over 3 to 6 months, but some increased uptake can last up to 1 year, even in uncomplicated stress fractures with uneventful healing (80). For this reason, bone scans are not particularly useful for monitoring healing and do not merit frequent repeating.

A grading system, based on the scintigraphic appearance, allows classification into milder or more severe stress fractures, recognizing that these stress injuries occur along a continuum of bony involvement (Table 21-1) (78). The minimally symptomatic grade 1 or grade 2 stress fractures typically resolve more quickly and completely. The grading system can assist in prescribing the requisite rest and rehabilitation intervals (27).

Single-photon emission CT (SPECT scanning) is used when lumbosacral stress fractures are suspected. The camera rotates about the patient, generating 3-D images of radioisotope uptake. This modality is particularly useful for investigating suspected pars interarticularis and sacral stress fractures (10,27).

MRI

MRI scans provide identical sensitivity and superior specificity compared to bone scintigraphy for evaluating stress fractures

TABLE 21-1 Bone Scintigraphy and MRI Grading Scale

Grade	Bone Scan	MRI
1	Small, ill-defined cortical area of mildly increased activity	Periosteal edema: mild to moderate on fat-suppressed T2 or STIR images; marrow is normal on T1 and fat-suppressed T2 or STIR images
2	Better-defined cortical area of moderately increased activity	Periosteal edema: moderate to severe on fat-suppressed T2 or STIR images; marrow edema on fat-suppressed T2 or STIR images
3	Wide to fusiform, cortical-medullary area of highly increased activity	Periosteal edema: moderate to severe on fat-suppressed T2 or STIR images; marrow edema on T1 and fat-suppressed T2 or STIR images
4	Transcortical area of intensely increased activity	Periosteal edema: moderate to severe on fat-suppressed T2 or STIR images; marrow edema on T1 and fat-suppressed T2 or STIR images; fracture line clearly visible

Adapted and reprinted with permission from Fredericson M, Bergman G, Hoffman KL, et al. Tibial stress reaction in runners: correlation of clinical symptoms and scintigraphy with a new magnetic resonance imaging grading system. *Am J Sports Med* 1995;23(4):472–481.

(82,83). The improved specificity derives from the comprehensive anatomic visualization provided from this modality, allowing for precise localization of the injury and differentiation from other possible conditions. The bony tissue, with comparatively few mobile protons, is not represented in significant detail. Instead, the MRI scan accentuates reactive edema in the soft tissues and marrow surrounding a stress injury. This soft tissue response is seen best in edema-sensitive sequences such as fat-suppressed T2-weighted and short tau inversion recovery (STIR) scans. Areas of edema appear as high-signal intensity sites on these sequences (27,84).

A grading system that corresponds to the scintigraphic grading system addresses the typical progression of stress injury documented on MRI scans (Table 21-1) (85). Earliest injuries demonstrate increased signal intensity first in the periosteum, and then also in the marrow on STIR and T2 images, while the T1 scans are normal. In grade 3 injuries, decreased marrow signal occurs with the T1 sequence, while the STIR and T2 sequences yield even higher-intensity marrow changes. Grade 4 stress fractures feature a low-signal fracture line on both sequences, continuous with the cortex and medullary space (84,85) (Fig. 21-2).

Although plain x-rays and bone scintigraphy accurately diagnose stress fractures in most patients, MRI scans are increasingly advocated as the study of choice (27,76,82) because they do not involve exposure to ionizing radiation and require much shorter imaging times than bone scintigraphy. The specificity of MRI scans significantly exceeds that of scintigraphy (86); for this reason, straightforward cases can be investigated reliably without MRI, but more difficult diagnostic dilemmas or problematic cases may well warrant MRI scanning.

CT

CT scans provide excellent bony anatomic detail. The delineation of fracture line orientation is assisted with 3-D CT information, which may improve treatment decisions for certain bones such as the tarsal navicular (87,88). Longitudinal fracture lines in diaphyseal locations can also be elucidated. Pars and sacral stress fractures are also well characterized with CT scans (10).

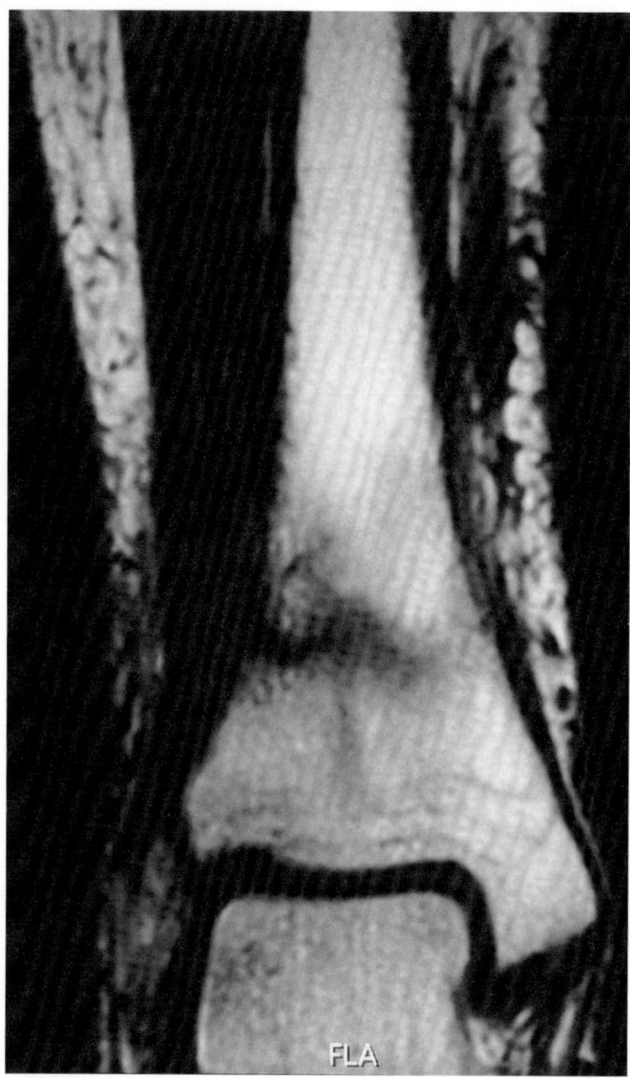

FIGURE 21-2 Coronal T1-weighted MR image of a grade 4 distal tibia stress fracture with visible fracture line and surrounding marrow edema.

TREATMENT RATIONALE

The fundamental principle of initial management is modified rest to allow the bone remodeling process to equilibrate. The inciting strain must be eliminated in order to break the cycle of accelerated resorption, allowing new bone formation to catch up and adequately repair the focus of stress fracture (10,26). Earlier initiation of rest, when the resorption-formation mismatch is minimal, allows a brief period of activity restriction to suffice (89). For athletes, alternative training should continue, provided regimens can be devised that unload the area of stress fracture. For nonathletes, a brief rest period is usually well tolerated and adequate to reverse the process.

Different stress fracture sites mandate certain specific management approaches, but the overarching message of activity modification and rest applies to every site. During this first treatment phase, remediable risk factors should be addressed. The training errors or changes that precipitated the stress fracture should be identified and corrected (18). Braces or other forms of immobilization are seldom needed. No controlled study strongly supports adjunctive measures akin to external electrical stimulation or ultrasound (52,90–92). For high-level athletes, early pool running programs prove highly successful at maintaining baseline fitness during the rest phase (93,94).

Second-phase rehabilitation begins when pain is substantially diminished or absent (10,26). For lower-extremity injuries, this time frame is roughly 2 weeks after painless walking is resumed (18,85). The training program emphasizes progressive aerobic conditioning with specified rest times to permit bone compensation for the slowly increasing strains (42,93). Provided that the progression does not reproduce the patient's pain, activity reintroduction proceeds steadily. Cross training is advisable to reduce the likelihood of recurrence (93). Surgery is seldom contemplated or required for managing most stress fractures.

CURRENT TREATMENT OPTIONS

Lower Extremity

Femoral Neck

Early recognition of femoral neck stress fractures prevents catastrophic consequences. Younger patients typically present with inferior or medial neck lesions, commonly known as *compression-side stress fractures*. Older patients are prone to superior, tension-side fractures, and these are more likely to fail and displace with continued activity (95–97). With either lesion, patients complain of activity-related diffuse groin or anterior hip pain and have pain at the limits of hip rotation on examination. MRI scans may be more accurate than scintigraphy in this region and provide differential information for other causes of hip pain such as tendonitis, bone cysts, or avascular necrosis of the femoral head (86).

Stage 1 or 2 injuries without a cortical crack are treated with a modified rest protocol beginning with an initial period of non-weight bearing until pain resolves. Stage 3 compression side injuries, demonstrating a nondisplaced cortical crack, are still stable and can be managed nonoperatively (Fig. 21-3) (97). Tension-sided stage 3 injuries with a nondisplaced crack can be managed similarly with complete unloading and frequent clinical and radiographic follow-up to document healing (97,98). Due to the long-term functional consequences of a displaced femoral neck fracture, however, some investigators support stabilization with cannulated screw fixation for this injury (99). Stage 4 injuries demonstrate widening of the cortical crack or even frank displacement of the completed fracture. These injuries demand operative stabilization. Nondisplaced complete fractures are stabilized with multiple screws. Fluoroscopic-guided curettage of the tension-side fracture site has been advocated. In young people with displaced fractures, emergent open reduction with internal fixation is mandatory (97,100). A recent series of displaced femoral neck stress fractures in military recruits associates delayed surgery and varus malreduction with an increased risk of avascular necrosis and poor function (101). In older patients, consideration can be given to hip arthroplasty depending on the individual situation.

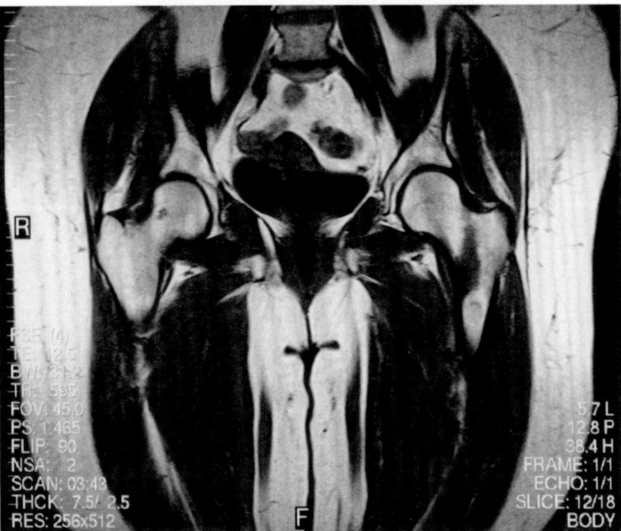

FIGURE 21-3 Coronal T1-weighted pelvis MR image of a 50-year-old female runner demonstrates a grade 3 left compression-side femoral neck stress fracture. The darker marrow signal represents edema.

Femoral Shaft

In most athletes, femoral diaphyseal stress fractures occur proximally in the medial or posteromedial cortex (5,102) (Fig. 21-1). Vague activity related anterior thigh pain is the typical complaint, and vigorous stressing on physical examination can reproduce the pain (95). These lesions occur in sites of compressive stress, are stable, and heal with modified rest protocols. Only catastrophic complete failures require reamed intramedullary stabilization.

Tibia

Tibial stress fractures are the most commonly reported among the many lower-extremity stress fractures (52). Other overuse injuries may simultaneously present or require elimination from the differential diagnosis. Inflammation of the aponeurotic tenoperiosteal origins of the tibialis posterior, and soleus and fascial attachments to the posterior medial border of the tibia produces pain previously termed *shin splints* and characterized as *medial tibial stress syndrome*. Pain from this inflammatory situation typically occurs along the medial border of the tibia, improves after warm up, and is worse in the morning. Exertional compartment syndromes of the anterior or deep posterior compartments present with muscle aching and subjective tightness that increase shortly after exercise begins. No bony tenderness usually accompanies this condition. Tibial stress fracture pain is progressive, with a gradual onset exacerbated by exercise and worse with impact, ultimately occurring while simply walking, or even at rest or at night. Tenderness is localized and bony (103).

The majority of tibial stress fractures are posteromedial compression injuries and usually occur in the proximal or distal thirds (103,104). When a fracture has developed, transverse orientation is typical (Fig. 21-2), but longitudinal stress fractures are also reported (105). These fractures respond well to cessation of the repetitive loading activity, which almost always is distance running, along with complete leg rest using crutches until the pain subsides (103). Some work suggests adjunctive treatment with a pneumatic brace may facilitate earlier functional return to activity by accelerating the initial time to pain-free walking (106,107). Surgery is not required for this condition, but return to activity can take up to 3 months (26).

The more unusual but significantly more vexing tibial stress fracture appears in the middle-third of the anterior cortex. This tension-side injury results from repetitive stress of jumping or leaping, as seen in basketball players and ballet dancers. Bone pain is easily demonstrated, and palpable periosteal thickening may be present if the process is chronic. These fractures frequently progress to nonunion, and complete fractures are also reported (104,108). In chronic cases, a transverse, wedge-shaped defect in the anterior cortex, dubbed the *dreaded black line*, is often seen in conjunction with cortical hypertrophy (26) (Fig. 21-4). Tissue obtained from these sites shows limited biologic potential, consistent with a pseudarthrosis (109,110).

Initial conservative treatment requires prolonged modified rest, with or without cast or brace immobilization (111); however, even over 4 to 6 months, many fractures with chronic changes and anterior fissures or cracks will remain symptomatic and nonunited. Some investigators have shown healing benefits from adjunctive electrical stimulation or ultrasound in nonoperative protocols (90–92), whereas others demonstrate no benefits from these modalities (108). Transverse drilling of the nonunion sites reportedly stimulates healing and speeds time to return to activity (18,26,109). Reamed intramedullary nailing works well for recalcitrant cases, and now has some support as the initial treatment of choice for the anterior cortical stress fracture nonunion (112,113).

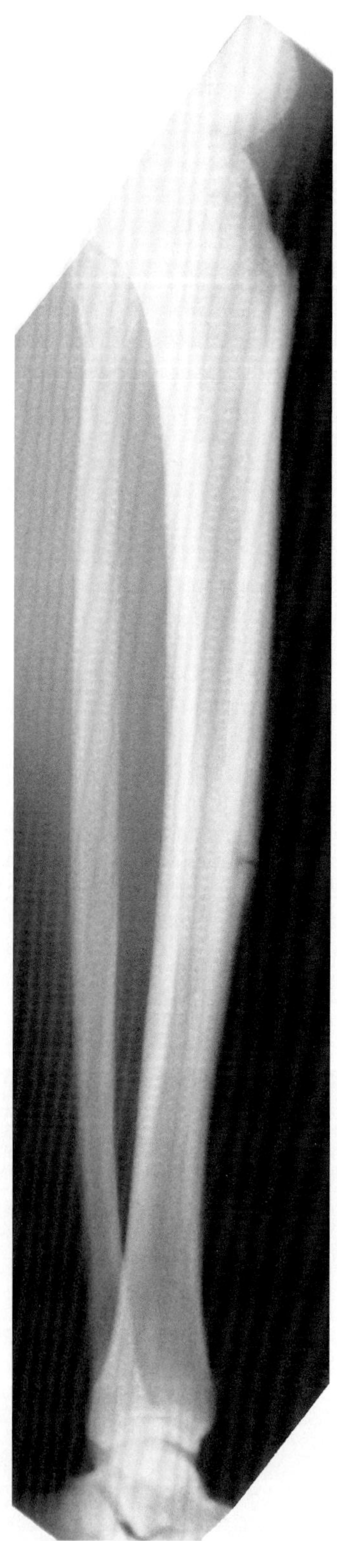

FIGURE 21-4 Lateral radiograph of the left tibia of a collegiate track athlete demonstrates anterior cortical hypertrophy and the dreaded black line of an anterior tension-side stress fracture.

Medial Malleolus

Participants in repetitive running and jumping activities are at risk for developing medial malleolus stress fractures characterized by bony tenderness and ankle effusion. The typically vertically oriented fracture line originates at the junction between the malleolus and plafond directly above the medial border of the talus, which is postulated to be the cyclic force transmitter (104,114). For grade 1 and 2 injuries, impact avoidance in a cast or pneumatic brace achieves return to function in 6 to 8 weeks. For grade 3 and 4 stress fractures, similar conservative measures are appropriate, but healing may take 4 to 5 months. More aggressive intervention is also supported depending on the injury chronicity and the demands of the patient. Drilling may enhance healing (115). Screw fixation for displaced fractures, nonunion, chronic cases, and elite performers allows early motion and may promote earlier return to activity (103,104).

Tarsal Navicular

Repetitive running and jumping activity places sprinters, hurdlers, middle-distance runners, football players, basketball players, ballet dancers, and other athletes at risk for tarsal navicular stress fracture (52,116). Insidious onset vague medial arch pain usually accompanies dorsal navicular tenderness to palpation (117). The stress fracture occurs in the sagittal plane in the relatively avascular central third of the bone, originating at the proximal dorsal articular surface and extending in a plantar distal direction (104,118). Plain x-rays often fail to demonstrate the navicular stress fracture (119). Although bone scintigraphy is sensitive, CT or MRI scans pro-

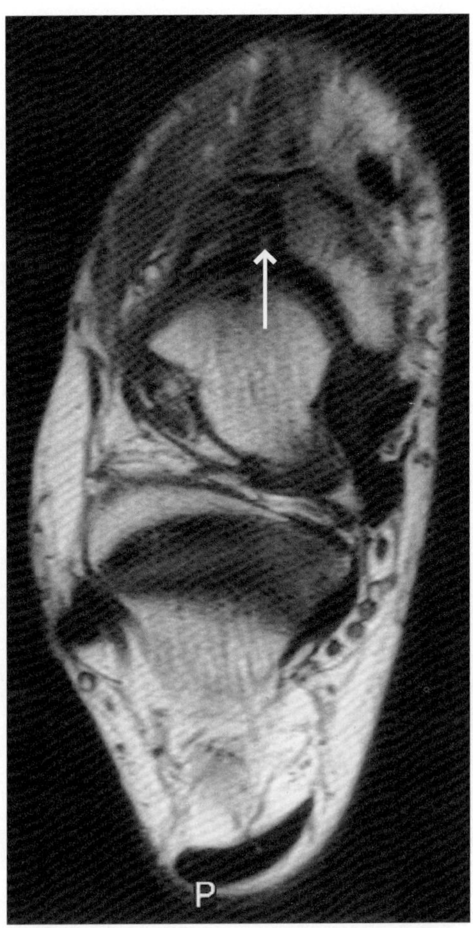

FIGURE 21-5 T1-weighted MR image of the right ankle of a collegiate basketball player shows a navicular stress fracture (arrow) originating at the talonavicular joint surface.

vide specific information regarding fracture completeness and orientation (104) (Fig. 21-5).

Among patients with an early diagnosis, 6 weeks of non–weight-bearing cast immobilization yields high union rates (118,120). Conversely, less than 25% of patients treated with weight-bearing immobilization heal, and the risk of delayed union and recurrence is also much higher (118,120–123). After the initial period of strict non-weight bearing, graduated return to activity is pursued, provided the physical examination reveals no navicular tenderness (117). In cases of displaced fractures, delayed unions, and nonunions, surgical stabilization is undertaken (104). Compression screw fixation alone usually provides adequate stability. Often, the dorsal cortex is not visibly disrupted, so placing supplemental bone graft may require more extensive dissection except in cases of complete, displaced stress fractures or nonunions (121,123). Non-weight bearing after fixation is advised.

Metatarsals

Metatarsal stress fractures are common in distance runners and ballet dancers (117). The second metatarsal neck is the most likely site for stress fracture, but all metatarsals are susceptible. Gradually worsening forefoot pain exacerbated by running or dancing herald the diagnosis, especially when accompanied by focal bony tenderness. For short-lived complaints, initiating modified rest without imaging studies usually leads to symptom resolution. For uncertain diagnoses or chronic complaints, imaging modalities provide clarification. A second metatarsal plantar base stress fracture recognized only in female ballet dancers appears to be secondary to the *en pointe* position and responds to rest and activity modification (124).

Stress fracture of the proximal diaphysis of the fifth metatarsal, common in basketball players, often are slow to heal and can have high recurrence rates (125,126). The problematic site is in the proximal 1.5 cm of the diaphysis, where cortical hypertrophy commonly occurs in running and jumping athletes, rendering the zone relatively avascular with a narrow medullary canal (127). Treatment choices are predicated on the stage of the lesion as described by Torg (125,128). Patients with acute fractures often acknowledge a 2- to 3-week prodromal history of activity-related lateral foot pain. These acute injuries show clear fracture lines with no medullary sclerosis and little or no cortical hypertrophy. Healing in most acute fractures ensues with a 6- to 8-week course of non–weight-bearing cast immobilization (128–131). Closed treatment with full weight bearing appears to predispose to nonunion and refracture (126). Surgical management of acute stress fractures, especially in athletes, is recommended by some physicians to avoid prolonged healing. Sliding bone graft procedures (132–134) and intramedullary compression screw fixation (135,136) techniques usually result in satisfactory healing within 3 months (137).

Patients with a history of previous injury and recurrent symptoms will have radiographic evidence of delayed union or nonunion. Delayed unions demonstrate a wider fracture completely through the medial and lateral cortices with some medullary sclerosis (Fig. 21-6). A very wide gap with periosteal new bone formation and complete medullary sclerosis characterizes the appearance of established nonunions (125,128). Delayed unions may heal with prolonged non–weight-bearing cast immobilization, but functional recovery often requires 6 months (128,130). Most active patients with delayed union and virtually all with an established nonunion recover faster with surgical management. Torg advises sclerotic bone debridement and inlay bone grafting (128). Other investigators propose a sliding bone graft (132) or compression screw fixation (136,138) (Fig. 21-6). For those averse to surgery, electrical stimulation has been shown to be effective (139).

Other Sites

Stress fractures are reported in most of the remaining bones in the lower extremity. Rare patella stress fractures, usually transverse but occasionally longitudinal, respond to extension immobilization for 4 weeks followed by progressive rehabilitation (103,140,141). Runners and jumpers are susceptible to this injury. Failure to improve and acute displacement are indications for open management with tension band stabilization

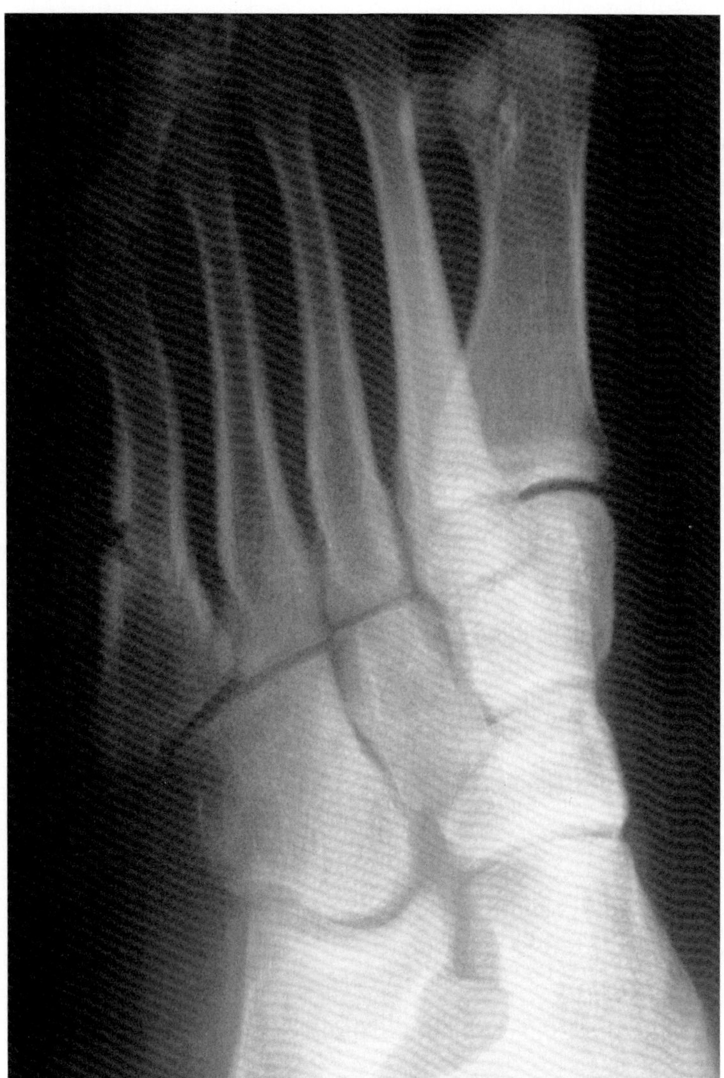

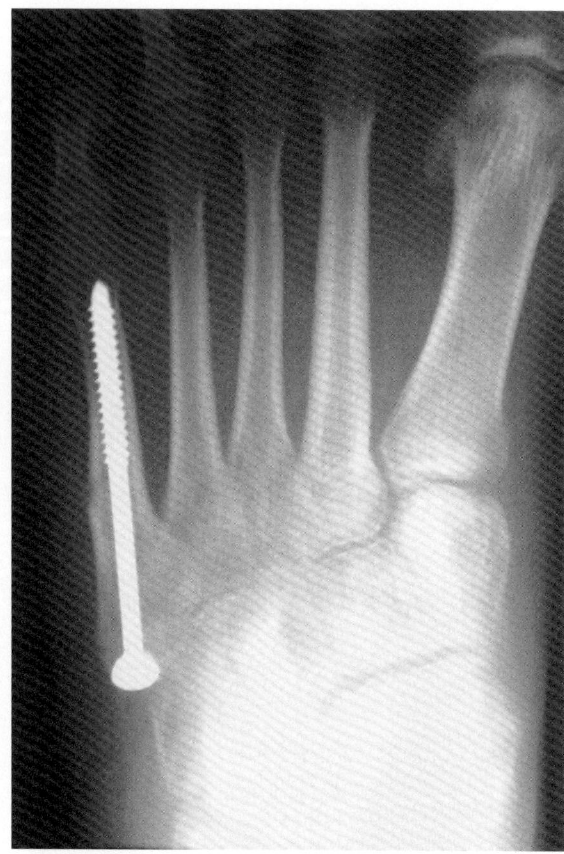

FIGURE 21-6 Middle-aged recreational runner with a several-month history of worsening activity-related lateral foot pain. **A.** Intermediate delayed union fifth metatarsal stress fracture with a complete fracture, some widening of the cortical gap, and moderate medullary sclerosis. **B.** Radiographic appearance 3 months after medullary drilling, bone grafting, compression screw stabilization, and an initial period of non-weight bearing.

(142). Fibula stress fractures occur typically in runners 1 to 2 inches above the ankle joint line, are much less common than tibial injuries, and usually respond to modified rest protocols (18,143). Talar neck stress fractures are rare. Stress fractures of the lateral process of the talus are encountered on occasion, and a 6-week period of non-weight bearing helps to control symptoms (18,117). Surgical stabilization or excision may be considered for recalcitrant or displaced cases (144,145). Calcaneal stress fractures occur typically transversely through the tuberosity in soldiers, runners, ballet dancers, and jumpers (117). Conservative treatment measures are always sufficient. Similarly, a few reports of cuboid and cuneiform stress fractures describe successful modified rest treatment protocols (146, 147).

Upper Extremity

Stress fractures in non–weight-bearing bones result from repetitive strains associated with recurrent loading activities such as rowing, swimming, and throwing. The possibility of stress fracture should be considered in athletes primarily involved in upper extremity sports who complain of gradual onset bony pain associated with the activity. Physical examination typically reveals bony tenderness to palpation and stressing. Imaging modalities are useful for clarifying the diagnosis. Modified rest and training technique corrections or alterations almost always result in early healing and return to activity (148).

Most humerus stress fractures occur in baseball pitchers, although other reports detail this finding in athletes ranging from tennis players to weight lifters (148). All of these athletes can be managed with modified rest and gradual activity resumption. One report describes progression of humerus stress fractures to spontaneous shaft fractures in men in a baseball league (149). The risk factors for complete fracture included age over 30 years, prolonged layoff from pitching before resuming participation, no regular exercise program, and prodromal arm pain.

In older adolescents and young adults involved in throwing sports or gymnastics, the presentation of gradually increasing elbow pain with activity mandates consideration of an olecranon stress fracture (148). Some patients who complain less of prodromal symptoms and more of acute elbow pain related to a particularly strong throwing effort may have tip avulsion fractures involving up to the proximal third of the olecranon. Surgical excision of the fractured tip allows early return to sports (150). Patients with classical stress fractures complain of longer-duration pain that recurs when throwing resumes. These fractures are usually transverse and in the middle third of the olecranon. Among baseball players, the olecranon is the most common site for stress fracture. Adolescent gymnasts can also develop this type of stress fracture (151). For nondisplaced fractures, immobilization and progressive return to activity are recommended. When displaced or delayed in healing, tension band fixation is effective (150–152).

Stress fractures of the ulna may occur in baseball and softball pitchers, tennis players, weight lifters, and volleyball players. Repetitive strains from underhanded softball pitching and two-handed tennis backhand strokes represent the typical inciting stresses. The athletes complain of bony pain with activity and even after the activity. Depending on the stage of injury, x-rays may show periosteal bone formation or a small cortical fracture. All reports document healing with modified rest for 4 to 6 weeks and progressive resumption of activity (148,153).

Stress injuries to the distal radial physis are common in young gymnasts (154), but radial shaft stress fractures in young adults are less common. Bilateral shaft stress fractures have been seen in a gymnast who doubled her weekly training time (155). Athletes in any sport who begin a high-stress weight program are at risk for developing a radial stress reaction. The typical modified rest protocol should be instituted for the radius. If weight training is the inciting stress, but the athlete's primary sport does not repetitively load the radius, continued participation in the sport usually presents no additional risk.

Repetitive strains to the metacarpals, particularly the second and fifth, can lead to stress fracture (153). Patients describe a change in training volume and technique. Tennis players may be susceptible at the second metacarpal because the racquet provides a fulcrum (156). Rest from the activity will yield healing and return to the sport within 4 weeks, provided technique errors and training overload are altered.

Pelvis

Stress fractures of the pubic rami occur not uncommonly in female distance runners, most of whom have associated risk factors. When present, groin pain prevents further training, and single-leg stance reproduces the pain. Deep palpation of the bone in these characteristically thin individuals typically elicits significant pain. Plain films and bone scintigraphy are usually diagnostic. An 8- to 12-week modified training regimen allows graduated return to activity (157).

Sacral stress fractures predominantly develop in female distance runners, but are also reported in their male counterparts. Most patients have prodromal low back and buttock pain. Physical examination demonstrates localized tenderness to palpation and stress of the sacroiliac region. SPECT scanning has been the investigation of choice, but MRI scanning now provides more specificity. Implementing initial protected weight bearing followed by a progressive activity regimen reliably leads to uneventful healing (158,159).

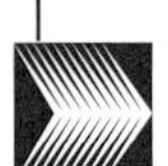

AUTHOR'S PREFERRED TREATMENT

A modified rest protocol successfully addresses the majority of stress fractures, and this initial conservative approach should be considered for all stress fractures and implemented for most. Patients with certain high-risk or problematic stress fractures may benefit from early surgical intervention, however.

Grade 3 or grade 4 tension-side femoral neck stress fractures should be stabilized with multiple screw fixation to promote healing and prevent displacement. Because the patients who develop this injury are usually runners, care must be taken to place the screws in good position and avoid lateral entry points below the midportion of the level of the lesser trochanter to minimize the risk of iatrogenic subtrochanteric fracture from stress risers. Acutely displaced femoral neck stress fractures require urgent open reduction and internal fixation in the typical younger, active population.

Anterior tibial stress fractures with an established transverse cortical lucency have limited healing potential even with activity modification. For patients who fail the rest and rehabilitation protocol, or for those unwilling or unable to modify their activities for perhaps as long as 1 year, reamed intramedullary nailing predictably leads to healing of the stress fracture in a shorter time course. Inadequate data make predicting long-term functional outcomes after nailing uncertain, regarding return to unrestricted sport or military activity.

For acute tarsal navicular stress fractures, an initial 6-week period of non–weight-bearing cast immobilization is the treatment of choice. For patients with delayed diagnosis or delayed union, compression screw stabilization provides high union rates. Displaced fractures and established sclerotic nonunions require open reduction internal fixation and supplemental bone graft.

Acute fifth metatarsal stress fractures treated with strict non–weight-bearing cast immobilization seldom require further intervention. The intermediate delayed union injury is preferentially managed with intramedullary compression screw placement after the medullary canal at the fracture site has been adequately drilled to remove fibrous tissue and sclerotic bone (Fig. 21-6). The established nonunion requires open debridement of the fracture gap with placement of graft, combined with intramedullary screw placement.

ACKNOWLEDGMENTS

The author thanks Doug Beall, MD, and Weyton Tam, MD, for providing the figures in this article and W. Bentley Edmonds, MD, Don McGinnis, MD, and Brock Schnebel, MD, for providing cases and sports medicine expertise.

REFERENCES

1. Briethaupt MD. Fur pathologie des menschlichen fusses. *Medizinische Zeitung* 1855;24: 169–177.
2. Devas MB, Sweetnam R. Stress fractures of the fibula: a review of 50 cases in athletes. *J Bone Joint Surg* 1956;38B:818–829.
3. Shaffer RA. Incidence and prevalence of stress fractures in military and athletic populations. In: Burr DB, Milgrom C, eds. *Musculoskeletal fatigue and stress fractures*. Boca Raton: CRC Press, 2001:1–14.
4. Bennell KL, Malcolm SA, Thomas SA, et al. The incidence and distribution of stress fractures in competitive track and field athletes. A twelve-month prospective study. *Am J Sports Med* 1996;24:211–217.
5. Johnson AW, Weiss CB, Jr, Wheeler DL. Stress fractures of the femoral shaft in athletes—more common than expected. A new clinical test. *Am J Sports Med* 1994;22: 248–256.
6. Almeida SA, Williams KM, Shaffer RA, et al. Epidemiological patterns of musculoskeletal injuries and physical training. *Med Sci Sports Exerc* 1999;31:1176–1182.
7. Gilbert RS, Johnson HA. Stress fractures in military recruits—a review of twelve years' experience. *Mil Med* 1966;131:716–721.
8. Jones BH, Cowan DN, Tomlinson JP, et al. Epidemiology of injuries associated with physical training among young men in the army. *Med Sci Sports Exerc* 1993;25: 197–203.
9. Kelly EW, Johnson SR, Cohen ME, et al. Stress fractures of the pelvis in female navy recruits: an analysis of possible mechanisms of injury. *Mil Med* 2000;165:142–146.
10. Carpenter RD, Matheson GO, Carter DR. Stress fractures and stress injuries in bone. In: Garrick JG, ed. *Orthopaedic knowledge update: sports medicine*, 3rd ed. Rosemont, IL: American Academy of Orthopaedic Surgeons, 2004:273–283.
11. Chamay A, Tschants P. Mechanical influence in bone remodeling: experimental research on Wolff's law. *J Biomech* 1972;2:173–180.
12. Brukner P, Bennell K, Matheson G. The pathophysiology of stress fractures. In: *Stress fractures*. Victoria: Blackwell Science, 1999:1–13.
13. Buckwalter JA, Glimcher MJ, Cooper RR, et al. Bone biology. *J Bone Joint Surg* 1995; 77–A:1276–1289.
14. Jones BH, Harris J, Vinh TN, et al. Exercise-induced stress fractures and reactions of bone. Epidemiology, etiology and classification. *Exerc Sports Sci Rev* 1989;17:379–422.
15. Sterling JC, Edelstein DW, Calvo RD, et al. Stress fractures in the athlete: diagnosis and management. *Sports Med* 1992;14:336–346.
16. Frost HM. Some ABC's of skeletal patho-physiology vs. microdamage physiology. *Calcif Tissue Int* 1991;49:229–231.
17. Sallis RE, Jones K. Stress fractures in athletes: How to spot this underdiagnosed injury. *Post Grad Med* 1991;89:185–192.
18. Lassus J, Tulikoura I, Konttinen Y, et al: Bone stress injuries of the lower extremity: a review. *Acta Orthop Scan* 2002;73:359–368.
19. Uhthoff HK, Jaworski ZG. Periosteal stress-induced reactions resembling stress fractures: a radiologic and histologic study in dogs. *Clin Orthop* 1985;199:284–291.
20. Frost HM. Wolff's law and bone's structural adaptation to mechanical usage: an overview for clinicians. *Angle Orthod* 1994;64:175–188.
21. Burr DB. Remodeling and the repair of fatigue damage. *Calcif Tissue Int* 1993;53(Suppl 1):S75–S81.
22. Maitra RS, Johnson DL. Stress fractures. Clinical history and physical examination. *Clin Sports Med* 1997;16:259–274.
23. Schaffler MB. Bone fatigue and remodeling in the development of stress fractures. In: Burr DB, Milgrom C, eds. *Musculoskeletal fatigue and stress fractures*. Boca Raton: CRC Press, 2001:161–182.
24. Greaney RB, Gerber FH, Laughlin, RL et al. Distribution and natural history of stress fractures in US Marine recruits. *Radiology* 1983;146:339–346.
25. Ekenman I. Physical diagnosis of stress fractures. In: Burr DB, Milgrom C, eds. *Musculoskeletal Fatigue and Stress Fractures*. Boca Raton: CRC Press, 2001:271–278.
26. Reeder MT, Dick BH, Atkins JK, et al. Stress fractures: current concepts of diagnosis and treatment. *Sports Med* 1996;22:198–212.
27. Brukner P, Bennell K, Matheson G. Diagnosis of stress fractures. In: *Stress fractures*. Victoria: Blackwell Science, 1999:83–96.
28. Bennell K, Grimston S. Risk factors for developing stress fractures. In: Burr DB, Milgrom C, eds. *Musculoskeletal fatigue and stress fractures*. Boca Raton: CRC Press, 2001:15–33.
29. Grimston SK. An application of mechanostat theory to research design: a theoretical model. *Med Sci Sports Exerc* 1993;25:1293–1297.
30. Frost HM, Skeletal structural adaptations to mechanical usage (SATMU): redefining Wolff's Law. *Anat Rec* 1990;226:403–413.
31. Bennell KL, Malcolm SA, Khan KM, et al. Bone mass and bone turnover in power athletes, endurance athletes and controls: a 12-month longitudinal study. *Bone* 1997; 20:477–484.
32. Giladi M, Milgrom C, Simkin A, et al. Stress fractures: identifiable risk factors. *Am J Sports Med* 1991;19:647–652.
33. Bennell KL, Malcolm SA, Thomas SA, et al. Risk factors for stress fractures in track and field athletes: a 12 month prospective study. *Am J Sports Med* 1996;24:810–818.
34. Crossley K, Bennell KL, Wrigley T, et al. Ground reaction forces, bone characteristics and tibial stress fracture in male runners. *Med Sci Sports Exerc* 1999;31:1088–1093.
35. Bennell K, Grimston S. Factors associated with the development of stress fractures in women. In: Burr DB, Milgrom C, eds. *Musculoskeletal fatigue and stress fractures*. Boca Raton: CRC Press, 2001: 35–54.
36. Lauder TD, Dixit S, Pezzin LE, et al. The relation between stress fractures and bone mineral density: evidence from active-duty army women. *Arch Phys Med Rehab* 2000; 81:73–79.
37. Beck TJ, Ruff CB, Mourtada FA, et al. Dual-energy x-ray absorptiometry derived structural geometry for stress fracture prediction in male U.S. Marine Corps recruits. *J Bone Miner Res* 1996;11:645–653.
38. Shaffer RA, Brodine SK, Almeida SA, et al. Use of simple measures of physical activity to predict stress fractures in young men undergoing a rigorous physical training program. *Am J Epidemiol* 1999;149:236–242.
39. Winfield AC, Moore J, Bracker M, et al. Risk factors associated with stress reactions in female marines. *Mil Med* 1997;162:698–702.
40. Cline AD, Jansen GR, Melby CL. Stress fractures in female army recruits–implications of bone density, calcium intake, and exercise. *J Am Coll Nutr* 1998;17:128–135.
41. Worthen BM, Yanklowitz BA. The pathophysiology and treatment of stress fractures in military personnel. *J Am Podiatric Med Assoc* 1978;68:317–325.
42. Scully TJ, Besterman, G. Stress fracture—a preventable training injury. *Mil Med* 1982; 147:285–287.
43. Reinker KA, Ozburne, SA. A comparison of male and female orthopaedic pathology in basic training. *Mil Med* 1979;144:532–536.
44. Proztman RR. Physiologic performance of women compared to men. *Am J Sports Med* 1979;7:191–195.
45. Pester S, Smith PC. Stress fractures in the lower extremities of soldiers in basic training. *Orthop Rev* 1992;21:297–303.
46. Taimela S, Kujala UM, Osterman K. Stress injury proneness: a prospective study during a physical training program. *Int J Sports Med* 1990;11:162–165.
47. Brunet ME, Cook SD, Brinker MR, et al. A survey of running injuries in 1505 competitive and recreational runners. *J Sports Med Phy Fitness* 1990;30:307–315.
48. Kadel NJ, Teitz CC, Kronmal RA. Stress fractures in ballet dancers. *Am J Sports Med* 1992;20:445–449.
49. Hughes LY. Biomechanical analysis of the foot and ankle for predisposition to developing stress fractures. *J Orthop Sports Phys Therapy* 1985;7:96–101.
50. Giladi M, Milgrom C, Stein M, et al. External rotation of the hip. A predictor of risk for stress fractures. *Clin Orthop Related Res* 1987;216:131–134.
51. Simkin A, Leichter I, Giladi M, et al. Combined effect of foot arch structure and an orthotic device on stress fractures. *Foot Ankle* 1989;10:25–29.
52. Matheson GO, Clement DB, McKenzie JE, et al. Stress fractures in athletes. A study of 320 cases. *Am J Sports Med* 1987;15:46–58.
53. Giladi M, Milgrom C, Stein M, et al. The low arch, a protective factor in stress fractures. A prospective study of 295 military recruits. *Orthop Rev* 1985;14:709–712.
54. Montgomery LC, Nelson FR, Norton JP, et al. Orthopedic history and examination in the etiology of overuse injuries. *Med Sci Sports Exerc* 1989;21:237–243.
55. Friberg O. Leg length asymmetry in stress fractures. A clinical and radiological study. *J Sports Med* 1982;22:485–488.
56. McMahon TA, Greene PR. The influence of track compliance on running. *J Biomech* 1979;12:893–904.
57. Steele JR, Milburn PD. Effect of different synthetic sport surfaces on ground reaction forces at landing in netball. *Int J Sport Biomech* 1988;4:130–145.
58. Lloyd T, Triantafyllou SJ, Baker ER, et al. Women athletes with menstrual irregularity have increased musculoskeletal injuries. *Med Sci Sports Exerc* 1986;18:374–379.
59. Barrow GW, Saha S. Menstrual irregularity and stress fractures in collegiate female distance runners. *Am J Sports Med* 1988;16:209–216.
60. Skarda ST, Burge MR. Prospective evaluation of risk factors for exercise-induced hypogonadism in male runners. *West J Med* 1998;169:9–13.
61. MacDougall JD, Webber CE, Martin J, et al. Relationship among running mileage, bone density, and serum testosterone in male runners. *J Appl Physiol* 1992;73:1165–1170.
62. Hetland ML, Haarbo J, Christiansen C. Low bone mass and high bone turnover in male long distance runners. *J Clin Endocrinol Metab* 1993;77:770–775.
63. Smith R, Rutherford OM. Spine and total body bone mineral density and serum testosterone levels in male athletes. *Eur J Appl Physiol* 1993;67:330–334.
64. Barrow GW, Saha S. Menstrual irregularity and stress fractures in collegiate female distance runners. *Am J Sports Med* 1988;16:209–216.
65. Otis CL, et al. American College of Sports Medicine position stand. The female athlete triad. *Med Sci Sports Exerc* 1997;29:i–ix.
66. Johnson C, Powers PS, Dick R. Athletes and eating disorders: the National Collegiate Athletic Association study. *Int J Eating Disorders* 1999;26:179–188.
67. Picard CL. The level of competition as a factor for the development of eating disorders in female collegiate athletes. *J Youth Adolescence* 1999;28:583–595.
68. Lauder TD, et al. Abnormal eating behaviors in military women. *Med Sci Sports Exerc* 1999;31:1265–1271.
69. Frusztajer NT, Dhuper S, Warren MP, et al. Nutrition and the incidence of stress fractures in ballet dancers. *Am J Clin Nutr* 1990;51:779–783.
70. Bennell KL, Malcolm SA, Thomas SA, et al. Risk factors for stress fractures in female track-and-field athletes: a retrospective analysis. *Clin J Sports Med* 1995;5:229–235.
71. Nattiv A, Puffer JC, Green GA. Lifestyles and health risks of collegiate athletes–a multicenter study. *Clin J Sports Med* 1997;7:262–272.

72. Hulkko A, Orava S. The role of age in the development of stress and fatigue fractures. In: Burr DB, Milgrom C, eds. *Musculoskeletal fatigue and stress fractures*. Boca Raton: CRC Press, 2001:55–71.
73. Bennell KL, Brukner PD. Epidemiology and site specificity of stress fractures. *Clin Sports Med* 1997;16:179–196.
74. Bennell KL, Matheson GO, Meeuwisse W, et al. Risk factors for stress fractures. *Sports Med* 1999;28:91–122.
75. Goldberg B, Pecora C. Stress fractures: a risk of increased training in freshmen. *Physician Sportsmed* 1994;22:68–74.
76. Chisin R. The role of various imaging modalities in diagnosing stress fractures. In: Burr DB, Milgrom C, eds. *Musculoskeletal fatigue and stress fractures*. Boca Raton: CRC Press, 2001:279–293.
77. Milgrom C, Giladi M, Stein M, et al. Stress fractures in military recruits. *J Bone Joint Surg* 1985;67B:732–735.
78. Zwas TS, Elkanovitch R, Frank G. Interpretation and classification of bone scintigraphic findings in stress fractures. *J Nucl Med* 1987;28:452–457.
79. Schneider R. Radionuclide techniques. In: Resnick D, Kransdorf MJ, eds. *Bone and joint imaging*, 3rd ed. Philadelphia: Elsevier/Saunders, 2005:86–117
80. Ammann W, Matheson GO. Radionuclide bone imaging in the detection of stress fractures. *Clin J Sports Med* 1991;1:115–122.
81. Rupani HD, Holder LE, Espinola DA, et al. Three-phase radionuclide bone imaging in sports medicine. *Radiology* 1985;156:187–196.
82. Resnick D, Goergen TG. Physical injury: concepts and terminology. In: Resnick D, Kransdorf MJ, eds. *Bone and joint imaging*, 3rd ed. Philadelphia: Elsevier/Saunders, 2005:789–830.
83. Kaplan PA, Helms CA, Dussault R, et al. Osseous trauma. In: *Musculoskeletal MRI*. Philadelphia: WB Saunders, 2001:151–167.
84. Deutsch AL, Coel MN, Mink JH. Imaging of stress injuries to bone: radiography, scintigraphy and MR imaging. *Clin Sports Med* 1997;16:275–290.
85. Fredericson M, Bergman AG, Hoffman KL, et al. Tibial stress reaction in runners: correlation of clinical symptoms and scintigraphy with a new magnetic resonance imaging grading system. *Am J Sports Med* 1995;23:472–481.
86. Shin AY, Morin WD, Gorman JD, et al. The superiority of magnetic resonance imaging in differentiating the cause of hip pain in endurance athletes. *Am J Sports Med* 1996; 24:168–176.
87. Khan KM, Fuller PJ, Brukner PD, et al. Outcome of conservative and surgical management of navicular stress fracture in athletes. *Am J Sports Med* 1992;20:657–666.
88. Kiss ZA, Khan KM, Fuller PJ. Stress fractures of the tarsal navicular bone: CT findings in 55 cases. *Am J Roentgen* 1993;160:111–115.
89. Milgrom C, Friedman E. Early diagnosis and clinical treatment of stress fractures. In: Burr DB, Milgrom C, eds. *Musculoskeletal fatigue and stress fractures*. Boca Raton: CRC Press, 2001:295–303.
90. Brand JC Jr, Brindle T, Nyland J, et al. Does pulsed low intensity ultrasound allow early return to normal activities when treating stress fractures? A review of one tarsal navicular and eight tibial stress fractures. *Iowa Orthop J* 1999;19:26–30.
91. Benazzo F, Mosconi M, Beccarisi G, et al. Use of capacitive coupled electric fields in stress fracture in athletes. *Clin Orthop 1995*;310:145–149.
92. Rettig AC, Shelbourne KD, McCarroll JR, et al. The natural history and treatment of delayed union stress fractures of the anterior cortex of the tibia. *Am J Sports Med* 1988; 16:250–255.
93. Brukner P, Bennell K, Matheson G. Diagnosis of stress fractures. In: *Stress fractures*. Victoria: Blackwell Science, 1999: 97–105.
94. Gehring MM, Keller BA, Brehm BA. Water running with and without a flotation vest in competitive and recreational runners. *Med and Science in Sports and Exercise* 1997; 29:1374–1378.
95. Brukner P, Bennell K. Matheson G. Stress fractures of the pelvis and thigh. In: *Stress fractures*. Victoria: Blackwell Science, 1999:139–146.
96. Fullerton LR. Femoral neck stress fractures. *Sports Med* 1990;9:192–197.
97. Fullerton LR, Snowdy HA. Femoral neck stress fractures. *Am J Sports Med* 1988;16: 365–377.
98. Clough TM. Femoral neck stress fracture: the importance of clinical suspicion and early review. *Br J Sports Med* 2002;36:308–309.
99. Egol KA, Frankel VH. Problematic stress fractures. In: Burr DB, Milgrom C, eds. *Musculoskeletal fatigue and stress fractures*. Boca Raton: CRC Press, 2001:305–319.
100. Visuri T, Vara A, Meurman KO. Displaced stress fractures of the femoral neck in young male adults: a report of twelve operative cases. *J Trauma* 1988;28:1562–1569.
101. Lee CH, Huang GS, Chao KH, et al. Surgical treatment of displaced stress fractures of the femoral neck in military recruits: a report of 42 cases. *Arch Orthop Trauma Surg* 2003;123:527–533.
102. Hershman EB, Lombardo J, Bergfeld JA. Femoral shaft stress fractures in athletes. *Clin Sports Med* 1990;9:111–119.
103. Brukner P, Bennell K, Matheson G. Stress fractures of the lower leg. In: *Stress fractures*. Victoria: Blackwell Science, 1999:147–161.
104. Boden BP, Osbahr DC. High-risk stress fractures: evaluation and treatment. *J Am Acad Orthop Surg* 2000;8:344–353.
105. Keating JF, Beggs I, Thorpe GW. Three cases of longitudinal stress fracture of the tibia. *Acta Orthop Scand* 1995;66:41–42.
106. Whitelaw GP, Wetzler MJ, Levy AS, et al. A pneumatic leg brace for the treatment of tibial stress fractures. *Clin Orthop* 1991;270:302–305.
107. Swenson EJ, DeHaven KE, Sebastienelli WJ, et al. The effect of a pneumatic leg brace on return to play in athletes with tibial stress fractures. *Am J Sports Med* 1997;25: 322–328.
108. Green NE, Rogers RA, Lipscomb AB. Nonunions of stress fractures of the tibia. *Am J Sports Med* 1985;13:171–176.
109. Orava S, Karpakka J, Hulkko A, et al. Diagnosis and treatment of stress fractures located at the mid-tibial shaft in athletes. *Int J Sports Med* 1991;12:419–422.
110. Rolf C, Ekenman I, Tornqvist H, et al. The anterior stress fracture of the tibia: an atrophic pseudoarthrosis. *Scand J Med Sci Sports* 1997;7:249–252.
111. Taube RR, Wadsworth LT. Managing tibial stress fractures. *Physician Sports Med* 1993; 21:123–128.
112. Chang PS, Harris RM. Intramedullary nailing for chronic tibial stress fractures: A review of five cases. *Am J Sports Med* 1996;24:688–692.
113. Plasschaert VF, Johansson CG, Micheli LJ. Anterior tibial stress fracture treated with intramedullary nailing: a case report. *Clin J Sports Med* 1995;5:58–62.
114. Shelbourne KD, Fisher DA, Rettig AC, et al. Stress fractures of the medial malleolus. *Am J Sports Med* 1988;16:60–63.
115. Orava S, Karpakka J, Taimela S, et al. Stress fracture of the medial malleolus. *J Bone Joint Surg Am* 1995;77:362–365.
116. Brukner P, Bradshaw C, Khan K, et al. Stress fractures: a review of 180 cases. *Clin J Sports Med* 1996;6:85–89.
117. Brukner P, Bennell K, Matheson G. Stress fractures of the foot and ankle. In: *Stress Fractures*. Victoria: Blackwell Science, 1999:163–186.
118. Torg JS, Pavlov H, Cooley LH, et al. Stress fractures of the tarsal navicular: a retrospective review of twenty-one cases. *J Bone Joint Surg* 1982;64A:700–712.
119. Khan KM, Brukner PD, Kearney C, et al. Tarsal navicular stress fractures in athletes. *Sports Med* 1994;17:65–76.
120. Khan KM, Fuller PJ, Brukner PD, et al. Outcome of conservative and surgical management of navicular stress fracture in athletes. *Am J Sports Med* 1992;20:657–666.
121. Fitch KD, Blackwell JB, Gilmour WN. Operation for nonunion of stress fracture of the tarsal navicular. *J Bone Joint Surg* 1989;71B:105–110.
122. Orava S, Hulkko A. Delayed unions and nonunions of stress fractures in athletes. *Am J Sports Med* 1988;16:378–382.
123. Lee S, Anderson RB. Stress fractures of the tarsal navicular. *Foot Ankle Clinics* 2004;9: 85–104.
124. O'Malley MJ, Hamilton WG, Munyak J, et al. Stress fractures at the base of the second metatarsal in ballet dancers. *Foot Ankle International* 1996;17:89–94.
125. Torg JS, Balduini FC, Zelko RR, et al. Fractures of the base of the fifth metatarsal distal to the tuberosity: classification and guidelines for non-surgical and surgical management. *J Bone Joint Surg* 1984;66A:209–214.
126. Josefsson PO, Karlsson M, Redlund-Johnell I, et al. Closed treatment of Jones fracture: good results in 40 cases after 11–26 years. *Acta Orthop Scand* 1994;65:545–547.
127. Dameron TB Jr. Fractures of the proximal fifth metatarsal: selecting the best treatment option. *J Am Acad Orthop Surg* 1995;3:110–114.
128. Torg JS. Fractures of the base of the fifth metatarsal distal to the tuberosity: a review. *Contemp Orthop* 1989;19:497–505.
129. Clapper MF, O'Brien TJ, Lyons PM. Fractures of the fifth metatarsal: analysis of a fracture registry. *Clin Orthop* 1995;315:238–241.
130. Zogby RG, Baker BE. A review of nonoperative treatment of Jones' fracture. *Am J Sports Med* 1987;15:304–307.
131. Acker JH, Drez D Jr. Nonoperative treatment of stress fractures of the proximal shaft of the fifth metatarsal (Jones' fracture). *Foot Ankle* 1986;7:152–155.
132. Dameron TB Jr. Fractures and anatomical variations of the proximal portion of the fifth metatarsal. *J Bone Joint Surg* 1975;57A:788–792.
133. Hens J, Martens M. Surgical treatment of Jones fractures. *Orthop Trauma Surg* 1990; 109:277–279.
134. Zelko RR, Torg JS, Rachun A. Proximal diaphyseal fractures of the fifth metatarsal: treatment of the fractures and their complications in athletes. *Am J Sports Med* 1979; 7:95–101.
135. Kavanaugh JH, Brower TD, Mann RV. The Jones fracture revisited. *J Bone Joint Surg* 1978;60A:776–782.
136. DeLee JC, Evans JP, Julian J. Stress fracture of the fifth metatarsal. *Am J Sports Med* 1983;11:349–353.
137. Mindrebo N, Shelbourne D, van Meter CD, et al. Outpatient percutaneous screw fixation of the acute Jones fracture. *Am J Sports Med* 1993;21:720–723.
138. Lawrence SJ, Botte MJ. Jones' fractures and related fractures of the proximal fifth metatarsal. *Foot Ankle* 1993;14:358–365.
139. Holmes GB Jr. Treatment of delayed unions and nonunions of the proximal fifth metatarsal with pulsed electromagnetic fields. *Foot Ankle* 1994;15:552–556.
140. Teitz CC, Harrington RM. Patellar stress fracture. *Am J Sports Med* 1992;20:761–765.
141. Mata SG, Grande MM, Ovejero AH. Transverse stress fracture of the patella. *Clin J Sports Med* 1996;6:259–261.
142. Orava S, Taimela S, Kvist M, et al. Diagnosis and treatment of stress fracture of the patella in athletes. *Knee Surg Sports Trauma Arthrosc* 1996;4:206–211.
143. Monteleone GP Jr. Stress fractures in the athlete. *Sports Med* 1995;26:423–432.
144. Black KP, Ehlert KJ. A stress fracture of the lateral process of the talus in a runner. *J Bone Joint Surg* 1994;76:441–443.
145. Bradshaw C, Khan K, Brukner P. Stress fracture of the body of the talus in athletes demonstrated with computer tomography. *Clin J Sports Med* 1996;6:48–51.
146. Mahler P, Fricker P. Case report: cuboid stress fracture. *Excel* 1992;8:147–148.
147. Khan KM, Brukner PD, Bradshaw C. Stress fracture of the medial cuneiform bone in a runner. *Clin J Sports Med* 1993;3:262–264.
148. Brukner P. Stress fractures of the upper limb. *Sports Med* 1998;26:415–424.
149. Branch T, Partin C, Chamberland P, et al. Spontaneous fractures of the humerus during pitching: a series of 12 cases. *Am J Sports Med* 1992;20:468–470.
150. Nuber GW, Diment MT. Olecranon stress fractures in throwers: a report of two cases and a review of the literature. *Clin Orthop* 1992;278:58–61.
151. Maffulli N, Chan D, Aldridge MJ. Overuse injuries of the olecranon in young gymnasts. *J Bone Joint Surg* 1992;74:305–308.

152. Wilkerson RD, Johns JC. Nonunion of an olecranon stress fracture in an adolescent gymnast: a case report. *Am J Sports Med* 1990;18:432–434.
153. Brukner P, Bennell K. Matheson G. Stress fractures of the upper limb. In: *Stress fractures*. Victoria: Blackwell Science, 1999:107–117.
154. Carter SR, Aldridge MJ. Stress injury of the distal radial growth plate. *J Bone Joint Surg* 1988;70:834–836.
155. Ahluwalia R, Datz FL, Morton KA, et al. Bilateral fatigue fractures of the radial shaft in a gymnast. *Clin Nuc Med* 1994;19:665–667.
156. Murakami Y. Stress fracture of the metacarpal in an adolescent tennis player. *Am J Sports Med* 1988;16:419–420.
157. Noakes TD, Smith JA, Lindenberg G, et al. Pelvic stress fractures in long distance runners. *Am J Sports Med* 1985;13:120–123.
158. Brukner P, Bennell K, Matheson G. Stress fractures of the trunk. In: *Stress fractures*. Victoria: Blackwell Science, 1999:119–138.
159. Eller DJ, Katz DS, Bergman AG, et al. Sacral stress fractures in long-distance runners. *Clin J Sport Med* 1997;7:222–225.

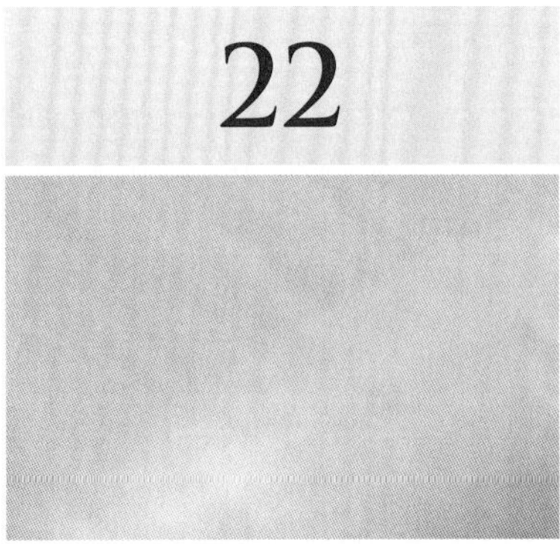

PERIPROSTHETIC FRACTURES

Robert H. Cofield, John W. Sperling, Bernard F. Morrey, Shawn W. O'Driscoll, and Jay D. Mabrey

PART 1
PERIPROSTHETIC FRACTURES OF THE ELBOW AND SHOULDER

ROBERT H. COFIELD, JOHN W. SPERLING, BERNARD F. MORREY, AND SHAWN W. O'DRISCOLL

PERIPROSTHETIC FRACTURES ABOUT THE ELBOW

Although periprosthetic fractures about various joint replacement devices is a frequent topic of discussion, to date there has been little attention of this subject referable to the elbow (1,2). Yet the complication is being observed with increasing frequency and carries with it some very specific treatment considerations.

Incidence

Based on our experience with 1,072 linked Coonrad-Morrey implant procedures, a fracture was documented before, during, or subsequent to surgery in approximately 13%. The complication was recorded with 68 of 748 primary (9%) and in 73 of 324 (23%) revision procedures. At the elbow, the anatomic site of the lesion involves the humerus in 71 (7%) and the ulna in 70 (7%). At Mayo we have developed a classification system based on our experience of approximately 1,200 elbow joint replacements of varying designs performed from 1973 through 2003. Analysis of treatment and prognosis is based on assessment of the 1,072 Coonrad-Morrey devices inserted from 1983 through 2003. During this period of time 70% of the implants were primary replacements (Table 22-1).

Classification

At the elbow, experience would suggest that it is most useful to consider these fractures according to three anatomic locations of either the humerus or ulna: metaphyseal (Type I), stemmed shaft (Type II), and beyond the stem (Type III) (Fig. 22-1). The

TABLE 22-1 Frequency of Fractures by Anatomic Location

Fracture Occurrence by Procedure Type			
	Primary (748) No/%	Revision (324) No/%	Total
Humerus	39/5%	32/10%	71/1,072 (7)
Ulna	29/4%	41/13%	70/1,072 (7)
Total	68/9%	73/23%	141/1,072 (14)

full implication of this classification is best appreciated in the context of the occurrence, management, and outcome of each fracture type. Consistent with the Vancouver system, the fracture is further characterized as associated with a well-fixed (A) or a loose (B) stem. The circumstances in which the fractures occur, frequency, treatment, and prognosis for each fracture type is shown in Table 22-2.

Type I Metaphyseal (Periarticular)

Periarticular fractures about the elbow account for about 80% of all periprosthetic fractures and may involve either the distal humerus or the proximal ulna. As at the hip, Type A fractures are treated on their own merit, but revision is performed in Type B fractures as by definition the implant is loose.

Type I Humerus (Condylar Fractures)

Temporal Occurrence. Condylar fractures may occur before surgery in severe mutilans rheumatoid arthritis (Mayo Type IV radiographic classification), intraoperatively, or even spontaneously after surgery (Fig. 22-2). Intraoperative fractures are associated with preparation of the metaphyseal region for the implant. If the collateral ligaments are attached, manipulation of the forearm can fracture the weakened supracondylar column with muscle contracture. In those with thin or porotic supracondylar structures, it is also possible to sustain a spontaneous fracture of either the medial or the lateral condylar region after surgery without specific trauma.

Frequency. Review of the 68 fractures associated with 748 primary procedures reveals 39 involved the humerus. Of these, approximately 60% involved the medial or lateral supracondylar column and occurred most commonly intraoperatively in pa-

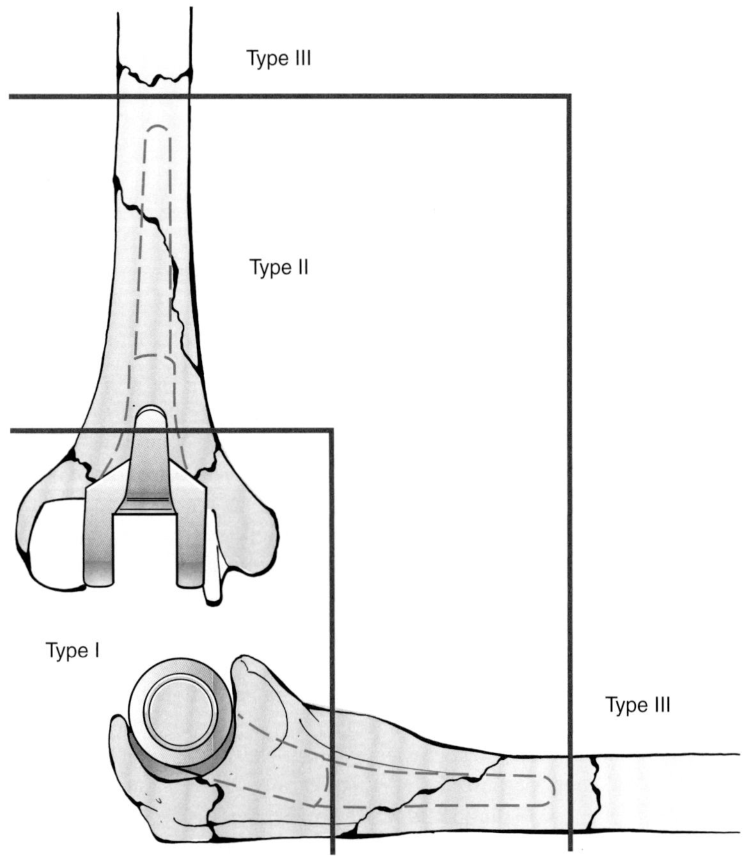

FIGURE 22-1 The Mayo classification of periprosthetic fractures defines fractures of the metaphysis as type I, fractures involving bone occupied by the stem or by the implant as a type II, and fractures beyond the tip of the implant as type III. The classification further subdivides these fractures based on whether or not the prosthesis is well fixed, or the implant is loose.

TABLE 22-2 **Considerations and Implications of Periprosthetic Fracture of the Elbow**

Type	Temporal Occurrence	Frequency	Implant Design				Outcome
			Prognostic Implications		Treatment		
			Coupled	Uncoupled	Coupled	Uncoupled	
Type I (periarticular)							
Humeral Condyle	Intraoperative	3%	None (wear?)	Instability, Wear?	Resect/ignore	Stabilize	Satisfactory
	Postoperative	<1%	None	Possible instability			
Coronoid	Intraoperative	Very rare	Loose flex strength	Strength, loose?	Circumferential		Little data
Olecranon	Intraoperative	2%	Loose ext strength	Strength, loose?	Tension band fixation		Satisfactory >90% (Marra)
	Postoperative						
Type II							
Diaphysis (stem involved)	Operative	Rare	Must stabilize		ORIF, strut graft, longer stem?		
	Postoperative	<2%	Must stabilize or revise				Satisfactory 85% (Sanchez-Sotelo, Kamineni)
	Loose stem				Immobilize, ORIF – strut graft		
					Impaction graft		
Type III							
Diaphysis (stem not involved)	Postoperative	<3%	Depends on loose or fixed stem		Loose: revise as above		Usually satisfactory
	Trauma Loose stem				Fixed: immobilize, ORIF; strut graft		Satisfactory 85%

tients with rheumatoid arthritis after the distal humerus had been prepared for prosthetic placement.

Implication and Treatment. There are minimal implications regarding treatment or prognosis with the linked Coonrad-Morrey device with a fracture of either condyle as the fixation of this implant is not compromised. If associated with deformity, this may be associated with accelerated wear of the articulation. Further, an intact condyle is essential for the linked GSB III device, which is designed to achieve stability by fixation to the humeral condyles. Hence, a repair or reconstruction of the condyles is necessary in this setting. The same is true for uncoupled devices requiring osseous integrity of the condyles for implant stability or ligamentous integrity for joint stability.

If the fracture occurs during a linked procedure and the musculature is functional, then the condyle is simply sutured back to the implant with nonabsorbable suture. If the fragment is very thin and osteoporotic, and particularly if the musculature is not substantial, then the fragment is excised and the common flexor or extensor tendon is sutured to the margin of the triceps. Open reduction and internal fixation is arduous and unnecessary for linked devices.

For unlinked devices a fractured condyle is uncommon but the occurrence is quite significant for an implant design that requires the integrity of the condyle for implant fixation. Most such implants require a supracondylar column for implant fixation and for articular stability, so fixation is considered necessary.

Result. Union occurs in approximately 50% of patients but this is not relevant with the linked implant. Displacement of more

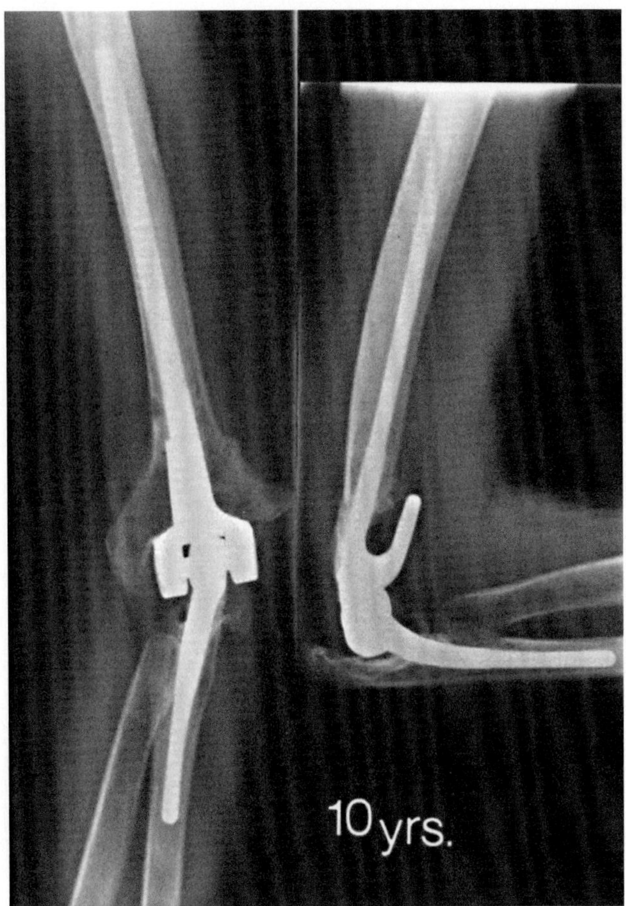

FIGURE 22-2 This patient developed a stress fracture of the medial epicondyle approximately 6 months after surgery. At 10 years the fracture has healed. Notice that this event has not caused excessive articular stress as minimal bushing wear is present.

than a few millimeters is uncommon. There is little data on this topic with unlinked devices. We have not observed clinically relevant grip strength alteration after the fracture.

Type I Ulna

The periarticular fracture of the ulna may involve the olecranon or coronoid, but fracture of the latter is quite uncommon.

Coronoid Fracture

Temporal Considerations. Coronoid fracture occurs intraoperative with preparation of the canal or at insertion of the implant. It is seen if the preparation for resurfacing the implant is too aggressive, or in those in whom the bone is resorbed from the arthritic process. An absent or severely compromised anterior proximal segment of ulna and coronoid may occur with a loose ulnar component, especially in those with extensive osteolysis.

Frequency. This is a very rare fracture occurring during surgery only once in our experience.

Implications and Treatment. If the fracture displaces and involves the canal it can compromise ulnar stem fixation. Treatment is by circumferential fixation using a wire or heavy suture. Screws and plates are unnecessary. If there is any question regarding the stability, then an assisted flexion splint is also prescribed. In the revision setting, osteolysis may dictate reconstruction of the proximal ulna with an allograft ulnar or fibular strut graft secured with circumferential wire.

Results. Undisplaced fractures occurring at primary surgery should not compromise outcome. Outcome of the strut graft is dependent on the overall extent of the osteolytic process, specifically whether the brachialis attachment has been compromised. In our experience, strut reconstruction has been successfully integrated in 85% to 90% of instances with stable short-term ulnar stem fixation (3).

Olecranon

Temporal Pattern. Intraoperative. In rheumatoid patients the olecranon may be markedly thinned and will sometimes fracture spontaneously. However, in the vast majority of instances the olecranon fractured prior to the procedure (Fig. 22-3). Some implant designs may also thin the olecranon in a manner that predisposes to fracture. For linked implants in which the olecranon is not directly addressed, there is slightly less chance of intraoperative fracture. If the triceps tendon is left attached, as in instances of distal humeral bone loss, care must be taken to avoid excessive stress or force on the olecranon during forearm manipulation.

Postoperative Fracture. Patients with posttraumatic arthritis and especially with rheumatoid arthritis can sustain an olecranon fracture just as any other patient population group. Those with rheumatoid arthritis are somewhat more vulnerable due to the compromised integrity of the olecranon from the resorptive process. We have seen patients who have fractured the olecranon with strong extension of the elbow, the fracture occurring from the force generated by muscle contracture. An absent or spontaneous fracture of the olecranon can also occur in the face of extensive osteolysis seen with a loose ulnar implant.

Frequency. This occurs second in frequency to the condylar fracture of the humerus and accounts for approximately two-thirds of all ulnar fractures.

Implication and Treatment. Fracture of the olecranon has significant implications referable to management at the time of implant replacement as well as functional implications depending on displacement. If the fracture has occurred before or during the surgery then the fracture can be mobilized as an osteotomy to facilitate exposure. Reattachment using two K-wires and the AO figure-of-eight tension band technique is performed at the completion of the procedure. It is not possible or necessary to plate

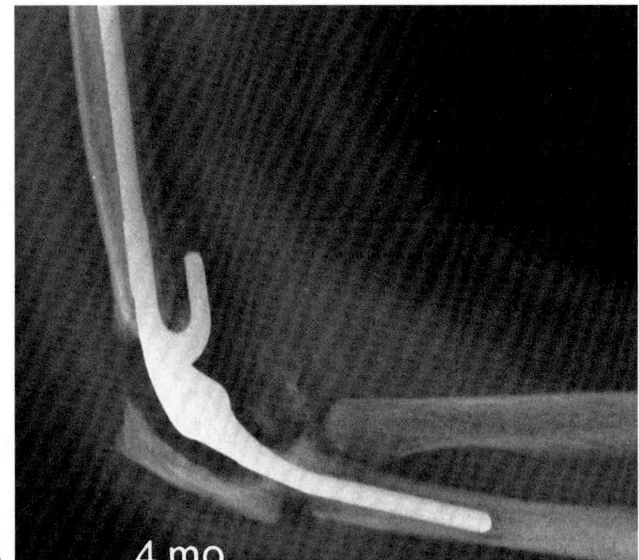

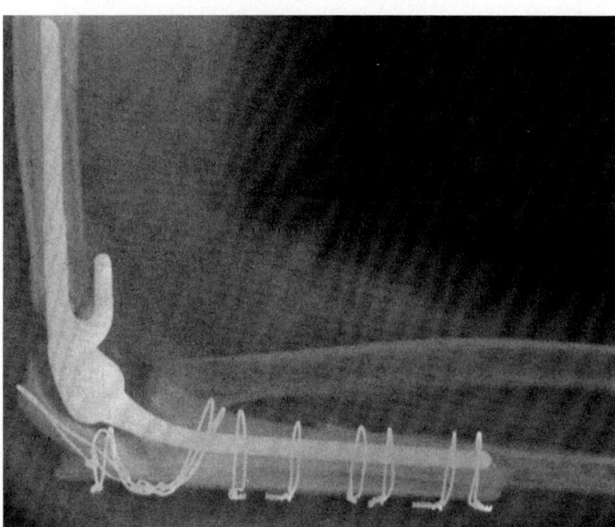

A B

FIGURE 22-3 A. Fracture of a tenuous olecranon following joint replacement in a patient with gross deformity. **B.** The deficiency was addressed by a strut graft augmentation of the anterior and posterior ulna with the fragment being secured with wires with the fracture being incorporated into the strut graft reconstruction.

this fracture in most patients undergoing elbow joint replacement. The specific technique that we employ involves placing the K-wires in the proximal fragment before cementing the implant. They are advanced along the canal with the trial ulnar component in place; they are then withdrawn to remain in the olecranon fragment. When the cement is soft and the ulnar component has been inserted and articulated with the humeral component, the K-wires are then cemented in place along with the medullary stem of the ulnar component. This stabilizes the wires and lessens the likelihood of them backing out. The fracture is reduced or fitted over the wires and an additional figure-of-eight wire is carefully placed making sure that the ulnar implant is not notched with the distal drill hole and the wire knot is not on the subcutaneous border of the ulna.

If the fracture occurs postoperatively, the treatment is generally nonoperative anticipating that sufficient fibrosis or osseus healing will occur. An extension assist brace is used after 3 weeks of immobilization. If the fracture displaces more than 2 cm and if there is a marked functional impairment, then open reduction and internal fixation is carried out just as with any other olecranon fracture. Care again must be taken to insert the K-wires in such a way as to avoid notching the implant. In those with olecranon deficiency due to osteolysis, reconstruction with a strut graft is recommended (3). This has the function of not just stabilizing the implant, but also restoring the integrity of the triceps function. We avoid plates because there is no purchase for the screws distally, and the plate is far too bulky over the olecranon in this patient type.

Results. We have assessed 22 olecranon fractures occurring with total elbow replacement treated at Mayo (4). Nonunion occurred in 50% but displacement of more than 1 cm did not occur. The Mayo Elbow Performance score and subjective outcome was no different in the group with healing compared to the patients with a stable nonunion.

Diaphyseal (Type II) Fractures

As at the hip, fractures of the diaphysis may involve a well-fixed (A) or loose (B) stem of the implant device.

Temporal Pattern. Fracture of bone around the stem may occur intraoperatively but it is very rare except for a revision procedure. If this occurs in primary joint replacement, it is due to cortical penetration during preparation of the canal. Alternatively, this can occur at the time of insertion of implants with stems of 15 cm or more, especially if the humerus has a prominent bow. We have not witnessed one such a fracture to date in our practice.

Fractures that occur around the stem of the implant in the postoperative period are due to significant violence or are associated with a loose implant. High-energy fractures are typically spiral, more comminuted, and occur from a torque or twisting motion of the forearm referable to the brachium. If the implant is loose, the fracture may be more transverse, usually at or around the tip of the stem (Fig. 22-4).

Incidence. Operative fractures are extremely uncommon. Postoperative Type A fractures are also not common. By far the most common Type II fracture is a subtype B, occurring in the presence of a loose device. In some instances this is an incidental

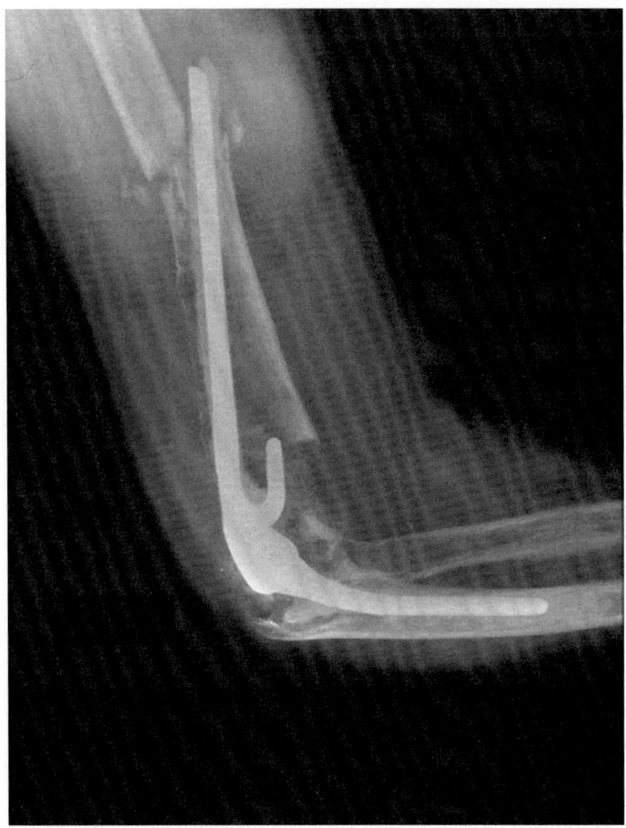

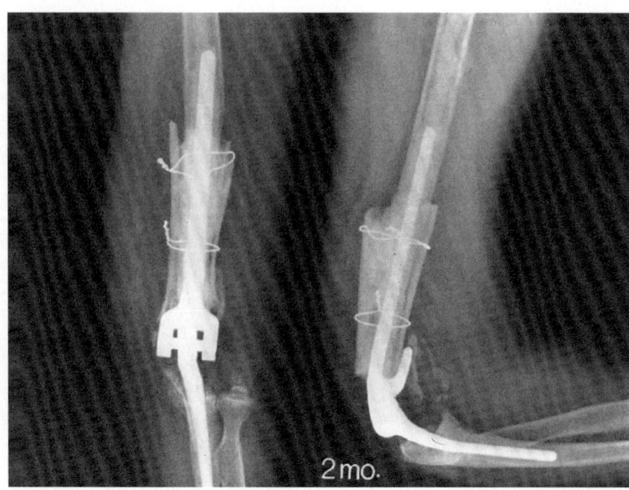

FIGURE 22-4 **A.** A Type IIB fracture in which the cortex is distorted and a frank transverse type fracture is noted just proximal to the tip of the implant. **B.** This type of fracture is well managed by dual cortical struts and cerclage wires.

feature of the pathology. In other circumstances, it may have spontaneously healed causing a deformity of the canal or be so extensive as to compromise subsequent implant fixation posing a major problem of planning and prognosis (Fig. 22-5).

Implications. For the linked implant as well as for the unlinked device, any fracture of the diaphysis involving the stem must be stabilized. The treatment logic is exactly the same as that well documented for similar processes occurring with hip replacement (5,6). If the fracture is associated with a loose elbow implant then, as with the femoral fractures, the implant revision is planned to bypass the fracture ideally by two bone diameters thereby serving as a means of helping to treat or stabilize the fracture itself.

Good quality bone may sometimes be considered amenable to a cerclage or circumferential type fixation. However, a cortical strut graft with cerclage fixation is the most reliable means of management (3,7). A plate with screws and cerclage is preferred by some. Postoperatively, if fixation is considered rigid, the elbow is not immobilized for long periods of time. A coaptation or hinged brace is used with compression of the brachium helping to stabilize the fracture and the elbow joint is allowed passive motion with a continuous passive motion machine (CPM) immediately after surgery. Active motion in the splint begins at 4 weeks.

Results. The intraoperative fractures at the time of revision are usually quite satisfactorily treated since a fresh implant can help stabilize the fracture. Similarly, fractures managed in association with revision are well managed at both the ulna and humerus with cortical struts. Our experience with 11 humeral and 22 ulnar struts reveal a success rate of fracture healing and a functional joint of approximately 90% at 3 to 5 years at both anatomic sites (3,7).

Diaphyseal (Type III) Fractures

Occurrence. Fractures proximal to the humeral or distal to the ulnar stem are not common. In our experience, these have all been postoperative fractures, usually associated with a loose device or specific trauma.

Frequency. The Type III fracture occurs in less than 2% of instances and may be from minimal trauma. When this occurs, as with Type II, it is usually associated with a loose stem. In most circumstances the fracture is only minimally displaced and mildly angulated.

Implications and Treatment. The significance and management differs considerably depending upon whether or not the implant stem is stable or loose. Fractures of the humerus are quite proximal and are difficult to control by splint or cast. If not displaced initially, they may become so in time unless effectively managed. Care with managing casts is advised in the

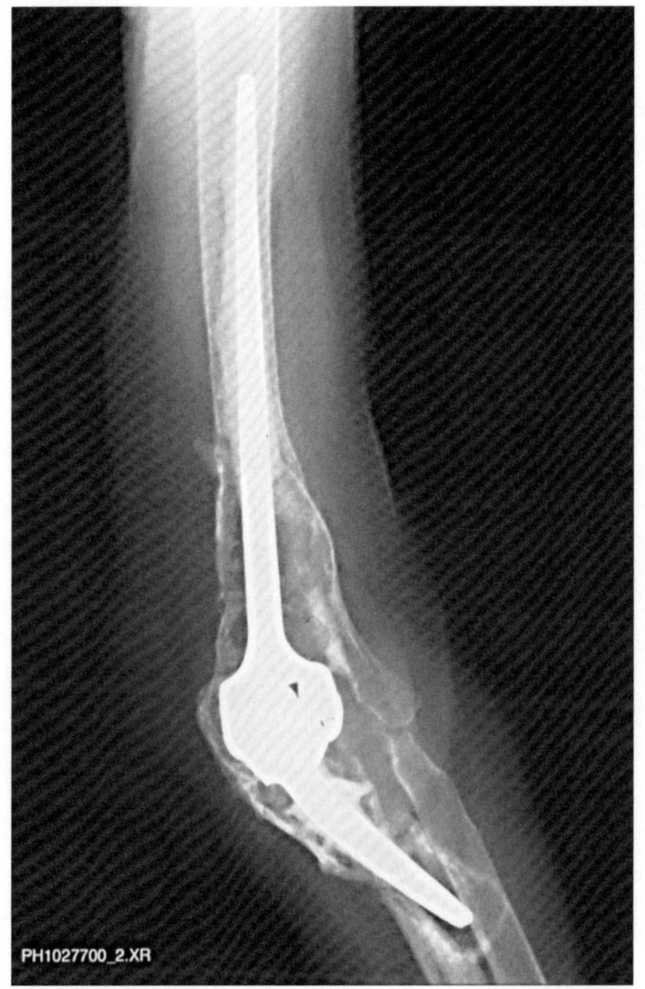

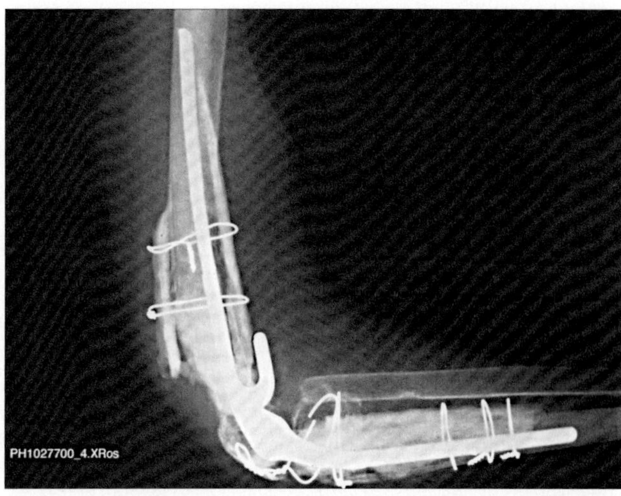

FIGURE 22-5 **A.** Osteolysis with a Type IIB fracture of the ulna and a healed fracture of the lateral aspect of the distal humerus. **B.** Fractures such as these are best managed by dual cortical onlay struts and impaction grafting.

elderly with poor muscle tone. Fractures of the ulna will also tend to angulate but are easier to control with nonoperative measures.

If the implant is stable and the fracture minimally displaced, humeral fractures are treated with a compressive splint. If the fracture angulates or displaces then strut grafts are used to bridge the fracture and are secured with cerclage wire. Half screws cemented into a single cortex may be used proximal or distal to the stem (Fig. 22-6). If the stem is not well fixed then the implant is revised. A longer-stemmed device is used as an intramedullary alignment and assists in the fixation. Struts or plates and screws are employed in all instances. Even with extensive Type B osteolysis, these techniques are preferable to prosthetic allograft composite revision (8).

Results. The results of fractures of these types are generally good and usually heal. Cast immobilization has resulted in a satisfactory outcome in most instances if adequate reduction can be obtained and maintained. Displaced fractures have also been successfully treated with open reduction and internal fixation. The functional result is good if the fracture heals.

Complications

The complications associated with the management of periprosthetic fractures are similar to those that might be anticipated with the primary elbow joint replacement. These include infection, ulnar or radial nerve paresthesias or palsy, wound healing problems, and triceps insufficiency as those with the major functional implications. Sanchez-Sotelo et al (7) documented four complications associated with humeral strut grafting in 11 periprosthetic fractures of the humerus. Most were neural, with one partial radial nerve palsy and two partial ulnar nerve palsies. No patient had a complete palsy and all improved to some extent including adequate motor function. No tendon transfers were necessary. One additional patient in Sanchez-Sotelo's experience developed triceps insufficiency after the surgery for the periprosthetic fracture. There were no infections in that group.

Complications documented to be associated with management of ulnar periprosthetic fractures are very limited. Seven of the 22 strut grafts reported by Kamineni and Morrey (3) involved patients with periprosthetic fractures. In this group a single patient did develop a fracture distal to the graft. Kamineni and Mor-

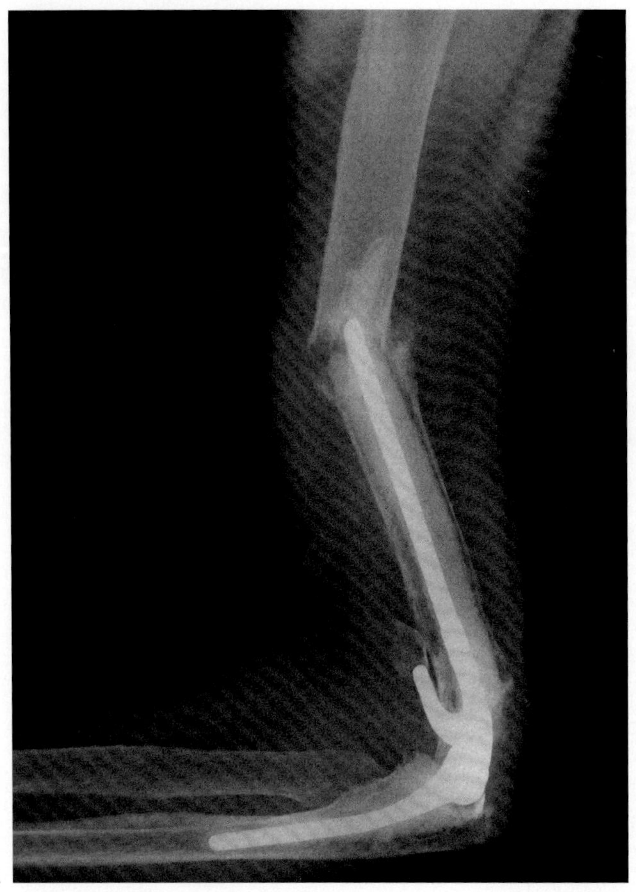

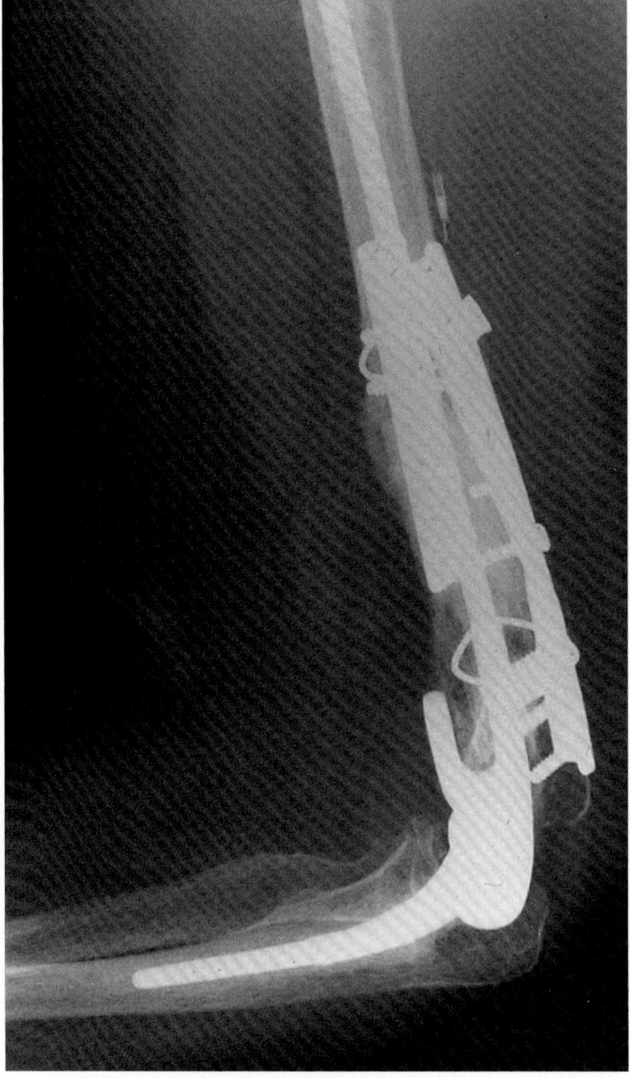

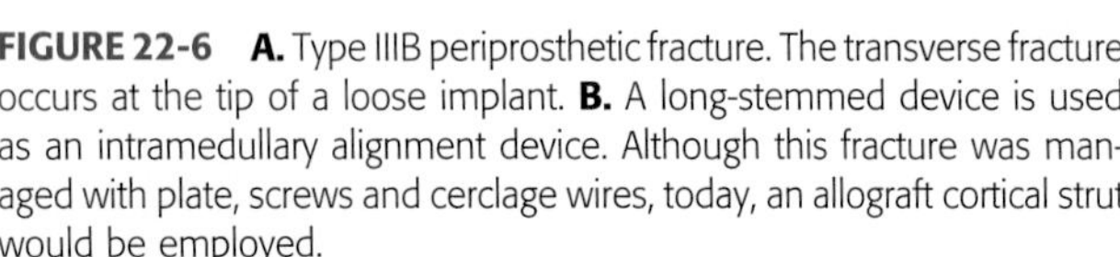

FIGURE 22-6 **A.** Type IIIB periprosthetic fracture. The transverse fracture occurs at the tip of a loose implant. **B.** A long-stemmed device is used as an intramedullary alignment device. Although this fracture was managed with plate, screws and cerclage wires, today, an allograft cortical strut would be employed.

rey also documented a lack of incorporation of the graft in 5% to 10%. There were no infections and no neural complications associated with the periprosthetic fracture of the ulna.

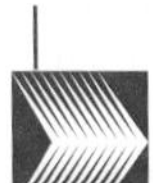

AUTHORS' PREFERRED TREATMENT

In all instances revision for a periprosthetic fracture includes replacing the bearings of the implant unless the implant has been inserted less than 2 years.

The Humerus

We utilize a Bryan-Morrey approach for exposure of humeral periprosthetic fractures. The elbow is disarticulated by removing the anterior aspect of the medial and lateral epicondyles and the articulation is disengaged. The ulnar nerve is immediately identified and protected. If it is symptomatic it is decompressed. The radial nerve is identified. Typically, however, the exposure of the humerus is subperiosteal from the posteromedial aspect of the triceps to posterolateral keeping the radial nerve anterior with its muscular investment. A humeral strut is used for periprosthetic fractures using the curvature of the strut to enhance stability. If the bone is of good quality, a single strut is employed. In osteoporotic patients two struts are employed in order to avoid the wire cutting through the osteoporotic bone. Typically two circumferential wires are employed above and below the fracture.

The Ulna

For ulnar periprosthetic fractures the bone is exposed subperiosteally. If necessary the articulation is exposed as mentioned above. A fibular or ulnar allograft is employed for the strut. Two 16-gauge circumferential wires are employed proximal and two distal to the fracture site. If there is evidence of an atrophic bone end, then bone grafting with allograft cancellous bone is employed.

Summary

The full spectrum of periprosthetic fracture at the elbow is well defined by the proposed classification system. Implications of treatment and results naturally follow from the fracture type.

For Type II and III fractures, principles of management are similar for periprosthetic fractures of the hip and long bones. For Type I fractures the management is dependent on implant type at the humerus, and a satisfactory outcome simply requires healing of the olecranon fragment in a minimally displaced position.

PERIPROSTHETIC FRACTURES ABOUT THE SHOULDER

The literature contains a small number of publications on this topic (9–17). The experience reported in the literature indicates that these fractures can be difficult to heal. Achieving union of the periprosthetic fracture while maintaining glenohumeral motion has proven to be challenging in this patient population.

Boyd reported on the results of seven periprosthetic humerus fractures (9). Only one of the seven fractures healed with nonoperative management. Each of the fractures was centered about the tip of the prosthesis. In addition, two patients developed an associated radial nerve palsy at the time of the fracture or during the early course of nonoperative treatment.

Campbell (12) reported on a multicenter series of periprosthetic humeral fractures. Each of the five postoperative fractures healed with nonoperative management. Four of these were distal to the tip of the humeral stem. Worland (15) reported on six patients with periprosthetic fractures at an average of 43 months after shoulder arthroplasty. Five patients with fractures about the stem were either treated with immediate operative management or failed nonoperative management and required surgery for union. There was one patient with a fracture distal to the tip of the humeral stem that healed with nonoperative management.

Wright and Cofield reported on the outcome of nine periprosthetic humerus fractures (16). Four fractures healed with nonoperative treatment. The authors suggested that operative treatment should be considered for short oblique or transverse fractures that occur at the level of prosthesis tip. In addition, they recommended the use of autologous bone graft at the time of surgery.

Kumar reviewed the outcome of 16 periprosthetic humerus fractures (14). Six fractures in this study healed with nonoperative treatment at a mean of 180 days. Five of 10 fractures requiring operative management had failed to heal at a mean of 123 days with nonoperative care. The remaining five fractures underwent immediate operative intervention. All fractures in this study healed.

Krakauer and Cofield (13) identified 38 fractures occurring during or subsequent to shoulder arthroplasty over an 18-year period. Intraoperatively, the humeral shaft was involved in nine cases, the greater tuberosity in five, the proximal humeral metaphysis in two, the glenoid in four, and the coracoid process in two. Postoperative fractures involved the humeral shaft in 15, and the coracoid process in one. Rheumatoid arthritis was the most common diagnosis. Their results suggested that intraoperative humeral shaft fractures could be successfully managed by using a long-stemmed implant with supplementary cerclage added if additional stability was needed. Of the 15 postoperative humeral shaft fractures, 11 were initially treated with a cast or brace. This treatment led to union in six. A trial of closed treatment was recommended if satisfactory reduction could be obtained and maintained. Three of four intraoperative glenoid fractures precluded placing a glenoid component. Greater tuberosity fractures occurring intraoperatively were sutured in place, and except in one case where nonunion developed did not impact the clinical outcome. Coracoid process fractures were also not clinically significant.

Incidence and Etiology

Periprosthetic fractures after shoulder arthroplasty are relatively uncommon. They have been reported to occur with an incidence of between 1.6% (7 of 436 shoulder arthroplasties) (9) and 2.3% (6 of 252 shoulder arthroplasties) (15).

Several reports have discussed possible factors that might increase the risk of periprosthetic fracture (11,14). Possible risk factors for fracture may include osteopenia and cortical thinning from osteolysis (12,14). In addition, reaming of the inner cortex at the time of arthroplasty may predispose to the fracture at a later time. A fall on the affected upper extremity has been reported as the most frequent cause of the fracture. Periprosthetic fractures also have been reported to occur after motor vehicle accidents, forceful use of the upper extremity, and during manipulation under general anesthesia (14).

Principles of Management

Diagnosis

It is useful to examine the prefracture x-rays to evaluate for cortical penetration at the time of reaming during arthroplasty, alignment of the prosthesis, cortical erosion over time, prosthetic loosening, and presence of osteolysis.

On the fracture x-rays, the degree of osteopenia can be judged according to Campbell (12). Osteopenia is graded on the basis of the ratio of combined width of mid-diaphyseal cortices to the diameter of the diaphysis. It is graded as normal if the ratio is greater than 50%, mildly osteopenic if the ratio is between 25% and 50%, and severely osteopenic if ratio is less than 25%. The degree of angulation, amount of displacement, and fracture configuration should be evaluated.

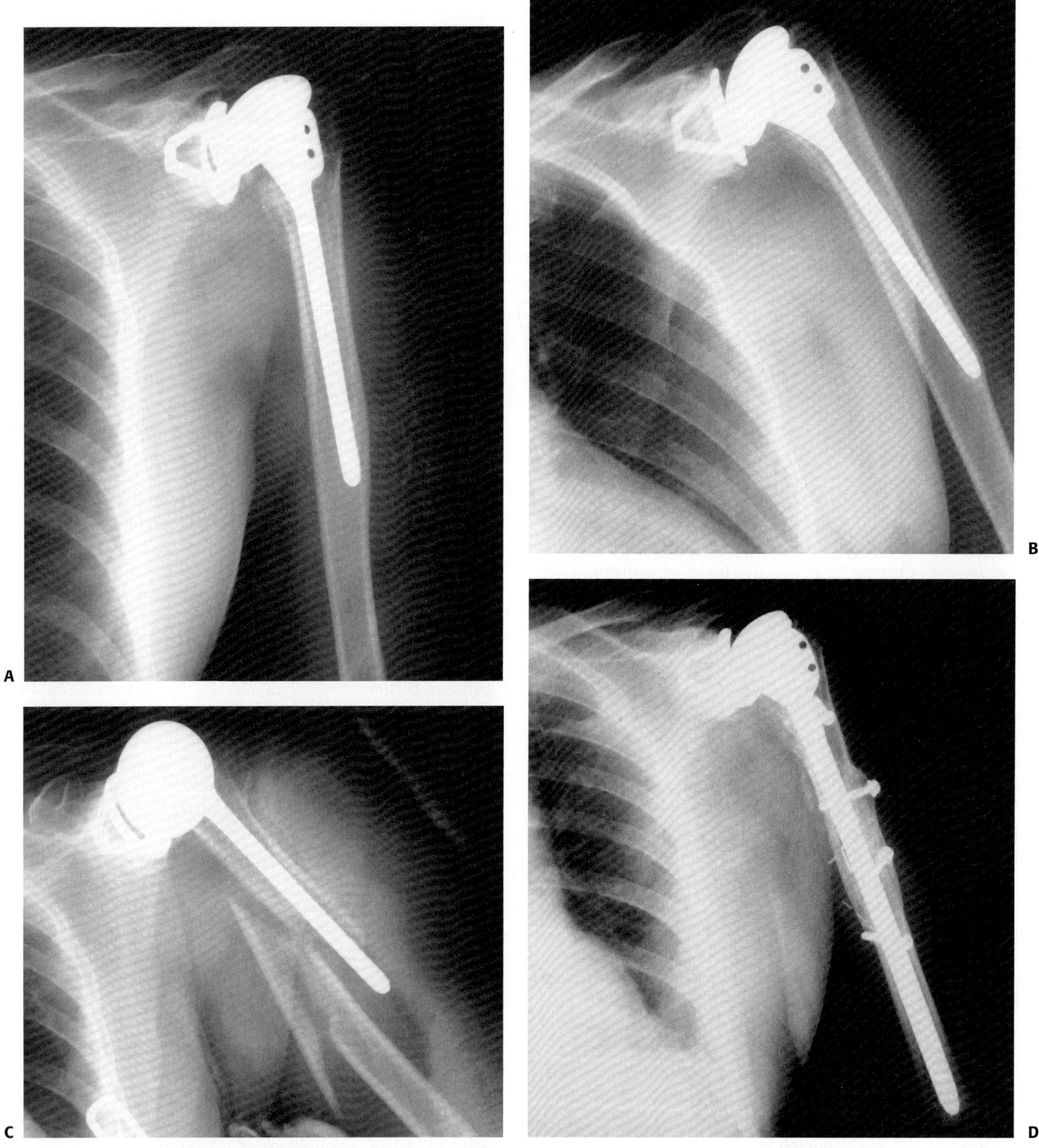

FIGURE 22-7 A total shoulder arthroplasty with an uncemented humeral component. In **(A)** there is no identifiable problem, although the uncemented humeral implant may be relatively undersized relative to the width of the humeral shaft. In **(B)**, 2 years later it is apparent the humeral component has shifted in position indicative of loosening. One year after the x-ray in **(B)** the patient had a severe fall sustaining a comminuted humeral shaft fracture **(C).** The fracture was treated with revision of the humeral component to a long-stem press-fitted component with heavy nonabsorbable suture cerclage of the butterfly fragment and allograft cancellous bone chips. Union did not occur by 1 year after surgery. A free fibular transfer was then added to achieve healing **(D).**

The determination should be made whether the humeral component is tightly fixed or loose. For uncemented components, it is quite helpful to understand the surface characteristics of the implant in place, the extent of tissue ingrowth coating or texturing. Some implants only have this proximally, some have it proximally and distally, and some have none at all. With uncemented components, if there is no texturing whatsoever, fracturing about the component is likely to be associated with prosthetic loosening as the implant would need to be firmly fixed both proximally and distally in order to remain stable. For those implants with proximal or proximal and distal ingrowth coatings or texturings, the implant may be stable proximally with some fracturing about the lower end of the implant that does not necessarily indicate prosthetic loosening. With extension of a periprosthetic fracture up along the stem of the implant, unless one is highly certain about stability of the implant proximally related to the texturing or ingrowth surfaces, the proximal extent of the fracture itself may clearly indicate implant loosening. In uncemented or cemented components, one may identify lucent lines at the implant-bone or cement-bone interface. If the lucent lines are 1.5 to 2 mm or greater in thickness and surround the implant, one would be seriously concerned that loosening of the implant is present. A similar line extending entirely along one side of the implant or substantive osteolysis of the humeral shaft adjacent to the implant would also likely indicate prosthetic loosening. In addition to assessing the above components of periprosthetic loosening, one should, if at all possible, evaluate whether there has been a subtle shift in component position over time, by use of sequential x-rays (Fig. 22-7). When a noncemented component is present it may be impossible to know whether or not loosening has occurred and as such, the surgeon will have to be prepared to approach both the fracture and the shoulder at the time of surgery. Evaluating for osteolysis is critical. Osteolysis may be absent, present to a minor degree, or be quite severe making reconstruction exceedingly difficult. This lysis may be occurring because of joint surface malfunction with plastic or metal wear that must also be corrected. In addition, by physical examination and x-ray, it is important to assess shoulder joint mobility, for if the shoulder is stiff, one will typically need to address attention to the shoulder joint at the time of fracture fixation to achieve range of motion and lessen stress about the fracture or nonunion site in the humeral shaft (Fig. 22-8).

Fracture Classification

There have been several fracture classifications described for periprosthetic fractures. At our institution, fractures are classified ac-

A

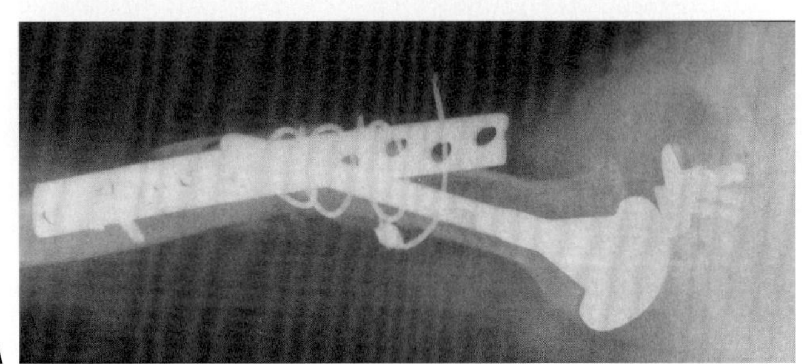

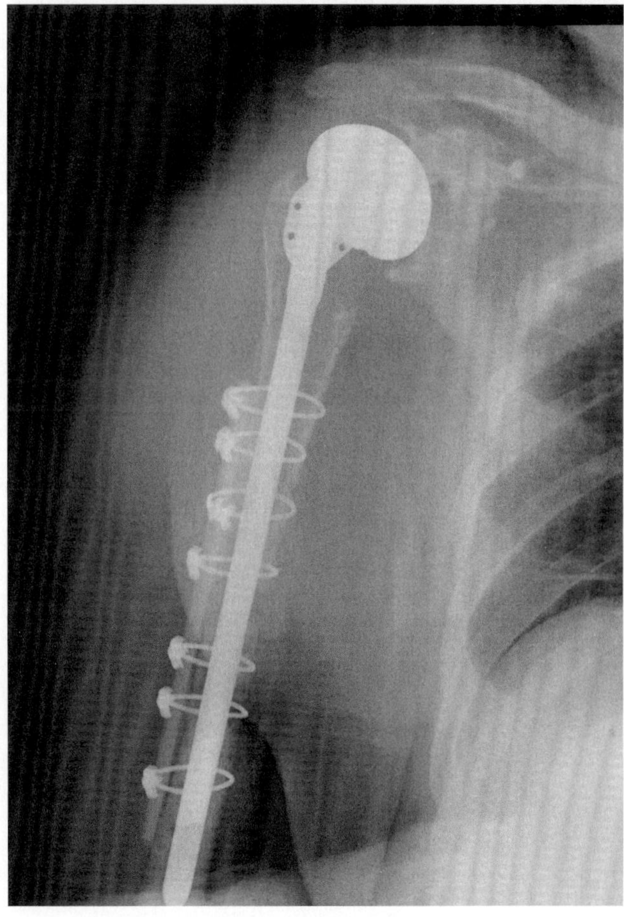

B

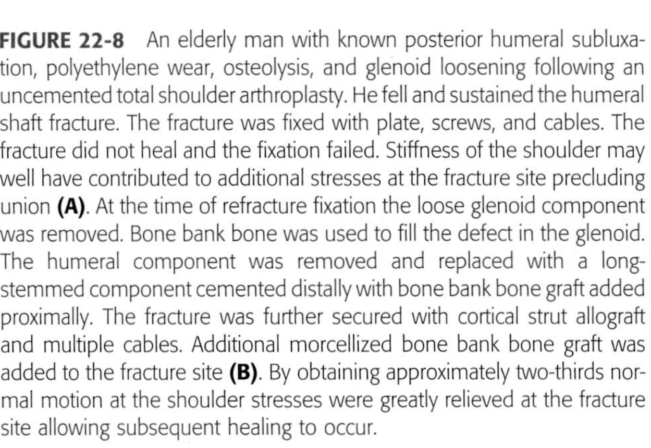

FIGURE 22-8 An elderly man with known posterior humeral subluxation, polyethylene wear, osteolysis, and glenoid loosening following an uncemented total shoulder arthroplasty. He fell and sustained the humeral shaft fracture. The fracture was fixed with plate, screws, and cables. The fracture did not heal and the fixation failed. Stiffness of the shoulder may well have contributed to additional stresses at the fracture site precluding union **(A)**. At the time of refracture fixation the loose glenoid component was removed. Bone bank bone was used to fill the defect in the glenoid. The humeral component was removed and replaced with a long-stemmed component cemented distally with bone bank bone graft added proximally. The fracture was further secured with cortical strut allograft and multiple cables. Additional morcellized bone bank bone graft was added to the fracture site **(B)**. By obtaining approximately two-thirds normal motion at the shoulder stresses were greatly relieved at the fracture site allowing subsequent healing to occur.

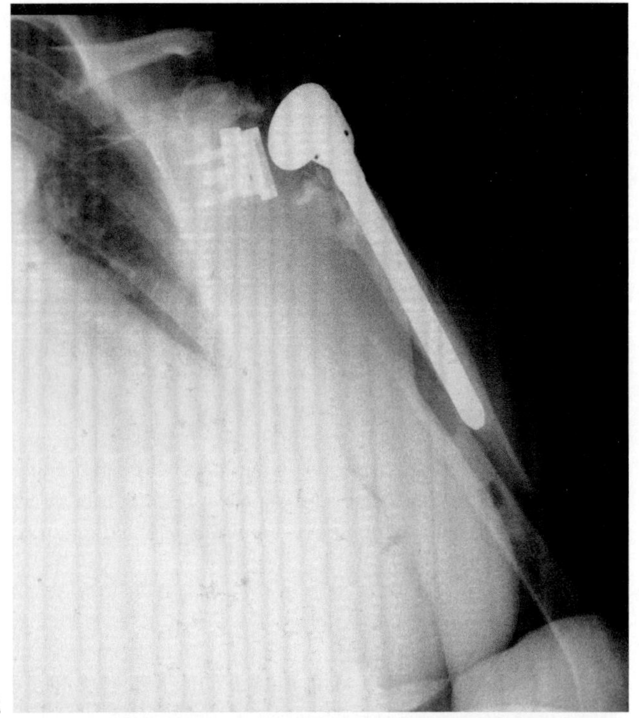

A

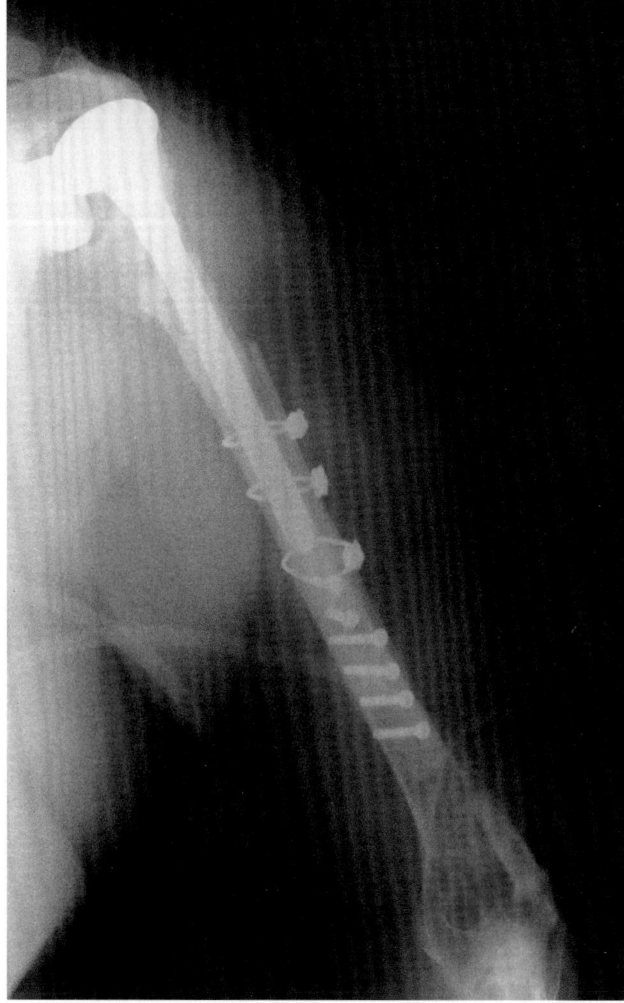

B

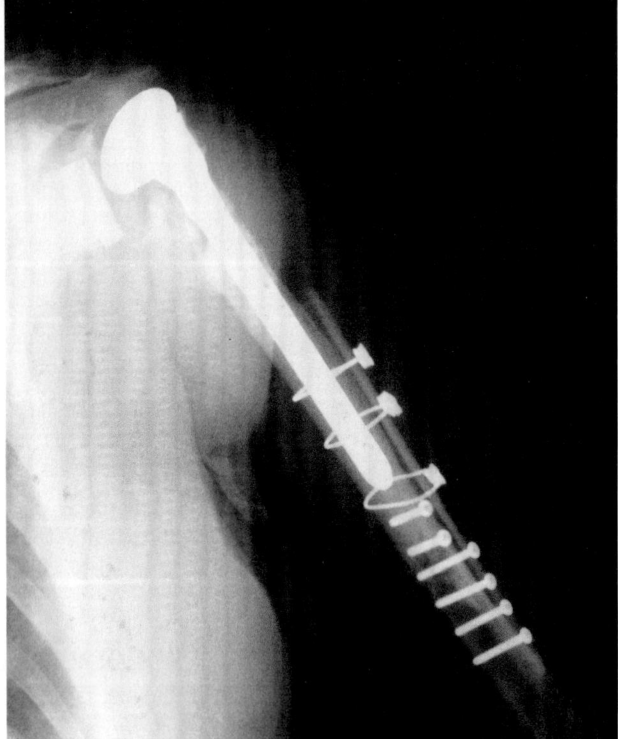

C

FIGURE 22-9 A Type A fracture though bone and cement. The fracture occurred at the tip of the implant with extension both proximally and distally. The humeral component is cemented and well fixed. This patient was treated successfully with open reduction and fixation of the spiral fracture with a cortical strut allograft, screws, and cables. The fracture healed by 4 months following surgery even though the strut allograft did not incorporate to the humeral shaft. Ideally, one additional cable could have been placed at the proximal end of the cortical strut allograft. X-ray **(A)** is soon after the fracture, **(B)** is immediately after operative treatment, and **(C)** is at 4 months following surgery.

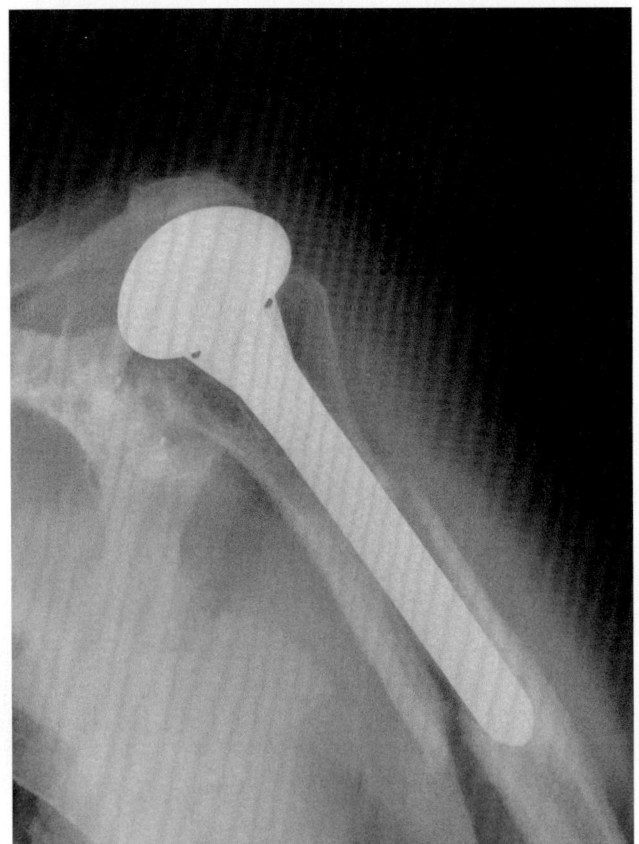
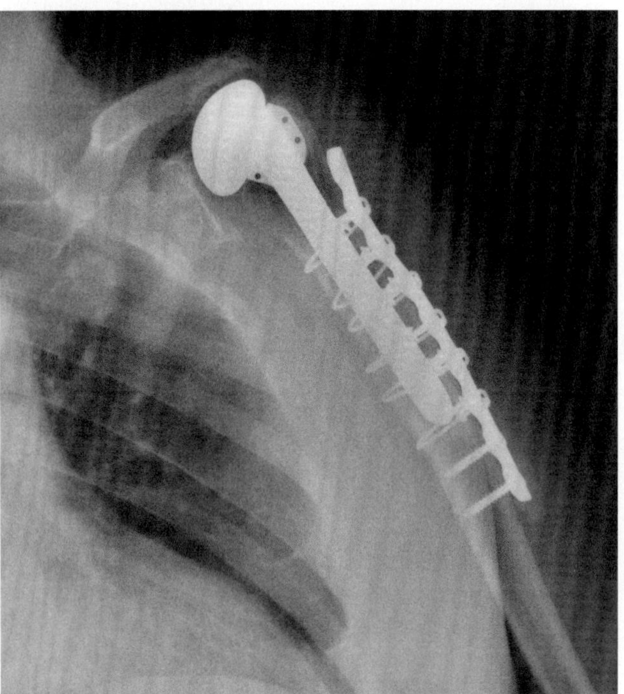

FIGURE 22-10 Active 67-year-old man with known rotator cuff tearing following total shoulder arthroplasty, but who had excellent shoulder function. He fell off a boat striking his arm during the fall. The fracture was treated nonoperatively for 3 months **(A)**, but did not progress toward healing. The fracture was then openly reduced and internally fixed with plate, screws, pins, and cerclage cables **(B)**. Within 3 months the fracture went on to solid union. The humeral component was well fixed at the time of surgery and thus revision of the humeral component was not necessary. However, with an uncemented humeral component it is often difficult to tell before fracture fixation whether a component is loose or not. One would need to be prepared to revise this humeral component to a long-stemmed humeral component as a part of the fracture fixation process.

cording to the system of Wright and Cofield (16). Fractures are defined in relation to their location with respect to the distal tip of the humeral implant. Type A are fractures at the prosthesis tip and extend proximally (Figs. 22-9 and 22-10). Type B are fractures at the prosthesis tip without extension or with a minimal amount of extension proximally and a variable amount of extension distally (Fig. 22-11). Type C fractures are those distal to the tip of the prosthesis (Figs. 22-12 and 22-13).

Surgical and Applied Anatomy

For shoulder arthroplasty we prefer a long deltopectoral exposure. Typically the skin incision is made over the anterior deltoid 2 to 3 cm lateral to the upper portion of the deltopectoral groove and ends over the anterior aspect of the deltoid insertion distally. A small skin flap is developed, the deltoid is retracted laterally and the cephalic vein is left in place medially and usually undisturbed. Occasionally (approximately 5% of cases) we use an anteromedial approach to the shoulder. This approach includes the deltopectoral approach allowing the cephalic vein to fall medially and a release of the clavicular and anterior acromial attachments of the deltoid. The deltoid attachment of the clavicle is J-shaped. To release the deltoid over the clavicle, an incision is made at the top of the clavicle, and the fibrous attachment of the deltoid is carefully stripped from the top, the front, and a portion of the undersurface of the clavicle, maintaining fibrous tissue to aid in deltoid reattachment. A portion of the acromioclavicular joint capsule is included with the deltoid at the time of release, and the deltoid is then carefully incised from bone over the anterior acromion. The combination of the deltopectoral exposure and this proximal deltoid release then allows one to turn the deltoid laterally in a progressive fashion and perform careful dissection of the deltoid from the underlying structures. The deltoid is then reattached through

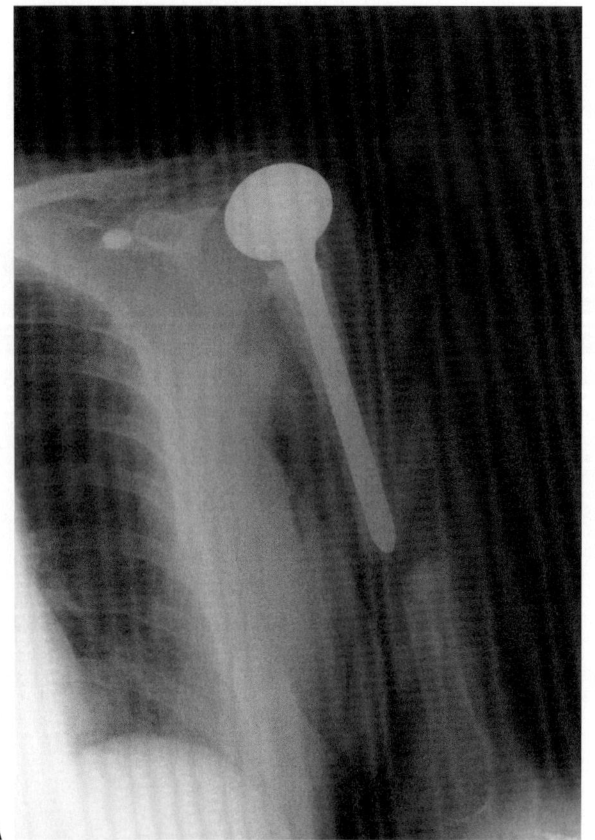

A

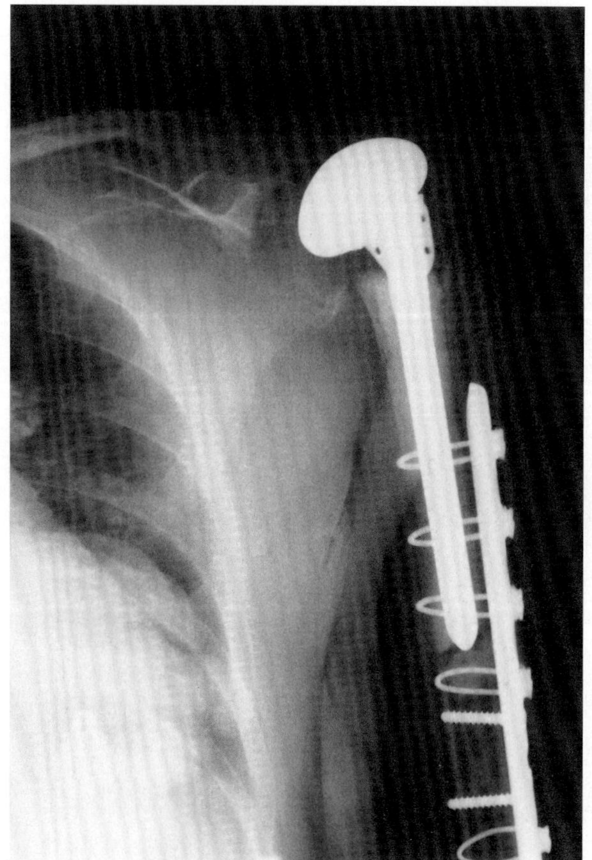

B

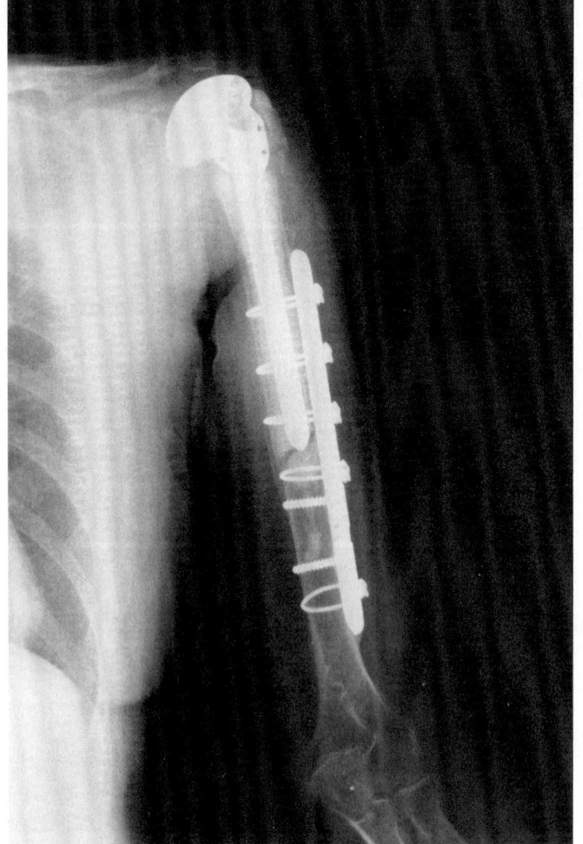

C

FIGURE 22-11 Illustration of a Type B fracture at the tip of the prosthesis through the cement mantle. This did not progress toward healing with nonoperative management. The component was well fixed and the patient was treated successfully with open reduction, internal fixation with a plate, screws, and multiple cables, and posterior iliac crest bone graft. **A.** Two months following fracture. **B.** Immediately after operative treatment. **C.** Fracture progressing toward healing with callus bridging the fracture gap. In **(A)** and **(B)** one can see that some callus had formed at the fracture site precluding perfect anatomic reduction and also in retrospect, recognize that a slightly longer plate with one additional cable proximally would have been preferred.

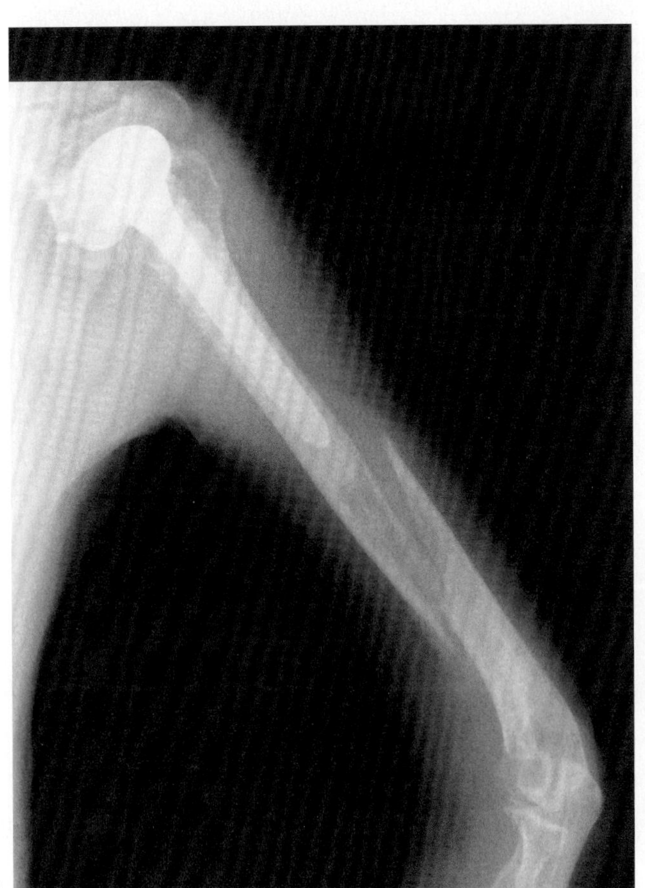

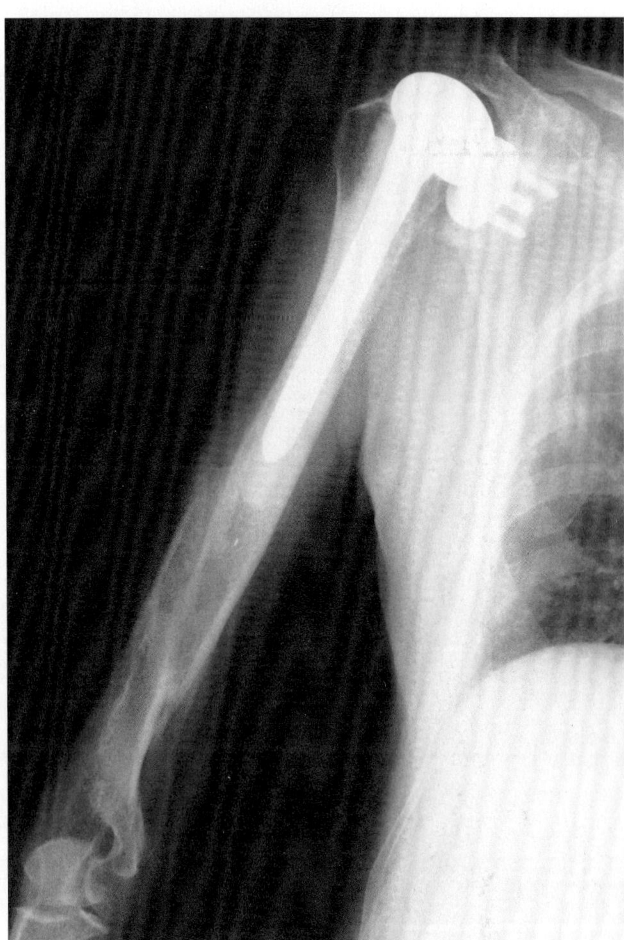

FIGURE 22-12 A Type C fracture distal to the humeral component. Although not in a perfect position, the fracture was thought to be reasonably reduced and stable and went on with nonoperative treatment to union. X-ray **(A)** shows the oblique distal humeral fracture soon after the injury, and **(B)** shows the healed fracture.

the bone of the acromion, through the capsule of the acromioclavicular joint, through suture to the trapezius and trapezial fascia, and most medially through drill holes in the clavicle.

When fracturing of the humeral shaft has occurred during surgery, or when periprosthetic humeral shaft fracture has occurred after surgery and one wishes to approach both the shoulder joint and the humeral shaft, this incision is extended distally following the anterolateral aspect of the humerus, again allowing the cephalic vein to remain medially (Fig. 22-14) (18). The fascia on the anterolateral aspect of the arm is then incised. The biceps is pushed medially and the brachialis is also pushed medially to avoid becoming confused by a lateral overhang of the brachialis relative to the humeral shaft. The brachialis is then incised approximately 1 to 1.5 cm medial to its lateral most aspect, leaving this small buffer of tissue between the bone on the lateral aspect of the surgical exposure and the radial nerve. By approaching this somewhat more lateral than is typically recommended, one has this buffering tissue yet has the availability to readily identify the radial nerve throughout the length of the exposure.

The fracture is then exposed by elevating the brachialis medially, elevating a portion of the anterior aspect of the deltoid insertion laterally, and for proximal extending fractures, a portion of the pectoralis major insertion may need to be elevated but we try to avoid disrupting the entire pectoralis major insertion as it, of course, performs important functions and is somewhat difficult to secure to its original site with fixation devices in place.

Enough exposure of the humeral shaft should be present (when a long-stemmed implant is not being used) so that one has space for four fixation points above and below the fracture, either four screws or cerclage cables, or some combination thereof on each side of the fracture. A lesser amount of exposure and fixation proximally and distally may be needed if the fracture is extremely oblique or spiral in shape.

Current Treatment Options

It seems useful to say a few words about prevention of periprosthetic shoulder fractures (19). Fractures of the lesser tuberosity

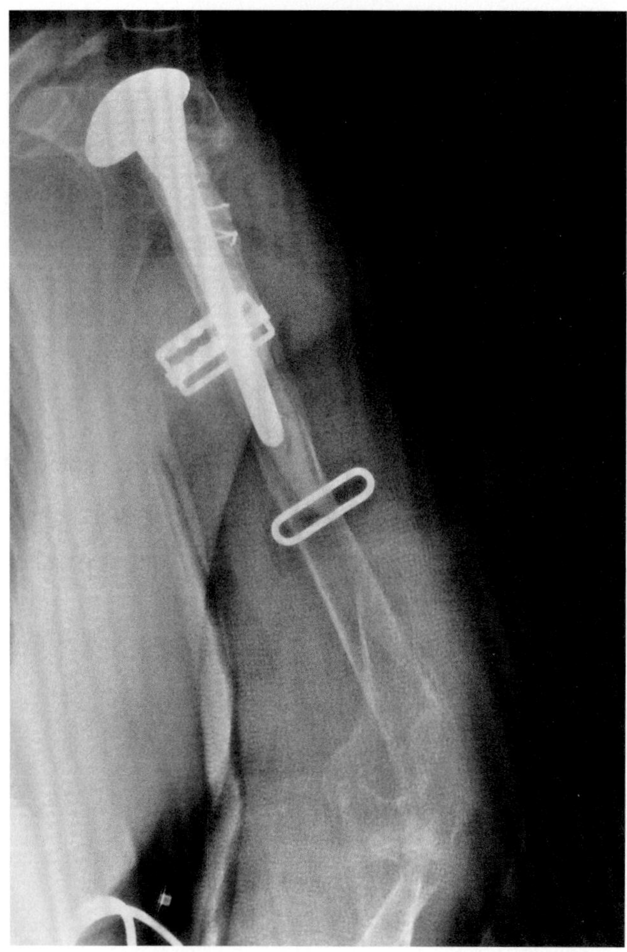

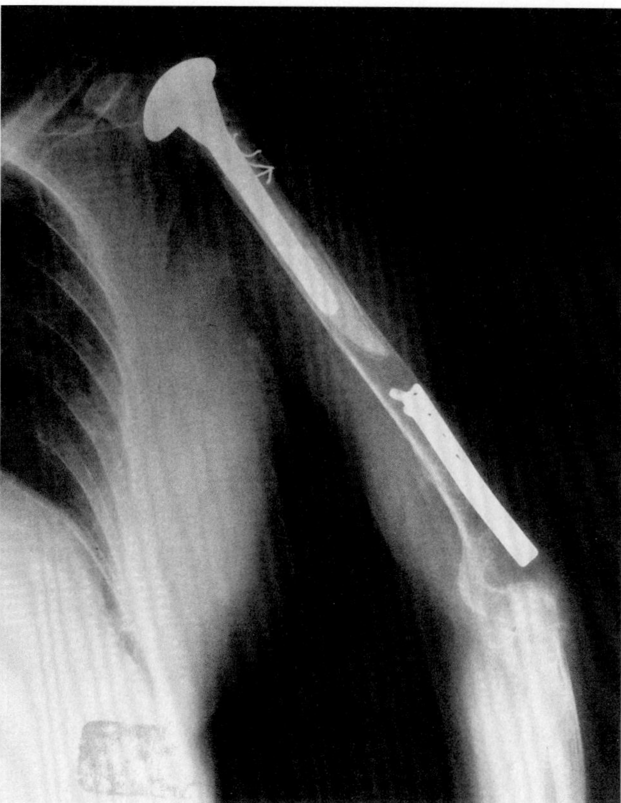

FIGURE 22-13 A distal humeral fracture, Type C, similar to the fracture illustrated in Figure 22-12. However, this fracture was felt to be grossly unstable and underwent immediate open reduction and internal fixation. The fracture soon after injury **(A)** and the reduction and fixation with subsequent healing **(B)**.

have been considerably diminished by having the availability of trial humeral stems without associated heads that can be maintained in the humeral canal during posterior retraction of the proximal humerus during glenoid preparation. If there are substantive cysts in the greater tuberosity that will weaken the greater tuberosity measurably, it may be useful to perform the anteromedial surgical exposure rather than the long deltopectoral exposure to avoid torsional stress on the tuberosity during performance of the index procedure. With better knowledge of surgical exposure, it is very unlikely to obtain a coracoid process fracture. However, if one does occur, re-suturing the fracture tip to the surrounding tissues—pectoralis minor tendon and coracoacromial ligament—is all that seems necessary. Fracture of the glenoid usually occurs when the glenoid is extremely osteopenic, such as in the patient with rheumatoid arthritis. When placing a retractor on the glenoid to direct the proximal humerus posteriorly, it is often useful in these situations to rest the retractor on the upper portion of the axillary border of the scapula rather than directly on the posterior glenoid rim.

By far the most important periprosthetic fracture occurring is that to the humeral shaft. There are several steps that can help prevent fracture of the humeral shaft including multiplanar preoperative x-rays with magnification markers if one is uncertain about the amount of magnification that occurs on x-rays (typically about 8%). Preoperative templating is possible for many systems. Complete soft-tissue releases will avoid substantial stress on the humerus during performance of arthroplasty. Scar within the subacromial and subdeltoid regions should be completely released. If there is contracture of the superior or posterior capsule, these capsular attachments are most efficaciously released surrounding the glenoid outside or above the biceps anchor attachment and then along the glenoid rim posteriorly. Almost always there is significant inferior shoulder joint contracture and this is most easily released by performing capsule release around the neck of the humerus, staying on the bone and carefully avoiding injury to the axillary nerve. Also with anterior shoulder contractures, releases are performed typically along the glenoid rim. With all these soft tissues fully released, the humerus can then be brought gently forward with minimal torsion applied to the bone. If the shaft is extremely osteopenic, again one might consider an anteromedial approach rather than only the deltopectoral approach to help avoid further stress on positioning the humerus during performance of the arthroplasty. It is also useful to have considerable flexibility

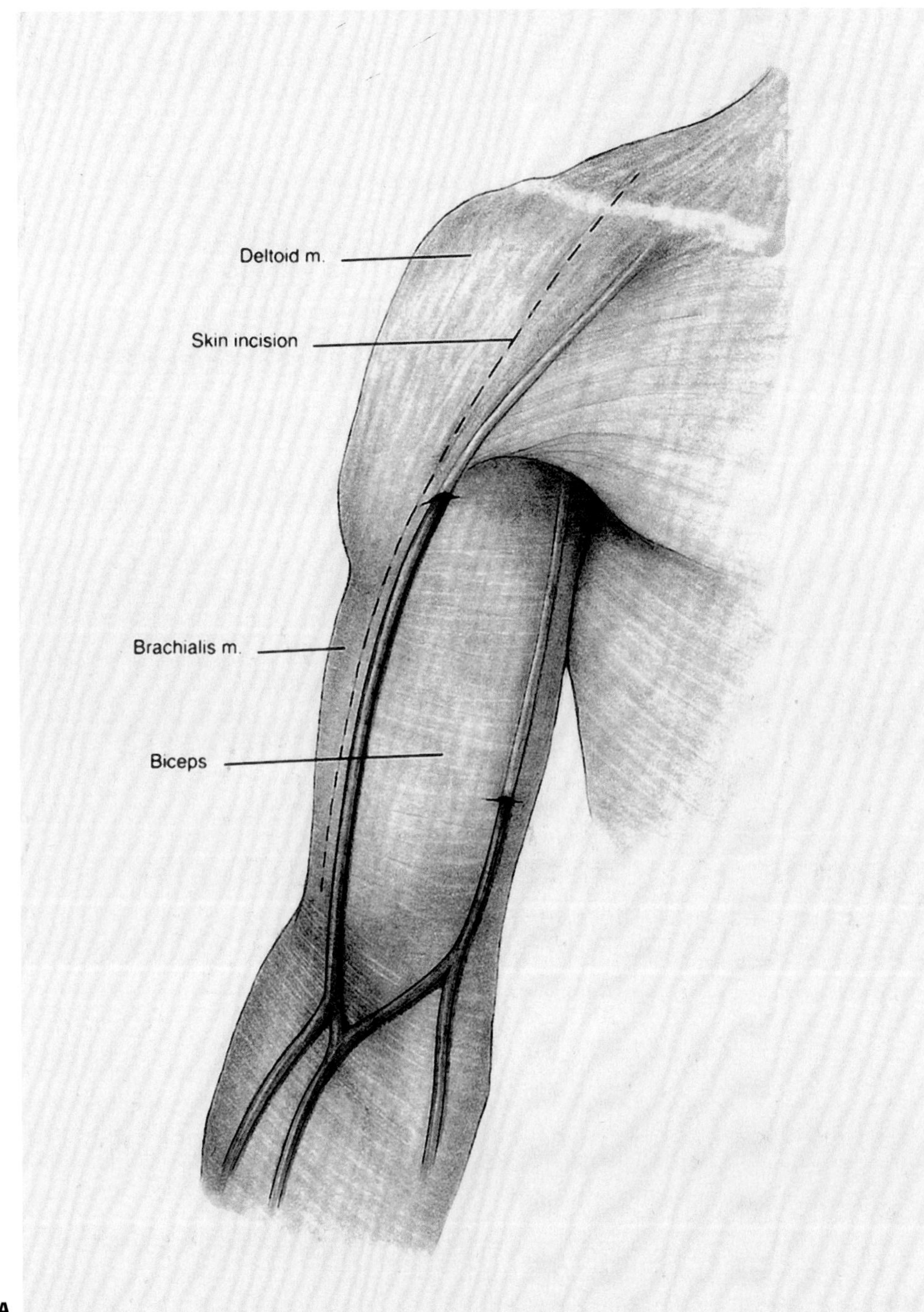

A

FIGURE 22-14 The anterolateral approach to the humeral shaft. **A.** Illustrates an anterolateral arm incision extended distally from a deltopectoral or anteromedial shoulder incision that is useful when an intraoperative humeral shaft fracture occurs. If the fracture occurs in the postoperative period the more distal portion of the incision is used for fracture reduction and fixation unless the shoulder also needs to be approached to exchange the humeral component. *(continues)*

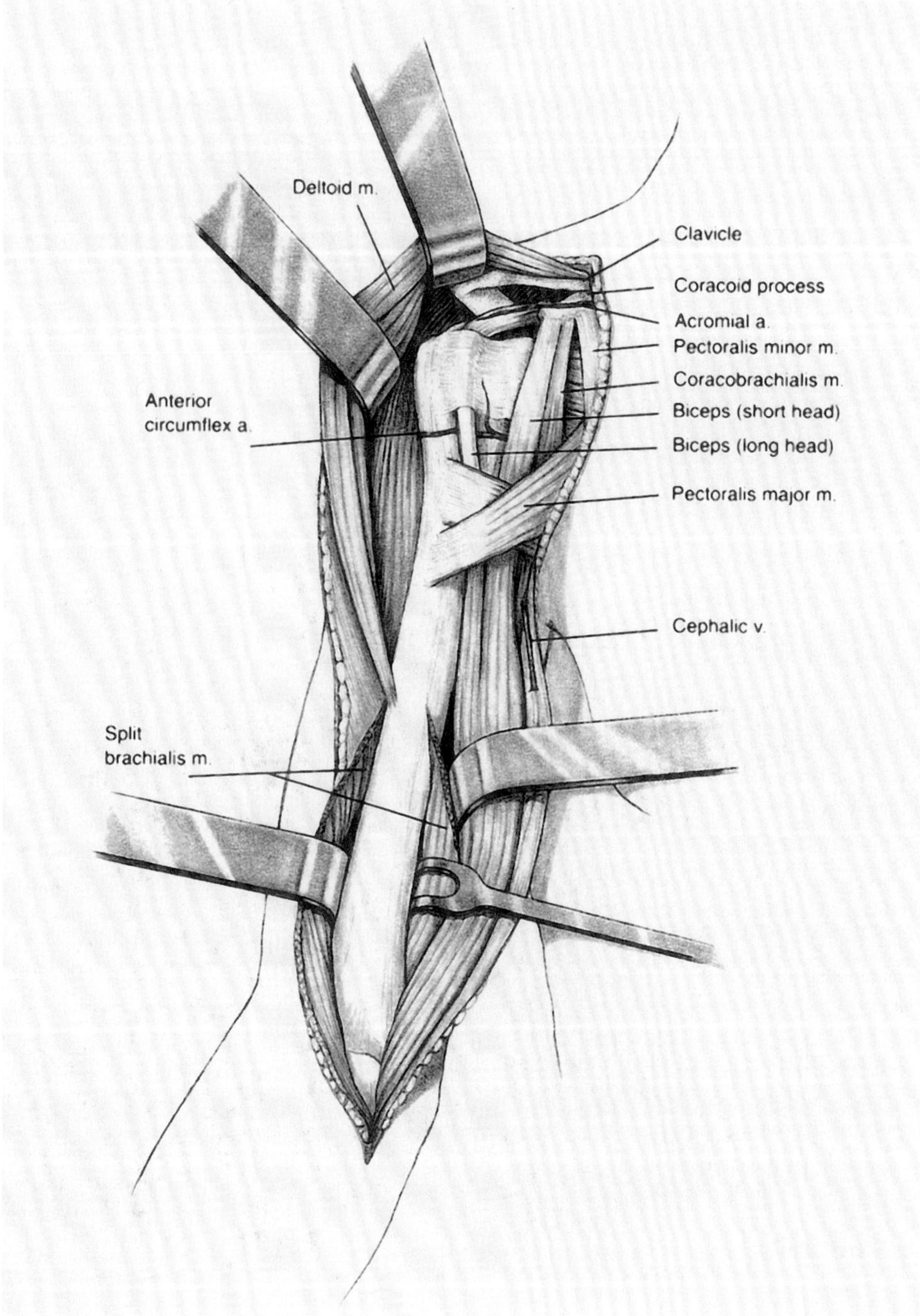

B

FIGURE 22-14 (*continued*) We prefer to allow the cephalic vein to fall medially with the proximal portion of the incision and continue to allow the vein to fall medially when the incision is extended distally. The biceps is retracted medially and the brachialis is also pushed medially so that a thinner portion of the brachialis may be incised longitudinally approximately 1 to 1.5 cm medial to its lateral-most aspect **(B)**. (*continues*)

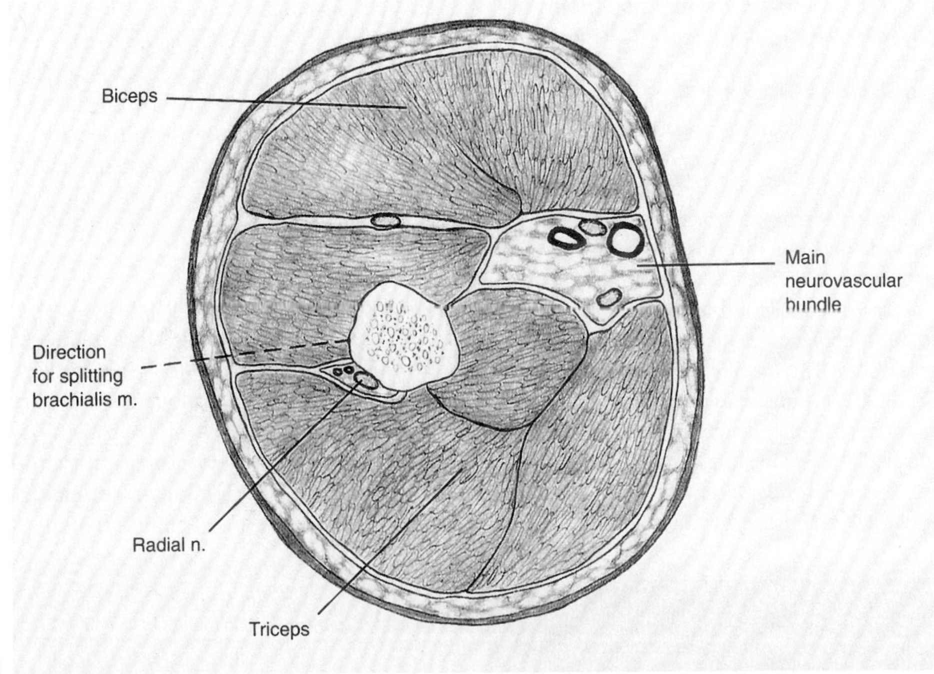

FIGURE 22-14 (*continued*) This leaves a narrow buffer of tissue between the bone on the lateral aspect of the exposure and the radial nerve. In addition, this also allows one to visualize the radial nerve at any point during the exposure should one wish to do so **(C)**. (From Cofield RH. Total shoulder replacement: managing bone deficiencies. In: Craig EV, ed. *The shoulder*, 2nd ed. Philadelphia: Lippincott Williams & Wilkins, 2004: 549–575.)

in the implant system so that one is not forcing an implant in place that is too tight. During humeral canal preparation it is important to avoid perforation of the canal by ensuring correct alignment of the instrumentation during bone preparation. Intraoperative x-rays will sometimes be needed in this regard, particularly in old fracture cases with some degree of malunion. If for some reason there is a cortical defect in the humeral shaft, this should be bypassed by a stem that is at least 4 to 5 cm distal to the defect.

Before addressing the humeral shaft fracture, it is important to mention some of the other fractures that occur around shoulder implants. Nondisplaced lesser tuberosity fractures often occur before routine placement of the trial component during the procedure. In this occasion, when repairing the subscapularis, one passes sutures (usually a nonabsorbable No. 2), through the subscapularis, through or around the lesser tuberosity, and into sound bone slightly more lateral on the proximal humerus. Issues with lesser tuberosity healing have almost never arisen. Should the greater tuberosity crack during placement of an arthroplasty, it is important to recognize how significant it is for the greater tuberosity to heal in good position. As such, even though the fracture is undisplaced, it seems sensible to secure it in its position with multiple large (usually a nonabsorbable No. 5) sutures to help ensure that displacement will not occur in the postoperative period and that healing will readily occur. Rarely, glenoid fractures occur during preparation. When this happens the bone is usually extremely osteopenic, and we have not been successful in placing a glenoid component in this circumstance but have bone grafted any defects that occurred during preparation and have then allowed this to heal with placement of a humeral head implant alone. One can envision that occasionally a crack in the glenoid may occur that is large enough that screw fixation may be possible with or without support by a buttress plate on the glenoid neck. However, in practice this rarely occurs (never in our experience).

To achieve a satisfactory outcome following periprosthetic humeral shaft fracture, the fracture must heal and the humeral implant must be secure within the bone. When undertaking operative intervention, the fracture must be stable, the implant must be secure, and there must be enough bone present to achieve a successful result. When extensive osteolysis is present, it will be necessary to add morcellized bone allograft and often strut allografts to support the reconstructed humerus. In the presence of a rather focal nonunion in the humeral shaft, a posterior iliac crest autograft is preferred.

When a humeral shaft fracture is felt to occur intraoperatively, x-rays are obtained. If the fracture is quite oblique the fracture site is exposed. A longer-stemmed implant is used to stabilize the fracture and additional stability is obtained with cerclage cables after the fracture is exposed. We would often use a noncemented humeral stem in this instance. If the fracture is nearly transverse or transverse, we prefer a longer-stem cemented component cemented both proximally and distally with bone bank allograft placed around the fracture site. In this setting, it is not usually necessary to use plates or cortical strut allografts.

For humeral shaft fractures occurring in the postoperative period, there are multiple considerations, the first is the fracture location. The second is whether the fracture occurred only through bone or through bone and bone cement; third is the alignment of the fracture including fracture displacement; fourth is whether or not the humeral prosthesis is loose; and fifth is analysis of the extent of bone lysis. Occasionally a crack develops through an area of osteolytic bone without displacement. It seems prudent to consider allowing this to heal before undertaking revision surgery. The specific indications for operative treatment would include a substantively displaced and unstable fracture, a fracture through bone and cement greatly limiting the area of bone available for healing, a transverse fracture at the tip of the prosthesis with displacement, or a displaced fracture surrounding a loose prosthesis with or without the presence of substantive osteolysis. Surgical treatment for periprosthetic fractures with associated radial nerve palsy is controversial. Some authors have noted that radial nerve palsy may be an indication for operative treatment. Boyd et al (9) reported on two of seven fractures treated with surgery due to radial nerve palsy. In each of these cases, radial nerve deficits were thought to be secondary to persistent motion of fracture fragments.

Fracture Location

The literature demonstrates that fractures located distal to the prosthesis tip are similar to closed humerus fractures and may respond favorably to nonoperative treatment. In the study by Campbell et al (12), four of five patients treated successfully by functional bracing were distal to the prosthesis tip and likely type C fractures. In the study by Kumar (14), two of three type C fractures healed successfully with nonoperative management.

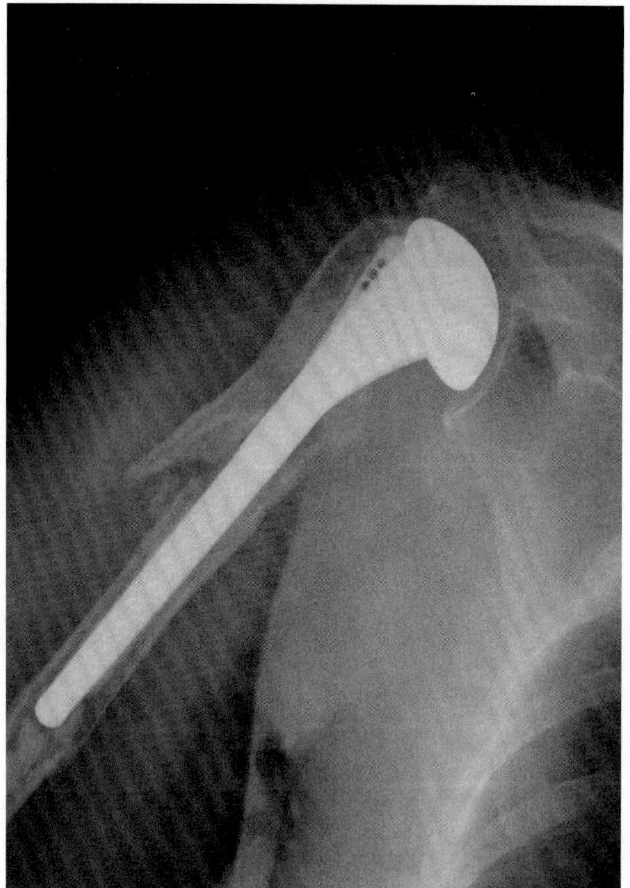

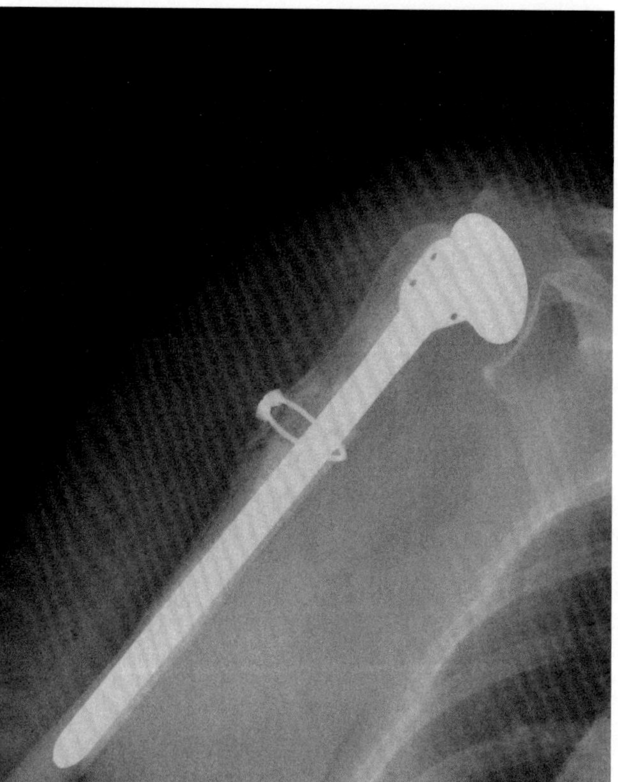

FIGURE 22-15 A humeral head prosthesis was used during treatment of a comminuted proximal humeral fracture with distal humeral extension. The shoulder joint functioned reasonably well following surgery, however, the more distal extension of the fracture did not heal and the prosthesis loosened with bone lysis **(A)**. This was revised to a long-stemmed humeral component cemented distally and press-fitted proximally with the addition of bone bank allograft to fill any interstices that were present between the osteolytic bone of the proximal humeral fragment and the implant. The fracture was further secured with a cerclage cable and the fracture went on to a union with maintenance of secure humeral implant fixation **(B)**.

One fracture distal to the prosthesis tip was also treated successfully by nonoperative means by Worland et al (15).

However, fractures located at the prosthesis tip (type A and type B) behave differently. In the literature, there are several cases of fractures at the tip of the prosthesis that did not heal with nonoperative management. This includes five cases in a series of seven by Boyd et al (9) and one case by Bonutti et al (10). In the series by Kumar et al (14), four of five type B fractures treated nonoperatively failed to heal and eventually required surgery. Among the three type A fractures treated nonoperatively in that series, two healed and one required multiple surgeries, including a free fibula transfer to heal.

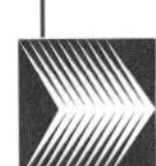

AUTHORS' PREFERRED TREATMENT

In fractures with a loose humeral prosthesis, it seems most practical to exchange this implant for a longer-stemmed implant. There are then four options relative to intramedullary fixation. One can use press-fitting proximally and distally, cementing proximally and distally, press-fitting proximally with cement distally, and cementing proximally with press-fitting distally. We tend to use press-fitting proximally and distally if there is good quality of the humeral bone, a tight fit can be achieved and there is substantial obliquity at the fracture site that will be amenable to adjunctive fixation with tensioned cables to avoid the prospect of rotational instability (Fig. 22-15). We tend to use cement proximally and distally when the bone proximally is good to fair and the bone distally is good in the presence of a largely transverse fracture. We tend to use press-fitting proximally and cement distally when the bone proximally is fair to poor and the bone distally is good—in the presence of a fracture that is rotationally stable by its shape or can be made stable by external support using a plate with cerclage cables and pins, or less commonly a strut allograft with cables. It is very unusual that we would elect to cement proximally and press-fit distally as there are currently no prostheses readily available that will allow for bone ingrowth fixation distally as there are for the femur. Of note, when there is a small amount of osteolysis proximally, cement or bone graft may be used. When there is extensive osteolysis proximally, usually bone graft is packed around the implant within the cortical shell that remains. Rarely the osteolysis may be so extensive that an allograft prosthetic composite might be necessary (Fig. 22-16).

If the implant is secure and the joint is reasonably mobile, one can approach the fracture site alone for fracture fixation. In this circumstance we prefer a plate with screws, pins and cerclage cables. Morcellized allograft will be added to the fracture site if an established nonunion is not present. If an established nonunion is present, we prefer posterior iliac crest autograft bone to graft the site. A metal plate is especially useful when the fracture is transverse or nearly transverse as rotational stability can be attained through the use of the screws, pins and cerclage. If the fracture is oblique about the implant and inherent stability can be achieved by reduction of the fracture and cerclage, we would tend to do this alone in the acute setting but in the chronic setting add a strut allograft in addition to the autograft morcellized bone. We have not found it necessary to add both a metal plate and a strut allograft; although, an occasional situation might be envisioned where this could be useful, particularly in larger individuals.

Rarely in an older individual with extreme osteolysis and pre-existing significant cuff deficiency, it may seem best to use a proximal humeral tumor prosthesis cemented distally to deal with the usually rather transverse humeral fracture and the extensive proximal osteolysis in the absence of substantive rotator cuff attachments.

Below are guidelines listed by fracture type as they have typically been presented in the literature and with which we would concur.

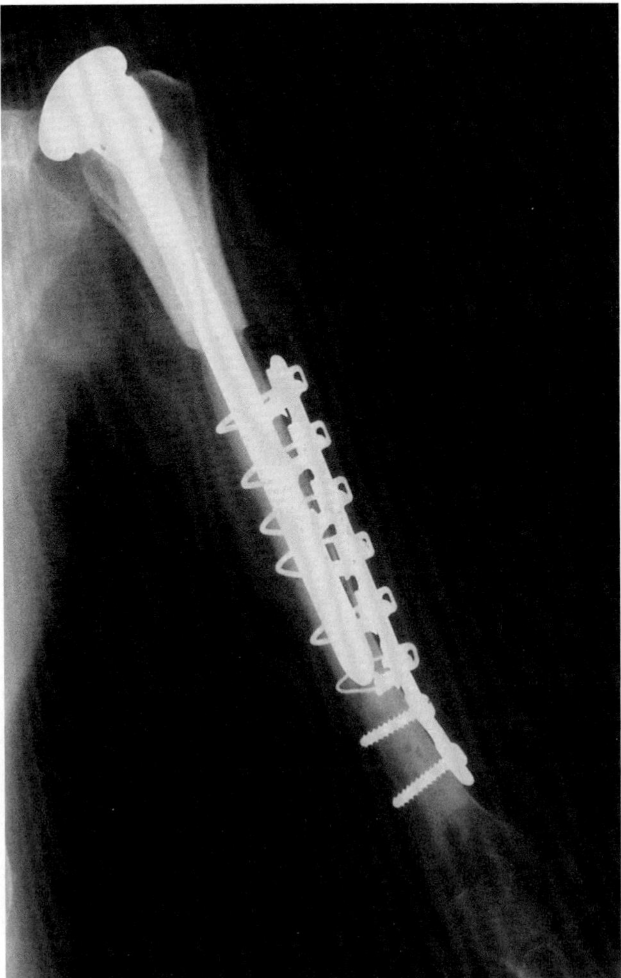

FIGURE 22-16 An allograft prosthetic composite was performed in a patient with a humeral shaft fracture but also with extensive osteolysis of the proximal fragment associated with humeral component loosening and nonunion at the fracture site that included significant distal extension of the fracture.

Type A

The literature and our own experience does not clearly indicate the need for surgery in type A fractures. In our series, three of six type A fractures healed with nonoperative management, one failed nonoperative management, and two were treated with immediate operative management (16). When there is substantial overlap between the length of fracture and humeral stem, the humeral component has a significant likelihood of being loose. Type A fractures with a loose humeral component should be treated operatively. Loose-components should be revised with a long-stem component that spans the fracture length by several cortical diameters. In our practice, we use bone graft in most operative cases to augment healing (allograft in acute cases and posterior iliac crest autograft in cases with delayed healing or nonunion). In addition, one may consider supplementary fixation with a cortical strut allograft or a plate and screws/cables to obtain secure fixation.

Type B

For Type B fractures with good alignment and a well-fixed humeral component, one may consider a trial of nonoperative treatment. However, in our experience and in a review of the literature, Type B fractures treated nonoperatively have a high propensity to fail to heal and eventually require surgery. Type B fractures that have not progressed toward union by 3 months are recommended for operative intervention.

For patients with a Type B fracture and a well-fixed humeral component, our current practice is to use a plate or strut graft with screw fixation in the distal portion and cerclage fixation in the proximal portion. Bone graft is also used in order to maximize the healing potential. Our experience shows this to be a good alternative to revising a well-fixed prosthesis.

In Type B fractures with a loose humeral component, one should consider revision with a cemented long-stem component and posterior iliac crest bone graft to the fracture site. Currently, there is no information on the relative efficacy of cortical strut allograft or plate fixation to provide adjunctive fixation together with insertion of a long-stem arthroplasty. However, additional adjuncts such as cortical struts or a plate have been described to improve fixation in revision total hip arthroplasty with a periprosthetic fracture (17).

Type C

Among those with a Type C fracture with a well-fixed humeral component, similar to a closed distal humerus fracture, a trial of nonoperative treatment is recommended if an acceptable closed reduction can be obtained with the use of a plastic orthosis.

Since it is essential to obtain humeral shaft bone healing (in most reconstructive options) to obtain a successful outcome, we tend to be quite conservative in our postoperative care. Within days after surgery the hand, forearm, and elbow are gently exercised with active movement. Typically, passive external rotation outward to neutral and in elevation to 100° is also started early; however, it is important to avoid stress at the fracture site when doing this and also to continue with a passive program until healing has been ensured. When a long-stemmed implant has been cemented both proximally and distally and the fracture is rotationally stable, we usually begin an active-assisted motion program at 4 to 6 weeks after the soft tissues have been allowed to heal. However, this situation is much less typical than deferring active-assisted motion until bone healing, as previously mentioned.

Complications

Complications have not been currently defined for periprosthetic shoulder fractures. However, one can readily imagine that radial nerve injury may occur at the time of surgery. Of course, it is best to avoid the nerve by careful dissection and exposure at the time of fracture fixation. The surgeon must be sure at the time of surgery that the radial nerve is not compromised, and should radial nerve palsy appear following surgery, observation would be usually all that is necessary in addition to intermittent wrist splinting as one can be virtually assured that function will recover.

This is a rather large procedure, particularly if it is necessary to operate on both the shoulder and the humeral shaft. As such, swelling of the arm, forearm, and hand can be anticipated. This is managed by elevation, elastic support, and the gentle active-motion program as outlined above.

An occasional acute infection might develop that would be managed by thorough debridement and irrigation, maintenance of the implanted internal fixation, and the use of antibiotics.

The largest concern, of course, is failure of humeral shaft healing. If fixation is secure but there is no apparent healing by 6 months, we would consider autogenous posterior iliac crest bone grafting at that time. On one occasion, even this did not suffice and a vascularized fibular transfer was employed to effect union at the fracture site in the presence of a long-stem implant that was well fixed proximally but somewhat unstable distally.

Controversies

The literature does not clearly indicate the need for surgery in Type A fractures—when the implant is not loose. A trial of nonoperative treatment may be considered for well-aligned Type B fractures with a well-fixed humeral component. However, as noted in the literature, Type B fractures have a high propensity to fail nonoperative treatment and eventually require surgery. Therefore, one should consider operative intervention for Type B fractures that have not progressed toward union by 3 months. If the humeral component is well fixed, open reduction and internal fixation may be performed. If the humeral component is loose, revision with a long stem is recommended. A trial of nonoperative treatment is recommended for well-reduced Type C fractures.

REFERENCES

1. Gschwend N, Simmen BR, Matejovsky Z. Late complications in elbow arthroplasty. *J Shoulder Elbow Surg* 1996;5(2):86.
2. O'Driscoll SW, Morrey BF. Periprosthetic fractures about the elbow. *Orthop Clinics North Am* 1999;30(2):319–325.
3. Kamineni S, Morrey BF. Proximal ulnar reconstruction with strut allograft in revision total elbow arthroplasty. *J Bone Joint Surg* 2004;86(6):1223–1229.
4. Marra G, Morrey BF, Gallay SH, et al. Fracture and nonunion of olecranon in total elbow arthroplasty (*submitted for publication*).
5. Garbuz DS, Masri BA, Duncan CP. Periprosthetic fractures of the femur: principles of prevention and management. *Instr Course Lect* 1998;47:237–242.
6. Lewallen DG, Berry DJ. Periprosthetic fracture of the femur after total hip arthroplasty: treatment and results to date. *Instr Course Lect* 1998;47:243–249.
7. Sanchez-Sotelo J, O'Driscoll SW, Morrey BF. Periprosthetic humeral fractures after total elbow arthroplasty: treatment with implant revision and strut allograft augmentation. *J Bone Joint Surg* 2002;84(9):1642–1650.
8. Morrey BF, Mansat P, Adams RA. Allograft-prosthesis-composite for revision of catastrophic failure of total elbow arthroplasty. *J Bone Joint Surg* 2004,86(4):724.
9. Cameron B, Iannotti JP. Periprosthetic fractures of the humerus and scapula: management and prevention. *Orthop Clin North Am* 1999;30:305–318.
10. Bonutti PM, Hawkins RJ. Fracture of the humeral shaft associated with the total replacement arthroplasty of the shoulder. *J Bone Joint Surg* 1992;74:617–618.
11. Boyd AD Jr, Thornhill TS, Barnes CL. Fractures adjacent to humeral prostheses. *J Bone Surg Am* 1992;74:1498–1504.
12. Campbell J, Moore R, Iannoti J, et al. Periprosthetic humeral fractures: mechanism of fractures and treatment options. *J Shoulder Elbow Surg* 1998;7:406–413.
13. Krakauer JD, Cofield RH. Periprosthetic fractures in total shoulder replacement. *Operative Techniques in Orthopaedics* 1994;4:243–252.
14. Kumar S, Sperling JW, Haidukewych GJ, et al. Periprosthetic humeral fractures after shoulder arthroplasty. *J Bone Joint Surg* 2004;86(4):680–689.
15. Worland RL, Kim DY, Arredondo J. Periprosthetic humeral fractures: management and classification. *J Shoulder Elbow Surg* 1999;8:590–594.
16. Wright T, Cofield RH. Humeral fractures after shoulder arthroplasty. *J Bone Joint Surg* 1995;77:1340–1346.
17. Incavo SJ, Beard DM, Pupparo F, et al. One stage revision of periprosthetic fractures around loose cemented total hip arthroplasty. *Am J Orthop* 1998;27:35–41.
18. Cofield RH. Total shoulder replacement: managing bone deficiencies. In: Craig EV, ed. *The shoulder*, 2nd ed. Philadelphia: Lippincott Williams & Wilkins, 2004:549–575.
19. Lewallen DG, Berry DJ. Periprosthetic fractures associated with hip arthroplasty. In: Morrey BF, ed. *Joint replacement arthroplasty*, 3rd ed. Philadelphia: Churchill Livingstone, 2003:902–919.

PART 2
PERIPROSTHETIC FRACTURES ABOUT TOTAL HIP AND TOTAL KNEE REPLACEMENTS

JAY D. MABREY

EDUCATIONAL OBJECTIVES

There are four educational objectives set forth for the reader upon completion of this chapter. First, for every case, the reader will identify the risk factors associated with and contributing to periprosthetic fractures of the hip and knee. Second, the reader will execute a complete evaluation of an individual case, including assessing prefracture patient function and deciding if he or she possesses the skills and tools to successfully treat the problem. Third, the reader will apply current classification schemes to determine implant stability and judge the adequacy of available bone stock. And fourth, the reader will develop, document, and carry out an appropriate treatment plan based upon these findings.

GOALS OF TREATMENT

Fractures about total joint replacements add a new level of complexity in terms of operative fixation due to the simple presence of the metal implants. Successful repair relies on a combination of the surgeon's trauma and reconstructive skills (1). Well-fixed implants interfere with standard intramedullary or screw/plate techniques whereas loose implants are often accompanied by significant bone loss. My goals of treatment of periprosthetic

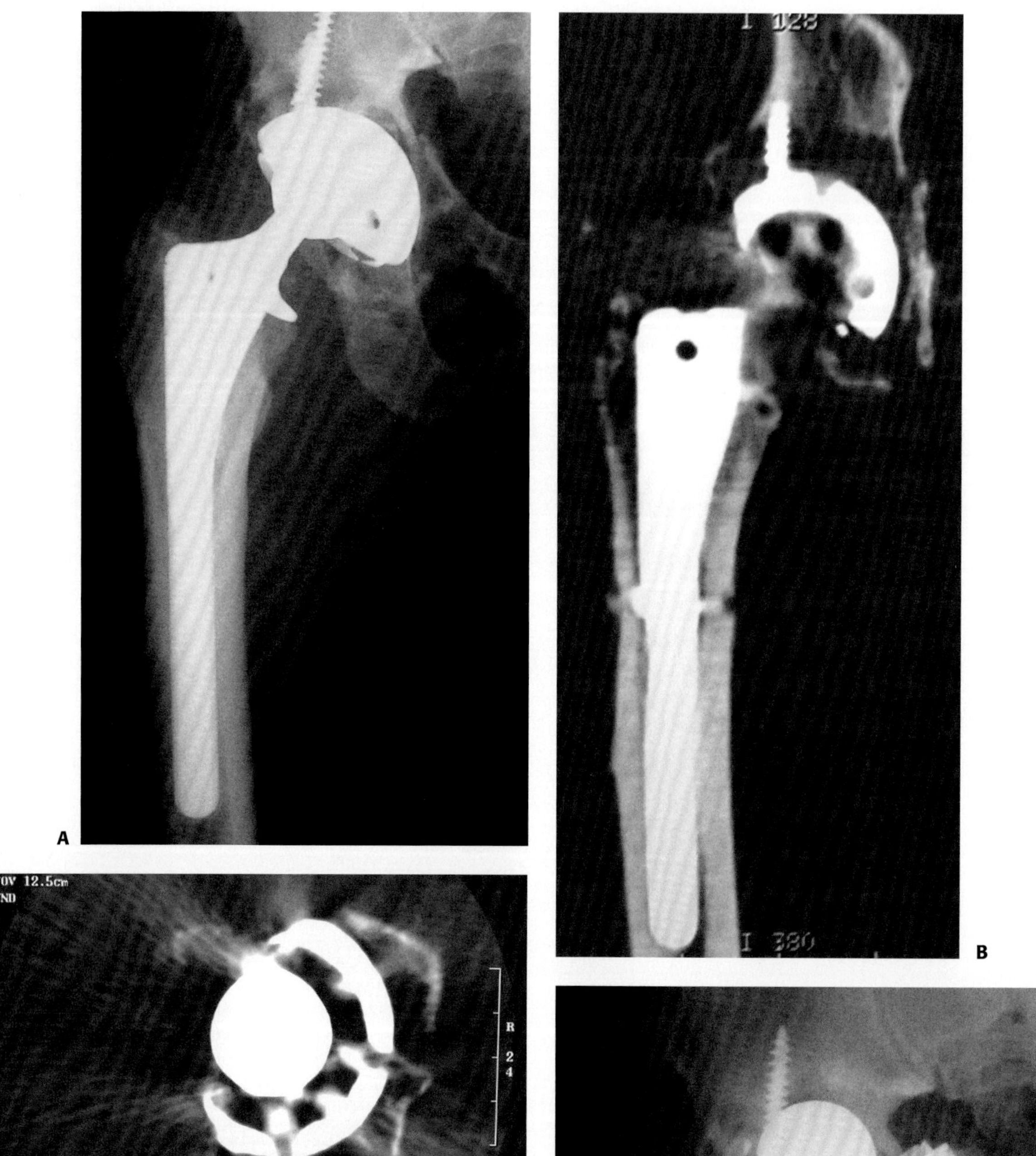

FIGURE 22-17 **A.** Anteroposterior x-ray of a total hip demonstrating severe polyethylene wear. **B.** Coronal reconstruction of computerized tomography scan of same hip demonstrating severe periacetabular osteolysis and fracture of medial wall of acetabulum. **C.** Transverse section of CT scan demonstrating severe osteolysis. **D.** Delay in treatment authorization by insurance company resulted in complete fracture through medial acetabular wall.

fractures include: (a) restoration of anatomic alignment, (b) maintenance or re-establishment of adequate bone stock, (c) creation of a stable prosthesis, (d) early mobilization of the patient, (e) early union of the fracture, and (f) return of the patient to prefracture function or better.

DIAGNOSIS OF PERIPROSTHETIC FRACTURES

Diagnosis of periprosthetic fractures relies upon one or more techniques: direct observation, clinical suspicion, and radiographic evaluation. Direct observation of periprosthetic fractures most likely occurs as the surgeon is revising a failed arthroplasty, through either a change in the pitch of a chisel on bone or a mallet striking an implant. Markedly displaced fractures about implants are obvious through the abrupt onset of pain and deformity, but clinical suspicion of a periprosthetic fracture is necessary in patients with nondescript complaints of pain about a component, especially one associated with osteolysis. Radiographic evaluation of all suspected periprosthetic fractures should include plain views of each bone including full-length views of long bones, complete pelvic films for fractures about total hips, and comparison with previous studies.

Cross-sectional imaging has not been routinely used in the evaluation of bone and soft tissues around metal implants because of "beam hardening" artifacts in computed tomography (CT) and "metal susceptibility" artifacts in magnetic resonance imaging (MRI) (2). Software packages on CT scanners have gone through several generations and can now reduce beam hardening artifacts with ease (Fig. 22-17A–C). MRI is catching up in its ability to scan around metallic implants. White et al (2) improved depiction of periprosthetic tissue by using thinner sections, increased frequency-encoding gradient strength, and fast spin-echo sequences. In one case of mechanical loosening evaluated with cross-sectional imaging, White et al (2) were able to demonstrate that the stem was penetrating the proximal cortex of the femur. The authors suggested that other types of periprosthetic fractures might also be detected (2) Olsen et al (3) reported on a similar study of MRI evaluation of periprosthetic tissues and dubbed the process the "Metal Artifact Reduction Sequence" or MARS.

Epidemiology

In 2002, the National Hospital Discharge Survey (4) recorded 193,000 discharges for total hip arthroplasty, up from 119,000 in 1990 (5). The true incidence of periprosthetic fractures about the hip is difficult to cull from the literature for a variety of reasons (6) including differences in the length of follow-up, demographics, whether revision surgeries are included, and whether the fractures occur intra- or postoperatively.

With the number of total hip revisions increasing from 24,000 in 1990 (5) to 31,000 in 2000 (7), it is inevitable that the number of periprosthetic hip fractures will continue to increase. Meek et al (8) studied 211 consecutive patients undergoing revision hip arthroplasty with a diaphyseal fitting cementless stem and reported that 64 patients sustained an intraoperative fracture of the femur. Out of 45 consecutive revisions using a long, straight-stem prosthesis, Zalzal and colleagues (9) recorded 7 intraoperative fractures for an incidence of 17.5%. Berry (6) reported 1,249 periprosthetic fractures among the 30,329 total hips performed at the Mayo Clinic from 1969 to 1999. Intraoperative fracture rates were 1% for primary and 7.8% for revision total hip arthroplasties. Postoperative fracture rates were 1.1% for primary and 4% for revision hips (6). Crockarell et al (10) conducted a literature review limited to those studies that listed the total number of hips and periprosthetic fractures and reported a fracture prevalence of 224 out of 17,644 arthroplasties or 1.27%. The Norwegian Arthroplasty Register recorded 1,042 hip revisions in 1998, of which only 41 (3.9%) were due to fracture of the femur (11).

Etiology

Traumatic events, while often cited as a leading cause of periprosthetic fractures, are more often than not the last factor in a long chain of events leading up to the fracture. The majority of periprosthetic fractures about the hip are reported to occur after relatively minimal trauma, such as a fall or a twisting motion with the fracture arising from one or more areas or weakness or stress concentration (Fig. 22-18). These falls are often associated with other developments that may accompany the aging process, such as Parkinsonism, myasthenia gravis, and simply poor balance.

Revision surgery of total hip prostheses often bears a similar blame for periprosthetic fractures as does trauma. In many revision cases, the surgeon operates in a situation where the risk of fracture is heightened for a variety of reasons. This includes loss of intramedullary blood supply from the original procedure (12), and previous screw holes and altered bone morphology (13).

The tools and techniques unique to revision surgery also impact upon the increased fracture risk. Impaction grafting with smooth stems in revision surgery carries a perioperative risk of about 5% (14,15). Large, porous-coated diaphyseal stems fare no better. Meek et al (8) reported 64 fractures in 211 revision cases utilizing this technique for a rate of nearly 30%. Long, straight stems carry a similar risk with Zalzal et al (9) documenting 7 fractures in 33 revision cases (18%).

Periprosthetic fractures of the hip associated with osteolysis have occurred around the acetabulum, greater trochanter, and femoral diaphysis (16–18), and it is a problem of increasing significance (16,19). Routine monitoring of patients and treating their periprosthetic osteolysis before fracture is not only easier on the patient, it is far less expensive than treating the resulting fracture (6,20).

The number of minimally invasive total hip arthroplasties is rapidly increasing, due in no small part to consumer demand. With so many surgeons applying a new technique to an old proven procedure, there is a potential for increased intraoperative fractures. Berger (21) reported only 1 calcar fracture out of the first 100 two-incision hips in his initial series. Goldstein et al (22) recorded none in the 85 patients who underwent a single-incision technique, whereas Woolson and colleagues

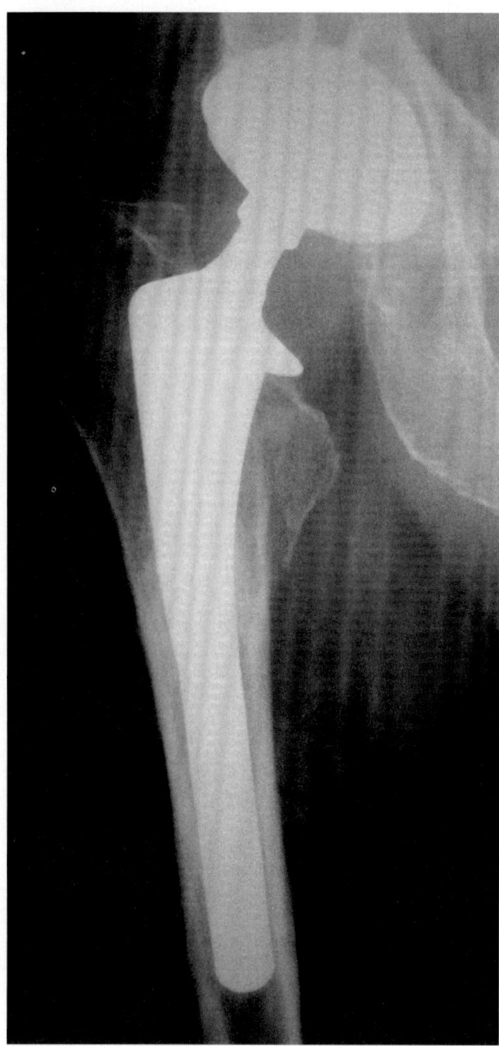

FIGURE 22-18 Vancouver A_L fracture sustained after patient pivoted on involved leg at his ranch. Case was successfully treated with partial weight-bearing.

noted 2 fractures in 50 patients undergoing a similar small-incision posterior approach (23).

PERIPROSTHETIC FRACTURES OF THE FEMUR

Classification

Development of Vancouver Classification

Although multiple classification schemes have been proposed over the last several years (24–34), the Vancouver Classification (Fig. 22-19) as originally proposed by Duncan and Masri (35) has become the standard for assessing and reporting periprosthetic femur fractures with its inclusion of fracture configuration, implant stability, and bone quality (1,36). Brady et al (37) tested the merit of the Vancouver Classification before its widespread adoption, and confirmed that it was both reliable and valid and could be recommended for guiding treatment and outlining prognosis (38).

Intraoperative

Masri, Meek, and Duncan (39) recently expanded the Vancouver Classification, which was originally developed to describe postoperative fractures, to also include intraoperative fractures. It is important to note that while the intraoperative classification is structured similarly to the postoperative scheme, they remain separate entities.

The intraoperative Vancouver Classification divides the femur into three zones: Type A fractures include the proximal metaphysis and do not extend into the diaphysis; Type B fractures are diaphyseal; and Type C fractures extend beyond the longest revision stem and include fractures about the distal metaphysis. A subclassification of each type reflects the nature of the fracture in that region: Subtype 1 represents a simple cortical perforation; Subtype 2 is an undisplaced linear crack; and Subtype 3 is a displaced, or unstable fracture (Table 22-3) (39). Treatment options for those fractures recognized intraoperatively and those noted only once the patient is in the recovery room or later are listed in Tables 22-4 and 22-5.

Postoperative

The Vancouver Classification for fractures occurring postoperatively consists of three major types based upon the location of the fracture: Type A are confined to the trochanteric region, Type B occur around or just distal to the femoral component, and Type C are distal enough to the stem that their treatment is considered independent of the hip replacement. Type A are subdivided into fractures about the greater trochanter, A_G, which are frequently associated with osteolysis and remain stable; and Type A_L, fractures about the lesser trochanter, which are more likely to lead to instability about the implant. The Type B are categorized according to the amount of remaining bone stock and the implant stability. B1 and B2 fractures have good bone stock but while the implant remains solidly fixed in the B1 type, it is loose in the B2 type. B3 fractures occur around loose implants that also suffer from severe bone stock deficiency, from either comminution, osteopenia, or osteolysis (Table 22-6) (39).

Current Treatment Options

The Vancouver Postoperative Classification is widely accepted and now the standard for reporting on periprosthetic femoral fractures in total hip arthroplasty. Fractures about the greater trochanter, A_G, may remain relatively undisplaced due to the continuity of the soft-tissue sleeve between the abductors and the vastus lateralis (16). As these fractures are often a result of osteolysis, Berry (16) cautions against taking down the fracture and fixing it and suggests grafting the osteolytic area with bone graft while leaving the soft-tissue sleeve intact. Of 118 hips that underwent revision hip arthroplasty for an acute Vancouver type B fracture, Springer et al (40) reported 7 as type B1, 76 as type B2, and 35 as type B3. All were treated with femoral revision and the long-term survival for these hips was 90% at 5 years and almost 80% at 10 years (40). Twelve Vancouver

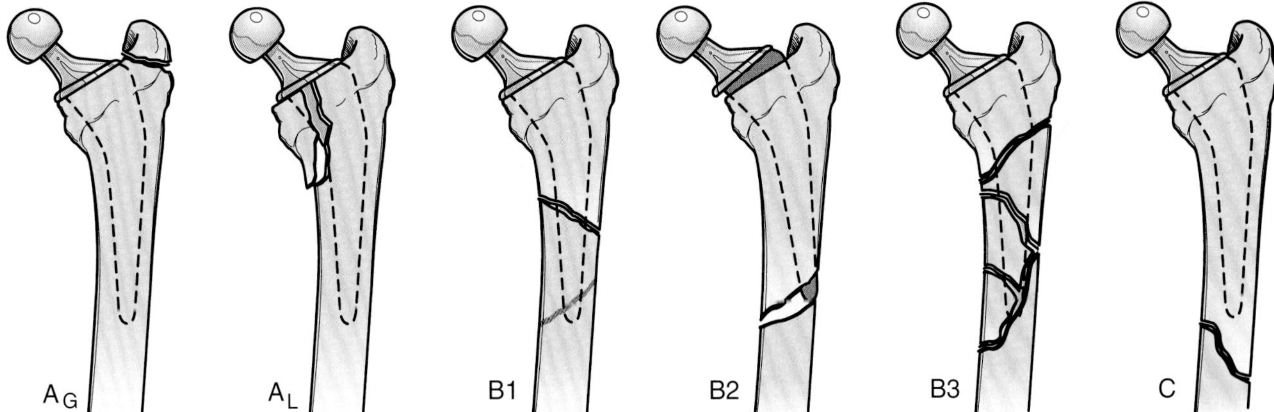

FIGURE 22-19 Vancouver classification scheme for periprosthetic fractures about total hip arthroplasties. (Modified from Duncan CP, Masri BA. Fractures of the femur after hip replacement. In: Jackson D, ed. *Instructional course lectures 44*. Rosemont, IL: American Academy of Orthopaedic Surgeons, 1995:293–304.)

B2 fractures treated with a conical Wagner revision stem (Sulzer, Switzerland) were followed for an average of 5 years and all had a stable prosthesis and solid fracture union with more than half reporting an excellent outcome (41). Barden et al (42) treated 19 patients with Vancouver B3 fractures using long revision stems and onlay strut allografts with only one early refracture at the stem tip, while the remaining 18 healed without deformity or shortening. Vancouver C fractures are not as widely reported in the literature as the Type B. Tsiridis et al (43) did note three Vancouver Type C fractures as part of a larger series of 16 periprosthetic fractures treated with Dall-Miles plates and cables. Two of the three Type C fractures healed, whereas the third went on to nonunion (43).

Techniques for the treatment of periprosthetic femoral fractures fall into two main categories: (a) allograft bone struts or metal fixation plates; (b) revision prostheses. It is not unusual for surgeons to employ a combination of these techniques in challenging cases. Struts and plates alone are more suitable for Vancouver B1 or C fractures whereas revision components are more appropriate for B2 and B3 fractures. Table 22-6 summarizes the advantages and disadvantages of the techniques that are described here.

Cerclage/Struts/Plates

Strut Grafts. Haddad et al (44) studied 40 Vancouver B1 periprosthetic fractures treated with cortical onlay strut allografts with or without a plate. Thirty-nine of the 40 fractures united with strut/host union typically seen within the first 12 months. No evidence of femoral loosening was evident in any patient and all but one of the surviving patients returned to their preoperative functional level within 1 year. There were 4 malunions, all of which had less than 10 degrees of malalignment, and there was only 1 deep infection.

Haddad et al (44) make four important technical points:

1. As many cables/wires as necessary should be used to establish stable fixation.
2. The struts must be contoured to provide maximum graft/host contact.
3. Preservation of the blood supply of the femur is critical and the linea aspera should not be stripped of its soft-tissue attachments.
4. Autograft or morselized allograft applied at the strut/host junction enhances healing.

Strut grafts also work well with more severe fractures. Eighteen of 19 comminuted Vancouver B3 fractures treated by Barden and colleagues (42) with onlay strut allografts healed without deformity and shortening. Barden and his group (45) have also reported on a series of 13 patients who had refractured after being treated for a Vancouver B3 fracture. In these cases they were not originally treated with large onlay grafts. All refractures and nonunions in their series healed without further treatment.

Additional measures may be necessary to ensure healing. Strut grafts may weaken after implantation (46,47), which can lead to failure in cases of delayed union. A combination of strut grafts with plate fixation is appropriate, especially if a tight interference fit by the femoral component cannot be achieved (1). Strut grafts should also be considered in patients who are noncompliant, or in cases where the grafts can not extend a minimum of 10 cm distal to the fracture (45,48,49).

In the future, additional measures may enhance and accelerate healing. Cook et al (50) interposed recombinant human osteogenic protein between onlay strut allograft and femur in 14 adult dogs. Healing was dramatically enhanced and rapid formation of new bone and graft incorporation occurred at all sites with osteogenic protein compared to contralateral controls.

Plates. Dennis et al (51) studied two fixation techniques about Vancouver B1 fractures using matched human femora: plate fixation with proximal cable and distal bicortical screw fixation compared to two allograft struts and cables. The constructs were loaded to failure after undergoing 10,000 loading cycles. The

TABLE 22-3 Vancouver Intraoperative Classification Scheme

Vancouver Intraoperative Fracture Classification

Location	Metaphyseal			Diaphyseal			Distal to Implant		
Stability	Cortical perforation	Undisplaced crack	Displaced or unstable	Cortical perforation	Undisplaced crack	Displaced or unstable	Cortical perforation	Undisplaced crack	Displaced or unstable
Classification	A1	A2	A3	B1	B2	B3	C1	C2	C3
Treatment options	Bone graft	Cerclage	Diaphyseal stem	Bypass with longer stem	Cerclage and bypass with longer stem	Reduction, cerclage, cortical strut	Bone graft and bypass with cortical strut	Cerclage with or without cortical strut	Locking plate and cerclage cables
	Observe		Trochanteric fixation	Cortical strut if at tip of longest stem	Cortical strut or plate & screws				

From Masri BA, Meek RM, Duncan CP. Periprosthetic fractures evaluation and treatment. *Clin Orthop* 2004;(420):80–95, with permission.

TABLE 22-4 **Treatment Options for Intraoperative Periprosthetic Femur Fractures**

Site	Greater Trochanter		Proximal Femur			Distal Femur	
Recognized Fracture							
Stability	Stable	Unstable	Stable	Unstable		Stem stable	Stem unstable
Treatment	Observe	Claw/plate	Cerclage	Cerclage		Cerclage and strut	Long stem with cerclage and strut
Reassessment	Stable	Stable	Stable	Now stable	Still unstable	Stable	Stable
Revised treatment	None	None	None	None	Revise to fully porous stem	None	None
Unrecognized Fracture							
Fracture stability	Stable	Unstable	Unstable	Stable			
Implant stability	Stable	Unstable	Stable	Unstable			
Treatment	Protected weight-bearing until union	Revise to long stem and cable plate and strut graft	Cable plate and strut	Revise to long stem and internal fixation			

From Masri BA, Meek RM, Duncan CP. Periprosthetic fractures evaluation and treatment. *Clin Orthop* 2004;(420):80–95, with permission.

TABLE 22-5 **Vancouver Postoperative Fracture Classification**

Location	Lesser Trochanter	Greater Trochanter	About the Stem			Distal to Stem
Stem fixation	Well-fixed	Well-fixed	Well-fixed	Loose	Loose	Ignore implant and revise if necessary after fracture has healed
Bone stock	Good	Good	Good	Good	Poor	
Classification	A-L	A-G	B1	B2	B3	C
Treatment options	Symptomatic treatment unless substantial medial cortex involved	Symptomatic treatment. Intervene only to treat pain, weakness, limp or instability	Cerclage, cortical struts and plate	Revision to long stem	Revision and augmentation with allograft or tumor prosthesis	Fix fracture first

From Masri BA, Meek RM, Duncan CP. Periprosthetic fractures evaluation and treatment. *Clin Orthop* 2004;(420):80–95, with permission.

TABLE 22-6 Treatment Options for Periprosthetic Fractures about Total Hip Arthroplasties

Treatment Option – THA	Advantages	Disadvantages
Strut grafts	– High union rate – Easily contoured – Low elastic modulus	– May weaken after implantation – Variable availability – Graft/host interaction – Not as strong as plates
Plates		
Dynamic compression	– Readily available – Minimal skill set – Stronger than strut graft – Reduced stress shielding	– Requires dissection to plate length – Weaker than locking/LISS plates
Mennen	– No transcortical fixation	– Mixed success in healing fractures – Requires extensive dissection – Prone to fracture or bend – Poor longitudinal support
LISS	– Minimal dissection – Preserves blood supply – Rigid internal fixation – Use with/without cables – Unicortical screws	– Cannot alter contour of titanium plates – More expensive than dynamic plate – Requires special training
Locking plate	– Rigid internal fixation – Use with/without cables – Unicortical screws	– Changing contour negates use of guide
Dall-Miles plates	– Readily available – High union rate when used with cortical struts	– High failure rate when used alone, especially in Vancouver B3 fracture
Revision prosthesis – femur		
Tapered stem	– Bypasses proximal femur – Avoids stress concentration at tip	– May subside after implantation
Locking stem	– Distal fixation – May allow earlier weight-bearing	– Screw breakage – May require screw removal
Proximally coated		– Poor distal stability
Extensively coated	– High success rate – Initial stability usually good	– Straight stem design may concentrate forces at tip during insertion – Bowed design may provide less circumferential contact
Allograft composite	– Replaces lost proximal bone – Good rotational stability with step cut	– Difficulty in accommodating larger prostheses
Impaction grafting	– May be useful in cases involving severe osteolysis	– May subside after implantation – Technically challenging
Revision prosthesis – acetabulum		
Multihole cup	– Readily available – Good initial stability	– Increased risk of vascular injury with multiple screws
Reconstruction cage	– Spans larger defects – Accommodates bone graft	– Increased dissection

plate/screw/cable fixation tolerated 1,295 Nm to failure whereas the allograft construct tolerated only 950 Nm, concluding that this type of plate construct was superior to the use of allograft. They came to a similar conclusion comparing five plate constructs against allograft stabilization (52). It should be noted, however, that this was bench research with limited cyclic loading and without the benefit of ongoing healing.

The first reports of minimally invasive plate fixation of femoral fractures in 1997 (53,54) suggested that in comminuted fractures, this technique was superior to open reduction because it preserved the periosteal blood supply. Cadaveric studies with fresh human cadavers and blue silicone dye confirmed the advantage in maintaining arterial femoral vascularity and perfusion (55).

Abhaykumar et al (56) treated 6 Vancouver B1 periprosthetic fractures about hip femoral stems with standard nonlocking plates using a minimally invasive technique and reported that all fractures healed within 6 months. The authors suggested that this limited approach preserved the fracture hematoma, reduced wound problems and periosteal stripping, and improved the chances of the fractures healing (56).

The latest addition to the minimally invasive plate technique is the LISS (less invasive stabilization system) (Synthes, Paoli, PA) plates that employ an external guide rigidly fixed to one end of the plate. This allows the use of screws that precisely lock into the plate, rather than the standard hemispherical head. These locking screws then provide increased rigidity to the construct and allow the use of unicortical screws adjacent to the femoral stem (Fig. 22-20A,B).

Mennen plate fixation for periprosthetic fractures has been

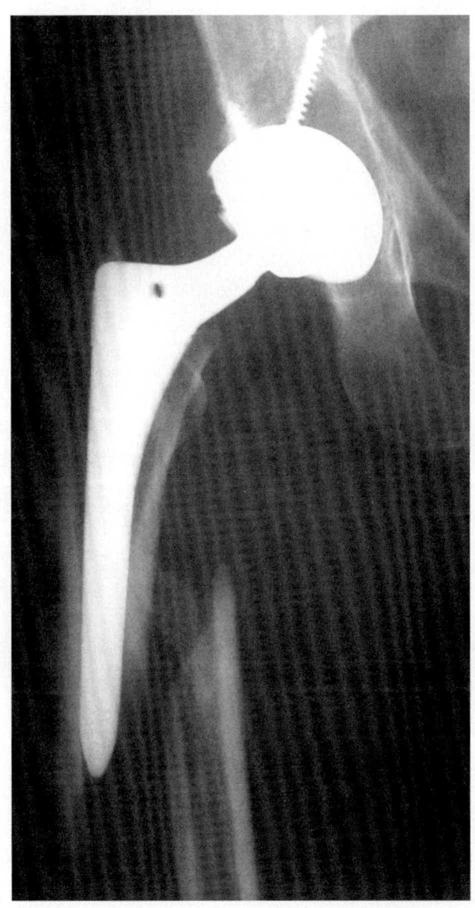

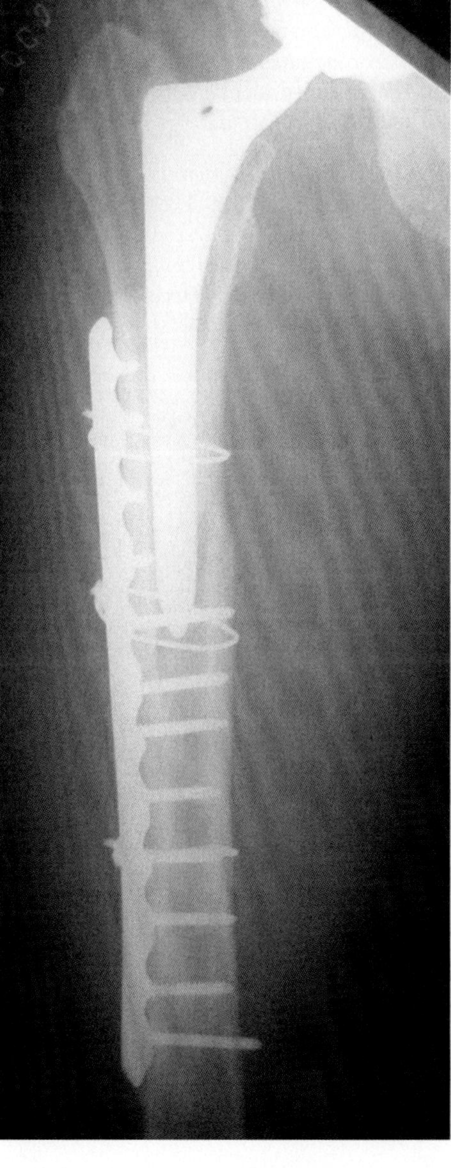

FIGURE 22-20 **A.** Vancouver B1 fracture. **B.** Treatment consisted of a long locking plate which allowed rigid screw fixation about the stem. Cables were for provisional stabilization.

employed in Europe for several years but rarely, if at all, in the United States. This plate consists of a central longitudinal ridge with a row of finger-like projections on each side that are compressed onto the bone to form a raised plate (57). Reports are mixed on its success in treating periprosthetic fractures of the femur. Noorda et al (58) compiled a series of 36 periprosthetic femoral fractures treated with Mennen plate fixation. Ten of those treated had a nonunion and varus bending of the plate. The plate fractured in 8 of those 10. All 8 fractured plates were successfully treated with a long-stem revision prosthesis and a compression plate. The authors concluded that the use of the Mennen plate was not recommended for the treatment of periprosthetic femoral fractures (58). Ahuja and Chatterji (59) reported a 75% complication rate in 16 periprosthetic fractures treated with the Mennen plate and noted that it was "unable to counter the medial compressive forces on the femur leading to a varus collapse of the fracture" (59). Kligman et al (57) compared Mennen plate fixation with nonoperative traction in the treatment of periprosthetic femoral fractures and proclaimed the Mennen plate superior to nonoperative management. Radcliffe and Smith (60) recommended Mennen plate fixation for cases where the patient was too frail to undergo revision.

Dall-Miles Plates. The Dall-Miles plate system is designed for hybrid screw and cable fixation. Haddad et al (61) utilized the Dall-Miles plate on femoral fractures about 4 total hips. In addition to the plates they also used dual cortical onlay strut grafts, achieving union in all 4 cases within 12 to 18 weeks (61). Shah and McCabe (62) treated 9 periprosthetic femoral fractures with the Dall-Miles system without using strut grafts and reported similar results (Fig. 22-21A–C). Venu et al (63) reported similar results with Dall-Miles plate systems in 12 fractures about total hips. Ten of the 12 united with two going to nonunion. Tsiridis et al (43) critically reviewed their experience with the Dall-Miles system in 16 periprosthetic femoral fractures and reported that 2 of the 3 Vancouver B1 fractures failed through the plate. They concluded that the Dall-Miles plate and cable system alone was insufficient and that treatment should "be supplemented with additional intramedullary or extramedullary fixation" (43).

Revision Prosthesis

Fractures about the stem often are associated with either a previous stress riser or a loose prosthesis. Intraoperative fractures in this region typically occur during revision surgery and are treated with a long-stem prosthesis that bypasses the cortical defect by two cortical diameters. Note that existing data supports this only for cemented stems (64) and that smooth, uncemented stems provide no protection against torsional fractures (65) although one would expect that fluted or extensively porous-coated stems could afford some protection. The critical concept here is to achieve both torsional and longitudinal stability with the implant in the distal fragment and not rely upon the empirical standard of two cortical diameters.

A variety of implants are available to revise periprosthetic femoral fractures:

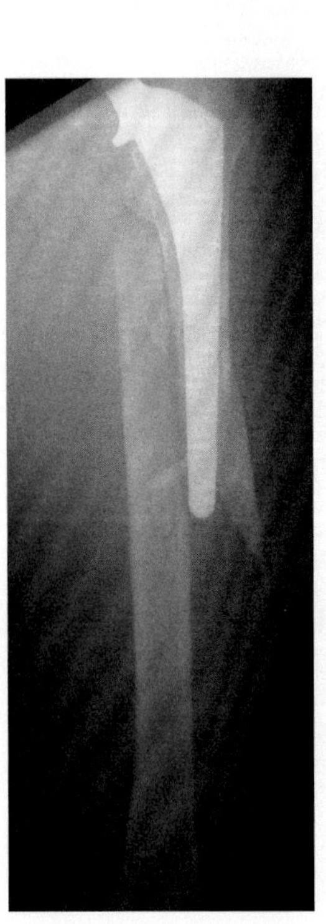

A

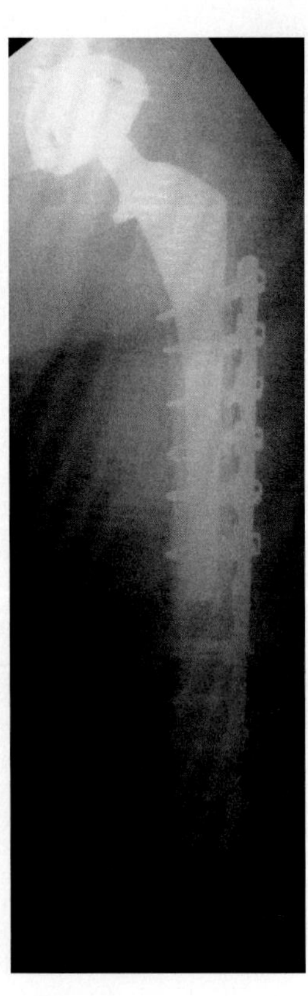

B

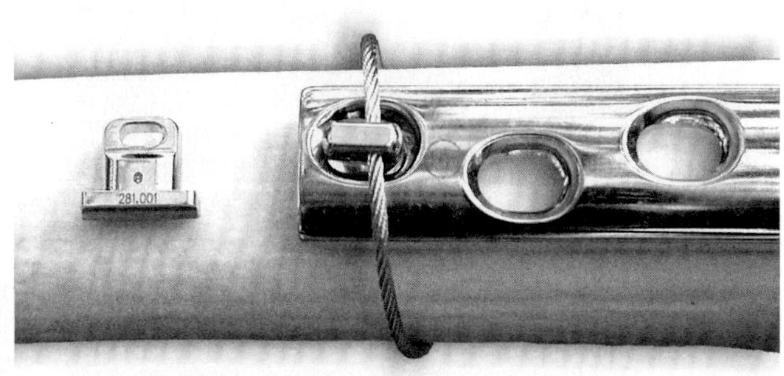

C

FIGURE 22-21 **A.** Vancouver B1 fracture. **B.** Treatment consisted of open reduction and plating with a Dall-Miles cable plate and grommets. **C.** Grommet for stabilization of cable about plate. The grommets prevent slippage of the cable along the plate and reduce fretting of the cable.

1. Tapered stems
2. Locking stems
3. Proximally coated stems
4. Extensively porous coated stems
5. Allograft composites
6. Impaction grafting stems

Again, the key to success with most of these implants appears to be immediate stable fixation. Without it, the implant may fail to incorporate and the fracture failed to heal (Fig. 22-22A,B).

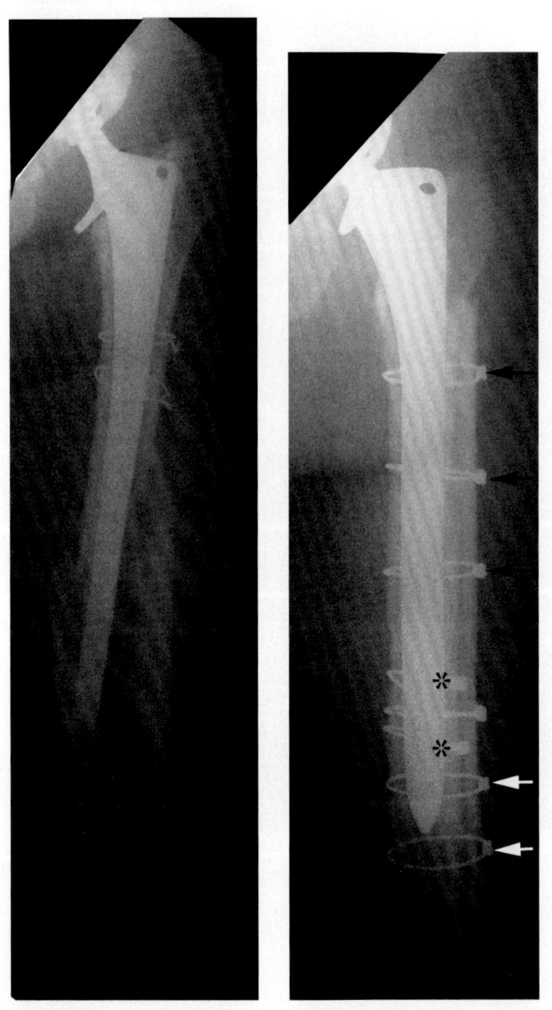

FIGURE 22-22 A. Vancouver B2 fracture involving a loose long-term prosthesis. **B.** Treatment consisted of a fully porous coated stem augmented with a contoured femoral allograft strut secured with cables. This x-ray demonstrates two important principles in the application of cerclage cables or wires. First, the more distal of the two inner cables marked with an asterisk (*) was placed around the intact distal fragment to reduce hoop stresses during insertion of the fully coated stem. The more proximal of the two cables was then added after insertion to stabilize the reduction. Second, the six outer cables marked with arrows should be spaced every three or four centimeters to distribute the load along the graft.

Tapered Stems. The Wagner revision stem (Zimmer, Warsaw, IN) is a cementless, grit-blasted conical femoral stem made of titanium alloy. It is designed to gain fixation in a conically reamed intact distal femoral shaft with rotational stability provided by eight sharp longitudinal ridges distributed evenly around the shaft (Fig. 22-23) (41). It is not uncommon for the prosthesis to subside after implantation with some series reporting greater than 10 mm of shortening in one-fifth of the patients treated with the prosthesis during revision arthroplasty (66).

Ko et al (41) reported on 12 patients with Vancouver B2 fractures treated with a Wagner revision stem. At an average of 6 years follow-up, all patients had a stable prosthesis and fracture union. Outcomes in 7 were reported as excellent, 3 good, and 2 poor. Only 2 of their patients experienced 5 mm of subsidence.

Subsidence of the Wagner stem was eliminated in one series with the use of Dall-Miles cables to contain hoop stresses at the site of femoral osteotomy (67). Of the 129 Wagner revision stems reported by Bohm et al (66) 44 (34%) had subsidence greater than 5 mm and 26 (20%) had subsidence greater than 10 mm.

The Link MP revision stem (Exactech Inc., Gainesville, FL) utilizes a similar tapered and fluted stem to gain distal fixation but has a modular design that allows for independent fitting of the diaphysis with a stem of varying lengths and diameters (68). Kwong et al (68) reported an average stem subsidence of 2 mm in a series of 143 patients treated with the device, 14 of which were periprosthetic fractures.

Locking Stem. The distal locking stem offers an alternative mode of fixation. The stem relies on two or more distal fixation screws placed either with an external jig or freehand under fluoroscopic control. The screws usually provide fixation until the fracture is healed and then are removed to promote proximal load transmission.

Rigby et al (69) treated 9 patients with periprosthetic fractures utilizing the Kent prosthesis (Biomet Europe, The Netherlands), a distally locked stem with 6 to 16 transverse fixation holes. No implant failures were reported and the majority of the patients were able to ambulate without pain. Stossel and Haddad (70) reviewed their results with 145 Kent Hip Prostheses, 37 of which were periprosthetic fractures. The majority of those patients had substantial improvement in their hip pain and the median time to full weight-bearing was only 2 days.

Probst et al (71) treated 21 periprosthetic fractures with the Prosthesis Nail, a hybrid hip prosthesis and intramedullary nail that allows immediate full weight-bearing. All periprosthetic fractures healed, although one 350-lb patient broke the distal locking screw. Eingartner et al (72) reported fracture healing in all 12 of their periprosthetic fractures treated with the BiContact stem (Aesculap, Tuttlingen, Germany), also with distal locking screws, although they suggested partial weight-bearing for 12 weeks.

Lewallen and Berry (73) note that an interlocking screw design for a revision prosthesis may not be sufficient if the stem does not demonstrate inherent initial stability without the screw

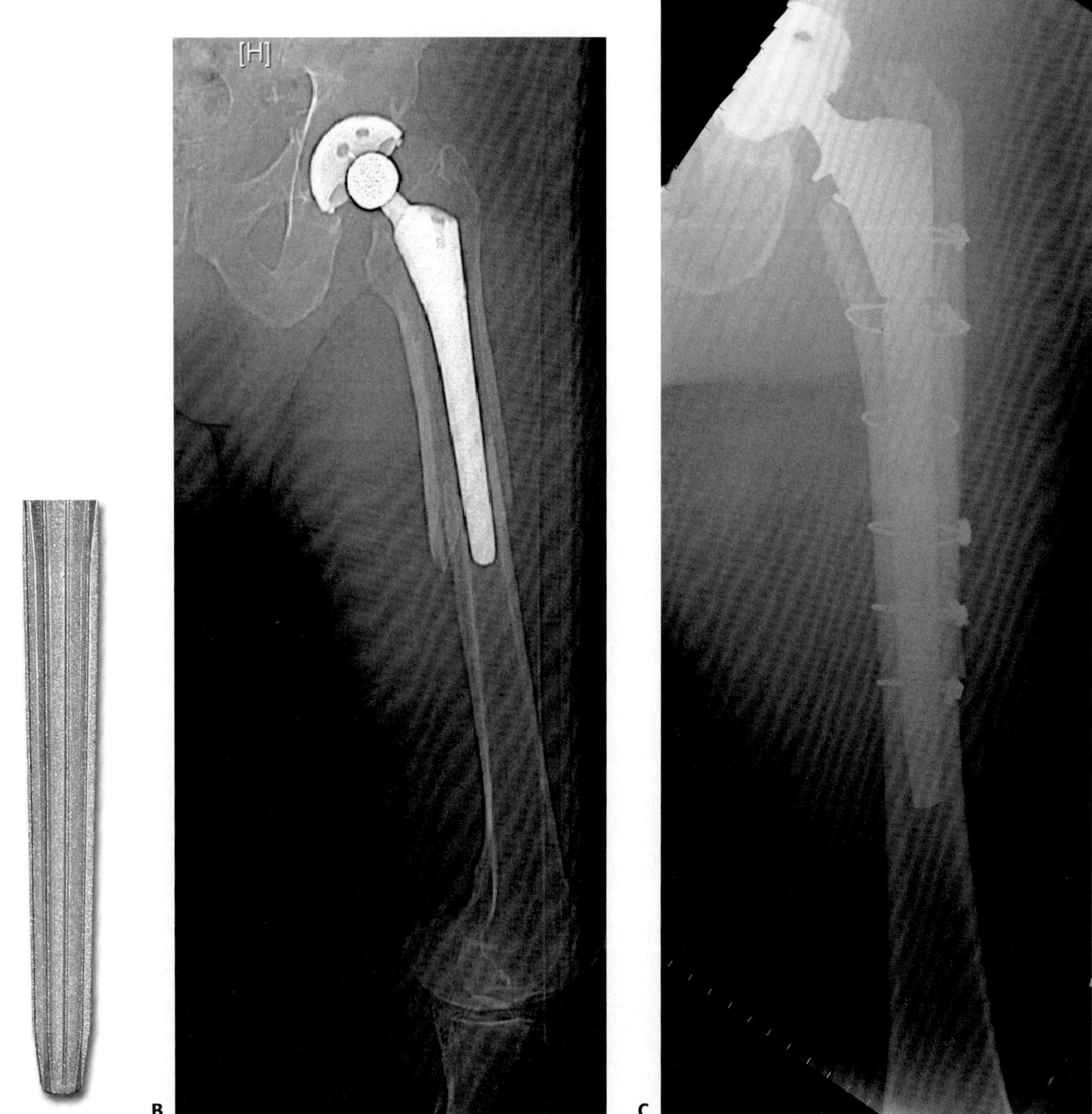

FIGURE 22-23 **A.** Close-up of Wagner tapered stem demonstrating stabilizing ridges. **B.** A 75-year-old male sustained this Vancouver B2 fracture in a fall on a cruise ship. **C.** Postreduction and fixation of the fracture with a modular tapered stem augmented with a lateral femoral strut graft. (Images courtesy of William K. Jackson, MD, Baylor University Medical Center, Dallas, Texas.)

fixation. They suggest a "validated revision stem design that has a proved record of long-term success in patients who have substantially compromised bone stock," supplemental cancellous and cortical bone graft, and removal of the screws after fracture healing (73).

Proximally Coated Stem. Proximally porous coated uncemented stems may not provide the degree of distal stability needed to ensure timely healing of periprosthetic fractures. Springer et al (40) reported that 12 of 28 periprosthetic fractures treated with proximally porous coated stems in their series demonstrated radiographic loosening while another three stems were re-revised for nonunion. Only 36% of these hips had a well-fixed, unrevised stem with a healed fracture (40).

Extensively Porous Coated. In contrast to their experience with proximally coated stems, extensively porous coated implants proved to be the most successful technique in the series reported by Springer (40). Seventy-seven per cent of the 30 periprosthetic fractures treated with this stem had healed with well-fixed unrevised components. Success is most likely attributed to the initial and long-term fixation achieved by the scratch fit of the component in the diaphysis. Scratch fit differs from simple press fit in that the leading edge of the porous coating on a cylindrical implant during insertion will displace a small amount of bone along the entire length of cortical contact, adding additional stability, like a cork in a bottle. Press fit places the bone and metal surfaces in apposition without any significant deformation, much like a round wooden peg in a round hole of the same size. MacDonald et al (74) treated 14 periprosthetic fractures with a canal-filling, extensively porous coated implant (Solution, DePuy, Warsaw, IN) and supplemental cortical struts grafts, achieving stable bone ingrowth in 12. All successful cases obtained distal diaphyseal fixation with at least 4 to 6 cm of intimate intramedullary cortical contact (Fig. 22-22B).

Allograft Composites. Allograft-prosthesis composite implants are particularly useful in the treatment of Vancouver B3 periprosthetic fractures. The long-stem femoral component is typically cemented into a proximal femoral allograft, which can be step-cut to provide rotational stability (75). Strut allografts may be used to provide additional support and stability. Thirteen of 15 cases treated with this technique achieved good pain relief and returned to their prefracture level of function (Fig. 22-24A,B) (75).

Impaction Grafting. Impaction grafting of Vancouver B3 fractures is uncommon, but has been employed in cases involving

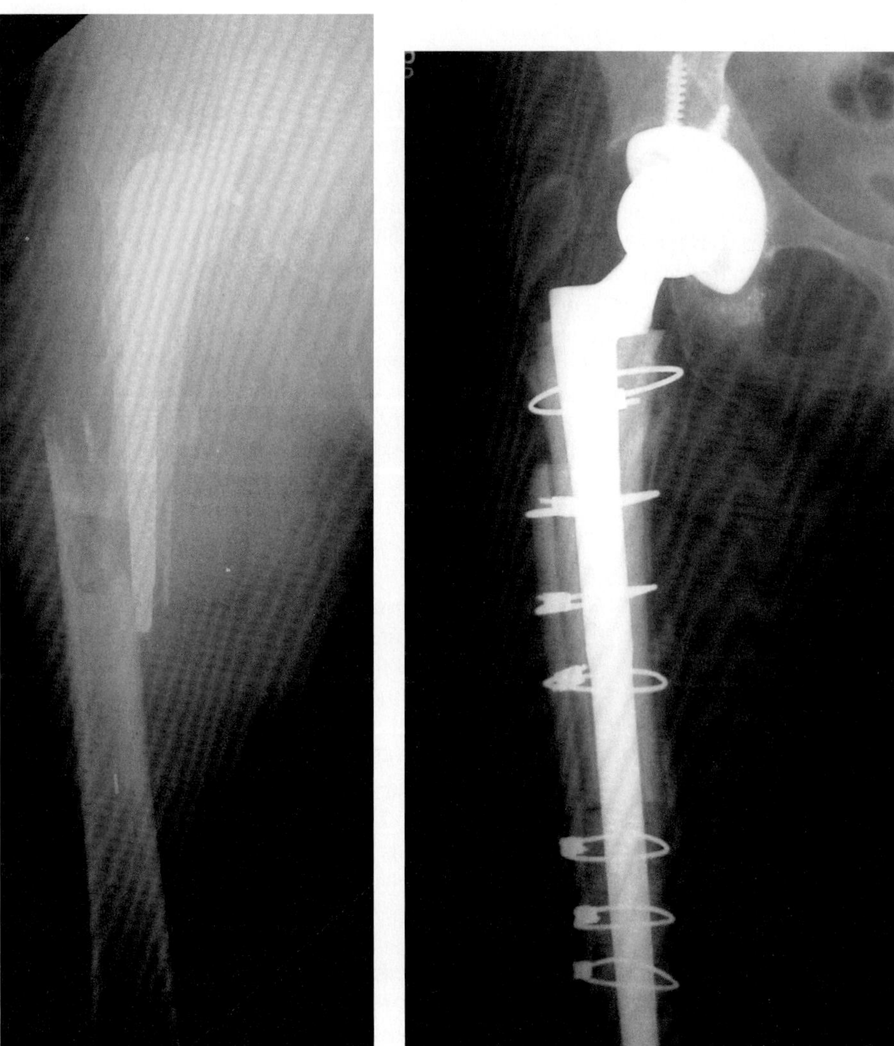

FIGURE 22-24 **A.** Vancouver B3 fracture. **B.** Treatment utilized an S-ROM stem (DePuy/Johnson & Johnson, Warsaw, IN) without its sleeve, cemented into a proximal femoral allograft. Construct was then telescoped into thin existing sleeve of bone. The remaining bone from the allograft was converted into struts and the entire construct was stabilized with cables.

significant proximal osteolysis. Of the four periprosthetic fractures treated with long-stem Exeter components and allograft impaction grafting by van Biezen et al (76) two subsided significantly, but healed. However, all three Vancouver B3 fractures treated by Barden (42) healed without subsidence using the same implant and a similar technique. Although others have also reported encouraging results (1), the technique of impaction grafting around a long-stem revision component remains challenging and should be used only by those already successful with the technique in primary hip replacement.

PERIPROSTHETIC FRACTURES OF THE ACETABULUM

Epidemiology

Acetabular fractures associated with total hip arthroplasty are far less common than femoral fractures and are associated primarily with uncemented components. McElfresh and Coventry (77) reported only one acetabular fracture among 5,400 arthroplasties performed with cement. In contrast, Sharkey et al (78) reported 13 acetabular fractures that occurred during insertion of an uncemented component. Petersen and Lewallen identified 11 patients with uncemented cups that sustained postoperative periprosthetic acetabular fractures at an average of 6 years postoperatively (79). Berry et al (80) reported 31 cases of pelvic discontinuity discovered in more than 3,500 consecutive acetabular revisions for an incidence of only 0.9%. Peterson and Lewallen (79) noted only 16 periprosthetic acetabular fractures out of 23,850 total hip arthroplasties performed from 1971 to 1991 at the Mayo Clinic.

Etiology

Intraoperative

Intraoperative fractures of the acetabulum are due to either poor sizing or poor bone quality. In vitro studies created fractures in cadaveric acetabulae when underreamed by as little as 2 mm (81). A clinical report by Sharkey et al (78) of 13 acetabular fractures associated with insertion of an uncemented component noted that 11 of the patients were female and that only 6 had a preoperative diagnosis of osteoarthritis, while 2 had rheumatoid arthritis, 3 had osteonecrosis, 1 had a hip fracture nonunion, and 1 had developmental dysplasia, suggesting that osteoporosis or the absence of sclerotic bone were contributing factors.

Postoperative

Of the 11 patients with postoperative periprosthetic acetabular fractures reported by Peterson and Lewallen (79) 8 were due to blunt trauma and 3 occurred spontaneously. It should be noted that the authors specifically excluded pelvic discontinuity secondary to osteolysis. Sanchez-Sotelo et al (18) did report 3 cases of acute acetabular fracture about uncemented components in association with osteolytic lesions of the pelvis. Loosening of the acetabular component was responsible for 7 transacetabular nonunions leading to pelvic discontinuity (Fig. 22-17D) (82).

Classification of Periprosthetic Acetabular Fractures

Periprosthetic acetabular fractures are categorized according to a straightforward classification based on component stability proposed by Petereson and Lewallen (79): Type 1 fractures have a stable acetabular component and in Type 2 fractures the cup is unstable. Of the eight Type 1 fractures described, four involved the medial wall, two fractured through the posterior wall, one fractured the anterior wall and one was transverse. Of the three Type 2 fractures, one was through the posterior wall, the second involved the medial wall, and the third was transverse. Six of the eight Type 1 fractures united as did one of the two Type 2 fractures. Six of the eight Type 1 fractures and both Type 2 fractures subsequently underwent revision of the component (79).

Treatment

Intraoperative

The best treatment for intraoperative fractures of the acetabulum is to avoid them. Avoid overreaming the acetabulum, especially in cases involving osteoporotic bone. With minor cracks and an otherwise stable implant, the surgeon may elect to add additional screws to the construct (83).

If the cup is unstable, additional stabilization of the pelvis may be necessary. The initial prosthesis should be removed, the fracture stabilized with as many bicortical screws as necessary, and additional contoured plate fixation added if appropriate. The newly stabilized acetabulum should then be reamed line to line for a new multihole component, carefully impacted, and then stabilized with as many screws as necessary. Weight-bearing is restricted to toe-touch for 3 months (84).

Postoperative

Postoperative fractures about the acetabulum do not fare well. Of the 10 surviving patients in Peterson and Lewellan's report (79), 8 eventually underwent revision of the acetabular component for pain, loosening, or nonunion. This included 4 patients in whom the original fracture about the acetabular component had healed without operative intervention (79).

Treatment of postoperative fractures about the acetabulum falls into three main categories: (a) simple fracture with stable pelvis; (b) fracture with pelvic discontinuity but adequate bone stock; and (c) fracture associated with loss of bone stock. This last category ranges from long-term loosening of the prosthesis to osteolysis-induced fracture.

Simple fractures associated with a stable pelvis include such cases as the five patients with fracture of the medial wall in Peterson and Lewallen's series (79). If the rim of the acetabulum remains stable, the cup can be revised with medial bone graft and a larger hemispherical cup with multiple holes and screws followed by several weeks of touch-down weight-bearing.

Larger medial defects may require the use of a reconstruction ring or cage.

Fracture with pelvic discontinuity but adequate bone stock is more likely to occur as a result of blunt trauma than osteolysis or loosening. In this case, if stabilization of the pelvis after removal of the original cup restores the bony anatomy, a multihole cup and bone graft may suffice. If there is any question about the bone quality, a reconstruction cage may be indicated. Eggli et al (82) treated seven pelvic discontinuities in acetabular revisions with a three step process: (a) mechanical stabilization of both columns; (b) bony reconstruction with allograft and autograft chips to achieve a contained defect; and (c) fixation of the cup with a reconstruction ring or cage. At final follow-up, all components were stable and the fracture healed (82). Berry et al (80) used several techniques to reconstruct 27 cases of pelvic discontinuity associated with total hip arthroplasty including a Burch-Schneider cage in 13, a single posterior plate in 7, and dual plates in 7. Two hips were treated with resection arthroplasty. Overall, worse results were seen in those cases with more severe bone loss and in those patients previously treated with irradiation (80).

Periprosthetic acetabular fractures associated with osteolysis can be challenging (Fig. 22-17B). In the best of cases, if the implant remains functional in the face of a fracture through osteolytic bone, it is possible to delay the surgery while the fracture heals and then revise the implant (16,18). Acute fractures through large osteolytic lesions will require bone graft in conjunction with a reconstruction cage.

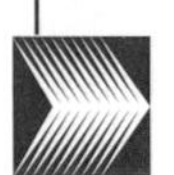

AUTHOR'S PREFERRED TREATMENT

Prevention

Avoidance of periprosthetic fractures begins with careful preoperative planning including recent full-length, biplanar x-rays. During surgical exposure, "finesse over force" (85) is the order of the day. Careful retraction, retaining previous fracture fixation implants until dislocation of the hip, and appropriate soft-tissue releases will reduce forces applied to the femur. In difficult primary hips and many revision arthroplasties, extended trochanteric osteotomy improves exposure and reduces fracture risk (86).

Primary total hips following developmental dysplasia of the hip may be at risk for femoral fracture due to the proximal femoral deformities associated with the condition (87) or acetabular fracture from overreaming (88,89).

Postoperative prevention of periprosthetic fractures begins with appropriate x-rays in the postanesthesia care unit to pick up any unrecognized intraoperative fractures. On a long-term basis, one recent study reported that the cyclic administration of etidronate postoperatively to total hip patients stabilized bone mineral density (BMD) in the proximal femur whereas BMD continued to decrease in the control total hip patients not receiving the drug (90).

Surgical Procedure

Femur

Fractures with a stable femoral component are excellent candidates for locking plate and cable technology. A long spiral fracture may lend itself to fixation with just a locking plate, however a more transverse or comminuted fracture requires the addition of a contoured femoral strut held in place with cables. Quartered struts allow for less dissection and better fit than simple half struts. Key here is to avoid too much dissection about the fracture site unless necessary. This preserves local blood supply.

A few basic principles guide my placement of cables along the femur and the strut allograft and are illustrated in Figure 22-22B. First, when inserting an interference fit stem into the distal shaft of the femur, I always place a cable close to the distal fracture line to reduce hoop stresses during insertion of the stem. This can be temporarily tightened during insertion and then re-used for fixation of the graft or, as in this case, slid up to the level of the fracture and used to provide initial stabilization while the large allograft is manipulated into place. For the case illustrated in Figure 22-22B, a second provisional cable was added before application of the graft. When applying the cables along the length of the allograft, I find that spacing them evenly every 3 to 4 cm provides appropriate stability. Obviously the final spacing will vary somewhat given the difficulties in passing the cable guide around the femur and through the linea aspera while trying to maintain as much of an intact soft-tissue envelope.

Preoperative computerized tomography of the implant/bone interface will confirm if the component is well fixed or not. I've found these scans also useful in delineating the extent of fracture lines that may not be visible on plain x-rays.

Difficulty arises in those situations where the component appears loose, but the patient's medical condition may benefit from a limited surgical approach with locking plates and cerclage cables. My preference is to stabilize the fracture and allow it to heal while also working toward improving the patient's medical status.

Acetabulum

Key to treating fractures of the acetabulum is reestablishing a stable base for the revision component. This usually requires stabilization with contoured pelvic reconstruction plates. Do not attempt to reduce and stabilize the fracture with multiple screws in a multihole cup. Three-dimensional reconstructions of thin slice computerized tomography scans are extremely helpful in developing a successful treatment plan in these cases.

Pearls and Pitfalls

Prexisting Fracture of the Femur

In stark contrast to total hip revision performed for acute periprosthetic fractures, healed fractures of the proximal femur present a different

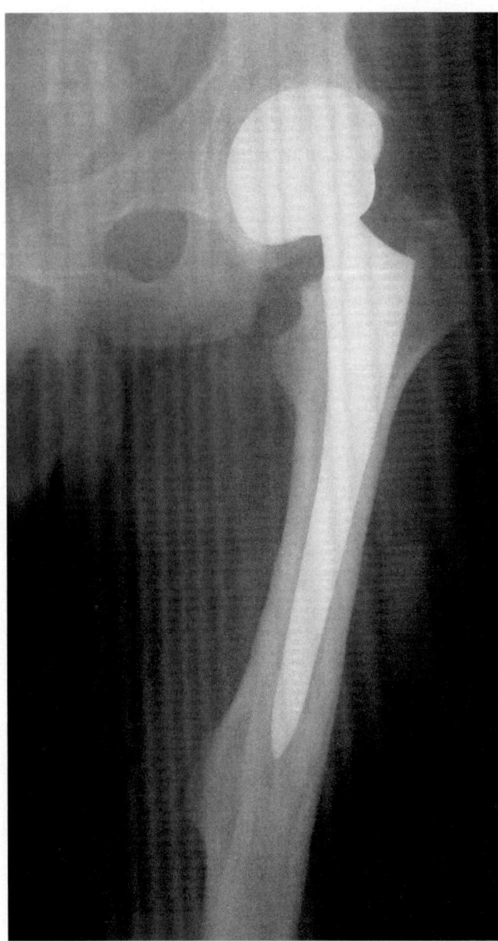

FIGURE 22-25 Primary total hip in patients with healed femoral shaft fracture from childhood. Multiplanar x-rays and careful templating preoperatively, and intraoperative x-rays were key in avoiding any complications.

set of challenges (Fig. 22-25). The advantage of a stable femur about the healed fractures is countered by retained hardware, stress risers, and malunion. Berry (91) has proposed a classification scheme for proximal femoral deformities that describes the site of the deformity (greater trochanter, femoral neck, metaphysis, diaphysis), geometry of the deformity (torsional, angular, translational, and size), and the etiology of the deformity (DDH, Paget's, osteotomy, and fracture). Referring to an early study by Mehlhoff et al (92), he notes that total hips performed for failed intertrochanteric fractures had poorer hip scores when compared to primary total hip arthroplasties (THA) (91). Mehlhoff et al (92) noted that medial displacement of the femoral shaft and bone loss were contributory factors to intraoperative complications and postoperative dislocations. However, they did report that results for THA for failed femoral neck fractures were comparable to primary joints (92).

Using the Norwegian Arthroplasty Register, Skeide et al (93) compared more than 3,800 total hip arthroplasties performed because of previous hip fracture with nearly 20,000 primary total hips for osteoarthritis. They noted that the fracture patients had a risk of revision 1.35 times higher than the arthritis patients with most of these occurring for dislocation or femoral shaft fracture.

Acute Femoral Neck Fracture

For the sake of completeness, I have included the following section on the treatment of acute femoral neck fractures with total hip replacement. Although I do believe there is a place for total hip arthroplasty (THA) in hip fracture patients with significant preexisting arthritis, I do not routinely perform THA for femoral neck fracture alone, preferring instead to treat displaced femoral neck fractures with hemiarthroplasty, details of which may be found elsewhere in this book.

McKinley and Robinson (94) conducted a matched pairs study of 107 patients who had undergone a salvage total hip arthroplasty for failed internal fixation of an intracapsular hip fracture and compared them with 107 patients in whom primary total hip replacement was used to treat the same type of fracture. The revision group of total hips had a higher complication rate, dislocation rate, and revision rate than the primary total hips performed for fracture (Table 22-7). In response to a letter to the editor from Padman and Shaw (95), the authors noted that the group of failed femoral neck fractures was drawn from a cohort of only 475 femoral neck fractures chosen to undergo a femoral head–sparing procedure. McKinley and Robinson reported that during the same time frame of their study, they performed more than 3,500 hemiarthroplasties for displaced femoral neck fractures, the results of which were not listed (95).

Mishra et al (96) treated 51 consecutive patients with displaced subcapital femoral neck fractures with cemented total hip replacements. All patients were socially independent, mobile, and mentally alert with 90% being female. The dislocation rate was 2% and the authors reported function to be comparable to elective total hip replacement for osteoarthritis.

The Cochrane Collaboration, named for the British epidemiologist, Archie Cochrane, is an international nonprofit and independent organization that produces and disseminates systematic reviews of health care interventions and promotes the search for evidence in the form of clinical trials and other studies of interventions. Parker and Gurusamy, as part of a Cochrane review of total hip arthroplasty for treatment of a proximal femur fracture (97), concluded that its role was uncertain, in part because of underreporting of outcomes. In one study of 46 patients with displaced intracapsular femoral neck fractures treated with cemented hemiarthroplasty in 23 and cemented Charnley total hips in the rest, the author concluded that the total hip patients performed better than the hemiarthroplasties (98). Three of the hemiarthroplasties were revised versus none of the Charnleys. One hundred twenty-six consecutive cemented total hip arthroplasties performed for acute fracture of the femoral neck were followed for a minimum of 10 years with an overall survivorship of 94% at 10 years (99). Ten percent of these hips dislocated but the authors noted THAs advantages of "reliable relief of pain and restoration of function" (99). The reader should be cautioned that this dislocation rate is substantially greater than the 0.85% rate reported by contemporary total joint surgeons (100).

Post Fracture Arthritis of the Acetabulum

Total hip arthroplasty in the treatment of posttraumatic arthritis of the acetabulum is a challenge secondary to extensive scarring, retained hardware, heterotopic bone, and residual deformity of the acetabulum (Fig. 22-26A,B) (101,102). Berry and Halasy (103) evaluated

TABLE 22-7 Early Complications within the First Year after Arthroplasty in Patients with Failed Internal Fixation Compared with Patients Undergoing Primary Arthroplasty for Fracture

Complication	Group 1 (107 Patients)	Group 2 (107 Patients)
Wound hematoma	2	1
Superficial infection*	12	3
Deep infection	8	2
Early dislocation*	21	9
Fracture of prosthesis	5	2
Deep venous thrombosis	3	3
Pulmonary embolus	1	2

Group 1: failed reduction and internal fixation for displaced femoral neck fracture revised to cemented total hip arthroplasty.
Group 2: primary cemented total hip arthroplasty for displaced femoral neck fracture.
* Denotes significant difference between groups ($p < 0.05$).
From McKinley JC, Robinson CM. Treatment of displaced intracapsular hip fractures with total hip arthroplasty: comparison of primary arthroplasty with early salvage arthroplasty after failed internal fixation. *J Bone Joint Surg Am* 2002;84(11):2010–2015, with permission.

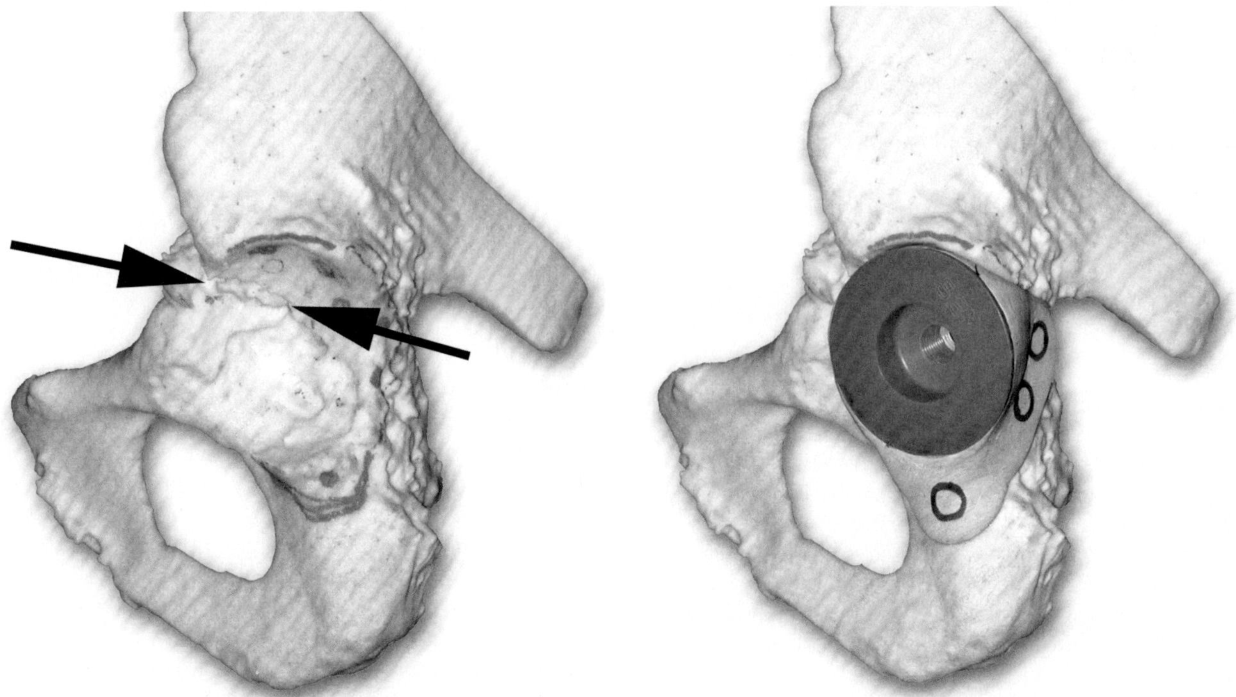

FIGURE 22-26 **A.** Full-sized plastic model reconstructed from CT scan demonstrating nonunion of transverse fracture. **B.** Custom component trial developed from CT data. Circles represent placement of fixation holes. Additional holes are behind cup.

33 patients with posttraumatic arthritis of the acetabulum who underwent implantation of an uncemented acetabular component. Only two of the shells were revised for loosening of the cup while another two underwent revision for osteolysis. Clinical follow-up was available for 14 patients with 15 hips at a minimum of 10 years postsurgery. Eight had no pain and 6 had mild pain and 13 walked without support (103). Weber et al (102) reported on a nearly 10-year follow-up in 66 patients who had undergone total hip arthroplasty for posttraumatic arthritis. Forty-four cups were inserted with cement and 22 without. Nine of the cemented cups were revised for loosening whereas none of the uncemented cups were revised or had signs of loosening (Fig. 22-27A–D).

Acute Fracture

Mears and Velyvis (104) reported good to excellent Harris Hip Scores in 45 out of 57 patients (79%) treated with total hip arthroplasty for acute fracture of the acetabulum. Average follow-up exceeded 8 years and the average age of the patients at the time of surgery was 69 years. The acetabular cups subsided an average of 2 mm vertically and 3 mm medially, all within the first 6 weeks after surgery. No cups showed any evidence of loosening and the only cup revision was for correction of malalignment in a patient with recurrent dislocations.

Posterior wall fractures with impaction involving 50% of the acetabulum are treated with a structural autograft taken from the femoral head and anchored into the defect with screws. The acetabulum is then reamed, any gaps are packed with remaining autograft, and a hemispherical cup oversized by 2 mm is impacted and stabilized with screws. Transverse fractures are stabilized with a braided cable passed in a figure-of-eight fashion in the inner surface of the quadrilateral plate (105).

Moushine et al (106) reported on early follow-up of 18 elderly patients treated with cable fixation and acute total hip arthroplasty. Their technique relies on using a single Dall-Miles cable to form a figure-of-eight resting on the center of the quadrilateral surface as previously described (106). Tensioning the cable provides the necessary compression to stabilize the acetabulum and permit implantation of an uncemented cup. Twelve of the patients were rated as excellent results and the remaining 6 as good at an average of 36 months postoperatively. Fourteen of the cups migrated an average of 2.3 mm and all fractures healed (106).

Infected Fractures

Infection following treatment of a periprosthetic fracture of the femur has been reported as a complication in several series (10,44,40) but primary treatment of a periprosthetic fracture that is infected is confined to case reports (108,109). The PROSTALAC (prosthesis of antibiotic-loaded acrylic cement) has been used successfully in the treatment of several cases of infected total hip arthroplasties associated with proximal femoral bone loss (109). The long stem version of the PROSTALAC may prove useful in the treating infected fractures in the future.

Hartford and Goodman (107) reported three cases of infected periprosthetic fracture treated with locked intramedullary nailing as an interim or salvage technique. In two cases, the locked nail was successfully revised to a total hip once cultures were sterile. The third fracture healed and the 81-year-old patient remained satisfied with her resection arthroplasty (107).

More recently, Schwab et al (108) reported one case of an infected periprosthetic fracture of the femur treated with an intramedullary device comprised of three packs of antibiotic-laden cement hand-molded around an Ender's nail. The patient remains infection-free 5 years after revision of the cement nail to a hybrid total hip replacement (108).

Complications

Nonunion of Periprosthetic Fractures

Fortunately, the majority of periprosthetic fractures about the hip go on to heal, but there is a small percentage of cases that go on to nonunion. Crockarell et al (10) in their review of periprosthetic fractures in the literature reported only 9 nonunions associated with the 224 periprosthetic fractures. Thus, only 4% of the periprosthetic fractures reported in the literature went on to nonunion (10). At their own institution, these same authors recorded 23 nonunions out of a total of 807 patients with a periprosthetic fracture about a total hip arthroplasty, and noted a 52% complication rate. Treatment for 16 patients included retaining the proximal femur, unfortunately only 10 of those healed with the first procedure (10).

In a later report from the same institution, Springer et al (40) reported 4 fracture nonunions out of 118 hips that underwent revision arthroplasty for a Vancouver Type B periprosthetic femoral fracture. Of note is that the authors reported no nonunions among the 30 hips revised with a fully porous coated prosthesis (40).

Attention to basic principles is important in achieving union in periprosthetic fractures. Six out of 16 Vancouver B1 and B3 fractures treated with Dall-Miles plates went on to either nonunion or to fracture through the plate (43). The authors advocated the continued use of the plates but emphasized the need for a long-stem revision prosthesis if the stem was unstable and the use of cortical strut grafts with the plates if the stem was well-fixed (43).

PERIPROSTHETIC FRACTURES ABOUT TOTAL KNEES

Principles of Management

Epidemiology

In a retrospective review of all 212 knee revisions performed at one institution from 1997 through 2000, Sharkey et al (110) reported that periprosthetic fracture accounted for 2.8% of the procedures (Table 22-8). Berry (6) analyzed nearly 30 years of data from the Mayo Clinic Joint Registry, and recorded a fracture incidence of 3% for primary and revision knees combined (Table 22-9). The 2000 National Hospital Discharge Survey reported total knee revisions were up from 12,000 in 1990 (5) to 28,000 in 2000 (7). Even taking Sharkey's lower estimate and extrapolating it to these data gives a rough estimate of 784 periprosthetic fractures per year at a cost of nearly $20 million if one assumes a conservative cost estimate of $25,000 per revision.

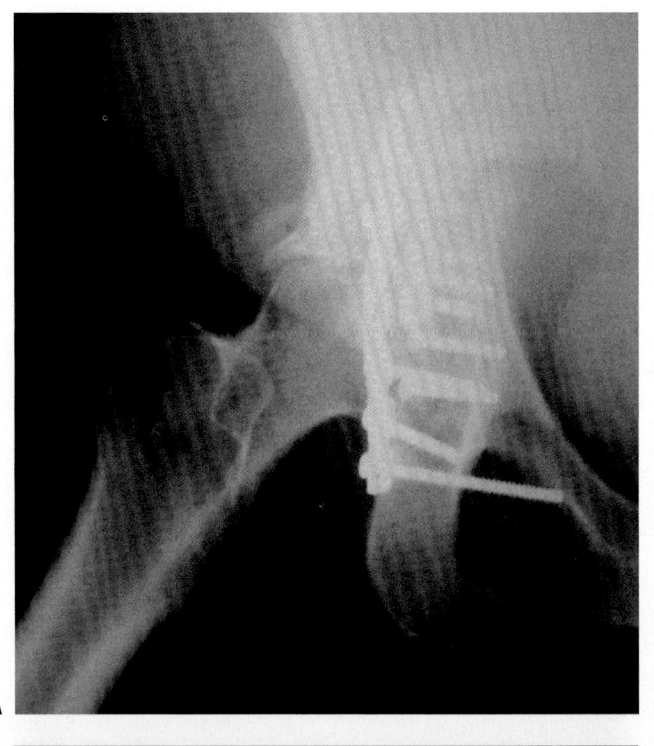

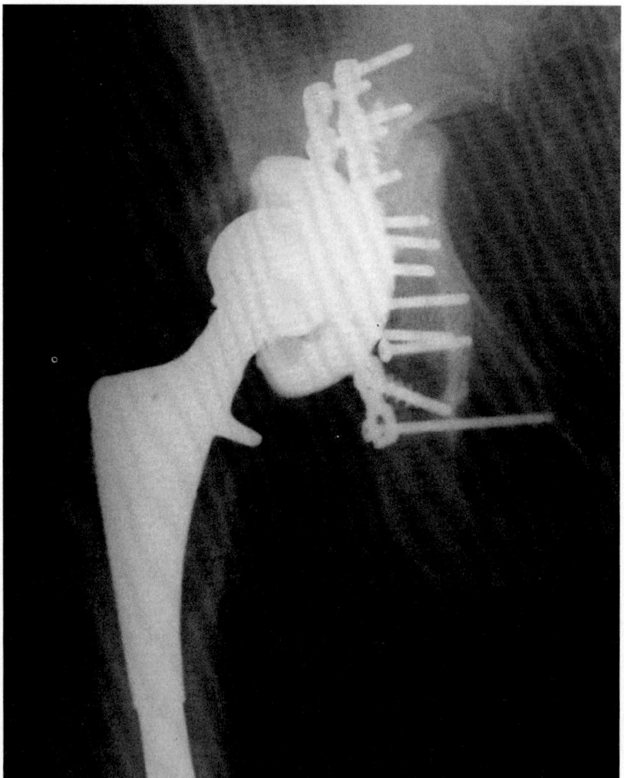

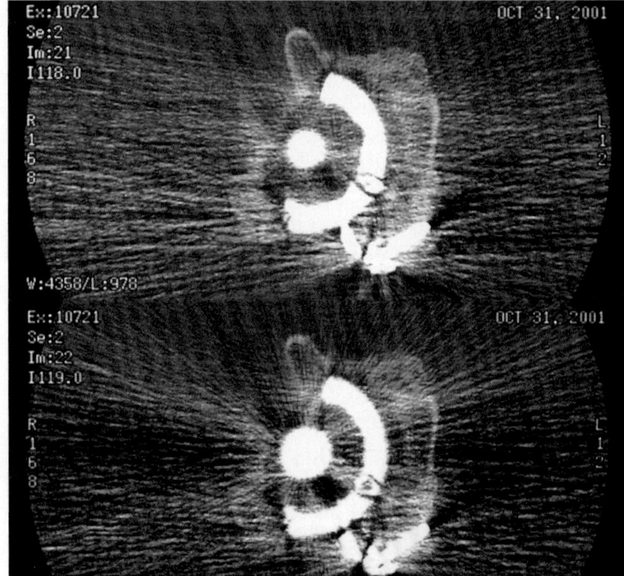

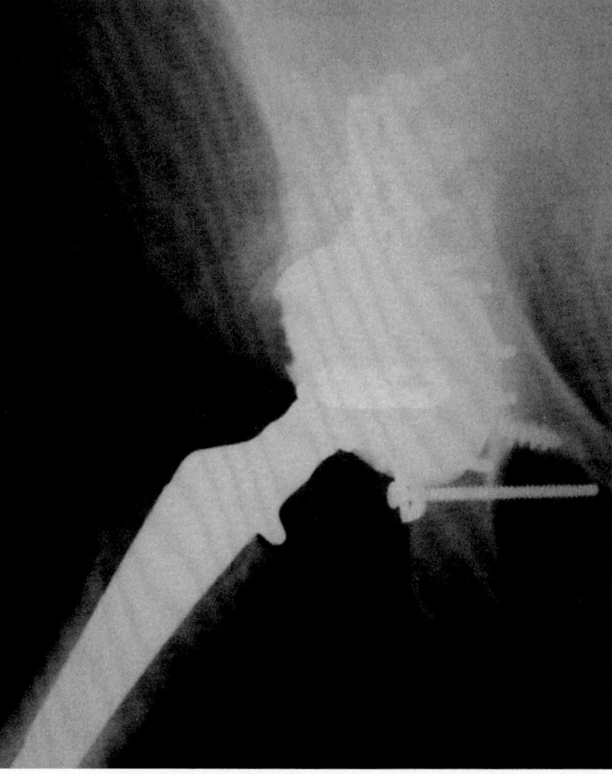

FIGURE 22-27 **A.** Traumatic arthritis of acetabulum following ORIF for acute fracture. **B.** Uncemented cup failed due to lack of bony ingrowth. **C.** Computed tomography of acetabulum confirming absence of non-union. **D.** Successful revision to larger hemispherical cup, multiple screws, and application of platelet derived growth factor and demineralized bone matrix.

TABLE 22-8 Overall Reasons for Revision Surgery Percentage

Polyethylene wear	25.0
Loosening	24.1
Instability	21.2
Infection	17.5
Arthrofibrosis	14.6
Malalignment or malpositioned	11.8
Extensor mechanism deficiency	6.6
Avascular necrosis patella	4.2
Periprosthetic fracture	2.8
Isolated patellar resurfacing	0.9

From Sharkey PF, Hozack WJ, Rothman RH, et al. Insall Award paper. Why are total knee arthroplasties failing today? *Clin Orthop* 2002;404:7–13.

Etiology

Systemic Factors

Osteopenia. Osteopenia is a major contributing factor to periprosthetic fractures in total knee arthroplasty (111–114). Patients with rheumatoid arthritis (112,115,116), especially those taking corticosteroids, are at increased risk for fracture. Petersen, et al (117) measured bone mineral density (BMD) in various regions of the distal femur in 29 patients who were 1 year out from total knee arthroplasty (TKA), noting a significant bone loss of between 19% and 44% compared to the initial values. They suggested that a decrease of this magnitude in BMD in the anterior distal femur 1 year after TKA may be an important determinant of periprosthetic fracture and later failure of the femoral component (117). In a follow-up study, Petersen's group (118) measured significant stress shielding anteriorly in the distal femur in total knee patients examined 2 years after surgery. They reported similar and progressive decreases in BMD below the tibial components of 25 patients at 3 years' follow-up (119). Wang et al (120) found similar significant postoperative decreases in bone mineral density in the distal femur and proximal tibia in a control group of 48 women who had undergone total knee arthroplasty. In their accompanying study group who took alendronate for 6 months postoperatively, bone mineral density significantly improved. They, too, suggested that this might reduce the rate of periprosthetic fractures after total knee arthroplasty (120).

Related to osteoporosis, stress fractures about the femur or tibia may develop in patients who have been inactive for an extended period when they are suddenly mobilized following total knee arthroplasty (121). These patients may complain of a sudden onset of pain about the knee during rehabilitation and require appropriate x-rays and additional studies to rule out stress fracture. Stress fracture of the proximal femur following total knee arthroplasty, although a rare complication, can be a diagnostic challenge when it occurs (122–128). These patients may complain of tenderness about the groin within weeks of resuming full weight-bearing after surgery (124,125). Bone scans and x-rays may demonstrate a stress fracture of the femoral neck (124) or in rarer instances, the subtrochanteric region of the hip (125). Protected weight-bearing and observation is

TABLE 22-9 Fracture Incidence About Total Knee Arthroplasties from the Mayo Clinic Registry

	Total No. of Cases	Femur %	Tibia %	Patella %	Total %
Intraoperative primary	16,906	23 (0.1)	13 (0.67)	0 (0)	36 (0.2)
Intraoperative revision	2,904	24 (0.8)	25 (0.8)	8 (0.2)	57 (1.9)
Postoperative primary	16,906	161 (0.9)	75 (0.4)	117 (0.7)	353 (2.1)
Postoperative revision	2,904	48 (1.6)	26 (0.9)	53 (1.8)	127 (4.4)
Total	19,810*	256 (1.3)	139 (0.7)	178 (0.9)	573 (2.8)

* Total of all primary and all revision cases.

From Berry DJ. Epidemiology: hip and knee. *Orthop Clin North Am* 1999;30(2):183–190, with permission.

usually successful although some of these cases have progressed to complete fracture (125).

Neurologic Disorders. More than one-third of the patients presented by Culp and colleagues (113) had a preexisting neurologic disorder, such as seizure, cerebral ataxia, or Parkinson's disease. These patients may have been predisposed to fracture secondary to disuse osteoporosis, ataxic gait, or osteoporosis resulting from prolonged phenytoin (Dilantin) use. Giori and Lewallen (129) reported 2 supracondylar periprosthetic femoral fractures out of 16 total knees performed in 15 patients with polio. Neither case demonstrated anterior notching on postoperative x-rays.

Local Factors

Osteolysis. The severe bony destruction resulting from osteolysis, if not a direct cause of periprosthetic fractures about the knee, certainly serves as an important precursor to fracture. Peters et al (130) reported on a series of 57 revision knee arthroplasties and listed osteolysis as the reason for revision in 7% of their cases and supracondylar femur fracture in 4%. Fehring et al (131) reported a similar incidence of 7% osteolysis in their series of 279 patients with early total knee failure.

Bony Defects. Osteotomy of the tibial tubercle can provide excellent exposure for a very stiff primary or revision knee, although the technique lowers the structural integrity of the proximal tibia. Ritter et al (132) reported on two cases of proximal tibial fracture out of a total of nine tibial tubercle osteotomies. In both cases, the fractures occurred from 1 to 2 months after surgery and both healed without further operative intervention.

Procedural Factors

Anterior Notching. Anterior notching of the femur during initial preparation for implantation has been implicated as a risk factor in periprosthetic fractures about total knee arthroplasties for several years. Recently, Lesh et al (133) reviewed 164 supracondylar periprosthetic femoral fractures reported in the literature and noted that more than 30% were associated with notching. However, they added that many had other risk factors for fracture, such as rheumatoid arthritis, osteopenia, steroid use, neurological disorder, and revision arthroplasty (133).

Notching of the femur does have a measurable adverse effect on the bone under load. Shawen et al (134) implanted femoral components into 13 matched pairs of cadaver femora with one side receiving a 3-mm deep anterior notch. Torsional load to failure for the notched specimens averaged 99 Nm while the controls required almost 144 Nm to fracture. In addition to the notching, the authors also reported that the distal femoral bone density of their specimens also correlated strongly with torsional load to failure (134). In a similar study conducted with 12 matched cadaveric femora, Lesh et al (133) created anterior notches in one of the pair and subjected the constructs to either a bending or torsional load. Again, notching significantly reduced load to failure in both bending and torsional modes.

Prosthesis Design. Thompson et al (135) reported 7 cases of periprosthetic fracture of the tibia involving the uncemented version of the low contact stress (LCS) total knee. In each case the hole for the conical stem of the tibial component was reamed without impaction and no trial component was placed prior to insertion of the final implant. The authors modified their treatment protocol and avoided uncemented tibial baseplates with this system. In my own experience with the LCS, this has happened just once and involved a cemented tibia. This was a case with hard, sclerotic bone that did not yield to the press fit of the cone. The fracture was noted in the operating theater and fixed with an L-plate and screws.

On the femoral side, Rorabeck and Taylor (136) note an increased risk of intraoperative fracture associated with posterior stabilized implants that remove bone from the intercondylar region. Fracture is more likely to occur if the component is not centered between the condyles. Typically, the medial condyle is more likely be involved (136).

Revision Arthroplasty. Osteolysis or loosening of a total knee implant may also lead to fracture during the revision procedure itself (121). Even revision of well-fixed components, as in cases of infected arthroplasty, may lead to intraoperative fracture if careful preoperative planning and intraoperative execution is not observed.

A summary of risk factors relevant to fractures about contemporary total knee arthroplasties is listed in Table 22-10.

Diagnosis of Periprosthetic TKA Fractures

Periprosthetic fractures about total knee arthroplasties may be hidden by the overlying femoral or tibial implant. This is further exacerbated by the secondary radiographic changes about loosened implants. As always, prefracture or presymptom x-rays are very helpful, especially when combined with current x-rays taken at multiple angles around the knee. Computerized tomography has been employed to evaluate fractured polyethylene about total knee components (137) so it is reasonable to consider it for the evaluation of fractures. Olsen and colleagues (3) have reported on the technique of "metal artifact reduction sequence" or MARS, which can significantly reduce the scatter of MRI signals about metal implants. It could prove useful in diagnosing the more subtle stress fracture about a total knee.

Classification of Periprosthetic TKA Fractures

Femur

The most widely used classification scheme for periprosthetic femur fractures about total knees is that proposed by Lewis and Rorabeck (138,139) that takes into account both fracture

TABLE 22-10 Contemporary Risk Factors for Periprosthetic Fractures about Total Knee Arthroplasties

Systemic	Osteoporosis – primary or secondary		
	Rheumatoid arthritis		
	Neurologic disorders (Parkinson's, epilepsy, polio)		
Local	Cortical defect	Femur	Previous ORIF Notching Fracture malunion
		Tibia	Bone-patellar tendon-bone donor site Tibial tunnel for anterior cruciate ligament reconstruction Fracture malunion
	Adjacent hardware	Femur	Distal total hip or hemi stem Dynamic hip screw plate Intramedullary hip screw stem
		Tibia	High tibial osteotomy fixation Plateau fixation plates
	Osteolysis		
Procedural	Anterior femoral notching Tibial tubercle osteotomy Medialized box cut in PCL substituting designs Conical tibial baseplate stem Overresection of patella		

displacement and prosthesis stability. The principal factor that makes this classification so useful is its assessment of the stability of the implant. Type I femoral fractures are essentially nondisplaced and the bone/prosthesis interface remains intact. In Type II fractures, the interface remains intact, but the fracture is displaced. Finally, Type III fractures all have a loose or failing prosthesis in the face of either a displaced or nondisplaced fracture (Table 22-11 and Fig. 22-28).

Tibia

Periprosthetic tibial fractures are classified according to Felix et al (140,141) based upon three factors:

1. Location of the fracture
2. Stability of the implant
3. Whether the fracture occurred intraoperatively or postoperatively

Type I fractures occur in the tibial plateau, Type II are adjacent to the stem, Type III are distal to the prosthesis, and Type IV fractures involve the tubercle. The stability of the implant is then used to further classify the fractures: subtype A is a well-fixed implant, subtype B is loose, and subtype C are intraoperative fracture (Table 22-12 and Fig. 22-29).

Patella

Goldberg et al (142) proposed a four-part classification system for patellar fractures based upon 36 fractures in 35 patients. The scheme is based upon the location of the fracture, disruption of implant fixation, dislocation of the patella, and the status of the extensor mechanism (Table 22-13). An updated algorithm for treatment of patellar fractures about total knee arthroplasties is presented in Table 22-14 based upon work presented by Ortiguera and Berry (143).

TABLE 22-11 Supracondylar Periprosthetic Fracture Classification and Treatment Algorithm

Classification	Type I	Type II	Type III	Type III
Fracture displacement	Undisplaced	Displaced	Undisplaced	Displaced
Implant	Well fixed	Well fixed	Loose or failing (significant polyethylene or metal wear)	
Bone quality	Good	Good Poor	Good Poor Good	Poor
Treatment options	Closed treatment brace	Internal fixation: Intramedullary rod 95 degree dynamic condylar screw plate Standard condylar plate Locking condylar plate LISS	Stemmed revision Internal fixation Bone graft	Allograft composite Rotating-hinge prosthesis

After Rorabeck CH, Taylor JW. Classification of periprosthetic fractures complicating total knee arthroplasty. *Orthop Clin North Am* 1999;30(2):209–214; and Rorabeck CH, Taylor JW. Periprosthetic fractures of the femur complicating total knee arthroplasty. *Orthop Clin North Am* 1999;30(2):265–277.

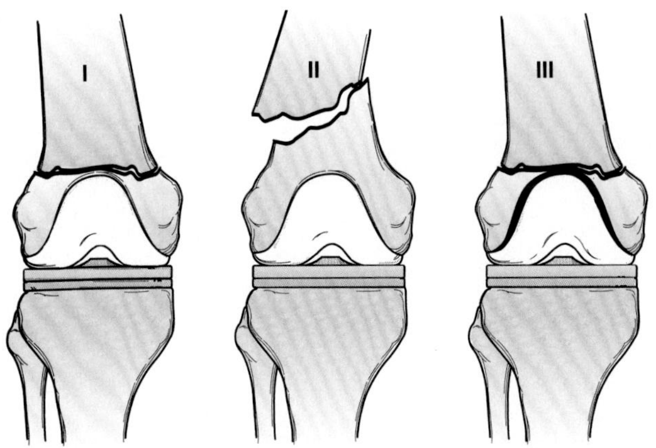

FIGURE 22-28 Classification scheme for periprosthetic fractures about the femoral component of the knee. Type I fractures are minimally displaced with an intact prosthesis bone interface; Type II fractures are displaced but maintain an intact bone prosthesis interface; and Type III fractures may be displaced or nondisplaced, but have a loose femoral component. (Modified from Lewis PL, Rorabeck CH. Periprosthetic fractures. In: Engh GA, Rorabeck CH, eds. *Revision total knee arthroplasty*. Baltimore: Williams & Wilkins, 1997:275–295.)

Current Treatment Options

Like fractures about total hips, the techniques for the treatment of periprosthetic fractures about total knees falls into two main categories: (a) plating techniques and (b) revision prostheses. As noted earlier, it is not unusual for surgeons to employ a combination of these techniques in challenging cases. Table 22-15 summarizes the advantages and disadvantages of the techniques that are described here.

Specific Techniques for Femoral and Tibial Fractures

Plating. The Less Invasive Stabilization System (LISS) (Synthes, Paoli, PA) applies the principles of rigid external fixation to the technique of internal plate stabilization while allowing for a minimal fracture site dissection (Fig. 22-30A,B) (144). Details of the technique are discussed elsewhere in this book. The percutaneous insertion of the plate and screws preserves the soft-tissue envelope, minimizes blood loss, and may obviate the need for additional bone graft (145).

Althausen et al (144) reported on five supracondylar femur fractures about total knee replacements treated with LISS. No shortening was noted and all cases healed in physiologic valgus.

TABLE 22-12 Tibial Fracture Classification and Treatment Algorithm

Main Category	Type I			Type II			Type III			Type IV		
Fracture position	*Tibial Plateau*			*Adjacent to Stem*			*Distal to Prosthesis*			*Tibial Tubercle*		
Subcategory:												
A – Prosthesis well-fixed	A	B	C	A	B	C	A	B	C	A	B	C
B – Prosthesis loose												
C – Intraoperative												
Classification	IA	IB	IC	IIA	IIB	IIC	IIIA	IIIB	IIIC	IVA	IVB	IVC
Incidence*		50%	11%	5%	10%	7%	14%	1%	1%	2%		
Treatment options	Nondisplaced: Bracing and limited weight-bearing Displaced: Reduction, screw fixation or locking plate; LISS	Revision; Impaction grafting of allograft chips into cavitary defects	Screw fixation; locking plate	Locking plate; LISS	Revision with long stem; locking plate fixation	Bypass with longer stem; locking plate fixation	LISS; locking plate	Revision with long stem; locking plate fixation	Bypass with long stem	Intact extensor mechanism: brace immobilization in extension. Disrupted extensor mechanism: repair	Revision of components; fracture fixation	Repair

Reflecting a combination of techniques from original article by Stuart and Hansen[141] and more recently developed techniques.

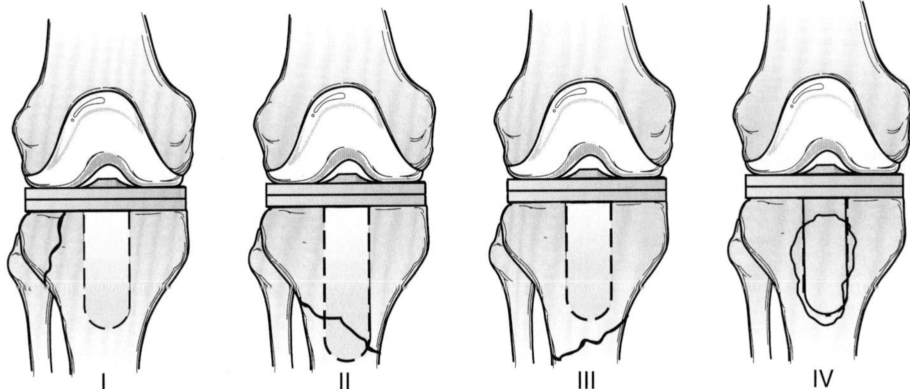

FIGURE 22-29 Classification scheme for periprosthetic fractures about the tibial component of the knee. Type I fractures involve only a portion of the metaphysis. Type II fractures occur about the stem of the tibial component. Type III fractures occur distal to the stem, and Type IV fractures involve the tibial tubercle. (Modified after Felix NA, Stuart MJ, Hanssen AD. Periprosthetic fractures of the tibia associated with total knee arthroplasty. *Clin Orthop* 1997;(345):113–124.)

Falck et al (145) were among the first to report on the use of the LISS to treat periprosthetic fractures about total knees. Treating three periprosthetic TKA fractures between June 1997 and June 1999 as part of a larger series of fractures, they noted no major difficulties were encountered and reduction was readily achieved using manual devices. Postoperatively, the authors noted that the LISS allowed faster mobilization of patients (145). Schutz et al (146) reported on the use of the LISS in treating 12 periprosthetic fractures of the femur out of a total series of 116 fractures treated between December 1996 and November 1998. Fracture healing occurred in 90% of all cases and the authors attributed most complications with healing as being directly related to the severity of the original trauma (146).

TABLE 22-13 Patellar Classification

Type I	Marginal fracture Extensor mechanism intact Implant/bone interface intact
Type II	Disruption of extensor mechanism or Implant/bone interface
Type III	Fracture of inferior pole of patella A – With patellar ligament disruption B – Nondisplaced
Type IV	Fracture associated with patellar dislocation

From Goldberg VM, Figgie HE, Inglis AE, et al. Patellar fracture type and prognosis in condylar total knee arthroplasty. *Clin Orthop* 1988;(236):115–122, with permission.

Bong et al (147) compared fracture stability of short retrograde intramedullary nails with LISS about posterior cruciate retaining total knees in a matched cadaveric study. Although both systems performed well, they suggested that the retrograde nail had the advantage in torsional stability in fractures with significant comminution.

Reflecting a trend among traumatologists toward minimally invasive techniques, O'Toole et al (148) treated 9 periprosthetic fractures about total knees and another 5 with hip and knee arthroplasties with LISS plating. All patients were female and averaged 80 years of age. Allograft bone was employed in only one case and the authors reported no complications associated with their treatment of fractures about TKAs. Ricci et al (149) treated 13 consecutive supracondylar femur fractures about well-fixed femoral components with the Locking Condylar Plate (Synthes, Paoli, PA). All cases employed indirect reduction and none used bone graft. There were no infections or revisions in this group that included 12 women. Seven of 13 cases did not employ locking screws proximal to the fracture. Two cases sustained broken screws but healed without intervention. Both broken screws occurred in the group that did not use proximal locking screws; there were no screw failures among those that did use proximal locking screws.

Before the development of LISS, traditional plating techniques, such as supracondylar blade plates and condylar

TABLE 22-14 Treatment Recommendations for Patellar Fracture after TKA

Classification	*Type I* (Implant/Extensor mechanism intact)	*Type II* (Implant/Extensor mechanism disrupted)	*Type IIIa* (Implant loose, good bone stock)	*Type IIIb* (Implant loose, poor bone stock)
Treatment regimen	Non-operative	Extensor mechanism repair + partial or complete patellectomy vs. ORIF	Operative treatment if sufficiently symptomatic	
			Patelloplasty with component revision vs. component resection	Patellar component removal with patelloplasty or complete patellectomy

From Ortiguera CJ, Berry DJ. Patellar fracture after total knee arthroplasty. *J Bone Joint Surg Am* 2002;84(4):532–540, with permission.

compression screws, had been utilized for many years to successfully treat periprosthetic TKA fractures (150–152). Ayers notes that the nonlocking condylar buttress plate is even more versatile than the fixed angle plates as it allows multiple point fixation and works quite well with comminuted fractures (150).

IM Nailing. Retrograde intramedullary nailing of supracondylar periprosthetic TKA fractures has been employed successfully for several years (Fig. 22-31) (153–157). The primary advantage of the technique lies in the need for only limited dissection of fracture fragments with preservation of blood supply. Disadvantages include the need to violate the joint space and the potential problems encountered with posterior stabilized components that have a closed box over the intercondylar notch (Table 22-16) (156).

In a direct comparison of intramedullary nails with LISS plates in the treatment of supracondylar fractures about TKAs, Wick et al (157) found both techniques useful. They treated nine fractures with IM nails and nine with LISS plates, noting that the LISS plates were preferred in cases involving osteoporotic bone (157).

Revision. Circumferential, uncontained bone loss about distal femoral periprosthetic fractures is a challenge to reconstruct. In such cases, use of a stemmed allograft composite can maintain limb length, joint stability, and knee motion (158). In 10 cases of periprosthetic TKA fractures treated with distal femoral allograft constructs, mean flexion was 100°, and 9 patients achieved union and were able to bear full weight (158) In these cases, the stemmed implant was cemented to the allograft first and then the stem was cemented into the host femur, carefully avoiding interposition of cement between graft and host bone. The authors employed two surgical teams for the procedure: one to revise the knee and the second to prepare and shape the allograft composite.

Rotating platform hinge knee replacement was employed as the primary treatment for nine acute periprosthetic total knee fractures and 10 nonunions of periprosthetic fractures (159). The authors noted that this procedure was reserved as a last ditch effort toward salvage of the knee and that it comprised only a small percentage of their knee replacement experience. Improvement in knee scores was reflected primarily by the significant pain relief achieved by the patients and not gains in functionality (Fig. 22-32A–C) (159).

Casting. Casting of nondisplaced and minimally displaced fractures about total knee replacements is possible when the alignment of the fracture is easily maintained with closed reduction (Fig. 22-33A,B) (150). Potential risks of casting and bracing include pressure sores in older patients and arthrofibrosis of the joint if it is kept immobile too long.

Amputation. Amputation above the knee as a treatment modality for periprosthetic TKA fractures is mentioned primarily for completeness. Sixty-three per cent of the 67 above knee amputations performed about TKAs in the series from Sierra et al (160) were for reasons unrelated to the knee replacement, usually peripheral vascular disease. Of those that were the majority were for uncontrolled infection; only 2 out of 25 were for periprosthetic fracture. The authors also noted that the functional outcome after amputation above a TKA was poor.

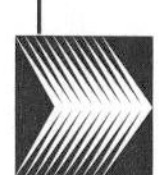

AUTHOR'S PREFERRED TREATMENT

Surgical Procedure

For periprosthetic fractures about femoral or tibial components in which the components remain well-fixed, I prefer to use locking plate technology. The external jig allows for as little dissection as necessary.

Loose prostheses require revision, either with modular components that can replace missing bone or allograft composites. I prefer to reserve hinged constrained components for the most severe cases and instead prefer to use semiconstrained components such as the Constrained Condylar Knee (Zimmer, Inc., Warsaw, IN).

TABLE 22-15 Treatment Options for Periprosthetic Fractures About Total Knee Arthroplasties

Treatment Options	Advantages	Disadvantages
Strut graft	– High union rate – Easily contoured – Low elastic modulus	– May weaken after implantation – Variable availability – Graft–host interaction – Not as strong as plates
Plates		
LISS	– Minimal dissection – Preserves blood supply – Rigid internal fixation – Use with/without cables – Unicortical screws – Multiple distal fixation screws	– Can't alter contour of titanium plates – More expensive than dynamic plate – Requires special training
Locking plate	– Rigid internal fixation – Use with/without cables – Unicortical screws – Multiple distal fixation screws	– Changing contour negates use of guide – More expensive than dynamic plate
Fixed blade	– Readily available – Rotational stability in sagittal plane	– Limited ability to place blade more distally – Difficult to change alignment – Possibility of fragmenting periprosthetic bone
Dynamic condylar	– Readily available	– Limited distal fixation options – Large screw removes distal bone
Dynamic compression	– Readily available – Minimal skill set – Stronger than strut graft – Reduced stress shielding	– Requires dissection to plate length – Weaker than locking or LISS plates
Revision components		
Femur-long stem	– Bypasses fracture – Fluted provides rotational stability	– Requires femoral revision – Requires adequate distal bone
Tibia-long stem	– Bypasses fracture – Fluted provides rotational stability	– Requires tibial revision – Requires adequate distal bone
Constrained	– Initial stability	– Requires femoral and tibial revision
Oncology reconstruction	– Initial stability – Accommodates extensive bone loss	– Requires femoral and tibial revision – Extensive dissection
Allograft composite	– Accommodates extensive bone loss – Easily contoured and shaped	– Limited availability – Additional dissection for stabilization
Intramedullary nail	– Limited dissection	– Less stability in comminuted fractures – Difficulty passing through intercondylar notch with some knee designs – Subsidence – Limited distal fixation – Stress concentration at tip if total hip stem is present
Amputation	– Definitive, but last resort treatment	– Significant functional deficit
Casting	– Nonoperative – Appropriate for nondisplaced fractures in low-demand patients	– Lengthy recovery – Displacement of fracture

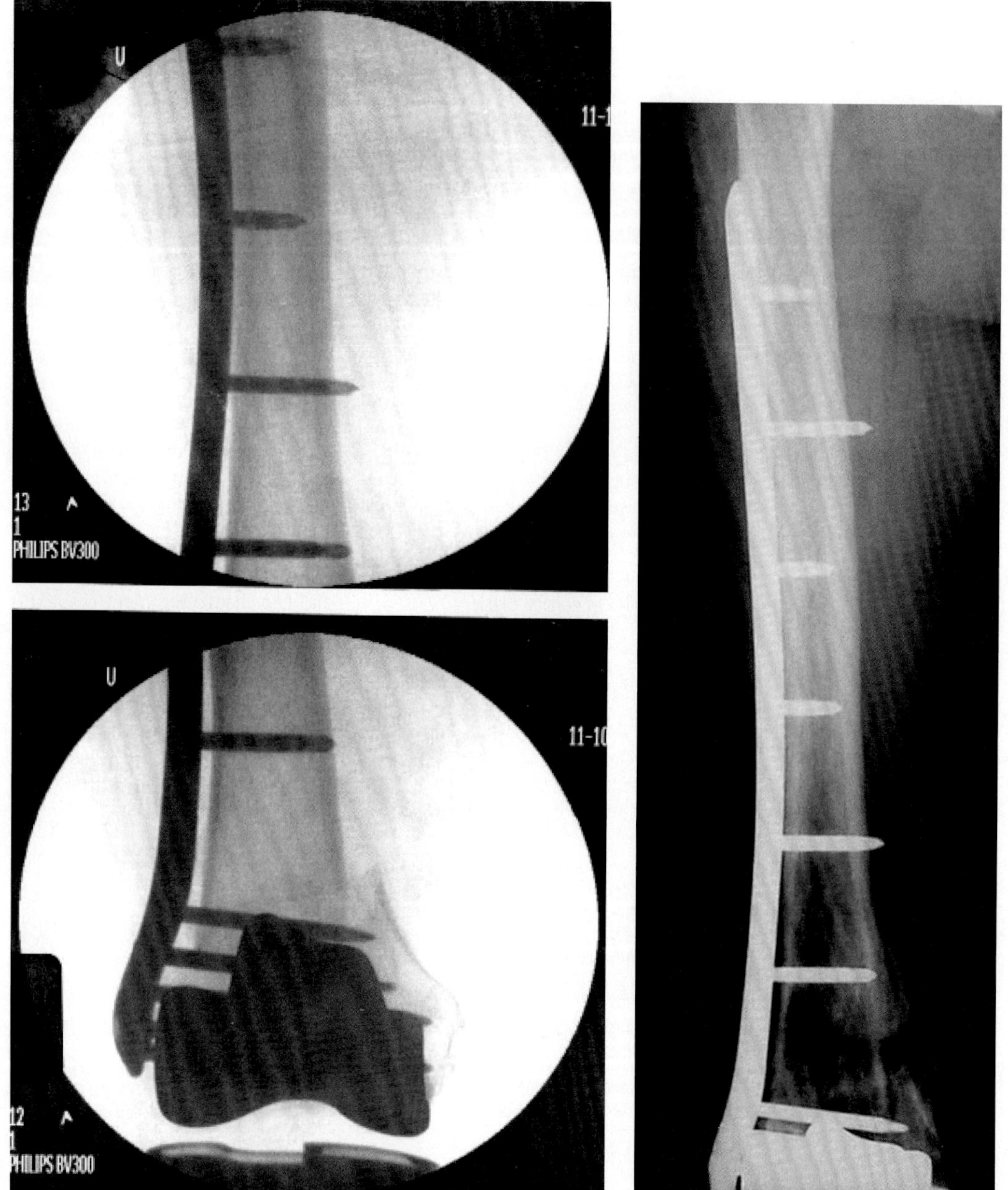

FIGURE 22-30 **A.** Intraoperative fluoroscopy of LISS applied to a Type II fracture. **B.** Six months postoperatively, the fracture has healed. Noted that all screws in this case were locked. (Courtesy of Dr. Paul Freudigman, Baylor University Medical Center, Dallas, Texas.)

Pearls and Pitfalls

TKA after Fracture

As with the total hips described earlier, total knee replacement following a healed fracture about the joint is challenging (Fig. 22-34). Weiss et al (161) reviewed 62 patients with a previous fracture of the tibial plateau, 38 of which had been treated with open reduction and internal fixation, who subsequently underwent total knee replacement. The authors concluded that these patients achieved substantial improvement in function and relief of pain, but noted a very high postoperative complication rate of 26%. They noted the most common complications included soft-tissue healing, intraoperative disruption of the extensor mechanism, and postoperative stiffness (161). There were only two infections in this series. Saleh et al (162) also noted that TKA after fracture of the proximal tibia yielded a significant decrease in pain and increase in function, but at a price. Unlike the study by Weiss (154), all 15 of the patients in their study had undergone open reduction and internal fixation. Five cases had an uncontained bone defect of the lateral plateau requiring bone grafting, 2 had unu-

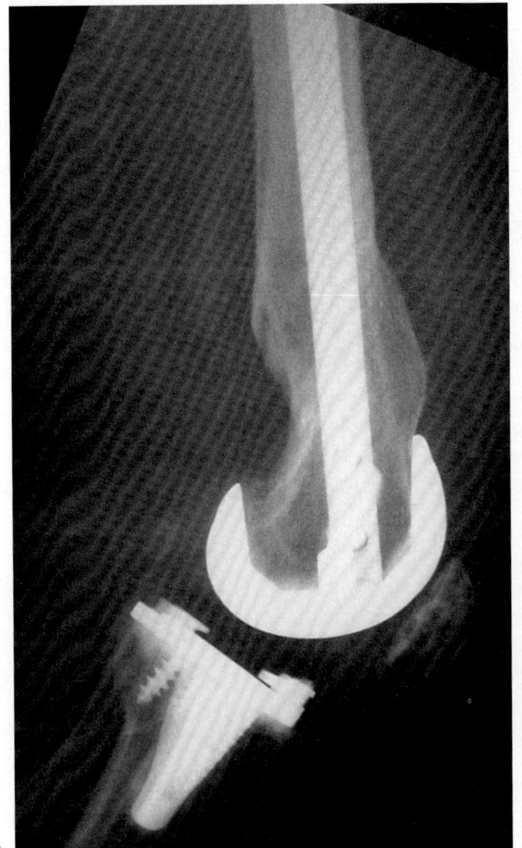

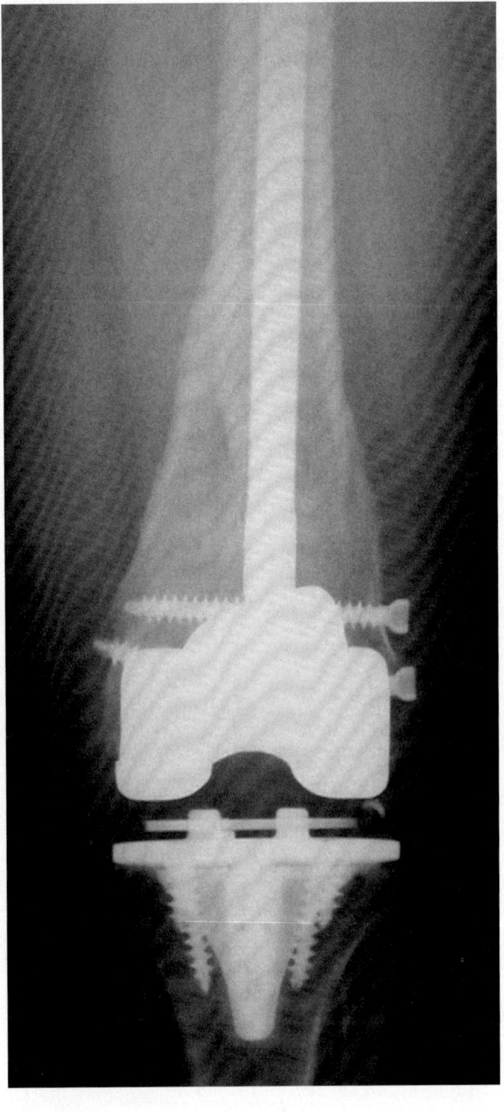

FIGURE 22-31 A,B. Lateral and anteroposterior views of healed Type II fracture treated with a retrograde intramedullary nail.

nited fracture fragments, and 5 required lateral retinacular release for exposure. Postoperatively, 3 cases became infected, 2 sustained disruption of the patellar tendon, and 3 required manipulation under anesthesia (162).

Total knee replacement following healed distal femoral fractures is not well documented in the literature, but one can surmise that the same problems with exposure and scarring will be encountered. Nelson et al (163) reported on 11 cases of TKA after distal femoral varus osteotomy. The authors noted that the procedure was technically demanding because of the difficulty in determining intramedullary alignment. Extramedullary guidance and intraoperative fluoroscopy are helpful in these cases.

Fracture between Total Hip and Total Knee Stems

There is a small but growing population of patients who have undergone multiple total joint replacements in the same extremity. When this leaves the tips of the knee and hip prostheses in close proximity, stress concentrations in this region may lead to fracture between the components. In those cases with adequate bone stock and well-fixed components, a combination of contoured femoral strut graft and locking/cable plates can be used. When the bone stock is poor and/or one or both components are loose, then total femoral replacement is an option.

CONTROVERSIES/FUTURE DIRECTIONS

Locking plate technology has significantly improved the management of periprosthetic fractures about total hip and total knee arthroplasties. The latest systems now offer short, unicorti-

TABLE 22-16 Intercondylar Diameters

Device Manufacturer	Knee Implant Model	Smallest Intercondylar Diameter in mm
Biomet	AGC sizes 55–80	17.0–22.0
	Maxim PCR sizes 55–80	13.0–15.0
	Maxim PCS open box sizes 55–80	14.0
	Ascent PCR sizes XS–XXL	17.0–23.0
	Ascent PCS open box sizes XS–XXL	20.0
Kirschner	Performance	14.0
DePuy/Johnson & Johnson	AMK Cruciate Retaining 1488, 1688 sizes 1–5	14.2–21.5
	AMK 1489 Series sizes 1–5	14.5–20.6
	AMK Congruency Posterior Stabilized 1956 sizes 1–5	13.2–17.2
	AMK Posterior Stabilized (diverging box) 1866	13.25
	AMK Universal 1489	14.5
	AMK Coordinate Ultra	Closed box
	LCS sizes Small–Large+	13.6–22.0
	LCS Complete sizes Small–Large+	14.4–21.9
	PFC Sigma Cruciate Retaining	17.4
	PFC Sigma Posterior Stabilized	11.9
	PFC Sigma TC3 Cruciate Substituting	11.9
	PFC Modular Cruciate Retaining	19.9
	PFC Modular Cruciate Substituting	9.3
	PFC TC3	Closed box
Wright Medical	Advantim PCR	19.0
	Advantim Open Housing Posterior Stabilized	16.0
	Advantim Closed Housing Posterior Stabilized	Closed box
	Advance Medial Pivot (PCR)	18.0
	Advance Posterior Stabilized	Closed box
	Axiom (PCR) sizes 55–85	14.0–22.0
	Axiom (Posterior Stabilized) sizes 55–85	16.0–24.0
Howmedica/Osteonics	PCA sizes Small–X-large	12.0–16.0
	Duracon	18.5
	Omnifit	Closed box
	Scorpio CR sizes 3–13	17.0–21.0
	Scorpio PS sizes 3–13	17.0–21.0
	Scorpio TS	Closed box
Centerpulse (Intermedics/Sulzer)	Natural, NKII	14.0
	Apollo PCR	18.5
	Apollo Posterior Stabilized	Closed box
Zimmer	Insall/Burstein I sizes 55–72	15.5–18.8
	Insall/Burstein II sizes 54–74	15.3–21.0
	Miller/Galante I sizes Small–Large++	10.6–17.4
	Miller/Galante II sizes 1–8	11.9
	Nex Gen LPS sizes A–H Open Box	14.1– 21.6
Smith & Nephew	Genesis	20.0
	Genesis II	16.5

From Su ET, DeWal H, Di Cesare PE. Periprosthetic femoral fractures above total knee replacements. *J Am Acad Orthop Surg* 2004;12(1):12–20, with permission.

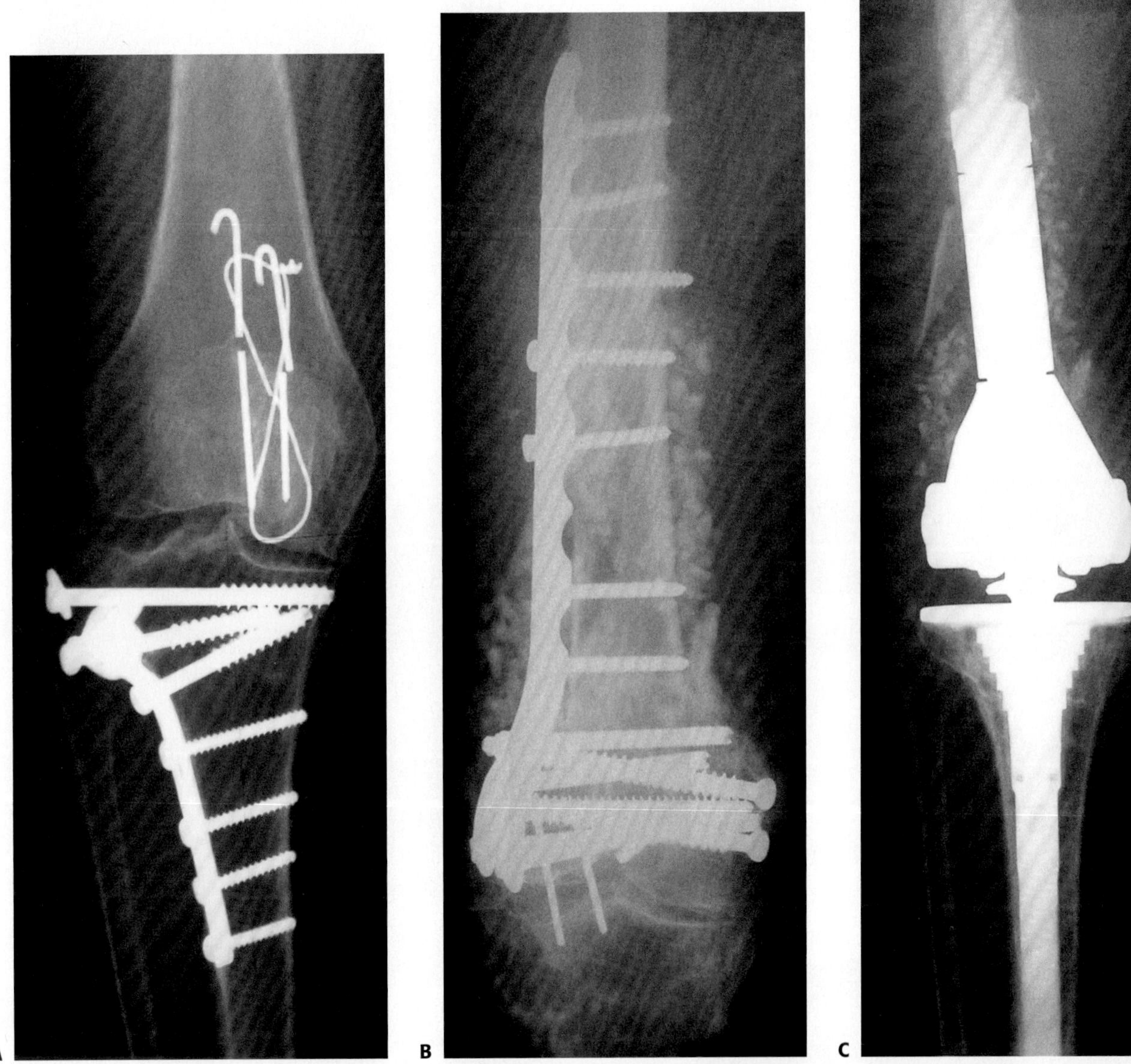

FIGURE 22-32 **A.** Preoperative x-ray of patient undergoing routine hardware removal in preparation for standard total knee replacement at a later date. **B.** Patient did well following hardware removal, but fell several weeks later, sustaining a comminuted supracondylar femur fracture. ORIF was performed at another facility. **C.** Subsequent painful nonunion of fracture led to implantation of rotating hinge prosthesis with resolution of pain.

cal screws for fixation about intramedullary stems. Biomechanical studies should be able to tell us if this fixation is as stable, or more so, than contemporary cable fixation.

Recombinant human bone morphogeneic protein may provide additional healing potential in difficult fractures. The reader is referred to additional discussion on rhBMP within this book.

Intraoperative computer-aided surgery still has a way to go before it becomes routinely useful in the treatment of periprosthetic fractures. Some biplanar fluoroscopic guidance systems may prove useful in applying LISS technology to more extensive periprosthetic fractures.

Preoperative planning with computer assistance will increase significantly as more hospital systems adopt picture archiving and communications systems (PACS). Software algorithms that can both eliminate metal artifacts from computerized tomogra-

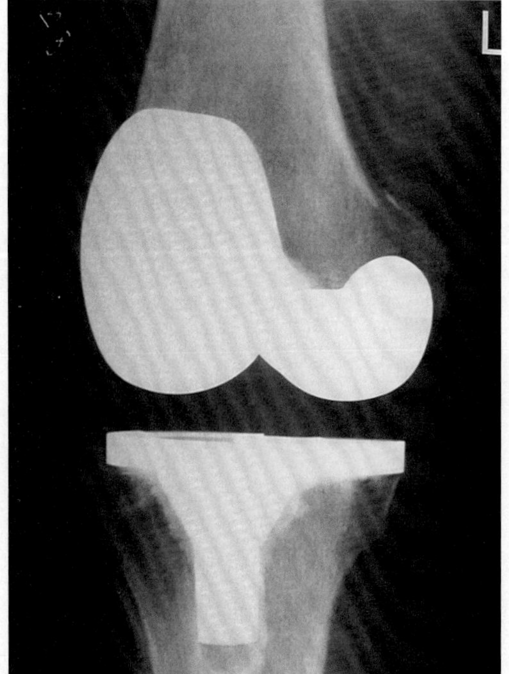

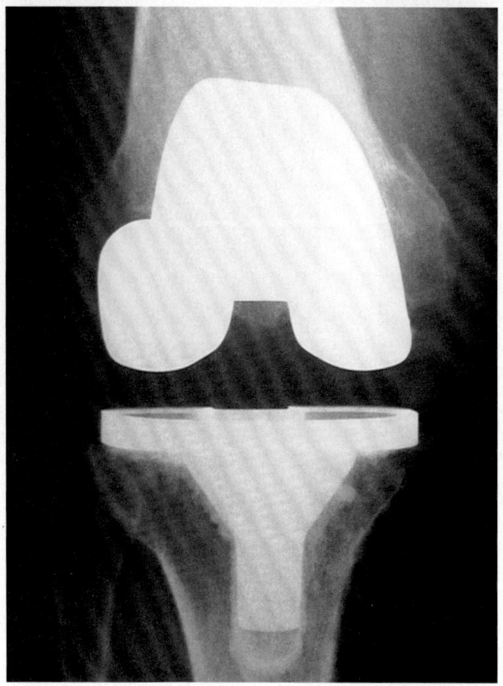

FIGURE 22-33 A,B. Oblique and anteroposterior radiographs of a total knee demonstrating a minimally displaced medial condyle fracture. Case was treated with limited weight-bearing and hinged knee brace for 8 weeks. Patient is now fully functional and pain free.

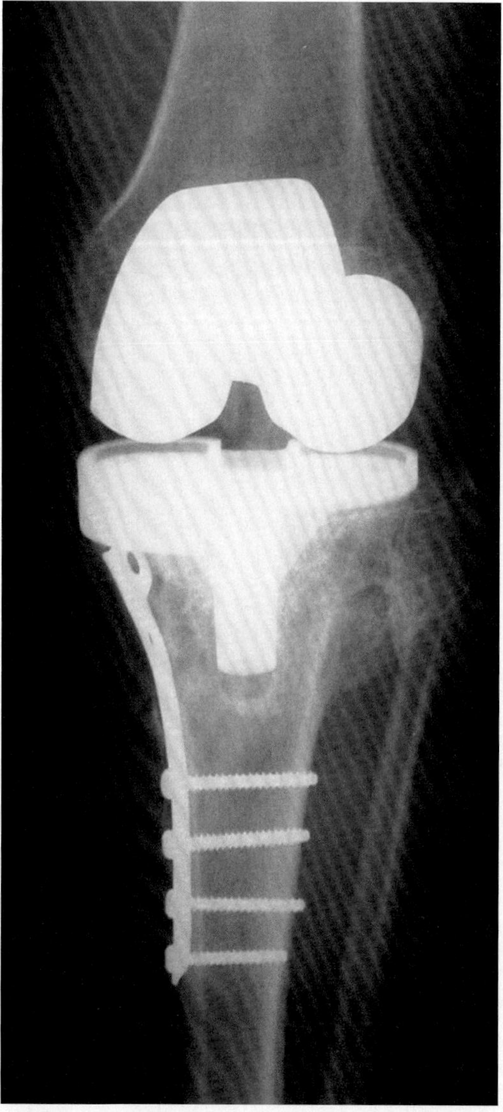

FIGURE 22-34 Total knee arthroplasty performed for painful post-traumatic arthritis following a comminuted fracture of the tibial plateau. An augmentation wedge and a tibial tray with an offset stem were necessary to accommodate bony deformity. The medial plate was left in situ to avoid additional dissection.

phy scans and then reconstruct those images into useful three-dimensional models will prove particularly useful in periacetabular fractures.

REFERENCES

1. Tsiridis E, Haddad FS, Gie GA. The management of periprosthetic femoral fractures around hip replacements. *Injury* 2003;34(2):95–105.
2. White LM, Kim JK, Mehta M, et al. Complications of total hip arthroplasty: MR imaging-initial experience. *Radiology* 2000;215(1):254–262.
3. Olsen RV, Munk PL, Lee MJ, et al. Metal artifact reduction sequence: early clinical applications. *Radiographics* 2000;20(3):699–712.

4. DeFrances CJ, Hall MJ. 2002 National Hospital Discharge Survey. *Adv Data* 2004; 21(342):1–29.
5. Graves EJ. Detailed diagnoses and procedures, national hospital discharge survey, 1990. *Vital Health Stat 13* 1992;113:1–225.
6. Berry DJ. Epidemiology: hip and knee. *Orthop Clin North Am* 1999;30(2):183–190.
7. Kozak LJ, Hall MJ, Owings MF. National Hospital Discharge Survey: 2000 annual summary with detailed diagnosis and procedure data. *Vital Health Stat 13* 2002;(153): 1–194.
8. Meek RM, Garbuz DS, Masri BA, et al. Intraoperative fracture of the femur in revision total hip arthroplasty with a diaphyseal fitting stem. *J Bone Joint Surg Am* 2004;86-A(3):480–485.
9. Zalzal P, Gandhi R, Petruccelli D, et al. Fractures at the tip of long-stem prostheses used for revision hip arthroplasty. *J Arthroplasty* 2003;18(6):741–745.
10. Crockarell JR Jr, Berry DJ, Lewallen DG. Nonunion after periprosthetic femoral fracture associated with total hip arthroplasty. *J Bone Joint Surg Am* 1999;81(8):1073–1079.
11. Havelin LI, Engesaeter LB, Espehaug B, et al. The Norwegian Arthroplasty Register: 11 years and 73,000 arthroplasties. *Acta Orthop Scand* 2000;71(4):337–353.
12. Koval KJ, Meek R, Schemitsch E, et al. An AOA critical issue. Geriatric trauma: young ideas. *J Bone Joint Surg* Am 2003;85(7):1380–1388.
13. Blatter G, Fiechter T, Magerl F. [Peri-prosthesis fractures in total hip endoprostheses]. *Orthopade* 1989;18(6):545–551.
14. Mikhail WE, Wretenberg PF, Weidenhielm LR, et al. Complex cemented revision using polished stem and morselized allograft. Minimum 5-years' follow-up. *Arch Orthop Trauma Surg* 1999;119(5–6):288–291.
15. Robinson DE, Lee MB, Smith EJ, et al. Femoral impaction grafting in revision hip arthroplasty with irradiated bone. *J Arthroplasty* 2002;17(7):834–840.
16. Berry DJ. Periprosthetic fractures associated with osteolysis: a problem on the rise. *J Arthroplasty* 2003;18[3 Suppl 1]:107–111.
17. Dunbar MJ, Blackley HR, Bourne RB. Osteolysis of the femur: principles of management. *Instr Course Lect* 2001;50:197–209.
18. Sanchez-Sotelo J, McGrory BJ, Berry DJ. Acute periprosthetic fracture of the acetabulum associated with osteolytic pelvic lesions: a report of 3 cases. *J Arthroplasty* 2000;15(1): 126–130.
19. Harris WH. Wear and periprosthetic osteolysis: the problem. *Clin Orthop* 2001;393: 66–70.
20. Lavernia CJ. Cost-effectiveness of early surgical intervention in silent osteolysis. *J Arthroplasty* 1998;13(3):277–279.
21. Berger RA. Total hip arthroplasty using the minimally invasive two-incision approach. *Clin Orthop* 2003;(417):232–241.
22. Goldstein WM, Branson JJ, Berland KA, et al. Minimal-incision total hip arthroplasty. *J Bone Joint Surg Am* 2003;85[Suppl 4]:33–38.
23. Woolson ST, Mow CS, Syquia JF, et al. Comparison of primary total hip replacements performed with a standard incision or a mini-incision. *J Bone Joint Surg Am* 2004;86-A(7):1353–1358.
24. AAOS, Committee on the Hip. Classification and management of femoral defects in total hip replacement [exhibit]. New Orleans 1990.
25. Bethea IJS, DeAndrade JR, Fleming LL, et al. Proximal femoral fractures following total hip arthroplasty. Clin Orthop Rel Res 1982;170:95–106.
26. Cooke PH, Newman JH. Fractures of the femur in relation to cemented hip prostheses. J Bone Joint Surg 1988;70B:386–389.
27. Johansson JE, McBroom R, Barrington TW, et al. Fracture of the ipsilateral femur in patients with total hip replacement. *J Bone Joint Surg Am* 1981;63(9):1435–1442.
28. Kavanagh BF. Femoral fractures associated with total hip arthroplasty. *Orthop Clin North Am* 1992;23(2):249–257.
29. Mallory TH, Kraus TJ, Vaughn BK. Intraoperative femoral fractures associated with cementless total hip arthroplasty. *Orthopaedics* 1989;12(2):231–239.
30. Mont MA, Maar DC. Fractures of the ipsilateral femur after hip arthroplasty: a statistical analysis of outcome based on 487 patients. *J Arthroplasty* 1994;9(5):511–519.
31. Schwartz JJ, Mayer JG, Engh CA. Femoral fracture during non-cemented total hip arthroplasty. *J Bone Joint Surg Am* 1989;71(8):1135–1142.
32. Serocki JH, Chandler RW, Dorr LD. Treatment of fractures about hip prostheses with compression plating. *J Arthroplasty* 1992;7(2):129–135.
33. Stuchin SA. Femoral shaft fracture in porous and press-fit total hip arthroplasty. *Orthop Rev* 1990;19(2):153–159.
34. Tower SS, Beals RK. Fractures of the femur after hip replacement: the Oregon experience. *Orthop Clin North Am* 1999;30(2):235–247.
35. Duncan CP, Masri BA. Fractures of the femur after hip replacement. In: Jackson D, ed. *Instructional Course Lectures 44*. Rosemont, IL: American Academy of Orthopaedic Surgeons, 1995:293–304.
36. Schmidt AH, Kyle RF. Periprosthetic fractures of the femur. *Orthop Clin North Am* 2002;33(1):143–152, ix.
37. Brady OH, Garbuz DS, Masri BA, et al. The reliability and validity of the Vancouver classification of femoral fractures after hip replacement. *J Arthroplasty* 2000;15(1): 59–62.
38. Garbuz DS, Masri BA, Esdaile J, et al. Classification systems in orthopaedics. *J Am Acad Orthop Surg* 2002;10(4):290–297.
39. Masri BA, Meek RM, Duncan CP. Periprosthetic fractures evaluation and treatment. *Clin Orthop* 2004;(420):80–95.
40. Springer BD, Berry DJ, Lewallen DG. Treatment of periprosthetic femoral fractures following total hip arthroplasty with femoral component revision. *J Bone Joint Surg Am* 2003;85-A(11):2156–2162.
41. Ko PS, Lam JJ, Tio MK, et al. Distal fixation with Wagner revision stem in treating Vancouver type B2 periprosthetic femur fractures in geriatric patients. *J Arthroplasty* 2003;18(4):446–452.
42. Barden B, von Knoch M, Fitzek JG, et al. Periprosthetic fractures with extensive bone loss treated with onlay strut allografts. *Int Orthop* 2003;27(3):164–167.
43. Tsiridis E, Haddad FS, Gie GA. Dall-Miles plates for periprosthetic femoral fractures. A critical review of 16 cases. *Injury* 2003;34(2):107–110.
44. Haddad FS, Duncan CP, Berry DJ, et al. Periprosthetic femoral fractures around well-fixed implants: use of cortical onlay allografts with or without a plate. *J Bone Joint Surg Am* 2002;84(6):945–950.
45. Barden B, Ding Y, Fitzek JG, et al. Strut allografts for failed treatment of periprosthetic femoral fractures: good outcome in 13 patients. *Acta Orthop Scand* 2003;74(2): 146–153.
46. Brady OH, Garbuz DS, Masri BA, et al. The treatment of periprosthetic fractures of the femur using cortical onlay allograft struts. *Orthop Clin North Am* 1999;30(2):249–257.
47. Chandler HP, King D, Limbird R, et al. The use of cortical allograft struts for fixation of fractures associated with well-fixed total joint prostheses. *Semin Arthroplasty* 1993; 4(2):99–107.
48. Chandler H, Tigges R. The role of allografts in the treatment of periprosthetic femoral fractures. *J Bone Joint Surg Am* 1997;79:1422–1432.
49. Haddad FS, Masri BA, Garbuz DS, et al. Femoral bone loss in total hip arthroplasty: classification and preoperative planning. *Instr Course Lect* 2000;49:83–96.
50. Cook SD, Barrack RL, Santman M, et al. The Otto Aufranc Award. Strut allograft healing to the femur with recombinant human osteogenic protein-1. *Clin Orthop* 2000;(381): 47–57.
51. Dennis MG, Simon JA, Kummer FJ, et al. Fixation of periprosthetic femoral shaft fractures: a biomechanical comparison of two techniques. *J Orthop Trauma* 2001;15(3): 177–180.
52. Dennis MG, Simon JA, Kummer FJ, et al. Fixation of periprosthetic femoral shaft fractures occurring at the tip of the stem: a biomechanical study of 5 techniques. *J Arthroplasty* 2000;15(4):523–528.
53. Krettek C, Schandelmaier P, Miclau T, et al. Minimally invasive percutaneous plate osteosynthesis (MIPPO) using the DCS in proximal and distal femoral fractures. *Injury* 1997;28[Suppl 1]:A20–A30.
54. Wenda K, Runkel M, Degreif J, et al. Minimally invasive plate fixation in femoral shaft fractures. *Injury* 1997;28[Suppl 1]:A13–A19.
55. Farouk O, Krettek C, Miclau T, et al. Minimally invasive plate osteosynthesis and vascularity: preliminary results of a cadaver injection study. *Injury* 1997;28[Suppl 1]: A7–A12.
56. Abhaykumar S, Elliott DS. Percutaneous plate fixation for periprosthetic femoral fractures—a preliminary report. *Injury* 2000 Oct;31(8):627–630.
57. Kligman M, Otramsky I, Roffman M. Conservative versus surgical treatment for femoral fracture after total or hemiarthroplasty of hip. *Arch Orthop Trauma Surg* 1999;119(1–2): 79–81.
58. Noorda RJ, Wuisman PI. Mennen plate fixation for the treatment of periprosthetic femoral fractures: a multicenter study of thirty-six fractures. *J Bone Joint Surg Am* 2002; 84(12):2211–2215.
59. Ahuja S, Chatterji S. The Mennen femoral plate for fixation of periprosthetic femoral fractures following hip arthroplasty. *Injury* 2002;33(1):47–50.
60. Radcliffe SN, Smith DN. The Mennen plate in periprosthetic hip fractures. *Injury* 1996; 27(1):27–30.
61. Haddad FS, Marston RA, Muirhead-Allwood SK. The Dall-Miles cable and plate system for periprosthetic femoral fractures. *Injury* 1997;28(7):445–447.
62. Shah NH, McCabe JP. Dall Miles cable and plate system for periprosthetic femoral fracture. *Eur J Orthop Surg Traumatol* 2002;12:137–139.
63. Venu KM, Koka R, Garikipati R, et al. Dall-Miles cable and plate fixation for the treatment of peri-prosthetic femoral fractures-analysis of results in 13 cases. *Injury* 2001; 32(5):395–400.
64. Larson JE, Chao EYS, Fitzgerald RH Jr, et al. Bypassing femoral cortical defects with cemented intramedullary stems. *J Orthop Res* 1991;9:414.
65. Mabrey JD, Foote J, Kose N, et al. Smooth uncemented femoral stems do not provide torsional stability of femurs with cortical defects. *Orthop Trans* 1998;22(1):236–237.
66. Bohm P, Bischel O. Femoral revision with the Wagner SL revision stem: evaluation of one hundred and twenty-nine revisions followed for a mean of 4.8 years. *J Bone Joint Surg Am* 2001;83(7):1023–1031.
67. Warren PJ, Thompson P, Fletcher MD. Transfemoral implantation of the Wagner SL stem. The abolition of subsidence and enhancement of osteotomy union rate using Dall-Miles cables. *Arch Orthop Trauma Surg* 2002;122(9–10):557–560.
68. Kwong LM, Miller AJ, Lubinus P. A modular distal fixation option for proximal bone loss in revision total hip arthroplasty: a 2- to 6-year follow-up study. *J Arthroplasty* 2003;18[3 Suppl 1]:94–97.
69. Rigby M, Bishay M, Chojnowski A, et al. Experience of the Kent hip prosthesis. *Injury* 1998;29(2):166.
70. Stossel CA, Haddad FS, Sexton SA. Cumulative survival of the Kent hip prosthesis—a distally locked femoral stem. Annual Proceedings; 2004 Mar 10; Rosemont, IL: American Academy of Orthopaedic Surgeons; 2004.
71. Probst A, Schneider T, Hankemeier S, et al. Der Prothesennagel - primär belastungsstabiles Implantat bei peri- und subprothetischen Frakturen des Femurs. *Unfallchirurg* 2003;106(9):722–731.
72. Eingartner C, Volkmann R, Putz M, et al. Uncemented revision stem for biological osteosynthesis in periprosthetic femoral fractures. *Int Orthop* 1997;21(1):25–29.
73. Lewallen DG, Berry DJ. Periprosthetic fracture of the femur—editorial response. *J Bone Joint Surg Am* 2000;82(3):446–447.
74. Macdonald SJ, Paprosky WG, Jablonsky WS, et al. Periprosthetic femoral fractures treated with a long-stem cementless component. *J Arthroplasty* 2001;16(3):379–383.
75. Wong P, Gross AE. The use of structural allografts for treating periprosthetic fractures about the hip and knee. *Orthop Clin North Am* 1999;30(2):259–264.

76. van Biezen FC, ten Have BL, Verhaar JA. Impaction bone-grafting of severely defective femora in revision total hip surgery: 21 hips followed for 41–85 months. *Acta Orthop Scand* 2000;71(2):135–142.
77. McElfresh EC, Coventry MB. Femoral and pelvic fractures after total hip arthroplasty. *J Bone Joint Surg* 1974;56(3):483–492.
78. Sharkey PF, Hozack WJ, Callaghan JJ, et al. Acetabular fracture associated with cementless acetabular component insertion: a report of 13 cases. *J Arthroplasty* 1999; 14(4):426–431.
79. Peterson CA, Lewallen DG. Periprosthetic fracture of the acetabulum after total hip arthroplasty. *J Bone Joint Surg Am* 1996;78(8):1206–1213.
80. Berry DJ, Lewallen DG, Hanssen AD, et al. Pelvic discontinuity in revision total hip arthroplasty. *J Bone Joint Surg Am* 1999;81(12):1692–1702.
81. Kim YS, Callaghan JJ, Ahn PB, et al. Fracture of the acetabulum during insertion of an oversized hemispherical component. *J Bone Joint Surg Am* 1995;77(1):111–117.
82. Eggli S, Muller C, Ganz R. Revision surgery in pelvic discontinuity: an analysis of seven patients. *Clin Orthop* 2002;398:136–145.
83. Berry DJ. Management of periprosthetic fractures: the hip. *J Arthroplasty* 2002;17[4 Suppl 1]:11–13.
84. Callaghan JJ. Periprosthetic fractures of the acetabulum during and following total hip arthroplasty. *Instr Course Lect* 1998;47:231–235.
85. Mitchell PA, Greidanus NV, Masri BA, et al. The prevention of periprosthetic fractures of the femur during and after total hip arthroplasty. *Instr Course Lect* 2003;52:301–308.
86. Aribindi R, Paprosky W, Nourbash P, et al. Extended proximal femoral osteotomy. *Instr Course Lect* 1999;48:19–26.
87. Scott RD, Turner RH, Leitzes SM, et al. Femoral fractures in conjunction with total hip replacement. *J Bone Joint Surg Am* 1975;57(4):494–501.
88. Crowe JF, Mani VJ, Ranawat CS. Total hip replacement in congenital dislocation and dysplasia of the hip. *J Bone Joint Surg Am* 1979;61(1):15–23.
89. Haddad FS, Masri BA, Garbuz DS, et al. Primary total replacement of the dysplastic hip. *Instr Course Lect* 2000;49:23–39.
90. Yamaguchi K, Masuhara K, Yamasaki S, et al. Cyclic therapy with etidronate has a therapeutic effect against local osteoporosis after cementless total hip arthroplasty. *Bone* 2003;33(1):144–149.
91. Berry DJ. Total hip arthroplasty in patients with proximal femoral deformity. *Clin Orthop* 1999;369:262–272.
92. Mehlhoff T, Landon GC, Tullos HS. Total hip arthroplasty following failed internal fixation of hip fractures. *Clin Orthop* 1991;(269):32–37.
93. Skeide BI, Lie SA, Havelin LI, et al. Total hip arthroplasty after femoral neck fractures. Results from the national registry on joint prostheses. *Tidsskr Nor Laegeforen* 1996; 116(12):1449–1451.
94. McKinley JC, Robinson CM. Treatment of displaced intracapsular hip fractures with total hip arthroplasty: comparison of primary arthroplasty with early salvage arthroplasty after failed internal fixation. *J Bone Joint Surg Am* 2002;84(11):2010–2015.
95. Padman M, Shaw DL. Primary compared with salvage arthroplasty for displaced intracapsular hip fractures. *J Bone Joint Surg Am* 2004;86(2):431.
96. Mishra V, Thomas G, Sibly TF. Results of displaced subcapital fractures treated by primary total hip replacement. *Injury* 2004;35(2):157–160.
97. Parker MJ, Gurusamy K. Arthroplasties (with and without bone cement) for proximal femoral fractures in adults. *Cochrane Database Syst Rev* 2004;(2):CD001706.
98. Rodriguez-Merchan EC. Displaced intracapsular hip fractures: hemiarthroplasty or total arthroplasty? *Clin Orthop* 2002;(399):72–77.
99. Lee BP, Berry DJ, Harmsen WS, et al. Total hip arthroplasty for the treatment of an acute fracture of the femoral neck: long-term results. *J Bone Joint Surg Am* 1998;80(1): 70–75.
100. Weeden SH, Paprosky WG, Bowling JW. The early dislocation rate in primary total hip arthroplasty following the posterior approach with posterior soft-tissue repair. *J Arthroplasty* 2003;18(6):709–713.
101. Jimenez ML, Tile M, Schenk RS. Total hip replacement after acetabular fracture. *Orthop Clin North Am* 1997;28(3):435–446.
102. Weber M, Berry DJ, Harmsen WS. Total hip arthroplasty after operative treatment of an acetabular fracture. *J Bone Joint Surg Am* 1998;80(9):1295–1305.
103. Berry DJ, Halasy M. Uncemented acetabular components for arthritis after acetabular fracture. *Clin Orthop* 2002;(405):164–167.
104. Mears DC, Velyvis JH. Acute total hip arthroplasty for selected displaced acetabular fractures: two to twelve-year results. *J Bone Joint Surg Am* 2002;84-A(1):1–9.
105. Mears DC, Shirahama M. Stabilization of an acetabular fracture with cables for acute total hip arthroplasty. *J Arthroplasty* 1998;13(1):104–107.
106. Mouhsine E, Garofalo R, Borens O, et al. Cable fixation and early total hip arthroplasty in the treatment of acetabular fractures in elderly patients. *J Arthroplasty* 2004;19(3): 344–348.
107. Hartford JM, Goodman SB. The use of femoral intramedullary nailing as an interim or salvage technique during complicated total hip replacement. *J Arthroplasty* 1998;13(4): 467–472.
108. Schwab JH, Pagnano M, Haidukewych GJ, et al. A technique for treating periprosthetic fractures of the femur associated with deep prosthetic infection. *J Arthroplasty* 2003; 18(2):211–215.
109. Younger AS, Duncan CP, Masri BA. Treatment of infection associated with segmental bone loss in the proximal part of the femur in two stages with use of an antibiotic-loaded interval prosthesis. *J Bone Joint Surg Am* 1998;80(1):60–69.
110. Sharkey PF, Hozack WJ, Rothman RH, et al. Insall Award paper. Why are total knee arthroplasties failing today? *Clin Orthop* 2002;(404):7–13.
111. Aaron RK, Scott RS. Supracondylar fracture of the femur after total knee arthroplasty. *Clin Orthop Rel Res* 1987;219:136–139.
112. Cain PR, Rubash HE, Wissinger HA, et al. Periprosthetic femoral fractures following total knee arthroplasty. *Clin Orthop* 1986;(208):205–214.
113. Culp RW, Schmidt RG, Hanks G, et al. Supracondylar fracture of the femur following prosthetic knee arthroplasty. *Clin Orthop* 1987;222:212–222.
114. Merkel KD, Johnson EW. Supracondylar fracture of the femur after total knee arthroplasty. *J Bone Joint Surg* 1986;68A(1):29–43.
115. Bogoch E, Hastings D, Gross A, et al. Supracondylar fractures of the femur adjacent to resurfacing and macintosh arthroplasties of the knee in patients with rheumatoid arthritis. *Clin Orthop Rel Res* 1988;229:213–220.
116. Hirsh DM, Bhalla S, Roffman M. Supracondylar fracture of the femur following total knee replacement. Report of four cases. *J Bone Joint Surg Am* 1981;63(1):162–163.
117. Petersen MM, Lauritzen JB, Pedersen JG, et al. Decreased bone density of the distal femur after uncemented knee arthroplasty. A 1-year follow-up of 29 knees. *Acta Orthop Scand* 1996;67(4):339–344.
118. Petersen MM, Olsen C, Lauritzen JB, et al. Changes in bone mineral density of the distal femur following uncemented total knee arthroplasty. *J Arthroplasty* 1995;10(1): 7–11.
119. Petersen MM, Nielsen PT, Lauritzen JB, et al. Changes in bone mineral density of the proximal tibia after uncemented total knee arthroplasty. A 3-year follow-up of 25 knees. *Acta Orthop Scand* 1995;66(6):513–516.
120. Wang CJ, Wang JW, Weng LH, et al. The effect of alendronate on bone mineral density in the distal part of the femur and proximal part of the tibia after total knee arthroplasty. *J Bone Joint Surg Am* 2003;85(11):2121–2126.
121. Engh GA, Ammeen DJ. Periprosthetic fractures adjacent to total knee implants: treatment and clinical results. *Instr Course Lect* 1998;47:437–448.
122. Cameron H. Femoral neck stress fracture after total knee replacement: A case report. *Am J Knee Surg* 1992;5:41–43.
123. Cracchiolo A. Stress fractures of the pelvis as a cause of hip pain following total hip and knee arthroplasty. *Arthritis Rheum* 1981;24(5):740–742.
124. Hardy DC, Delince PE, Yasik E, et al. Stress fracture of the hip. An unusual complication of total knee arthroplasty. *Clin Orthop* 1992;281:140–144.
125. Kumm DA, Rack C, Rutt J. Subtrochanteric stress fracture of the femur following total knee arthroplasty. *J Arthroplasty* 1997;12(5):580–583.
126. Lesniewski PJ, Testa NN. Stress fracture of the hip as a complication of total knee replacement. Case report. *J Bone Joint Surg Am* 1982;64(2):304–306.
127. Palance Martin D, Albareda J, Seral F. Subcapital stress fracture of the femoral neck after total knee arthroplasty. *Int Orthop* 1994;18:308–309.
128. Rawes ML, Patsalis T, Gregg PJ. Subcapital stress fractures of the hip complicating total knee replacement. *Injury* 1995;26(6):421–423.
129. Giori NJ, Lewallen DG. Total knee arthroplasty in limbs affected by poliomyelitis. *J Bone Joint Surg Am* 2002;84-A(7):1157–1161.
130. Peters CL, Hennessey R, Barden RM, et al. Revision total knee arthroplasty with a cemented posterior-stabilized or constrained condylar prosthesis: a minimum 3-year and average 5-year follow-up study. *J Arthroplasty* 1997;12(8):896–903.
131. Fehring TK, Odum S, Griffin WL, et al. Early failures in total knee arthroplasty. *Clin Orthop* 2001;(392):315–318.
132. Ritter MA, Carr K, Keating EM, et al. Tibial shaft fracture following tibial tubercle osteotomy. *J Arthroplasty 1996*;11(1):117–119.
133. Lesh ML, Schneider DJ, Deol G, et al. The consequences of anterior femoral notching in total knee arthroplasty. A biomechanical study. *J Bone Joint Surg Am* 2000;82(8): 1096–1101.
134. Shawen SB, Belmont PJ Jr, Klemme WR, et al. Osteoporosis and anterior femoral notching in periprosthetic supracondylar femoral fractures: a biomechanical analysis. *J Bone Joint Surg* Am 2003;85(1):115–121.
135. Thompson NW, McAlinden MG, Breslin E, et al. Periprosthetic tibial fractures after cementless low contact stress total knee arthroplasty. *J Arthroplasty* 2001;16(8): 984–990.
136. Rorabeck CH, Taylor JW. Periprosthetic fractures of the femur complicating total knee arthroplasty. *Orthop Clin North Am* 1999;30(2):265–277.
137. Clarke HD, Math KR, Scuderi GR. Polyethylene post failure in posterior stabilized total knee arthroplasty. *J Arthroplasty* 2004;19(5):652–657.
138. Lewis PL, Rorabeck CH. Periprosthetic fractures. In: Engh GA, Rorabeck CH, eds. *Revision total knee arthroplasty*. Baltimore: Williams & Wilkins, 1997:275–295.
139. Rorabeck CH, Taylor JW. Classification of periprosthetic fractures complicating total knee arthroplasty. *Orthop Clin North Am* 1999;30(2):209–214.
140. Felix NA, Stuart MJ, Hanssen AD. Periprosthetic fractures of the tibia associated with total knee arthroplasty. *Clin Orthop* 1997;345:113–124.
141. Stuart MJ, Hanssen AD. Total knee arthroplasty: periprosthetic tibial fractures. *Orthop Clin North Am* 1999;30(2):279–286.
142. Goldberg VM, Figgie HE, Inglis AE, et al. Patellar fracture type and prognosis in condylar total knee arthroplasty. *Clin Orthop* 1988;236:115–122.
143. Ortiguera CJ, Berry DJ. Patellar fracture after total knee arthroplasty. *J Bone Joint Surg Am* 2002;84(4):532–540.
144. Althausen PL, Lee MA, Finkemeier CG, et al. Operative stabilization of supracondylar femur fractures above total knee arthroplasty: a comparison of four treatment methods. *J Arthroplasty* 2003;18(7):834–839.
145. Falck M, Hontzsch T, Weise K. LISS (less invasive stabilization system) als minimal invasive Alternative bei distalen Femurfrakturen. *Trauma Berufskrankh* 1999;1: 402–406.
146. Schutz M, Muller M, Krettek C, et al. Minimally invasive fracture stabilization of distal femoral fractures with the LISS: a prospective multicenter study. Results of a clinical study with special emphasis on difficult cases. *Injury* 2001;32[Suppl 3]:SC48–SC54.
147. Bong MR, Egol KA, Koval KJ, et al. Comparison of the LISS and a retrograde-inserted supracondylar intramedullary nail for fixation of a periprosthetic distal femur fracture proximal to a total knee arthroplasty. *J Arthroplasty* 2002;17(7):876–881.

148. O'Toole RV, Chandler A, Hwang R, et al. *Use of the LISS to treat periprosthetic femur fractures below hip or above knee arthroplasty or both.* Rosemont, IL: Orthopaedic Trauma Association, 2004:239–240.
149. Ricci WM, Loftus T, Cox C, et al. *Locked plates combined with minimally invasive insertion technique is the treatment of choice for periprosthetic supracondylar femur fractures above a total knee arthroplasty.* Rosemont, IL: Orthopaedic Trauma Association, 2004:241–242.
150. Ayers DC, Dennis DA, Johanson NA, et al. Common complications of total knee arthroplasty. *J Bone Joint Surg Am* 1997;79(2):278–311.
151. Healy WL, Siliski JM, Incavo SJ. Operative treatment of distal femoral fractures proximal to total knee replacements. *J Bone Joint Surg Am* 1993;75(1):27–34.
152. Zehntner MK, Ganz R. Internal fixation of supracondylar fractures after condylar total knee arthroplasty. *Clin Orthop* 1993;293:219–224.
153. Fitzek JG, Wessinghage D. [Intramedullary nailing of peri-prosthetic fractures following total knee joint replacement]. *Aktuelle Traumatol* 1990;20(5):248–253.
154. Murrell GA, Nunley JA. Interlocked supracondylar intramedullary nails for supracondylar fractures after total knee arthroplasty. A new treatment method. *J Arthroplasty* 1995;10(1):37–42.
155. Smith WJ, Martin SL, Mabrey JD. Use of a supracondylar nail for treatment of a supracondylar fracture of the femur following total knee arthroplasty. *J Arthroplasty* 1996; 11(2):210–213.
156. Su ET, DeWal H, Di Cesare PE. Periprosthetic femoral fractures above total knee replacements. *J Am Acad Orthop Surg* 2004;12(1):12–20.
157. Wick M, Muller EJ, Kutscha-Lissberg F, et al. [Periprosthetic supracondylar femoral fractures: LISS or retrograde intramedullary nailing? Problems with the use of minimally invasive technique]. *Unfallchirurg* 2004;107(3):181–188.
158. Kassab M, Zalzal P, Azores GM, et al. Management of periprosthetic femoral fractures after total knee arthroplasty using a distal femoral allograft. *J Arthroplasty* 2004;19(3): 361–368.
159. Springer BD, Hanssen AD, Sim FH, et al. The kinematic rotating hinge prosthesis for complex knee arthroplasty. *Clin Orthop* 2001;(392):283–291.
160. Sierra RJ, Trousdale RT, Pagnano MW. Above-the-knee amputation after a total knee replacement: prevalence, etiology, and functional outcome. *J Bone Joint Surg Am* 2003; 85-A(6):1000–1004.
161. Weiss NG, Parvizi J, Trousdale RT, et al. Total knee arthroplasty in patients with a prior fracture of the tibial plateau. *J Bone Joint Surg Am* 2003;85-A(2):218–221.
162. Saleh KJ, Sherman P, Katkin P, et al. Total knee arthroplasty after open reduction and internal fixation of fractures of the tibial plateau: a minimum five-year follow-up study. *J Bone Joint Surg Am* 2001;83(8):1144–1148.
163. Nelson CL, Saleh KJ, Kassim RA, et al. Total knee arthroplasty after varus osteotomy of the distal part of the femur. *J Bone Joint Surg Am* 2003;85(6):1062–1065.

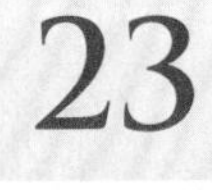

COMPUTER-AIDED ORTHOPAEDIC SURGERY IN SKELETAL TRAUMA

Meir Liebergall, Rami Mosheiff, and Leo Joskowicz

Computers are becoming pervasive in all fields of human endeavor, and medicine is no exception. Starting with the advent of computed tomography (CT) in the 1970s, computer-based systems have become the standard of care in many clinical fields, most notably in radiology, radiation therapy, neurosurgery, and orthopaedics. These systems assist the surgeon in planning, executing, and evaluating the surgery, often improving existing procedures and at times enabling new procedures that could not have been realized without them.

The first computer-based systems for surgery were developed in the mid 1980s for neurosurgery. The key characteristic of these systems is an *integration of preoperative information with intraoperative execution*. Traditionally, preoperative film x-ray, CT, and magnetic resonance imaging (MRI) showing the patient's condition and the planned approach are brought into the operating room to guide the surgeon. However, when performing surgical actions, it is not possible to determine exactly where the surgical tools and implants are with respect to these images, especially when direct line-of-sight is limited, such as in keyhole, minimally invasive, and percutaneous surgery. Often, intraoperative images, such as fluoroscopic x-rays, are acquired to monitor the location of tools, implants, and anatomy. The surgeon must then mentally recreate the spatio-temporal situation from these images and decide on a course of action. This integration is qualitative and imprecise, as is the surgeon's hand-eye coordination, requiring significant skills, experience, and judgment, which varies from surgeon to surgeon.

Computer-assisted surgery (CAS) systems perform this integration automatically and accurately, thereby providing the surgeon with a precise, more complete, and up-to-date view of the intraoperative situation (1). By incorporating real-time tracking of the location of instruments and anatomy, and their precise relation to preoperative and intraoperative images, the systems create a new modality akin to continuous imaging. In this sense,

CAS systems are like navigators based on Global Position Systems (GPS) found in cars that help drivers find their way to a desired destination. While driving, the system shows the exact location of the car at all times on a computerized map and provides turn-by-turn directions ahead of time.

In orthopaedics, the first commercial CT-based navigation systems were introduced in the mid 1990s for spinal surgery (2). Several years later, fluoroscopic x-ray based systems were developed for total hip and total knee replacement (3). Today, a variety of image-free and image-based systems exist for planning and executing a variety of orthopaedic procedures, including primary and revision total hip and total knee replacement, ACL reconstruction, spinal pedicle screw insertion, and trauma (3–6).

Computer-assisted surgery has already become an integral part of the orthopaedic trauma surgery setup. The rapid development in the use of computers in this field provides many feasible options at all stages of treatment of the orthopaedic trauma patient, from preoperative planning to postoperative evaluation. The role of computerization in the treatment of trauma patients is not only to improve the possibilities in the preplanning stage but also to shorten it, an advantage that could be crucial for patients' morbidity in a trauma setup. Although computerized imaging equipment can be moved into the admitting area and/or the trauma unit of the emergency room, this may involve adaptation of an existing setup, requiring administrative changes and incurring high costs. Another option is the use of comprehensive imaging provided by the improvement of conventional image intensifiers in achieving accurate three-dimensional (3D) information in a minimal period of time inside the operating room. The ISO-C 3D is the first harbinger of this tendency.

Recently, computerized navigation has made a breakthrough in expanding the use of computerized aided surgery from the preplanning to the intraoperative stage. This integrates well with the current tendency toward minimal invasive surgery. CAS technology brings important digitized information into the operating room, enabling the accomplishment of two main goals: minimal invasive surgery and maximal accuracy. Moreover, both surgeon and patient enjoy a significant reduction in the amount of radiation exposure usually associated with orthopaedic trauma surgery. The main modality, which is currently in various stages of application and has been adapted to trauma surgery, is fluoroscopy-based navigation. Although this technology might be viewed by some as only improved fluoroscopy, it is undoubtedly this feature that has allowed computer-based navigation systems to become a pioneer in the process of CAS integration in the orthopaedic trauma operating room.

TECHNICAL ELEMENTS

Computer-Assisted Orthopaedic Surgery in Skeletal Trauma (CAOS-ST) systems consist of preoperative planning (when available and feasible) and intraoperative navigation. We next describe the technical principles of each and the existing types of navigation systems.

Computerized Preoperative Planning and Model Construction

Preoperative planning for skeletal trauma surgery is usually accomplished using film x-rays and film CT. The drawbacks of this current practice are that anatomical measurements are either approximate or cannot be obtained; fixation plates and implant templates are usually not available; their size, position, and orientation can only be approximately determined; and spatial views are unavailable. Consequently, only a few alternatives can be explored.

Digital x-ray and CT data open the door for better planning. Digital x-ray images can be correlated and anatomical measurements, such as anteversion angle and leg length can be performed on them. Digital templates of fixation and implant devices can be superimposed on the x-ray images to explore a variety of alternatives.

For CT data, preoperative planning allows for 3D measurements and spatial visualization of complex structures and fractures. It allows the construction of computer *models*, such as bone *surface mesh*, anatomical axes, and osteotomy planes. Bone fragment models and implants can be visualized in 3D and manipulated to analyze "what-if" scenarios. Figure 23-1 illustrates these concepts in the preoperative planning of distal radial malunion correction (7,8).

Principles of Navigation and Guidance

The goal of *navigation* is to provide precise, real-time visual feedback of the spatial location of surgical instruments and anatomical structures that cannot be directly observed. In current practice, this information is obtained by repeated use of x-ray fluoroscopy, which produces a time frozen two-dimensional view, is not updated in real time, and results in cumulative radiation to the surgeon, staff, and patient. The goal of *guidance* is to indicate to the surgeon in real time, via images, graphics, or sound, the best course of action during surgery.

Navigation systems show the current location of surgical instruments with respect to images of the anatomy, either a preoperative CT or intraoperative fluoroscopic x-ray images, and continuously update the image as the instruments and bone structures move. The resulting display, called *navigation images*, is equivalent to continuous intraoperative imaging without radiation.

Navigation requires *tracking*, *registration*, *visualization*, and *validation*. Tracking determines in real time the location of moving objects in space. Registration establishes a common reference frame between the moving objects and the images. Visualization creates navigation images showing the location of moving objects with respect to the anatomy. Validation ensures

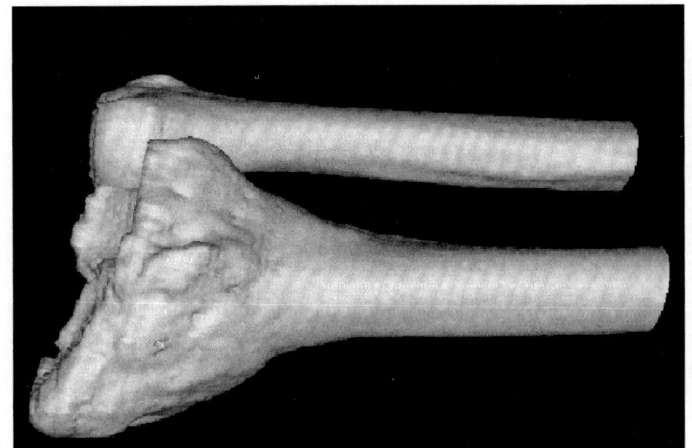

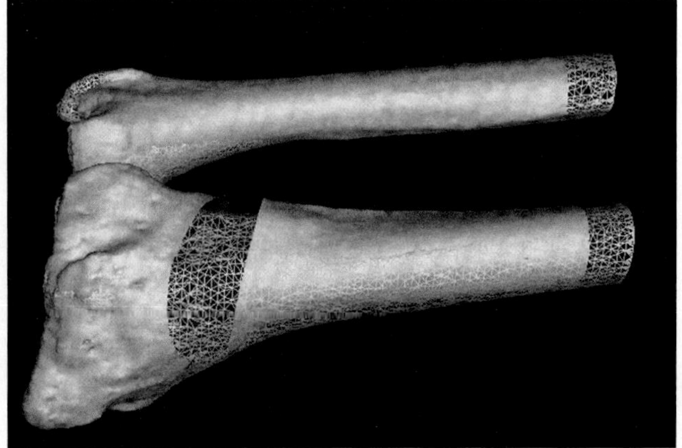

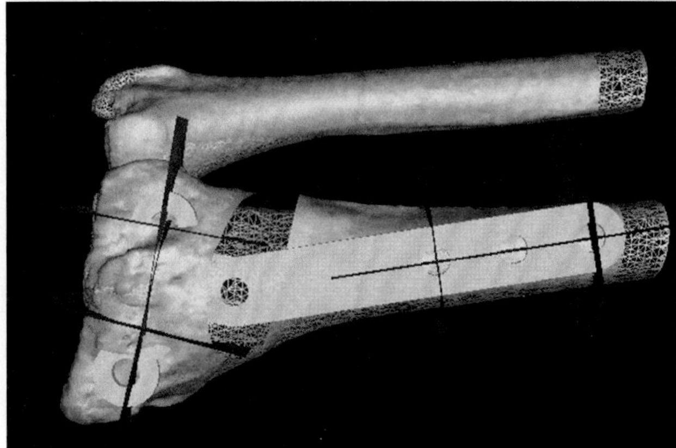

FIGURE 23-1 Preoperative planning for distal radius malunion correction. **A.** Three-dimensional view of the malunion reconstructed from the original CT. **B.** Mirror model of the healthy contralateral distal radius (superimposed green mesh) and the planned osteotomy. **C.** Fixation plate and guide planes in their desired location. (Images courtesy of Prof. R. Ellis).

that the updated images match the clinical intraoperative situation.

The key advantage of navigation is that it obviates the need for repeated x-ray fluoroscopy. However, it requires additional procedures, including setting up the navigation system and attaching trackers to both instruments and bone structures of interest, and additional surgeon training.

System Components and Mode of Operation

A navigation system consists of a computer unit, a tracking unit, and tracker mounting hardware. Figure 23-2 shows the equipment setup in the operating room. A rolling cart usually holds the computer unit and the *tracking base unit*. The cart is placed next to the patient, so that the surgeon conveniently sees the display. Tracking requires a *position sensor* and one or more *trackers*. The position sensor determines the spatial location of the trackers at any moment in time. By attaching trackers to surgical tools and bone structures, their relative spatial position can continuously be followed and updated in the computer display. Trackers are rigidly mounted on tools and bones with *tracker mounting jigs*, which are mechanical jigs similar to screws and clamps. Since the trackers and their mounting jigs come in contact with the patient, they must be sterilized. The position sensor is either mounted on the cart, is part of a separate unit, or is attached to the ceiling or to a wall. It is aimed at the surgical field so that the expected tracker motions are within its working area throughout surgery. The position sensor location can be changed during surgery as needed. When fluoroscopic x-ray images are used for navigation, the computer unit is also connected to a C-arm and imports images acquired with it. The C-arm is usually fitted with its own tracker to determine its relative location with respect to the tracked objects and imaged anatomy.

The tracking base unit receives and integrates the signals from the position sensor and the trackers. The computer integrates the signals from the base unit with fluoroscopic x-ray or CT images and instrument models (registration), and creates one or more views for display (visualization). The navigated images are updated in real time by the computer as the instruments and anatomy move. The *tool calibration unit* is used to obtain the geometric data of surgical tools fitted with trackers, e.g., the tool tip's offset. This geometric data is used to create the instrument model for display.

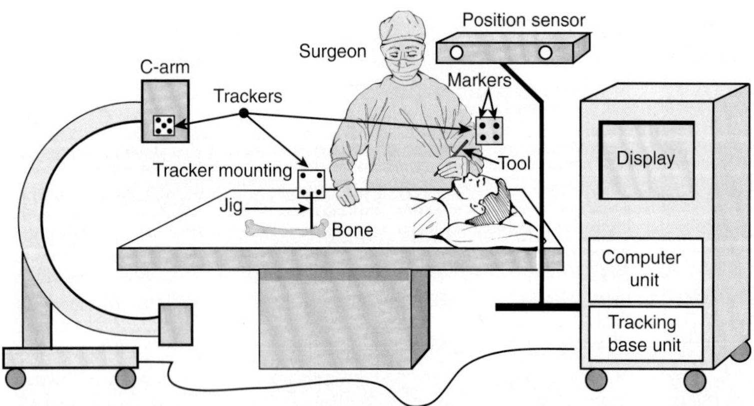

FIGURE 23-2 Equipment setup in the operating room. A navigation system consists of a computer unit, a tracker unit, and tracker mounting hardware. The computer unit consists of a computer, a keyboard and a mouse, and a display monitor or a touch screen. The tracking unit consists of a tracking base unit, a position sensor, one or more trackers, and a tool calibration unit (optional).

Tracking

A tracking system obtains the position and orientation of trackers by measuring spatially dependent physical properties, which can be optical, magnetic, acoustic, or mechanical. Currently, two types of tracking technologies are available for medical applications: optical and magnetic, with optical being by far the most commonly used (Fig. 23-3).

Optical Tracking. In optical tracking, the position sensor consists of two or more *optical cameras* that detect light emitted or reflected by *markers*. Each camera measures the distance of the markers from it. Since the base distance between the optical cameras is known, the position of the marker with respect to the camera's base line can be computed by a method known as triangulation. A *tracker* consists of three or more markers mounted on a rigid base (Fig. 23-3A). The tracker's position and orientation is determined by the markers' positions relative to each other and by their sensed position with respect to the position sensor. A key requirement is the maintenance of an unobstructed *line of sight* between the position sensor and the trackers.

Optical tracking systems can be *active*, *passive*, or *hybrid*. *Active tracking* uses active markers, which are light-emitting diodes (LEDs) that are "strobed" (turned on and off) in tandem by the base unit. LEDs emit infrared light that is detected by the cameras. The cameras capture is synchronized with the LED strobing so that the identity of the lighting marker is known. Active trackers consist of three of more wired LEDs mounted on a rigid base and connected by a cable or by a wireless link (tetherless communication) to the tracking base unit. Each active tracker has a unique identifier. Active trackers are built so that they can be sterilized many times.

Passive Tracking. Passive tracking uses passive markers, which can be reflective spheres or printed patterns (Fig. 23-3B). Reflective spheres reflect the infrared light generated by the position sensor, which is then detected by the cameras. Unlike the active markers, passive markers are not controlled by the tracking base unit and are "seen" simultaneously by the cameras. Passive trackers consist of three or more passive markers. The identity of the passive tracker is determined by the configuration of the markers on the rigid mounting base. Consequently, no two passive trackers can have the same marker configuration. The tracking base unit must know the tracker configuration. Because the markers lose their reflectance with sterilization and touch, they must be replaced after a few uses.

Hybrid Tracking. Hybrid tracking incorporates both active and passive tracking. Hybrid tracking systems track both passive and active trackers simultaneously, thus providing the advantages of both technologies. Table 23-1 summarizes the advantages and disadvantages of active (wired and tetherless) and passive trackers. Neither technology is always superior to the other in all categories. Therefore, the anatomy, the surgical instruments, and the clinical situation determine the choice of trackers.

In terms of physical characteristics, tracker sizes are comparable. Passive trackers are lightest, while tetherless active trackers are heaviest because of the battery required to activate the circuitry and the LEDs. Passive trackers are more rugged than active ones because they have no electronics. Tetherless trackers are more convenient because there are no cables in the way. In terms of functionality, active trackers have an advantage in that they indicate on the tracker itself (via a light indicator) when the line-of-sight is maintained; passive tracker obstruction can only be shown on the display. Active trackers are automatically recognized as soon as they are plugged in. Passive trackers are the most reliable, because there are no electric connections; tetherless active trackers are the least reliable because of possible communication interferences and their short battery life (LEDs require substantial power to illuminate them). In terms of performance, active trackers are somewhat more accurate than pas-

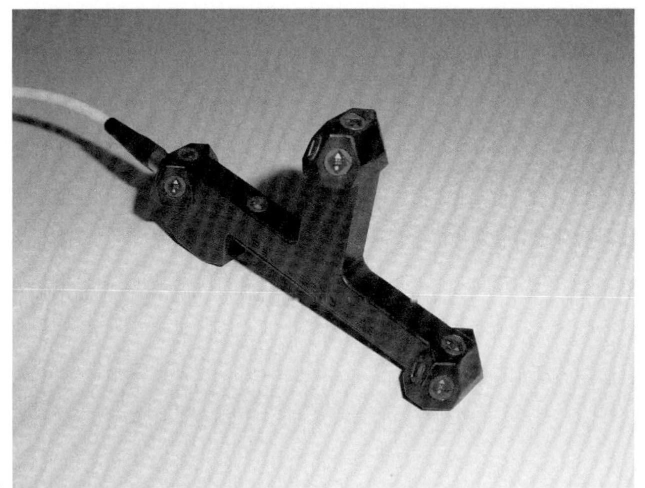

A

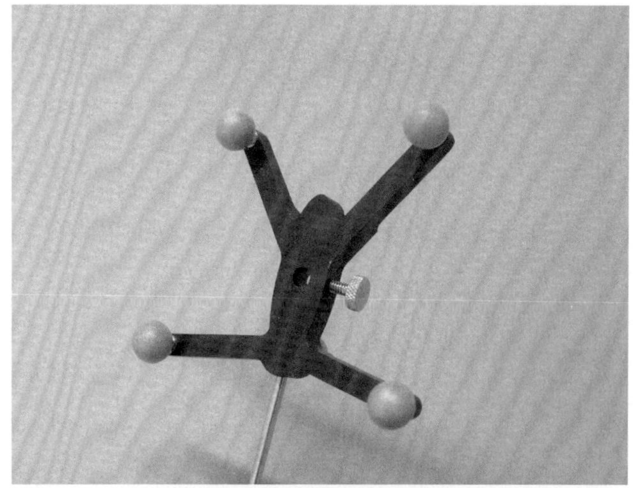

B

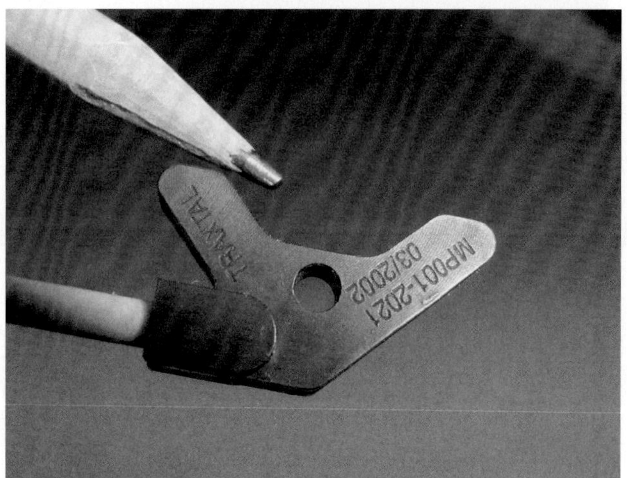

C

FIGURE 23-3 Trackers. **A.** Active optical tracker. **B.** Passive optical tracker. **C.** Magnetic trackers. (Courtesy of Traxtal Technogies, Toronto, Canada).

sive trackers but they are also more sensitive to their orientation with respect to the cameras. In terms of cost, it is highest for active tetherless tracking due to the additional electronics, and lowest for passive trackers, which have no electronics at all. The running cost of active wired tracking is the lowest, because there are no batteries or reflective spheres to replace. The amortized cost over time of the wired active trackers is best.

Magnetic Tracking. Magnetic tracking works by measuring variations of generated magnetic fields. The position sensor consists of a magnet that generates a uniform magnetic field and a sensor that measures its phase and intensity variations. Trackers consist of one or more miniature coils mounted on a rigid base that generate a local magnetic field from an electric current, which can be alternating or pulsed direct (Fig. 23-3C). Both the position sensor and the trackers are connected to the tracking base unit. The tracker magnetic field modifies the sensor's magnetic field characteristics according to its position in space. The location of the tracker is computed from the relative variations of the sensor's intensity and its phase magnetic field. A key requirement is the maintenance of a uniform magnetic field, which is altered by the proximity of magnetic fields from other electric devices and by nearby ferromagnetic objects.

Magnetic trackers are usually much smaller, lighter, and cheaper than optical trackers and their functionality is similar to that of active optical trackers (Table 23-1). However, the accuracy of existing magnetic tracking systems is less than that of optical tracking systems. Their main advantages are that they are small and do not require a direct line-of-sight, and therefore they are useful in percutaneous procedures. However, they require careful control of the environment in which they operate, because the nearby presence of ferrous objects and electrical instruments in the operating room influence their measurements.

Tracking Technical Issues

The best way to think about a tracking system is as a 3D measurement instrument, also called a coordinate measuring machine. A 3D measurement instrument provides a stream of spatial location measurements in a given range, accuracy, and rate

TABLE 23-1 Comparison of Tracking Technologies

	Optical			
Characteristic	Active Wired	Active Tetherless	Passive	Magnetic
Physical				
Size	0	0	0	+
Weight	0	–	+	+
Ruggedness	0	–	+	+
Ergonomics	–	0	+	–
Functional				
Activation indicator	+	+	N/A	+
Integrated switch	+	+	N/A	+
Tool recognition	+	+	N/A	+
Reliability	0	–	+	0
Performance				
Orientation dependency	–	–	+	–
Accuracy	+	+	0	–
Cost				
Upfront cost	0	–	+	+
Running cost	+	–	0	+
Amortized cost	0	–	+	+

Scores (1, 0, 2) are relative: 1 indicates most favorable, 0 neutral, and 2 least favorable. N/A indicates that the feature is not available.

(frequency). It measures the *location* of an object (a tracker) with respect to a fixed coordinate frame centered at the position sensor's origin. The location of an object in space, its position and orientation, is uniquely determined by six parameters: three translational (vertical, horizontal, and depth) and three rotational (roll, yaw, and pitch).

Tracking systems measure the position of markers in a predefined volume in space, called the *tracking work volume*. Its shape is usually simple, such as a sphere, a pyramid, or a cube, depending on the type of position sensor technology used. The distance between the position sensor and the tracking work volume center is fixed.

Accuracy is defined as the measure of an instrument's capability to approach a true or absolute value. Accuracy is a function of both *bias* and *precision* (Fig. 23-4). Bias is a measure of how closely the mean value in a series of replicate measurements approaches the true value. Precision is a measure of how closely the values within a series of replicate measurements agree with each other. It has no units and indicates the relative degree of repeatability. *Repeatability* is a measure of *resolution* and *stability*. Resolution is the smallest discernable difference between two measurements. Stability refers to making identical measurements at a steady state and over a sufficiently long period of time. *Frequency* is the number of overall measurements per second. Static accuracy refers to measurements obtained when the trackers are at rest, whereas

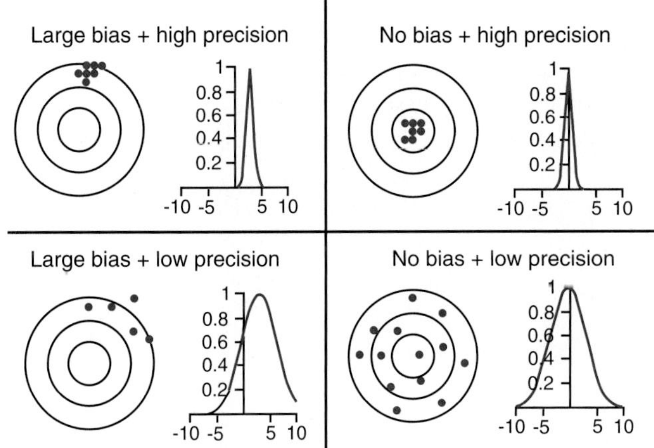

FIGURE 23-4 Accuracy and bias. Accuracy is a combination of precision and bias. High accuracy requires no bias and high precision (upper right image). The concentric circles represent the distance from the true value (the common center of the circles); the dots represent actual measurements.

dynamic accuracy refers to measurements obtained as the trackers move.

The factors influencing tracking accuracy are:

- Position sensor accuracy: for optical tracking, the number of cameras, the distance between them, and their resolution. For magnetic tracking, the intensity of the magnetic field and the resolution of the magnetic sensor.
- Marker accuracy: for optical tracking, the type of LEDs or sphere size and reflectance. For magnetic tracking, the strength of the coil magnetic field.
- Tracker accuracy: depends on the marker accuracy, number of markers, their configuration, and the distance between them.
- Tracking system accuracy: depends on all the above, and on the relative position and orientation of the position sensor with respect to the trackers.

Note that accuracy is not uniform within the tracking work volume. It is usually highest at the center, with decay toward the boundaries of the tracking work volume. Therefore, the position sensor should always be placed as close as possible to the center of the expected operating volume. It is often useful to distinguish between position and orientation accuracy. Statistics on accuracy include average, minimum, maximum, and root-mean-square (RMS) error. Table 23-2 summarizes the typical characteristics of current tracking systems.

Tool and Bone Tracking. Tool and bone tracking are achieved by rigidly attaching trackers to them with mounting hardware (Fig. 23-5). To track a surgical tool, a tracker can be added to it or the tool can be custom designed, with markers integrated within the tool. To track the C-arm, a ring with several dozen markers is attached to its image intensifier. It is very important that the trackers do not move with respect to the tracked body during surgery, because relative movement cannot be detected and measured and will increase system error.

Registration

Registration is the process of establishing a common reference frame between objects and images. It is a prerequisite for creating a reliable image of the intraoperative situation, accurately showing the relative locations of the anatomy and the surgical tools of interest with respect to the preoperative and/or intraop-

TABLE 23-2 Typical Characteristics of Commercial Tracking Systems

	Optical		
Characteristic	Active	Passive	Magnetic
Work volume	Sphere 1 m^3 diameter	Sphere 1 m^3 diameter	Cube 0.5 × 0.5 × 0.5 m^3
Distance from center	2.25 m	1 m	0.55 m
Accuracy (RMS)	0.1–0.35 mm	0.35 mm	1–2 mm 0.8°–1.7°
Frequency	60–450 Hz	60–250 Hz	20–45 Hz
Interferences	Line-of-sight	Line-of-sight	Ferrous objects Magnetic fields
Number of tools	3	6	3

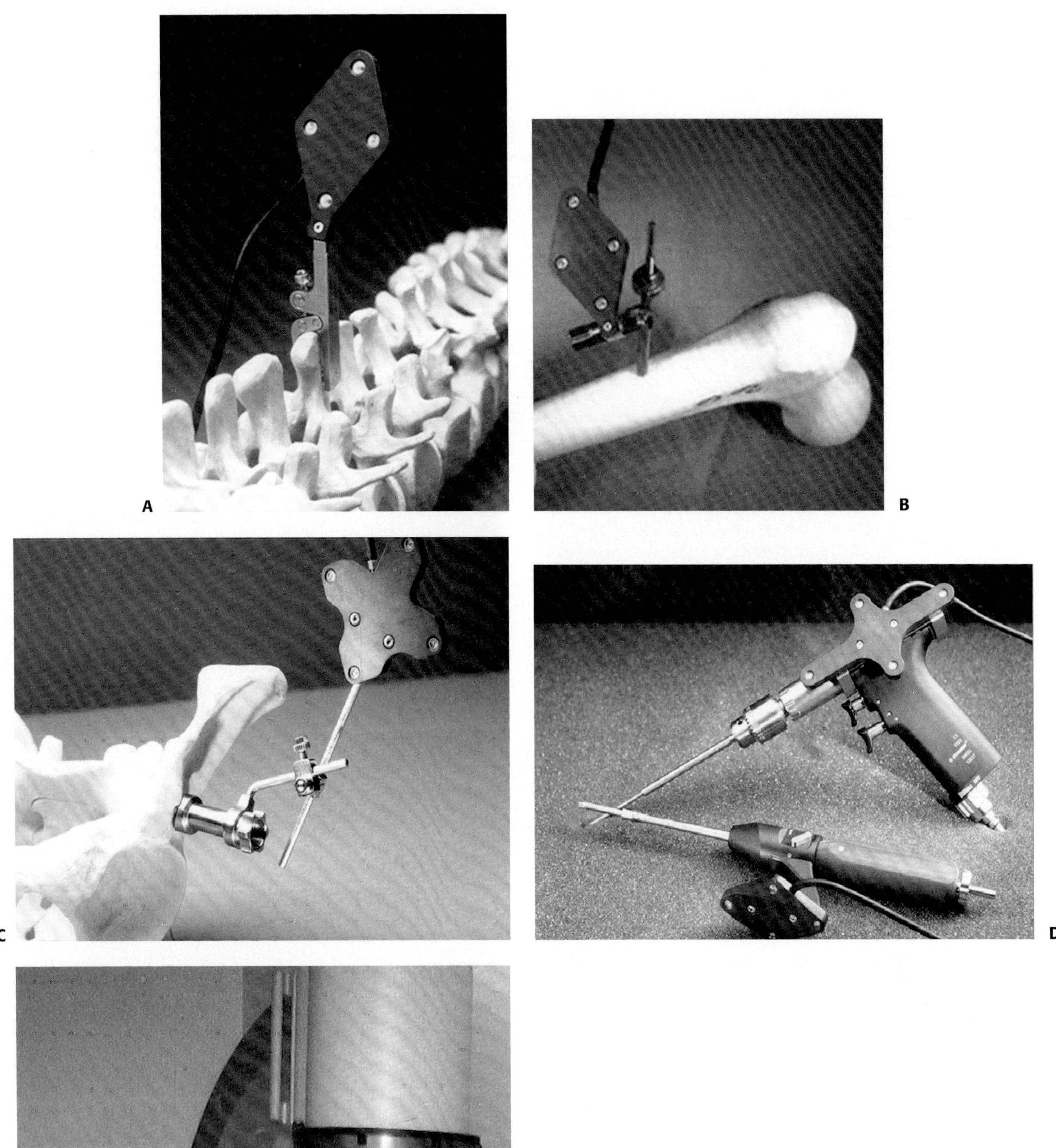

FIGURE 23-5 Trackers and mounting hardware. **A.** Bone clamp attached to spinous process. **B.** Bone screw attached to femur. **C.** Bone screw and extender attached to pelvis. **D.** Trackers on surgical drill and screwdriver. **E.** Ring tracker on C-arm image intensifier. (Photos courtesy of Medvision and Traxtal Technologies.)

erative images (9). Registration is achieved by *transformations* between the objects' *coordinate frames* at all times.

A coordinate frame serves as a reference within which the spatial locations (position and orientation) of objects can be described. Each object of interest has its own coordinate frame. The relative location of objects is described by a transformation T_B^A describing the location of *B*'s coordinate frame with respect to *A*. A transformation is a matrix describing the relationship between the three rotational and three translational parameters of the objects. The transformation is *static* (constant) when the relative locations of *A* and *B* do not change, or *dynamic* $T_B^A(t)$ (a function of time *t*) when one or both of the objects move. The relative locations of objects are obtained by *chaining* (composing) transformations. Thus, the location of *C* with respect to *A* is obtained from the location of *B* with respect to *A* and the location of *C* with respect to *B*, $T_C^A = T_B^A \cdot T_C^B$.

The goal is to compute the location of the surgical tools with respect to the displayed images $T_{tool}^{display}(t)$, as illustrated in Figure 23-6. This registration involves four types of transformations: (a) tracker transformations, (b) tool transformations, (c) image transformations, and (d) display transformations.

1. *Tracking transformations*: Tracking transformations $T_{tracker}^{sensor}(t)$ indicate the location of each tracker with respect to the position sensor coordinate system. They are provided in real time by the tracking system and can be static or dynamic, depending on whether the objects attached to the tracker move or not. The relative location of one tracker with respect to the other is obtained by chaining their transformations: $T_{tracker1}^{tracker2}(t) = T_{sensor}^{tracker1}(t) \cdot T_{tracker2}^{sensor}(t)$ where $T_{sensor}^{tracker1}(t) = (T_{tracker1}^{sensor}(t))^{-1}$ is the inverse transformation.
2. *Tool transformations*: tool transformations $T_{tool}^{t\_tracker}$ indicate the location of the tool coordinate frame with respect to the tracker. Since the tracker is rigidly attached to the tool, the transformations are static. They are provided at shipping time when the tracker and the tool come from the same manufacturer, i.e., precalibrated tools. Alternatively, they are computed shortly before surgery with a *tool calibration* procedure, which typically consists of attaching the tool to a tracked calibration object and computing with custom calibration software the transformation and the tool's geometric features, such as its main axis and its tip position.
3. *Image transformations*: image transformations T_{images}^{sensor} indicate the location of the images with respect to the position sensor. There are two types of transformations, T_{ct}^{sensor} and $(T_{X\text{-}ray}^{sensor})_i$, depending on the type of images used: one preoperative CT or several intraoperative fluoroscopic x-ray images. The transformation between the position sensor and the CT image T_{ct}^{sensor} is static and unknown, and must be computed with a *CT registration procedure*. The transformation between the position sensor and fluoroscopic x-ray images $(T_{X\text{-}ray}^{sensor})_i$, where *i* indicates each C-arm viewpoint, is computed from the transformation $(T_{i\_tracker}^{sensor})_i$ of the ring tracker attached to the C-arm image intensifier transformation and $(T_{X\text{-}ray}^{i\_tracker})_i$ the C-arm internal imaging transformation: $(T_{X\text{-}ray}^{sensor})_i = (T_{i\_tracker}^{sensor}) \cdot (T_{X\text{-}ray}^{i\_tracker})$. In older fluoroscopic units, this internal transformation is orientation-dependent, and thus must be computed for each C-arm viewpoint *i* (10).
4. *Display transformations:* display transformations $T_{ct}^{display}$ and $(T_{X\text{-}ray}^{display})_i$ indicate the location of the CT and fluoroscopic x-ray images with respect to the display shown to the surgeon. The transformations are determined by the viewpoint shown to the surgeon. Note that the transformation between the bone and the tracker $T_{bone}^{b\_tracker}$ is unknown and cannot be computed, since the exact location of the tracker mounting jig with respect to the bone is not known. Instead, the relative location of the tool with respect to the tool is used:

$$T_{tool}^{b\_tracker}(t) = T_{sensor}^{b\_tracker}(t) \cdot T_{t\_tracker}^{sensor}(t) \cdot T_{tool}^{t\_tracker}$$

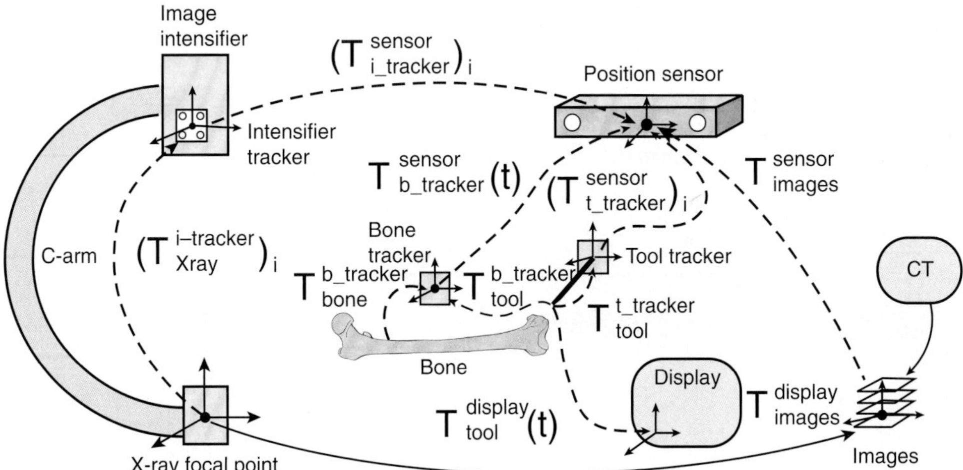

FIGURE 23-6 Coordinate frames and transformations between objects. The goal is to compute the location of the surgical tools with respect to the displayed images $T_{tool}^{display}(t)$.

In effect, the bone tracker becomes the reference coordinate frame, and is thus also called the *dynamic reference frame*.

The registration between the tool coordinate frame and the display coordinate frame $T_{tool}^{display}(t)$ is computed by chaining the transformations:

$$T_{tool}^{display}(t) = T_{image}^{display} \cdot T_{sensor}^{image} \cdot T_{t\_tracker}^{sensor} \cdot (t) \cdot T_{tool}^{t\_tracker}$$

For fluoroscopic x-ray images, there is one transformation $(T_{X\text{-}ray}^{sensor})_i$ and $(T_{tool}^{display})_i\ (t)$ for every C-arm viewpoint i.

Registration Accuracy. The accuracy of the registration depends on the accuracy of each transformation and on the cumulative effect of transformation chaining. Because the transformation includes rotation, the translational error is amplified as the distance from the reference frame increases (Fig. 23-7).

Tracking transformation accuracy depends upon the accuracy of the tracking system and on the location of the tracker with respect to the center of the position sensor work volume. Tool transformation accuracy depends upon the accuracy of the tool calibration procedure and on the relative location of the tracker with respect to the tool tip. Image transformation accuracy depends on the accuracy of the imaging modality used and on the tracking system's accuracy. For CT images, it depends on the resolution (slice spacing and pixel size) of the CT scan and on the accuracy of the CT registration procedure. For fluoroscopic x-ray images, it depends on the C-arm calibration and distortion correction procedures. Display transformation accuracy is always relatively very high, because it only involves numerical computations.

Note that any accidental shift in the location of the bone tracker with respect to the bone will introduce an error in the registration. It is therefore essential that the bone tracker remains rigidly secured to the bone at all times during navigation.

Visualization

Visualization creates updated images showing the location of moving objects with respect to the anatomy. The navigation images are created by merging the preoperative and intraoperative images with the tools and bone location information. The navigation images can be augmented with relevant procedure-dependent data, such as anteversion angle and distance from a predefined safe zone.

The type of navigation images created depends on the preoperative and intraoperative images that are used, on the surgical tools, and on the surgical procedure. In fluoroscopic-based navigation systems, the navigation images consist of fluoroscopic x-ray images from the C-arm typically used in conventional surgical procedure poses (anterior-posterior, lateral, oblique) with the surgical tools silhouette at its present location superimposed on them. For example, when the tool is a long cylinder (e.g., drill, pointer, or screwdriver), the tool's location and its prolongation are displayed in two different colors, to indicate what would be the tool's location if the current direction were followed. The number of images, tool silhouette, and additional navigation information are procedure-dependent.

In CT-based navigation systems, the navigation images typically consist of sagittal, coronal, and transverse CT cross sections, and a spatial view with the preoperative plan (e.g., fixation screws, fixation plate at their desired location) and the surgical tool's silhouette at its current location superimposed on them. Typically, the tool tip corresponds to the crosshair location in the CT cross sections.

Visualization software usually provides the surgeon with various image processing, viewpoint selection, and information display features such as contrast enhancement, viewpoint rotation and translation, window selection, and tool silhouette thickness and color control.

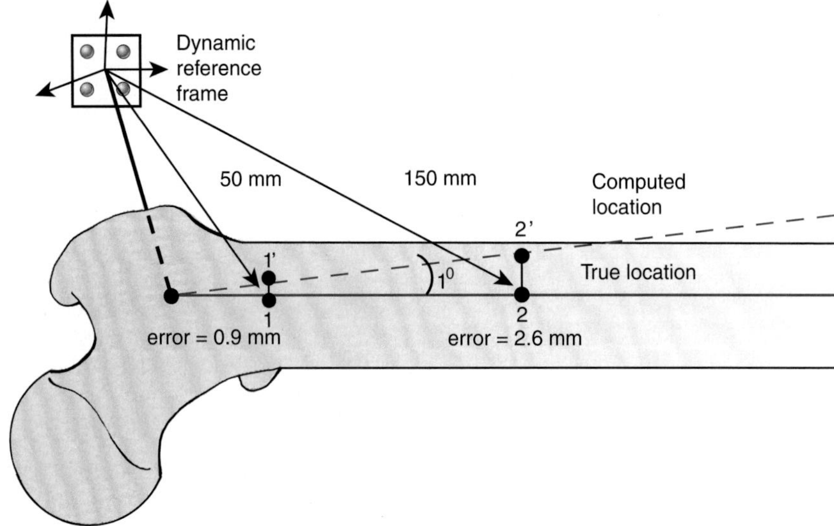

FIGURE 23-7 Influence of the angular error on the translational offset. A dynamic reference frame is attached to the proximal femur. With an angular transformation error of only 1°, a nearby target (1) 50 mm away from the origin of the bone coordinate frame will be offset by 0.9 mm (1′), which is acceptable in most situations. However, a further target (2) 150 mm away will be offset by 2.6 mm (2′), which may not be acceptable.

Validation

Validation is the task of verifying that the images and data used for intraoperative navigation closely correspond to the clinical situation. It is essential to verify and quantify the correlation, otherwise the data can mislead the surgeon and yield unwanted results. Validation is an integral part of the surgical protocol for navigation. It is done both before the surgery starts and at key points during the surgery.

There are three main types of verification:

1. *Tool's calibration verification*: verifies that the tool's geometric information is accurate. Sources of inaccuracy include deformations in the tools due to high-temperature sterilization, bending, wear and tear, tracker relative motion, and marker drift.
2. *Dynamic reference frame verification*: verifies that the bone tracker has not moved with respect to the bone to which it is attached.
3. *Registration accuracy verification*: verifies that the tool, implant, and bone fragment locations are indeed where they are shown in the navigation images. Over time, the registration accuracy depends on variations in the tool's calibration accuracy, on the dynamic reference frame's relative location with respect to the bone to which it is attached, on the tracking system's drift over time, and on the accumulation of small computational numerical errors.

The validation procedure depends on the type of surgery, the navigated surgical tools, and the images used. Tool calibration verification usually consists of verifying with a calibration jig that the tool tip is at its computed location. Dynamic reference frame and registration accuracy verification usually consist of verifying that the tracked bones and tools are indeed where the navigated images show that they are. This is done by acquiring one or more fluoroscopic x-ray images and comparing them with the navigation images. Alternatively, it is done by touching with the tip of a surgical tool known anatomical landmarks and verifying that the tool tip appears close to the landmark in the navigated image. Registration accuracy is quantified by measuring the drift between the actual and the computed location of tools and anatomical landmarks. When the registration accuracy is inadequate, the surgeon must repeat the registration process.

Navigation Systems

There are currently two types of navigation systems for computer-aided surgery in skeletal trauma: fluoroscopy-based and CT-based navigation systems.

Fluoroscopy-Based Systems

Fluoroscopy-based systems create navigation images by superimposing the surgical tool silhouette on conventional fluoroscopic images and updating its location in real time, thereby creating the impression of continuous fluoroscopy without the ensuing radiation. The resulting effect is called *virtual fluoroscopy*. Fluoroscopy-based systems are thus closest to the current practice of conventional fluoroscopy because the navigation images are in close proximity to the familiar fluoroscopic images with the advantage being that only a dozen fluoroscopic x-ray images are used, instead of tens or even hundreds.

There are two types of fluoroscopy-based navigation systems: systems that use conventional C-arm fluoroscopy and systems that use new 3D fluoroscopy, such as the ISO-3D C-arm (Siemens, Germany). Virtually any C-arm can be used, provided that the images are corrected for geometric distortion and the C-arm imaging properties are calibrated. The correction is usually done with an online C-arm calibration procedure that relies on imaged patterns of metallic spheres mounted on the C-arm ring tracker (the spheres appear as a grid of black circles in the images). Newer conventional and 3D C-arms do not require calibration.

Conventional C-arm Fluoroscopy. The surgical protocol is as follows: shortly before surgery, the rolling cart with the display, computer unit, and tracking base unit is positioned in the operating room so that the display can be easily seen by the surgeon. The position sensor is positioned so that it does not get in the way and its working volume is roughly at the center of where the surgical actions will take place. Next, the ring tracker is mounted on the C-arm's image intensifier and covered with a transparent plastic for sterility. The patient is then brought into the operating room and surgical preparations proceed as usual. Next, the surgeon validates the tool calibration and installs the dynamic reference frame with tracker mounting hardware. Touching known anatomical landmarks with the tip of a surgical tool and verifying that the tool tip appears close to the landmark in the navigated image validate the registration. Once the registration validation is successful, the navigated surgery begins. Later, at key points during surgery, e.g., before drilling a pilot hole or inserting a fixation screw, one or more validation fluoroscopic x-ray images can be acquired to verify that the navigated images correspond to the actual situation. The navigation procedure can be repeated with other tools and implants. At any time during the procedure, the navigation system can be stopped and the procedure can continue in the conventional manner.

3D Fluoroscopy. Three-dimensional fluoroscopy is a new imaging modality that allows the acquisition of CT-like images during surgery by taking about 100 fluoroscopic x-ray images at 1 degree intervals with a motorized isocentric C-arm. It can also be used as a conventional C-arm, with the added advantage that CT and fluoroscopic x-ray images acquired with it are already registered. Although the CT images are not of as high a quality as those obtained with a preoperative CT (the CT dose is about half of the radiation of a regular CT) and can only be used to image limbs, they accurately reflect the actual intraoperative situation. The navigation images consist of both CT images and fluoroscopic x-ray images. The advantages are that complex fractures can be better visualized and that CT images before and after reduction can be taken. In addition, CT images open the door for better intraoperative planning, and thus might advantageously blur the distinction between preoperative and intraoperative planning. The surgical protocol is very similar to the previous one for conventional fluoroscopy, with the additional step of acquiring the intraoperative CT images during surgery when necessary (11,12). Figure 23-8 shows an example of navigation with 3D fluoroscopy.

CT-Based Systems

CT-based systems create navigation images by superimposing on preoperative CT cross-sectional and spatial images the surgical tool silhouette and updating its location in real time. This type of navigation is only feasible when a CT data set is available.

The surgical protocol is as follows: any time between a few hours to a day before surgery, a CT is acquired and transferred to the computer within which the planning will be performed by the surgeon. With the help of preoperative planning and model construction software, the surgeon visualizes the clinical situation, takes measurements, and plans the target location of implants and fixation screws for navigation. The plan is then saved for use during surgery. Shortly before surgery, the rolling cart with the display, computer unit, and tracking base unit is positioned in the operating room so that the surgeon can easily see the display. The position sensor is positioned so that it does not get in the way and its working area is roughly placed at the center of where the surgical actions will take place. The preoperative plan is loaded into the computer unit. The patient is then brought into the operating room and surgical preparations proceed as usual. Next, the surgeon validates the tool calibration and installs the dynamic reference frame with tracker mounting hardware. Before the surgery starts, the preoperative CT is registered to the actual intraoperative anatomical site with a *CT registration procedure*. Touching known anatomical landmarks with the tip of a surgical tool and verifying that the tool tip appears close to the landmark in the navigated image validate the registration. Once the registration validation is successful, the navigated surgery begins. Later, at key points during the surgery, e.g., before drilling a pilot hole or inserting a fixation screw, one or more validation fluoroscopic x-ray images are taken to verify that the navigated images correspond to the actual situation. The navigation procedure can be repeated with other tools and implants. At all times during the procedure, the navigation system can be stopped and the procedure can continue as usual. Figure 23-9 shows images of a typical CT-based navigation system (13,14).

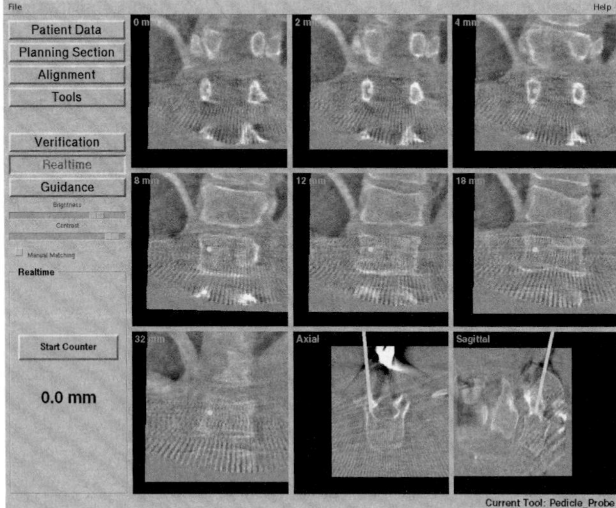

FIGURE 23-8 Pedicle screw insertion with 3D fluoroscopy. Screen view of 3-D fluoroscopy navigation during pedicle screw insertion in a fractured thoracic vertebra with the SIREMOBIL ISO-3D Mobile C-arm (Siemens, Germany). (Image courtesy of Prof. F. Gebhard).

A key step in the protocol is the CT registration procedure. The relationship between the CT and the intraoperative situation is established by automatically matching a set of points on the surface of the bone region to the corresponding points on the CT surface model. The intraoperative point set is obtained by touching the surface of the bone region of interest with a precalibrated tracked pointer and recording the location of a few dozen of these points by pressing on a foot pedal. The point set is then matched to a corresponding point set automatically extracted from the CT surface model of the same bone region. The points must be a representative sample of the bone surface, that is, they must be as far apart as is possible and cover the entire region of interest.

Comparison Between Fluoroscopy-Based and CT-Based Systems

Table 23-3 summarizes the advantages and disadvantages of navigation systems. Only CT-based systems allow for preoperative planning. Spatial visualization is only available with a CT data set, and is thus only available in CT-based and 3D fluoroscopy-based systems. No additional registration procedure is necessary for intraoperative imaging, as the position sensor provides a common reference frame for trackers and images. All navigation systems require additional setup procedures, which is a drawback in comparison with conventional practice. CT-based systems are not suitable for fracture reduction, as there is no way to determine bone fragment locations during and after reduction. 3D fluoroscopy-based systems can be used before and after reduction (but not during), provided that two images (before and after) are acquired. In fluoroscopy-based systems, reduction navigation is feasible when the bone fragments have trackers attached to them and new images are acquired at key points during reduction. Currently, CT-based navigation requires the surgeon to touch the surface of the bone; therefore it cannot be used for percutaneous procedures. In terms of radiation, the best option for the patient and the surgeon is fluoroscopy-based navigation. The indications for fluoroscopy-based systems are the widest, while 3D fluoroscopy-based and CT-based systems are best used with complex situations requiring spatial visualization. Currently, CT-based systems are mostly used for pelvic fracture fixation, whereas fluoroscopy-based systems are used for intramedullary nailing and fixation screw insertion.

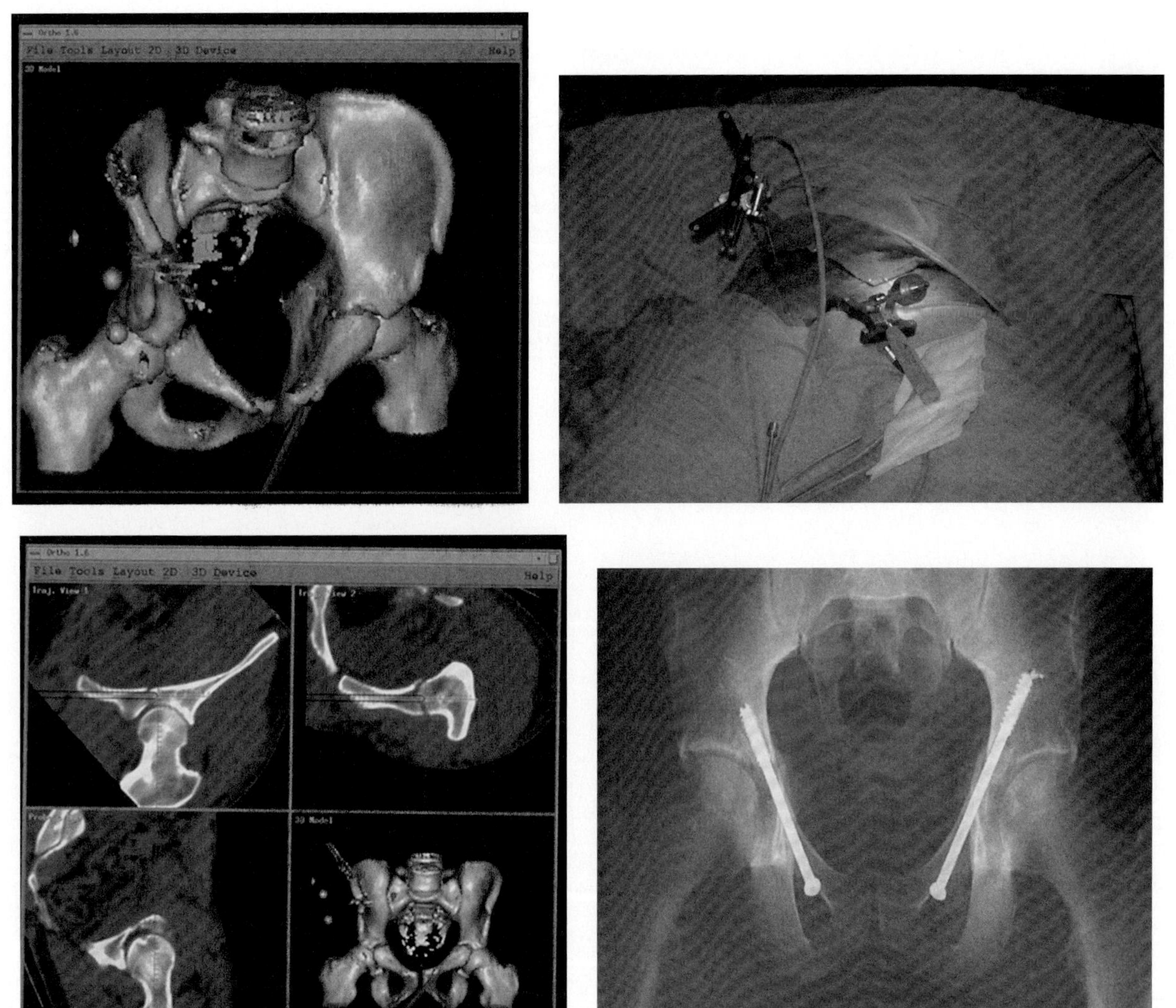

FIGURE 23-9 Retrograde anterior column screw. **A.** 3D model of the patient's pelvis built on the computer-guided surgery workstation (StealthStation, Sofamor-Danek, Memphis, TN). The position of a virtual drill guide for placement of a retrograde anterior column screw has been added to the virtual image. **B.** Intraoperative photograph taken during placement of the right retrograde anterior column screw (view from the foot of the bed). The reference frame attached to the external fixator is visible at upper left. Also visible is the navigated drill guide, chuck, and guide wire. **C.** The two upper images show a preoperative plan for placement of the left-sided retrograde anterior column screw. Two customized orthogonal planes relative to the drilling path are depicted, with a planned trajectory diameter of 7.0 mm. There is a small safe zone available between the planned position of the implant and the pelvic brim, as well as the articular surface of the acetabulum. The implant path is perpendicular to the fracture line, allowing lag screw reduction and fracture fixation. **D.** An AP pelvis image at 6 weeks postfixation shows accurate implant placement and early fracture healing without displacement. (Images courtesy of Dr. D. Kahle).

SURGICAL TECHNIQUES

Clinical Considerations

The concept of combining computer-aided procedures in the treatment of trauma patients should take into account the available innovative technologies along with the clinical situation and the decision-making process. The main goals of computer-aided surgery are minimal invasiveness and maximal accuracy in surgical procedures. Recent experience shows that if used appropriately, this combination has added value. While the first generation of computer-aided surgery employs computerized technology for current surgical concepts, it is clear that in the future the surgeon will be able to develop new ways of approaching surgical conditions.

There is no doubt that the timing and duration of procedures are of major concern in trauma management. Damage-control

TABLE 23-3 Comparison between the Conventional Technique and the Fluoroscopy-Based and CT-Based Navigation Systems

Characteristics	No Computerized Navigation	Fluoroscopy-Based		CT-Based
		Conventional	3-D Fluoroscopy	
Preoperative planning	No (−)	No (−)	No (−)	Yes (+)
3-D views	No (−)	No (−)	Yes (+)	Yes (+)
Registration	No (+)	No (+)	No (+)	Yes (−)
Additional OR setup	None (+)	Yes (−)	Yes (−)	Yes (−)
Reduction	Yes (+)	Yes (+)	Limited (−)	No (−)
Percutaneous	Yes (+)	Yes (+)	Yes (+)	No (−)
Radiation to surgeon	Yes (−)	Very limited (+)	Very limited (+)	None (+)
Radiation to patient	Yes (−)	Very limited (+)	Yes (−)	Yes (−)
Indications	Current practice	Wide range of procedures	Complex anatomy	CT available Partially open
Current use	All of trauma	Intramedullary nailing, screw fixation	In its beginnings	Pedicle screw insertion

(+) indicates an advantage, (−) indicates a disadvantage.

principles are considered the leading guidelines in the treatment of the severely injured patient. On the other hand, isolated skeletal trauma may be treated in a semi-elective fashion. Adding computer-assisted procedures to the trauma armamentarium is definitely influenced by, and affects, time-related factors. This is relevant to all stages of treatment of trauma patients, starting with the preplanning stage and up to the end of the surgery itself.

Currently, most surgeons believe that computer-aided surgery is a time-consuming and cumbersome procedure. The setup time of the system and the registration process prolong the preparation phase and might not suit acute trauma management considerations. Moreover, experienced surgeons believe that most surgical tasks can be carried out easily and sufficiently accurately without employing computer-related technologies. This conservative approach is well known in medical history whenever a new technology emerges. For example, a long time elapsed from the introduction of laparoscopic procedures until surgeons were ready to use them routinely.

We are currently in the learning phase for CAS systems, and therefore indications are still being selected for their use. Further assimilation of these promising technologies requires them to become easier to use and more user-friendly. The setup time for the computerized system will definitely be reduced in the modern surgical suite, where it will be built directly into the operating theater environment. Furthermore, the execution of some surgical tasks is faster and more accurate with CAS equipment, and will in the future allow procedures that are currently considered almost impossible. For example, the placement of a sacroiliac screw in the fixation of pelvic and acetabular fractures becomes a fast and accurate procedure with minimal radiation utilizing a navigation system (13,14). A second example is placement of a retrograde percutaneous posterior column screw, which previously has been considered an almost impossible task to perform, becomes an available option with computer assistance (15,16).

Which Type of CAOS-ST System Is Appropriate for Which Procedure?

The best indications for using CAOS-ST systems in trauma care are percutaneous surgical procedures in which added imaging can provide essential information that will contribute to reducing invasiveness and increasing accuracy (17). Clearly, the fixation of nondisplaced fractures is most suitably carried out with navigation systems, although often the indication for internal fixation is questionable. On the other hand, because available systems can only follow tracked bony fragments, they are not suitable for treating displaced multiple fragment fractures, such as comminuted articular fractures where careful anatomic reduction is required. Therefore, the main indications for using CAOS-ST systems are intermediate clinical situations where displaced fractures are amenable for closed reduction. A reduced fracture is a prerequisite for the use of computerized navigation systems.

In general, navigation systems function best in static or stable situations. For example, using a fracture reduction table or an external fixator eliminates the movement between fragments and creates a temporary situation in which there is little or no movement at the fracture site. Following fracture reduction, a guide wire or a fixation tool can be inserted using the navigation system according to specific clinical guidelines.

The required accuracy is a key factor for deciding whether or not to use a CAOS-ST system. For example, the accuracy needed for pedicular screw insertion is by far greater than that of hip fracture fixation with cannulated screws. Accuracy is directly influenced by the cost of inaccuracy. For example, the cost of inaccuracy in spinal surgery is much higher than in intramedullary nailing.

Computerized navigation has been shown to increase placement accuracy and reduce variability as compared with manual placement. In a recent study, the accuracy of cannulated screw placement in hip fracture fixation was evaluated (18). After verifying stable reduction on a fracture table, the reference tracker was attached to the anterior superior iliac crest. The reference frame was not attached to the affected bone in order to improve working convenience during the procedure and to eliminate morbidity. It was found that the accuracy of the procedure was much better than that of nonnavigated procedures. The navigation system enabled the surgeon to place screws with optimal alignment including configuration, parallelism, and scattering. This experience demonstrates that stable reduction creates a stable situation for navigation systems, and that the reference tracked frame may be fixed on such occasions to an adjacent bone as well as to an external fixator or even to the operating table.

After reduction/stabilization of the fracture, the process of registration is performed. In a simple situation such as the one described above, basic fluoroscopic images are sufficient. With the advent of new technologies such as 3D fluoroscopy, more complex surgical tasks are amenable to CAOS-ST systems. For example, in a displaced tibial plateau fracture that is reduced by means of ligamentotaxis, three-dimensional accuracy of the reduction can be evaluated intraoperatively using 3D fluoroscopy and followed by navigated closed internal fixation.

Preparing for Surgery

Before surgery, the decision as to whether the procedure is suitable for CAOS-ST is determined by the surgeon's knowledge and capabilities. In most trauma cases, fluoroscopy-based navigation is the method of choice.

It is very important to plan and prepare the operating room in order to create a surgeon-friendly environment and to enable proper tracking without interference (Fig. 23-10). Adding CAOS-ST equipment (computer, monitor, position sensor, and trackers) to an already crowded room requires careful planning. The computer screen should be positioned so that the surgeon can see it without any effort, because, as in arthroscopic procedures, most of the time the surgeon will watch the screen rather than the operative site. Easy access to the computer's control panels is also important and is usually realized with a sterile touch screen. When using optical tracking, maintaining an unobstructed line-of-sight between the position sensor and the trackers is very important. Thus, the location of the position sensor with respect to the surgeon, nurses, and patient must be carefully examined.

For the initial phase, the minimal required free field of vision is determined by the location of the ring tracker attached to the C-arm, the reference frame tracker attached to the patient's anatomy, and by the optical camera. During the navigation phase, tracked surgical instruments replace the ring tracker, and the tracking space changes accordingly. Continuous tracking of the patient's anatomy and of the surgical instrument is required. Verification and validation are extremely important at every stage in order to achieve optimal accuracy. Tracking the surgical instrument is relatively simple and precise, whereas tracking anatomy, especially in trauma surgery, is more problematic.

The registration and tracking of the patient's anatomy is usually the main cause of inaccuracy. The first obstacle is attaching the rigid frame to the patient. The problem of inserting a stable screw into the bone fragment is well known from the field of external fixators. Screw or pin grip depends on their design and on bone quality. For each procedure, the location needs to be selected according to local morbidity (soft tissue access and crucial anatomic structures), convenience during the procedure (line-of-sight and free surgical site), and stability of anatomical frame fixation. The stability of the screw holding the anatomically referenced tracked frames depends on bone quality and soft tissue interference. Subcutaneous locations, such as the iliac crest or the medial aspect of the tibia, are preferable.

Newly designed frames contain more than one screw as well as several soft tissue adaptors. In the future, newly designed bone trackers are expected to be much smaller and will be able to transfer accurate information to the computer using several innovative technologies rather than optical transmission. Improvement of bone tracking technology as well as the ability of tracking more than one bone fragment will significantly enhance the surgeon's surgical performance in the treatment of fractures.

Basic Procedures Under Navigation

The clinical situations in which computerized navigation is mostly used are now presented. For each clinical application, both the rationale and the contribution of these systems will be discussed. The aim of this section is to expose the reader to the first generation of computerized navigation systems. The

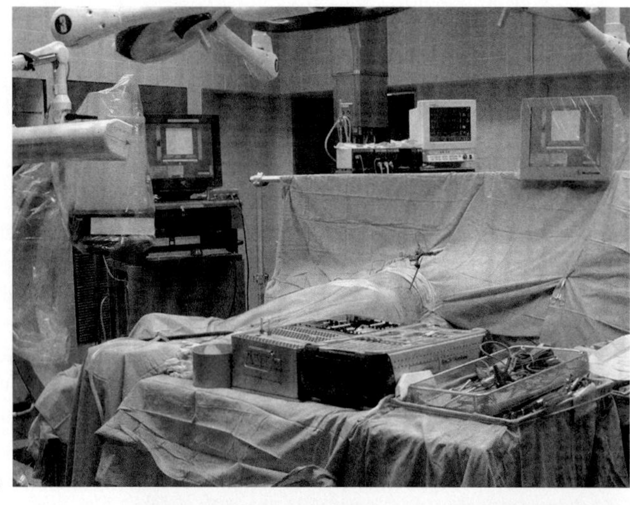
A

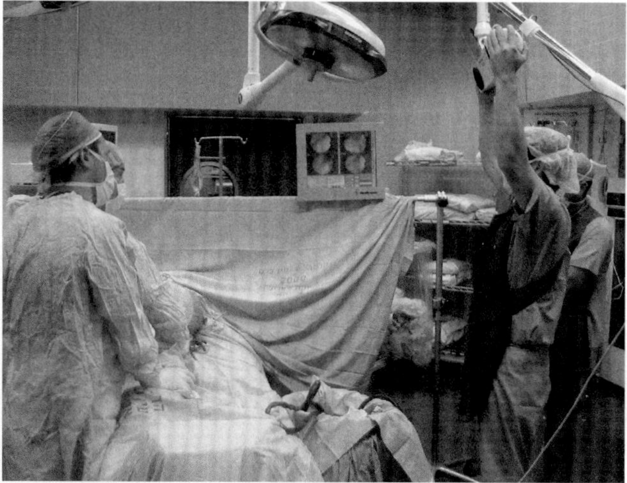
B

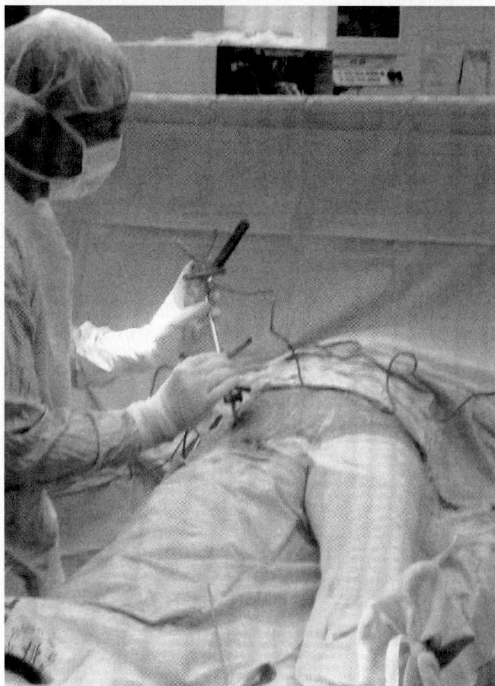
C

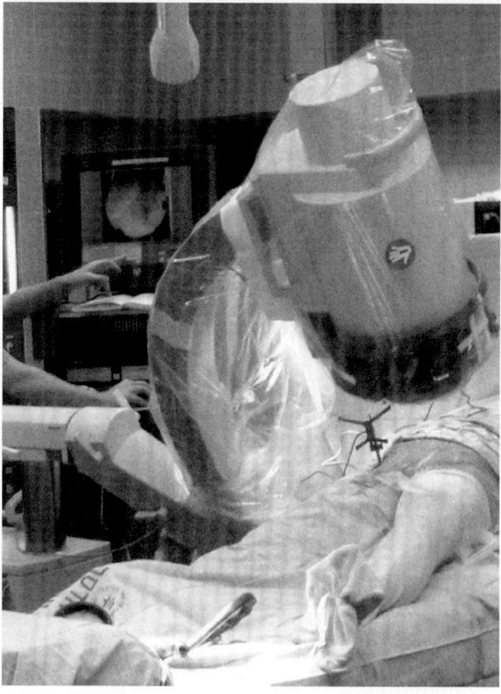
D

FIGURE 23-10 Operating room setup. **A.** View of the operating room showing locations of the computer unit, position sensor, and bone-mounted reference frame. **B.** Reorientation of the position sensor during surgery. **C.** Surgical tool calibration. **D.** Acquisition of fluoroscopic images. *(continues)*

specific indication for each surgical procedure is beyond the scope of this discussion. Although all the surgical procedures discussed are based on optical infrared tracking, similar principles apply to other current and future tracking technologies.

When using fluoroscopy-based navigation, the first step is to mount the ring tracker on the C-arm and drape it for sterility. Next, the dynamic reference frame is attached to the patient's anatomy and several (typically between one and four) essential fluoroscopic images are acquired. The optimal images are stored in the computer and will be activated during the navigation process. It should be noted that for all of the clinical examples to be discussed, the preliminary fluoroscopic views can be taken while the operating team stands at a distance of 2 m or more from the radiation source, thus almost eliminating the team's radiation exposure. However, a significant amount of radiation is still being delivered to both the patient and the surgical team during fracture reduction, particularly to the surgeon's hands.

The next stage relates to the activation of the designated surgical tool (i.e., wires, awls, drill bits, etc.), which is to be attached to a tracker commonly referred to as the *instrument*

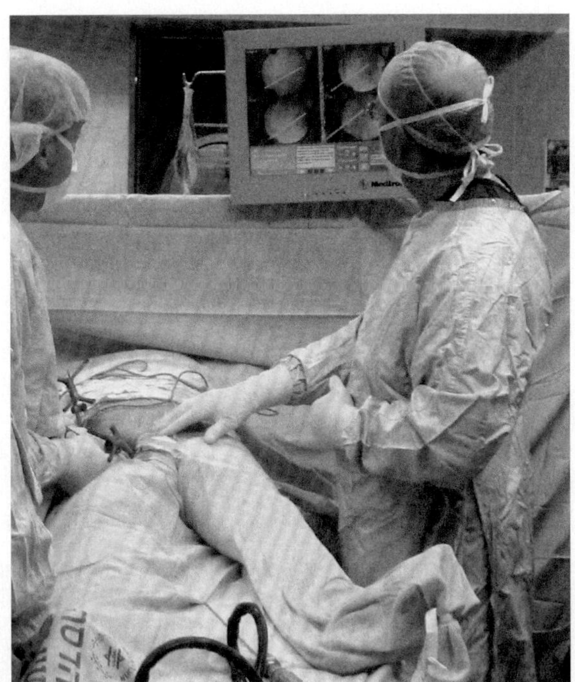

FIGURE 23-10 *(continued)* **E.** Navigation with fluoroscopy-based system.

tracker. The contour of the instrument in its current location is displayed on the previously activated fluoroscopic images, thereby creating the effect of virtual fluoroscopy.

Removal of Surgical Hardware and Shrapnel

The simplest indication for using CAOS-ST systems are situations in which foreign bodies retained in bone or soft tissue, such as surgical hardware or penetrating injuries with retained metals, such as shrapnel, nuts, and bolts, need to be removed. It is not necessary to track foreign bodies as they usually remain in place and do not drift. They can be reached with a navigated tool by following the tool's location with respect to them, in the activated fluoroscopic images. Given the simplicity of the procedure, we recommend that this be the first surgical procedure using computerized navigation systems to be performed by inexperienced surgeons (19,20).

The main indication for metal/hardware removal is local discomfort, although other indications include infection or risk of toxicity. The removal of missiles retained in an inaccessible location poses a major problem for the trauma surgeon, because they can be hazardous to the integrity of adjacent internal structures.

Fluoroscopy-based navigation is the method of choice for these situations. Unlike CT-based systems, it requires very short preoperative preparation, making it appropriate in emergency situations as well, where its effectiveness has already been proven, even during the urgent stages of treatment. Thanks to the high accuracy of fluoroscopy-based navigation, its utilization in complex and dangerous situations where a foreign body is located in the proximity of structures such as blood vessels and/or nerves is promising. In comparison to other conventional techniques, the use of fluoroscopic-based navigation has allowed us to minimize soft-tissue dissection.

Surgical Technique. Tracked reference frames are rigidly attached to the patient's adjacent bone and to a calibrated pointer. Several fluoroscopic images of the required anatomical site are acquired and stored in the computer. The accurate spatial location of the foreign object can be seen in the images displayed on the computer's screen (Fig. 23-11). The surgeon then plans the most accurate and safest minimal surgical approach to the foreign body that needs to be removed. Once the fluoroscopic images have been activated, the location of the guided probe with respect to the patient's anatomy is continuously displayed and updated on all of the fluoroscopic images. This enables accurate determination of the entry point and spatial advancement of the probe toward the foreign body.

Cannulated Screw Insertion

The second indication for the use of CAOS-ST systems is the insertion of cannulated screws. This surgical procedure sometimes requires high accuracy and unusually large radiation exposure for the surgeon and for the patient. Both can be successfully addressed with fluoroscopy-based navigation.

For the acetabulum, internal fixation of slipped capital femoral epiphysis is a procedure that can greatly benefit from computerized navigation. The use of computerized navigation makes this a simple task to perform while using minimal radiation (21). The internal fixation of intracapsular fractures of the femoral neck is considered straightforward, although accurate performance requires high proficiency on the one hand and large exposure to radiation on the other. Recently, a prospective comparison between patients who underwent internal fixation of intracapsular fracture of the femoral neck by means of cannulated screws, with and without the assistance of a navigation system, was performed (18). This study revealed that computerized navigation increased the accuracy of screw placements in all measured parameters. Having acquired proficiency with the computerized system, the surgeon is ready to move on to the next level that includes the percutaneous fixation of pelvic and acetabular fractures.

Internal pelvic fracture fixation is a challenging task for the orthopaedic trauma surgeon. The pelvis is a complex, three-dimensional bone, crowded with susceptible structures in a relatively small space. Therefore, surgical fixation of displaced traumatic fractures should be meticulously performed under strict visual control, since the "safe zones" are narrow. In many cases, closed reduction and percutaneous fixation is feasible and provides enough stability to allow immediate patient mobilization. The conventional image intensifier is most frequently used in percutaneous pelvic fixation. However, it only provides a two-dimensional image and requires multiple images in different projections (AP, lateral, inlet, outlet, Judet, or roll-over views)

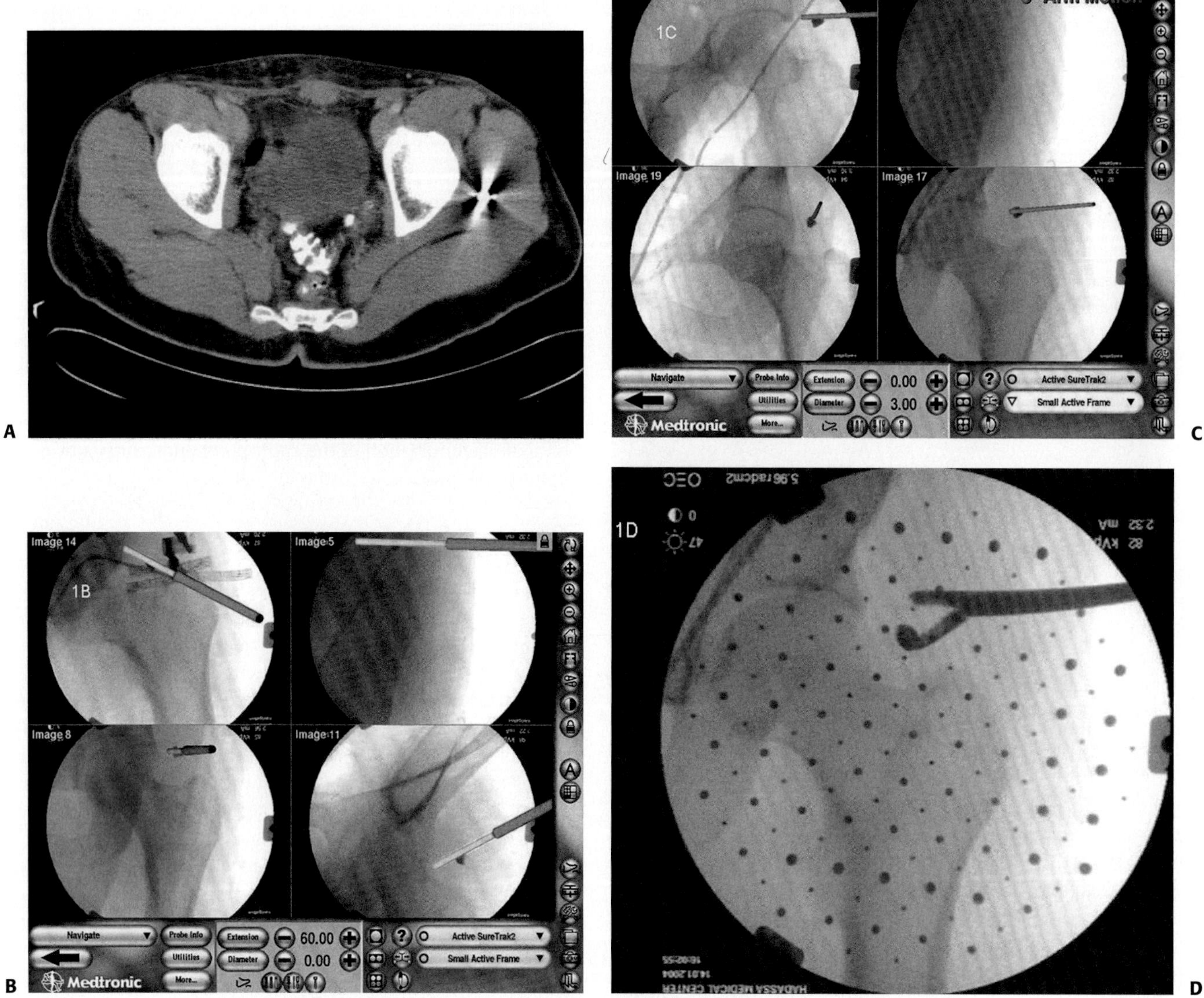

FIGURE 23-11 Shrapnel removal. **A.** Preoperative CT scan showing shrapnel that is intended to be removed due to its proximity to the left hip joint. **B.** Four acquired images displayed on the system's screen, showing the location of the missile allowing immediate presurgery planning of percutaneous surgical approach. The darker line represents the surgical tool and the virtual lighter line assists in determining the point of entry and direction of surgical tool. **C.** The surgical tool, represented by the darker line, arrives at the missile. **D.** Verification fluoroscopy followed by removal of missile.

to determine the correct point of entry and the direction of the screw. Furthermore, the use of conventional fluoroscopy makes the procedure long and tedious and exposes both the patient and the medical team to prolonged radiation (13,14). Fluoroscopy-based navigation systems have the potential to significantly reduce radiation exposure and operative time, while allowing the surgeon to achieve maximum accuracy (16,22,23).

The indications for percutaneous pelvic and acetabular surgery are controversial and are not discussed here. At this stage, a selected population with traumatic pelvic and acetabular fractures can be treated percutaneously under three conditions: (a) cases with minimally displaced pelvic and acetabular fractures; (b) displaced fractures with feasible closed reduction; and (c) complex fractures in which a combination of closed and open reduction is necessary. Even in open pelvic surgery the insertion of several screws is very challenging and demands the assistance of guiding systems such as fluoroscopy or navigated fluoroscopy.

It is important to note that the percutaneous approach to fracture fixation of the pelvis is still evolving and is undergoing many improvements and developments in which computerized technology may be of great assistance. For example, for preplanning, the use of standard axial CT data to create computer reconstructed 3D images and/or models may replace the standard radiographic assessment of pelvic and acetabular fractures (24). Similarly, 3D fluoroscopy technology allows the surgeon to obtain immediate and accurate 3D reconstructions in the operating room. By integrating these images into navigation systems, preplanning becomes easier and more accurate, and allows for direct, truly spatial surgical navigation. It enables the precise evaluation of closed reduction (using a fracture table, external fixator and/or other fixation instruments) prior to the insertion of the navigated screws. These new technologies may change the classic approach to pelvic and acetabular fractures.

Surgical Technique. For both acetabular and pelvic surgery, the dynamic reference frame can be rigidly attached to the patient's iliac crest. Several fluoroscopic images of the pelvis (inlet, outlet, Judet, or roll-over views) are acquired and saved in the system's computer. No further fluoroscopic imaging is necessary, except for verification fluoroscopy prior to the insertion of the cannulated screw, or in the case of reduced fracture the crossing of the fracture site.

During surgery, following the activation of the fluoroscopic images, the surgeon can accurately determine the entry point and direction of each screw. At the same time, by means of a virtual line, the correct length and diameter of the screw can be calculated (Fig. 23-12). After satisfactory virtual alignment and length have been achieved, the conventional guide wire

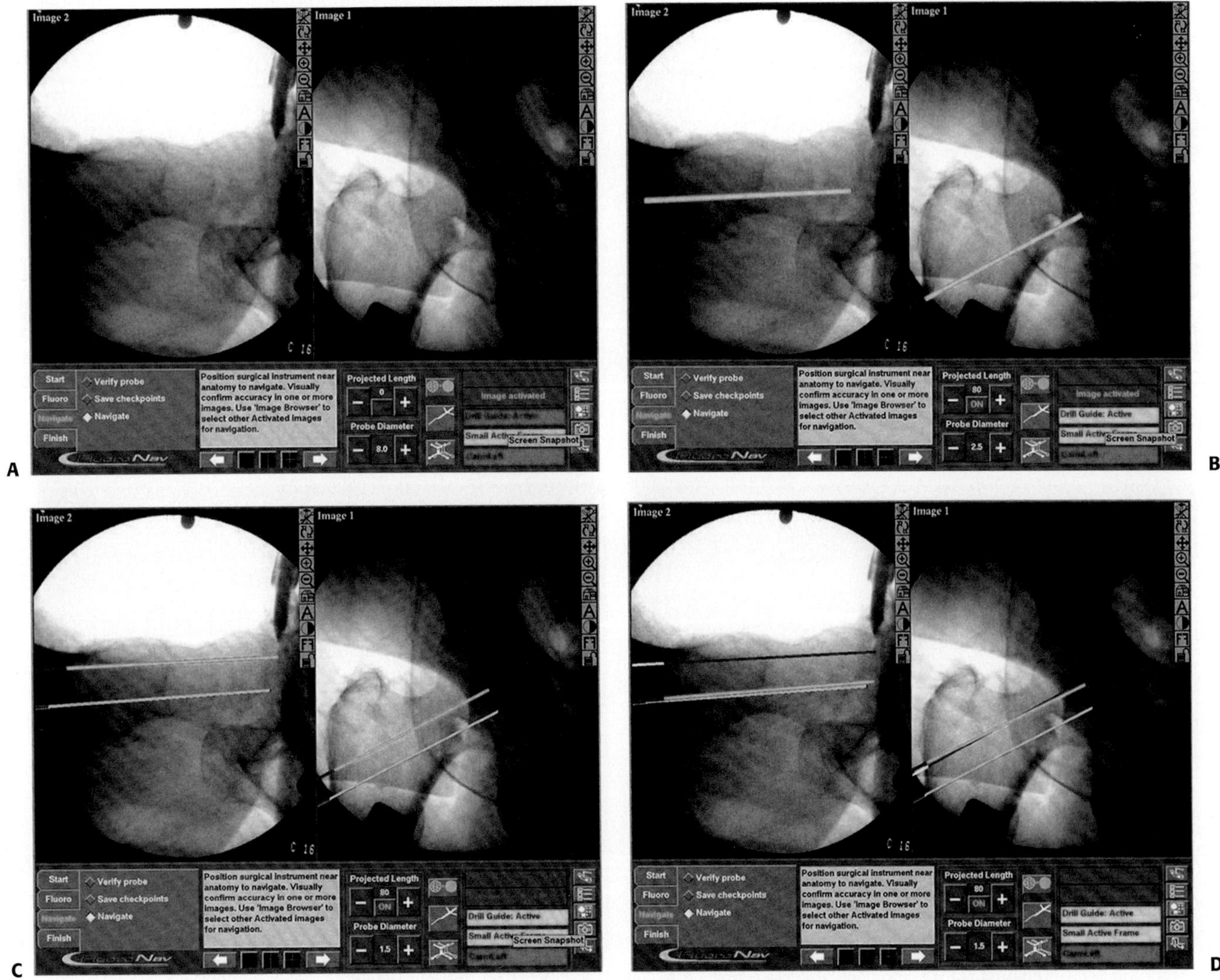

FIGURE 23-12 Cannulated screws. **A.** AP and lateral views of a reduced intra-capsular fracture of the femoral neck displayed on the computer's screen. **B–D.** Insertion of the three guide wires without additional radiation.

pertaining to the cannulated screw system is driven through the drill guide. Before insertion of a self-drilled cannulated screw, the position of the guide wire should be verified by fluoroscopy. When the insertion of several screws in the same area is required, such as in the fixation of fractures or dislocations in the sacroiliac zone, the acquired fluoroscopic views can be used for the insertion of more than one screw (Figs. 23-13 and 23-14).

In pelvic surgery, serious complications might arise from the surgical procedure and intervention rather than from the initial injury. Therefore, it is only natural that percutaneous minimal surgical approaches are sought in order to overcome the difficulties that arise in relation to fractures in the complex anatomy of the pelvis and acetabulum.

Figure 23-9 illustrates the placement of a retrograde anterior column screw with a CT-based navigation system.

Intramedullary Nailing

Intramedullary nailing is the preferred surgical option in many long bone fracture cases. Although it is a routine procedure performed by most trauma surgeons, it is not devoid of technical pitfalls and complications. Achieving accurate and successful results with conventional techniques involves exposure to significant amounts of radiation for both patients and surgeons.

Fluoroscopy-based navigation can be helpful in closed intramedullary nailing by increasing precision, minimizing soft tissue damage, and significantly decreasing radiation exposure (25–27). Several surgical goals can be achieved by using computerized navigation systems. The insertion of instruments based on real-time information becomes possible and significantly increases the accuracy of nail placement. Determining the exact point of entry of the nail is critical since it is one of the main sources of morbidity in intramedullary nailing. Computerized navigation systems help to precisely locate the nail entry point, thus minimizing soft tissue dissection. This is particularly helpful in special cases such as with obese patients where anatomic landmarks are obscured. Working with several images simultaneously, can also decrease unnecessary drill holes, tissue damage, and cartilage perforation, because all targeting is done prior to the introduction of the actual instrument. The insertion of locking screws into certain nails can be a potential hazard for neurovascular structures (28,29). In addition, improvement in nailing techniques is achieved by the facilitation of Poller screw insertion. When precisely placed, better angular correction of metaphyseal fractures is achieved. Precision of length measurement can also decrease the complications associated with nailing, such as protrusion of the nail's or the screw's ends.

Surgical Technique. The use of a fluoroscopy-based surgical navigation system can be implemented at different stages of intramedullary nailing: the nail entry point, nail and screw measurements, freehand locking, or placement of auxiliary screws. In each stage, the reference frame should be attached to the tracked bone fragment (either proximal or distal), depending on the specific procedure.

1. Nail entry point: The actual point of entry is determined by the use of simultaneous virtual fluoroscopic views (mostly AP and lateral). Prior to incision, the tracked drill guide is drawn next to the skin. Its position is adjusted by viewing its virtual trajectory superimposed on the activated fluoroscopic images to minimize the surgical exposure. The entry point location is established while moving the

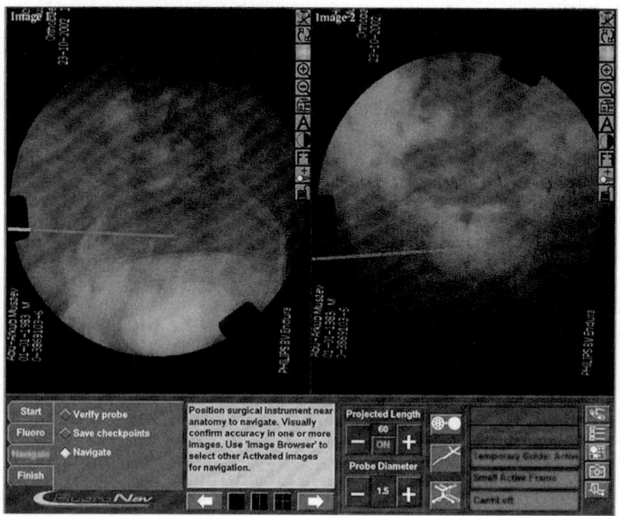

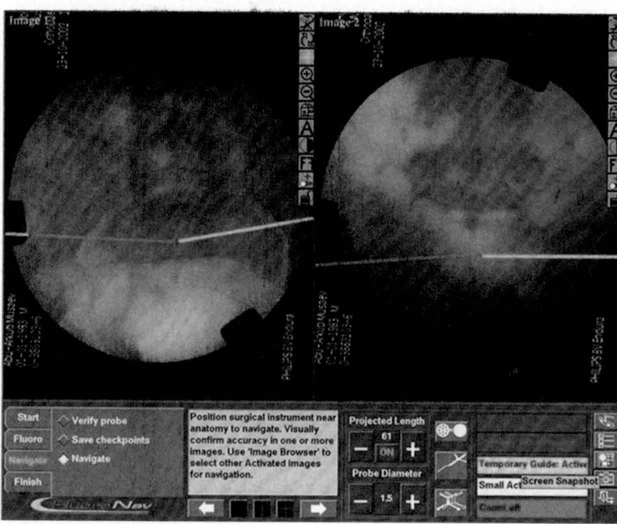

FIGURE 23-13 Bilateral sacroiliac screws. **A,B.** Typical intraoperative display of computer screen during bilateral insertion of two sacroiliac screws. The live spatial position of the drill guide is presented simultaneously on two views (inlet and outlet) with a virtual continuation representing the track of the guidewire.

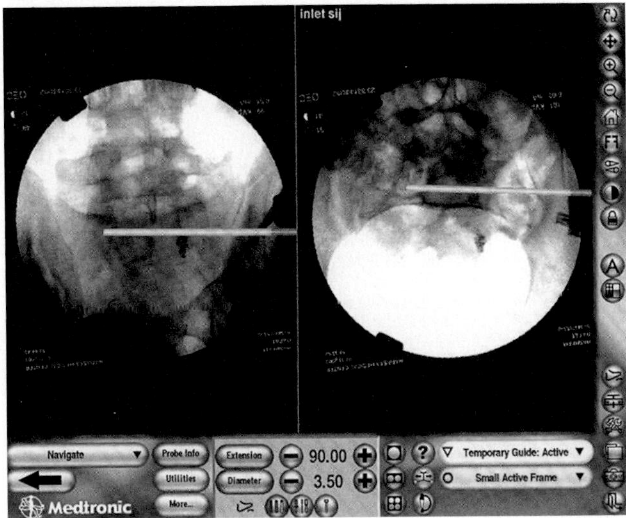

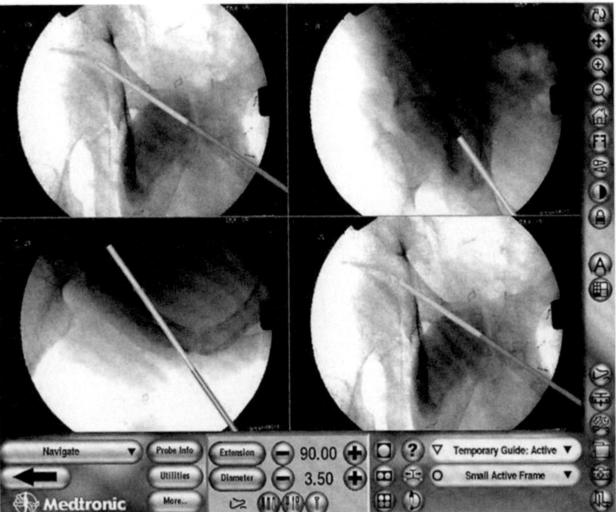

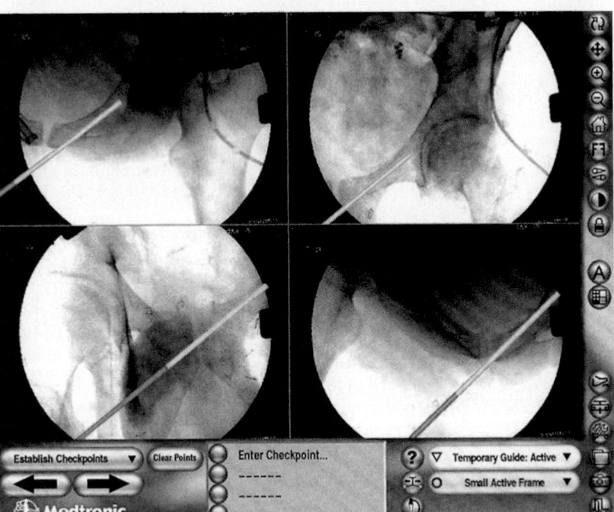

FIGURE 23-14 Sacroiliac and pubic ramus screw. An intraoperative display of computer screen during insertion of a sacroiliac screw and two intramedullary pubic ramus screws.

tracked drill guide to an optimal position (Fig. 23-15). No further fluoroscopy is needed and a verification fluoroscopic image is taken only after insertion of the guide wire. After this task is performed, a cannulated awl or a larger cannulated drill is inserted, according to the manufacturer's instructions through this guide in order to open the medullary canal.

2. Nail and screw measurements: Nail length and width can be determined by means of two x-rays of the adjacent points between which the nail head will be placed. The reference frame should be moved from the proximal to the distal part of the fracture prior to acquiring images of the distal part. These images are stored in the computer and displayed simultaneously on the screen. By placing the tracked drill guide at the point of entry, a virtual projected beam is extended from this point toward the estimated end of the nail in the distal fragment. The length of the beam on the screen indicates the required length (Fig. 23-15A). The length of the required screw can then easily be obtained by measuring the length of the virtual beam on the image.
3. Freehand locking: This technique is relatively easy to perform and involves minimal radiation exposure. The bone tracker is fixed closed to the location of the locking screws. Using the "perfect circle" technique, an AP of the locking hole, in which the holes almost resemble circles, is acquired. An additional lateral view may be taken in order to determine the screw length measurement. The tracked drill guide is then drawn toward the locking screw area and is navigated until a circle within the hole appears on the computer screen (Fig. 23-16B,C). This is followed by drilling through the tracked drill guide and inserting the locking screw. Sometimes, such as in the case of the tibial nail, the same AP and lateral views can be used for insertion of two or even three adjacent locking screws.
4. Placement of auxiliary screws: Poller screws are important tools for correcting bone alignment while nailing metaphy-

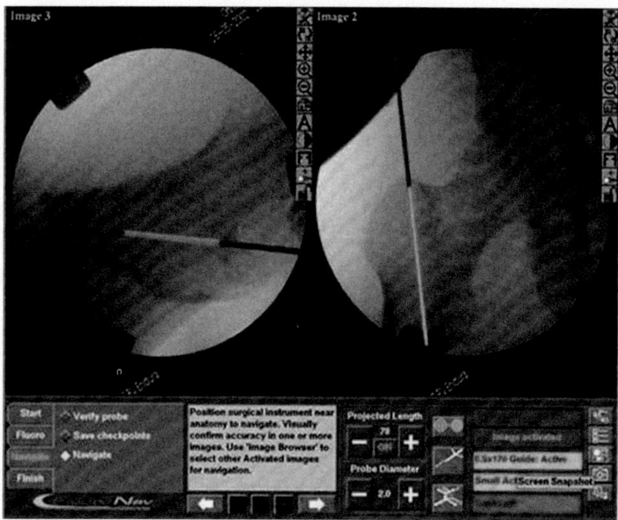

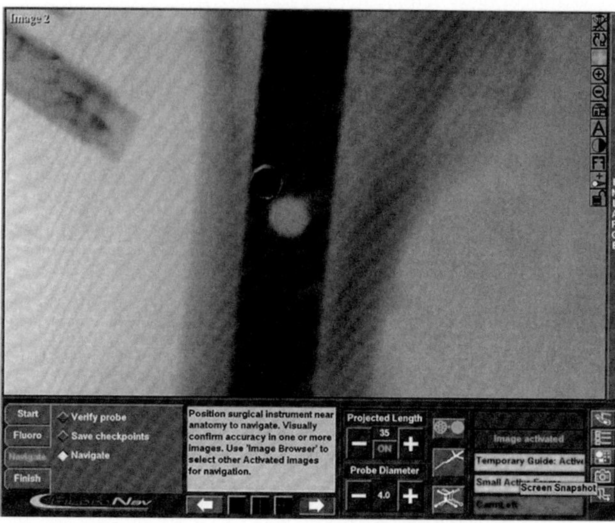

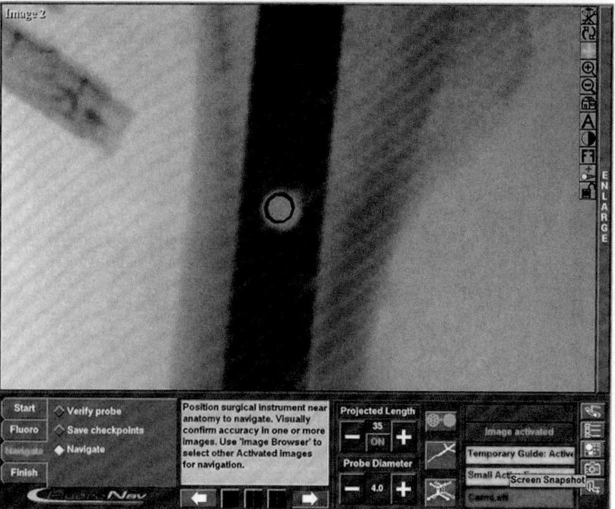

FIGURE 23-15 Intramedullary nailing. **A.** Typical computer display employed during antegrade femoral intramedullary nail consisting of simultaneous AP and lateral views, where the darker line represents the guide's insertion point at the precise entry point in the piriform fossa and lighter line represents the nail's direction. **B,C.** Proximal locking hole in the retrograde femoral nail. Notice the hole as a perfect circle enabling a precise aiming of the locking screw.

seal fractures. Precise placement of these screws can now be performed using a technique similar to that of locking screws. Virtual fluoroscopy based on AP and lateral images, enables easy and precise positioning of Poller screws. For "miss a nail" screws, additional AP and lateral images of the proximal femur are obtained following the insertion of the intramedullary nail. The goal is then to insert the cross-neck screw without interfering with the intramedullary nail. The navigation system enables the surgeon to determine the precise position of the "miss a nail" cross-neck screws, and to navigate safely through the narrow safe zone (Fig. 23-16).

Fracture Reduction: Tracking Two or More Rigid Bodies

Current commercial navigation systems do not support fracture reduction because they are unable to track the position of two independent anatomic sites, such as fracture fragments. However, for long bone fractures, tracking a reduction tool can help circumvent this limitation.

The approach is to attach a dynamic reference frame to one bone fragment and insert a long, straight calibrated reduction tool into the canal of the other fragment. The reduction tool is calibrated intraoperatively shortly before its use, and then displayed on previously acquired images. Since the axis of the reduction tool roughly coincides with the axis of the fragment canal, fragment axis alignment and reduction are possible by following the position of the tracked reduction tool with respect to the other fragment's relative location.

Surgical Technique. The patient is positioned in a supine position on a radiolucent table; skeletal traction usually simplifies closed reduction. Preparation for the nailing procedure and the location of the entry point can be performed conventionally or by using fluoroscopy-based navigation as previously described. After locating the entry point, the proximal fragment is reamed up to the diameter of the tracked intramedullary fracture alignment device. This device is then inserted into the medullary

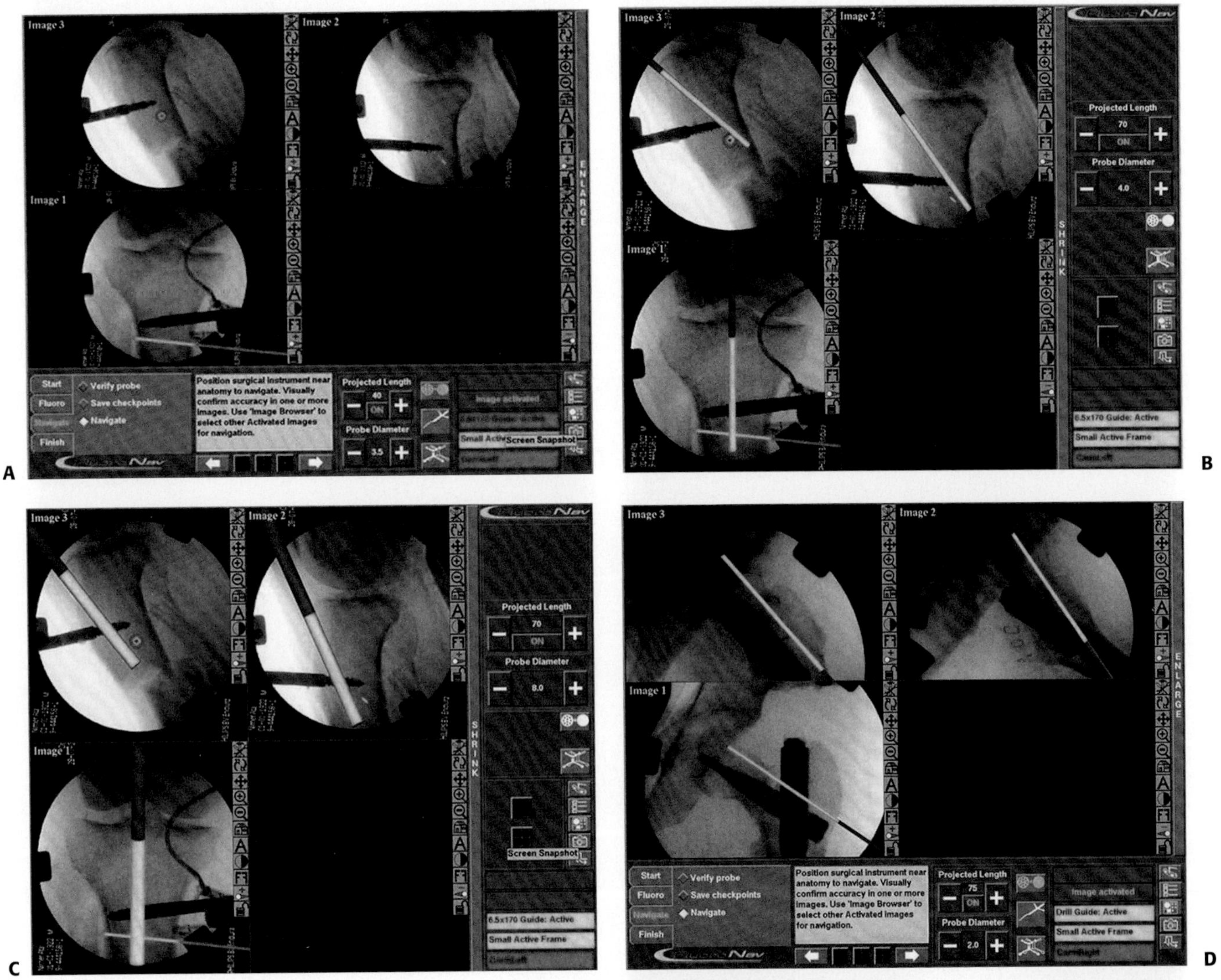

A

B

C

D

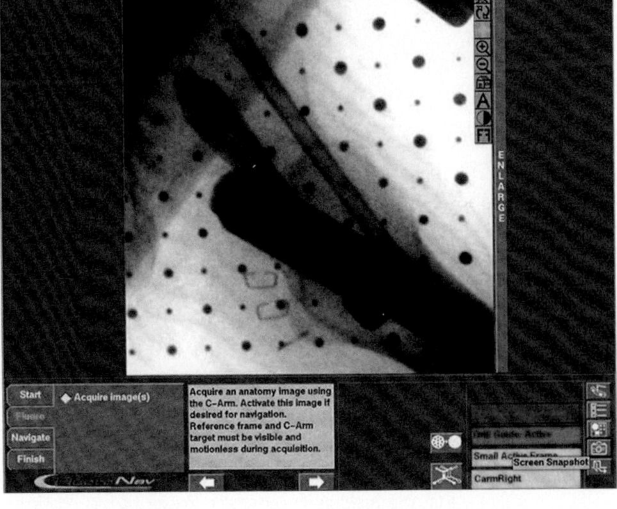

E

FIGURE 23-16 Intramedullary nailing: Poller and miss-a-screw. **A.** Poller screw planning for reduction of a proximal tibial fracture. The circle demonstrates the planned position of the Poller screw. The lighter line is the virtual nail. The surgeon can predict the relationship between the two. **B,C.** Insertion process of Poller screw. **D,E.** "Miss a nail" screw through a femoral neck fracture after insertion of a femoral nail with a spiral blade. **D.** Planning the "miss a nail" route with the navigation system displayed as a lighter line. **E.** Fluoroscopic image after nail insertion. Notice the parallelism between the planned and the real route of the nail.

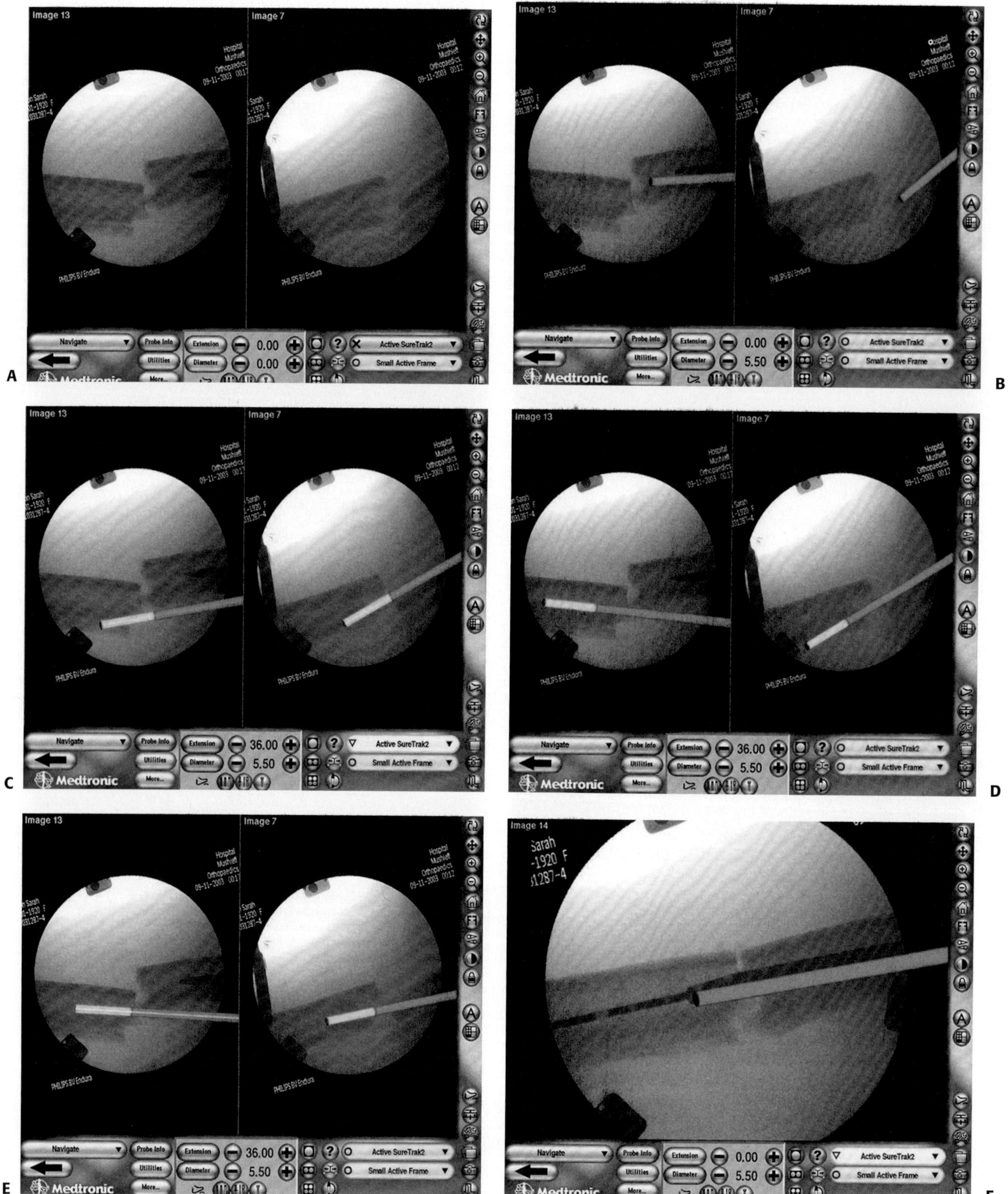

FIGURE 23-17 Fracture reduction. **A–E.** During the navigation process, the fracture is manipulated by the intramedullary fracture alignment device that has been inserted into the proximal fragment (represented by a darker line). Its virtual extrapolation (represented by a lighter line) is aimed toward the distal fragment. Note that the residual fluoroscopic image of the proximal fragment on the computer screen is not tracked and should be ignored. **(F)** Verification image of the aligned fracture after the insertion of guide wire. The overlapping of the verified location of the guide wire and the virtual image confirms the accuracy of the procedure.

canal of the proximal fragment, and advanced to the fracture site. At a later stage it will be used as a "joystick" for fracture reduction. The bone tracker is now moved into the distal segment of the fracture. Two fluoroscopic images (AP and lateral) of the distal fragment are taken and stored in the computer.

The position sensor tracks the intramedullary fracture alignment device based on the instrument tracker, and the distal fragment based on the bone tracker. Since the intramedullary device is located inside the proximal fragment, its image represents both the device and the bone around it as a single unit. Seemingly, the image seen on the computer screen displays the tracked instrument only, but it actually represents the proximal fragment surrounding it. This eliminates the need to fix a reference frame to the proximal fragment. The actual fracture reduction is then carried out by manipulating the proximal fragment, using the tracked intramedullary alignment device and directing its virtual image on the computer screen toward the medullary canal of the distal fragment. While performing navigation, the images seen on the computer screen during the reduction process are the virtual images of the device and the distal fragment. The fracture is reduced when both images are aligned on previously taken AP and lateral views (Fig. 23-17). At this point the reduction has been accomplished.

The above technique overcomes some of the drawbacks of the existing computer navigation systems. It is based on tracking standard available equipment for fracture reduction, thus eliminating the need for two separate bone trackers on fracture fragments. In the future, customized tracked instruments based on these principles will further improve and facilitate computer-assisted intramedullary nailing (30–33).

COMPLICATIONS AND CONTROVERSIES

The most frequent clinical and technical complications that lead to navigation errors and failure are as follows:

1. *Loss of line-of-sight*

   An unobstructed view between the optical camera and the trackers at all times is the basic requirement of optical navigation. Loss of line-of-sight occurs when the view between the optical camera and one or more of the trackers is obstructed by the surgeon or another member of the surgical team, by the patient's body, by the fluoroscopy C-arm, by the overhead lamps, or by any other object in the vicinity of the surgical field. When there is not line-of-sight, the tracker that is not seen either disappears from the display or the entire display freezes. Navigation resumes as soon as the obstruction disappears.

   Loss of line-of-sight can be remedied by moving the object causing the interference, by repositioning the optical camera, or by changing the surgical team's location around the patient. In some situations, due to the surgical approach, it is not possible to see all of the trackers at once. In this case, partial navigation is possible with the visible trackers. In some surgical situations, maintenance of the line-of-sight is not possible and therefore navigation should be avoided. As discussed previously, the surgeon can control some of the obstacles by appropriate placement of the trackers and the camera. Practically, this step should be considered as an integral part of the preplanning stage of CAOS-ST.

2. *Shift of the dynamic reference frame rigid bone mounting*

   Maintaining a rigid attachment between the bone tracker and the bone throughout surgery is essential in order to guarantee registration accuracy. The shift is usually the result of bone fixation loosening, poor jig fixation, unintentional pushing or hitting the tracker and its mounting jig. An undetected shift will result in inaccurate navigation images that might mislead the surgeon and lead to undesired results and complications. To avoid this situation, the surgeon should ensure that the tracker mounting jig is securely fixated to the bone structure.

   The only way to detect dynamic reference frame motion is by validation. Validation is done either by acquiring one or more fluoroscopic x-ray images and comparing them with the navigation images, or by touching with the tip of a surgical tool known anatomical landmarks and verifying that the tool tip appears close to the landmark in the navigated image. Validation should be performed at key points during surgery and always when in doubt.

3. *Tool decalibration*

   Tool decalibration occurs when the geometric data of the tracked tool does not match its actual geometry. Tool decalibration is caused by tool wear and tear, such as tip bending, frame deformation due to repeated sterilization, or tool tracker shift. To avoid this situation, the surgeon should verify the tool calibration before surgery, at key points during the surgery, and always when in doubt. Tool decalibration cannot automatically be detected. The surgeon must perform a tool calibration verification procedure, which usually involves the use of custom calibration hardware and software.

4. *Navigation of images' inaccuracy*

   Inaccuracy of navigation images is the mismatch between the displayed images and the intraoperative situation. The inaccuracy is the result of errors in the registration chain. The main causes of the errors include the shift of the dynamic reference frame, tool decalibration, and the shift of the C-arm tracker ring. Secondary causes include tracking system drift over time and navigation at the edge of the position sensor working volume. Other causes are related to the images themselves. For CT images, they include poor contrast, low slice resolution, insufficient radiation dose, large spacing between slices, patient motion during the CT scan, and blooming artifacts due to the presence of metallic objects. For fluoroscopic x-ray images, they include poor image resolution, poor contrast due to insufficient or excessive radiation, inappropriate viewpoints, and patient motion during image acquisition.

   The surgeon must realize that the acquired images serve

as the basis for the entire navigated surgical procedure (34). Therefore, optimization of these images (contrast, field, viewing angle, etc.) is crucial and should be done during the image acquisition stage, before moving on to surgery. Note that navigation images' inaccuracy can be observed by the surgeon but cannot automatically be detected. It requires performing validation tests for C-arm ring and dynamic reference frame shift, tool decalibration, restarting of the tracking system, repositioning of the position sensor, and the acquisition of new images.

5. *System robustness issues*

   Robustness is the ability of a system to perform its intended tasks with a minimum number of failures over time. The more robust the system, the more acceptable it will be for the surgeon. Robustness depends upon both the software and hardware components. Software failures include: flaws (bugs) in the computer operating system (e.g., Windows), flaws in the custom-designed software, and flaws in the tracking base unit controller. At best, software flaws can be temporarily overcome by restarting the system. At worst, they require preempting navigation and reporting the flaw to the company. Hardware failures include failure of the computer unit, poor cable connections, and failure of the tracking unit.

6. *Verification of surgical tool and implant spatial position*

   The surgeon should always remember to make a distinction between the virtual and nonvirtual situations displayed on the computer screen. This is of great importance especially because in trauma surgery the surgeon is used to working under fluoroscopic guidance that provides a true view of the surgical site instead of a virtual display in CAOS-ST procedures. For example, a perfect virtual position of a guide wire may be a false presentation of the real situation because during the insertion of the real guide wire it may slip or bend and point at a wrong position, without being detected or shown on the augmented image. There are several ways to tackle this critical obstacle. The best is to use rigid guide wires to prevent bending. Moreover, the first obstacle is penetrating the cortical bone in the right location. Experience and/or the use of rigid drills can usually overcome this problem. In addition, it is also very important to perform real-time fluoroscopic verification at critical or questionable time points during the surgical procedure.

7. *Adaptation to different surgical techniques*

   The main addition in computer-assisted navigation compared with conventional fluoroscopic trauma surgery is the bone-mounted reference frame. The significant ramifications of the loosening of the reference frame have previously been described. The actual location of this frame can interfere during the surgical procedure. For example, while inserting the reference frame screw into the bone diaphysis during intramedullary nailing, it should not penetrate the medullary canal. In addition, during the insertion of a locking screw the reference frame might be in the way and prevent either an accurate line-of-sight or the proper positioning of certain surgical instruments (such as drills). The surgeon must choose between placing the frame close to the operative site in order to increase accuracy of the procedure and to improve triangulation or placing the frame where it establishes a convenient working distance.

PERSPECTIVES

Technical Perspectives

Navigation systems are limited by technical elements. Currently, their main limitations, in decreasing order of importance, and perspectives for improvements are as follows:

1. *Support for implants and instrumentation*

   Navigation systems are designed to be used with specific tools, implants, and hardware from specific manufacturers. The choice of supported instruments and implants depends on the decisions made by the navigation and instrument companies, which are dictated mostly by commercial interests. Often, the software module only accepts models from one manufacturer. In some cases, tools from other manufacturers can be incorporated following a tool calibration procedure. Currently, only a handful of instruments and implants are supported.

2. *Support for surgical procedures*

   Navigation systems require software modules (software surgical protocols) that implement the surgical protocol for navigation for specific procedures. Without the custom software module for the surgical procedure, the navigation system cannot be used, although in principle it is technically feasible in procedures other than those for which they were designed. Currently, only a handful of procedures are supported.

3. *Improvements in the tracking technology*

   Current optical-tracking technology has several drawbacks, including line-of- sight, size of trackers, cables, number of trackers, accuracy, and cost. Magnetic tracking offers a variety of potential advantages, including: no line-of-sight requirement, reduced tracker size, and reduced cost. Although the technology is not as yet ready for routine clinical use, it is likely that most of the obstacles will be overcome in the near future, offering the possibility of tracking bone fragments and easing tracker fixation to the bone, thus significantly reducing or eliminating dynamic reference frame shift and opening the door for navigation during reduction.

4. *Image-based CT registration*

   Current CT-based navigation systems require the surgeon to acquire points on the surface of the anatomy of interest in order to perform the registration between the CT data set and the intraoperative situation. This precludes its use in percutaneous procedures, is time-consuming, error-prone, and produces suboptimal registration results. An alternative is to use fluoroscopic x-ray images instead of points harvested from the bone surface. This type of registration, called anatomy-based CT to fluoroscopic x-ray registration, has been demonstrated in the laboratory and will soon be available in navigation systems.

5. *Planning*
   Current intraoperative planning is either nonexistent or limited at best. Intraoperative definition of goals, such as screw path safety zone and insertion axis, can greatly help the surgeon perform the surgery. The blurring of the distinction between preoperative and intraoperative planning opens the door for better, more adaptive planning and consequently better and more consistent results.
6. *Spatial visualization without CT*
   A drawback of fluoroscopy-based navigation systems is that they do not show spatial views of the intraoperative situation, which can only be produced when CT data is available. To overcome this limitation, the following has been proposed: to acquire several fluoroscopic x-ray images and adapt a closely related CT or generic anatomical model to match the patient-specific fluoroscopic x-ray images. This approach, called atlas-based matching, is currently under investigation.

Clinical Perspectives

The use of computerized navigation systems in orthopaedic trauma surgery is rather new. The four main contributions to trauma surgery are:

1. Facilitates minimal invasive surgery (MIS) by reducing the soft tissue damage and thus shortening the postoperative rehabilitation process.
2. Improves the accuracy of implant and screw placement compared with that obtained with conventional methods and reduces outcome variability.
3. Significantly reduces radiation exposure to both the patient and the surgeon.
4. Creates a powerful educational and quality control tool.

Most of the contributions achieved so far are in the preplanning stage. If we take, for instance, the imaging field, it is clear that computerized imaging supplies a better three-dimensional understanding that may influence the planning of the surgical procedure. Undoubtedly, this new technology can and should change our way of thinking in relation to other stages of surgical treatment.

It is quite obvious that computerized navigation systems are continuously advancing and offer additional possibilities. Although these systems are taking their first steps, it seems that they have already managed to change the setting in trauma centers. The CT suite can be transformed into an operating room, or alternatively, the modern high-tech fluoroscope can now be altered to produce three-dimensional images. Basically, these modern available technologies on one hand, and surgeons' preferences and compliance on the other, will in the future determine the setup of the operating room, where it will be situate. The next generation of computerized navigation systems will be characterized not only by improved accuracy but also in diminishing the robustness and improving working convenience in the computerized environment. When these changes finally take place it is expected that computerized technology will be of assistance not only in navigation but also in the execution of the surgical procedure by means of robots (35).

If the trauma surgeon can overcome the difficulties entailed in integrating the new technology in spite of its initial cumbersomeness, we may experience a revolution in surgical approaches and education.

GLOSSARY

General

CAS: Computer-Aided Surgery. The planning and execution of a surgery with the help of a computer system. Synonyms: **Computer-Assisted Surgery**, **Computer-Integrated Surgery**, **CIS**, **Image-Guided Surgery**, **IGS**, **surgical navigation**.

CAOS: Computer-Aided Orthopaedic Surgery. The planning and execution of an orthopaedic surgery with the help of a computer system.

CAOS-ST: Computer-Aided Orthopaedic Surgery for Skeletal Trauma. The planning and execution of skeletal trauma orthopaedic surgery with the help of a computer system.

Planning

Model: a computer representation of the relevant characteristics (e.g., shape, location, main axis) of an object of interest (e.g., a bone, bone fragment, surgical instrument, implant, fixation plate, cutting plane). Synonyms: **digital template**.

Preoperative planning: the process of creating a computerized plan for the purposes of surgery.

Surface mesh: a geometric description of a bone surface consisting of a collection of interconnected points, usually extracted from CT data. Synonyms: **surface model.**

Navigation

CT-based navigation: navigation with images created by superimposing on a preoperative CT cross sections and spatial images the surgical tool silhouette and updating its location in real time.

Fluoroscopy-based navigation: navigation with images created by superimposing on conventional fluoroscopic images the surgical tool silhouette and updating its location in real time, thereby creating the impression of continuous fluoroscopy without the ensuing radiation. Synonyms: **virtual fluoroscopy, augmented fluoroscopy**.

Guidance: the process of indicating in real time to the surgeon, via images, graphics, or sound, the best course of action during surgery.

Navigation: the process of determining the spatial location of surgical instruments and anatomical structures in real time for the purposes of guiding surgical gestures during surgery.

Navigation images: images created by a navigation system for the purposes of navigation. Synonyms: **active display, navigation display, real-time visualization**.

Navigation system: a system that shows the current location of surgical instruments with respect to images of the anatomy and continuously updates this image as the instruments and bone structures move. It requires tracking, registration, visualization, and validation. Synonyms: **surgical navigator**, **guidance system**.

Tracking

Line-of-sight: a basic requirement of optical tracking systems in which there must be no occluding objects between the position sensor and the trackers.

Marker: basic element recognized by the position sensor; can be an LED or a reflective sphere. Synonym: **infrared light-emitting diode, IRED**.

Position sensor: a system that determines the spatial location of the trackers at any moment in time. It is an *optical camera* for optical systems and a *magnetic field generator* for magnetic systems. Synonym: **localizer**.

Tracked pointer: a pointer with a tracker used for pointing and probing during navigation. Synonyms: **digitizing probe**.

Tracker: a rigid body with markers that are recognized by the position sensor. Synonym: **optical localizer**, **3-D localizer**, **sensor, marker carrier**.

Tracker mounting jigs: mechanical jigs, such as screws and clamps, used to rigidly attach trackers to surgical instruments and bone structures, whose purpose is to mechanically fix their positional relationship. Synonym: **attachment.**

Tracking: the process of determining in real time the spatial location of moving objects. Synonym: **localization**.

Tracking base unit: the unit that controls and processes the information from the position sensor and the trackers. Synonym: **tracking data acquisition unit**.

Tracking system: a system that obtains the position and orientation of trackers by measuring spatially dependent physical properties, such as optical and magnetic properties. Synonym: **localization system**.

Tracking technology: the physical means by which the location of trackers is measured. Tracking technology is optical or magnetic. *Optical tracking* is *active* (light-emitting diodes), *passive* (reflective spheres), or *hybrid* (both active and passive), also called *semi-active*. Synonym: **localization technology**.

Tracking work volume: volume of space covered by the position sensor in which measurements can be made. Synonym: **measurement volume**.

Accuracy

Accuracy: the measure of an instrument's capability to approach a true or absolute value. Static accuracy refers to measurements that do not change over time, whereas dynamic accuracy refers to time-varying measurements. Accuracy is a function of both bias and precision.

Bias: a measure of how closely the mean value in a series of replicate measurements approaches the true value.

Frequency: the number of overall measurements per second. Static accuracy refers to measurements obtained when the trackers are at rest, while dynamic accuracy refers to measurements obtained as the trackers move. Synonyms: **rate, frame rate, display rate**.

Precision: a measure of how closely the values within a series of replicate measurements agree with each other.

Repeatability: a measure of resolution and stability. Resolution is the smallest discernable difference between two measurements. Stability refers to measurements made at steady state and over a sufficiently long period of time.

Registration

Coordinate frame: a fixed reference within which the spatial locations of objects can be described. Each object of interest has its own coordinate frame. Synonyms: **coordinate system**, **COS**.

CT registration: the process of establishing a common reference frame between the preoperative CT images and the intraoperative situation. Synonyms: **point registration, surface registration, contact registration**.

Dynamic reference frame: the tracker attached to the bone used to track the bone motions to determine the relative location of the bone with respect to the tool. Synonyms: **reference**, **reference base**, **dynamic reference base**, **DRB**, **dynamic referencing**.

Location: the six parameters determining the position and orientation of an object in space. Synonyms: **placement, degrees-of-freedom, DOF**.

Registration: the process of establishing a common reference frame between objects and images. Synonyms: **alignment**.

Registration chain: a series of transformations that relate the locations of objects in space.

Tool calibration: the process of computing the transformation and the tool's geometric features, such as its main axis and its tip position. Tool calibration verification is the process of comparing the actual and computed calibration. The *tool calibration unit* is the device used for calibrating tools.

Transformation: a mathematical description of the relation between the locations of two objects. Transformations are static (constant) when the relative locations of the objects do not change, dynamic otherwise. There are four types of transformations: *tracking transformations, tools transformations, image transformations,* and *display transformations*.

Visualization

Silhouette: the projection of the contours of a 3-D object onto a plane.

Viewpoint: the location from which navigation images are created.

Visualization: the process of creating, manipulating, and displaying images showing the location of objects in space.

Validation

Validation: the process of verifying that the navigation images match the clinical intra-operative situation. There are three types of validation: *tool calibration validation, dynamic reference frame validation,* and *registration accuracy validation*. Synonym: **verification**.

REFERENCES

1. Taylor R, Lavallee S, Burdea C, et al. *Computer-integrated surgery: technology and clinical applications*. Boston: The MIT Press, 1995.
2. Lavallee S, Sautot P, Troccaz J, et al. Computer-assisted spine surgery: a technique for accurate transpedicular screw fixation using CT data and a 3-D optical localizer. *Comput Aided Surg (formerly J Image Guid Surg)* 1995;1(1):65–73.
3. Nolte LP, Ganz R. *Computer assisted orthopaedic surgery*. Bern: Hogrefe and Huber Publishers, 1999.
4. Hazan E. Computer aided orthopaedic surgery: special issue. *Tech Orthop* 2003;18(2).
5. Liebergall M, Mosheiff R, Segal D. Navigation in orthopedic trauma. *Oper Tech Orthop* 2003;13(2):64–72.
6. Nolte L, Beutler T. Basic principles of CAOS. *Injury* 2004;35[Suppl 1]:6–16.
7. Ellis R, Tso CY, Rudan JF, et al. Computer aided high tibial open wedge osteotomy. *Injury* 2004;35[Suppl 1]:S-A68–S-A78.
8. Keppler P, Gebhard F, Grutzner P, et al. A surgical planning and guidance system for high tibial osteotomy. *Comput Aided Surg* 1999;4(5):264–274.
9. Hajnal J, Hill D, Hawkes D. *Medical image registration*. Boca Raton: CRC Press, 2001.
10. Livyatan H, Yaniv Z, Joskowicz L. Robust automatic C-arm calibration for fluoroscopy-based navigation: a practical approach. *Proceeding. 5th International Conference on Medical Computing and Computer-Aided Intervention. Lecture Notes in Computer Science* 2488, Springer 2002;2:60–68.
11. Euler E, Heining T, Fischer T, et al. Initial clinical experiences with the SIREMOBIL Iso-3^D. *Electromedica* 2002;70(1):48–51.
12. Grutzner PA, Hebecker A, Waelti H, et al. Clinical study for registration-free 3D navigation with the SIREMOBIL Iso-3^D mobile C-arm. *Electromedica* 2003;71(1):6–15.
13. Kahler DM. Computer-assisted closed techniques of reduction and fixation. In: Tile M, Helfet D, Kellam J, eds. *Surgery of the pelvis and acetabulum*. Philadelphia: Lippincott Williams & Wilkins, 2003:604–615.
14. Kahler DM. Computer assisted fixation of acetabular fractures and pelvic ring disruptions. *Tech Orthop* 2000;10(1):20–24.
15. Crowl AC, Kahler DM. Closed reduction and percutaneous fixation of anterior column acetabular fractures. *Comput Aided Surg* 2002;7(3):169–178.
16. Mosheiff R, Khoury A, Weil Y, et al. First generation of fluoroscopic navigation in percutaneous pelvic surgery. *J Orthop Trauma* 2004;18(2):106–111.
17. Stockle U, Krettek C, Pohlemann T, et al. Clinical applications—pelvis. *Injury* 2004; 35[Suppl 1]:46–56.
18. Ben-David D, Mosheiff R, Weil Y, et al. The role of computerized navigation in fixating femoral neck fractures. *4th Annual Meeting of CAOS–International Proceedings*, 2004, Chicago:118–120.
19. Weil Y, Liebergall M, Khoury A, et al. The use of computerized fluoroscopic navigation for removal of pelvic screws. *Am J Orthop* 2004;33(8):384–385.
20. Mosheiff R, Weil Y, Khoury A, et al. The use of computerized navigation in the treatment of gunshot and shrapnel injury. *Comput Aided Surg* 2004;9:39–44.
21. Weil Y, Mosheiff R, Simanovsky N, et al. The use of fluoroscopy based navigation systems for placement of screws in slipped femoral capital epiphysis—a novel surgical technique. *23rd Annual Meeting of the Israeli Orthopaedic Association*, 2003, Tel Aviv: 122–125.
22. Hinsche AF, Giannoudis PV, Smith RM. Fluoroscopy based multi-planar image guidance for insertion of sacroiliac screws. *Clin Orthop* 2002;395:135–144.
23. Gautier E, Bachler R, Heini PF, et al. Accuracy of computer-guided screw fixation of the sacroiliac joint. *Clin Orthop* 2001;393:310–317.
24. Borrelli J, Peele M, Ricci WM, et al. Validation of CT-reconstructed images for the evaluation of acetabular fractures. Proceedings of the American Academy of Orthopedic Surgery 2004, San Francisco: 610.
25. Hazan E, Joskowicz L. Computer-assisted image-guided intramedullary nailing of femoral shaft fractures. *Tech Orthop* 2003;18(2):191–201.
26. Joskowicz L, Milgrom C, Simkin A, et al. FRACAS: a system for computer-aided image-guided long bone fracture surgery. *Comput Aided Surg* 1999;3(6):271–288.
27. Kahler DM. Virtual fluoroscopy: a tool for decreasing radiation exposure during femoral intramedullary nailing. *Stud Health Technol Inform* 2001;81:225–228.
28. Slomczykowski MA, Hofstetter R, Sati M, et al. Novel computer-assisted fluoroscopy system for intraoperative guidance: feasibility study for distal locking of femoral nails. *J Orthop Trauma* 2001;15:122–131.
29. Suhm N, Jacob AL, Nolte LP, et al. Surgical navigation based on fluoroscopy: clinical application for computer-assisted distal locking of intramedullary implants. *Comput Aided Surg* 2000;5(6):391–400.
30. Mosheiff R, Weil Y, Peleg E, Liebergall M. Computerized navigation for closed reduction during femoral intermedullary nailing. *4th Annual Meeting of CAOS–International Proceedings*, 2004, Chicago: 386–388.
31. Hofstetter R, Slomczykowski M, Krettek C, et al. Computer-assisted fluoroscopy-based reduction of femoral fractures and anteversion correction. *Comput Aided Surg* 2000;5(5): 311–325.
32. Hufner T, Pohlemann T, Tarte S, et al. Computer-assisted fracture reduction of pelvic ring fractures: an in vitro study. *Clin Orthop* 2002;399:231–239.
33. Schmucki D, Gebhard F, Grutzner P, et al. Computer aided reduction and imaging. *Injury* 2004;35 [Suppl 1]:96–104.
34. Langlotz F. Potential pitfalls of computer aided orthopedic surgery. *Injury* 2004;35[Suppl 1]:17–23.
35. Taylor RH. Medical robotics: special issue. *IEEE Trans. on Robotics and Automation* 2003; 19(5).

SECTION

TWO

UPPER EXTREMITY

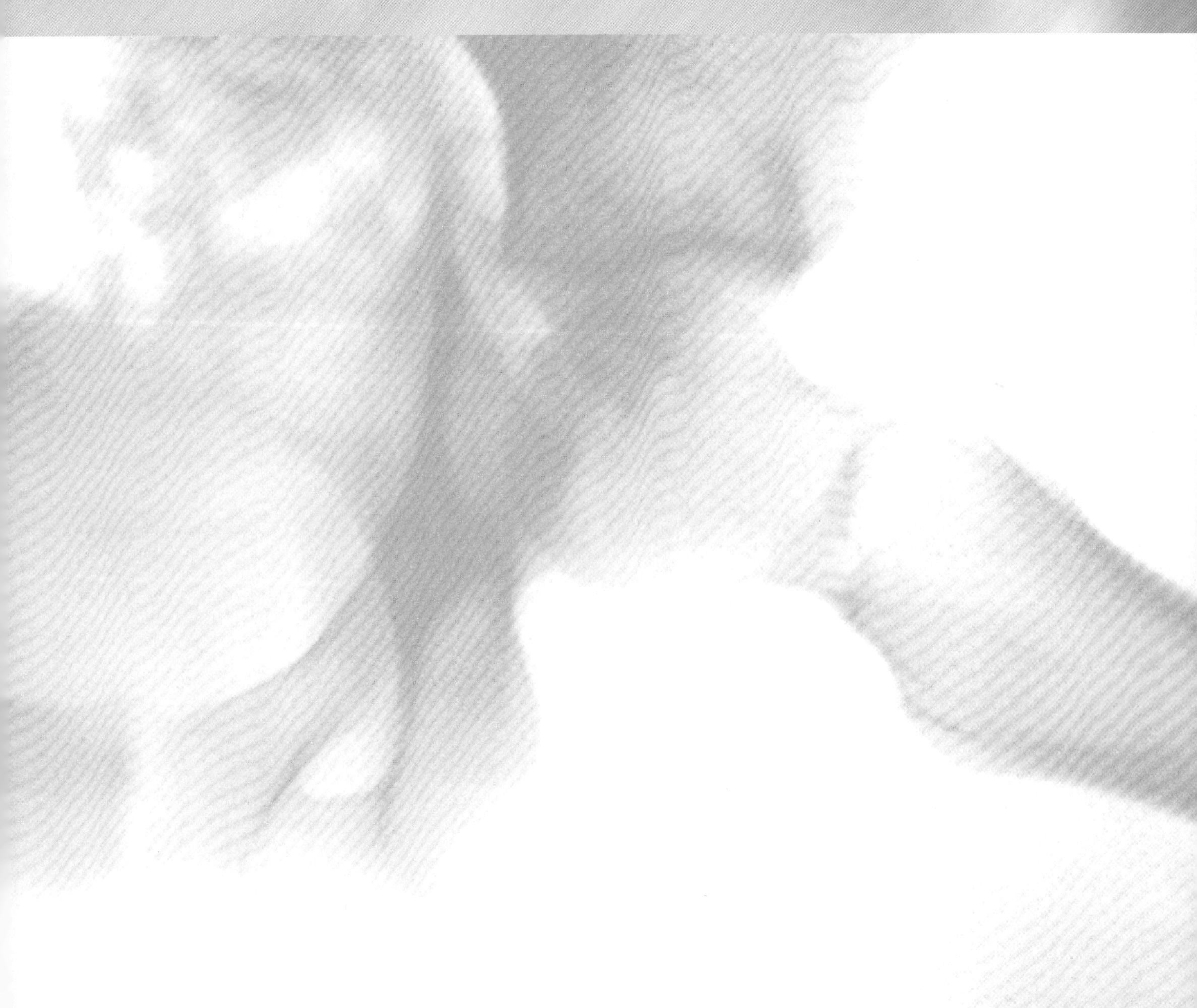

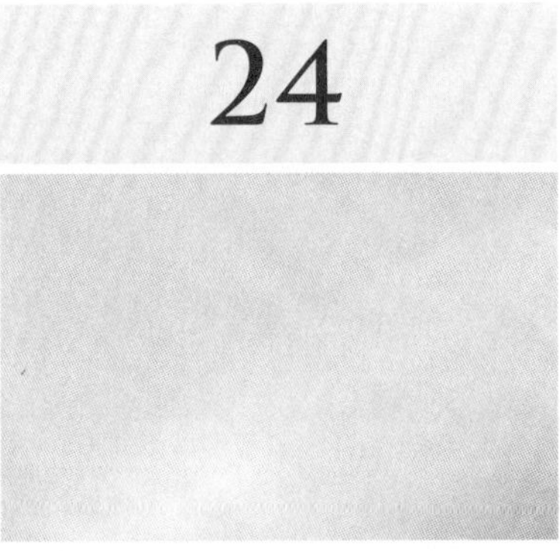

FRACTURES AND DISLOCATIONS OF THE HAND

Mark H. Henry

Fractures and dislocations of the hand are some of the most frequently encountered orthopaedic injuries. The 1998 United States National Hospital Ambulatory Medical Care Survey found phalangeal (23%) and metacarpal (18%) fractures to be the second and third most common hand and forearm fractures following radius fractures (1). They constitute anywhere from 1.5% to 28% of all emergency department visits depending on survey methods (1–3). In a stable population of 215,000 persons, 1,300 hand fractures per year occurred (representing 17.5% of all fractures throughout the body) (4). Phalangeal fractures comprised 46% of the hand fractures, metacarpal fractures 36%, and fifth metacarpal neck fractures 9.7%. Another series of 1,358 fractures reported the distribution as 57.4% proximal phalanx, 30.4% middle phalanx, and 12.2% metacarpal (5). Of 502 phalangeal fractures, 192 were at the proximal phalanx (P1), 195 at the middle phalanx (P2), and 115 at the distal phalanx (P3) (6). Expenses to society run between $3,000 and $22,000 per injured patient when accounting for costs of medical treatment combined with lost productivity in the workplace (7). Male to female ratios run from 1.8:1 to 5.4:1 with higher ratios seen in the age groups associated with the greatest incidence (sports injuries in the early 3rd decade and workplace injuries in the 5th decade).

The potential for functional loss that can occur is often under appreciated. The most common complication is stiffness. Only a few patterns of dislocation lead to residual instability. Fractures, however, can easily result in malunion. Some practitioners perceive a direct trade off between stiffness and either residual instability or malunion. This is not necessarily the case. As the understanding of these difficult injuries improves along with new surgical techniques, it is becoming increasingly possible to achieve good hand function while avoiding complications for most isolated fractures and dislocations. Major hand trauma is another matter.

PRINCIPLES OF MANAGEMENT

Perhaps one of the most fundamental principles of management is that the negative effects of surgery on the tissues should not exceed the negative effects of the original injury. Accordingly, nonoperative treatment plays a significant role in the management of fractures and dislocations of the hand. A corollary to this principle is that even though fractures and dislocations are fundamentally skeletal injuries, most of the difficult decision making centers on management of the soft tissues. The injured part must not be considered in isolation. The multiple joints of the hand are maintained in a delicate balance by the intrinsic and extrinsic tendon systems such that a disturbance in one set of tissues will often significantly affect others.

Mechanism of Injury

The history of the mechanism of injury should reveal the magnitude, direction, point of application, and type of force that caused the injury. A high degree of variation in mechanism of injury accounts for the broad spectrum of patterns seen in skeletal trauma sustained by the hand. Axial load or "jamming" injuries are frequently sustained during ball sports or sudden reaches made during everyday activities such as to catch a falling object. Patterns frequently resulting from this mechanism are shearing articular fractures or metaphyseal compression fractures. Axial loading along the upper extremity must also make one suspicious of associated injuries to the carpus, forearm, elbow, and shoulder girdle. Diaphyseal fractures and joint dislocations usually require a bending component in the mechanism of injury, which can occur during ball handling sports or when the hand is trapped by an object and unable to move with the rest of the arm. Individual digits can easily be caught in clothing, furniture, or workplace equipment to sustain torsional mechanisms of injury, resulting in spiral fractures or more complex dislocation patterns. Industrial settings or other environments with heavy objects and high forces lead to crushing mechanisms that combine bending, shearing, and torsion to produce unique patterns of skeletal injury and significant associated soft tissue damage.

Fracture Reduction

Reduction maneuvers should not cause added tissue trauma. If the injury is reducible at all, gentle manipulation will accomplish the reduction far more successfully than forceful longitudinal traction. The principle is relaxation of deforming forces through proximal joint positioning such as metacarpophalangeal (MP) joint flexion to relax the intrinsics or wrist flexion to relax the digital flexor tendons. Often a gentle back and forth rotatory maneuver is necessary to free a bony prominence from soft tissue entrapment. The mobile distal part is then reduced to the stable proximal part.

Splinting

Splints should immobilize the minimum number of joints possible and allow unrestricted motion of all other joints. One controversial point concerns the need to immobilize the wrist. Setting appropriate length tension relationships in the extrinsic motors (in cases where they are deforming forces) is most easily accomplished through immobilization of the wrist in 25 to 35 degrees of extension. This is extremely helpful in patients with low pain tolerance who tend to place the hand in a characteristic dysfunctional posture of wrist flexion–MP joint extension–interphalangeal (IP) joint flexion (the "wounded paw" position). Other patients who are capable of avoiding this position on their own often do not need wrist immobilization. A simple splint that is useful for injuries ranging from the carpometacarpal (CMC) joints proximally to P1 fractures distally consists of a single slab of plaster or fiberglass applied dorsally. With a foundation at the forearm, the splint runs out to the level of the proximal interphalangeal (PIP) joints distally with the wrist extended and MP joints fully flexed (Fig. 24-1C). Full motion of the IP joints should be encouraged throughout the healing process. The total duration of immobilization should rarely exceed 3 to 4 weeks. Hand fractures are stable enough by this time to tolerate active range of motion (AROM) with further remodeling by 8 to 10 weeks (8).

Signs and Symptoms

Symptoms associated with a fracture or dislocation of the hand include pain, swelling, stiffness, weakness, deformity, and loss of coordination. Numbness and tingling signify associated nerve involvement (either direct injury to the nerve or as a secondary effect of swelling). Signs include tenderness, swelling, ecchymosis, deformity, crepitus, and instability. A better skeletal examination can often be obtained with the aid of anesthesia applied directly at the injury site or regionally. Isolated MP joint dislocations and metacarpal fractures can be treated with direct injection of anesthetic into the injury site. More distal injuries are easily anesthetized with a digital block. More global pain relief can be obtained through nerve blocks performed at the wrist to include the median nerve, ulnar nerve, and dorsal cutaneous branches of the radial and ulnar nerves. Addition of 1 cc of hyaluronidase (Wydase) to the 1% lidocaine solution enhances the completeness of the anesthetic and minimizes local edema formation. Addition of 1 cc of 10% bicarbonate solution will reduce the acidity of the lidocaine and the pain associated with injection. The time following administration of the anesthetic can be used to cleanse any superficial wounds and to prepare splinting supplies. Pain-free demonstration of tendon excursion and fracture and ligament stability can then be performed. At the conclusion of the anesthetized skeletal exam, the injury can be promptly reduced and splinted.

An important factor in many treatment algorithms is the presence of rotational deformity. The examiner must understand the appropriate method of assessment. The bones of the hand are short tubular structures. Malrotation at one bone segment is best represented by the alignment of the next more distal segment. This alignment is best demonstrated when the intervening joint is flexed to 90 degrees (Fig. 24-2). Comparing nail plate alignment is an inadequate method of evaluating rotation. Other unique physical examination findings will be discussed in association with specific injuries.

Associated Injuries

Open Injuries

The integument is easily damaged, and open fractures are common. Open wounds should not be probed in the emergency department; doing so only drives the surface contaminants deeper and rarely yields useful information. The need for prophylactic antibiotics in open hand fractures is controversial. Ancef remains the standard for most fractures. Aminoglycosides are added for contaminated wounds and penicillin for soil or farm environments. No hard evidence exists to support continuation beyond the initial 24 hours.

The distal phalanx directly supports the nail matrix. With substantial displacement of the dorsal cortex, matrix disruption should be expected and direct repair planned. Reconstruction of residual open wounds overlying skeletal injury sites requires the use of flaps. Frequently transposition flaps will suffice. Less frequently, pedicle or free flaps will prove necessary. The greatest challenge in the hand, and particularly the digit, is to achieve both thin and supple tissue coverage. A fascial flap covered with a split thickness skin graft provides this combination of features but may not facilitate subsequent reconstructive surgeries as well as a cutaneous flap (Fig. 24-3).

Tendons

Closed extensor tendon ruptures at points of insertion near joints may accompany dislocations. Prime examples are terminal tendon ruptures sustained in association with distal interphalangeal (DIP) joint injuries and central slip ruptures sustained in association with PIP joint injuries. Initial examination of the traumatized hand must include a survey that inventories each potential tendon injury. Apart from these, tendon damage usually only occurs with high energy crush mechanisms or in open combined injuries.

Nerves and Vessels

Apart from open combined injuries, these tissues are rarely injured as part of simple fractures and dislocations of the hand. In major open hand trauma, there is usually a significant zone of injury. Appropriate treatment includes excision of the devitalized tissues in the zone of injury including nerve and vessel tissues followed by reconstruction with autogenous grafts or adjacent transfers.

Combined Injuries

The term *combined injuries* refers to the association of a hand fracture with injury to at least one of the soft tissues listed above. These are most often open injuries with the soft tissue component of greatest significance being the injury to flexor tendons, extensor tendons, or both. The occurrence of this combined pattern of injury directly impacts the treatment strategy for the fracture

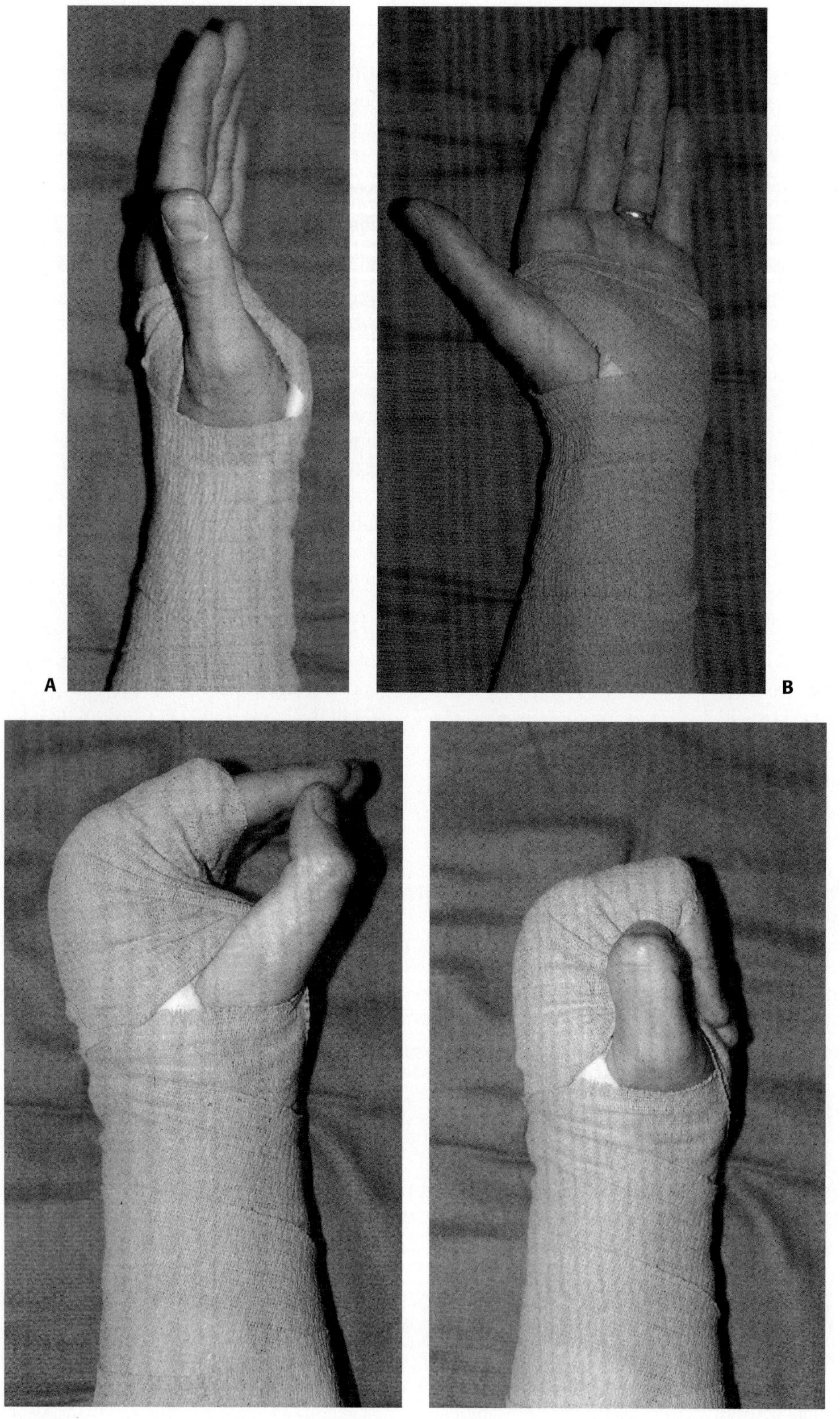

FIGURE 24-1 If a two-piece splint is chosen, the first slab of fiberglass is applied to the volar wrist in extension **(A)**, taking care to only go to the proximal rather than the distal wrist crease **(B)**. **C.** The second part, which can be used by itself, is applied dorsally with the MP joints in full flexion. **D.** The PIP joints should be left free for motion rehabilitation.

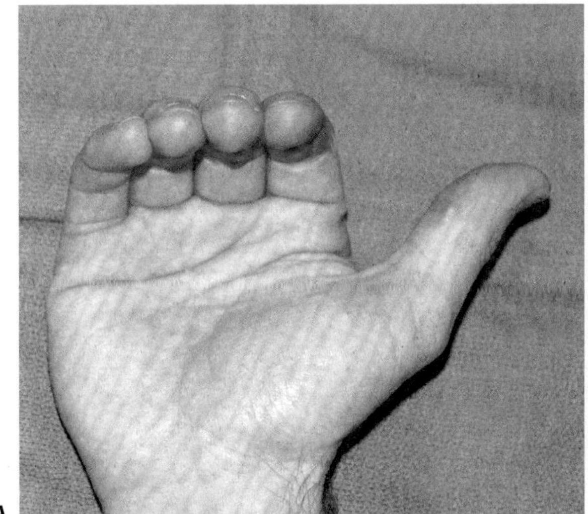

A

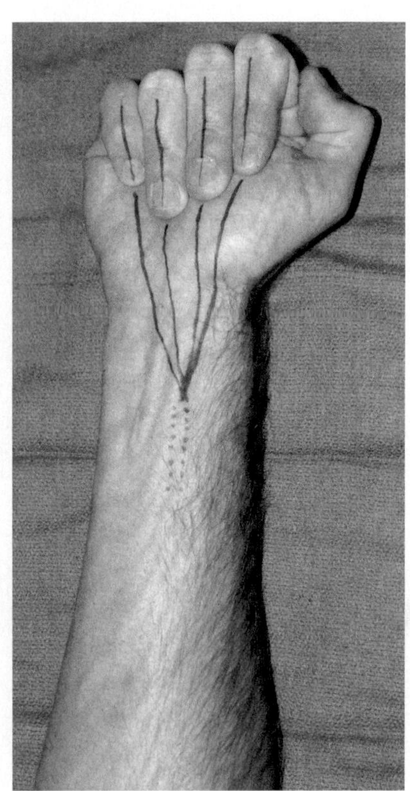

B

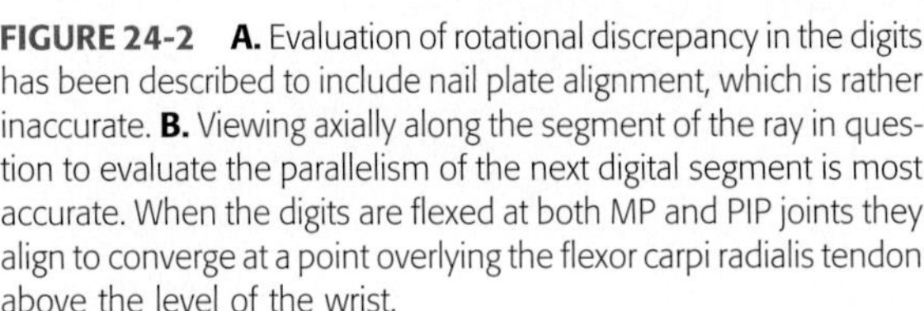

FIGURE 24-2 **A.** Evaluation of rotational discrepancy in the digits has been described to include nail plate alignment, which is rather inaccurate. **B.** Viewing axially along the segment of the ray in question to evaluate the parallelism of the next digital segment is most accurate. When the digits are flexed at both MP and PIP joints they align to converge at a point overlying the flexor carpi radialis tendon above the level of the wrist.

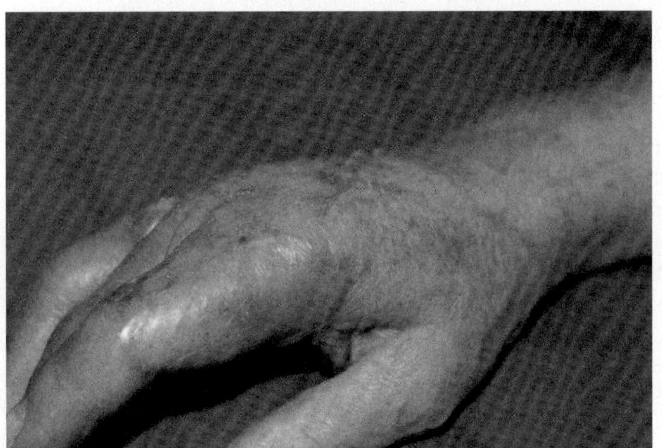

A

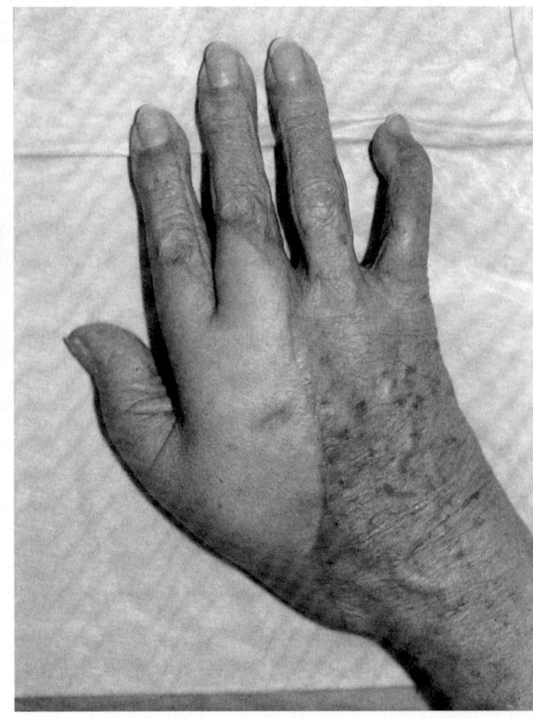

B

FIGURE 24-3 Thin supple coverage of open hand trauma wounds can be accomplished with thinner fascial flaps covered with a split thickness skin graft **(A)** or bulkier cutaneous or fasciocutaneous flaps **(B)**. (*continues*)

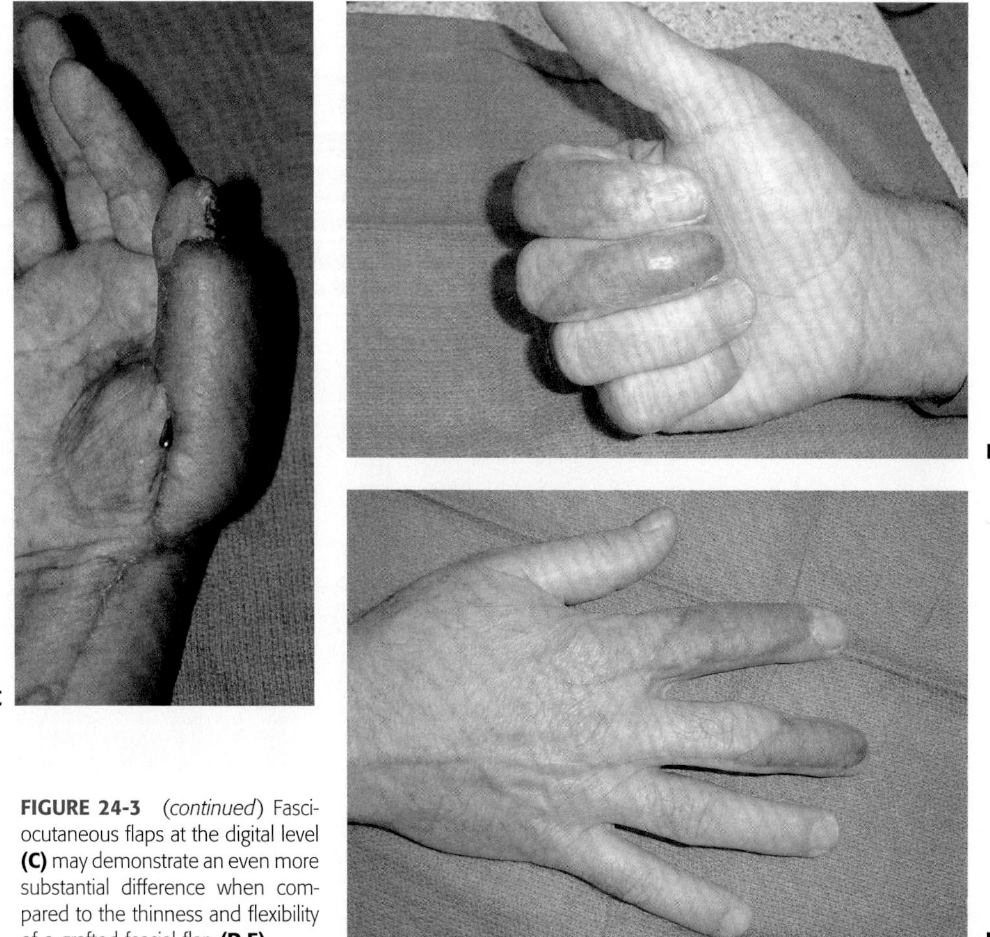

FIGURE 24-3 *(continued)* Fasciocutaneous flaps at the digital level **(C)** may demonstrate an even more substantial difference when compared to the thinness and flexibility of a grafted fascial flap **(D,E)**.

itself. Many fracture patterns in their own right as an isolated injury would be best cared for nonoperatively or with closed reduction and internal fixation using smooth stainless steel Kirschner wires (K-wires). The open wound leading to the fracture site automatically changes the surgical approach to open reduction. The presence of an adjacent tendon repair site necessitates achieving skeletal stability sufficient to withstand the forces of an immediate tendon glide rehabilitation program. This often means the use of rigid internal fixation (Fig. 24-4). The remainder of this chapter describes the most appropriate techniques for managing fractures and dislocations of the hand as isolated injuries since this is how they present 98.6% of the time (9). The term, combined injuries, will be found associated with the more stable fixation options as part of the indications for treatment tables when listed throughout the chapter.

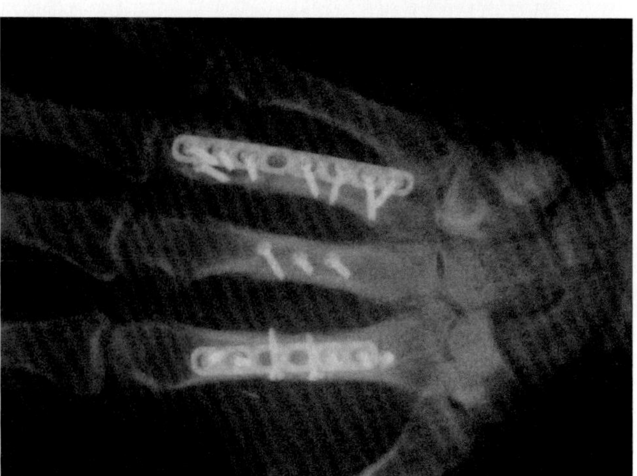

FIGURE 24-4 Major open hand trauma frequently requires the most stable forms of fixation to facilitate an aggressive early motion rehabilitation program focusing on tendon gliding.

Massive Hand Trauma

The comprehensive planning required for treatment of massive hand trauma merits a textbook in its own right and is beyond the scope of this chapter. Excellent reviews are available from Levin and Condit (10) and Freeland and Jabaley (11). The majority of the complex decision-making in these injuries occurs with respect to the strategy chosen for the soft tissues (Fig. 24-5). Clinical evaluation of these injuries is quite difficult because the patient is often unable or unwilling to do very much with respect to an interactive examination. Much of the determination regarding the extent of injury is made intra-operatively. Retrospective analysis has correlated the return to work with the initial results of the Hand Injury Scoring System, which considers injury to the integument, skeleton, motor system, and nerves (12). Good-quality radiographs are rarely obtained initially and usually consist of semi-oblique views of the hand with a high degree of bone overlap. Every effort should be made within the scope of total patient management to obtain additional x-ray views that can be set up properly so that associated injuries are not missed. More often than not the opportunity for these views first presents itself in the operating room. A very easy pitfall is to draw attention to the most obvious radiographic findings without taking the time to search for more subtle injuries. X-ray evidence of foreign matter embedded in the hand should be sought as well as its absence at the conclusion of the debridement.

The Gustilo classification of open fractures has been modified for the hand by reducing the 10 cm wound length threshold to 2 cm. The validity of the classification is supported by 62.5% normal hand function found after type I injuries compared to 21% following type III fractures (13). Another series found 92% poor results associated with grade III B and C injuries (14). From a series of 200 open hand fractures, Swanson (15) differentiated type II wounds from type I wounds by three criteria: contamination at initial presentation, open for more than 24 hours before treatment, or in patients with systemic illness. Type II wounds are not recommended for primary closure.

Both internal and external fixation may be appropriate in massive hand injuries. Standard indications for external fixation include gross contamination of the original wound, segmental bone loss or comminution, or the lack of availability of good soft tissue coverage (16–23). The biomechanics of external fixation in the hand are the same as elsewhere in the body with pin diameter constituting the chief determinant of fixator stiffness (23,24). Four pins are sufficient for hand applications. Twenty-seven patients with external fixation had a single pin tract infection and 91% primary healing by an average of 7 weeks (25). Another series found a 7.5% incidence of mechanical failure through clamp loosening with pin reactions seen in 2.5% of cases at the phalangeal level and in 9.8% of cases at the metacarpal level (21). A given hand injury may best be fixed by all internal, all external, or a combination of the two methods of fixation. An improved understanding and wider array of elegant soft tissue coverage techniques have overcome previous concerns regarding exposure of hardware with internal fixation.

Whenever the injury involves the first web space (especially with crush injuries) the thumb and index metacarpals should be pinned into abduction to prevent contracture (26). No matter how the injury is managed, the strategy should plan for rehabilitation to begin, unobstructed by bulky external dressings, by

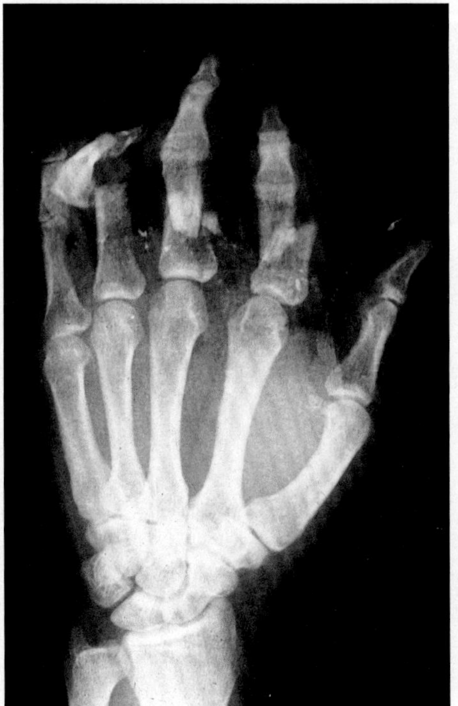
A

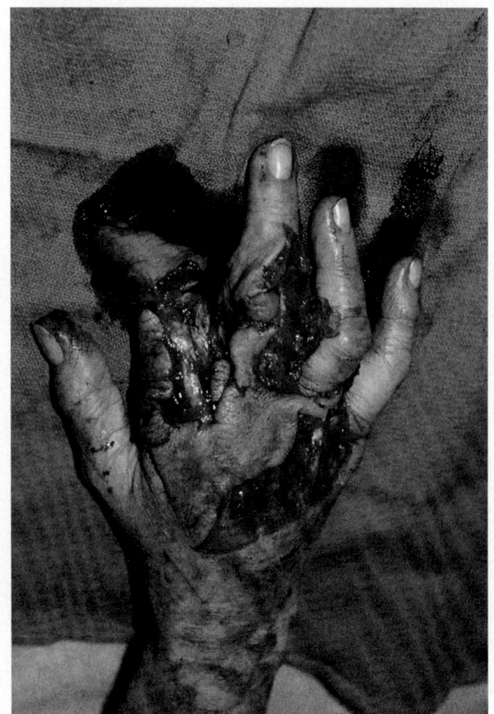
B

FIGURE 24-5 Massive crush trauma to the hand usually causes its most devastating effects, not to the skeletal elements themselves, but rather diffusely through devitalization of the soft tissues covering the bone.

72 hours after surgery. Seventy-two metacarpal and phalangeal fractures with severe associated soft tissue injury were treated with plates and screws yielding 46% good, 32% fair, and 22% poor results by the American Society for Surgery of the Hand (ASSH) criteria of total active motion (TAM) (27). The overall results for treatment of these severe injuries are most closely related to the soft tissue component rather than the status of the skeletal injury. In 245 open injuries studied prospectively, extensor tendon injury alone had 50% poor results, but flexor tendon or multiple soft tissue injuries produced 80% poor results (28). A series of 140 open fractures demonstrated better results at the metacarpal compared to the phalangeal level with the worst outcomes occurring for injuries at the P1 and PIP level, especially when associated with an overlying tendon injury (14).

Bone Loss

Segmental bone loss is a frequent finding in massive hand injuries. Once the wound has been rendered clean through either a single or multiple debridements, bone grafting is appropriate using corticocancellous iliac crest, shaped and sized to match the curvature of the missing segment. If only mild comminution is present without loss of structural stability, cancellous graft alone is sufficient (29). Stable fixation is achieved with either internal plate (Fig. 24-6) or external fixator application. Delayed

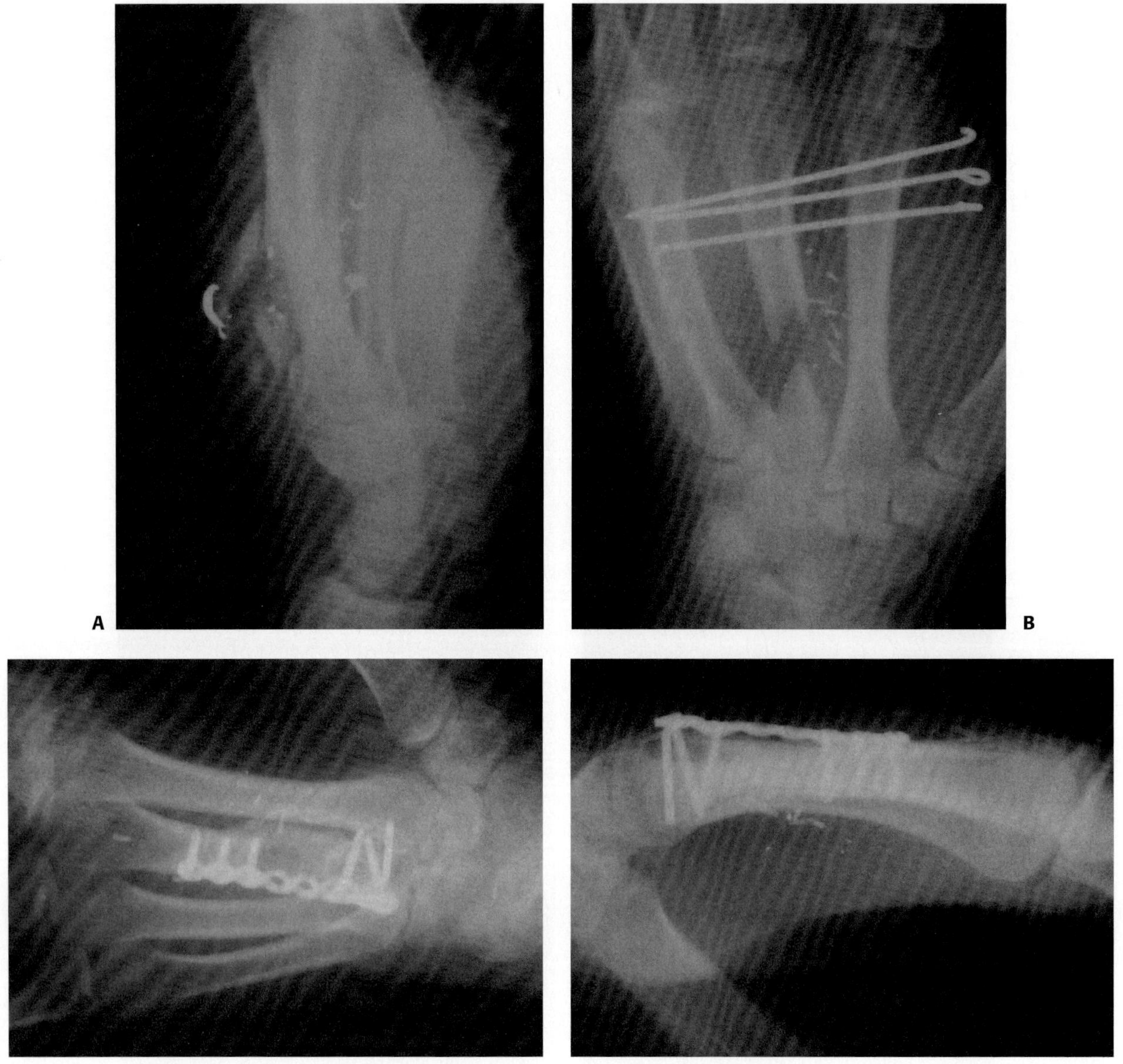

FIGURE 24-6 When segmental bone loss occurs **(A)**, shortening may be prevented by temporary stabilization **(B)**. Subsequent internal fixation **(C,D)** and bone grafting can restore the original anatomic parameters of the skeletal unit.

primary bone grafting following debridement is safe with no deep infections reported in two series of 21 and 64 fractures (29,30). If delayed bone grafting is planned, a temporary spacer may be used to preserve the volume that will later be occupied by the graft (Fig. 24-7). A series of 28 patients suffering gunshot wounds with bone loss were treated by early stable fixation resulting in 100% union and TAM of 200 degrees (213 degrees for extra-articular injuries and 169 degrees for intra-articular injuries) (29). Bone loss that includes the articular surface represents an entirely different and much more difficult problem. Strategies that have been advocated include autografts of metatarsal head, second, and third CMC joints, immediate Silastic prosthetic replacement, osteoarticular allografts, primary arthrodesis, and free vascularized composite whole toe joint transfer (31–35). A series of seven osteochondral rib grafts healed by 2 months and yielded a PIP joint range of motion (ROM) of 64 degrees (36).

Rationale

The fundamental rationale for treatment in fractures and dislocations of the hand is to achieve sufficient stability of the bone or joint injury to permit early motion rehabilitation without resulting in malunions for fractures or residual instability for dislocations. The correct treatment option is the least invasive technique that can accomplish these goals. When multiple injuries are present, one must determine treatment for the primary injury around which the management of the other injuries will be based. There are essentially five major treatment alternatives: immediate motion, temporary splinting, closed reduction and internal fixation (CRIF), open reduction and internal fixation (ORIF), and immediate reconstruction. The general advantages of entirely nonoperative treatment are assumed to be lower cost and avoidance of the risks and complications associated with surgery and anesthesia. The generally presumed disadvantage is that stability is less assured than with some form of operative fixation. Closed reduction and internal fixation is expected to prevent overt deformity but not to achieve an anatomically perfect reduction. Pin tract infection is the prime complication that should be mentioned to patients is association with CRIF. Open treatments are considered to add the morbidity of surgical tissue trauma, titrated against the presumed advantages of the most anatomic and stable reduction.

Treatment Selection

Critical elements in selecting between nonoperative and operative treatment are the assessments of rotational malalignment and stability (Fig. 24-8). If carefully sought, rotational discrepancy is relatively easy to determine (37). Defining stability is somewhat more difficult. Some authors have used what seems to be the very reasonable criterion of maintenance of fracture reduction when the adjacent joints are taken through at least 30% of their normal motion (28,38,39). Contraction of soft tissues begins approximately 72 hours following injury. Motion should be instituted by this time for all joints stable enough to tolerate rehabilitation (40). Elevation and elastic compression promote edema control (41). The more aggressive the surgeon's management of the injury has been, the more aggressive must be the rehabilitation. Low-energy isolated injuries have far less risk of stiffness than those created by high-energy trauma with large zones of injury.

Diagnosis and Classification

The diagnosis of a fracture or dislocation of the hand should be made in accordance with the fundamental principles of patient

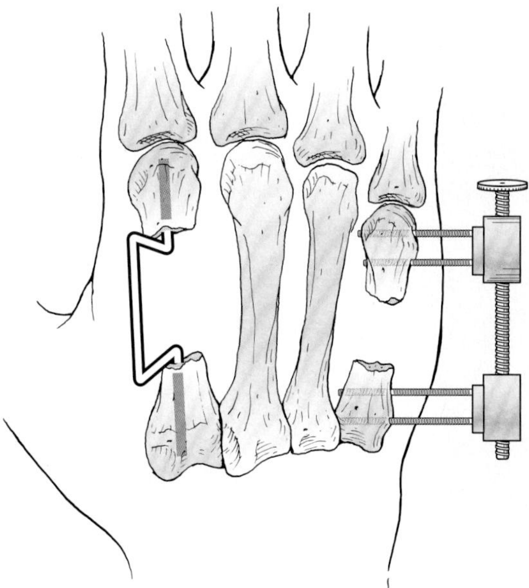

FIGURE 24-7 When extensive contamination precludes the use of internal fixation or bone reconstruction is to be done at a later date, the use of spacer wires or the application of an external fixator with distraction and compression capabilities can be useful.

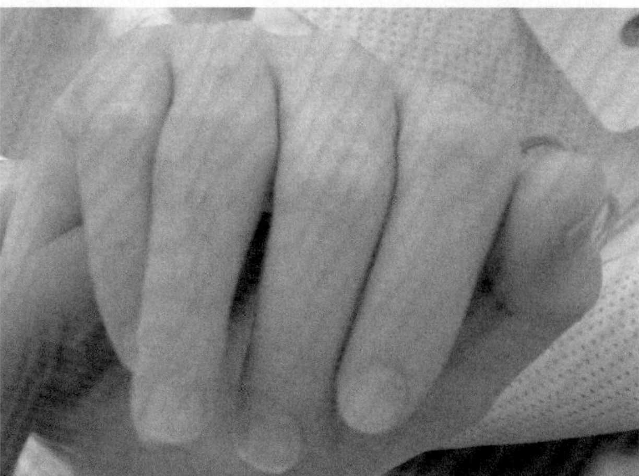

FIGURE 24-8 Pronation of the ring finger proximal phalanx is easily demonstrated by the angular discrepancy of the middle phalanges viewed with the PIP joints flexed 90 degrees.

evaluation and management. A well-taken history should be followed by a thorough examination that is followed by imaging studies. The set of combined information from these three sources creates a profile of the individual patient's unique problem that then leads to all subsequent management decisions. The history should include a description of the environment where the injury occurred. If the injury is open, expected contaminants from different environments would dictate different choices for prophylactic antibiotics. A clear history of the mechanism of injury should be obtained. The patient should be questioned regarding visible deformity immediately following injury and whether any immediate reduction maneuvers were performed at the site of injury or subsequently in an emergency department. The degree and duration of swelling should be described with specific reference to exact location. The patient's current symptoms and chief complaint are essential and often the best clues to uncovering associated injury patterns. Physical examination includes assessment of all tissue layers beginning with the integument and including flexor and extensor tendons, nerves, vessels and ultimately the skeletal structure.

Imaging

Plain radiographic evaluation includes at least two projections with the beam centered at the level of interest (Fig. 24-9). A third oblique view is often quite instructive, revealing displacement not evident on the standard PA or lateral. Rarely are other imaging studies necessary in evaluating fractures and dislocations of the hand. In complex periarticular fractures, such as "pilon" fractures of the base of P2, computed tomography (CT) scans assist some surgeons with operative planning. Foreign bodies may not always be detected by standard radiographic projections. Russell et al (42) provides guidelines for visualizing different types of material. Glass or gravel is best seen with soft tissue technique. CT scans may detect plastic, glass, and wood (43). Ultrasound can detect objects that lack radioopacity (44). Magnetic resonance imaging (MRI) remains a more expensive backup for all types of foreign materials.

Classification

Unfortunately, the literature regarding these injuries has not been written in accordance with any defined classification scheme, and true comparisons are difficult to make. Descriptions of fractures have been based largely on the location within the bone (head, neck, shaft, base) and further modified by the direction of the fracture plane (transverse, spiral, oblique, comminuted) and the measurable degree of displacement. Dislocations have been described by the direction the distal segment travels (dorsal, volar, rotatory) and further modified by the capacity (simple) or incapacity (complex) for closed reduction. In the sections that follow regarding each injury, it will be assumed that the above-stated designations are in effect unless specific exceptions are noted.

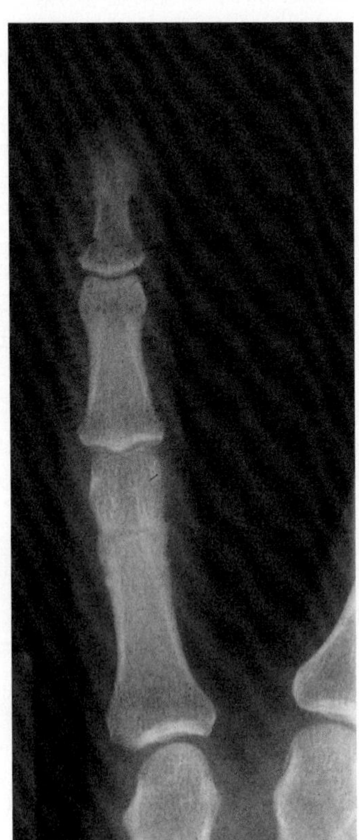

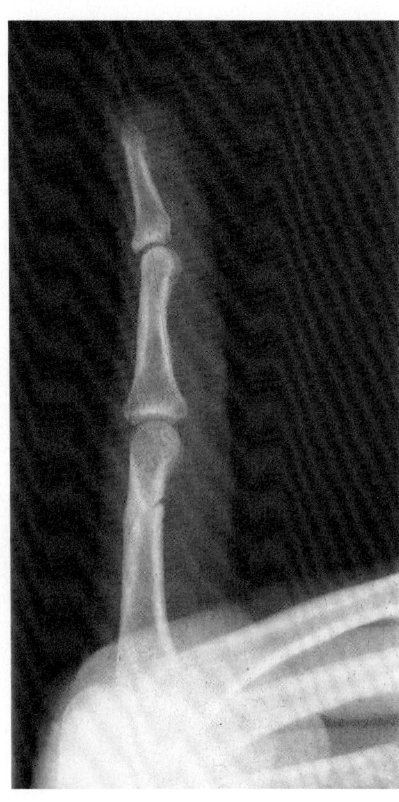

FIGURE 24-9 Fractures in the digit itself are best demonstrated by isolated digital radiographs **(A,B)** with the beam centered at the level of injury.

DISTAL PHALANX FRACTURES

As the terminal point of human contact with the environment, the distal phalanx experiences stress loading with nearly every use of the hand. The soft tissue coverage is limited and local signs of fracture can usually be detected at the surface. When distal phalanx (P3) fractures accompany a nail bed injury, hematoma can be seen beneath the nail plate. When the seal between the nail plate and the hyponychium is also broken, the fracture is open and should be treated as such. The mechanism of injury often involves crushing, and the soft tissue injury is frequently of greater significance for long-term prognosis than the fracture. When one is suspicious of a distal phalanx fracture, x-rays should be taken as isolated views of the injured digit.

Surgical and Applied Anatomy

Unique features of the distal phalanx include the ligaments that pass from the distal margin of the widened lateral base to the expanded proximal margins of the tuft. The small branches of the proper digital artery that supply the dorsal arcade just proximal to the nail fold pass under these ligaments very close to the base of the shaft of the distal phalanx. The tuft is an anchoring point for the specialized architecture of the digital pulp, a honeycomb structure of fibrous septae that contain pockets of fat in each compartment. The proximal part of the pulp is thicker and more mobile than the distal pulp (45). The proximal portion of a tuft fracture may become entrapped in the septae of the pulp and prove irreducible (46). The dorsal surface of the distal phalanx is the direct support for the germinal matrix and sterile matrix of the nail. The bone volarly and the nail plate dorsally create a three layered sandwich with the matrix in the middle (Fig. 24-10).

Fractures in the distal phalanx can be conceived of as occurring in three primary regions: the tuft, the shaft, and the base (Fig. 24-11). Relative incidences of fracture patterns have been suggested as 63% shaft or tuft, 36% longitudinal, and 18% basal (47). The two mechanisms of injury experienced most frequently are a sudden axial load (as in ball sports) or crush injuries. Crush fractures of the tuft are usually stable injuries held in place by the fibrous network of the pulp volarly and the splinting effect of the nail plate dorsally. Proximally the digital flexor and terminal extensor tendons insert on the volar and dorsal bases of the distal phalanx. Since these are the last tendon attachments in the digit, all fracture planes occurring distal to these tendon insertions have been separated from any internal deforming forces. Volar and dorsal base fractures are unstable, with the entire force of a tendon pulling the small base fragment away from the remainder of the bone. Controlling rotation in these small pieces may be particularly difficult. Dorsal base intra-articular fractures due to the shearing component of an axial load injury should be distinguished from avulsion fractures occurring under tension from the terminal tendon. The latter are smaller fragments with the fracture line perpendicular to the line of tensile force in the tendon whereas the former

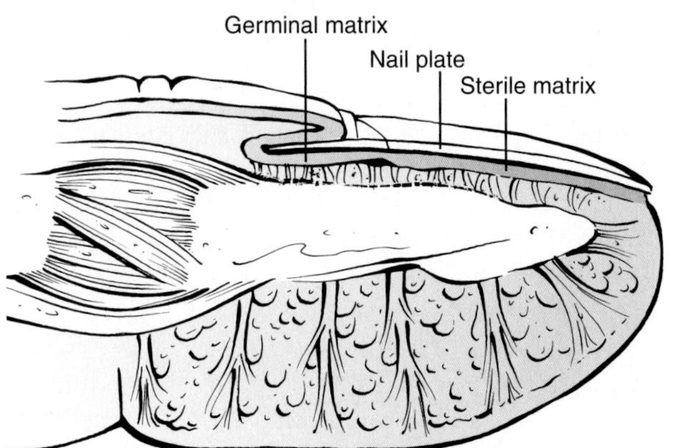

FIGURE 24-10 An intimate relationship exists between the three layers of the dorsal cortex of the distal phalanx, the nail matrix (both germinal and sterile), and the nail plate.

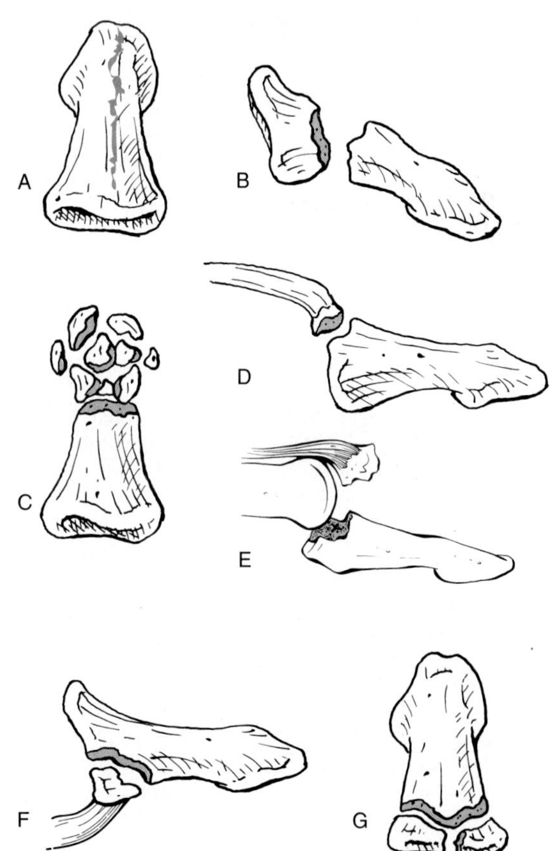

FIGURE 24-11 Fracture patterns seen in the distal phalanx include **(A)** longitudinal shaft, **(B)** transverse shaft, **(C)** tuft, **(D)** dorsal base avulsion, **(E)** dorsal base shear, **(F)** volar base, and **(G)** complete articular.

are larger fragments comprising a significant (>20%) portion of the articular surface with the fracture line being perpendicular to the articular surface. These are very different injuries with different treatment requirements (48). In a similar fashion, the majority of bone flakes at the volar base of P3 are really flexor digitorum profundus (FDP) tendon ruptures occurring through bone. A small percentage of volar base fractures, especially when large in size, are not FDP avulsions but rather shearing fractures that are amenable to extension block splinting (49).

Current Treatment Options

Current treatment options are listing in Table 24-1. Most distal phalanx fractures can be treated with digital splints (Fig. 24-12). The splint should leave the PIP joint free but usually needs to cross the DIP joint simply to gain enough foundation to provide adequate stability. Aluminum and foam splints or plaster of Paris are common materials chosen. The significance of lingering symptoms with fractures of the distal phalanx remains under appreciated. In a series of 98 fractures surveyed at 6 months, 39 still had numbness, 32 had cold sensitivity, 38 had abnormal nail growth, and 70% still had functionally disabling symptoms (47).

Tuft Fractures

If the dorsal surface of the distal portion of the phalanx that supports the nail matrix has a significant step-off, especially with a concomitant nail plate avulsion, the fracture should be restored to a level surface and pinned to render support to the surgical repair of the nail matrix. Conversely, if the nail plate has maintained its seal at the hyponychium and the dorsal surface of the distal phalanx is level, formal removal of the plate to perform a nail matrix repair is not necessary despite any measured percentage of hematoma occupying the area under the nail. Matrix defects should be split-thickness grafted from the adjacent or a distant nail bed. Following repair, the dorsal nail fold should be stented to prevent adherence to the matrix but still allow fluid drainage (50). The patient should be warned of the potential for nail deformity and the time required (4–5 months) for regrowth.

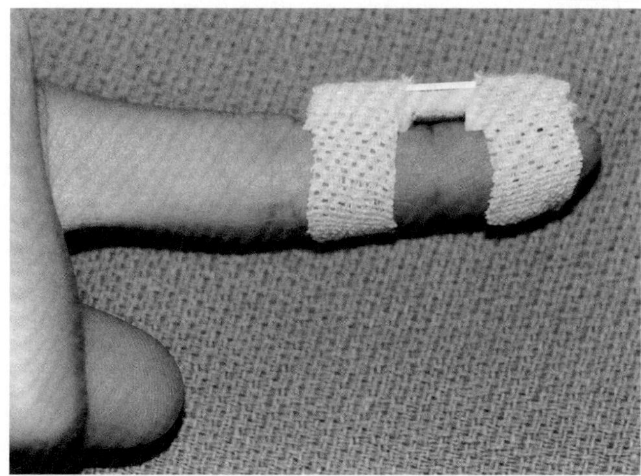

FIGURE 24-12 Dorsal splinting of the distal phalanx and the DIP joint is easily accomplished with an aluminum and foam splint. Cutting out the foam over the dorsal nail fold skin relieves direct pressure where the skin is at greatest risk for ischemic necrosis.

TABLE 24-1 Distal Phalanx Fractures

Treatment Option	Pros	Cons
Splinting	Minimal treatment-related complications; this is the maximum treatment needed for tuft fractures with level cortex under nail matrix	Not precise enough to control an angulated shaft fracture or displaced articular fracture
CRIF	Capable of maintaining the dorsal cortex level to support the nail, extension block pinning for dorsal base fractures restores articular congruence	Pin tract infection rate is significant owing to distal location in hand and retention of pins for at least 4 weeks
ORIF	Part of open fracture management	High rate of complications related to hardware and wound healing with generally unsatisfactory results

CRIF, closed reduction and internal fixation; ORIF, open reduction and internal fixation.

Shaft Fractures

Most shaft fractures have limited enough displacement that nonoperative management is appropriate. Active motion of the DIP joint can be pursued from the outset since the forces of the FDP and the terminal extensor tendon are not acting across the fracture site. Only externally applied forces such as pinch will deform the fracture (Fig. 24-13). Shaft fractures with wide displacement are headed for a nonunion without closer approximation of the fragments. Closed reduction and internal fixation is usually sufficient for these unless there is interposed tissue blocking the reduction (Fig. 24-14). K-wire fixation may also be preferable (0/5 malunions) compared to splinting (3/18 flexion malunions) when the fracture is transverse, extra-articular and located at the base of the distal phalanx (51).

Dorsal Base Fractures—CRIF

Although entirely closed management has been stated to do well even in those joints with volar subluxation and comminution, CRIF is the treatment of choice for true displaced dorsal base fractures comprising over 25% of the articular surface (Fig. 24-15) (52). A variety of closed pinning techniques are

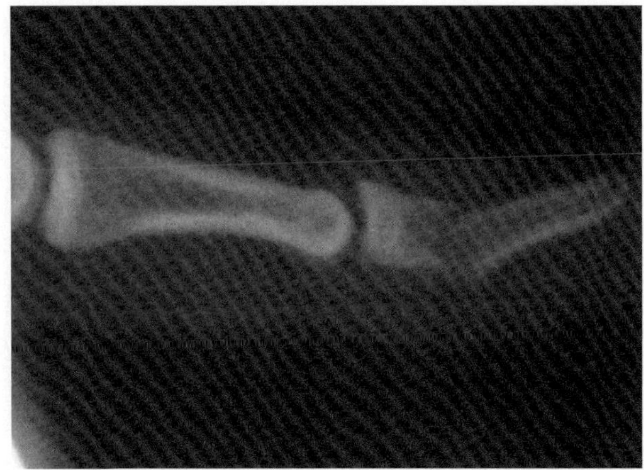

FIGURE 24-13 Transverse shaft fractures in the distal phalanx are subject to apex volar angulation when pinch forces are applied to the pulp, distal to the fracture line.

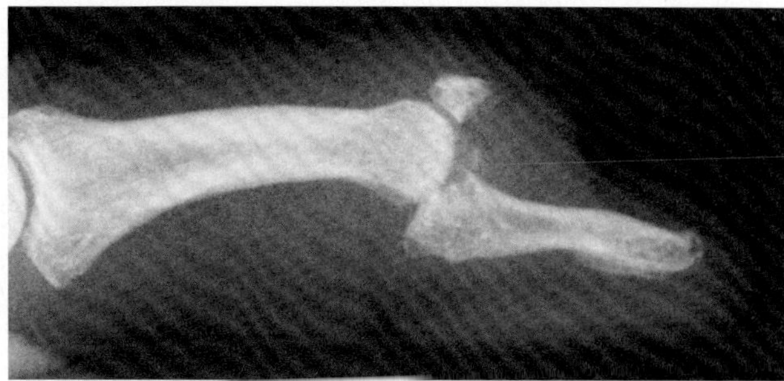

FIGURE 24-15 Dorsal base fractures from axial impaction with shearing rather than traction avulsion injury may demonstrate subluxation of the volar fragment and rotation into extension of the smaller dorsal fragment. These features are consistent with operative management of the injury.

possible, but the mainstay is extension block pinning (Figs. 24-16 and 24-17) (53). In a series of 86 patients, union was achieved in 4 to 6 weeks following wire removal at 4 weeks and the institution of passive extension rehabilitation (54,55). Twenty-three patients treated with extension block pinning for fragments comprising an average of 40% of the joint surface had flexion of 77 degrees with a 4-degree extensor lag and two losses of reduction (56). The difficulty in comparing the published outcomes for these injuries is that the literature has usually failed to distinguish between dorsal fractures that are merely bony variants of terminal tendon injuries and those that are the more significant intra-articular fractures discussed in this section.

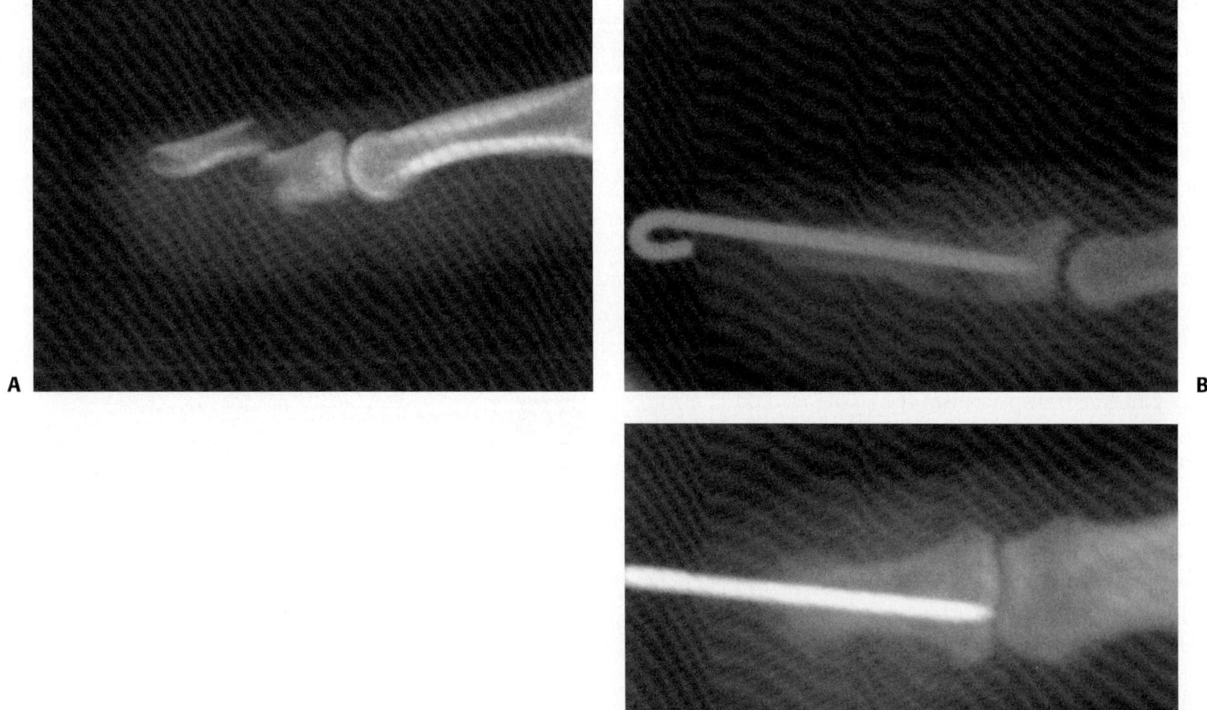

FIGURE 24-14 Closed reduction and internal fixation of **(A)** displaced and unstable shaft fractures in the distal phalanx should **(B)** produce a level dorsal cortex and **(C)** avoid distraction at the fracture site.

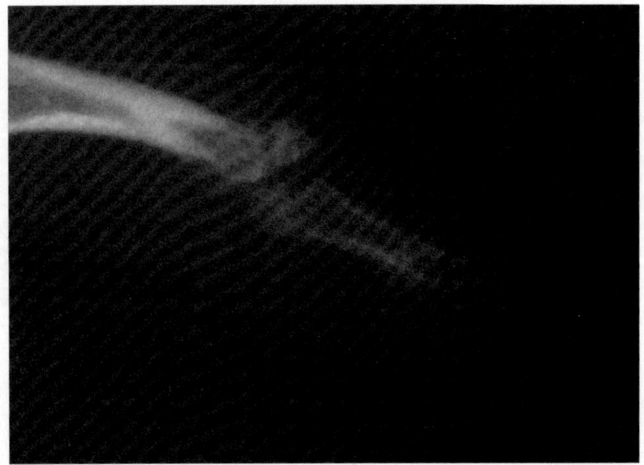

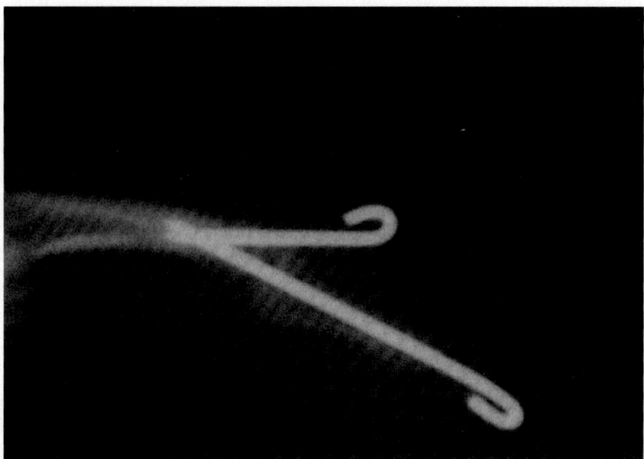

A B

FIGURE 24-16 Dorsal base shearing articular fractures **(A)** can be stabilized by the extension block pinning technique using two 0.045-inch K-wires **(B)**.

Dorsal Base Fractures—ORIF

Dorsal base fractures may rarely require open reduction and internal fixation. Advocates for ORIF of dorsal base fractures have been able to show some benefit in selected cases. Lubahn cites subluxation with incongruence and a dorsal base fracture involving 30% to 40% of the articular surface as an indication for ORIF (57). In his series of 30 patients comparing double K-wire fixation to nonoperative management, the ORIF group had extensor lags of 0 to 20 degrees, ROM of 55 degrees, and no dorsal prominence. The nonoperative group had extensor lags of 20 to 30 degrees, ROM of 35 degrees, and dorsal prominence of the fragment (58). Thirty-six patients in another series treated with ORIF using two K-wires had a final mean ROM of 2 to 69 degrees (59). Thirty-three patients with K-wire ORIF had a mean arc of 4 to 67 degrees of final motion (60). Cadaveric testing of dorsal base fracture fixation techniques favored tension band suture over tension band wire, figure-of-8 wire, or K-wire fixation (61). However, 31 of 51 dorsal base P3 fractures had a poor result both clinically and radiographically with tension band fixation, noting skin breakdown, superficial and deep infection, and secondary fragment displacement (62). One method of avoiding such complications (0/19) might be the 5 weeks of external fixation employed in 19 patients resulting in 70 degrees of flexion with a 2-degree average extensor lag (63).

Volar Base Fractures

Open reduction and internal fixation is the treatment of choice for highly displaced volar base fractures that have a large intra-articular fragment and loss of FDP functional integrity (64). If the volar FDP fragment is large enough, it may be fixed with a compression screw. Extension block pinning is another rarely employed alternative. The remaining small bone flakes located at the volar base of the distal phalanx are in fact tendon avulsions and should be treated in accordance with modern principles of flexor tendon reinsertion.

Rehabilitation

Healing at this level of the digit is often prolonged. Transverse shaft fractures may take 3 to 4 months before being able to resist maximum pinch force. For stable tuft and longitudinal fractures, splints may be removed and functional use of the hand instituted as soon as tolerated by the patient's symptoms. Dorsal base fractures usually have the K-wires removed by 4 weeks with continued external protection for 2 to 3 more weeks when using traditional pinning techniques. The dorsal base extension block method works through the institution of passive extension exercises beginning at 4 weeks and coinciding with wire removal. The more distal the injury is in the digit, the more hypersensitivity to surface contact the patient is likely to have. Desensitization through progressively more stimulating contact is the earliest component of the rehabilitation program, with the goal of reincorporating the fingertip into as many activities of daily living as possible.

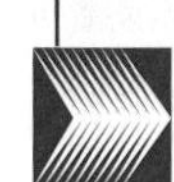

AUTHOR'S PREFERRED TREATMENT

Tuft Fractures

Most tuft fractures can be splinted in a simple aluminum and foam splint for a duration determined by the patient's symptoms alone. The time course for healing of the associated soft tissue injury may well determine the total duration of disability far more than that of the fracture itself. When the seal of the nail plate with the hyponychium has been broken and the tuft fracture is displaced, this represents an open fracture that should be treated on the day of injury with direct nail bed repair. If the distal fragment is of substantial size, the dorsal cortex of the distal phalanx that supports

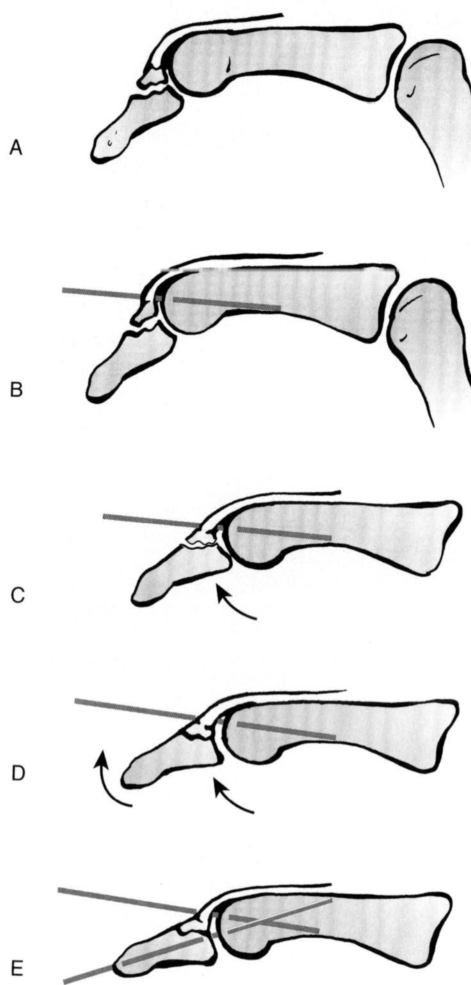

FIGURE 24-17 The steps of the extension block pinning method begin with **(A)** hyperflexion of the DIP joint to draw the smaller dorsal fragment volarly where it is **(B)** blocked from returning into further extension by the first 0.045-inch K-wire. The larger volar fragment is then reduced **(C)** first at the articular surface to meet the dorsal fragment followed by **(D)** extension of the shaft to approximate the metaphysis, and maintained by the **(E)** second K-wire.

the nail bed will provide a more level surface if pinned with a longitudinal 0.045- or 0.035-inch K-wire for 4 to 6 weeks.

Shaft Fractures

Longitudinal sagittal plane shaft fractures of the distal phalanx can be treated entirely nonoperatively if minimally displaced or by CRIF with transverse 0.028- to 0.035-inch K-wires being used for the rare displaced fracture. For unstable transverse shaft fractures, the surrounding tissues usually impart enough rotational stability that a single axial wire is sufficient. Depending on the size of the phalanx, either a 0.045- or 0.035-inch Kirschner wire is appropriate. Care should be taken to avoid penetration of the nail matrix tissues with the wire. If the fracture is at mid-shaft level or more distal, the wire will provide enough stability if driven to the subchondral base of the distal phalanx only. Fractures occurring at the meta-diaphyseal junction may need the wire passed across the DIP joint to achieve sufficient stability. Distraction at the shaft fracture site can easily occur and should be avoided to diminish the possibility of nonunion. Nonunions can be treated by bone grafting through a volar midline approach. The custom is to leave the pin emerging from the hyponychium for ease of removal later in the office. The distal phalanx heals slowly, often taking up to 8 weeks or longer. Fortunately, DIP joint rehabilitation may proceed since the fracture is only deformed by external application of pinch forces.

Dorsal Base Fractures

Dorsal base intra-articular shear fractures produce a triangular dorsal fragment that is extended and translated by the pull of the terminal tendon. With proper collateral ligament damage, the larger articular fragment that is in continuity with the remainder of the phalanx may sublux volarly. Open reduction and internal fixation adds excessive surgical trauma to a delicate set of tissues and the dorsal fragment is usually too small to accommodate fixation devices passing directly through it without experiencing comminution. The injury is best addressed by extension block pinning. The DIP joint is hyperflexed, drawing the dorsal fragment volarly to reach its natural position in relation to the head of P2. A 0.045-inch K-wire is inserted at the dorsal margin of the fragment (but not through the fragment) to block it from returning to the retracted position under the influence of the terminal extensor tendon (Fig. 24-17). The remainder of the distal phalanx consisting of the volar articular fragment and shaft is then extended to meet the blocked smaller fragment and restore articular congruity. A second 0.045-inch K-wire is passed from P3 across the DIP joint into P2. The wires are retained for 4 weeks. Upon removal, passive extension exercises further compress the two fragments and assist in the final stages of cancellous bone healing. The treatment can still be executed up to 4 to 5 weeks after the initial injury, but early callus formation between the two fragments must be dispersed or satisfactory approximation will not be achieved.

Pearls and Pitfalls

When performing the extension block pinning technique for dorsal base fractures, achieving a truly congruent joint is difficult. There are two typical problems: rotation of the smaller fragment into extension under the influence of the terminal extensor tendon and cantilevering of the volar articular-shaft fragment. A method to overcome the first problem is to use another K-wire percutaneously to hold pressure on the dorsal cortex of the small fragment while placing the extension block wire. The flat side of the wire rather than the sharp tip should be used for this reduction maneuver. The surgeon holding the distal phalanx shaft fragment manually and applying the extension force for reduction creates the second problem. Instead of achieving a con-

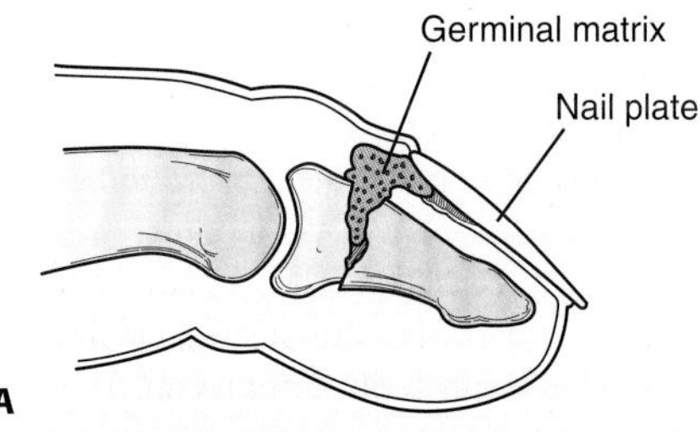

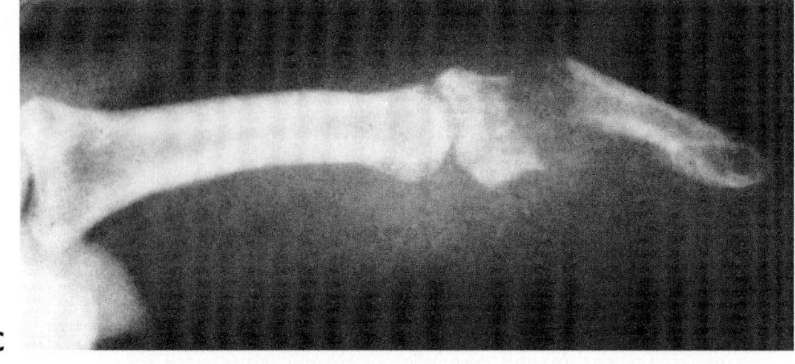

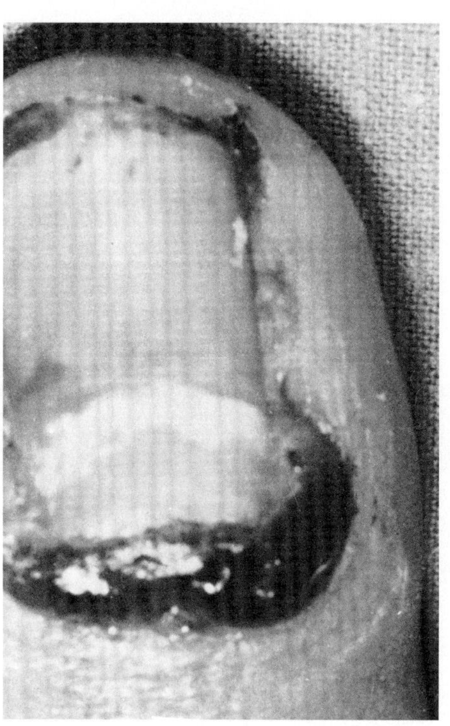

FIGURE 24-18 **A.** Transverse fractures occurring at the root of the nail can entrap the germinal matrix in the fracture site. Clues to this clinical scenario appear **(B)** at the base of the nail in a **(C)** widened fracture resistant to reduction.

gruent joint reduction, the larger fragment cantilevers and reduces at the metaphyseal level but leaves an incongruent articular gap. Placing an instrument handle such as a Freer elevator transversely across the volar base just distal to the flexion crease and using the instrument to apply the extension force directly at the level of the joint can overcome this second problem. The reduction will first occur congruently at the joint and then secondarily at the metaphysis.

Nail Matrix

Matrix tissue may fold into any dorsal opening of a fracture site, particularly at the base of the germinal matrix (Fig. 24-18). If attempted reduction of a distal phalanx fracture with a visible dorsal cortical gap on the lateral radiograph is not forthcoming, this possibility must be considered and extrication performed to prevent both nonunion and nail deformity. Suturing the nail matrix can be difficult. Friable nail matrix tissue is easily torn as the needle is pushed rather than rolled along its axis during repair, a problem that is compounded by the needle tip's tendency to catch on the dorsal cortex during the bottom of the stroke. These problems are overcome by using a special 7-0 chromic suture with a spatula tipped needle that can be passed with a rolling motion of the fingers when loaded on a Castro-Viejo needle driver.

DISTAL INTERPHALANGEAL AND THUMB INTERPHALANGEAL JOINT DISLOCATIONS

Dislocations at the distal interphalangeal (DIP) and thumb interphalangeal (IP) joints suffer from under appreciation and late presentation. Injuries are considered chronic after 3 weeks (65). Pure dislocations without tendon rupture are rare, usually result from ball-catching sports, are primarily dorsal in direction, and may occur in association with PIP joint dislocations (Fig. 24-19). Transverse open wounds in the volar skin crease are frequent (Fig. 24-20). Injury to a single collateral ligament or to the volar plate alone at the DIP joint is rare (66).

Surgical and Applied Anatomy

The DIP/IP joint is a bicondylar ginglymus joint stabilized on each side by proper and accessory collateral ligaments and the

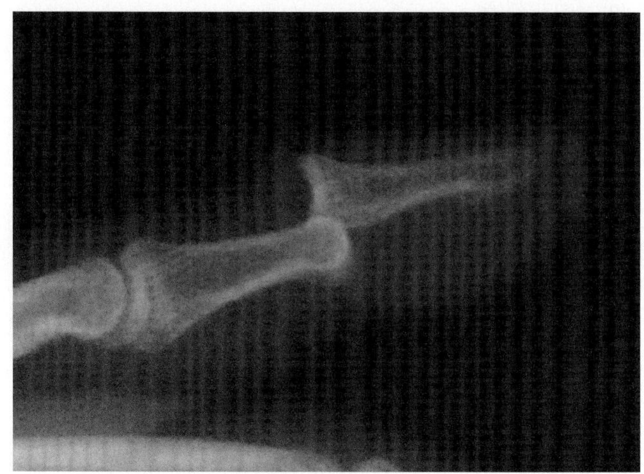

FIGURE 24-19 Dislocations of the DIP joint are nearly always dorsal.

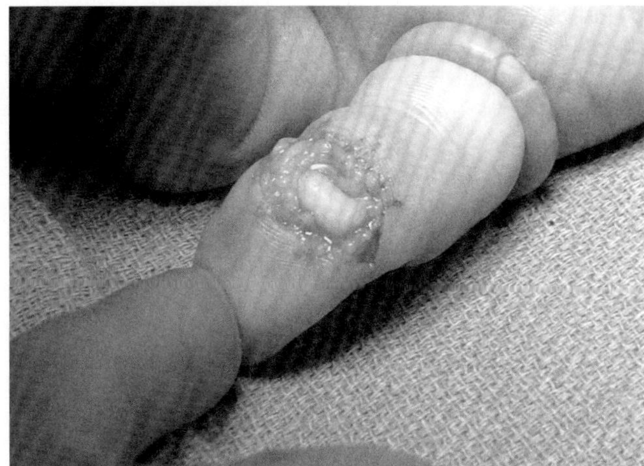

FIGURE 24-20 Dorsal DIP dislocations are often open with a transverse rent in the flexion crease from tearing rather than direct laceration. The wound should be debrided prior to reduction if possible.

volar plate (Fig. 24-21). The proper collateral ligaments insert on the lateral tubercles at the base of P3, which also serve as the origin for the lateral ligaments to the tuft (67). The accessory collateral ligaments attach distally to the lateral margins of the volar plate. The volar plate of the DIP joint has a proximal attachment weakly confluent with the distal extent of the flexor digitorum superficialis (FDS) tendon but has no strong checkrein ligaments like those at the PIP joint. This is in keeping with the clinical observation of proximal volar plate detachment with dorsal dislocation (68). The joint is inherently stable owing to articular congruity and the dynamic balance of flexor and extensor tendons. However, the DIP/IP joint is not as inherently stable as the PIP joint and depends to a greater degree on ligaments for stability.

The DIP joints have complex motion patterns involving axial rotation that are different for each finger and designed to ensure conformity when the hand surrounds an object (67). The capacity for passive DIP hyperextension is unique to modern humans, but the role this plays in the etiology of dislocation is unclear (45). Irreducible dorsal dislocations are thought to occur through a variety of different anatomic circumstances (Fig. 24-22). Reasons include a trapped volar plate, the FDP trapped behind a single condyle of P2 (marked lateral displacement), P2 buttonholed through the volar plate or through a rent in

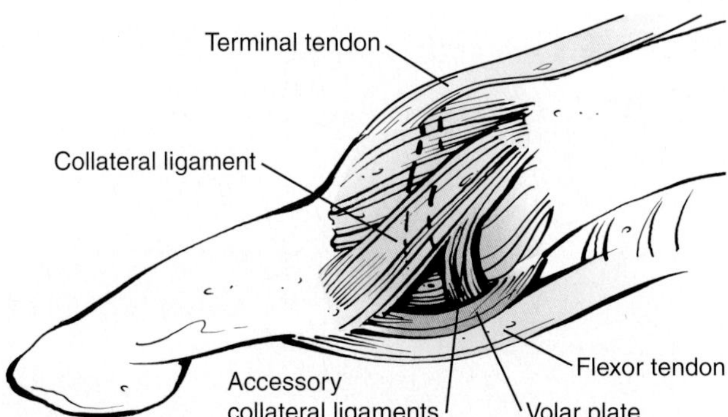

FIGURE 24-21 The balanced forces of the terminal extensor tendon and the long flexor tendon dynamically stabilize The DIP joint. The proper and accessory collateral ligaments and the volar plate provide static stability.

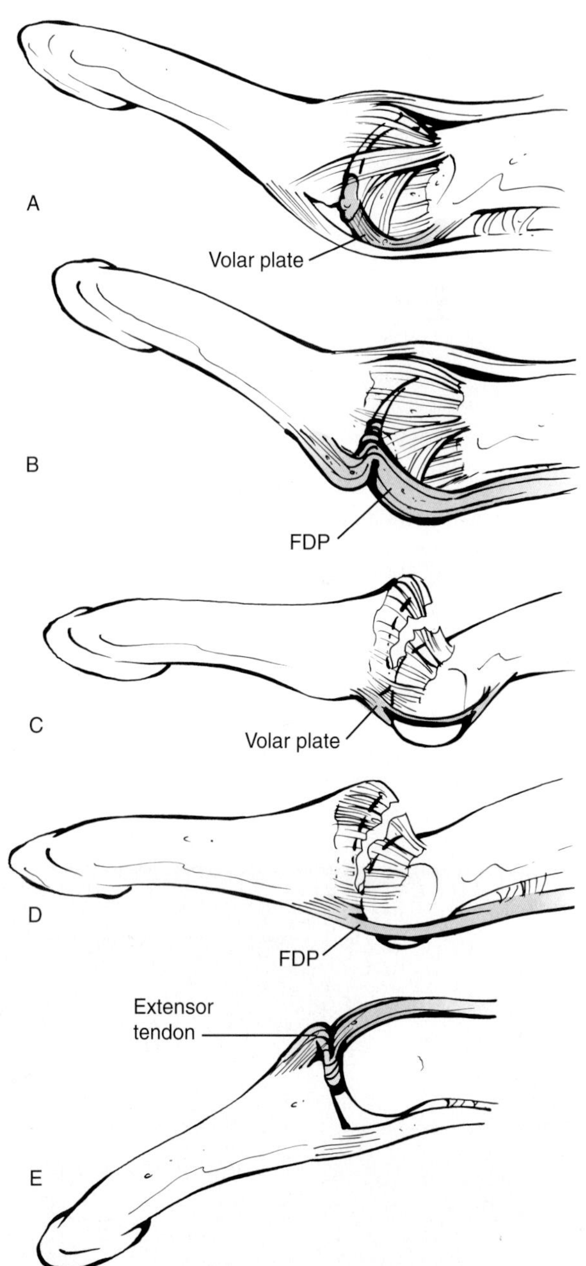

FIGURE 24-22 Irreducible dislocations of the DIP joint occur due to **(A)** volar plate entrapment, **(B)** the FDP trapped behind a single condyle of P2, **(C)** P2 buttonholed through the volar plate, **(D)** P2 through a rent in the FDP, **(E)** the extensor tendon displaced around the head of P2.

TABLE 24-2 Distal Interphalangeal Joint and Thumb Interphalangeal Joint Dislocations

Treatment Option	Pros	Cons
Splinting	Minimizes treatment-related complications	In a noncompliant patient will not prevent re-dislocation
CRIF	Prevents re-dislocation during early collateral ligament healing	Pin tract infection and stiffness
ORIF	Part of open dislocation management, and essential for irreducible dislocations	Introduces wound healing complications, and stiffness may be a more significant problem

CRIF, closed reduction and internal fixation; ORIF, open reduction and internal fixation.

the FDP (69,70). Volar dislocations may also be irreducible with the extensor tendon displaced around the head of P2 (71). Thumb sesamoids or the volar plate may render an IP joint dislocation irreducible (72,73).

Current Treatment Options

Nonoperative Management

Current treatment options are listing in Table 24-2. Reduced dislocations that are stable may begin immediate AROM. The rare unstable dorsal dislocation should be immobilized in 20 degrees of flexion for up to 3 weeks prior to instituting AROM. The duration of the immobilization should be in direct proportion to the surgeon's assessment of joint stability following reduction. Complete collateral ligament injuries should be protected from lateral stress for at least 4 weeks. When splinting at the level of the DIP/IP joint, extreme caution must be exercised with regard to the vascularity of the dorsal skin between the extension skin crease and the dorsal nail fold. It is not only direct pressure but merely the angle of hyperextension that can "wash out" the blood supply to this skin potentially resulting in full-thickness necrosis. This complication is thought to occur at an angle representing 50% of the available passive hyperextension of the DIP joint and can be identified by blanching of the skin (74).

CRIF

It is possible that the degree of instability post-reduction is great enough to require a brief period (3–4 weeks) of 0.045-inch K-wire stabilization across the joint (Fig. 24-23). The necessity of added stabilization occurs primarily when aggressive rehabilitation is required for adjacent hand injuries.

Open Reduction

Delayed presentation (over 3 weeks) of a subluxated joint may require opening to resect scar tissue and allow tension free reduction to occur, resulting often in 10-degree fixed flexion contractures and loss of 10 to 30 degrees of the flexion range (75). Open dislocations require thorough debridement to prevent infection. The need for fixation with a K-wire should be based on the assessment of stability and is not necessarily required for all open dislocations. The wire may be placed either longitudinally or on an oblique path. The duration of pinning should not be longer than 4 weeks and the wire may be left through the skin for easy removal. The advantage of longitudinal pinning is the absence of any

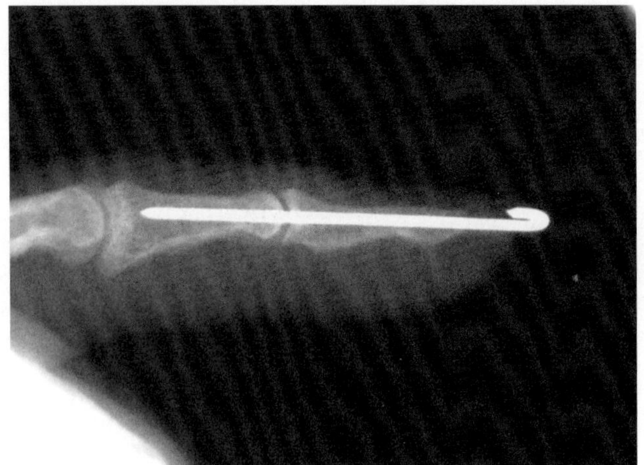
A

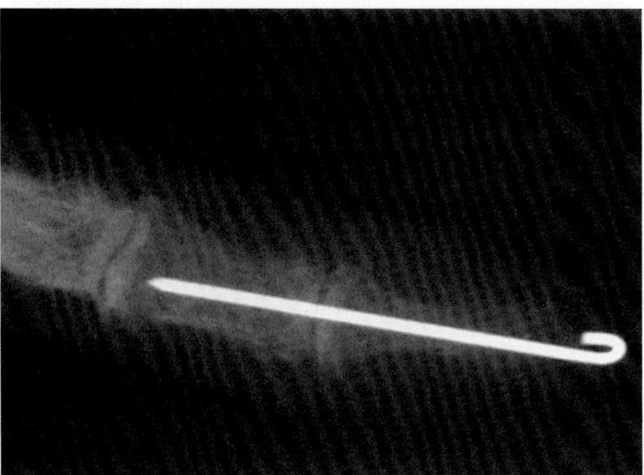
B

FIGURE 24-23 Closed reduction and internal fixation of the DIP joint should assure **(A)** a congruent articulation in neutral on the lateral view, and **(B)** neutral pin placement on the AP view.

lateral wire protrusion to contact adjacent digits. The advantage of oblique pinning is the ability to remove both sections of wire should breakage across the joint occur. When open reduction of the joint is required, a transverse dorsal incision at the distal joint crease from mid-axial line to mid-axial line provides ample exposure. Should additional exposure be required mid-axial proximal extensions can be made.

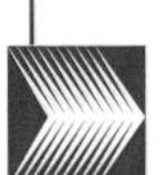

AUTHOR'S PREFERRED TREATMENT

Closed reduction and splinting is the preferred treatment for most injuries. Should added pin stabilization prove necessary due to recurrent instability, a single longitudinal 0.045-inch K-wire is sufficient. Closed reduction may appear impossible. Interposed tissue is usually the cause and may include volar plate, collateral ligament or tendon. Longitudinal traction rarely is successful in overcoming the blockade. Instead proximal joint positioning to relax the involved tendons and gentle rotation may allow the interposed tissue to slip out of the joint.

Open Reduction

My preferred incision for the DIP/IP joint is dorsal and transverse (Fig. 24-24). The most distal of the major extensor creases corresponds to the joint level. Proximal extensions of 5 mm made in the mid-axial lines create a small trapdoor effect that gives ample exposure for any procedure. The terminal extensor tendon or extensor pollicis longus should be protected. Using a single prong skin hook is a gentle method to control the tendon without grasping and crushing its fibers with forceps while working to achieve reduction. One must search for small chondral or osteochondral injuries primarily for the purpose of removing the fragments from the joint to avoid subsequent third body wear.

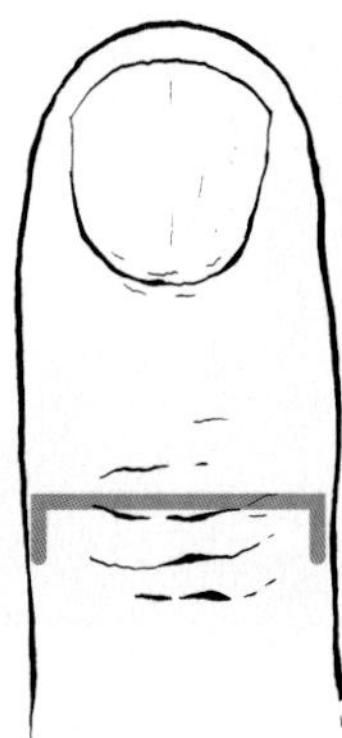

FIGURE 24-24 The safest surgical approach to the DIP joint with respect to skin blood supply is transverse in the distal extensor crease with mid-axial proximal extensions as needed not exceeding 5 mm.

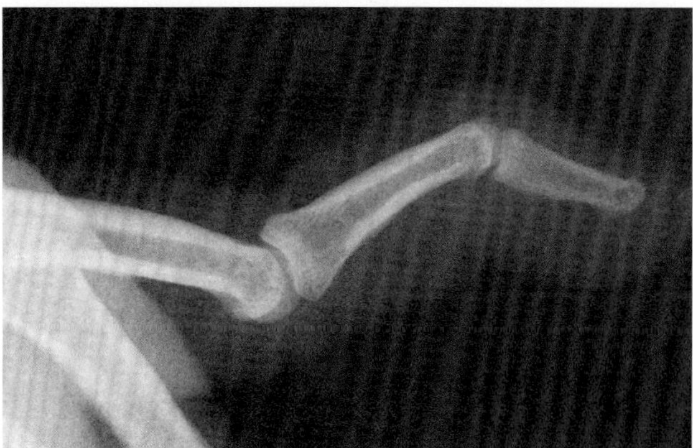

FIGURE 24-25 Terminal tendon retraction results in transfer of all extensor force to the central slip. In the setting of associated PIP joint volar plate laxity, a swan-neck deformity results.

Pearls and Pitfalls

Two primary complications of open surgery in this region are wound complications and hypersensitivity. Dissecting and preserving longitudinal venous channels during the surgery facilitates venous drainage of the narrow skin flap between the wound and the dorsal nail fold. There is usually one major group of veins directly in the midline overlying the extensor tendon and one major group at each dorsolateral corner. The lateral venous groups are accompanied by the distal branches of the dorsal digital nerves. Transection of these small nerve branches with the subsequent formation of small neuromas adherent to the wound may be one reason for the high incidence of hypersensitivity in this region. The initial surgical incision should be just through dermis only, followed by careful longitudinal dissection of these neurovascular structures under magnification before proceeding with the remainder of the surgery. An additional nonoperative pitfall is the development of imbalance following splinting, perhaps as a result of failure to monitor the physical examination at each time point during healing (Figs. 24-25 and 24-26).

MIDDLE PHALANX FRACTURES

This section is intentionally biased to concentrate on the intra-articular fractures that occur at the base of the middle phalanx

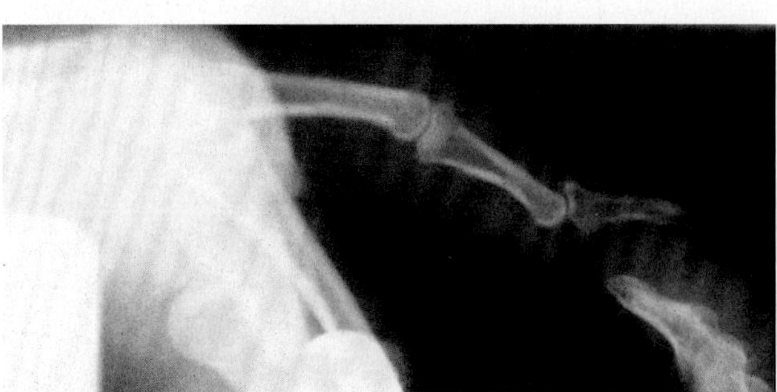

FIGURE 24-26 Dorsal instability is a rare complication following DIP dislocation attributable to poor volar plate healing.

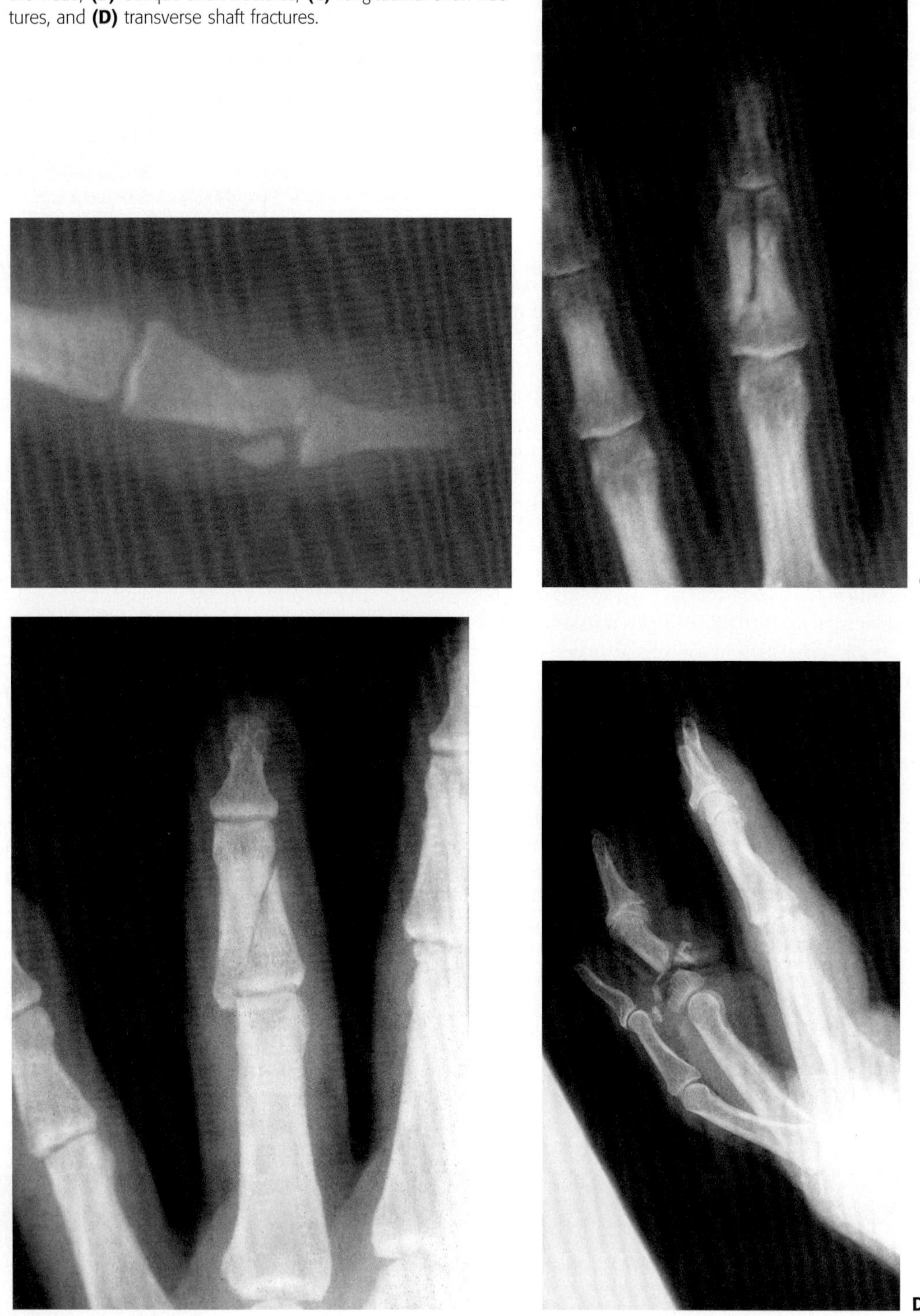

FIGURE 24-27 Fracture patterns of P2 other than the specific base patterns discussed later include **(A)** intra-articular fractures of the head, **(B)** oblique shaft fractures, **(C)** longitudinal shaft fractures, and **(D)** transverse shaft fractures.

(P2). These are perhaps the most functionally devastating of all fractures and dislocations of the hand and the most technically difficult to treat. Many other fracture patterns that occur in the middle phalanx are the same as those patterns seen in the proximal phalanx. Distinction between the middle and proximal phalanges when reporting on these patterns is rare in the published literature, and the majority of the published data on this subject is covered in the section on proximal phalanx fractures later in this chapter.

Surgical and Applied Anatomy

Fractures of the middle phalanx can be grouped by the anatomic regions of head, neck, shaft, and base (Fig. 24-27). Tendon insertions that play a role in fracture deformation include the central slip at the dorsal base and the terminal tendon acting through the DIP joint. The flexor digitorum superficialis has a long insertion along the volar lateral margins of the shaft of P2 from the proximal ¼ to the distal ¼. Fractures at the neck of P2 will usually angulate apex volar as the proximal fragment is flexed by the FDS and the distal fragment extended by the terminal tendon (Fig. 24-28). Those at the base will usually angulate apex dorsal as the distal fragment is flexed by the FDS and the proximal fragment is extended by the central slip Despite the theoretical resolution of these force vectors, actual P2 fractures are less predictable and subject to any variety of displacement patterns. Axial loading patterns of injury may produce unicondylar or bicondylar fractures of the head or intra-articular fractures of the base. Base fractures can be divided into partial articular fractures of the dorsal base, volar base, and lateral base or complete articular fractures that are usually comminuted and often referred to as "pilon" fractures. "Pilon" fractures are unstable in every direction including axially.

Although the complete articular fractures are the most challenging ones to return to good function, the force vectors of volar base fractures are perhaps more interesting. Fractures at the volar base of P2 can be particularly unstable in direct relation to the percentage of articular surface involved. When the volar small fragment constitutes greater than around 40% of the articular surface, this fragment carries the majority of the proper collateral ligament insertion in addition to the accessory ligament and volar plate insertions (Fig. 24-29). The dorsal fragment and remainder of P2 will thus sublux proximally and dorsally with displacement driven by the pull of the FDS and the central slip (Fig. 24-30). The joint then hinges rather than glides, pivoting on the fracture margin of the dorsal fragment and destroying articular cartilage on the head of P1.

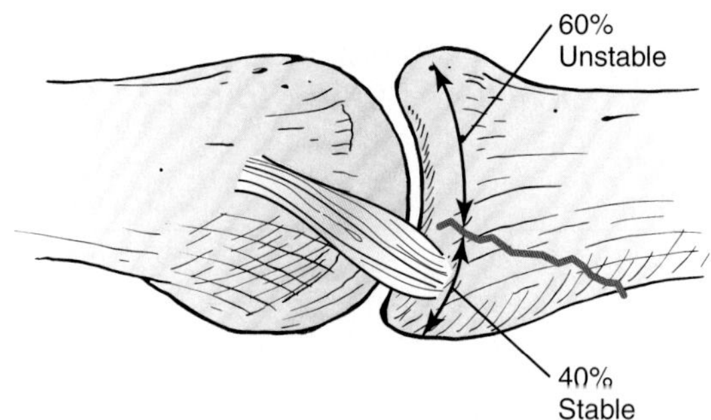

FIGURE 24-29 When the volar fragment of the base of P2 comprises more than 40% of the joint surface, the collateral ligaments attach to the volar rather than the dorsal fragment, rendering the dorsal fragment with the shaft unstable in extension.

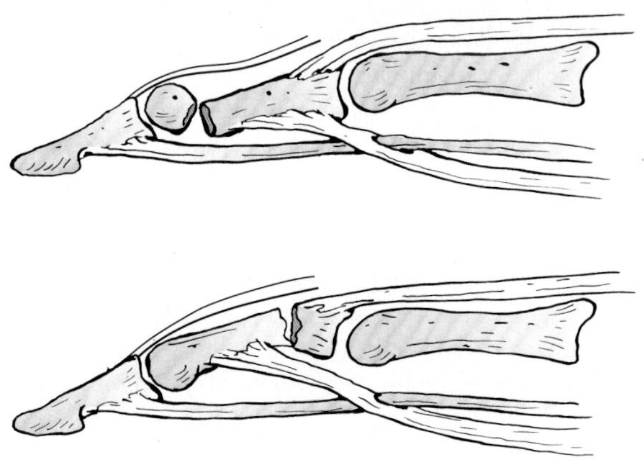

FIGURE 24-28 The insertions of the FDS, the FDP and the components of the extensor apparatus typically cause fractures in the distal ¼ of P2 to angulate apex volar and in the proximal ¼ of P2 to angulate apex dorsal.

Current Treatment Options

Static Splinting

Current treatment options are listed in Table 23-3 through 23-5. Many P2 fractures can be effectively managed entirely nonoperatively. The presence of comminution alone does not necessitate surgery. When crushing is the mechanism of injury, the

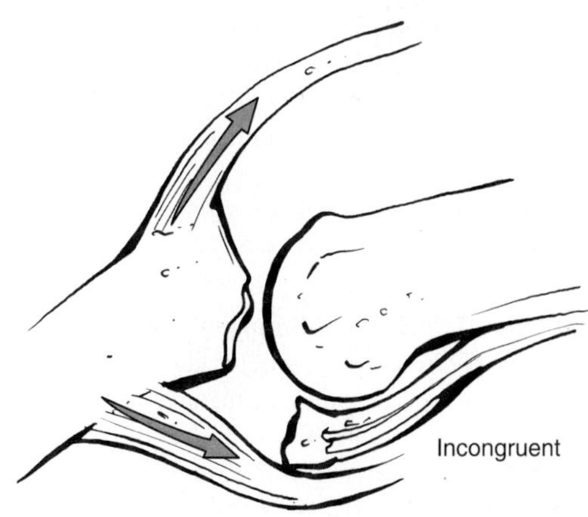

FIGURE 24-30 The central slip of the extensor and the FDS serve as prime deforming forces for dorsal subluxation in volar base P2 fractures.

TABLE 24-3 Middle Phalanx Fractures Not Involving the PIP Joint

Treatment Option	Pros	Cons
Splinting	Simple	Only effective in fractures with inherent stability and minimal displacement
CRIF	Treatment of choice for most unstable head, neck and shaft fractures	Pin tract infection
ORIF with screws only	Compression achieved between condyles in fractures of the head, controls rotation effectively	Stiffness, extensor lag of DIP joint, not effective in the presence of comminution
ORIF with plates and screws	Necessary in open fractures and for internal fixation with bone loss or a high degree of comminution	Stiffness, extensor lag of DIP joint, need for hardware removal

PIP, proximal interphalangeal; CRIF, closed reduction and internal fixation; ORIF, open reduction and internal fixation; DIP, distal interphalangeal.

periosteal envelope may remain relatively intact as long as fracture displacement is not significant. Degree of displacement is more related to inherent stability than the direction or number of fracture planes. Nevertheless, certain patterns are more stable than others. Transverse fractures are more stable than long oblique or spiral fractures, both of which tend to shorten and either laterally deviate or rotate to cause interference patterns with neighboring digits. Splinting is confined to the digit alone with dorsally applied aluminum and foam or custom orthoplast splints. Motion rehabilitation should be initiated by 3 weeks post-injury with interim splinting until clinical signs of healing are present (but not longer than 6 weeks) (76). Side strapping to an adjacent digit usually provides sufficient protection from external forces after the first 3 weeks.

Dynamic Extension Block Splinting

A nonoperative technique used specifically for volar base fractures is extension block splinting. Fractures at the volar base of P2 that involve less than 40% of the articular surface can usually be managed effectively with extension block splinting (77). In a series of 27 patients treated with extension block splinting (beginning as flexed as 60 degrees with advancement of 10 degrees per week for a total of 5 weeks), the final PIP joint ROM was 87 degrees (78). The key to success with this treatment is absolute maintenance of a congruent reduction, avoiding the hinge motion that occurs with dorsal and proximal subluxation of the large fragment (Fig. 24-31) (77,78). Correct application of a dorsal extension block splint requires maintenance of contact between the dorsum of the proximal phalangeal segment and the splint (Fig. 24-32). If the digit is allowed to "pull away" from the splint volarly, the PIP joint can extend beyond the safe range, subluxate, and negate the desired effect of the splint. Once the splint is in place, weekly follow-up with a true lateral radiograph of the PIP joint is mandatory to monitor the advancement of extension at a rate of around 10 degrees per week.

TABLE 24-4 Volar Base Fracture Dislocations of the Middle Phalanx at the PIP Joint

Treatment Option	Pros	Cons
Extension block splinting	Treatment of choice for most <40% articular surface volar base fractures	Requires careful assessment of congruence and follow-up, not effective in most >40% articular surface volar base fractures
Extension block pinning	Specific strategy for dorsal base fractures and select volar base fractures that reduce spontaneously with PIP joint flexion	Useful only in these specific patterns Pin tract infection
Volar plate arthroplasty	Specific strategy for subset of volar base fractures involving between 30%–60% of articular surface	Numerous specific anatomic requirements must be met for procedure to be effective; surface is not hyaline cartilage
Osteochondral reconstruction	Bone to bone healing, true hyaline cartilage restoration, recreates volar lip buttress effectively	Technically complex; graft resorption and collapse are possible

PIP, proximal interphalangeal.

Condylar Fractures of the Head

Displaced unicondylar or bicondylar fractures of the head of P2 require a transverse wire be placed across the condyles to maintain a level distal articular surface at the DIP joint. A second wire passed obliquely to the diaphysis of the opposite cortex will pre-

TABLE 24-5 "Pilon" Complete Articular Fractures of the Base of the Middle Phalanx

Treatment Option	Pros	Cons
Splinting	No hardware-related complications	Only effective for minimally displaced, inherently stable fractures
CRIF	No added stiffness of open procedure	Pin tract infection; no early motion if pinned across the joint; if not pinned across the joint, congruent reduction may not be controlled
ORIF	Most precise reduction of articular surface; no pin tracts	Even with a condylar blade plate may still not control metaphyseal collapse or maintain joint congruence; hardware-related complications
Dynamic traction	Maintains joint congruence, protects against metaphyseal collapse, and permits early active motion	Technically complex Pin tract infection

CRIF, closed reduction and internal fixation; ORIF, open reduction and internal fixation.

vent lateral migration of the condyle along the smooth shaft of the first wire and thus create an articular gap (Fig. 24-33). This second wire also controls the rotation of the fragment in the sagittal plane that can occur with single wire fixation alone. If the patient presents late or soft tissue lies interposed in the fracture plane between condyles, achieving an accurate closed reduction is unlikely and open reduction may be required. Once opened, the opportunity for threaded lag screw fixation exists as opposed to smooth sided K-wire fixation (Fig. 24-34). If the condylar fragment does not have a diaphyseal extension, then the location for lag screw placement is directly through the collateral ligament, which may negate the screw's theoretical advantage over two diverging K-wires in terms of early motion.

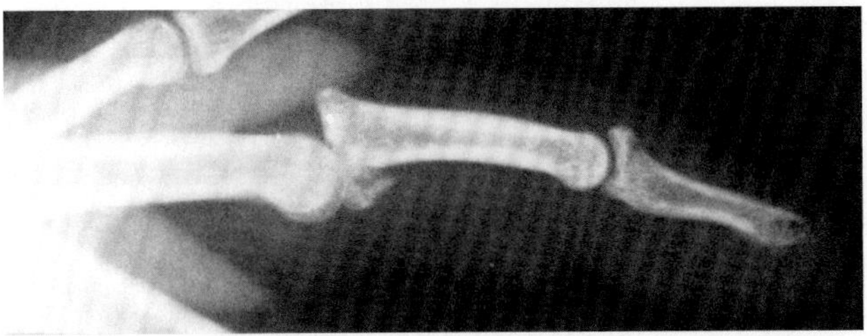

FIGURE 24-31 When dorsal subluxation of P2 volar base fractures occurs, the cancellous bed exposed at the base of P2 articulates against the cartilage on the head of P1 with hinge motion rather than gliding motion.

Unstable Shaft Fractures

Closed reduction and internal fixation is usually accomplished with 0.045- or 0.035-inch K-wires depending on patient size (Fig. 24-35). Kirschner wires that cross in the middle of the shaft produce a less stable pattern of fixation particularly if the fracture is located at the level of the wires' crossing. For transverse or short oblique patterns, K-wire placement other than the crossing pattern may be difficult to achieve without violating either the DIP or PIP joint or directly penetrating a tendon. Long oblique or spiral shaft fractures are amenable to relatively transverse placement of K-wires without joint or tendon penetration (Fig. 24-36). When rotational alignment cannot be effectively restored closed, interfragmentary lag screw fixation is usually quite effective for spiral fractures. When comminution or axial instability is present, a limited number of P2 fractures may actually be most appropriately treated with plate and screw fixation.

Temporary Transarticular Pinning for Partial Articular Base Fractures

Extension block pinning is an effective strategy for dorsal and volar base fractures (Fig. 24-37). An average PIP joint ROM of 91 degrees was achieved following CRIF of dorsal base fractures despite an extensor lag of over 10 degrees in five of nine patients (79). Extension block pinning for 3 weeks or even longer to treat volar base fractures has been used with success in limited numbers of patients (80,81). Ten patients with 16-year follow-up of transarticular pins for 3 weeks with 2 additional weeks of extension block splinting achieved an average 85-degree arc of motion with an 8-degree flexion contracture and no severe degenerative changes (82).

Volar Base Fractures

Another closed fixation strategy uniquely designed for volar base fractures is a force couple device proposed by Agee (83) that works to dynamically reduce the tendency for dorsal subluxation of P2 (84). The construct involves three K-wires and a rubber band, resulting in 83% of normal ROM in 16 patients. Interested readers are referred to Agee's (83) original article and that of Buchanan (84). Acute volar base fractures involving more than 40% of the joint surface and those with sub-acute or chronic residual subluxation can be treated with volar plate arthroplasty (Fig. 24-38) (85–87). Eaton and Malerich report PIP joint ROM of 95 degrees for acute injuries and 78 to 87 degrees when treated after 6 weeks (88). Seventeen patients followed at 11.5 years demonstrated a TAM of 85 degrees when operated on within 4 weeks of injury and 61 degrees when operated on later than 4 weeks from injury (89). A series of 56 patients with volar base fracture-dislocations treated by either volar plate arthroplasty (23/56) or ORIF (33/56) yielded at 46-

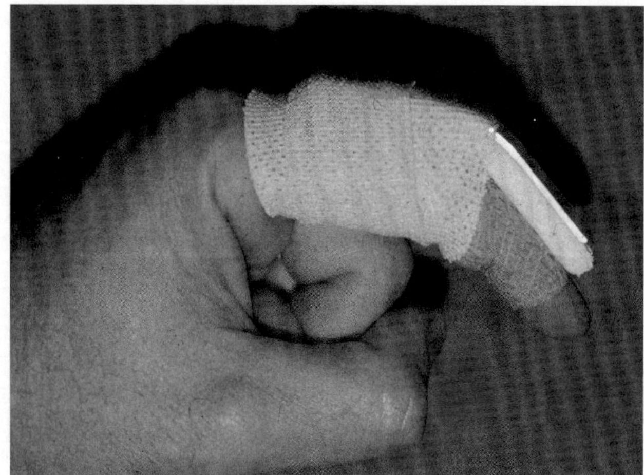

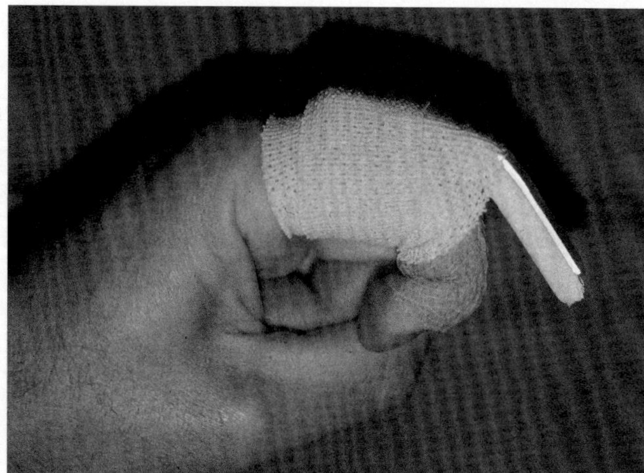

FIGURE 24-32 Extension block splinting requires that the dorsal surface of the PIP joint and proximal phalanx not be capable of pulling away from the splint.

months follow-up minimal pain in 83% but radiographic evidence of degenerative changes in 96% (90). An interesting alternative procedure offered by Weiss (91) and performed through the same "shotgun" volar exposure as a volar plate arthroplasty is that of cerclage wiring of the base of P2, which resulted in an average of 89 degrees of normal ROM for 12 patients. A few volar base (as well as dorsal base) fractures with a single large fragment can be managed by placement of one or two compression screws if great care is taken not to comminute the fragment (92). When comminution is excessive, restoration of the volar buttress with true hyaline cartilage is possible using a hemi-hamate osteochondral autograft. Thirteen patients treated with this strategy at an average of 45 days post-injury for comminution of the volar 60% of the P2 base had an average 85-degree arc of motion at 16-months follow-up (93).

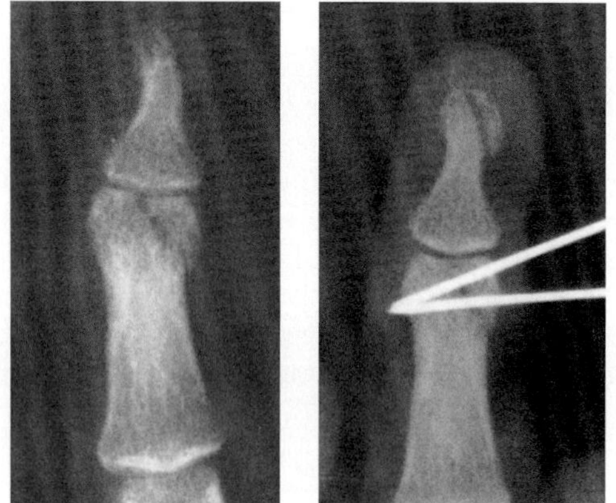

FIGURE 24-33 **A.** Unicondylar fractures at the head of P2 tend to slide along the interface producing an articular gap and/or step-off. **B.** Reduction and maintenance of the articular surface requires K-wires that converge or diverge to prevent sliding along the smooth surface of a single wire with resultant fracture displacement.

"Pilon" Fractures

The most functionally devastating injuries to the PIP joint are "pilon" fractures that involve the complete articular surface combined with metaphyseal compaction and bone loss. These are highly unstable injuries refractory to standard surgical techniques. Although adverse events such as pin tract infections may intercede, the primary complication is stiffness with long-term arcs of motion reported around 80 degrees (83,88,94,95). Unique forms of treatment have been devised for these injury patterns involving "dynamic traction" (94,96–101). The general principle is to establish a foundation at the center of rotation in the head of P1. From this foundation, traction (adjustable or elastic) is applied along the axis of P2 to hold the metaphyseal component of the fracture out to length while allowing early motion to remodel the articular surface (Fig. 24-39). In a comparative study between dynamic traction, ORIF, and splinting, Stern found the results (70- to 80-degree arc of motion and quality of articular surface restoration) to be similar between

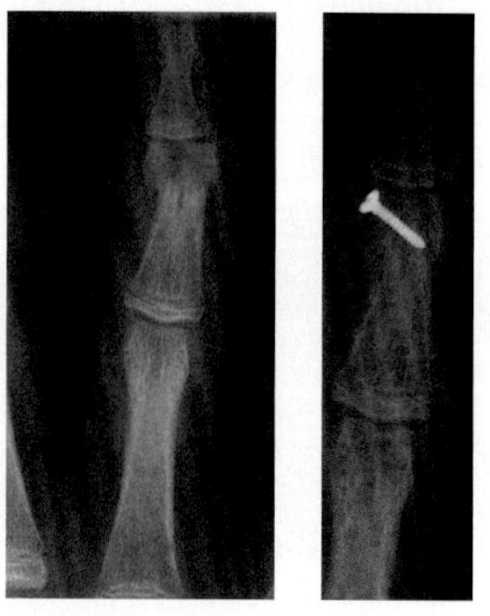

FIGURE 24-34 Lag screw fixation of **(A)** unicondylar fractures at the head of P2 can be performed with **(B)** a single screw only.

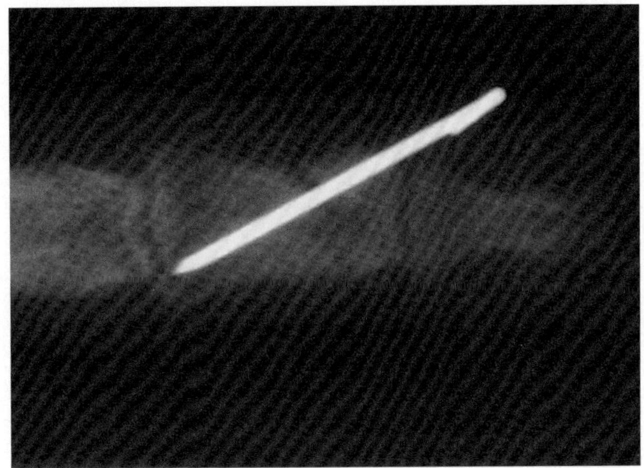

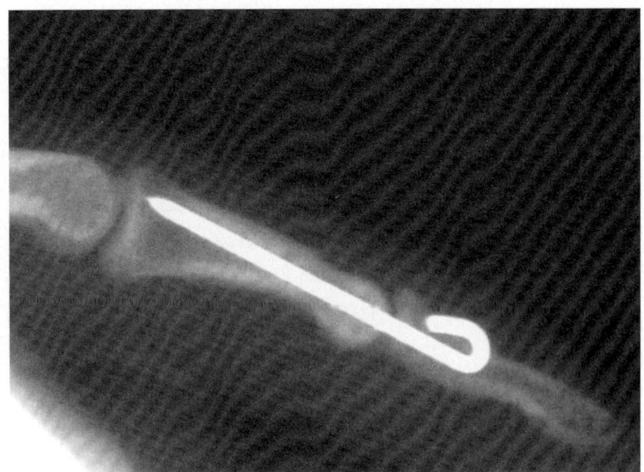

FIGURE 24-35 Fractures of the neck and shaft of P2 can be pinned with a single oblique pin only when local soft tissues and the geometry of the fracture itself add some inherent stability. Correct placement is from the **(A)** collateral recess distally to the opposite corner of the metaphyseal base and with **(B)** restoration of the natural neck to shaft curvature on the lateral.

dynamic traction and ORIF but the complications to be less with traction (102). Dynamic traction with pins and rubber bands in 14 patients followed for 2.5 years produced average PIP motion of 74 degrees and a TAM of 196 degrees (103). Dynamic fixation with wires but not elasticity in eight patients yielded final average motion of 12 to 88 degrees following wire removal at 6 weeks (104). Using a dorsal spring mechanism, 19 of 20 patients were subjectively satisfied and had a TAM of 226 degrees (105). The results are best when the patients begin treatment acutely compared with those undergoing delayed application of the devices (94,98,106). Many devices are available. Surgeons should choose the one with which they are most familiar. Although one of the original dynamic traction systems designed by Schenck called for passive motion, most of the subse-

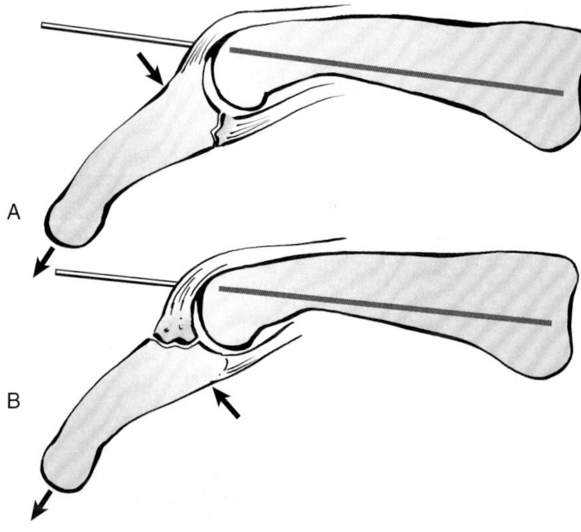

FIGURE 24-37 Extension block pinning is a closed strategy for managing **(A)** volar base fractures of P2, and **(B)** dorsal base fractures of P2.

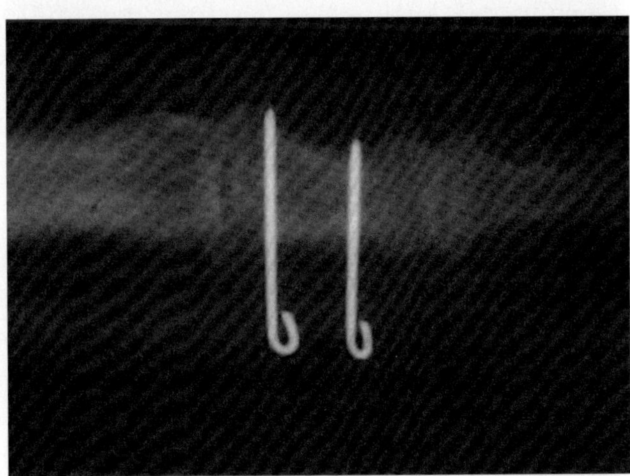

FIGURE 24-36 When the fracture planes are primarily longitudinal, transverse pinning avoids tethering near the joints.

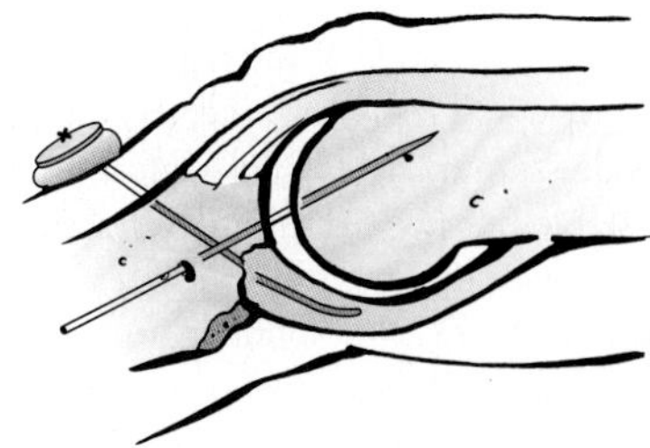

FIGURE 24-38 A volar plate arthroplasty is secured by pinning the PIP joint in flexion with the volar plate advanced distally, securing it to the margin of the articular defect with trans-osseous sutures passed to a dorsal tie-over.

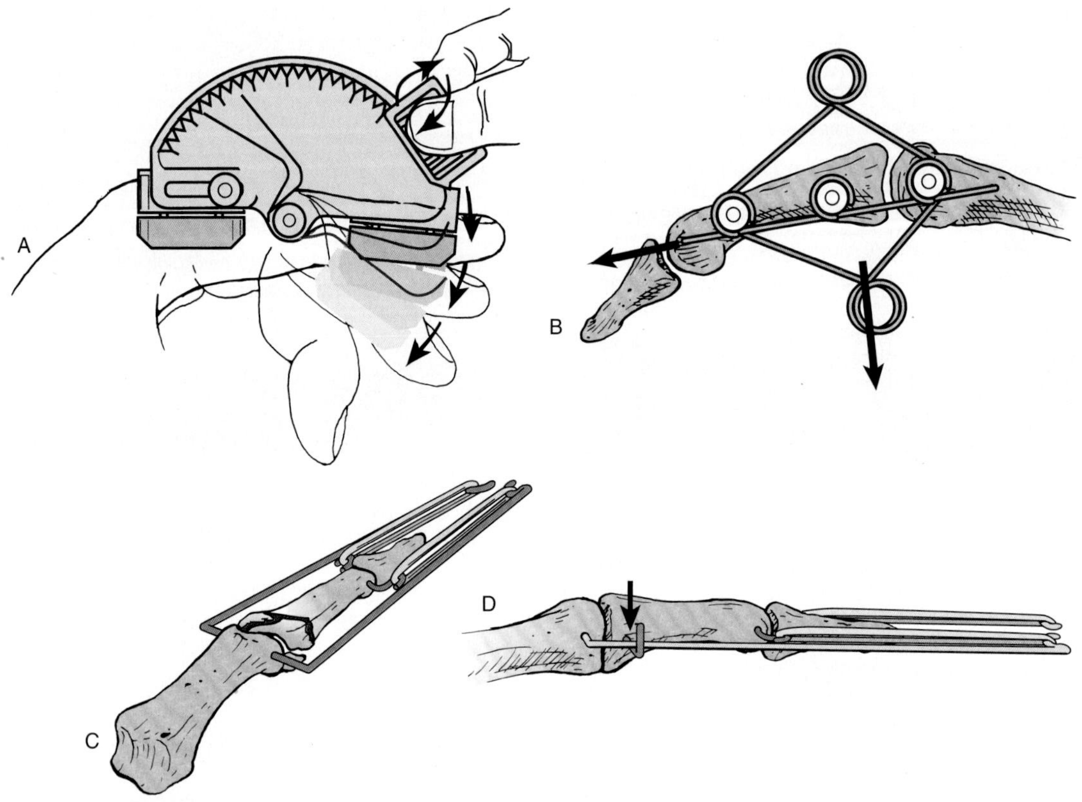

FIGURE 24-39 Strategies for managing "pilon" fractures at the base of P2 include **(A)** an adjustable unilateral hinged external fixator with distraction capabilities, **(B)** a wire spring construct, **(C)** the original configuration of pins and rubber bands, and **(D)** the same foundation augmented with an additional transverse wire across the metaphyseal base of P2 to resist dorsal subluxation.

quent ones have relied on active motion (95,101,107). Active motion with the device in place should be checked with fluoroscopy to ensure congruent motion rather than hinge motion is occurring at the PIP joint. For this reason, these cases should be done under digital block, and the need for AROM by the patient should be explained prior to the procedure.

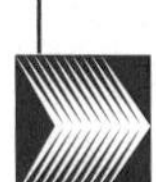

AUTHOR'S PREFERRED TREATMENT

Stable fractures are preferably treated by limited digital splints for 3 weeks or less and protected early motion thereafter with side strapping to an adjacent digit until clinically healed. Unstable but not comminuted fractures of the shaft can be treated well by temporary (3 weeks) closed pinning (Fig. 24-40). There are a few spiral fractures for which closed reduction will not achieve satisfactory control of rotation such that lag screw fixation with 1.3 mm screws is preferable to closed pinning techniques. These treatment strategies are also used in proximal phalanx fractures and more detail may be found in that subsequent section of this chapter.

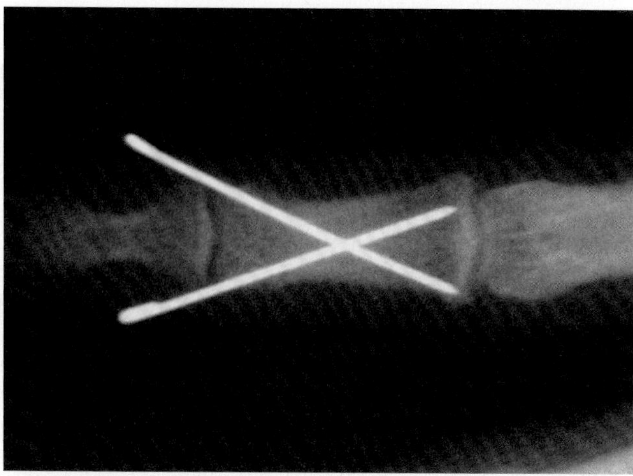

FIGURE 24-40 The relative biomechanical inferiority of K-wires crossing at the mid-shaft of the phalanx is offset by the lesser demands placed on P2 during rehabilitation than on P1 and the advantage of avoiding articular penetration to achieve a closed pinning.

Dorsal Base Fractures

When a dorsal base fracture presents early, extension block pinning is an excellent treatment. The principles are all the same as described above for extension block pinning of dorsal base fractures in the distal phalanx. At the base of P2, the larger dorsal fragment (compared to the base of P3) is easier to work with and manipulate, but the PIP joint (compared to the DIP joint) imposes greater demands for a perfect congruent joint reduction due to its more important role in overall digital function. The volar articular and shaft fragment is almost always subluxated proximally and volarly. When more than 10 to 14 days have passed since injury, it can be quite difficult (due to early soft tissue contracture) to achieve a closed reduction of this fragment relative to the head of P1. It is for these reasons that late presenting dorsal base fractures are often better managed with ORIF to ensure the clearance of consolidating hematoma from between the fragments and exact approximation of the articular reduction (Fig. 24-41). In this setting, fixation with two 1.3 mm lag screws affords enough stability to pursue early motion. Use of the countersink tap is important to minimize dorsal prominence of the screw heads and to avoid pressure concentration that might comminute the still relatively small dorsal fragment. Even though the surgical procedure occurs distal to extensor zone IV, a priority still must be placed on active extensor tendon excursion during rehabilitation to avoid a long-term extensor lag. Intra-operative assessment of the stability of the fixation will guide the progression of rehabilitation to ensure against fixation failure, recognizing the small size of the thread purchase in cancellous rather than cortical bone at the metaphyseal base of P2.

Volar Base Fractures—Closed Treatment

Volar base fractures constituting less than 25% to 30% of the joint surface rarely require surgery unless presenting late with an incongruent joint. When seen acutely, these fractures are well managed with extension block splinting that begins around 40 degrees and advances 10 to 15 degrees per week for the first 3 weeks. If the extension block splint cannot be eliminated in 3 weeks' time, this treatment strategy may not be appropriate. Fractures constituting more than 25% but less than 40% of the joint surface pose a difficulty in treatment planning as they constitute an intermediate group where the disadvantages of the two primary options are relatively well matched. It is difficult to predict in advance how the disadvantages will play out over the course of treatment for an individual patient. The disadvantage of extension block splinting or pinning is that with a greater amount of joint surface involved, the blocking must begin at a higher angle and take longer to achieve full extension. A permanent fixed flexion contracture is the consequence to be avoided. This must be compared to the overall tendency for loss of joint motion associated with open reduction and internal fixation or open reconstruction.

Volar Base Fractures—ORIF

When the volar fragment(s) constitute greater than 40% of the joint surface, an open procedure offers the greatest assurance of achieving a congruent joint as a final result. The distinction between open reduction and internal fixation for one or two relatively large fragments or open reconstruction for highly comminuted multiple fragments cannot often be made until the time of surgery. One should always be prepared for both possibilities in the pre-operative planning discussions with the patient. Dorsal base fractures usually provide a single fragment of reasonable size for direct lag screw fixation. Volar base fractures are not so easy. One or two large fragments that facilitate lag screw fixation are the exception rather than the rule. In this case, two 1.3mm lag screws are appropriate. Placement is side by side with one

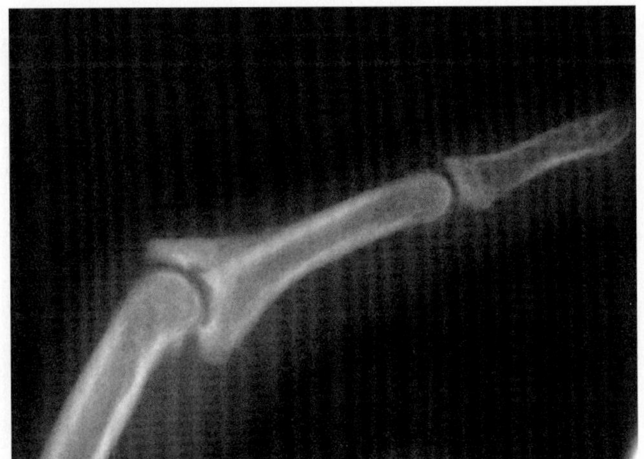
A

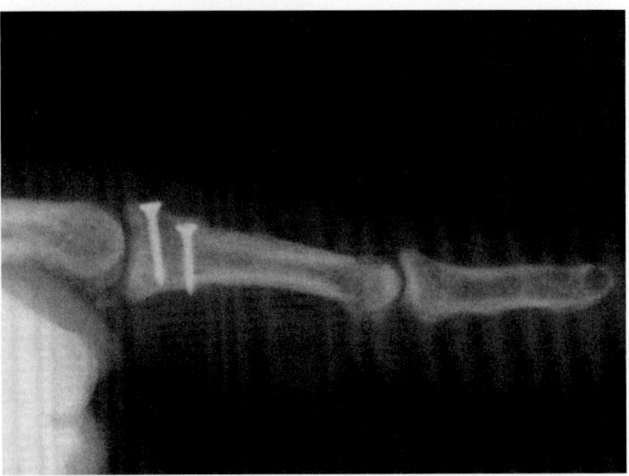
B

FIGURE 24-41 A. Dorsal base fractures allow the volar articular fragment and the attached shaft of P2 to sublux volarly and proximally. **B.** A congruent joint is restored with sufficient stability to initiate early rehabilitation by lag screw fixation.

screw in the radial half of the base fragment and other in the ulnar half. If two separate radial and ulnar volar base fragments are found, this strategy is still acceptable provided that the fragment diameter is at least three times the screw diameter and compression can be achieved without causing fragment comminution. The countersink tap is useful in this regard. The operative approach is the same as described for reconstruction of a collection of comminuted fragments.

Volar Base Fractures—Osteochondral Reconstruction

A Bruner incision is made using one limb over P1 and a second over P2. The flexor tendon sheath is reflected as a single rectangular flap hinging on its lateral margin between the distal margin of the A2 pulley and the proximal margin of the A4 pulley. The FDS and FDP are retracted laterally to either side, and the collateral ligament origins are dissected as a sleeve from the lateral surfaces of the head of P1. Release of the volar plate allows complete hyperextension of the PIP joint with presentation of both joint surfaces towards the surgeon. This is the so-called "shotgun" approach and its variations center around management of the volar plate. This approach is also used for volar plate arthroplasty and ORIF. In the former procedure, the volar plate is released distally so that it may be advanced to replace the defect in the volar articular surface. In the latter, it should remain attached to the fragments as an important source of blood supply. When performing a reconstruction of irreparable comminution, the volar plate may be released along its distal margin. The defect in the volar articular surface may range anywhere from 40% up to almost 90%, often with irregular margins. A small saw or burr should be used to straighten the irregular margins into sharp orthogonal cuts that define a clear bed of cancellous bone in the metaphysis that can be accurately measured for reconstruction. The articular surface at the base of P2 has a sagitally oriented ridge that interdigitates with the recession between the two condyles at the head of P1. This relationship is important not only for preserving joint congruence but for maintaining stability in the setting of the collateral ligament releases. An excellent geometric match has been found in the distal articular surface of the hamate at the ridge that separates the ring from the small finger CMC joints. The measurements taken from the defect at the base of P2 are transposed to the hamate and a small saw and osteotomes are used to remove the osteochondral graft from its donor site. The graft is then exactly trimmed to match the defect and secured with two 1.3-mm lag screws (Fig. 24-42). The joint is checked clinically and radiographically for maintenance of congruence through a full range of motion. The flexor sheath is re-approximated with 6-0 monofilament sutures and the PIP joint splinted for protection. Immediate active motion rehabilitation is begun within days of surgery.

Open Reduction with Internal and External Fixation (ORIEF) of "Pilon" Fracture

Complete articular fractures of the base of P2 may be treated by entirely closed reduction and stabilization. If significant metaphyseal bone loss is present or if the articular fragments at the base of P2 do not reduce sufficiently with traction alone, a small incision can be made through which cancellous bone graft can be added to fill the metaphyseal void and to assist in supporting a reduction of the articular fragments (108). Transverse 0.035-inch K-wires may be placed at the subchondral level to maintain the articular relationships. The fracture as a whole must then be reduced at the metaphyseal level and undergo stabilization sufficient to withstand the rigors of early motion that must accompany articular fractures. It is at this point that the significant variations in technique

A 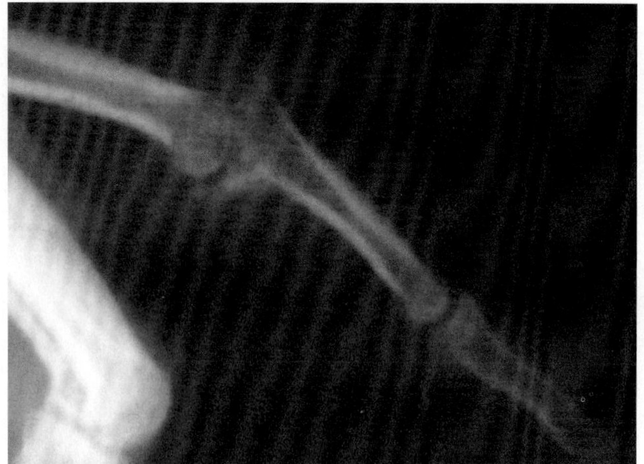

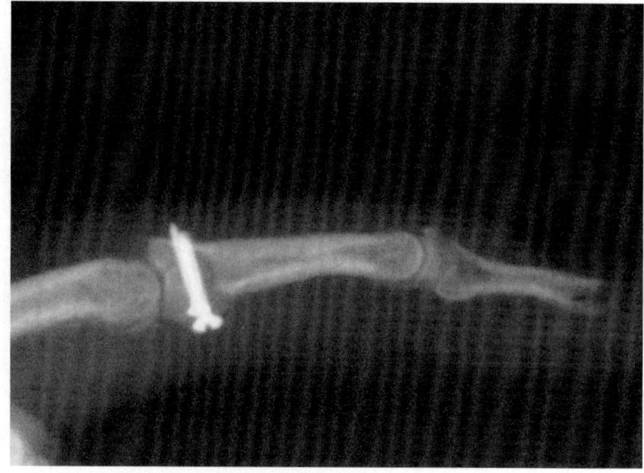 B

FIGURE 24-42 Volar base fractures with **(A)** comminution of a substantial portion of the articular surface and subluxation can be **(B)** reconstructed with an osteochondral graft from the hamate with particular emphasis placed on recreating the volar lip buttress and a truly congruent reproduction of the radius of curvature.

arise along with different devices available for stabilization. My preference is for an off-the-shelf unilateral hinged external fixator with a manual adjustment for longitudinal traction. The device itself allows either free AROM with a gear disengaged or passive range of motion (PROM) with the gear engaged (Fig. 24-43). Motion rehabilitation is initiated immediately and continued until final healing. The patient's performance of hourly motion exercises often causes significant pin irritation to the point of necessitating an early removal prior to the planned 4 weeks.

Pearls and Pitfalls

Volar Base Fracture Dislocations

There are two critical steps in performing volar base osteochondral graft reconstructions. The first is to establish sharp and flat borders in the metaphyseal defect to receive and inset the graft stably with broad cancellous surfaces for rapid bone healing. The second critical step is trimming the graft to fit this bed. The common pitfall is to set the graft's articular surface perpendicular to the neutral axis of the bone. This fails to reestablish the volar buttress and a truly congruent joint surface. If the graft is cut correctly, once inset it should replicate the buttressing function of the native volar base and prevent dorsal dislocation.

"Pilon" Fractures

When fixing a "pilon" fracture with the unilateral hinged fixator, repeated checks on orientation of the device as a whole are needed to prevent progression to malunion. The majority of the mistakes cause the hinge on the device to rotate along a different axis than the joint itself.

Common errors are to have the device translated farther from the neutral axis of the bone at the P1 level than the P2 level or to have the pins entering the phalanges obliquely rather than in the true mid-axial plane. Above all, the surgery should be performed under a local anesthetic with the patient demonstrating true active PIP joint motion under fluoroscopy to judge the maintenance of congruence throughout the range of motion. Finally, there must be no tension in the skin around the pins, as the hourly motion performed in rehabilitation will enhance pin tract infections.

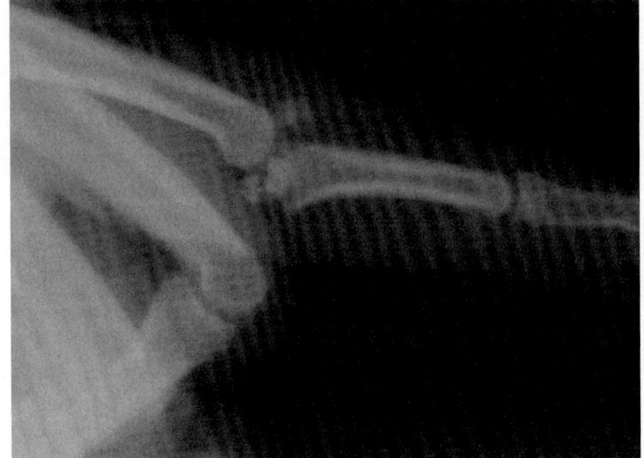

A

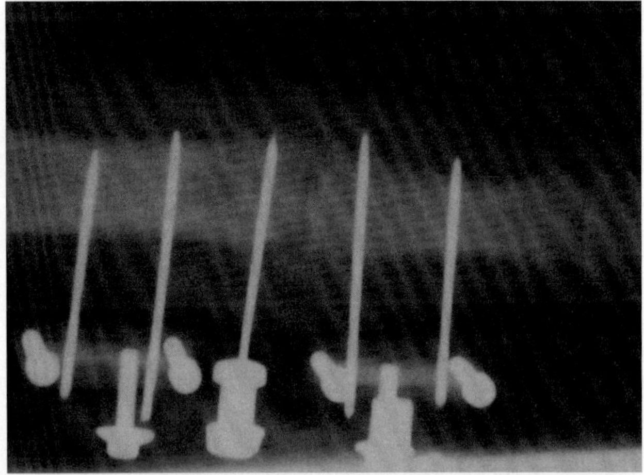

B

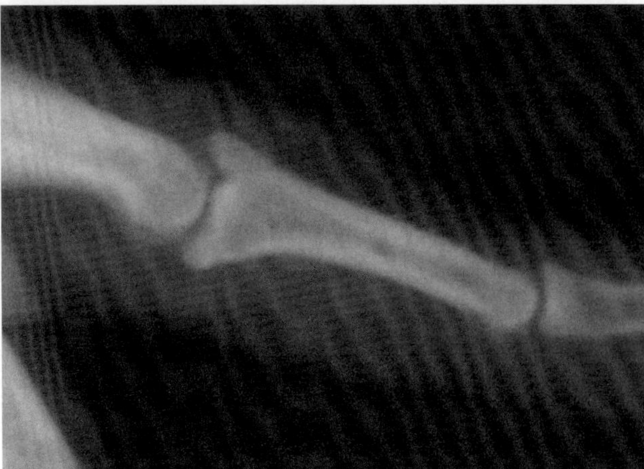

C

FIGURE 24-43 Comminuted complete articular fractures at the base of P2 **(A)** can be treated with a hinged external fixator **(B)** to the point of restoration of a congruent joint with smooth gliding motion **(C)**.

PROXIMAL INTERPHALANGEAL JOINT DISLOCATIONS

Dislocations of the proximal interphalangeal (PIP) joint have a high rate of missed diagnoses that are passed off as "sprains." Although a large number of incomplete injuries occur (especially in ball-handling sports), complete disruptions of the collateral ligaments and the volar plate are also frequent (50% occur in the long finger followed in frequency by the ring finger) (109). Since dramatic swelling is often present even with minor injuries to the PIP joint, this sign may often get dismissed by initial examiners of the patient who in fact has a more serious injury. One series of 15 volar dislocations went an average of 11 weeks before appreciation of the correct diagnosis through referral (110). Careful palpation for localized tenderness may direct attention to one of the collateral ligaments, the volar plate, or the insertion of the central slip. The capacity for active PIP extension against resistance from a starting position of PIP flexion confirms the integrity of the central slip. Limitation of passive DIP flexion while the PIP joint is held in extension may appear several weeks following the initial injury and signify a developing boutonnière deformity. Congruence on the lateral radiograph is the key to detecting residual subluxation. Correct axial rotational alignment is demonstrated when both P1 and P2 are seen in a true lateral projection on the same film.

Residual instability is quite rare in pure dislocations as opposed to fracture-dislocations where it is the chief issue at stake. It manifests as hyperextension laxity following volar plate injuries managed with an inadequate initial degree of extension blocking. Correction of hyperextension instability can be performed with either delayed reattachment of the volar plate or a capsulotenodesis reconstruction (111). In pure dislocations, stiffness is the primary concern. Stiffness can occur following any injury pattern and responds best at the late stage to complete collateral ligament excision (112). Chronic missed dislocations require open reduction with a predictable amount of subsequent stiffness (110,113). In a series of 15 open dorsal PIP dislocations, only seven patients had a satisfactory outcome. Factors associated with poor outcome were treatment in the emergency department, failure to administer antibiotics, failure to repair the volar plate, fracture at the base of P2, and associated injuries in the hand (114). Patients should be counseled to expect permanent residual enlargement of the joint and for the final resolution of stiffness and aching to take as long as 12 to 18 months (115).

Surgical and Applied Anatomy

The head of P1 is quite different from that of the metacarpal. There is no cam effect. The head is bicondylar, and the collateral ligaments originate from the center axis of joint rotation. Nevertheless, the accessory collateral ligaments and volar plate are lax in flexion and will become contracted if immobilized in that position (116). At the volar base of P2, there are tubercles for the confluence of the proper and accessory collateral ligaments with the volar plate. This junction is referred to as the "critical corner." This three-sided box design provides excellent inherent joint stability (Fig. 24-44). The volar plate anatomy is unique at the PIP joint with the presence of strong check-rein ligaments that originate inside the margins of the A2 pulley confluent with the C1 pulley fibers and the oblique retinacular ligament (111). The distal insertion of the volar plate is strong only at its lateral margins (117). A concept found consistently in 70 cadavers was the existence of a dorsal plate of articulating fibrocartilage on the joint surface of the central slip that may aid in stabilization, prevent central slip attenuation, and increase the extensor moment arm (118). Although primarily a hinge, the PIP joint accommodates 7 to 10 degrees of lateral deviation and slight axial rotation (68,116). The normal range of motion may be up to 120 degrees of flexion. In contrast to the other small joints of the hand, PIP joint volar plate disruptions usually occur distally (117,119). The proper collateral ligaments are the primary stabilizers to lateral stress, and greater than a 20-degree opening signifies complete disruption (120,121). Collateral ligament disruption is usually proximal, but the fibers traditionally stay positioned over their anatomic origin for subsequent healing (120).

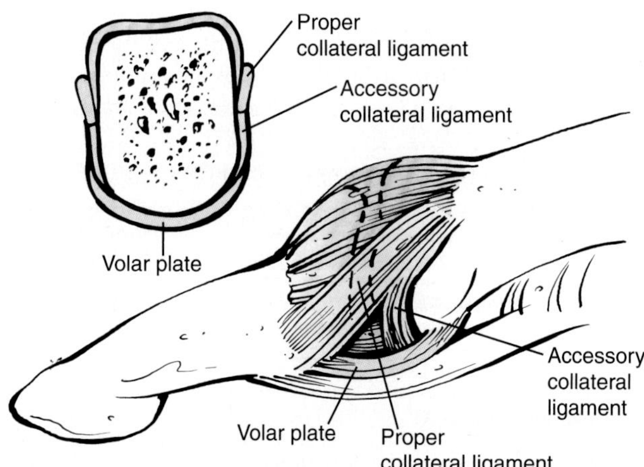

FIGURE 24-44 The PIP joint receives static stability from the proper and accessory collateral ligaments and the volar plate, supplemented by the dynamic stability of the dorsal plate and other balanced tendon forces acting across the joint.

Recognized patterns of dislocation other than complete collateral ligament injury are dorsal dislocation, pure volar dislocation, and rotatory volar dislocation (Fig. 24-45). Dorsal dislocations involve volar plate injury (usually distally and with or without a small flake of bone). For pure volar dislocations the pathologic findings are consistently damage to the volar plate, one collateral ligament, and the central slip (110). Rotatory volar dislocation occurs as the head of P1 passes between the central slip and the lateral bands, which can form a noose effect and prevent reduction (Fig. 24-46) (122). Irreducible dislocations obstructed by the volar plate or flexor tendons are uncommon injuries.

Current Treatment Options

Dorsal Dislocations—Nonoperative Management

Current treatment options are listed in Table 24-6. Isolated volar plate injuries had 95% good or excellent results with only 7 to

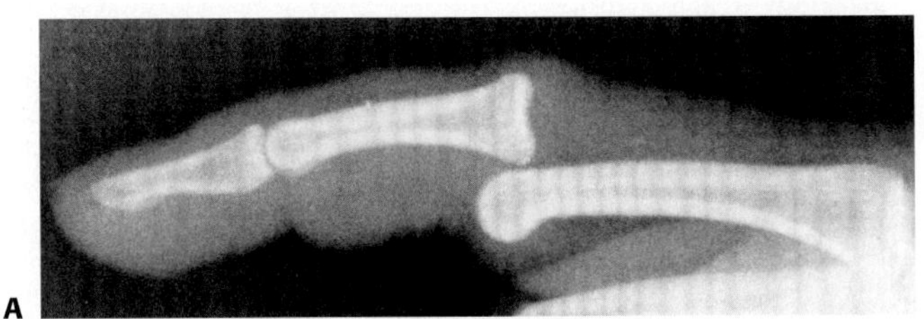

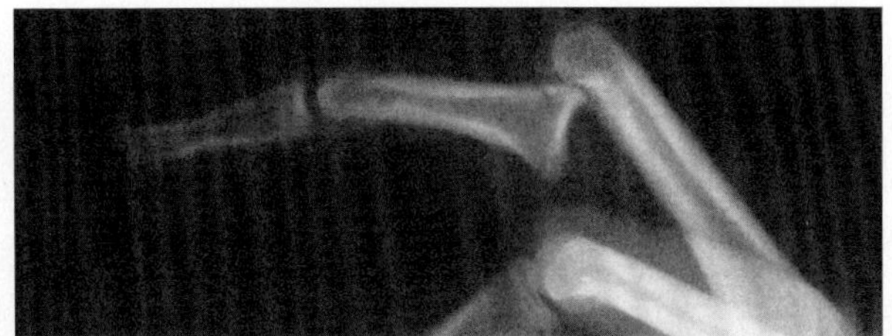

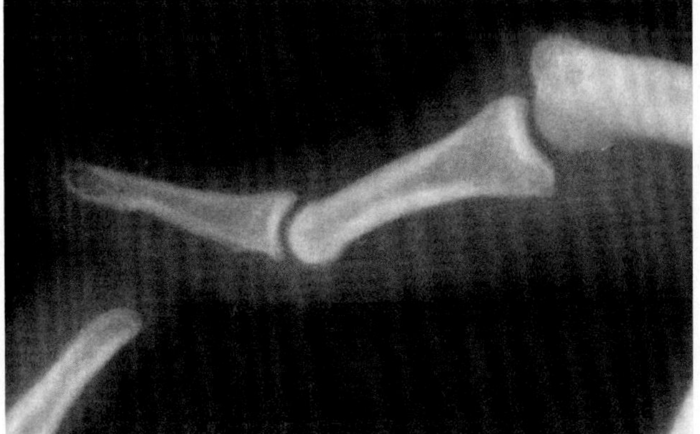

FIGURE 24-45 Three variants of PIP dislocation are seen. The most common are dorsal **(A)**, pure volar with central slip disruption **(B)**, and volar rotatory (note that P2 is seen as a true lateral whereas P1 is seen in oblique profile) **(C)**.

10 days of splinting followed by 6 weeks of "buddy taped" (strapped to an adjacent digit) AROM (123). If subluxation is not present at full extension, immediate mobilization allowed full functional return by 6.8 weeks compared to 10.9 weeks when started with extension block splinting (124). Fortunately, the majority of hyperextension injuries remain congruent even at full extension and do not require extension block splinting (Fig. 24-47). However, one must consider that the distal volar plate is poorly vascularized, and a lack of early healing may lead to chronic hyperextension laxity (117). Lower profile digitally based splints or buddy taping may effectively prevent the full extension that could threaten sound volar plate healing (125). When formal extension block splinting is chosen (usually only in the situation of fracture-subluxation), the rate of progression each week is determined by the severity of the initial injury but should reach full extension no later than 4 weeks from injury.

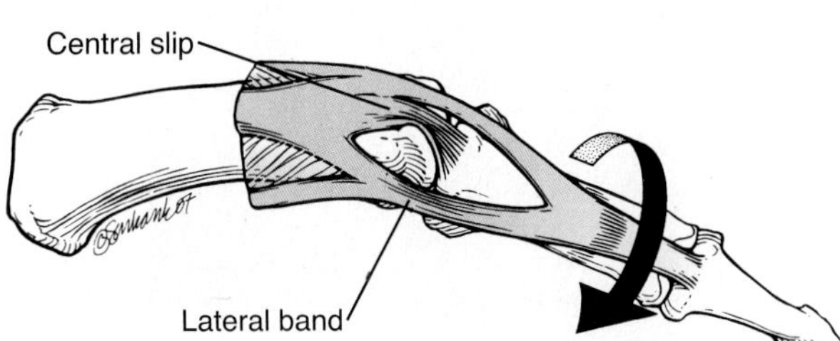

FIGURE 24-46 In volar rotatory dislocations, the head of P1 protrudes between the intact central slip and one lateral band, which create a noose effect preventing reduction especially if longitudinal traction is applied.

Pure Volar Dislocations—Nonoperative Management

With pure volar dislocations, central slip disruption occurs and will result in a boutonnière deformity if not treated properly. Careful examination consisting of PIP extension against resistance from a starting position of full flexion will prevent missing the diagnosis of a central slip disruption. Limitation of passive DIP flexion is an early sign of a developing boutonnière. Even

TABLE 24-6 Proximal Interphalangeal Joint Dislocations

Treatment Option	Pros	Cons
Splinting	Least stiffness	Requires patient cooperation
CRIF	Reliably maintains reduction	Rarely indicated, pin tract infection, stiffness
ORIF	Part of open dislocation management; required for irreducible dislocations	Added stiffness

CRIF, closed reduction and internal fixation; ORIF, open reduction and internal fixation.

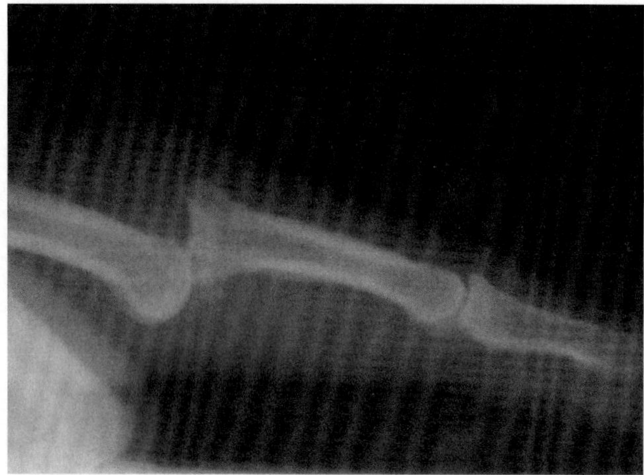

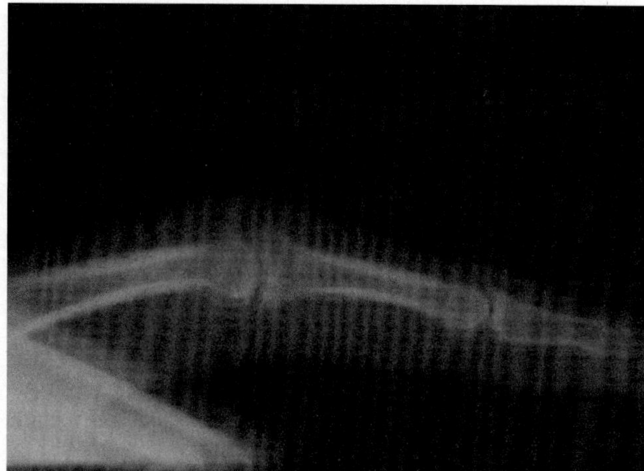

FIGURE 24-47 **A.** Dorsal PIP joint dislocations frequently demonstrate a small bone flake at the volar base of P2 representing the distal volar plate avulsion that usually **(B)** reduces spontaneously with the remainder of the congruent articulation.

when identified late, the treatment of choice is extension splinting at the PIP joint with immediate active DIP flexion exercises. Active DIP flexion pulls the whole extensor mechanism (including the ruptured central slip) distally through the intact lateral bands. The duration of PIP extension splinting is usually 4 to 6 weeks with a transitional period of night splinting for several weeks to follow.

Rotatory Volar Dislocations—Nonoperative Management

Rotatory volar dislocations where the head of P1 is trapped between the central slip and lateral band may be difficult to reduce owing to the noose effect exerted by these two soft tissue structures. The key to reduction (if it is possible at all) is to relax both structures. Wrist extension relaxes the extrinsic component, and full MP flexion relaxes the intrinsic component. A gentle rotating maneuver that avoids excessive longitudinal traction stands the highest chance of success. A few of these dislocations remain irreducible even in the most skilled hands. When a reduction can be achieved, early mobilization is then instituted with buddy taping to an adjacent digit (usually the more radial) in an attempt to prevent stiffness.

Open Reduction

There are two indications for open treatment of PIP joint injuries: an open injury or an irreducible dislocation. Lateral dislocations may also be irreducible due to interposition of a torn collateral ligament (Fig. 24-48) (126). A mid-axial (or dual mid-axial) incision allows for management of both dorsal and volar dislocations (127,128). Controversy remains as to the need for direct repair of complete collateral ligament ruptures and volar plate injuries (108). Direct repair is probably only functionally necessary in the long term for the radial collateral ligament of the index finger. Chronic reconstruction of collateral ligament deficiency is an even more technically demanding procedure

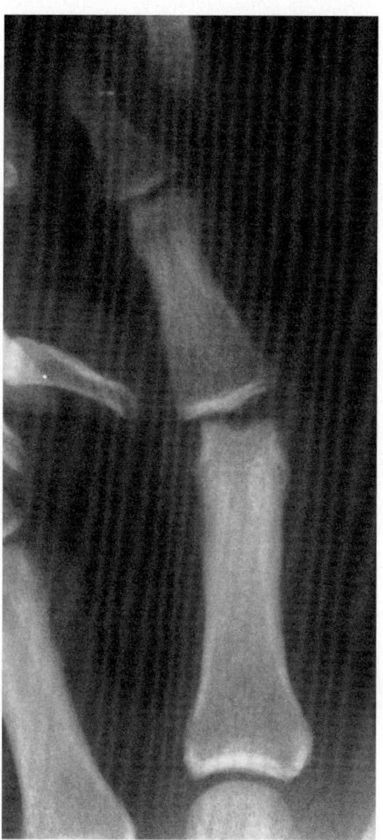

FIGURE 24-48 Entrapment of a collateral ligament can prevent reduction of the PIP joint; lateral stress examination demonstrates the high degree of instability in this situation.

with a high propensity for generating stiffness but may be accomplished by a variety of techniques.

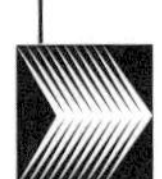

AUTHOR'S PREFERRED TREATMENT

Once reduced, rotatory volar dislocations, isolated collateral ligament ruptures, and dorsal dislocations congruent in full extension on the lateral radiograph can all begin immediate AROM with adjacent digit strapping. Dorsal dislocations that are subluxated on the extension lateral radiograph require a few weeks of extension block splinting before progressing (this is an almost unheard of situation with pure dislocation and no fracture component). Volar dislocations with central slip disruptions require 4 to 6 weeks of PIP extension splinting followed by nighttime static extension splinting for 2 additional weeks. The DIP joint should be unsplinted and actively flexed throughout the entire recovery period.

Open dorsal dislocations usually have a transverse rent in the skin at the flexion crease. Debridement of this wound should precede reduction of the dislocation (114). Any joint debris should be cleared out to prevent third body wear. The "critical corner" warrants particular attention. For closed irreducible joints, unilateral or bilateral mid-axial incisions allow excellent access to both volar and dorsal structures without violating the extensor mechanism. Post-operative management follows the same time courses stated above for nonoperative management based on the injury pattern and severity.

Pearls and Pitfalls

Straight longitudinal traction is almost never the answer to accomplishing a reduction and certainly is the surest way to fail at the PIP joint. Relaxation of the most powerful tendon forces acting across the joint is the key to facilitating a smooth reduction that does not cause additional hyaline cartilage damage. Post-reduction clinical and radiographic assessment is crucial with an emphasis on the lateral radiograph in full extension to assess congruence. The patient should be able to move the finger through a near full range of motion under the influence of the digital block used to accomplish the reduction. Open dislocations should be taken seriously for their high rate of complications and debrided prior to reduction.

PROXIMAL PHALANX (P1) FRACTURES

Proximal phalanx (P1) fractures include intra-articular fractures of the head, extra-articular fractures of the neck and shaft, and both extra-articular and intra-articular fractures of the base (Fig. 24-49). Further describing the pattern of the fracture as transverse, short oblique, long oblique or spiral for shaft fractures and partial or complete articular for intra-articular fractures (along with the degree and direction of displacement) provides the necessary information on which to base treatment decisions. A specific fracture pattern that risks extreme PIP limitation is that of the proximal phalangeal neck, where a volar spike of bone from the proximal fracture fragment impinges into the sub-capital recess volar to the neck of P1 (Fig. 24-49B). If the fracture heals in this position, full PIP flexion is prevented through obstruction of the space for volar plate in folding. This pattern is best identified on an individual digital lateral view and warrants operative treatment to prevent a functionally disabling malunion.

Surgical and Applied Anatomy

Local Soft Tissue Relationships

Fracture of the proximal phalanx may well be one of the most frustrating orthopaedic injuries to manage (129,130). The prime reason is the local soft tissue anatomy. While the metacarpal has only a cord-like extensor tendon running well dorsal to it, the proximal phalanx is closely invested by a sheet-like extensor mechanism with a complex array of decussating collagen fibers (Fig. 24-50). Surgical disturbance of the fine balance between these fibers can permanently alter the long-term function of the digit. The operative approach to P1 can be either dorsal or lateral. The dorsal approach may be technically simpler but transgresses the extensor mechanism. The lateral mid-axial approach allows the fracture to be fully exposed and hardware placed in its proper lateral position (if hardware is indicated) without directly violating the extensor mechanism. If prominent hardware is to be placed, the intrinsic tendon on that side (usually ulnar) may be resected. Finally, one must understand the phalanx to be highly elliptical (in fact tunnel shaped) in cross section, rather than cylindrical, with a thicker dorsal cortex (131).

Deforming Forces

At the proximal phalangeal level, both intrinsic and extrinsic tendon forces deform the fracture (132). They result in a predictable apex volar deformity for transverse and short oblique fractures. These forces can in fact be used with benefit during rehabilitation. If the MP joints are maximally flexed, the intrinsic muscle forces acting through the extensor mechanism overlying P1 create a tension band effect that helps to maintain fracture reduction (Fig. 24-51). Active PIP joint motion will heighten this effect and forms the basis for nonoperative fracture management. Spiral and long oblique fractures tend to shorten and rotate rather than angulate. These fractures also have more complex patterns of deformity that are not so easily controlled through the joint positioning just described.

There should be 12 degrees of extensor lag at the PIP joint for each millimeter of shortening and 1.5 degrees of extensor lag for each degree of apex palmar fracture angulation (133).

Biomechanics of Fixation

The biomechanics of internal fixation for phalangeal fractures have been well studied, reiterating the weakness of crossed K-wires and the strength of compression lag screws (134,135).

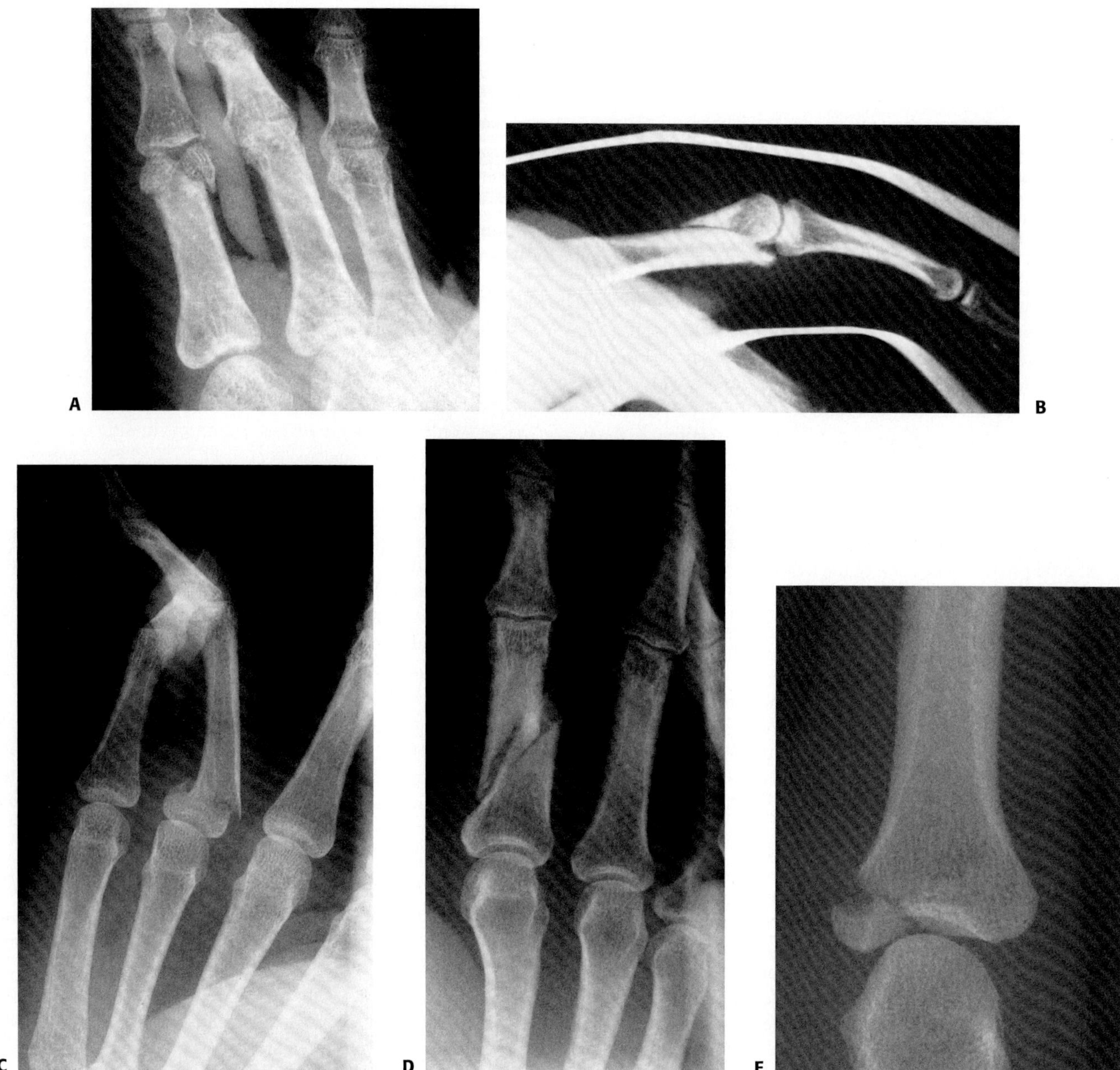

FIGURE 24-49 Fracture patterns appearing in P1 include **(A)** complete articular fractures of the head, **(B)** sub-capital fractures with impingement in the volar plate recess, **(C)** transverse fractures of the shaft or base, **(D)** oblique fractures of the shaft, and **(E)** articular fractures of the base.

Modes of failure in a four-point bending model on transverse osteotomies confirmed existing information, with screws and plates failing through the propagation of new fracture planes, intra-osseous wires failing through cutout or untwisting, and K-wires failing by bending or sliding out at the bone interface (136). Studies have shown the biomechanical inefficiency of dorsally applied plates in an apex volar bending model that correlated with the clinical forces experienced at the P1 level (137,138). In an interesting cadaver study, the effect of plate application on PIP joint flexion demonstrated a limitation by all plates but less so for the laterally applied mini-condylar plate than the dorsal straight or H-plate (138).

Current Treatment Options

Nonoperative Management

Current treatment options are listed in Table 24-7. Nonoperative management is the preferred treatment for most phalangeal fractures (Barton suggests 75%), which fall into the categories

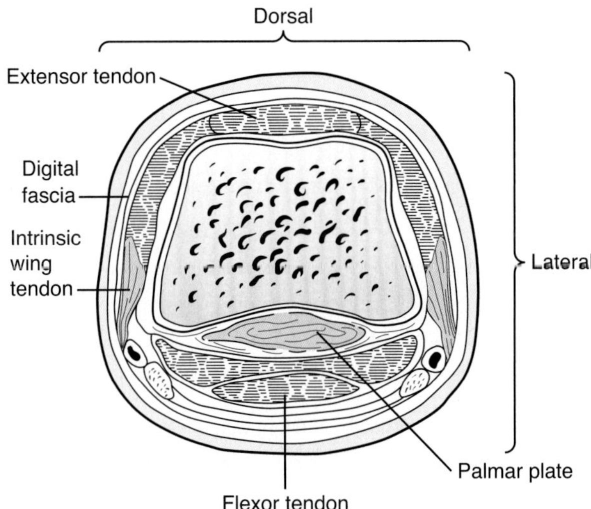

FIGURE 24-50 The proximal phalanx is closely invested by the sheet of the zone IV extensor tendon dorsally, the blending of the intrinsic wing tendons laterally and volarly, and the flexor tendons and flexor sheath direct volarly.

of minimally displaced-stable and reducible-stable (139). Transverse fracture patterns will generally prove to be stable after reduction compared to oblique, spiral, or comminuted fractures. Stable proximal phalangeal fractures are ideal candidates for dorsal splinting in MP joint flexion (140). This is particularly true in the proximal 6 to 9 mm of the proximal phalangeal base, where local soft tissue attachments confer an additional degree of stability (141). Nonoperative management has proven clinically effective in these base fractures (96% excellent/good) but also at the shaft level (80% excellent/good) (142). Only 4 of 45 patients treated in intrinsic plus splints failed to achieve full motion by 6 weeks (143). The splint should be able to be discontinued at 3 weeks and followed by AROM without resistance. Stable, nondisplaced fractures may even be treated by a program of immediate AROM, protected only with adjacent digit strapping. A series of 147 patients with stable transverse fractures had over 90% good to excellent results with entirely nonoperative means (144). The take-home message for nonoperative management is that a carefully formed splint and/or adjacent digit strapping can effectively maintain an existing and reasonably stable reduction. What splints and strapping cannot accomplish is a reduction in their own right. In case this fact is not appreciated at the initial encounter, all patients undergoing nonoperative management should be seen back in the office at a week to verify maintenance of reduction.

Closed Reduction Internal Fixation

This is the treatment of choice for the category of reducible but unstable isolated fractures, both extra-articular and some intra-articular (145). A higher degree of care must be exercised when pursuing CRIF in the phalanges compared to the metacarpals due to the close investment by the broad extensor mechanism. Entry sites should be chosen carefully to minimize tethering of the extensor mechanism. In the proximal two-thirds of P1, this is virtually impossible. As one approaches the distal one-third, a direct lateral approach can be made volar to the interosseous tendon. For long oblique and spiral fractures, three K-wires (0.045 or 0.035 inch) are placed perpendicular to the fracture plane (Fig. 24-52). For short oblique and transverse fractures, longitudinal pins are placed through the MP joint (Fig. 24-53). Trocar-tipped K-wires rather than diamond-tipped or self-cut wires should be used (146). The wire should be passed through the soft tissues down to bone prior to activating the wire driver. Pins should be cut off outside the skin and bent to prevent migration. Absolute parallelism of the K-wires for oblique fractures risks the fracture displacing as it slides along the wires. Some degree of convergence or divergence of the wires will help to prevent this consequence of using smooth wires. Wires may even be placed through the metacarpal head itself and then longitudinally down the phalanx, accepting lack of motion at the MP joint for the 3-week duration of pinning.

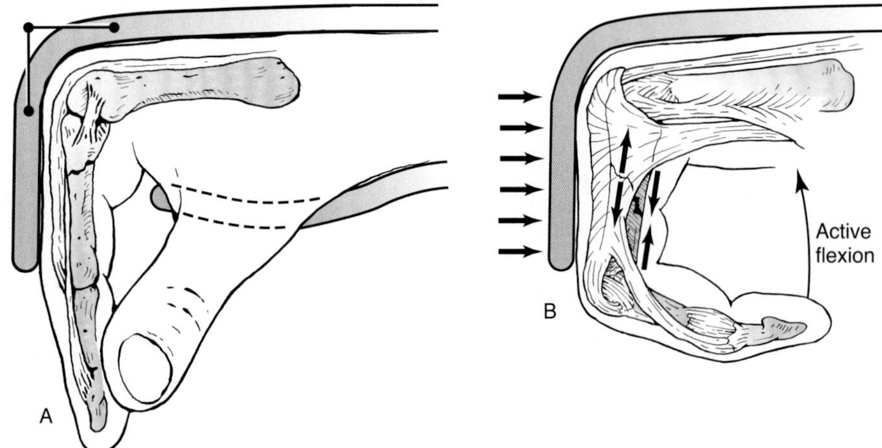

FIGURE 24-51 Flexing the MP joints fully causes the extensor apparatus to function as a tension band to a transverse fracture in the P1 shaft, helping to reduce the deformity when the PIP joint is actively flexed.

TABLE 24-7 Proximal Phalanx Fractures

Treatment Option	Pros	Cons
Splinting	Treatment of choice for stable and minimally displaced fractures; no added surgical stiffness	Does not effectively control rotation, noncompliant patients with unstable fractures
CRIF	Very effective for simple two-part fractures, especially transverse and short oblique	Pin tract infection, may not control the rotation of spiral fractures effectively
ORIF lag screws	Controls rotation accurately for spiral fractures	Added surgical stiffness especially at PIP joint Extensor lag
ORIF plates and screws	Necessary for comminution or bone loss	Added hardware bulk often necessitating removal with stiffness proportionate to surgical dissection
ORIF composite wiring	Simple supplies easily obtained. May be the only method possible with some fragment patterns, including comminution	K-wires protrude to interfere with tendons; need for hardware removal; not effective in presence of segmental bone loss

CRIF, closed reduction and internal fixation; ORIF, open reduction and internal fixation; PIP, proximal interphalangeal.

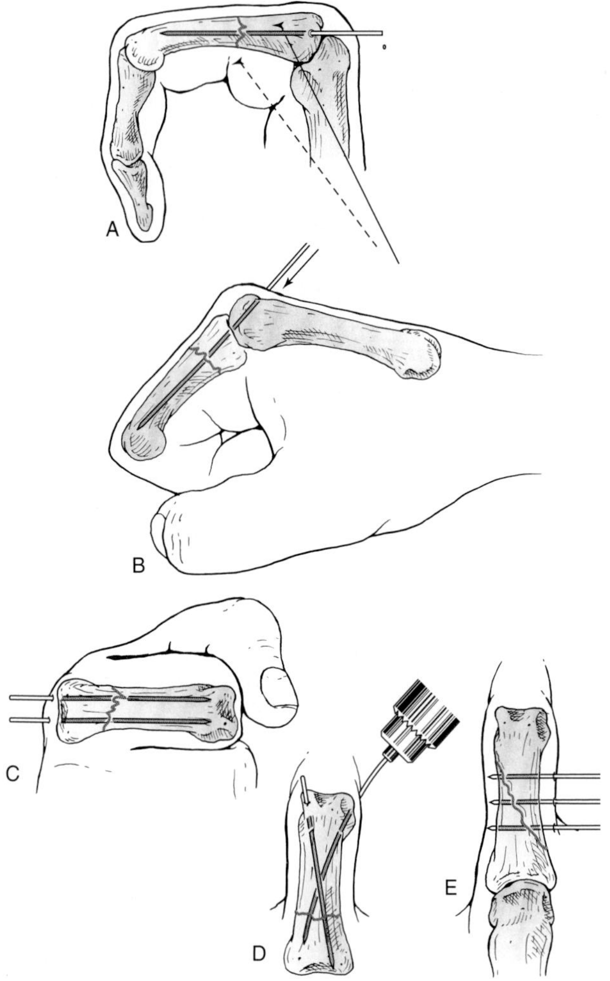

FIGURE 24-52 Closed reduction and internal fixation of P1 shaft fractures can be accomplished **(A)** longitudinally through the MP joint but not the metacarpal head, **(B)** or through the metacarpal head, **(C)** with the wires for either of these options running parallel in the phalanx, or **(D)** entering at the collateral recess and crossing, or **(E)** transverse.

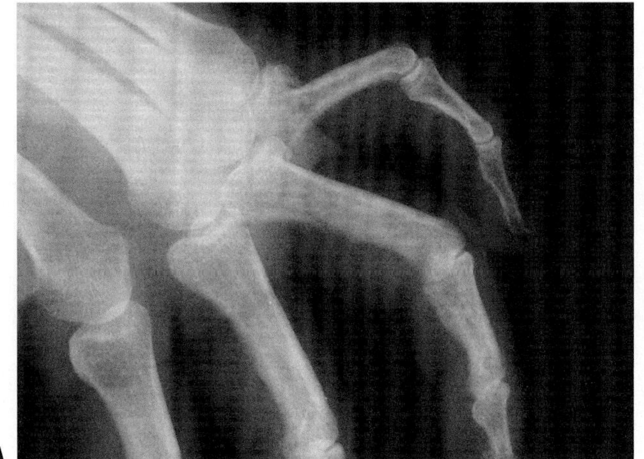

A

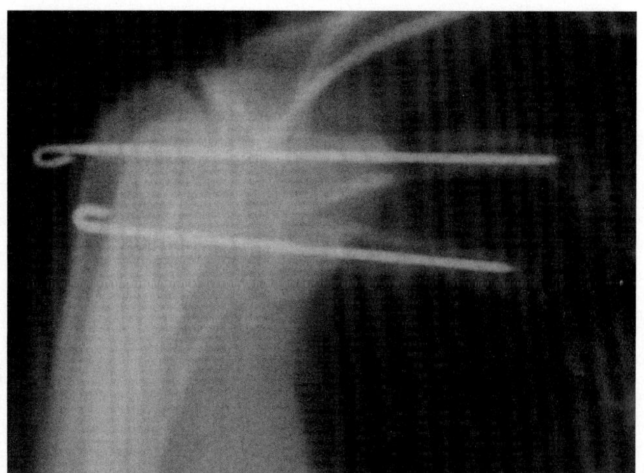

B

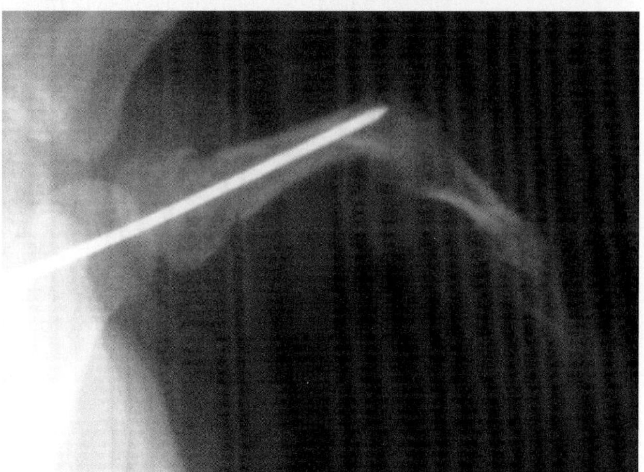

C

FIGURE 24-53 Transverse fractures at the base of P1 **(A)** have inherent soft tissue stability once reduced and can be stabilized by a single wire per fracture (passing through the metacarpal head) **(B)**. **C.** This is best demonstrated on an oblique view.

Commercially available devices have been specially designed for closed intramedullary rodding of the phalanx (Fig. 24-54). Routinely, pins should be removed by 3 weeks. When this is done, any final limitations of motion are most likely due to the injury itself rather than the pins. Eighteen of 21 patients who had 26 fractures achieved normal motion when pins were removed at 3 weeks followed by active motion with adjacent digit strapping for 3 additional weeks (147). Similar results were seen in 29 spiral oblique and 25 transverse fractures where pins were removed at 4 weeks yielding an average TAM of 245 degrees (148). Twelve patients achieved an average TAM of 265 degrees with double longitudinal pins placed across the MP joint (149). However, another series of 100 closed fractures treated within 5 days of injury and pins retained for 3 weeks had a TAM of >215 degrees in only 61%, a TAM of <180 degrees in 10%, and six pin tract infections (150). The procedure of CRIF is made more difficult than it may initially appear by the challenge of obtaining a truly accurate reduction by closed means. An interesting alternative applicable to even closed fractures is the use of closed reduction and external fixation for 4 weeks, which resulted in an average of 84% of normal TAM in 11 patients (151).

Open Reduction and Internal Fixation

ORIF is the technique of choice for severe open fractures with multiple associated soft tissue injuries and for patients with multiple fractures (within the same hand or polytrauma victims). It is also the technique of choice for intra-articular fractures with displacement in P1. Two excellent reviews have concentrated on the management of intra-articular fractures in particular (152,153). In a series of 38 distal unicondylar fractures of P1, 5 of 7 initially nondisplaced and unfixed fractures and 4 of 10 fixed with a single K-wire went on to displace (154). Displaced fractures at the intra-articular base of P1 with more than 20% articular involvement should be internally fixed (155,156). Using a volar A1 pulley approach, 10 patients had fixation of lateral base fractures with full motion recovery, good stability, and over 90% contralateral grip strength (157). The role of ORIF for an isolated extra-articular fracture of the phalanx is clearly defined only for the rare irreducible fracture. Spiral fractures may benefit from ORIF with lag screws to achieve precise control over rotation, provided that surgeons experienced in this specific technique can minimize soft tissue disruption. Most surgeons will be more comfortable with CRIF for those fractures that can be reduced. The 40-month follow-

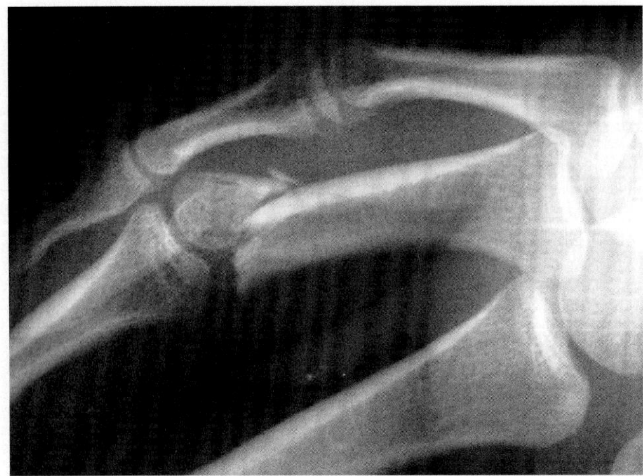

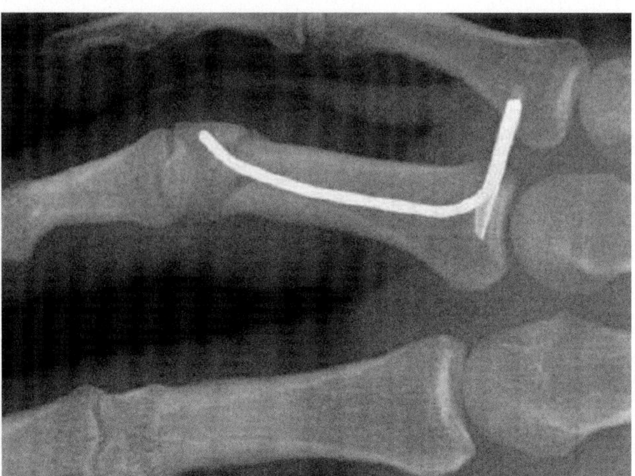

FIGURE 24-54 Proximal phalanx fractures **(A)** can be stabilized by closed placement of a specially designed device that achieves three-point fixation with a rotational locking sleeve proximally **(B)**.

up of 32 patients prospectively randomized for percutaneous pinning versus lag screw fixation for long oblique and spiral shaft fractures found no differences in function, pain scores, malunion, range of motion, or grip strength, but with a mean loss of active extension of 8 degrees in the pinning group and 27 degrees in the screw fixation group (158). ORIF with screws and or plates is considerably more technically demanding than in the metacarpal for a number of reasons including the proximity of the extensor mechanism, the origins of the fibro-osseous flexor tendon sheath, and the size and consistency of the bone. More than just the technical complexity of ORIF is the problem of the post-operative response of the surrounding soft tissues to the surgical dissection.

Options for ORIF include intra-osseous wiring, composite wiring, screw only fixation, or screw and plate fixation (Figs. 24-55 and 24-56) (147,162,167). The familiarity of the surgeon

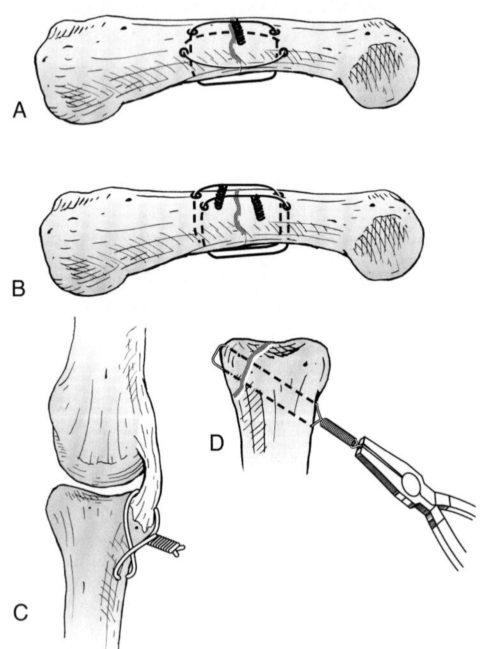

FIGURE 24-55 A malleable intraosseous wire alone can be applied in its strongest configuration of **(A)** two loops at 90 degrees from each other, **(B)** two parallel loops, **(C)** a figure-of-8 tension band, and **(D)** a single loop to compress a smaller fragment against the larger fragment.

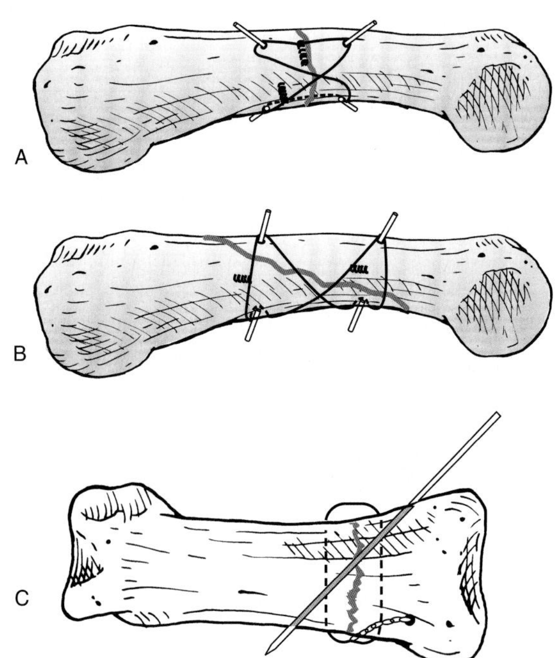

FIGURE 24-56 Composite wiring techniques may involve any configuration or combination of nonflexible fixation with a malleable intraosseous wire that is twisted to achieve compression across the fracture site.

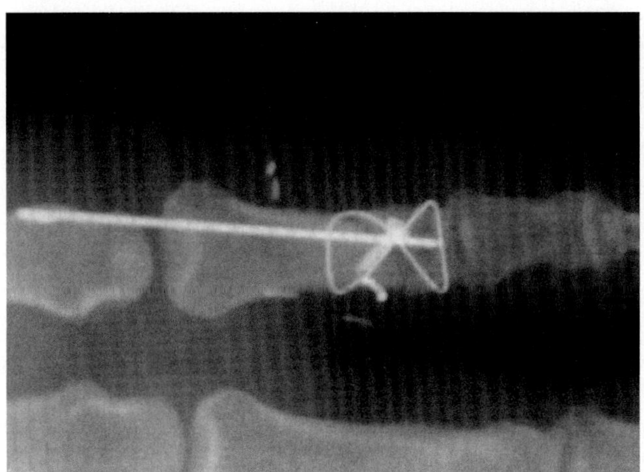

FIGURE 24-57 Composite fixation can be achieved by any combination of materials that best address the individual biomechanics of the specific fracture pattern.

with the specific technique is probably the most important factor for the selection of a method (Fig. 24-57). Fractures in 21 patients internally fixed with composite wiring techniques resulted in an average TAM of 215 degrees without complications (162). Intra-osseous wiring with 26-gauge wire in 150 patients was accomplished with no wire breakage (166). Of 30 patients followed for 2.3 years after tension band wiring, 17 had a TAM over 195 degrees and 13 had a TAM of between 130 to 195 degrees (168). More recently, attention has increasingly turned to the use of screw and plate technology (Fig. 24-58). Melone compared his personal experience of condylar fractures fixed with K-wires (TAM = 192 degrees) to those fixed with screws (TAM = 216 degrees), which was mirrored by his experience with diaphyseal fractures treated with K-wires (TAM = 213 degrees) compared to screw fixation (TAM = 229 degrees) (148). Another series of screw only treatment in 36 fractures (40% of which were complicated by open injury, associated soft tissue injury, or comminution) resulted in a TAM of more than 220 degrees in 24 cases, with only two patients having a TAM of less than 180 degrees (169). Even the use of plates and screws can produce excellent results in proximal phalangeal fractures (170). The relative bulkiness of plates at the phalangeal level compared to the metacarpals often results in the need for removal despite the excellent results initially achieved (171,172). The results of internal fixation are intimately related to the associated injuries present. In a prospective series of 284 digital fractures and the follow-up series of 52 unstable fractures, the chief determinants of outcome were associated soft tissue injury (49% to 57% poor outcome), open fracture, and comminution to the degree that these factors overrode the method of fixation (38,39). When these poor prognostic factors are associated with other variables such as initial articular displacement and a high degree of comminution, outcomes are further compromised (173). The gravest danger, however, occurs when the surgeon elects ORIF but is then unable to secure rigid fixation of the fracture. In this situation, the patient has been subjected to the "worst of both worlds," and a poor outcome can be reliably predicted.

Intra-articular Fractures

Two patterns are seen distally at the phalangeal head, unicondylar (partial articular fracture) or bicondylar (complete articular fracture). The condylar fragments are extremely small, can be fragile, and receive their blood supply from the attached collateral ligament. Fixation of a single condyle is most rigid when accomplished with a compression screw placed transversely, entering near the collateral ligament origin (Fig. 24-59). This can be quite challenging technically, and the bone stock may only tolerate K-wire or composite wiring techniques (Fig. 24-60). Tri-plane fractures of the head of the proximal phalanx are well managed with 1.5-mm lag screws (174). Complete articular

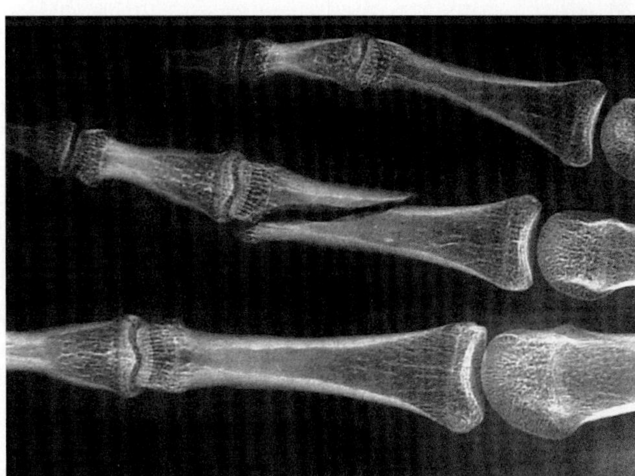

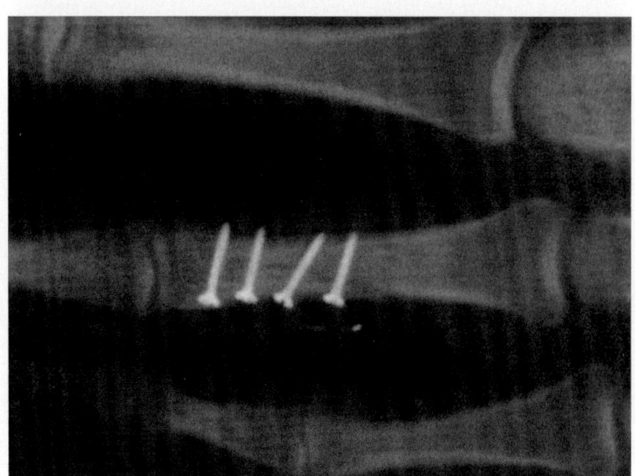

FIGURE 24-58 **A.** Long oblique fractures of the shaft with shortening can achieve **(B)** an exact reduction and stability sufficient to withstand early motion through lag screw fixation only.

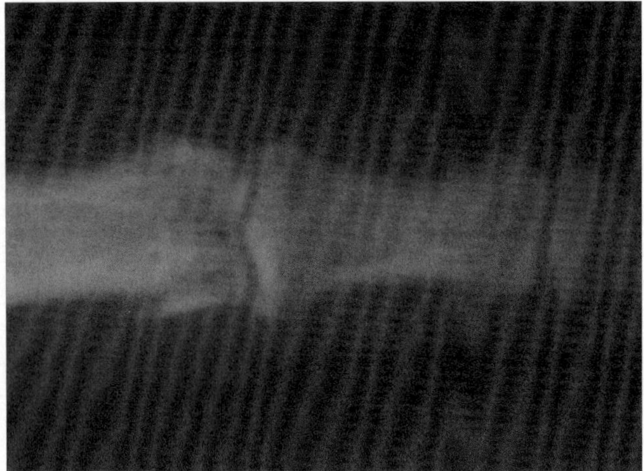

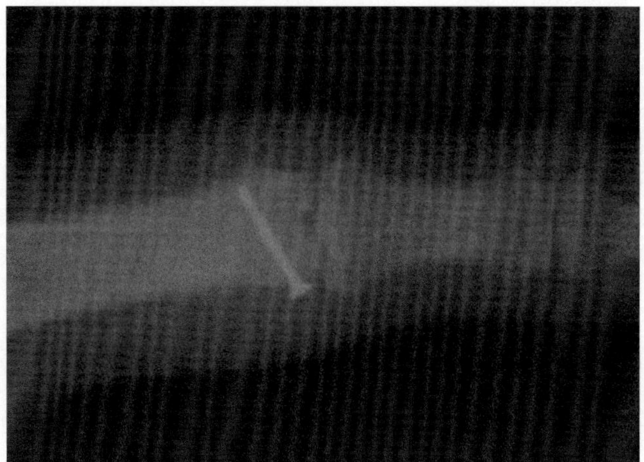

FIGURE 24-59 **A.** Unicondylar fractures at the head of P1 benefit from compression between the articular fragments through **(B)** lag screw fixation.

fractures can be fixed with screws only if one of the two condyles has an extended spike. If not, mini-condylar plate fixation may be necessary for excellent rigidity. Again, the bone stock may not tolerate the application of this device, and wiring techniques remain an alternative strategy.

The final articular fractures are those seen at the lateral corner of the phalangeal base, which are particularly amenable to the technique of tension band wiring. An alternative is a volar approach to the lateral base P1 fractures using single lag screw fixation to achieve full motion in 3 weeks (175). A specific subset of proximal phalangeal base fractures that are purely impactions by nature may be treated by supporting the impacted fragments with packed cancellous bone only; in one series of 10 patients followed for 32 months there was no secondary displacement and an average flexion of 88 degrees (176).

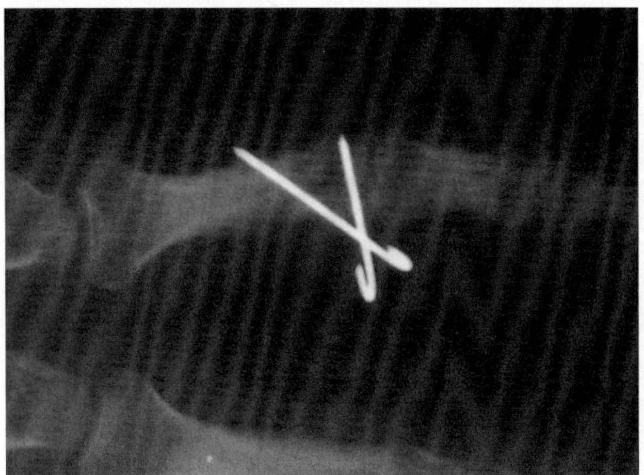

FIGURE 24-60 When a unicondylar fracture at the head of P1 has a proximal shaft extension on the smaller fragment, K-wire fixation in a diverging pattern can prevent migration of the fragment that would otherwise occur with a single smooth sided K-wire as the only fixation.

Rehabilitation

Nonoperative management should restrict splinting to 3 weeks followed by AROM that can include adjacent digit strapping if necessary. Similarly, CRIF should allow for pin removal at 3 weeks, with AROM beginning no later than this time. If ORIF is chosen, AROM should begin within 72 hours of surgery and edema control should be foremost in the treatment plan using cohesive elastic bandages (177). Active range of motion alone may be insufficient to counteract extensor lag at the joint distal to the site of fixation. Rapidly accelerating the extensor tendon concentrically without resistance best limits local adhesion formation (Fig. 24-61). These exercises can be supplemented with the use of electrical stimulation during outpatient therapy sessions. Night splinting with the PIP joint in extension can be helpful but will not in and of itself overcome a lag.

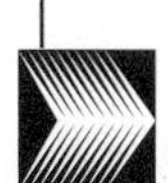

AUTHOR'S PREFERRED TREATMENT

Closed Reduction Internal Fixation

Closed reduction internal fixation is my preferred treatment for all isolated, closed transverse and short oblique fractures of the proximal phalanx (Fig. 24-62). Longitudinal pinning with two wires passing through the metacarpal head with the MP joint flexed 80 to 90 degrees has yielded reliable results. In larger patients, two 0.045-inch wires can both be fit through the medullary canal. In smaller patients, one 0.045-inch and one 0.035-inch wire may be more compatible. The wires are placed one each on either side of the thick central extensor tendon dorsal to the MP joint, thus passing through the sagittal band fibers. The wires are then passed through the base fragment, across the fracture site, and down the distal shaft of the phalanx to the head. Care must be taken to not power drill the wires through the subchondral

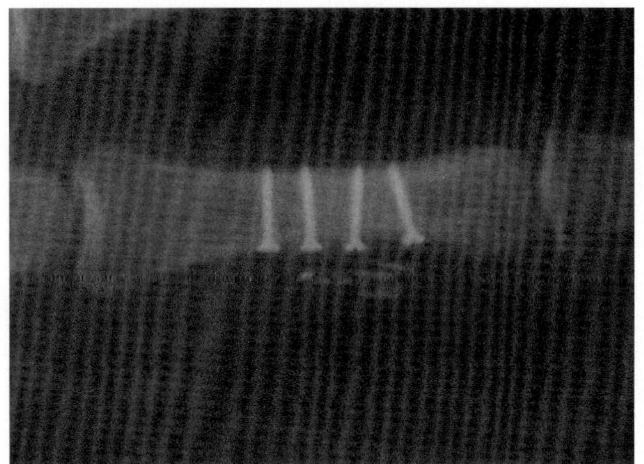

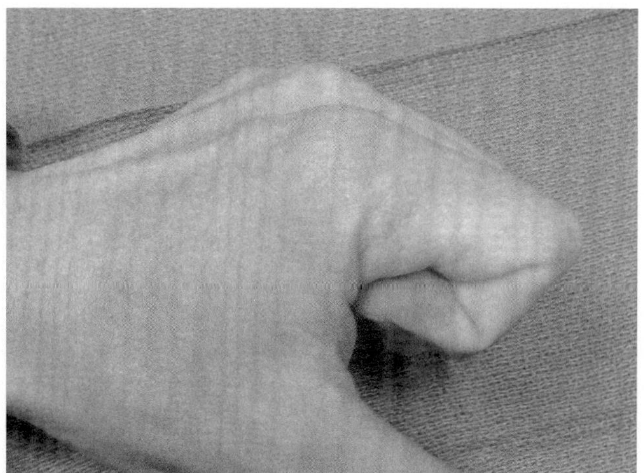

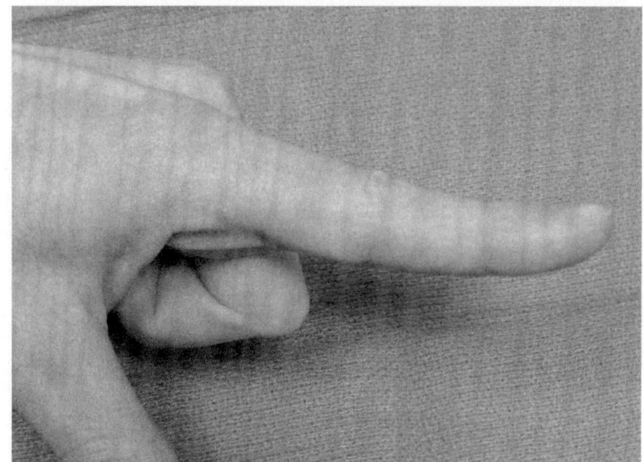

FIGURE 24-61 Following **(A)** lag screw fixation of a shaft fracture in P1, **(B)** complete PIP joint flexion, and **(C)** PIP joint hyperextension are achievable with an aggressive special therapy program of resisted zone IV extensor tendon pre-load followed by sudden release with follow-through.

bone of the phalangeal head, creating a pin tract into the PIP joint. If such a passage exists, the wire may migrate distally into the PIP joint during early rehabilitation and cause hyaline cartilage damage in the base of P2. Instead, the wire may be drilled up to but not into the subchondral bone. After crimping the wires dorsally, they may be manually impacted a few millimeters further into subchondral bone, conferring an added degree of stability.

Closed pinning is also a valuable technique for nondisplaced fractures at the head of P1. Both a transverse pin connecting the two condyles as well as an oblique pin from the condyle to the opposite diaphyseal cortex should be used for a unicondylar fracture (Fig. 24-60). For bicondylar fractures, two such oblique pins are needed. The oblique pins are best cut outside the skin proximally rather than distally as the pins passage through the peri-articular soft tissues interferes with PIP joint motion. Closed pinning also represents a reasonable treatment option for nondisplaced long-oblique or spiral fractures that are suspected of subsequent displacement when subjected to the stress of motion rehabilitation. However, practically I have not found this fracture pattern to exist. I see either truly nondisplaced fractures that I expect to remain stable and treat nonoperatively or displaced long oblique and spiral fractures that I prefer to treat with open reduction.

Open Reduction and Internal Fixation with Lag Screws

This is my preferred treatment for long oblique and spiral fractures of the shaft and displaced partial articular fractures (Fig. 24-63). I have found it difficult through closed means alone to correct all the shortening and rotation of long oblique and spiral fractures. There is a natural trade off between the undeniable added surgical trauma of the open approach and the benefits of an anatomically precise reduction. When lag screws alone are used for fixation, full motion rehabilitation can begin immediately. This is not the case with K-wires and their attendant risk of pin tract infection. Performing the open fixation gently and precisely to minimize soft tissue trauma and realize the theoretical benefits of the procedure is more easily described than executed. The first principle is to carefully evaluate fracture geometry. In

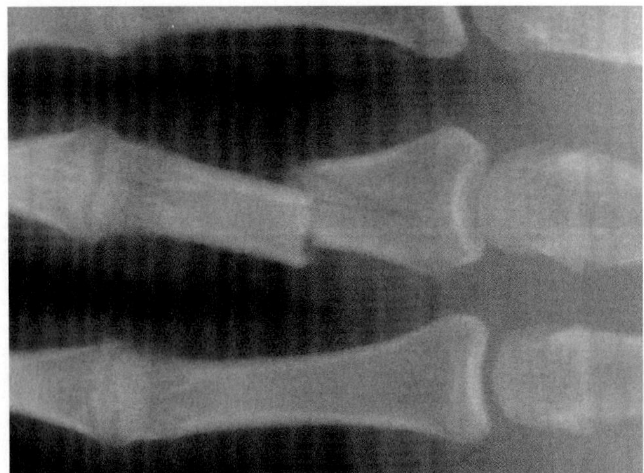

A

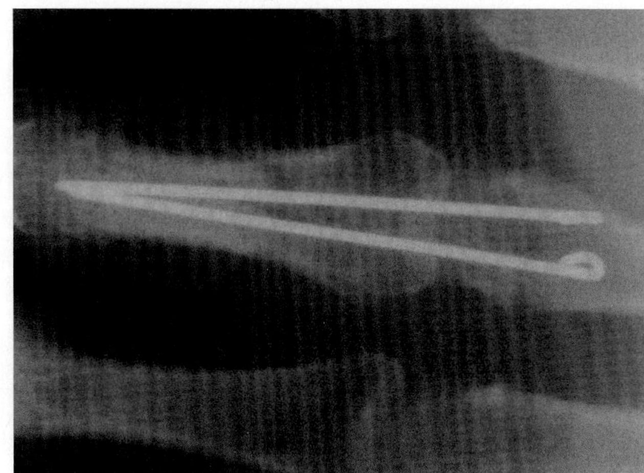

B

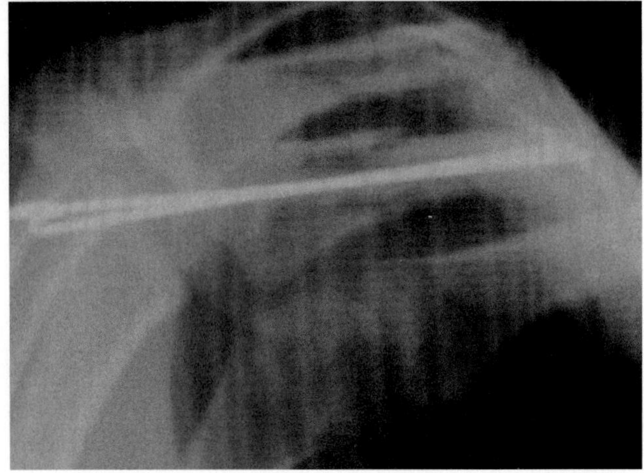

C

FIGURE 24-62 Transverse P1 fractures of the mid-shaft **(A)** are not as inherently stable as those at the base and are best stabilized by two rather than one K-wire **(B)** passing through the metacarpal head with the MP joint in flexion **(C)**.

a simple two-fragment diaphyseal fracture, there will be inherent stability between the bone edges once the fracture has been reduced. The role of internal fixation is then to exploit this inherent stability by further compressing the fracture line. Fixation involving the use of lag screws achieves the maximum compression possible. One must always heed the ground rules for screw only fixation: fracture length is at least two times the bone diameter, and fragment width is at least three times the screw diameter. For all of the above techniques, adherence to strict principles is mandatory; multiple passes are not well tolerated by the phalanx. Screws of 1.3- to 1.5-mm diameters are appropriate for P1. Biomechanically, it is desirable to have at least one screw perpendicular to the neutral axis of the bone. The remaining screws should be perpendicular to the fracture plane. In a spiral fracture, there will be one screw that satisfies both these requirements simultaneously and is termed the "ideal" screw. In an oblique fracture this will not be the case.

Plates at the Phalangeal Level

Plates at the phalangeal level are not desirable due to their bulk and propensity for tendon adherence, and I avoid using them whenever possible. This is my treatment of choice for fractures with comminution and bone loss and complete articular fractures of the phalangeal head that are unstable (Fig. 24-64). Remembering that the biomechanics of P1 fractures create an apex palmar sagittal plane deformity, the plate would (impossibly so) have to be applied to the volar surface of the bone to have its optimum tension band effect. Lateral placement is then the next most desirable option, which corresponds well to the surgical access that is least harmful to the soft tissues (178). More proximally in P1, the ulnar intrinsic tendon can be completely resected to improve access and obviate snapping over the edge of the plate. When plates are used, one should attempt to place screws as perpendicular to the surface of the plate as possible. The heads of obliquely placed screws have a very prominent edge (Fig. 24-65). Plates should also be painstakingly contoured to ensure both the lowest profile as well as proper biomechanical function (preload, dynamic compression, buttress, etc.). If more than 50% cross-sectional area of the bone is comminuted or lost, bone graft will be required.

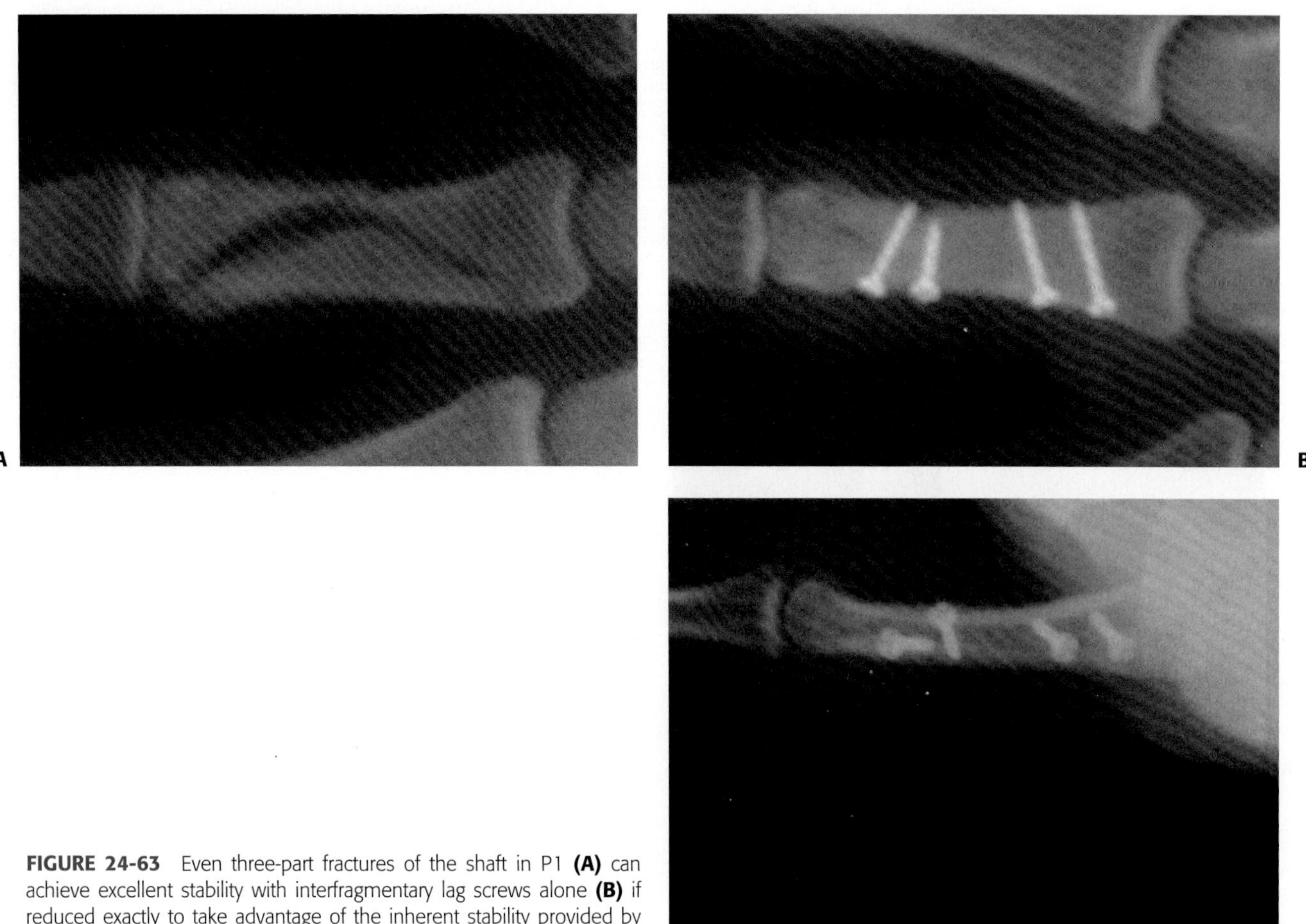

FIGURE 24-63 Even three-part fractures of the shaft in P1 **(A)** can achieve excellent stability with interfragmentary lag screws alone **(B)** if reduced exactly to take advantage of the inherent stability provided by interdigitation of the fracture surfaces **(C)**.

Pearls and Pitfalls

The pearls of CRIF are captured in the Author's preferred treatment section. The details of the difficult open fixation procedures at the proximal phalanx level will be covered here. I prefer to operate on closed fractures around post-injury day 5 when even adult periosteum will thicken dramatically in response to injury and can be surgically manipulated as a tissue flap. Post-traumatic swelling will have begun to subside by this time. A true mid-axial incision is in the neutral tension lines of the skin and brings the approach down to the volar leading edge of the intrinsic wing tendon. One of the most important principles of open fixation of a P1 fracture is to not create planes of surgical dissection either superficial or deep to the zone IV extensor

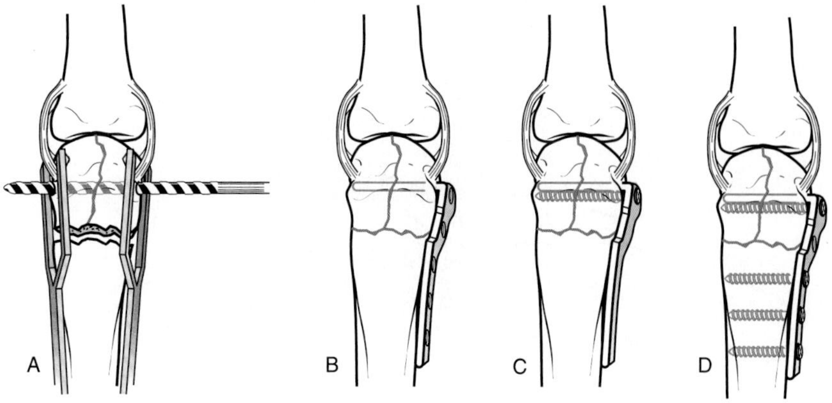

A B C D

FIGURE 24-64 **A.** After reduction of the condylar fragments to each other and the shaft, the hole for the condylar blade is drilled and its depth is measured. **B.** The blade is cut to size and inserted to evaluate the accuracy of the plate contouring. The condylar screw is inserted **(C)**, along with the shaft screws **(D)**.

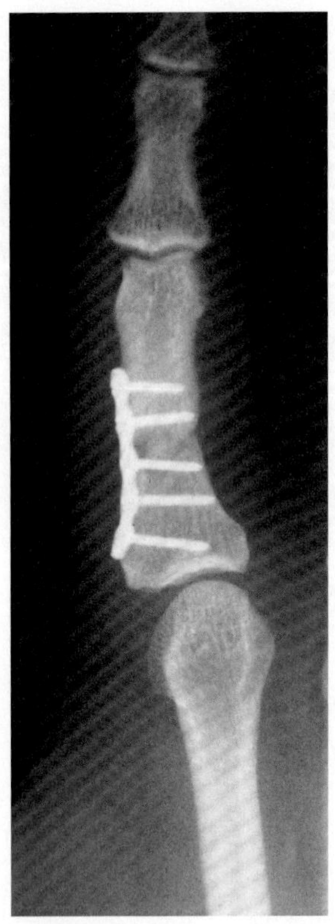

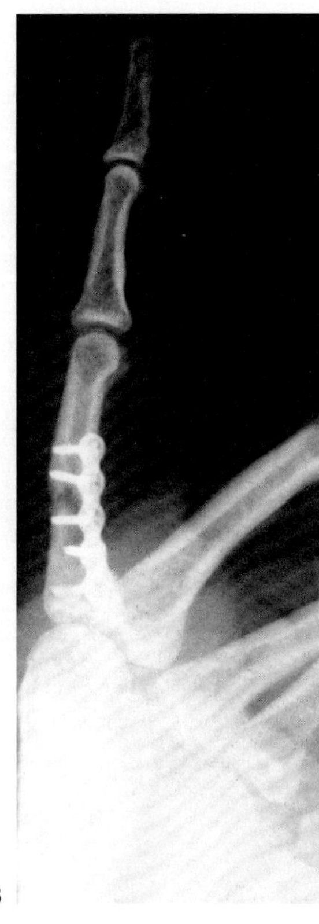

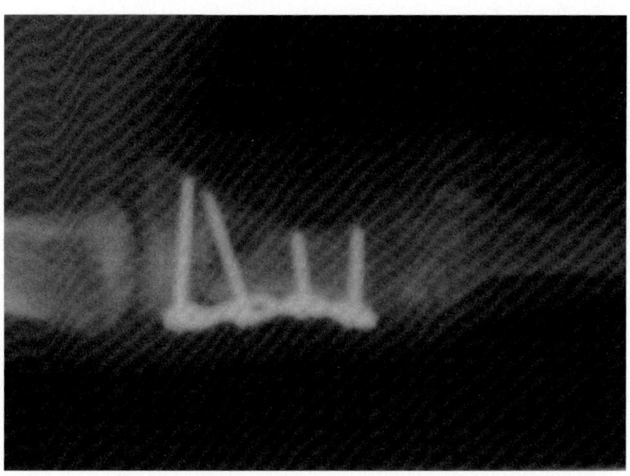

FIGURE 24-65 Plate fixation in P1 **(A)** must be contoured meticulously to restore the normal anatomic shape of the bone **(B)**. **C.** The condylar blade plate can be used at the metaphyseal base of a proximal phalanx also. An oblique screw is often advantageous to achieve an extra point of compression in the metaphyseal fragment, but doing so leaves the screw head proud.

tendon (Fig. 24-66). The only dissection that should occur at the subcutaneous level is to identify dorsal cutaneous nerve branches passing obliquely from the proper digital nerves and to mobilize them effectively to avoid neuromas. Other than this, the approach should be a single tissue flap from skin through periosteum to bone. A sharp blade is needed to carefully preserve the periosteum for later repair using fine monofilament resorbable sutures. This creates an additional gliding layer of protection for the extensor mechanism. A fine tipped curette must be used on the fracture interface to clear all clot and soft tissue or a truly anatomic interdigitated reduction will not be possible. Although provisional fixation of the fracture with K-wires has been recommended by others, I have found that the absoluteness of a perfect reduction is not well maintained by smooth wires, which invariably allow the reduction to slip a little bit. This ensures that the drill path will not be exactly in the desired location and that final placement of the screw or plate will thus be imperfect. I prefer to hold the reduction manually with either a bone clamp specialized for the short tubular bones of the hand or Brown-Adson forceps. Caution must be used to drill at lower speeds as high speeds can introduce an eccentric "whip" to the tip of these small drill bits, resulting in a larger drill path than desired. I strongly prefer a "pencil grip" micro drill over a "pistol grip" driver for the sake of accuracy in drilling a straight path.

The steps for screw only fixation after reduction and provisional stabilization are core drilling followed by countersinking the near bone surface (Fig. 24-67). Countersinking not only recesses the screw head but also distributes the force of compression, lessening the chance of propagating a new fracture line. Measuring for screw length is done next, and the time for the scrub technician to procure the correct screw can be used to drill the gliding hole. Self-tapping screws are a little difficult to start into bone as some axial load is necessary to get

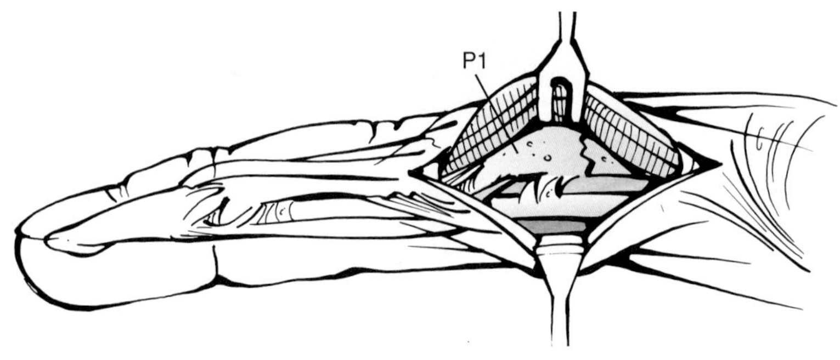

FIGURE 24-66 The lateral approach to P1 should not create layers of dissection around the extensor tendon but rather pass volar to the leading edge of the intrinsic wing tendon and through periosteum to bone, leaving skin, extensor tendon, and periosteum as a single tissue flap for retraction.

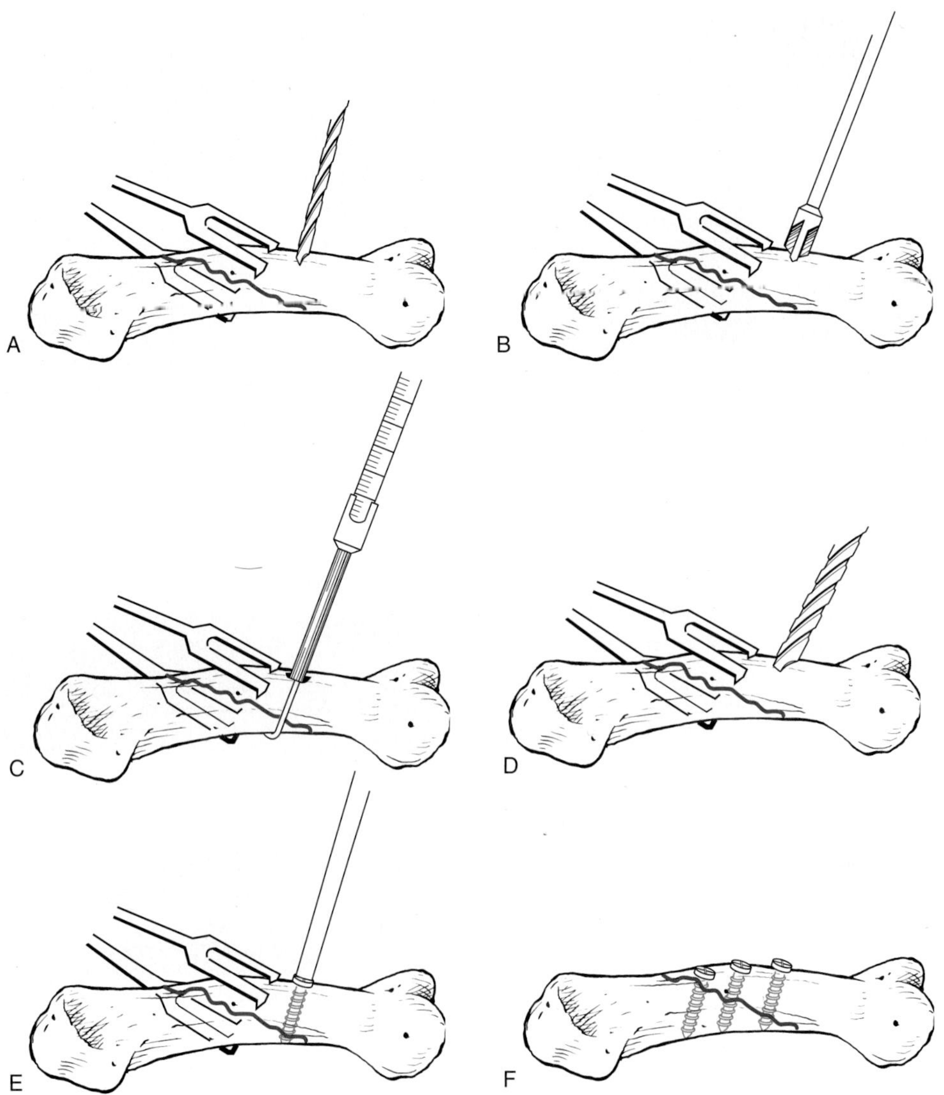

FIGURE 24-67 After stabilized reduction of a shaft fracture, lag screw fixation is accomplished by **(A)** drilling with the smaller core bit, **(B)** countersinking the near cortex, **(C)** measuring the correct length, **(D)** drilling the gliding hole, **(E)** tightening the lag screw with two finger tip pressure, and **(F)** ensuring all distances between screws and fracture edges are sufficient to avoid propagation of new fracture lines under the pressure of screw tightening.

them to bite, but application of this load off the true axis will toggle the screw. A fine touch must be learned over the course of many cases using these implants. Screws are tightened with a "chuck" pinch on the screwdriver using three fingers, not with the more forceful "key" pinch that may shear the head off the shaft of the screw. All plates must be meticulously and often painstakingly contoured prior to application (Fig. 24-68). One must not hesitate to remove a plate and re-contour it after the first two screws have been placed if it is clear that the shape is not correct. Application of an incorrectly contoured plate guarantees an imperfect fracture reduction. A common error is with plates ending near the metaphyseal flare that must have a small bend at the last hole to accommodate the curvature of the bone at this level.

METACARPOPHALANGEAL JOINT DISLOCATIONS

Dorsal dislocations are the most common metacarpophalangeal (MP) joint dislocations. Simple dislocations are reducible and present with a hyperextension posture. They are really subluxations, as some contact remains between the base of P1 and the metacarpal head (Fig. 24-69). The volar plate stays volar or distal to the metacarpal head. Reduction should be achieved with simple flexion of the joint; excessive longitudinal traction on the finger should be avoided. Wrist flexion to relax the flexor tendons may assist reduction. The other variety of MP joint dislocation is a complex dislocation, which

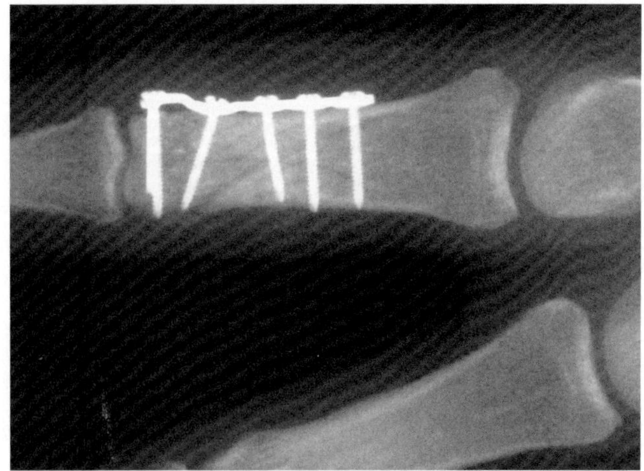

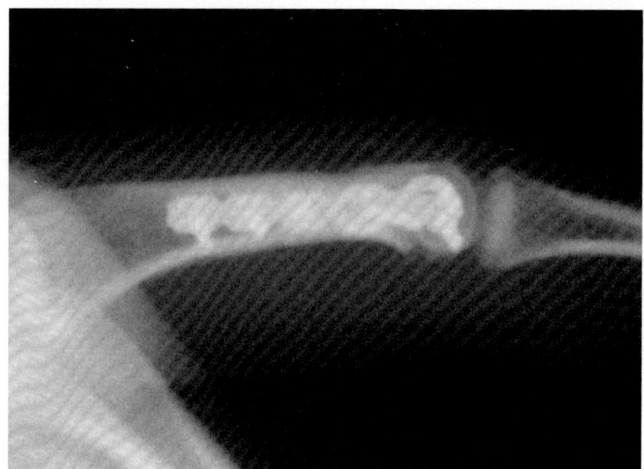

FIGURE 24-68 Comminuted fractures involving the head and shaft of P1 **(A)** can be stabilized for early motion with a condylar blade plate **(B)** placed laterally in the mid-axial plane.

is by definition irreducible, most often due to volar plate interposition (Fig. 24-70). Complex dislocations occur most frequently in the index finger. Longitudinal traction can convert a simple to a complex dislocation. A pathognomonic x-ray sign of complex dislocation is the appearance of a sesamoid in the joint space (Fig. 24-71). Concomitant injuries include small chip fractures on the dorsum of the metacarpal head that have been sheared off in complex dislocations by the volar base of P1. Other difficult fractures to detect are bony collateral ligament avulsions.

Most dorsal dislocations will be stable following reduction

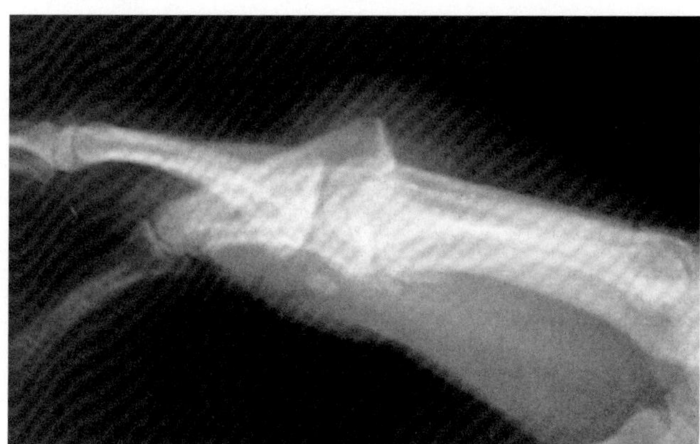

FIGURE 24-70 The typical complex dorsal dislocation of the MP joint presents with complete overriding of the phalanx on the metacarpal.

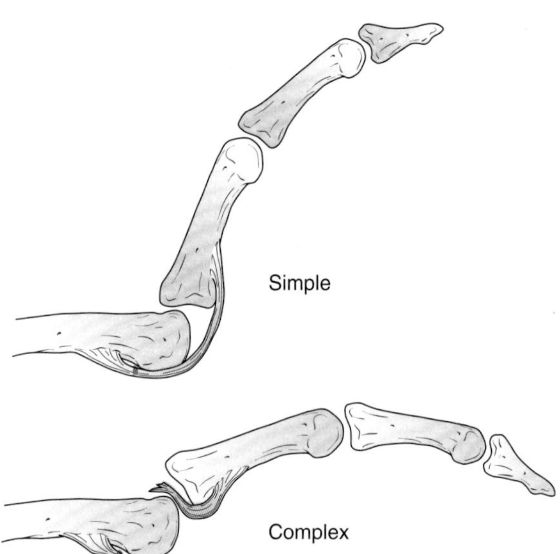

FIGURE 24-69 Simple MP joint dislocations are spontaneously reducible and usually present in an extended posture with the articular surface of P1 sitting on the dorsum of the metacarpal head. Complex dislocations have bayonet apposition with volar plate interposition that prevents reduction.

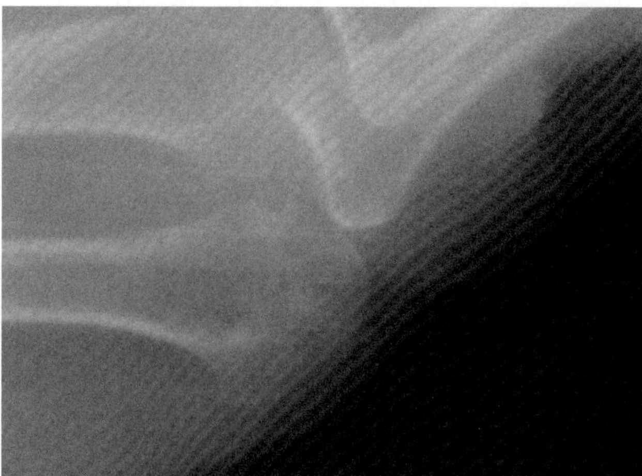

FIGURE 24-71 A pathognomonic radiographic sign of a complex MP joint dislocation is a sesamoid (representing the volar plate) seen residing in a widened joint space.

and do not need surgical repair of the ligaments or volar plate. Volar dislocations are rare but are particularly unstable (179,180). Volar dislocations risk late instability and should have repair of the ligaments (179). Obstructions to reducing volar dislocations include the volar plate, collateral ligament, and dorsal capsule. Open dislocations may be either reducible or irreducible (181,182). Multiple dorsal subluxations as well as dislocations have been reported (183,184). The unusual combination of dislocation and an associated P1 fracture has been cited (185). Isolated collateral ligament injuries are more common on the radial aspect of the small finger followed by the index. A differential diagnosis to consider with swelling at the MP joint level following injury is rupture of the sagittal bands, which requires protection in extension for 4 weeks.

Thumb MP Joint Ligament Injuries

Complete rupture of the ulnar collateral ligament (UCL) of the thumb MP joint is a common injury that less frequently may accompany a full MP joint dislocation (Fig. 24-72). Circumferential palpation of the MP joint can often localize pain to the UCL, radial collateral ligament (RCL), volar plate, or combinations of these. Following joint injection with local anesthetic, stress testing in full extension and 30-degrees of flexion (eliminates false negative conclusion of stability in setting of ruptured proper collateral ligament but intact volar plate) should reveal any instability (Fig. 24-73). If clinical uncertainty remains, stress radiographs may also be performed (Fig. 24-74). The role of MRI in the diagnosis of the Stener lesion (distally ruptured ulnar collateral ligament blocked from healing by the interposed adductor aponeurosis) still remains undefined, but continues to show promise (186–189). Arthrography has been suggested as an inexpensive method for identifying the Stener lesion, but the accuracy of the technique is insufficient to use for surgical decision-making (190). In a series of 24 patients, a palpable tender mass on the ulnar side of the MP joint was used as the sole diagnostic criterion for the Stener lesion. Operative treatment was performed for those felt to have the lesion and nonoperative management for those who did not, resulting in a single case of long-term instability (191).

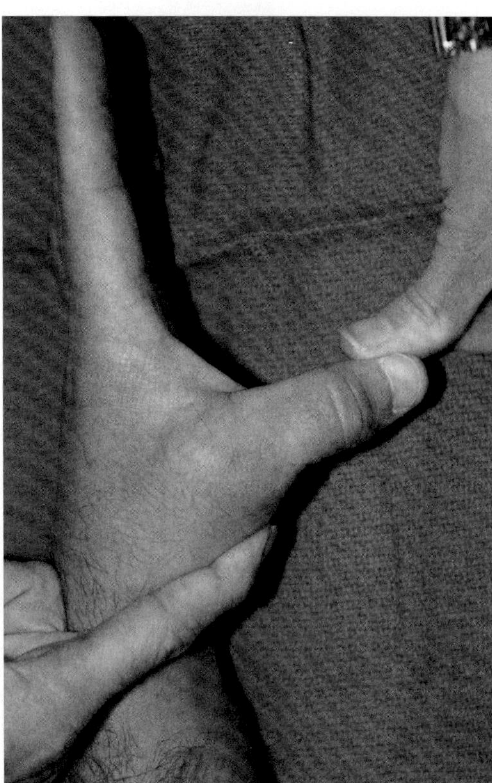

FIGURE 24-73 Clinical stress testing of the ulnar collateral ligament in 30 degrees of flexion prevents reaching a false-negative conclusion when an intact volar plate obscures the instability of a complete proper ulnar collateral ligament rupture.

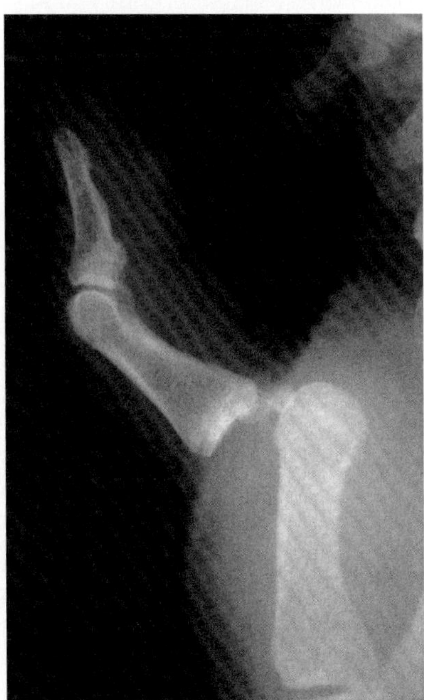

FIGURE 24-72 Metacarpophalangeal joint dislocation in the thumb, like the fingers, is typically dorsal.

The term *gamekeeper's thumb,* which more appropriately applies to chronic attrition injuries, has largely been supplanted by *skier's thumb* owing to the prominent role played by this sport in the etiology of acute UCL injuries (192,193). The interaction between the thumb and first web space with ski pole grips has been blamed for the association of UCL ruptures in this sport. Unfortunately, alterations in ski pole grip designs have not lessened the incidence of injury (192–194). Not all fracture fragments seen on the ulnar aspect of the MP joint represent the anatomic insertion of the UCL. Some of these fragments may be attached to the volar plate insertion, separate from the collateral ligament (188,195). The differential diagnosis of sesamoid fracture must also be considered when volar tenderness is present.

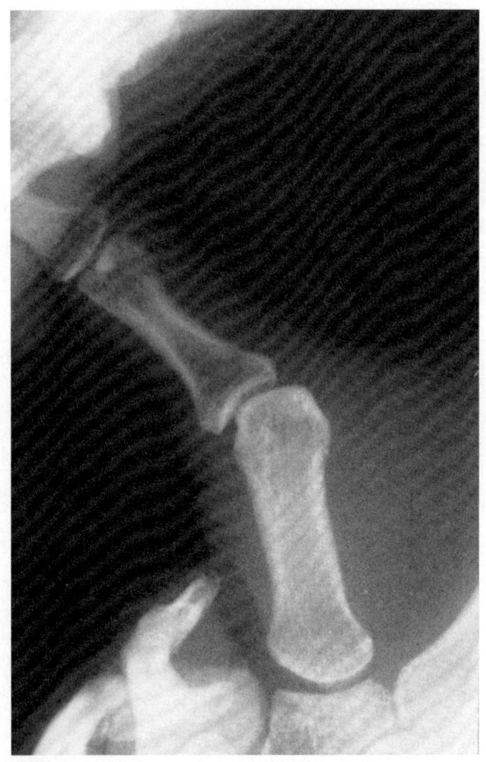

FIGURE 24-74 Radiographic stress testing is also useful when there is clinical uncertainty.

Oblique views may be helpful in this respect when considering the frequent incomplete ossification of the sesamoids (196–198). Special mention should be made of irreducible dislocations (199). Irreducible volar dislocations have been reported with the radial condyle of the metacarpal trapped in a rent dorsal to the accessory collateral–volar plate complex (197). Other causes of volar trapping may involve the EPL and EPB (200). The FPL may block reduction of a dorsal dislocation (201).

Surgical and Applied Anatomy

The anatomy of the MP joint is like the same three-sided box previously presented for the PIP joint, composed of the proper collateral ligaments, the accessory collateral ligaments and the volar plate (Fig. 24-75). The radial and ulnar proper collateral ligaments are the primary stabilizers to motion in all planes including distraction, dorsopalmar translation, abduction-adduction, and supination-pronation (202). The accessory collateral ligaments supplement adduction-abduction. The volar plates are connected to each other by the deep transverse inter-metacarpal ligament (203). The MP collateral ligaments have an origin dorsal to the center axis of joint rotation. This feature combines with two others (a greater width of the metacarpal head volarly and a greater distance from the center of rotation to the volar articular surface than the distal articular surface) to maximize tension in the true collateral portion of the ligament when the joint is in full flexion. Consequently, stress testing to determine the presence of instability must be performed in full flexion.

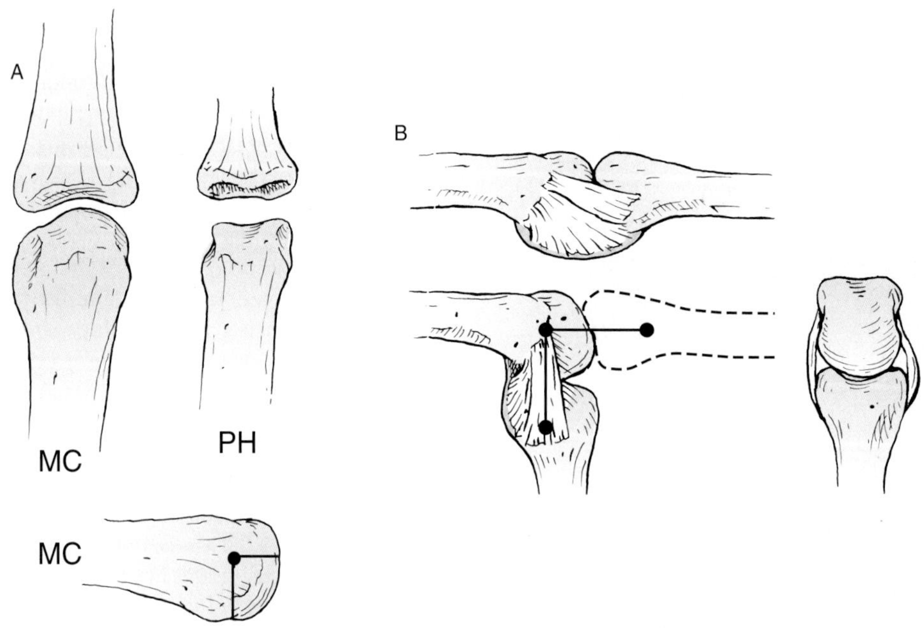

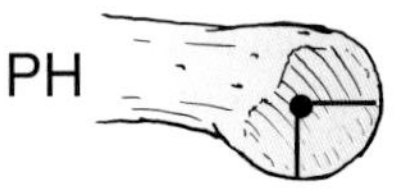

FIGURE 24-75 The anatomy of the MP joint differs from that of the PIP joint in the unicondylar vs. bicondylar head, the cam effect in the sagittal plane unique to the metacarpal, and the collateral origin offset dorsally from the center of rotation in the metacarpal.

Access for open reduction of complex dislocations is a topic of great controversy (204). Central MP joints can be approached either dorsally or volarly. Although the volar plate is the most commonly noted structure in the prevention of reduction, the flexor tendons, lumbricals, deep transverse inter-metacarpal ligaments, juncturae tendinae, and dorsal capsule have all been implicated (205). In a series of 10 operatively treated ruptures, most were distal with the ligament occasionally trapped between the intrinsic tendon and the sagittal band, including two associated dorsal interosseous ruptures at the phalangeal insertion (206).

Thumb MP Joint

The thumb MP joint, in addition to its primary plane of flexion and extension, allows abduction-adduction and a slight amount of rotation (pronation with flexion). With a one-sided collateral ligament injury, the phalanx tends to subluxate volarly in a rotatory fashion, pivoting around the opposite intact collateral ligament. The range of flexion and extension has a wide natural variation that may be related to the flatness of the metacarpal head and may also play a role in predisposition to injury for those with less motion (207). The ulnar collateral ligament may have a two-level injury consisting of a fracture of the ulnar base of P1 with the ligament also ruptured off the fracture fragment (208). Of particular importance is the proximal edge of the adductor aponeurosis that forms the anatomic basis of the Stener lesion. The torn UCL stump comes to lie dorsal to the aponeurosis and is thus prevented from healing to its anatomic insertion on the volar, ulnar base of the proximal phalanx (Fig. 24-76). The true incidence of the Stener lesion remains unknown due to widely disparate reports. The abductor pollicis brevis also sends fibers to the extensor mechanism, but a discrete edge capable of preventing healing of the radial collateral ligament does not exist; therefore, there is no correlate to a Stener lesion on this side of the joint. Radial collateral ligaments injuries were found to occur at the phalangeal insertion in 13 of 38 cases and at the metacarpal origin in 25 of 38 (209).

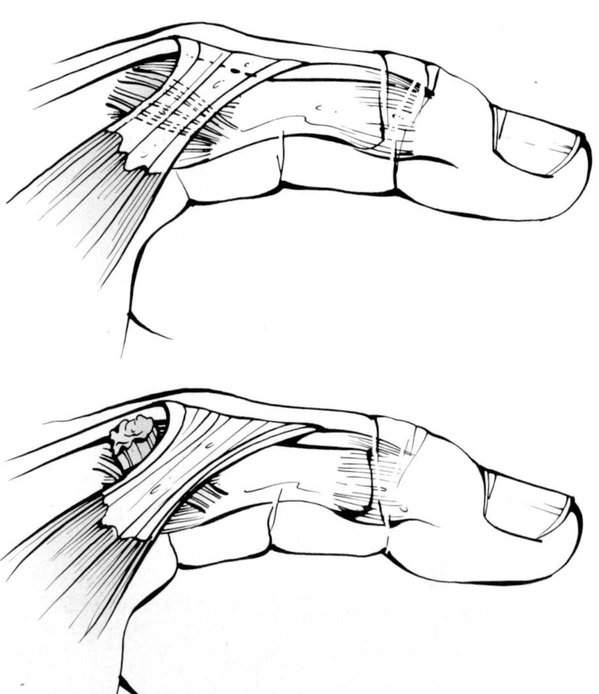

FIGURE 24-76 The Stener lesion: the adductor aponeurosis proximal edge functions as a shelf that blocks the distal phalangeal insertion of the ruptured ulnar collateral ligament of the thumb MP joint from returning to its natural location for healing after it comes to lie on top of the aponeurosis.

Current Treatment Options

Nonoperative Management—Fingers

Current treatment options are listed in Table 24-8. For reducible dorsal dislocations and collateral ligament injuries, nonoperative management is the treatment of choice. Collateral ligament injuries should be immobilized in incomplete flexion (50 degrees) for 3 weeks followed by AROM while the digit is strapped to an adjacent digit to resist lateral deviation stress. Dorsal dislocations will normally prove stable during early AROM. Only in an exceptional case would the use of extension block splinting of 20 degrees or so for 2 to 3 weeks be required. In a high-demand patient the radial collateral ligament of the index MP joint should be considered for operative repair.

TABLE 24-8 Metacarpophalangeal Joint Dislocations

Treatment Option	Pros	Cons
Splinting	No added surgical stiffness	Does not guarantee anatomic ligament healing at critical locations
Open ligament repair	Restores stability in cases treated early; important for Stener lesion and possibly for torn radial collateral of index	Added surgical stiffness
Open ligament reconstruction	Restores stability in cases treated late when functional instability is a clinical problem	Surgical stiffness may be greater following reconstruction compared to repair in some cases

Nonoperative Management—Thumb

Nonoperative management is the mainstay of treatment for thumb MP joint injuries. Only the complete UCL injury with a Stener lesion and volar dislocations require more aggressive treatment (190,210,211). Forty-two patients with UCL tears were treated for 6 weeks with an orthosis taken off three times daily for AROM. The overall series had reduction of instability from 17 degrees to 2.3 degrees; 12% of the patients were suspected of having Stener lesions and completed treatment with a mean of 12.6 degrees of instability that did not, however, correlate with clinical symptoms (190). Another series of 40 patients with UCL injuries were treated with either a cast or a splint that allowed uniplanar flexion-extension motion. The results were the same but the patients preferred the motion splint (211). Despite these descriptions of early motion treatment, the standard is 4 weeks of static MP joint immobilization with the IP joint left free. Management in the presence of a fracture at the ulnar base of P1 is more controversial. Nine patients with less than 2 mm displacement of such a fragment treated nonoperatively all had chronic pain with pinch strength rated at 36% of normal. Following operative treatment, pinch improved to 89% of normal with symptom resolution (212). Conversely, 28 patients with ulnar base fractures but with a joint clinically assessed as stable to stress testing were managed nonoperatively resulting in equivalent grip and pinch strengths to the contralateral side and 93% pain free despite a 60% rate of fibrous union (213). Radial collateral ligament disruptions and pure dorsal dislocations can be successfully managed by a 4-week period of MP joint immobilization. Sesamoid fractures also are managed primarily by 3 to 4 weeks of immobilization in partial flexion (197,198,214).

Open Reduction—Fingers

Volar dislocations, complex dorsal dislocations, and collateral ligament disruptions associated with large bone fragments should be treated with open reduction and repair (Fig. 24-77) (215). Some advocate repair of finger MP collateral ligament

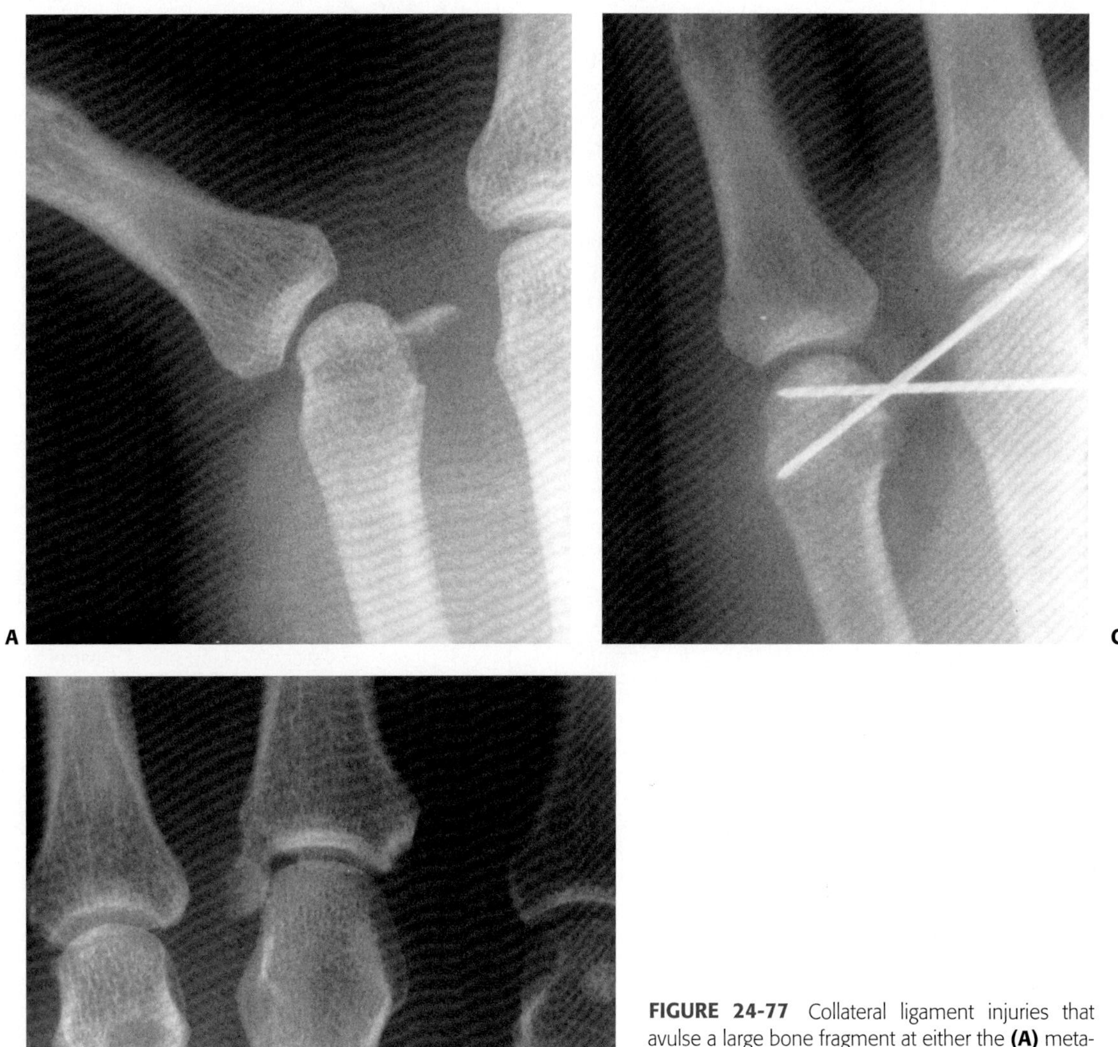

FIGURE 24-77 Collateral ligament injuries that avulse a large bone fragment at either the **(A)** metacarpal head or **(B)** phalangeal base can be stabilized by **(C)** direct bone fixation.

injuries with reports of a Stener-type lesion involving the sagittal band (216,217). Radial collateral ligament injuries repaired late risk a higher incidence of pinch weakness and should be attended to promptly. Open repair or reconstruction with a free tendon graft may also be required in chronic cases with persistent symptoms after nonoperative management (218). Volar MP dislocations should have repair of the collateral ligaments and volar plate to prevent late instability (179). Either a dorsal or a volar approach is acceptable, and the one that provides access to the major pathology should be chosen based on the individual patient's preoperative findings (219). Dorsally, a midline longitudinal incision provides good access to manage any associated osteochondral fractures. One may have to split the volar plate longitudinally and draw it around the sides of the metacarpal head to accomplish a reduction. The volar approach avoids splitting the volar plate but risks injury to digital nerves which are tented over the deformity and lying directly under the dermis. From the front, the volar plate can be pulled back out of the joint and reduced without splitting it.

The duration of immobilization should be in direct proportion to the surgeon's assessment of instability following reduction. While most injuries may begin AROM immediately, those that demonstrate an extra degree of instability during the post-reduction assessment should be immobilized in partial flexion for 3 weeks. Whether simple or complex, the dislocations should be immobilized in only partial (50-degree) flexion to allow ligament healing under appropriate tension. After 3 weeks, AROM is progressed until 6 weeks, when full passive motion including hyperextension is allowed.

Open Reduction—Thumb

Surgical management of thumb MP joint injuries is largely limited to UCL disruptions with a Stener lesion and volar or irreducible MP dislocations (179,200,201,220). The results of acute repair of the *radial* collateral ligament equal that of chronic reconstructions. This makes a very weak case for early operative repair considering that no Stener lesion exists on the radial side of the joint (221). Determining the presence of a Stener lesion on the ulnar side of the joint remains an inexact science; therefore, open management can be argued to be the treatment of choice for all widely unstable ulnar-sided disruptions. Pure ligamentous mid-substance ruptures can be repaired by direct suture. The usual site of disruption is distally at the phalangeal insertion where bone anchors can be used for ligament reinsertion (222–225). Thirty-six patients with suture anchor repairs healed with loss of 10 degrees of MP joint motion and 15 degrees of IP joint motion (225). Over-tensioning should be avoided as insertion sites malpositioned volarly or distally on the proximal phalanx will cause loss of motion (226). Arthroscopic reduction of the Stener lesion has been reported in eight patients (227). With bony avulsion fragments, tension band wire, intra-osseous wire, or fragment excision with pullout suture may all be used at the surgeon's discretion (62,228,229).

Ligament Reconstruction

Cases presenting late with residual instability (after degeneration of the tendon substance has occurred) may require reconstructive methods (230,231). Adductor advancement at the ulnar side of the thumb was shown in a comparative series to be the least attractive of the options, allowing only 65% normal MP motion (232). An intermediate option is mobilization and advancement of a U-shaped flap of residual capsule-ligament distally to the phalangeal insertion. The strongest reconstruction is with a free tendon graft (233). Twenty-six patients with tendon reconstruction for the thumb UCL followed for 4.5 years had 85% normal ROM and key pinch strength equal to the opposite side at 20 pounds (234). High-grade radial collateral ligament tears that are widely unstable may benefit from direct soft tissue advancement and repair with 38 patients at 10-month follow-up achieving 92% of normal pinch, 87% of which were symptom free (209).

Associated Osteochondral Injuries to the Metacarpal Head or a Base of P1 Fracture

Careful inspection of the dorsal aspect of the metacarpal head should identify any chondral or osteochondral fractures. There are three strategies to manage these fractures. If the fragment is small and extremely unstable, it should be excised. If the fragment has a large subchondral bone base, it can be fixed with a countersunk screw. If fixation is not possible but the fragment can be stably trapped in its bed by the congruent opposing joint surface, it can be further restrained with fine resorbable sutures. For collateral ligament injuries associated with bone fragments, there are two options. If the bone fragment is both large and solid enough to receive definitive fixation, ORIF may be performed with a tension band wire or lag screw. If the bone fragment is too small or too comminuted, the bone can be excised and the end of the ligament reinserted to the cancellous bed of either the metacarpal head or the base of the proximal phalanx. This can be accomplished with a mini-bone anchor (many models are currently available) or by transosseous suture. Surgery may not always be necessary to achieve grip and key pinch strength in avulsion fractures of the lateral base of P1. For example, 27 of 30 nonoperatively treated patients achieved clinical stability despite a 25% incidence of radiographic nonunion, but with only 19 of 30 reporting no pain (235).

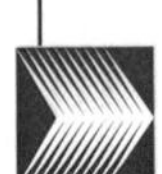

AUTHOR'S PREFERRED TREATMENT

Careful review of the published literature regarding both finger and thumb MP joint ligament injuries indicates that the clinical assessment of instability is paramount in planning subsequent treatment. Local anesthetic injection into the MP joint allows vigorous stress testing of the ligament to be performed without fighting the patient or causing undue pain. Testing in extension and flexion reveals both the absolute value of deviation as well as the discrepancy compared to the uninjured side. The feel at the end point is also a significant piece of information. A greater than 15-

degree difference side to side and a soft end point are stronger indicators of complete ligament disruption than the absolute value of the joint angle when stressed. The integrity of the volar plate should be assessed along with the appearance of rotatory subluxation. I use a combination of the clinical degree of instability and the presence of a palpable Stener lesion to choose direct repair of the thumb UCL, the index RCL, and large bony avulsion injuries. Thumb radial collateral ligament and other finger MP joint injuries are managed nonoperatively. Volar dislocations risk late instability if not surgically repaired. When the patient presents late, direct repair is rarely possible. The simplest reconstruction is then to create a proximally based flap of retracted ligament and advance it back to the anatomic insertion at the volar base of the proximal phalanx. This tissue is not always of sufficient quality. When that is the case, a free tendon graft (plantaris or palmaris longus) reconstruction can be placed through drill holes (233). With appropriate rehabilitation, these patients can still achieve normal motion.

Open Reduction of Finger MP Dislocations

The border digits, the index and small fingers, can easily be approached with a mid-axial incision that offers all the advantages that are contested for both volar and dorsal approaches. Cartilage injuries on the metacarpal head can be well visualized, the digital nerves are easily protected, and the volar plate can be guided back into its correct position. For the long and ring fingers I prefer a transverse incision made at the level of the distal portion of the metacarpal head. This level can reliably be found at the dorsal apex of the sloping V shape of the web commissure. The sagittal bands do not need to be divided but rather retracted distally to access the joint. The volar plate can be reduced without dividing it through a combination of wrist flexion to relax the extrinsic flexor tendons and MP hyperextension. A freer elevator then guides the volar plate to the distal surface of the metacarpal head prior to attempting to reduce the joint itself. For the radial collateral ligament of the index, an absorbable 1.3-mm bone anchor can be used for repair of insertional ruptures and a 4-0 absorbable monofilament suture for midsubstance ruptures. Pinning of the joint is not necessary in fingers as adjacent digit strapping provides enough blockade to excessive coronal plane deviation to protect the healing repair.

Thumb MP Collateral Ligament Repair

The operative technique consists of a chevron incision over the ulnar aspect of the MP joint ensuring adequate volar exposure at the base of the proximal phalanx. Care must be taken with the superficial branches of the radial nerve to avoid neuroma formation. There is usually one large branch passing through the surgical field that is best mobilized dorsally. An incision in the adductor aponeurosis is made just ulnar to the EPL tendon with a cuff being left for repair. Reflection of this layer reveals the joint capsule and torn

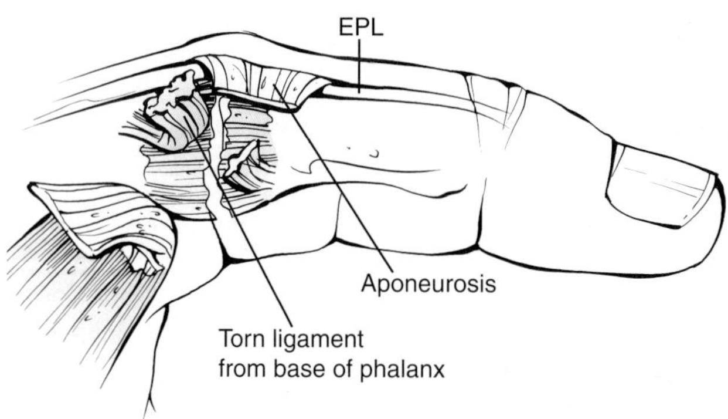

FIGURE 24-78 The approach to the ulnar side of the MP joint must protect dorsal digital nerve branches, leave a cuff for aponeurosis repair to the EPL, and provide adequate exposure to reach the true volar location of the tubercle at the base of the phalanx that represents the anatomic point of proper collateral ligament insertion or the "critical corner."

collateral ligament (Fig. 24-78). While all patterns of disruption have been reported, the most frequent is that of distal avulsion from the base of the proximal phalanx. Often there is a transverse rent in the dorsal capsule and evidence of volar plate injury as well. Direct repair is easiest with an absorbable 1.3-mm bone anchor placed at the true insertion site on the volar lateral tubercle to restore normal anatomy and reduce the rotatory subluxation of the joint. The repair may include a suture through the volar plate margin to recreate the "critical corner." The joint is pinned with a 0.045-inch K-wire prior to tying the anchor sutures to prevent inadvertent ulnar deviation and early rupture of the repair during the first 4 weeks post-operatively. A large bone fragment carrying the point of ligament insertion can be stabilized with one or two lag screws (Fig. 24-79). The IP joint

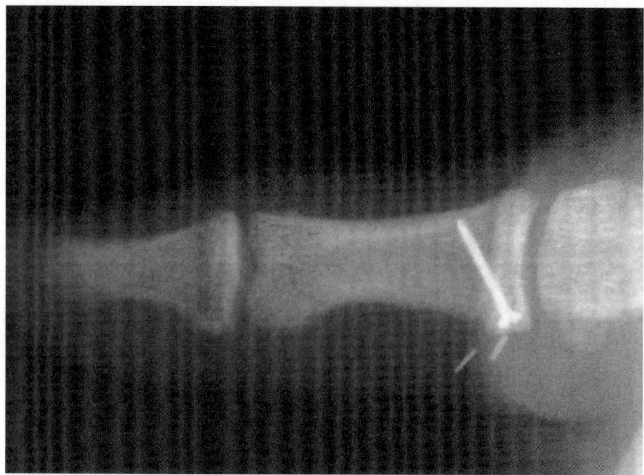

FIGURE 24-79 When a substantial bone fragment accompanies an ulnar collateral ligament injury to the MP joint, lag screw compression provides excellent stability through direct bone healing provided that there is not a multilevel injury of the ligament separating from the bone fragment as well.

should be left free for motion at all times. Motion at the MP joint can begin in a protected fashion at 4 weeks following pin removal and then in an unprotected fashion by 6 weeks. Power pinch activities that stress the ligament in the coronal plane of the thumb should be avoided for up to 3 months after repair.

Free Tendon Graft Reconstruction of Thumb UCL

The approach to the ulnar base of the thumb is the same as for simple repair. The correct anatomic sites of ligament origin at the metacarpal head and insertion at the phalangeal base should be easily discernable with remnants of the original ligament fibers. Drill tunnels are made from each of these points obliquely directed away from the joint with a 2.5-mm bit. Free tendon graft may be harvested by conventional methods from either the palmaris longus (within the operative field) or the plantaris (more appropriate size match). The tendon is passed through each of the drill holes and out the opposite cortex where it may be grasped for tensioning of the reconstruction (Fig. 24-80). The joint is pinned with a 0.045-inch K-wire prior to setting final tension. The graft tension may be secured any number of ways, but a simple method involves the use of two absorbable 1.3-mm bone anchors. One anchor is drilled adjacent to each bone tunnel, further away from the joint. The tendon graft is captured by the sutures from the anchor at the margin of the bone tunnel thus fixing the tension in the graft between these two points.

Pearls and Pitfalls

Hypersensitivity and small cutaneous neuroma formation are often considered the banes of hand surgery. Although never totally avoidable, these unwanted complications can be minimized by a thorough knowledge of the branching patterns of the cutaneous nerves and meticulous attention to detail at the time of surgery. The dorsal digital nerve along the ulnar side the thumb MP joint is at high risk of injury. It should be mobilized dorsally for the procedure and checked each time before drilling. Perhaps the greatest risk is during closure of the adductor aponeurosis along the margin of the EPL tendon. It is quite easy to simply capture the nerve branch with one of these sutures if it is not visualized to be clear with each suture pass.

First web space contracture can easily occur following immobilization of any hand injury and especially when the injury is located in the first web space. Since the first web is located at the level of the MP joint, all positioning forces designed to prevent contracture act on the proximal phalanx and across the MP joint. The value of pinning the thumb MP joint with a 0.045-inch K-wire during the 4-week period of immobilization in a thumb spica splint is that the splint may be appropriately molded to abduct the thumb and avoid contracture.

METACARPAL FRACTURES

Fracture patterns may be broken down for the sake of discussion into those of the metacarpal head, neck, and shaft. Intra-articular fractures of the metacarpal base are covered in the next section on CMC joint fracture dislocations. Metacarpal head fractures present in a variety of patterns requiring different treatment strategies aimed at restoring a smooth congruent joint surface. McElfresh and Dobyns divided metacarpal head fractures into ten categories, finding comminuted and oblique sagittal patterns to be the most common (236). Transverse metacarpal neck and shaft fractures will typically demonstrate apex dorsal angulation (Fig. 24-81). The normal anatomic neck to shaft angle of 15 degrees should be recalled when radiographically assessing the amount of angulation in sub-capital fractures. Radiographic assessment of apex dorsal angulation has a high inter-observer and intra-observer variability (237). Pseudoclawing is a term used to describe a dynamic imbalance manifested as a hyperextension deformity of the MP joint and a flexion deformity of the PIP joint (Fig. 24-82). This occurs as a compen-

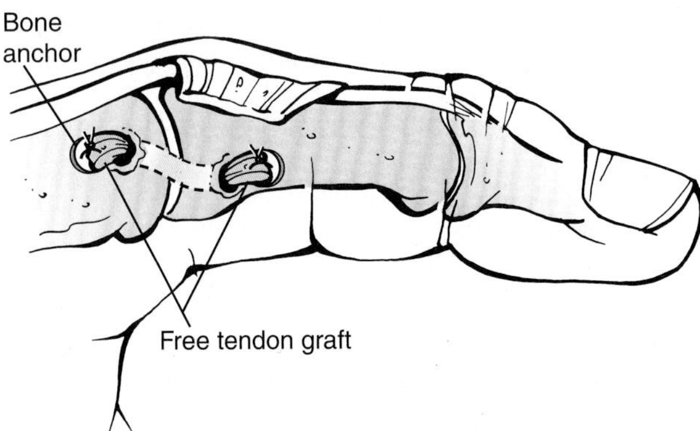

FIGURE 24-80 Free tendon graft reconstruction of the thumb MP ulnar collateral ligament uses the same surgical approach as for direct ligament repair. Drill holes are made obliquely through the metacarpal and the phalanx from the points of anatomic ligament attachment so that a free tendon graft can be passed and tensioned. The graft may be secured by bone anchors adjacent to the bone tunnels.

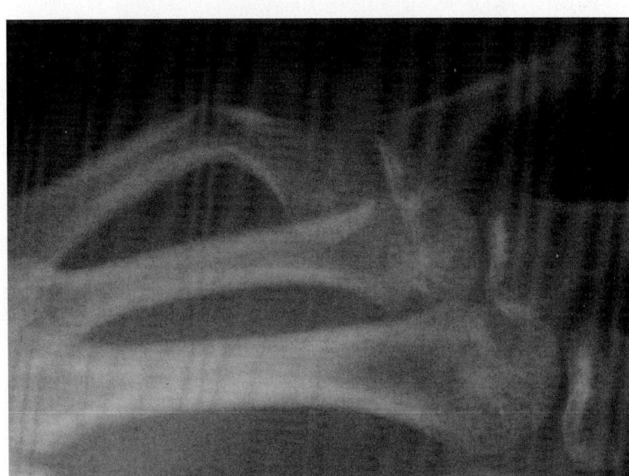

FIGURE 24-81 Transverse metacarpal shaft and neck fractures angulate apex dorsal, deformed by the pull of the intrinsics.

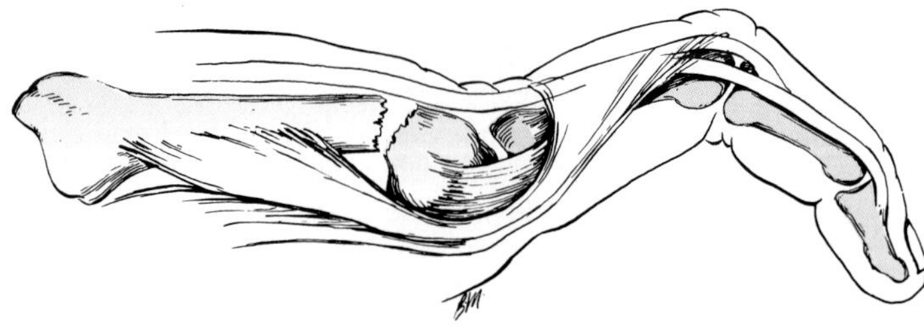

FIGURE 24-82 Pseudoclawing is an imbalance of compensatory MP joint hyperextension and PIP joint flexion that occurs on attempted digital extension in proportion to the degree of apex dorsal angulation at the metacarpal fracture site and represents one indication for surgery.

satory response to the apex dorsal angulation of the metacarpal fracture (usually at the neck) and represents a clinical indication for correcting the fracture angulation. Oblique and spiral fractures tend to shorten and rotate more than angulate (Fig. 24-83). As with all hand fractures, evaluation of rotation remains one of the most critical assessments to avoid a functionally disabling malunion. Ten degrees of malrotation (which risks as much as 2 cm of overlap at the digital tip) should represent the upper tolerable limit (238,239). The problem of overlapping bone shadows has led to the development of a number of specialized radiographic views (Fig. 24-84). The Brewerton view and a view described by Mehara and Bhan may show otherwise occult fractures at the metacarpal bases (240). The reverse oblique projection allows a more accurate estimation of angulation at the second metacarpal neck (241). The skyline view may show vertical impaction fractures of the metacarpal head not appreciable in any other projection (242).

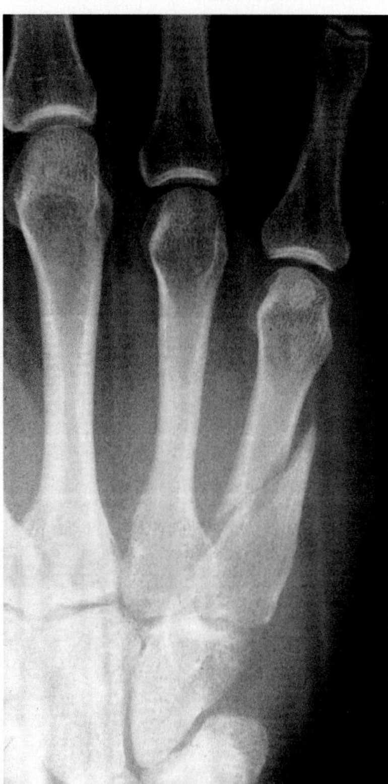

FIGURE 24-83 Long oblique and spiral fractures of the metacarpal shaft tend to shorten and rotate more than angulate.

Surgical and Applied Anatomy

The metacarpals are the key skeletal elements participating in the formation of the three arches of the hand (Fig. 24-85). There are two transverse arches that exist at the CMC and MP joints. The metacarpals themselves are longitudinally arched with a fairly broad convex dorsal surface. Intramedullary geometry is highly variable but with a consistently 20% thicker volar cortex (243). Surgical access to the metacarpals is easily achieved through incisions placed over the inter-metacarpal valleys and curved distally to avoid entering the digital web commissures.

The metacarpals are held tightly bound to each other by strong interosseous ligaments at their bases and by the deep transverse inter-metacarpal ligaments distally. These connections help to maintain the transverse arches of the hand, but flattening can occur with multiple metacarpal fractures or crushing injuries. Shortening of individual metacarpal fractures is limited by these same ligaments (more effectively for the central metacarpals than for the border metacarpals) (244). For each 2 mm of metacarpal shortening there should be 7 degrees of extensor lag (245). One of the weakest points in the metacarpal is the volar aspect of the neck, where comminution is often present (Fig. 24-86). In the sagittal plane the primary deforming forces are the intrinsic muscles, which can be counteracted through MP joint flexion, an important component of the reduction maneuver for metacarpal fractures. Correction of apex dorsal angulation and rotational control are achieved indirectly by grasping the finger to exert control over the distal metacarpal fragment. Flexion of the PIP joint for reduction, as has been long recommended, is an unnecessary maneuver that actually encumbers the reduction process by tensioning the intrinsics (Fig. 24-87).

The biomechanics of fixation for metacarpal fractures has spawned a large body of literature (246–253). The majority consists of cadaver studies testing different fixation constructs in materials testing machines using transverse or oblique osteotomies, cantilever, torsion, three- or four-point bending, and producing load-displacement data. The inherent flaw in this whole approach is that the stiffness of the implant is not the important factor for the surgeon to consider. More important is the implant's fatigue failure properties in response to cyclic stress. Nevertheless, the conclusions reached by nearly all the authors support the following: (a) the interfragmentary lag

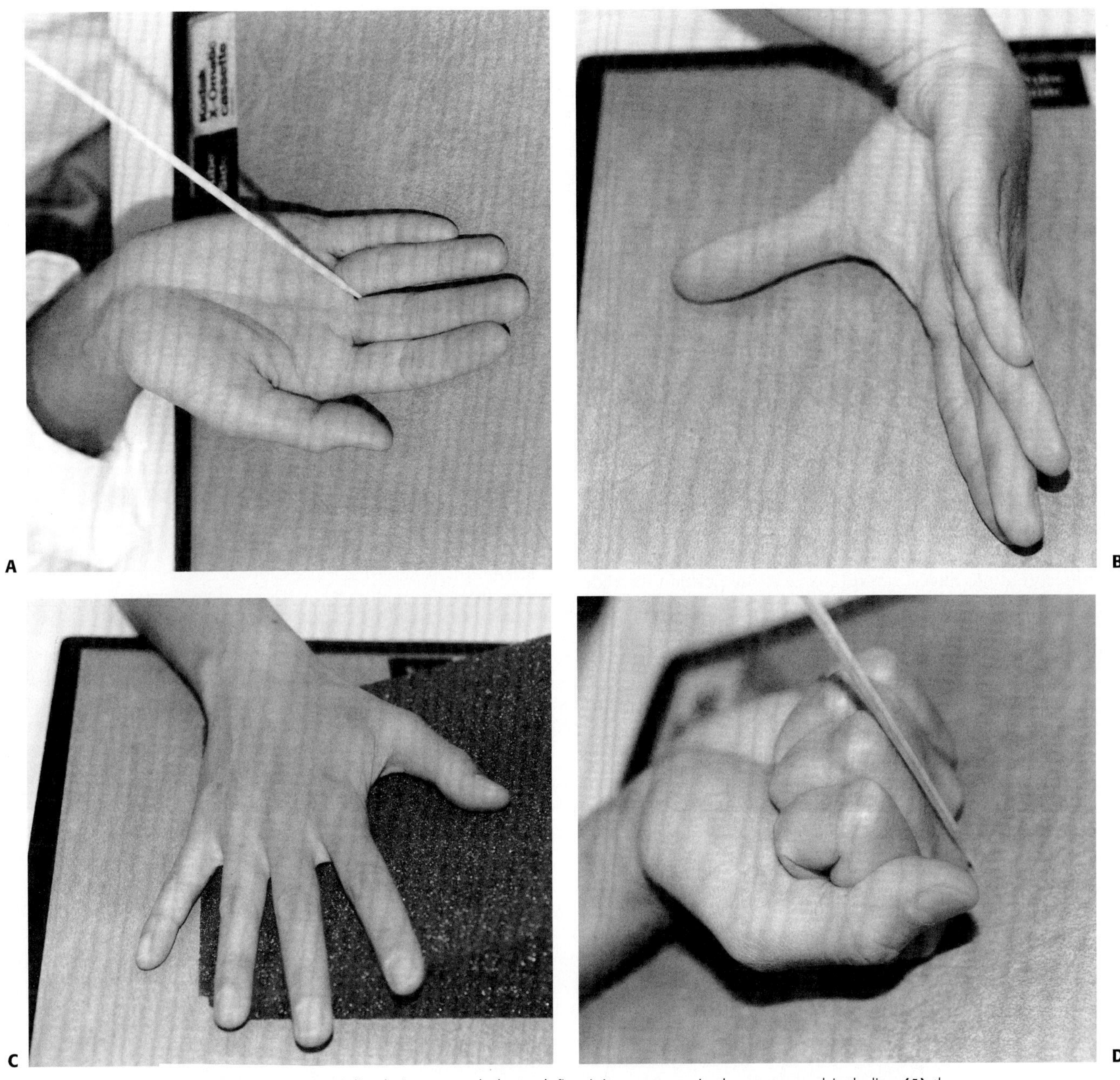

FIGURE 24-84 Specialized views may help to define injury patterns in the metacarpal including **(A)** the Brewerton view for the metacarpal bases, **(B)** the Mehara view for the index CMC relationships, **(C)** the reverse oblique view for angulation in the index metacarpal neck, and **(D)** the skyline view for vertical impaction fractures of the metacarpal head.

screw is, biomechanically, one of the most effective tools available to the surgeon (when applied alone or with a plate, it can even resist nearly the same failure loads as intact bone); (b) self-tapping screws are as strong as standard screws that require a separate step of advance tapping; (c) plates function most effectively as tension bands (which dictates dorsal placement for metacarpal fractures); (d) intra-osseous wire constructs placed in orthogonal planes (90 degrees/90 degrees) are not improved with the addition of K-wires and are the only intra-osseous wire constructs that can compete with plates and screws; and (e) all other intra-osseous wire designs are less rigid than screws and/or plates but stronger than K-wires alone, which tend to slide through bone and loosen. None of this research actually generates the answer for which fixation constructs can be loaded immediately after surgery with specific types of rehabilitation or work stress.

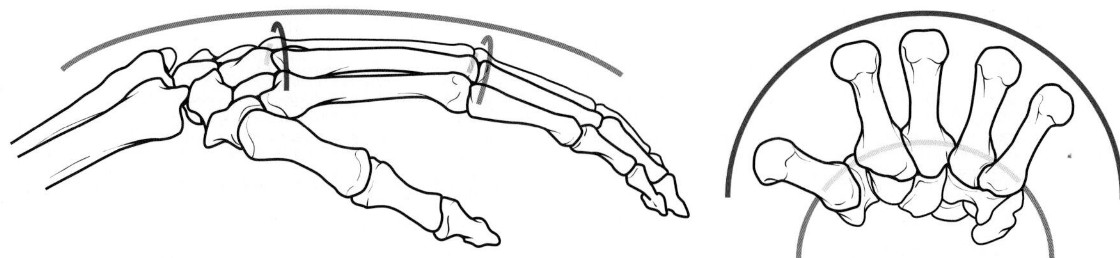

FIGURE 24-85 The three arches of the hand are the longitudinal arch and two transverse arches (one at the metacarpal bases and the other at the metacarpal neck level).

Current Treatment Options

Nonoperative Management

Current treatment options are listed in Table 24-9. Many metacarpal neck and shaft fractures can be treated nonoperatively. Intra-articular fractures of the head and base may also be treated nonoperatively provided the fracture plane is both stable and minimally displaced. Metacarpal fractures with significant rotation or shortening cannot be effectively controlled through entirely nonoperative means. An externally applied splint exerts indirect (but not direct) control over fracture position through positioning and reduction of myotendinous deforming forces (Fig. 24-88). A splint is able to preserve a fracture position that is inherently stable but is not capable of reducing and maintaining an unstable position. The stability of a metacarpal fracture is determined primarily by the adjacent structures (periosteum, adjacent metacarpals, deep transverse inter-metacarpal, and proximal interosseous ligaments) as well as the degrees of initial displacement and comminution. Splinting should be directed at pain control and neutralization of deforming forces. Surface contact should be as broad as possible with an appropriate amount of padding. The splint may be discontinued as soon as the patient can comfortably perform ROM with the hand and not later than 3 weeks. Interphalangeal joint motion should begin immediately following injury. A dorsal splint in full MP joint flexion meets the patient's needs well but may be more than is required. In 100 metacarpal fractures a hand-based cast allowed earlier return to work and produced 9 degrees less angulation than a more encompassing splint (254). Even less restrictive methods of "functional bracing" have been advocated. A brace functioning as a three-point clamp around the hand achieved final angulation of 15 degrees compared to 31 degrees with an ulnar gutter splint in an article by its originators (255). Other authors reported three cases of dorsal skin necrosis when attempting to use this device (256). Compared to simple adjacent digit strapping in 73 patients, a molded metacarpal brace for less than 40 degree angulated fractures of the small finger metacarpal neck yielded similar clinical results with less pain for the brace group (257). Extending this concept, several au-

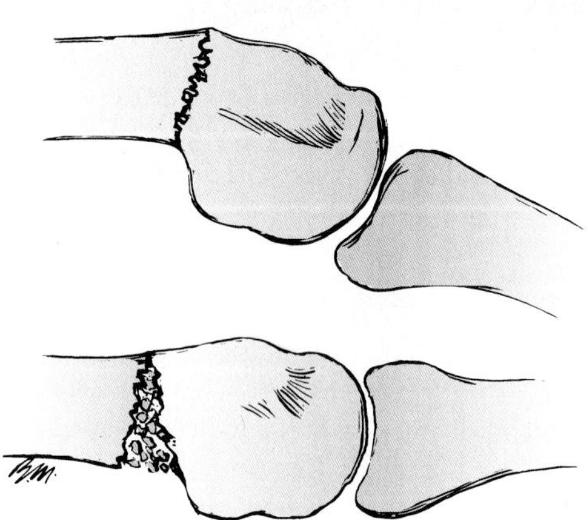

FIGURE 24-86 Fractures of the metacarpal neck frequently experience volar comminution and lack the inherent stability to resist apex dorsal angulation.

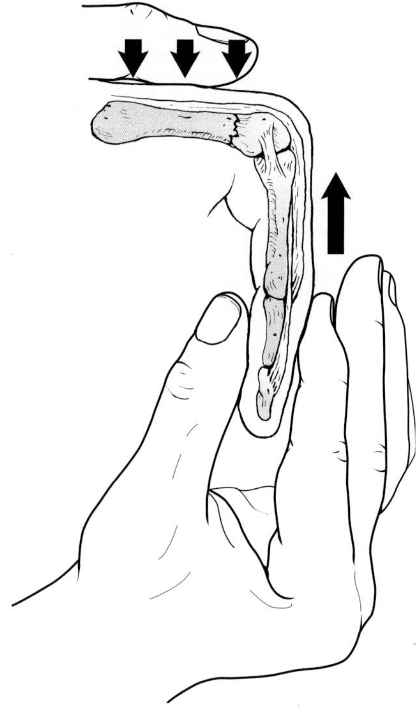

FIGURE 24-87 Reduction of metacarpal fractures can be accomplished by using the digit to control the distal fragment but the PIP joint should be extended rather than flexed.

TABLE 24-9 **Metacarpal Fractures Not Involving the CMC Joints**

Treatment Options	Pros	Cons
Splinting	No added surgical stiffness	Will not maintain reduction of an inherently unstable fracture Poor control of rotation
CRIF	Treatment of choice for most single metacarpal fractures	Transverse method cannot be used for adjacent fractures at the same level in one column
Intramedullary fixation	Can be used for multiple adjacent fractures without opening the fracture site	Rotational control is not exact Tendon irritation proximally
ORIF with screws only	Effective control of rotation for spiral fractures Independent of adjacent fracture patterns	Not effective in presence of comminution or segmental bone loss
ORIF with plates and screws	Bridges segmental bone loss or comminution	Hardware related complications Added surgical stiffness

CMC, carpometacarpal; CRIF, closed reduction and internal fixation; ORIF, open reduction and internal fixation.

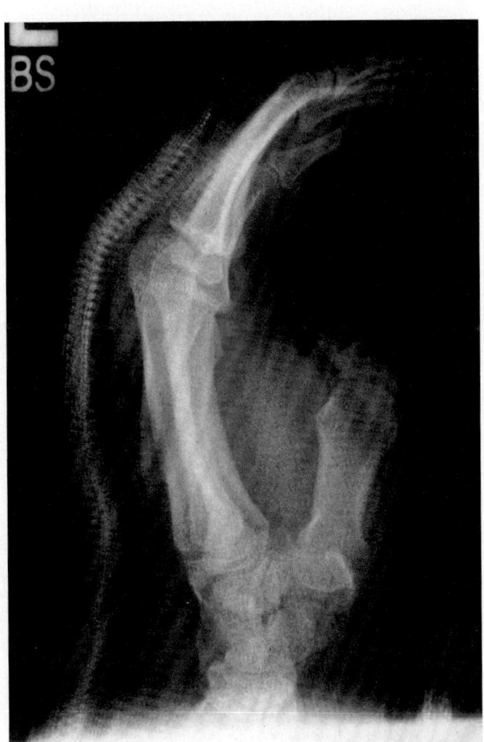

A

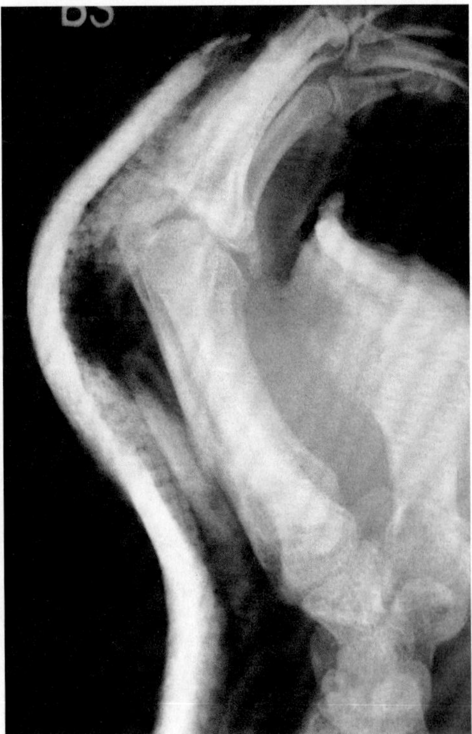

B

FIGURE 24-88 When the MP joints are inadequately flexed **(A)**, the metacarpal shaft fracture angulates apex dorsal with the spike from the distal fragment easily visible. When the MP joints are fully flexed **(B)**, the angulation is substantially improved.

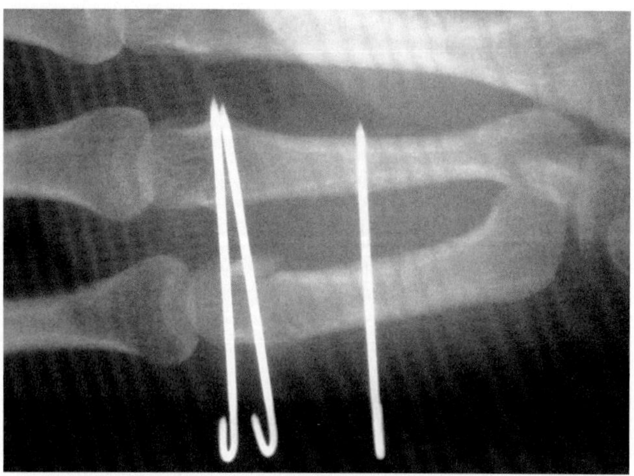

FIGURE 24-89 Closed reduction and internal fixation is effective for metacarpal neck fractures despite the smaller size of the head fragment and the need to achieve separation of the two wires that pass through it for control of fragment rotation in the sagittal plane.

thors have advocated functional mobilization for metacarpal fractures without splinting at all (258–261). Stable fractures (defined as <50% displacement, <40 degrees angulation, and fracture obliquity <60 degrees) treated with a compression glove had better early motion and less early swelling than those treated with 2 weeks of initial splinting (long-term results showed no differences) (261).

Defining the acceptable limits of deformity for each injury location is the subject of much controversy. Functionally, pseudoclawing is unacceptable. Also, the patient may be troubled by the appearance of a dorsal prominence at the fracture site or a shift in the metacarpal head from its dorsally visible position toward the palm. Only rarely will the shift toward the palm create a functional problem. Each patient may have different degrees of deformity that he or she is willing to tolerate. A correlation between deformity and symptoms has not been clearly established (262). Greater degrees of angulation are tolerable in neck fractures than in shaft fractures. Greater angulation is tolerable in the ring and small metacarpals than in the index and long metacarpals due to the increased mobility of the ulnar-sided CMC joints. Biomechanically significant decay in flexor tendon efficiency due to slack in the flexor digiti minimi and third volar interosseous occurs with angulations over 30 degrees in the fifth metacarpal neck, the site of greatest allowable angulation (263,264).

Closed Reduction and Internal Fixation

Closed reduction and internal fixation is the mainstay of treatment for isolated metacarpal fractures not meeting the criteria for nonoperative treatment (Fig. 24-89). CRIF may be used for both extra-articular and intra-articular fractures provided that the fracture is anatomically reducible and stable to the stress of motion with only K-wire fixation (Fig. 24-90). A related treatment is closed reduction and external fixation, which for 19 patients resulted in 95% total active motion (TAM) by 4 weeks (151). CRIF is the minimum treatment necessary for metacarpal base fractures that cannot be held reduced by nonoperative means (265).

Intramedullary Fixation

Intramedullary fixation strategies are best matched with transverse and short oblique fracture patterns and include a single large-diameter rod such as a Steinmann pin, an expandable intramedullary device, multiple pre-bent K-wires or specially manufactured devices inserted at the metacarpal base designed to achieve three-point intramedullary fixation (Figs. 24-91 and 24-92) (266–273) . A single Steinmann pin may be inserted open through the fracture site with the two fragments then impacted over it (Fig. 24-93). Rotational control is achieved by

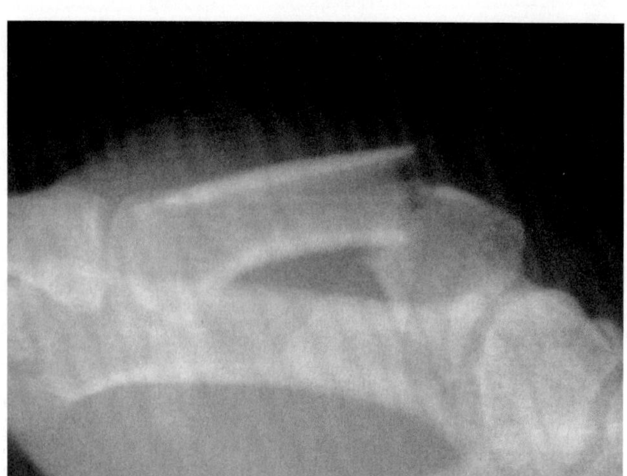

A

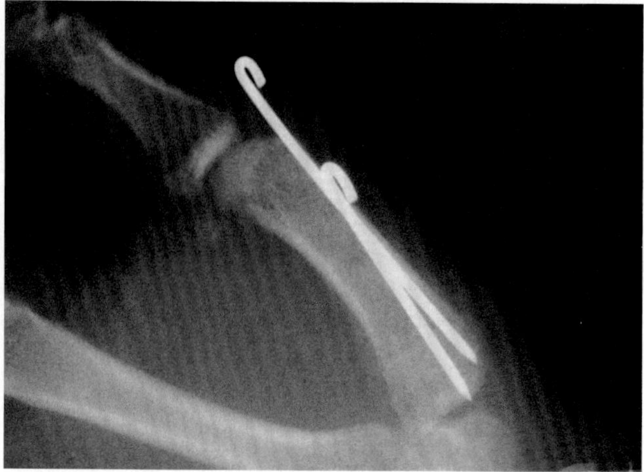

B

FIGURE 24-90 Extra-articular fractures of the thumb metacarpal **(A)** can be effective managed by **(B)** retrograde longitudinal pinning across the fracture into the base fragment.

FIGURE 24-91 Fractures of the metacarpal at the same level that cannot be treated by transverse pinning **(A)** can be stabilized by a specially manufactured device shaped for three-point fixation and closed intramedullary application with a rotational locking sleeve used proximally **(B)**. This device is also effective in oblique fracture patterns **(C)** and fractures near the base **(D)**.

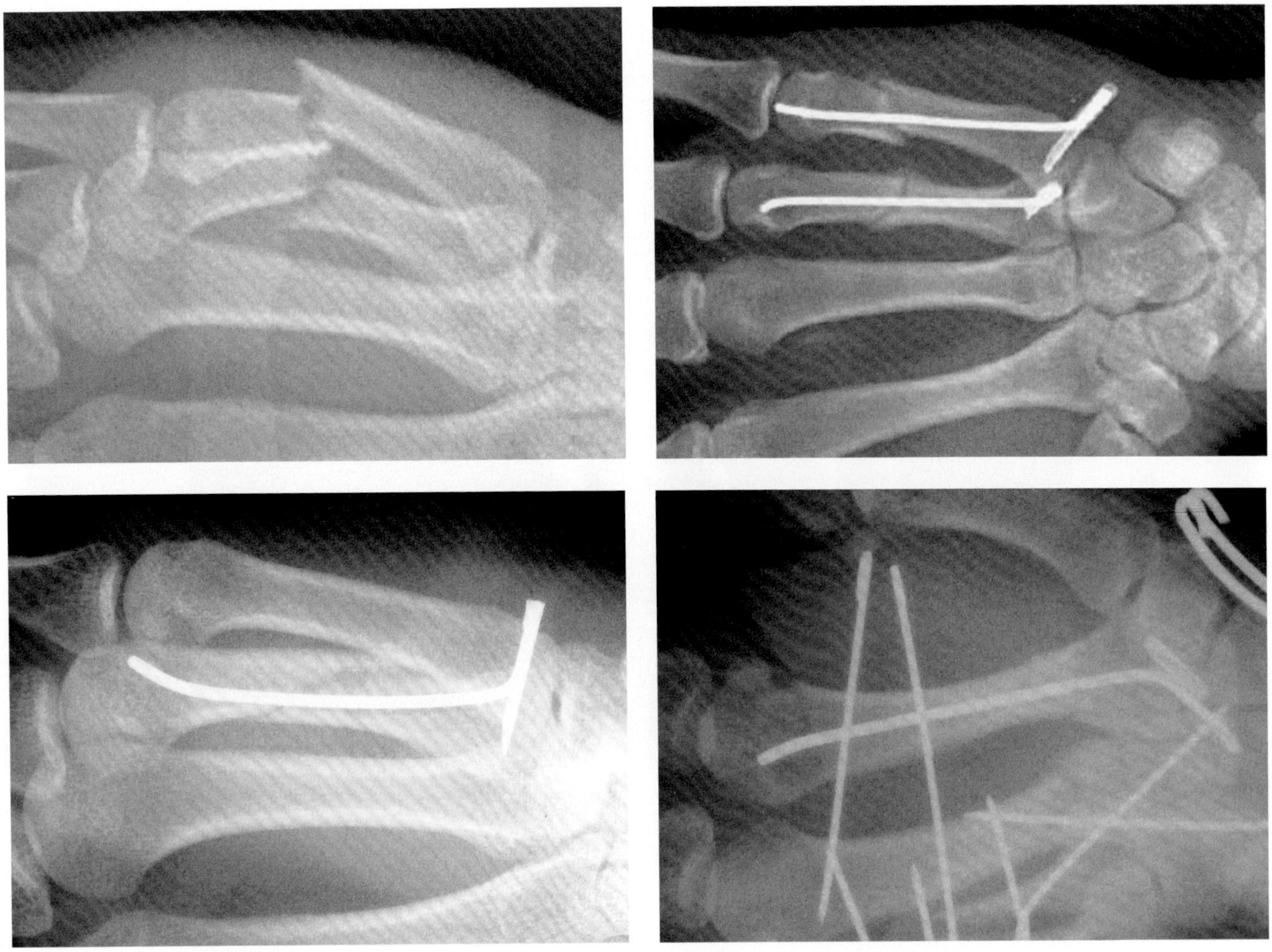

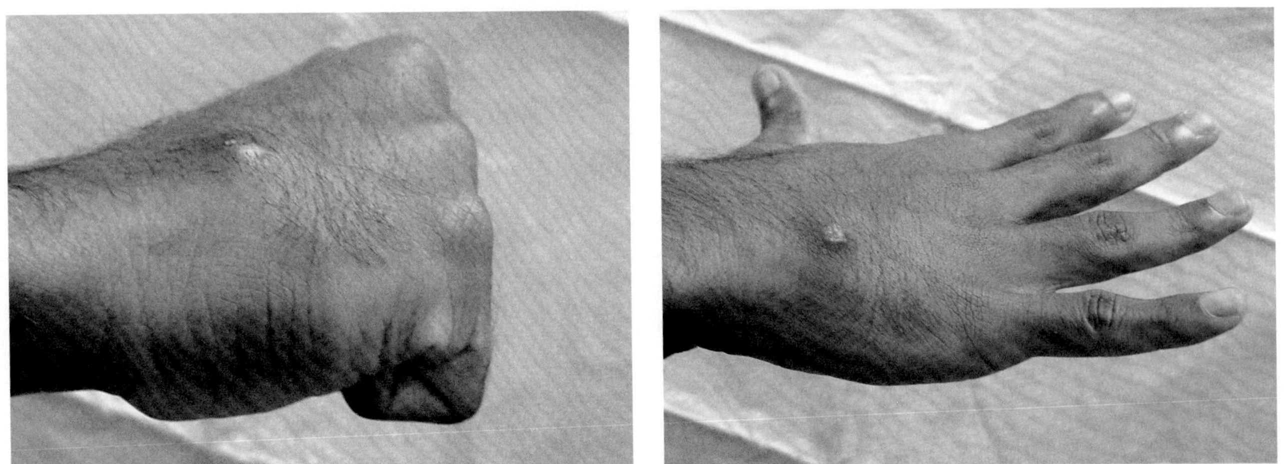

FIGURE 24-92 Full motion **(A)** in flexion and even **(B)** hyperextension can be achieved through early motion rehabilitation following antegrade intramedullary fixation of metacarpal fractures.

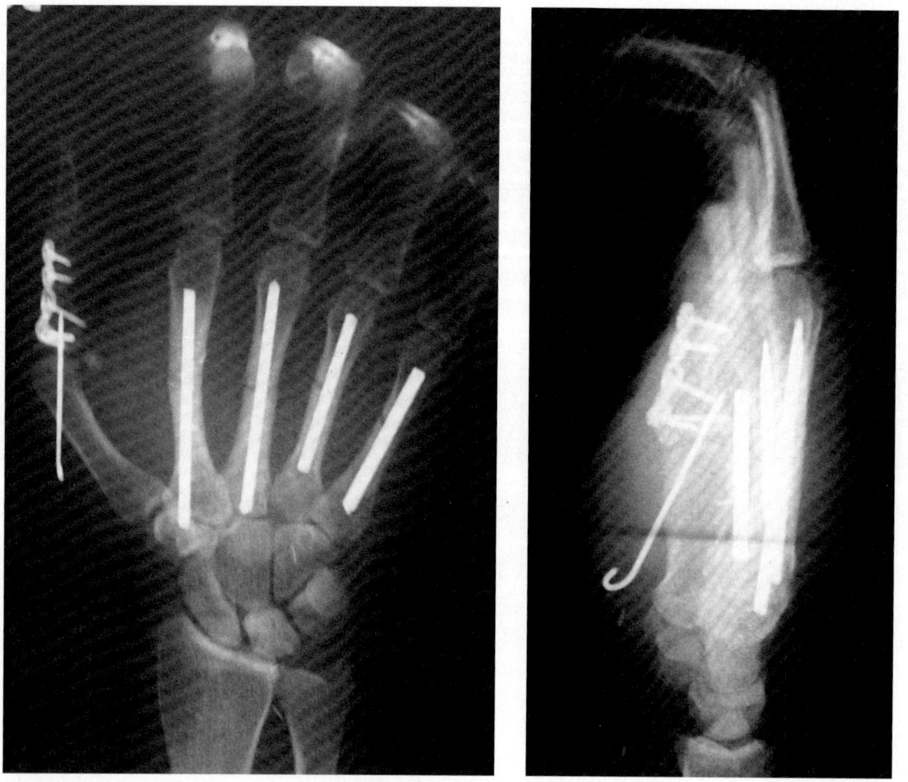

FIGURE 24-93 When crush trauma produces a series of open fractures of the metacarpal shafts all at the same level, a rapid method of stabilization that facilitates soft tissue surgery and revascularization is open intramedullary rodding of the fractures using Steinmann pins cut to length.

fracture fragment interlock, and early motion can be started immediately. Also designed to be inserted open through the fracture site is an expandable intramedullary device indicated for mid-diaphyseal transverse or short oblique fractures (272). The strategy of multiple, stacked pre-bent wires has received broader acceptance than the other two strategies, perhaps owing to the closed technique for introduction (267,270,271,273). The wires are to be pre-bent such that three-point contact is obtained dorsally at the proximal and distal ends of the metacarpal and volarly at the mid-diaphysis (Fig. 24-94). This bow opposes the natural dorsal convexity of the metacarpal and is the basis for the apparently secure fixation achieved with this technique. The pins are to be stacked into the canal, filling it and imparting improved rotational control, as many as three to five 0.045-inch K-wires may be required. Excellent results with multiple wires have been reported primarily for fractures at the metacarpal neck level (270,271). One series of 20 patients with 5-year follow-up reported essentially no complications (271). The other series of 66 patients with 4.5-year follow-up noted eight incomplete reductions (average 18 degree deformity) and 12 patients with MP joint extensor lags of 10 to 15 degrees (270).

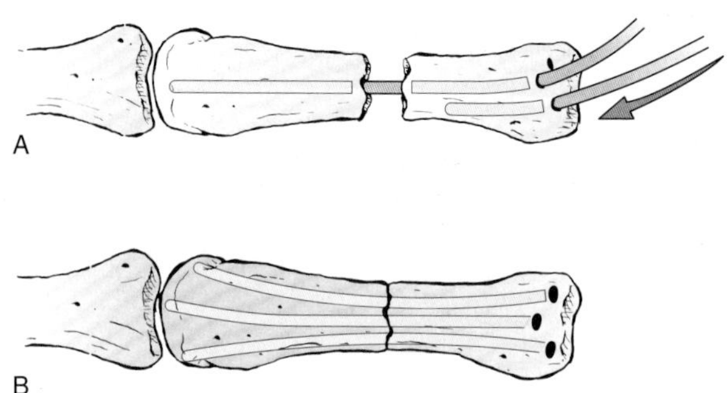

FIGURE 24-94 An alternative antegrade intramedullary fixation strategy includes multiple 0.045-inch K-wires "stacked" into the canal in an attempt to achieve both rotational and angular control over the fracture.

Open Reduction and Internal Fixation

ORIF is the treatment of choice for intra-articular fractures that cannot be reduced and held by closed means (267). Internal fixation is also required for multiple fractures without inherent stability and for open fractures especially when associated with tendon disruptions (274). Internal fixation can be accomplished with intra-osseous wiring, composite wiring, screws only, or screws and plates (Figs. 24-95 and 24-96) (160,275,276). Wiring techniques have traditionally held the advantage over plate and screw application in terms of technical ease and availability of materials. However, with the modular plating systems now available specifically for use in hand surgery, equally low-profile

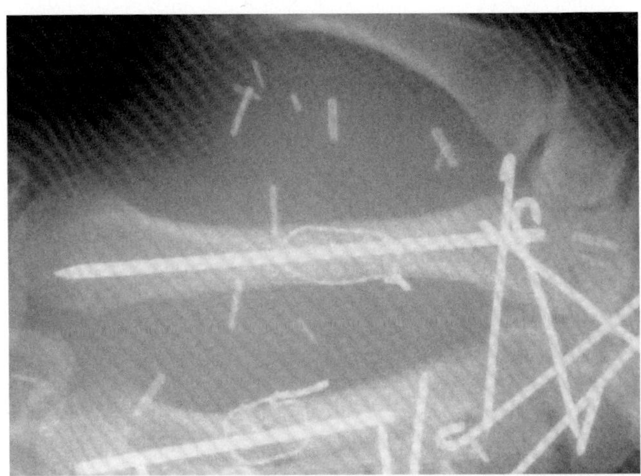

FIGURE 24-95 When rotational control is not sufficient with intramedullary fixation alone, composite wiring is useful and also adds a compressive force across the fracture site.

fixation can be achieved with greater rigidity (Fig. 24-97) (167). The most important consideration is that the surgeon should choose the method of internal fixation with which he is the most comfortable. In a series of 33 fractures internally fixed using composite wiring by surgeons very skilled and familiar with this technique, the average TAM was 256 degrees with no complications (162). Similarly a series of 27 patients treated with plates and screws had an average TAM of 252 degrees (170).

Metacarpal Head Fractures

For partial articular metacarpal head fractures screw only fixation is the treatment of choice. If sufficient interlock of bone spicules occurs, a single 1.3 to 1.5 mm countersunk screw can control rotation of the fragment. If interlock is not effective, two screws are preferred even if this means downsizing the screw diameter to accommodate both of them in the fragment without causing comminution. For complete articular head fractures the condylar blade plate is usually required, but it is the most technically demanding plate to apply (Fig. 24-98). This plate is applied laterally with the blade dorsal and the condylar screw hole volar. The drill hole for the blade is round but the blade is rectangular in cross-sectional area. This makes manual insertion of the blade into its hole difficult, and a fine touch is required to not further comminute the metacarpal head fragments. More importantly, the exact angle of the drill path for the blade must be determined in advance relative to the cortical surface of the more proximal shaft against which the plate will be applied. The condylar screw hole of the plate usually needs to be bent to avoid prominence on its volar edge.

Rehabilitation

The importance of early motion must be considered in direct proportion to the magnitude of the injury or the surgical procedure performed (277). The more tissue damage that is present, the more aggressive must be the motion program. One frequently overlooked factor that greatly confounds progress in therapy is edema control. External compression wraps to the zone of injury with cohesive elastic bandages work to minimize the presence of edema from the outset. When internal fixation has been required, one must anticipate the development of an extensor lag at the MP joint. Specific attention should be given to extensor tendon gliding in zone VI to overcome a developing lag. Rapid tendon activation has been successful in breaking free developing adhesions between the peritendinous tissues and their surroundings (Fig. 24-99). Patients should be allowed to use the hand for light activities throughout the healing period. Light resistance activities can begin at 6 weeks. Extremely forceful use patterns should be deferred until 3 months (8).

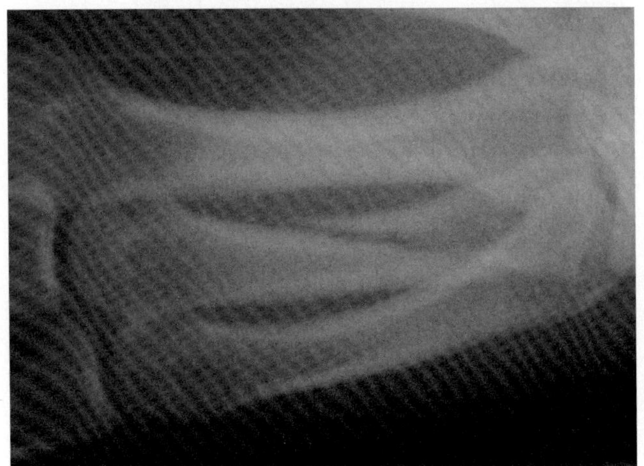

A

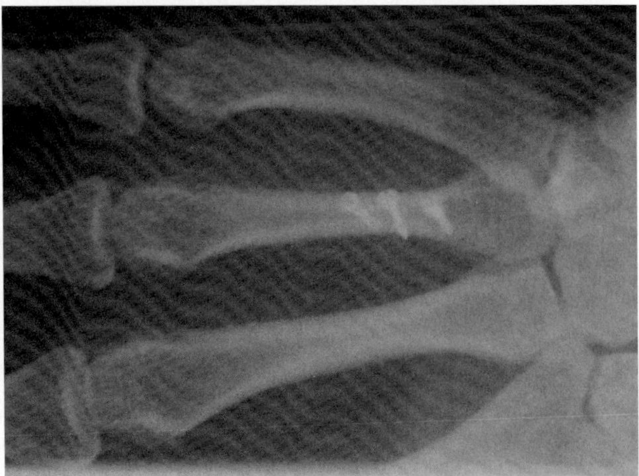

B

FIGURE 24-96 Spiral fractures of the shaft **(A)** that prove difficult to control in rotation and length can be anatomically restored **(B)** with interfragmentary lag screw fixation.

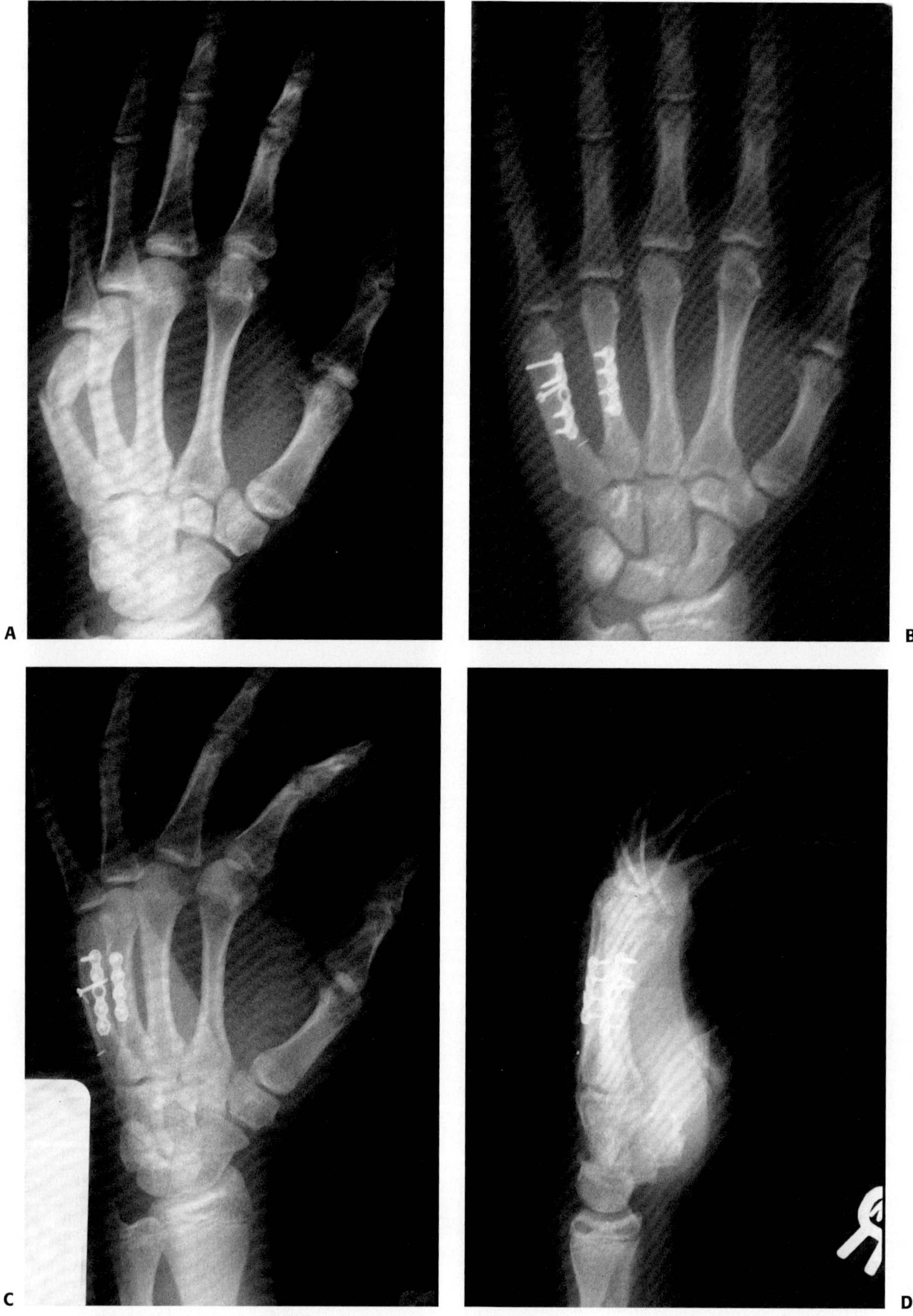

FIGURE 24-97 When adjacent metacarpal fractures occur at the same level **(A)** especially in association with significant soft tissue trauma, **(B)** ORIF with plates and screws can provide **(C)** restoration of the original anatomy and **(D)** a stable foundation for early motion rehabilitation.

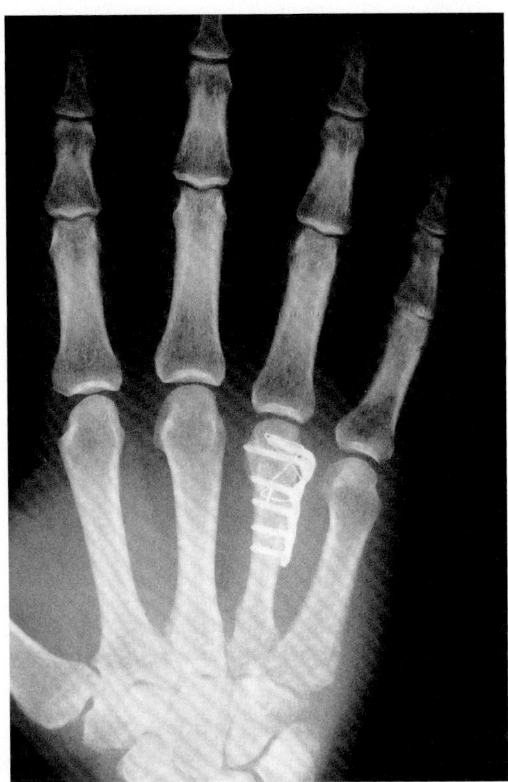

FIGURE 24-98 Difficult fractures of the metacarpal head may benefit from stabilization with the fixed angle support of a condylar blade plate.

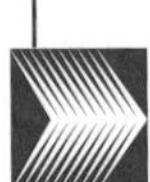

AUTHOR'S PREFERRED TREATMENT

Nonoperative Management

Many extra-articular and some intra-articular fractures, which are categorized as stable by virtue of having over 30% normal ROM without motion at the fracture site, can be managed with entirely nonoperative means using temporary splinting. Patients with entirely nondisplaced fractures that have excellent inherent stability do not require any external immobilization at all and can begin immediate AROM, usually with the added protection of adjacent digit strapping. Patients with stable metacarpal shaft fractures can be returned to nearly all light activities in a hand-based splint that is continued for a maximum of 3 weeks. Stable neck and intra-articular head fractures are more effectively protected by support that covers from the PIP level to the forearm with the MP joints in full flexion. At least one adjacent digit is included with the affected ray. Interphalangeal joint motion should begin immediately with all strategies.

Closed Reduction and Internal Fixation

Transverse pinning to adjacent metacarpals is my treatment of choice for all unstable closed metacarpal fractures except multiple adjacent fractures at the same level that include a border digit (Fig. 24-100). The biomechanics of the transverse pinning strategy is that of external fixation. Four points of control with 0.045-inch K-wires are needed. The two points closest to the fracture site on either side should be as close as possible. The two farthest from the fracture site should be as far apart as possible. The CMC ligaments are stout enough that adjacent metacarpal relationships at the base are secure enough to qualify as the most proximal point of fixation such that only one pin is required proximal to the fracture site. The distal most pin should avoid transgression of the sagittal bands if at all possible. This must be titrated clinically against the goal of placing the point of fixation as far from the fracture site as possible. The transverse pinning strategy works equally well for central (long and ring) and border (index and small) metacarpals. If the four finger metacarpals are conceived of as occurring in two columns (a radial column for index and long and an ulnar

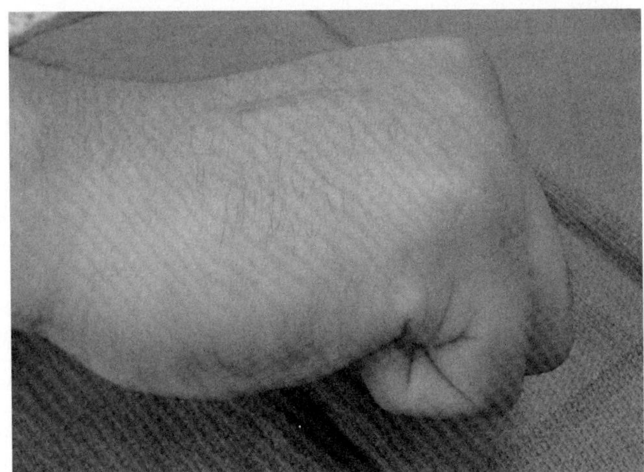

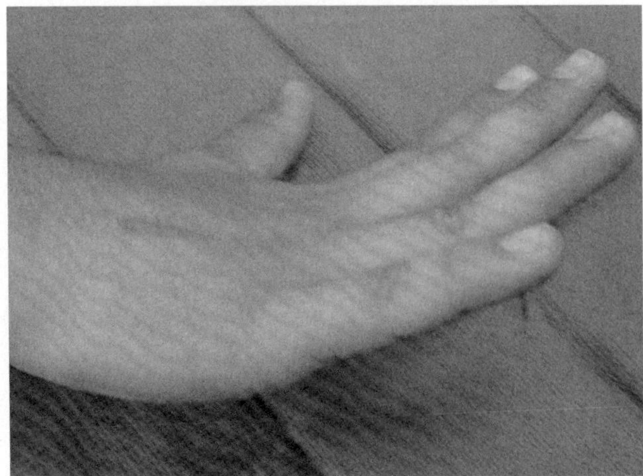

FIGURE 24-99 Even following ORIF, when a properly designed rehabilitation program is administered, **(A)** complete flexion and **(B)** hyperextension is possible.

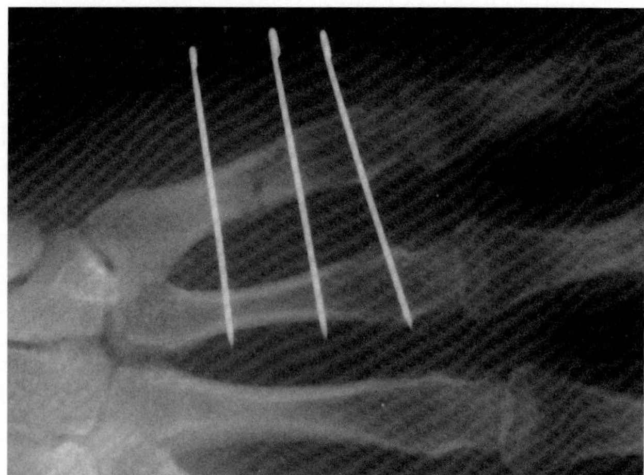

FIGURE 24-100 Transverse closed reduction internal fixation functions under the same biomechanical principles as external fixation. Note the distal wire is placed just proximal to the collateral recess of both bones and has also avoided tethering the sagittal bands.

column for ring and small) then most combinations of multiple metacarpal fractures can still be fixed with this strategy. The strategy can always be used if there is only one fracture per column. If both metacarpals in the column are fractured, but at different levels, they can be used to reciprocally stabilize each other (Fig. 24-101). The specific requirement for reciprocal stabilization to be effective is that there is a zone in the diaphysis of both bones where two pins with adequate spacing from each other can be placed (distal to one fracture site and proximal to the other). At the conclusion of the procedure, one has the choice of leaving the pins protruding through the skin or cutting them off beneath the skin. I have rarely seen problems with pins left through the skin for 4 weeks or less, which is the duration required for the treatment of metacarpal fractures. The hand is initially splinted in full MP flexion to resist the development of contracture. Early motion can proceed while the pins are still in place.

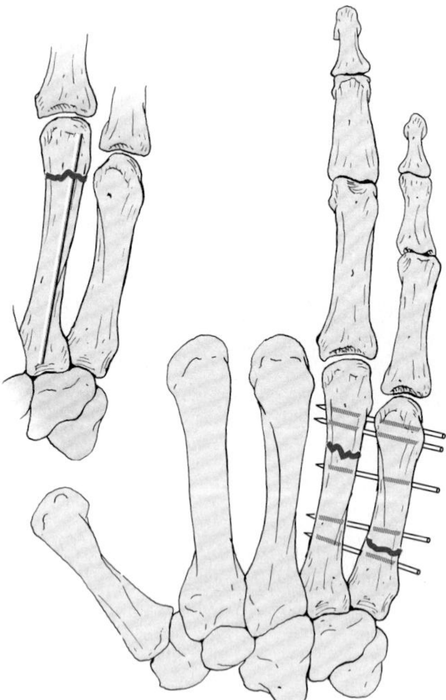

FIGURE 24-101 Reciprocal transverse stabilization of adjacent metacarpal fractures is possible when the levels of the two fractures are separated enough to be able to place two pins that fall distal to the first fracture and proximal to the second such that the first metacarpal is sufficiently stabilized to in turn provide stability to the other metacarpal.

Open Reduction and Internal Fixation

Open reduction and internal fixation is my treatment of choice for open fractures and multiple fractures not meeting the criteria for reciprocal transverse stabilization. When fracture plane interlock between bone spicules is present, intraosseous wiring, composite wiring, screw only, or screw and plate fixation may all be considered. I prefer screw only fixation for long-oblique or spiral fractures (Fig. 24-102). In order to select screw only fixation, the ratio of the length of the oblique or spiral fracture plane to the bone diameter must be at least 2:1. Furthermore, to avoid comminution, the desired location of the screws must pass through an area in the bone spike where the screw outer diameter is less than one-third the width of the spike. The screw sizes most appropriate for a metacarpal are between 1.5 and 2.0 mm. Multiple open transverse or short oblique fractures of the mid-diaphysis (from crushing injuries) are nicely managed with intra-medullary pins. Rotational control can be supplemented with a composite wire loop. When interfragmentary compression cannot be achieved owing to the presence of comminution or bone loss, plates and screws are indicated. As with all techniques of internal fixation, it is essential to cover the hardware with periosteal closure to provide a separate gliding layer. I prefer to operate 3 to 5 days following injury so that the periosteum will have thickened in response to injury and can be both dissected as a discrete tissue flap and closed with solid suture purchase. Unlike over the proximal phalanx, the extensor tendons at this level are discrete cords, and placement of the hardware away from them should be possible in most cases. Placement of the plate dorsally puts it on the tension cortex of the bone, but in this position it interferes most directly with the extensor tendons. Placement of the plate in a true lateral position allows sagittal plane forces to be resisted by the width of the plate rather than its thickness, but is rarely technically possible. A dorsolateral position offers a reasonable compromise and is the preferred location. All the technical comments made in the section on proximal phalangeal fractures apply equally here.

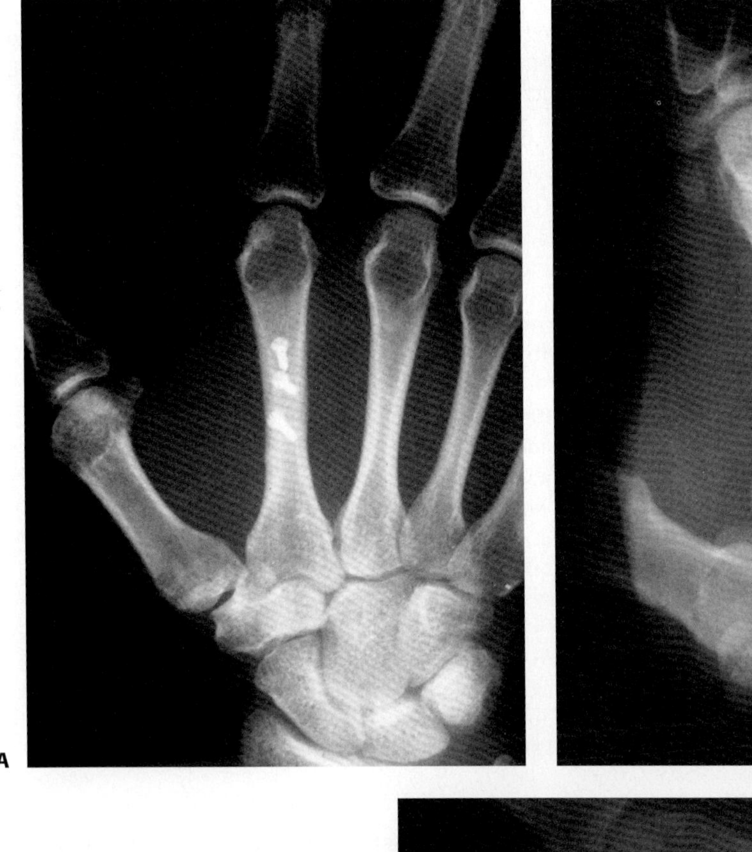

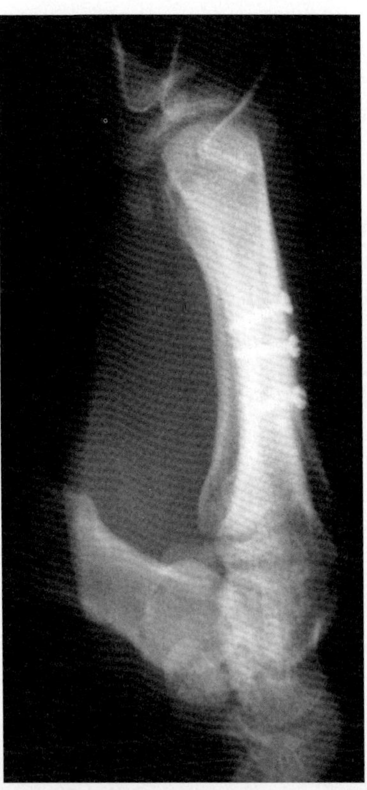

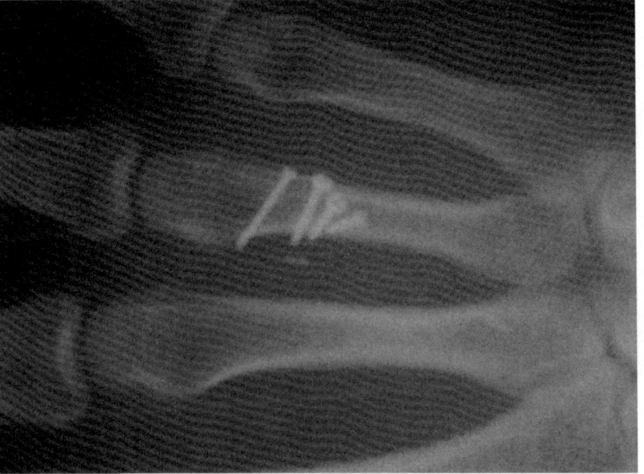

FIGURE 24-102 ORIF with interfragmentary lag screws is typically performed using **(A)** 2 mm screws in spiral fractures of the metacarpal shaft with **(B)** countersinking of the heads, but may be accomplished with **(C)** 1.5 mm screws that still allow immediate motion rehabilitation.

Pearls and Pitfalls

The metacarpal is the most proximal bone in the ray. Rotational malunions here will be the most obvious and functionally disabling. In large part, the management of metacarpal fractures is all about ensuring that rotation is correct. Length and angulation are, of course, not to be forgotten. The assessment of rotation both pre-operatively and intra-operatively merits discussion. In both cases, the examiner should not touch the digit during the assessment. A pre-operative patient that is awake may require an anesthetic block to relieve enough pain so that he or she is capable of flexing sufficiently to demonstrate the rotational status of the digit. In the anesthetized patient, tenodesis driven by full range wrist motion produces sufficient flexion and extension of the digit that rotational alignment can be accurately judged.

When performing transverse pinning of metacarpals, intra-operative imaging will effectively demonstrate depth of pin penetration and coronal plane fracture orientation. Metacarpal overlap obscures any individual metacarpal lateral view. Ensuring that the pins have penetrated all four cortices cannot be judged radiographically and must be determined by feel at the time of placement. If the reduction is difficult to obtain closed or tends to slip as the pins are driven, the case does not have to be converted to a full open reduction. A small instrument such as a dental pick or micro-elevator can be placed percutaneously at the fracture site to directly control reduction while proceeding with the otherwise entirely closed pinning.

CARPOMETACARPAL JOINT DISLOCATIONS AND FRACTURE DISLOCATIONS

Dislocations at the finger carpometacarpal (CMC) joints are usually high-energy injuries with involvement of associated structures, often neurovascular (Fig. 24-103) (278). Particular care must be given to the examination of ulnar nerve function, especially motor, due to its close proximity to the fifth CMC joint (279,280). Frequently the pattern is one of fracture dislocation involving the metacarpal bases, the distal carpal bones, or both (281). Overlap on the lateral x-ray obscures accurate depiction of the injury pattern, and most authors recommend at least one variant of an oblique view (282). The Brewerton view may be helpful in this respect, profiling individual metacarpal bases. A special view has been described for the second metacarpal base (240). When fracture dislocations include the dorsal cortex of the hamate, CT or polytomography may be necessary to fully evaluate the pathoanatomy (283). Another pattern to recognize is dislocation of one CMC joint with fracture of an adjacent metacarpal base. Shortening can be evaluated by noting a disruption in the normal cascade seen distally at the MP joints. Volar CMC dislocations are rare (279,284). All five CMC joints simultaneously dislocated and a divergent dislocation have been reported (285,286).

Pure Thumb CMC Dislocations

Most thumb carpometacarpal dislocations are dorsal and are thought to occur through axial loading of a partially flexed thumb (Fig. 24-104). Motorcyclists may be uniquely prone to sustaining this rare injury and to having the injury missed on initial evaluation (287). The injury will often be reduced prior to being seen by the surgeon. Clinical diagnosis is then based on identifying the residual instability. Differentiating complete from incomplete ligament rupture is essential, as initial operative treatment is appropriate only for complete disruptions. Instillation of local anesthetic into the joint may be required to allow an unimpeded examination. Manual stress testing compared to the contralateral side should allow diagnosis in most cases. The injury has also been reported in concert with MP dislocation, fracture of the trapezium, and with small avulsion fractures from the metacarpal base (288–292).

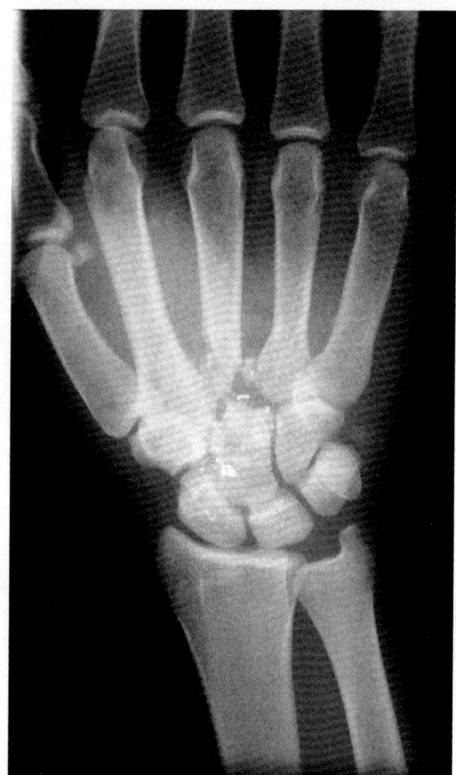

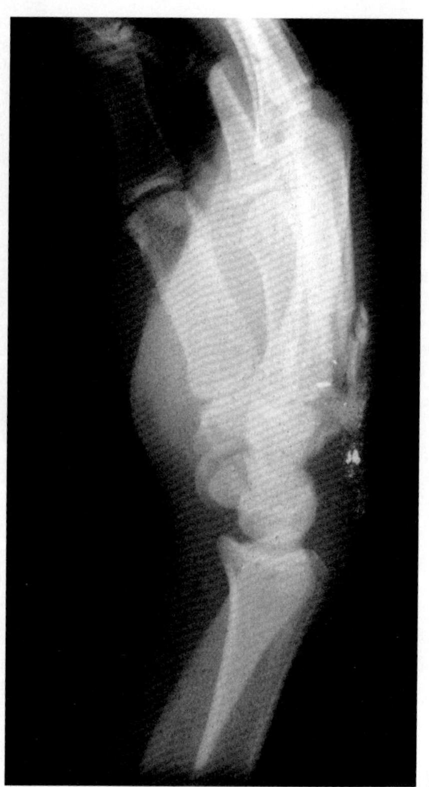

FIGURE 24-103 Fractures of CMC joints **(A)** are typically high-energy injuries with **(B)** comminution of both the metacarpal base and the distal carpal row.

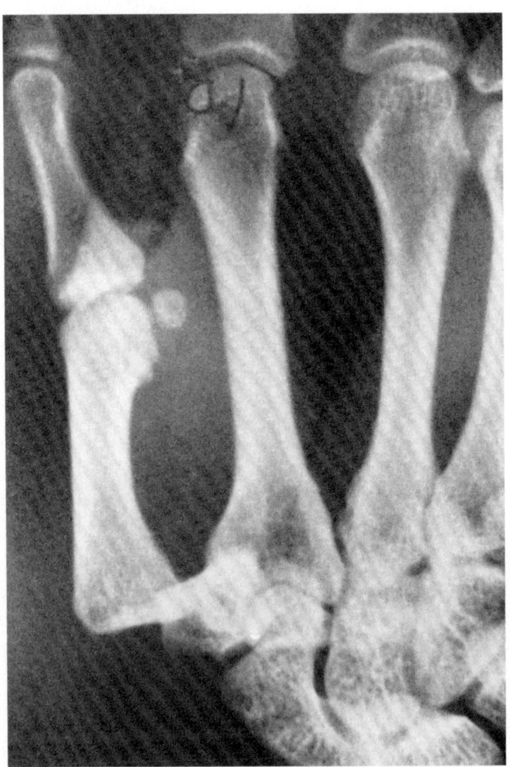

FIGURE 24-104 Pure dislocations of the thumb CMC joint are rare injuries and typically occur dorsoradially.

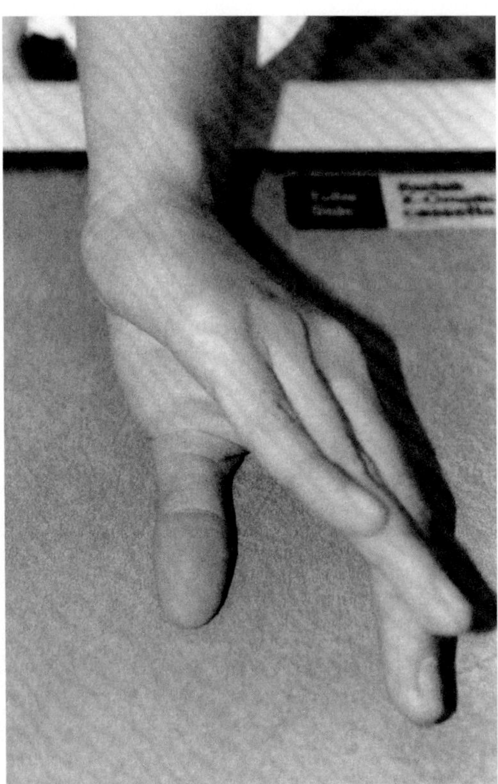

FIGURE 24-106 The thumb does not reside in the same plane as the rest of the hand. A true AP of the thumb can be obtained with the Robert's view.

Thumb CMC Fracture Dislocations

The majority of thumb metacarpal base fractures are intra-articular (Fig. 24-105). The majority of thumb CMC joint injuries are fracture dislocations rather than pure dislocations. The smaller fracture fragment at the thumb metacarpal volar base is deeply placed and not palpable. Terms associated with these fracture dislocations are Bennett's (partial articular), and Rolando's (complete articular) fractures. Specific x-rays must be obtained in the true AP and lateral plane of the thumb (not a series of hand x-rays) if injuries along this axis are to be correctly identified (Fig. 24-106).

Surgical and Applied Anatomy

Finger CMC Joints

Stability at the finger CMC joints is provided by a system of four ligaments. There is a high degree of variation with dorsal, multiple palmar, and two sets of interosseous ligaments (only one between long and ring) (293,294). The interosseous ligaments are the strongest and have a V-configuration oriented with the base of the V oriented toward the fourth metacarpal. Range of motion of the index and long CMC joints is limited to less than 5 degrees, with 15 degrees at the ring, and up to

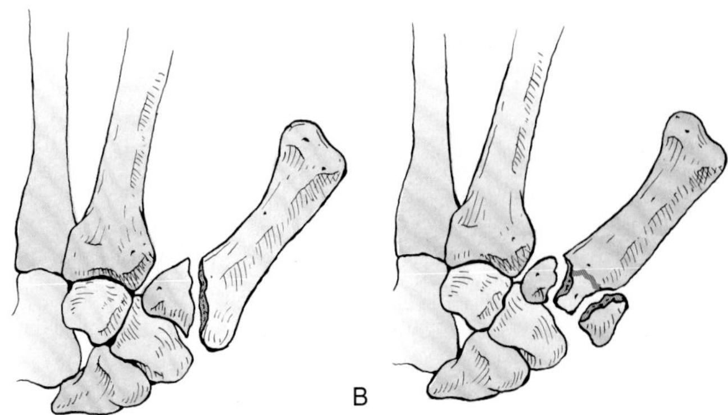

FIGURE 24-105 The most recognized patterns of thumb metacarpal base intra-articular fractures are **(A)** the partial articular Bennett's fracture and **(B)** the complete articular Rolando's fracture.

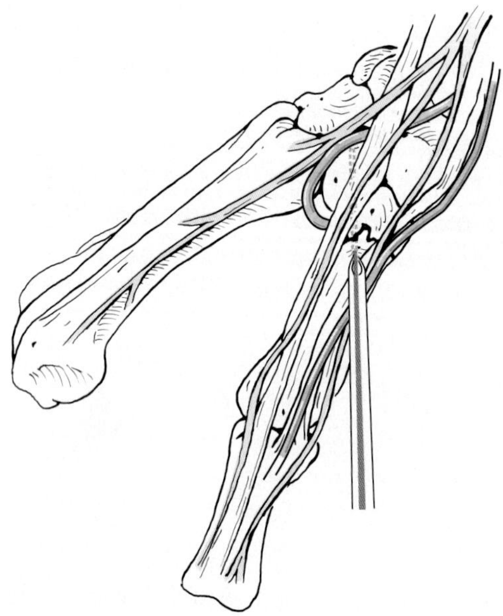

FIGURE 24-107 The radial artery, branches of both the superficial radial and lateral antebrachial cutaneous nerves, and the thumb extensor tendons all pose soft tissue risks for damage during closed pinning strategies around the thumb metacarpal base.

25 to 30 degrees at the small finger (295–297). Small finger CMC motion is reduced 28% to 40% when the ring finger is immobilized (298). The axis of motion is located near the base of the metacarpal. The index metacarpal has a particularly stable configuration through its wedge-shaped articulation with the trapezoid. The small finger CMC joint is the only joint not having a gliding configuration but instead is a modified saddle-shaped joint. The increased mobility on the ulnar side of the hand may predispose to its noted greater frequency of injury. Critical soft tissue relationships to appreciate during treatment of injuries to the CMC joints are the position of the motor branch of the ulnar nerve directly in front of the fifth CMC joint and the deep palmar arch in front of the third CMC joint. Of all hand fractures and dislocations, injury at the CMC level requires the highest degree of vigilance regarding associated neurologic injury. The high-energy mechanism of these injuries and profound degrees of swelling may lead to worsened outcomes through residual long-term nerve compression (283).

Thumb CMC Joints

Branches of both the lateral antebrachial cutaneous and superficial radial nerve ramify throughout the region of the thumb base on the radial side (Fig. 24-107). Three tendons pass through this region: the abductor pollicis longus (APL), extensor pollicis brevis (EPB), and extensor pollicis longus (EPL). The radial artery passes beneath the APL and EPB on its course to the first web space and lies just proximal to the CMC joint. The joint anatomy includes reciprocal saddle-shaped surfaces of the distal trapezium and proximal metacarpal. The axis of this concavo-convex joint is then itself curved in a third plane with the convexity lateral. The normal ROM at the thumb CMC joint is around 53 degrees flexion-extension, 42 degrees abduction-adduction, and 17 degrees pronation-supination (299). There is consensus as to which ligaments are anatomically present at the trapeziometacarpal joint (Fig. 24-108). They are the superficial anterior oblique, deep anterior oblique (beak), ulnar collateral, inter-metacarpal, posterior oblique, and dorsoradial ligaments (300,301). A point of confluence exists at the palmar ulnar tubercle of the first metacarpal base. There is disagreement regarding the primary stabilizing ligament in preventing dislocation between the deep anterior oblique and the dorsoradial ligament. Although the deep anterior oblique was previously considered the primary stabilizer, more recent research favors the dorsoradial ligament. In cadaveric dissection, the degree of arthritis correlated most closely with attenuation of the anterior

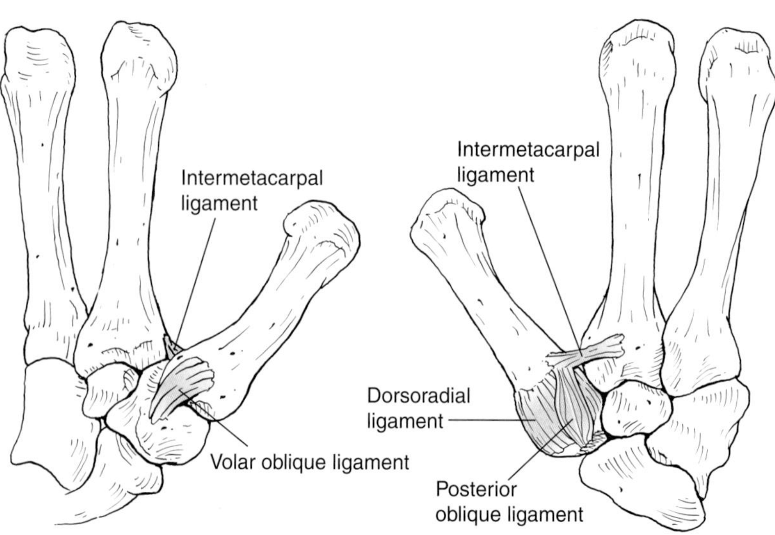

FIGURE 24-108 The primary stabilizing ligaments of the thumb CMC joint include the deep anterior oblique, dorsoradial, posterior oblique, and intermetacarpal ligaments. The superficial anterior oblique and ulnar collateral ligaments are not primary stabilizers.

oblique ligament (301). The dorsoradial ligament is the shortest ligament in the group and the first to become taut with dorsal or dorsoradial subluxation (300). Selective ligament sectioning showed the dorsoradial ligament's deficiency to lead to the greatest degree of subluxation (302). Dorsal dislocation usually occurs through rupture of the dorsal ligaments with a sleeve-type avulsion of the anterior oblique ligament as it peels off the volar surface of the first metacarpal (303,399). Supination may also play a significant role in the mechanism of this injury. Deformation of fractures at the base of the thumb metacarpal occurs with a complex motion (Fig. 24-109). The distal metacarpal is adducted and supinated by the adductor pollicis. At the same time, the APL pulls the metacarpal radially and proximally. Reduction maneuvers must attempt to counteract each of these forces. Probably the most difficult aspect of the reduction to maintain through splinting is the radial displacement of the base.

Current Treatment Options

Nonoperative Management

Current treatment options are listed in Table 24-10. Closed reduction is usually possible early but may be difficult later following injury. Dorsal finger CMC fracture dislocations cannot usually be held effectively with external means alone (283,304,305). Although usually acceptable as the least invasive method of treatment for most injuries, entirely nonoperative management of pure thumb CMC dislocations does not provide sufficient stability for accurate healing of the ligaments. In a series of 12 patients treated with closed reduction (three had additional percutaneous pins) only seven could be documented to have a fully satisfactory outcome (290).

It is not possible through external means to completely maintain control over the reduction of a widely displaced intra-articular fracture dislocation at the base of the thumb throughout the entire period of healing. However, the necessity of achieving anatomic union in these fractures has been questioned in the literature. In a series of 25 fractures followed at 9.6 years, 5 had malrotation, 16 had a separation of over 1 mm at the articular surface, and 23 had varus angulation (306). None of these findings could be definitively correlated to the 15 mildly symptomatic patients, limited movement in 21 patients, or radiographic signs of arthritis in three patients. A series of 17 patients followed for 26 years all had decreased range of motion and pinch strength and some degree of arthritis radiographically, but only seven complained of symptoms (307). Although no one study is definitive, the risk of significant malunion when managing an initially widely displaced intra-articular fracture is too great to warrant entirely nonoperative management.

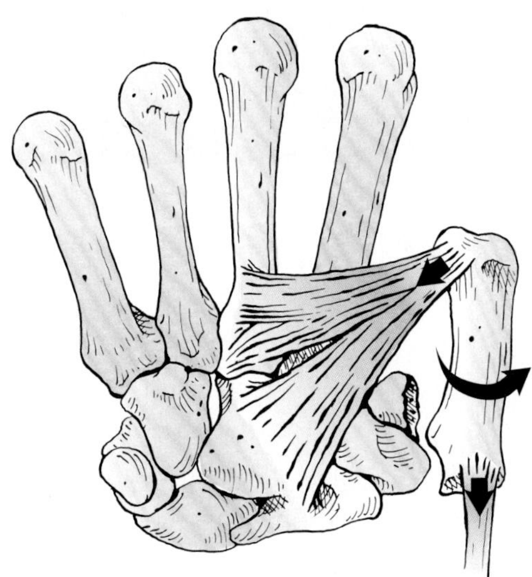

FIGURE 24-109 Displacement of Bennett's fractures is driven primarily by the abductor pollicis longus and the adductor pollicis resulting in flexion, supination, and proximal migration.

TABLE 24-10 Carpometacarpal Joint Dislocations and Fracture Dislocations

Treatment Options	Pros	Cons
Splinting	Avoidance of surgical complications	Only capable of maintaining reduction of inherently stable, minimally displaced fractures
CRIF	Avoids open surgical tissue trauma Able to maintain reduction of those injuries that can be accurately reduced closed	Many CMC fracture dislocation patterns cannot be accurately reduced closed Poor results for pure thumb CMC dislocations
ORIF	Allows direct control and visualization of reduction Direct ligament repair for pure thumb CMC dislocations	Added surgical tissue trauma

CRIF, closed reduction and internal fixation; CMC, carpometacarpal; ORIF, open reduction and internal fixation.

Finger CMC Dislocations and Fracture Dislocations—Operative Management

For those injuries that can be accurately reduced, CRIF is the treatment of choice (265,278,283,304). The technique involves restoration of anatomic length to the shortened and dislocated metacarpals through the combined application of traction and direct pressure at the metacarpal bases. Manual reduction is then followed by placement of 0.045-inch K-wires across the metacarpal shaft and into either the carpal bones or into adjacent stable metacarpals (Fig. 24-110). Adequacy of reduction as well as stability should be evaluated both radiographically and clinically. Actual radiographs in addition to fluoroscopic images should be obtained while in the operating room for confirmation. Pins should remain for 6 weeks. Residual instability rather than stiffness from prolonged immobilization is the risk with this injury. Nine of 10 patients treated with CRIF ultimately achieved full motion (304). Initially open fractures and those with tissue interposition preventing reduction will require ORIF. Open reduction is much more likely to be required in cases presenting late and may be accomplished as long as 3 months after the initial injury (Fig. 24-111). The stabilization strategy is the same as for CRIF with the open part of the procedure being used strictly for reduction purposes (283,308–310). Excellent long-term stability without pain is achieved in the majority of cases. In more severe cases, immediate arthrodesis of the CMC joints may be required (311).

Thumb CMC Pure Dislocations—Operative Management Surprisingly even the results of CRIF have not been sufficient to consistently prevent long-term symptoms of instability and arthritis in pure thumb CMC dislocations. In a series of eight dislocations pinned for 6 weeks and immobilized for a total of 7.4 weeks, four required ligament reconstruction (three for symptomatic instability and one for progression of early post-traumatic arthritis) (312). Based on these poor results, the same authors subsequently treated the next nine patients with early ligament reconstruction, resulting in no late symptoms, full motion, and normal grip strength (312).

Open repair and pinning led to instability in two out of four patients who then needed later tendon reconstruction (313). Thus, other authors have also chosen to treat complete dislocation of the thumb CMC joint not with open ligament repair but rather tendon graft reconstruction (Fig. 24-112) (314,315). The method of Eaton using the split flexor carpi radialis (FCR) tendon has produced 95% excellent and good results with 90% normal pinch strength and no evidence of arthritis at 7-year follow-up in 50 patients who presented with symptomatic instability (316). This group of patients may or may not be directly representative of those patients who have the definite diagnosis of acute complete thumb CMC joint dislocation. However, it is known that the good and excellent results decrease to 74% if the procedure is done as a reconstruction for late symptomatic

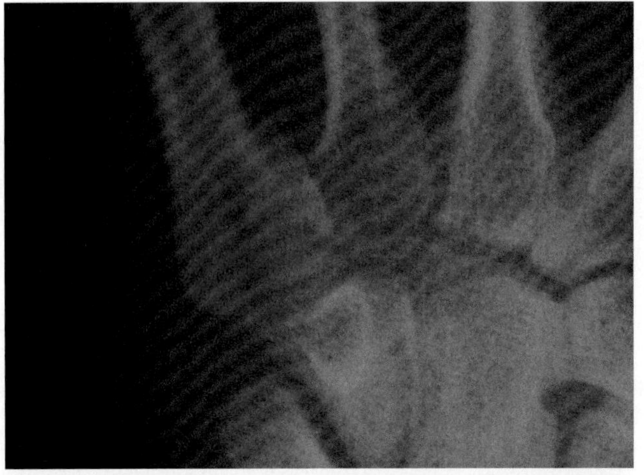
A

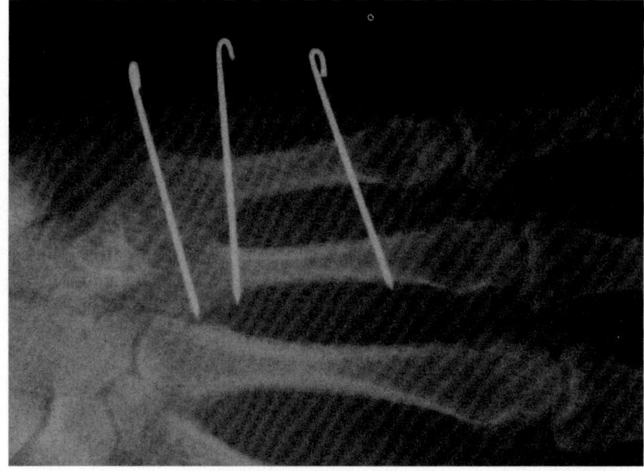
B

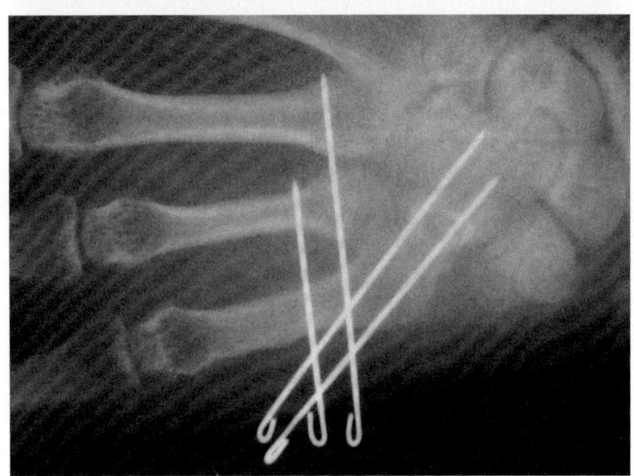
C

FIGURE 24-110 Small finger CMC fracture dislocations **(A)** can be brought back out to length and stabilized by **(B)** transverse pinning to the ring finger metacarpal with subchondral pins maintaining the articular reduction and further stabilized with **(C)** additional pinning across the CMC joint into the distal carpal row.

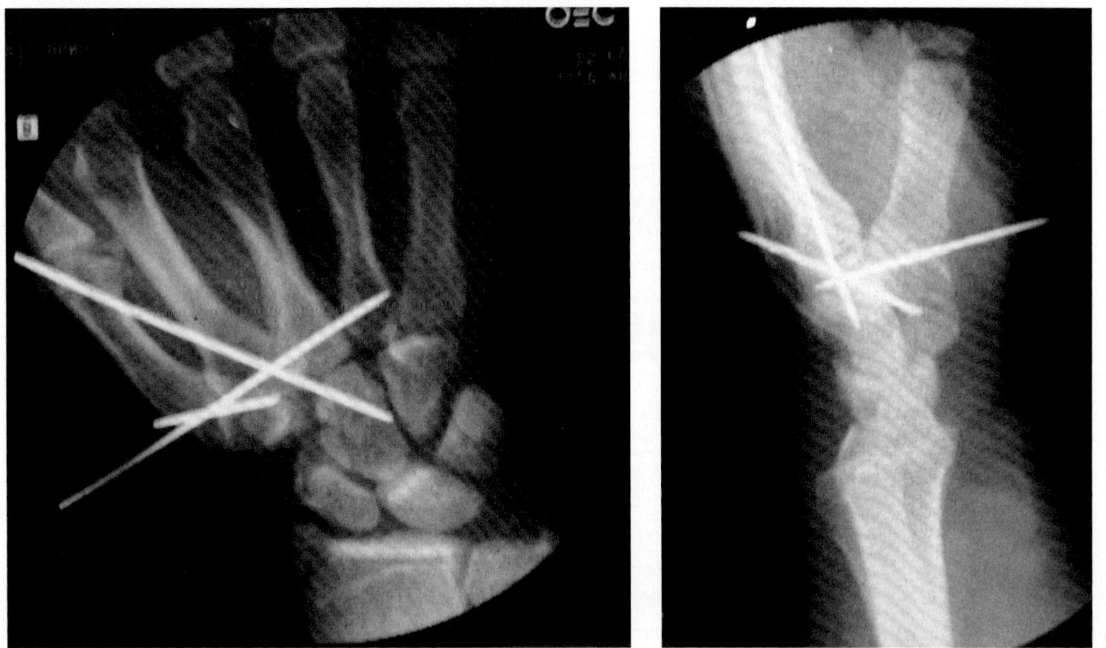

FIGURE 24-111 Open reduction of finger CMC dislocations includes **(A)** stabilization between metacarpal bases to preserve adjacent relationships as well as **(B)** fixation across the CMC joints to the distal row to prevent dorsal subluxation from recurring.

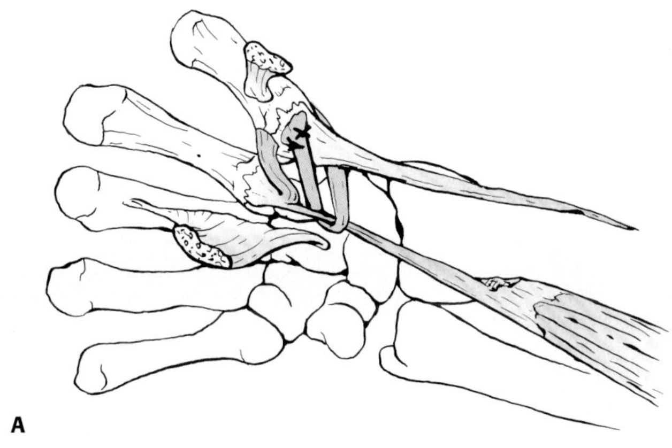

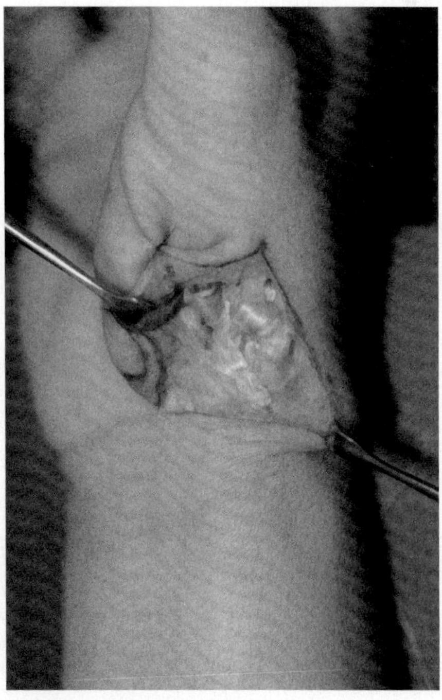

FIGURE 24-112 Reconstruction of the thumb CMC ligaments can be performed with **(A)** a split flexor carpi radialis graft woven through a bone tunnel in the thumb metacarpal base, exiting the dorsal cortex, passing deep to the abductor pollicis longus, around the intact remaining FCR, and back to the volar radial aspect of the metacarpal base. **B.** This procedure is accomplished through a traditional Wagner approach.

instability (316). Other authors have been equally satisfied with this procedure (312).

Thumb CMC Fracture Dislocations—Operative Management

Closed reduction and internal K-wire (0.045-inch) stabilization is the treatment of choice for nearly all Bennett's fractures and some Rolando's fractures (Fig. 24-113). A series of 32 patients followed for 7 years with intra-articular step-offs of less than 1 mm found no difference between closed pinning and open reduction and internal fixation for Bennett's fractures with the exception of a higher incidence of adduction contracture in the pinning group (317). Advocates of internal fixation may choose to manage less comminuted Rolando's fractures and some Bennett's fractures with ORIF (292,318–320). The series by Foster and Hastings (319) of 18 patients using screws alone and 32 patients with plates and screws progressing to a 100% union rate with 0% infection and no need for hardware removal demonstrates what is possible in the hands of a master surgeon. When there are reasonably large fragments that will support purchase of at least one solid screw per fragment, one may consider plate and screw stabilization of Rolando's fractures (Fig. 24-114). However, ORIF of a Rolando's fracture is not for the occasional hand surgeon. Comminution is the rule rather than the exception, and restoration of normal anatomy is quite difficult. The combination of limited internal fixation and external fixation to support the length and unload the articular reduction may be helpful in complex Rolando's fractures (321,322). A series of 10 patients managed this way and followed at 35 months showed 88% contralateral key pinch with nine of 10 patients having good or fair overall satisfaction (321). While some series have deemphasized the role of anatomic reduction in improving long-term results, others have stressed its role (323). Eighteen patients followed at 10.7 years showed a clear correlation between the quality of reduction and post-traumatic arthritis (324). A similar series with over 7-year follow-up demonstrated a clear correlation between radiographic post-traumatic arthritis and greater than 1-mm step-off in the final reduction (325). Twenty-one patients achieved 80% of normal grip strength despite radiographic signs of degeneration in 16 of 21 that did not correlate to clinical outcome (326). Thirty-one patients followed at 7.3 years demonstrated a correlation of both radiographic signs of osteoarthritis and (more importantly) symptoms of pain with the final residual displacement when healing occurred with more than a 2 mm articular step-off (327).

Rehabilitation

Immobilization should last from 6 to 8 weeks in an orthoplast splint. The primary problem with finger CMC joint injuries is residual instability not joint stiffness. The MP joints should be left free throughout the aftercare period with attention paid to excursion of the common digital extensor tendons. For thumb CMC joint injuries, immobilization is continued for 6 weeks in a thumb spica splint. The IP joint should be left free throughout the post-operative period. Following cast removal the patient undergoes a standard progression of ROM exercises that graduates as tolerated into functional use by 8 to 10 weeks. Forceful pinch loading is avoided for 3 months after surgery.

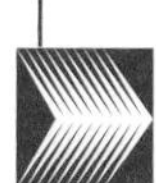

AUTHOR'S PREFERRED TREATMENT

Finger CMC Joint Pure Dislocations

Pure dislocations rarely occur without fracture of either the metacarpal bases or carpal bones of the distal row. However, the absence of such fractures creates an opportunity for successful management by closed reduction and internal fixa-

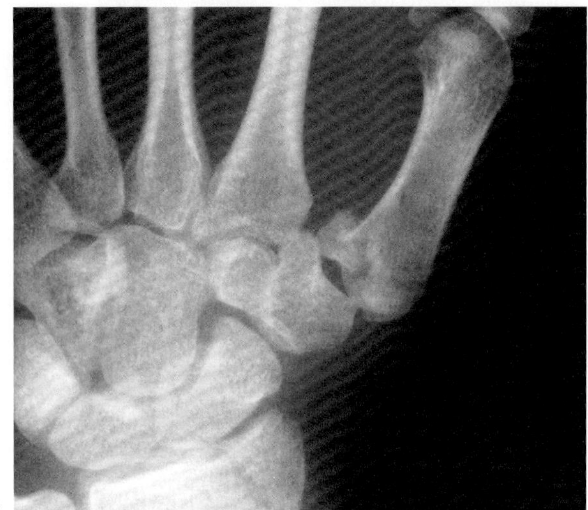

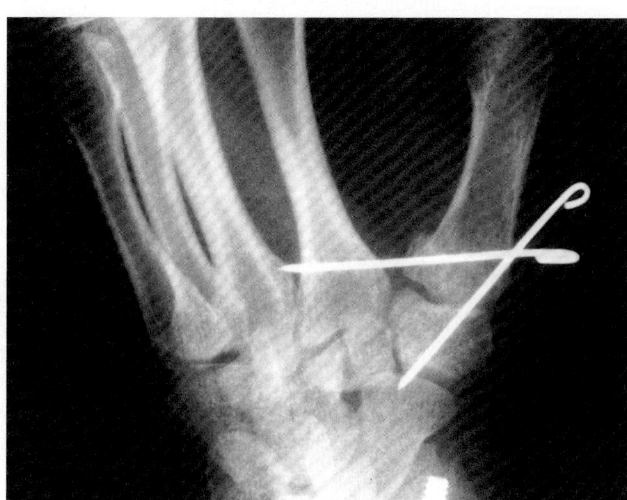

FIGURE 24-113 Bennett's fractures **(A)** can be stabilized with closed pinning to the index metacarpal base and across the CMC joint into the trapezium **(B)**.

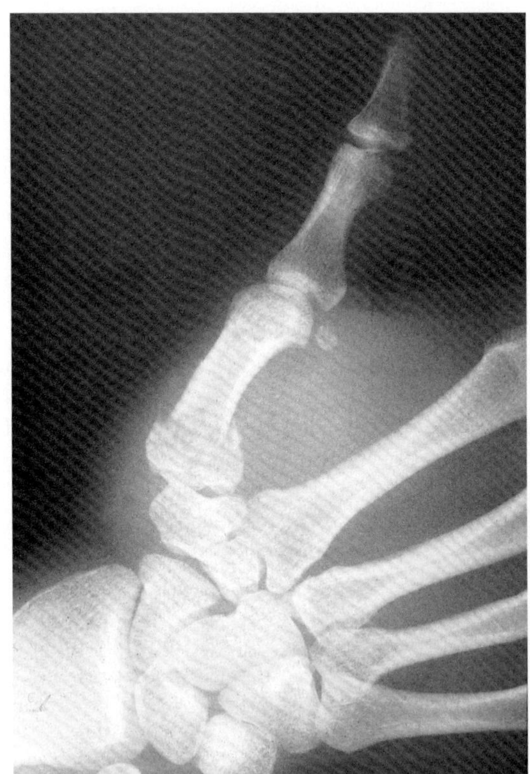

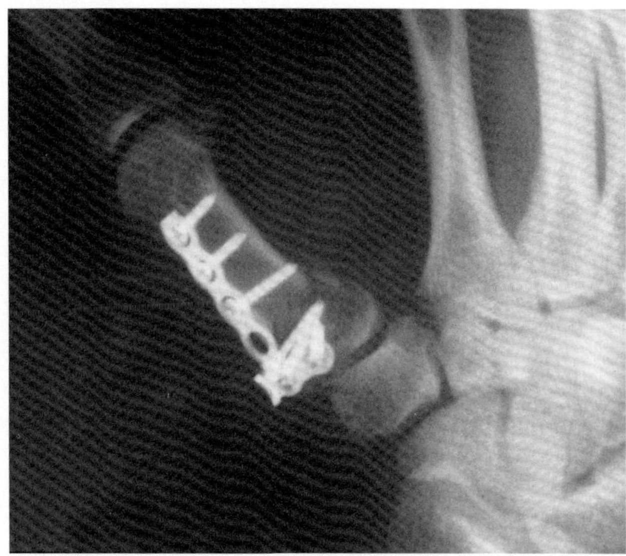

FIGURE 24-114 **A.** Rolando's fractures can be stabilized with a small (2 mm) condylar buttress plate. **B.** Drilling eccentrically to the lateral margins of the screw holes in the condylar fragments will add transverse compression between the articular fragments.

tion. The metacarpal bases must both be felt to engage their articulations fully and demonstrate complete congruence on radiographs. This is one injury pattern where the added time invested in obtaining true radiographs rather than fluoroscopy alone is worthwhile to assure this congruence. Only when the x-ray beam passes tangentially through the joint can an accurate assessment be made. It is practical to use the fluoroscope to determine the angle of projection that best demonstrates the reduction and then try to reproduce the shot with the plain radiograph. K-wires are retained for 6 weeks outside the skin with an additional 2 weeks of splint protection before initiating rehabilitation to the CMC joints and the wrist. All other joints remain mobile throughout the post-operative period.

Finger CMC Joint Fracture Dislocations

If accurate closed reduction can be achieved, CRIF is an excellent choice. Cases seen many days after injury or those with tissue interposition will likely require ORIF to achieve accurate reduction. The approach may be dictated by the presence of an open traumatic wound. Otherwise a transverse incision at the level of the joint is best. Branches of the superficial radial nerve and dorsal cutaneous branch of the ulnar nerve must be identified and protected not only from the surgical approach to reach the injury site but also during pin placement. The common extensor tendons overlie the central metacarpal bases, and the wrist extensor tendons insert on the border metacarpals. Incision of the extensor retinaculum increases the lateral mobility of these tendons, allowing the surgeon to work around them. Bone and cartilage fragments too small for fixation but large enough to create third body wear in the joint should be removed. Fixation is founded in 0.045-inch K-wire passage from the metacarpal bases across the CMC joints into the distal carpal row. If adjacent metacarpals are stable without CMC joint injury, transverse stabilization between metacarpal bases is an excellent addition. Evaluation of the dorsal cortices of the hamate and capitate should be performed on each case as these are often also fractured. Large bone fragments should be restored to their cancellous beds and fixed with countersunk compression screws. Small bone fragments should be excised. Index or long finger CMC joints with extensive articular cartilage damage are good candidates for primary arthrodesis. Motion in the ring and small finger CMC joints should be preserved if possible but arthrodesis remains an acceptable method of management as a last resort.

Thumb CMC Joint Pure Dislocations

The literature simply does not support CRIF as a valid treatment for this injury despite basic principles that should allow this method to produce satisfactory results. Although some articles suggest that one needs to perform immediate free tendon graft reconstruction of complete thumb CMC dislocations, this has not been my experience. I have found stable and pain-free motion in a growing series of thumb CMC dislocations managed by open ligament repair (Fig. 24-115). The consistent surgical findings are a sleeve-like avulsion of the deep anterior oblique ligament from the volar surface of the metacarpal and a rupture of the dorsoradial and posterior oblique ligaments. The rupture has usually been distally from the metacarpal insertion. The procedure is easily accomplished by inserting a series of 1.3-mm bone anchors around the margin of the metacarpal base and using the sutures for anatomic repair of the dorsal ligaments. The joint should be pinned in a reduced position prior to tying down the dorsal ligaments. The deep anterior oblique ligament comes to lie flush with the metacarpal surface when the joint is reduced and stabilized. Pins are retained for 6 weeks with thumb CMC joint motion being instituted at that time. Light pinch is also allowed with progression to power pinch by 3 months post-operatively.

Thumb CMC Joint Fracture Dislocations

The majority of these can be treated with CRIF, most of the remainder augmented with small openings to control small articular fragments or pack bone graft into the metaphysis, and the final minority with full ORIF. The soft tissue anatomy of this region should be taken into account when placing pins. The drill should not be activated until the pin is solidly placed down to bone. Bennett's fractures can be stabilized with either one or two pins. The primary pin reduces and stabilizes the shaft of the metacarpal to the trapezium. An alternative to trapezium pinning is to pin the thumb to the index metacarpal or to both (328,329). A second pin may be placed across the two fragments to prevent the development of an articular step-off, but this pin will not hold the fracture surfaces opposed. Many surgeons do not even use this second pin.

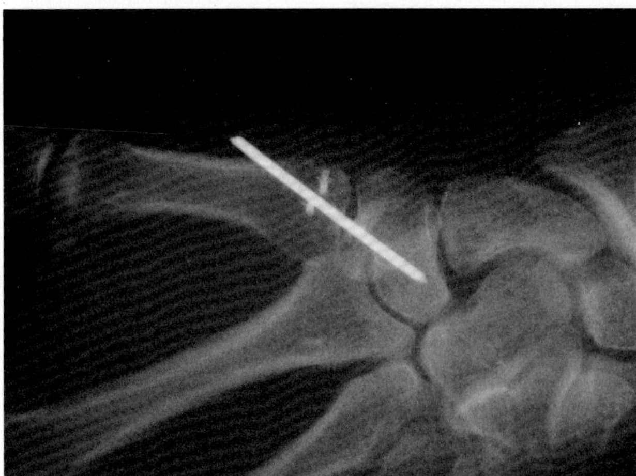

FIGURE 24-115 Pure thumb CMC dislocations can be repaired by direct ligament reinsertion of the dorsoradial and posterior oblique ligaments to the metacarpal base with bone anchors and temporary pinning.

The goals of treatment in a Rolando's fracture are different. The primary aim is to provide distraction to allow healing through the often-comminuted metaphyseal zone. This is best accomplished by pinning (two 0.062-inch K-wires) to the index metacarpal rather than to the trapezium. It is in the complete articular cases with comminution that making a small opening to place an elevator into the metaphysis may prove useful. The articular fragments can be molded against the distal surface of the trapezium and kept there by either packing bone graft in behind them or with additional smaller caliber (0.035 inch) pins placed transversely at the subchondral level to maintain articular congruity. The advantage of plate and screw stabilization of an intra-articular fracture in general is usually to allow early motion of the joint for the sake of cartilage nutrition and preservation of long-term range of motion. The small fragments at the base of the thumb metacarpal are more at risk of devascularization with a widely open procedure that includes periosteal stripping to place a small titanium plate. I have not experienced that long-term loss of motion is a problem at the trapeziometacarpal joint following 6 weeks of pin immobilization for these fractures. I have observed that the presence of the plate results in tendon adherence for the EPB and EPL and can cause long-term loss of motion of both the MP and IP joint, which is a clinically relevant problem.

If ORIF is chosen for a select case, a Wagner incision along the glabrous/nonglabrous border of the thumb base may be curved in a volar and transverse direction to expose the thenar muscle group. Reflection of these muscles reveals the joint capsule volar to the insertion of the APL. Arthrotomy reveals the intra-articular fracture, and subperiosteal dissection along the shaft allows for placement of a plate in Rolando's fractures. Stable internal fixation of Rolando's fractures is only possible when the fragments are large enough to accept the purchase of individual screws. The 2 mm condylar plate with two condylar holes is the most appropriate. Eccentric drilling of the condylar holes can add transverse compression between the articular base fragments. If ORIF is chosen for a Bennett's fracture, a smaller version of the same approach is used to allow sufficient access to compress the reduction and place an interfragmentary lag screw from dorsal to volar.

Pearls and Pitfalls

Treatment of both finger and thumb CMC joint injuries provides ample opportunity for the occurrence of two complications frequent in hand surgery: injury to cutaneous nerves and pin tract infections. The injury to cutaneous nerves is likely to occur by a pin rather than during dissection and particularly when approaching the radial side of the thumb base. Pins are retained longer here (6 weeks) than for stabilization of metacarpal (removed by 4 weeks) or phalangeal (removed by 3 weeks) fractures. There is thus more time for a pin tract infection to develop. The pearls and pitfalls for finger CMC joint fracture dislocations are contained in two statements: be sure the joint is fully reduced and do not miss associated carpal bone fractures of significant size.

Comminuted fractures of the thumb CMC joint are indeed difficult injuries to treat but are made much simpler by approaching their management as follows. Conceive of where the shaft of the thumb metacarpal lies when correctly positioned in a functional position relative to the rest of the hand and pin it there with two 0.062-inch K-wires. Then make the articular surface of the metacarpal base congruent with supportive bone graft and/or small subchondral wires through a limited opening. What originally appeared as an impossible undertaking now becomes a relatively simple two-step process.

COMPLICATIONS

Published complication rates associated with rigid internal fixation are high and often attributable to the complex nature of the injuries for which this treatment method is selected (3,172,330). In a series of 41 metacarpal and 27 phalangeal fractures, complications of related to hardware (45%), extensor lag (19%), and infection (12%) were seen (330). Increased complications were associated with intra-articular/peri-articular locations with extension to the shaft, open injuries, associated soft tissue injury, and the need for bone graft. Another series had an overall complication rate of 29% with three nonunions and two patients with a TAM of less than 190 degrees (172). Only 27% of 54 patients with phalangeal fractures were asymptomatic at 5 months post-injury, but this proportion increased to 66% at long-term follow-up (331). As long as 18 months may be required for soreness and stiffness to abate following an MP joint dislocation. In 490 severe phalangeal fractures there were 31 (6%) nonunions, 44 (9%) malunions, and 8 (2%) infections (332).

In 200 open hand fractures there were nine deep infections, 18 malunions, 17 delayed unions or nonunions, 23 fixation-related complications, and two late amputations (15). These complications were usually associated with Swanson type II wounds (14% compared to 1.4% in type I wounds) but not with the use of internal fixation, high-energy injury, large wound size, or associated soft tissue injury.

Infection

Despite the excellent vascularity of the hand, infection still occurs, being reported twice each in series of 52 and 65 open fractures (39,333). An 11% infection rate occurred in 146 open hand fractures, all in Gustilo type II or III injuries, and in association with a crushing component to the injury (13). Preoperative wound cultures were of no help, and *Staphylococcus aureus* was the most commonly isolated species. The role of antibiotics in reducing the infection rate in noncontaminated open wounds with intact vessels has not been supported by prospective studies (334,335). The exception to this may be open distal phalangeal fractures where a 30% infection rate without antibiotics was reduced to less than 3% with a two-dose regimen of a first-generation cephalosporin (336). Conversely, 198 patients were randomized in a double blind placebo controlled study with flucloxacillin for open distal phalangeal fractures with seven superficial and no deep infections developing (three with antibiotic, four without) (337).

Stiffness

Perhaps the most feared complication and certainly one of the most common following a fracture or dislocation of the hand is stiffness. Stiffness is a product of the magnitude of the original trauma, the age and genetic composition of the patient, the duration of immobilization, the position of immobilization, and the invasiveness of any surgical intervention. The primary factors influencing stiffness are associated soft tissue injury and the age of the patient (28,38,173,338). Too often the position of immobilization violates the fundamental principles of splinting ligaments at full length and balancing tendon forces that act across the fracture site. First web space contractures are common and can be minimized by pinning or splinting the thumb metacarpal in maximum abduction. Active versus passive motion discrepancies most commonly appear in the form of an extensor lag. The overlying extensor tendon becomes adherent to the fracture site and its subsequent failure of excursion produces an extensor lag at the next most distal joint. This is most common at the PIP joint following fractures of P1 with adherence of the flat and broad extensor tendon in zone IV. Stiffness remains the number one complication of proximal phalangeal fractures (with rates exceeding 50%), and the most frequent feature is the PIP joint extensor lag (172,339). Fixed flexion contractures of 10 to 30 degrees can develop when treating condylar fractures at the PIP joint (169). Only 11% of phalangeal fractures fixed with plates had a TAM of more than 220 degrees (339). One of the chief concerns with operative management of thumb MP ligament disruptions has been the loss of motion that, in most series, occurs to a mild degree (235,340). However, one series of 19 patients had no loss of motion following acute ligament repair with 4 to 6 weeks of postoperative cast immobilization. Loss of motion may be more significant in patients undergoing late reconstructions as occurred in 21 patients from a series of 70 after free tendon graft (235).

Hypersensitivity

The size and structure of the hand provides for very little padding between the surface and a complex array of small caliber nerve branches. There are very few locations for either surgical incisions or percutaneous pins where small nerve branches are more than a centimeter away. Hypersensitivity is a frequently seen consequence of the mechanism of injury itself. Crush injuries are almost invariably accompanied by some degree of hypersensitivity. When surgical management is performed soon after the injury, the procedure itself is often erroneously blamed for causing the hypersensitivity. Some areas are at higher risk than others. Neuroma formation through direct injury or nerve encasement in postoperative scar should be guarded against when one is operating along the ulnar side of the thumb MP joint with its high concentration of small dorsal digital nerve branches (341,232). Treatment is based on a combination of specific medications to reduce nerve pain such as gabapentin (Neurontin) and amitryptyline (Elavil) and a progressive contact desensitization therapy program. Gentle surface contact essentially trains the sensitive nerve fibers to tolerate that level of stimulation before then progressing to more intense stimulation. Eventually, the patient works his or her way up to normal use of the hand over a period of weeks. In the meantime, over stimulation of the nerve pain by traction and motion must be avoided even if this means slower progress in the motion program. Failure to heed this principle will result in progression from straightforward hypersensitivity to complex regional pain syndromes and a downward spiral of worsening pain and function that far exceeds the simple early reduction in motion.

Malunion and Deformity

Malunion is a frequently encountered complication in hand fractures owing to a lack of understanding regarding hand biomechanics, to an unfounded belief that all hand fractures do well with nonoperative treatment, or to a noncompliant patient. Sagittal plane malunion with apex volar at the P1 level usually occurs due to failure to splint the hand in the position of full MP flexion that will correct the dynamic imbalance across the fracture site (Fig. 24-116). Rotational malunion is usually the result of improper choice of nonoperative treatment when direct fixation was needed to control rotation. Spiral fractures are difficult to correctly reduce closed, and rotational malunions can easily result from CRIF especially at the level of the proximal phalanx. Nail plate alignment is an inadequate method of assessing rotation, which should be judged by parallelism of the short tubular bone segment distal to the injured one with the intervening joint flexed to 90 degrees. Corrective osteotomy is more successful at the metacarpal level than the phalangeal level (Fig. 24-117) (342). Correction of a sagittal plane or multidirectional malunion is best accomplished at the site of the original fracture (343–346). Significant stiffness often accompanies the malunion. Concomitant tenocapsulolysis can be performed if rigid fixation of the osteotomy is achieved. The alternative is to break the solution down into two parts: stage one achieves correction of the skeletal deformity through osteotomy and stage two improves motion through tenocapsulolysis. These patients achieve the greatest gains in motion even though the measured final range may be less than that of other patients with less severe injuries (159,347). Tenolysis alone improves extensor lag, but when dorsal capsulotomy is required to regain flexion, lag may actually increase (348). For mild to moderate malunions, a thorough evaluation of its effect on function must be made and weighed carefully against the predicted degree of digital stiffness created by the osteotomy procedure itself and the hardware used. The choice to perform an osteotomy may be influenced by remembering that 12 degrees of extensor lag is generated for each millimeter of shortening and that sagittal plane malunion itself induces lag in a nonlinear relationship (349). Intra-articular osteotomy is an extremely demanding undertaking and should be restricted to carefully selected patients. Surgery may be performed as late as several months after the initial injury through the original fracture plane, and restoration of as much as 95 to 100 degrees of PIP motion has been reported (350,351).

Malunions of a metacarpal fracture usually present as an apex dorsal sagittal plane deformity. Patients may complain of the cosmetic deformity, pain at the dorsal prominence, or grip discomfort with a prominent metacarpal head in the palm (352). Patients should be counseled to evaluate their deformity and decide if their dissatisfaction is sufficient to warrant undergoing corrective osteotomy. The osteotomy should be delayed until tissue homeostasis has been achieved unless an opportunity for early intervention (<4 weeks) exists. Correction is best achieved through the site of the original fracture with rigid internal fixa-

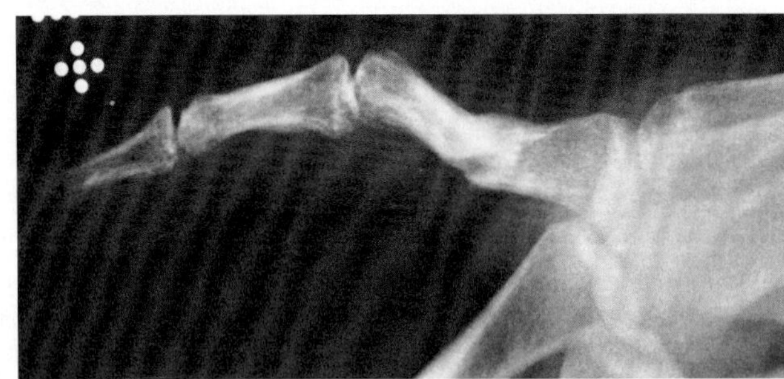
A

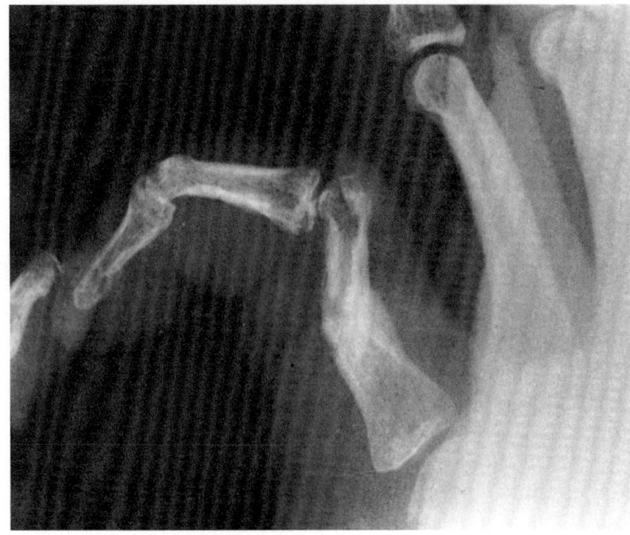
B

FIGURE 24-116 Malunion of P1 fractures is typically apex volar with a compensatory loss of extension at the PIP joint correctable only with osteotomy.

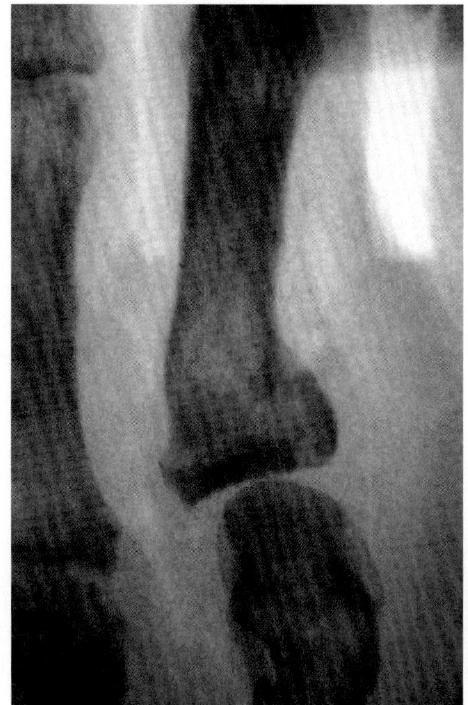

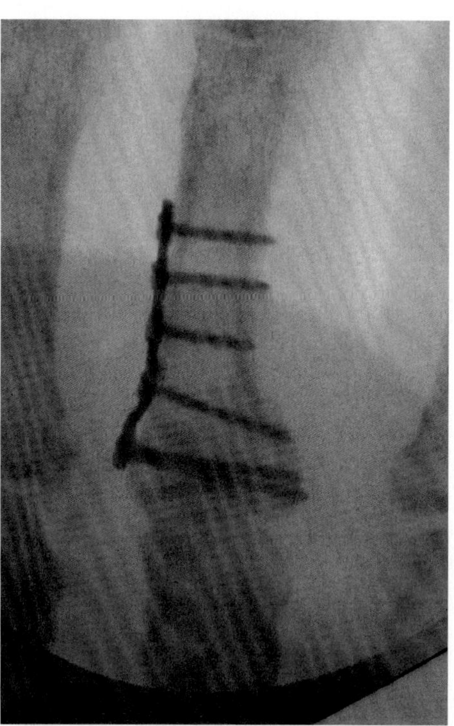

FIGURE 24-117 Corrective osteotomies are best performed at the site of the original deformity to optimize the anatomic relationships and biomechanics between bone, joint, and tendon structures.

tion and immediate motion. One such series of 30 patients led to a 30-degree improvement in ROM (360). In choosing between opening wedge, closing wedge, pivot osteotomy, or oblique osteotomy, the exact pattern of deformity needs to be assessed and the osteotomy designed to most closely restore normal anatomy (352). This will demand a different cut for each patient, but the simpler the intended osteotomy, the more likely the surgeon can effect a good result. Shortening must be considered if a closing wedge is planned. An extensor lag at the MP joint of 7 degrees can be predicted for every 2 mm of shortening (245). Rotational malunion in a metacarpal may also occur, causing digital overlap. Osteotomy can be performed at the site of original injury or at the metacarpal base. Rotational osteotomy performed at the base of the metacarpal offers broader cancellous surfaces for healing and can correct up to 25 to 30 degrees of rotation (353). If the plane of deformity is more complex than pure rotation, it may be wiser to attempt multiplanar correction through the original fracture site.

Intra-articular osteotomy at the metacarpal head has infrequent indications, as correction of an intra-articular malunion is extremely difficult. Nevertheless, when performed diligently in a well-selected patient by a skilled surgeon, restoration of as much as 0- to 90-degree ROM is possible (350). In long-term follow-up, intra-articular malunion at the metacarpal base leads to osteoarthritis (65%), decreased grip (49%), and pain (38%) (354). Arthrodesis is the preferred solution for these problems even for the fifth metacarpal. It reliably improves grip strength with the elimination of pain. Compensatory triquetrohamate motion may alleviate the effect of arthrodesis on the mobility of the ulnar side of the hand.

Nonunion

Nonunion is a rare complication in hand fractures with the exception of distal phalanx fractures, when CRIF has caused distraction, or fractures treated with open reduction and internal fixation where excessive periosteal stripping has occurred (355). Tuft fractures of the distal phalanx rarely achieve osseous union, going on instead to a fibrous union that eventually usually becomes relatively pain free. Transverse shaft fractures of the distal phalanx left without support too early may result in an apex volar malunion or nonunion after being repeatedly subjected to pinch forces. Symptomatic nonunion of a transverse shaft fracture can be treated through a palmar midline approach with cortical peg bone grafting (356). Compression screws also are effective but the diameter relative to that of the sagittal plane dimension of the P3 shaft risks both fracture extension and damage to the overlying nail apparatus (357). Four nonunions were seen in a series of 52 unstable hand fractures of which 61.5% were open and at a rate of 2.5% in another series of open fractures (28,39). A treatment for phalangeal nonunion consisting of Herbert screw placement through the distal joint has been proposed in four patients (91). If no bone loss is present, simple compression across a hypertrophic nonunion site with a short plate should be sufficient to achieve healing. If bone loss is present, a longer plate and corticocancellous or cancellous bone graft may be required. Avascular necrosis of the metacarpal head remains a concern in peri-articular fractures, as an independent blood supply may be absent in 35% of cases (358).

Residual Instability

Residual instability following dislocation is rare distally, but more common proximally. All five carpometacarpal joints are quite subject to recurrent instability particularly with pure dislocation patterns rather than fracture dislocations. The reason is that in pure dislocation, all the ligaments are ruptured and require ligament to bone or ligament to ligament healing. Fracture dislocations usually occur with one or more key stabilizing ligaments attached to the smaller fragment that remains at the joint while the larger articular fragment dislocates. If properly reduced and stabilized, bone to bone healing will restore joint stability. Re-dislocation occurred in 6 of 56 dorsal fracture dislocations of the PIP joint (90). Chronic instability following closed treatment of a complete MP joint radial collateral ligament injury may need to be treated surgically (215,218). A small population of patients exists with chronic hyperextension laxity at the thumb MP joint that may be either passive (volar plate only) or active (involving the intrinsics) and may in a few instances require surgical advancement for reconstruction and restoration of stability (194,197,359,360). Late symptomatic (painful) instability after CMC fracture dislocation can be evaluated with lidocaine injection into the joint. If relief is provided, arthrodesis is a reliable way to eliminate the pain (361). The fifth CMC joint may be fused in 20 to 30 degrees of flexion with little long-term loss of hand motion, apparently through increased compensatory triquetrohamate motion.

Post-traumatic Arthritis

As in other locations throughout the body, intra-articular fractures and residual joint instability may cause accelerated hyaline cartilage wear and lead to post-traumatic arthritis. A poor correlation exists between the radiographic appearance of post-traumatic arthritis and clinical loss of function and pain. Patients should be managed for the arthritis on the basis of clinical deficits and not based on radiographic abnormality. Post-traumatic arthritis of the thumb MP joint can be successfully managed by arthrodesis with excellent overall hand function (172). Few other joints in the hand can be fused as successfully other than the index and long finger CMC joints. Finger MP and PIP joint fusions result in tremendous loss of function (362).

Hardware Complications

Kirschner wires are appropriate tools for performing internal fixation of hand fractures and occasionally for stabilizing dislocations. Consequently, pin tract infections are apt to occur. Infections are rare when pins are left in for less than 4 weeks and usually respond well to removal of the pin with administration of oral antibiotics. Another hardware complication is simply irritation of adjacent tissues such as overlying tendons by the presence of prominent hardware. Given the delicate and thin tissues in the hand, even implants measuring only several millimeters thick are enough to produce persistent symptoms for many patients. In one series 7 of 57 patients required plate removal (363). In a series of 51 ORIF cases for dorsal base fractures of the distal phalanx, there were 24 complications including dorsal skin breakdown, superficial and deep infection, re-displacement, fragment resorption, nail growth abnormalities, and 20 re-operations for hardware removal (62). It is for these reasons that open procedures in this region are discouraged.

Tendon Rupture

Tendon ruptures can occur in association with dislocations of the joint adjacent to the site of tendon insertion. Failure to recognize this associated injury may occur with an inadequate examination. The consequence is usually a deformity posture such as mallet finger at the DIP joint or a boutonnière deformity at the PIP joint. Open reconstructions of chronic terminal tendon ruptures with either local tissues or free tendon grafts have not proven particularly successful. For disabling terminal tendon deficiencies in a high angle of flexion, arthrodesis of the DIP joint is a permanent and durable solution to the problem. The loss of motion associated with arthrodesis is not as well tolerated at the PIP joint where every effort should be made to restore active extension. Mild deformities especially when identified reasonably early may respond to a program of PIP extension splinting and DIP joint flexion exercises. Success is dependent on the natural tendency of collagen-based scar to contract. For more substantial deficiencies surgical reconstruction with local tissues or free tendon graft may be required once passive motion has first been regained through either rehabilitation or a previously staged surgical capsulectomy.

Nail Matrix

Nail deformities can occur when a crush mechanism of injury includes the zone of the nail or when fixation hardware damages the delicate matrix tissues. Temporary or permanent passage of fixation devices through the region of the germinal matrix should be avoided, and sterile matrix penetration should be either temporary or by suture material. A rare but troublesome complication is entrapment of the germinal matrix in a transverse fracture gap (which can occur with a reasonably normal external appearance of the digit) that both prevents fracture healing and results in permanent nail deformity.

CONTROVERSIES AND FUTURE DIRECTIONS

Decision Making

There is not a great deal of controversy surrounding the technical methods of reduction and fixation for fractures and dislocations of the hand. Controversy is much greater when it comes to deciding how specific fractures and dislocations should be managed. Most surgeons understand and accept the basic principle that the least invasive method should be employed that will result in stable, anatomically correct healing and still permit enough motion rehabilitation to achieve a useful and functional final result. The problem lies in the fact that the data simply doesn't exist anywhere in the published literature to definitively link specific treatment strategies to the many different fracture patterns that exist. Each of the various small bones in the hand (P3, P2, P1, metacarpal) responds to treatment differently. There are numerous varieties of just the fracture pattern alone in each of these bones, not to mention the associated soft tissue injuries that impact final outcome substantially. No study has used rigorous enough statistics to separate all the groups and stratify the results. The same holds true for dislocations.

The area where decision-making becomes particularly difficult is that of coordinating more complex reconstructions that involve multiple tissues. When the original management of skeletal trauma to the hand yields unsatisfactory results, secondary surgery may be required. The timing and order of events is very much a matter of individual surgeon experience and preference. The foundation for good hand function is a stable inner skeletal structure and a well-vascularized and supple outer envelope of integument. These are the first steps to be accomplished in any reconstruction. The next step is to ensure passively supple joints that are also stable. This infrastructure is then powered by three groups of tendons responsible for active motion in the hand: the extrinsic extensors, the extrinsic flexors, and the intrinsics. Good motion facilitates interaction with the environment, a function that also requires sensibility. Reconstructive surgery of nerves is well timed to coincide with tendon procedures. Three stages have been outlined here, but this does not necessarily mean that three distinct surgical procedures are required. Judging which combinations of procedures will yield the best results is the province of an experienced revision hand surgeon. In general, procedures that require the same type of rehabilitation may be combined whereas those that have disparate therapy goals should be separated as distinct surgical events. When a series of surgical procedures is staged, tissue homeostasis after the former procedure should be achieved prior to executing the subsequent procedure.

Malunions and Nonunions

Malunions are managed with corrective osteotomy. Each aspect of the deformity must be well understood from angular to rotational to length considerations. The decision is whether to place the osteotomy at the site of original deformity or to make a compensatory osteotomy that produces reciprocal deformities. Fundamentally, it is best to make the correction at the site of the original deformity. The problem is hardware interference with soft tissues. The plate and screws usually necessary to stabilize the correction may not fit well at the site of original deformity. Another consideration is the healing potential of metaphyseal as compared to diaphyseal regions particularly if the diaphyseal bone has been stripped of its blood supply during prior procedures. A popular location for rotational corrections in particular is the metacarpal base for the above reasons. Nonunions are treated no differently than anywhere else in the body. Hypertrophic nonunions may be addressed by compression alone using a dynamic compression plate. Nonunions with bone loss or inadequate vascular supply require supplementary bone grafting in addition to stable fixation.

Post-traumatic Arthritis

The only alternative to arthrodesis apart from microvascular whole joint transfer was previously implantation of a Swanson-type one piece silicone prosthesis with the attendant high rates of prosthetic fracture and generation of silicone debris leading to osteolysis. Since the last edition of this text, new prosthetic implants have become available for total joint replacement of the MP and PIP joints. There are models with metal on polyethylene bearing surfaces as well as polycarbonate on polycarbonate bearings. Long-term data in high numbers for post-traumatic arthritis are not yet available. Rates of loosening, osteolysis from debris, and prosthetic breakage will determine if these models offer a new opportunity for improved hand motion and function to those with post-traumatic arthritis in the MP and PIP joints.

Managing Skeletal Loss

Skeletal loss can occur at either peri-articular locations or in the diaphysis. Diaphyseal loss is by far the more straightforward issue. Current controversies relate to the choice of purely cancellous graft with bridge plating as opposed to corticocancellous grafts. Additional controversy exists regarding the timing of bone grafting for open fractures. The traditions have been corticocancellous grafts with delay. New trends are for immediate grafting after extensive debridement and using purely cancellous graft (364). Osteoarticular defects can be replaced with nonvascularized osteoarticular autografts as long as the defect only involves at most one half of a joint (365). Partial toe joint osteochondral grafts to the PIP joint resulted in significant motion loss in 3 of 5 cases and resorption in one (366). Nonvascularized whole joint transfers are unsuccessful. If an entire joint requires autogenous replacement, a vascularized whole joint transfer from the foot is required. The most common sites requiring partial osteoarticular grafts are single condyles at the head of P1 and the volar base of P2. Toe PIP joints provide well matched condyle donor sites. The dorsal portion of the hamate provides an excellent donor site for the volar base of P2.

Associated Wounds

Achieving stable wound coverage is a prerequisite to any other reconstruction. It is often performed at the same time as skeletal reconstruction and should be performed prior to most other reconstructions except first stage tendon grafting. Methods of wound reconstruction include primary closure, secondary closure, split or full thickness skin grafts, transposition flaps, pedicle flaps, and free flaps. The simplest strategy that provides for optimum gliding of subjacent structures without contracture formation should be chosen. The challenge for more complex wounds that require flap reconstruction in the hand is finding tissue that is both supple and thin. Current trends are for earlier applications within 72 hours of increasingly thinner flaps. A useful strategy involves fascial flaps that are covered with split thickness skin grafts. The lateral arm flap inverted to orient the muscular surface to receive the skin graft has performed particularly well in this respect. The fascia overlying the serratus anterior is thin with a reliable, large, and long pedicle. One criticism of skin grafted fascial flaps is that they are slightly more difficult to operate through at the time of further revision compared to cutaneous flaps. The current trend in microsurgery for perforator flaps has spawned a number of cutaneous flaps thin enough for use around the hand, wrist, and forearm, but not the digits.

Bioabsorbable Implants

Polylactic acid in vitro degradation showed maintenance for 8 weeks comparable to titanium but loss of strength over 12 weeks under four point bending stress (367). Testing in 112 fresh-frozen cadavers of 2-mm poly-L/DL-lactide plates demonstrated an overall stability comparable to 1.7 mm titanium plates (368,369). Studies such as these appear in the literature, but the regular use of bioabsorbable implants in the hand simply has not caught on clinically. One concern may be reports of sterile abscess formation around implants of the same materials used in other orthopaedic applications. The soft tissues of the hand have little tolerance for any process that might cause additional inflammation at the site of skeletal trauma. At the same time, there is no doubt that the physical presence of a plate (even when 1.3 to 2.0 mm in thickness) along the surface of a short tubular bone can create significant problems for tendon adherence and obstructed motion. Time will tell if the promise offered by bioabsorbable implants to alleviate these hardware-related complications can be realized.

CONCLUSION

Fractures and dislocations of the hand represent a diverse group of injuries that share a common theme in management. The hand is a delicate organ that requires both stability and flexibility—function follows form. Although rough guidelines can be drawn from the published literature, it remains the responsibility of individual surgeons to judge which fractures and dislocations can be managed by each of the various methods discussed in this chapter. There are three basic treatment options for most fractures and dislocations of the hand: splinting, closed reduction and internal fixation, and open reduction and internal fixation. Many fractures and the majority of dislocations of the hand have enough inherent stability to be managed nonoperatively. Testing for inherent stability in the office setting using active motion under the protection of injectable anesthetics should demonstrate those fractures and dislocations that can safely be managed without surgery. Malrotated, multiple, high-energy, and open fractures are usually treated operatively. CMC dislocations and fracture dislocations (unlike MP and PIP joint injuries) are usually treated operatively. The majority of operatively treated hand fractures and dislocations are closed and isolated injuries for which closed reduction and internal fixation is usually an appropriate method. The exceptions to this where open reduction internal fixation is required are noted throughout the chapter. A few select injury patterns such as intra-articular P2 base fractures have specific and unique treatments that must be remembered and used according to the indications described. Once underway with treatment, one should stay focused on edema control and promoting early motion. The final steps to a successful outcome lie in avoiding complications such as nerve hypersensitivity and pin tract infections. When complications do occur, the key is in planning a well thought out correction in terms of risk benefit analysis and staging. Finally, patients should be counseled regarding expectations, which are that fractures and dislocations of the hand produce swelling, stiffness, and aching that frequently take more than a year to overcome.

REFERENCES

1. Chung KC, Spilson SV. The frequency and epidemiology of hand and forearm fractures in the United States. *J Hand Surg* 2001;26:908–915.
2. Lamb D. Training in hand surgery. *J Hand Surg* 1990;15B:148–150.
3. Packer GJ, Shaheen MA. Patterns of hand fractures and dislocations in a district general hospital. *J Hand Surg* 1993;18B:511–514.
4. Hove LM. Fractures of the hand. Distribution and relative incidence. *Scand J Plast Reconstr Surg* 1993;27:317–319.
5. Ip WY, Ng KH, Chow SP. A prospective study of 924 digital fractures of the hand. *Injury* 1996;27:279–285.
6. Van Onselen EBH, Karim RB, Hage JJ, et al. Prevalence and distribution of hand fractures. *J Hand Surg* 2003;28B:491–495.
7. Gaul JS. Identifiable costs and tangible benefits resulting from the treatment of acute injuries of the hand. *J Hand Surg* 1987;12A:966–970.
8. Brennwald J. Fracture healing in the hand. A brief update. *Clin Orthop Relat Res* 1996; 327:9–11.
9. DeJonge JJ, Kingma J, Van der Lei B, et al. Phalangeal fractures of the hand. An analysis of gender and age related incidence and aetiology. *J Hand Surg* 1994;19B:168–170.
10. Levin LS, Condit DP. Combined injuries soft tissue management. *Clin Orthop Relat Res* 1996;327:172–181.
11. Freeland AE, Jabaley ME. Stabilization of fractures in the hand and wrist with traumatic soft tissue and bone loss. *Hand Clin* 1988;4:425–436.
12. Campbell DA, Kay SPJ. The Hand Injury Severity Scoring System. *J Hand Surg* 1996; 21B:295–298.
13. McLain RF, Steyers C, Stoddard M. Infections in open fractures of the hand. *J Hand Surg* 1991;16A:108–112.
14. Duncan RW, Freeland AE, Jabaley ME, et al. Open hand fractures: an analysis of the recovery of active motion and of complications. *J Hand Surg* 1993;18A:387–394.
15. Swanson TV, Szabo RM, Anderson DD. Open hand fractures: prognosis and classification. *J Hand Surg* 1991;16A:101–107.
16. Cziffer E. Static fixation of finger fractures. *Hand Clin* 1993;9:639–650.
17. Drenth DJ, Klasen HJ. External fixation for phalangeal and metacarpal fractures. *J Bone Joint Surg* 1998;80B:227–230.
18. Freeland AE. External fixation for skeletal stabilization of severe open fractures of the hand. *Clin Orthop Relat Res* 1987;214:93–100.
19. Parsons SW, Fitzgerald AW, Shearer JR. External fixation of unstable metacarpal and phalangeal fractures. *J Hand Surg* 1992;17B:151–155.
20. Putnam MD, Walsh TM IV. External fixation for open fractures of the upper extremity. *Hand Clin* 1993;9:613–623.
21. Schuind F, Cooney WP, Burny F, et al. Small external fixation devices for the hand and the wrist. *Clin Orthop Relat Res* 1993;293:77–82.
22. Schuind F, Donkerwolke M, Burny F. External minifixation for treatment of closed fractures of the metacarpal bones. *J Orthop Trauma* 1991;5:146–152.
23. Seitz WH Jr, Froimson AI, Brooks DB, et al. External fixator pin insertion techniques: biomechanical analysis and clinical relevance. *J Hand Surg* 1991;16A:560–563.

24. Stuchin SA, Kummer FJ. Stiffness of small bone external fixation methods: an experimental study. *J Hand Surg* 1984;9:718–724.
25. Ashmead D, Rothkopf DM, Walton RI, et al. Treatment of hand injuries by external fixation. *J Hand Surg* 1992;17A:956–964.
26. Lees VC, Wren C, Elliot D. Internal splints for prevention of first web space. *J Hand Surg* 1994;19B:560–562.
27. Chen SH, Wei FC, Chen HC, et al. Miniature plates and screws in acute complex hand injury. *J Trauma* 1994;37:237–242.
28. Chow SP, Pun WK, So YC, et al. A prospective study of 245 open digital fractures of the hand. *J Hand Surg* 1991;16B:137–140.
29. Gonzalez MH, McKay W, Hall RF. Low velocity gunshot wounds of the metacarpal: treatment by early stable fixation and bone grafting. *J Hand Surg* 1993;18A:267–270.
30. Freeland AE, Jabaley ME, Burkhalter WE, et al. Delayed primary bone grafting in the hand and wrist after traumatic bone loss. *J Hand Surg* 1984;9A:22–28.
31. Bury TF, Stassen LPS, Van der Werken C. Repair of the proximal interphalangeal joint with a homograft. *J Hand Surg* 1989;14A:657–658.
32. Hagan HJ, Hastings H II. Use of a step cut osteotomy for immediate posttraumatic proximal interphalangeal joint fusion. *J Hand Surg* 1990;15A:374–376.
33. Ishida O, Ikuta Y, Kuroki H. Ipsilateral osteochondral grafting for finger joint repair. *J Hand Surg* 1994;19A:372–377.
34. Nagle DJ, Ekenstam FW, Lister GD. Immediate silastic arthroplasty for non salvageable intraarticular phalangeal fractures. *Scand J Plast Reconstr Surg* 1989;23:47–50.
35. Rose EH. Reconstruction of central metacarpal ray defects of the hand with a free vascularized double metatarsal and metatarsophalangeal joint transfer. *J Hand Surg* 1984;9A:28–31.
36. Hasegawa T, Yamano Y. Arthroplasty of the proximal interphalangeal joint using costal cartilage grafts. *J Hand Surg* 1992;17B:583–585.
37. Smith NC, Moncrieff NJ, Hartnell N, et al. Pseudorotation of the little finger metacarpal. *J Hand Surg* 2003;28B:395–398.
38. Pun WK, Chow SP, So YC, et al. A prospective study on 284 digital fractures of the hand. *J Hand Surg* 1989;14A:474–481.
39. Pun WK, Chow SP, So YC, et al. Unstable phalangeal fractures. Treatment by AO screw and plate fixation. *J Hand Surg* 1991;16A:113–117.
40. Crosby CA, Wehbe MA. Early motion protocols in hand and wrist rehabilitation. *Hand Clin* 1996;12:31–41.
41. Margles SW. Early motion in the treatment of fractures and dislocations in the hand and wrist. *Hand Clin* 1996;12:65–72.
42. Russell RC, Williamson DA, Sullivan JW, et al. Detection of foreign bodies in the hand. *J Hand Surg* 1991;16A:2–11.
43. Bauer AR Jr, Yutani D. Computed tomographic localization of wooden foreign bodies in children's extremities. *Arch Surg* 1983;118:1084–1086.
44. Gilbert FJ, Campbell RSD, Bayliss AP. The role of ultrasound in the detection of non radiopaque foreign bodies. *Clin Radiol* 1990;41:109–112.
45. Shrewsbury MM, Johnson RK. Form, function and evolution of the distal phalanx. *J Hand Surg* 1983;8:475–479.
46. Al-Qattan MM, Hashem F, Helmi A. Irreducible tuft fractures of the distal phalanx. *J Hand Surg* 2003;28B:18–20.
47. DaCruz DJ, Slade RJ, Malone W. Fractures of the distal phalanges. *J Hand Surg* 1988; 13B:350–352.
48. Lubahn JD, Hood JM. Fractures of the distal interphalangeal joint. *Clin Orthop Relat Res* 1996;327:12–20.
49. Hamer DW, Quinton DN. Dorsal fracture subluxation of the distal interphalangeal joint of the finger and the interphalangeal joint of the thumb treated by extension block splintage. *J Hand Surg* 1992;17B:591–594.
50. Dove AF, Sloan JP, Moulder TJ, et al. Dressings of the nailbed following nail avulsion. *J Hand Surg* 1988;13B:408–410.
51. Al-Qattan MM. Extra-articular transverse fractures of the base of the distal phalanx (Seymour's fracture) in children and adults. *J Hand Surg* 2001;26B:201–206.
52. Schneider LH. Fractures of the distal interphalangeal joint. *Hand Clin* 1994;10: 277–285.
53. Pegoli L, Toh S, Arai K, et al. The Ishiguro extension block technique for the treatment of mallet finger fracture: indications and clinical results. *J Hand Surg* 2003;28B:15–17.
54. Inoue G. Closed reduction of mallet fractures using extension block Kirschner wire. *J Orthop Trauma* 1992;6:413–415.
55. Ishiguro T, Yabe Y, Itoh Y, et al. Extension block with Kirschner wire for fracture dislocation of the distal interphalangeal joint. *Tech Hand Upper Ext Surg* 1997;1: 95–102.
56. Hofmeister EP, Mazurek MT, Shin AY, et al. Extension block pinning for large mallet fractures. *J Hand Surg* 2003;28:453–459.
57. Lubahn JD. Mallet finger fractures: a comparison of open and closed technique. *J Hand Surg* 1989;14A:394–396.
58. Lubahn JD. Dorsal fracture dislocations of the proximal interphalangeal joint. *Hand Clin* 1988;4:15–24.
59. Stark HH, Gainor BJ, Ashworth CR, et al. Operative treatment of intraarticular fractures of the dorsal aspect of the distal phalanx of digits. *J Bone Joint Surg* 1987;69A:892–896.
60. Takami H, Takahashi S, Ando M. Operative treatment of mallet finger due to intraarticular fracture of the distal phalanx. *Arch Orthop Trauma Surg* 2000;120:9–13.
61. Damron TA, Engber WD, Lange RH, et al. Biomechanical analysis of mallet finger fracture fixation techniques. *J Hand Surg* 1993;18A:600–607.
62. Bischoff R, Buechler U, De Roche R, et al. Clinical results of tension band fixation of avulsion fractures of the hand. *J Hand Surg* 1994;19:1019–1026.
63. Kaleli T, Ozturk C, Ersozlu S. External fixation for surgical treatment of a mallet finger. *J Hand Surg* 2003;28B:228–230.
64. Bynum DK, Gilbert JA. Avulsion of the flexor digitorum profundus: anatomic and biomechanical considerations. *J Hand Surg* 1988;13A:222–227.
65. Thayer DT. Distal interphalangeal joint injuries. *Hand Clin* 1988;4:1–4.
66. Lineaweaver W, Mathes SJ. Distal avulsion of the palmar plate of the interphalangeal joint of the thumb. *J Hand Surg* 1988;13A:465–467.
67. Gigis PI, Kuczynski K. The distal interphalangeal joints of the human fingers. *J Hand Surg* 1982;7:176–182.
68. Craig SM. Anatomy of the joints of the fingers. *Hand Clin* 1992;8:693–700.
69. Ghobadi F, Anapolle DM. Irreducible distal interphalangeal joint dislocation of the finger: a new cause. *J Hand Surg* 1994;19:196–198.
70. Simpson MB, Greenfield GQ. Irreducible dorsal dislocation of the small finger distal interphalangeal joint: the importance of roentgenograms—case report. *J Trauma* 1991; 31:1450–1454.
71. Inoue G, Maeda N. Irreducible palmar dislocation of the distal interphalangeal joint of the finger. *J Hand Surg* 1987;12:1077–1079.
72. Failla JM. Irreducible thumb interphalangeal joint dislocation due to a sesamoid and palmar plate: a case report. *J Hand Surg* 1995;20:490–491.
73. Sabapathy SR, Bose VC, Rex C. Irreducible dislocation of the interphalangeal joint of the thumb due to sesamoid bone interposition: a case report. *J Hand Surg* 1995;20: 487–489.
74. Rayan GM, Mullins PT. Skin necrosis complicating mallet finger splinting and vascularity of the distal interphalangeal joint overlying skin. *J Hand Surg* 1987;12A:548–552.
75. Horiuchi Y, Itoh Y, Sasaki T, et al. Dorsal dislocation of the DIP joint with fracture of the volar base of the distal phalanx. *J Hand Surg* 1989;14B:177–182.
76. Cannon NM. Rehabilitation approaches for distal and middle phalanx fractures of the hand. *J Hand Ther* 2003;16:105–116.
77. Dobyns JH, McElfresh EC. Extension block splinting. *Hand Clin* 1994;10:229–237.
78. Hamer DW, Quinton DN. Dorsal fracture subluxation of the proximal interphalangeal joints treated by extension block splintage. *J Hand Surg* 1992;17B:586–590.
79. Rosenstadt BE, Glickel SZ, Lane LB, et al. Palmar fracture dislocation of the proximal interphalangeal joint. *J Hand Surg* 1998;23A:811–820.
80. Twyman RS, David HG. The doorstop procedure. A technique for treating unstable fracture dislocations of the proximal interphalangeal joint. *J Hand Surg* 1993;18B: 714–715.
81. Viegas SF. Extension block pinning for proximal interphalangeal joint fracture dislocations: preliminary report of a new technique. *J Hand Surg* 1992;17A:896–901.
82. Newington DP, Davis TRC, Barton NJ. The treatment of dorsal fracture-dislocation of the proximal interphalangeal joint by closed reduction and Kirschner wire fixation: a 16-year follow up. *J Hand Surg.* 2002;27B:537–540.
83. Agee JM. Unstable fracture dislocations of the proximal interphalangeal joint: treatment with the force couple splint. *Clin Orthop Relat Res* 1987;214:101–112.
84. Buchanan RT. Mechanical requirements for application and modification of the dynamic force couple method. *Hand Clin* 1994;10:221–228.
85. Bilos ZJ, Vender MI, Knutson K. Fracture subluxation of the proximal interphalangeal joint treated by palmar plate advancement. *J Hand Surg* 1994;19A:189–196.
86. Durham Smith G, McCarten GM. Volar plate arthroplasty for closed proximal interphalangeal joint injuries. *J Hand Surg* 1992;17B:422–428.
87. Malerich MM, Eaton RG. The volar plate reconstruction for fracture dislocation of the proximal interphalangeal joint. *Hand Clin* 1994;10:251–260.
88. Eaton RG, Malerich MM. Volar plate arthroplasty of the proximal interphalangeal joint: a review of 10 years' experience. *J Hand Surg* 1980;5:260–268.
89. Dionysian E, Eaton RG. The long-term outcome of volar plate arthroplasty of the proximal interphalangeal joint. *J Hand Surg* 2000;25:429–437.
90. Dietch MA, Kiefhaber TR, Comisar R, Stern PJ. Dorsal fracture dislocations of the proximal interphalangeal joint: surgical complications and long-term results. *J Hand Surg* 1999;24:914–923.
91. Weiss APC. Cerclage fixation for fracture dislocation of the PIP joint. *Clin Orthop Relat Res* 1996;327:21–28.
92. Green A, Smith J, Redding M, et al. Acute open reduction and rigid internal fixation of proximal interphalangeal joint fracture dislocation. *J Hand Surg* 1992;17A:512–517.
93. Williams RMM, Kiefhaber TR, Sommerkamp TG, et al. Treatment of unstable dorsal proximal interphalangeal fracture/dislocations using a hemi-hamate autograft. *J Hand Surg* 2003;28:856–865.
94. Morgan JP, Gordon DA, Klug MS, et al. Dynamic digital traction for unstable comminuted intra articular fracture dislocations of the proximal interphalangeal joint. *J Hand Surg* 1995;20A:565–573.
95. Suzuki Y, Matsunaga T, Sato S, et al. The pins and rubbers traction system for treatment of comminuted intraarticular fractures and fracture dislocations in the hand. *J Hand Surg* 1994;19B:98–107.
96. Syed AA, Agarwal M, Boome R. Dynamic external fixation for pilon fractures of the proximal interphalangeal joints: A simple fixator for a complex fracture. *J Hand Surg* 2003;28B:137–141.
97. Hastings H II, Ernst MJ. Dynamic external fixation for fractures of the proximal interphalangeal joint. *Hand Clin* 1993;9:659–674.
98. Inanami H, Ninomiya S, Okutsu I, et al. Dynamic external finger fixator for fracture dislocation of the proximal interphalangeal joint. *J Hand Surg* 1993;18A:160–164.
99. Murray KA. Active traction splintage for proximal interphalangeal joint injuries. *Ann Plast Surg* 1995;35:15–18.
100. Patel MR, Joshi BB. Distraction method for chronic dorsal fracture dislocation of the proximal interphalangeal joint. *Hand Clin* 1994;10:327–337.
101. Schenck RR. The dynamic traction method. Combining movement and traction for intraarticular fractures of the phalanges. *Hand Clin* 1994;10:187–198.
102. Stern PJ, Roman RJ, Kiefhaber TR, et al. Pilon fractures of the proximal interphalangeal joint. *J Hand Surg* 1991;16A:844–850.

103. Majumder S, Peck F, Watson JS, et al. Lessons learned from the management of complex intra-articular fractures at the base of the middle phalanges of fingers. *J Hand Surg* 2003;28B:559–565.
104. Hynes MC, Giddins GEB. Dynamic external fixation for pilon fractures of the interphalangeal joints. *J Hand Surg* 2001;26B:122–124.
105. Fahmy NRM, Harvey RA. The "S" quattro in the management of fractures in the hand. *J Hand Surg* 1992;17B:321–331.
106. Krakauer JD, Stern PJ. Hinged device for fractures involving the proximal interphalangeal joint. *Clin Orthop Relat Res* 1996;327:29–37.
107. Chinchalkar SJ, Gan BS. Management of proximal interphalangeal joint fractures and dislocations. *J Hand Ther* 2003;16:117–128.
108. Wolfe SW, Katz LD. Intra articular impaction fractures of the phalanges. *J Hand Surg* 1995;20A:327–333.
109. Jesperson B, Nielsen NS, Bonnevie BEB, et al. Hyperextension injury to the proximal interphalangeal joint or to the metacarpophalangeal joint of the thumb—a clinical study. *Scand J Plast Reconstr Surg Hand Surg* 1998;32:317–321.
110. Peimer CA, Sullivan DJ, Wild DR. Palmar dislocation of the proximal interphalangeal joint. *J Hand Surg* 1984;9A:39–48.
111. Bowers WH, Wolf JW Jr, Nehil J, et al. The proximal interphalangeal joint volar plate. I. An anatomical and biomechanical study. *J Hand Surg* 1980;5:79–88.
112. Diao E, Eaton RG. Total collateral ligament excision for contractures of the proximal interphalangeal joint. *J Hand Surg* 1993;18A:395–402.
113. Freeland AE, Roberts TS. Percutaneous screw treatment of spiral oblique finger proximal phalangeal fractures. *Orthopaedics* 1991;14:384–388.
114. Stern PJ, Lee AF. Open dorsal dislocations of the proximal interphalangeal joint. *J Hand Surg* 1985;10A:364–370.
115. Liss FE, Green SM. Capsular injuries of the proximal interphalangeal joint. *Hand Clin* 1992;8:755–768.
116. Liebovic SJ, Bowers WH. Anatomy of the proximal interphalangeal joint. *Hand Clin* 1994;10:169–178.
117. Bowers WH. The proximal interphalangeal joint volar plate. II. A clinical study of hyperextension injury. *J Hand Surg* 1981;6:77–81.
118. Slattery PG. The dorsal plate of the PIP joint. *J Hand Surg* 1990;15B:68–73.
119. Rhee RY, Reading G, Wray RC. A biomechanical study of the collateral ligaments of the proximal interphalangeal joints. *J Hand Surg* 1992;17A:157–163.
120. Kiefhaber TR, Stern PJ, Grood ES. Lateral stability of the proximal interphalangeal joint. *J Hand Surg* 1986;11A:661–669.
121. Minamikawa Y, Horii E, Amadio PC, et al. Stability and constraint of the proximal interphalangeal joint. *J Hand Surg* 1993;18A:198–204.
122. Inoue G, Maeda N. Irreducible palmar dislocation of the proximal interphalangeal joint of the finger. *J Hand Surg* 1990;15A:301–304.
123. Incavo SJ, Mogan JV, Hilfrank BC. Extension splinting of palmar plate avulsion injuries of the proximal interphalangeal joint. *J Hand Surg* 1989;14A:659–661.
124. Phair IC, Quinton DN, Allen MJ. The conservative management of volar avulsion fractures of the PIP joint. *J Hand Surg* 1989;14B:168–170.
125. Soelberg M, Gebuhr P, Klareskov B. Interphalangeal dislocations of the fingers treated by an elastic double finger bandage. *J Hand Surg* 1990;15B:66–67.
126. Stern PJ. Stener lesion after lateral dislocation of the proximal interphalangeal joint—indication for open reduction. *J Hand Surg* 1981;6:602–604.
127. Crick JC, Conners JJ, Franco RS. Irreducible palmar dislocation of the proximal interphalangeal joint with bilateral avulsion fractures. *J Hand Surg* 1990;15A:460–463.
128. Inoue G, Maeda N. Irreducible palmar dislocation of the proximal interphalangeal joint of the finger. *J Hand Surg* 1990;15A:301–304.
129. Kozin SH, Thoder JJ, Lieberman G. Operative treatment of metacarpal and phalangeal shaft fractures. *J Am Acad Orthop Surg* 2000;8:111–121.
130. Lee SG, Jupiter JB. Phalangeal and metacarpal fractures of the hand. *Hand Clin* 2000; 16:323–332.
131. Shulter Ellis FP, Lazar G. Internal morphology of human phalanges. *J Hand Surg* 1984; 9A:490–495.
132. Agee JM. Treatment principles for proximal and middle phalangeal fractures. *Orthop Clin North Am* 1992;23:35–40.
133. Vahey JW, Wegner DA, Hastings H. Effect of proximal phalangeal fracture deformity on extensor tendon function. *J Hand Surg* 1998;23:673–681.
134. Black DM, Mann RJ, Constine RM, et al. The stability of internal fixation in the proximal phalanx. *J Hand Surg* 1986;11A:672–677.
135. Viegas SF, Ferren EL, Self J, et al. Comparative mechanical properties of various Kirschner wire configurations in transverse and oblique phalangeal fractures. *J Hand Surg* 1988;13A:246–253.
136. Massengill JB, Alexander H, Langrana N, et al. A phalangeal fracture model—quantitative analysis of rigidity and failure. *J Hand Surg* 1982;7:264–270.
137. Lins RE. A comparative mechanical analysis of plate fixation in a proximal phalanx fracture model. *J Hand Surg* 1996;21A:1059–1064.
138. Nunley JA, Kloen P. Biomechanical and functional testing of plate fixation devices for proximal phalangeal fractures. *J Hand Surg* 1991;16A:991–998.
139. Barton NJ. Conservative treatment of articular fractures in the hand. *J Hand Surg* 1989; 14A:386–390.
140. Burkhalter WE. Closed treatment of hand fractures. *J Hand Surg* 1989;14A:390–393.
141. Widgerow AD, Ladas CS. Anatomical attachments to the proximal phalangeal base—a case for stability. *Scand J Plast Reconstr Surg Hand Surg* 2001;35:85–90.
142. Reyes FA, Latta LL. Conservative management of difficult phalangeal fractures. *Clin Orthop Relat Res* 1987;214:23–30.
143. Ebinger T, Erhard N, Kinzl L, et al. Dynamic treatment of displaced proximal phalangeal fractures. *J Hand Surg* 1999;24:1254–1262.
144. Maitra A, Burdett Smith P. The conservative management of proximal phalangeal fractures of the hand in an accident and emergency department. *J Hand Surg* 1992;17B: 332–336.
145. Eaton RG. Closed reduction and internal fixation versus open reduction and internal fixation for displaced oblique proximal phalangeal fractures. *Orthopaedics* 1989;12: 911–916.
146. Namba RS, Kabo M, Meals RA. Biomechanical effects of point configuration in Kirschner wire fixation. *Clin Orthop Relat Res* 1987;214:19–22.
147. Green DP, Anderson JR. Closed reduction and percutaneous fixation of fractured phalanges. *J Bone Joint Surg* 1973;55A:1651–1654.
148. Melone CP Jr. Rigid fixation of phalangeal and metacarpal fractures. *Orthop Clin North Am* 1986;17:421–435.
149. Hornbach EE, Cohen MS. Closed reduction and percutaneous pinning of fractures of the proximal phalanx. *J Hand Surg* 2003;26B:45–49.
150. Belsky MR, Eaton RG, Lane LB. Closed reduction and internal fixation of proximal phalangeal fractures. *J Hand Surg* 1984;9A:725–729.
151. Shehadi SI. External fixation of metacarpal and phalangeal fractures. *J Hand Surg* 1991; 16A:544–550.
152. Freeland AE, Benoist LA. Open reduction and internal fixation method for fractures at the proximal interphalangeal joint. *Hand Clin* 1994;10:239–250.
153. Hastings H II, Carroll C IV. Treatment of closed articular fractures of the metacarpophalangeal and proximal interphalangeal joints. *Hand Clin* 1988;4:503–528.
154. Weiss APC, Hastings H II. Distal unicondylar fractures of the proximal phalanx. *J Hand Surg* 1993;18A:594–599.
155. Light TR, Bednar MS. Management of intraarticular fractures of the metacarpophalangeal joint. *Hand Clin* 1994;10:303–314.
156. Margles SW. Intraarticular fractures of the metacarpophalangeal and proximal interphalangeal joints. *Hand Clin* 1988;4:67–74.
157. Kuhn KM, Khiem DD, Shin AY. Volar A1 pulley approach for the fixation of avulsion fractures of the base of the proximal phalanx. *J Hand Surg* 2001;26:762–771.
158. Horton TC, Hatton M, Davis TRC. A prospective randomized controlled study of fixation of long oblique and spiral shaft fractures of the proximal phalanx: closed reduction and percutaneous Kirschner wiring versus open reduction and lag screw fixation. *J Hand Surg* 2003;28B:5–9.
159. Buchler U, Gupta A, Ruf S. Corrective osteotomy for post traumatic malunion of the phalanges in the hand. *J Hand Surg* 1996;21B:33–42.
160. Ford DJ, El Hadidi S, Lunn PG, et al. Fractures of the metacarpals: treatment by AO screw and plate fixation. *J Hand Surg* 1987;12B:34–37.
161. Freeland AE, Benoist LA, Melancon KP. Parallel miniature screw fixation of spiral and long oblique and phalangeal fractures. *Orthopaedics* 1994;17:199–200.
162. Greene TL, Noellert RC, Belsole RJ, et al. Composite wiring of metacarpal and phalangeal fractures. *J Hand Surg* 1989;14A:665–669.
163. Jupiter JB. Discussion of application of maxillofacial miniplating and microplating systems to the hand. *Plast Reconstr Surg* 1993;92:708–709.
164. Liebovic SJ. Internal fixation sets for use in the hand. A comparison of available instrumentation. *Hand Clin* 1997;13:531–540.
165. Rayhack JM, Bottke C. Intraosseous compression wiring of displaced articular condylar fractures. *J Hand Surg* 1990;15A:370–373.
166. Zimmerman NB, Weiland AJ. Ninety nine intraosseous wiring for internal fixation of the digital skeleton. *Orthopaedics* 1989;12:99–104.
167. Diwaker HN, Stothard J. The role of internal fixation in closed fractures of the proximal phalanges and metacarpals in adults. *J Hand Surg* 1986;11B:103–108.
168. Safoury Y. Treatment of phalangeal fractures by tension band wiring. *J Hand Surg* 2001; 26B:50–52.
169. Ford DJ, Ed Hadidi S, Lunn PG, et al. Fractures of the phalanges: results of internal fixation using 1.5 mm and 2 mm AO screws. *J Hand Surg* 1987;12B:28–33.
170. Dabezies EJ, Schutte JP. Fixation of metacarpal and phalangeal fractures with miniature plates and screws. *J Hand Surg* 1986;11A:283–288.
171. Hastings H II. Unstable metacarpal and phalangeal fracture treatment with screws and plates. *Clin Orthop Relat Res* 1987;214:37–52.
172. Stern PJ, Wieser MJ, Reilly DG. Complications of plate fixation in the hand skeleton. *Clin Orthop Relat Res* 1987;214:59–65.
173. Shibata T, O'Flanagan SJ, Ip FK, et al. Articular fractures of the digits: a prospective study. *J Hand Surg* 1993;18B:225–229.
174. Chin KR, Jupiter JB. Treatment of triplane fractures of the head of the proximal phalanx. *J Hand Surg* 1999;24:1263–1268.
175. Shewring DJ, Thomas RH. Avulsion fractures from the base of the proximal phalanges of the fingers. *J Hand Surg* 2003;28B:10–14.
176. Strickler M, Nagy L, Buchler U. Rigid internal fixation of basilar fractures of the proximal phalanges by cancellous bone grafting only. *J Hand Surg* 2001;26B:455–458.
177. Freeland AE, Hardy MA, Singletary S. Rehabilitation for proximal phalangeal fractures. *J Hand Ther* 2003;16:129–142.
178. Field LD, Freeland AE, Jabaley ME. Midaxial approach to the proximal phalanx for fracture fixation. *Contemp Orthop* 1992;25:133–137.
179. Moneim MS. Volar dislocation of the metacarpophalangeal joint. Pathologic anatomy and report of two cases. *Clin Orthop Relat Res* 1983;176:186–189.
180. Wood MB, Dobyns JH. Chronic, complex volar dislocation of the metacarpophalangeal joint. Report of three cases. *J Hand Surg* 1981;6:73–76.
181. al-Quattan MM, Murray KA. An isolated complex dorsal dislocation of the MP joint of the ring finger. *J Hand Surg* 1994;19B:171–173.
182. Araki S, Uchiyama M, Nishimura T, et al. Irreducible open dislocation of the metacarpophalangeal joint of the small finger. *J Hand Surg* 1992;17A:1146–1147.
183. Ramirez Ruiz G, Combali Aleu A, Valer Tito A, et al. Simultaneous subluxation of the metacarpophalangeal joints of all four fingers: a case report. *J Hand Surg* 1985;10A: 78–80.

184. Wright CS. Compound dislocations of four metacarpophalangeal joints. *J Hand Surg* 1985;10B:233–235.
185. Viegas SF, Heare TC, Calhoun JH. Complex fracture dislocation of a fifth metacarpophalangeal joint: case report and literature review. *J Trauma* 1989;29:521–524.
186. Harammati N, Hiller N, Dowdle J, et al. MRI of the Stener lesion. *Skeletal Radiol* 1995; 24:515–518.
187. Hinke DH, Erickson SJ, Chamoy L, et al. Ulnar collateral ligament of the thumb: MR findings in cadavers, volunteers, and patients with ligamentous injury (gamekeeper's thumb). *AJR Am J Roentgenol* 1994;163:1431–1434.
188. Louis DS, Buckwalter KA. Magnetic resonance imaging of the collateral ligaments of the thumb. *J Hand Surg* 1989;14A:739–741.
189. Spaeth HJ, Abrams RA, Bock GW, et al. Gamekeeper thumb: differentiation of nondisplaced and displaced tears of the ulnar collateral ligament with MR imaging. *Radiology* 1993;188:553–556.
190. Pichora DR, McMurty RY, Bell MJ. Gamekeeper's thumb: a prospective study of functional bracing. *J Hand Surg* 1989;14A:567–573.
191. Abrahamson SO, Sollerman C, Lundborg G, et al. Diagnosis of displaced ulnar collateral ligament of the metacarpophalangeal joint of the thumb. *J Hand Surg* 1990;15A: 457–460.
192. Derkash RS, Matyas JR, Weaver JK. Acute surgical repair of the skier's thumb. *Clin Orthop Relat Res* 1987;216:29–33.
193. Van Dommelen A, Zvirbulis RA. Upper extremity injuries in snow skiers. *Am J Sports Med* 1989;17:751–753.
194. Posner MA, Retailloud J. Metacarpophalangeal joint injuries of the thumb. *Hand Clin* 1992;8:713–732.
195. Hintermann B, Holzach PJ, Schutz M, et al. Skier's thumb—the significance of bony injuries. *Am J Sports Med* 1993;21:800–804.
196. Dong PR, Seeger LL, Shapiro MS, et al. Fractures of the sesamoid bones of the thumb. *Am J Sports Med* 1995;23:336–339.
197. Ishizuki M, Nakagawa T, Ito S. Hyperextension injuries of the metacarpophalangeal joint of the thumb. *J Hand Surg* 1994;19B:361–367.
198. Patel MR, Pearlman HS, Bassini L, et al. Fractures of the sesamoid bones of the thumb. *J Hand Surg* 1990;15A:776–781.
199. Ostrowski DM. Irreducible dorsoulnar dislocation of the proximal phalanx of the thumb. *J Hand Surg* 1991;16A:121–124.
200. Miyamoto M, Hirayama T, Uchida M. Volar dislocations of the metacarpophalangeal joint of the thumb—a case report. *J Hand Surg* 1986;11B:51–54.
201. Hughes LA, Freiberg A. Irreducible MP joint dislocation due to entrapment of FPL. *J Hand Surg* 1993;18B:708–709.
202. Minami A, An K, Cooney WP, et al. Ligament stability of the metacarpophalangeal joint. A biomechanical study. *J Hand Surg* 1985;10A:255–260.
203. Al Quattan MM, Robertson GA. An anatomical study of the deep transverse metacarpal ligament. *J Anat* 1993;182:443–446.
204. Barry K, McGee H, Curtin J. Complex dislocation of the metacarpophalangeal joint of the index finger: a comparison of the surgical approaches. *J Hand Surg* 1988;13B: 466–468.
205. Patel MR, Bassini L. Irreducible palmar metacarpophalangeal joint dislocation due to juncture tendinum interposition: a case report and review of the literature. *J Hand Surg* 2000;25:166–172.
206. Delaere OP, Suttor PM, Degolla R, et al. Early surgical treatment for collateral ligament rupture of metacarpophalangeal joints of the fingers. *J Hand Surg* 2003;28:309–315.
207. Shaw SJ, Morris MA. The range of motion of the metacarpophalangeal joint of the thumb and its relationship to injury. *J Hand Surg* 1992;17B:164–166.
208. Giele H, Martin J. The two-level ulnar collateral ligament injury of the metacarpophalangeal joint of the thumb. *J Hand Surg* 2003;28B:92–93.
209. Coyle MP. Grade III radial collateral ligament injuries of the thumb metacarpophalangeal joint: treatment by soft tissue advancement and bony reattachment. *J Hand Surg* 2003;28:14–20.
210. Campbell JD, Feagin JA, King P, et al. Ulnar collateral ligament injury of the thumb. Treatment with glove spica cast. *Am J Sports Med* 1992;20:29–30.
211. Sollerman C, Abrahamsson S, Lundborg G, et al. Functional splinting versus plaster cast for ruptures of the ulnar collateral ligament of the thumb. A prospective randomized study of 63 cases. *Acta Orthop Scand* 1991;62:524–526.
212. Dinowitz M, Trumble T, Hanel D, et al. Failure of cast immobilization for thumb ulnar collateral ligament avulsion fractures. *J Hand Surg* 1997;22A:1057–1063.
213. Sorene ED, Goodwin DR. Non-operative treatment of displaced avulsion fractures of the ulnar base of the proximal phalanx of the thumb. *Scand J Plast Reconstr Surg Hand Surg* 2003;37:225–227.
214. Gibeault JD, Saba P, Hoenecke H, et al. The sesamoids of the metacarpophalangeal joint of the thumb: an anatomical and clinical study. *J Hand Surg* 1989;14B:244–247.
215. Doyle JR, Atkinson RE. Rupture of the radial collateral ligament of the metacarpophalangeal joint of the index finger: a report of three cases. *J Hand Surg* 1989;14B:248–250.
216. Ishizuki M. Injury to collateral ligament of metacarpophalangeal joint of a finger. *J Hand Surg* 1988;13A:456–460.
217. Schubiner JM, Mass DP. Operation for collateral ligament ruptures of the metacarpophalangeal joints of the fingers. *J Bone Joint Surg* 1989;71B:388–389.
218. Zemel NP. Metacarpophalangeal joint injuries in fingers. *Hand Clin* 1992;8:745–753.
219. Williams JS Jr, Kamionek S, Weiss AC, et al. The surgical approach in non border digit complex dislocations of the metacarpophalangeal joint. *Orthop Rev* 1994;23:601–605.
220. Downey DJ, Moneim MS, Omer GE. Acute gamekeeper's thumb. Quantitative outcome of surgical repair. *Am J Sports Med* 1995;23:222–226.
221. Durham JW, Khuri S, Kim MH. Acute and late radial collateral ligament injuries of the thumb metacarpophalangeal joint. *J Hand Surg* 1993;18A:232–237.
222. Boulas HJ, Herren A, Buchler U. Osteochondral metatarsophalangeal autografts for traumatic articular metacarpophalangeal defects: a preliminary report. *J Hand Surg* 1993;18A:1086–1092.
223. Husband JB, McPherson SA. Bony skier's thumb injuries. *Clin Orthop Relat Res* 1996; 327:79–84.
224. Rehak DC, Sotereanos DG, Bowman MW, et al. The Mitek bone anchor application to the hand, wrist and elbow. *J Hand Surg* 1994;19A:853–860.
225. Weiland AJ, Berner SH, Hotchkiss RN, et al. Repair of acute ulnar collateral ligament injuries of the thumb metacarpophalangeal joint with an intraosseous suture anchor. *J Hand Surg* 1997;22A:585–591.
226. Bean CHG, Tencer AF, Trumble TE. The effect of thumb metacarpophalangeal ulnar collateral ligament attachment site on joint range of motion: an in vitro study. *J Hand Surg* 1999;24:283–287.
227. Ryu J, Fagan R. Arthroscopic treatment of acute complete thumb metacarpophalangeal ulnar collateral ligament tears. *J Hand Surg* 1995;20A:1037–1042.
228. Kozin SH, Bishop AT. Tension wire fixation of avulsion fractures at the thumb metacarpophalangeal joint. *J Hand Surg* 1994;19:1027–1031.
229. Saetta JP, Phair IC, Quinton DN. Ulnar collateral ligament repair of the metacarpophalangeal joint of the thumb: a study comparing two methods of repair. *J Hand Surg* 1992;17B:160–163.
230. Fairhurst M, Hansen L. Treatment of "Gamekeeper's thumb" by reconstruction of the ulnar collateral ligament. *J Hand Surg* 2003;27B:542–545.
231. Arnold DM, Cooney WP, Wood MB. Surgical management of chronic ulnar collateral ligament insufficiency of the thumb metacarpophalangeal joint. *Orthop Rev* 1992;21: 583–588.
232. Osterman AL, Hayken GD, Bora FW. A quantitative evaluation of thumb function after ulnar collateral repair and reconstruction. *J Trauma* 1981;21:854–861.
233. Breek JC, Tan AM, Van Thiel TPH, et al. Free tendon grafting to repair the metacarpophalangeal joint of the thumb. Surgical techniques and a review of 70 patients. *J Bone Joint Surg* 1989;71B:383–387.
234. Glickel SZ, Malerich M, Pearce SM, et al. Ligament replacement for chronic instability of the ulnar collateral ligament of the metacarpophalangeal joint of the thumb. *J Hand Surg* 1993;18A:930–941.
235. Kuz JE, Husband JB, Tokar N, et al. Outcome of avulsion fractures of the ulnar base of the proximal phalanx of the thumb treated nonsurgically. *J Hand Surg* 1999;24: 275–282.
236. McElfresh EC, Dobyns JH. Intraarticular metacarpal head fractures. *J Hand Surg* 1983; 8:383–393.
237. Leung YL, Beredjiklian PK, Monaghan BA, Bozentka DJ. Radiographic assessment of small finger metacarpal neck fractures. *J Hand Surg* 2002;27:443–448.
238. Royle SG. Rotational deformity following metacarpal fracture. *J Hand Surg* 1990;15B: 124–125.
239. Seitz WH Jr, Froimson AI. Management of malunited fractures of the metacarpal and phalangeal shafts. *Hand Clin* 1988;4:529–536.
240. Mehara AK, Bhan S. Rotatory dislocation of the second carpometacarpal joint: case report. *J Trauma* 1993;34:464–466.
241. Lane CS, Kennedy JF, Kuschner SH. The reverse oblique x ray film—metacarpal fractures revealed. *J Hand Surg* 1992;17A:504–506.
242. Eyres KS, Allen TR. Skyline view of the metacarpal head in the assessment of human fight bite injuries. *J Hand Surg* 1993;18B:43–44.
243. Lazar G, Shulter Ellis FP. Intramedullary structure of human metacarpals. *J Hand Surg* 1980;5:477.
244. Eglseder WA, Juliano PJ, Roure R. Fractures of the fourth metacarpal. *J Orthop Trauma* 1997;11:441–445.
245. Strauch RJ, Rosenwasser MP, Lunt JG. Metacarpal shaft fractures: the effect of shortening on the extensor tendon mechanism. *J Hand Surg* 1998;23:519–523.
246. Bickley BT, Hanel DP. Self tapping versus standard tapped titanium screw fixation in the upper extremity. *J Hand Surg* 1998;23A:308–311.
247. Black DM, Mann RJ, Constine RM, et al. Comparison of internal fixation techniques in metacarpal fracture. *J Hand Surg* 1985;10A:466–472.
248. Firoozbakhsh KK, Moneim MS, Howey T, et al. Comparative fatigue strengths and stabilities of metacarpal internal fixation techniques. *J Hand Surg* 1993;18A: 1059–1068.
249. Mann RJ, Black D, Constine R, et al. A quantitative comparison of metacarpal fracture stability with five different methods of internal fixation. *J Hand Surg* 1985;10A: 1024–1028.
250. Matloub HS, Jensen PL, Sanger JR, et al. Spiral fracture fixation techniques. A biomechanical study. *J Hand Surg* 1993;18B:515–519.
251. Prevel CD. Comparative biomechanical stability of titanium bone fixation systems in metacarpal fractures. *Ann Plast Surg* 1995;35:6–14.
252. Prevel CD, Eppley BL, Jackson JR, et al. Mini and micro plating of phalangeal and metacarpal fractures: a biomechanical study. *J Hand Surg* 1995;20:44–49.
253. Fischer KJ, Bastidas JA, Provenzano DA, Tomaino MM. Low-profile versus conventional metacarpal plating systems: a comparison of construct stiffness and strength. *J Hand Surg* 1999;24:928–934.
254. Konradsen L, Nielsen PT, Albrecht Beste E. Functional treatment of metacarpal fractures. *Acta Orthop Scand* 1990;61:531–534.
255. Viegas SF, Tencer A, Woodard P, et al. Functional bracing of fractures of the second through fifth metacarpals. *J Hand Surg* 1987;12A:139–143.
256. Geiger KR, Karpman RR. Necrosis of the skin over the metacarpal as a result of functional fracture bracing. *J Bone Joint Surg* 1989;71A:1199–1202.
257. Harding IJ, Parry D, Barrington RL. The use of a moulded metacarpal brace versus neighbour strapping for fractures of the finger metacarpal neck. *J Hand Surg* 2001;26B: 261–263.

258. Braakman M. Functional taping of fractures of the fifth metacarpal results in a quicker recovery. *Injury* 1998;29:5–9.
259. Breddam M, Hansen TB. Subcapital fractures of the fourth and fifth metacarpals treated without splinting and reposition. *Scand J Plast Reconstr Surg Hand Surg* 1995;29: 269–270.
260. Ford DJ, Ali MS, Steel WM. Fractures of the fifth metacarpal neck: is reduction or immobilization necessary? *J Hand Surg* 1989;14B:165–167.
261. McMahon PJ, Woods DA, Burge PD. Initial treatment of closed metacarpal fractures. A controlled comparison of compression glove and splintage. *J Hand Surg* 1994;19B: 597–600.
262. Theeuwen GAJM, Lemmens JAM, van Niekerk JLM. Conservative treatment of Boxer's fracture: a retrospective analysis. *Injury* 1991;22:394–396.
263. Ali A, Hamman J, Mass DP. The biomechanical effects of angulated boxer's fractures. *J Hand Surg* 1999;24:835–844.
264. Birndorf MS, Daley R, Greenwald DP. Metacarpal fracture angulation decreases flexor mechanical efficiency in human hands. *Plast Reconstr Surg* 1997;99:1079–1083.
265. Rawles JG Jr. Dislocations and fracture dislocations at the carpometacarpal joints of the fingers. *Hand Clin* 1988;4:103–112.
266. Gonzalez MH, Igram CM, Hall RF. Flexible intramedullary nailing for metacarpal fractures. *J Hand Surg* 1995;20:382–387.
267. Gonzales MH. Intramedullary fixation of metacarpal and proximal phalangeal fractures of the hand. *Clin Orthop Relat Res* 1996;327:47–54.
268. Liew KH, Chan BK, Low CO. Metacarpal and proximal phalangeal fractures—fixation with multiple intramedullary Kirschner wires. *Hand Surg* 2000;5:125–130.
269. Orbay JL, Indriago I, Gonzales E, et al. Percutaneous fixation of metacarpal fractures. *Operative Tech in Plast Recon Surg* 2002;9:138–142.
270. Foucher G. "Bouquet" osteosynthesis in metacarpal neck fractures: a series of 66 patients. *J Hand Surg* 1995;20A:s86–90.
271. Manueddu CA, Della Santa D. Fasciculated intramedullary pinning of metacarpal fractures. *J Hand Surg* 1996;21B:230–236.
272. Nordyke MD, Lewis RC Jr, Janssen HF, et al. Biomechanical and clinical evaluation of the expandable intramedullary fixation device. *J Hand Surg* 1988;13A:128–134.
273. Varela CD, Carr JB. Closed intramedullary pinning of metacarpal and phalanx fractures. *Orthopaedics* 1990;13:213–215.
274. Freeland AE, Lineaweaver WC, Lindley SG. Fracture fixation in the mutilated hand. *Hand Clin* 2003;19:51–61.
275. Bosscha K, Snellen JP. Internal fixation of metacarpal and phalangeal fractures with AO minifragment screws and plates: a prospective study. *Injury* 1993;24:166–168.
276. Jabaley ME, Freeland A. Rigid internal fixation in the hand: 104 cases. *Plast Reconstr Surg* 1986;77:288–297.
277. McNemar TB, Howell JW, Chang E. Management of metacarpal fractures. *J Hand Ther* 2003;16:143–151.
278. Gurland M. Carpometacarpal joint injuries of the fingers. *Hand Clin* 1992;8:733–744.
279. O'Rourke PJ, Quinlan W. Fracture dislocation of the fifth metacarpal resulting in compression of the deep branch of the ulnar nerve. *J Hand Surg* 1993;18B:190–191.
280. Peterson P, Sacks S. Fracture dislocation of the base of the fifth metacarpal associated with injury to the deep motor branch of the ulnar nerve. *J Hand Surg* 1986;11A: 525–528.
281. Kumar R, Malhotra R. Divergent fracture-dislocation of the second carpometacarpal joint and the three ulnar carpometacarpal joints. *J Hand Surg* 2001;26:123–129.
282. Yoshida R, Shah MA, Patterson RM, et al. Anatomy and pathomechanics of ring and small finger carpometacarpal joint injuries. *J Hand Surg* 2003;28:1035–1043.
283. Garcia Elias M, Bishop AT, Dobyns JH, et al. Transcarpal carpometacarpal dislocations, excluding the thumb. *J Hand Surg* 1990;15A:531–540.
284. Thomas WO, Gottliebson WM, D'Amore TF, et al. Isolated palmar displaced fracture of the base of the index metacarpal: a case report. *J Hand Surg* 1994;19A:455–456.
285. Bergfield TG, Dupuy TE, Aulicino PL. Fracture dislocations of all five carpometacarpal joints: a case report. *J Hand Surg* 1985;10A:76–78.
286. Gunther SF, Bruno PD. Divergent dislocation of the carpometacarpal joints: a case report. *J Hand Surg* 1985;10A:197–201.
287. Johnson SR, Jones DG, Hoddinott HC. Missed carpometacarpal dislocation of the thumb in motorcyclists. *Injury* 1987;18:415–416.
288. Mody BS, Dias JJ. Carpometacarpal dislocation of the thumb associated with fracture of the trapezium. *J Hand Surg* 1993;18B:197–199.
289. Tolat AR, Jones MW. Carpometacarpal dislocation of the thumb associated with fracture of the trapezium. *Injury* 1990;21:411–412.
290. Watt N, Hooper G. Dislocation of the trapeziometacarpal joint. *J Hand Surg* 1987;12B: 242–245.
291. Garcia Elias M, Henriquez Lluch A, Rossignani P, et al. Bennett's fracture combined with fracture of the trapezium. A report of three cases. *J Hand Surg* 1993;18B:523–526.
292. Radford PJ, Wilcox DT. Holdsworth BJ. Simultaneous trapezium and Bennett's fractures. *J Hand Surg* 1992;17A:621–623.
293. Nakamura K, Patterson RM, Viegas SF. The ligament and skeletal anatomy of the second through fifth carpometacarpal joints and adjacent structures. *J Hand Surg* 2001;26: 1016–1029.
294. Dzwierzynski WW, Matloub HS, Yan J-G, et al. Anatomy of the intermetacarpal ligaments of the carpometacarpal joints of the fingers. *J Hand Surg* 1997;22:931–934.
295. Ashkenaze DM, Ruby LK. Metacarpal fractures and dislocations. *Orthop Clin North Am* 1992;23:19–33.
296. Gunther SF. The carpometacarpal joints. *Orthop Clin North Am* 1984;15:259–277.
297. Viegas SF, Crossley M, Marzke M, et al. The fourth carpometacarpal joint. *J Hand Surg* 1991;16A:525–533.
298. El-shennawy Maged, Nakamura K, Patterson RM, et al. Three-dimensional kinematic analysis of the second through fifth carpometacarpal joints. *J Hand Surg* 2001;26: 1030–1035.
299. Cooney WP, Lucca MJ, Chao EYS, et al. The kinesiology of the thumb trapezio metacarpal joint. *J Bone Joint Surg* 1981;63A:1371–1381.
300. Bettinger PC, Linscheid RL, Berger RA, Cooney WP, An K-N. An anatomic study of the stabilizing ligaments of the trapezium and trapeziometacarpal joint. *J Hand Surg* 1999;24:786–798.
301. Imaeda T, An K, Cooney WP, et al. Anatomy of trapeziometacarpal ligaments. *J Hand Surg* 1993;18A:226–231.
302. Van Brenk B, Richards RR, Mackay MB, et al. A biomechanical assessment of ligaments preventing dorsoradial subluxation of the trapeziometacarpal joint. *J Hand Surg* 1998; 23:607–611.
303. Strauch RJ, Behrman MJ, Rosenwasser MP. Acute dislocation of the carpometacarpal joint of the thumb: an anatomic and cadaver study. *J Hand Surg* 1994;19:93–98.
304. DeBeer JV, Maloon S, Anderson P, et al. Multiple carpometacarpal dislocations. *J Hand Surg* 1989;14B:105–108.
305. Mueller JJ. Carpometacarpal dislocations: report of five cases and review of the literature. *J Hand Surg* 1986;11A:184–188.
306. Cannon S, Dowd G, Williams DH, et al. A long term study following Bennett's fracture. *J Hand Surg* 1986;11B:426–431.
307. Livesley PJ. The conservative management of Bennett's fracture dislocation: a 26 year follow up. *J Hand Surg* 1990;15B:291–294.
308. Foster RJ. Stabilization of ulnar CMC dislocations or fracture dislocations. *Clin Orthop Relat Res* 1996;327:94–97.
309. Lawlis JR III, Gunther SF. Carpometacarpal dislocations: long term follow up. *J Bone Joint Surg* 1991;73A:52–58.
310. Schortinghuis J, Klasen HJ. Open reduction and internal fixation of combined fourth and fifth carpometacarpal fracture dislocations. *J Trauma* 1997;42:1052–1055.
311. Hanel DP. Primary fusion of fracture dislocations of central carpometacarpal joints. *Clin Orthop Relat Res* 1996;327:85–93.
312. Simonian PT, Trumble TE. Traumatic dislocation of the thumb carpometacarpal joint: early ligamentous reconstruction versus closed reduction and pinning. *J Hand Surg* 1996;21A:802–806.
313. Shah J, Patel M. Dislocation of the carpometacarpal joint of the thumb. A report of four cases. *Clin Orthop Relat Res* 1983;175:166–169.
314. Brunelli G, Monini L, Brunelli F. Stabilisation of the trapeziometacarpal joint. *J Hand Surg* 1989;14B:209–212.
315. Magnusson A, Bertheussen K, Weilby A. Ligament reconstruction of the thumb carpometacarpal joint using a modified Eaton and Littler technique. *J Hand Surg* 1985;10B: 115–116.
316. Eaton RG, Lane LB, Littler JW, et al. Ligament reconstruction for the painful thumb carpometacarpal joint: a long term assessment. *J Hand Surg* 1984;9A:692–699.
317. Lutz M, Sailer R, Zimmerman R, et al. Closed reduction transarticular Kirshner wire fixation versus open reduction internal fixation in the treatment of Bennett's fracture dislocation. *J Hand Surg* 2003;28B:142–147.
318. Breen TF, Gelberman RH, Jupiter JB. Intraarticular fractures of the basilar joint of the thumb. *Hand Clin* 1988;4:491–501.
319. Foster RJ, Hastings H II. Treatment of Bennett, Rolando and vertical intraarticular trapezial fractures. *Clin Orthop Relat Res* 1987;214:121–129.
320. Liebovic SJ. Treatment of Bennett's and Rolando's fractures. *Tech Hand Upper Ext Surg* 1998;2:36–46.
321. Buchler U, McCollam SM, Oppikofer C. Comminuted fractures of the basilar joint of thumb: combined treatment by external fixation, limited internal fixation, and bone grafting. *J Hand Surg* 1991;16A:556–560.
322. Proubasta IR. Rolando's fracture of the first metacarpal. Treatment by external fixation. *J Bone Joint Surg* 1992;74B:416–417.
323. Langhoff O, Anderson K, Kjaer Petersen K. Rolando's fracture. *J Hand Surg* 1991;16B: 454–459.
324. Timmenga EJF, Blokhuis TJ, Maas M, et al. Long term evaluation of Bennett's fracture. A comparison between open and closed reduction. *J Hand Surg* 1994;19B:373–377.
325. Thurston AJ, Dempsey SM. Bennett's fracture: a medium to long term review. *Aust NZ J Surg* 1993;63:120–123.
326. Bruske J, Bednarski M, Niedzwiedz Z, et al. The results of operative treatment of fractures of the thumb metacarpal base. *Acta Orthop Belg* 2001;67:368–373.
327. Kjaer Peterson K, Langoff O, Andersen K. Bennett's fracture. *J Hand Surg* 1990;15B: 58–61.
328. Dartee DA, Brink PRG, Van Houtte HP. Iselin's operative technique for thumb proximal metacarpal fractures. *Injury* 1992;23:370–372.
329. Van Niekerk JLM, Ouwens R. Fractures of the base of the first metacarpal bone: results of surgical treatment. *Injury* 1989;20:359–361.
330. Ouellette EA. Use of the minicondylar plate in metacarpal and phalangeal fractures. *Clin Orthop Relat Res* 1996;327:38–46.
331. O'Rourke SK, Gaur S, Barton NJ. Long term outcome of articular fractures of the phalanges: an eleven year follow up. *J Hand Surg* 1989;14B:183–193.
332. Van Oosterom FJT, Brete GJV, Ozdemir C. Treatment of phalangeal fractures in severely injured hands. *J Hand Surg* 2001;26B:108–111.
333. Buchler U, Gupta A, Ruf S. Corrective osteotomy for post-traumatic mal-union of the phalanges of the hand. *J Hand Surg* 1996;21B:33–42.
334. Peacock KC, Hanna DP, Kirkpatrick K, et al. Efficacy of perioperative cefamandole with postoperative cephalexin in the primary outpatient treatment of open wounds of the hand. *J Hand Surg* 1988;13A:960–964.
335. Suprock MD, Hood JM, Lubahn JD. Role of antibiotics in open fractures of the finger. *J Hand Surg* 1990;15A:761–764.

336. Sloan JP, Dove AF, Maheson M, et al. Antibiotics in open fractures of the distal phalanx? *J Hand Surg* 1987;12B:123–124.
337. Stevenson J, McNaughton G, Riley J. The use of prophylactic flucloxacillin in treatment of open fractures of the distal phalanx within an accident and emergency department: A double-blind randomized placebo-controlled trial. *J Hand Surg* 2003;28B:388–394.
338. Strickland JW, Steichen JB, Kleinman WB, et al. Phalangeal fractures, factors influencing digital performance. *Orthop Rev* 1982;11:39–50.
339. Page SM, Stern PJ. Complications and range of motion following plate fixation of metacarpal and phalangeal fractures. *J Hand Surg* 1998;23A:827–832.
340. Bostock S, Morris MA. The range of motion of the MP joint of the thumb following operative repair of the ulnar collateral ligament. *J Hand Surg* 1993;18B:710–711.
341. Helm RH. Hand function after injuries to the collateral ligaments of the metacarpophalangeal joint of the thumb. *J Hand Surg* 1987;12B:252–255.
342. Gollamudi S, Jones WA. Corrective osteotomy of mal united fractures of phalanges and metacarpals. *J Hand Surg* 2000;25B:439–441.
343. Lester B, Mallik A. Impending malunions of the hand. Treatment of subacute, malaligned fractures. *Clin Orthop Relat Res* 1996;327:55–62.
344. Pichora DR, Meyer R, Maeser VR. Rotational step cut osteotomy for treatment of metacarpal and phalangeal malunion. *J Hand Surg* 1991;16A:551–555.
345. Trumble T, Gilbert M. In situ osteotomy for extraarticular malunion of the proximal phalanx. *J Hand Surg* 1998;23A:821–826.
346. Van der Lei B, de Jonge J, Robinson PH, et al. Correction osteotomies of phalanges and metacarpals for rotational and angular malunion: a long term follow up and a review of the literature. *J Trauma* 1993;35:902–908.
347. Wray RC Jr, Glunk R. Treatment of delayed union, nonunion and malunion of the phalanges of the hand. *Ann Plast Surg* 1989;22:14–18.
348. Creighton JJ Jr, Steichen JB. Complications in phalangeal and metacarpal fracture management. *Hand Clin* 1994;10:111–116.
349. Vahey JW, Wegner DA, Hastings H II. Effect of proximal phalangeal fracture deformity on extensor tendon function. *J Hand Surg* 1998;23A:673–681.
350. Duncan KH, Jupiter JB. Intraarticular osteotomy for malunion of metacarpal head fractures. *J Hand Surg* 1989;14A:888–893.
351. Light TR. Salvage of intraarticular malunions of the hand and wrist. The role of realignment osteotomy. *Clin Orthop Relat Res* 1987;214:130–135.
352. Thurston AJ. Pivot osteotomy for the correction of malunion of metacarpal neck fractures. *J Hand Surg* 1992;17B:580–582.
353. Menon J. Correction of rotary malunion of the fingers by metacarpal rotational osteotomy. *Orthopaedics* 1990;13:197–200.
354. Kjaer Peterson K, Jurik AG, Peterson LK. Intraarticular fractures at the base of the fifth metacarpal. A clinical and radiographic study of 64 cases. *J Hand Surg* 1992;17B:144–147.
355. Jupiter JB, Koniuch MP, Smith RJ. The management of delayed union and nonunion of the metacarpals and phalanges. *J Hand Surg* 1985;10A:457–466.
356. Itoh Y, Uchinishi K, Oka Y. Treatment of pseudarthrosis of the distal phalanx with the palmar midline approach. *J Hand Surg* 1983;8:80–84.
357. Weiss APC. Intramedullary Herbert screws for treatment of phalangeal nonunion. *Tech Hand Upper Ext Surg* 1997;1:41–47.
358. Wright TC, Dell PC. Avascular necrosis and vascular anatomy of the metacarpals. *J Hand Surg* 1991;16A:540–544.
359. Posner MA, Langa V, Ambrose L. Intrinsic muscle advancement to treat chronic palmar instability of the metacarpophalangeal joint of the thumb. *J Hand Surg* 1988;13A:110–115.
360. Schuurman AH, Bos KE. Treatment of volar instability of the metacarpophalangeal joint of the thumb VY volar capsulodesis. *J Hand Surg* 1993;18B:346–349.
361. Carroll RE, Carlson E. Diagnosis and treatment of injury to the second and third carpometacarpal joints. *J Hand Surg* 1989;14A:102–107.
362. Clendenin MB, Smith RJ. Fifth metacarpal hamate arthrodesis for posttraumatic osteoarthritis. *J Hand Surg* 1984;9A:374–378.
363. O'Sullivan ST, Limantzakis G, Kay SP. The role of low-profile titanium miniplates in emergency and elective hand surgery. *J Hand Surg* 1999;24B:347–349.
364. Stahl S, Lerner A, Kaufman T. Immediate autografting of bone in open fractures with bone loss of the hand: a preliminary report. Case reports. *Scand J Plast Reconstr Surg Hand Surg* 1999;33:117–122.
365. Ishida O, Ikuta Y, Kuroki H. Ipsilateral osteochondral grafting for finger joint repair. *J Hand Surg* 1994;19:372–377.
366. Gaul JS. Articular fractures of the proximal interphalangeal joint with missing elements: repair with partial toe joint osteochondral autografts. *J Hand Surg* 1999;24:78–85.
367. Bozic KJ, Perez LE, Wilson DR, et al. Mechanical testing of bioresorbable implants for use in metacarpal fracture fixation. *J Hand Surg* 2001;26:755–761.
368. Waris E, Ashammakhi N, Happonen H, et al. Bioabsorbable miniplating versus metallic fixation for metacarpal fractures. *Clin Orthop Relat Res* 2003;410:310–319.
369. Waris E, Ashammakhi N, Raatikainen T, et al. Self-reinforced bioabsorbable versus metallic fixation systems for metacarpal and phalangeal fractures: a biomechanical study. *J Hand Surg* 2002;27:902–909.

FRACTURES AND DISLOCATIONS OF THE CARPUS

Christian Gaebler

The carpus is a complex unit of bony articulations that transfers the force and motion of the hand to the supporting forearm and upper extremity. It allows a wide range of motion in two major planes and with its adjacent radioulnar joints permits a substantial rotatory arc around the longitudinal axis of the forearm. Unlike a simple hinge joint, such as the elbow, the wrist involves a delicate interaction between eight carpal bones that are divided into two carpal rows (1–3). While the main motions are flexion–extension and radioulnar deviation, the primary axis of motion of the carpal bones resides within the head of the capitate, which is not a singular point, but rather an oblique screw axis for combined motions of wrist extension/flexion and radial/ulnar deviation (4–6). To produce this natural movement, individual carpal bones not only turn up and down and back and forth, but also spin and roll about their own axes.

GENERAL, TOPOGRAPHIC, SURGICAL, AND APPLIED ANATOMY

Bones and Joints

The carpus is composed of eight bones in two rows (Fig. 25-1). The articular surfaces of the joints that make up the wrist have important roles in subsequent integrated movements of the wrist. The eight carpal bones are influenced by the shape of the distal radius, the distal ulna, and the triangular fibrocartilage complex (TFCC).

The proximal row consists of the scaphoid, the lunate, and the triquetrum. The proximal carpal row is regarded by many authors as an "intercalated segment" between the radius and the distal row, the keystone in the coordination of motions of the wrist as well as in the control of forces that are transmitted from the hand to the forearm and vice versa. To cope with such an important role, the three proximal row bones continuously need to adapt their position and orientation to guarantee the necessary joint congruency between the radius and distal row. Articular joint congruency depends on joint geometry and the integrity of the ligaments that connect the three bones to each other and to the surrounding bones, as the proximal carpal row has no direct tendon attachments (2,3,7,8).

The pisiform is a sesamoid bone enclosed in the sheath of the flexor carpi ulnaris tendon; accordingly, it does not belong directly to the proximal carpal row. It may stabilize the proximal

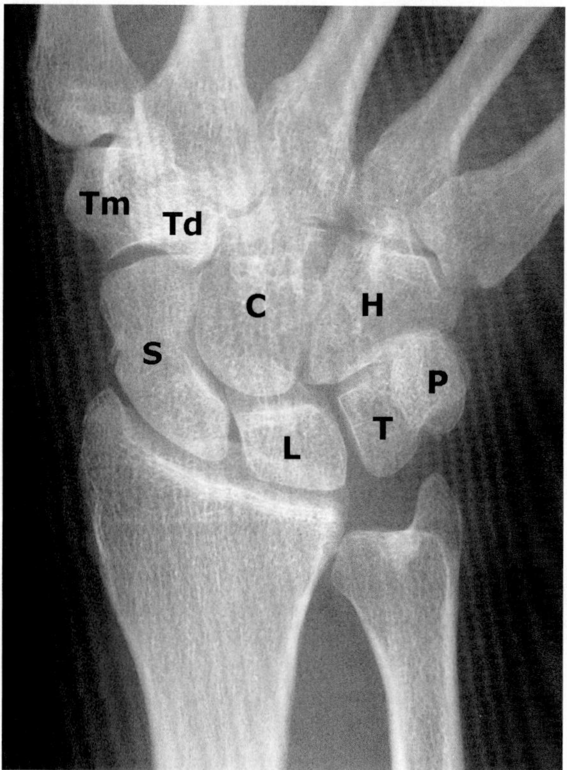

FIGURE 25-1 The wrist is composed of two rows of bones that provide motion and transfer forces: scaphoid (S), lunate (L), triquetrum (T), pisiform (P), trapezium (Tm), trapezoid (Td), capitate (C), hamate (H).

carpal row indirectly by acting on the triquetrum via the pisotriquetral joint.

The distal row, which is more stable and moves as a unit, consists of the trapezium, the trapezoid, the capitate, and the hamate. The distal row forms a rigid, supportive transverse arch upon which the five metacarpals of the hand are supported. The trapezium articulates with the first metacarpal, the trapezoid with the second, and the capitate with the third one. The capitate and trapezoid are tightly connected to the metacarpals, whereas there is 30 degrees to 40 degrees of flexion–extension and rotation at the metacarpotrapezial joint. The hamate articulates with the fourth and fifth metacarpal.

Ligaments of the Wrist

The carpal bones are supported by both extrinsic and intrinsic ligaments (8–10).

Extrinsic Ligaments

Extrinsic ligaments link the carpal bones to the radius, ulna, and metacarpals and are attached to roughened areas on the dorsal and palmar surfaces. The transverse carpal ligament is an extrinsic ligament that connects the scaphoid tuberosity and trapezial ridge with the hamate and pisiform to provide structural integrity to the proximal carpal arch. It also constrains the flexor tendons.

The deeper extrinsic ligaments are intracapsular ligaments best observed from within the radio- and midcarpal joints. From an external view, the ligaments appear as condensations of the fibrous capsule (Fig. 25-2) and are difficult to distinguish through the superficial adventitia. They are, however, quite prominent from the intra-articular aspect of the joint (1).

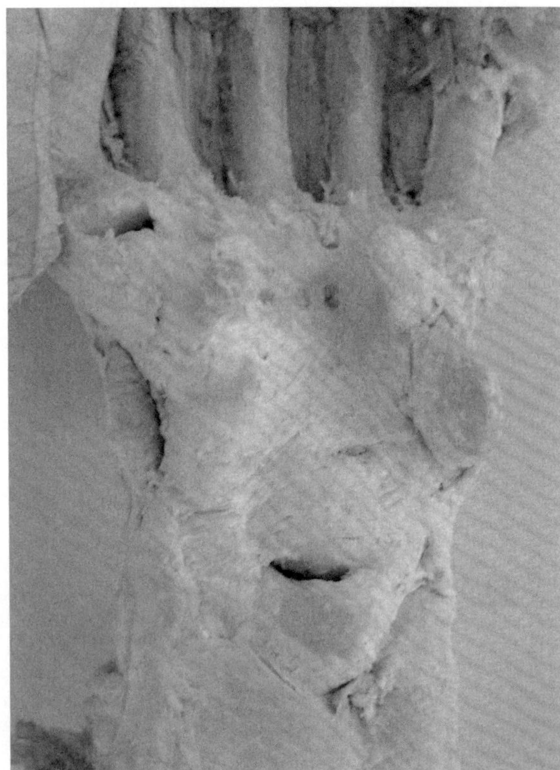

FIGURE 25-2 It is difficult to distinguish the extrinsic ligaments from the fibrous capsule, however, they are quite prominent from the intra-articular aspect of the joint.

Palmar Wrist Ligaments. The palmar wrist ligaments originate laterally from a radial-palmar facet of the radial styloid and are directed in a distal ulnar direction, where they meet ligaments originating medially from the TFCC and the distal ulna.

The stronger and more oblique radial ligaments prevent the carpus from translating ulnarly on the medially angulated slope of the distal radius. The palmar extrinsic ligaments consist of two V-shaped ligamentous bands: one is proximal and connects the forearm to the proximal carpal row; one is distal and connects the forearm to the distal carpal row. The distal limb of the palmar extrinsic ligaments consists of the radioscaphocapitate ligament laterally and the ulnocapitate ligament medially (Fig. 25-3). The proximal limb consists of the radiolunatotriquetral and radioscaphoid ligaments laterally and the ulnolunate und ulnotriquetral ligaments medially.

The radioscaphoid ligament that inserts into the tuberosity of the scaphoid is the radial expansion of the radioscaphocapitate ligament, which courses over the palmar concavity of the scaphoid proximal to the tuberosity before inserting on the palmar aspect of the keel and neck of the capitate (1). It appears to act as a sling across the waist of the scaphoid over which the scaphoid rotates and it usually does not have a ligamentous insertion into the scaphoid itself.

The distal portions of the radio- and ulnocapitate ligaments do not attach to the head of the capitate, but form a support sling commonly referred to as the "arcuate ligament." Between these two rows of ligaments is a thinned area termed the "Space of Poirier" (11). This area expands when the wrist is dorsiflexed and disappears in palmar flexion. A rent develops during dorsal dislocations, and it is through this interval that the lunate displaces into the carpal canal.

The extrinsic palmar radiolunate (RL) ligaments have been subdivided into short and long radiolunate ligaments. The radioscapholunate ligament originates from the palmar aspect of the ridge between the scaphoid and lunate fossae and inserts into the scapholunate interosseus ligament (12,13). The radioscapholunate ligament acts as a neurovascular supply to the scapholunate interosseus membrane and it is not a true extrinsic ligament of the wrist.

Dorsal Wrist Ligaments. The dorsal ligaments of importance are the radio- and scaphotriquetral (dorsal intercarpal) ligaments, which describe a V-shape from the dorsal aspect of the distal radius near Lister's tubercle to the triquetrum and then back to the dorsal scaphoid rim. The radial capsule is thickened and fused with the radioscaphoid ligament, while the ulnodorsal capsule is augmented by the floors of the fifth and sixth dorsal compartments. There are no true collateral ligaments (1).

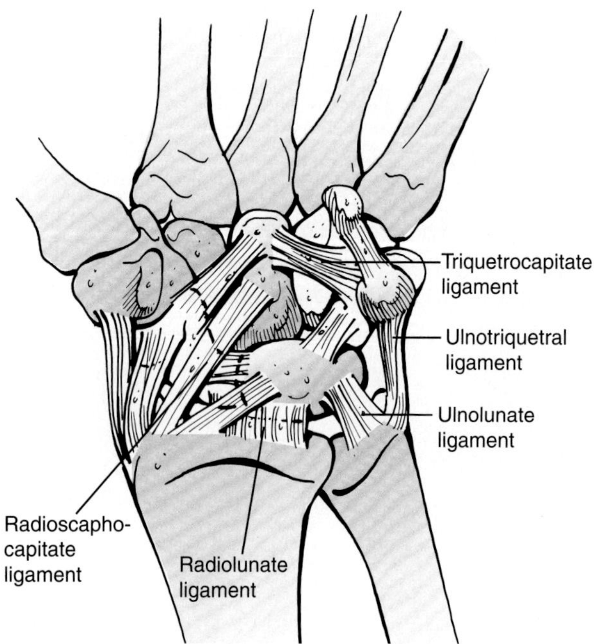

FIGURE 25-3 The palmar capsule consists of two major ligamentous inclusions: the radiolunate ligament is the deeper of the two, which proceeds to the triquetrum and composes in effect the radiolunotriquetral ligament. The more distal and superficial component is often referred to as the arcuate ligament or distal V. The radial component of this ligament is the radioscaphocapitate ligament. The ulnar component of the arcuate ligament is the triquetrocapitate ligament.

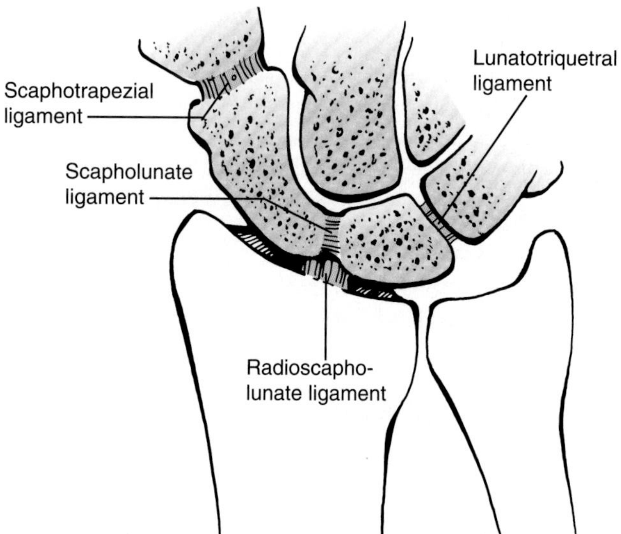

FIGURE 25-4 The intra-articular intrinsic ligaments connect adjacent carpal bones.

Another group of extrinsic ligaments support the midcarpal joint and couple the distal carpal bones to each other. On the radial side of the wrist, a V-shaped scaphotrapezial ligament extends from the scaphoid tuberosity to the palmar tubercle of the trapezium. Adjacent to it medially are the scaphocapitate and palmar capitotrapezial ligaments and the capitotrapezoidal ligament. On the ulnar side of the wrist, the triquetrocapitate and the triquetrohamate ligaments are a continuation of the ulnotriquetral ligament (1).

Intrinsic Ligaments

The intrinsic ligaments interconnect individual carpal bones, particularly the scaphoid, lunate, and triquetrum. They are collections of relatively short fibers that bind the bones of either the proximal or distal rows to each other (8–10). In the proximal carpal row, the ligaments are intra-articular, connecting the scaphoid to the lunate and the lunate to the triquetrum (Fig. 25-4). There is a contiguous blending of the interosseous ligaments with the joint articular cartilage.

Laterally, the strong scapholunate interosseous ligament (SLIL) has been shown to consist of three components: palmar, central, and dorsal. The scapholunate ligament (SL) has an important role in carpal stability. The dorsal SL ligament is the key SL joint stabilizer. It is formed by a thick collection of fibers and transversely oriented, linking the dorsomedial edge of the scaphoid to the dorsolateral rim of the lunate. The palmar SL ligament, a secondary SL stabilizer, is formed by longer, more obliquely oriented fibers. The long fibers of the palmar portion of the scapholunate interosseous membrane allow the scaphoid flexibility as it rotates on the lunate. The dorsal third of the ligament is the strongest, while the palmar ligament has more laxity. The central third appears to be a fibrocartilaginous membrane, which blends with the adjacent cartilage of scaphoid and lunate. The membrane is thicker palmarly, as it incorporates a richly vascularized expansion from the radioscapholunate ligament (1,9,14–16).

The lunatotriquetral interosseous ligament (LTIL) is similarly formed from two interosseous ligaments (palmar and dorsal) connecting the proximal edges of triquetrum and lunate. It interdigitates with the dorsal radiotriquetral ligament and palmar ulnotriquetral, ulnolunate, and radiolunatotriquetral insertions. The palmar third of the LT ligament is stronger than the dorsal third being supported by strong palmar ulnocarpal ligaments. Its fibers are tighter through all ranges of motion than the SL ligaments, making for a closer kinematic relationship (1,9,10).

Neurovascular Anatomy

The innervation and blood supply of the wrist and carpus come from the regional nerves and vessels. Circulation of the wrist is obtained through the radial, ulnar, and anterior interosseous arteries and the deep palmar arch. The extraosseous arterial pattern is formed by an anastomotic network of three dorsal and three palmar arches connected longitudinally at their medial and lateral borders by the radial and ulnar arteries (Fig. 25-5). In addition to transverse and longitudinal anastomoses, there are dorsal to palmar interconnections between the dorsal and palmar branches of the anterior interosseous artery (17–19).

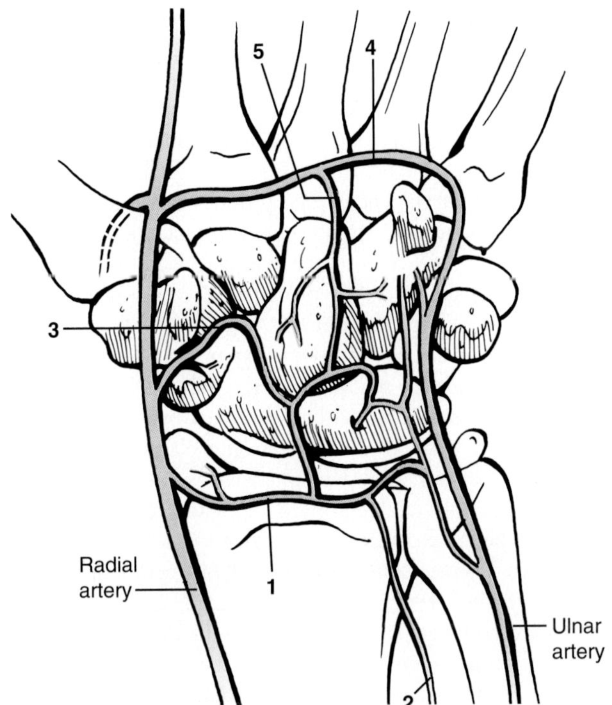

FIGURE 25-5 Schematic drawing of the arterial supply of the palmar aspect of the carpus. Circulation of the wrist is obtained through the radial, ulnar, and anterior interosseous arteries and the deep palmar arch: (1) palmar radiocarpal arch, (2) palmar branch of anterior interosseous artery, (3) palmar intercarpal arch, (4) deep palmar arch, (5) recurrent artery.

The intrinsic blood supply to the carpal bones is an important factor in the incidence of osteonecrosis (ON) after trauma (19). Studies (17,18,20) show three patterns of intraosseous vascularization:

1. The scaphoid, capitate, and about 20% of all lunates are supplied by a single vessel and thus are at risk for osteonecrosis.
2. The trapezium, triquetrum, pisiform, and 80% of lunates receive nutrient arteries through two nonarticular surfaces and have consistent intraosseous anastomoses. ON is therefore rare.
3. The trapezoid and hamate lack an intraosseous anastomosis and, after fracture, can have avascular fragments.

These observations extend previous work, which showed that the blood supply to most carpal bones enters the distal half, leaving the proximal half at risk. There is no interval, for example, by which the scaphoid can be approached without endangering some of the branches that supply its circulation. The lunate blood supply is constantly endangered by common dorsal approaches to the wrist, but the blood supply from the palmar radiocarpal arch is usually sufficient to maintain its blood supply. With fracture dislocations of the wrist, the palmar radiolunate ligament usually remains intact because the dislocation is distal through the space of Poirier.

Mechanism of Injury

The most common mechanism of injury is an axial compression force applied with the wrist in hyperextension, in which the palmar ligaments are placed under tension and the dorsal joint surfaces are compressed and subject to shear stresses (1,8,21). Depending on the degree of radial or ulnar deviation, a ligament or bone injury or a combination of both will result. A scaphoid fracture appears to occur when the wrist is dorsiflexed past 95 degrees and radially deviated by 10 degrees. In this position, the proximal pole of the scaphoid is securely held by the radius and the proximal radioscaphocapitate ligament while the distal pole of the bone is carried dorsally by the trapeziocapitate complex (Fig. 25-6). The radioscaphoid ligament is relaxed by the radial deviation and cannot alleviate the tensile stresses accumulating on the radiopalmar aspect of the scaphoid. The fracture then propagates dorsally and can be transverse, oblique, or comminuted depending on the direction of the applied loads (22).

The most common injury is a fall on the outstretched hand, when the individual straightens the arm for protection, and the

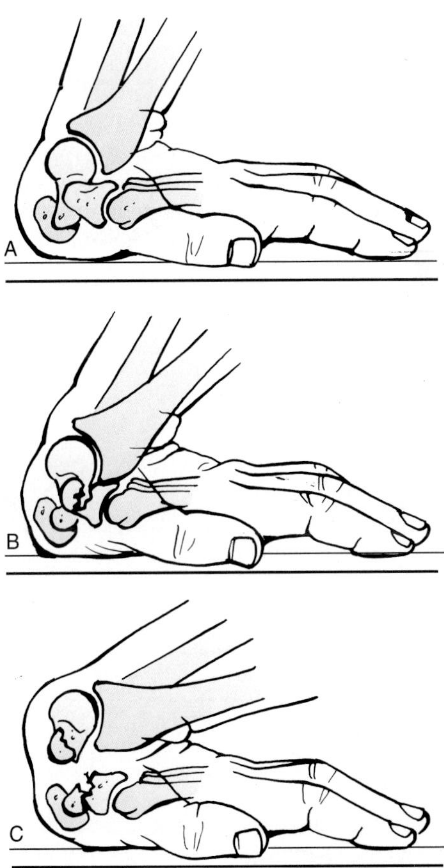

FIGURE 25-6 The most common mechanism of injury is an axial compressive force applied with the wrist in hyperextension. **A–C.** The drawings show the fracture mechanism of the scaphoid where the proximal pole of the scaphoid is trapped between the radius and the tense palmar extrinsic ligaments—and the full force is concentrated at the waist of the scaphoid.

body weight and exterior forces are concentrated across the wrist. Other mechanisms include palmar flexion, as occurs in an over-the-handlebars motorcycle accident, or twisting injuries in sports where the hand is forcefully rotated against the stationary body. Ligament tears involve more substantial force to the hand. High-energy forces result in carpal bone fractures or ligamentous disruptions of both intrinsic and extrinsic ligaments and perilunate dislocations. The majority of these injuries occur around the lunate, which as the carpal keystone is held most securely to the distal radius. Several authors have shown (1,23) that many injuries to the wrist appear to be sequential variants of perilunate dislocation. Minor injuries, such as sprains, result from low-energy forces.

Kinematics

The global motion of the wrist is composed of flexion extension, radioulnar deviation at the radiocarpal joint, and axial rotation around the distal radioulnar joint (DRUJ) (3). The radiocarpal articulation acts as a universal joint allowing a small degree of intercarpal motion around the longitudinal axis related to the rotation of individual carpal bones. The forearm accounts for about 140 degrees of rotation. Radiocarpal joint motion is primarily flexion–extension of nearly equal proportions (70 degrees) and radial and ulnar deviation of 20 degrees and 40 degrees, respectively. This amount of motion is possible as a result of complex arrangements between the two carpal rows. During flexion and extension, each carpal row angulates in the same direction with nearly equal amplitude and in a synchronous fashion (3,6,24,25) (Fig. 25-7). Much of the wrist's versatility, however, is due to the intercalated three-bone system of the proximal carpal row. During radioulnar deviation the proximal row exhibits a secondary angulation in the sagittal plane to the synchronous motion occurring in the coronal plane. Radial deviation induces flexion of the obliquely situated scaphoid as the trapezium approaches the radius. Through the dorsal aspect of the scapholunate ligament, this motion is transmitted sequentially to the lunate and triquetrum, which flex approximately 25 degrees (1,3,16). As the carpus moves back to neutral and onto full ulnar deviation the proximal row extends and supinates with respect to the radius.

The scaphoid can be observed to extend with ulnar deviation but it is the proximal migration of the hamate that forces the triquetrum to displace palmarly and extend, bringing the lunate with it. This rotation, by varying the length and contour of the proximal carpal row, allows for extensive excursion of the wrist while maintaining stability around a longitudinal axis. This has been described as the "variable geometry" of the proximal carpal row. When this mechanism is disrupted by fracture or ligamentous injury, the wrist becomes destabilized. The usual arcs of motion are no longer synchronous, and the intercarpal contact patterns change. A snap, catch, or clunk can be appreciated with motion of the wrist, particularly when under compressive load. Instability leads, in time, to degenerative changes as a consequence of increased shear forces and abnormal contact between individual carpal bones.

Normally, in the coronal plane, the center of rotation of the wrist is located within a small area in the capitate neck. A line drawn through the axis of rotation parallel with the anatomical

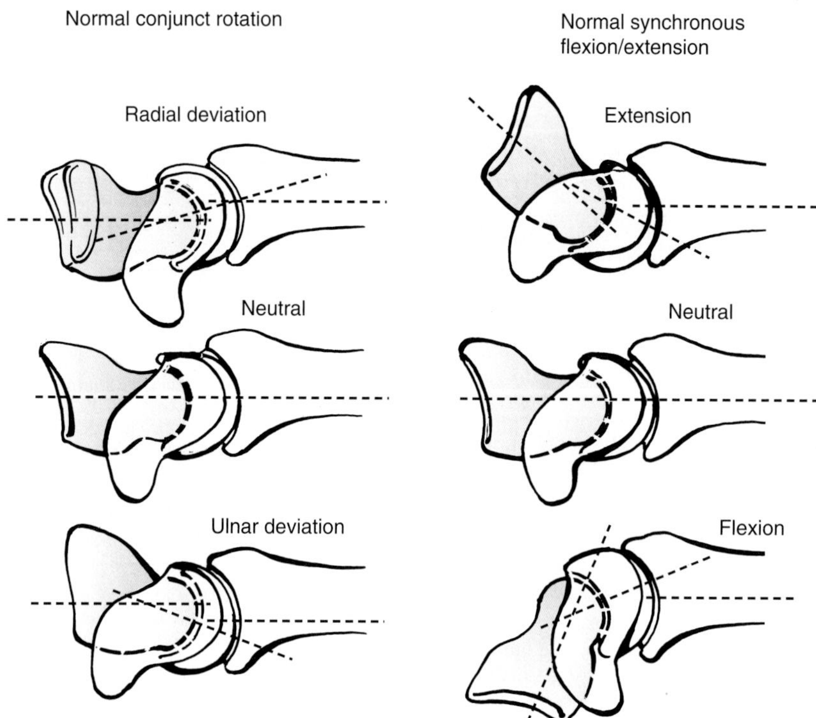

FIGURE 25-7 Conjunct rotation of the entire proximal row occurs in flexion during radial deviation (*upper left*). The axes of the radius and carpal rows are collinear in neutral (*middle left*), and the proximal row extends with ulnar deviation (*lower left*). Angulatory excursions of the proximal and distal rows are essentially equal in amplitude and direction during extension (*upper right*) and flexion (*lower right*). This has been described as synchronous angulation.

axis of the forearm will, with the hand in neutral position, pass through the head and base of the third metacarpal, the capitate, the radial aspect of the lunate, and the center of the lunate fossa of the radius (6). In the sagittal plane with the wrist in neutral flexion–extension, a line passing through the longitudinal axis of the capitate, lunate, and radius will show these to be nearly superimposed or colinear. The scaphoid axis lies at 45 degrees to this line and passes between the lunate and capitate in a fashion that provides optimal stability to the midcarpal joint. The scaphoid acts as a stabilizing strut or column to support the central column. By virtue of its obliquity, the scaphoid will flex when under compression and exerts a similar force on the lunate. The lunate, however, is also under the influence of the triquetrum, which inherently prefers to extend. For this reason, the lunate may be thought of as being in a state of dynamic balance between two antagonists. It tends to lie in the position of least mechanical potential energy (1).

Volar Intercalated Segment Instability and Dorsal Intercalated Segment Instability

When the dynamic balance is interrupted, the lunate will tend to flex with loss of ulnar support from the triquetrum (Fig. 25-8). When the lunate slips into a statically fixed position of flexion >15 degrees, volar intercalated segment instability (VISI) is present. VISI is typical of lunatotriquetral dissociation (LTD), nondissociative carpal instability, and a carpal instability complex in which associated instabilities are also present.

When the lunate slips into fixed extension >10 degrees dorsal intercalated segment instability (DISI) is present. The relative alignment of the scaphoid to the lunate, which is usually about 45 degrees, is important. When this exceeds 70 degrees, the ligamentous linkage between the scaphoid and lunate is usually inoperative. The lunate then generally adopts an extended position (i.e., DISI) and maintains this position even during radial deviation thus interrupting the normal rotation and the spatial adaptability of the proximal row. The same is true when the lunate is fixed in flexion in a VISI deformity. The wrist will not extend even during ulnar deviation. A DISI deformity is rarely seen in acute scaphoid fractures when it indicates gross carpal instability. It is more often seen in association with scaphoid pseudarthrosis and scapholunate dissociation, where it indicates the degree of carpal collapse deformity that has occurred. In advanced cases, the capitolunate joint becomes subluxed and may show signs of degenerative arthritis (26).

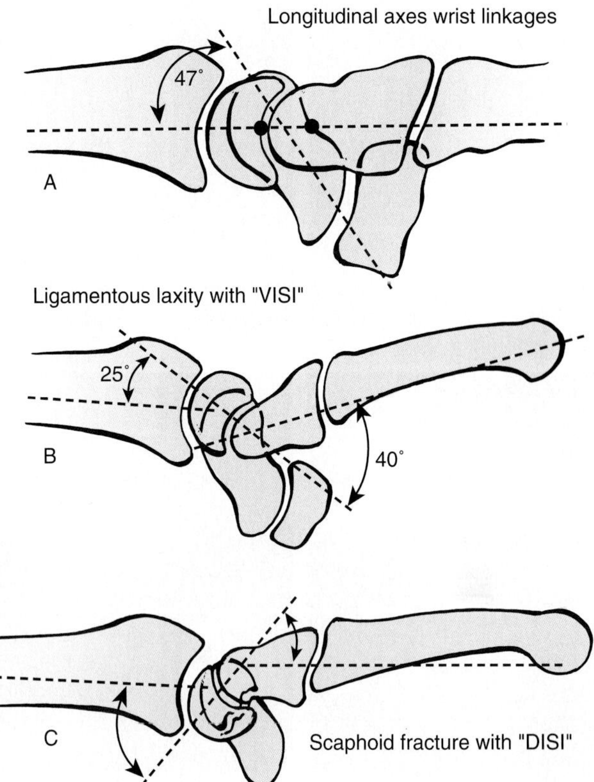

FIGURE 25-8 Schematic drawing of carpal instability. **A.** Normal longitudinal alignment of the carpal bones with the scaphoid axis at a 47 degree angle to the axes of the capitate, lunate, and radius. **B.** VISI deformity is usually associated with disruption of the lunatotriquetral ligament. **C.** DISI deformity is associated with scapholunate ligament disruption or a displaced scaphoid fracture.

IMAGING OF THE CARPUS

Radiographic Examination

It is not easy to differentiate clinically if a fall on the outstretched hand led to an injury of the wrist or to an injury of the carpus. The two most important views to diagnose an injury are the posteroanterior (PA) and lateral x-rays, each taken in the exactly neutral position. For further diagnosis of carpal and mainly scaphoid fractures, the author suggests radial oblique (supinated PA) and ulnar oblique views (Fig. 25-9). These four standard views detect most of the carpal injuries (27). If there is the suspicion of carpal instability, additional views in maximal radial and ulnar deviation are recommended. Further views can be done in maximal flexion and extension.

In the normal carpus, with the wrist in neutral position, the longitudinal axes of the long finger metacarpal, capitate, lunate, and the radius all fall in the same line. The longitudinal axis of the scaphoid can be drawn through the midpoints of its proximal and distal poles. Using these axes, it is possible to measure angles that define the positions of the carpal bones. For example, the scapholunate angle averages 45 degrees and ranges from 30 degrees to 60 degrees in normal wrists. An angle greater than 70 degrees suggests instability, and one greater than 80 degrees is almost certain proof of carpal instability. A capitolunate angle of more than 20 degrees is also strongly suggestive of carpal instability.

Gilula's lines (three smooth radiographic arcs) should be examined on the PA view. Disruption of these arcs indicates ligamentous instability (28). The assessment of Gilula's line continuity should be a standard in the evaluation of all PA wrist

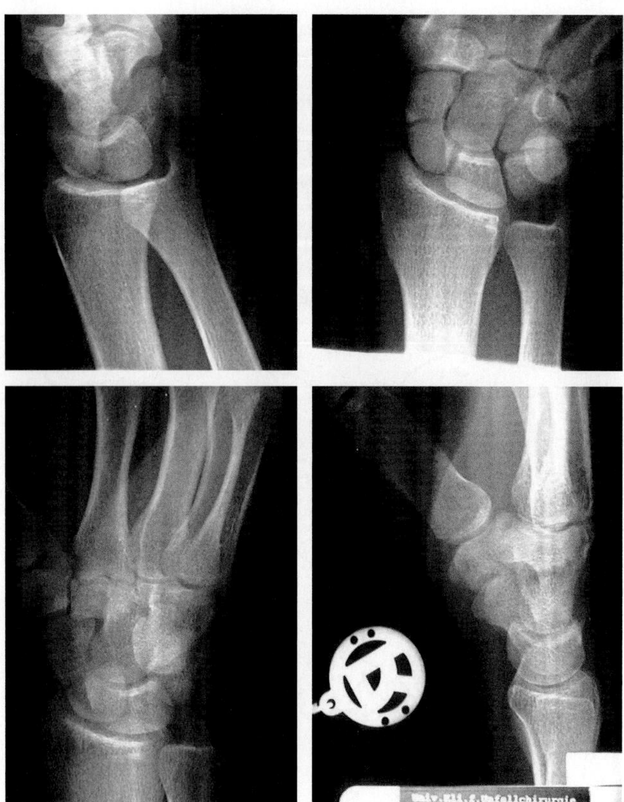

FIGURE 25-9 The four scaphoid views (PA, true lateral, radial oblique, ulnar oblique) detect most of carpal fractures. A fisted PA view can be helpful in detecting scaphoid fractures.

x-rays to prevent a missed diagnosis of a perilunate dislocation (Fig. 25-10).

DISI and VISI patterns are diagnosed easily by lateral x-rays. The DISI pattern is most commonly observed with displaced scaphoid fractures and scapholunate dissociation (SLD), while the VISI pattern is more likely to be associated with lunotriquetral dissociation (LTD).

SLD and LTD are diagnosed by PA views. The normal x-ray should show a constant space between scaphoid, lunate, and triquetrum, which is maintained throughout the range of motion. The joint space between scaphoid and lunate is usually 1 to 2 mm. With SLD, an increasing gap appears, which may in time be wide enough to accept proximal migration of the entire capitate head. A spread of more than 3 mm is considered abnormal, and a gap greater than 5 mm is confirmatory of an SL injury. In addition, the scaphoid flexes palmarward, which gives it less of an elongated profile on the PA view and projects the cortical waist of the scaphoid as an overlapping ring of bone inside the scaphoid projection "the cortical ring sign." The lunate also moves into a DISI position, which can be visualized on the PA view by the increasing overlap of the capitate silhouette by a lunate horn producing a wedge shape (Fig. 25-10B). With LTD, a gap between the two bones is not usually evident, but a break in the normal carpal arc of the proximal carpal row can be seen.

Carpal height ratio, which is carpal height divided by the length of the third metacarpal, is used to quantify carpal collapse. One method of measuring carpal height is to determine the distance between the base of the third metacarpal and the articular surface of the distal radius using a line bisecting the middle of the radius and metacarpal. The carpal height ratio, however, is of little significance in assessing ligament damage in wrist hyperextension injuries.

Special Imaging Techniques

Arthrography, magnetic resonance (MR) wrist arthrography, video radiography, and arthroscopy can assist in the diagnosis of carpal ligament injuries (1,29). Computed tomography (CT) scans are helpful in evaluating carpal fractures, malunion, nonunion, and bone loss. Three dimensional imaging is of use in planning reconstructive procedures for malunions and nonunion. Macroradiography does not show any advantage in diagnosing carpal fractures, particularly scaphoid fractures compared with normal x-rays (30).

Bone scans can be helpful in confirming occult fractures and avulsion injury (31,32). However, MRI scans are more sensitive in detecting occult fractures and ON of the carpal bones (33,34) as well as in detecting soft-tissue injuries, including ruptures of the scapholunate ligament and TFCC injuries.

Imaging Pearls and Pitfalls

Pearls

- Standard scaphoid views detect most carpal injuries.
- A DISI pattern is most commonly observed with displaced scaphoid fractures and scapholunate dissociation.
- A VISI pattern is more likely to be associated with lunotriquetral dissociation.
- MRI scans are useful in detecting occult fractures, ON of the carpal bones, and ligamentous injuries.

Pitfalls

- Perilunate dislocations are easily missed if the continuity of Gilula's line is not assessed.

SCAPHOID FRACTURES

Acute fractures of the scaphoid were first recognized in 1889 by Cousin and Destot before the discovery of x-rays. They were also well described by Mouchet and Jeanne in 1919. Fractures of the scaphoid are common and account for about 50% to 80% of carpal injuries (Table 25-1) (1). Scaphoid fractures predominantly occur in young, active individuals. The position of the scaphoid on the radial side of the wrist, as the proximal extension of the thumb ray, makes it vulnerable to injury. The

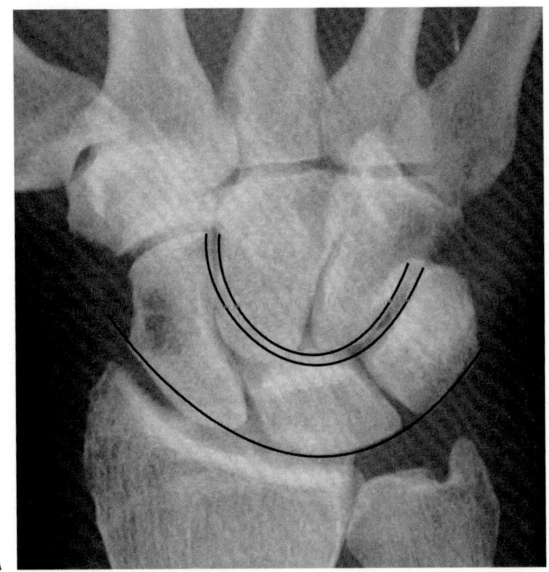
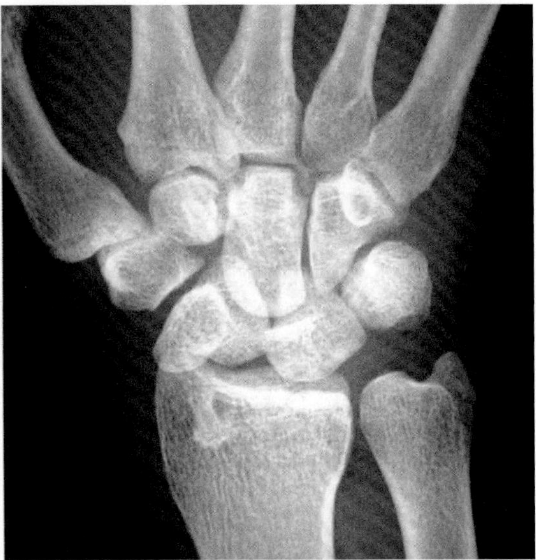

FIGURE 25-10 Gilula's lines. **A.** PA views show three smooth Gilula arcs in a normal wrist. These arcs outline proximal and distal surfaces of the proximal carpal row and the proximal cortical margins of capitate and hamate. **B.** Arc I is broken, which indicates an abnormal lunotriquetral joint due to a perilunate dislocation. Additional findings are the *cortical ring sign* produced by the cortical outline of the distal pole of the scaphoid and a trapezoidal shape of the lunate.

annual incidence of carpal fractures in the United States was reported at more than 678,000 in 1995, of which at least 70% (47,000) represent fractures of the scaphoid (35,36). Fractures of the scaphoid are second only to fractures of the distal radius among fractures of the upper extremity but have an obviously different demographic profile. Unlike distal radius fractures, scaphoid fractures are common among young men with a peak incidence in the second and third decades (37,38). The average time for healing of a nondisplaced scaphoid fracture in a cast is 8 to 12 weeks, accounting for a considerable loss of time and productivity in this young and active population (1,34,39–44).

TABLE 25-1 Relative Incidence of Carpal Bone Fractures*

Bone	Incidence
Scaphoid	68.2%
Triquetrum	18.3%
Trapezium	4.3%
Lunate	3.9%
Capitate	1.9%
Hamate	1.7%
Pisiform	1.3%
Trapezoid	0.4%

* Gelberman RH, Panagis JS, Taleisnik J, et al. The arterial anatomy of the human carpus: Part I. The extraosseous vascularity. *J Hand Surg* 1983;8-A:367–376.

Anatomy

The scaphoid is one of the smallest bones of the human body. It is an irregularly shaped tubular bone, twisted and bent into an S-shape (Fig. 25-11), It resembles a deformed peanut or a boat (from the Greek word for boat, *skaphos*). It lies entirely within the wrist joint, with more than 80% of its surface being covered by articular cartilage (26), which reduces its capacity for periosteal healing and increases its tendency for delayed union and nonunion. The scaphoid is located in a 45 degree plane to the longitudinal and horizontal axes of the wrist.

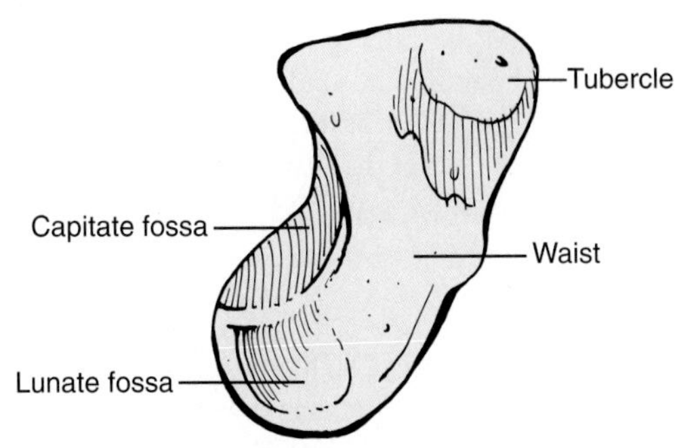

FIGURE 25-11 Schematic drawing of the scaphoid.

The scaphoid is concave on its ulnar surface, where it articulates like a socket with the spherical head of the capitate. Proximally there is a small, semilunar facet for articulation with the lunate. The proximal third of the radial surface is convex and articulates with the radius. Distal to this articulation is the waist, grooved on its palmar surface by the radioscaphocapitate ligament, which acts as a sling across the waist of the scaphoid although it has no connection to the bone itself. Taleisnik (10) suggested that the radioscaphocapitate ligament provided a fulcrum for the scaphoid. The scaphoid is ridged across its nonarticular dorsoradial surface, along which the critical dorsal ridge vessels traverse. The ridge acts as an insertion point for both the dorsal component of the scapholunate interosseous ligament (15), as well as the intercarpal ligament (45). The distal pole is pronated, flexed, and ulnarly angulated with respect to the proximal pole and presents separate articular surfaces to the trapezium and trapezoid distally (46).

The stability of the scaphoid depends to a great extent on the short intrinsic ligaments (Fig. 25-4) that attach it to the lunate and distally to the trapezium and trapezoid. Motion in these joints is restricted by the strong ligaments, which permit a degree of rotation proximally and a degree of gliding distally (26). These ligaments merge with the extrinsic ligaments and capsule, which are loose enough to allow free motion of the scaphoid within the wrist. Otherwise, the scaphoid has no ligamentous or tendinous attachments and acts with the rest of the proximal carpal row as an "intercalated segment."

Biomechanics

The scaphoid acts as a link across the midcarpal joint, connecting the proximal and distal carpal rows. Any shear strain that occurs across the midcarpal joint is transferred through the scaphoid, and may cause fractures and dislocations. Through its stout proximal and distal ligamentous connections, the scaphoid serves to coordinate and smooth the motions of the proximal and distal rows, and it has been likened to a slider-crank mechanism that stabilizes an inherently unstable dual link system as the midcarpal joint tends to assume a lunate-extended posture unless constrained by an intact scaphoid (8,47). The kinematic effect of an unstable scaphoid fracture is a dissociation of the proximal and distal carpal rows that permits the natural tendency of the two carpal rows to fail by collapsing. This is demonstrated clinically by the collapse pattern seen with chronic scaphoid nonunion, a condition called "scaphoid nonunion advanced collapse" appearing as DISI (7,47,48). Under axial load, the two halves of the scaphoid collapse into a flexed or "humpback" posture (49,50).

Vascularity

The scaphoid receives most of its blood supply from two major vascular pedicles (18,51). One enters the scaphoid tubercle and supplies its distal 20% to 30% and the other arises from the dorsal scaphoid branch of the radial artery (Fig. 25-12). The dorsal ridge vessels enter through numerous small foramina along the spiral groove and dorsal ridge. This source accounts for about 80% of the blood supply. Several studies have shown no vascular supply or only a single perforator proximal to the waist of the scaphoid (40,51,52). Because of its unusual retrograde vascular supply, the scaphoid has a high risk of nonunion and ON after fracture. Temporary interruption of the blood supply to the proximal fragment is virtually certain with proximal pole fractures but, if stabilized, the proximal pole has the capacity to revascularize and heal (47,53,54).

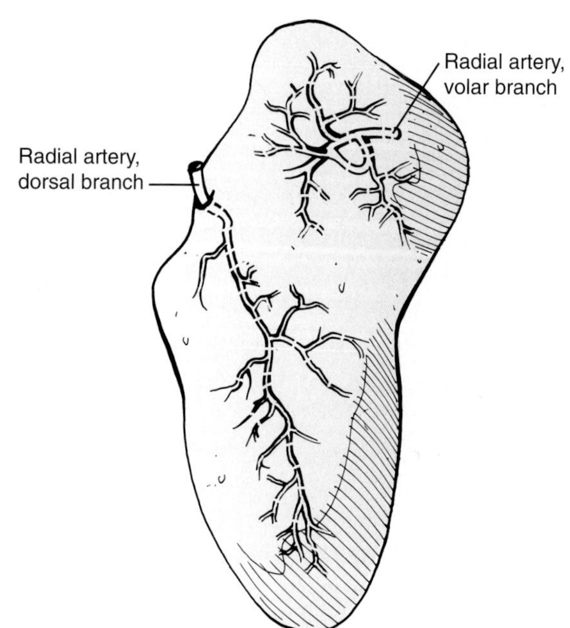

FIGURE 25-12 The vascular supply of the scaphoid is provided by two vascular pedicles.

Fracture Mechanism and Functional Anatomy

Scaphoid fractures are common in young men due to falls, athletic injuries (particularly heavy falls when tackling during a game of football), or motor vehicle accidents as it requires a considerable amount of force to break the scaphoid bone. In most patients, a clear history of a fall on the outstretched hand can be elicited.

The mechanism of fracture is usually considered to be bending with compression dorsally and tension on the palmar surface, owing to forced dorsiflexion of the wrist. When the wrist is extended beyond 95 degrees, the proximal pole of the scaphoid is tightly held between the capitate, the dorsal lip of the radius, and the taut palmar capsule. Fracture of the scaphoid occurs at the waist, which is exposed to the maximal bending movement (22). However, scaphoid fractures can be caused by several other mechanisms (39). The force must be sufficient to produce at least a transient subluxation of the joint. This is only one step away from the classic transscaphoid perilunate fracture

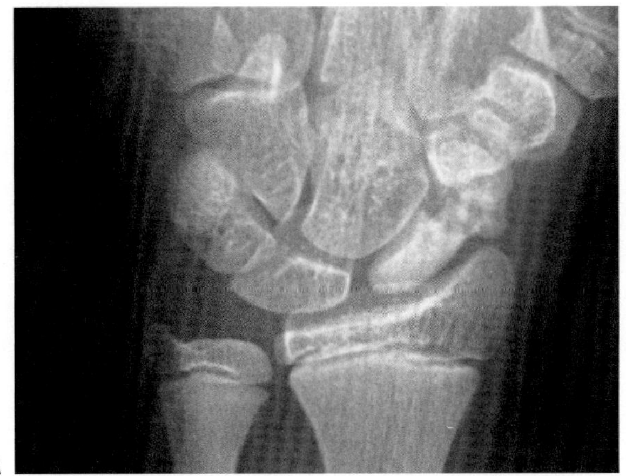
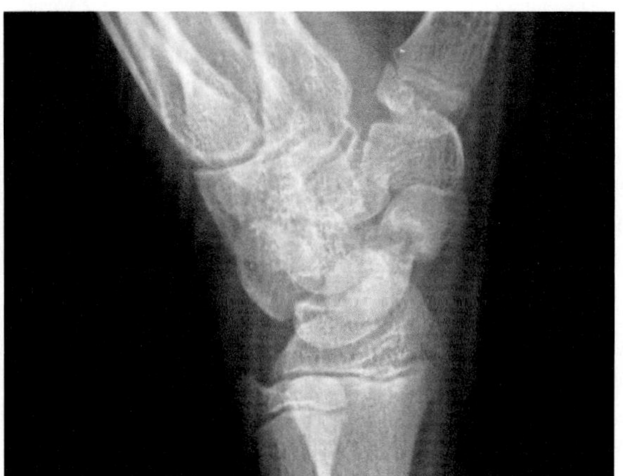

FIGURE 25-13 Symptomatic scaphoid nonunion in a 12-year-old boy due to a fall 2 months before.

dislocation that results from more severe trauma. Thus, there must be a subtle difference between the degree of force required to produce an occult fracture, a complete but stable fracture, or an unstable fracture of the scaphoid. Herbert (26) states that since the line of the midcarpal joint crosses the proximal pole in radial deviation and the distal pole in ulnar deviation, the wrist deviation at the time of injury might determine the line of fracture. Fractures of the waist are usually the result of shear forces across the scaphoid. Fractures of the tubercle, like radial styloid fractures, appear to be caused by either compression or avulsion (41). Small proximal pole fractures can be caused by an avulsion of the attachment of the scapholunate ligament.

Scaphoid fractures in children are uncommon, because the physis of the distal radius usually fails first. However, scaphoid fractures can occur in children and x-rays are mandatory to diagnose this injury (Fig. 13A,B). Concomitant fractures of the distal radius have been reported. Most fractures heal with cast at an average of 6 to 8 weeks; however, nonunion and ON can occur (55–57). In the elderly, the distal radial metaphysis usually fractures before the scaphoid.

Fractures of the scaphoid result in significant functional disability as well as time off work, loss of earnings, and interference with recreational activities. Common problems with the fractured scaphoid are diagnosis (58) and posttraumatic complications include pain, dysfunction, malunion, delayed union, and nonunion.

Malunion occurs because the distal pole of the fractured scaphoid tends to flex and the proximal scaphoid extends with the proximal carpal row, initially causing a dorsal fracture gap followed by the humpback deformity (Fig. 25-14) (7). Despite the lack of direct tendon attachments, joint compressive forces, trapezium-scaphoid shear stress, and capitolunate rotation moments all act on the fractured scaphoid. The scaphoid often assumes an anteverted position, the lunate and triquetrum

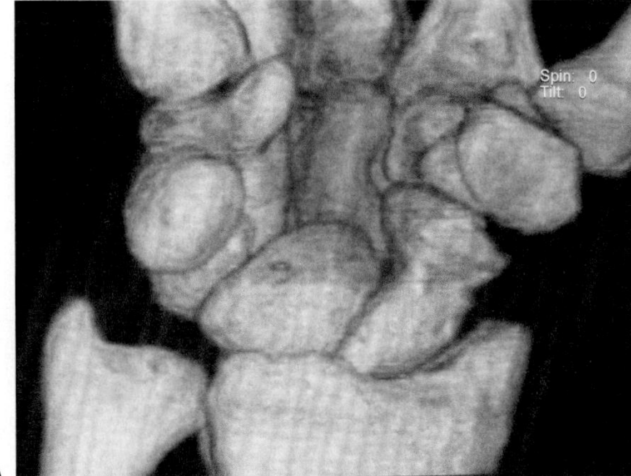

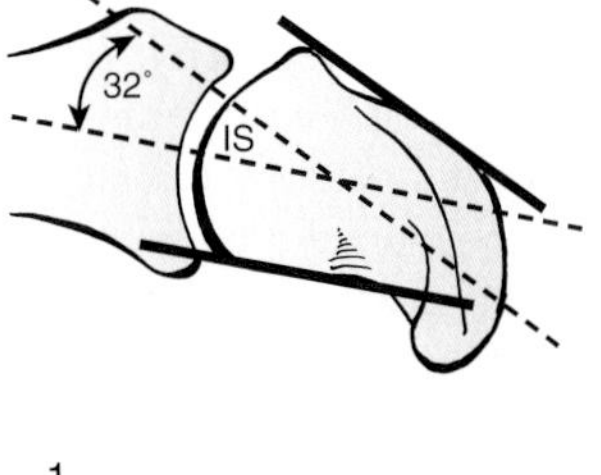

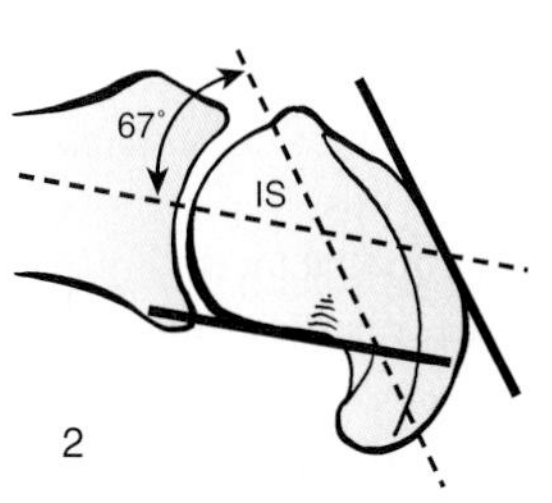

FIGURE 25-14 **A.** CT scan of a scaphoid fracture that has healed with a humpback deformity. **B.** Schematic drawing of scaphoid: (1) Normal scaphoid, (2) Humpback deformity. The normal intrascaphoid angle (IS) is 30 degrees ± 5 degrees. The humpback deformity angle measure 67 degrees and the normal scaphoid 32 degrees.

subluxate forward and rotate dorsally, and the capitate and hamate subluxate dorsally and proximally, producing the DISI deformity (Fig. 25-8C) (26). As a consequence of these mechanical factors, as well as the critical vascularity of the scaphoid bone, scaphoid fractures have a high tendency toward delayed union and nonunion. Nonunion of the scaphoid is a severe problem, causing arthritis secondary to abnormal loading on the articular surfaces of the midcarpal joint, severe pain, and weakness.

Signs and Symptoms

Patients with scaphoid injuries usually complain of wrist pain after a fall on the outstretched hand. The diagnosis of a scaphoid fracture is made from the clinical history with about 90% of patients recalling a hyperextension injury, the clinical examination where the index of suspicion is raised, and by proper radiographic examination, which confirms the diagnosis. The importance of obtaining an accurate history cannot be overestimated, because both treatment and prognosis depend on the type of fracture and fracture mechanism (26). It is important to inquire carefully about previous trauma and not to treat a nonunion as if it was an acute fracture. Although tenderness in the anatomic snuffbox has been described as a classic finding in scaphoid fractures, it is an overly sensitive test that is notoriously inaccurate when used in isolation (59,60). Swelling and pain are usually apparent in acute fractures; however, these symptoms can be minimal. After 24 hours, there is often diffuse pain and swelling. Parvizi et al (60) showed that a combination of snuffbox tenderness, scaphoid tubercle tenderness, and pain with axial compression yielded a sensitivity of 100%. These authors found that any one of these tests in isolation was inadequate.

In sports injuries, it is not uncommon for the wrist injury to go unnoticed, with 25% of lunate and perilunate fracture dislocations being missed on initial examination in one multicenter study (61). Bruising tends not to be present except in fracture dislocations. However, swelling is often extreme occasionally leading to acute compartment syndrome. Range of motion is reduced, and there is usually pain at the extremes of motion. Clearly, these same physical findings may also be seen with ligamentous injuries of the wrist, and thus, whenever there are any findings suggestive of a scaphoid fracture, the patient should be treated for a suspected scaphoid fracture. Loss of wrist extension is also typical for ununited scaphoid fractures associated with carpal collapse deformity and palmar capsular contracture. Missed diagnosis is not uncommon and often results in additional morbidity from secondary changes, including nonunion, collapse deformity, and degenerative arthritis.

Radiographic Examination

Because of the inconsistency of clinical signs, the diagnosis of scaphoid fracture is usually made by x-ray. Radiographic diagnosis of a scaphoid fracture requires four x-rays—these being a posteroanterior view with the hand in a fist to extend the scaphoid, a lateral view, a radial oblique (supinated PA) view, and an ulnar oblique view (Fig. 25-9). These four views detect most scaphoid fractures (26,27,44,62). Comparative views of the opposite uninjured wrist are often helpful. It is difficult to diagnose scaphoid fractures on the lateral x-ray although this x-ray is essential to diagnose perilunate fracture dislocations and to evaluate the overall alignment of the carpus.

Barton (63) describes three common reasons as to why scaphoid fractures are incorrectly diagnosed.

1. A dark line may be formed by the dorsal lip of the radius overlapping the scaphoid.
2. The presence of a white line formed by the proximal end of the scaphoid tuberosity.
3. The dorsal ridge of the scaphoid may appear bent on the semisupinated view.

Motion views of the wrist (flexion–extension and radial and ulnar deviation) may demonstrate fracture displacement, which indicates an unstable scaphoid fracture. Since the scaphoid flexes in radial deviation and extends in ulnar deviation, the length of bone should be assessed by comparing ulnar and radial deviation views in both wrists. Assuming that the two views are identical, any difference in length must indicate a scaphoid deformity resulting from either a fracture or ligament injury (26). When instability of the scaphoid is suspected, careful analysis of the lateral x-ray for intrascaphoid angulation or a dorsally tilted lunate is recommended.

It is a well-known fact that undisplaced scaphoid fractures may not be visible on the initial set of x-rays, although it has been shown that this is rarely the case if they are evaluated by experienced observers (27,39). Clinical studies (64) have shown that scaphoid and pronator fat stripe signs are poor predictors of the presence or absence of underlying occult fractures. If there is clinical suspicion but x-rays are negative, a scaphoid cast is applied, and another set of scaphoid views is performed after 10 days (Fig. 25-15) (27). As most of the patients with suspected scaphoid fractures are young and active, early diagnosis is important. Macroradiography (30) and ultrasound (65) have a sensitivity of <50% in detecting occult scaphoid fractures. MRI scans are the most effective way of diagnosing scaphoid fractures (Fig. 25-16) (34,66). It has been shown that an MRI performed as early as 48 hours after the injury has a sensitivity and specificity approaching 100% and may have the potential to save as much as $7,200 per 100,000 inhabitants by avoiding loss of productivity owing to unnecessary cast immobilization (34). Technetium 99m bone scans (32,52,67) also have a high sensitivity in diagnosing occult fractures of the carpus. CT scans have the advantage of speed and can produce high-resolution fine-cut images of the scaphoid in multiple planes (68). Three-dimensional reconstructions of these scans can be helpful for planning operative procedures of scaphoid reconstruction.

Differentiation between an acute scaphoid fracture and a scaphoid nonunion is important for planning treatment, and good x-rays should distinguish between the two (1), although

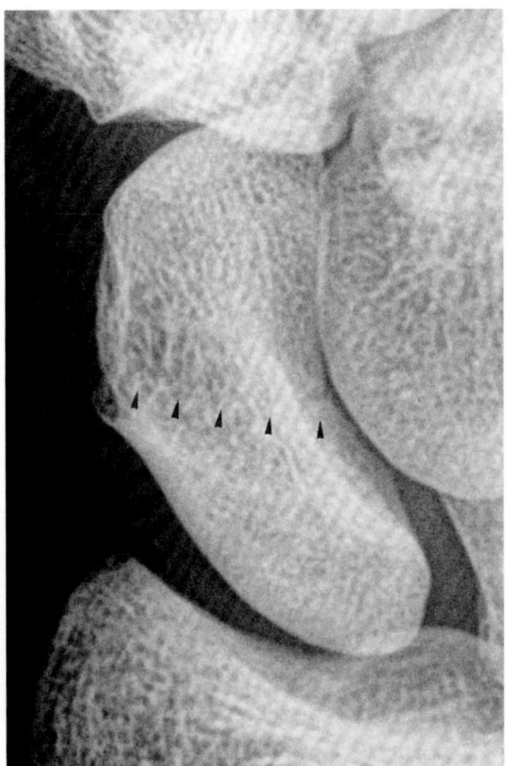

FIGURE 25-15 An occult fracture was detected 10 days after a fall on the outstretched hand. This fracture was not visible on the initial set of x-rays.

an MRI scan may be helpful. Not uncommonly, a second injury will draw attention to a minimally symptomatic nonunion that has been aggravated by the recent event. The acute scaphoid fracture is represented by a single line through the bone, occasionally with dorsoradial comminution and dorsal angulation. Late presentation of a fracture or an established nonunion may show resorption at the fracture site, subchondral sclerosis, and displacement on both the PA and lateral x-rays. The longer the time since injury, the greater the cystic resorption, the denser the sclerosis, the more prominent the shortening of the scaphoid, and the greater the loss of carpal height (26). Secondary degenerative changes are usually present by 10 to 15 years.

Associated Injuries

Fractures of the distal radius are not uncommon and injuries such as perilunate dislocation and transscaphoid perilunate fracture dislocations may occur. Whatever the mechanism of scaphoid fracture, it is important to remember that an x-ray never reveals the true degree of joint and ligament damage that inevitably accompanies this injury (26).

Classification

Classification by anatomical location has many proponents, some of whom attempt to correlate fracture union rate with the site of injury (Fig. 25-17). Waist fractures account for 80% of scaphoid fractures, with a further 15% being in the proximal pole, 4% in the tuberosity, and 1% being distal articular fractures. Herbert and Fisher (69) proposed a classification intended to identify those fractures most applicable for operative fixation (Table 25-2) (Fig. 25-18). They recommended early operative management of all acute fractures of the scaphoid waist or proximal pole, because of the incidence of displacement or nonunion.

The blood supply of the scaphoid is critical in regard to fracture location. Gelberman's work (18,20,51) confirmed earlier studies by demonstrating that the major blood supply comes from the scaphoid branches of the radial artery, which enter the dorsal ridge and supply 70% to 80% of the bone, including the proximal pole. The second major group of vessels enters the scaphoid tubercle, perfusing only the distal 20% to 30% of the bone. In fractures through the waist and proximal third,

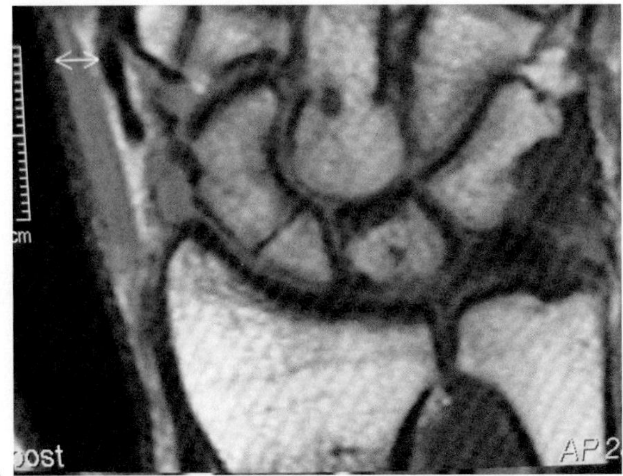

A

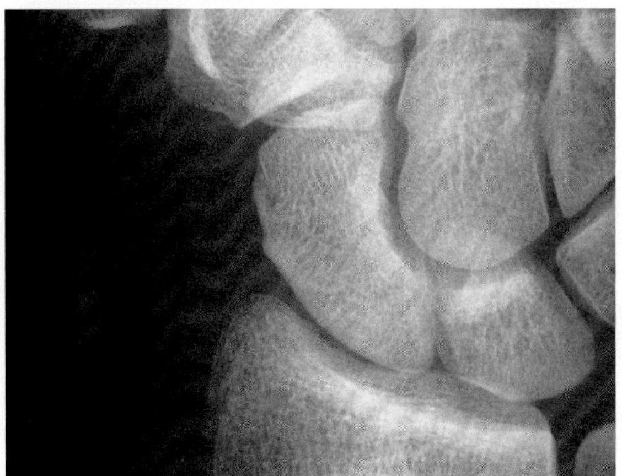

B

FIGURE 25-16 **A.** The MRI scan demonstrates a clear fracture line of the scaphoid (proximal pole). **B.** It is difficult to identify the proximal fracture by native x-rays.

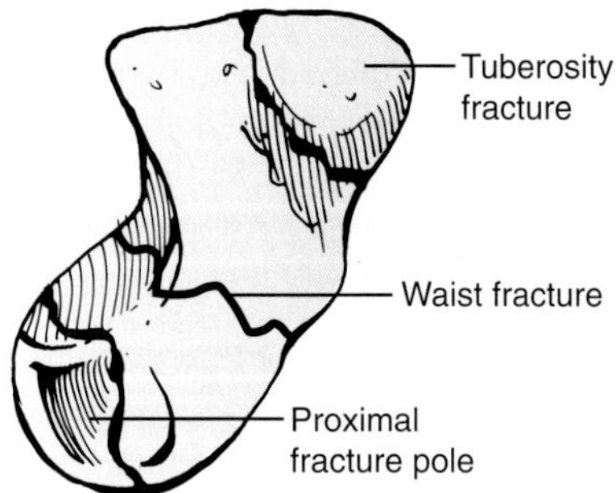

FIGURE 25-17 Classification of scaphoid fractures by anatomical location.

revascularization will occur only with fracture healing. One can reasonably assume that with proper treatment nearly 100% of tuberosity and distal third scaphoid fractures will heal as will 80% to 90% of waist fractures, but only 60% to 70% of proximal pole fractures will heal (1,26). Similarly union in oblique or shear fractures has been shown to be delayed in comparison to horizontal fractures. Comminuted or distracted osteochondral fractures have the poorest rate of union. The healing time for these different fracture types ranges from 4 to 6 weeks for tuberosity fractures, 6 to 8 weeks for occult and stable fractures, 10 to 12 weeks for distal third and waist fractures, and 12 to 20 weeks for comminuted and proximal pole fractures.

Occult Scaphoid Fractures

Undisplaced fissures and fractures of the scaphoid might not be visible on the initial set of radiographs. Patients with wrist injuries are usually seen in the emergency department by less experienced doctors who are aware of the dangers of missing a scaphoid fracture and who know that up to 30% of all scaphoid fractures might not be detected on initial x-rays (27,39,70). Knowledge of the poor outcome of undiagnosed and untreated scaphoid fractures ending in pseudarthrosis of the scaphoid and severe radiocarpal arthritis leads to a tendency to overtreatment. To avoid missing a few occult fractures of the scaphoid, some patients are immobilized for prolonged periods of time without a diagnosis being made before being seen by a senior surgeon (38,63).

Diagnosis of Occult Scaphoid Fractures

It has been demonstrated that radionuclide (32,67) and MRI scans (34,71) are reliable methods of diagnosing occult fractures of the scaphoid. MRI has a higher sensitivity and specificity in the diagnosis of occult fractures of the scaphoid compared to other methods of diagnosis and might even be more cost effective than repeated clinical examinations and x-rays (34). However, most countries do not have the facilities to refer patients with supposedly minor injuries for an MRI scan. The literature states that there is low inter- and intraobserver reliability in diagnosing occult scaphoid fractures on plain x-rays (31,32). Scaphoid fractures and other injuries to the wrist might not be

TABLE 25-2 Classification of Scaphoid Fractures

Type A: Stable acute fractures

Features:
- Fracture appears incomplete (only one cortex involved)
- Union normally rapid
- Minimal treatment required

Type A1: Fracture of tuberosity

Type A2: Incomplete fracture through waist

Type B: Unstable acute fractures

Features:
- Fracture likely to displace in plaster
- Delayed union common
- Internal fixation is the treatment of choice

Type B1: Distal oblique fracture

Type B2: Complete fracture of waist

Type B3: Proximal pole fracture

Type B4: Transscaphoid-perilunate fracture dislocation of carpus

Type B5: Comminuted fractures

Type C: Delayed union

Features:
- Widening of the fracture line
- Development of cysts adjacent to the fracture
- Relative density of the proximal fragment

Type D: Established nonunion

Type D1: Fibrous union

Features:
- Common after conservative treatment
- Relatively stable
- Little or no deformity
- Variable cystic change
- Likely to progress to pseudarthrosis in time
- Surgery is normally required

Type D2: Pseudarthrosis

Features:
- Usually unstable
- Progressive deformity
- Leads to development of osteoarthritis
- May result following untreated fibrous union (Type D)
- Surgery is normally required

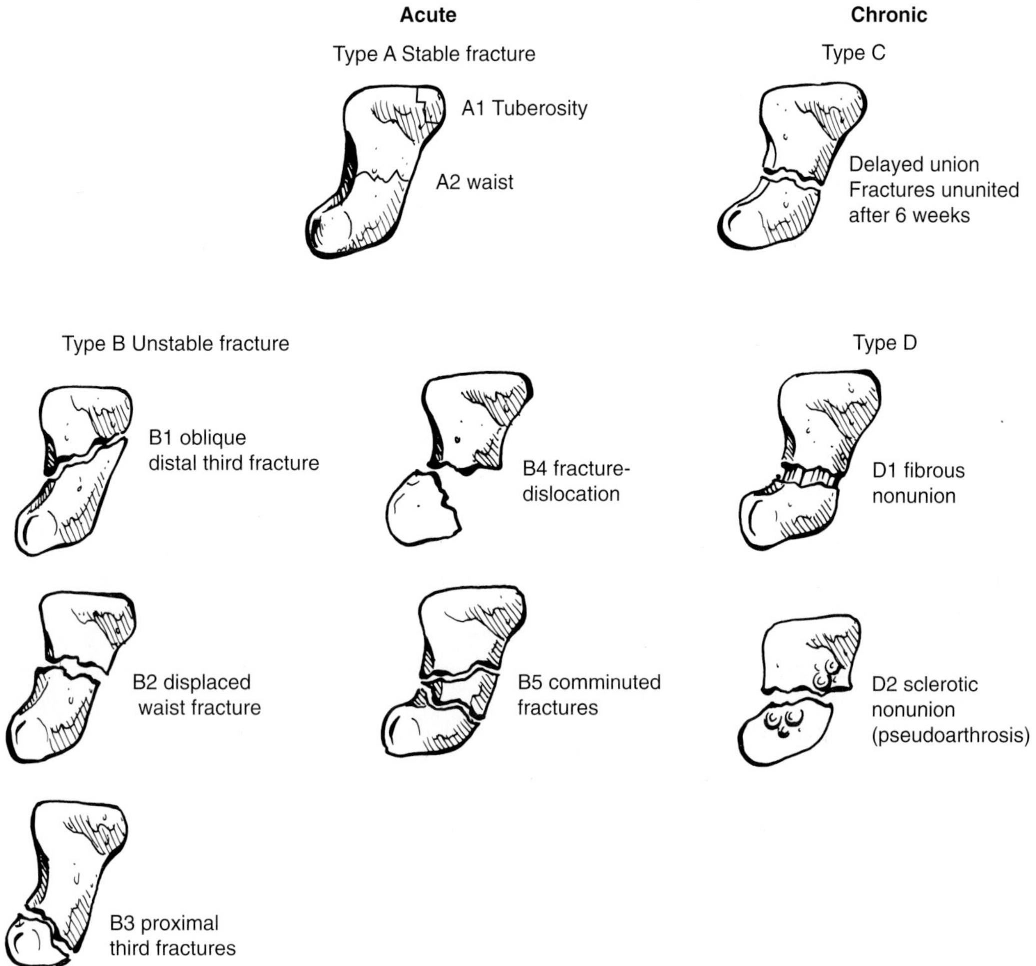

FIGURE 25-18 Schematic drawing of Herbert and Fisher's classification of fractures of the scaphoid.

very painful initially, although persisting pain clearly indicates an injury. The diagnosis is usually made by a combination of clinical and radiological findings (26), which means that the evaluation of x-rays even by experienced radiologists can lead to poor diagnostic results (31). If an occult fracture of the scaphoid or severe concomitant wrist injury is suspected but not visible on initial x-rays, the wrist should be immobilized for 10 days in a forearm cast or splint, and the patient should be seen then by an experienced surgeon and a repeat scaphoid series obtained. However, a prospective study has shown that 70% of all "occult" scaphoid fractures and 60% of avulsion fractures are visible on the initial set of x-rays (27). There is little doubt that MRI scans are the most reliable method of diagnosing occult carpal and wrist fractures at an early stage (34,66). However, it has been shown that repeated clinical examinations and x-rays can also detect occult fractures of the scaphoid and associated wrist injuries in a reasonable time (27). N'Dow et al (70) showed that patients with suspected injuries to the scaphoid and wrist were often seen for months by junior staff and unnecessarily immobilized for the same time. It is therefore advised that a protocol be adopted where senior members of staff see these patients at the first follow-up and at least once again after 6 weeks.

Because of its high sensitivity and specificity, MRI is the "gold standard" in the diagnosis of occult fractures of the wrist. However, if MRI is not available, adequate clinical follow-up and radiography should lead to the correct diagnosis. It is important to include the radius and proximal aspects of the metacarpals in the scaphoid series to evaluate possible injuries to these bones. Fractures of the radius, ulna, and the metacarpals occur in 13% of all cases (27).

Only 30% of all scaphoid fractures are really occult, but 85% of all other carpal fractures are true occult fractures (27). About 66% of carpal avulsion fractures and distal radial fractures are detectable on the initial set of scaphoid views (27). A few more might be diagnosed by more views, but up to 16 x-rays as suggested by Trojan (44) would seem to be an unnecessary waste of time, money, and potentially harmful. The literature suggests that there may be up to 34% of other wrist injuries where an occult scaphoid fracture is initially suspected (69,72).

However, the author (27) found a higher rate of these injuries. Of all the injuries detected, only 25% were scaphoid fractures. The other 75% consisted of carpal fractures other than the scaphoid (13%), avulsion fractures of extrinsic ligaments (12.5%), fractures of the distal radius (12%), bone bruises (10%), other fractures (26.5%), and soft-tissue injuries (26%).

MR imaging is cost effective compared to repeated clinical and radiographic follow-up examinations (34). However, many countries provide MRI scans only for emergency situations or do not have MRI facilities at all. The results of a prospective study showed that repeat clinical and radiographic examinations are adequate (27). They will reveal occult fractures of the scaphoid and other occult fractures of the wrist but have the disadvantage that STI remains undetected except for ruptures of the scapholunate ligament, resulting in scapholunate dissociation.

Current Treatment Options

Occult Fractures

Early diagnosis of an occult scaphoid fracture is important. If MRI scans prove the diagnosis, cast immobilization should be used. Above elbow casts and scaphoid casts are not required and a simple Colles forearm cast should be used for 4 to 6 weeks. Check x-rays should be obtained at the time of cast removal. If there are still clinical and radiological signs of a scaphoid fracture, another cast is applied for two more weeks.

If MRI is not available and there is clinical suspicion of an occult fracture of the scaphoid, a Colles cast should be applied. Most nonunions are caused by the patient or surgeon suspecting a simple wrist sprain and undertaking no further diagnosis or treatment. The solution is a simple clinic policy. Patients with a suspected occult scaphoid fracture and negative x-rays are treated by the application of a Colles cast for 10 to 14 days. After this time, the cast is removed and a further scaphoid series undertaken. In most cases, a correct diagnosis is then made and appropriate treatment undertaken.

Fractures of the Tubercle (Type A1)

These are benign fractures and represent an avulsion injury. Although some authors suggest that splinting is adequate, the author prefers cast immobilization for 4 weeks. This injury represents a soft-tissue injury and requires time to heal properly. X-rays can show persistent displacement and fibrous union causing no disability, although these findings are more commonly seen in fractures treated without immobilization.

Undisplaced Scaphoid Fractures (Type A2)

Conservative Treatment. Undisplaced scaphoid fractures are usually stable. However, it is not always easy to decide whether this is the case. Thus radiological follow-up is mandatory, and surgery may be necessary if the fracture displaces. If there is doubt about the fracture type and the presence of displacement, a CT scan is recommended with the treatment being based on the findings.

As most authors suggest that cast immobilization is the method of choice for the primary treatment for undisplaced fractures of the scaphoid, the important questions to be answered are: which joints should be immobilized, and what type of cast should be applied?

Above-Elbow Casts. Some authors still advocate the use of above-elbow casts in scaphoid fractures citing union rates of 95%. However, studies have shown no advantage to the use of above-elbow casts (39,73). In fact, Kuhlmann et al (74) in a prospective study found the above-elbow cast harmful, as it blocked the normal rotation of forearm bones and transferred any rotational movement to the radiocarpal joint where it caused movement at the fracture.

Scaphoid Casts. Before 1942, Böhler proposed the use of an unpadded dorsal backslab, but in 1942, he changed the cast to include the proximal phalanx of the thumb (39). This method of treatment quickly became accepted and is still used in many hospitals. However, Trojan (44), one of Böhler's pupils, assessed most of the patients treated by Böhler and found no advantage in the use of the scaphoid cast and advocated its use only for highly unstable and proximal pole fractures.

Colles Cast. Yanni et al (75) found that, provided the wrist was neither ulnar deviated nor extended, the position of the thumb had no influence on the fracture gap. Clay and coworkers, in a large prospective randomized study, showed that there was no difference in union rates whether the thumb was immobilized or not (76). For this reason the use of Colles or forearm casts, rather than scaphoid casts is advocated.

There is a general consensus that most stable scaphoid fractures unite in 6 to 8 weeks with cast immobilization However, bone consolidation can take 12 to 16 weeks, and some fractures will not have healed even after this time. Apart from the fact that vertical and proximal fractures have a worse prognosis than other scaphoid fractures, there is unfortunately no reliable way of predicting the outcome in undisplaced fractures (39).

Herbert and Fisher (69) believed the incidence of nonunion to be about 50% and they advocated internal fixation of scaphoid fractures with a newly designed screw. However, the idea of internal fixation was not new. McLaughlin (77) published the first results in 1954, followed by Streli (72) in 1970. The development of percutaneous techniques has improved operative treatment for both patient and surgeon, minimizing the operative risks and nonunion rates (78–80). The author (40) showed in a randomized study that percutaneous screw fixation of undisplaced fractures gives significantly better results and a significantly lower rate of nonunion together with shorter times to return to work and sports when compared to conservative treatment. These findings have been corroborated by other surgeons (78,81,82).

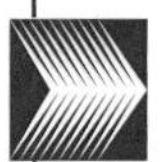

AUTHOR'S PREFERRED TREATMENT

Undisplaced Scaphoid Fractures (Type A2)

Cast Immobilization

The author recommends a Colles cast for nondisplaced stable scaphoid fractures in low-demand patients, with the wrist in neutral deviation and neutral flexion–extension for 8 to 12 weeks until there is radiographic union. The decision to treat patients conservatively is based on the fact that a CT scan shows no displacement. Careful clinical and radiographic follow-up examinations at the time of cast removal are essential. It is recommended that the patient be reviewed 6 weeks after cast removal for clinical and radiological examination and then every 3 months until the outcome is clear. Patients should be seen for a final check up after 1 year.

Percutaneous Screw Fixation

In all other patients with acute scaphoid fractures, the author prefers percutaneous screw fixation. This includes the majority of young high-demand patients. The method is relatively easy and, if the patient is compliant, it allows postoperative treatment without cast immobilization. The advantage of this minimally invasive method is early return to sports and work in a population which is usually young and active (40,78). No serious complications are expected when the surgical procedure is performed carefully. Of all the screws available the author prefers the Acutrak® screw (Acumed, Inc., Beaverton, Oregon, USA), which has some key features that make it different from other cannulated screws (Fig. 25-19J). It was developed to produce interfragmentary compression while eliminating the exposed head. The thread pitch varies at a constant rate along the length of the screw. This accumulation of pitch differentials results in gradual compression at the fracture site. The taper on the outer profile of the screw causes the threads to constantly purchase new bone. This minimizes thread damage and improves pull-out strength. Biomechanical studies have shown that the Acutrak® variable pitch, tapered, headless, compression screw performed significantly better and provided superior fixation than did the Herbert compression screw, and it was often better than the AO lag screw (63,83–86). Another screw with superior compression capacities is the TwinFix screw (Stryker®), which allows compression after the screw has been inserted into the bone.

The operative procedure is simple and fast but a good three-dimensional understanding of the anatomy of the scaphoid is required (Fig. 25-19A–N). There are no major vessels, nerves, or tendons endangered by the minimal invasive approach to the scaphoid. The injured hand is surgically cleaned and put on a radiolucent table. The important step is the proper insertion of the guide wire. It helps to remember that the scaphoid lies in a 45 degree plane to the longitudinal and horizontal axes of the wrist. A 4 to 5 mm skin incision is made about 1 cm distal and radial to the scaphoid tubercle. The author always opens the joint space between scaphoid and trapezium with an 11 scalpel blade and inserts a small guide sleeve, which facilitates the insertion of a guide wire, at the correct entry point on top of the scaphoid tubercle. The author usually inserts the guide wire at a 45 degree angle at both planes, visualizing the anteroposterior plane with a fluoroscope. Inserting the guide wire and determining its position are the key points of the procedure. Unstable scaphoid fractures have a tendency to rotate when the drill bit and screw are inserted. A second wire is mandatory in these cases to secure the fracture site and avoid rotational deformity. The length of the screw is then checked and the bone is drilled. The author always checks the drilling maneuver as well as screw insertion by fluoroscopy, making sure that no rotation occurs. The screw should be chosen 3 mm shorter than measured to avoid prominence. Postoperatively a bandage is applied with no cast being required. Sports activities that do not involve the wrist are allowed immediately. Other sports, such as tennis, are allowed 4 weeks after the operation if check x-rays are satisfactory and more strenuous sports are allowed 6 weeks after the operation.

Unstable and Displaced Fractures (Type B2)

Displaced fractures of the scaphoid as well as proximal pole and oblique fractures require different treatment from that of nondisplaced fractures. A displaced fracture, by definition, is one with more than 1 mm of step-off or more than 60 degrees of scapholunate or 15 degrees of lunatocapitate angulation as observed on either plain x-rays or CT scans. The degree of instability may vary and thus there are different choices for fracture treatment.

One has to be aware that unstable fractures of the scaphoid have a high incidence of delayed union and nonunion. The routine use of cast immobilization in displaced scaphoid fractures therefore represents incorrect treatment. There are only a few indications for closed reduction and cast management of displaced scaphoid fracture. Patients who undergo conservative treatment have to be carefully selected and will include patients with metabolic diseases, noncompliant patients, and those patients with significant medical comorbidities. Closed reduction involves three-point pressure on the tubercle of the distal scaphoid in a palmar direction combined with dorsal pressure over the capitate and dorsal support of the distal radius, which helps reduce and maintain the dorsolunate angulation. An acceptable reduction includes alignment with less than 1 mm of displacement and a scapholunate angle of not more than 60 degrees.

Herbert questioned the efficacy of closed treatment as he was convinced, as most orthopedic surgeons are, that for sound bone union to take place, the fracture fragments must be in close apposition so that soft-tissue interposition or synovial fluid cannot affect healing. He believed that if closed treatment is used for complete fractures osseous, union may be the result more of luck than skill (26).

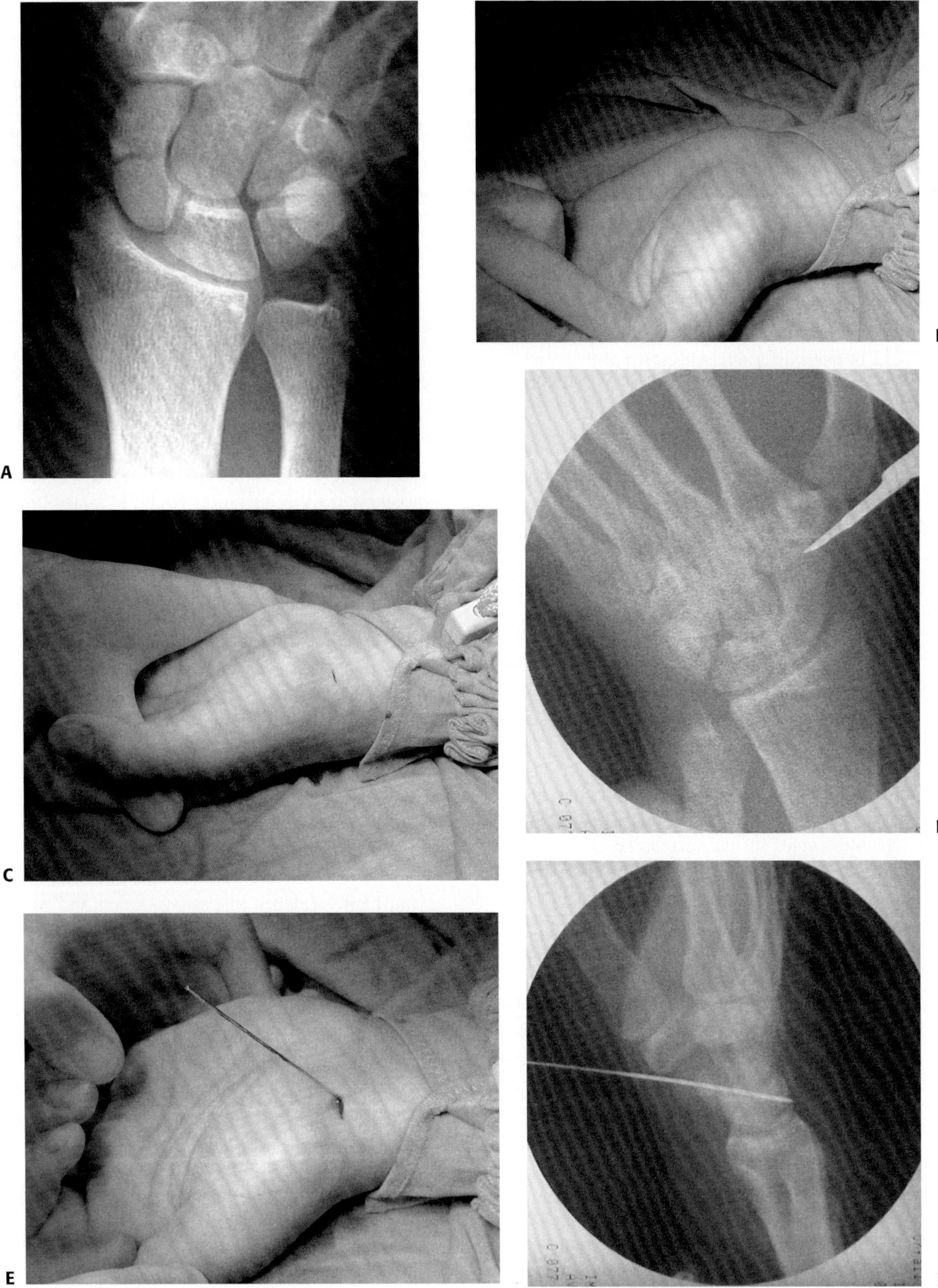

FIGURE 25-19 Percutaneous stabilization of scaphoid fracture. **A.** PA view of scaphoid fracture in an athlete. **B.** The wrist should be dorsiflexed before insertion of the K-wire. **C.** A 4 to 5 mm incision is sufficient for insertion of the screw. The incision should be placed in skin crease to avoid visible scars. **D.** The joint space between scaphoid and trapezium is opened under fluoroscopy. **E.** The K-wire is inserted in a 45 degree angle at both planes. *(continues)*

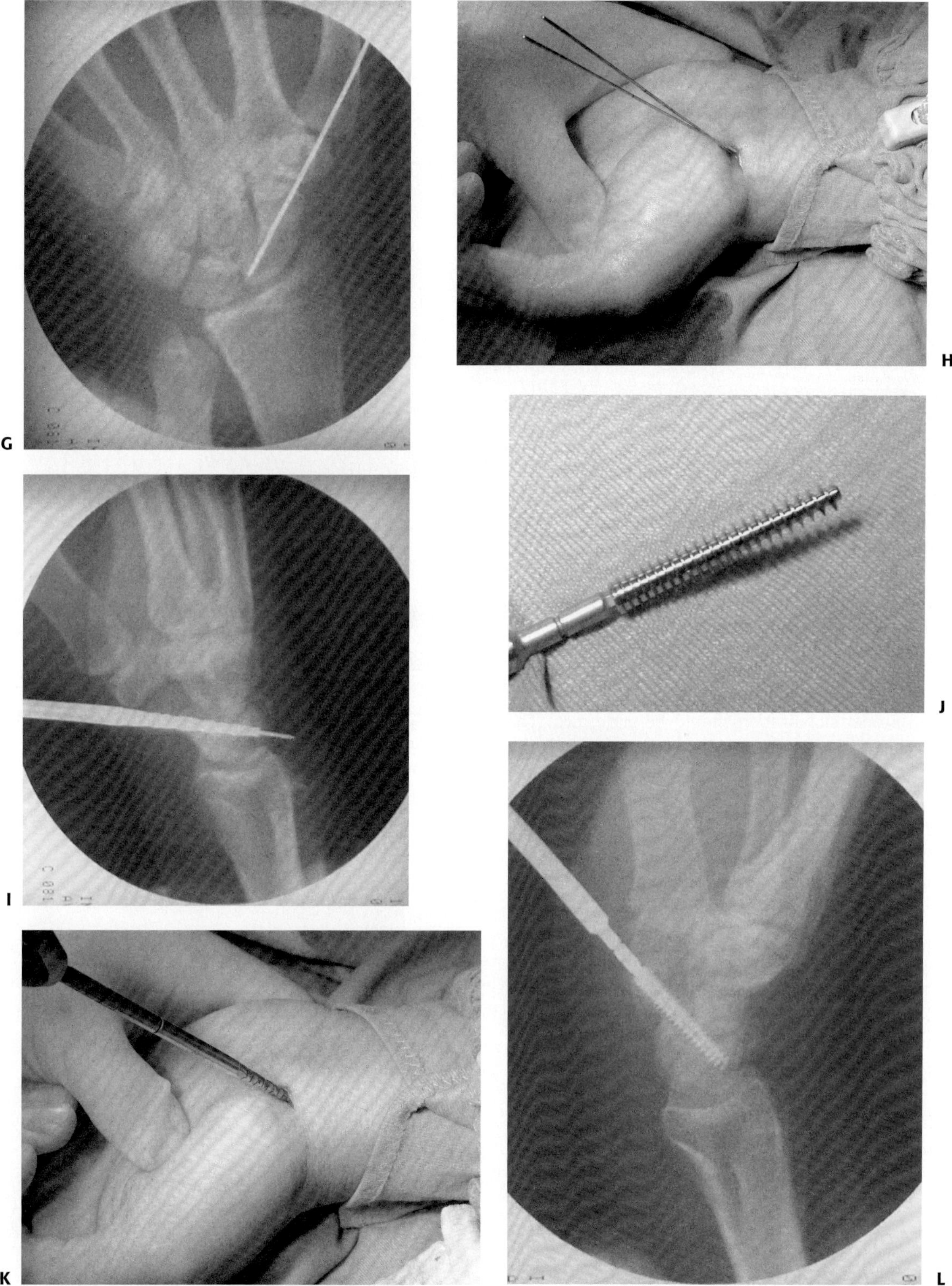

FIGURE 25-19 *(continued)* **F,G.** The position of the K-wire is checked by fluoroscopy. **H.** A second K-wire is required in unstable scaphoid fractures to prevent rotation of the fracture fragments. **I.** The drill is inserted. **J.** A variable pitch scaphoid screw. **K.** Insertion of scaphoid screw. **L.** Check insertion of screw by fluoroscopy to avoid rotation of fracture fragments. *(continues)*

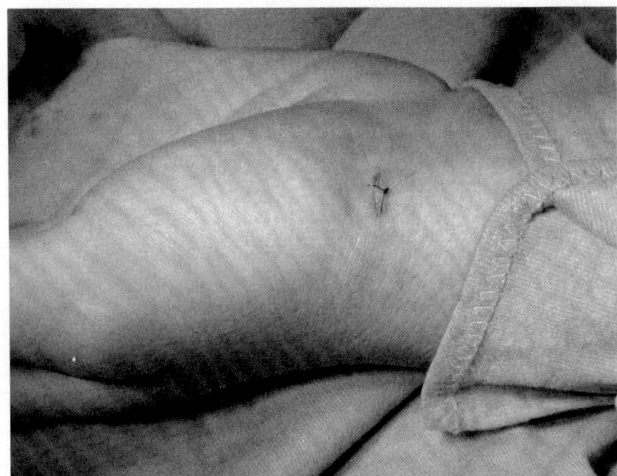

M

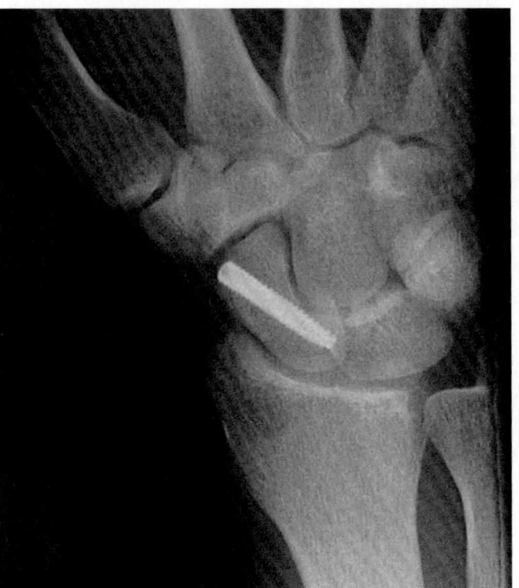

N

FIGURE 25-19 *(continued)* **M.** Closure of wound with one suture. **N.** Postoperative x-ray shows a good compression of the fragments—the fracture gap is no longer visible.

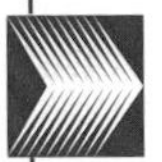

AUTHOR'S PREFERRED TREATMENT

Unstable and Displaced Fractures (Type B2)

As most of these fractures occur in a young, healthy, active population proper stabilization should be performed. The author prefers percutaneous screw fixation as previously described (Fig. 25-19A–N). If reduction cannot be achieved, two pins should be inserted, one in each fragment, and these pins used as joy sticks to reduce the fracture. A temporary K-wire can be inserted to maintain the reduction and the guide wire for the screw is then introduced. For acute displaced fractures that cannot be reduced percutaneously, the author recommends open reduction and compression screw fixation of the scaphoid as soft-tissue interposition is not uncommon and often results in fibrous instead of osseous union (26,36,87,88). K-wire fixation alone is not advisable as the rate of nonunion is high. The author always tries to keep the incision small, reduce the fracture after removing synovium or capsule from the fracture site, stabilize the fracture with a temporary K-wire, and then insert the guide wire by a percutaneous approach distal to the skin incision. In comminuted fractures, immediate bone grafting may be required.

Postoperative Colles cast immobilization for 4 weeks is recommended in cases of displaced fractures.

Proximal Pole Fractures (Type B3)

Proximal pole fractures (Type B3) should be treated operatively as they rarely unite without surgery.

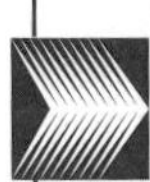

AUTHOR'S PREFERRED TREATMENT

Proximal Pole Fractures

The author stabilizes these fractures percutaneously using a dorsal approach (Fig. 25-20). With this technique it is much easier to get a proper purchase on the small proximal fragment (89).

An open technique is required for the exposure of displaced small proximal pole fractures, nonunions of the prox-

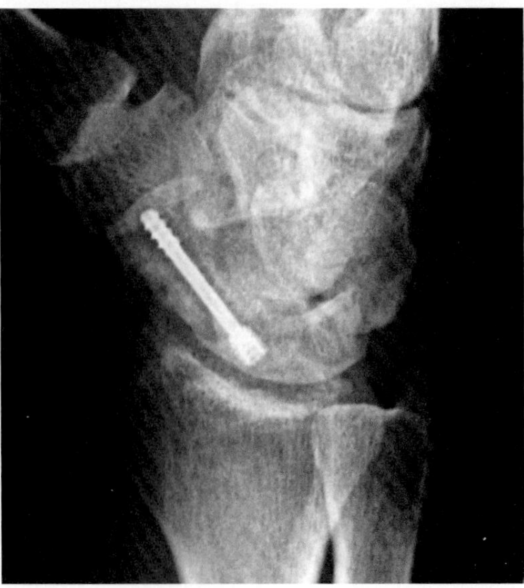

FIGURE 25-20 Healed proximal pole fracture 6 months after dorsal approach.

imal pole, and for exposure of injuries to the scapholunate ligament. The author prefers a straight 3 to 4 cm incision centered over the back of the wrist after checking the level of the scapholunate junction with the fluoroscope. The extensor pollicis longus tendon is mobilized radially after incision of the retinaculum. The dorsal capsule is then incised and the scaphoid exposed. Care is taken to avoid injury to the dorsal ridge vasculature during the approach. The fragments are reduced manually or with the assistance of Kirschner wire joysticks. Nonunions are curetted and the cavity is packed with cancellous bone graft. A compression screw is then used after inserting a temporary K-wire to prevent rotation. The dorsal wrist capsule should always be repaired. If ON is present a vascularized bone graft can be considered. An osteotomy of the proximal pole should not be tried.

Scaphoid Nonunion

Most patients with nonunion have either not been immobilized at all or only for a week or two (39,90). However, there are other patients who develop nonunions after a prolonged period of cast immobilization. The surgeon should discuss the advantages and disadvantages of both operative and conservative treatment with the patient. Some patients decide to undergo conservative treatment with Colles cast fixation and they require careful clinical and radiological follow-up. If there are no signs of union after 8 weeks, another Colles cast is applied for 4 weeks. If there are no signs of union after 12 weeks, operative intervention should be discussed. Some patients will still decide to maintain cast immobilization for another 4 weeks. If there are still no signs of union after 16 weeks, the patient has to understand that union is unlikely. In these cases, carpal malalignment is rare.

The operative procedure consists of an open procedure. The fracture is exposed and fibrous tissue removed. The author usually leaves the dorsal structures intact, which gives a good indication of the length of the scaphoid. Cancellous bone is harvested from distal radius. The two fragments of the scaphoid are fixed with a compression screw, which is inserted percutaneously as previously described.

Stable Nonunions (Herbert Type D1)

It is essential to differentiate between stable and unstable scaphoid nonunions. The stable scaphoid nonunion is characterized by a firm fibrous nonunion that prevents deformity from occurring. The length and shape of the scaphoid remain well preserved and the risk of osteoarthritis is minimal. X-rays show an indistinct fracture line with variable cystic changes affecting the adjacent bone fragments. The patients are usually relatively symptom-free unless the wrist is subjected to further trauma, which often leads to an unstable nonunion with all of the associated problems of carpal collapse, osteoarthritis, pain, and weakness (26). Although there are patients who seem to have an asymptomatic, stable nonunion of the scaphoid for many years, most patients will become symptomatic when the stable nonunion progresses to an unstable one and osteoarthritis occurs.

The indication to treat patients with a stable nonunion is the fact that treating fibrous nonunions is usually straightforward and gives good results, whereas patients with unstable nonunions often have persistent postoperative problems due to the osteoarthritic changes of the radiocarpal joint. The earlier patients are operated the lower the incidence of secondary osteoarthritis. The standard palmar approach should be used for all reconstructions, except those involving small proximal pole fractures (26).

Slade and coworkers (91) reported a series of stable scaphoid nonunions that were treated by percutaneous screw fixation with good results. Their indications were nonunions that were well aligned and without extensive sclerosis or bone resorption at the nonunion site. It seems that selected nonunions might require only rigid fixation, preferably undertaken percutaneously to minimize devascularization.

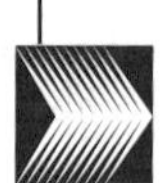

AUTHOR'S PREFERRED TREATMENT

Stable Nonunions (Herbert Type D1)

The author prefers an open palmar approach using a straight incision as opposed to the curved incision described by Russe (92). The incision is based over or radial to the flexor carpi radialis just above the scaphoid. Inexperienced surgeons should check the level of incision with the fluoroscope. The sheath of the flexor carpi radialis tendon is incised and the tendon retracted ulnarly. Directly beneath the tendon lies the palmar capsule of the wrist, just above the scaphoid. The capsule should be incised longitudinally. There are no neurovascular structures at risk as the radial neurovascular bundle lies radially. The superficial palmar branch of the radial artery is distal at the end of incision and needs to be ligated in cases of wider exposure of the distal scaphoid. It is important to remove the fibrous tissue and sclerotic bone. Occasionally, it may be necessary to identify the site of nonunion with a fluoroscope as the articular cartilage can look intact in stable nonunions. The author usually leaves the dorsal cartilage in place. This provides a hinge and facilitates assessment of scaphoid length. In most cases of stable nonunion, cancellous bone graft from either the distal radius (for small defects) or the iliac crest (preferable because of its superior osteogenic and mechanical properties) is packed into the defect. If cancellous bone graft is taken from the distal radius the incision is lengthened proximally. In larger defects, a corticocancellous bone block may be required to achieve normal length of the scaphoid (Fig. 25-21). Some authors prefer a Russe inlay graft. However, simple cancellous bone grafting in combination with a compression screw will suffice in most cases. Postoperative immobilization in Colles cast is maintained for 6 weeks.

The nonunion gap is exposed and debrided and the fracture fragments are mobilized. The author usually tries to leave a cartilage hinge posteriorly to provide a fulcrum around which the fragments may be hinged open, although this is often not possible in older, unstable scaphoid fractures. If the hinge is released in an effort to regain all of the scaphoid length, the fracture fragments will become extremely unstable and difficult to align. Furthermore, the gap between the two fragments may be too great for the scaphoid to revascularize the proximal pole (95).

The wrist is forcibly extended and the two fragments gently distracted with small spreaders. This maneuver usually achieves adequate correction of the carpal deformity and a satisfactory improvement of wrist extension. Provided that reasonable correction is achieved and that the wrist extends to at least 45 degrees, most patients achieve satisfactory clinical results (26). The fracture surfaces are excised with a small osteotome. The cuts need to be parallel to each other and perpendicular to the long axis of the scaphoid to ensure that the graft is stable when it is locked into position. Reduction is maintained with a Kirschner wire. The width and depth of the defect is measured and a graft of the exact size is removed from the iliac crest with an osteotome. Oscillating saws should not be used as thermal necrosis of the graft can occur. With the wedge graft in place and the scaphoid reduced and held with a Kirschner wire, a compression screw is inserted (Fig. 25-21). Internal fixation with K-wires alone is usually not successful as compression is required to achieve union. However, if the graft shows a tendency to rotate, additional fixation with a K-wire may be required. If a longstanding DISI deformity is present with a radiolunate angle greater than 20 degrees, additional pinning of the lunate to radius for 6 to 8 weeks is advised (96). Postoperative immobilization in a Colles cast is maintained for 8 to 12 weeks.

Vascularized bone grafts from the distal radius (radial artery) or distal ulna (ulnar artery) have also been described (100). The author prefers the pronator quadratus graft (Fig. 25-23). If there is marked DISI angulation of the lunate, it is best to reduce the lunate and proximal scaphoid by flexing the wrist and pinning the lunate in a reduced position through the radial styloid. An alternative procedure is to use multiple Kirschner wires as described by Fernandez (96). It may be difficult to completely correct carpal instability in long-standing cases, and these patients may be better served by various salvage procedures. Union rates in most series seem to be about 80% (39). The use of CT scans to evaluate fracture healing is recommended to keep the time of immobilization as short as possible.

A partial radial styloidectomy should be performed in all patients with radiological signs of stage I radioscaphoid arthritis, this being arthritis that is limited to the scaphoid and radial styloid. This is undertaken to relieve pain arising from arthritic joints or osteophyte impingement. Even if the pain is not too severe, this procedure should be performed prophylactically as problems are quite likely to arise with an arthritic joint (Fig. 25-24). If there are no radiological signs of arthritis, a styloidectomy should not be undertaken at the same time as scaphoid reconstruction as lengthening of the scaphoid due to reconstruction often relieves symptoms.

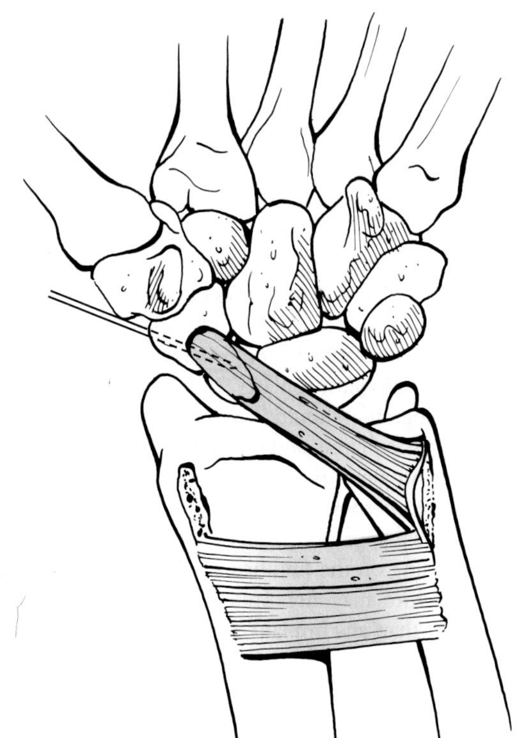

FIGURE 25-23 Pronator quadratus graft.

Salvage Procedures for Scaphoid Nonunion

Excision of Part or All of the Scaphoid. A very small fragment can be excised with impunity. However, most surgeons are aware that if it is more than 8 mm long, the results are poor and the wrist feels weak (39).

Wrist Denervation. Wrist denervation (101) is often helpful as it is combined with significant pain relief. However, pain relief can be temporary.

Proximal Row Carpectomy. The results of excising the scaphoid, lunate, and triquetrum have been disappointing in some series (26), which is why the author prefers wrist arthrodesis in cases of panscaphoid arthritis and severe pain.

Scaphoid Prosthesis. In selected patients with panscaphoid osteoarthritis, total replacement of the scaphoid is worth considering (102). If the scaphoid must be excised, it seems reasonable to replace it with something! Silicone implants induced progressive silicone arthritis in many cases (103), and the technique was abandoned 20 years ago. Other methods of replacement,

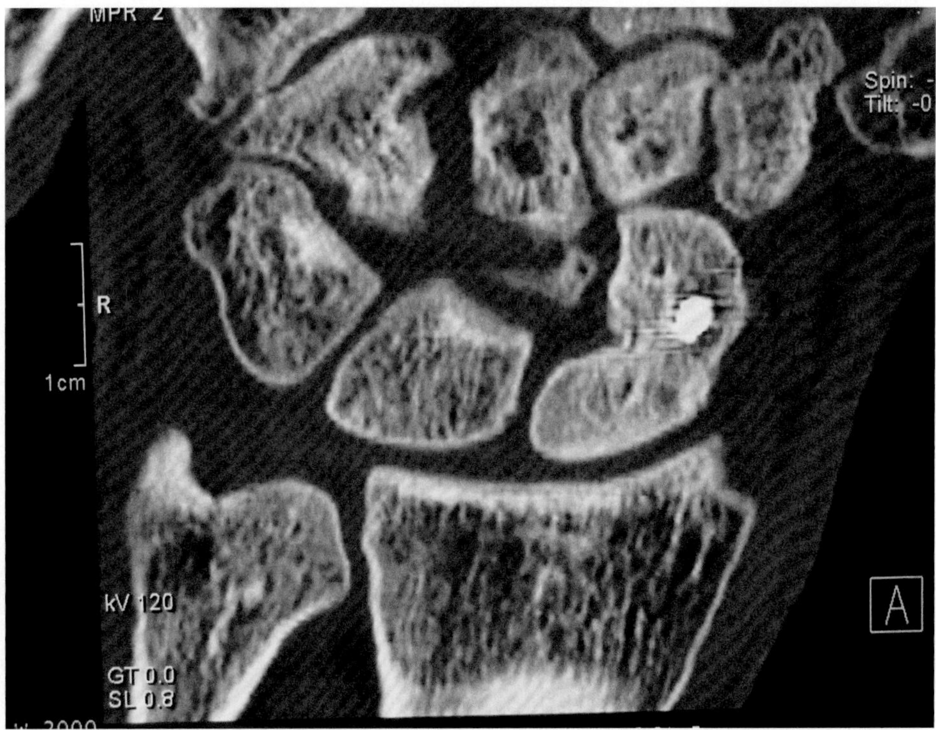

FIGURE 25-24 Radial styloidectomy for pain relief in a patient who showed arthritic changes due to scaphoid nonunion.

such as cadaveric bones and titanium implants, are currently in clinical trials. However, unless the midcarpal joint is stable and painless, this procedure should be combined with a fusion across the midcarpal joint (26). Without this fusion, progressive carpal subluxation is likely to occur. The fusion is unlikely to trouble patients as most have long-standing carpal collapse deformity with secondary osteoarthritis. It is important to correct the midcarpal subluxation as much as possible in order to improve the range of dorsiflexion. Unless at least 30 degrees of extension are maintained after surgery, the patient will almost certainly continue to experience pain when the wrist is loaded (26). Young and active patients are likely to complain of continued pain after this procedure and wrist arthrodesis is therefore preferable in these patients.

Wrist Arthrodesis. Unstable nonunion of the scaphoid can lead to increasing midcarpal and radiocarpal osteoarthritis secondary to increasing carpus collapse. If this is not treated, there is increasing pain and weakness, and wrist motion becomes restricted to the extent that reconstructive surgery is no longer feasible and wrist fusion is required. Pain is the main factor to be taken into consideration when deciding for or against wrist arthrodesis. Arthrodesis is an accepted surgical treatment option for patients with markedly restricted and painful wrist motion. Instability and deformity of the wrist affect hand function significantly, but pain diminishes both strength and dexterity. Wrist arthrodesis achieves good pain relief (26,104), especially in younger patients with high functional demands. It can be difficult to convince patients with severe pain but good wrist function, that the optimal treatment might be a wrist fusion. However, the pain relief associated with a successful fusion results in significant improvement of hand function and grip strength. Preoperatively, it is easy to supply the patient with a dorsal splint to simulate arthrodesis to see if this helps wrist function and symptoms.

Operative Technique. The wrist should always be fused in about 30 degrees of dorsiflexion, with neutral deviation. After a straight midline incision dorsally to the third metacarpal and radius, the extensor retinaculum is divided, the third extensor compartment is opened, the extensor tendons retracted, the wrist capsule is the opened longitudinally, and the joint surfaces of all carpal bones and the radius excised. An osteotome is used to remove Lister's tubercle. Cancellous bone is used to graft the resulting defects. There are elegant arthrodesis plates supplied by several companies but the author prefers the AO/ASIF titanium arthrodesis plate in these cases. A Colles cast is applied for 4 weeks.

Scaphoid Malunion

Fractured scaphoids are prone to triplane angulation due to the joint compressive forces at the scaphotrapezial and radioscaphoid joints. The proximal fragment has a tendency to extend, deviate radially and supinate relative to the distal fragment. This is why CT scans are suggested in unstable scaphoid fractures before operative treatment. The collapse of the scaphoid in the sagittal plane causes DISI pathology and increases the chances of wrist arthrosis even if the scaphoid finally heals (49).

Although the malunited scaphoid fracture is a recognized entity that causes altered carpal kinematics and abnormal load distribution, which may cause premature wrist arthrosis, the reported number of patients treated with early osteotomy is surprisingly small. Restoration of normal scaphoid anatomy in malunion aims to reduce or postpone the incidence of osteoarthritis and to improve function of the wrist (96). Lynch et al (105) reported a technique of corrective osteotomy that corrects the intrascaphoid angles, restores palmar length to the scaphoid, and reduces DISI deformity of the carpus. Indications for osteotomy are pain, weakness, limited range of motion, and deformity of the scaphoid detected on x-rays and evaluated by CT scans. This method seems to have a role in the prevention or slowing of the onset of arthritis in young patients with high functional demands (105).

Osteonecrosis of the Scaphoid (Preiser's Disease)

Osteonecrosis (ON) of the scaphoid can occur as a late complication of scaphoid fractures, especially those involving the proximal pole. Occasionally ON may occur without a fracture, either as a complication of scapholunate ligament injury or as an idiopathic condition known as Preiser's disease (106). The term Preiser's disease is associated with ON of the scaphoid without fracture or trauma although it should be noted that the ON described by Preiser probably occurred in fractured scaphoids as all of his patients had a well-documented history of trauma. The typical symptoms for of ON are increasing pain and stiffness of the wrist. X-rays usually show a small, deformed proximal pole fragment with cystic changes and areas of sclerosis. It is mandatory in all cases of scaphoid nonunion to exclude ON by MRI scans before surgery is undertaken as the diagnosis of ON alters the treatment options.

The treatment of ON often involves arthroscopic debridement and drilling of the lesion. This is a minimally invasive technique that seems to provide pain relief for a long period of time in patients with Preiser's disease (107). If arthroscopic debridement and nonoperative treatment methods, such as rest, splintage, and electrical stimulation are unsuccessful and ON progresses with the scaphoid showing collapse similar to that seen in a nonunion, a vascularized bone graft is recommended (108,109). The bone graft can be harvested dorsally through the second dorsal compartment of the distal radius, anteriorly in the form of a pronator quadratus graft, or from the second metacarpal.

The author recommends harvesting a pronator quadratus graft. The scaphoid is approached anteriorly and the nonunion site is excavated. Kirschner wires are positioned using a retrograde technique and the vascularized bone graft is inserted. Care is taken to protect the vascular pedicle and additional cancellous bone may be packed around the vascular graft. With the graft in place, a guide wire is drilled percutaneously from the dorsal surface across the nonunion site and a compression screw inserted. A radial styloidectomy may be required because the width of the scaphoid is usually increased. Cast immobilization is continued until CT scans show osseous healing.

Scaphoid Fractures: Pearls and Pitfalls

Pearls

- Occult scaphoid fractures are easily detected by MRI scans.
- Percutaneous stabilization of scaphoid fractures significantly reduces the rate of nonunion, as well as reducing the time lost from work and sports.
- Proximal pole fractures can also be stabilized percutaneously by a dorsal approach.

Pitfalls

- Scaphoid fractures are easily missed in children. This can result in nonunion and serious problems.
- Malalignment of scaphoid fractures is often undiagnosed. CT scans are helpful.
- Conservative treatment often ends in delayed healing. An aggressive operative approach is recommended.

LUNATE FRACTURES

The lunate is the fourth most fractured carpal bone after the scaphoid, triquetrum, and trapezium (Table 25-1). Isolated fractures of the lunate are often unrecognized (110). Some authors think that unrecognized and untreated fractures of the lunate lead to Kienböck's disease. This opinion was based on the work of Verdan (111), who applied strong forces to cadaver bones and observed that the resulting fractures were not visible on standard x-rays but only on histology. A major argument against this hypothesis are the MRI findings of Schiltenwolf et al (112) who postulated that early venous congestion of the lunate was responsible for the pathogenesis of Kienböck's disease but found no fractures. The lunate necrosis after perilunate dislocation is probably due to impairment of the arterial vasculature (113).

Kienböck's disease is an eponym for idiopathic avascular osteonecrosis of the lunate. It usually has an insidious onset without a history of injury; however, diagnosis is sometimes made after a simple fall that fractures the necrotic bone (Fig 25-25). Osteonecrosis may be the result of interruption of the vascular supply to the lunate (112), which shows no radiographic evidence of injury until sclerosis and osteochondral collapse are seen. The condition is more common in patients with an ulnar minus variant.

Anatomy

The lunate sits like a keystone in the proximal carpal row in the well-protected concavity of the lunate fossa of the radius, anchored on either side by the interosseous ligaments to the scaphoid and triquetrum with which it articulates. Distally, the convex

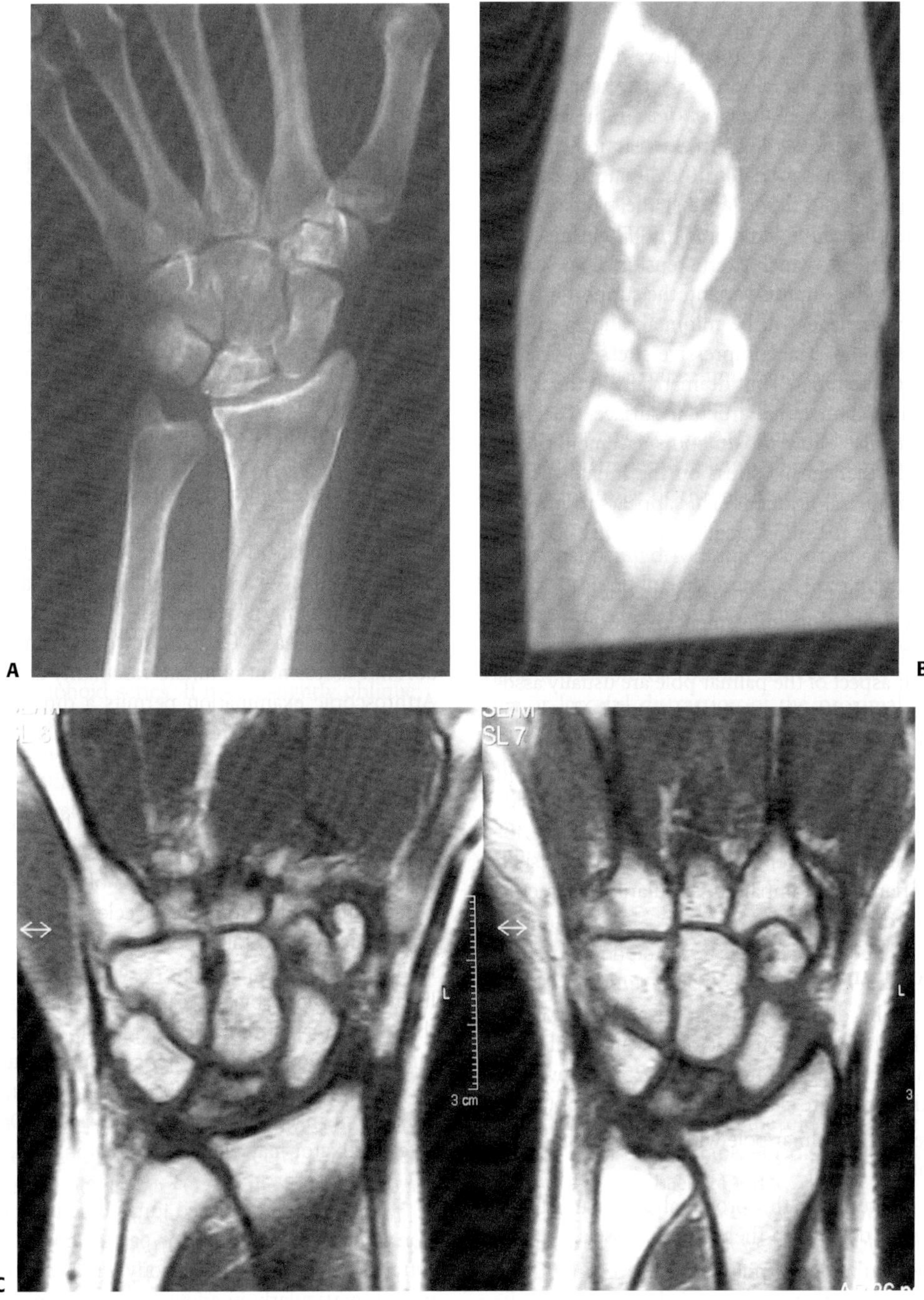

FIGURE 25-25 **A.** AP x-ray of a 25-year-old woman after a sking accident. It shows a sclerotic lunate and an ulnar negative variance. **B.** A CT scan demonstrates a fracture of the sclerotic lunate. **C.** An MRI scan demonstrates decreased vascularity of the lunate.

capitate head fits into the concavity of the lunate. The joint reaction force from the capitate and radius squeezes the lunate ulnarly. The proximal horn of the hamate has a variable articular facet on the distal ulnar surface of the lunate, and ulnar deviation increases the degree of contact of these two bones. The vascular supply of the lunate is primarily through the proximal carpal arcade both dorsally and palmarly. However, the literature suggests that 7% to 26% of lunates may have a single volar or dorsal blood supply and are therefore vulnerable to ON because of disruption of extraosseous blood supply (17). Several authors (1,18,20) have shown the intralunate anastomoses to be of three main types. The degree of cross flow between the systems is variable.

similar displacement of the triquetrum ulnarly during radioulnar deviation, which is also painful.

It must be remembered that some patients have ligamentous laxity. This may be associated with the ability to subluxate the midcarpal joint by displacing the carpometacarpal unit on the distal radius. Tendon displacements with audible snaps are easily produced by some persons but are seldom symptomatic. Distraction can be a good clue to a "lax wrist" or a damaged area, particularly when viewed under fluoroscopic imaging with static traction of approximately 25 pounds applied. Stress loading the wrist with compression and motion from radial to ulnar deviation may simulate midcarpal instability and produce a "catch-up clunk" as the proximal row of carpal bones snap from a flexion to extension.

Radiocarpal Instability

The most common injuries at the radiocarpal joint are fracture-dislocations of the distal radius and carpus, these being palmar and dorsal Barton's fracture-dislocations, radial styloid fracture-dislocations, and die-punch fracture-dislocations. Less common are the pure ligamentous radiocarpal injuries (Fig. 25-27), which may cause the wrist to translate in an ulnar, dorsal, or palmar direction. True dislocations without fracture of the bony margins are rare, and they may sometimes spontaneously reduce, making it even more difficult to demonstrate them. However, they are occasionally seen unreduced with the carpus lying dorsal, palmar, or ulnar to the radius (1).

Diagnosis of these injuries is made from a history of appropriate trauma followed by the usual initial findings of swelling, deformity, tenderness, and pain. Swelling and tenderness are most noticeable dorsally at the radiocarpal level and are aggravated by wrist motion. Deformity may be an ulnar, dorsal, or palmar shift of the carpus. This may be visible on standard x-rays although provocative stress may be required to demonstrate dynamic radiocarpal instability (1).

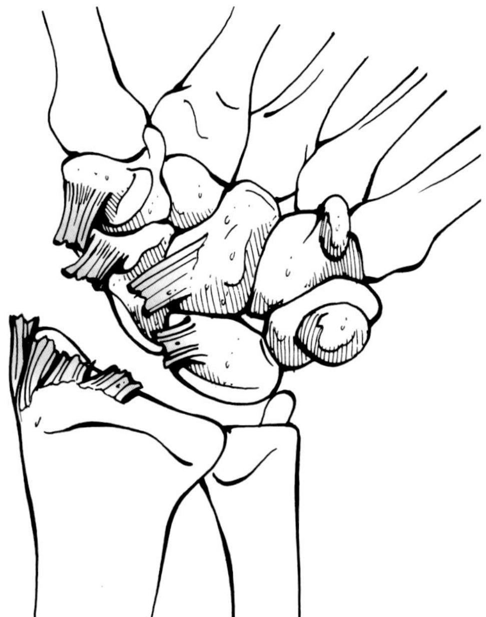

FIGURE 25-27 Radiocarpal dislocation with torn radiocarpal ligaments. This injury requires K-wire stabilization and direct repair of the radiocarpal ligaments.

Ulnar translation is the most frequent radiocarpal instability (1). It may occur acutely, develop gradually, or be observed as a late sequela of a perilunate dislocation. It may occur after an injury at the radiocarpal level, where the radiocarpal ligaments are avulsed from their origins, or after perilunate injury. Clinically, the carpus and hand are offset in an ulnar direction. The radiographic appearance is often dramatic, with the lunate positioned just distal to the ulna and a large space between the radial styloid and the scaphoid. If perilunate destabilization is also involved, the lunate and triquetrum slide ulnarly opening a gap between scaphoid and lunate. In some cases, the ulnar shift is subtle, and a decrease in the ulnocarpal index may provide the only clue to diagnosis. Ulnar translation is also commonly seen in diseases, such as rheumatoid arthritis, and in developmental deformities, such as Madelung's deformity. It may occur with an increase in the radial to ulnar slope of the distal radius.

Dorsal translation of the carpus together with ulnar translation can be seen in two modes: one a true instability secondary to ligament damage, the other an apparent instability due to a carpal shift in response to a change in position of the distal radial articular surface. Pure dorsal translation usually occurs after a loss of the normal palmar slope of the distal radius from a flexion angle to an extension angle. The latter is a common problem after collapse of a distal radius fracture (1).

Treatment of Radiocarpal Instability

Dislocations of the radiocarpal joint require immediate reduction because the associated deformity may compromise adjacent neurovascular structures. Although reduction is usually possible, maintaining it is often difficult. The author believes that open treatment should be considered in most carpal dislocations. In the acute situation, palmar and dorsal ligamentous repair together with temporary percutaneous K-wire stabilization for 6 to 8 weeks is necessary to avoid late displacement and loss of carpal reduction. If the carpal shift is the result of the dorsal radial articular surface, the best management is complete reduction and immobilization of the distal radial fracture by Kirschner wires or appropriate condylar or T-plates (1). One should be certain that the reduction also results in realignment of the carpus because additional carpal ligament injury may have occurred.

Late cases of deformity after distal radius fracture may require corrective osteotomy and bone graft to restore the position of the articular surface. Late identification of ulnar translation deformity or dorsal or palmar translation deformity has responded poorly to ligamentous repair. The most certain method of controlling possible recurrence of deformity is to carry out a partial or total radiocarpal arthrodesis. Radiolunate fusion is an appropriate technique for this situation; however, the variation of joint damage may indicate radioscaphoid fusion in some cases and radioscapholunate fusion in others. The latter is usually indicated in the combination of radiocarpal and perilunate instability (1).

Carpal Instabilities: Pearls and Pitfalls

Pearls

- Dissociative instability involves disruption of the ligaments or bone structure between the lunate and an adjacent carpal bone.
- Nondissociative instabilities include subluxations or incomplete dislocations of the entire carpus with or without a distal radial fracture.
- Perilunate dislocation patterns include a considerable spectrum of sprains, fracture dislocations, and instabilities.
- Scapholunate dissociation is the commonest pattern of carpal instability.
- A capitolunate or radiolunate angle >20 degrees confirms scapholunate instability.
- Lunatotriquetral dissociation may result in disruption of Gilula's lines on x-ray.
- There are four types of midcarpal instability and the direction of subluxation may be palmar or dorsal.

Pitfalls

- A scapholunate dissociation without a dorsiflexed lunate is probably not traumatic.
- In scapholunate dissociation, the results of K-wire treatment are unpredictable. Ligamentous repair should be undertaken if closed reduction is unsuccessful on serial x-rays.
- In chronic scapholunate instability, partial or complete wrist fusion may be needed.
- Sixteen percent to 25% of perilunate dislocations are missed initially.
- Open repair of the lunatotriquetral ligament is only possible in acute injury.
- X-rays in midcarpal instability may be normal or may show a VISI or DISI deformity.

SCAPHOLUNATE DISSOCIATION

Scapholunate (SL) dissociation or rotatory subluxation of the scaphoid is the most frequent pattern of carpal instability. It may occur alone or in association with wrist fractures (1,134–139). Most injuries result from excessive wrist extension and ulnar deviation with intracarpal supination such as occurs with a fall onto the outstretched pronated hand. SL dissociation includes a spectrum of injuries ranging from grade I sprains through all grades of ligament destabilization of a single scapholunate interosseous ligament (SLIL) to injuries of multiple ligaments up to scaphoid dislocation (eponyms: SL-dissociation, SL-instability, rotatory subluxation of scaphoid, DISI). A variety of ligament injuries are associated with SL dissociation. The involved ligaments include the SLIL, the radioscapholunate ligament (RSLL), the radioscaphocapitate ligament (RSCL), the scaphotrapezial ligament complex (STLC), the dorsal radiocarpal ligament (DRCL), and the dorsal intercarpal ligament (DICL). Disruption of the SLIL results in separation of the motion between the scaphoid and lunate in the acute phase and the development of persisting widening of the SL joint as a late clinical consequence (140) (Fig. 25-28).

The clinical consequences of the injury depend on the tightness or laxity of the capsule-ligamentous system of the wrist and the presence of any associated palmar radiocarpal or midcarpal ligament damage. Without treatment, this injury leads to advanced scapholunate collapse and progressive, painful arthritis of the wrist (Fig. 25-28). SL injuries in children are rare (122) and should be treated operatively.

History and Clinical Signs

The diagnosis may be made from the clinical history, which is usually consistent with a dorsiflexion ulnar deviation injury with stress loading of the extended carpus. This combination of position and axial compression causes injury to the SLIL and palmar wrist ligaments (14,137). Particularly vulnerable are the radioscaphocapitate (RSC) and radiolunate ligaments, which are under maximum tension in dorsiflexion and ulnar deviation. Mayfield described this injury pattern as the four stages of progressive perilunate instability with SL instability occurring in stage I. Stages II through IV progress around the lunate, eventually leading to lunate dislocation (Fig. 25-29) (141). Previous or repetitive injury, or the presence of acute or chronic synovitis, modifies the degree of stress required to the point that the index

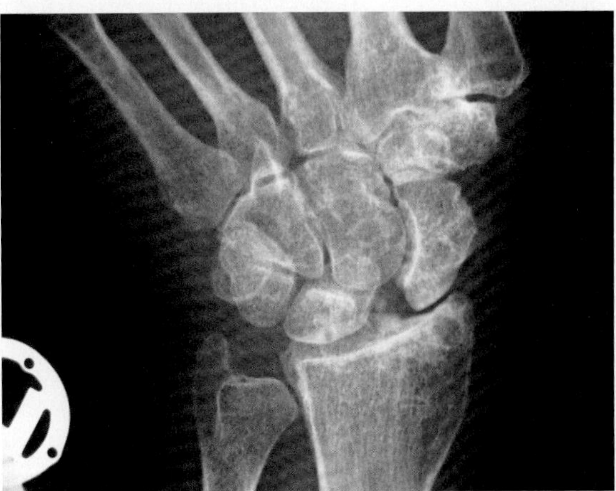

FIGURE 25-28 SL-dissociation in a 60-year-old woman who was treated conservatively resulting in progressive carpal collapse and painful arthritis.

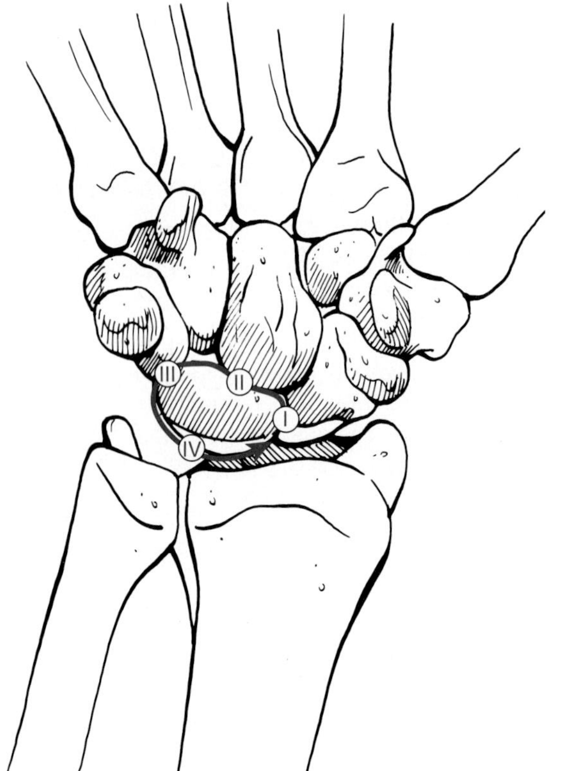

FIGURE 25-29 Mayfield's stages of progressive perilunate instability. Stage I results in SL instability. Stages II–IV result in progressively worse PL instability.

event may be fairly trivial, such as slamming a car door or catching a basketball (1).

The clinical symptoms are swelling and tenderness over the scapholunate area. Associated radial styloid fractures may cause pain over the radial styloid. A neurovascular examination is imperative, as acute carpal tunnel syndrome can occur with carpal fractures and dislocations (137). The degree of associated stability may be such that only provocative stress will reveal the classic findings. An easy provocative maneuver is a vigorous grasp that induces pain; another indication is decreasing repetitive grip strength. The patient may also demonstrate pain during flexion–extension or radioulnar deviation.

Provocative stress is often accompanied by a click in the region of the proximal scaphoid and sometimes by a visible deformity dorsally. A positive Watson test (a combination of pain and a palpable clunk when the wrist is brought from ulnar deviation into radial deviation while pressure is applied to the palmar aspect of the scaphoid tubercle) is highly suggestive of SL instability (Fig. 25-30A). This test is not absolutely specific for SLD, because it may reposition the entire proximal carpal row if the row, rather than the individual scaphoid, is unstable. In addition, in individuals with lax ligaments there may be false-positive signs of dorsal subluxation of the scaphoid that are not pathological. Generalized ligamentous laxity may be present, as many wrists with an SL injury have some form of preexisting ligamentous laxity (1,10,137,141).

Imaging

The four standard views of the carpus are mandatory in the diagnosis of scapholunate instability. SL injuries may be associated with fractures of the radius or carpus especially in younger patients. X-rays of patients with fractures of the distal radius should be evaluated closely for evidence of ligamentous injury. The incidence of SLD in combination with fractures of the radius is about 10% (138). A greater arc injury is associated with radial styloid fractures and SL ligament disruption (137). Gilula's lines should be examined to evaluate ligamentous instability (Fig. 25-10A). The appearance of the lunate should also be assessed. The lunate projects as a quadrilateral shape on the posteroanterior x-ray in normal wrists. Malrotation of the lunate makes it appear more triangular this being commonly seen in perilunate dislocations.

A scapholunate gap >3 mm suggests, and a gap >5 mm confirms, a SLD if there is a positive cortical ring sign (Fig. 25-10B). This increased space between scaphoid and lunate has been named the Terry Thomas sign (142) after the smile of the British comedian (Fig. 25-30B). However, the techniques used to measure the diastasis have not been uniform (Fig. 25-30C). Generally, it is suggested that the SL gap should be compared to the uninjured opposite extremity (10,143). An SL diastasis without a dorsiflexed lunate is most likely nontraumatic (137). Similar findings may be apparent on views of the contralateral extremity.

The SL angle is an angle created by the long axis of the scaphoid and a line perpendicular to the capitolunate joint. The long axis of the scaphoid is determined by a line tangential to the palmar convex surfaces of the proximal and distal poles of the scaphoid. The transverse axis of the lunate is a perpendicular line drawn to the line connecting the dorsal and palmar lips of the lunate (Fig. 25-30D). Normal SL angles range from 30 degrees to 60 degrees. The lateral radiographic appearance of a scapholunate angle >60 degrees suggests SL instability and if the angle >80 degrees the x-ray appearance confirms SL instability (1,8,28,61,137). The radiolunate angle describes the tilt of the lunate with respect to the radius. A capitolunate or radiolunate angle >15 degrees is suspect, but if greater than 20 degrees, it confirms SL instability. Carpal height ratio (Fig. 25-30E), which is carpal height divided by the length of the third metacarpal, is used to quantify carpal collapse. A DISI deformity with a dorsally angulated lunate and a flexed position of the scaphoid is a typical consequence of SL dissociation. Another sign suggestive of SL instability is the cortical ring sign (Fig. 25-10B), which suggests that the scaphoid is flexed. The distal tubercle of the scaphoid is seen end-on on a posteroanterior projection of the wrist (10,143).

If these findings are not present, the provocative maneuvers discussed earlier may cause them to appear. If scapholunate instability cannot be seen with clenched-fist views or radioulnar

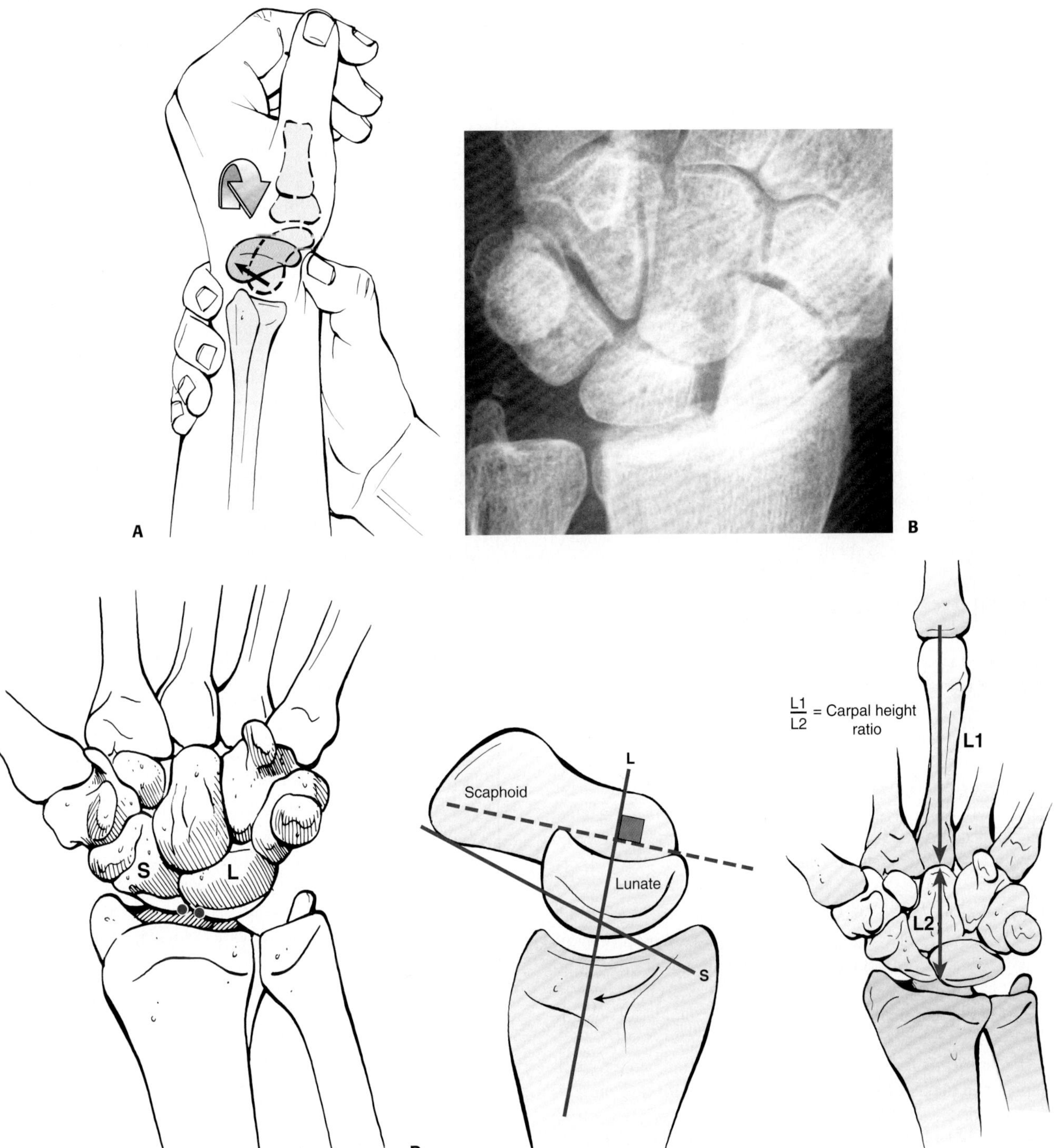

FIGURE 25-30 Watson test. **A.** Pressure applied to the palmar aspect of the scaphoid tubercle while moving the wrist from an ulnar to radial deviation. A positive test elicits a combination of pain and a palpable clunk or snapping. **B.** X-ray of patient with old SL instability, Terry Thomas sign, and progressive arthritic deformation of the radiocarpal joint. **C.** Measurement of the scapholunate gap from the proximal ulnar corner of the scaphoid to the proximal radial corner of the lunate. **D.** The SL angle is created by the long axis of the scaphoid and a line perpendicular to the capitolunate joint. **E.** Carpal height ratio.

stress x-rays, then fluoroscopy or cineradiography using standard and provocative stress motions should be performed. Arthrography has a high rate of false-positive and false-negative results and is therefore not recommended. Arthroscopy can be used to determine the extent of ligament disruption and the presence of radioscaphoid arthritis, as well as to classify and treat SL injuries (144). MRI is helpful in discriminating the extent of ligament injury.

Classification

The classification of SL instability considers whether the injury is acute or chronic and whether it is static or dynamic, this being helpful for planning further treatment procedures. Static deformity does not occur with isolated injury to the dorsal SL ligament (15). Static instability, which means that the injury can be identified on plain posteroanterior and lateral x-rays occurs when the dorsal scapholunate interosseous ligament (DSLIL) is injured along with the palmar ligaments, particularly the radiolunate ligaments and the RSC ligament. Dynamic instability, which cannot be determined with plain x-rays but may be apparent on stress x-rays or fluoroscopy, is thought to result from isolated injury to the DSLIL (137,145).

Current Treatment Options

Different treatment options need to be considered based on the duration of injury, extent of ligamentous involvement, and the presence of associated carpal instabilities. The patient with an injury <4 weeks old is considered to have an acute tear. If it is >4 weeks but <24 weeks, it is a subacute tear. If it is >6 months from injury, the tear is chronic and may be reducible or irreducible. Depending on the mechanism of injury and amount of force across the wrist, the scapholunate ligament may be accompanied by injuries to the palmar radiocarpal and lunatotriquetral ligament or the TFCC.

Acute Scapholunate Dissociation

Patients with partial ligament tears without carpal instability may be treated conservatively with cast immobilization. Cast immobilization is ineffective in unstable cases (139) because the scaphoid requires wrist extension to maintain reduction and the lunate requires wrist flexion.

If the carpus is easily reduced and reduction can be maintained, percutaneous K-wires in combination with cast immobilization for 8 weeks can be used. One K-wire is placed from the scaphoid to the lunate and another from the scaphoid to the capitate. Some authors recommend arthroscopic visualization and reduction followed by percutaneous pinning. Pins can be placed into the scaphoid and lunate and used as joysticks to reduce the SL joint. Whipple (146) reported an 85% success rate in maintaining SL reduction in patients with an SL interval that was greater than the unaffected wrist by 3 mm or less and whose injuries were less than 3 months old. Results were less satisfactory in patients with a wrist injury that was older than 3 months.

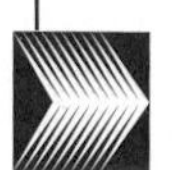

AUTHOR'S PREFERRED TREATMENT

Acute Scapholunate Dissociation

Owing to the unpredictable results with percutaneous pin fixation, the author believes that ligament repair should be considered in all acute scapholunate injuries unless the carpus is easily reduced anatomically by closed techniques and remains reduced in sequential x-rays without carpal malalignment. An increasing scapholunate angle exceeding 60°, a lunatocapitate angle exceeding 15°, or an increasing scapholunate gap >3 mm are indications for operative intervention. Anatomical restoration of the scapholunate complex by open ligament repair is a realistic goal when the patient presents early. Soft-tissue repair and reconstruction are popular because they attempt to restore the normal kinematics of the wrist. Arthroscopy of the wrist can assist in confirming the diagnosis and determining the location and extent of ligamentous damage. The technique of repair changed considerably with the introduction of intraosseous suture retaining anchors allowing ligament attachment directly to the bone (Fig. 25-31) (147,148).

The primary goals of the treatment of SL dissociation are stabilization of the carpal bones in their proper alignment and the maintenance of wrist mobility. The earlier ligament repair takes place the easier it is to perform a direct repair. The results of direct ligament repair are superior to ligament reconstruction (149). Experimental studies have shown that reduction of the displaced SL joint is essential to the recovery of wrist kinematics after SLD (140). Open reduction and internal fixation can undertaken through a dorsal approach centered over Lister's tubercle, reflecting the dorsal wrist capsule to preserve the dorsal intercarpal and dorsal radiotriquetral ligaments, using a radial based capsular flap. The radial capsule is reflected from the scaphoid to its waist. The open technique allows direct visualization of the injured ligament, reduction, and ligament repair. Most often the SL ligament is found to be torn off the scaphoid and still attached to the lunate. In rare cases, avulsion from the lunate or an oblique tear will be seen.

Reduction of the lunate and scaphoid is performed with Kirschner-wire "joysticks" inserted in a dorsal to palmar direction. The rim of the proximal scaphoid is freshened to subcortical bone with a fine rongeur to facilitate ligament healing. Ideally, high-speed burrs should be avoided as thermal necrosis may occur. When the ligament remains attached to the lunate intraosseous anchors are inserted into the waist of the scaphoid. The anchors are placed in such a position that the suture lies in a slightly oblique direction in order to resist the rotational forces between scaphoid and lunate (Fig. 25-31) (150). The sutures attached to the anchors are placed in the scapholunate ligament in a palmar to dorsal direction. If anchors are not available, drill holes in the scaphoid are required to allow direct attachment of the ligament onto the scaphoid. When the sutures are positioned, the scaphoid and lunate are reduced with joysticks

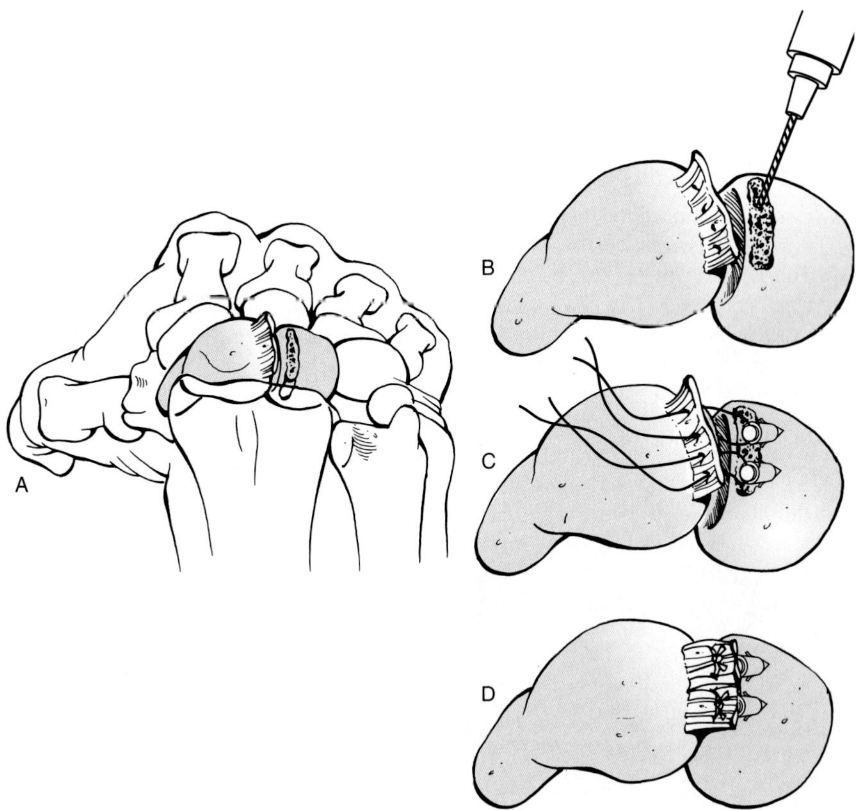

FIGURE 25-31 A–D. Ligament repair for SL instability. Anchors are placed into the lunate (or scaphoid—depending on where the SLIL has ruptured) and the ligament is sutured back into position.

and held in the reduced position with K-wires. One K-wire is placed from the scaphoid to the lunate and another from the scaphoid to the capitate. They are removed 6 weeks after operation. The sutures are tied and the capsule repaired. Results of open ligament repair by a dorsal approach are very good (150,151).

Scapholunate injuries occurring in combination with distal radius fractures should be operatively treated as the results of conservative treatment are unacceptably poor (139).

Subacute Ligament Tear

For subacute scapholunate ligament tears, the addition of local tissue may be necessary if the scapholunate ligament has retracted or is deficient (1). Blatt's technique (152) (see Fig. 25-33) reflects a proximally based dorsal capsular flap onto the scapholunate interspace, and this is sutured tautly to the dorsal scaphoid to act as a tether to the proximal pole. This flap can be added to the ligament repair process described earlier by placing nonabsorbable sutures from the lunate ligament remnant into the capsular tissue and then out through the scaphoid. An alternative method is to use a strip of tendon from the radial wrist extensors (extensor carpi radialis longus or extensor carpi radialis brevis), but tendon tissue is not an ideal ligament replacement, and capsular tissue is preferred (1).

In both subacute and severe acute scapholunate tears, palmar extrinsic ligament attenuation may be found (1). Use of the arthroscope intraoperatively helps to identify these conditions and plan appropriate incisions (146). A palmar approach with direct ligament repair by nonabsorbable sutures can be performed. If there is deficient tissue in the subacute case, part of the flexor carpi radialis can be used to augment the repair process by placing drill holes through the proximal scaphoid and radial half of the lunate and passing one half of the flexor carpi radialis tendon in a circular fashion to reinforce the dorsal and palmar ligaments. The radioscaphocapitate and radiolunate ligaments may be advanced into the gap. With a large, complete scapholunate ligament tear associated with a wide scapholunate gap of 5 mm or more, palmar ligament repair is usually needed (1). A carpal tunnel incision extended slightly radially is performed, and the damaged area is identified with a probe inserted from a separate dorsal incision. The interval between the radioscaphocapitate ligament and long radiolunate ligament is developed. Sutures may then be placed with intraosseous anchors into the scaphoid proximal pole or remnants of the interosseous membrane, which are then used to pull the radiolunate ligament against the proximal pole to hold the overreduction of the proximal scaphoid, which is stabilized by Kirschner wires. The purpose of this palmar repair is to bring the dorsally subluxed and rotated proximal scaphoid in apposition with the palmar intracapsular ligaments.

Whether the approach is dorsal or palmar or combined, tight repair of the capsular structures is required for subacute dissociation. Internal fixation for a period of 8 weeks is preferred supplemented with a supportive Colles cast. After cast removal, an orthoplast splint is worn as muscle strength and joint motion are restored. Return to work or sports is best delayed for a minimum of 6 months, with continued protection being used during sports activities.

Chronic Scapholunate Instability

The major concerns with chronic scapholunate instability are whether the ligaments can be directly repaired, whether any residual carpal dislocation is reducible, and whether the joint has developed arthritis. When possible, restoration of normal carpal anatomy by repair and reconstruction of the support ligaments of the wrist remains the preferred treatment. This requires there be sufficient local tissue for a repair and a correctable carpal instability. When the patient presents with a fixed carpal deformity and the rotational subluxation of the scaphoid or dorsal angulated lunate (DISI) cannot be reduced, or when local degenerative changes or work demands that require heavy lifting or repetitive stress loading are present, the alternative of partial or complete fusion of the wrist may be preferred (1). There are many techniques described to treat chronic scapholunate instability (1,152–154). Weiss et al (155) showed that, in patients with a suspected intercarpal ligament tear and normal x-rays, arthroscopy was useful for both diagnosis and treatment. Current techniques for ligament reconstruction include repair with the dorsal capsular flap procedure, a palmar ligament reefing procedure, and combined dorsal and palmar procedures that add flexor or extensor tendon tissue to the repair site. The goal of each of these repair techniques involves the addition of local tissue to provide a collagen framework for future stability (1,152,154). Soft-tissue reconstructions have several theoretical advantages that make them attractive alternatives to other procedures. In contrast to arthrodeses, soft-tissue reconstructions preserve more intercarpal motion (154).

Several procedures have been designed to restrict rotatory subluxation of the scaphoid by creating a dorsal tether (Fig. 25-32) (152,154,156,157). A commonly used method of dorsal capsulodesis is the Blatt type of capsular reconstruction (152). Results of Blatt's capsulodesis are acceptable (152), although some clinical series have not reported favorable outcomes, which might

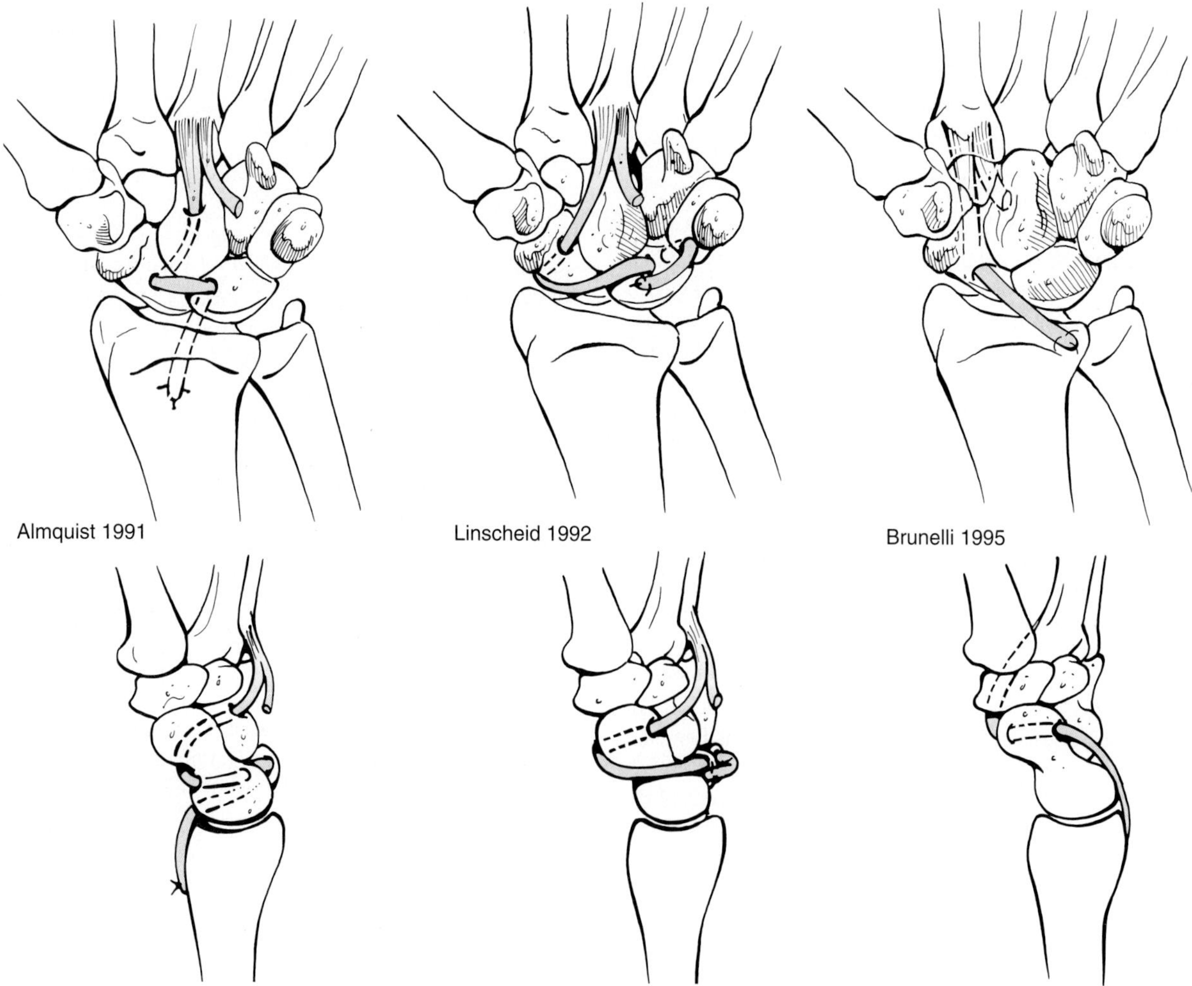

FIGURE 25-32 Tendon weaves and reconstructions proposed by various authors.

be related to patient selection (158). Szabo and Slater (154,157) described the dorsal intercarpal ligament capsulodesis (DILC), which is a soft-tissue reconstruction procedure based on the dorsal intercarpal ligament of the wrist. The theoretical advantage of this method is that it avoids a tether between the distal radius and scaphoid. This keeps the proximal carpal row linked as a functional unit. Clinical results seem to be encouraging (154).

Wyrick et al (148) evaluated SL ligament repair and dorsal capsulodesis for static SLD and found that no patients were free of pain at follow-up. The experience of Wyrick and others suggests that dorsal capsulodesis is more suited for patients with dynamic instability than for those with static instability (134). Dynamic instability is characterized by normal x-rays of the unloaded wrist but by a typical step-off between scaphoid and lunate when evaluated arthroscopically. Axial loading of the wrist can produce a widening of the SL gap in dynamic instability. Static instability is characterized by a widening of the SL gap in an unloaded wrist and an SL angle >60 degrees. Arthroscopy in such a case is grossly abnormal and there is usually a communication between the radiocarpal and midcarpal joints. Static instability requires an intercarpal arthrodesis.

Tendon weave procedures and tenodeses (Fig. 25-32) have been attempted with variable success. Wrist extensor or flexor tendon augmentation procedures require placement of drill holes in bone. In this procedure, drill holes are carefully placed in a dorsal-to-palmar direction through the scaphoid and lunate. Tendon strips are then passed through these holes to attempt a reconstruction of the SLIL. The large holes required to pass tendon grafts often lead to carpal fractures. An alternative technique is to take part of an extensor or flexor tendon and pass it through the capitate, scaphoid, lunate, and distal radius (121). Another technique is the reconstruction of the dorsal part of the SL ligament using a bone-ligament-bone autograft. However, clinical results are not particularly convincing (159).

The palmar approach for scapholunate ligament repair (Conyers' technique) is performed through a carpal tunnel incision (1). A probe or needle passed dorsal to palmar is helpful in locating the ligament tear and palmar ligament intervals. Flaps of radioscaphocapitate and long radiolunate ligaments are reflected laterally and medially. The cartilage surfaces of the scaphoid and lunate are denuded to subchondral bone to encourage a strong syndesmosis. The scaphoid and lunate are then reduced and pinned with threaded wires that are left in place for at least 8 weeks. The palmar ligaments are carefully repaired. Motion is delayed 10 to 12 weeks to encourage adequate strength of the syndesmosis.

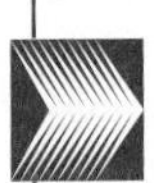

AUTHOR'S PREFERRED TREATMENT

Chronic Scapholunate Instability

The author prefers the Blatt technique of capsule reconstruction (152) using dorsal capsulodesis for the treatment of chronic SLD (Fig. 25-33). For the Blatt type of capsule reconstruction, a long rectangular flap, about 1.5 cm wide, based on the dorsal aspect of the distal radius, is used. The distal edge of capsule is sutured to the distal pole of the scaphoid once the scaphoid is placed in a reduced position. A K-wire can be passed into the dorsum of the lunate to be used as a joystick to reduce any DISI. The scaphoid is reduced by pressure on the scaphoid tubercle and then transfixed to the capitate by another K-wire. The dorsal surface of the scaphoid is roughened with a fine rongeur just distal to the center of rotation. The dorsal flap of wrist capsule is sutured under tension with intraosseous anchors distal to the scaphoid center of rotation so that it tethers the proximal pole in the scaphoid fossa. The flap is sutured to reinforce the local tissue of the scapholunate interval. For a distally based flap, one can raise a rectangular capsular flap, leaving the distal end of the flap attached to the scaphoid (160).

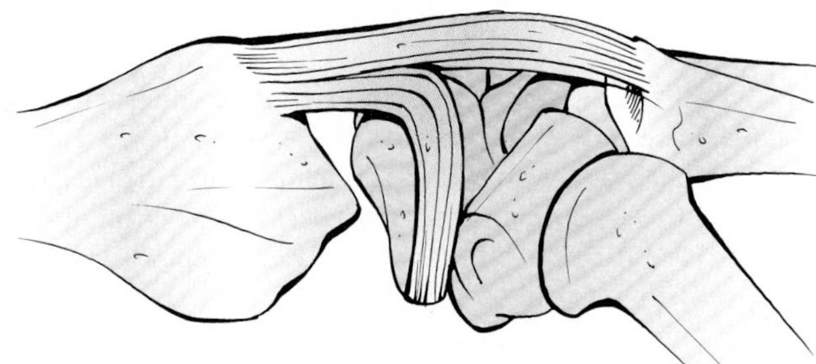

FIGURE 25-33 Blatt type of dorsal capsulodesis. The scaphoid is reduced and the capsular flap is secured to the distal pole with an anchor.

After scapholunate ligament reconstruction, immobilization in a Colles cast is recommended for 8 weeks. The K-wires are removed at 8 weeks. Splint immobilization for an additional 4 weeks is suggested to allow for tissue healing with gradual stress loading. Supporting splints are best worn intermittently for 6 months to prevent sudden stress to the wrist and to allow further collagen maturation (1).

Scaphotrapeziotrapezoidal Fusion

The decision regarding the need for intercarpal fusion for SLD is based on the length of time from the original injury, the degree of ligament disruption, and the ability to reduce the carpal instability. The expectations of the patient are also important. The presence of radiocarpal and midcarpal arthritis should influence the decision toward intercarpal fusion. Arthroscopic examination of both midcarpal and radiocarpal joints may determine the extent of scapholunate ligament and articular cartilage damage and therefore assist in determining treatment (144). Of the partial wrist fusions performed for wrist instability, the scaphotrapeziotrapezoidal (triscaphe) (STT) fusion has had the widest clinical application (1,161,162). The purpose of this procedure is to stabilize the distal scaphoid and thereby hold the proximal pole more securely within the scaphoid fossa of the distal radius (94). This operation can be performed through a transverse incision centered over the scaphotrapeziotrapezoidal joint or through the universal longitudinal incision.

If either STT fusion or the equivalent scaphocapitate fusion is undertaken, it is important to reduce the palmar-flexed scaphoid, close the scapholunate interval, and maintain carpal height. X-ray control is recommended. The ideal flexion angle of the scaphoid is 45°. Fixation of the STT or scaphocapitate joints is performed with K-wires, screws, or staples. Bone graft from the distal radius or iliac crest is placed between the decorticated distal scaphoid and the proximal surfaces of the trapezium and trapezoid (STT fusion) or between the medial articular surface of the scaphoid and the lateral surface of the capitate (scaphocapitate fusion). Once scaphoid alignment is achieved, cancellous bone graft is inserted and Kirschner wires are placed to support the fusion area. Prereduction placement of Kirschner wires into the scaphoid facilitates correct orientation after reduction (1). Clinical studies have shown that STT fusion is reliable and effective, giving pain relief and reasonable functional results (162).

Immobilization after intercarpal fusion is usually for 8 weeks in a scaphoid cast, followed by a support splint for 4 to 6 weeks. CT scans of the wrist can help determine the degree of consolidation at the fusion site.

Four-Corner Fusion

Young active patients with chronic SL instability and severe arthritis can be treated with excision of the scaphoid and a four-corner fusion with arthrodesis of the capitate, lunate, hamate, and triquetrum.

PERILUNATE DISLOCATIONS AND FRACTURE-DISLOCATIONS

Of all wrist dislocations, the perilunate is the most common. Most patients are usually young males, as the bone stock of the distal radius and the scaphoid needs to be strong enough to resist the amount of torque that is involved in these dislocations. Perilunate dislocations are characterized by a progressive disruption of most capsular and ligamentous connections of the lunate to the adjacent carpal bones and radius. Ligament disruption typically begins radially and propagates around or through the lunate to the ulnar side of the carpus (Fig. 25-34). Ligament disruption may be associated with different carpal fractures around the lunate. The distal row dislocates in a dorsal or dorsoradial direction followed by the entire scaphoid and triquetrum in pure perilunate dislocations or just by the distal portion of these bones in perilunate fracture dislocations. Scapholunate (SL) or lunatotriquetral (LT) dissociation often persist even after relocation of the perilunate injury. Recurrence of carpal instability is common whether the injury involves the "lesser arc" injury through ligamentous tissue or the "greater arc" injury through bone, or some combination of the two. The most common pattern of perilunate instability is the transscaphoid perilunate fracture dislocation (1,31,61,163,164).

Pathomechanics

Most dorsal perilunate injuries occur as a consequence of a fall from a height on the outstretched hand or from motor vehicle accidents. At the time of impact, the hand is typically extended and ulnarly deviated (23). The axial compressive load twists the joint beyond the limits of extension and ulnar deviation, adding a progressive midcarpal supination stress that induces the progressive perilunate dissociation. Differences in bone stock, direction and magnitude of the deforming forces, or position of the wrist at the time of impact explain the different types of injuries that occur. These injuries are associated with marked carpal instability (10,23,141,164–167). There are also rare cases of reversed perilunate instability, when the wrist is pronated at the time of impact, thus adding an external force to the hypothenar region, forcing the wrist into extension and radial deviation. In such cases, the LT dissociation occur first followed by lunatocapitate dislocation and then SLD (164,168).

Signs and Symptoms

The diagnosis is established by a history of a hyperextension injury and persistent pain, swelling, and deformity often after a fall from a height or a motor vehicle accident. These high-energy injuries produce significant deformity and soft-tissue damage. Commonly, the clinical presentation includes median nerve injury, but ulnar neuropathy, arterial injury, and tendon damage may also be seen. The pattern of skeletal deformity is variable. The hand and distal carpal row usually remain intact, but the disruption pattern between distal and proximal carpal rows is quite variable. In the transscaphoid fracture dislocation, the distal scaphoid dislocates with the distal row leaving the proximal scaphoid and lunate in near-normal relationship to the forearm. When the perilunate ligaments rupture, the lunate usually remains within the radiocarpal joint and the remainder of the carpus dislocates, usually dorsally but occasionally in a volar direction. Occasionally, the lunate is displaced and rotated palmarly and the remainder of the carpus settles into a seminormal alignment with the distal radius. Rarely, even the palmar attachment of lunate is torn, allowing extrusion into the forearm or through the skin.

Radiographic Examination

The diagnosis is based on careful examination of the x-rays (Fig. 35A–C). The basic pattern can be discerned on standard posteroanterior and lateral x-rays. The typical radiographic appearance of a perilunate dislocation are: (a) The proximal and distal outlines of the proximal carpal rows (Gilula's arcs) present with a discontinuity that indicates a grossly altered intercarpal relationship; (b) the more the lunate is rotated the more it appears triangularly shaped; and (c) on the lateral view, the lunate no longer articulates with the head of the capitate, but appears palmarly rotated, the so-called "spilled teapot sign."

Approximately 20% of perilunate dislocations are misinterpreted on the initial x-rays leading to late treatment, which is

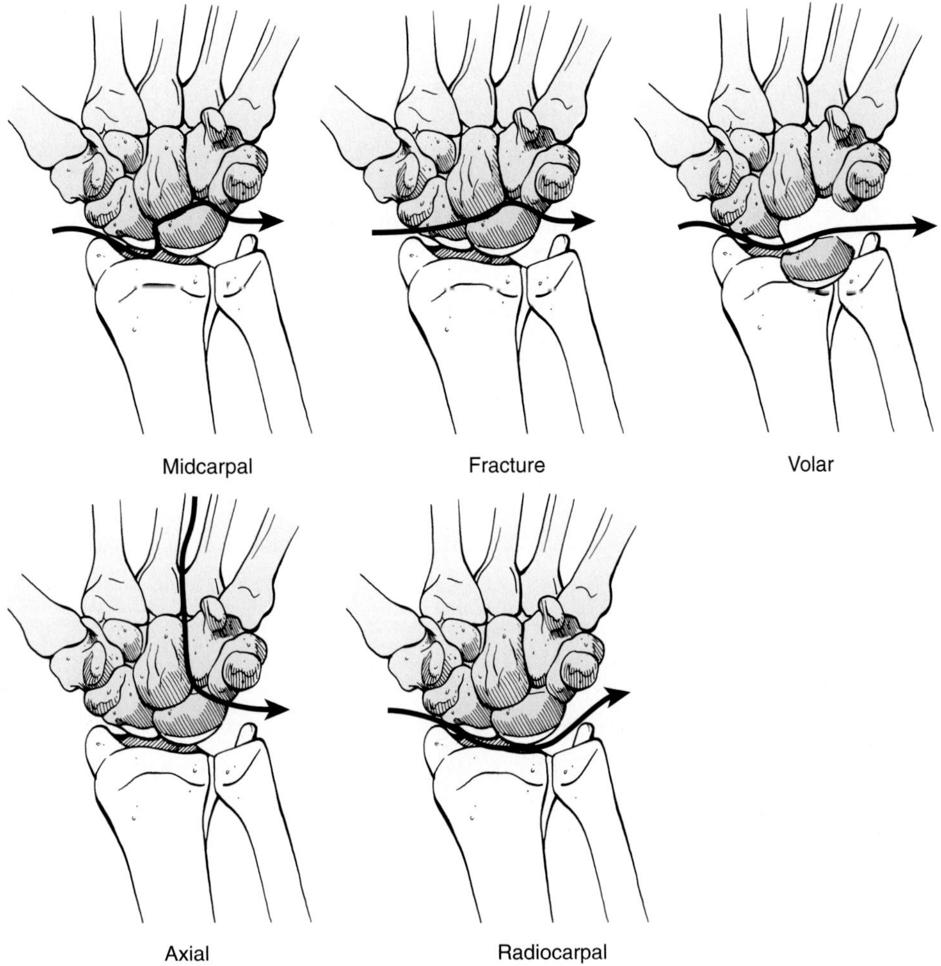

FIGURE 25-34 Different types of perilunate dislocations.

difficult and frequently less successful. It is usually the lesser arc dislocation that is missed because of the lack of an obvious osseous pathology and inexperience of the initial observer. Additional useful studies include tomography, CT scanning, and MRI. Arthrography and arthroscopy may have a useful role in determining the exact injury.

Classification

Mayfield et al (23,41) showed that the disruption of ligaments due to perilunate dislocation is not random but follows the progressive perilunate instability (PLI) pattern of joint derangement (Fig. 25-29). Four stages of PLI have been identified (18).

Stage I: Scaphoid Fracture or Scapholunate Dissociation, or Both

As the distal carpal row is violently extended, supinated, and ulnarly deviated, the STT and scaphocapitate ligaments are tightened, causing the scaphoid to extend. As the scaphoid extends, the SL ligaments transmit the forces to the lunate, which cannot rotate as much as the scaphoid, because it is constrained by the palmarly located RL and UL ligaments. As a consequence, a scaphoid fracture or a progressive tearing of the SL ligaments may occur, eventually leading to a complete SLD.

Stage II: Lunatocapitate Dislocation

If the extension–supination force on the wrist persists once the proximal carpal row has been dislocated the capitate may displace and eventually may dislocate dorsally. It is followed by the rest of the distal carpal row and the radialmost portion of the dislocated proximal carpal row. This may be the complete scaphoid or just its distal fragment.

Stage III: Lunatotriquetral Disruption

If the extension–supination force to the wrist persists, once the capitate is displaced, dorsally an LT dissociation or triquetrum-

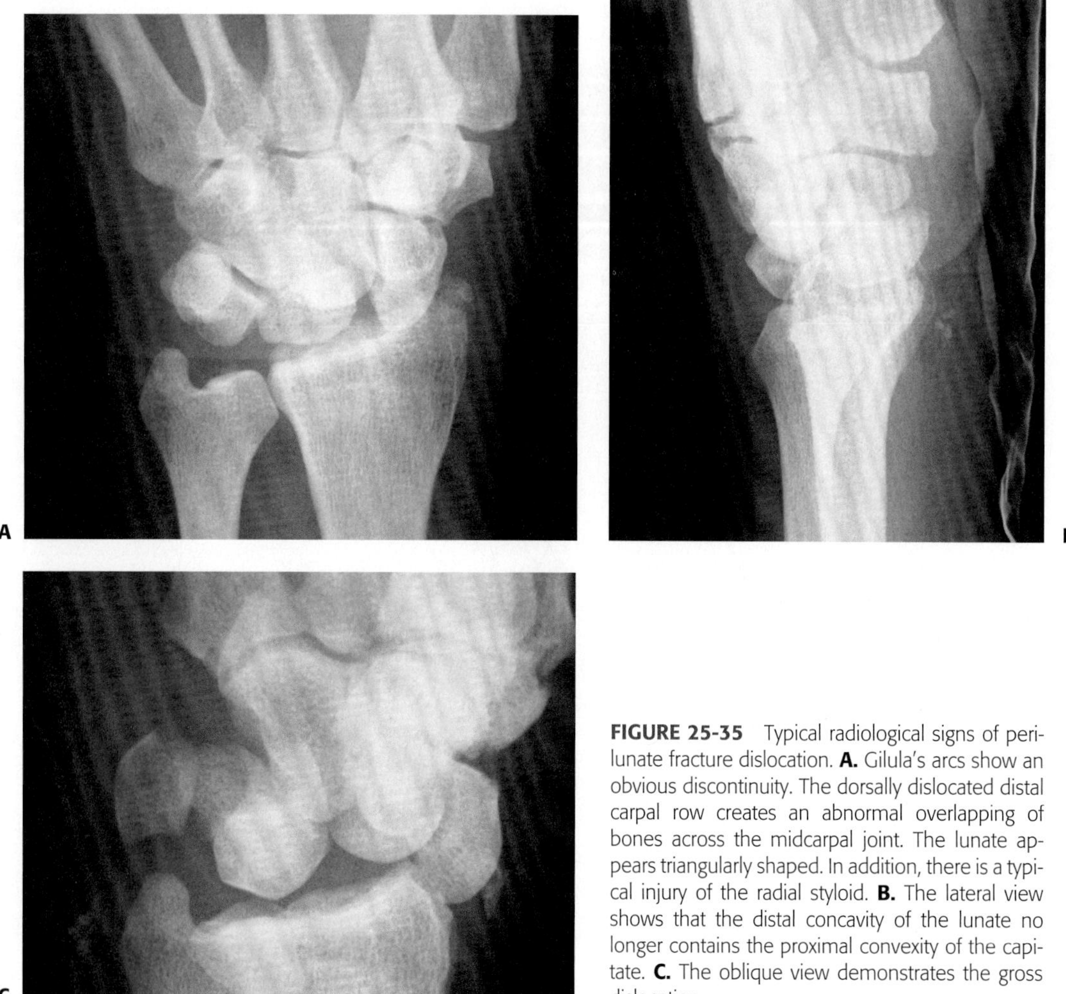

FIGURE 25-35 Typical radiological signs of perilunate fracture dislocation. **A.** Gilula's arcs show an obvious discontinuity. The dorsally dislocated distal carpal row creates an abnormal overlapping of bones across the midcarpal joint. The lunate appears triangularly shaped. In addition, there is a typical injury of the radial styloid. **B.** The lateral view shows that the distal concavity of the lunate no longer contains the proximal convexity of the capitate. **C.** The oblique view demonstrates the gross dislocation.

hamate-capitate ligament disruption may occur. LT dissociations are more common. Stage III is complete when the palmar LT ligament, including the medial expansions of the long RL ligament is completely disrupted, and the joint has displaced.

Stage IV: Perilunate Dislocation

If the extension–supination force to the wrist persists and the dorsally displaced capitate is pulled proximally, pressure is applied onto the dorsal aspect of the lunate, forcing it to dislocation in a palmar direction. Because the palmar ligaments are much stronger than the dorsal capsule, such a dislocation seldom involves a pure palmar displacement of the lunate, but rather a variable degree of palmar rotation of the bone into the carpal tunnel, using the intact palmar ligaments as a hinge. Lunate dislocation is the end stage of progressive perilunate dislocation.

Perilunate dislocations can be further subdivided into two subgroups (169):

A. Lesser-arc perilunate dislocations, which are characterized by pure ligamentous injuries around the lunate.

B. Greater-arc perilunate dislocations, which are characterized by a fracture of one or more of the bones around the lunate.

According to Witvoet and Allieu (170), the lunate may appear normally aligned (grade I), rotated palmarly <90 degrees (grade II), rotated palmarly >90 degrees but still attached to the radius by its palmar ligaments (grade III), or totally enucleated without any connection to the radius (grade IV).

In clinical practice, the prefix *trans* is used to refer to fractures, whereas the prefix *peri* is used to describe a dislocation (164). On the basis of this terminology, the amount of osseous and ligamentous injury as well as the amount of dislocation can be described exactly; thus, a transscaphoid, transcapitate dorsal perilunate dislocation grade IV implies the existence of a displaced fracture of the scaphoid and the capitate, with their distal fragments being dislocated dorsally together with the rest of the distal carpal row The lunate is rotated and totally enucleated without any connection to the radius.

Treatment

Lesser-Arc Injuries

These injuries are divided into (a) acute and reducible perilunate dislocations, (b) acute and irreducible perilunate dislocations, and (c) chronic perilunate dislocations.

Acute and Reducible Perilunate Dislocations. There are reductions that are so stable that it is difficult to determine whether a full perilunate-type dislocation took place, and there are others that reduce and can be maintained in near-normal alignment in casts and splints. Ideally, reduction should be undertaken in the emergency room. The most commonly used method of closed reduction is Tavernier's maneuver (17), which was discussed by Watson-Jones (171). It consist of locking the capitate into the distal concavity of the lunate by combined axial traction and flexion of the distal row, followed by reduction of the capitate-lunate unit onto the radius by an extension movement, while externally applying a localized dorsally directed force to the lunate to help reposition it (164). The earlier reduction is performed, the easier it is. Complete relaxation under general or regional anesthesia is required. Local anesthesia is not sufficient. Successful closed reduction requires adequate imaging with good, standardized posteroanterior and lateral x-rays of the wrist or special imaging techniques. An SL angle that is >80 degrees or an asymmetric SL gap, or both, indicates poor reduction and poor a prognosis if not corrected. It is also important to confirm ligamentous stability with stress-test imaging, MRI, arthroscopy, or open exploration.

The rare injuries that reduce to a normal alignment by closed reduction can be treated with a scaphoid cast with the wrist placed in neutral. They require monitoring on a daily basis for the first week and on a weekly basis thereafter. Cast immobilization of 12 weeks is required. However, the results of closed reduction and cast immobilization are unpredictable. Loss of reduction with cast loosening is common (1).

The literature recommends the use of percutaneous K-wire fixation to stabilize the carpus after closed reduction. This reduces the incidence of later loss of reduction and enhances the healing capability of the intrinsic ligaments by maintaining complete immobility (164). If possible, pin fixation should be performed using arthroscopy. Perilunate dislocations that are stable after reduction require only two pins for fixation. One transverse pin is placed from the scaphoid into the lunate (this can also pinned through the radius into the lunate to neutralize the RL alignment) and a second pin is placed from the scaphoid into the capitate. The pins are usually removed at 8 weeks but wrist immobilization in a scaphoid cast should be maintained for a total of 12 weeks after reduction (164).

Acute and Irreducible Perilunate Dislocations. The majority of perilunate injuries fall into the irreducible or unstable group. If reduction is not optimal or reduction cannot be achieved at all, then open exploration and repair is indicated (172). The author believes that open reduction should be undertaken in all cases where there is the slightest doubt about the reduction. Significantly better results have been reported after open reduction and ligament repair compared to closed reduction and percutaneous pinning (61,164).

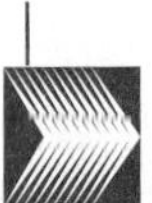

AUTHOR'S PREFERRED TREATMENT

Acute and Irreducible Perilunate Dislocations

The author prefers a dorsal approach because it gives good exposure of the proximal carpal row and midcarpal joint (Fig. 36A–C). If there are neurovascular problems, an additional palmar approach allows access for median nerve decompression, vascular repair if required and repair of the damaged palmar carpal ligaments. This allows both intra-articular and extra-articular damage to be assessed and treated adequately (1,164,173). The surgery is similar to that for treatment of scapholunate dissociation except that an extended carpal tunnel release is performed. The palmar capsule should be examined either along its attachments to the radial rim or through the frequently damaged space of Poirier. The dorsal capsule is usually opened along its origin from the dorsal radial rim, as well as longitudinally in the space between the second and fourth extensor compartments, and the proximal carpal row is examined. If a scaphoid fracture is present, it can be reduced through the dorsal approach, temporarily stabilized with K-wires, and fixed with a cannulated screw. After the scaphoid is reduced, the lunate is reduced to the neutral position using a K-wire as a joystick. The normal scapholunate relationship is restored, while a K-wire is placed through the scaphoid percutaneously, from radial to ulnar, to stabilize the scapholunate joint. A second wire is placed through the scaphoid into the capitate. The LT relationship is restored next and stabilized with another K-wire from ulnar to radial. Torn ligaments can be repaired through the palmar and dorsal incisions. Intraosseous bone anchors are used to repair the scapholunate and lunotriquetral ligaments.

It is important to assess all elements of the injury, restore the normal bony anatomy, and repair soft-tissue damage. The reduction and internal K-wire fixation should be centered around the lunate. The lunate must be aligned and pinned first to the distal radius to neutralize the RL alignment. The LT joint is then reduced and fixed by a second K-wire. Ligaments are repaired as needed. The capitolunate joint alignment is then evaluated and correct colinear alignment is assessed. Lastly the scapholunate joint is reduced and held with K-wires. Many of the patients have an associated radial styloid fracture, which should be reduced anatomically and stabilized with K-wires or a compression screw.

ated with the radius, but the radial one-half of the carpus begins to dislocate dorsally away form the radius and lunate. The soft-tissue disruption propagates proximally, disrupting the LTIL, and often extending proximally into the palmar radioulnar ligament of the TFCC. This dissociates the triquetrum from the lunate (4,8,21,23,141,177).

Diagnosis

Diagnosis of LTD involves a history of specific injury with ulnar-sided wrist pain aggravated by activity. Tenderness is present directly over the LT joint, and ballottement of the unstable triquetrum may be possible. Many patients even state that they sense a "clunk" in their wrist with radial-ulnar deviation (177). Stress loading of the LT joint (compression, ballottement, or shear) helps to confirm the diagnosis (1). The most sensitive test to diagnose LT dissociation is the lunatotriquetral shear test. This is performed by applying a dorsally directed pressure to the pisiform (which is directly palmar to the triquetrum) and a palmarly directed pressure to the lunate (just distal to the palpable dorsoulnar corner of the distal radius). This maneuver results in a shearing vector across the lunotriquetral joint and results in crepitation or clicking, reproducing the patient's pain.

Radiographic diagnosis is more difficult than the diagnosis of SLD because the subtle findings are less obvious and the provocative, stress-induced deformity is less frequent (1). As in all conditions of the wrist, imaging studies should be considered as confirmatory rather than diagnostic (177). True LTD may result in a disruption of Gilula's lines. A static VISI deformity implies an injury to the LT ligament because there is dissociation between lunate and triquetrum, and the usual pattern is for the lunate to follow the scaphoid into flexion while the triquetrum extends (1). Wrist arthrography is not a reliable diagnostic tool but videofluoroscopy can be helpful. Arthroscopy has become the most important diagnostic tool for confirming the presence and degree of LTD. Radiocarpal and midcarpal arthroscopy allows visualization of the scaphoid-trapezoid-trapezium joint, midcarpal extrinsic ligaments, the capitohamate joint, and the articular surfaces of the carpal bones. Arthroscopic staging is applicable to SL, LT, and all other ligamentous dissociations (144).

Treatment

Acute LTD with minimal deformity is ideally treated with a well-molded Colles cast using closed reduction and percutaneous internal fixation of the lunate to the triquetrum if there is displacement. If conservative measures fail, surgical intervention can be considered (177).

LTD with angular deformity or following unsatisfactory results from previous treatment may need open treatment, particularly in the subacute or acute phase (1). Arthroscopy can be helpful in acute injuries to guide closed reduction and percutaneous pinning. It is suggested that the arthroscope be placed in the radial midcarpal portal for this procedure because the alignment of the LT joint is much easier to evaluate from this perspective (177).

Open reduction, repair of lax or damaged ligaments, and temporary internal fixation with percutaneous wires across the triquetrum and lunate, and left in place for 6 to 8, weeks, is recommended for isolated LT ligament tears, if arthroscopy fails. All ligaments that seem to be concerned with LT stability should be reattached. An open repair should be attempted only when there are sufficiently strong ligament remnants present, when the ligament remnants have a reasonable healing potential, and when the LT relationship is easily reduced. These criteria limit the application of open repair techniques to acute injuries (177).

The interosseous ligament repair is usually done through a dorsal approach. Care should be taken to avoid injury to the dorsal sensory branch of the ulnar nerve or to branches of the superficial radial nerve. The fifth extensor compartment is opened and an ulnar-based retinacular flap is elevated. The ligament is more likely to be stripped from the triquetrum. Intraosseous bone anchors with attached sutures are used for reconstruction. Capsular flaps are useful for reinforcing the dorsal portion of such a repair or augmenting the dorsal radiotriquetral and dorsal scaphotriquetral ligaments. For late presentations with complete ligament disruption and no tissue for repair, ligament reconstruction using part of the extensor carpi ulnaris tendon is recommended (1).

If it appears that soft-tissue repair cannot control the tendency to recurrent deformity, LT fusion may be indicated. It is mandatory to correct the VISI deformity. Treatment of the painful wrist may be accompanied with denervation procedures. Concomitant ulnar shortening procedures should be considered (especially with ulnar plus variance) to tighten the palmar ulnocarpal ligaments in addition to LT fusion or ligament reconstruction (1). More aggressive treatments are proximal row carpectomy and total wrist arthrodesis in patients with radiological signs of arthrosis.

MIDCARPAL INSTABILITY

Anatomy and Kinematics

The midcarpal joint can be regarded as a combination of three different types of articulations (178):

- Radially, there is a universal joint that is composed of the distal surface of the scaphoid and the concavity that is formed by the trapezium, the trapezoid, and the radial aspect of the capitate.
- In the center, there is a ball-and-socket type of joint, with the socket lying proximally being formed by the distal surfaces of the scaphoid and lunate. The ball lies distally being formed by the head of the capitate and, variably, the proximal pole of the hamate.
- Finally, on the ulnar side of the midcarpal joint, the triquetrohamate articulation is helicoid, or screw shaped, in con-

figuration. A helicoid facet represents a surface that is generated by the rotation of a plane or a twisted curve about a fixed line, so that each point of the curve traces out a circular helix with the fixed line as the axis. The surfaces of the triquetrohamate joint are only in full contact when the wrist is ulnarly deviated.

The kinematics of the midcarpal joint are controlled by several anatomic structures including the bones and the intrinsic and extrinsic ligaments. The intrinsic ligaments are not always well differentiated and seem to form a continuous palmar capsule that spans the entire width of the midcarpal joint space. However, it is possible to discern two V-shaped ligamentous bands that converge centrally toward the capitate. These bands are formed by the intrinsic palmar midcarpal ligaments, the extrinsic radiocarpal and ulnocarpal ligaments, the radioscaphocapitate ligament, and the short and long radiolunate ligaments. The extrinsic dorsal intercarpal ligament originates from the dorsal aspect of the triquetrum, crosses the midcarpal joint almost transversely in a radial direction, and inserts mainly onto the waist of the scaphoid, the trapezium, and the trapezoid. Despite the fact that there are no attachments to the capitate or hamate, the dorsal intercarpal ligament is capable of holding the head of the capitate and proximal pole of the hamate in position during wrist flexion. The palmar distal V-shaped ligament, consisting of the radiocapitate and ulnocapitate ligaments, also does not attach to the head of the capitate but forms a support sling commonly referred to as the arcuate ligament. Together, these bands allow for maximum range of motion at the level of the midcarpal joint with maximum midcarpal stability (1,178,179).

Pathology

Midcarpal instability (MCI) does not refer to one specific pathology, but to a number of conditions (179,180). MCI is characterized by a loss of normal alignment between the bones in the proximal and distal carpal rows when they are placed under physiologic and pathologic loads owing to ligament injuries of the wrist. Carpal instabilities have been classified into dissociative (CID) and nondissociative (CIND) ones, which have already been discussed in the section dealing with carpal instabilities. MCI is a form of CIND and is difficult to diagnose.

There are four types of MCI (178):

MCI Type I

The so-called palmar MCI, which is secondary to an injury to the palmar midcarpal ligaments, includes the scaphotrapeziotrapezoid ligaments or the triquetrohamate and triquetrocapitate ligaments, or both. The direction of subluxation is palmar.

MCI Type II

The so-called dorsal MCI is a type I MCI in combination with an injury to the radioscaphocapitate ligament. The direction of subluxation is dorsal.

MCI Type III

This is characterized by hyperlaxity of the midcarpal and radiocarpal (dorsal and palmar) ligaments. The direction of subluxation is dorsal or palmar.

MCI Type IV

The so-called extrinsic MCI is due to a malunited radius with dorsal (less commonly palmar) angulation with adaptive deformity of the carpus, inducing progressive stretching of the radiocapitate ligaments, thus reproducing the typical symptoms of a dorsal MCI. The direction of subluxation is dorsal (rarely palmar).

Diagnosis

The history and the physical findings differ little between radiocarpal and midcarpal types of CIND. Some patients recall a history of recent hyperextension injury and a localized area of tenderness. However, many patients do not recall a significant trauma. Frequently, MCI is associated with congenital ligamentous laxity and a hypermobile wrist. Either VISI or DISI deformity or alternating patterns may occur at either level. In the early stages, these patterns of deformity may be so subtle that they are difficult to detect. Nearly all patients with MCI present with painful clunking on the ulnar side of the wrist during activities that involve active ulnar deviation. Many of these patients have had asymptomatic wrist clunking for many years.

The diagnosis is made by the midcarpal stress test. A painful and characteristic clunk (catch-up clunk) can be produced by applying an axial load to a pronated and slightly flexed wrist, which is then brought into ulnar deviation. The "catching-up" occurs when the smooth transition during ulnar deviation lags behind until late in ulnar deviation, when the proximal row suddenly clunks into a reduced extended posture (135,178). The contralateral wrist should be examined in similar fashion, as 50% of patients with MCI may also have a contralateral clunk that is not yet symptomatic (181).

As MCI is a dynamic condition, plain x-rays are often normal. However, they can show a moderate or even severe VISI deformity (type I MCI) or a DISI deformity (type II MCI). An extrinsic MCI (type IV) shows significant angulatory malunion with an adaptive Z-shaped deformity of the carpus (178). Videofluoroscopy, while moving the compressed carpus through the normal range of motion and applying ulnar deviation to the pronated wrist, shows a dramatic and sudden shift at the midcarpal joint, when the proximal row suddenly clunks into a reduced extended posture (1,178).

Imaging findings are also almost identical for radiocarpal or midcarpal CIND and drawing a careful distinction between these uncommon and unusual injuries is difficult. Comparison of video motion patterns of the symptomatic wrist to the normal contralateral wrist is often useful (1). These difficulties are compounded by the fact that ligament insufficiency, which is usually posttraumatic but occasionally congenital (181), may be present at both radiocarpal and midcarpal levels. Visualizing both joints and the intervening proximal carpal row by arthroscopy (75) or surgery gives the final opportunity to decide where the instability is most noticeable. Inflammatory synovitis and clear ligament laxity are the diagnostic signs. Even then, one may have to judge from subtle deviations from the norm, because the attenuation may not be obvious (1).

Treatment

Conservative treatment is usually used initially as many patients with MCI, especially the milder variety, respond well to nonoperative management. Many of these wrist problems occur in individuals with congenitally or posttraumatically lax wrists and who can control the subluxation tendency to some degree by muscle contraction. In such instances, external support to limit the provocative wrist motion together with musculotendinous training may suffice. In addition, patients may be treated with NSAIDs or steroid injections, or modification of their employment may be suggested (1,178).

For those with relatively normal joint surfaces but in whom conservative treatment has failed, surgery aims to prevent pathologic motion at the midcarpal joint and to stabilize the proximal carpal row. If a specific lesion can be identified, such as damage to radial arcuate (radioscaphocapitate) ligament, the ulnar palmar arcuate (triquetrocapitate) ligament, or the scaphotrapeziotrapezoidal ligament, direct soft-tissue reconstruction is indicated with temporary percutaneous fixation (1,178).

In type I MCI with VISI instability (VISI-CIND), four-quadrant fusion (lunate-capitate-triquetrum-hamate) is the gold standard (178). In type II MCI, the interligamentous sulcus between the radioscaphocapitate and the long radiolunate ligaments is closed with strong sutures constructing a radiocarpal tether between radius and proximal carpal row that limits proximal row excursion. If manual reduction is incomplete or there is rapid recurrence after reduction, localized fusion of the midcarpal joint is the best treatment (1,178,182). In type III MCI, radiocarpal fusion is more likely to control the unstable proximal carpal row but proximal row carpectomy is a satisfactory salvage procedure.

In type IV MCI, a corrective open-wedge osteotomy and bone grafting in combination with plate fixation of the radius is the treatment of choice. If there is associated instability of the distal ulna, DRUJ problems, or fixed deformity of the carpus, then further surgical alternatives, such as ulnar shortening, DRUJ stabilization, or midcarpal joint fusion, may need to be undertaken at the same time (1,178).

Axial Instabilities

Axial (longitudinal) instabilities are a type of carpal instability in which the injury affects longitudinal support or alignment of the wrist rather than transverse alignment of the proximal and distal carpal rows. Crush injuries that flatten the hand cause this "axial" instability. Axial instabilities have been separately categorized from other carpal injuries (Fig. 25-37). They represent longitudinal fracture-dislocations of the wrist and, for the most part, are caused by high-energy injuries. Traumatic causes have included an exploding truck tire, crushing under heavy objects, and high-pressure machine compression. The basic pathophysiology is collapse of the carpal arch, often with tearing or avulsion of the bony origins of the transverse carpal ligament. The focus of this injury is usually in the distal carpus and adjacent metacarpals, occasionally extending either distally into the intermetacarpal area or proximally through the proximal carpal row (1). The most common pattern is separation of either radial or ulnar "columns" of the carpus with their metacarpal rays from the central carpus. From a review of the more common patterns, a proposed nomenclature is axial-radial, axial-ulnar, or a combination of the two fracture-dislocations. The carpal elements involved are usually indicated by the term "peri" if the discontinuity is primarily ligamentous, as in peritrapezial or peritrapezoidal-trapezial. If the discontinuity is through bone, the term "trans" is employed, as in transtrapezial or transtrapeziotrapezoidal. The accompanying soft-tissue disruption is often of more importance than the bone and joint disruption. Neurovascular injury is frequent, sometimes to the point of nonviability of the digits (1).

Diagnosis is established by the history of a force propagating in the sagittal plane, with a dorsal to palmar crush, often with evidence of severe soft-tissue damage, swelling, and open wounds. Standard x-rays should confirm the diagnosis, although the carpal malalignment may be subtle and escape notice. A high index of suspicion is needed. Provocative stress x-rays, CT scanning, or MRI should be obtained preoperatively. Evidence of neurological, vascular, musculotendinous, and ligamentous damage is usually present, often to a severe degree. Instances of median neuropathy are less than expected, probably because the carpal tunnel is usually decompressed by the injury (1).

Treatment

A complete assessment is needed in these injuries for planning of both soft-tissue and joint repair. Urgent surgical intervention is often indicated to salvage neurovascular function and restore skeletal alignment. Massive swelling may necessitate decompression of compartments not already decompressed by the injury. Traction can help reduce the axial displacement. Fractures and dislocations, once reduced, can be maintained by Kirschner wires and lag screws. Transcarpal or metacarpal K-wire fixation is usually necessary to prevent redisplacement. Early active motion of the hand helps prevent adhesions of the flexor and extensor tendons. Rehabilitation is often prolonged, and the prognosis depends mainly on the severity of soft-tissue damage (1).

FUTURE DIRECTIONS

Significant progress has been made in the understanding and detection of carpal fractures and instabilities in the last decade,

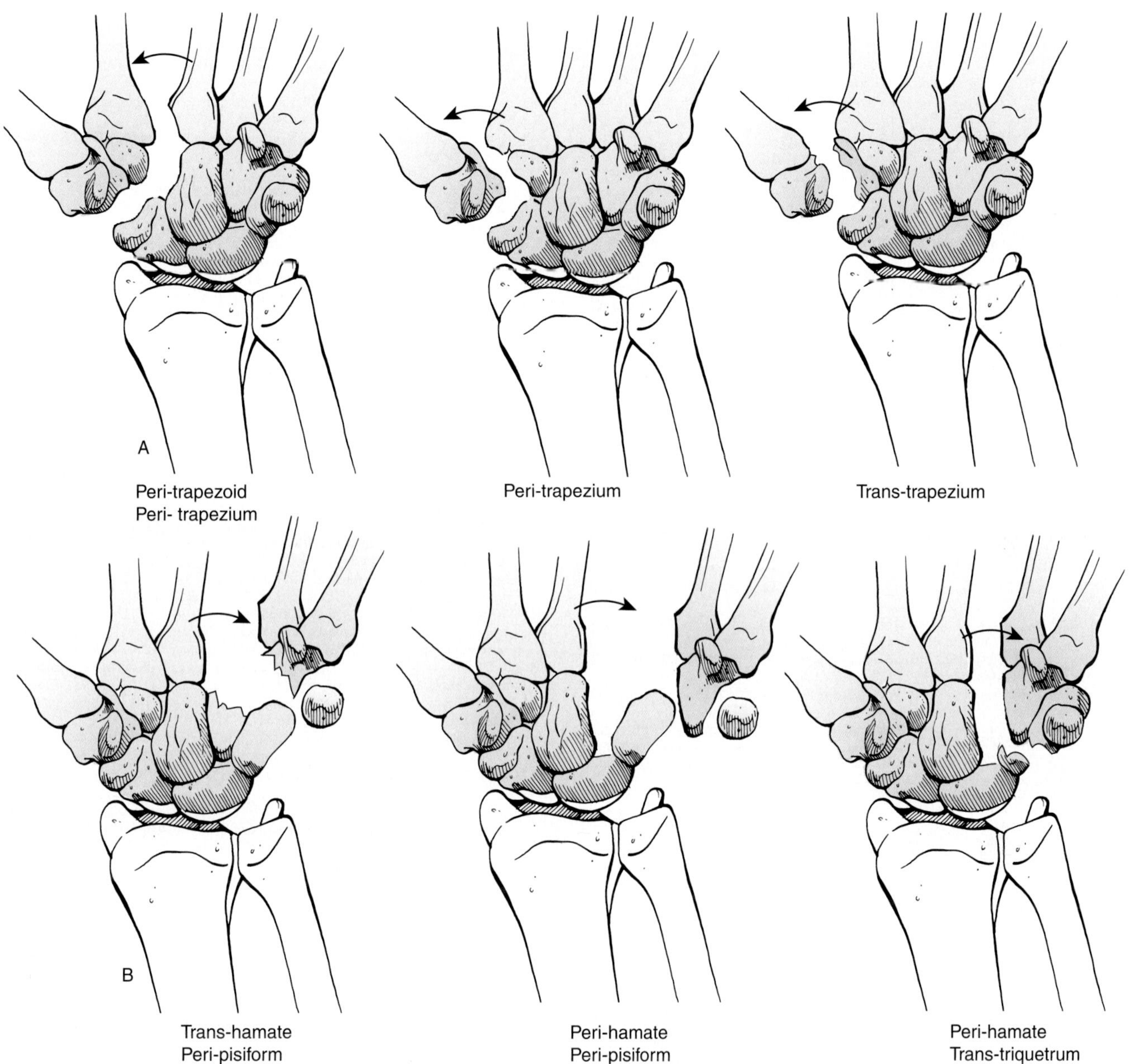

FIGURE 25-37 Axial disruptions of the carpus. **A.** Axial radial disruptions of the carpus. **B.** Axial ulnar disruptions.

mainly because of better imaging techniques. Unfortunately, the dissemination of knowledge has lagged behind, and it is important that surgeons appreciate the importance of early diagnosis and treatment of these relatively common injuries.

Hopefully, improved imaging and surgery will allow better prediction of the evolution of individual carpal instabilities and therefore determine the requirement for operative treatment at an earlier stage. It is likely that improved surgical methods will be devised to treat these problems. The use of closed, fluoroscopically controlled, and arthroscopically controlled techniques will increase and the results of treatment should improve. It is interesting to speculate whether an increasingly aging society will affect the diagnosis and management of carpal problems. Currently, they mainly occur in younger patients, but with altering patient demographics, will this continue?

REFERENCES

An asterisk denotes a Level 1 evidence-based reference.

1. Cooney WP, Linscheid RL, Dobyns JH. Fractures and dislocations of the wrist. In: Rockwood CA, Green DP, Bucholz RW, Heckman JD, eds. *Rockwood and Green's Fractures in adults*. Philadelphia: Lippincott-Raven, 1996:745–867.

2. Kauer JMG. The mechanism of carpal joint. *Clin Orthop* 1986;202:16–26.
3. Linscheid RL. Kinematic considerations of the wrist. *Clin Orthop* 1986;202:27–39.
4. Cooney WP, Garcia-Elias M, Dobyns JH, et al. Anatomy and mechanics of carpal instability. *Surg Rounds Orthop* 1989;1:15–24.
5. Kauer JMG. Functional anatomy of the wrist. *Clin Orthop* 1980;149:9–20.
6. McMurtry RY, Youm Y, Flatt AE, et al. Kinematics of the wrist: II. Clinical Applications. *J Bone Joint Surg* 1978;60-A:955–961.
7. Fisk GR. Carpal instability and the fractured scaphoid. *Ann R Coll Surg Engl* 1970;46: 63–76.
8. Linscheid RL, Dobyns JH, Beabout JW, et al. Traumatic instability of the wrist: diagnosis, classification, and pathomechanics. *J Bone Joint Surg* 1972;54-A:1612–1632.
9. Mayfield JK, Johnson RP, Kilcoyne RK. The ligaments of the human wrist and their functional significance. *Anat Rec* 1976;186:417–428.
10. Taleisnik J. The ligaments of the wrist. *J Hand Surg* 1976;1:110–118.
11. Poirier P, Charpy A. *Traite d'anatomie humaine (arthrolgie)*. Paris: Massonh et Cie, 1897.
12. Kuenz CL. *Les geodes du semi-lunaire* (Thesis). Lyon, 1923.
13. Testut L, Latarget A. *Traite d'anatomie humaine*. Paris: Doin, 1949.
14. Berger RA, Blair WF, Crowninshied RD, Flatt AE. The scapholunate ligament. *J Hand Surg* 1982;7-A:87–91.
15. Berger RA. The gross and histologic anatomy of the scapholunate interosseous ligament. *J Hand Surg* 1996;21-A:170–178.
16. Logan SE, Nowak MD, Gould PL, Weeks PM. Biomechanical behaviour of the scapholunate ligament. *Biomed Sci Instrum* 1986;22:81–85.
17. Gelberman RH, Gross MS. The vascularity of the wrist. Identification of arterial patterns at risk. *Clin Orthop* 1986;202:40–49.
18. Panagis JM, Gelberman RH, Taleisnik J, et al. The arterial anatomy of the human carpus II. The intraosseous vascularity. *J Hand Surg* 1983;8:375–382.
19. Taleisnik J, Kelly PJ. Extraosseous and intraosseous blood supply of the scaphoid bone. *J Bone Joint Surg* 1966;48-A:1125–1137.
20. Gelberman RH, Panagis JS, Taleisnik J, et al. The arterial anatomy of the human carpus: Part I. The extraosseous vascularity. *J Hand Surg* 1983;8-A:367–376.
21. Linscheid RL, Dobyns JH. The unified concept of carpal injuries. *Ann Chir Main Memb Super* 1984;3:35–4.
22. Weber ER, Chao EY. An experimental approach to the mechanism of scaphoid waist fractures. *J Hand Surg* 1978;3:142–148.
23. Mayfield JK, Kilcoyne RK, Johnson RP. Carpal dislocations: pathomechanics and progressive perilunate instability. *J Hand Surg* 1980;5:226–241.
24. Brumbaugh RB, Crowninshield RD, Blair WF, Andrews JG. An in-vivo study of normal wrist kinematics. *J Biomech Eng* 1982;104:176–181.
25. Erdman AG, Mayfield JK, Dorman F, et al. Kinematic and kinetic analysis of the human wrist by stereoscopic instrumentation. *J Biomech Eng* 1979;101:124–133.
26. Herbert TJ. *The fractured scaphoid*. St. Louis: Quality Medical Publishing, 1990.
*27. Gaebler Ch, Kukla Ch, Breitenseher MJ, et al. Diagnosis of occult scaphoid fractures and other wrist injuries: Are repeated clinical examinations and plain radiographs still state of the art. *Langenbeck's Arch Surg* 2001;386:150–154.
28. Gilula LA, Weeks PM. Post-traumatic liagmentous instabilities of the wrist. *Radiology* 1978;129:641–651.
29. Braun H, Krenn W, Schneider S, et al. Direkte MR-Arthrographie des Handgelenkes–Wertigkeit im Nachweis von Komplett- und Partialdefekten der intrinsischen Ligamente und des TFCC im Vergleich zur Arthroskopie. *Fortschr Röntgenstr* 2003; 175:1515–1524.
*30. Gaebler C, Kukla C, Breitenseher MJ, et al. Limited diagnostic value of macroradiography in scaphoid fractures. *Acta Orthop Scand* 1998;69:401–403.
*31. Tiel-van-Buul MMC, vanBeek EJR, Borm JJJ, et al. Radiography and scintigraphy of suspected scaphoid fracture. A long-term study in 160 patients. *J Bone Joint Surg* 1993; 75-B:61–65.
32. Tiel-van-Buul MMC, vanBeek EJR, Borm JJJ, et al. The value of radiographs and bone scintigraphy in suspected scaphoid fracture. A statistical analysis. *J Hand Surg* 1993; 18-B:403–406.
*33. Gaebler C, Kukla C, Breitenseher MJ, et al. Die diagnostische Sicherheit von 0,2 Tesla dedizierten MRT Niederfeldgeräten in der Traumatologie. *Swiss Surgery* 1998;4: 175–179.
34. Gaebler C, Kukla C, Breitenseher M, et al. Magnetic resonance imaging of occult scaphoid fractures. *J Trauma* 1996;41:73–76.
35. Leslie IJ, Dickson RA. The fractured carpal scaphoid. Natural history and factors influencing outcome. *J Bone Joint Surg* 1981;63-B:225–230.
36. Osterman AL, Mikulics M. Scaphoid nonunion. *Hand Clin* 1988;4:437–455.
37. Larsen CF, Brondum V, Skov O. Epidemiology of scaphoid fractures in Odense, Denmark. *Acta Orthop Scand* 1992;63:216–218.
38. Rettig AC. Elbow, forearm and wrist injuries in the athlete. *Sports Med* 1998;25: 115–130.
39. Barton NJ. Twenty questions about scaphoid fractures. *J Hand Surg* 1992;17-B: 289–310.
*40. Gaebler C, Court-Brown C, Vecsei V, et al. Percutaneous screw fixation of acute scaphoid fractures versus conservative treatment: a prospectively randomised study of 60 patients. Oral presentation at European Trauma Conference, Vienna, Austria, 2002.
41. Prosser AJ, Brenkel IJ, Irvine GB. Articular fractures of the distal scaphoid. *J Hand Surg* 1988;19B:87–91.
42. Ruby LK, Stinson J, Belsky MR. The natural history of scaphoid non-union: a review of fifty cases. *J Bone Joint Surg* 1985;67-A:428–432.
43. Taleisnik J. Fractures of the scaphoid. In: Taleisnik J, ed. *The wrist*. New York: Churchill Livinstone, 1985:105–148.
44. Trojan E. Der Kahnbeinbruch der Hand, Habilitationsschrift, Eigenverlag, Druck Brüder Hollinek, Wien, 1961.
45. Moritomo H, Viegas SF, Nakamura K, et al. The scaphotrapezio-trapezoidal joint. Part I: an anatomic and radiographic study. *J Hand Surg* 1999;25-A:899–910.
47. Wolfe SW. Fractures of the carpus: scaphoid fractures. In: Berger RA, Weiss APC, eds. *Hand surgery*, vol 1. Philadelphia, London, Tokyo: Lippincott Williams & Wilkins, 2004:381–408.
48. Smith BS, Cooney WP. Revision of failed bone grafting for nonunion of the scaphoid. Treatment options and results. *Clin-Orthop* 1996;327:98–109.
49. Amadio PC, Berquist TH, Smith DK, et al. Scaphoid malunion. *J Hand Surg* 1989; 14-A:679–687.
50. Sanders WE. Evaluation of the humpback scaphoid by computed tomography in the longitudinal axial plane of the scaphoid. *J Hand Surg* 1988;13-A:182–187.
51. Gelberman RH, Menon J. The vascularity of the scaphoid bone. *J Hand Surg* 1980;5: 508–513.
52. Obletz BE, Halbstein BM. Non-union of fractures of the carpal navicular. *J Bone Joint Surg* 1938;20-A:424–428.
53. Gelberman RH, Wolock BS, Siegel DB. Fractures and non-unions of the carpal scaphoid. *J Bone Joint Surg* 1989;71-A:1560–1565.
54. Mack GR, Bosse MJ, Gelbermannh RH, et al. The natural history of scaphoid nonunion. *J Bone Joint Surg* 1984;66A:504–509.
55. Duteille F, Dautel G. Non-union fractures of the scaphoid and carpal bones in children: surgical treatment. *J Ped Orthop* 2004;B:13:34–38.
56. Günal Ý, Öztuna V, Özcelik A, et al. Medium-term results of trapezio-lunate external fixation of scaphoid fractures. *J Hand Surg* 2002;27B:5:410–412.
57. Vahvanen V, Westerlund M. Fracture of the carpal scaphoid in children. A clinical and roentgenological study of 108 cases. *Acta Orthop Scand* 1980;51:909–913.
*58. Gaebler C, Kukla C, Breitenseher M, et al. Magnetic resonance imaging of occult scaphoid fractures. *J Trauma* 1996;41:73–76.
59. Freeland P. Scaphoid tubercle tenderness: a better indicator of scaphoid fractures? *Arch Emerg Med* 1989;6:46–50.
*60. Parvizi J, Wayman J, Kelly P, et al. Combining the clinical signs improves diagnosis of scaphoid fractures. A prospective study with follow-up. *J Hand Surg* 1998;23-B: 324–327.
61. Hertzberg G, Comtet JJ, Linscheid RL, et al. Perilunate dislocations and fracture dislocations: a multicenter study. *J Hand Surg* 1993;18-A:768–779.
62. Breitenseher MJ, Gaebler C. Trauma of the wrist. *Eur J Radiol* 1997;25:129–139.
63. Beadel GP, Ferreira L, Johnson JA, et al. Interfragmentary compression across a simulated scaphoid fracture–analysis of 3 screws. *J Hand Surg* 2004;29A:273–278.
64. Annamalai G, Raby N. Scaphoid and pronator fat stripes are unreliable soft tissue signs in the detection of radiographically occult fractures. *Clin Radiol* 2003;58:798–800.
65. Munk B, Bolvig L, Kroner K, et al. Ultrasound for diagnosis of scaphoid fractures. *J Hand Surg* 2000;25-B:369–371.
*66. Breitenseher MJ, Metz VM, Gilula LA, et al. Radiographically occult scaphoid fractures: value of mr imaging in detection. *Radiology* 1997;203:245–250.
67. Brismar J. Skeletal scintigraphy of the wrist in suggested scaphoid fracture. *Acta Radiol* 1988;29:101–107.
*68. Roolker W, Tiel-van-Buul MM, Ritt MJ, et al. Experimental evaluation of scaphoid X-series, carpal box radiographs, planar tomography, computed tomography, and magnetic resonance imaging in the diagnosis of scaphoid fracture. *J Trauma* 1997;42: 247–253.
69. Herbert TJ, Fisher WE. Management of the fractured scaphoid using a new bone screw. *J Bone Joint Surg* 1984;66B:114–123.
70. N'Dow J, N'Dow K, Maffulli N, et al. The suspected scaphoid fracture. How useful is a unit policy? *Bull Hosp Joint Dis* 1998:57:93–95.
71. Imaeda T, Nakamura R, Miura T, Makino N. Magnetic resonance imaging in scaphoid fracture. *J Hand Surg* 1992;17-B:20–27.
72. Streli R. Perkutane Verschraubung des Handkahnbeines mit Bohrdrahtkompressionsschraube. *Zentralbl Chir* 1970;95:1060–1078.
73. Alho A, Kankaanpaa U. Management of fractured scaphoid bone: a prospective study of 100 fractures. *Acta Orthop Scand* 1975;46:737–743.
74. Kuhlmann JN, Boabighi A, Kirsch JM, et al. An experimental study of plaster immobilization for fractures of the carpal scaphoid. A clinical investigation. *Rev Chir Orthop Reparatrice Appar Mot French* 1987;73:49–56.
75. Yanni D, Lieppins P, Laurence M. Fractures of the carpal scaphoid. A critical study of the standard splint. *J Bone Joint Surg* 1991;73B:600–602.
76. Clay NR, Dias JJ, Costigan PS, et al. Need the thumb be immobilized in scaphoid fractures? A randomized prospective trial. *J Bone Joint Surg* 1991;73B:828–832.
77. McLaughlin HL. Fracture of the carpal navicular (scaphoid) bone. Some observations based on treatment by open reduction and internal fixation. *J Bone Joint Surg* 1954; 36A:765–774.
*78. Haddad FS, Goddard NJ. Acute percutaneous scaphoid fixation. A pilot study. *J Bone Joint Surg* 1998;80B:95–99.
79. Rettig AC, Weidenbener EJ, Gloyeske R. Alternative management of midthird scaphoid fractures in the athlete. *Am J Sports Med* 1994:22:711–714.
80. Wozasek GE, Moser KD. Percutaneous screw fixation for fractures of the scaphoid. *J Bone Joint Surg* 1991:73B:138–142.
81. Papaloizos MY, Fusetti C, Christen T, et al. Minimally invasive fixation versus conservative treatment of undisplaced scaphoid fractures: a cost-effectiveness study. *J Hand Surg* 2004;29B:2:116–119.
*82. Yip HSF, Wu WC, Chang RYP, et al. Percutaneous cannulated screw fixation of acute scpahoid wrist fracture. *J Hand Surg* 2002;27B:1:42–46.
83. Galladay GJ, Jebson PJL, Louis DS. The versatility of a new variable pitch screw system in hand, wrist and elbow surgery. American Association for Hand Surgery Meeting 1998.

84. Hoy G, Powell G. Scaphoid fixation using the Acutrak screw. Presented 25th Sept. 1996, Australian/New Zealand Hand Surgery Meeting, Cairns, Australia.
85. Toby EB, Butler TE, McCormack TJ, et al. A comparison of fixation screws for the scaphoid during application of cyclical bending loads. *J Bone Joint Surg* 1997;79A: 1190–1197.
86. Wheeler DL, McLoughlin SW. Biomechanical assessment of compression screws. *Clin Orthop* 1998;350:237–245.
87. Kujala S, Raatikinen T, Kaarela O, et al. Successful treatment of scaphoid fractures and nonunions using bioabsorbable screws: report of six cases. *J Hand Surg* 2004;29A: 68–73.
88. Wilton TJ. Soft tissue interposition as a possible cause of scaphoid non-union. *J Hand Surg* 1987;12B:50–51.
89. Slade JF, Jaskwhich D. Percutaneous fixation of scaphoid fractures. *Hand Clin* 2001; 17:553–574.
90. Langhoff O, Andersen JL. Consequences of late immobilization of scaphoid fractures. *J Hand Surg* 1988;13-B:77–79.
91. Slade JF, Geissler WB, Gutow AP, Merrell GA. Percutaneous internal fixation of selected scaphoid nonunions with an arthroscopically assisted dorsal approach. *J Bone Joint Surg* 2003;86-A[Suppl 4]:20–32.
92. Russe O. Fracture of the carpal navicular: diagnosis, nonoperative treatment and operative treatment. *J Bone Joint Surg* 1960;42A:759–765.
93. Fisk GR. The wrist. *J Bone Joint Surg* 1984;66:396–407.
94. Watson HK, Ballet FL. The SLAC wrist: scapholunate advanced collapse pattern of degenerative arthritis. *J Hand Surg* 1984;9:358–365.
95. Trumble T, Nyland W. Scaphoid nonunions–pitfalls and pearls. *Hand Clin* 2001;17: 611–624.
96. Fernandez DL, Eggli S. Scaphoid non-union and malunion–how to correct deformity. *Hand Clin* 2001;17:631–646.
97. Green DP. The effect of avascular necrosis on Russe bone grafting for scpahoid nonunion. *J Hand Surg* 1985;10-A:597–605.
98. Eggli S, Fernandez DL, Beck T. Unstable scaphoid fracture non-union: a medium-term study of anterior wedge grafting procedures. *J Hand Surg* 2002;27B:1:36–41.
99. Hull WJ, House JM, Gustilo RB, et al. The surgical approach and source of bone graft for symptomatic non-union of the scaphoid. *Clin Orthop* 1976;115:241–247.
100. Steinmann SP, Bishop AT. A vascularized bone graft for repair of scaphoid nonunion. *Hand Clin* 2001;17:647–653.
101. Buck-Gramcko D. Denervation of the wrist joint. *J Hand Surg* 1977;2:54–61.
102. Vender MI, Watson HK, Black DM, Strickland JW. Acute scaphoid fracture with scapholunate gap. *J Hand Surg* 1989;14-A:1004–1007.
103. Haussmann P. Long-term results after silicone prosthesis replacement of the proximal pole of the scaphoid bone in advanced scaphoid non-union. *J Hand Surg* 2002;27B:5: 417–423.
104. Houshian S, Schröder HA. Wrist arthrodesis with the AO titanium wrist fusion plate: a consecutive series of 42 cases. *J Hand Surg* 2001;26B:4:355–359.
105. Lynch NM, Linscheid RL. Corrective osteotomy for scaphoid malunion: technique and long-term follow-up evaluation. *J Hand Surg* 1997;22A:35–43.
106. Preiser G. Zu einer typischen posttraumatischen und zur Spontanfraktur führenden Osteitis des Naviculare Carpi. *Fortschr Roentgenstr* 1910;15:189.
107. Menth-Chiari WA, Poehling GG. Preiser's disease: arthroscopic treatment of avascular necrosis of the scaphoid. *Arthroscopy* 2000;16:208–213.
108. Pao VS, Chang J. Scaphoid nonunion: diagnosis and treatment. *Plast Reconstr Surg* 2003;112:1666–1675.
109. Waters PM, Stewart SL. Surgical treatment of nonunion and avascular necrosis of the proximal part of the scaphoid in adolescents. *J Bone Joint Surg* 2002;84-A:6:915–920.
110. Cetti R, Christensen SE, Reuther K. Fracture of the lunate bone. *Hand* 1982;14:80–84.
111. Verdan C. Les fractures ignorées du semi-lunaire. *Ann Chir Main* 1982;1:248–249.
112. Schiltenwolf M, Martini AK, Eversheim S, et al. Die Bedeutung des intraossären Druckes für die Pathogenese des Morbus Kienböck. *Handchir Mikrochir Plast Chir* 1996;28: 215–219.
113. Sennwald GR. Carpal bone fractures other than the scaphoid. In: Berger RA, Weiss APC, eds. *Hand surgery*, vol I. Philadelphia, London, Tokyo: Lippincott Williams & Wilkins, 2004:409–423.
114. Teisen H, Hjarback J. Classification of fresh fractures of the lunate. *J Hand Surg* 1989; 13-B:458–462.
115. De Beer JdeV, Hudson DA. Fractures of the triquetrum. *J Hand Surg* 1987;12-B:52–53.
116. Garcia-Elias M. Dorsal fractures of the triquetrum. Avulsion or compression fractures? *J Hand Surg* 1987;12-A:266–268.
117. Linscheid RL, Dobyns JH. Wrist sprains. In: Tubiana R, ed. *The hand*, vol II. Philadelphia: WB Saunders, 1985:970–985.
118. Lacey JD, Hodge JC. Pisiform and hamulus fractures: easily missed wrist fractures diagnosed on a reverse oblique radiograph. *J Emer Med* 1998;16:445–452.
119. Arner M, Hagberg L. Wrist flexion strength after excision of the pisiform bone. *Scand J Plast Reconstr Surg* 1984;18:241–245.
120. Rettig ME, Dassa GL, Raskin KB, et al. Wrist fractures in the athlete. Distal radius and carpal fractures. *Clin Sports Med* 1998;17:469–489.
121. Almquist EE, Bach AW, Sack JT, et al. Four-bone ligament reconstruction for treatment of chronic complete scapholunate separation. *J Hand Surg* 1991;16-A:322–327.
122. Alt V, Sicre G, Schad A. Intraligamentäre Naht einer skapholunären Bandläsion bei einem 9-jährigen Kind. *Unfallchirurg* 2002;105:943–945.
123. Garcia-Elias M. Carpal bone fractures (excluding scaphoid fractures). In: Watson HK, Weinberg J, eds. *The wrist*. Philadelphia: Williams & Wilkins, 2001:173–186.
124. Cordrey LJ, Ferrer-Torrels M. Management of fractures of the greater multangular. *J Bone Joint Surg* 1969;42-A:1111–1118.
125. Calandruccio JH, Duncan SF. Isolated nondisplaced capitate waist fracture diagnosed by magnetic resonance imaging. *J Hand Surg* 1999;24-A:856–859.
126. Fenton RL. The naviculo-capitate syndrome. *J Bone Joint Surg* 1956;38-A:681–684.
127. Vance RM, Gelberman RH, Evans EF. Scaphocapitate fractures. *J Bone Joint Surg* 1980; 62-A:271–276.
128. Freeman BH, Hay EL. Nonunion of the capitate: a case report. *J Hand Surg* 1985;10-A:187–190.
129. Foucher G, Schuind F, Merle M, et al. Fractures of the hook of the hamate. *J Hand Surg* 1985;10-B:205–210.
130. Rettig A. Athletic injuries of the wrist and hand. Part I: traumatic injuries of the wrist. *Am J Sports Med* 2003;31:1038–1048.
131. Zemel NP, Stark HH. Fractures and dislocations of the carpal bones. *Clin Sports Med* 1986;5:709–724.
132. Boulas HJ, Milek MA. Hook of the hamate fractures. Diagnosis, treatment, and complications. *Orthop Rev* 1990;19:518–529.
133. Watson HK, Rogers WD. Nonunion of the hook of the hamate: an argument for bone grafting the non-union. *J Hand Surg* 1989;14:486–490.
134. Baratz ME, Dunn MJ. Ligament injuries and instability of the carpus: scapholunate joint. In: Berger RA, Weiss APC, eds. *Hand surgery*, vol I. Philadelphia, London, Tokyo: Lippincott Williams & Wilkins, 2004:460–479.
135. Cohen MS. Ligamentous injuries of the wrist in the athlete. *Clin Sports Med* 1998;17: 533–552.
136. Lewis DM, Osterman AL. Scapholunate instability in athletes. *Clin Sports Med* 2001; 20:131–139.
137. Mudgal CS, Jones WA. Scapho-lunate diastasis: a component of fractures of the distal radius. *J Hand Surg* 1990;15-B:503–505.
138. Schwendenwein E, Wozasek GE, Hajdu S, Vécsei V. Okkulte skapholunäre Dissoziation bei distaler Radiusfraktur. *Wiener Klin Wochenschr* 2003;115:580–583.
139. Tang JB, Shi D, Gu YQ, et al. Can cast immobilization successfully treat scapholunate dissociation associated with distal radius fractures? *J Hand Surg* 1996;21A:583–590.
140. Tang JB, Ryu J, Omokawa S, et al. Wrist kinetics after scapholunate dissociation: the effect of scapholunate interosseous ligament injury and persistent scapholunate gaps. *J Orthop Res* 2002;20:215–221.
141. Mayfield JK. Pattern of injury to carpal ligaments: a spectrum. *Clin Orthop* 1984;187: 36–42.
142. Frankel VH. The Terry-Thomas sign. *Clin Orthop* 1986;20:50–56.
143. Cautilli GP, Wehbe MA. Scapholunate distance and cortical ring sign. *J Hand Surg* 1991;16-A:501–503.
144. Hofmeister EP, Dao KD, Glowacki KA, Shin AY. The role of midcarpal arthroscopy in the diagnosis of disorders of the wrist. *J Hand Surg* 2001;26A:407–414.
145. Ruby LK. Carpal instability. *J Bone Joint Surg* 1995;77-A:476–487.
146. Whipple TL. The role of arthroscopy in the treatment of scapholunate instability. *Hand Clin* 1995;11:37–40.
147. Wilhelm K, Kettler M, Strassmair M. SL. Bandrekonstruktion mit Mitek-Fadenankerdübeln. Erste klinische Ergebnisse. *Unfallchirurg* 2001;104:127–130.
148. Wyrick JD, Youse BD, Kiefhaber TR. Scapholunate ligament repair and capsulodesis for the treatment of static scapholunate dissociation. *J Hand Surg* 1998;23-B:776–780.
149. Hahn P, Krimmer H, Prommersberger KJ, et al. Die skapholunäre Dissoziation. Ergebnisse nach Bandnaht und Bandplastik. *Handchir Mikrochir Plast Chir* 1999;31:346–350.
150. Bickert B, Sauerbier M, Germann G. Scapholunate ligament repair using the Mitek™ bone anchor. *J Hand Surg* 16;25B:2:188–192.
151. Lavernia CJ, Cohen MS, Taleisnik J. Treatment of scapho-lunate dissociation by ligamentous repair and capsulodesis. *J Hand Surg* 1992;17-A:354–359.
152. Blatt G. Capsulodesis in reconstructive hand surgery: dorsal capsulodesis for the unstable scaphoid and volar capsulodesis following excision of the distal ulna. *Hand Clin* 1987;3:81–102.
153. Schweizer A, Steiger R. Long-term results after repair and augmentation ligamentoplasty of rotatory subluxation of the scaphoid. *J Hand Surg* 2002;27A:674–684.
154. Szabo RM, Slater RR, Palumbo CF, et al. Dorsal intercarpal ligament capsulodesis for chronic, static scapholunate dissociation: clinical results. *J Hand Surg* 2002;27A: 978–984.
155. Weiss AP, Sachar K, Glowacki KA. Arthroscopic debridement alone for intercarpal tears. *J Hand Surg* 1997;22-A:344–349.
156. Lutz M, Kralinger F, Goldhahn J, et al. Dorsal scapholunate ligament reconstruction using a periostal flap of the iliac crest. *Arch Orthop Trauma Surg* 2004;124:197–202.
157. Slater RR, Szabo RM, Bay BK, et al. Dorsal intercarpal ligament capsulodesis for scapholunate dissociation: biomechanical analysis in a cadaver model. *J Hand Surg* 1999;24A: 232–239.
158. Deshmukh SC, Givissis D, Belloso D, et al. Blatt's capsulodesis for chronic scapholunate dissociation. *J Hand Surg* 1999;24B:2:215–220.
159. Kalb K, Markert S. Erste Erfahrungen mit der Osteoligamentoplastik und Kapsulodese nach Cuénod zur Behandlung der chronischen skapholunären Dissoziation. *Handchir Mikrochir Plast Chir* 2003;35:310–316.
160. Herbert TJ, Hargreaves IC, Clarke AM. A new surgical technique for treating rotatory instability of the scaphoid. *J Hand Surg* 1996;21-B:75–77.
161. Crosby EB, Linscheid RL, Dobyns JH. Scaphotrapezial trapezoidal arthrosis. *J Hand Surg* 1978;3:223–234.
162. Meier R, Prommersberger KJ, Krimmer H. Teil-Arthrodesen von Skaphoid, Trapezium und Trapezoideum (STT-Fusion). *Handchir Mikrochir Plast Chir* 2003;35:323–327.
163. Cooney WP, Bussey R, Dobyns JH, et al. Difficult wrist fractures. Perilunate fracture-dislocations of the wrist. *Clin Orthop* 1987;214:136–147.
164. Garcia-Elias M. Perilunate injuries including fracture dislocations. In: Berger RA, Weiss APC, eds. Hand surgery, vol I. Philadelphia, London, Tokyo: Lippincott Williams & Wilkins, 2004:511–523.

165. Harrington P, Quinlan WB. Palmar lunate trans-scaphoid, trans-triquetral fracture-dislocation. *J Hand Surg* 1999;24B:4:493–496.
166. Masmejean EH, Romano SJ, Saffar PH. Palmar perilunate fracture-dislocation of the carpus. *J Hand Surg* 1998;23B:2:264–265.
167. Pandit R. Proximal and palmar dislocation of the lunate and proximal scaphoid as a unit in a case of scaphocapitate syndrome—A 32-month follow-up. *J Hand Surg* 1998; 23B:2:266–268.
168. Reagan DS, Linscheid RL, Dobyns JH. Lonotriquetral sprains. *J Hand Surg* 1984;9-B: 502–514.
169. Johnson RP. The acutely injured wrist and its residuals. *Clin Orthop* 1980;149:33–44.
170. Witvoet J, Allieu Y. Lesions traumatiques fraiches. *Rev Chir Orthop* 1973;59[Suppl]: 98–125.
171. Watson-Jones R. *Fractures and joint injuries*, 3rd ed. Edinburgh: Churchill Livingstone, 1943:568–577.
172. Green DP, O'Brian ET. Open reduction of carpal dislocations: indications and operative techniques. *J Hand Surg* 1978;3A:250–265.
173. Sotereanos DG, Mitsionis GJ, Giannakopoulos PN, et al. Perilunate dislocation and fracture dislocation: a critical analysis of the volar-dorsal approach. *J Hand Surg* 1997; 22A:49–56.
174. Herzberg G, Forissier D. Acute dorsal trans-scaphoid perilunate fracture-dislocations: medium-term results. *J Hand Surg* 2002;27B:6:498–502.
175. Apergis E, Darmanis S, Kastanis G, et al. Does the term scaphocapitate syndrome need to be revised? A report of 6 cases. *J Hand Surg* 2001;26B:5:441–445.
176. Strohm PC, Laier P, Müller CA, et al. Erstbeschreibung des beidseitigen Auftretens einer seltenen Verletzung. *Unfallchirurg* 2003;106:339–342.
177. Berger RA. Lunotriquetral joint. In: Berger RA, Weiss APC, eds. *Hand surgery*, vol I. Philadelphia, London, Tokyo: Lippincott Williams & Wilkins, 2004:495–509.
178. Ritt MJPF. Midcarpal instability. In: Berger RA, Weiss APC, eds. Hand surgery, vol I. Philadelphia, London, Tokyo: Lippincott Williams & Wilkins, 2004:525–532.
179. Ono H, Gilula LA, Evanoff BA, et al. Midcarpal instability: is capitolunate instability pattern a clinical condition? *J Hand Surg* 1996;21B:2:197–201.
180. Apergis EP. The unstable capitolunate and radiolunate joints as a source of wrist pain in young women. *J Hand Surg* 1996;21B:4:501–506.
181. Wright TW, Dobyns JH, Linscheid RL, et al. Carpal instabilities non-dissociative. *J Hand Surg* 1994;19-A:763–773.
182. Johnson RP, Carrera GF. Chronic capitolunate instability. *J Bone Joint Surg* 1986;68-A:1164–1176.

FRACTURES OF THE DISTAL RADIUS AND ULNA

David S. Ruch

HISTORICAL PERSPECTIVE

The optimal management of distal radius fractures has changed dramatically over the previous two decades from almost universal use of cast immobilization to a variety of highly sophisticated operative interventions. Few prospective studies confirm the benefit of this increasingly aggressive operative approach, however. Surgeons are increasingly faced with the dilemma of when to consider operative management and when cast immobilization is the optimal treatment. Although some patients still seem to confirm Abraham Colles' famous remarks that the casted wrist "will at some remote period again enjoy perfect freedom in all of its motions and be completely exempt from pain," (1) an increasing preponderance of published studies supports the need for operative intervention in a growing number of patients. In addition to apparent discrepancies regarding surgical interventions, there are other equally disparate studies regarding multiple facets of this fracture. There are conflicting data about the long-term relationship regarding radiographic parameters and patient-reported outcomes. Fernandez and Trumble as well as others have reported that as little as 1 mm of articular incongruity is associated with a worse functional outcome (2). Catelano et al have indicated that although there is a correlation between articular incongruity and radiographic arthrosis, there is not a correlation with self-reported function (3). Age is also a confounding variable in determining the need for operative management. Young and Rayan indicated that in elderly patients (mean age 72 years), the radiographic outcome did not correlate with functional outcome despite significant collapse and incongruity (4). By contrast, Madhok indicated that 26% of elderly patients still experience functional impairment after nonoperative management at 1 year following closed treatment (5). Even when operative intervention is clearly indicated, there is still controversy over the use of external fixation versus one of the growing number of internal fixation devices. This chapter examines the presumably known variables including the epidemiology, mechanism of injury, and classification systems as well as the current trends in nonoperative and operative management, and the complications and pitfalls of each.

EPIDEMIOLOGY

Distal radius fractures represent approximately one-sixth of all fractures treated in emergency departments. Data extracted from the National Hospital Ambulatory Medical Care Survey indicate that in 1998, there were approximately 644,985 fractures of the distal radius treated in the United States. The incidence of this injury appears to be both gender and age specific (6). There are three main peaks of fracture distribution: the first peak is in children ages 5 to 14, the second is in males under age 50, and the third peak is in females over the age of 40 years. There seems to be a growing incidence of these fractures in all three groups with the sharpest increase seen in both elderly females and younger adult males (7–9). More importantly, these studies suggest that the difference in the two peak incidences indicates that these fractures represent two very different injuries: one, an insufficiency fracture in elderly patients, and the other is a traumatic injury in younger males. The differences in these injuries and corresponding groups may account for some of the discrepancies noted in the literature.

Current data suggest that distal radius fractures in the elderly may represent an insufficiency fracture associated with all of the risk factors for osteoporosis (9). The age-adjusted incidence rates of distal radius fractures for women were 165 in 1986 and 211 in 1995, indicating a steady rise over 10 years (6). In females, the incidence rises sharply after the age of 40 from approximately 36.8/10,000 to 115/10,000 at age 70 (10,11). In males aged 35 years and older, the incidence is approximately 9/10,000 and remains constant until a slight rise at age 70 (10,11). The data also indicate that this is one of the most common osteoporotic fractures with a strong correlation with femoral neck bone mineral density (12). The sharpest increase in incidence occurs in elderly females, and has been linked to estrogen withdrawal and reduced bone mineral density (13,14). In addition, just as studies have indicated an increased mortality rate associated with hip and vertebral fractures, there is evidence to suggest a higher mortality rate after distal radius fractures, particularly in elderly males (15).There is also a growing incidence of wrist fractures in males under the age of 49, but epidemiologic studies suggest that the injury in younger adults is not as strongly related to gender, but occurs more equally between the sexes (6,16). Further, the injury in this population is related to higher-energy injuries (21% of all fractures) rather than to simple falls. These data suggest that one should regard radius fractures in this population differently from those in elderly patients (16,17). The majority of fractures in the elderly are extra-articular, whereas there is a much higher incidence of intra-articular fractures in younger patients (18). There is also a difference in the mechanism of injury between the groups. The majority of osteoporotic fractures occur as the result of a fall, while the majority of injuries in the younger patients are secondary to motor vehicle accidents and sports (17,19,20). This may also explain the growing trend seen in hospital admissions for this injury in younger patients, as these patients, on the whole, are being treated increasingly with operative intervention.

Risk factors for distal radius fractures in the elderly have been studied extensively. Decreased bone mineral density, female gender, ethnicity, heredity, and early menopause have all been shown to be risk factors for this injury (13,21–23). Although the relationship between bone density and risk of distal radius fracture is not as powerful as is seen with hip and spine fractures, it is clearly evident in the epidemiological literature (9,24). Furthermore, late onset of menopause and estrogen replacement may help protect against injury in this group.

DIAGNOSIS

Physical Examination

The majority of the external physical findings seen with this fracture may be related to the fact that the fractured radius has shortened relative to the intact strut of the ulna. This relationship accounts for the radially deviated and dorsally prominent distal forearm described by Dupuytren, Goyrand (25), and Colles (1). The degree of dorsal angulation and the presence of the prominent palmar proximal fragment result in significant displacement of the median nerve. This displacement of the nerve and the associated hematoma in the carpal tunnel may result in symptoms of an acute carpal tunnel syndrome. The acute shortening of the radius relative to the ulna may manifest as an open wound palmarly and ulnarly where the intact ulna buttonholes through the skin. Finally, the degree of radial shortening accounts for the significant distal radioulnar joint injuries seen with the fractured radius. A cadaveric study demonstrated that shortening of the radius relative to the intact ulna of over 5 mm must result in disruption of the distal radioulnar joint (DRUJ) ligaments (19).

After injury, in addition to examination of the radius, a thorough assessment of the affected ipsilateral shoulder and elbow is required, especially for associated fractures of either the radial head or supracondylar humerus. These injuries have significant implications regarding (a) the high degree of energy imparted to the fracture and (b) rehabilitation challenges with injuries to both the elbow and the wrist. Ipsilateral radial head and distal radial fractures may indicate that sufficient energy has been imparted to result in an Essex-Lopresti lesion (26). An effort should also be made to identify an ipsilateral scaphoid fracture, which may direct the surgeon to consider operative versus nonoperative management. Although there are no prospective studies in the literature, there may be a benefit to rigid internal fixation of the scaphoid to permit early motion of both injuries (27,28).

Attention should then be directed to soft tissue considerations. Open fractures typically result in soft tissue injury palmarly and ulnarly where the distal ulna emerges as the radius displaces dorsally. Direct blows and rotational injuries may result in dorsal soft tissue injuries. A thorough evaluation of the extrinsic flexor and extensors is indicated. Particular attention should be directed to the extensor pollicis longus, which may be injured acutely at Lister's tubercle or may present with a late spontaneous rupture.

Finally, attention is directed to the neurological complications. Median nerve injury—either acute or chronic— is a common cause of functional impairment and chronic pain secondary to complex regional pain syndrome. Examination should include a subjective evaluation of the patient's pain and an objective assessment of median nerve function. Subjectively, the patient should be monitored for pain out of proportion to the injury and also for "burning pain," which is often associated with nerve injury. Reduction of the fracture and limb elevation typically will improve this type of pain. Objectively, sensibility in the median innervated digits must be assessed and monitored before and after reduction as well as after immobilization. An abnormal sensory examination despite reduction and immobilization may be secondary to (a) direct contusion, (b) mechanical deformation of the nerve, or (c) abnormal pressure within the carpal tunnel. Neurapraxia typically appears at presentation and is associated with only moderate pain with gradual improvement over time. Mechanical deformation of the nerve typically improves with reduction and limb elevation. Symptoms due to increased pressure within the carpal canal may not improve and require more aggressive treatment. This diagnosis is similar to a compartment syndrome involving the median nerve, and urgent treatment may be required to avoid long-term dystrophic symptoms. Patients with acute carpal tunnel syndrome typically complain of burning pain, which may be out of proportion to the usual symptoms secondary to these injuries. Fracture reduction and immobilization often does not improve these symptoms, and patients may continue to report worsening pain. As in many conditions involving injured nerves, the pain does not improve significantly with narcotic treatment. The degree of neurologic impairment does not improve objectively, and often two-point discrimination actually worsens. Treatment in this situation should include establishing a diagnosis of acute carpal tunnel syndrome with early decompression of the carpal canal.

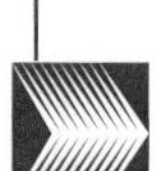

AUTHOR'S PREFERRED TREATMENT

Before reduction and immobilization, the patient's pain is quantified numerically, and the two-point sensation is assessed in both the median and the ulnar nerve distributions. After satisfactory radiographic and clinical reduction of the deformity, the examination is again performed to provide a baseline for subsequent serial examinations. The upper extremity is elevated above the level of the heart, and oral narcotics are administered. Any worsening of the patient's symptoms from this point on requires repeat pain measurements and assessment of sensory and motor function. The immobilization is loosened down to the skin, and ice packs may be applied. If no relief is seen within 6 hours, an immediate carpal tunnel release should be performed. We prefer a longitudinal incision, which permits proximal identification of the median nerve and subsequent release of the antebrachial fascia and transverse carpal ligament. Note that the bony deformity, hematoma, and edema make visualization difficult, and an extensile approach may be necessary to avoid iatrogenic nerve injury. Any hematoma is evacuated, and a silastic drain may be necessary to avoid reaccumulation. In general, it is not necessary to release Guyon's canal at this time. The exception to this rule occurs when there is obvious extrusion of the palmar lunate facet to impinge on the ulnar nerve. Finally, if there is clinical evidence of a compartment syndrome of the hand, then the compartment pressures in the adductor and dorsal interosseous muscles must be checked, and the compartments need to be decompressed when elevated pressures are found.

Imaging Studies

The standard series of posteroanterior (PA), lateral, and oblique x-ray views is useful to visualize a suspected distal radius fracture. Additional views may be obtained as needed to assess for displacement or additional injuries.

PA View

For extra-articular fractures assess (a) radial shortening/comminution and (b) ulnar styloid fracture location (tip/waist/base). For intra-articular fractures assess (a) depression of the lunate facet, (b) gap between scaphoid and lunate facet, (c) central impaction fragments, and (d) interruption of the proximal carpal row.

Lateral View

For extra-articular fractures assess (a) palmar tilt, (b) extent of metaphyseal comminution, (c) displacement of the volar cortex, (d) the scapholunate angle, and (e) position of the DRUJ. For intra-articular fractures assess (a) depression of the palmar lunate facet, (b) depression of the central fragment, and (c) the gap between palmar and dorsal fragments. It is critical to recognize that rotating the radial styloid in relation to the shaft of the radius alters one's ability to accurately assess the true palmar tilt of the radius. Johnson and Szabo found that rotation of the radius on the lateral view resulted in a change in the apparent palmar tilt. A 5-degree rotational change produces a 1.6-degree change in palmar tilt on the conventional lateral view and a 1.0 degree change on the 15-degree lateral view (29).

Oblique View

For extra-articular fractures assess radial comminution. For intra-articular fractures assess (a) the radial styloid for split or depression and (b) depression of the dorsal lunate facet.

Tilted Lateral View

The tilted lateral view (30) is a lateral view taken with a pad under the hand to incline the radius 22% toward the beam. It eliminates the shadow of the radial styloid and provides a clear tangential view of the lunate facet. It is useful to assess (a) residual depression of the palmar lunate facet and (b) possible hardware penetration into the articular surface.

Anteroposterior and Lateral Traction Views

Anteroposterior (AP) and lateral traction views are taken with manual traction or finger traps applied after reduction. They indicate whether external fixation may reduce the fracture sufficiently or whether direct reduction will be required. Furthermore, examination of the proximal carpal row may indicate the presence of incongruity consistent with interosseous ligament injury.

AP and Lateral Contralateral Wrist

AP and lateral contralateral wrist x-rays may be indicated before surgery to assess the patient's normal ulnar variance and scapholunate angle, both of which vary between patients.

Other Studies

In 1986, Knirk and Jupiter correlated patient outcome with residual intra-articular incongruity. They found a 91% incidence of radiographically apparent arthrosis with any measurable intra-articular step-off and a 100% incidence with more than 2 mm of articular step-off (31). Subsequent investigators also emphasized the relationship of as little as 1 mm or more of articular incongruity with a worse clinical outcome (32,33). Although these studies indicate the importance of restoring articular congruity, other investigators question the ability of plain x-rays to consistently show incongruity of less than 2 mm. Data on healed fractures indicate that clinicians measuring step and gap deformity on a random x-ray film will differ by more than 3 mm at least 10% of the time. Repeat step or gap measurements by the same observer are also expected to differ by more than 2 mm at least 10% of the time (34). In addition, significant discrepancy regarding intra- and interobserver reliability has been demonstrated in the measurement of standard radiographic criteria regarding the management of these fractures. For extra-articular fractures, the mean standard deviation between surgeons was 3.2 degrees for radial angle, 3.6 degrees for conventional lateral palmar tilt, and 2.1degrees for 15 degrees of lateral palmar tilt (29).

In an effort to improve the accuracy of measurement of articular congruity, some surgeons have proposed the use of computerized tomography (CT) to assess intra-articular fractures. Clinical data suggest that CT demonstrates intra-articular extension more accurately than plain x-rays (35). CT has been shown to be superior in defining step-off and gaps in the articular surface of the distal radius when compared with plain x-rays. Cole et al found that there was greater reproducibility of measurements with CT and a poor correlation between radiographic measurements and CT measurements (36). CT also allows more accurate measurement of gap formation between palmar and dorsal fragments and has also been documented to be superior for imaging the sigmoid notch. In one study comparing plain x-rays to CT, the investigators found that in 20 consecutive fractures, plain x-rays documented notch involvement in only 35% of the fractures compared with 65% found on CT. Finally, CT may improve the reliability of classification of these fractures by accurately determining the presence of articular involvement (37). It seems that plain x-rays do not reliably permit measurements at the level of 1 mm, but the clinical significance of these studies remains unknown. The majority of clinical outcome studies have relied on plain x-rays both to assess the injury and the treatment outcomes.

CLASSIFICATION

There is perhaps no other fracture in the orthopaedic literature that has garnered so many eponyms over time than fractures of the distal radius. Classifications of fractures as "Colles," "Barton's," "Smith's," "Chauffeur's," and "Reverse Barton's" continues to be presented despite the investigators' failure to read the original descriptions. The resultant conflicting understanding of each eponym creates difficulty in assessing outcomes after treatment.

To remedy this situation, several classification systems have been proposed. To present a complete record of each would be exhaustive and probably inadequate. Some proposed classifications seem to be more of an attempt to stress the significance of a fracture's particular feature rather than to provide a more global approach. There are, however, some classification patterns that have withstood the test of time and continue to be useful in the understanding of these fractures.

Gartland and Werley (38) proposed a classification system that assessed the three basic components of these injuries: (a) metaphyseal comminution; (b) intra-articular extension; and (c) displacement of the fragments. Their classification system has been accompanied by one of the first clinically useful outcomes scores (Fig. 26-1):

- Group I: Simple Colles' fracture with no involvement of the radial articular surfaces
- Group II: Comminuted Colles' fractures with intra-articular extension without displacement
- Group III: Comminuted Colles' fractures with intra-articular extension with displacement
- Group IV: Extra-articular, undisplaced

Frykman (39) established a classification that incorporated individual involvement of the radiocarpal and radioulnar joints (Fig. 26-2 and Table 26-1). Melone emphasized the effect of the lunate's impaction on the radial articular surface to create characteristic fracture fragments (Fig. 26-3) (40):

- Type I: Stable fracture without displacement. This pattern has characteristic fragments of the radial styloid and a palmar and dorsal lunate facet
- Type II: Unstable "die punch" with displacement of the characteristic fragments and comminution of the anterior and posterior cortices
- Type IIA: Reducible
- Type IIB: Irreducible (central impaction fracture)
- Type III: "Spike" fracture. Unstable. Displacement of the articular surface and also of the proximal spike of the radius
- Type IV: "Split" fracture. Unstable medial complex that is severely comminuted with separation and/or rotation of the distal and palmar fragments
- Type V: Explosion injury

AO Classification (the comprehensive classification of fractures of long bones) emphasizes the increasing severity of the bony injury:

- Type A: Extra-articular fracture. Subgroups are based upon angulation and comminution

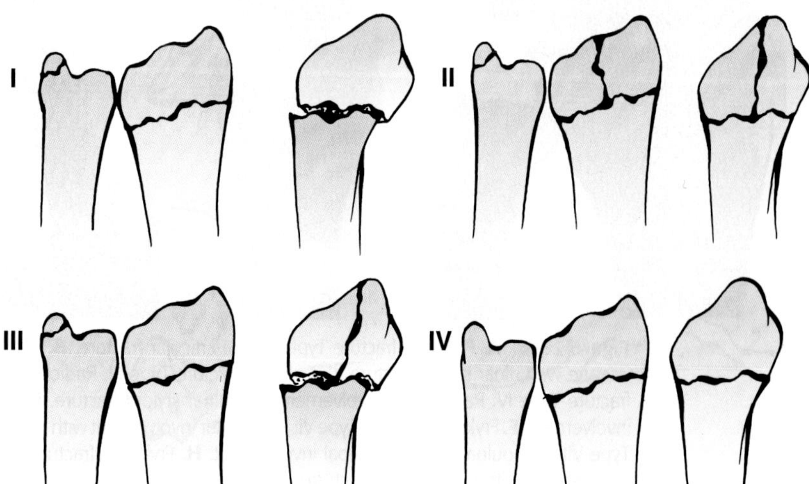

Figure 26-1 Gartland and Werley classification system.

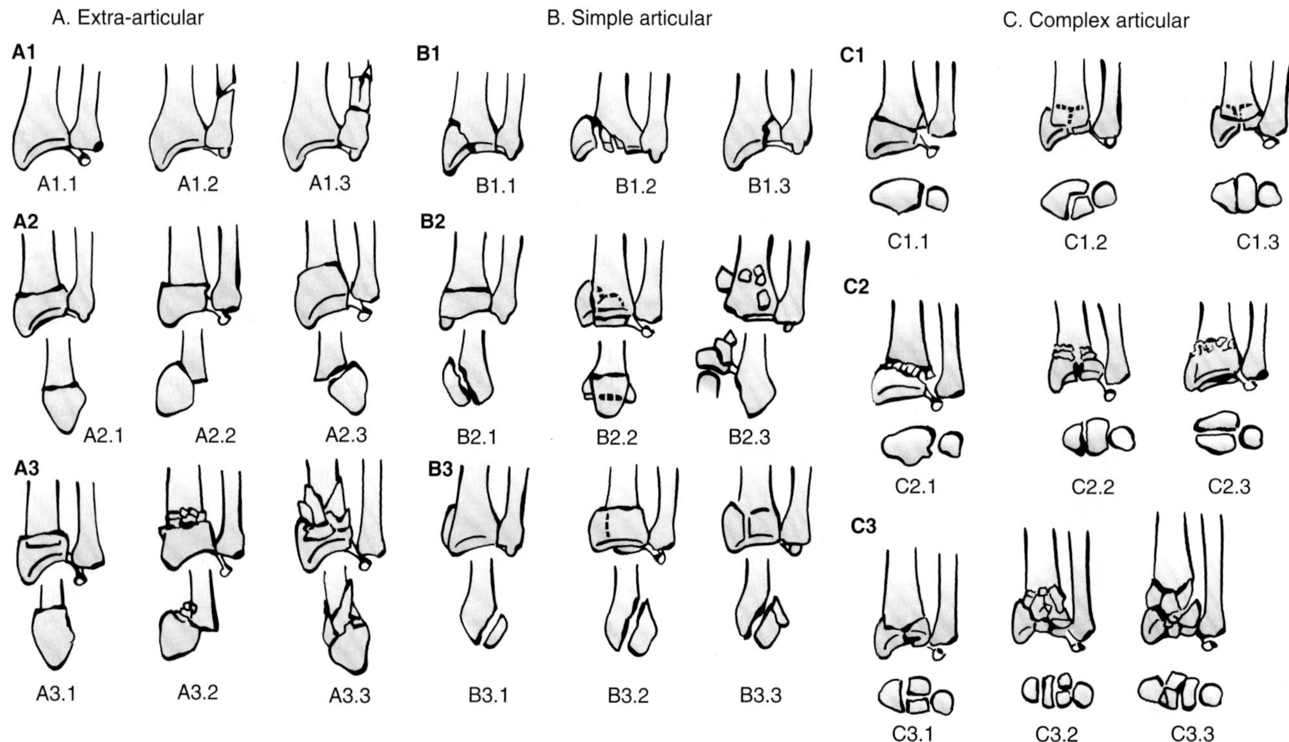

Figure 26-4 AO classification.

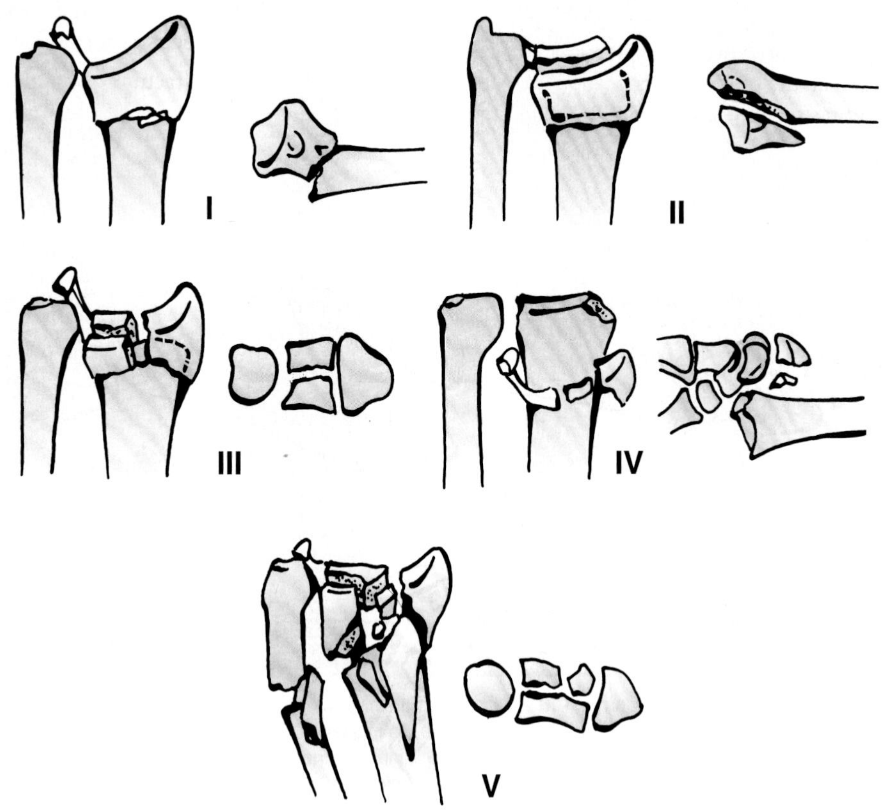

Figure 26-5 Fernandez classification.

- Type V: Combined injuries with significant soft tissue involvement due to the high-energy nature of these fractures.

There is also a separate grouping of the possible associated distal radioulnar joint lesions (44).

RATIONALE FOR TREATMENT

The treatment goal of these fractures is a wrist that provides sufficient pain-free motion and stability to permit vocational and avocational activities without the propensity for future degenerative changes. Although this goal may be easily accepted, there is very little consistency regarding the radiographic features that will afford this result.

Intra-Articular Incongruity

Radiocarpal articular congruity remains the most clinically significant radiographic parameter regarding both functional outcome and future degenerative changes. The threshold for acceptable amounts of radiographic congruity remains somewhat controversial. Knirk and Jupiter retrospectively evaluated 43 young adults at 6.7 years and found that any degree of articular incongruity was associated with radiographically apparent arthritis. If 2 mm of incongruity were present, there was a 100% incidence of degenerative changes on plain x-rays (31). Trumble et al evaluated 52 intra-articular fractures and found that the strongest correlation with outcome was articular congruity. Note that both of these studies documented the significance of lunate facet residual depression after lunate impaction (die punch) fractures as the cause of residual articular incongruity. Cadaver studies (45) using pressure-sensitive film document increases in contact stresses with step-offs as small as 1 mm (Fig. 26-6).

Although these investigators and others have noted the radiographic changes seen after incomplete reduction of articular congruity, their functional significance is debated (32,33). Catellano et al examined 26 operatively treated intra-articular

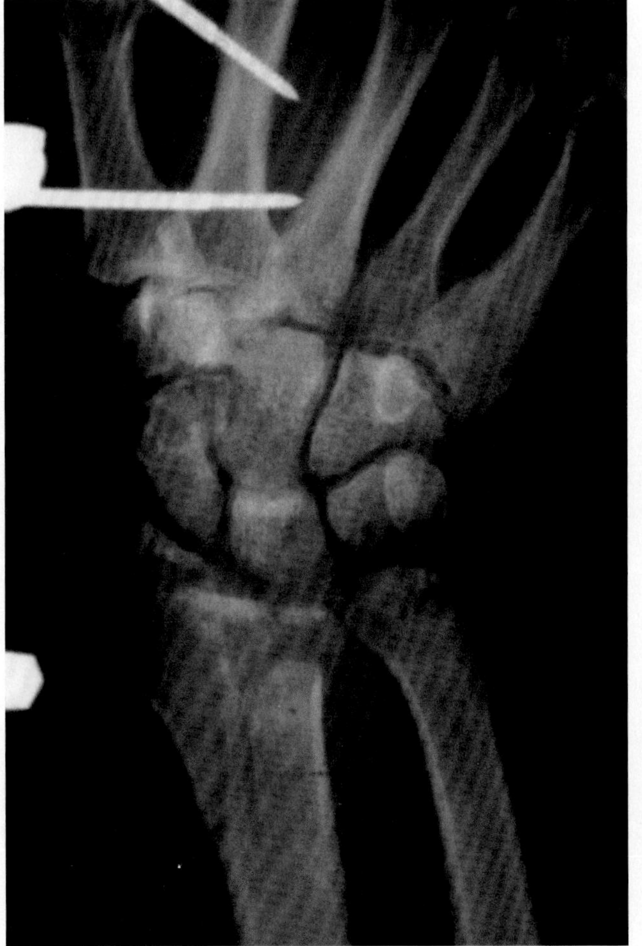

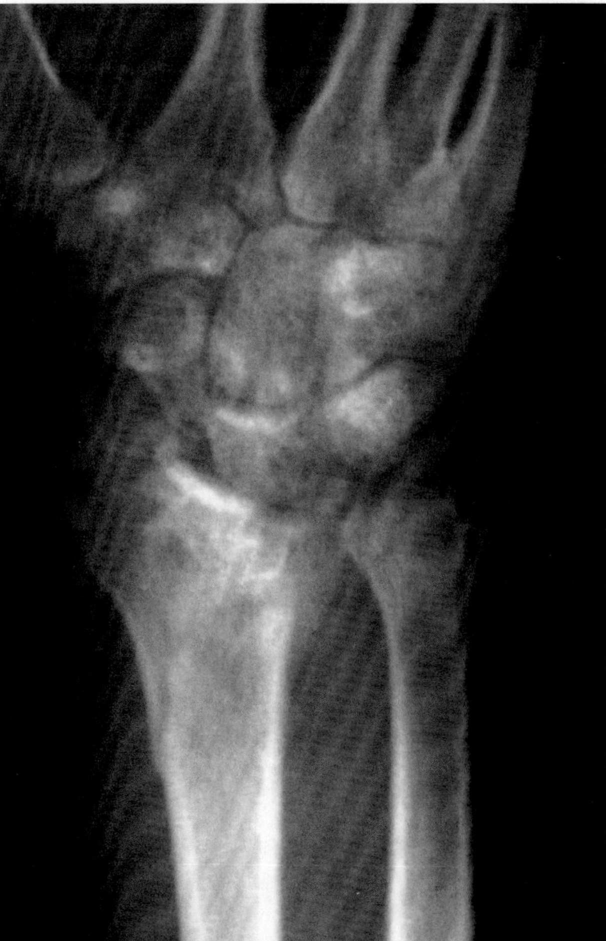

A B

Figure 26-6 **A.** There is incongruity of the radiocarpal joint despite attempted external fixation of the radius. The radiographic result **(B)** shows significant arthrosis at 2 years, necessitating a fusion of the wrist.

fractures at a mean of 7.1 years. They found that despite radiographically apparent arthrosis, there was no correlation between residual articular congruity and the functional outcome. They also found that step-off in the articular surface is more significant than gapping between fragments of the same height (3). Similarly with extra-articular fractures, Tsukazaki et al examined 83 consecutive patients and a found poor correlation between final angulation and functional outcome at 2 years (46). The discrepancy in these data combined with limitations in the ability to visualize step-offs of less than 2 mm on plain x-rays makes definitive recommendations difficult to mandate (34).

Palmar Tilt

Clinical studies have implicated the loss of the normal 11 to 12 degrees of palmar tilt as having a significant effect on functional outcome. Gartland and Werley concluded that residual dorsal tilt has a more direct effect on outcome than residual radial deviation, radial shortening, or loss of integrity of the radioulnar joint (38). In a retrospective review, Kopylov (33) found that loss of as little as 12 degrees from the normal tilt resulted in an 80% increased risk of radiographically apparent arthritis. McQueen examined 30 patients with extra-articular fractures and found that loss of 12 degrees or more of the normal palmar tilt resulted in functional impairment when compared with fractures that healed at neutral or with a positive palmar tilt (47). Porter felt that loss of function did not occur until at least 20 degrees of palmar tilt was lost (48). Why the loss of palmar tilt results in functional impairment is not entirely clear. McQueen concluded that angulation of the distal radius resulted in carpal malalignment that closely correlated with functional outcome (49). Taleisnik indicated that the dorsal shift of the proximal carpal row results in a clinically apparent midcarpal instability with ulnar deviation. The symptoms of instability resolved with corrective osteotomy of the radius (50).

The reason for the loss of function is probably multifactorial; however, cadaveric data have provided some potential explanations. The changes in palmar tilt affect not only radiocarpal mechanics, but also radioulnar mechanics. Short et al found that as little as a 10-degree loss of palmar tilt causes the area of maximum load on the radius to become more concentrated and to shift dorsally. This change in load concentration may explain the clinical findings relating dorsal tilt to radiographically apparent degenerative changes at long-term follow-up (51). In addition, the change in palmar tilt increases the tension on the palmar and dorsal radioulnar ligaments resulting in an increased load required for forearm rotation (52).

Radial Length

Collapse of the lunate facet results in radiocarpal incongruity, and collapse of the radial metaphysis results in radioulnar incongruity. In a series of cadaver studies, Adams found that radial shortening resulted in the most significant changes in the kinematics of the radioulnar joint when compared with loss of radial inclination and palmar tilt (19). Clinical studies have also indicated a strong correlation between radial length and loss of strength. McQueen found that more than 2 mm of radial shortening resulted in symptomatic loss of strength (49). Jenkins found that not only was shortening of more than 4 mm associated with loss of strength, but it also correlated with pain (53). Sologaard retrospectively analyzed a series of 269 fractures and concluded that reduction of the distal radius should primarily aim at the correction of radial length (54). Their findings were corroborated by Batra and Gupta who noted that the most important factor affecting functional outcome was radial length followed by palmar tilt (55).

Radial Inclination

Cadaver data indicate that the carpus shifts ulnarly in response to loss of radial inclination, thereby resulting in increased load on the triangular fibrocartilage complex (TFCC) and the ulna. This effect is not as severe as other deformities, but clinical studies show a correlation between decreased radial inclination and decreased grip strength (53). In addition, long-term follow-up indicates that this increases the risk of degenerative changes by 90% (33).

It is significant to note that these deformities frequently do not occur in isolation (56). The typical malunion is a 3D deformity that is visualized using 2D plain x-rays. While the radius is shortened with an apparent loss of palmar tilt, there is also a rotational component that is typically not visualized and may prove to be significant. It is difficult, therefore, to separate out the effect of one of these deformities from the others when assessing their impact on outcome.

Carpal Malalignment

The role of ligamentous injuries in subsequent radiographic outcomes is only recently becoming apparent as more and more studies are documenting significant associated ligament injuries during arthroscopically assisted treatment (57–60).

Although some degree of lateral scapholunate angle widening due to palmar flexion of the scaphoid may be acceptable, it appears that a dorsiflexed lunate (a static DISI deformity) is associated with a worse outcome (55,61). The critical shift is in the radiolunate angle, as it indicates a shift of contact forces dorsally on the radius in the intermediate column. There is as yet no defined threshold for this angle; however, greater than 25 degrees has been correlated with a worse outcome (55). The currently acceptable radiographic parameters for a healed radius fracture in an active, healthy patient are listed in Table 26-2.

SURGICAL AND APPLIED ANATOMY

Although the surgical anatomy of the distal radius remains relatively significant, pitfalls lie in interpretation of the bony architecture using 2D imaging, including fluoroscopy. In addition,

TABLE 26-2 Acceptable Radiographic Parameters for Healed Radius Fracture in an Active, Healthy Patient

Radial length	Within 2 to 3 mm of the contralateral wrist
Palmar tilt	Neutral tilt (0°)
Intra-articular step-off	<2 mm
Radial angle	<5° loss

the complex ligamentous anatomy of both the extrinsic and intrinsic aspects of the radiocarpal and distal radioulnar joints compounds the challenge.

Bony Anatomy

The distal radius consists of the (a) metaphysis, (b) scaphoid facet, (c) lunate facet, and (d) sigmoid notch. The metaphysis is flared distally in both the AP and the lateral planes with thinner cortical bone lying dorsally and radially (Fig. 26-7).

The significance of the thinness of these cortices is that the fractures typically collapse dorsoradially. In addition, the bone with the greatest trabecular density lies in the palmar ulnar cortex (62). The fact that this bone is thicker even in osteoporotic cadaver specimens may explain the success of internal fixation techniques, which take advantage of this superior bone

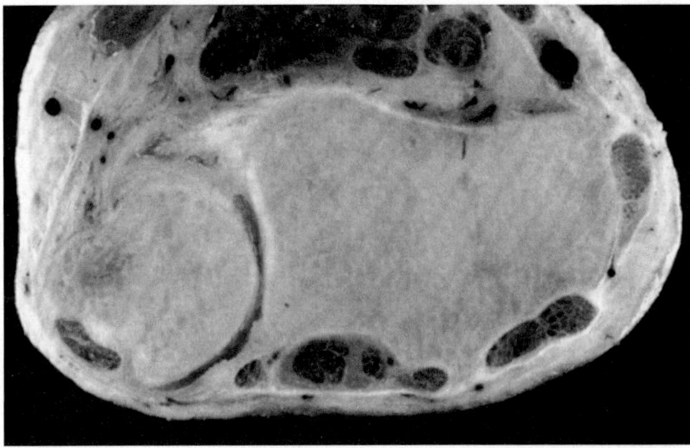

Figure 26-8 The cross-sectional anatomy of the radius immediately below the radiocarpal joint. Note that the radial styloid angles palmarly and that the extensor tendons are in immediate contact with the bone, while palmarly, a layer of fat protects the flexors from the bone. (Courtesy of Professor Golano, Barcelona, Spain.)

(63). Distally, the radius has a somewhat trapezoidal shape. The radial styloid rotates palmarly 15 degrees off the axis of the radius, which makes capture difficult from a dorsal approach (Figs. 26-8 and 26-9).

In the AP plane, the strongest bone is found under the lunate facet of the radius. The line of force passes down the long finger axis through the capitolunate articulation and contacts the radius at this location. The "palmar ulnar corner" is often referred to as the keystone of the radius. It serves as the attachment for the palmar distal radioulnar ligaments and also for the stout radiolunate ligament. Displacement of this fragment is associated with palmar displacement of the carpus and also with loss

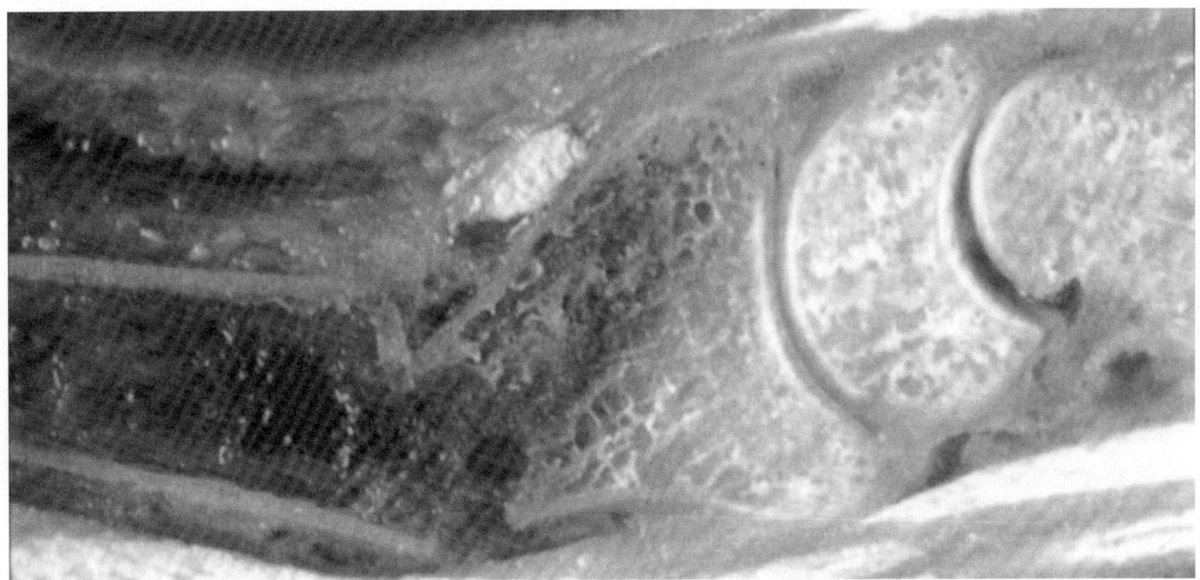

Figure 26-7 The cross-sectional anatomy of the radius with comminution dorsally and radially. Note the tendency to dorsal collapse is the result of dorsal comminution and the collapse at the midcarpal joint. (Courtesy of Professor Golano, Barcelona, Spain.)

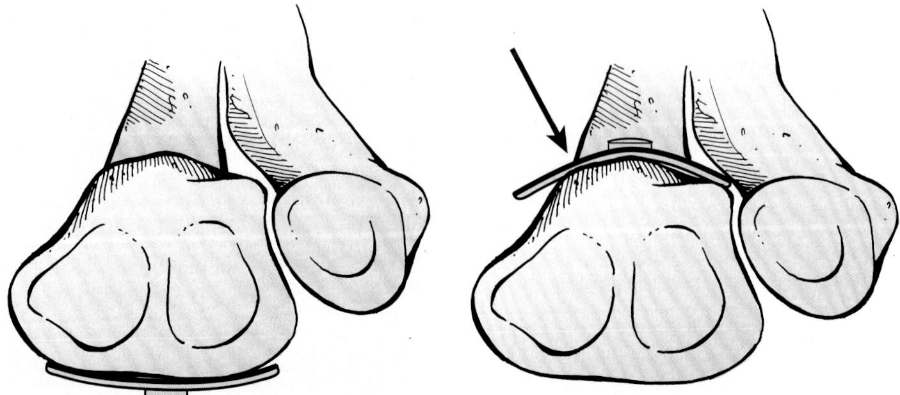

Figure 26-9 Cross-sectional anatomy of the radial metaphysis. Note that the dorsal surface is much more irregular than the palmar surface. The V-shape dorsally caused by Lister's tubercle (arrow) makes it difficult to contour a plate to fit the dorsum of the radius. (Reprinted with permission from A Papadonikolakis.)

of forearm rotation (64). Figure 26-10 shows residual depression of the lunate facet. The result is loss of rotation as well as a step-off in the articular surface.

Ligamentous Anatomy

The extrinsic ligaments of the wrist play a major role in the use of indirect reduction techniques. The palmar extrinsic ligaments are attached to the distal radius, and these ligaments are relied on to reduce the components of a fracture using closed methods. There are two factors about these ligaments that make them significant for reduction. First, the orientation of the extrinsic ligaments from the radial styloid is oblique relative to the more vertical orientation of the ligaments attached to the lunate facet. Figures 26-11 and 26-12 show the palmar and dorsal extrinsic ligamentous anatomy in the wrist.

The second significance of the ligamentous anatomy is due to the relative strengths of the thicker palmar ligaments when compared with the thinner dorsal ligaments. In addition, the dorsal ligaments are oriented in a relative "Z" orientation, which allows them to lengthen with less force than the more vertically oriented palmar ligaments. The significance is that distraction will result in the palmar ligaments becoming taut before the dorsal ligaments. Thus, the palmar cortex is brought out to length before the dorsal cortex. It is for this reason that it is difficult to achieve reduction of the normal 12 degrees of palmar tilt using distraction alone (see Fig. 26-12).

Applied Anatomy

Rikkli et al interpreted the wrist as consisting of three distinct columns, each of which is subjected to different forces and must be addressed as discrete elements. Figure 26-13 demonstrates the "columnar" approach to managing intra-articular fractures of the radius.

The radial column consists of the scaphoid fossa and the radial styloid. Due to the radial inclination of 22 degrees, impaction of the scaphoid on the articular surface results in a shear moment on the radial styloid causing failure laterally at the radial cortex. The radial column, therefore, is best stabilized by buttressing the lateral cortex.

The intermediate column consists of the lunate fossa and the sigmoid notch of the radius. The intermediate column may be considered the cornerstone of the radius because it is critical for both articular congruity and distal radioulnar function. Failure of the intermediate column occurs as a result of impaction of the lunate on the articular surface with dorsal comminution. A direct buttress of the dorsal ulnar aspect of the radius stabilizes the column.

The ulnar column consists of the ulna styloid, but also should include the TFCC and the ulnocarpal ligaments.

NONOPERATIVE MANAGEMENT

Closed reduction and cast immobilization has historically been the mainstay of treatment for these fractures. The difficulty in treating patients with immobilization lies in the ability to accurately predict the fracture's position at final union. Cast immobilization is indicated in (a) stable fractures in which the expected radiographic outcome achieves the goals of treatment outlined earlier and (b) low-demand elderly patients in whom future functional impairment is less of a priority than immediate health concerns and/or operative risks.

Stable Fractures

In order to understand the definition of *stability*, it is useful to consider the mechanical loads that caused the bone to fail and present with the initial radiographic images (prereduction x-rays). A fall on the outstretched hand may result in (a) a metaphyseal bending fracture, (b) a lunate impaction fracture, or (c) an articular shear fracture. The stability of the avulsion fractures is based on the prognosis of the ligamentous injury,

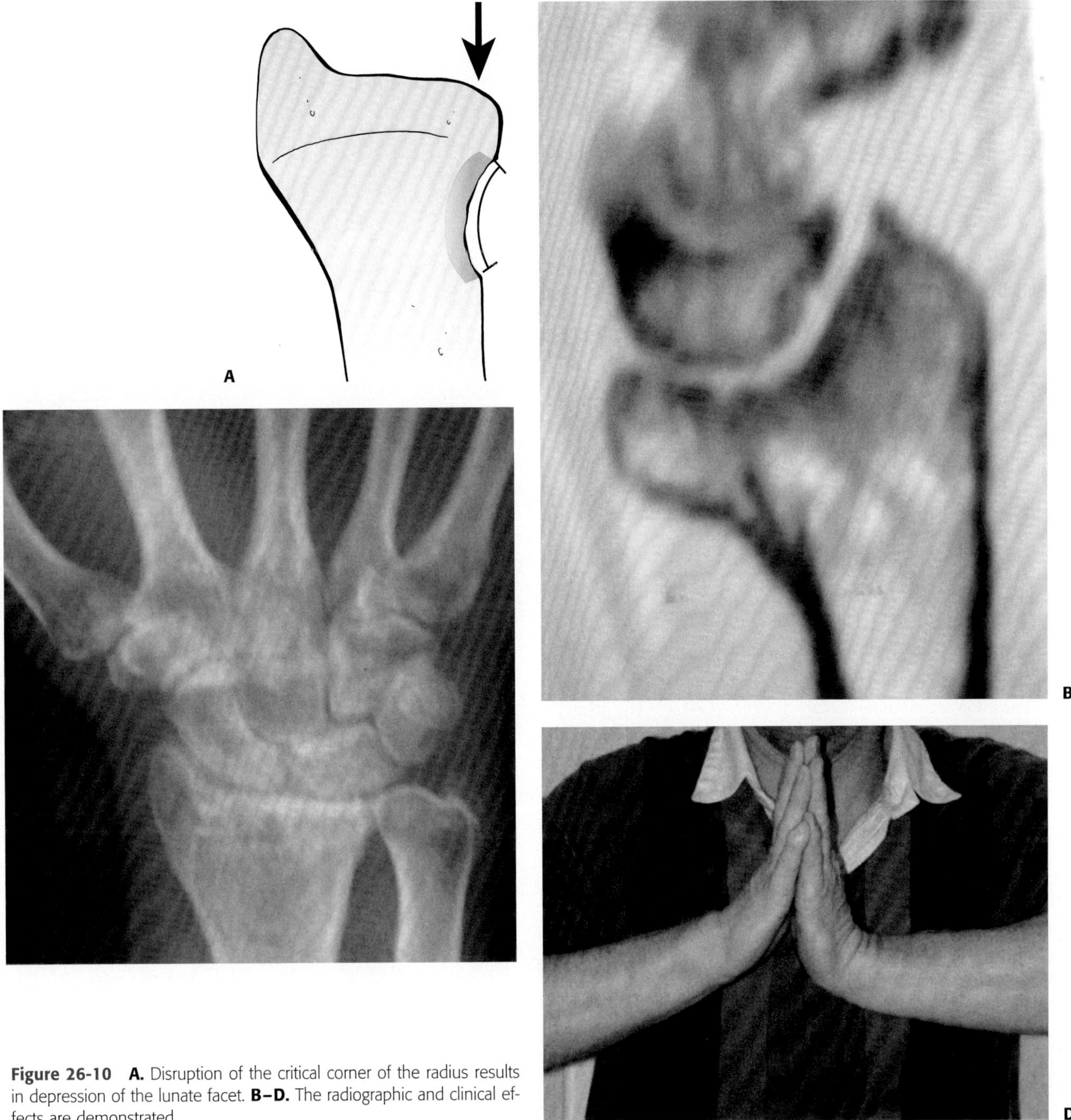

Figure 26-10 **A.** Disruption of the critical corner of the radius results in depression of the lunate facet. **B–D.** The radiographic and clinical effects are demonstrated.

and combined injuries are generally too unstable to be treated with cast immobilization.

A metaphyseal bending fracture that failed under tension must be able to resist axial load and dorsal displacement. A cast with a dorsal mold may prevent dorsal displacement; however, a cast does not resist collapse due to an axial load. Resistance to collapse depends on an intact palmar buttress. Several investigators have documented that when comminution extends into the palmar buttress, collapse occurs even in the face of cast immobilization (65,66). The critical degree to which the comminution extends from the dorsal cortex to the palmar cortex as viewed on the lateral x-ray lies somewhere between two-thirds and three-quarters of the radial metaphysis (67) (Fig. 26-14). Lunate impaction fractures typically result secondary to

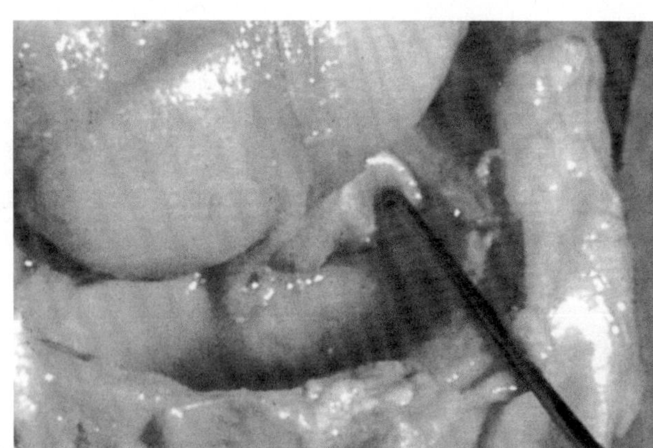

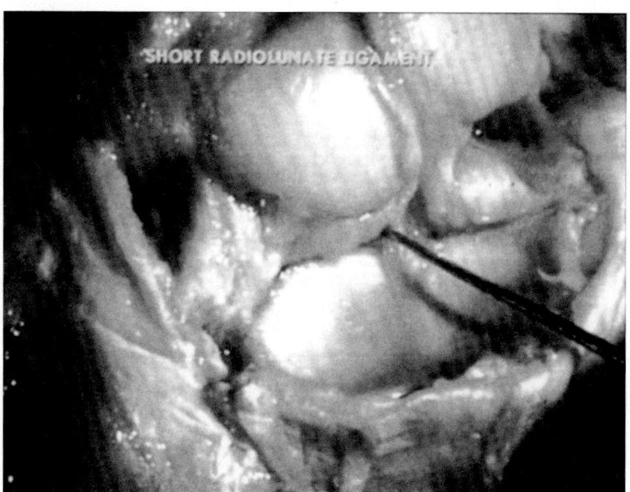

Figure 26-11 **A,B** show the thick palmar radial extrinsic ligaments when viewed from the back. Note that these ligaments are oriented obliquely off the radial styloid **(A)** and vertically off the lunate facet **(B).** Application of ulnar deviation to restore radial length with cast immobilization or external fixation results in a distraction of the radial styloid, but does little to reduce the lunate face.

axial load. Although cast immobilization prevents dorsal displacement, it does not resist axial loads and cannot resist redisplacement of the lunate facet over time.

Several factors have been associated with redisplacement after closed manipulation of a distal radius fracture.

- The initial displacement of the fracture (68–70). The greater the degree of the initial displacement is (especially radial shortening), the more energy was imparted to the fracture, resulting in a higher likelihood that closed treatment will be unsuccessful (71).
- The age of the patient. Fractures in elderly patients with osteopenic bones tend to displace particularly late (54).
- The extent of metaphyseal comminution (the metaphyseal defect) as evidenced by either plain x-rays or CT (65).
- Finally, displacement after closed treatment is a predictor of instability, and repeat manipulation is unlikely to result in a successful radiographic outcome (70,72).

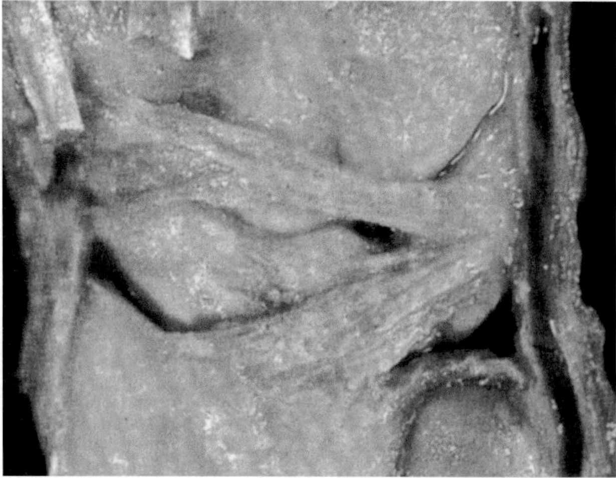

Figure 26-12 The dorsal ligaments of the wrist have a "Z" configuration, which allows for elongation. Compared with the palmar ligaments, the dorsal ligaments must stretch farther to achieve reduction of the palmar tilt.

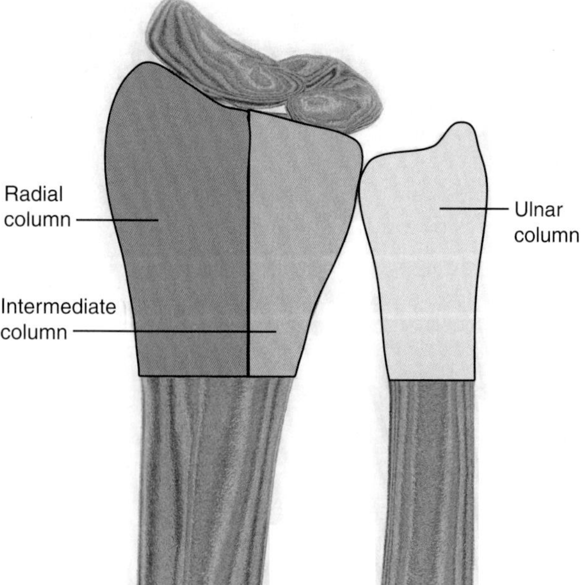

Figure 26-13 The three columns of the wrist.

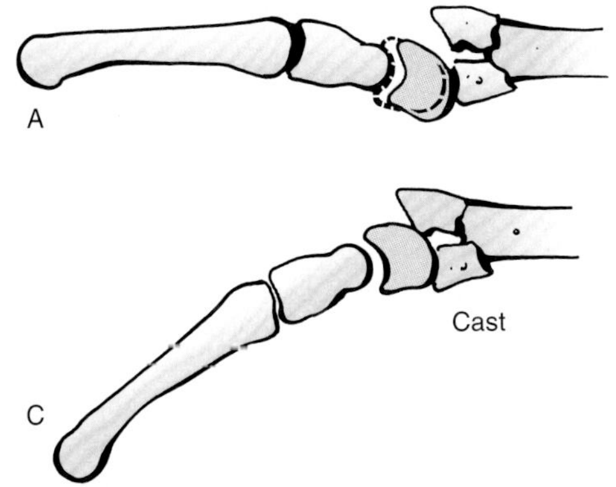

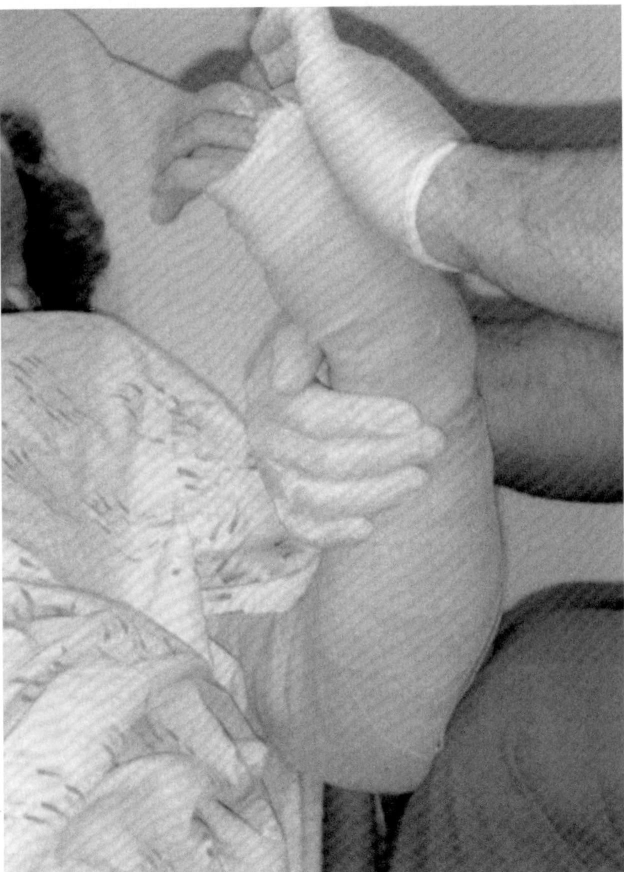

Figure 26-14 **A.** The fate of the lunate facet with attempted closed treatment of an intra-articular fracture. Palmar flexion **(B),** which is used to restore palmar tilt, results in depression of the volar lunate facet **(C).**

Patient Considerations

The decision regarding cast treatment versus operative management of a comminuted unstable fracture must also incorporate host factors including physical demands, health status, independent lifestyle, vocation, avocation, and comorbidities. With the use of regional anesthesia and the results of several cohort series of elderly patients having a favorable outcome with surgery, it has become more difficult to identify patients in whom nonoperative treatment is indicated.

The literature reflects the controversy regarding nonoperative management. Young et al reported that at 7 years, there was overall good function with nonoperative management, and no apparent advantage was seen with external fixation (73). Young and Rayan indicated that in patients over the age of 60, radiographic appearance at union had a poor correlation with patient-reported outcomes (74,75). Other investigators noted persistent disability after nonoperative management and have proposed more aggressive treatment in elderly patients to avoid collapse (76,77). Future prospective randomized studies will need to address whether patient needs and expectations should affect the operative indications.

Closed Reduction Technique

Successful reduction of a displaced fracture requires adequate pain relief to overcome muscle spasm. Hematoma block with supplemental intravenous sedation or Bier block provides adequate anesthesia in most settings. The use of finger traps may prove useful in managing completely displaced fractures and may assist in the application of a cast or splint.

Manipulation starts with longitudinal traction and then direct pressure is applied on the displaced radial metaphyseal fragment. Great care must be taken to avoid tearing the skin, particularly in elderly patients with parchment-like skin. Reduction may be confirmed using sonography, fluoroscopy, or with plain x-rays after the maneuver (78).

The position of immobilization of the radius is critical after reduction. The splint or cast should provide a dorsal buttress to prevent collapse, but excessive palmar flexion of the radius should be avoided. Palmar flexion of an uninjured wrist to 60 degrees has been shown to cause a significant elevation of pressure in the carpal tunnel. When palmar flexion is combined with the swelling seen in a distal radius fracture, the elevation of pressure may result in an acute carpal tunnel syndrome (79). The exact amount of palmar wrist flexion that places the median nerve at risk depends on the degree of swelling, any pre-existing carpal tunnel syndrome, and the presence of an associated hematoma. It appears likely that a position of the wrist at greater than 30 degrees of palmar flexion places the patient at an increased risk of an acute carpal tunnel syndrome (80). Agee has indicated that not only does the palmarly flexed position of the wrist predispose the patient to median nerve symptoms, but it also places tension on the extrinsic extensor tendons, thereby preventing complete digital flexion (81).

The optimal position of immobilization of the radioulnar joint is controversial. Several investigators have proposed immobilization in supination (82). This position restores stability to the distal radioulnar joint and theoretically allows the injured DRUJ complex to heal in the appropriate position. Other studies have indicated that the injury pattern determines the outcome, and they found no significant long-term difference between immobilization in supination and other degrees of forearm rotation (56).

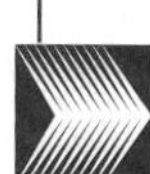

AUTHOR'S PREFERRED TREATMENT

A careful examination of the patient is performed with particular attention to (a) skin quality and integrity, (b) median and ulnar nerve function as measured by two-point discrimination, and (c) continuity of the extrinsic digital flexor and extensor tendons, most importantly those to the thumb.

Routine administration of Bier blocks has not been practical at our institution. Therefore, we still rely on administering an intravenous narcotic and a hematoma block. The block is performed with 10 mL of 1% lidocaine without epinephrine using an 18-gauge needle inserted after betadine preparation and alcohol rinse. The hematoma is evacuated, and the lidocaine is injected slowly until resistance is met. Extravasation of the lidocaine in the vicinity of the median nerve is common; therefore, care should be taken to accurately assess the function of the median nerve before administering the hematoma block.

The distal metaphysis is reduced by increasing the degree of the deformity and then applying longitudinal traction. The distal metaphyseal fragment can be reduced on the shaft only when sufficient traction has been applied. The goal is to reapproximate the palmar cortex. When the palmar cortex is reestablished, the cast has only to resist dorsal angulation. Once the palmar cortex is realigned, the forearm is placed in 30 degrees of supination. This position serves to prevent dorsal subluxation of the distal ulna relative to the intact radius. Shortening of the radius relative to the ulna results in disrupting the distal radioulnar joint ligaments. In the absence of radioulnar joint stability, the ulna subluxes dorsally relative to the radius when the forearm is placed in pronation. This tendency is increased with ulnar deviation of the fracture. Whereas full supination may result in palmar subluxation of the radius, 30 degrees of supination has not seemed to result in functional impairment. Finally, palmar tilt is restored using gentle pressure on the distal fragment. Care is taken to avoid excessive palmar flexion of the radiocarpal joint, which can result in an acute carpal tunnel syndrome. We find it useful to have a portable fluoroscopy unit present to verify the reduction. Immobilization is performed in a sugartong plaster splint with the forearm in approximately neutral to 30 degrees of supination.

Postreduction x-rays are obtained at 7, 14, and 21 days. The postreduction x-rays must be compared with the initial postreduction x-rays to accurately determine redisplacement.

OPERATIVE TREATMENT

Timing

The optimal timing of the surgical intervention depends on the associated soft tissue factors and the proposed surgical procedure (Table 26-3). As in all operative fracture treatment, optimally, the surgeon should provide adequate soft tissue coverage of the implants and all vital soft tissue structures. In the case of acute fractures, the fracture should be reduced by closed means as soon as possible to minimize complications, and operative stabilization should be performed either acutely or when the swelling is sufficiently diminished to prevent soft tissue complications. One exception is arthroscopically assisted reduction and stabilization in which operative treatment is delayed for at least 3 to 5 days to avoid significant extravasation of irrigation fluid into the surrounding soft tissue (60).

Pins and Plaster

Adding percutaneous pins to provide additional stability is one of the earliest forms of internal fixation. The technique is minimally invasive and inexpensive. It relies on the ability to reduce the distal segment and to maintain the reduction while the pins are applied. For the larger segments, 0.62-inch Kirschner wires (K-wires) may be used, while 0.45-inch K-wires may be used to fix the intermediate column and for subchondral fragment support. The radial styloid is pinned to the proximal shaft in a reduced position. Once the lateral cortex is reconstituted, the intermediate column (lunate facet) is pinned from dorsal ulnar to proximal radial. Finally, the central impaction fragments can be supported using subchondral transverse wires. Outcome studies reveal successful management of extra-articular and simple articular fractures with this technique (83).

The major disadvantage with adding percutaneous pins lies in the need for associated cast immobilization to neutralize the

TABLE 26-3 Indications for Operative Intervention

Comminuted displaced intra-articular fracture
Open fractures
Associated carpal fractures
Associated neurovascular injury/tendon injury
Failed conservative treatment
Bilateral fractures
Impaired contralateral extremity

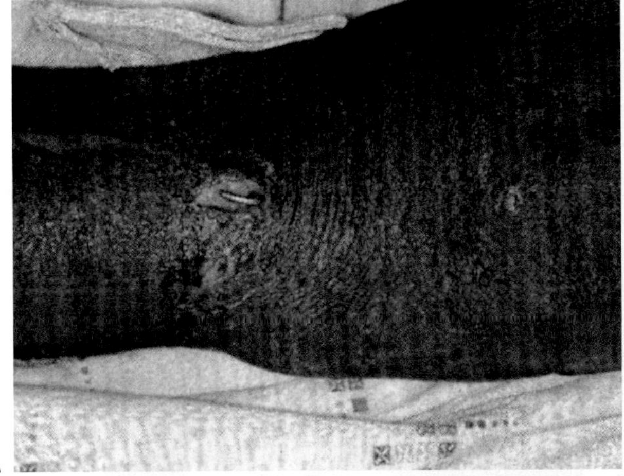

A

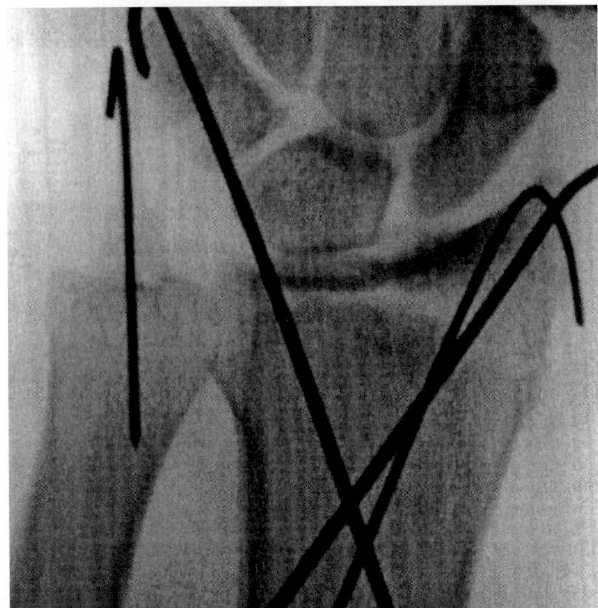

B

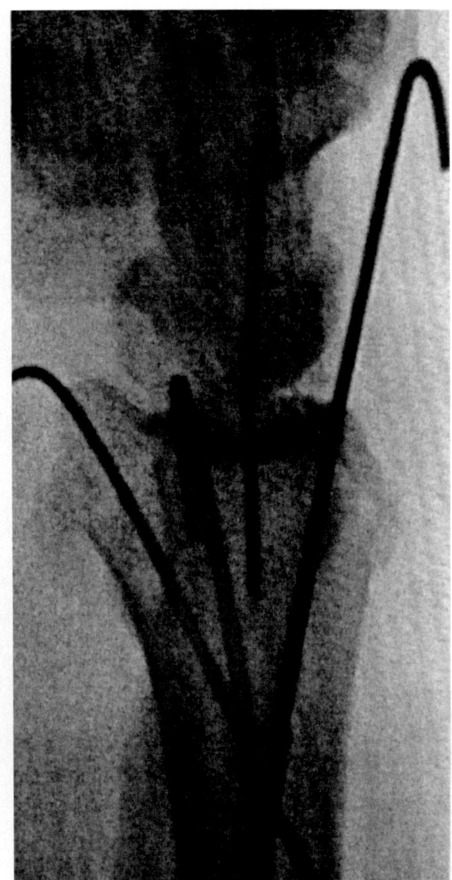

C

Figure 26-15 Comminuted radius fracture in a polytrauma patient treated with percutaneous pinning technique.

flexion-extension moments at the wrist, as the fixation using this technique is often insufficient to prevent displacement. Thus, the technique does not eliminate the causes of so-called fracture disease that lead to digital swelling and stiffness. In addition, the pins may become superficially infected, as pin care is difficult with the cast in place (84).

A second difficulty with percutaneous pinning is that biomechanically, it relies on fixation to the proximal shaft. This results in an oblique orientation of the pins, which does little to prevent collapse of the fragments. Figure 26-15 demonstrates percutaneous pinning of intra-articular fractures of the radius.

Kapandji "Intra-Focal" Pinning

Kapandji described a technique of trapping the major fragment by buttressing to prevent displacement. The wires are inserted both radially and dorsally directly into the fracture site. The wires are then levered up and directed into the proximal intact opposite cortex. The fragments are buttressed from displacing dorsally or proximally. In addition to being relatively simple and inexpensive, this technique has been shown to be very effective, particularly in elderly patients (85–88) (Fig. 26-16).

One difficulty with this technique, however, is the tendency to translate the distal fragment in the opposite direction of the pin. This is particularly problematic if the pins are placed dorsally resulting in palmar displacement of the distal fragment, thereby preventing the palmar cortex from reducing anatomically.

EXTERNAL FIXATION

Although percutaneous pinning, plaster immobilization, and Kapandje pinning remain effective techniques for extra-articu-

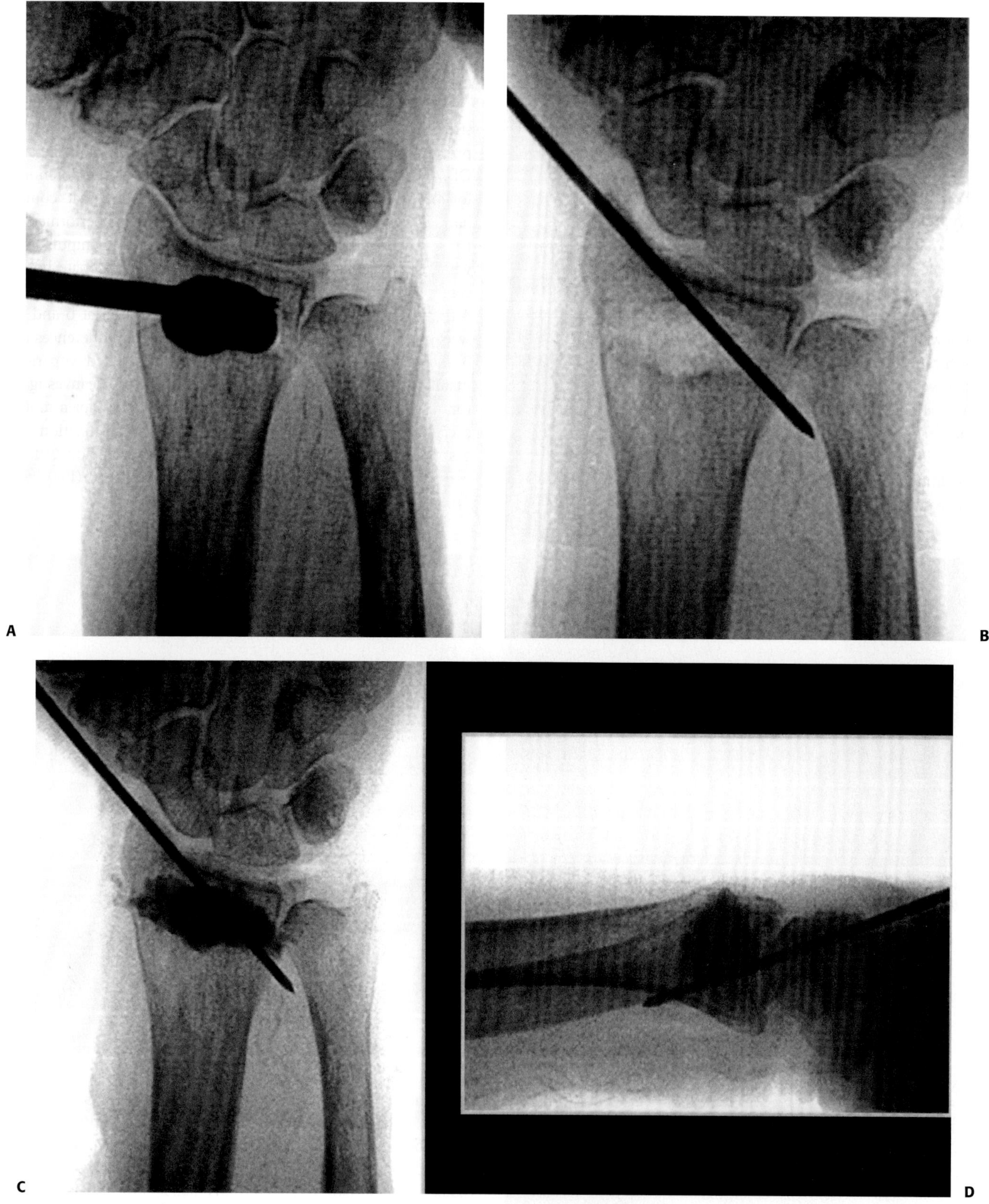

Figure 26-18 Cement augmentation of a distal radius metaphyseal fracture. **A.** First, the defect is compartmentalized using a balloon stent. Next, the fracture is stabilized with a K-wire **(B),** and then the defect is filled with injectable calcium phosphate cement **(C,D).** (Courtesy of Mark Cohen, MD.)

Adjunctive K-Wire Fixation

The use of adjunctive percutaneous pins has also been introduced to improve the stability of external fixation and to prevent loss of reduction. Cadaver studies have shown that supplemental wires increase the stability of the construct to nearly that of dorsal plating (107). The use of crossed wires engaging the contralateral cortex substantially further increases the construct's rigidity. The major complication seen with the use of pins is iatrogenic injury to the superficial radial nerve. The nerve emerges proximally through the brachioradialis and arborizes distally. This risk of injury may be lessened by making a small 5-mm incision and spreading with a hemostat down to bone. Several investigators have documented the clinical efficacy of this technique in preventing loss of reduction and achieving excellent clinical outcomes (32,108) (Fig. 26-19).

Complications

The use of external fixation to treat distal radius fractures has reported complication rate ranging from 6% to 60% depending on how "major" and "minor" complications are reported (109–111). Many complications of distal radius fractures are seen regardless of the treatment, and some are directly related to treatment with an external fixator and/or supplemental pins (112).

Overdistraction

Overdistraction during external fixation has been implicated in producing worse digital motion, worse functional outcomes, and worse strength and pain scores after fracture treatment (113). There is no threshold limit for distraction, but it appears that there is a correlation between increasing carpal height index and worse functional outcomes (114). The fact that there is no threshold for overdistraction makes it difficult to demonstrate a strict causal relationship as evidenced by one study that documented distraction of 5 mm to 8 mm across the radiocarpal and midcarpal joints without a negative outcome (115). Overdistraction of the wrist, particularly if it is combined with palmar flexion, results in relative shortening of the extrinsic extensor tendons and may prevent full active and passive digital motion. Prolonged loss of full flexion combined with the swelling after a wrist fracture can result in permanent loss of metacarpophalangeal motion. Therefore, it is critical to look for this complication after the procedure is completed. The diagnosis is suspected when there is a gap across the midcarpal joint upon fluoroscopic assessment during the procedure and confirmed when full passive digital motion is difficult to achieve.

Overdistraction is usually attributable to a failure to recognize the limitations of external fixation alone in managing highly comminuted fractures. In extra-articular fractures, external fixation in isolation does not typically restore the physiological 12 degrees of palmar tilt. Cadaver studies indicate that the thicker and vertically oriented palmar ligaments become taut before the thinner and "Z"-configured ligaments dorsally. Pure distraction results in the palmar ligaments tightening before the dorsal ligaments and a failure to achieve palmar tilt (99,116). Clinical studies also indicate that loss of palmar tilt is common after external fixation alone without supplemental grafting or pinning (97,116–118). In addition, external fixation in isolation may not elevate the intra-articular component of the fracture. Central impaction fragments have no capsuloligamentous attachments; therefore, distraction alone will not elevate these fragments. The palmar lunate facet may not reduce with distraction alone, and ulnar deviation actually allows the lunate to settle relative to the radial styloid due to the oblique orientation of the extrinsic radial ligaments. This complication may be avoided by recognizing the limitations of the technique and making use of more direct reduction tools to achieve a congruent articular surface and physiologic palmar tilt.

Cutaneous Nerve Injury

Injury to the superficial radial nerve may be seen after open pin insertion, percutaneous half pin insertion, or with the use of supplemental K-wires. The incidence varies; however, several series report transient dysethesias in 16% to 21% of cases (119–121). In an effort to lessen this complication, several investigators have recommended open rather than percutaneous half pin insertion (97,122,123).

The use of adjunctive K-wires offers increased rigidity, but may also result in the increased likelihood of injury to associated soft tissue structures, particularly branches of the superficial radial nerve. These smaller branches have been shown to be at risk with percutaneous introduction of pins in the distal radius or the carpus (124). These injuries tend to be transient with resolution by 6 months, but they may also precipitate a complex regional pain syndrome. Biomechanically, the pins are best placed radially; however, the more dorsal the pin placement is, the safer they are from iatrogenic cutaneous nerve injury (Fig. 26-20).

Pin Tract Infections

The true incidence of pin tract infections is unknown due in part to failure to define whether such an entity is a transient cellulitis, or a deeper infection with or without bony involvement. For K-wires, the incidence ranges from 6% to as high as 33% (125). For external fixation pins, the incidence has been reported to range from 1% to 8% (97,126). Because the instance of pin tract infection is relatively low, studies comparing predrilling to direct drilling of the pins are generally underpowered, and the relationship of predrilling to the infection rate has not been established (105).

Nonbridging External Fixation

In an effort to have direct control of the distal fragment and to avoid crossing the radiocarpal joint, several nonbridging external fixation devices have been introduced. Theoretically, these devices permit the surgeon to directly control palmar tilt, which is difficult with bridging external fixation (99,116). In addition, the early freedom of wrist motion may improve functional outcomes (127).

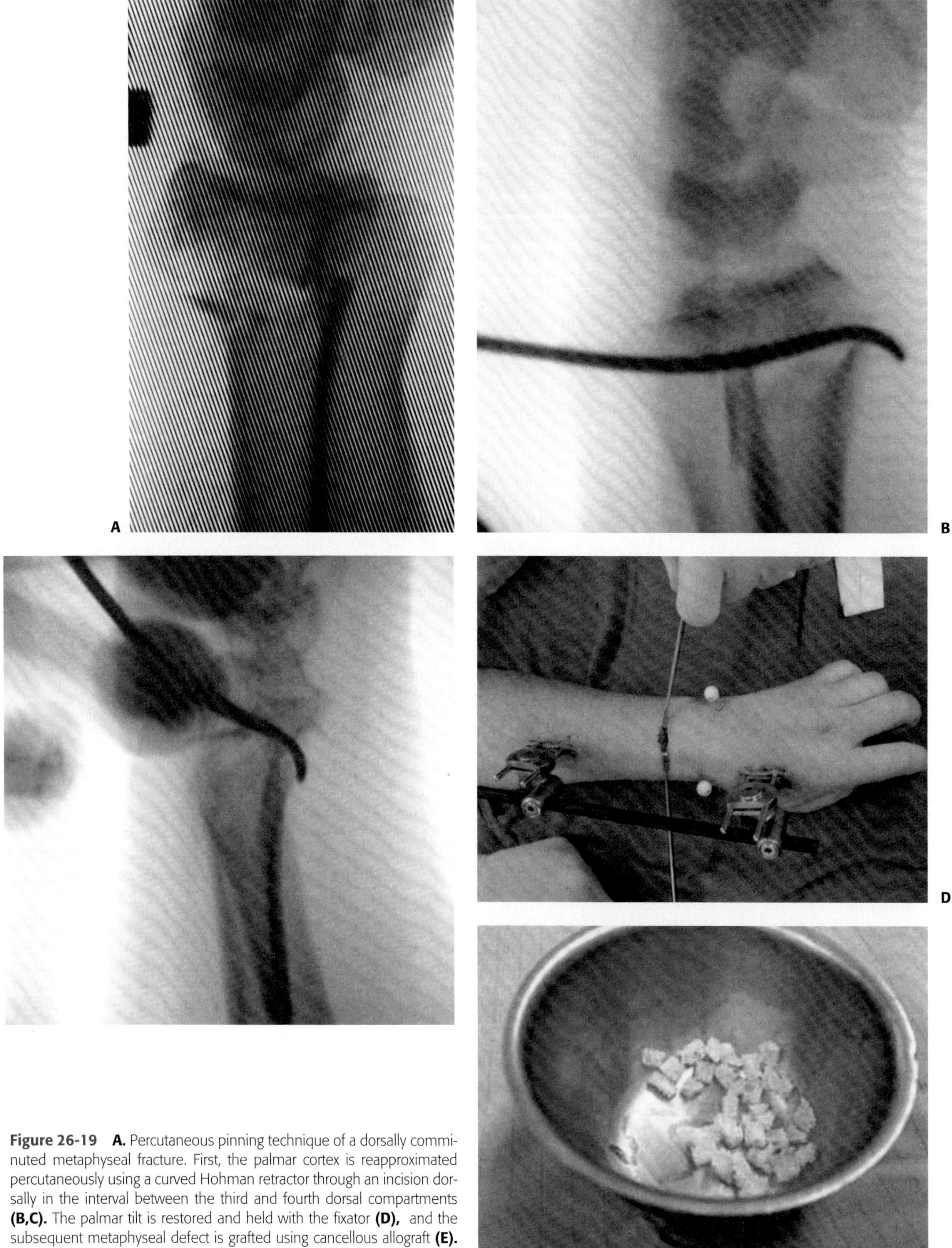

Figure 26-19 **A.** Percutaneous pinning technique of a dorsally comminuted metaphyseal fracture. First, the palmar cortex is reapproximated percutaneously using a curved Hohman retractor through an incision dorsally in the interval between the third and fourth dorsal compartments **(B,C).** The palmar tilt is restored and held with the fixator **(D),** and the subsequent metaphyseal defect is grafted using cancellous allograft **(E).** *(continues)*

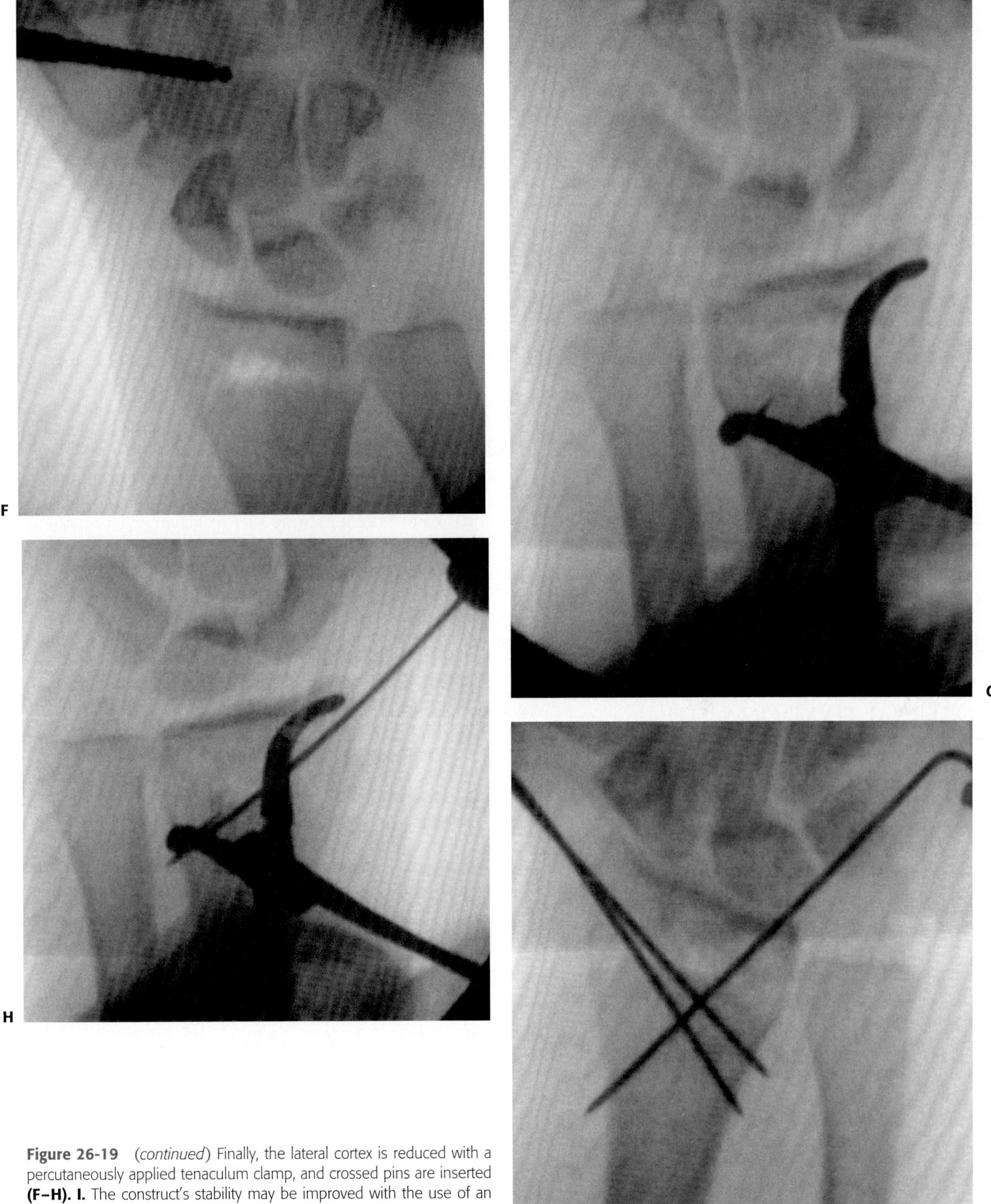

Figure 26-19 *(continued)* Finally, the lateral cortex is reduced with a percutaneously applied tenaculum clamp, and crossed pins are inserted **(F–H). I.** The construct's stability may be improved with the use of an additional pin applied radially.

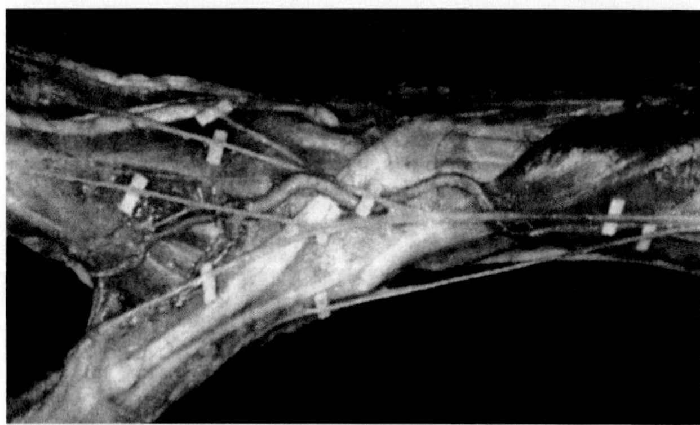

Figure 26-20 The anatomy of the superficial radial nerve at the distal radius. Note that the majority of the branches lie palmar to the second dorsal compartment. (Courtesy of Professor Golano, Barcelona Spain.)

COMBINED INTERNAL EXTERNAL FIXATION

Hybrid External Fixation

Several investigators have documented improved mechanical stability and control over palmar tilt by inserting pins into the distal metaphyseal fragment and attaching them directly to the external fixator (118,128–130). Direct control over the distal fragment may eliminate some of the loss of reduction seen with external fixators, including the loss of palmar tilt and radial collapse (Fig. 26-21).

COMBINED OPEN REDUCTION AND INTERNAL FIXATION WITH EXTERNAL FIXATION

This technique has been shown to be effective when the articular fragments are felt to be too small and too numerous for internal fixation with plate-screw constructs, and yet the fracture does not reduce anatomically with standard techniques. This method has been used primarily for high-energy injuries with comminution both dorsally and palmarly. The technique permits internal fixation of the comminuted fragments palmarly, and the use of the external fixation device prevents collapse on the side opposite the plate. Several cohort series have documented success with this technique (93,110,131). The underlying principle is to create an intact palmar buttress using a plate and then to avert dorsal collapse by tensioning across it using an external fixator. The procedure was felt to prevent the need for combined plate fixation and its associated extensive soft tissue stripping (132).

Operative Technique

The operative technique is most often used when external fixation has been performed and when persistent incongruity of the palmar lunate facet is shown. It is critical to reduce and stabilize this facet to obtain both articular congruity and distal radioulnar joint stability. A 5-cm skin incision is made ulnar to the flexor tendons, which are gently retracted to expose the intermediate column. The lunate facet is elevated and then held in position with a palmar plate. Once the plate is fixed proximally, it creates an intact palmar buttress across which tension can be applied (Fig. 26-22).

When the dorsal cortex is out to length, the distal screws may be placed. The radial column may be stabilized with either the radial limb of the plate or with percutaneously applied K-wires.

Arthroscopically Assisted Reduction and External Fixation of Intra-Articular Fractures

Although many investigators have shown the importance of articular congruity in the outcome after distal radius fractures, there is concern regarding whether we can adequately visualize the articular surface intraoperatively (43,133–136). Despite the reported significance of a residual step-off of 1 mm or more, several investigators have documented difficulty in the reliable measurement of articular step-offs of 1 mm, using conventional x-rays or intraoperative fluoroscopy (137–139). Arthroscopy has demonstrated residual displacement of articular fragments in 33% to 71% of fractures after reduction under fluoroscopy (137,140). The technique has also been extremely useful in documenting a wide variety of chondral lesions, interosseous ligament injuries, and avulsions of the triangular fibrocartilage (57–59,141,142). The incidence of interosseous ligament injuries associated with intra-articular fractures appears to be approximately 50% for scapholunate ligament injuries and 20% for lunotriquetral injuries (60,139). Triangular fibrocartilage injuries occur in approximately 40% of fractures, and direct chondral injury occurs in up to 30% of fractures (141).

Arthroscopy has been invaluable in enhancing existing knowledge of associated soft tissue lesions in distal radius fractures, but there is still question whether the technique provides outcomes superior to conventional techniques. Doi et al performed a prospective randomized study comparing the results of 34 patients treated using arthroscopically guided reduction; 48 patients were treated with open reduction and internal fixation (143). The results indicated superior radiographic and functional outcomes with the arthroscopically guided procedure. A second matched control study comparing arthroscopically assisted external fixation with fluoroscopically assisted external fixation, however, documented no significant differences between groups with the exception of forearm rotation and ulnar-sided symptoms (60). The investigators concluded that although arthroscopy provides superior imaging of the articular surface, external fixation permits some collapse during fracture union, which may detract from the subsequent radiographic outcome measurements.

Operative Technique

The decision regarding which fractures would benefit most from arthroscopically assisted reduction and external fixation

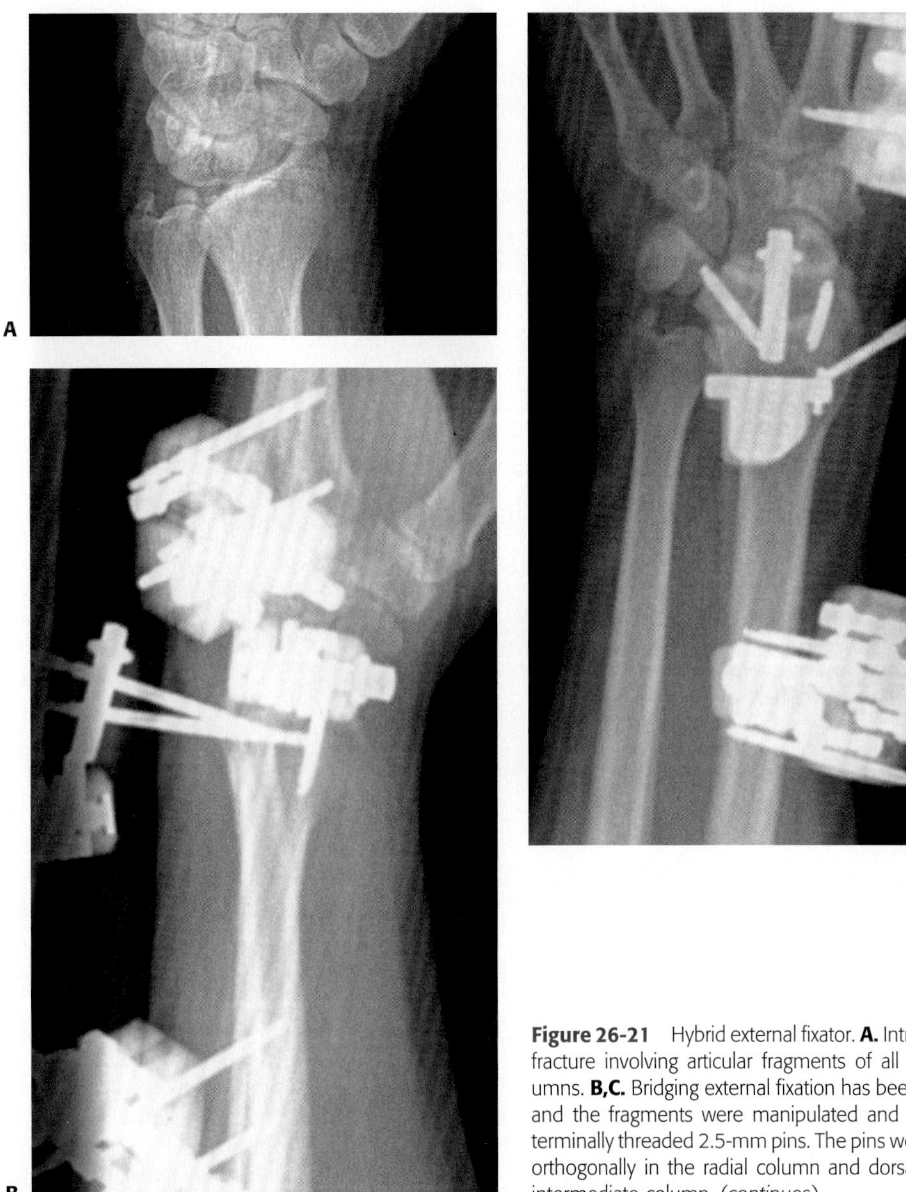

Figure 26-21 Hybrid external fixator. **A.** Intra-articular fracture involving articular fragments of all three columns. **B,C.** Bridging external fixation has been applied, and the fragments were manipulated and fixed with terminally threaded 2.5-mm pins. The pins were placed orthogonally in the radial column and dorsally in the intermediate column. (*continues*)

is controversial. In general, fractures with extensive metaphyseal comminution might be best managed with formal open reduction and internal fixation to prevent subsequent collapse. In patients with a large ulnar styloid fracture fragment and distal radioulnar instability, open reduction and internal fixation of the ulnar styloid fragment may be required, and arthroscopy may not add substantially to the care. Fractures that may benefit most from adjunctive arthroscopy are (a) complex articular fractures without metaphyseal comminution, particularly those with central impaction fragments and (b) fractures with evidence of substantial interosseous ligament or TFCC injury without a large ulnar styloid fragment (a fracture at the base of the styloid).

Timing

Ideally, the procedure is performed between 5 and 15 days postinjury. When fragments are significantly displaced, there may be associated palmar and dorsal rents in the capsule. This situation permits extravasation of irrigation fluid into the surrounding soft tissue, which is exacerbated with the use of a pump. Waiting 5 to 7 days minimizes this complication.

The external fixator may be applied before or after reduction

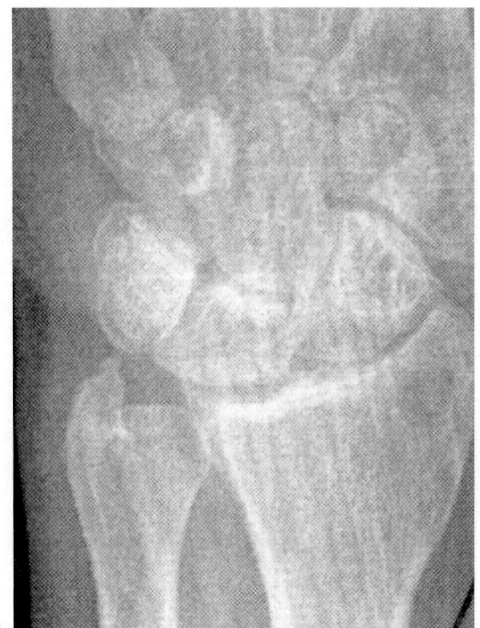

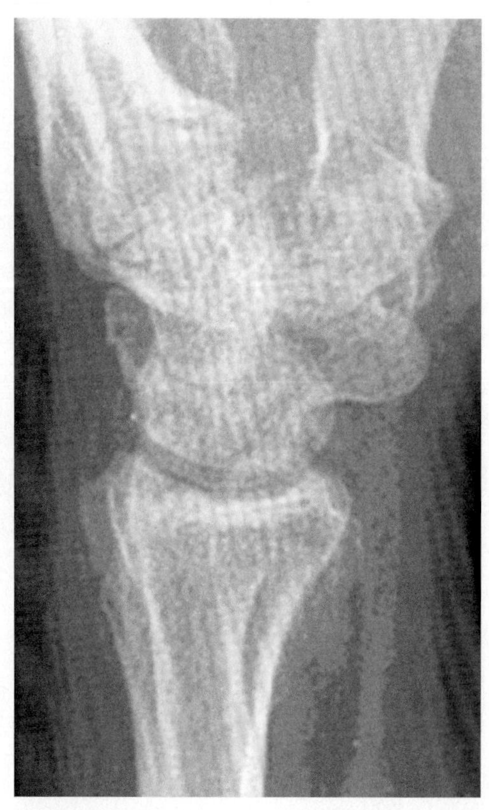

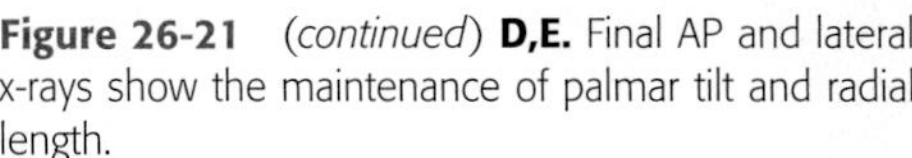

Figure 26-21 *(continued)* **D,E.** Final AP and lateral x-rays show the maintenance of palmar tilt and radial length.

of the articular surface; however, there are advantages to having the fixator in place before the arthroscopy. First, the extra-articular portion is reduced and out to length, thereby providing a template for elevating the depressed segments of the articular surface. Secondly, the external fixator provides excellent distraction of the joint for the arthroscopy.

After the external fixator has been placed, the metaphyseal defect must be addressed. Through a small 2-cm incision, the dorsal metaphyseal comminution may be exposed, and the defect may be partially filled with graft. One should avoid interposing graft between the major fragments of the articular surface. The window is left exposed to allow for manipulation during the arthroscopy. A provisional reduction is obtained and verified fluoroscopically. Additionally, prepositioned K-wires in the major fragments are useful to facilitate stabilization once the reduction has been effected.

The first step of the procedure is to irrigate the clot and other debris from the joint and perform a diagnostic arthroscopy through the 3-4 portal. This portal is best used for the purposes of instrumentation, while the 6-R or 6-U portals permit superior visualization of the fracture (60). Careful inspection of the scapholunate and lunotriquetral ligaments as well as the TFCC is performed both for prognostic and therapeutic purposes. Any disruptions of the interosseous ligaments may require further inspection through the midcarpal portals. Pathology is addressed from the radial side, proceeding ulnarly. Incomplete ligament injuries may be stable, and debridement can be performed if indicated. Subluxation from complete ligament injuries is reduced and pinned using K-wires. Next, the articular surface is reduced and pinned. It is critical to have a landmark for length and tilt in order to reduce the articular surface correctly. K-wires are placed in each of the major fragments, and their depth of penetration is verified at the end to avoid overpenetration palmarly. Ulnarly, the lunotriquetral interosseous ligament is treated with pinning or debridement. Finally, the TFCC may be repaired back to the extensor carpi ulnaris subsheath. If distal radioulnar joint instability has been treated surgically, the forearm is placed in 30 degrees of supination for a total of $3\frac{1}{2}$ weeks, after which range of motion is initiated (Fig. 26-23).

OPEN REDUCTION AND INTERNAL FIXATION

During 1950 to 1985, more than 450 articles were published on distal radius fractures. Of these, 60 dealt with internal fracture fixation. By contrast, the last 15 years have produced over 2,000 articles on distal radius fractures, 400 of which focused on internal fixation (144). There are many potential advantages to internal fixation of periarticular fractures including direct fixation of articular fragments, early range of motion of the joint, and avoidance of constrictive dressings or casts. Despite these potential advantages, the technique has been considered technically difficult, and a number of soft tissue complications have been noted with the use of plate fixation (145).

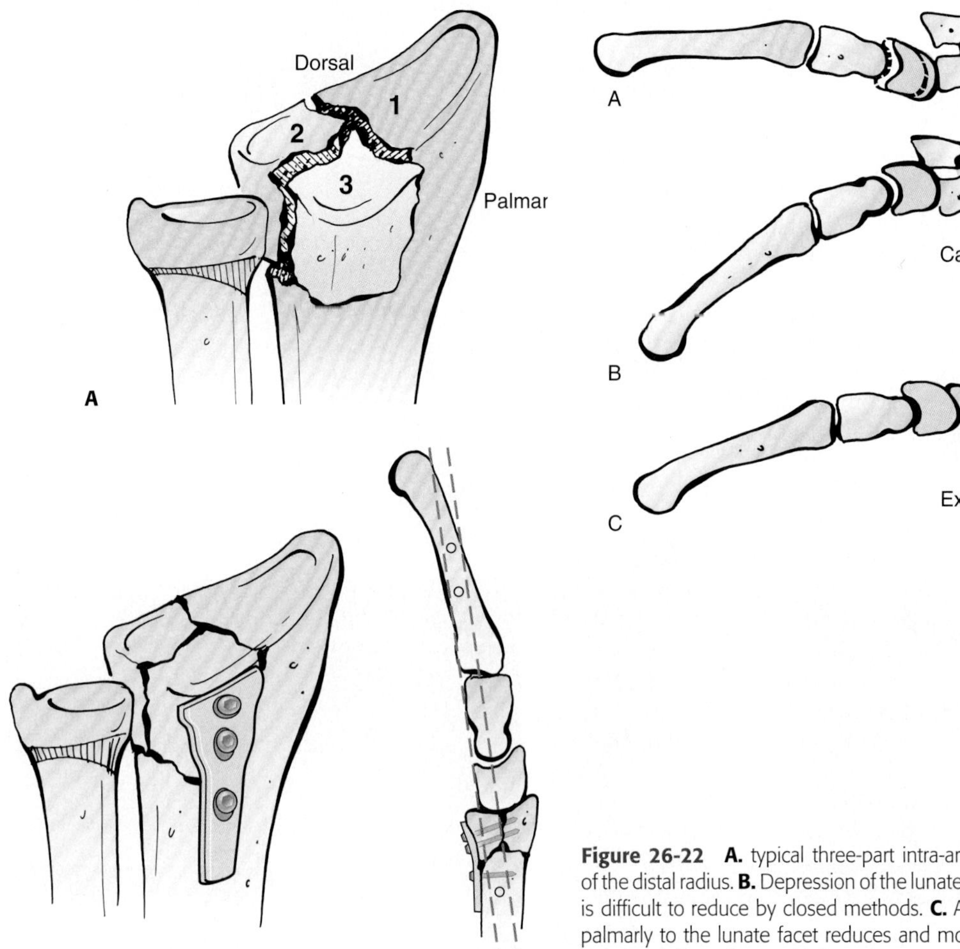

Figure 26-22 **A.** typical three-part intra-articular fracture of the distal radius. **B.** Depression of the lunate facet palmarly is difficult to reduce by closed methods. **C.** A plate applied palmarly to the lunate facet reduces and mortars both the DRUJ and the radiocarpal joint.

Dorsal Plate Application

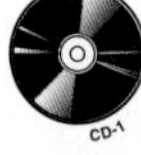

Internal fixation using a dorsal plate has several theoretical advantages. Technically familiar to most surgeons, the approach avoids the neurovascular structures on the palmar side. Further, the fixation is on the compression side of most distal radius fractures and provides a buttress against collapse. Initial reports of the technique demonstrated successful outcomes with the theoretical advantages of earlier return of function and better radial anatomy restoration than was seen with external fixation (146–151).

Despite the initial success with the technique, there were increasing reports of extensor tendon ruptures due to prominent hardware, particularly at Lister's tubercle (150,152–154), The more distally the plate is applied on the dorsum of the wrist, the more proximally the distal screws need to be directed to avoid articular penetration. This oblique orientation of the screws allows the distal fragment to displace palmarly. The palmar displacement of the fragment is particularly problematic because it results in incongruity at the distal radioulnar joint and dorsal prominence of the hardware with the tendency for extensor tenosynovitis or tendon rupture (Fig. 26-24).

More proximal fractures with larger distal fragments allow superior purchase in the distal fragment while permitting screw placement from proximal to distal, thereby engaging the palmar fragment and preventing it from collapsing palmarly.

Operative Technique

A longitudinal incision is centered over the fracture in line with the ulnar aspect of Lister's tubercle. The extensor retinaculum is incised in a Z-plasty manner, which allows for one limb to be placed over the plate and the second limb to be repaired over the extensor tendons to prevent bowstringing of the tendons with wrist extension. The extensor pollicis longus tendon is dislocated from its position at the tubercle and subperiosteal dissection is performed radially and ulnarly. Care should be taken to preserve all of the dorsal fragments for re-establishment of radial length. Traction is then applied by either an assistant or by the use of finger traps with weights suspended off the end of the table. Care should be taken to ensure that the patient's hand is not pronated relative to the forearm. The metaphyseal void can then be filled with graft, and the articular surface can be assessed. In the case

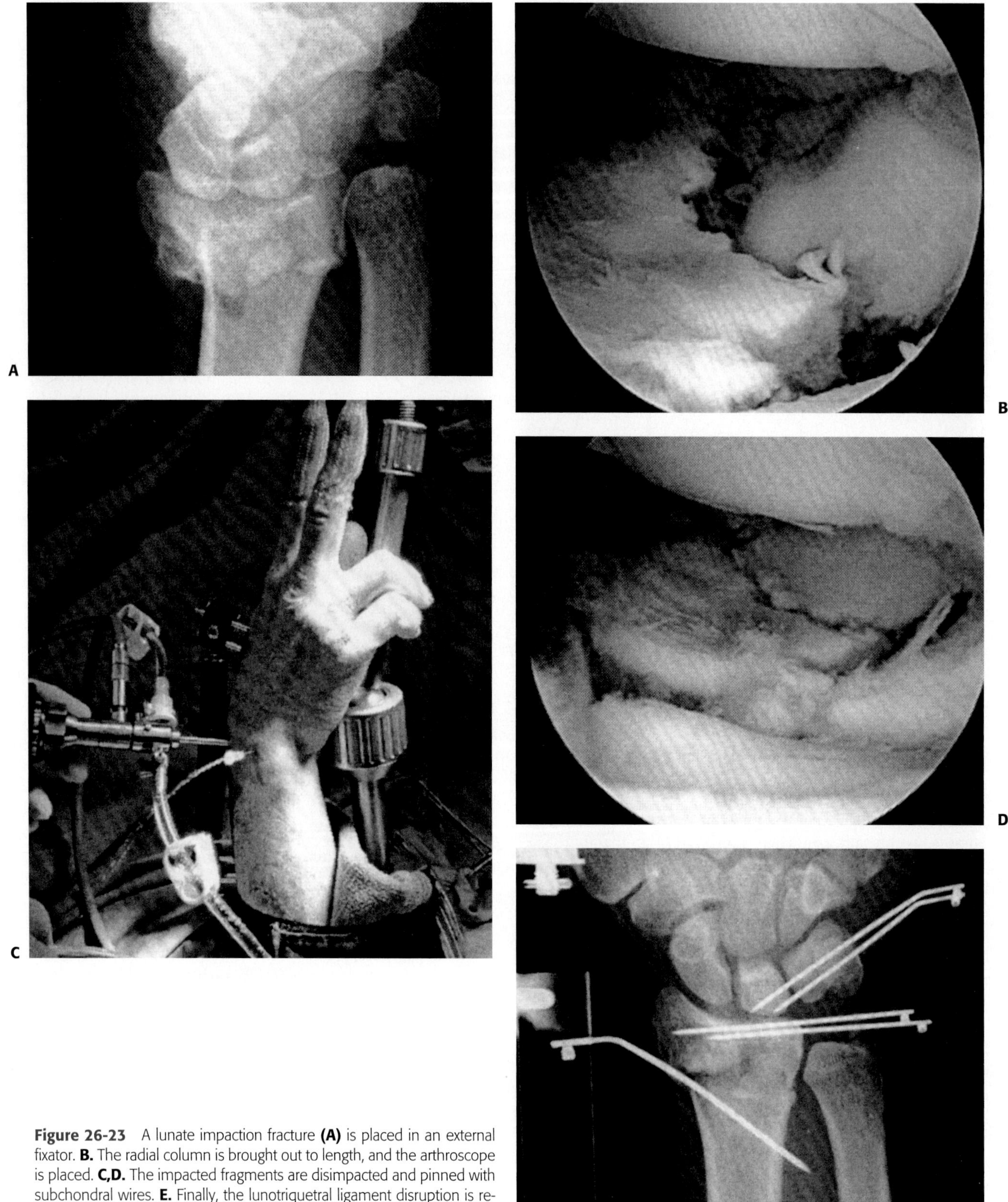

Figure 26-23 A lunate impaction fracture **(A)** is placed in an external fixator. **B.** The radial column is brought out to length, and the arthroscope is placed. **C,D.** The impacted fragments are disimpacted and pinned with subchondral wires. **E.** Finally, the lunotriquetral ligament disruption is reduced and pinned.

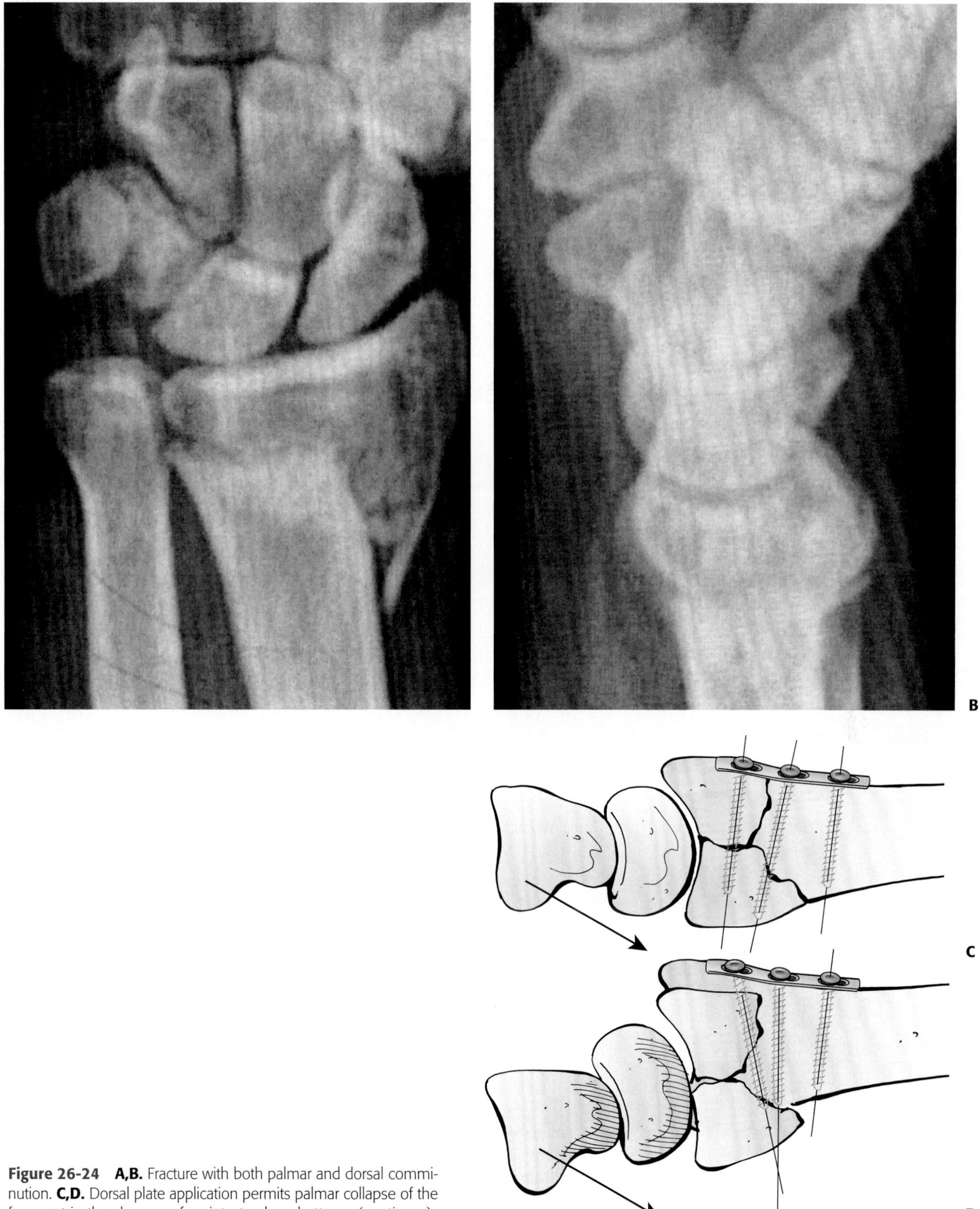

Figure 26-24 A,B. Fracture with both palmar and dorsal comminution. **C,D.** Dorsal plate application permits palmar collapse of the fragment in the absence of an intact palmar buttress. (*continues*)

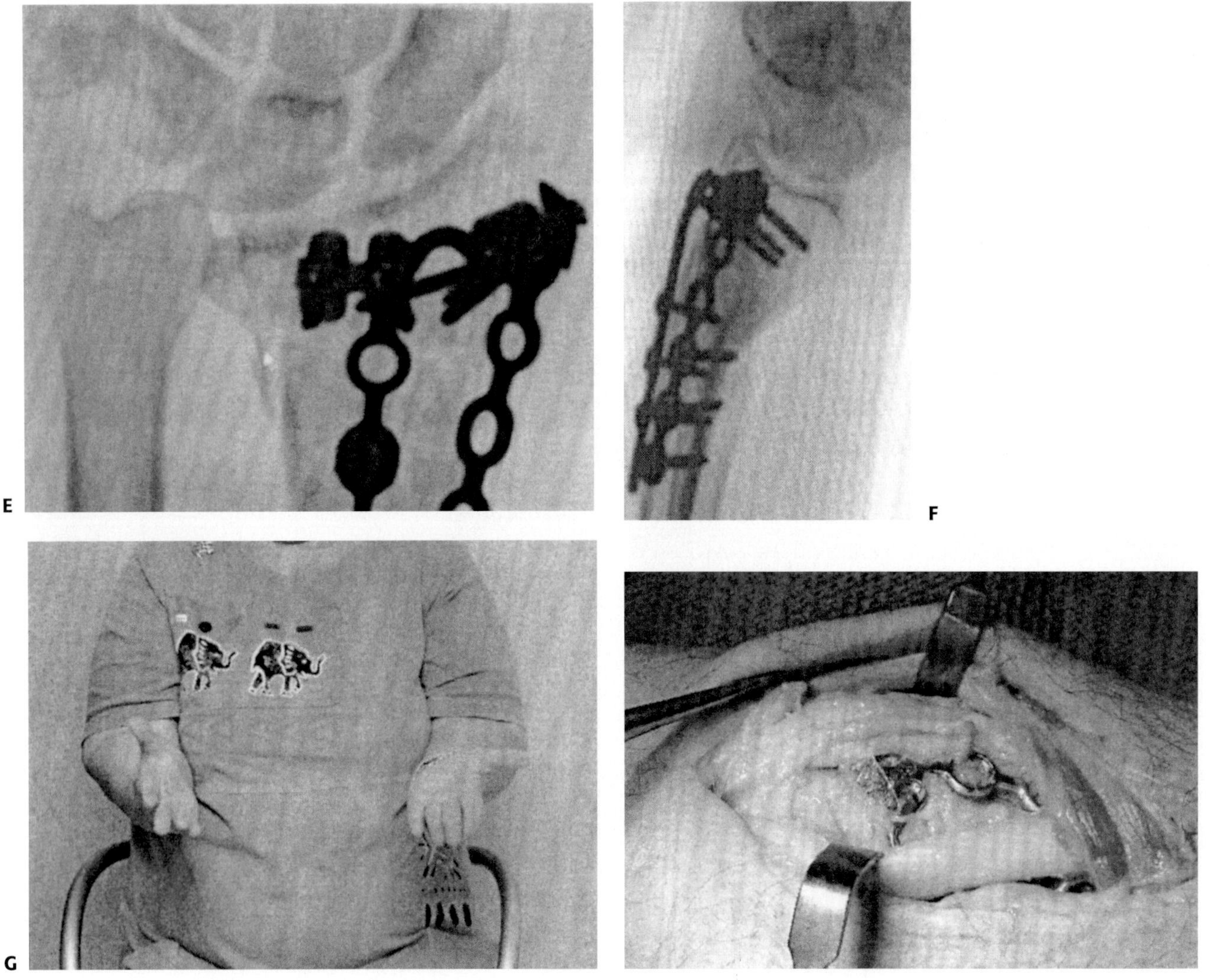

Figure 26-24 *(continued)* **E–G.** The palmar displacement of the metaphyseal fragment relative to the distal ulna results in radioulnar incongruity and loss of rotation. **H.** Hardware is now more prominent relative to the extensor tendons, resulting in extensor tenosynovitis and tendon rupture.

of residual incongruity of the articular surface, the joint may be directly assessed by extending the periosteal dissection distally, but care must be taken to avoid injury to the scapholunate interosseous ligament. Skin hooks can be placed under the capsular flaps and the articular surface can be visualized and reduced. Generally speaking, it is preferable to achieve the reduction by supporting the articular surface with supplemental graft and preventing subsequent displacement with screws placed through the distal aspect of the plate. If an arthrotomy is not performed, the articular surface should be visualized using a 20-degree inclined fluoroscopy view to assess for palmar displacement of the lunate facet and screw penetration into the articular surface. It is critical to ascertain whether the palmar cortex is aligned and does not displace palmarly with plate application. It is also advantageous to position the plate such that the screws are oriented perpendicular to the radial shaft, rather than directed from distal to proximal (Figs. 26-24E,F). In cases when there is extensive palmar comminution, supplemental fixation may be necessary. The addition of K-wires or a screw through the radial styloid to engage the proximal cortex of the radius is helpful to prevent palmar collapse.

Due to concerns over extensor tendon rupture from prominent dorsal hardware, multiple investigators have proposed the stabilization of dorsally displaced fractures through a palmar approach (155–159) (Figs. 26-25 and 26-26) While the position of the plate on the side opposite the displacement does not permit a direct buttress against dorsal displacement, the screw position in the distal fragment directly buttresses collapse. The addition of screw locking fixation in the distal fragment further

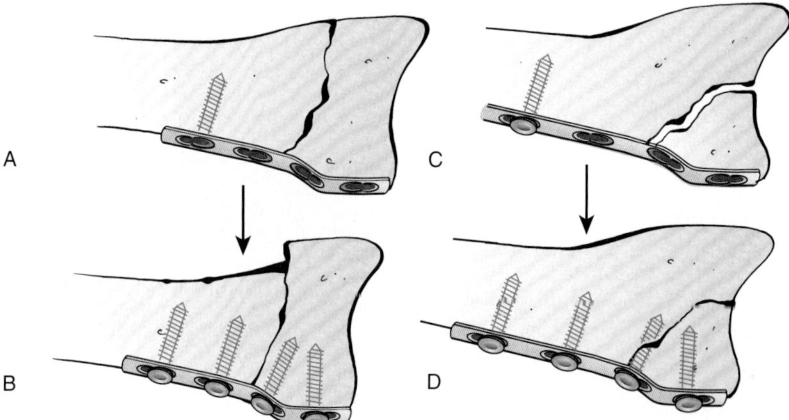

Figure 26-25 Palmar plating. The use of a palmar plate was originally reserved for articular shear fractures. **A,B.** Use of a palmarly applied undercontoured plate allows compression of the volar lip back to the intact dorsal buttress. **C,D.** In the absence of an intact dorsal buttress, undercontouring the plate will result in dorsal displacement of the entire articular surface.

prevents dorsal displacement of the distal fragment. One concern over these locking plates is the potential for articular penetration with distal plate position on the palmar surface of the radius. The more distal the plate placement on the radius is, the more the screws need to angle back proximally to avoid penetration into the lunate fossa (Fig. 26-27).

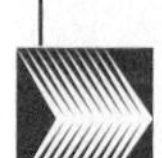

Palmar plates may be applied through either a flexor carpi radialis (FCR)/radial artery interval or through a midline flexor tendon/ulnar neurovascular bundle interval. The FCR/radial artery approach is preferable for fixation of dorsally displaced fractures with dorsal comminution and fixation of partial articular fractures (articular shear fractures). The skin incision is centered over the FCR with care being taken to avoid injury to the palmar cutaneous branch of the median nerve, which lies ulnar to the tendon. The radial artery is mobilized, and dissection is carried radially by releasing the brachioradialis tendon from the radial styloid. Using this approach, the comminution on the dorsum of the radius can be visualized, and graft can be placed. Articular depression can also be seen by pronation of the radius away from the rest of the articular surface. The depressed articular surface may be visualized from within the fracture site, which allows for subarticular graft placement. The pronator quadratus muscle is released from its radial attachment and should be preserved to place over the plate at the conclusion of the case. The main limitation of this approach is in the visualization of the palmar ulnar corner of the radius.

The second surgical approach to the palmar radius is the flexor tendon/ulnar neurovascular bundle interval. The skin incision is centered over the ulnar border of the palmaris longus, the flexor tendons are mobilized radially, and the ulnar neurovascular bundle is taken ulnarly. With this approach, the pronator quadratus is released from the ulna. The incision may be extended distally to release the transverse carpal ligament, particularly if the patient had any median nerve symptoms preoperatively. This incision is preferred when the majority of the comminution is at the palmar lunate facet. Note that the location of the skin incision does not preclude the surgeon from developing the interval between the FCR and the radial artery through the same incision. This incision permits the development of both intervals if there is any question regarding the adequacy of the reduction.

Once the approach has been performed, the next step is to obtain an anatomic reduction of both the radial and the intermediate columns. The decision of which column to reduce first lies in which cortex can be anatomically reduced and fixed using a K-wire. Once the columns have been aligned, the fracture may be fixed to the palmar plate. First the plate is temporarily fixed to the shaft preferable with either a unicortical screw or a screw in a sliding hole in the plate. The lateral view is useful to determine if screws placed through the plate are going to penetrate the articular surface. A combination of traction and palmar flexion usually reduces the metaphyseal fragment to the plate, and then the remaining screws may be placed (Fig. 26-28).

AUTHOR'S PREFERRED TREATMENT

As has been noted throughout this chapter, there are a wide variety of techniques that may be applied successfully to nearly every fracture. A dogmatic approach is not appropriate and cannot be supported by the literature. Evidence that compares different options indicates that the most important aspect of outcome is to achieve the radiographic measures of a successful outcome in the least invasive method possible.

Metaphyseal Bending Fractures

Metaphyseal bending fractures typically arise as the result of a fall on the outstretched hand. The fracture is usually a lower-energy injury and may be considered as either a stable or an

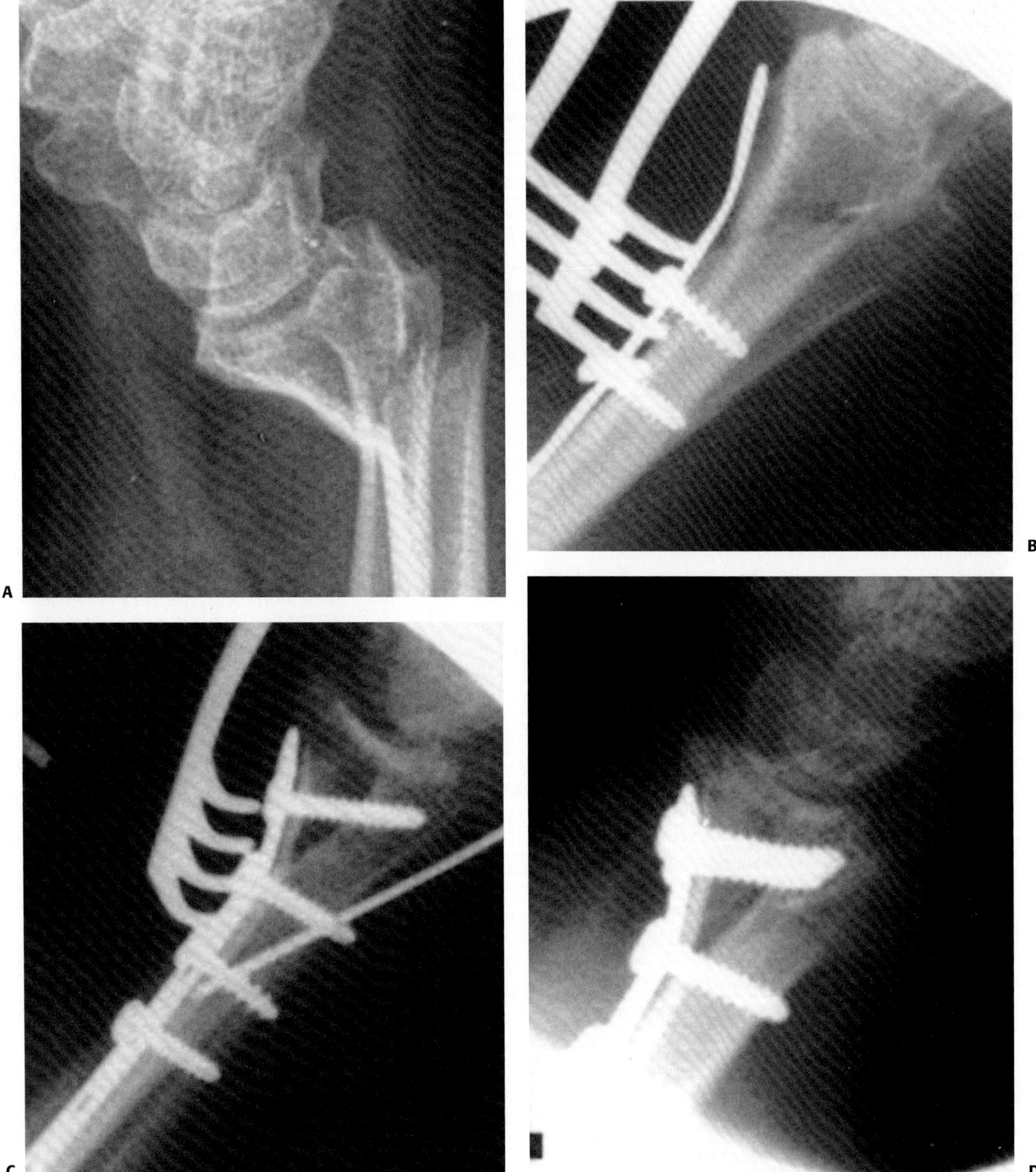

Figure 26-26 A,B. Sequential tightening of an undercontoured plate to the distal radius. Note that the technique requires an intact dorsal cortex; otherwise, the technique will push the distal radius dorsally. To prevent this, a temporary pin may be placed to provide a dorsal buttress while the plate is applied. The pin is then removed after the screws have been tightened **(C,D).**

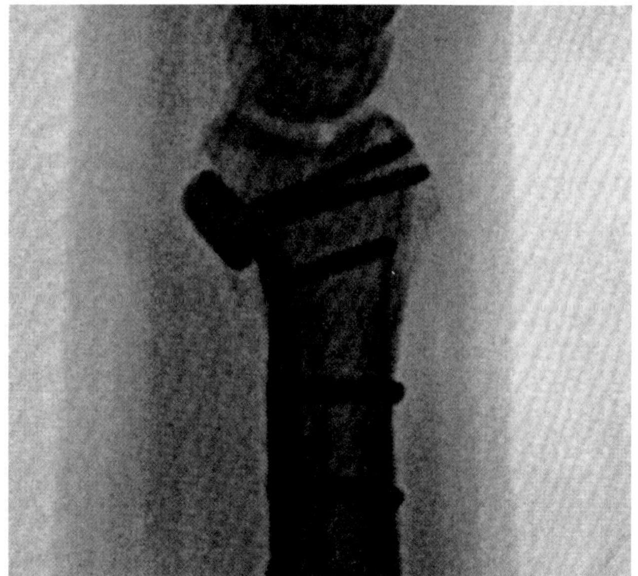

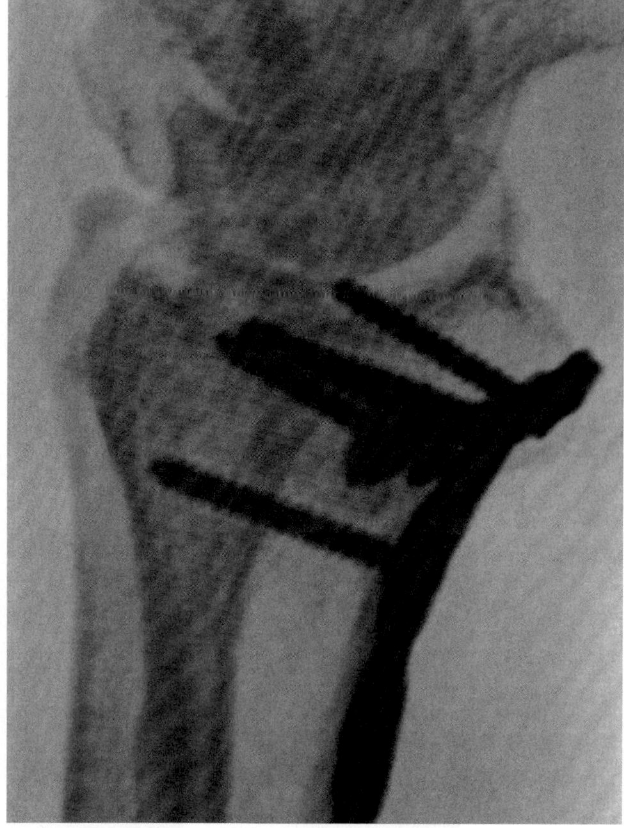

Figure 26-27 Palmar plate fixation of a distal radius fracture. Note the anatomy of the volar lip of the radius distally. The more distal the placement of the plate is, the more likely the screw will penetrate the articular surface.

unstable fracture. Stable fractures are characterized by (a) minimal metaphyseal void with no palmar comminution, (b) an intact palmar cortex after reduction, and (c) good quality bone stock without osteoporosis or osteopenia secondary to advanced age or metabolic bone disease.

Unstable fractures create two long-term problems: shortening of the radius relative to the intact ulna and loss of palmar tilt at the radiocarpal joint. Shortening of the radius relative to the ulna during the injury disrupts the distal radioulnar joint ligaments. Adams demonstrated that shortening the radius relative to the intact ulna of more than 5 mm must, by definition, disrupt the TFCC or cause avulsion of the ulnar styloid (160). The resultant distal radioulnar joint instability may be responsible for the ulnar-sided pain noted in follow-up by several investigators (142,161). Further, the residual shortening results in long-term ulnar impaction syndrome with resultant pain with ulnar deviation and strong grip.

Unstable bending fractures of the radial metaphysis are ideally suited for open reduction and internal fixation. Internal fixation of metaphyseal bending fractures has become increasingly popular due primarily to the ability to (a) directly control and maintain physiologic palmar tilt, (b) prevent collapse with external fixation, and (c) avoid bridging the radiocarpal joint. The distal fragment typically has sufficient size and integrity to provide adequate purchase and may be approached from either a dorsal or a volar approach. Palmar plating is preferred, as the screws directly buttress against collapse and loss of palmar tilt. With smaller and more distal fragments, a dorsal plate has to be positioned distally on the dorsum of the radius making extensor tendon injury more likely.

A flexor carpi radialis/radial artery approach is preferred. If a carpal tunnel release is indicated, then it is performed through a separate distal palmar incision, and the wrist crease is not crossed. The interval is extended up to the transverse palmar branches of the radial artery to attain full exposure of the radial styloid. The brachioradialis tendon is released, and the exposure is carried around dorsally. A combination of allograft and demineralized bone matrix is placed in the comminuted area to fill the metaphyseal void.

The ulnar corner is visualized by release of the pronator quadratus muscle, and the ulnar corner is aligned. A large tenaculum clamp may be useful to maintain the alignment of the ulnar corner while a K-wire is placed obliquely through the lunate facet to engage the proximal radius. The same procedure can be performed on the radial cortex, and a second pin may be placed.

The palmar plate is positioned next. As the plates are precontoured to match the volar angulation, it is critical that the track the screws will take in the distal fragment is templated on an inclined view. Often, the plate is placed slightly too distally. Thus, it is helpful to leave sufficient room in the oblique hole in the plate to permit proximal positioning of the plate without

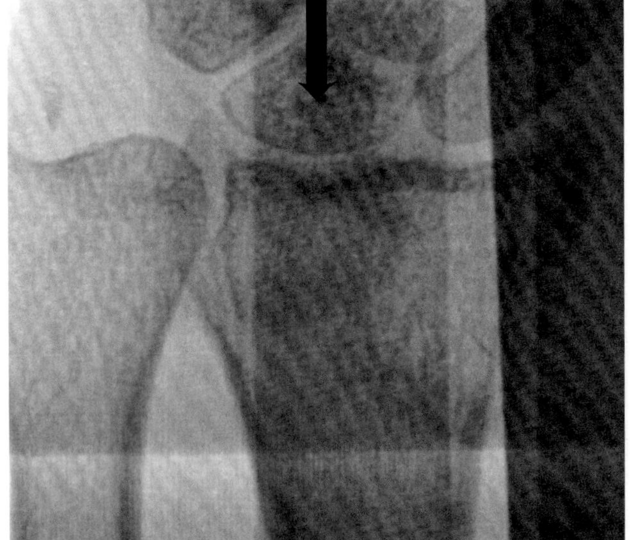

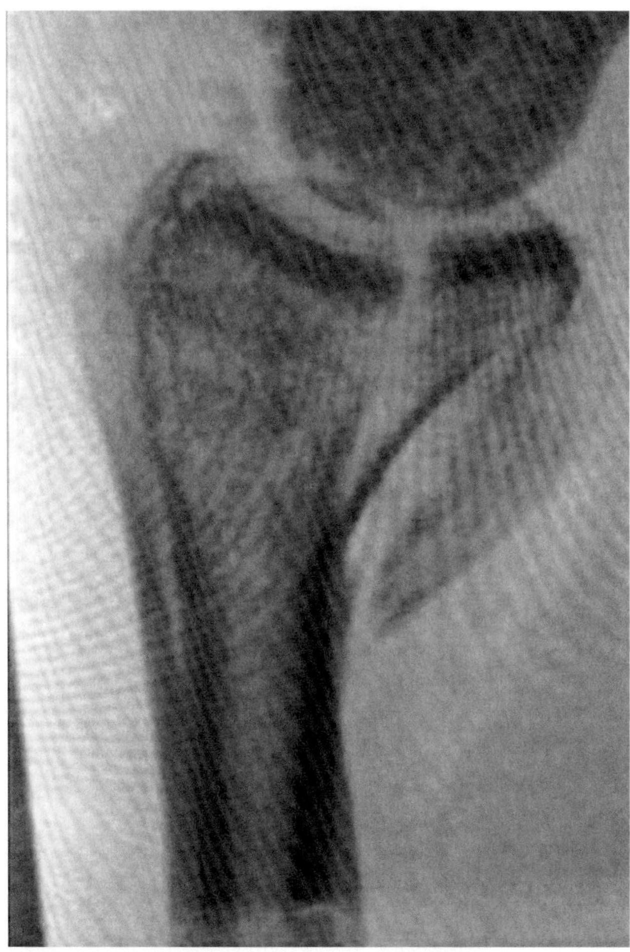

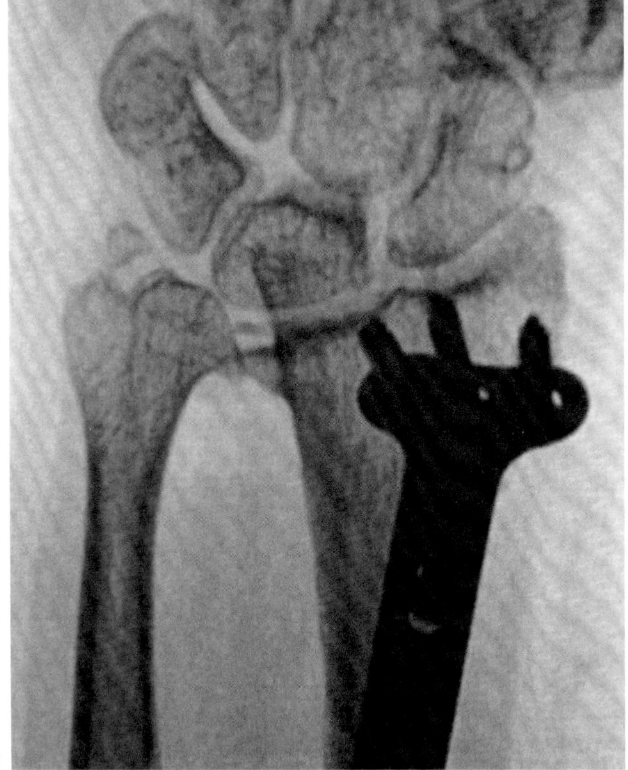

Figure 26-29 A,B. Articular shear fractures may have a nondisplaced fracture line between the scaphoid and the lunate facets, which can displace if the plate is not placed sufficiently ulnarly to support the lunate facet. **C.** Note the late effect of a depressed lunate facet on both the distal radioulnar joint and the radiocarpal joint.

Compression Fractures of the Articular Surface

The optimal management of lunate impaction fractures is one of the most controversial topics in wrist fracture surgery. The most critical point in treating these injuries is to understand the mechanism of the injury and recognize the fragments. Melone emphasized the role of the lunate in the creation of intra-articular fractures (162). As the lunate impacts the articular surface, it splits the lunate fossa into two characteristic fragments with the potential for a third "central impaction" fracture. The scaphoid impacts the radial styloid and results in a shearing force, which typically does not split the styloid into a palmar and a dorsal fragment. When faced with these fractures, the surgeon is required to identify each fragment and assess for displacement. Once the fragments have been identified, the decision must be made whether to stabilize the displaced fragments based on the fragment size and the degree of the displacement.

In general terms, there are two methods for reducing and stabilizing displaced articular fragments: external fixation and internal fixation. Each technique has its advantages and its complications. In an attempt to directly compare each technique, one group of investigators prospectively randomized patients into either internal fixation or external fixation. The external fixation group demonstrated superior outcomes provided that they were able to achieve satisfactory radiographic parameters at the time of the end of treatment. The investigators concluded that the goal should be to achieve satisfactory radiographic parameters using the least invasive technique possible (163). In general terms, it can be concluded that each individual surgeon will have a level of comfort regarding his or her preferred technique. External fixation is an exceedingly useful technique for treating a variety of radius fractures; however, it is critical to understand that certain fracture patterns will require more invasive treatment methods. In the case of lunate impaction fractures, the lunate must be assessed before obtaining patient consent. If the lunate facet is split into a palmar and a dorsal fragment, traction alone may not reduce the critical volar ulnar corner. The surgeon and the patient must understand that if indirect reduction of this fragment does not occur with traction, then direct reduction will be required.

In one study of 132 patients treated with external fixation, 15 (11%) required limited open techniques to achieve reduction (164). Direct reduction may be performed either through a limited open or an extensile approach. Smaller fragments may be fixed with wires, whereas fragments that extend more proximally may require plate stabilization. Because volar plating may actually address all the components of the fracture, the surgeon may elect to use a locked volar plate only and forego external fixation. Extensive preoperative planning and templating is critical due to the multitude of variables.

The preferred method of anesthesia is axillary block; a tourniquet is used. A 3-cm dorsoradial skin incision is made at the distal third of the radius. Careful dissection is performed to avoid injury to the dorsal sensory portion of the radial nerve, which emerges from under the brachioradialis tendon 7.5 to 11.0 cm proximal to the tip of the radial styloid (Fig. 26-30).

The drill holes are placed in the interval between the extensor carpi radialis brevis and longus. This position places the extensor carpi radialis longus between the pin and the sensory branch of the radial nerve. Predrilling and hand placement of the pins may prevent overheating of the cortical bone and subsequent pin site problems. To avoid interference with thumb retroflexion, the distal pins should be placed 45 degrees off the sagittal plane at the adductor tubercle of the index metacarpals. The fracture is then reduced manually in the following sequence: (a) longitudinal traction is applied to achieve radial length, and the fracture is assessed for the presence of a metaphyseal defect; (b) palmar translation (not palmar flexion) of the carpus; and (c) ulnar deviation. If there is evidence of significant radioulnar instability, the fracture is reduced in supination to avoid displacing the radial metaphysis palmar to the distal ulna as ulnar deviation is applied. The most critical element to this technique is to anatomically align the palmar cortex on the lateral view. It is especially useful to incline the radius 15 to 20 degrees to the fluoroscopy beam to check the alignment. In order to prevent collapse during healing and permit early removal of the external fixator, the metaphyseal void may be filled with a bone graft or a bone graft substitute at this time. It may be useful to temporarily overdistract the fracture to enlarge the defect. The majority of graft substitutes do not permit complete packing of the defect, and temporary overdistraction will allow better filling of the void. As traction is decreased, the material will be compacted. The metaphyseal comminution permits "opening" of the fracture through a 2-cm wound dorsally immediately proximal to the fracture. Small right angle retractors may facilitate exposure of the thin metaphyseal dorsal cortical fragments. One or more of these fragments may be removed after marking its distal aspect with a marking pen to indicate its correct orientation for reinsertion. This opens the fracture and exposes the metaphyseal defect to allow irrigation of the clot from the fracture site. For extra-articular fractures, the graft is packed radially and distally with care being taken to avoid displacing the palmar cortex.

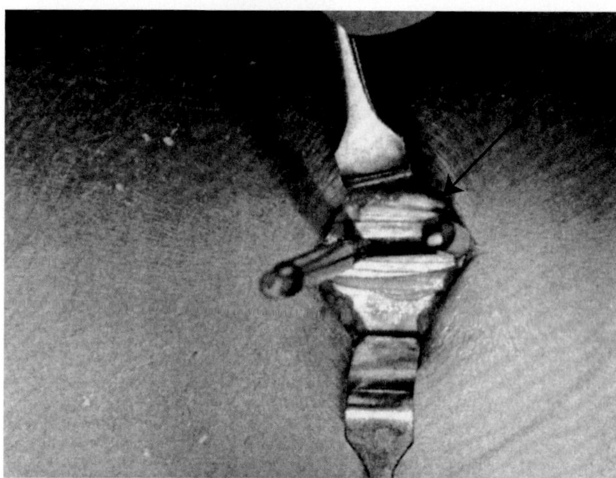

Figure 26-30 Pin position between the extensor carpi radialis longus and brevis. Note the proximity of the radial nerve's dorsal sensory branch (*arrow*). Iatrogenic injury to this nerve is a frequent cause of neurogenic pain after external fixation and may be minimized by open rather than percutaneous pin insertion.

Supplemental graft is critical in external fixation of most compression fractures, particularly those with a central impaction component. After irrigating out the clot, a tamp can be used to gently elevate the compressed segments. Start palmarly and work dorsally. It is theoretically useful to elevate some of the native cancellous bone up with the fragments to create a uniform subchondral surface for the intermediate column. The supplemental graft can then be packed in the resultant defect. The dorsal cortical "window" can be replaced with care being taken to create a smooth surface for the extensor tendons.

Intra-Articular Fractures

After reduction of the radial metaphysis, it is critical to evaluate the lunate facet on the inclined lateral view with traction in place. If traction fails to reduce the palmar facet, then direct reduction will be required through an open rather than a percutaneous approach.

Two-Part Intra-Articular Fractures

In the case of a two-part intra-articular fracture, the radial cortex may be reduced with longitudinal traction and slight ulnar deviation. The radial cortex is stabilized using two percutaneously placed 0.45- or 0.62-inch K-wires. Once the radial cortex is out to length, the lunate fossa may be pinned in a reduced position. If there is minimal comminution, a large tenaculum clamp may be placed percutaneously between the dorsal ulnar corner and the newly fixed radial cortex. After verifying that the lunate fossa is out to length and that there is no step-off between the scaphoid and the lunate facets, transverse wires may be placed under the subchondral surface.

Three-Part Intra-Articular Fractures

In the case of three-part intra-articular fractures, the radial column again is reduced first. The lunate fossa should then be assessed on a tilted lateral view. If the palmar lunate facet is reduced after grafting and applying traction, transverse subchondral wires may again be placed; care must be taken to direct at least one of the wires to support the palmar lunate facet.

When x-rays reveal that the palmar lunate facet is still depressed after application of traction and placing graft material, a direct reduction is performed. A skin incision is placed longitudinally at the ulnar aspect of flexor tendons but radial to the ulnar neurovascular bundle. The flexor tendons are retracted radially and the ulnar neurovascular bundle is retracted ulnarly to expose the critical palmar ulnar fragment. If the fracture lies distally and does not involve the thick cortical support of the lunate facet, then the fragment may be fixed with two K-wires leaving the wire emerging dorsally for later removal. The more common fracture pattern results in extension below the level of the sigmoid notch. The proximal extension typically results in a triangular-shaped fragment of cortical bone, which will require buttress fixation using a plate-screw construct. If the surgeon plans to leave the external fixation in place and if the radial column is well stabilized, then a small 2.0- or 2.4-mm plate may be applied to the intermediate column.

It is critical when applying this plate to make sure that the dorsal lunate facet is out to length when the distal screws are placed. Failure to reduce the dorsal lunate facet will result in an intra-articular step-off as the distal screws are placed. Once the intermediate column is fixed, the radial side is reassessed to ensure that there is no step-off. The radial pins may need to be readjusted to reflect the reduced position to the intermediate column.

Four-Part Fractures

When the articular surface is comminuted into four parts or greater, it becomes even more critical to support the articular surface with a bone graft or a bone graft substitute. Placing the graft from the dorsum may result in the ability to restore a relatively congruous articular surface from below.

Once the graft has been placed, it is critical to evaluate for displacement of the palmar radial and ulnar facets. The central impaction fragment may be reduced percutaneously from the dorsal side using the subchondral graft and wires, although the palmar articular facets remain a problem. If tilted x-rays reveal displacement palmarly, then the surgeon should make a limited or an extensile palmar approach. After stabilization of the intermediate column with a small buttress plate, lateral x-rays may still reveal some articular step-off palmarly, which reflects the split in the radial styloid. The radial column is visible through the midline incision, but it may not be stabilized by a smaller 2.0- or 2.4-mm plate buttressing the lunate facet. At this time, the surgeon can either apply a more conventional "T" plate or maintain the reduction with percutaneously applied K-wires exiting radially.

Supplemental Fixation

In an effort to directly fix the fractured segments and avoid the loss of palmar tilt and radial length after external fixation, several investigators have recommended supplemental fixation with or without the use of adjunctive bone graft (108).

When fixation is completed, it is critical to evaluate the tension in the extrinsic extensor tendons by assessing passive metacarpophalangeal motion. Overdistraction results in excessive tension on the digital extensors. The metacarpal phalangeal joints may be passively flexible, but with excessive tension, the digits "spring" back into extension when the digit is released. If there is any doubt, the traction can be let off, and the passive motion can be reassessed. If the motion is improved after releasing some distraction, fixation should be secured in this position.

Internal Fixation of Intra-Articular Fractures

The approach to internal fixation of intra-articular fractures is determined by the location and the degree of displacement of the intra-articular component. The degree of comminution determines the decision of approach and fixation. In general terms, for fractures that are primarily comminuted either palmarly or dorsally, the most direct approach may be performed. When the comminution involves both the palmar and the dorsal cortices, the use of a palmar locked plate is preferred.

It is helpful to have both the injury film and the postreduction films to determine the approach and the implant selection. AP, lateral, and oblique x-rays after reduction should be viewed to determine any displacement of the radial styloid and the palmar and dorsal lunate facets. Any question of central impaction is assessed with CT. Typically, the intermediate column is assessed for residual displacement first. Residual displacement of the palmar lunate cortex should be addressed with the palmar plate. Comminution of the intermediate column should be addressed first, and the displaced palmar lunate cortex should be approached through the flexor tendon/ulnar neurovascular bundle interval (Fig. 26-31A,B). Residual displacement of the radial styloid should be addressed with a separate plate or with percutaneous wires (Fig. 26-31C–F). For residual dorsal displacement with the palmar cortex reduced, a dorsal approach to the intermediate column should be used with an incision between third and fourth compartments (Fig. 26-32A,B). Separate fixation of the radial column may be needed to avoid dorsal impingement at Lister's tubercle (Fig. 26-32C–E).

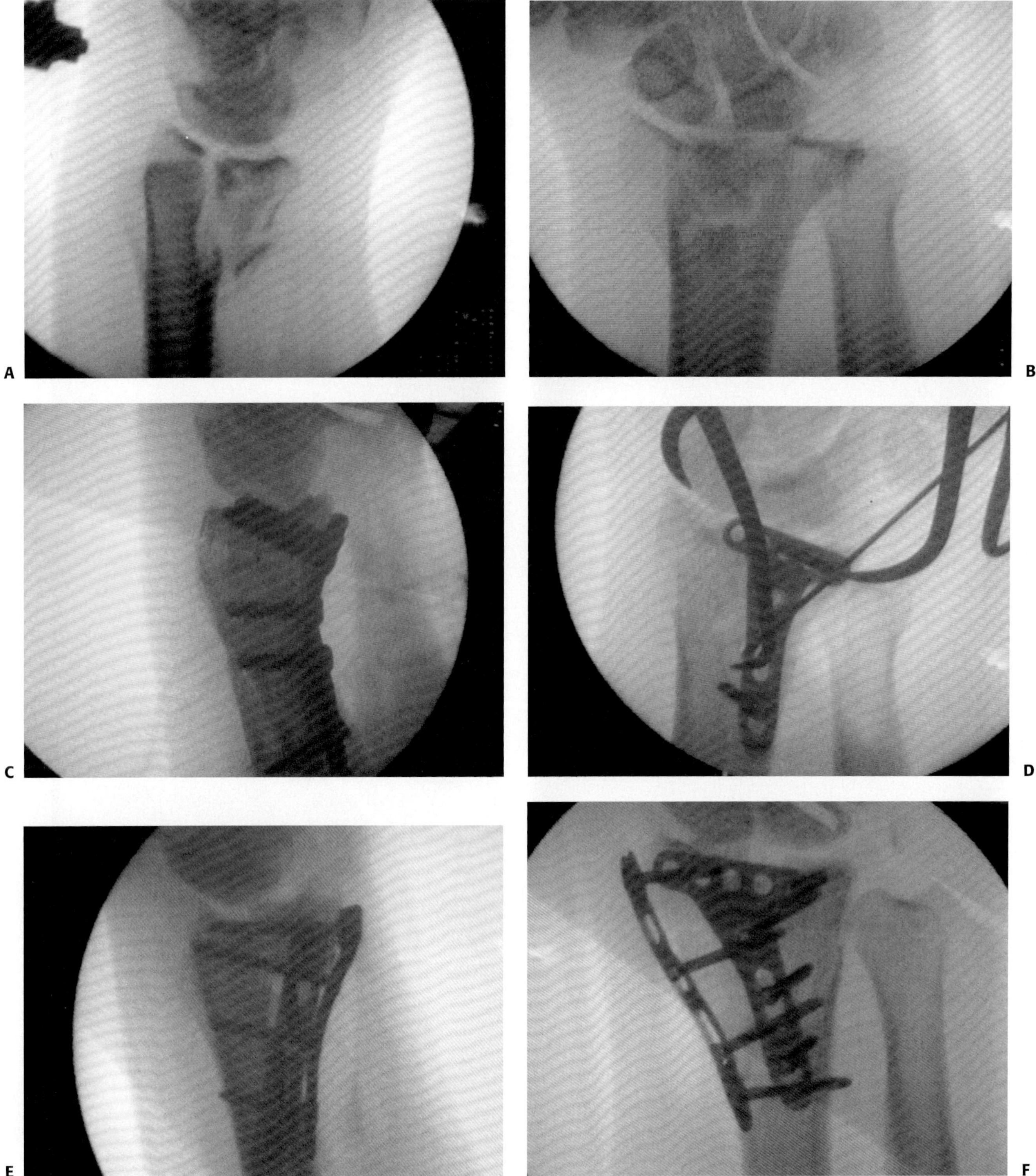

Figure 26-31 **A,B.** Lateral and PA fluoroscopy views after reduction in traction of a highly comminuted intra-articular fracture. Note that the dorsal cortex comes out to length while the palmar cortex remains displaced. **C,D.** Following application of a palmar plate, there is still some residual comminution of the radial styloid. The radial styloid (particularly distally) may require adjunctive fixation with either a second plate or K-wires. **E,F.** For this case, a separate radial column plate was used to create the final construct.

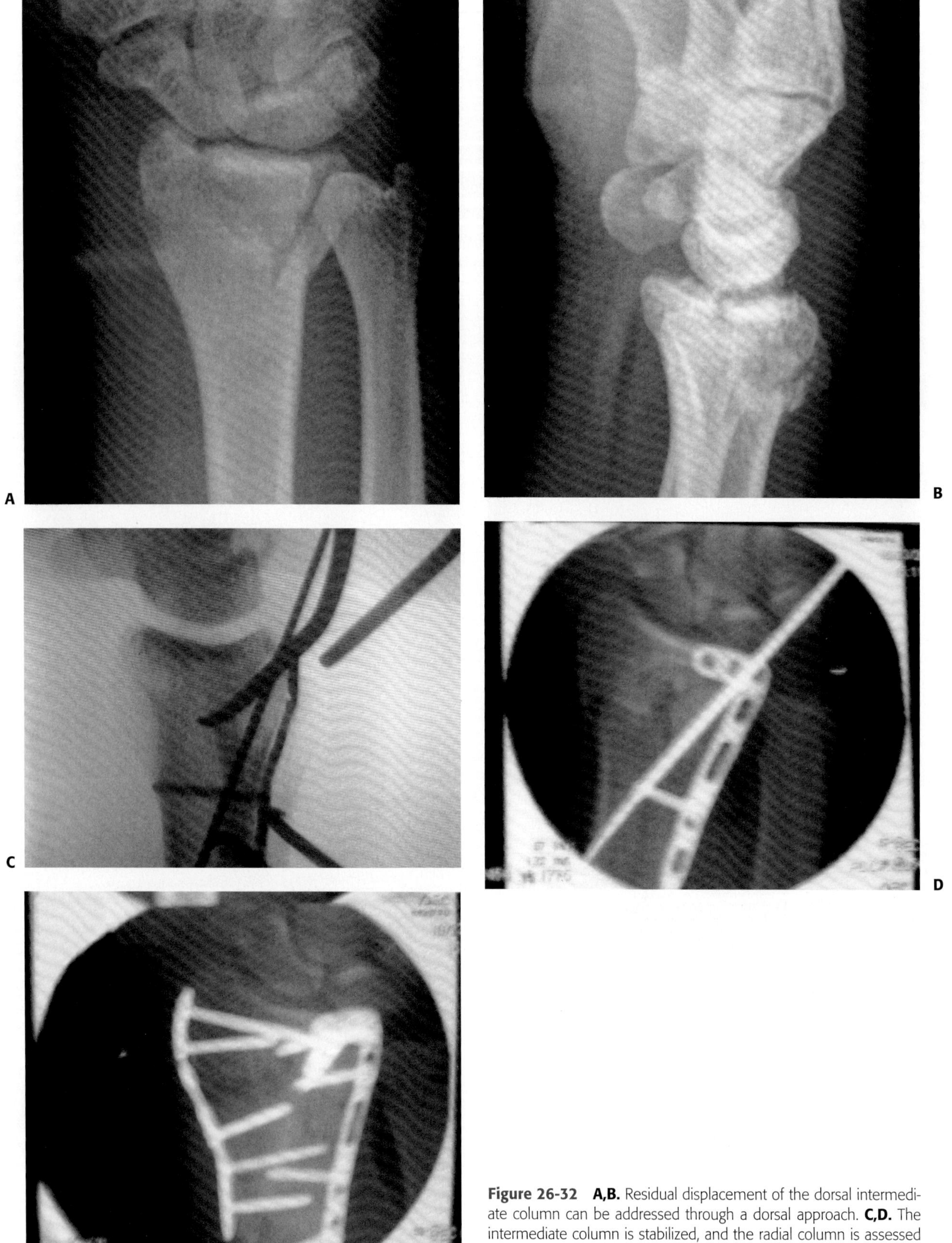

Figure 26-32 **A,B.** Residual displacement of the dorsal intermediate column can be addressed through a dorsal approach. **C,D.** The intermediate column is stabilized, and the radial column is assessed for palmar displacement and rotation. **E.** If necessary, a second radial plate is applied.

ASSOCIATED INJURIES

Radial styloid fractures, isolated volar or dorsal lip fractures, and ulnar styloid fractures serve as markers of high-energy ligament injuries about the wrist.

Radial Styloid Fractures

Depressed radial styloid fractures are associated with a high incidence of scapholunate ligament injuries; the scaphoid displaces relative to the lunate. A shear injury between the two bones ruptures the scapholunate interosseous ligament. Treatment should be geared toward the ligamentous injury and should include stabilization of the radial styloid. For acute injuries, a dorsal ligament repair with reattachment of the dorsal extrinsic ligaments may be performed. A cannulated screw or K-wires may be used to stabilize the fracture.

Volar Lip Injuries

The management of volar lip injuries depends on the size of the fragment relative to the remaining portion of the lunate facet. Smaller ulnar-sided fragments indicate a distal radioulnar joint injury, and treatment may be geared toward reducing and stabilizing the distal radioulnar joint. Larger fragments indicate true palmar radiocarpal instability and should be assessed for residual palmar displacement of the lunate relative to the radiocarpal joint (165–168). Stabilization of these fragments may be difficult. Smaller fragments may be neutralized by placing a wire through the fragment and through a drill hole in the radius. The fragments are then sutured to the radius. Larger fragments may be fixed with a plate/screw construct. As these fragments represent the insertions of the volar extrinsic ligaments, there is a growing trend to repair, rather than excise, these fragments.

Dorsal Lip Injuries

Avulsion injuries of the dorsal lip of the radius indicate intercarpal ligament injuries rather than radiocarpal instability. The most commonly encountered injury is an avulsion of the dorsal radiolunotriquetral ligament attached to a fragment of the distal radius. More distal injuries arise from lunotriquetral interosseous disruptions.

Normally, if the injury arises from the dorsum of the radius, then both the radiocarpal joint and the scaphoid should be assessed for stability. External fixation may be used to stabilize the radiocarpal joint, and percutaneous pinning may be used to fix the intercarpal instability.

Ulnar Styloid Fractures

Fractures of the ulnar styloid occur in approximately 60% to 70% of distal radius fractures (169–173). It is well accepted that the distal ulna is a common source of symptoms after injury. The disability that arises directly from the fracture versus the associated injury to the triangular fibrocartilage complex remains controversial (174–177). Adams documented in cadaver studies that displacing the radius relative to the ulna 5 mm or more must result in a fracture of the ulnar styloid or a disruption of the TFCC (19). The disruption may occur at the base of the ulnar styloid, the ulnar insertion of the distal radio-ulnar ligaments, or the radial insertion of the TFCC complex.

The indications for treatment of these injuries remain controversial. Although it is accepted that displacement of the radius results in acute joint disruption, whether these injuries require treatment is unknown. Lindau documented that persistent radioulnar instability was a risk factor for a poor outcome independent of radiographic appearance. Clinically apparent instability was present in 26 of 76 patients at 1 year postinjury. Instability of the distal radioulnar joint was associated with a worse wrist score and doubled the score on the visual analog pain scale (178). Fixation of the ulnar styloid and/or repair of the TFCC has been reported to have good outcomes, but it is uncertain as to which injuries require acute repair (173,179). The indications for treatment of ulnar styloid fractures are evolving. Currently, a fracture at the base of the ulnar styloid with both significant displacement and/or gross palmar dorsal translation of the radius relative to the ulna represents an indication for treatment.

One special circumstance is a large displaced ulnar styloid fragment, which may appear to be lined up in the AP plane; however, when the lateral view is examined, the styloid fragment is actually displaced palmarly in relation to the distal ulna. Often, this problem is only recognized late when the patient has difficulty achieving wrist supination either actively or passively. The treatment for such a displaced fragment both acutely and subacutely is reattachment of the styloid to the distal ulna.

The distal ulna is approached through a longitudinal incision over the extensor carpi ulnaris. Transverse branches of the ulnar nerve are preserved. Often, the extensor carpi ulnaris subsheath is still attached to the fragment. The fragment typically will reduce with supination of the wrist and will displace with pronation. It is helpful to maintain the wrist in supination while repairing the styloid to the distal ulna. For large fragments, the simplest and most secure fixation may be with a cannulated headless screw. For smaller fragments, 0.28-inch K-wires and a 24-gauge tension band may be applied. Care must be taken to bury the hardware, as it is often prominent in this region and may require removal later.

Geissler has documented that significant TFCC injuries may occur with ulnar styloid fractures (180). Reattaching the ulnar styloid alone may not result in restoration of stability in this situation. Therefore, it is critical to reassess the stability of the DRUJ after repair of the styloid.

An alternative to internal fixation is to reduce the distal radioulnar joint by supinating the forearm. Immobilizing the wrist in supination allows the soft tissue to heal in a reduced position and may prevent late instability of the radioulnar joint (Fig. 26-33).

Fractures of the distal ulnar metaphysis occur much less commonly (181). In one report of 320 fractures, the distal ulnar metaphysis was fractured in 7% of cases, and the most common fracture pattern was an extra-articular fracture of the ulnar metaphysis. Although nonoperative management may be successful, care should be taken to immobilize the radioulnar joint in a reduced position and look for radiographic evidence of impingement. Late heterotopic bone formation is common and will result in significant loss of rotation with this fracture pattern.

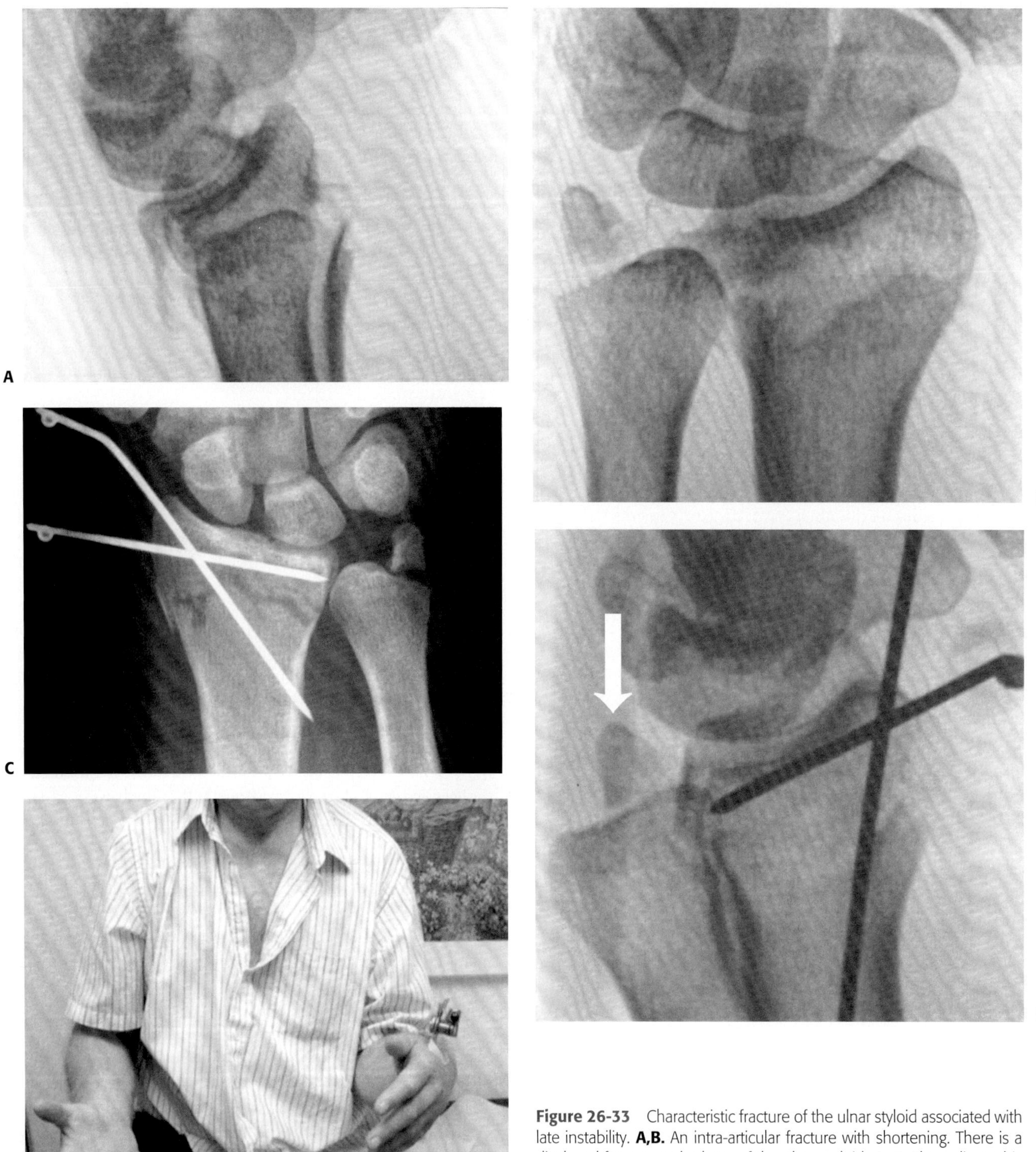

Figure 26-33 Characteristic fracture of the ulnar styloid associated with late instability. **A,B.** An intra-articular fracture with shortening. There is a displaced fracture at the base of the ulnar styloid. **C–E.** The radiographic and clinical appearance of the patient's wrist 2 weeks after external fixation in the clinic. Note that the patient is unable to supinate due to the dorsal displacement of the ulna relative to the radius. Radiographically, there is the characteristic palmar position of the ulna styloid relative to the remainder of the ulna. *(continues)*

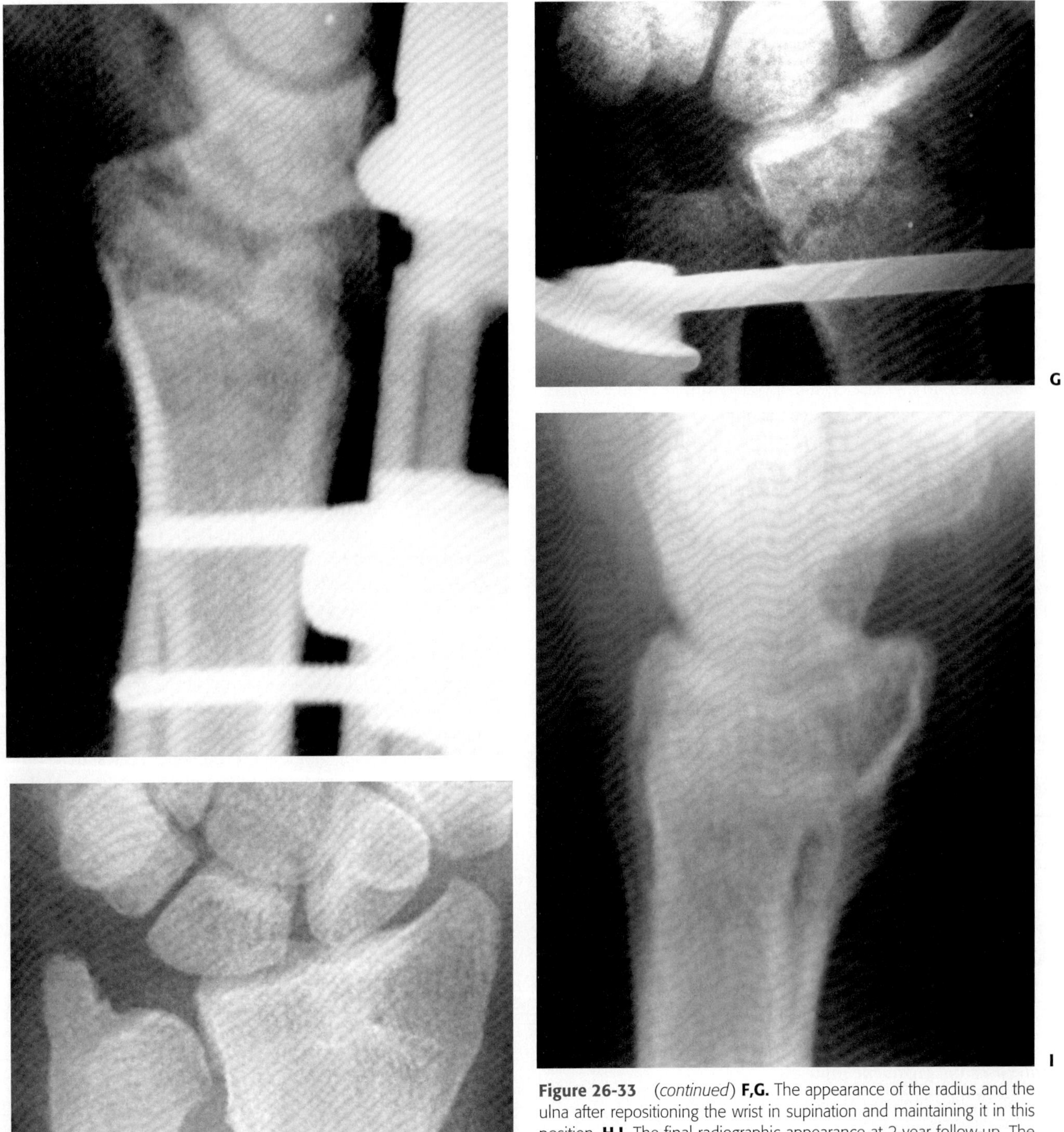

Figure 26-33 (*continued*) **F,G.** The appearance of the radius and the ulna after repositioning the wrist in supination and maintaining it in this position. **H,I.** The final radiographic appearance at 2-year follow-up. The patient regained full pronation and supination.

Combined (High-Energy) Injuries

Combined injuries represent fractures with components of several other fracture types. These injuries characteristically (a) are high energy, (b) have significant comminution often with proximal extension, and (c) may have significant soft tissue injuries. The management of these injuries is often complex and may require several steps. It is useful to treat them in a stepwise fashion by first achieving rigid skeletal stabilization and then addressing the soft tissue injuries.

Simple articular fractures with diaphyseal extension are best managed with a palmar plate. Using external fixation for the diaphyseal component will result in significant collapse before fracture union. Dorsal plates often will impinge where they intersect; for this reason, a palmar locking plate is preferred. When there is also extensive distal comminution, hybrid fixation may be necessary. In this case, a palmar plate is applied and a dorsal external fixator may be used to neutralize the displacement through the distal comminution. Extensive grafting may be necessary in order to prevent late collapse.

When an open dislocation of the distal radioulnar joint has occurred, it is generally the result of extreme shortening of the fractured radius relative to the intact ulna. In these cases, exploration reveals that the ulna has been stripped of the insertion of the DRUJ ligaments and the ulnocarpal ligaments. In some cases, with an associated large ulnar styloid base fracture, those ligaments may still be attached to the base of the ulnar styloid. Stability may be restored by repairing the ulnar styloid base back to the ulna's shaft, fixing it with either a headless screw or a tension band wire construct. When there is no associated ulnar styloid base fracture, the ligaments may reapproximate to the ulna provided that the DRUJ is reduced. For this reason, in patients with obvious DRUJ instability and no large ulnar styloid fracture, the forearm should be immobilized in supination to reduce the DRUJ for 4 weeks before permitting forearm rotation.

Soft Tissue Injuries

Adjunctive arthroscopy has shown that significant interosseous and distal radioulnar ligament injuries occur in association with both metaphyseal bending and intra-articular fractures.

Interosseous Ligament Injuries

Injury to the interosseous ligaments occurs in roughly 50% of all distal radius fractures and varies by fracture pattern (57,182). Geissler graded these injuries as follows: Grade I injuries have attenuation or hemorrhage of the ligament. Grade II injuries have incongruity of the ligament from the midcarpal portal, and the probe may be inserted between the bones. Grade III injuries show an incongruity from both the midcarpal and the radiocarpal portals, and the probe may be passed all the way through the articulation. Grade IV injuries have gross instability with manipulation, and the arthroscope (2.7 mm) may be passed from the radiocarpal to the midcarpal joints.

Scapholunate ligament injuries have been documented to occur in 30% to 50% of fractures, approximately twice as frequently as lunotriquetral injuries (57,182). They are seen most frequently in fractures that result in significant displacement of the lunate facet from the radial styloid (Fig. 26-34). Several studies examine the incidence of these injuries, but the natural history of these soft tissue lesions remains controversial. In one study of 50 patients with distal radius fractures, there were 27 partial or complete injuries to the scapholunate interosseous ligament. At 1-year follow-up, 18% demonstrated radiographic evidence of dissociation; however, none of the patients was symptomatic (57). In a second study examining 76 patients after fracture, radiographically apparent scapholunate instability was not associated with either pain or functional impairment (178). In a purely radiographic study of 95 fractures, dissociative ligamentous lesions were seen in 40 patients, 24 of which were noted to progress at 1-year follow-up. The results of this study again found no correlation between radiographic evidence of instability and symptoms at 1 year (183).

Triangular Fibrocartilage Injuries

Lesions of the triangular fibrocartilage (TFCC) occur in approximately 40% to 70% of distal radius fractures (58,59,142). The majority of these lesions are peripheral avulsions generally from the ulnar insertion compared to fewer central perforations. These lesions may occur with or without fracture of the ulnar styloid. In contrast to the interosseous ligament injuries, peripheral avulsions of the TFCC appear to be more likely to be symptomatic at short-term follow-up. Lindau documented that 10 of 11 peripheral avulsions of the TFCC had DRUJ instability and worse outcome scores than other ligamentous injuries at 1-year follow-up (184). Repair of these injuries has been documented to restore stability and provide excellent results, yet the indications for acute repair have yet to be elucidated (179).

COMPLICATIONS

Malunion

Malunion after distal radius fracture treatment continues to be a significant complication following nonoperative management. In addition, as the number of operatively treated cases increases, the incidence of collapse and malunion seen in previously treated fractures also increases. The effect of radial malunion has to be taken into consideration when weighing treatment options. Malunion of the radius results in alterations to (a) the radiocarpal joint, (b) the midcarpal joint, and (c) the radioulnar joint. The effect of these changes can be significant with regard to both immediate functional impairment and the development of late degenerative changes.

Radial malunion can have two potential effects on radiocarpal mechanics. First, the loss of palmar tilt shifts the carpus distally on the radius, thereby increasing contact stress on the dorsal lip of the radius. In addition, the loss of radial inclination

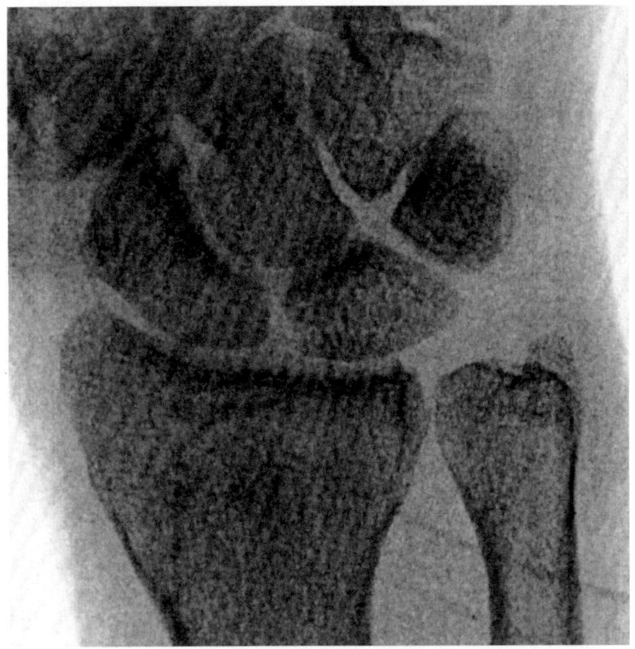

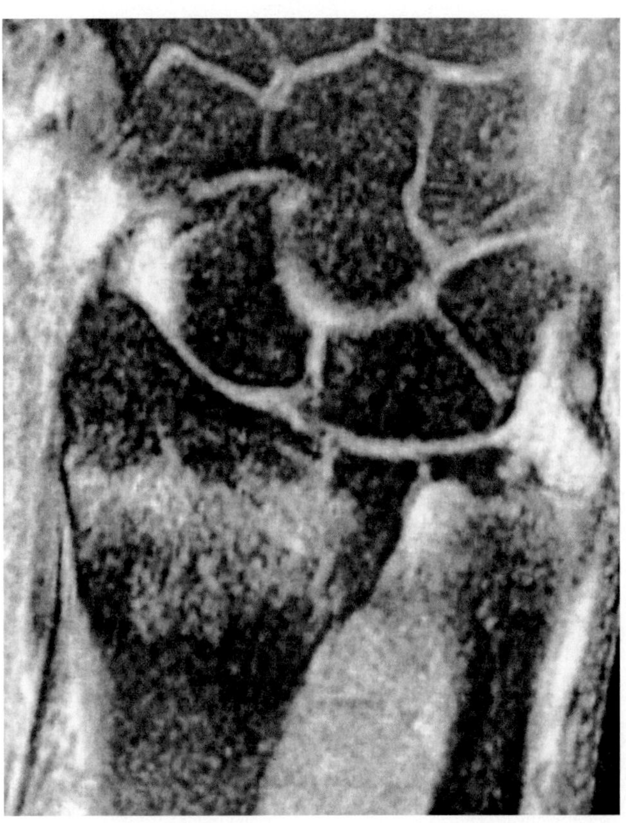

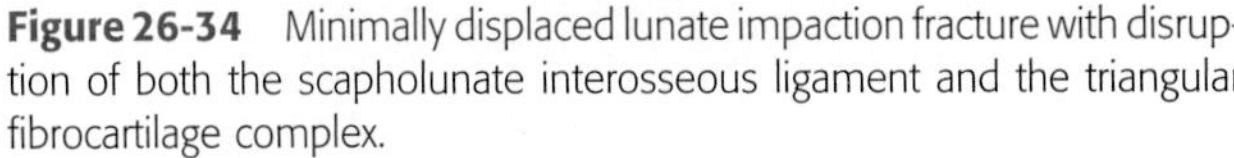

Figure 26-34 Minimally displaced lunate impaction fracture with disruption of both the scapholunate interosseous ligament and the triangular fibrocartilage complex.

results in increased stress at the radiolunate articulation (185–187). The increased contact stresses result in a higher likelihood for degenerative changes (33). Functionally, the shortening may account for the loss of grip strength that has been observed after malunion (185). There is also evidence that there is a functionally significant loss of motion at the radiocarpal joint after malunited extra-articular fractures (188). Finally, the extended position of the lunate and the scaphoid may result in a compensatory collapse at the midcarpal joint (see Fig. 26-7) (189).

Intra-articular incongruity similarly causes a significant change in contact stresses at the radiocarpal joint. It is of note that depression of the lunate facet results in significant increases in the contact forces at the radioscaphoid articulation. Clinical studies indicate that 2 mm of lunate depression results in degenerative changes and worse functional outcomes (33,135,190).

The impact of radial malunion on radioulnar mechanics has received significant attention. Dorsal angulation results in increased strain on the radioulnar ligaments (191–196). Because of this increased strain, extra force is required to achieve full rotation of the forearm. Loss of rotation in these cases seems to occur at approximately 30 degrees loss of palmar tilt. By contrast, in cases of severe angulation with significant shortening, the same loss of rotation is not seen. One explanation offered for this contradiction is that in cases of severe deformity, there are no longer any attachments of the distal radioulnar ligaments to constrain the joint. Unconstrained by soft tissue attachments, the joint enjoys its full mobility (191–196).

Corrective Osteotomy

The exact indications for osteotomy remain unknown. Cadaver studies have not examined the additive effects of radial shortening, loss of tilt, and associated ligamentous injuries. In general terms, the indications are based on (a) the patient's age, (b) the direction of (palmar vs. dorsal) and degree of deformity, (c) functional limitations, and (d) pain. In general terms, it is difficult to recommend surgical treatment of an asymptomatic deformity. Likewise, correction of the deformity has to offer a high likelihood of alleviating the patient's symptoms.

Normally, the osteotomy may be performed as early as the surgeon and the patient agree that there is a plateau in the patient's improvement. At one time, there was a feeling that the osteotomy should be delayed until the fracture callus had completely incorporated. This practice is probably not necessary, as taking down the callus and internal fixation may be technically easier and may not require bone graft when completed before the fracture is healed (197).

Although it is accepted that the deformity is 3D, standard

PA and lateral x-rays of both wrists are considered adequate for planning the osteotomy. The contralateral view is critical for assessing the radial length, radial inclination, palmar tilt, and carpal alignment. Special attention must be paid to the distal radioulnar joint to assess for congruency of the distal radioulnar joint and for potential arthritis of the distal ulna, which may require an associated resection.

Generally speaking, an opening wedge osteotomy is preferred when the distal radioulnar joint can be salvaged, and a closing wedge osteotomy is preferred with an associated hemiresection of the ulna, when the DRUJ cannot be reconstructed. For an intra-articular osteotomy, CT with 3D reconstructions may be necessary to determine the location of the intra-articular step-off in both planes. Finally, CT with superimposition of the proximal forearm may also be useful for correcting rotational deformities.

The typical deformity of the distal radius malunion has three components: (a) loss of radial inclination, (b) loss of palmar tilt, and (c) and pronation of the fracture fragment. The surgical technique depends on the location and the degree of the deformity.

Dorsal Displacement with Loss of Radial Inclination

The osteotomy is best performed at the site of the deformity. An opening-wedge osteotomy is typically performed, and a corticocancellous graft is usually placed. Note that with the use of more rigid implants, it may be satisfactory to use cancellous graft alone (198). Stabilization of the osteotomy has been described using K-wires, dorsal plates, palmar plates, and external fixators (199–210). Regardless of the stabilization method, the goal is to correct the deformity and achieve early union. In general, a trapezoidal defect is created after the osteotomy, and correction of both the palmar tilt as well as the radial inclination has been achieved. The void is filled and the bone is stabilized. Rotation is verified before fixation of the osteotomy.

Palmar Displacement of the Distal Fragment

Palmar displacement (apex volar angulation) is best approached via a palmar approach. An associated carpal tunnel release should be strongly considered if lengthening is to be achieved. The osteotomy is again performed at the previous fracture line. If radial inclination has been lost, the FCR/radial artery approach allows opening of the radial column and release of the contracted brachioradialis tendon. A corticocancellous graft is inserted, and a palmar plate is applied. It is critical to recognize that an apex palmar angulation is often associated with dorsal displacement of the ulna relative to the radius, leading to loss of rotation. Restoration of rotation must be assessed before finalizing the position of the distal fragment relative to the proximal diaphysis. The results of osteotomy to correct palmar angulation have been reported, and restoration of rotation is better than the restoration of extension (Fig. 26-35) (211,212).

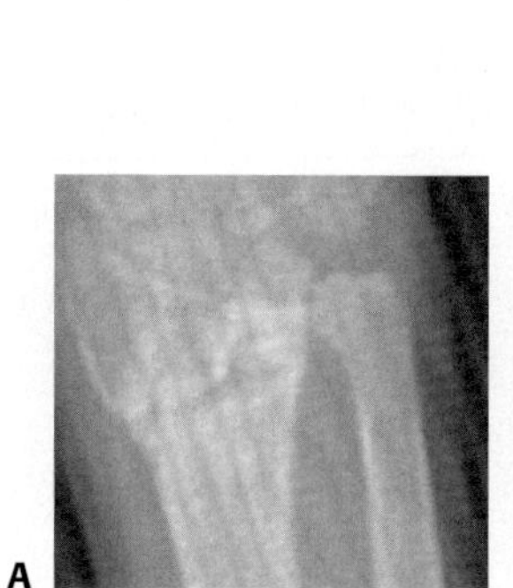
A

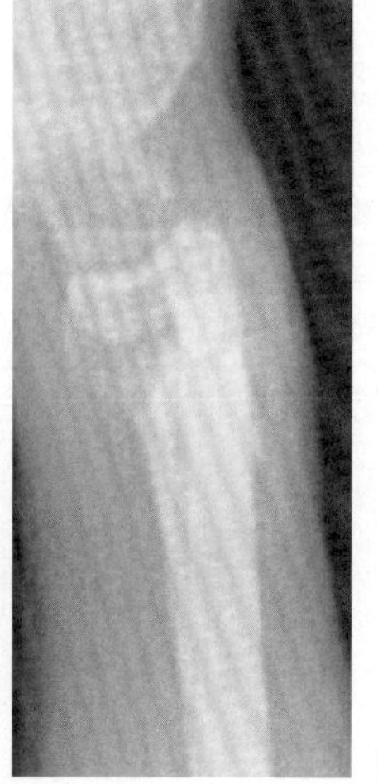
B

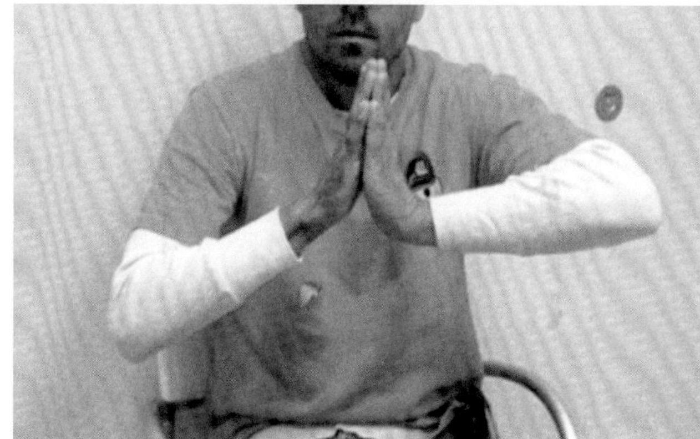
C

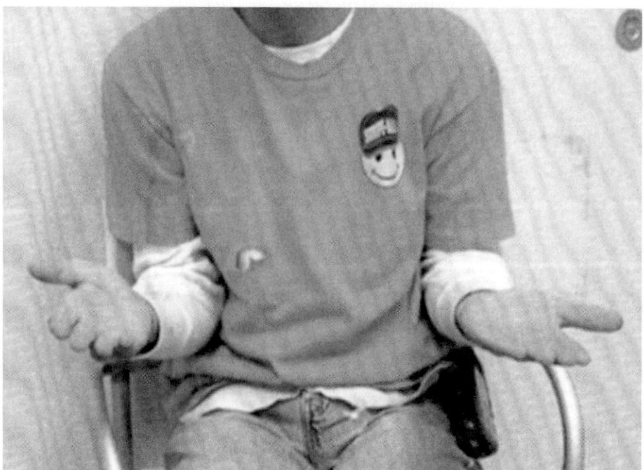
D

Figure 26-35 A,B. Palmar malunion after dorsal plating and collapse. **C,D.** Note the position of the ulna relative to the radius in the lateral plane while dorsiflexion was limited. The patient's chief complaint was loss of supination.

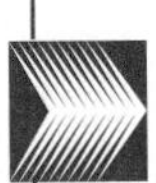

AUTHOR'S PREFERRED TREATMENT

In planning an osteotomy, it is critical to consider what the patient is seeking from the procedure from both a symptom and a functional perspective. Preoperative range of motion is critical to keep in mind, as some loss of the total arc of motion may be expected. Because extension is typically more critical than flexion, the surgeon may wish to template the wrist to a neutral palmar tilt rather to an anatomic 12 degrees of palmar tilt.

A second preoperative consideration is the distal radioulnar joint. It is important to note the presence of significant deformity or loss of articular cartilage on the distal ulna, which may preclude salvage of a reasonably functioning radioulnar joint. CT may be indicated to assess the potential for salvaging the distal radioulnar joint.

A third consideration is the need for bone graft or substitute to fill the defect after the deformity is corrected. If the distal radioulnar joint is not salvageable in elderly patients, consider using the distal ulna as a graft to avoid the need to harvest one from the iliac crest. If salvage of the DRUJ is precluded, complete restoration of radial length may not be as important as correcting the tilt in the sagittal plane. Restoring palmar tilt requires a triangular graft, whereas restoring overall radial length may require a trapezoidal graft.

Finally, the surgeon must decide if there are any adjunctive procedures that may be required in order to achieve a satisfactory outcome. Carpal tunnel symptoms preoperatively may be exacerbated by an acute change in the length of the radius or by carpal canal swelling (81). An opening wedge osteotomy may actually alleviate the deformity that causes the carpal tunnel symptoms, but it is critical to consider whether the patient will tolerate the acute swelling and the nerve lengthening associated with an osteotomy. Nerve decompression associated with correction of the deformity may prevent an acute carpal tunnel syndrome.

These considerations must be taken during discussion with the patient preoperatively. In templating the deformity, we are increasingly relying on tomography to assess the deformity in multiple planes. These deformities are three-dimensional, and the surgeon should have a low threshold for obtaining CT scans with reformatted images to look for significant rotational deformity and the presence of significant arthritis in the distal radioulnar joint (Fig. 26-36).
Typically, the deformity is approached from the collapsed side, which is dorsal in most cases. A longitudinal approach is performed, and the extensor retinaculum is preserved to permit later coverage of a plate. In cases of long-standing deformity or when significant shortening has occurred, it is critical to release the brachioradialis from its insertion on the distal radius. A Z-plasty can be performed if preoperative templating reveals the need for hardware distally over the styloid; however, this is usually unnecessary and the tendon may be left to heal back to the styloid. It is also helpful to visualize the dorsal ulnar corner of the radius and assess the distal radioulnar joint directly for articular changes, which could preclude salvage.

Under C-arm guidance on the lateral view, a pin is inserted proximal (preferably proximal to the proximal extent of the plate) and perpendicular to the radial shaft. A second pin is placed distally in the radial metaphysis parallel to the articular surface. In the case of severe or long-term deformity, it is helpful to use terminally threaded pins from a small external fixator. Once the osteotomy has been performed, the fixator can be used to maintain the radius in the reduced position while the bone graft and/or the plate is applied. An oscillating saw is then used to cut the bone. It is significant here again to assess whether correction should be limited to palmar tilt or whether it should include correcting radial length and inclination as well. If the correction is for palmar tilt, it is easier to leave the palmar cortex intact and hinge the distal fragment on the cortex. If length correction is to be achieved, the osteotomy must be completed. In this situation, adding the external fixator is particularly helpful. The graft material is harvested. I still prefer to use iliac crest graft particularly when radial length is required. In elderly patients or when the distal radioulnar joint is not salvageable, the ulnar head may be harvested and inserted in the defect; however, it is generally not sufficient for complex deformities. Preoperative templating may now be confirmed visually by directly measuring the defect when the pins are made parallel on the lateral plane. The iliac crest graft is harvested with an oscillating saw matching the measurements of the defect as precisely as possible.

Once the graft has been inserted, the plate can be applied. To correct radial length in the case of a trapezoidal graft, it may be helpful to maintain its position with crossed wires to prevent displacing the distal fragment proximally when the plate is applied. Once the plate has been applied and the position is confirmed radiographically, the retinaculum may be closed over the plate and the wounds can be closed. The stability of the construct and the distal radioulnar joint determine the length of immobilization (Fig. 26-37).

A palmar approach is used for volar collapse. The interval that is followed is generally the FCR/radial artery approach. The incision is taken down to the volar carpal branch of the radial artery. The pronator quadratus is detached and preserved to lay back down over the plate. A pin may be placed parallel to the articular surface, and a second pin is positioned perpendicular to the proximal shaft. The osteotomy may then be performed, and the articular surface may be manipulated back to the appropriate degree of tilt. In general, a small corticocancellous graft enhances the stability, but is not always necessary. A palmar plate is applied (Fig. 26-38).

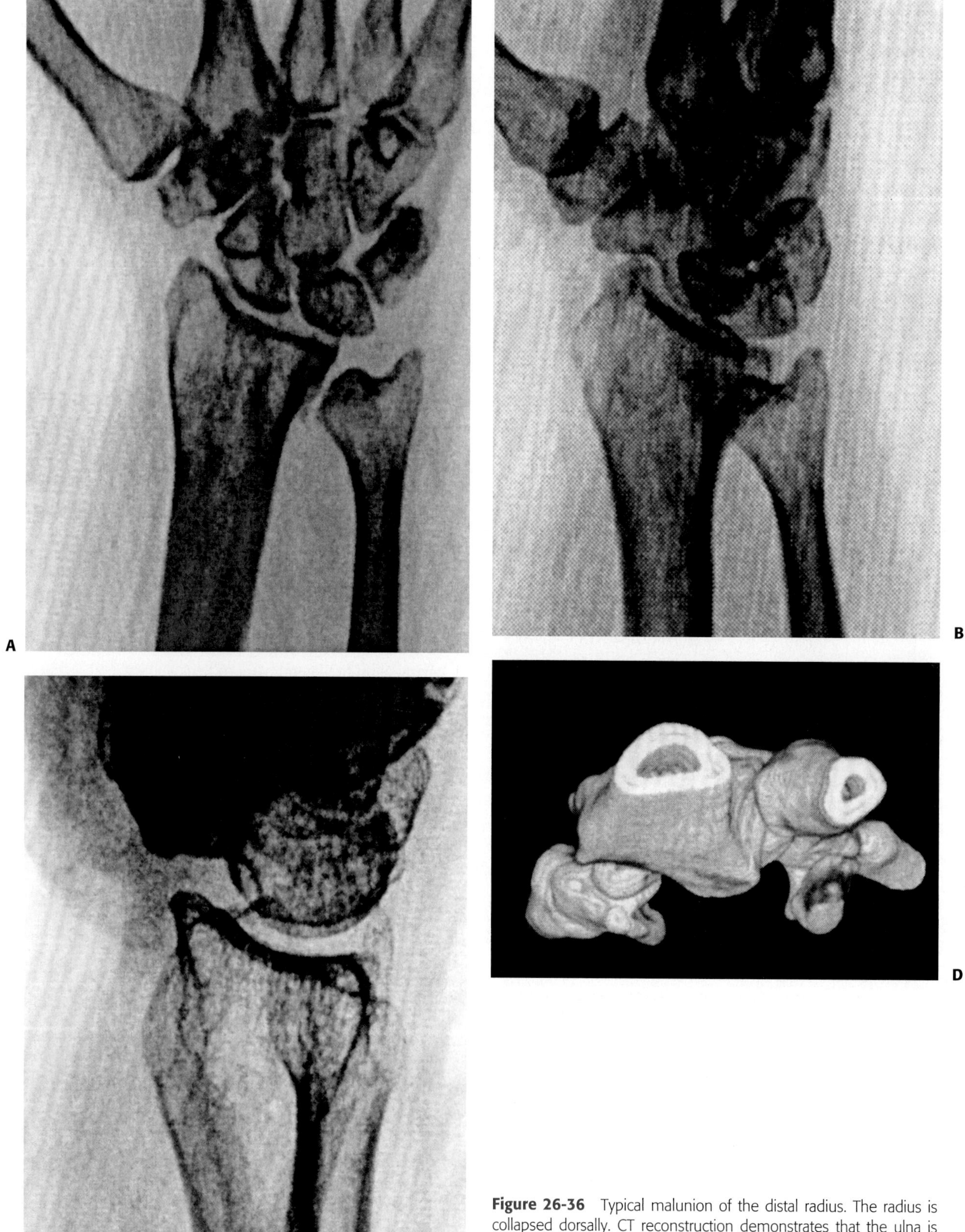

Figure 26-36 Typical malunion of the distal radius. The radius is collapsed dorsally. CT reconstruction demonstrates that the ulna is subluxated dorsally.

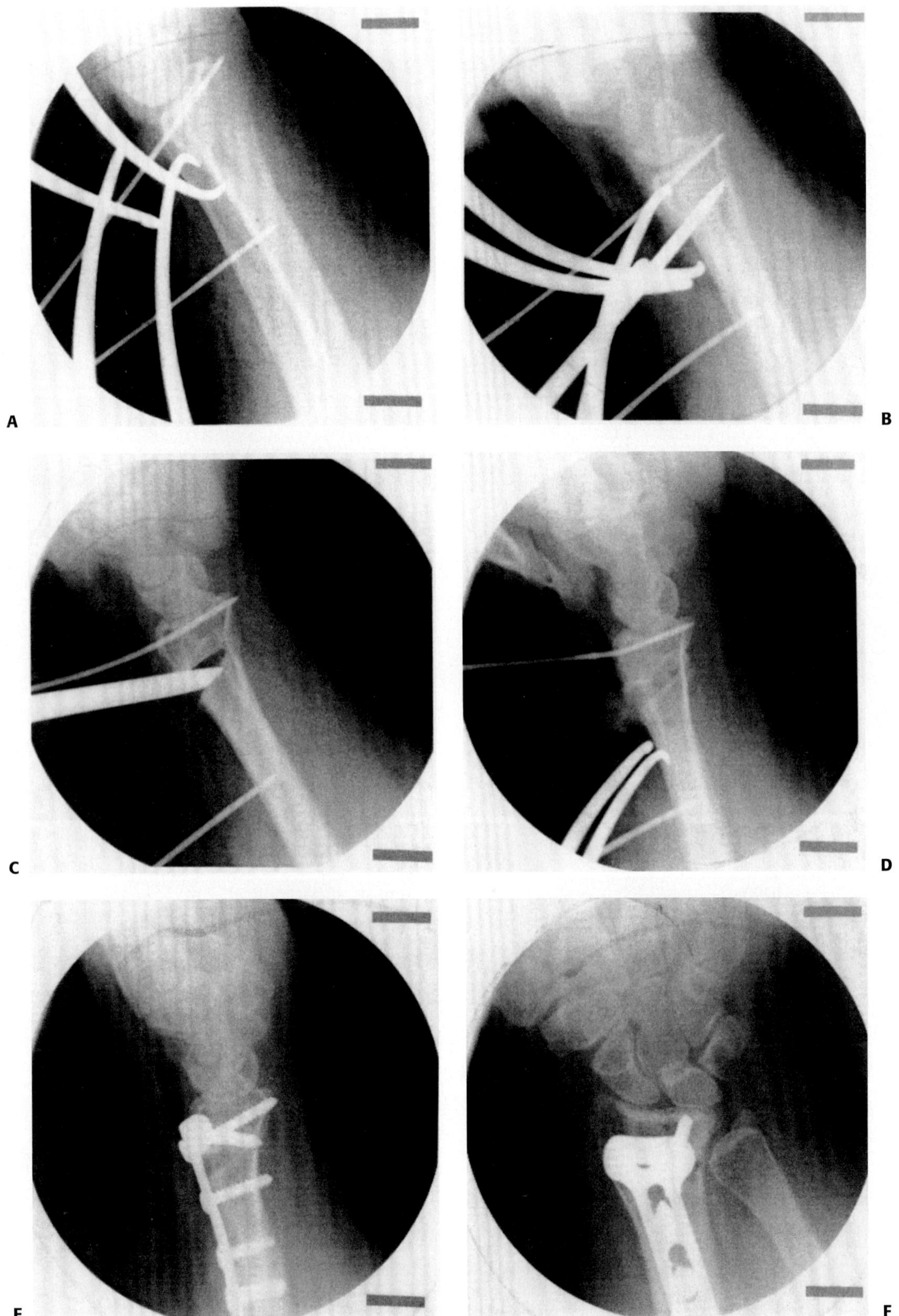

Figure 26-37 **A.** Technique of osteotomy for a dorsal malunion. Pins are placed parallel to the joint and perpendicular to the shaft. An oscillating saw is used to cut the dorsal cortex **(B)** while the palmar cortex is left intact. The fragment is levered into position **(C),** the bone graft is placed **(D),** and a dorsal plate is applied **(E,F).**

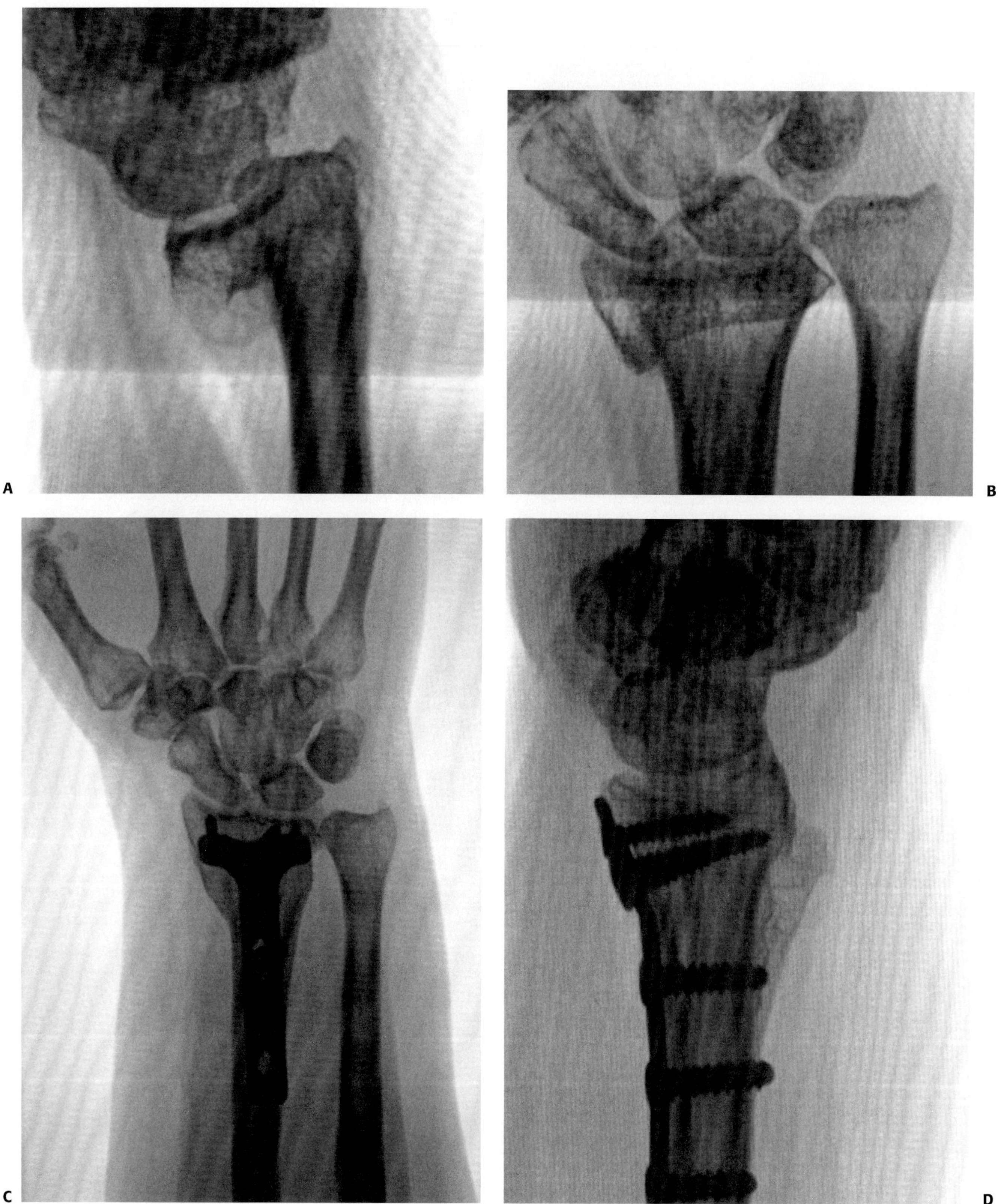

Figure 26-38 **A,B.** Palmar displacement of the distal fragment. This deformity is common with collapse after dorsal plating. There is a profound effect on supination, as the ulna becomes in essence "dislocated" dorsally due to the palmar displacement of the radius. **C,D.** The osteotomy is performed through a palmar approach and stabilized with a palmar plate.

Distal Radioulnar Joint Complications Associated with Malunions

Some fractures of the distal radius resulting in incongruity at the distal radioulnar joint may not be amenable to an osteotomy of the distal radius. In these cases, the treatment is directed at the distal ulna in an effort to either restore congruity (e.g., an ulnar shortening osteotomy) or to salvage function (e.g., arthroplasty).

Ulnar Shortening Osteotomy

In cases when the radius has shortened without significant loss of palmar tilt or radiocarpal incongruity, it may be preferable to perform an ulnar shortening osteotomy rather than a radial lengthening. The procedure, performed through a longitudinal approach to the ulna and fixed with a dynamic compression plate, has been extensively reported for ulnar abutment syndrome (Fig. 26-39) (213–216). Contraindications to the procedure are (a) ulnar translation of the radial metaphysis in association with the deformity, as shortening of the ulna results in excessive contact at the distal radioulnar joint and (b) excessive palmar tilt of the radius, as shortening of the ulna will still leave the ulna dorsally displaced relative to the radius.

Neurologic Injuries

Complications associated with the neurovascular structures at the wrist may be classified as injuries that occurred at the time of the fracture and those that arise late as a result of swelling, scarring, or deformity.

Median Nerve

Acute carpal tunnel syndrome may be seen with either intra- or extra-articular fractures (179). Risk factors are bleeding dyscrasias, open fractures, compressive dressings, and a prolonged period between injury and reduction. The pressure within the canal after a closed fracture treated conservatively has been shown to be at its highest during reduction and then to fall gradually during the next 12 hours (217). Chronic compressive neuropathy of the median nerve occurs in approximately 5% of conservatively treated fractures of the distal radius (223,224).

Ulnar Nerve

Ulnar nerve injuries occur far less commonly than median nerve injuries (218,219). This nerve may have more excursion and is located at an increased distance from the displacement of the radius (220). Acute injuries may be seen with displacement of the palmar lunate facet or with a palmar distal radioulnar joint dislocation. Late progressive ulnar nerve palsy has been reported due to open distal radioulnar joint injuries (220).

Complex Regional Pain Syndrome

Complex regional pain syndrome (CRPS) is estimated to occur in approximately 1% of all conservatively treated distal radius fractures and up to 5% of operatively treated fractures (218,219,221). It has been classified into types I and II. CRPS type I is secondary to an identifiable neurologic compression or injury. Examples may include an ulnar nerve axonotemesis or a superficial radial nerve injury secondary to direct trauma from an external fixator pin. CRPS type II has no identifiable neurological injury and would previously have been referred to a sympathetically mediated pain.

Treatment of CRPS depends on determining whether the patient has CRPS type I or CRPS type II. The key is to critically and exhaustively determine whether there is a treatable source (type I), which may partially or completely relieve the patient's symptoms.

The most common identifiable lesion associated with CRPS type I is injury to the median nerve. These injuries may be due to either direct trauma or an undiagnosed compressive neuropathy. Other potential causes are injury to the ulnar nerve, the superficial radial nerve, the intercarpal ligament, or the triangular fibrocartilage. In addition, delayed union, incomplete union, and nonunion may also contribute to symptoms.

Diagnostic studies are directed to defining the lesion. Peripheral nerve conduction studies including evaluating the compression points around the elbow are useful for establishing a treatable cause of CRPS. Care should be taken to evaluate the ulnar nerve as well, as it is often overlooked secondary to concerns regarding the median nerve. MRI may show an incomplete union, carpal injuries, or a triangular fibrocartilage injury. Finally, arthroscopic evaluation may reveal arthrofibrosis and/or triangular fibrocartilage injuries.

Surgical treatment of these lesions should be aimed at neurolysis for external compression of the median and ulnar nerve injuries. Injury to sensory branches of the superficial radial or dorsal ulnar nerve may require adjunctive grafting or barrier wrapping. If this is not an option, the neuroma may be resected proximally and the nerve stump can be buried in appropriate soft tissue. Treating an incomplete union may require the use of external bone stimulators or revision osteosynthesis.

The treatment of CRPS type II is multifaceted and is geared at restoring autonomic nervous system control as well as improving physical function. Its early recognition and the use of regional blockade combined with physical therapy may prove useful (222). Medical management is guided by the appearance of the hand and wrist. Early phases of the syndrome are often marked by erythema and swelling, while in later phases, they may appear cool and atrophic. For the warm, swollen erythematous hand, the treatment may include gabapentin, selective serotonin reuptake inhibitors, or clonidine hydrochloride. In later stages, the purpose of treatment may be to improve blood flow, using nifedipine or selective serotonin reuptake inhibitors.

Physical therapy is directed at mobilizing the wrist and digits. Focus is directed initially at the wrist to improve extension. As wrist extension improves, the digital flexors have greater mechanical advantage and are more likely to be effective. Adjunctive modalities such as dynamic or serial static splinting may prove effective at mobilizing the wrist and the metacarpophalangeal joints.

Figure 26-39 **A,B.** Malunion of the radius with loss of radial length and loss of forearm rotation. **C,D.** An ulnar shortening osteotomy eliminated the symptoms of impaction, and full rotation was restored.

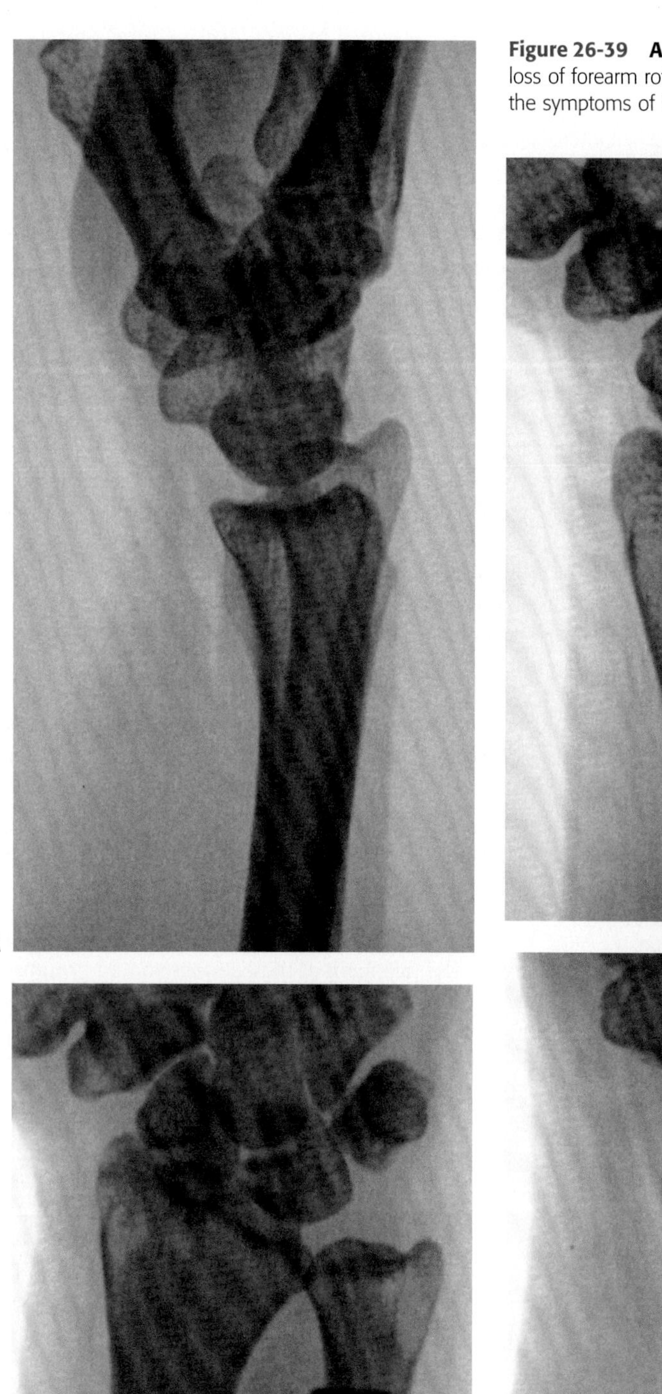

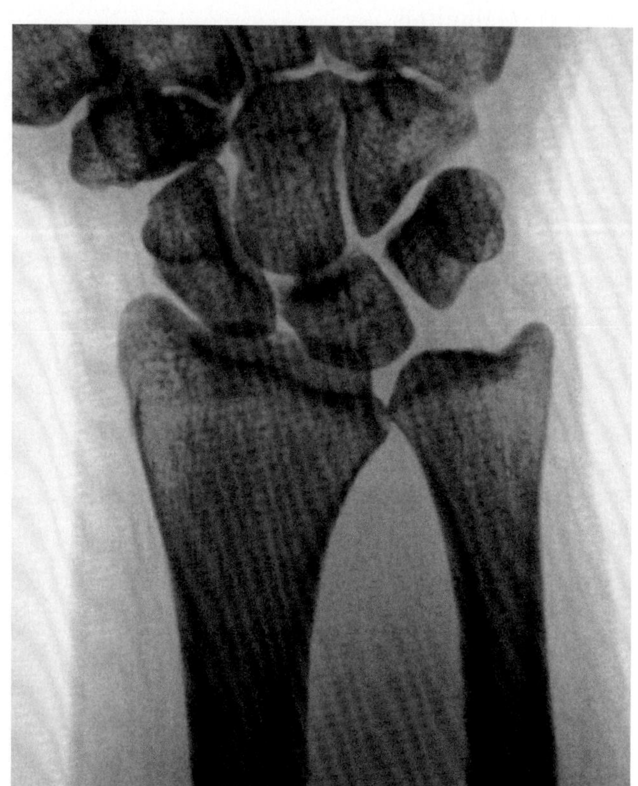

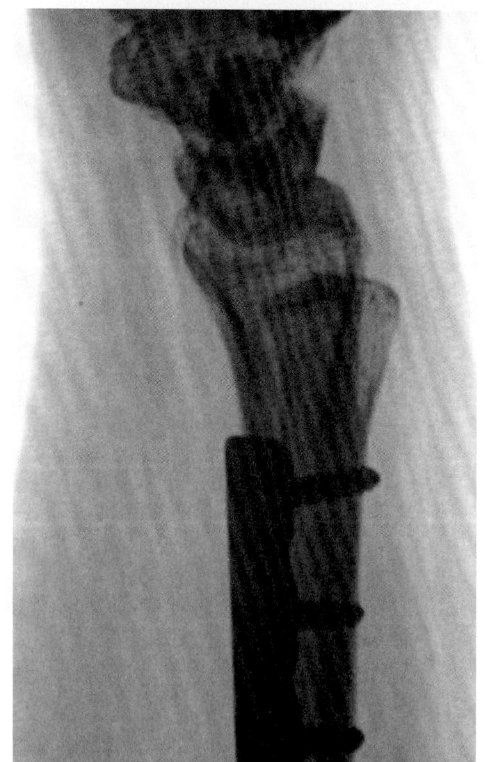

Recovery after CRPS treatment varies. In general, the prognosis for CRPS type I is better than that of CRPS type II. When the syndrome continues for more than 1 year, it is likely that residual impairment will be present. Regardless of the treatment afforded, it can be expected that patients will experience delayed recovery (218).

Tendon Injuries

The majority of flexor tendon injuries associated with distal radius fractures occur as a result of penetrating trauma and direct laceration. Closed ruptures, particularly of the extensor pollicis longus, have been extensively reported; however, rupture appears to be relatively uncommon in other tendons. These injuries may occur either acutely as a result of the initial trauma or late and can be related to either increased pressure within the compartment or due to attrition from either callus or hardware.

Late extensor pollicis longus rupture occurs in approximately 0.3% of distal radius fractures (223). Interestingly, these ruptures occur most frequently in minimally displaced fractures treated nonoperatively. The rupture is usually painless and occurs late at 6 weeks to 3 months after injury. Treatment is directed first at mobilizing the wrist and then performing an appropriate transfer.

In closed fractures, flexor tendon ruptures may occur either as a result of a rotational injury at the time of fracture or in a delayed fashion due to attrition (224). Late ruptures due to hardware impingement have been described particularly secondary to attrition of the flexor pollicis on prominent hardware radially (158).

REFERENCES

1. Colles A. On the fracture of the carpal extremity of the radius. *Edinburgh Med Surg* 1814;10:182–186.
2. Fernandez DL, Geissler WB. Treatment of displaced articular fractures of the radius. *J Hand Surg* 1991;16(3):375–384.
3. Catalano LW, Cole RJ, Gelberman RH, et al. Displaced intra-articular fractues of the distal aspect of the radius. Long-term results in young adults after open reduction and internal fixation. *J Bone Joint* 1997;79(9):1290–1302.
4. Young BT, Rayan GM. Outcome following nonoperative treatment of displaced distal radius fractures in low-demand patients older than 60 years. *J Hand Surg* 2000;25(1): 19–28.
5. Madhok R, Green S. Longer term functional outcome and societal implications of upper limb fractures in the elderly. *J R Soc Health* 1993;113(4):179–180.
6. Hagino H, Yamamoto K, Ohshiro H, et al. Changing incidence of hip, distal radius, and proximal humerus fractures in Tottori Prefecture, Japan. *Bone* 1999;24(3):265–270.
7. Swiontkowski MF. Increasing rates of forearm fractures in children. *JAMA* 2003;24; 290(24):3193.
8. Solgaard S, Petersen VS. Epidemiology of distal radius fractures. *Acta Orthop Scand* 1985;56(5):391–393.
9. Mensforth RP, Latimer BM. Hamann-Todd Collection aging studies: osteoporosis fracture syndrome. *Am J Phys Anthropol* 1989;80(4):461–479.
10. O'Neill TW, Cooper C, Finn JD, et al. Incidence of distal forearm fracture in British men and women. *Osteoporos Int* 2001;12(7):555–558.
11. Mallmin H, Ljunghall S. Incidence of Colles' fracture in Uppsala. A prospective study of a quarter-million population. *Acta Orthop Scand* 1992;63(2):213–215.
12. Nguyen TV, Center JR, Sambrook PN, et al. Risk factors for proximal humerus, forearm, and wrist fractures in elderly men and women: the Dubbo Osteoporosis Epidemiology Study. *Am J Epidemiol* 2001;153(6):587–595.
13. Mensforth RP, Latimer BM. Hamann-Todd Collection aging studies: osteoporosis fracture syndrome. *Am J Phys Anthropol* 1989;80(4):461–479.
14. Masud T, Jordan D, Hosking DJ. Distal forearm fracture history in an older community-dwelling population: the Nottingham Community Osteoporosis (NOCOS) study. *Age Ageing* 2001;30(3):255–258.
15. Rozental TD, Branas CC, Bozentka DJ, et al. Survival among elderly patients after fractures of the distal radius. *J Hand Surg Am* 2002;27(6):948–952.
16. Lindau TR, Aspenberg P, Arner M, et al. Fractures of the distal forearm in young adults. An epidemiologic description of 341 patients. *Acta Orthop Scand* 1999;70(2):124–128.
17. Cuenca J, Martinez AA, Herrera A, et al. The incidence of distal forearm fractures in Zaragoza (Spain). *Chir Main* 2003;22(4):211–215.
18. Schmalholz A. Epidemiology of distal radius fracture in Stockholm 1981-82. *Acta Orthop Scand* 1988;59(6):701–703.
19. Adams BD. Effects of radial deformity on distal radioulnar joint mechanics. *J Hand Surg* 1993;18(3):492–498.
20. Miller SW, Evans JG. Fractures of the distal forearm in Newcastle: an epidemiological survey. *Age Ageing* 1985;14(3):155–158.
21. Lester GE, Anderson JJ, Tylavsky FA, et al. Update on the use of distal radial bone density measurements in prediction of hip and Colles' fracture risk. *J Orthop Res* 1990; 8(2):220–226.
22. Mallmin H, Ljunghall S, Persson I, et al. Risk factors for fractures of the distal forearm: a population-based case-control study. *Osteoporos Int* 1994;4(6):298–304.
23. Mallmin H, Ljunghall S, Naessen T. Colles' fracture associated with reduced bone mineral content. Photon densitometry in 74 patients with matched controls. *Acta Orthop Scand* 1992;63(5):552–554.
24. Hui SL, Slemenda CW, Johnston CC, Jr. Age and bone mass as predictors of fracture in a prospective study. *J Clin Invest* 1988;81(6):1804–1809.
25. Goyrand G. Memoire sur les fractures de l'extremite inferieure du radius qui simulent les luxations du poignet. *Gaz Med* 1832;3:664–667.
26. Smith AM, Castle JA, Ruch DS. Arthroscopic resection of the common extensor origin: anatomic considerations. *J Shoulder Elbow Surg* 2003;12(4):375–379.
27. Hove LM. Simultaneous scaphoid and distal radial fractures. *J Hand Surg Br* 1994; 19(3):384–388.
28. Trumble TE, Benirschke SK, Vedder NB. Ipsilateral fractures of the scaphoid and radius. *J Hand Surg Am* 1993;18(1):8–14.
29. Johnson PG, Szabo RM. Angle measurements of the distal radius: a cadaver study. *Skeletal Radiol* 1993;22(4):243–246.
30. Lundy D, Quisling S, Lourie G, et al. Tilted lateral x-rays in the evaluation of intra-articular distal radius Fractures. *J Hand Surg* 1999;24(2):249–256.
31. Knirk J, Jupiter J. Intraarticular fractures of the distal end of the radius in young adults. *J Bone Joint Surg* 1986;68(5):647–659.
32. Geissler WB, Fernandez DL. Percutaneous and limited open reduction of the articular surface of the distal radius. *J Orthop Trauma* 1991;5(3):255–264.
33. Kopylov P, Johnell O, Redlund-Johnell I, et al. Fractures of the distal end of the radius in young adults: a 30-year follow-up. *J Hand Surg* 1993;18(1):45–49.
34. Kreder HJ, Hanel DP, McKee M, et al. X-ray film measurements for healed distal radius fractures. *J Hand Surg* 1996;21:31–39.
35. Johnston GH, Friedman L, Kriegler JC. Computerized tomographic evaluation of acute distal radial fractures. *J Hand Surg Am* 1992;17(4):738–744.
36. Cole RJ, Bindra RR, Evanoff BA, et al. Radiographic evaluation of osseous displacement following intra-articular fractures of the distal radius: reliability of plain radiography versus computed tomography. *J Hand Surg* 1997;22(5):792–800.
37. Flinkkila T, Nikkola-Sihto A, Kaaela O, et al. Poor interobserver reliability of AO classification of fractures of the distal radius. *J Bone Joint Surg* 1998;80:670–672.
38. Gartland J, Werley C. Evaluation of healed Colles' fractures. *J Bone Joint Surg* 1951; 33(4):895–907.
39. Frykman GK. Fractures of the distal radius including sequelae-shoulder-hand-finger syndrome, disturbance in the distal radio-ulnar joint and impairment of nerve function. *Acta Orthop Scand* 1967;(Suppl 108):7–153.
40. Melone CP. Distal radius fractures: Patterns of articular fragmentation. *Orthop Clin N Am* 1993;24(2):239–253.
41. Andersen DJ, Blair WF, Steyers CM Jr, et al. Classification of distal radius fractures: an analysis of interobserver reliability and intraobserver reproducibility. *J Hand Surg Am* 1996; 21(4):574–582.
42. Jupiter J, Fernandez DL. Comparative classification for fractures of the distal end of the radius. *J Hand Surg* 1997;22(4):563–571.
43. Fernandez DL. Fractures of the distal radius: operative treatment. *Instr Course Lect* 1993;42:73–88.
44. Fernandez DL, Jupiter JB. *Fractures of the distal radius*, 2nd ed. Berlin: Springer-Verlag; 2002.
45. Wagner WF, Tencer AF, Kiser P. Effects of intra-articular distal radius depression on wrist joint contact characteristics. *J Hand Surg* 1996;21(4):554–560.
46. Tsukazaki T, Takagi K, Iwasaki K. Poor correlation between functional results and radiographic findings in Colles' fracture. *J Hand Surg* 1993;18(5):588–591.
47. McQueen M, Caspers J. Colles' fracture: does the anatomical result affect the final function? *J Bone Joint Surg* 1988;70(4):649–651.
48. Porter M, Stockley I. Fractures of the distal radius. *Clin Orthopaed Rel Res* 1987;220: 241–252.
49. McQueen MM, Hajducka C, Court-Brown C. Redisplaced unstable fractures of the distal radius: a randomised, prospective study of bridging versus non-bridging external fixation. *J Bone Joint Surg* 1996;78(3):404–409.
50. Taleisnik J. Midcarpal instability caused by malunited fractures of the distal radius. *J Hand Surg* 1984;9(3):350–357.
51. Short WH, Palmer AK, Werner FW, et al. A biomechanical study of distal radial fractures. *J Hand Surg* 1987;12(4):529–534.
52. Kihara H, Palmer AK, Werner F, et al. The effect of dorsally angulated distal radius fractures on distal radiolunar joint congruency and forearm rotation. *J Hand Surg* 1996; 21:40–47.
53. Jenkins NH, Mintowt-Czyz WJ. Mal-union and dysfunction in Colles' fracture. *J Hand Surg Br* 1988;13:291–293.

54. Solgaard S. Classification of distal radius fractures. *Acta Orthop Scand* 1984;56: 249–252.
55. Batra S, Gupta A. The effect of fracture-related factors on the functional outcome at 1 year in distal radius fractures. *Injury* 2002;33:499–502.
56. van der LW, Ericson R. Colles' fracture. How should its displacement be measured and how should it be immobilized? *J Bone Joint Surg Am* 1981;63(8):1285–1288.
57. Lindau T, Arner M, Hagberg L. Intraarticular lesions in distal fractures of the radius in young adults. A descriptive arthroscopic study in 50 patients. *J Hand Surg Br* 1997; 22(5):638–643.
58. Geissler WB, Freeland AE, Savoie FH, et al. Intracarpal soft-tissue lesions associated with an intra-articular fracture of the distal end of the radius. *J Bone Joint Surg Am* 1996;78(3):357–365.
59. Richards RS, Bennett JD, Roth JH, et al. Arthroscopic diagnosis of intra-articular soft tissue injuries associated with distal radial fractures. *J Hand Surg Am* 1997;22(5): 772–776.
60. Ruch DS, Vallee J, Poehling GG, et al. Arthroscopic reduction versus fluoroscopic reduction in the management of intra-articular distal radius fractures. *Arthroscopy* 2004; 20(3):225–230.
61. Tang JB, Shi D, Gu YQ, et al. Can cast immobilization successfully treat scapholunate dissociation associated with distal radius fractures? *J Hand Surg Am* 1996;21(4): 583–590.
62. Gausepohl T, Worner S, Pennig D, et al. Extraarticular external fixation in distal radius fractures pin placement in osteoporotic bone. *Injury* 2001;32:SD79–SD85.
63. Orbay JL, Fernandez DL. Volar fixation for dorsally displaced fractures of the distal radius: a preliminary report. *J Hand Surg Am* 2002;27(2):205–215.
64. Apergis E, Darmanis S, Theodoratos G, et al. Beware of the ulno-palmar distal radial fragment. *J Hand Surg Br* 2002;27(2):139–145.
65. Flinkkila T, Nikkola-Sihto A, Raatikainen T, et al. Role of metaphyseal cancellous bone defect size in secondary displacement in Colles' fracture. *Arch Orthop Trauma Surg* 1999;119(5-6):319–323.
66. Zmurko MG, Eglseder WA Jr, Belkoff SM. Biomechanical evaluation of distal radius fracture stability. *J Orthop Trauma* 1998;12:46–50.
67. Zmurko M, Eglseder W, Belkoff S. Biomechanical evaluation of distal radius fracture stability. *J Orthop Trauma* 1998;12:46–50.
68. Jenkins NH. The unstable Colles' fracture. *J Hand Surg* 1989;14(2):149–154.
69. Solgaard S. Function after distal radius fracture. *Acta Orthop Scand* 1988;59(1):39–42.
70. Szabo RM. Extra-articular fractures of the distal radius. *Orthop Clin N Am* 1993; 24(2): 229–237.
71. Gurland M. Carpometacarpal joint injuries of the fingers. *Hand Clinics* 1992;8: 733–744.
72. Leung F, Ozkan M, Chow SP. Conservative treatment of intra-articular fractures of the distal radius—factors affecting functional outcome. *Hand Surg* 2000;5(2):145–153.
73. Young CF, Nanu AM, Checketts RG. Seven-year outcome following Colles' type distal radial fracture. A comparison of two treatment methods. *J Hand Surg Br* 2000;28(5): 422–426.
74. Young BT, Rayan GM. Outcome following nonoperative treatment of displaced distal radius fractures in low-demand patients older than 60 years. *J Hand Surg Am* 2000; 25(1):19–28.
75. Prokop A, Swol-Ben J, Rehm KE. Treatment methods for geriatric patients at the Traumatology Clinic at the University of Cologne —retrospective studies. *Chir Narzadow Ruchu Ortop Pol* 1996;61(3):315–318.
76. Jupiter JB, Ring D, Weitzel PP. Surgical treatment of redisplaced fractures of the distal radius in patients older than 60 years. *J Hand Surg Am* 2002;27(4):714–723.
77. Ark J, Jupiter JB. The rationale for precise management of distal radius fractures. *Orthop Clin N Am* 1993;24(2):205–210.
78. Chern TC, Jou IM, Lai KA, et al. Sonography for monitoring closed reduction of displaced extra-articular distal radial fractures. *J Bone Joint Surg Am* 2002;84:194–203.
79. Waters PM, Kolettis GJ, Schwend R. Acute median neuropathy following physeal fractures of the distal radius. *J Pediatr Orthop* 1994;14(2):173–127.
80. Bourrel P, Ferro RM. Nerve complications in closed fractures of the lower end of the radius. *Ann Chir Main* 1982;1(2):119–126.
81. Agee JM, Szabo RM, Chidgey LK, et al. Treatment of comminuted distal radius fractures: an approach based on pathomechanics. *Orthopedics* 1994;17(12):1115–1122.
82. Solgaard S, Bunger C, Sllund K. Displaced distal radius fractures. A comparative study of early results following external fixation, functional bracing in supination, or dorsal plaster immobilization. *Arch Orthop Trauma Surg* 1990;109(1):34–38.
83. Allain J, le Guilloux P, Le Mouel S, et al. Trans-styloid fixation of fractures of the distal radius. A prospective randomized comparison between 6- and 1-week postoperative immobilization in 60 fractures. *Acta Orthop Scand* 1999;70(2):119–123.
84. Weber SC, Szabo RM. Severely comminuted distal radial fracture as an unsolved problem: complications associated with external fixation and pins and plaster techniques. *J Hand Surg Am* 1986;11(2):157–165.
85. Rosenthal AH, Chung KC. Intrafocal pinning of distal radius fractures: a simplified approach. *Ann Plast Surg* 2002;48(6):593–599.
86. Saeki Y, Hashizume H, Nagoshi M, et al. Mechanical strength of intramedullary pinning and transfragmental Kirschner wire fixation for Colles' fractures. *J Hand Surg Br* 2001; 26(6):550–555.
87. Trumble TE, Wagner W, Hanel DP, et al. Intrafocal (Kapandji) pinning of distal radius fractures with and without external fixation. *J Hand Surg Am* 1998;23(3):381–394.
88. Walton NP, Brammar TJ, Hutchinson J, et al. Treatment of unstable distal radial fractures by intrafocal, intramedullary K-wires. *Injury* 2000;32(5):383–389.
89. Edwards GS Jr. Intra-articular fractures of the distal part of the radius treated with the small AO external fixator. *J Bone Joint Surg Am* 1991;73(8):1241–1250.
90. Fernandez DL, Jakob RP, Buchler U. External fixation of the wrist. Current indications and technique. *Ann Chir Gynaecol* 1983;72(6):298–302.
91. Huch K, Hunerbein M, Meeder PJ. External fixation of intra-articular fracture of the distal radius in young and old adults. *Arch Orthop Trauma Surg* 1996;115(1):38–42.
92. Christensen OM, Christiansen TC, Krasheninnikoff M, et al. Plaster cast compared with bridging external fixation for distal radius fractures of the Colles' type. *Int Orthop* 2001;24(6):358–360.
93. Bass RL, Blair WF, Hubbard PP. Results of combined internal and external fixation for the treatment of severe AO-C3 fractures of the distal radius. *J Hand Surg Am* 1995; 20(3):373–381.
94. Howard P, Stewart H, Hind R, et al. External fixation or plaster for severely displaced comminuted Colles' fractures? A prospective study of anatomical and functional results. *J Bone Joint Surg Br* 1989;71:68–73.
95. Jenkins N, Jones D, Mintowt-Czyz. External fixation and recovery of function following fractures of the distal radius in young adults. *Injury* 1988;19(3):235–238.
96. Chan BK, Leong LC, Low CO, et al. The use of the external fixator in the treatment of intra-articular fractures of the distal radius. *Singapore Med J* 1999;40(6):420–424.
97. Cooney WP. External fixation of distal radial fractures. *Clin Orthop* 1983;180:44–49.
98. Gausepohl T, Pennig D, Mader K. Principles of external fixation and supplementary techniques in distal radius fractures. *Injury* 2000;31:56–70.
99. Bartosh RA, Saldana MJ. Intraarticular fractures of the distal radius: a cadaveric study to determine if ligamentotaxis restores radiopalmar tilt. *J Hand Surg* 1990;15(1):18–21.
100. Dodds SD, Cornelissen S, Jossan S, et al. A biomechanical comparison of fragment-specific fixation and augmented external fixation for intra-articular distal radius fractures. *J Hand Surg Am* 2002;27:953–964.
101. Leung KS, So W, Chiu V, et al. Ligamentotaxis for comminuted distal radial fractures modified by primary cancellous grafting and functional bracing: Long-term results. *J Orthop Trauma* 1991;5(3):265–271.
102. Herrera M, Chapman CB, Roh M, et al. Treatment of unstable distal radius fractures with cancellous allograft and external fixation. *J Hand Surg Am* 1999;24:1269–1278.
103. Cannegieter DM, Juttmann JW. Cancellous grafting and external fixation for unstable Colles' fractures. *J Bone Joint Surg Br* 1997;79(3):428–432.
104. Leung K, Shen W, Leung P, et al. Ligamentotaxis and bone grafting for comminuted fractures of the distal radius. *J Bone Joint Surg* 1989;71:838–842.
105. Cassidy C, Jupiter JB, Cohen M, et al. Norian SRS cement compared with conventional fixation in distal radial fractures. A randomized study. *J Bone Joint Surg Am* 2003;85: 2127–2137.
106. Sanchez-Sotelo J, Munuera L, Madero R. Treatment of fractures of the distal radius with remodellable bone cement. *J Bone Joint Surg Br* 2000;82:856–863.
107. Dunning CE, Lindsay CS, Bicknell RT, et al. Supplemental pinning improves the stability of external fixation in distal radius fractures during simulated finger and forearm motion. *J Hand Surg* 1999;24:992–1000.
108. Seitz WH Jr, Froimson AI, Leb R, et al. Augmented external fixation of unstable distal radius fractures. *J Hand Surg Am* 1991;16:1010-1016.
109. Riis J, Fruensgaard S. Treatment of unstable Colles' fractures by external fixation. *J Hand Surg Br* 1989;14:145–148.
110. Rikli DA, Kupfer K, Bodoky A. Long-term results of the external fixation of distal radius fractures. *J Trauma* 1998;44:970–976.
111. Sanders RA, Keppel FL, Waldrop JI. External fixation of distal radial fractures: results and complications. *J Hand Surg Am* 1991;16:385–391.
112. Hutchinson DT, Strenz GO, Cautilli RA. Pins and plaster vs external fixation in the treatment of unstable distal radial fractures. A randomized prospective study. *J Hand Surg Br* 1995;20(3):365–372.
113. Kaempffe FA. External fixation for distal radius fractures: adverse effects of excess distraction. *Am J Orthop* 1996;25(3):205–209.
114. Kaempffe FA, Walker KM. External fixation for distal radius fractures: effect of distraction on outcome. *Clin Orthop* 2000;380:220–225.
115. Biyani A. Over-distraction of the radio-carpal and mid-carpal joints following external fixation of comminuted distal radial fractures. *J Hand Surg Br* 1993;18(4):506–510.
116. Combalia A. Over-distraction of the radiocarpal and midcarpal joints with external fixation of comminuted distal radial fractures. *J Hand Surg Br* 1996;21:289.
117. Dee W, Klein W, Rieger H. Reduction techniques in distal radius fractures. *Injury* 2000; 31(Suppl 1):48–55.
118. Braun RM, Gellman H. Dorsal pin placement and external fixation for correction of dorsal tilt in fractures of the distal radius. *J Hand Surg Am* 1994;19(4):653–655.
119. Bruske J, Niedzwiedz Z, Bednarski M, et al. Acute carpal tunnel syndrome after distal radius fractures—long term results of surgical treatment with decompression and external fixator application. *Chir Narzadow Ruchu Ortop Pol* 2002;67(1):47–53.
120. Kuner EH, Mellios K, Berwarth H. Treatment of complicated fracture of the distal radius with external fixator. Follow-up—complications—outcomes. *Unfallchirurg* 2002;105(3):199–207.
121. Hove LM, Furnes O, Nilsen PT, et al. Closed reduction and external fixation of unstable fractures of the distal radius. *Scand J Plast Reconstr Surg Hand Surg* 1997;31(2):159–164.
122. Eglseder WA, Hay M. Open half-pin insertion for distal radial fractures. *Mil Med* 1993; 158:708–711.
123. Hassan DM, Johnston GH. Safety of the limited open technique of bone-transfixing threaded-pin placement for external fixation of distal radial fractures: a cadaver study. *Can J Surg* 1999;42:363–365.
124. Habernek H, Weinstabl R, Schmid L. Anatomic studies of percutaneous bore wire osteosynthesis of the distal radius. *Unfallchirurgie* 1993;19(1):49–53.
125. Hargreaves DG, Drew SJ, Eckersley R. Kirschner wire pin tract infection rates: a randomized controlled trial between percutaneous and buried wires. *J Hand Surg Br* 2004; 29:374–376.

126. Hutchinson DT, Bachus KN, Higgenbotham T. External fixation of the distal radius: to predrill or not to predrill. *J Hand Surg Am* 2000;25:1064–1068.
127. van Dijk J, Laudy F. Dynamic external fixation versus non-operative treatment of severe distal radial fractures. *Injury* 1996;27(1):57–61.
128. Dunning CE, Lindsay CS, Bicknell RT, et al. Ilizarov hybrid external fixation for fractures of the distal radius: Part II. Internal fixation versus Ilizarov hybrid external fixation: stability as assessed by cadaveric simulated motion testing. *J Hand Surg Am* 2001; 26(2):218–227.
129. Markiewitz AD, Gellman H. Five-pin external fixation and early range of motion for distal radius fractures. *Orthop Clin N Am* 2001;32(2):329–335, ix.
130. Werber KD, Raeder F, Brauer RB, et al. External fixation of distal radial fractures: four compared with five pins: a randomized prospective study. *J Bone Joint Surg Am* 2003; 85:660–666.
131. Putnam MD, Fischer MD. Treatment of unstable distal radius fractures: methods and comparison of external distraction and ORIF versus external distraction-ORIF neutralization. *J Hand Surg Am* 1997;22:238–251.
132. Ruch DS, Yang C, Smith BP. Results of palmar plating of the lunate facet combined with external fixation for the treatment of high-energy compression fractures of the distal radius. *J Orthop Trauma* 2004;18:28–33.
133. Fernandez DL. Should anatomic reduction be pursued in distal radial fractures? *J Hand Surg Br* 2000;25:523–527.
134. Geissler WB, Fernandes D. Percutaneous and limited open reduction of intra-articular distal radial fractures. *Hand Surg* 2000;5:85–92.
135. Knirk JL, Jupiter JB. Intra-articular fractures of the distal end of the radius in young adults. *J Bone Joint Surg Am* 1986;68:647–659.
136. Trumble TE, Schmitt S, Vedder NB. Factors affecting functional outcome of displaced intra-articular distal radius fractures. *J Hand Surg* 1994;19:325–340.
137. Edwards CC, Haraszti CJ, McGillivary GR, et al. Intra-articular distal radius fractures: arthroscopic assessment of radiographically assisted reduction. *J Hand Surg Am* 2001; 26:1036–1041.
138. Catalano LW III, Cole RJ, Gelberman RH, et al. Displaced intra-articular fractures of the distal aspect of the radius. Long-term results in young adults after open reduction and internal fixation. *J Bone Joint Surg Am* 1997;79:1290–1302.
139. Kreder HJ, Hanel DP, McKee M, et al. X-ray film measurements for healed distal radius fractures. *J Hand Surg Am* 1996;21:31–39.
140. Auge WK, Velazquez PA. The application of indirect reduction techniques in the distal radius: the role of adjuvant arthroscopy. *Arthroscopy* 2000;16:830–835.
141. Lindau T, Adlercreutz C, Aspenberg P. Cartilage injuries in distal radial fractures. *Acta Orthop Scand* 2003;74:327–331.
142. Lindau T, Adlercreutz C, Aspenberg P. Peripheral tears of the triangular fibrocartilage complex cause distal radioulnar joint instability after distal radial fractures. *J Hand Surg Am* 2000;25:464–468.
143. Kazuteru D, Hattori Y, Otsuka K, et al. Intraarticular fractures of the distal aspect of the radius: arthroscopically assisted reduction compared with open reduction and internal fixation. *J Bone Joint Surg Am* 1999;81:1093–1110.
144. Ruch DS, Ginn TA. Open reduction and internal fixation of distal radius fractures. *Op Tech Ortho* 2000;13:138–143.
145. Schnur DP, Chang B. Extensor tendon rupture after internal fixation of a distal radius fracture using a dorsally placed AO/ASIF titanium pi plate. Arbeitsgemeinschaft fur Osteosynthesefragen/Association for the Study of Internal Fixation. *Ann Plast Surg* 2000; 44:564–566.
146. Hahnloser D, Platz A, Amgwerd M, et al. Internal fixation of distal radius fractures with dorsal dislocation: pi-plate or two 1/4 tube plates? A prospective randomized study. *J Trauma* 1999;47:760–765.
147. Herron M, Faraj A, Craigen MA. Dorsal plating for displaced intra-articular fractures of the distal radius. *Injury* 2003;34:497–502.
148. Jakob M, Rikli DA, Regazzoni P. Fractures of the distal radius treated by internal fixation and early function. A prospective study of 73 consecutive patients. *J Bone Joint Surg Br* 2000;82:340–344.
149. Konrath GA, Bahler S. Open reduction and internal fixation of unstable distal radius fractures: results using the trimed fixation system. *J Orthop Trauma* 2002;16:578–585.
150. Rozental TD, Beredjiklian PK, Bozentka DJ. Functional outcome and complications following two types of dorsal plating for unstable fractures of the distal part of the radius. *J Bone Joint Surg Am* 2003;85:1956–1960.
151. Ring D, Jupiter JB, Brennwald J, et al. Prospective multicenter trial of a plate for dorsal fixation of distal radius fractures. *J Hand Surg Am* 1997;22:777–784.
152. Lowry KJ, Gainor BJ, Hoskins JS. Extensor tendon rupture secondary to the AO/ASIF titanium distal radius plate without associated plate failure: a case report. *Am J Orthop* 2000; 29:789–791.
153. Lucas GL, Fejfar ST. Complications in internal fixation of the distal radius. *J Hand Surg Am* 1998;23:1117.
154. Zemel NP. The prevention and treatment of complications from fractures of the distal radius and ulna. *Hand Clin* 1987;3:1–11.
155. Constantine KJ, Clawson MC, Stern PJ. Volar neutralization plate fixation of dorsally displaced distal radius fractures. *Orthopedics* 2002;25:125–128.
156. Drobetz H, Kutscha-Lissberg E. Osteosynthesis of distal radial fractures with a volar locking screw plate system. *Int Orthop* 2003;27(1):1–6.
157. Kamano M, Honda Y, Kazuki K, et al. Palmar plating for dorsally displaced fractures of the distal radius. *Clin Orthop* 2002;397:403–408.
158. Lee HC, Wong YS, Chan BK, et al. Fixation of distal radius fractures using AO titanium volar distal radius plate. *Hand Surg* 2003;8:7–15.
159. Leung F, Zhu L, Ho H, et al. Palmar plate fixation of AO type C2 fracture of distal radius using a locking compression plate—a biomechanical study in a cadaveric model. *J Hand Surg Br* 2003;28:263–266.
160. Adams BD. Effects of radial deformity on distal radioulnar joint mechanics. *J Hand Surg Am* 1993;18:492–498.
161. Geissler WB, Fernandez DL, Lamey DM. Distal radioulnar joint injuries associated with fractures of the distal radius. *Clin Orthopaed Rel Res* 1996;327:135–146.
162. Melone CP, Melone C. Open treatment for displaced articular fractures of the distal radius. *Clin Orthop Rel Res* 1986;202:103–111.
163. Kreder HJ, Hanel DP, Agel J, et al. A randomized controlled trial of closed reduction and casting versus closed reduction and external fixation for distal radius fractures with metaphyseal displacement but without joint incongruity. Orthopaedic Trauma Association 18th Annual Meeting, October 13, 2002.
164. Jakim I, Pieterse HS, Sweet MB. External fixation for intra-articular fractures of the distal radius. *J Bone Joint Surg Br* 1991;73(2):302–306.
165. Chin KR, Jupiter JB. Wire-loop fixation of volar displaced osteochondral fractures of the distal radius. *J Hand Surg Am* 1999;24:525–533.
166. Mudgal CS, Psenica J, Jupiter JB. Radiocarpal fracture-dislocation. *J Hand Surg Br* 1999; 24:92–98.
167. Smith RS, Crick JC, Alonso J, et al. Open reduction and internal fixation of volar lip fractures of the distal radius. *J Orthop Trauma* 1988;2:181–187.
168. Takami H, Takahashi S, Ando M. Comminuted intra-articular fracture of the distal radius with rotation of the palmar medial articular fragment: case reports. *J Trauma* 1992;32:404–407.
169. Chidgey LK. Treatment of acute and chronic instability of the distal radio-ulnar joint. *Hand Clin* 1998;14:297–303.
170. Faierman E, Jupiter J. The management of acute fractures involving the distal radioulnar joint and distal ulna. *Hand Clin* 1998;14:213–229.
171. May MM, Lawton JN, Blazar PE. Ulnar styloid fractures associated with distal radius fractures: incidence and implications for distal radioulnar joint instability. *J Hand Surg Am* 2002;27:965–971.
172. Nicolaidis SC, Hildreth DH, Lichtman DM. Acute injuries of the distal radioulnar joint. *Hand Clin* 2000;16:449–459.
173. Shaw JA, Bruno A, Paul EM. Ulnar styloid fixation in the treatment of posttraumatic instability of the radioulnar joint: a biomechanical study with clinical correlation. *J Hand Surg* 1990;15:712–720.
174. Kaukonen JP, Karaharju EO, Porras M, et al. Functional recovery after fractures of the distal forearm. Analysis of radiographic and other factors affecting the outcome. *Ann Chir Gynaecol* 1988;77(1):27–31.
175. McClain EJ, Wissinger HA. The acute carpal tunnel syndrome: nine case reports. *J Trauma* 1976;16(1):75–78.
176. Roysam GS. The distal radio-ulnar joint in Colles' fractures. *J Bone Joint Surg Br* 1993; 75(1):58–60.
177. Geissler WB, Fernandez DL, Lamey DM. Distal radioulnar joint injuries associated with fractures of the distal radius. *Clin Orthop* 1996;327:135–146.
178. Lindau T, Hagberg L, Adlercreutz C, et al. Distal radiulnar instability is an independent worsening factor in distal radial fractures. *Clin Orthop Rel Res* 2000;376:229–235.
179. Ruch DS, Yang CC, Smith BP. Results of acute arthroscopically repaired triangular fibrocartilage complex injuries associated with intra-articular distal radius fractures. *Arthroscopy* 2003;19(5):511–516.
180. Geissler WB, Freeland AE, Savoie FH, et al. Intracarpal soft-tissue lesions associated with an intra-articular fracture of the distal end of the radius. *J Bone Joint Surg* 1996; 78:357–365.
181. Biyani A, Simison AJ, Klenerman L. Fractures of the distal radius and ulna. *J Hand Surg Br* 1995;20:357–364.
182. Geissler WB, Freeland AE, Savoie FH, et al. Intracarpal soft tissue lesions associated with an intra-articular fracture of the distal end of the radius. *J Bone Joint Surg Am* 1996;78(3):357–365.
183. Laulan J, Bismuth JP. Intracarpal ligamentous lesions associated with fractures of the distal radius: outcome at one year. A prospective study of 95 cases. *Acta Orthop Belg* 1999;65(4):418–423.
184. Lindau T, Hagberg L, Adlercreutz C, et al. Distal radioulnar instability is an independent worsening factor in distal radial fractures. *Clin Orthop* 2000;376:229–235.
185. Prommersberger KJ, Lanz U. Biomechanical aspects of malunited distal radius fracture. A review of the literature. *Handchir Mikrochir Plast Chir* 1999;31(4):221–226.
186. Pogue DJ, Viegas SF, Patterson RM, et al. Effects of distal radius fracture malunion on wrist joint mechanics. *J Hand Surg Am* 1990;15(5):721–727.
187. Porter M, Stockley I. Fractures of the distal radius. Intermediate and end results in relation to radiologic parameters. *Clin Orthop* 1987;220:241–252.
188. Kazuki K, Kusunoki M, Yamada J, et al. Cineradiographic study of wrist motion after fracture of the distal radius. *J Hand Surg Am* 1993;18(1):41–46.
189. Minami A, Ogino T. Midcarpal instability following malunion of a fracture of the distal radius. A case report. *Ital J Orthop Traumatol* 1986;12(4):473–477.
190. Missakian M, Cooney W, Amadio P, et al. Open reduction and internal fixation for distal radius fractures. *J Hand Surg Am* 1992;17:745–755.
191. Bade H, Lobeck F. Behavior of the joint surface of the distal radio-ulnar joint in malposition of the distal radius. *Unfallchirurgie* 1991;17(4):213–217.
192. Bronstein AJ, Trumble TE, Tencer AF. The effects of distal radius fracture malalignment on forearm rotation: a cadaveric study. *J Hand Surg Am* 1997;22(2):258–262.
193. Dumont CE, Thalmann R, Macy JC. The effect of rotational malunion of the radius and the ulna on supination and pronation. *J Bone Joint Surg Br* 2002;84:1070–1074.
194. Hirahara H, Neale PG, Lin YT, et al. Kinematic and torque-related effects of dorsally angulated distal radius fractures and the distal radial ulnar joint. *J Hand Surg Am* 2003; 28(4):614–621.
195. Moore DC, Hogan KA, Crisco JJ III, et al. Three-dimensional in vivo kinematics of the

distal radioulnar joint in malunited distal radius fractures. *J Hand Surg Am* 2002;27: 233–242.

196. Sato S. Load transmission through the wrist joint: a biomechanical study comparing the normal and pathological wrist. *Nippon Seikeigeka Gakkai Zasshi* 1995;69(7):470–483.
197. Jupiter JB, Fernandez DL. Complications following distal radial fractures. *J Bone Joint Surg* 2001;83:1244–1265.
198. Fernandez DL. Reconstructive procedures for malunion and traumatic arthritis. *Orthop Clin N Am* 1993;24:341–363.
199. Amadio PC, Botte MJ. Treatment of malunion of the distal radius. *Hand Clin* 1987;3: 541–561.
200. Arslan H, Subasi M, Kesemenli C, et al. Distraction osteotomy for malunion of the distal end of the radius with radial shortening. *Acta Orthop Belg* 2003;69(1):23–28.
201. Baillon R, Gris M, Tollet P, et al. Corrective osteotomy using Hoffmann II external fixators for extra-auricular malunion of the distal radius. *Acta Orthop Belg* 2001;67(5): 500–504.
202. Bora FW Jr, Osterman AL, Zielinski CJ. Osteotomy of the distal radius with a biplanar iliac bone graft for malunion. *Bull Hosp Jt Dis Orthop Inst* 1984;44(2):122–131.
203. Brown JN, Bell MJ. Distal radial osteotomy for malunion of wrist fractures in young patients. *J Hand Surg Br* 1994;19(5):589–593.
204. Fernandez DL. Malunion of the distal radius: current approach to management. *Instr Course Lect* 1993;42:99–113.
205. Flinkkila T, Raatikainen T, Kaarela O, et al. Corrective osteotomy for malunion of the distal radius. *Arch Orthop Trauma Surg* 2000;120:23–26.
206. Kwasny O, Fuchs M, Schabus R. Opening wedge osteotomy for malunion of the distal radius with neuropathy. 13 cases followed for 6 (1-11) years. *Acta Orthop Scand* 1994; 65:207–208.
207. Melendez EM. Opening-wedge osteotomy, bone graft, and external fixation for correction of radius malunion. *J Hand Surg Am* 1997;22:785–791.
208. Van Cauwelaert dW, De Smet L. Corrective osteotomy for malunion of the distal radius in young and middle-aged patients: an outcome study. *Chir Main* 2003;22:84–89.
209. Viso R, Wegener EE, Freeland AE. Use of a closing wedge osteotomy to correct malunion of dorsally displaced extra-articular distal radius fractures. *Orthopedics* 2000;23: 721–724.
210. Watson HK, Castle TH Jr. Trapezoidal osteotomy of the distal radius for unacceptable articular angulation after Colles' fracture. *J Hand Surg Am* 1988;13:837–843.
211. Linder L, Stattin J. Malunited fractures of the distal radius with volar angulation. *Acta Orthop Scand* 1996;67(2):179–181.
212. Linder L, Stattin J. Malunited fractures of the distal radius with volar angulation: corrective osteotomy in 6 cases using the volar approach. *Acta Orthop Scand* 1996;67: 179–181.
213. Gaebler C, McQueen MM. Ulnar procedures for post-traumatic disorders of the distal radioulnar joint. *Injury* 2003;34(1):47–59.
214. Hunt TR, Hastings H II, Graham T. A systematic approach to handling the distal radioulnar joint in cases of malunited distal radius fractures. *Hand Clin* 1998;14(2): 239–249.
215. Oskam J, Kingma J, Klasen HJ. Ulnar-shortening osteotomy after fracture of the distal radius. *Arch Orthop Trauma Surg* 1993;112(4):198–200.
216. Rodriguez Merchan EC, de la Corte H. Injuries of the distal radioulnar joint. *Contemp Orthop* 1994;29(3):193–200.
217. Dresing K, Peterson T, Schmit-Neuerburg KP. Compartment pressure in the carpal tunnel in distal fractures of the radius. A prospective study. *Arch Orthop Trauma Surg* 1994;113(5):285–289.
218. Bauman TD, Gelberman RH, Mubarak SJ, et al. The acute carpal tunnel syndrome. *Clin Orthop* 1981;156:151–156.
219. Hove LM. Nerve entrapment and reflex sympathetic dystrophy after fractures of the distal radius. *Scand J Plast Reconstr Surg Hand Surg* 1995;29(1):53–58.
220. Clarke AC, Spencer RF. Ulnar nerve palsy following fractures of the distal radius: clinical and anatomical studies. *J Hand Surg Br* 1991;16:438–440.
221. Dumont C, Fuchs M, Folwaczny EK, et al. Results of palmar T-plate osteosynthesis in unstable fractures of the distal radius. *Chirurg* 2003;74(9):827–833.
222. Koman LA, Poehling GG, Smith TL. Complex regional pain syndrome: reflex sympathetic dystrophy and causalgia. In: Green DP, Hotchkiss RN, Pederson WC, eds. *Green's operative hand surgery,* 4th ed. New York: Churchill Livingstone; 1999:636–666.
223. Hove LM. Delayed rupture of the thumb extensor tendon. A 5-year study of 18 consecutive cases. *Acta Orthop Scand* 1994;65(2):199–203.
224. Kato N, Nemoto K, Arino H, et al. Ruptures of flexor tendons at the wrist as a complication of fracture of the distal radius. *Scand J Plast Reconstr Surg Hand Surg* 2002;36(4): 245–248.

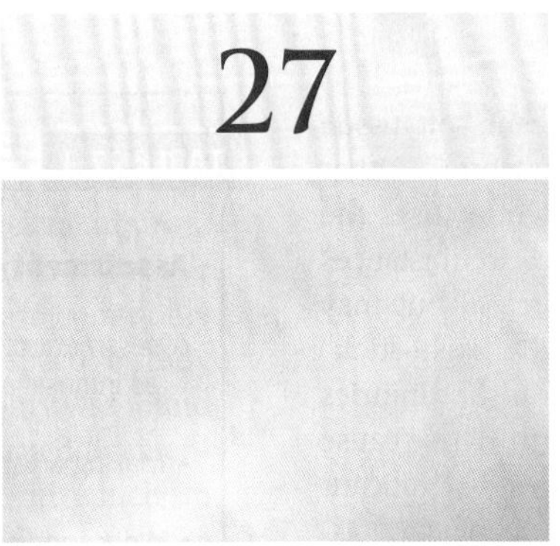

FRACTURES OF THE SHAFTS OF THE RADIUS AND ULNA

Ralph Hertel and Dominique A. Rothenfluh

Forearm fractures can be regarded as articular fractures as slight deviations in the spatial orientation of the radius and ulna will significantly decrease the forearm's rotational amplitude and thereby impair the positioning and function of the hand. Thus, the management of these fractures and their associated injuries deserve special attention as their treatment is not the same as the treatment of other diaphyseal fractures. Imperfect treatment of fractures of the radius and ulna diaphyses leads to a loss of motion as well as muscle imbalance and poor hand function.

This chapter gives an overview of the different treatment options. The inherent difficulties associated with the management of forearm fractures have long been recognized and several different strategies of treatment have been developed. The most significant impact on the treatment of forearm fractures was the development of compression plate osteosynthesis. Several studies will be presented which indicate that plate osteosynthesis provides a good treatment option which has a very predictable outcome. However, it is important to realize that the choice of implant is not the only parameter that governs outcome. It is important to evaluate the patient and to understand the type of surgery that is involved in the management of these fractures.

PRINCIPLES OF MANAGEMENT

Mechanism of Injury

Of the many mechanisms of injury that cause fractures of the radius and ulna, a direct blow is the most common. These are not infrequently associated with road traffic accidents and result

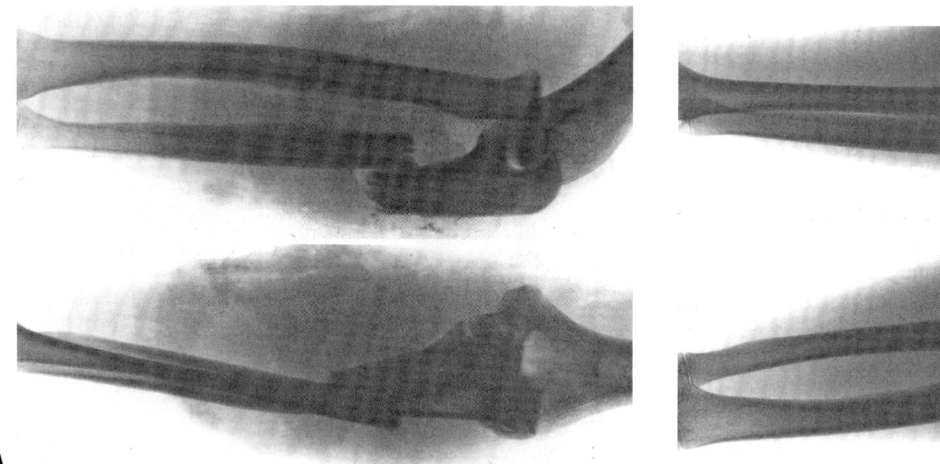

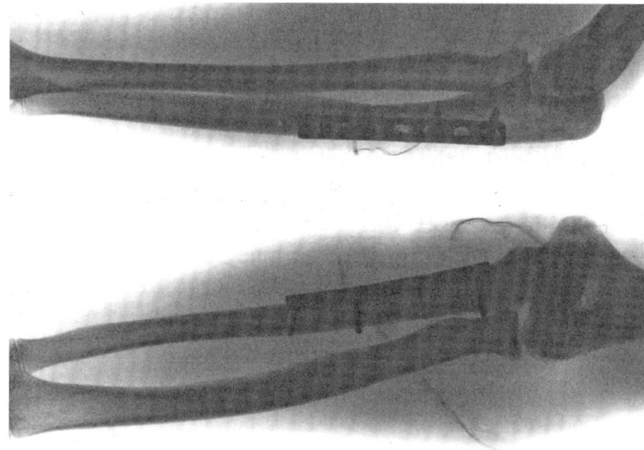

FIGURE 27-3 **A.** AP and lateral x-rays of a type 1 Monteggia fracture dislocation. **B.** Treated by compression plating using a LC-DCP.

Most authorities indicate that about 60% of Monteggia fracture dislocations are type I, 15% are type II, 10% are type III, and 10% are type IV. Type III lesions virtually only occur in children. Figure 27-3 shows pre- and postoperative x-rays of a Monteggia fracture dislocation.

The posterior Monteggia fracture dislocation (type II) has been studied in detail. Jupiter et al (10) recognized an anterior triangular or quadrilateral fracture fragment (Fig. 27-4) in proximity with the coronoid process in these fracture dislocations. A radial head fracture may often be found in association with the radial head dislocation. This injury combination represents a potentially unstable fracture pattern, which may lead to impaired forearm rotation as well as flexion and extension. Any fixation method has to counteract the tendency for anterior angulation to occur if the anterior cortex is not intact (10).

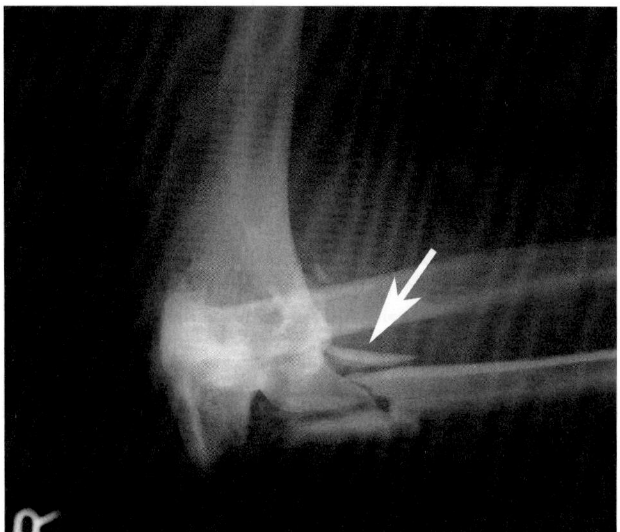

FIGURE 27-4 The arrow is pointing to the anterior quadrilateral fragment in this comminuted Monteggia fracture. This fragment must be looked for in noncomminuted fractures.

Neurovascular Injuries

Nerve injuries in closed forearm fractures are relatively uncommon. Although injuries to the median, ulnar, and radial nerves can occur injuries of the posterior interosseous nerve have been most commonly reported, particularly in association with Monteggia fracture dislocations (11,12). There have been a few reports of ulnar nerve injury following forearm fractures in children. In one report the injury resolved spontaneously with nonoperative management of the fracture (13). In another injury secondary ulnar nerve exploration was undertaken when no evidence of recovery was observed (14).

Most nerve injuries are neuropraxias commonly caused by contusion or compression. Rarely the nerve is trapped in the fracture or in scar tissue (14), or is transected by the fracture fragments (15). Neuropraxias generally resolve spontaneously (13). However, as most forearm fractures, and particularly Monteggia fracture dislocations, are treated operatively, we advocate exploration of the injured nerve if damage is suspected clinically prior to surgery. In open fractures nerve exploration should be carried out during the initial debridement.

Collateral circulation of the forearm in the presence of either isolated radial or ulnar arterial damage is usually sufficient to maintain viability of the hand and forearm. Viability may even be maintained if both the radial and ulnar arteries are damaged because the longitudinally orientated collateral vessels may still provide sufficient blood supply (16). If one major artery is intact and there is adequate perfusion to the hand, the damaged vessel does not have to be repaired. However, in combination with nerve injuries, it has been argued that recovery of the associated nerve lesion will be improved by an enhanced blood supply and vascular repair is therefore advocated (17).

Compartment Syndrome

A compartment syndrome of the forearm may develop following a fracture of the diaphyses of the radius and ulnar, but it may also follow soft tissue crush injuries and supracondylar humeral fractures as well as nontraumatic causes. Compartment syndrome is discussed further in Chapter 13. Swelling and significant pain may suggest a developing compartment syndrome. Passive stretch of the fingers generally elicits pain and is highly suggestive of the presence of a compartment syndrome. However, if there is a displaced closed forearm fracture, this finding may only be of limited use as all manipulation may be painful. The presence or absence of the radial pulse is not a reliable diagnostic sign (18). The presence of a palpable radial pulse never excludes a compartment syndrome of the forearm as the intra-compartmental pressures may have risen high enough to occlude muscle and nerve blood flow but may still be below the systolic blood pressure.

Although compartment pressure measurement is recommended for early diagnosis of compartment syndrome, the critical threshold pressure which indicates that fasciotomy is necessary is controversial and values between 30–45 mm Hg have been suggested (19–21). Whitesides et al (22) commented on the importance of the pressure differential between compartment pressure and the diastolic blood pressure. Ischemia was thought to begin when the pressure rose to within 10–30 mm Hg of the diastolic blood pressure. Generally, if there is a pressure difference of less than 10 mm Hg, muscle histology shows scattered areas of infarction and fibrosis, whereas if there is a difference of at least 20 mm Hg there are no such changes in the muscle (23). McQueen and Court-Brown (24) reported on a series of 116 patients with tibial fractures in which continuous monitoring of compartment pressures was carried out for 24 hours. Two patients had a differential pressure of below 30 mm Hg and underwent fasciotomy. Although absolute pressures above 30 mm Hg were observed in 53 patients in the first 12-hour period and in 28 patients in the second 12-hour period, none of these patients had any sequelae of acute compartment syndrome. Had they used absolute pressures of 30 mm Hg as a threshold, 53 patients would have had unnecessary fasciotomy.

The authors concluded that absolute compartment pressure is an unreliable indicator of the requirement for fasciotomy and that a pressure differential of less than 30 mm Hg between the diastolic blood pressure, and the compartment pressure indicates that immediate fasciotomy is required. However, we believe that the diagnosis of acute compartment syndrome should not be delayed by waiting for the differential pressure to drop below 30 mm Hg if clinical signs are present. In borderline cases when continuous monitoring is chosen, the indication for treatment is not just the absolute pressure or pressure differential but rather the evolution of the pressure differential over time. Increasing compartment pressures require action, and if there is any doubt about the presence of an acute compartment syndrome we advocate fasciotomy rather than temporizing, missing the diagnosis, and risking the serious sequelae of this condition.

Diagnosis and Classification

Forearm fractures are usually classified according to the location of the fracture, the fracture pattern, degree of displacement, degree of comminution, the involvement of the radio-ulnar joints, the amount of bone loss, and the degree of soft tissue injury in both closed and open fractures. The presence or absence of the associated injuries described above has significant implications on the method of treatment. Diagnostic algorithms therefore have to include not only x-rays of the forearm but also true antero-posterior and lateral x-rays of the wrist and elbow. Involvement of the proximal or distal radio-ulnar joints carries particular significance because effective therapy requires integrated treatment of both the fracture and the associated joint injury. Thus these injuries must be looked for. CT scans are usually only required for the assessment of radio-ulnar joint injury and not for the primary diagnosis of forearm fractures.

The most commonly used classification for forearm diaphyseal fractures is that of the AO group (25), which has also been adopted by the Orthopaedic Trauma Association (OTA). This classification is shown in Figure 27-5. As with all AO classifications this is an alpha-numeric classification. Type A fractures are simple fractures of the ulna, radius, or both bones. In A1 fractures there is a simple fracture of the ulna and the radius is intact. In A2 fractures there is a simple fractures of the radius and the ulna is intact. In both these groups, .1 refers to an oblique fractures, .2 to a transverse fracture, and .3 to a fracture associated with the dislocation. The A1.3 fracture represents a Monteggia fracture dislocation and the A2.3 fracture represents a Galeazzi fracture dislocation. In the A3 group, .1 refers to a radial fracture in the proximal third of the bone, .2 to a radial fracture in the middle third, and .3 to a radial fracture in the distal third.

Type B fractures are wedge fractures of either the ulna (B1), the radius (B2), or both the radius and ulna (B3). In groups B1 and B2, .1 refers to an intact wedge, .2 to a fragmented wedge, and .3 to an associated dislocation with B1.3 fractures being Monteggia fracture dislocations and B2.3 fractures being Galeazzi fracture dislocations. In the B3 group, B3.1 fractures have an ulnar wedge and a simple fracture of the radius, B3.2 fractures have a radial wedge and a simple fracture of the ulna, and B3.3 fractures have radial and ulnar wedges.

Type C fractures are complex fractures. C1 fractures are complex fractures of the ulna, C2 fractures involve the radius, and C3 fractures involve both the radius and ulna. In C1.1 fractures there is a bifocal fracture of the ulna with an intact radius, in C1.2 fractures there is a bifocal fracture of the ulna with a radial fracture, and in C1.3 fractures the ulnar fracture is irregular. In C2.1 fractures the radial fracture is bifocal and the ulna is intact. In C2.2 fractures the radial fracture is bifocal but the ulna is fractured, and in C2.3 fractures the radial fracture is irregular. In C3.1 fractures both bones show a bifocal fracture and in C3.2 fractures there is a bifocal fracture of one bone with an irregular fracture of the other. In the rare C3.3 fracture, both fractures are irregular or comminuted. It should be noted

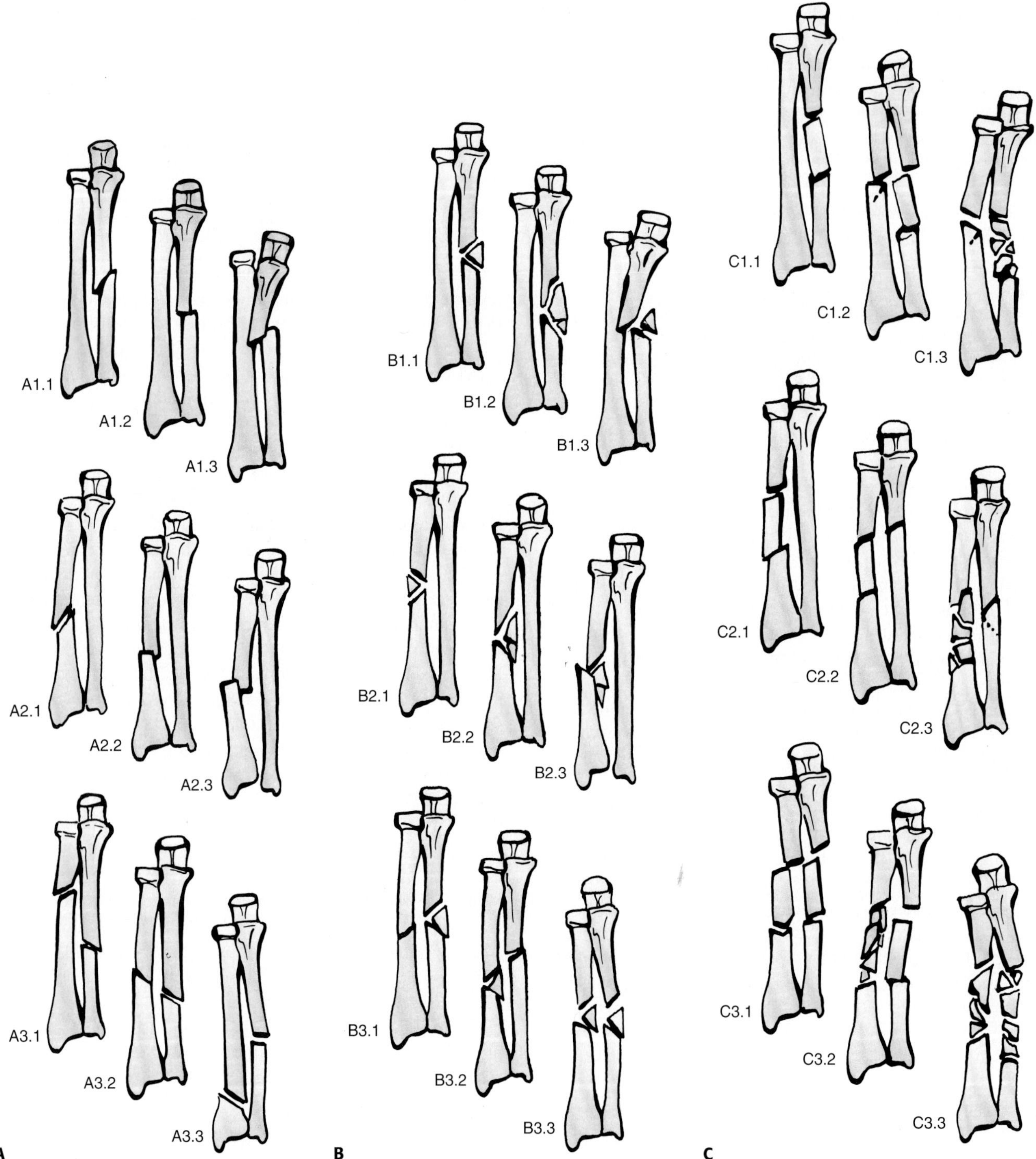

FIGURE 27-5 The AO (OTA) classification of radius and ulnar diaphyseal fractures. See text for details.

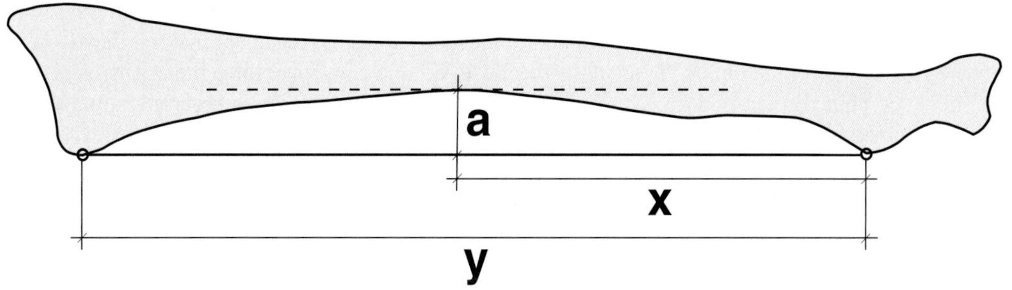

Maximum radial bow **a** (mm)

Location of maximum radial bow (%) $\frac{x}{y} \times 100$

FIGURE 27-6 The method of Schemitsch and Richards (30) for quantifying the maximum radial bow and its location relative to the length of the entire radius.

that while the AO (OTA) classification is useful for scientific and epidemiological purposes, it does not consider the full spectrum of lesions associated with radius and ulnar diaphyseal fractures.

Rationale for Treatment

Although the radius and ulna function as a unit, they only come into contact proximally and distally at the radio-ulnar joints. The proximal radio-ulnar joint consists of the radial head which articulates with the corresponding articular facet of the ulna and is fixed to it by the annular ligament, which itself serves as an extension of the ulnar articular surface. It is stabilized by the capsule of the elbow joint.

At the distal end the radius articulates with the ulna in a sigmoid notch which is stabilized mainly by the triangular fibrocartilage complex and the capsule of the wrist. The proximal and distal radio-ulnar joints articulate closely with their neighboring joints, the elbow, and wrist joints. The interosseous membrane spans the space between the radio-ulnar joints joining the radius and ulna. Its fibers run in an oblique fashion from distal ulna to proximal radials and they show a centrally thickened portion, 3.5 cm in width, that accounts for about 70% of actual stability of the forearm bones (26).

While the ulna is a straight bone which allows the radius to rotate around it, the anatomy of the radius is very complex (27–30). The rotation of the forearm depends on the ability of the radius to rotate around the ulna. Forearm rotation is vulnerable to any malalignment of the radius and accurate rotational as well as axial reduction is necessary.

To investigate the effect of angular malalignment on the subsequent loss of range of motion (ROM) of the forearm Matthews et al (28) tested forearm ROM with simulated fractures in cadavers. They showed that 10 degrees of angulation of one or both bones of the forearm resulted in a loss of ROM of 20 degrees of pronation and supination. With 20 degrees of angulation significant restriction in passive rotation of the forearm was observed, mediated either by direct radio-ulnar impingement or by extreme tension in the interosseous membrane. Tarr et al (29) found that loss of forearm rotation with a given deformity also depended on the location of the deformity. They observed a significantly greater loss of ROM in forearms with middle-third deformities than with distal-third deformities, with more supination being lost than pronation. They also observed a significant decrease of ROM with 15° of angulation. The greater decrease of ROM in middle-third deformities was attributed to the loss of the radial bow where the two forearm bones overlap at the extremes of pronation and supination. Schemitsch and Richards (30) undertook an outcome study correlating function with the radial bow. They described a method of quantifying the normal radial bow and reduction after fixation (Fig. 27-6). In the normal forearm, the maximal radial bow is reported to be about 15 mm and located at 60% of the radial length from the distal end (30). In patients who had rotation of the forearm of at least 80% of the opposite side, the normal radial bow differed on average by 1.5 mm and its location differed by 9% from that of the normal arm (Table 27-2). In patients with less satisfactory results, these differences were significantly greater.

Simple rotational deformities of either the radius or the ulna were reported to produce a loss of ROM equal to the extent of the rotatory deformity (29). However, in accordance with the findings stated above, simple rotational deformity of the radius results in a more pronounced loss of ROM in supination than

TABLE 27-2 Radial Bow*

Range of Motion (ROM)	Maximum Radial Bow	Location of Maximum Radial Bow
Normal	15.3 ± 0.3 mm	59.9 ± 0.7%
≥80% of normal ROM	15.3 ± 1.5 mm	59.9 ± 4.3%
<80% of normal ROM	15.3 ± 2.8 mm	59.9 ± 8.9%

* According to Schemitsch and Richards (30).

pronation (31). Dumont et al (31) reported that combined deformity in the same direction decreased the ROM similarly to that of an equivalent isolated rotatory deformity of the radius. The highest loss of ROM is observed in combined rotatory deformities in an opposite direction, with one bone in supination and the other in pronation. These investigations show the detrimental effects of incorrect axial and rotational alignment on forearm rotation, and they have implications for the method of treatment.

SURGICAL APPROACHES AND APPLIED ANATOMY

Surgical Approaches to the Radius

Anterior Approach (Henry)

CD-1

The anterior approach to the radius was first described by Henry (32). It allows a wide exposure of the anterior surface of the radius and exposes the bone over its entire length, if this is required. The approach can be extended across the elbow and into the hand. Care has to be taken not to harm the radial artery as it runs down the forearm under the brachioradialis muscle with the superficial branch of the radial nerve. The posterior interosseous nerve is vulnerable during deep dissection proximally if the radial neck needs to be accessed as the nerve winds round the radial neck within supinator muscle. The distal part of the approach is also used to access the distal radius for internal fixation of distal radial fractures, and the approach can also be easily extended if more proximal exposure is required.

Surgical Anatomy. The anterior part of the forearm is basically subdivided into two groups of muscles. Henry termed the group consisting of brachioradialis, extensor carpi radialis longus, and extensor carpi radialis brevis as the *mobile wad* (32). These muscles define the lateral aspect of the proximal forearm and are supplied by the radial nerve. The flexor-pronator group is found on the medial aspect and consists of three muscular layers supplied by the median and ulnar nerves. Superficially, from lateral to medial, the pronator teres, flexor carpi radialis, palmaris longus, and flexor carpi ulnaris muscles are found. The middle layer consists of flexor digitorum superficialis and the deep layer of flexor digitorum profundus, flexor pollicis longus and, more distally, pronator quadratus. To expose the forearm by a Henry approach, the inter-nervous plane between the radial and median nerves has to be found between the mobile wad, with brachioradialis lying most medially and pronator teres proximally and flexor carpi radialis distally in the flexor-pronator group.

Surgical Technique. The patient is placed supine on the operating table with the arm abducted on an arm board and the forearm supinated. Before the incision is made the mobile wad, with its medial border adjacent to the biceps tendon, and the styloid process of the radius should be palpated. A straight incision is made along the medial border of the mobile wad. The length and axial location of the incision depends on where and to what extent the bone needs to be exposed. The incision is carried down to the fascia while protecting the lateral cutaneous nerve. The fascia is incised and the inter-nervous plane between the radial and median nerves is developed. The radial artery lies just beneath, or just ulnar to the brachioradialis. It is exposed and retracted medially. The superficial branch of the radial nerve is retracted laterally (Fig. 27-7). Care has to be taken not to harm this nerve because it has a tendency to develop painful neuromata (Table 27-3).

Further dissection depends on what length of bone needs to be exposed to reduce and fix the fracture. In the middle third of the radius pronation of the arm exposes the insertion of

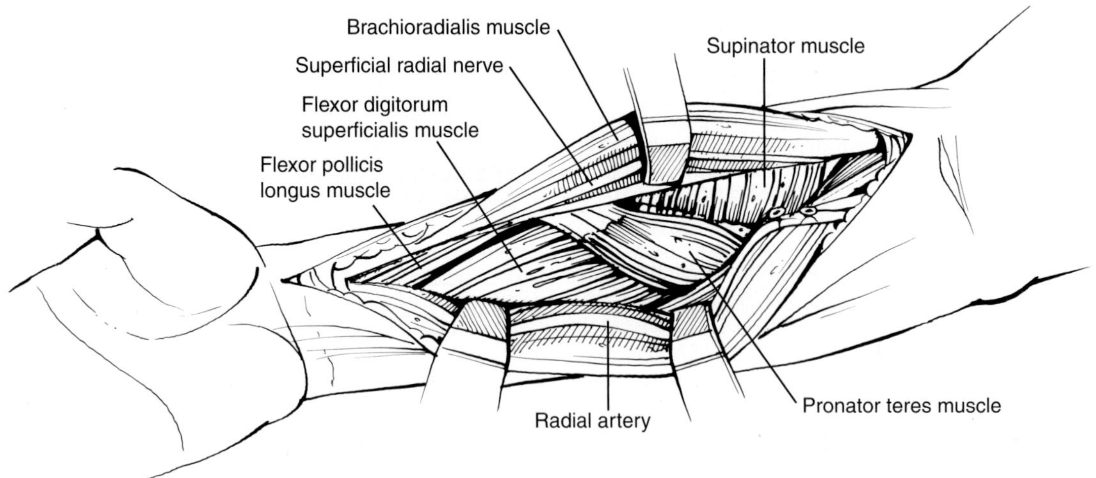

FIGURE 27-7 After the interval between brachioradialis and flexor carpi radialis is exposed and the radial artery retracted medially, supinator, pronator teres, flexor pollicis longus, and flexor digitorum superficialis can be seen.

TABLE 27-3 Pearls and Pitfalls of Surgery of Radius and Ulna Diaphyseal Fractures

Pearls

Anterior Approach (Henry)

The anterior approach is an extensile approach.

Avoid damage to the posterior interossoeus nerve by supinating the forearm.

Proximal dissection should be lateral to biceps tendon.

Dorsolateral Approach (Thompson)

Most suitable for fractures in the middle third of the forearm.

In 25% of patients the posterior interosseous nerve is in an extraperiosteal location.

Ulna Approach

Allows exposure of the entire length of the bone.

Pitfalls

Anterior Approach

The radial artery is vulnerable under brachioradialis.

The posterior interosseous nerve can be damaged during proximal dissection.

Damage to the superficial nerve may cause painful neuromata.

Dorsolateral Approach

The dorsolateral approach is not extensile and proximal and distal exposure is difficult.

If used for proximal fractures, the posterior interosseous nerve must be exposed.

Ulna Approach

Ulna nerve damage may occur in distal dissection.

pronator teres. Its tendon is detached from proximal to distal in order not to split the muscle. The flexor pollicis longus, pronator quadratus, and/or supinator muscles are also partially detached from their origin in order to provide adequate exposure to insert the plate. In general muscles should be detached extra-periosteally and the periosteum left intact where possible.

To gain access to the proximal third of the radius, the supinator muscle has to be partially or totally detached from the bone. The deep branch of the radial nerve, the posterior interosseous nerve, passes through supinator on its way to the dorsal compartment of the forearm. To avoid damage to this nerve the forearm is held in supination (Fig. 27-8). This maneuver is important as it exposes the insertion of supinator. It also displaces the nerve laterally and posteriorly away from the operative field. The muscle is then detached extra-periosteally and retracted laterally. The supinator, with the posterior interosseous nerve, must be handled with caution, especially when using retractors as it is easy to put excessive traction on the nerve. More proximally the dissection should always be carried out on the lateral side of the biceps tendon for anatomic reasons and not just to stay away from the radial artery and the median nerve. The radial recurrent vessels are ligated if necessary.

In the distal two-thirds the radius is mainly covered by flexor pollicis longus and pronator quadratus muscles. When extending the exposure to the distal end of the radius (Fig. 27-9), the surgeon must be aware that the radial artery is relatively fixed distally where it passes posteriorly after giving off the superficial palmar branch.

Dorsolateral Approach (Thompson)

This approach was originally described by Thompson in 1918: it provides access to the posterior aspect of the radius (33). It is particularly suited for fractures of the middle third of the radius. In our experience the approach is less well suited if extension to the distal third or the proximal third of the radius is required. In the distal third the abductor pollicis longus and extensor pollicis brevis muscles cross the surgical field. Although it is technically possible to tunnel the plate under the muscles after carefully lifting the muscles from their origins, we consider that the potential morbidity of this approach is too great. In the proximal third the approach is limited by supinator muscle with the enclosed posterior interosseous nerve. The dorsolateral approach requires exposure of the posterior interosseous nerve as it exits the supinator canal. The approach may be useful in posterior interosseous nerve palsy when the nerve needs to be explored. If this is the case, the supinator canal can be split in order to expose the entire length of the nerve.

Surgical Anatomy. The posterior muscles of the forearm can be split into three groups. On the radial side the mobile wad (32) consists of brachioradialis and extensor carpi longus and brevis. The mobile wad is supplied by the radial nerve. On the ulnar aspect of the forearm, the superficial extensors comprise extensor digitorum communis, extensor digiti minimi, extensor carpi ulnaris, and anconeus. The anconeus muscle does not extend the wrist but is an important dynamic stabilizer of the elbow. While the three extensor muscles are supplied by the posterior interosseous nerve the neural pedicle of anconeus originates directly from the radial nerve and travels in the triceps muscle to enter anconeus proximally deep to the lateral epicondyle. There are five deep muscles, three of which supply the thumb, these being abductor pollicis longus and extensor pollicis brevis and longus. The remaining two deep muscles are supinator and extensor indicis. All the deep muscles are sup-

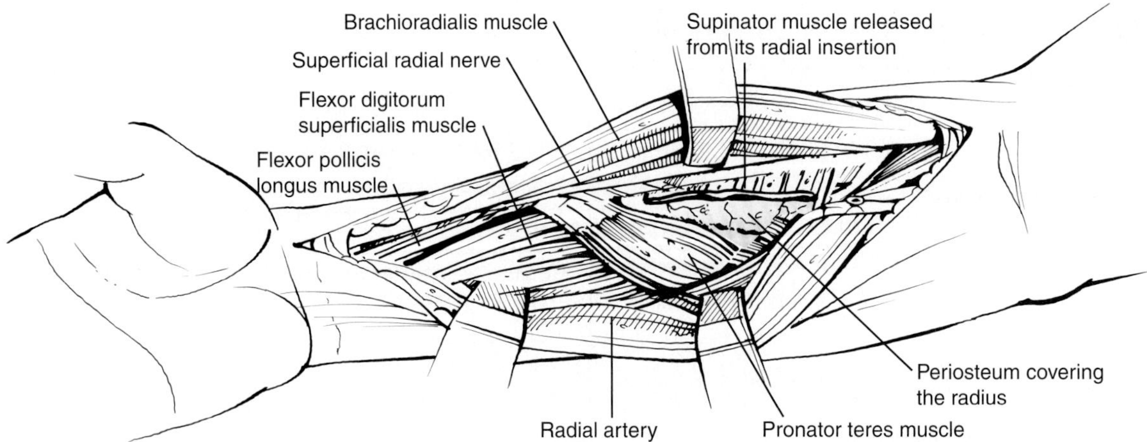

FIGURE 27-8 The insertion of supinator should be released with the patient's arm held in supination. The posterior interosseous nerve should be left within the muscle.

plied by the posterior interosseous nerve. Two inter-nervous planes can be found on the posterior aspect of the forearm, although they are not inter-nervous planes between two different nerves as they consist of planes between two branches of the radial nerve. There is a proximal inter-nervous plane between the mobile wad (radial nerve) and extensor digitorum communis (posterior interosseous nerve). A second inter-nervous plane is found between extensor carpi ulnaris (posterior interosseous nerve) and anconeus (branch of radial nerve). This is generally called the Kocher interval and is used to access the radial head.

The critical step in the dorsolateral approach is to identify and preserve the posterior interosseous nerve. The nerve is protected in the mass of supinator when the muscle is detached from the bone and retracted as it mainly travels within the substance of the muscle. However, in 25% of patients, the posterior interosseous nerve actually runs extra-periosteally (34,35) and is potentially at risk if the supinator is detached and re-

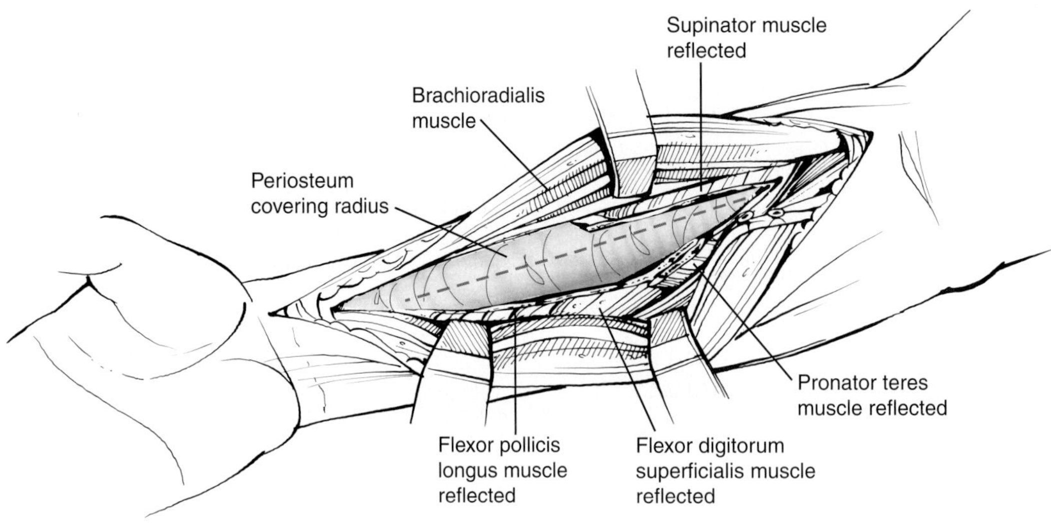

FIGURE 27-9 By continuing the dissection distally with the arm held in pronation, the entire radius is exposed. The dissection should be extraperiosteal in order not to strip the periosteum off the bone.

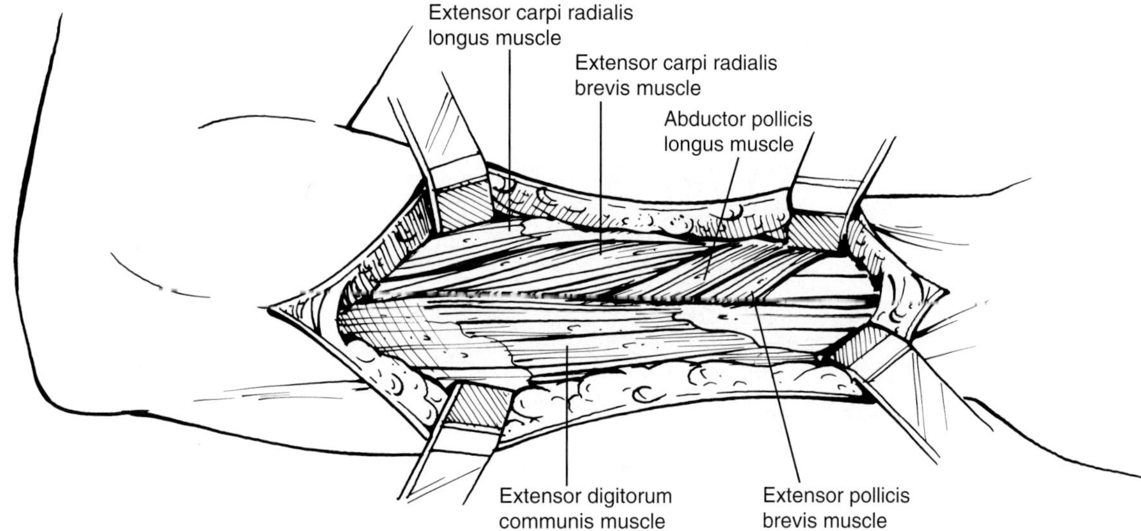

FIGURE 27-10 After incising the deep fascia, the interval between the extensor carpi radialis brevis and the extensor digitorum communis muscles should be identified.

tracted without prior identification and dissection of the nerve. Therefore, deep dissection of the proximal radius should always include prior identification of the posterior interosseous nerve.

Surgical Technique. The patient is placed supine on the operating table with the arm abducted on an arm board and the forearm pronated. Before the incision is made the mobile wad of Henry, the lateral epicondyle of the humerus, and Lister's tubercle are palpated. The skin is incised from the lateral epicondyle along the ulnar border of the mobile wad to Lister's tubercle, the length of the skin incision depending on the location of the fracture. The incision is deepened down to fascia which is incised in line with the skin incision. The interval between extensor carpi radialis brevis and extensor digitorum comminus is developed and followed distally to where abductor pollicis longus crosses (Figs. 27-10 and 27-11). If it is difficult to find the interval between the muscles, it can also be developed from distal to proximal where the abductor pollicis longus and extensor pollicis brevis cross. More proximally, the common aponeurotic origin of extensor carpi radialis brevis and longus is split, revealing the underlying supinator muscle (Fig. 27-12). Distal to abductor pollicis longus and extensor pollicis brevis, the interval between extensor carpi radialis brevis and extensor pollicis longus is developed which exposes the extraperiosteal posterolateral aspect of the distal radius (Fig. 27-13).

In the proximal two-thirds of the forearm, deep dissection to expose the bone involves identification and protection of the posterior interosseous nerve. In the proximal third the nerve can be identified where it exits supinator. If access to the radial nerve is required, the nerve is dissected through the substance of supinator while preserving its motor branches. Once the nerve is identified, the forearm is supinated to expose the anterior inser-

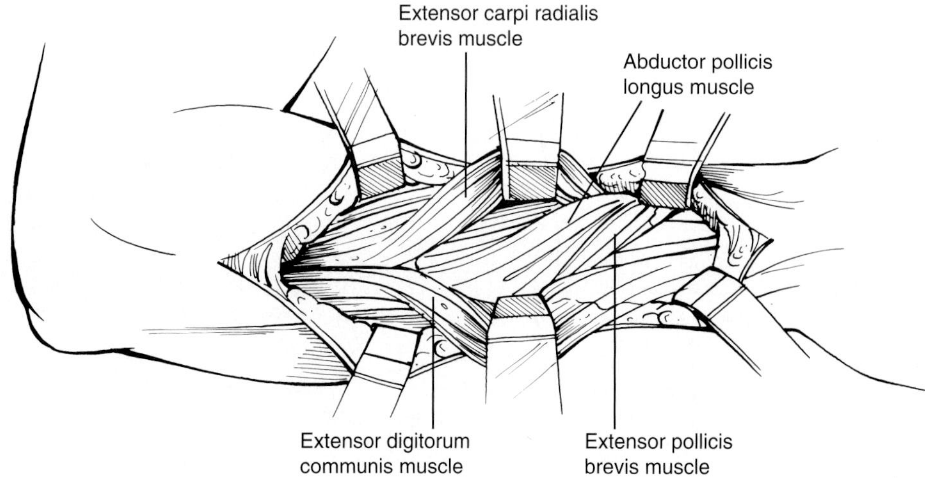

FIGURE 27-11 The interval between extensor carpi radialis brevis and extensor digitorum is developed.

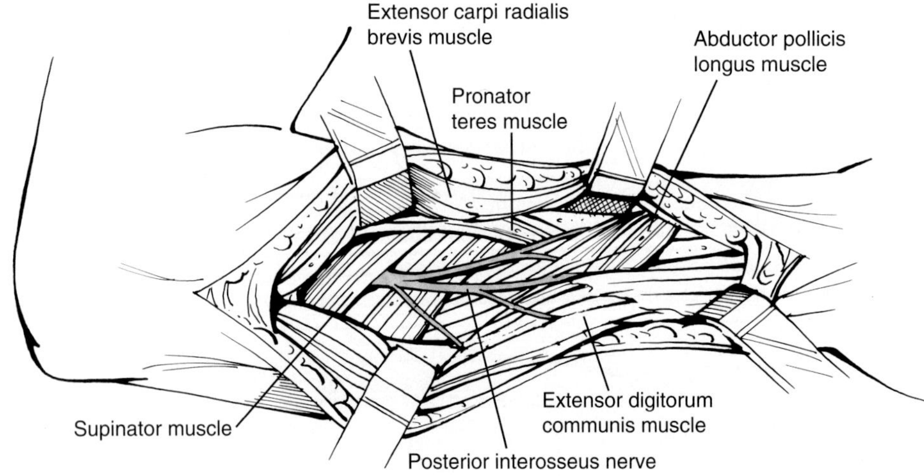

FIGURE 27-12 Further dissection of the interval proximally with splitting the aponeurotic origin of the extensors reveals supinator and the posterior interosseous nerve as it leaves the arcade of Frohse.

tion of supinator where it is detached extra-periosteally. The muscle can then be retracted to gain access to the proximal radius (Fig. 27-14). To undertake deep dissection distally into the middle third of the forearm, abductor pollicis longus and extensor pollicis brevis have to be detached extraperiosteally from the underlying radius and mobilized proximally and distally to gain access to bone (Fig. 27-14).

Surgical Approach to the Ulna

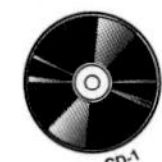

Exposure of the shaft of the ulnar is the most straightforward approach in the forearm. It permits exposure of the entire length of the bone. The approach relies on the plane between flexor and extensor carpi ulnaris. Careful dissection has to be carried out distally where the dorsal branch of the ulna nerve crosses the interval.

Surgical Anatomy

On the medial side the ulna is covered by flexor and extensor carpi ulnaris. Extensor carpi ulnaris is the most medial muscle supplied by the posterior interosseus nerve and flexor carpi ulnaris is the most medial muscle supplied by the ulnar nerve. The two muscles therefore form the borders of the inter-nervous plane used to approach the ulna. The ulnar nerve runs underneath flexor carpi ulnaris between flexor digitorum superficialis and profundus with the ulnar artery on its lateral side. Proximally, the nerve is fixed to flexor carpi ulnaris as it leaves the sulcus ulnaris and enters the flexor muscle between its humeral and ulnar origins. The ulnar nerve divides into four branches distally, one of which is the dorsal branch which runs across the surgical field distally. It may be encountered if dissection is continued to the distal end of the ulna.

Surgical Dissection

The patient is placed supine on the operating table with the arm abducted on an arm board. The forearm is held in a neutral position and the arm flexed at the elbow. Alternatively, the arm may be placed across the chest. For isolated fractures of the ulna a lateral decubitus position with the arm on an arm rest

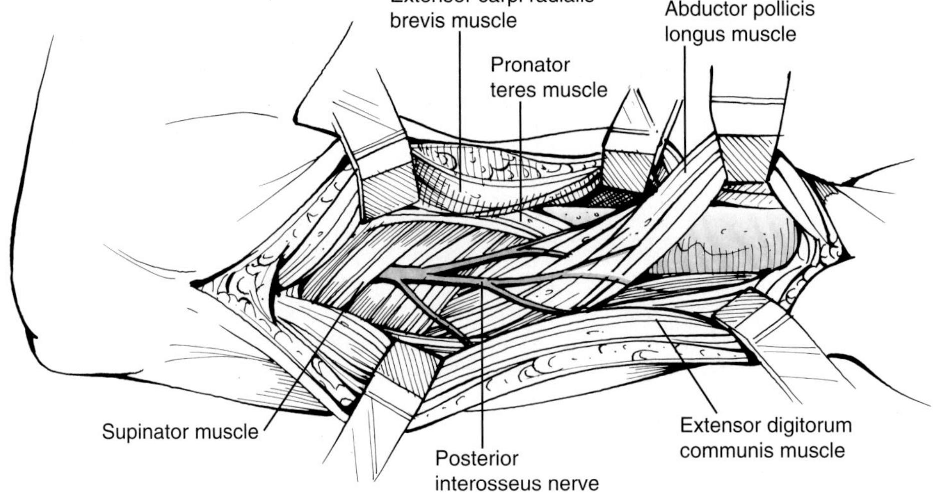

FIGURE 27-13 Development of the interval between extensor carpi radialis brevis and extensor pollicis longus reveals the radius distal to extensor pollicis brevis. Proximally, the nerve can be mobilized where it exits supinator if required. The posterior interosseous nerve should be identified and protected throughout the whole procedure.

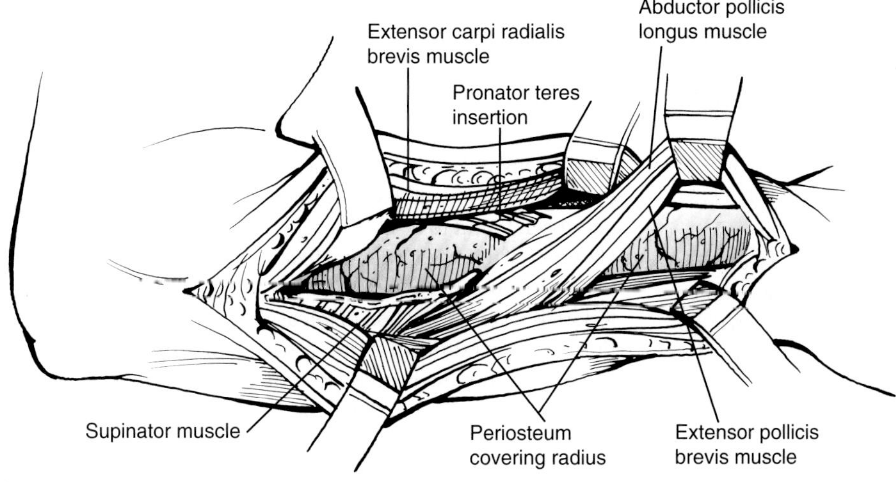

FIGURE 27-14 After identification of the posterior interosseous nerve, the forearm can be supinated in order to release supinator, which then exposes the proximal radius.

offers the best option. Before the incision is made the subcutaneous border of the ulna is palpated along its entire length and the surgeon can usually palpate the fracture. The incision is centered over the fracture site and is made longitudinally slightly anterior or posterior to the palpable subcutaneous crest. The length of the incision depends on the degree of exposure that is required. The incision is deepened down to fascia which is incised in line with the skin incision. Distally, care must be taken to identify and protect the dorsal branch of the ulnar nerve which passes onto the dorsal surface of extensor carpi ulnaris. The plane between extensor and flexor carpi ulnaris is developed to expose the underlying bone extraperiosteally. At the level of the olecranon the anconeus is found on the extensor side instead of extensor carpi ulnaris. The muscles are detached extraperiosteally depending on whether access to the anterior or posterior aspects of the bone is required. Anteriorly flexor carpi ulnaris has to be retracted carefully as the ulnar nerve and the ulnar artery run underneath between flexor digitorum superficialis and profundus. If the bone is exposed extraperiosteally by detaching and retracting flexor carpi ulnaris together with flexor digitorum profundus, the neurovascular structures are not endangered.

CURRENT TREATMENT OPTIONS

Several methods are available for treatment of fractures of the radius and ulna. While there are some indications for nonoperative management, operative treatment with internal fixation is generally acknowledged to be the most appropriate treatment method in most cases because it permits the most precise anatomic reduction of the fracture fragments. As functional outcome closely correlates with the restoration of anatomical alignment (28,29), particularly with reference to the maximum radial bow (30), the technique providing the most accurate restoration of the osseous anatomy will theoretically yield the best functional results. However, functional outcome also depends on how any associated injuries are managed and how soft tissue management and rehabilitation is carried out. Thus, all aspects of the injury have to be taken into account when selecting the most appropriate treatment method. Table 27-4 gives an overview of the advantages and disadvantages of the different treatment options.

Nonoperative Treatment

As the treatment of fractures of the radius and ulnar diaphyses is mainly operative, there are only a few indications for nonoper-

TABLE 27-4 Nonoperative vs Operative Treatment

Nonoperative Treatment	No control of fracture fragments High rate of secondary displacement Uncertain time to union Poor functional results in most cases
Intramedullary Nailing	Poor control of fracture fragments Anatomical re-alignment difficult More difficult to explore neurovascular structures High rate of nonunion High rate of unsatisfactory results
Open Reduction and Plate Osteosynthesis	Excellent control of fracture fragments Perfect anatomical re-alignment possible Possibility of treating concomitant injuries Can explore neurovascular structures Very low rate of nonunion Good to excellent functional results Very predictable outcome

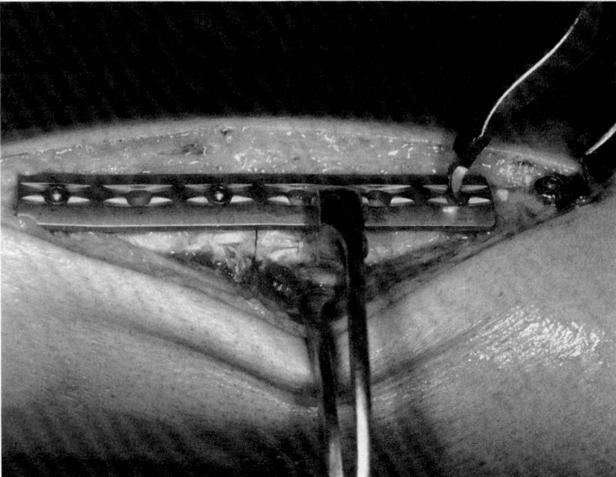

FIGURE 27-16 A typical indirect reduction with a PC-Fix plate. Note that the screw hole configuration doesn't allow inclination of the screws, thereby limiting the surgeons ability to place the screws for fragment fixation.

nation of the screws in the holes impossible and therefore lag screws cannot be used (Fig. 27-16). Although the use of unicortical screws was considered more biological, the fixation is less good and potentially more screws are required compared to the LC-DCP (Fig. 27-17).

The concept of the PC-Fix places maximum emphasis on the preservation of bone vascularity and the degree of stability of fixation is considered less important. However, a prospective clinical study by Leung and Chow (65) comparing union rates and functional outcome of the PC-Fix with the LC-DCP concluded that the two implants are equally effective for treatment of fractures of the radius and ulna diaphyses, despite their fundamental differences. Clinically the PC-Fix provides no advantage over the conventional LC-DCP, but it does require the surgeon to accept a different concept of plate fixation (72). It is however a step in the evolutionary process of improving the biomechanical and biological properties of fracture fixation. Information gained during the development and use of the PC-Fix led to the development of the locking compression plate (LCP). We believe that the investigation of Anderson et al (42) using conventional devices has set the standard whereby new devices must be measured and we believe that until other fixation devices prove to be superior, the 3.5 LC-DCP remains the gold standard for internal fixation of forearm fractures.

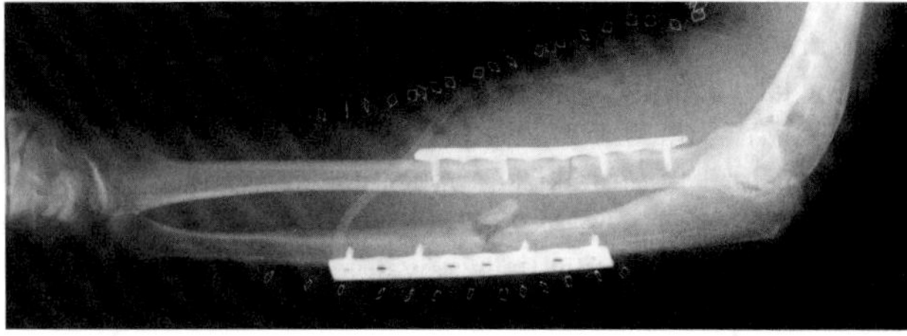

FIGURE 27-17 Postoperative x-ray of a fracture treated with a PC-Fix plate illustrates the parallel orientation of the unicortical screws.

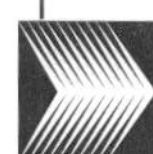

AUTHORS' PREFERRED TREATMENT

It is clear that the authors preferred method for the treatment of forearm diaphyseal fractures is plate osteosynthesis. Nonoperative treatment may be used for undisplaced fractures or in patients with significant comorbidities, but virtually all fractures are amenable to treatment with a 3.5-mm LC-DCP. However, it is important to realize that the selection of the implant is not the only factor to consider. It is important to have a treatment algorithm when considering the surgical treatment of any fracture, but the complexity of forearm fracture treatment makes this essential. A useful algorithm is:

1. Patient assessment
2. Selection of treatment method
3. Planning of surgery
4. Surgical approach
5. Reduction techniques
6. Postoperative treatment

Patient assessment and selection of the most appropriate treatment method have already been discussed.

Planning of Surgery

It is important to plan the surgical procedure. There are two different ways of doing this. Standard planning as suggested by the AO/ASIF group (73) consists of:

1. Drawing the fragments on transparent paper
2. Aligning the bones by superimposing the transparent sheets on each other
3. Adding a chosen implant template
4. Drawing the final outcome corresponding to the expected postoperative x-ray

This technique is helpful but does not really provide the surgeon will all the tools that allow him or her to deal with the various difficulties that might arise during surgery. An improvement on standard pre-operative planning is "strategic planning." Mast et al (74) have illustrated how important it is not just to have a final vision of what one is aiming at but rather to have a set of steps that helps the surgeon undertake good reduction and fixation.

Strategic Planning

The guidelines for strategic planning are shown in Table 27-6. This method of planning includes a timeframe and a problem list helping the surgeon to anticipate what to do

TABLE 27-6 Guideline for Strategic Planning

Aim?

- Anatomic reduction of all fragments or anatomic alignment of the shaft (length, axial alignment, and rotation)? With or without anatomic reduction of all fragments?

Position of the patient?

Tourniquet?

Approach?

How and when to treat associated ligamentous injuries.

Which side first? Ulna or radius?

Technique of reduction and alternatives?
- Direct or indirect?
- Distractor?

How and when to check adequacy of reduction.
- Image intensifier?
- X-ray?

Wound closure.
- Will it be possible? Swelling, compartment syndrome?
- What to do if closure is not possible?
- How to avoid exposure of the implant?

Required personnel, infrastructure, instruments, and implants? Availability?

and when. It also includes a set of alternatives in case problems arise. Strategic planning has greatly improved our ability to undertake surgery and to minimize potential harm to the patient.

Surgical Approach

The surgical approach must be selected according to the particular requirements imposed by the fracture and the associated soft tissue injury. If there is a compartment syndrome present, the approach should anticipate eventual difficulties in wound closure. The anterior Henry approach is the work horse for the radius; but the dorsolateral Thompson approach offers a useful alternative in specific situations, such as when a soft tissue lesion requires a dorsal approach for adequate debridement. Appropriate planning will often result in the use of an extensile approach, rather than one that can not be modified intraoperatively.

A number of basic surgical techniques should be followed. The surgeon should inflict minimal additional vascular damage to the bone and the soft tissues. This requires meticulous soft tissue preparation, exposing the bone by sharp extraperiosteal dissection and avoiding subperiosteal and circumferential exposure of the bone. To avoid soft tissue damage, it is preferable to use long incisions. Paradoxically, small key-hole incisions may inflict more vascular damage to the bone than longer incisions. Subcutaneous plate insertion is contraindicated in forearm fractures because of the presence of the neurovascular structures in the forearm and because of the presence of numerous muscle origins and insertions. The surgical techniques have already been described.

Reduction Techniques

Repeated attempts at reduction may cause substantial additional damage to the already devascularised bone. It is therefore important to plan how reduction can be achieved. We advocate the use of indirect reduction techniques (74) using the plate to obtain length, axial alignment, and rotation. Figure 27-18 shows the various steps that are required to obtain a straightforward reduction. These are:

1. The approximate application of a slightly pre-bent plate to the proximal or distal main fragment.
2. Slight over-distraction using a solitary screw in the other main fragment and a fracture distractor.
3. Reduction by minimal manipulation of the main fragments with no manipulation of any comminuted fragments.
4. After alignment has been obtained, tensioning of the plate with a tensioning device or clamp will permit compression between the main fragments.

Compression increases stability without damaging the vascularity of the bone and should be obtained when possible. It also helps to transfer more load through the bone and therefore unload the plate. If compression is applied, thinner plates can be used. It is important to use the concept of load sharing—not load bearing—as this provides stable fixation with a minimum of hardware. Standard plates tend to be less bulky than locking screw implants, and the reduced soft tissue compromise and mechanically better osteosynthesis associated with their use explains why locking screw implants do not perform better than conventional plates (65). Conventional plates can be regarded as a gliding splint which allows some seating of the fracture gap after marginal absorption has been produced by osteoclastic activity at the fracture site. Locking screw plates do not allow secondary seating of a fracture gap.

We prefer to use long conventional plates because alignment is easier to obtain and fixation can be achieved with less screws. Typically we use an 8-hole low-contact compression plate using two screws in the proximal and two screws in the distal fragment (Fig. 27-19).

Associated musculoskeletal injuries require special attention. In Galeazzi fracture dislocations anatomical reduction of the radius usually reduces the distal radio-ulnar joint. If

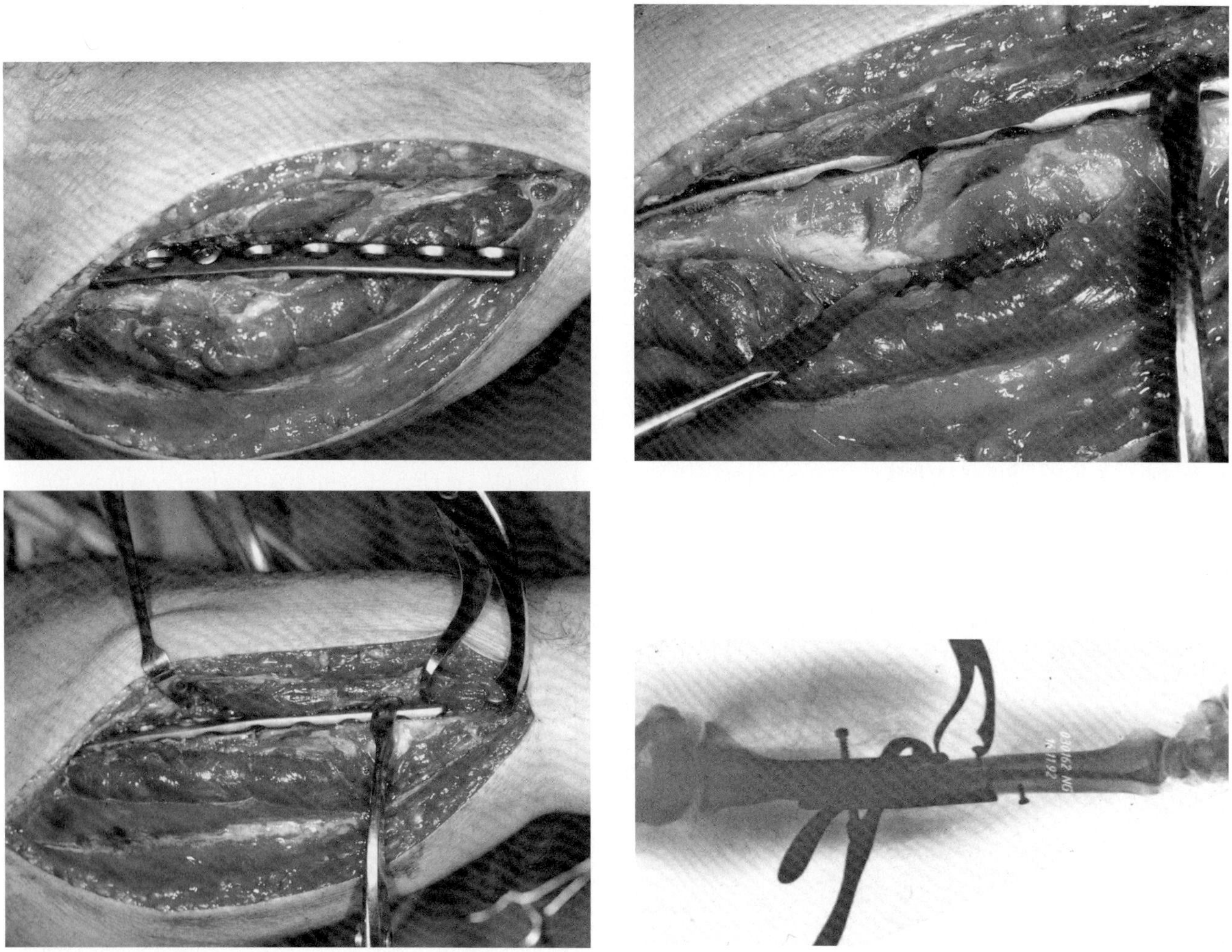

FIGURE 27-18 Reduction technique sequence. **A.** A pre-bent plate is approximately mounted on the proximal fragment to prepare for indirect reduction. **B.** The fragments are gently reduced with minimal manipulation of the main fragments and no manipulation of the accessory fragments and temporarily fixed to the plate with a clamp. **C.** Adequate alignment is obtained. **D.** Compression is applied between the main fragments by the use of a clamp or a tensioning device.

the joint is stable in forearm rotation, no additional treatment is required. Should there be a tendency for dorsal subluxation, the reason for this should be found. The radial fixation should be reevaluated as the radius may have been plated with rotational malalignment. If this is not the case, there may be interposition of the extensor tendons blocking reduction (7).

Additional stabilization of the distal radio-ulnar joint is rarely required. If it is required, it can be accomplished with a simple tension band wiring around the styloid process thus

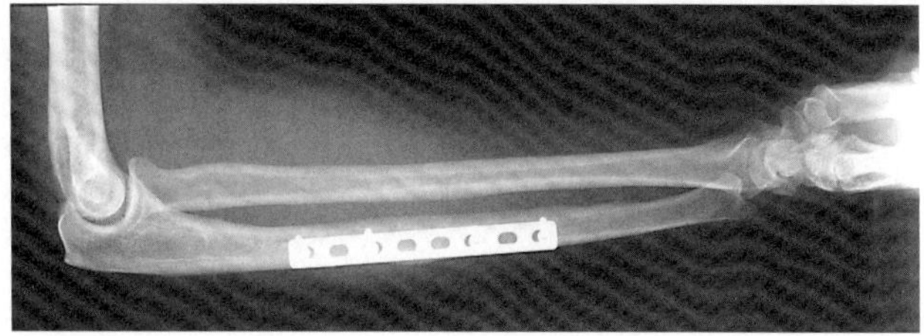
A

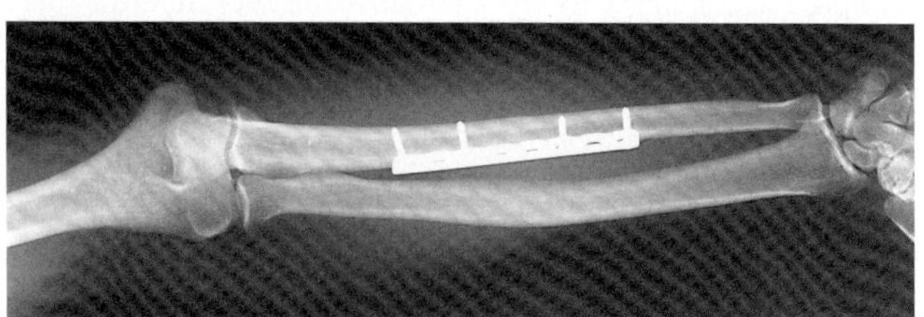
B

FIGURE 27-19 Osteosynthesis using an 8-hole low contact-dynamic compression plate (LC-DCP) with two screws on each side of the fracture.

retensioning the triangular fibro-cartilage complex. We do not advocate transfixion of the radius and ulna with Kirschner wires to maintain alignment, although the technique may be occasionally required (Fig. 27-15).

Similar arguments apply to the proximal radio-ulna joint. Anatomical reduction of the ulna should lead to articular realignment. If this is not the case, there may be interposition of the annular ligament. In young adults Monteggia fractures may not tear the annular ligament. Instead, the radial head may slip out of the intact ligament by axial traction. In this case, reduction of the fracture leads to interposition of the annular ligament and malalignment. In these circumstances, the annular ligament usually needs to be transected to allow proper reduction following which the ligament should be sutured.

In lesions of the interosseous membrane the general principles are:

1. Anatomic reduction of the forearm bones
2. Reduction and stabilization of the proximal and distal radio-ulnar joints
3. Reconstruction of the central oblique band of the interosseous membrane (26) using palmaris longus transplants in selected cases (75)

Postoperative Management

Closed diaphyseal forearm fractures treated with plate osteosynthesis are generally placed in a volar splint which supports the wrist in slight extension for the first week after surgery. The patient is encouraged to actively move the fingers through a full ROM several times a day. To prevent stiffness, the elbow and shoulder should also be fully exercised several times a day. After removal of the splint, forearm rotation is initiated and full movement allowed. The patient is encouraged to use the arm for activities of daily living that do not require significant loading. Lifting heavy weights, using the hand to perform mechanical tasks against resistance, and participating in sports should be avoided until union.

Radiologic signs of union can generally be observed by about 8 weeks. These include bridging callus at the fracture site without any evidence of loosening of the screws or plates. If x-rays show evidence of resorption around the screws, callus formation at the ends of the plate, loosening or fatigue fracture of the implant, surgeons should be suspicious that the primary osteosynthesis procedure may have been inadequate or the patient may not be complying with the postoperative regime. An infection may also be present. The postoperative management of open fractures is essentially similar. However, the soft tissue damage may delay functional rehabilitation and it may not be possible to initiate full mobilization of the arm until a local or distant flap has healed (76). The treatment of open fractures is discussed in Chapter 12.

Pearls and Pitfalls

Pearls

There is a high incidence of associated musculoskeletal injury.

Tense swelling in the forearm suggests compartment syndrome.

In type II Monteggia fracture dislocations, an anterior triangular or quadrilateral anterior fragment must be looked for on x-rays.

It is important to have a good treatment algorithm.

The results of using the 3.5-mm LC-DCP have not been bettered by more modern plates

Pitfalls

Subluxation of dislocation of the DRUJ may develop slowly.

Failure to restore the radial bow will restrict forearm rotation.

Intramedullary nailing frequently does not restore the radial bow.

In initially undisplaced fractures, nonoperative management can be associated with poor results.

Minimally invasive techniques are not recommended.

Early plate removal may cause refracture.

Narrowing of the interosseous space may cause radio-ulnar synostosis.

COMPLICATIONS

Compartment Syndrome

Compartment syndrome is an important complication (77). There are a number of initiating factors. One pathway is tissue hypoxia followed by swelling which further reduces the perfusion pressure at the capillary level, eventually leading to ischemic muscle and myonecrosis. Another more common pathway is direct or indirect muscle damage leading to muscle swelling followed by increased intracompartmental pressure, the pressure rising more quickly if the injury was not severe enough to tear the fascial compartments. Again, increased intracompartmental pressure will lead to reduced capillary blood flow, muscle ischemia, and myonecrosis. As the capillary blood flow will cease at a pressure much lower than the arterial blood flow, palpation of the pulses and the use of laser Doppler will not diagnose an impending compartment syndrome and will only diagnose the established compartment syndrome after it is too late to treat it successfully (21). The most useful clinical sign of acute compartment syndrome is increased pain, which can be tested by passively stretching the fingers in a flexor compartment syndrome or extending the fingers in an extensor compartment syndrome. Compartment syndromes are more common in young men, in patients with low-energy minimally displaced fractures, and in patients with bleeding disorders or who are anticoagulated (78). Further information on compartment syndrome is contained in Chapter 13.

The forearm is the most common site for compartment syndrome in the upper extremity. The three compartments of the forearm include the anterior (or flexor compartment), the posterior (or extensor compartment), and the mobile wad (including brachioradialis and extensor carpi radialis longus and brevis). Flexor digitorum profundus and flexor pollicis longus are the most severely affected muscles because of their deep location.

Initial management consists of removal of occlusive dressings with splitting or removal of a cast. If the symptoms do not resolve rapidly, fasciotomy is indicated. Fasciotomy of the forearm is performed through volar and/or dorsal approaches. The carpal tunnel should be included.

Malunion

As has already been discussed, exact anatomical realignment is crucial to restore forearm function. There is limited literature available on the treatment and outcome of corrected osteotomies after forearm fracture malunion. Trousdale and Linscheid (79) reported on a consecutive series of 27 corrective osteotomies undertaken an average of 73 months after fracture. In 20 patients the indication for surgery was functional loss of forearm rotation with an average arc of prosupination of 72 degrees ranging from 20 degrees to 120 degrees. Nine of these patients underwent the procedure within 12 months of the initial injury and 11 were treated later. The patients who were managed within the first 12 months regained an average of 79 degrees of forearm rotation, while those managed after the first 12 months regained only an average of 30 degrees. It seems therefore that early correction yields better results than late correction if osteotomy is required.

Nonunion

In general, fracture nonunion results from unstable fixation or a compromised blood supply secondary to the severity of the injury or poor surgical technique. As nonoperative management has only limited control of the fracture fragments and stability during healing, it is not surprising that it is associated with substantial rates of nonunion (39,80). Smith and Sage (54) published the results of early attempts at intramedullary fixation of forearm fractures. The use of Kirschner wires introduced with an open technique was associated with an increased risk of nonunion and the results were disappointing.

With the advent of plate osteosynthesis nonunions have been almost eliminated. Following the guidelines of the AO/ASIF group (61) who have promoted the concept of interfragmentary compression, the only fractures that are still associated with a high rate of nonunion are those with substantial bone loss or comminution (42,44,63,81). Although routine bone grafting is not advocated now as there is no evidence that bone grafted fractures have a higher union rate than nonbone grafted fractures (42,62), it is reasonable to bone graft fractures associated with bone loss and devitalized bone fragments. This has helped reduce the rate of nonunion.

In their series of 258 patients treated with compression plating Anderson et al (42) had nonunion rates of 2% to 3%. Chapman et al (44) stated that the nonunion rate should be less than 2% if the proper technique is used in compliant patients. With the exception of severely comminuted or open fractures associated with substantial bone loss and/or significantly traumatized soft tissues, nonunions are usually ascribed to technical errors nowadays. If a correct approach and proper soft tissue handling is employed, the rate of nonunion using compression plate osteosynthesis should be low. If it does occur, re-osteosynthesis with iliac crest cancellous bone grafting is recommended. Figure 27-20 shows an example of a nonunion that healed after re-osteosynthesis with cancellous bone grafting. Nonunion is discussed further in Chapters 8 and 18.

Infection

Nowadays infection after operative treatment of closed fractures is rare if proper surgical technique is employed. The reduction in infection rates has been mainly attributed to improved operative technique, implant development, and peri-operative antibiotic prophylaxis (42,44,82). If infection does occur, surgical treatment with an adequate debridement is recommended. Implant removal should not be undertaken, as in our experience eradication of the infection does not require plate removal and instead requires well-vascularised bone and soft tissues with stable internal fixation. We believe that fracture stability is important and therefore advocate aggressive surgical treatment combined with appropriate antibiotic treatment depending on the bacteria involved in the infection.

Infection rates between 0% to 3% have also been reported for open fractures treated immediately by open reduction and plate fixation (44,83–85). In these fractures, a thorough debridement is crucial for successful treatment. It should be carried out as an emergency procedure on the day of admission with flap reconstruction being performed if required (76). If this approach is employed, the infection rate is minimized; but if infection does occur, it requires an aggressive surgical approach with resection of all infected and devitalized soft tissues and reconstruction of any bone defects and flap cover as required. Infection is discussed further in Chapter 18.

Plate Removal and Refracture

Plate removal is not without complications (86). In addition to the operative complications of infection, hematoma or neurovascular damage, refracture after plate removal is not uncommon. The literature reports refracture rates from as low as 4% (44,63,87) up to 25% (88). Deluca et al (88) and Hidaka and Gustilo (89) have identified that an inadequate technique, delayed union or nonunion, and plate removal less than 1 year after injury are the most important causes of refracture (Table 27-7). Refracture has also been linked to local osteoporosis visible as a radiolucency under the plate. This was initially thought

TABLE 27-7 Risk Factors for Refracture

Inadequate technique
Delayed union/nonunion
Premature plate removal (<1 year after injury)

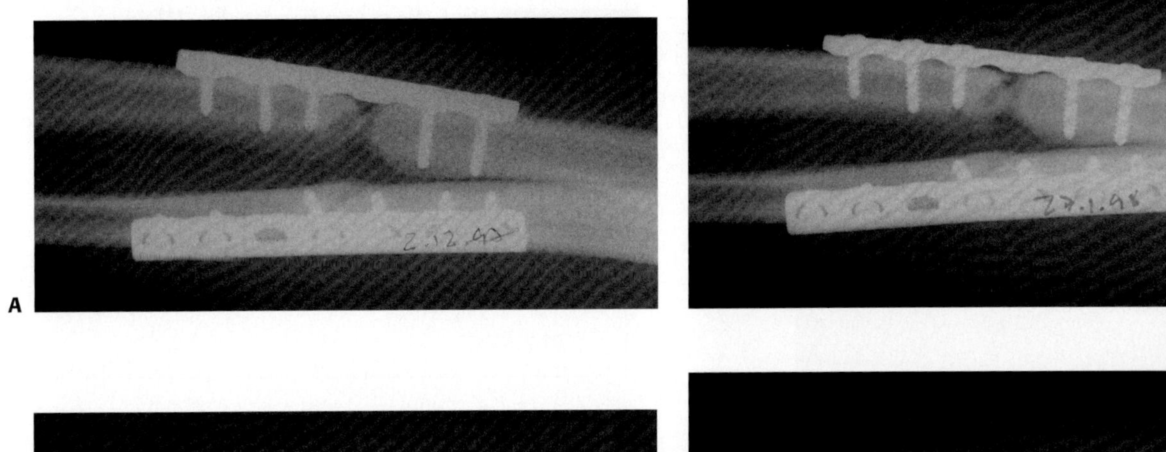

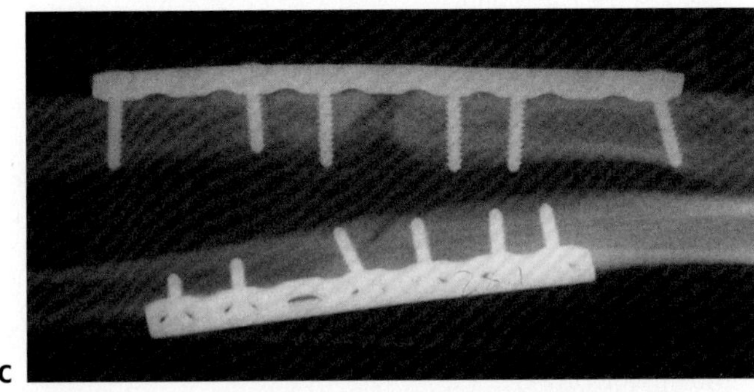

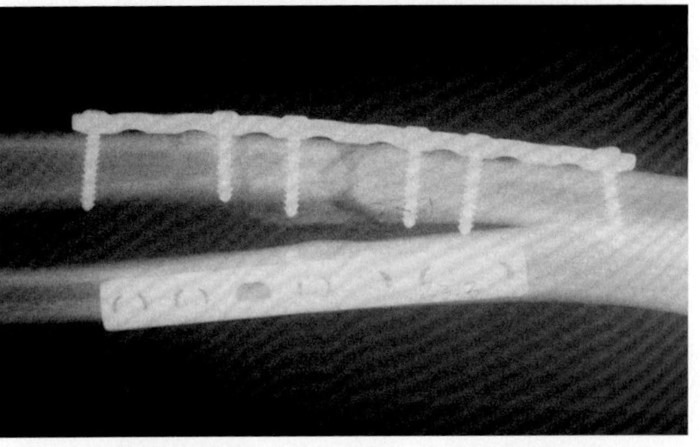

FIGURE 27-20 **A.** The fracture of the radius shows no union 3 months after surgery, while on the ulna callus formation is visible. **B.** After another 1.5 months, the fracture still showed no signs of healing. **C.** Re-osteosynthesis was performed by using a longer plate and compression together with cancellous bone grafting. **D.** Follow-up 2 months after revision surgery shows callus formation at the fracture site.

to be due to stress protection following application of the plate (88,90), but it has been demonstrated that the initial osteoporosis is the result of impaired local blood supply to the cortical bone under the plate. If plate removal is to be undertaken, it is therefore clear that the bone should be allowed to remodel before the plate is removed. It has been suggested that remodeling takes up to 21 months to complete (91,92). We do not advocate routine plate removal in the asymptomatic patient.

Radio-Ulnar Synostosis

Radio-ulnar synostosis, or crossed union between the radius and ulnar (Fig. 27-21), is rarely reported either because it rarely occurs or because it is an issue that is not addressed. However, it is an important problem as it may severely impair forearm function by limiting the rotational amplitude. In a review of 2,381 forearm fractures, an incidence of about 2% was reported (93); and it is suggested that the incidence is higher in type IV Monteggia fractures involving both bones of the forearm together with a radial head dislocation. Another study reported an incidence of 6.6% in a series of 167 patients, more than half of which were fractures of both bones of the forearm (94). In patients with co-existing head trauma, the incidence of radio-ulnar synostosis has been reported as high as 18% in a mixed group of nonoperative and operatively treated patients (95).

The most important risk factors for the development of radio-ulnar synostosis are summarized in Table 27-8 and include high-energy trauma open fractures (96,97), infection, head injuries (93,95), and where internal fixation is delayed by several weeks (93,94). Surgical factors include narrowing of the interosseous space by imperfect reduction, bone grafting, and overlong screws that transgress the interosseous space or may impinge in the proximal third of the forearm (38,98).

Restoration of forearm rotation after radio-ulnar synostosis has occurred involves surgical excision with interposition of silicone rubber, muscle, or fat grafts. The results of surgical excision in combination with these procedures are unfortunately not very encouraging with an average rotation of 55 degrees with a mean follow-up of 40 months (99). Combining surgical resection with low-dose radiation has yielded better results (100). Restoration of forearm rotation in the presence of a proximal-third synostosis is difficult because of a subsequent loss of rotational amplitude after the surgical procedure due to heterotopic ossification or scarring. Jupiter and Ring (101) reported on a series of 18 forearms in 17 patients. Using surgical resection with adjuvant radiotherapy an average forearm rotation of 139° was reported in patients who underwent surgery as early as 6 months after the injury. Recently Kamineni et al (102) published the results of a series of seven patients

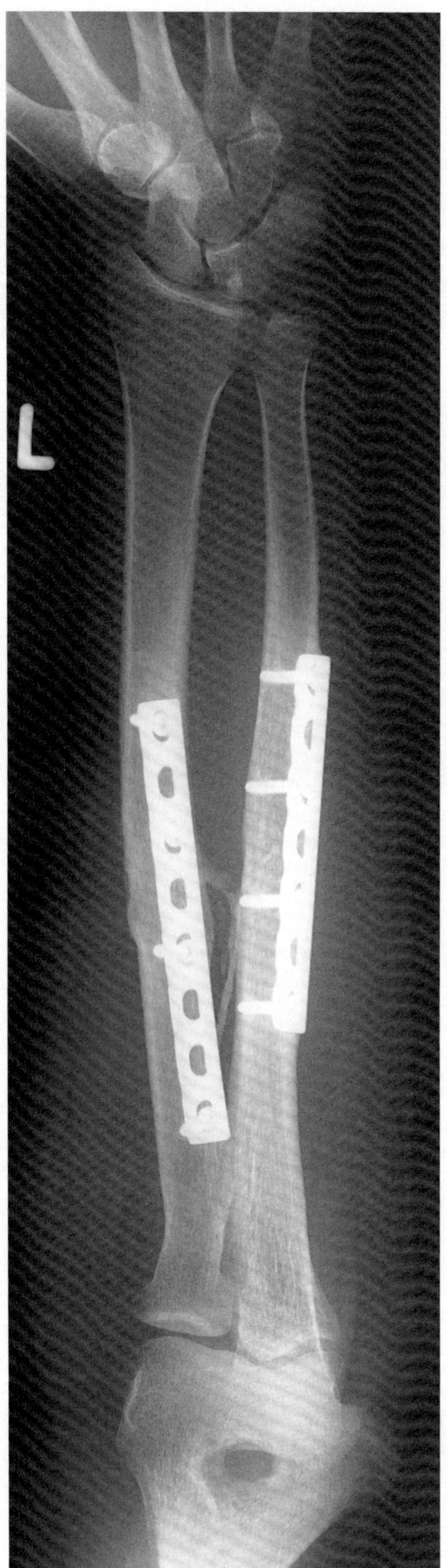

FIGURE 27-21 A radio-ulnar synostosis.

TABLE 27-8 Risk Factors for Radio-Ulnar Synostosis

General
- Open fractures
- Infection
- Multiply-injured patients with head trauma
- Delayed internal fixation

Surgical (less common)
- Narrowing the interosseous space by nonanatomic reduction
- Use of too long screws
- Bone grafting

with radio-ulnar synostosis who were treated by resection of a 1-cm section of the proximal radius distal to the synostosis. Initially the seven patients started with a mean fixed pronation of 5 degrees, but at an average follow-up of 80 months the mean forearm rotation was 98 degrees.

We believe that the use of a nontraumatic surgical technique and rehabilitation with early mobilization should prevent the development of radio-ulnar synostosis. However, if it occurs, there are surgical treatment options which provide an improvement in forearm rotation.

Neurovascular Complications

A number of neurovascular complications are iatrogenic and are caused either by the surgery, the use of a tourniquet, or positioning the patient on the table incorrectly. If an anterior Henry approach is used, the superficial radial nerve and the radial artery need to be protected and care has to be taken not to over-retract the nerve thereby causing a neuropraxia. The posterior interosseous nerve is at risk in both the anterior and dorsolateral Thompson approach and care must be taken when the supinator muscle is elevated subperiosteally, as the posterior interosseous nerve runs in this muscle and exits in the arcade of Frohse.

CONTROVERSIES AND FUTURE DIRECTIONS

Surgeons always seek to treat their patients better. Ideally it would be desirable to obtain a higher union rate, avoid any malalignment, and consistently obtain full function following treatment. These goals were largely addressed in the second half of the last century, and in expert hands good results should be obtained.

If results are poor, it is usually due to factors that are difficult to control, such as bone and soft tissue devascularization, contamination, and an impaired immune response. It is therefore unlikely that developing new implants is going to materially improve existing results.

Future developments should therefore perhaps focus on

other aspects, such as the type of surgery and the precise operative technique that is used. Theoretically it might be desirable to develop minimally invasive treatment techniques providing the injured patient with a less painful and more efficient method of restoring function quickly. As has already been pointed out, this is difficult if plate fixation is used and would seem to indicate that the future might lie with intramedullary nailing. Unfortunately the use of intramedullary nailing in the forearm is not as atraumatic as it would initially appear. Restoration of the normal bow of the radius and the shape of the ulna is not consistently achieved and rotational stability is poor particularly in AO (OTA) type B and type C fractures. It is certainly possible that even with improved intramedullary nails, minimally invasive surgery might be achieved at the expense of functional outcome. Minimally invasive osteosynthesis aims at minimizing damage to all soft tissues including those that immediately surround the bone, but it is unlikely that percutaneous plating is going to be as successful in forearm fractures as in other fractures because of the local anatomy. However, it is possible that improving reduction techniques will help to facilitate the surgery and may prove to be more beneficial than merely inventing new implants and plant introduction techniques (103).

ACKNOWLEDGMENT

The authors would like to acknowledge and thank Dr. Norman Espinosa for the illustrations he provided for our chapter.

REFERENCES

1. Griggs SM, Weiss AP. Bony injuries of the wrist, forearm, and elbow. *Clin Sports Med* 1996;15(2):373–400.
2. Goldberg HD, Young JW, Reiner BI, et al. Double injuries of the forearm: a common occurrence. *Radiology* 1992;185(1):223–227.
3. Galeazzi R. Ueber ein besonderes Syndrom bei Verletzungen im Bereich der Unterarmknochen. *Arch Orthop Unfallchir* 1934;35:557–562.
4. Rang M. *Anthology of Orthopaedics*. Edinburgh: E & S Livingstone; 1968.
5. Hughston JC. Fracture of the distal radial shaft: Mistakes in Management. *J Bone Joint Surg* 1957;39A:249–264.
6. Nicolaidis SC, Hildreth DH, Lichtman DM. Acute injuries of the distal radioulnar joint. *Hand Clin* 2000;16(3):449–459.
7. Bruckner JD, Lichtman DM, Alexander AH. Complex dislocations of the distal radioulnar joint. Recognition and management. *Clin Orthop* 1992;(275):90–103.
8. Monteggia GB. *Instituzioni Chirurgiche* Vol. 5. Milano: Maspero; 1814.
9. Bado JL. The Monteggia lesion. *Clin Orthop* 1967;50:71–86.
10. Jupiter JB, Leibovic SJ, Ribbans W, et al. The posterior Monteggia lesion. *J Orthop Trauma* 1991;5(4):395–402.
11. Morris AH. Irreducible Monteggia lesion with radial nerve entrapment. *J Bone Joint Surg* 1974;56A:1744.
12. Jessing P. Monteggia lesions and their complicating nerve damage. *Acta Orthop Scand* 1975;46:601–609.
13. Neiman R, Maiocco B, Deeney VF. Ulnar nerve injury after closed forearm fractures in children. *J Pediatr Orthop* 1998;18(5):683–685.
14. Stahl S, Rozen N, Michaelson M. Ulnar nerve injury following midshaft forearm fractures in children. *J Hand Surg (Br)* 1997;22(6):788–789.
15. Huang K, Pun WK, Coleman S. Entrapment and transection of the median nerve associated with greenstick fractures of the forearm: case report and review of the literature. *J Trauma* 1998;44(6):1101–1102.
16. Jupiter JB, Kleinert HE. Vascular injuries in the upper extremity. In: Tubiana R, ed. *The Hand*. Philadelphia: W.B. Saunders; 1988:593.
17. Levin LS, Goldner RD, Urbaniak JR, et al. Management of severe musculoskeletal injuries of the upper extremity. *J Orthop Trauma* 1990;4(4):432–440.
18. Eaton RG, Green WT. Volkmann's ischemia. A volar compartment syndrome of the forearm. *Clin Orthop* 1975;(113):58–64.
19. Blick SS, Brumback RJ, Poka A, et al. Compartment syndrome in open tibial fractures. *J Bone Joint Surg Am* 1986;68(9):1348–1353.
20. Hargens AR, Akeson WH, Mubarak SJ, et al. Kappa Delta Award paper. Tissue fluid pressures: from basic research tools to clinical applications. *J Orthop Res* 1989;7(6):902–909.
21. Matsen FA 3rd, Winquist RA, Krugmire RB Jr. Diagnosis and management of compartmental syndromes. *J Bone Joint Surg Am* 1980;62(2):286–291.
22. Whitesides TE, Haney TC, Morimoto K, et al. Tissue pressure measurements as a determinant for the need of fasciotomy. *Clin Orthop* 1975;(113):43–51.
23. Heckman MM, Whitesides TE Jr, Grewe SR, et al. Histologic determination of the ischemic threshold of muscle in the canine compartment syndrome model. *J Orthop Trauma* 1993;7(3):199–210.
24. McQueen MM, Court-Brown CM. Compartment monitoring in tibial fractures. The pressure threshold for decompression. *J Bone Joint Surg Br* 1996;78(1):99–104.
25. Müller ME, ed. *The Comprehensive Classification of Fractures of Long Bones*. Berlin: Springer-Verlag; 1990.
26. Hotchkiss RN, An KN, Sowa DT, et al. An anatomic and mechanical study of the interosseous membrane of the forearm: pathomechanics of proximal migration of the radius. *J Hand Surg (Am)* 1989;4(2 Pt 1): 256–261.
27. Sage FP. Medullary fixation of fractures of the forearm. A study of the medullary canal of the radius and a report of fifty fractures of the radius treated with a prebent triangular nail. *Am J Orthop* 1959;41-A:1489–1516.
28. Matthews LS, Kaufer H, Garver DF, et al. The effect on supination-pronation of angular malalignment of fractures of both bones of the forearm. *J Bone Joint Surg Am* 1982; 64(1):14–17.
29. Tarr RR, Garfinkel AI, Sarmiento A. The effects of angular and rotational deformities of both bones of the forearm. An in vitro study. *J Bone Joint Surg Am* 1984;66(1): 65–70.
30. Schemitsch EH, Richards RR. The effect of malunion on functional outcome after plate fixation of fractures of both bones of the forearm in adults. *J Bone Joint Surg Am* 1992; 74(7):1068–1078.
31. Dumont CE, Thalmann R, Macy JC. The effect of rotational malunion of the radius and the ulna on supination and pronation. *J Bone Joint Surg Br* 2002;84(7):1070–1074.
32. Henry AK. *Extensile Exposure*, 2nd ed. Baltimore: Williams & Wilkins; 1970.
33. Thompson JE. Anatomical methods of approach in operations on the long bones of the extremities. *Ann Surg* 1918;68:309.
34. Davies F, Laird M. The supinator muscle and the deep radial (posterior interosseous) nerve. *Anat Rec* 1948;101:243.
35. Hoppenfeld S, deBoer P. *Surgical Exposures in Orthopaedics: The Anatomic Approach*. Philadelphia: J. B. Lippincott; 1994.
36. Mackay D, Wood L, Rangan A. The treatment of isolated ulnar fractures in adults: a systematic review. *Injury* 2000;31(8):565–570.
37. Sarmiento A, Latta LL, Zych G, et al. Isolated ulnar shaft fractures treated with functional braces. *J Orthop Trauma* 1998;12(6):420–423; discussion 423–424.
38. Knight RA, Purvis GD. Fractures of both bones of the forearm in adults. *J Bone Joint Surg* 1949;31A:755–764.
39. Bolton H, Quinlan AG. The conservative treatment of fractures of the shaft of the radius and the ulna in adults. *Lancet* 1952;1:700.
40. Evans EM. Rotational deformities in the treatment of fractures of both bones of the forearm. *J Bone Joint Surg* 1945;27A:373.
41. Patrick J. A study of supination and pronation with especial reference to the treatment of forearm fractures. *J Bone Joint Surg* 1946;28B:737–748.
42. Anderson LD, Sisk D, Tooms RE, et al. Compression-plate fixation in acute diaphyseal fractures of the radius and ulna. *J Bone Joint Surg Am* 1975;57(3):287–287.
43. Rosacker JA, Kopta JA. Both bone fractures of the forearm: A review of surgical variables associated with union. *Orthopaedics* 1981;4:1353–1356.
44. Chapman MW, Gordon JE, Zissimos AG. Compression-plate fixation of acute fractures of the diaphyses of the radius and ulna. *J Bone Joint Surg Am* 1989;71(2):159–169.
45. Hadden WA, Reschauer R, Seggl W. Results of AO plate fixation of forearm shaft fractures in adults. *Injury* 1983;15(1):44–52.
46. Langkamer VG, Ackroyd CE. Internal fixation of forearm fractures in the 1980s: lessons to be learnt. *Injury* 1991;22(2):97–102.
47. Sarmiento A, Cooper JS, Sinclair WF. Forearm fractures. Early functional bracing—A preliminary report. *J Bone Joint Surg Am* 1975;57(3):297–304.
48. Sarmiento A, Latta LL. *Closed Functional Treatment of Fractures*. Berlin: Springer-Verlag; 1981.
49. DeLee JC. External fixation of the forearm and the wrist. *Orthop Rev* 1981;6:43–48.
50. Cooney WP 3rd, DK Smith. External fixation of the upper extremity. *Instr Course Lect* 1987;36:455–469.
51. Helber MU, Ulrich C. External fixation in forearm shaft fractures. *Injury* 2000;31(Suppl 1):45–47.
52. Flinkkila T, Ristiniemi J, Hyvonen P, et al. Nonbridging external fixation in the treatment of unstable fractures of the distal forearm. *Arch Orthop Trauma Surg* 2003;123(7): 349–352.
53. Putnam MD, Walsh TM 4th. External fixation for open fractures of the upper extremity. *Hand Clin* 1993;9(4):613–623.
54. Smith H, Sage FP. Medullary fixation of forearm fractures. *J Bone Joint Surg* 1957;39A: 91–98.
55. Aho AJ, Nieminen SJ, Salo U, et al. Antebrachium fractures: rush pin fixation today in the light of late results. *J Trauma* 1984;24(7):604–610.
56. Street DM. Intramedullary forearm nailing. *Clin Orthop* 1986;(212):219–230.
57. Schemitsch EH, Jones D, Henley MB, et al. A comparison of malreduction after plate and intramedullary nail fixation of forearm fractures. *J Orthop Trauma* 1995;9(1):8–16.
58. Jones DJ, Henley MB, Schemitsch EH, et al. A biomechanical comparison of two methods of fixation of fractures of the forearm. *J Orthop Trauma* 1995;9(3):198–206.

59. Van der Reis WL, Otsuka NY, Moroz P, et al. Intramedullary nailing versus plate fixation for unstable forearm fractures in children. *J Pediatr Orthop* 1998;18(1):9–13.
60. Lascombes P, Prevot J, Ligier JN, et al. Elastic stable intramedullary nailing in forearm shaft fractures in children: 85 cases. *J Pediatr Orthop* 1990;10(2):167–171.
61. Müller ME, Allgöwer M, Willenegger H. *Technique of Internal Fixation of Fractures*. New York: Springer-Verlag; 1965.
62. Wright RR, Schmeling GJ, Schwab JP. The necessity of acute bone grafting in diaphyseal forearm fractures: a retrospective review. *J Orthop Trauma* 1997;11(4):288–294.
63. Dodge HS, Cady GW. Treatment of fractures of the radius and ulna with compression plates. *J Bone Joint Surg Am* 1972;54(6):1167–1176.
64. Hertel R, Pisan M, Lambert S, et al. Plate osteosynthesis of diaphyseal fractures of the radius and ulna. *Injury* 1996;27(8):545–548.
65. Leung F, Chow SP. A prospective, randomized trial comparing the limited contact dynamic compression plate with the point contact fixator for forearm fractures. *J Bone Joint Surg Am* 2003;85-A(12):2343–2348.
66. Rüedi TP, Murphy WM. *AO principles of fracture management*. Stuttgart, New York: Thieme; 2000.
67. Perren SM, Klaue K, Pohler O, et al. The limited contact dynamic compression plate (LC-DCP). *Arch Orthop Trauma Surg* 1990;109(6):304–310.
68. Field JR, Hearn TC, Caldwell CB. Bone plate fixation: an evaluation of interface contact area and force of the dynamic compression plate (DCP) and the limited contact-dynamic compression plate (LC-DCP) applied to cadaveric bone. *J Orthop Trauma* 1997;11(5):368–373.
69. Gunst MA, Suter C, Rahn BA. [Bone perfusion after plate osteosynthesis. A study of the intact rabbit tibia with disulfin blue vital staining]. *Helv Chir Acta* 1979;46(1–2): 171–175.
70. Tepic S, Perren SM. The biomechanics of the PC-Fix internal fixator. *Injury* 1995; 26(Suppl 2):5–10.
71. Hertel R, Eijer H, Meisser A, et al. Biomechanical and biological considerations relating to the clinical use of the point contact-fixator—evaluation of the device handling test in the treatment of diaphyseal fractures of the radius and/or ulna. *Injury* 2001;32(Suppl 2):B10–14.
72. Miclau T, Remiger A, Tepic S, et al. A mechanical comparison of the dynamic compression plate, limited contact-dynamic compression plate, and point contact fixator. *J Orthop Trauma* 1995;9(1):17–22.
73. Muller ME, Allgower M, Schneider R, et al. *Manual of Internal Fixation: Techniques Recommended by the AO-ASIF Group*. Berlin, New York: Springer-Verlag; 1991.
74. Mast J, Jakob R, Ganz R. *Planning and Reduction Technique in Fracture Surgery*. Berlin, New York: Springer-Verlag; 1989.
75. Ruch DS, Chang DS, Koman LA. Reconstruction of longitudinal stability of the forearm after disruption of interosseous ligament and radial head excision (Essex-Lopresti lesion). *J South Orthop Assoc* 1999;8(1):47–52.
76. Hertel R, Lambert SM, Muller S, et al. On the timing of soft-tissue reconstruction for open fractures of the lower leg. *Arch Orthop Trauma Surg* 1999;119(1–2):7–12.
77. Brostrom LA, Stark A, Svartengren G. Acute compartment syndrome in forearm fractures. *Acta Orthop Scand* 1990;61(1):50–53.
78. McQueen MM, Gaston P, Court-Brown CM. Acute compartment syndrome. Who is at risk? *J Bone Joint Surg Br* 2000;82(2):200–203.
79. Trousdale RT, Linscheid RL. Operative treatment of malunited fractures of the forearm. *J Bone Joint Surg Am* 1995;77(6):894–902.
80. Brakenbury H, Corea JR, Blakemore ME. Nonunion of the isolated fracture of the ulnar shafts in adults. *Injury* 1985;12:371.
81. Teipner WA, Mast JW. Internal fixation of forearm fractures: Double plating versus single compression (tension band) plating. A comparative study. *Orthop Clin North Am* 1980;11:381.
82. Mih AD, Cooney WP, Idler RS, et al. Long-term follow-up of forearm bone diaphyseal plating. *Clin Orthop* 1994;(299):256–258.
83. Duncan R, Geissler W, Freeland AE, et al. Immediate internal fixation of open fractures of the diaphysis of the forearm. *J Orthop Trauma* 1992;6(1):25–31.
84. Jones JA. Immediate internal fixation of high-energy open forearm fractures. *J Orthop Trauma* 1991;5(3):272–279.
85. Moed BR, Kellam JF, Foster RJ, et al. Immediate internal fixation of open fractures of the diaphysis of the forearm. *J Bone Joint Surg Am* 1986;68(7):1008–1017.
86. Bednar DA, Grandwilewski W. Complications of forearm-plate removal. *Can J Surg* 1992;35(4):428–431.
87. Labosky DA, Cermak MB, Waggy CA. Forearm fracture plates: to remove or not to remove. *J Hand Surg (Am)* 1990;15(2):294–301.
88. Deluca A, Lindsey RW, Ruwe A. Refracture of bones of the forearm after the removal of compression plates. *J Bone Joint Surg Am* 1988;70(9):1372–1376.
89. Hidaka S, Gustilo RB. Refracture of bones of the forearm after plate removal. *J Bone Joint Surg Am* 1984;66(8):1241–1243.
90. Kettunen J, Kroger H, Bowditch M, et al. Bone mineral density after removal of rigid plates from forearm fractures: preliminary report. *J Orthop Sci* 2003;8(6):772–776.
91. Rosson JW, Petley GW, Shearer JR. Bone structure after removal of internal fixation plates. *J Bone Joint Surg Br* 1991;73(1):65–67.
92. Rosson JW, Shearer JR. Refracture after the removal of plates from the forearm. An avoidable complication. *J Bone Joint Surg Br* 1991;73(3):415–417.
93. Vince KG, Miller JE. Cross-union complicating fracture of the forearm. Part I: Adults. *J Bone Joint Surg Am* 1987;69(5):640–653.
94. Bauer G, Arand M, Mutschler W. Post-traumatic radioulnar synostosis after forearm fracture osteosynthesis. *Arch Orthop Trauma Surg* 1991;110(3):142–145.
95. Garland DE, Dowling V. Forearm fractures in the head-injured adult. *Clin Orthop* 1983; (176):190–196.
96. Maempel FZ. Post-traumatic radioulnar synostosis. A report of two cases. *Clin Orthop* 1984;(186):182–185.
97. Breit R. Post-traumatic radioulnar synostosis. *Clin Orthop* 1983;(174):149–152.
98. Botting TD. Posttraumatic radio-ulna cross union. *J Trauma* 1970;10(1):16–24.
99. Failla JM, Amadio C, Morrey BF. Post-traumatic proximal radio-ulnar synostosis. Results of surgical treatment. *J Bone Joint Surg Am* 1989;71(8):1208–1213.
100. Thurston AJ, Spry NA. Post-traumatic radio-ulnar synostosis treated by surgical excision and adjunctive radiotherapy. *Aust N Z J Surg* 1993;63(12):976–980.
101. Jupiter JB, Ring D. Operative treatment of post-traumatic proximal radioulnar synostosis. *J Bone Joint Surg Am* 1998;80(2):248–257.
102. Kamineni S, Maritz NG, Morrey BF. Proximal radial resection for posttraumatic radioulnar synostosis: a new technique to improve forearm rotation. *J Bone Joint Surg Am* 2002;84-A(5):745–751.
103. Leunig M, Hertel R, Siebenrock KA, et al. The evolution of indirect reduction techniques for the treatment of fractures. *Clin Orthop Relat Res* 2000;(375):7–14.

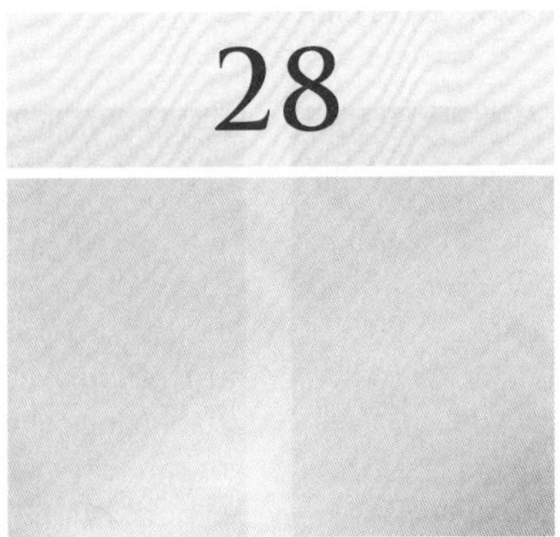

FRACTURES AND DISLOCATIONS OF THE ELBOW

David Ring

(34). It can be more straightforward to define a safe area intraoperatively by applying a plate as posteriorly as possible with the forearm in full supination (35) or as the area on the proximal radius corresponding to that area between Lister's tubercle and the radial styloid on the distal radius (Fig. 28-8) (36).

The anatomy of the radial head is difficult to replicate with a prosthesis (37). It has a slightly elliptical cross section and interdigitates precisely with both the lesser sigmoid notch and the lateral lip of the trochlea, not to mention the capitellar articular surface (10). The slight angulation of the proximal radius with respect to the shaft further complicates attempts to reconstruct or replace the radius.

The triceps have a very broad and thick insertion onto the posterior and proximal aspects of the olecranon. This is notable during the application of a plate that contours around this portion of the bone—if the center of the triceps insertion is not split and elevated from the bone, the proximal aspect of the plate will rest well off the bone. For complex olecranon fractures this compromise may sometimes be preferable to additional dissection of the soft tissue attachments.

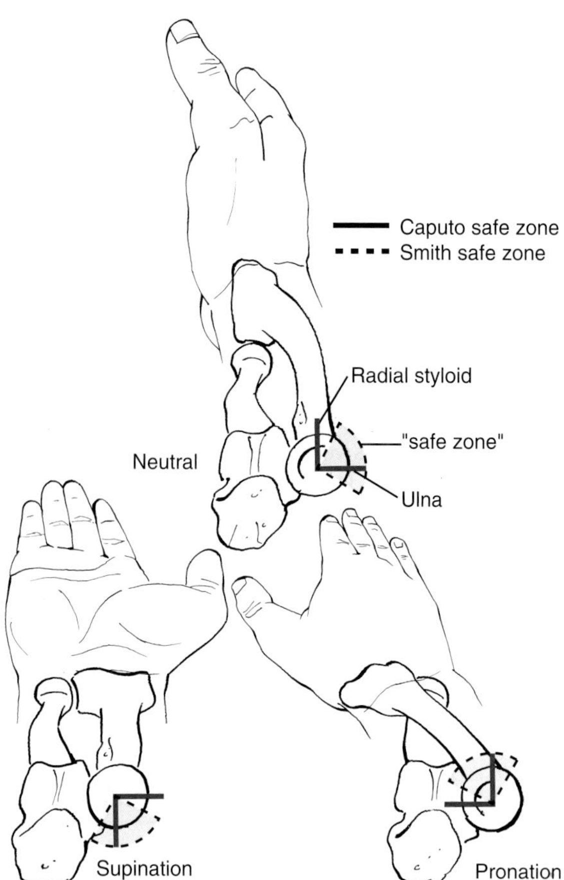

FIGURE 28-8 The nonarticular area of the radial head—or the so-called safe zone for the application of internal fixation devices—has been defined in various ways. Smith and Hotchkiss defined it based on lines bisecting the radial head made in full supination, full pronation, and neutral. Implants can be placed as far as half way between the middle and posterior lines and a few millimeters beyond half way between the middle and anterior lines. Caputo and colleagues recommend using the radial styloid and Lister's tubercle as intraoperative guides to this safe zone, but this describes a slightly different zone.

GENERAL FEATURES OF ELBOW INJURIES

Several features of elbow injuries are similar for very different injury types and are best considered in general before reviewing the specific injury types.

Mechanism

Elbow injuries occur in identifiable patterns that are determined by the injury forces or mechanism, the energy of the injury, and the quality of the underlying bone. Recognition of the injury pattern helps with management of the injury and counseling of the patient.

Signs and Symptoms

Patients with fractures and dislocations of the elbow present variable degrees of pain, swelling, and ecchymosis. In many cases there is also instability, crepitation, and deformity.

Associated Injuries

Relatively few of these injuries are associated with open wounds or acute neurovascular injury. Most elbow injuries occur in isolation with ipsilateral skeletal injuries and polytrauma being much less common.

Rationale

The key element of the treatment of elbow injuries is restoration of a congruent articular reduction. Malaligned articular surfaces or instability will restrict motion and cause arthrosis that is difficult to salvage (13,38). In contrast, a stiff but congruent elbow joint can often be restored to good function with secondary surgeries even when there is extensive heterotopic bone, an ununited fracture, or ulnar neuropathy (39–42). Although the majority of elbow injuries benefit from early active use and exercise, with complex articular fractures and very unstable elbows it can be better to err on the side of a healed and congruent but stiff elbow by delaying mobilization or even—in rare instances—cross-pinning the joint.

Recognition of the injury pattern leads directly to an understanding of the injury components. Appropriate treatment of each injury component will help avoid pitfalls and provide the best opportunity for recovery.

Rehabilitation

The hand is typically swollen and ecchymotic after an elbow injury and can become permanently stiff if confident active exercises are not encouraged.

Active exercises and gentle functional use of the arm for daily activities is usually initiated within a few days, most often the morning after surgery. The patient is encouraged to use his or her other hand, gravity, and pushing against other objects to help assist with elbow mobilization.

Passive manipulation by a therapist or family member is discouraged. There is a long-standing belief that this will contribute to heterotopic bone formation. It may also be more likely to loosen implants or impede healing. Finally, the patient must learn how to mobilize his or her own arm if the exercise program is to be effective.

In the treatment of traumatic elbow instability, when the x-ray shows slight sagging or subluxation of an otherwise concentrically reduced joint, this can usually be addressed by encouraging confident active motion of the elbow (9,43). This adds a dynamic muscular component of stability, which overcomes what is likely a type of pseudo-subluxation of the joint. More substantial subluxations should be treated operatively as they risk damage to the articular surface. Given the useful dynamic component of stability, combined with the fact that the elbow can dislocate in a cast when unstable, the value of casts or braces for enhancing elbow stability must be questioned—this author does not use them. The idea of an extension block brace is also common, but probably not usually necessary because patients usually struggle to regain extension.

For some elbow injuries—distal humerus fractures in particular—many surgeons prefer to immobilize the elbow in maximum extension overnight, before initiating active exercises (44). The rationale for this is that flexion is easier to regain than extension. Considering the following counterpoints, I no longer immobilize the elbow in extension: (a) even an overnight immobilization will make the patient stiff in that position and flexion is more important functionally than extension—if an anxious patient has trouble with exercises, they can often fail to regain flexion; (b) if the ulnar nerve is transposed, immobilization in extension will bring it to a more posterior position where it may be more vulnerable at subsequent operations; (c) the braces for elbow extension are much better than those for elbow flexion—I think it is easier to regain extension in a very stiff elbow. Elbow braces for stiffness can be either static progressive (a position of static stretch is applied and adjusted as the pain dissipates) or dynamic (a constant dynamic force is applied to the elbow). Some hinged external fixators incorporate a static progressive stretch mechanism.

When an LCL injury or an anteromedial facet coronoid fracture is repaired, it is useful to avoid shoulder abduction for a few weeks—so-called varus stress precautions (9).

The use of continuous passive elbow motion (using various devices) with or without continuous anesthesia via a brachial plexus catheter is gaining in popularity in spite of the lack of evidence that it improves elbow motion. It is not clear that the additional risk and cost are justified. I believe that active elbow motion is the key and that motivated patients will do better—I therefore shy away from passive treatments.

Complications

Stiffness and Heterotopic Ossification

Stiffness is a complication that is common to all elbow injuries (4). Some permanent loss of elbow motion is to be expected for all but the simplest injuries, usually it is a loss of extension. Severe loss of motion is often associated with heterotopic ossification, joint incongruity, ulnar neuropathy, or arthrosis. In the absence of these associated problems, a program of active-assisted exercises supplemented by static progressive or dynamic elbow splints can improve motion to a functional range in a large percentage of patients (45,46). With complex or unresponsive stiffness, operative release of the contracted capsule, the constricted ulnar nerve, heterotopic bone, and osteophytes can often improve motion (24). Passive manipulation of the elbow in an attempt to regain motion is generally discouraged for fear of causing heterotopic bone, inhibiting healing, or fracturing the arm.

The formation of heterotopic ossification can be reduced by the administration of a single local 700 Gy dose of radiation (47) and, to some degree, by nonsteroidal anti-inflammatory medications (48). Both of these interventions may also inhibit fracture healing. Radiation also has a potential cancer risk that must be respected. It is still recommended that these prophylactic measures be used selectively. Patients with head injuries, high-energy fracture-dislocations, and repeat surgery during the first few weeks of treatment are at the highest risk for substantial heterotopic ossification.

Ulnar Neuropathy

The ulnar nerve is vulnerable to constriction as it runs through the cubital tunnel fascia and Osbourne's fascia. Cubital tunnel syndrome—a gradually developing, chronic ulnar neuropathy—is quite common after elbow trauma (49), likely due to the swelling, bleeding, tissue injury and distortion, scar formation and tissue contracture, heterotopic ossification, and arthrosis that develop after injury. Consideration has been given to routine in situ decompression of the ulnar nerve for some fractures that seem to be particularly at risk, such as fracture-dislocations of the elbow. There is an ongoing debate about whether or not to perform a complete anterior subcutaneous transposition of the ulnar nerve when treating a fracture of the distal humerus, or whether a limited mobilization is sufficient to protect the nerve.

An ulnar neuropathy that develops after treatment of the injury can contribute to stiffness and pain in addition to affecting hand function (50). It is important to be aware of the importance of the ulnar nerve and always evaluate for symptoms and signs of ulnar nerve dysfunction, being particularly suspicious when stiffness or pain are greater than might otherwise be expected.

Acute ulnar nerve dysfunction with an intact nerve (due to either the injury or handling of the nerve during surgery) usually, but not always, recovers. In can take a very long time, in some cases a year or more to recover. Serial clinical examination and nerve conduction studies and electromyography can help determine if surgical intervention is worthwhile. Operative treatment is considered if serial neurophysiological testing does not demonstrate improvement or if there is obvious worsening of the deficit on examination.

Instability

Truly unstable elbows or flail elbows are usually related to bone loss or nonunion (51). Instability after a fracture-dislocation usually refers to residual malalignment and incongruity of the elbow (13,52). This will lead to arthrosis and must be addressed as soon as possible. Even a few weeks of elbow motion and use in a malaligned position can permanently damage the articular surfaces. At that point, only an interpositional arthroplasty or total joint arthroplasty can be considered—neither are great options in young, active individuals.

If the elbow articulation remains malaligned after operative treatment, additional surgery is necessary as soon as possible, even though early reoperation increases the risk of extensive heterotopic ossification. Operative treatment of persistent elbow malalignment consists of restoration of the stabilizing anatomy of the elbow (radial head, coronoid, collateral ligaments) and hinged external fixation to maintain concentric reduction during the initial treatment period (13,38,52). Although this is fortunately uncommon, it is my impression that patients in whom the trochlear notch is relatively spared do better than those with instability associated with large and complex coronoid fractures.

Nonunion

The metaphyseal bone around the elbow is well-vascularized and nonunions are relatively uncommon overall; however, several specific injuries are more prone to nonunions than others and require specific attention in treatment.

Whereas nonunion of the olecranon is very unusual, fractures of the proximal ulna with extensive metaphyseal comminution have been more problematic (53,54). Much of this seems to relate to inadequate fixation of the proximal, metaphyseal fragment, particularly in the setting of osteoporotic bone. Both in the treatment of fresh fractures and nonunions, it seems better to apply a long plate on the dorsal surface of the ulna that wraps around the olecranon process, thereby providing additional screw fixation (38,54,55). It is also important not to remove the muscular and periosteal attachments to the comminuted fragments in the metaphysis, but rather to bridge this area with a long plate and use the fragments as vascularized bone graft, rather than depending upon them for stability. In the setting of nonunion, debriding the fracture site of sclerotic, inflammatory, and devitalized tissues and applying a nonstructural cancellous bone graft has been very successful in our experience (55,56).

Nonunion of the radial head may be more common than previously recognized (30,57–59). Minimally displaced fractures involving the radial neck often fail to heal (57,58). We do not know the true incidence of nonunion because it rarely causes symptoms, we do not usually reevaluate the elbow radiographically, and ununited fractures of the radial head may eventually heal without additional intervention if followed for more than 2 years (57,59).

Complex fractures of the radial head that are repaired with a plate and screws are also prone to early failure and nonunion (30,59). Usually the reconstructed radial head has served well as a stabilizer of the elbow and, with the ligaments now healed, it can safely be resected without replacing it.

Nonunions of the distal humerus tend to occur at the supracondylar level. Osteochondral fracture fragments also occasionally fail to heal or develop avascular necrosis. Nonunion is usually related to inadequate fixation, over vigorous rehabilitation, or bone loss and devitalization of the fragments. It can be salvaged in most cases with ulnar nerve release, elbow capsular release, stable internal fixation, and autogenous cancellous bone grafting (60).

Infection

Infections are fortunately very uncommon after the operative treatment of elbow fractures. They are usually related to complex open injuries, devitalized fracture fragments, and immunocompromised patients. These infections are often treated with serial debridement, retention of implants, and parenteral antibiotics, particularly when the fracture is complex. Healing of the fractures can usually be achieved with this regimen (Fig. 28-9). Eventually, complete eradication of the infection usually requires implant removal.

Elbow mobility is typically allowed during treatment of infection. It can be assisted with external fixation or hinged external fixation when there is associated elbow instability or an unsupported fracture or nonunion.

Wound Problems

Wound problems are also very uncommon, due to the excellent blood supply. Most patients with wound edge necrosis or slight wound separation can be treated with dressing changes, but patients with exposed implants or an underlying total elbow arthroplasty should be treated operatively to obtain better skin cover. This can often be accomplished with local rotational flaps, pedicled flaps (such as a radial forearm flap), and on occasion a free microvascular tissue transfer (61,62). I follow the so-called reconstructive stepladder, using the simplest procedure that will address the problem.

Arthrosis

In spite of sometimes dramatic claims made by nutritional supplement and pharmaceutical companies, there is no cure for post-traumatic arthrosis. Patients must adapt to and live with the arthrosis or consider reconstructive procedures, none of which are perfect. Debridement of osteophytes and loose bodies and capsulectomy can be useful in the short term, and may be best used in conjunction with ulnar nerve release as ulnar neuropathy is a commonly associated problem (63).

Patients with severe articular damage or incongruity must

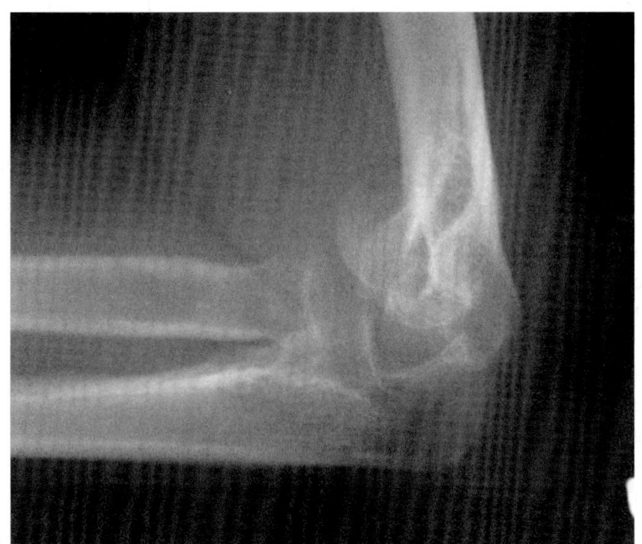

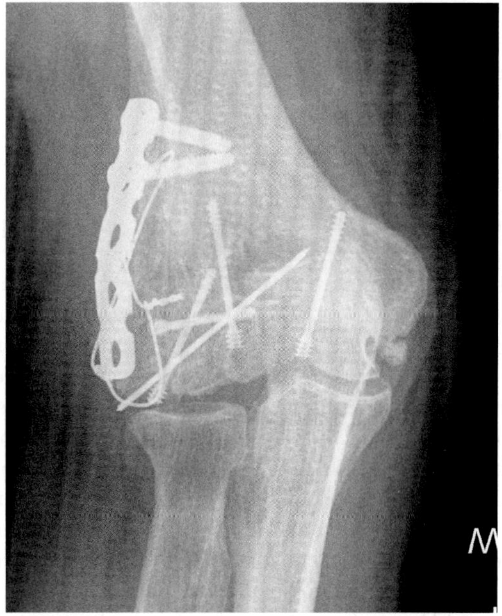

FIGURE 28-9 Infected upper-extremity fractures can often be treated with the implants in place. **A.** A severely immunocompromised patient (being treated for a life-threatening autoimmune skin disease) developed a deep infection after operative treatment of a very complex articular fracture of the distal humerus. **B.** Removal of the implants would have left the patient with no elbow joint, so the infection was treated with removal of loose hardware only, serial debridement, and parenteral antibiotics. This x-ray, 3 years later documents a healed fracture and absence of infection resulting in very good elbow function.

consider interpositional arthroplasty (64,65) or total elbow arthroplasty (66). Total elbow arthroplasty has a finite life span (with each revision becoming increasingly more difficult), is more prone to infection and major complications than knee or hip arthroplasty, and requires strict activity limitations (a 5 kg lifting limit). Total elbow arthroplasty is only suitable for older, low demand patients. Fascial interpositional arthroplasty is better suited for younger, more active patients. The material used for interposition has traditionally been the cutis layer of skin or fascia lata, but more recently allograft Achilles tendon has been used. Interpositional arthroplasty does not eliminate elbow pain and leaves the elbow somewhat unstable—it is best suited for patients with severe stiffness related to arthrosis (64,65).

DISTAL HUMERUS FRACTURES

Fractures of the distal humerus compromise joint function and durability, cause loss of motion, and occur in complex patterns that are challenging to treat operatively and prone to complications. Total elbow arthroplasty has been used increasingly for these fractures and the early results can be seductively good (67,68); however, given the limited durability and severe activity restrictions associated with total elbow arthroplasty, it may only be appropriate for very low demand elderly patients and patients with preexisting elbow arthritis. Effective treatment of fractures of the distal humerus requires accurate identification and secure internal fixation of all injury components.

Rationale

Healing of the fracture will restore stability to the upper limb. Maintenance of alignment—including the anterior tilt and translation of the distal articular surface, restoration of the medial and lateral lips of the trochlea, and avoidance of major articular incongruity—is necessary to maintain motion and limit the potential for arthrosis. The elbow is prone to stiffness with prolonged immobilization and the goal of treatment is secure fixation allowing immediate elbow mobilization. On the other hand, a healed, well-aligned fracture takes precedence, particularly with complex fractures, because capsular contracture can be addressed with subsequent surgery if needed, but early loss of fixation or articular damage may be irrecoverable. Operative treatment must be undertaken carefully and meticulously as it introduces the potential for several additional complications, particularly those related to handling of the ulnar nerve and the triceps mechanism. Furthermore, the combination of operative trauma and unstable internal fixation can do more harm than good.

Diagnosis and Classification

Standard x-rays will identify that the distal humerus has been fractured, but they are notoriously poor at demonstrating the complexity of the fracture—particularly at the articular surface. X-rays taken with axial traction applied to the limb can improve visualization of the fragments, but are usually not available until

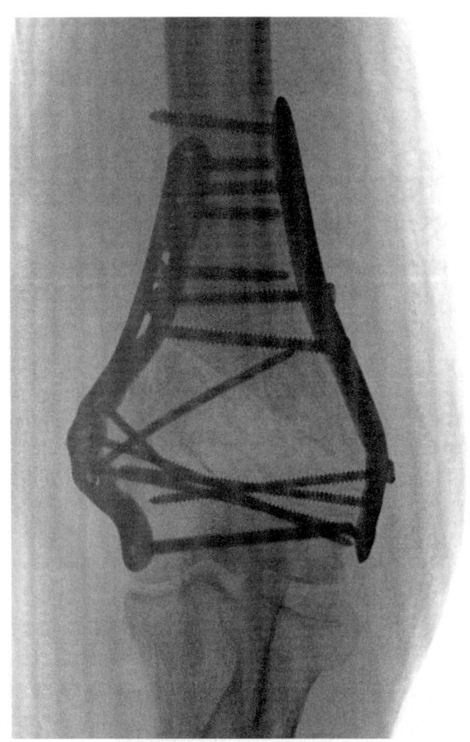

FIGURE 28-13 *(continued)* **E.** The use of parallel plates (one placed directly medial and one directly lateral) is appealing in several respects.

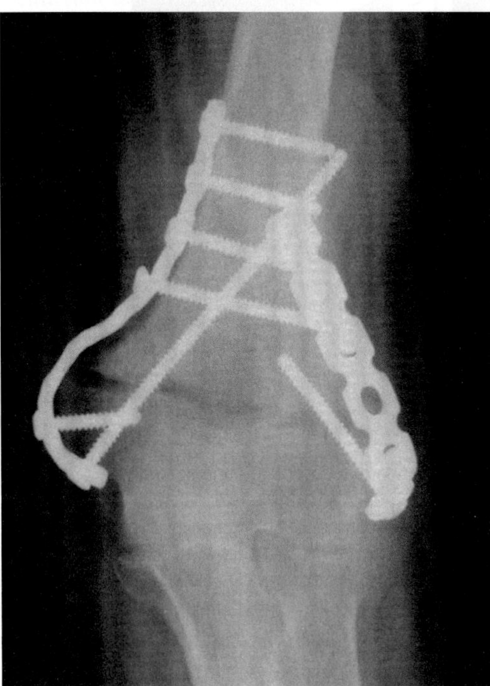

FIGURE 28-14 While the so-called home run screw—a long screw aimed up the medial or lateral column—is favored by some surgeons, it is important to remember to obtain adequate hold on the distal fragments as this nonunion demonstrates.

I have found it necessary to place the screw first and then bring the plate to the screw, finding that if I apply the plate first my screw position will be directed by the plate and will more likely be inadequate.

Tension-band wiring of columnar fractures of the distal humerus has been described in two studies (101,102). Although this might initially seem to violate the need for stable fixation in anatomical alignment, the reported results are reasonably good and I have found this technique to be a useful bailout in osteoporotic, fragmented fractures, particularly in the setting of an early reoperation for loss of fixation where repeat plate and screw fixation is not possible (Fig. 28-15).

Finally, distal humerus fractures often create entirely articular fragments that can only be secured with implants that are counter sunk beneath the articular surface (11,71). Small threaded Kirschner wires can be very useful in this regard because there is often limited bone opposite these fragments for internal fixation. The small threaded Kirschner wires can be placed through the edge of the fracture site connecting the subchondral bone of adjacent fragments (Fig. 28-11A). When the major articular fragments are reduced, the small wires are buried. For larger articular fragments with an opposite bony support, headless screws (the Herbert screw and variations, many of which are now cannulated) are useful. I would caution against the use of a countersunk threaded screw as these allow settling, which results in protrusion of the screw head into the joint—it is better if the head is threaded so that it cannot back out as easily.

Total Elbow Arthroplasty

The increasing use of total elbow arthroplasty for the treatment of complex fractures of the distal humerus (68,103–105) reflects surgeon dissatisfaction with open reduction and internal fixation in many cases. This approach became possible after the development of successful semi-constrained elbow arthroplasties that do not require the retention of collateral ligaments or other stabilizing structures. As a result, total elbow arthroplasty for fracture is one of the easiest types of total elbow arthroplasties to perform because the prosthesis can be inserted without releasing the triceps from the proximal ulna by working in the space created by resecting the distal fracture fragments, including the medial and lateral epicondyles (103).

The rapid recovery and excellent early results also increase the appeal of total elbow arthroplasty for fractures of the distal humerus (68). I believe that the results are seductively good, because the surgeon will gladly abandon tedious and challenging attempts to repair a complex distal humerus fracture and celebrate his or her decision by virtue of the more rapid return to function; however, the patient will now have to severely limit use of the limb, prepare for the eventual failure of the prosthesis, and occasionally experience a severe complication, such as a wound dehiscence or deep infection, which are much more difficult to treat after total elbow arthroplasty than after internal fixation.

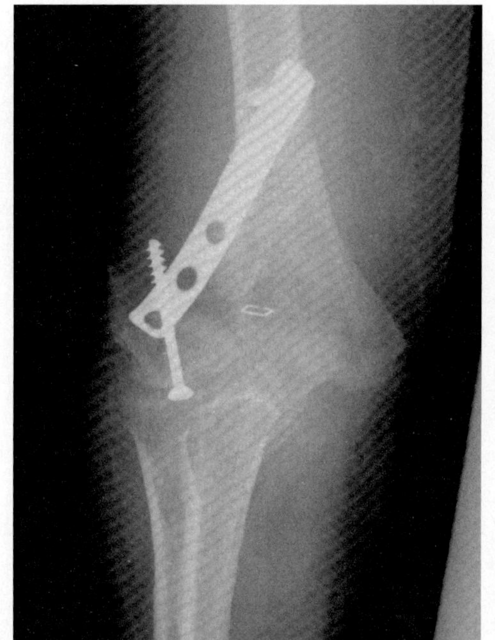

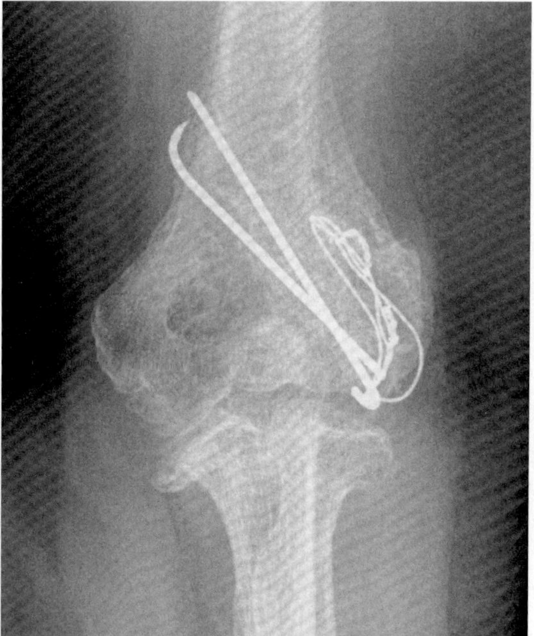

FIGURE 28-15 A 75-year-old woman presented after failed internal fixation of a lateral column fracture of the distal humerus. **A.** There was loose fixation and osteoporotic bone. There were also several drill holes and an attempt at application plates and screws led to additional fragmentation of the fracture. **B.** This problem was salvaged using a tension band wiring. The tension wire provided fixation of the lateral condylar fracture fragments through their soft-tissue attachments and did not rely on bone quality. Healing and good function were obtained.

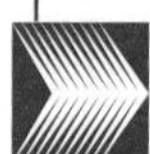

AUTHOR'S PREFERRED TREATMENT

I use the bag-of-bones technique for patients with extremely limited demands (for instance a patient with severe Alzheimer's disease or prior strokes that is nursing home bound and already dependent upon others for basic care); total elbow arthroplasty for older low-demand patients that remain somewhat independent, but do not use their arm for forceful or repetitive activities and are not expected to live more than 10 or 20 years after injury; patients with preexisting elbow disease such as rheumatoid arthritis (Fig. 28-16); and open reduction and internal fixation for all other injuries (Table 28-1). Although failed internal fixation can be salvaged, severe complications of total elbow arthroplasty (infection, severe wound problems, end-stage osteolysis, and triceps insufficiency) can be difficult to salvage (Fig. 28-17).

Although age is often used as a decision-making criterion, the more appropriate criteria are health, activity-level, and bone quality. As the duration and quality of life increase and the population of older-aged persons continues to expand, more and more of our patients remain active in sports or other vocations or avocations that require vigorous use of the elbow.

For operative exposure of bicolumnar fractures and complex articular fractures of the distal humerus, I prefer olecranon osteotomy. For simple articular and extra-articular fractures, I will often start by developing the Allonso-Llamas exposure and then cut the olecranon only if the fracture is more complex than anticipated or difficult to reduce. For most complex articular fractures (variations of the capitellum fracture), I use an extensile lateral exposure.

I favor the concept of parallel plating, but will use whatever plate configuration gives the best fixation. I attempt to repair small articular fragments and rarely discard them. I believe these provide support and assist with healing, but my primary reason for repairing them is to monitor and ensure accurate reduction of the major articular fragments. Fragments of the thin bone between the olecranon and coronoid facets are occasionally discarded, and small articular fragments that seem to be doing more harm than good in spite of attempts to repair them can also be discarded.

Access to articular fragments is one of the major advantages of the olecranon osteotomy, but these can be accessed through other exposures by rotating the fractured condyles posteriorly into the wound so that the olecranon does not impede access (Fig. 28-11A), or by using a fractured condyle or epicondyle to allow rotation or subluxation of the distal humerus away from the ulna. Many small articular fragments can be secured with headless screws to major fragments of the distal humerus, but others are better suited to repair with small threaded Kirschner wires inserted through the fracture surface and connecting the subchondral bone of adjacent fragments. Non-threaded Kirschner wires may be more risky as they have been known to migrate throughout the body. In my experience, most bicolumnar fractures have at least one small separate articular fragment or additional

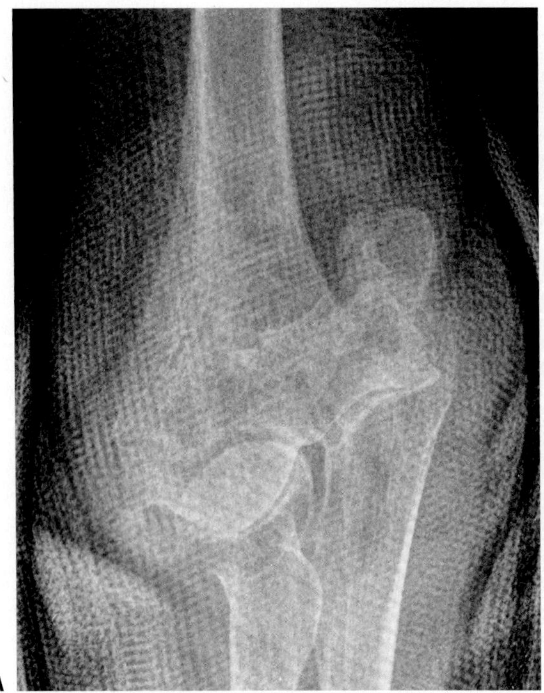

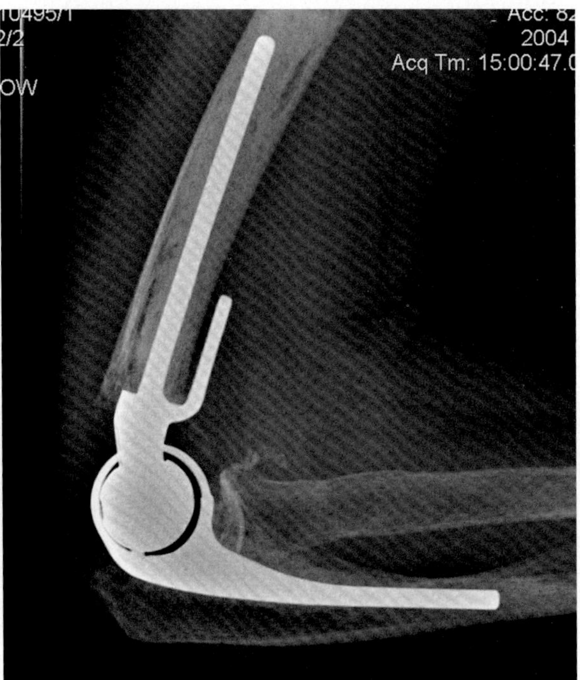

FIGURE 28-16 Total elbow arthroplasty is an increasingly popular treatment for distal humerus fractures, but this technique is best limited to a very specific set of patients. **A.** This fracture occurred in a patient with rheumatoid arthritis, preexisting elbow arthritis, and very poor bone quality from chronic corticosteroid use. **B.** A semi-constrained total elbow arthroplasty restored elbow function.

TABLE 28-1 **Pitfalls and Pearls for Fractures of the Distal Humerus**

Pitfalls	Pearls
• Failure to recognize complex articular fragmentation	• Anticipate common patterns of injury • Beware of coronal plane fracture lines and entirely articular fragments • Use traction x-rays and computed tomography, particularly with three-dimensional reconstructions • Achieve adequate exposure of the entire articular surface of the distal humerus
• Failure to adequately stabilize comminuted columnar fractures	• Either bridge comminution with a large plate or shorten column to gain stable contact
• Inadequate fixation of low columnar fractures	• Be familiar with how to utilize the nonarticular portions of the distal humerus • Use two orthogonal plates on a single column or a plate with several smaller screws distally • Place as many screws as possible in the distal fragments
• Complications related to exposure	• Put as much care and effort into the exposure and repair as in the fixation of the fracture
• Use of total elbow arthroplasty in healthy active individuals	• Limit the use of total elbow arthroplasty to older, low-demand patients and those with preexisting elbow joint damage

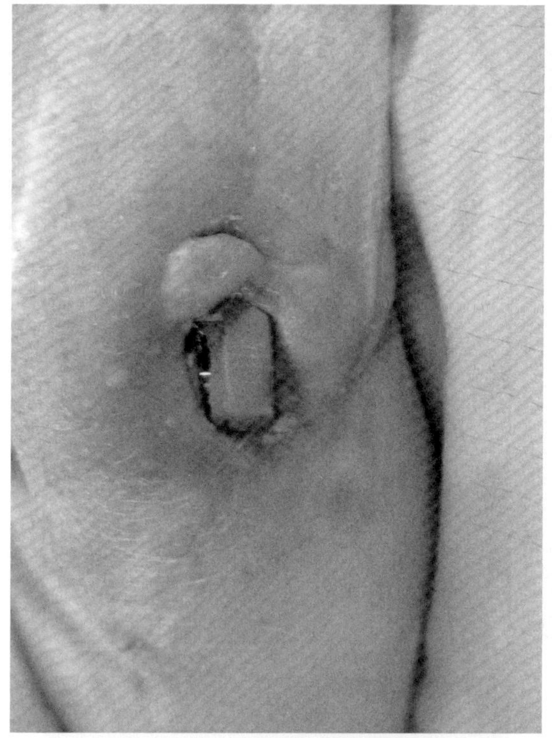
A

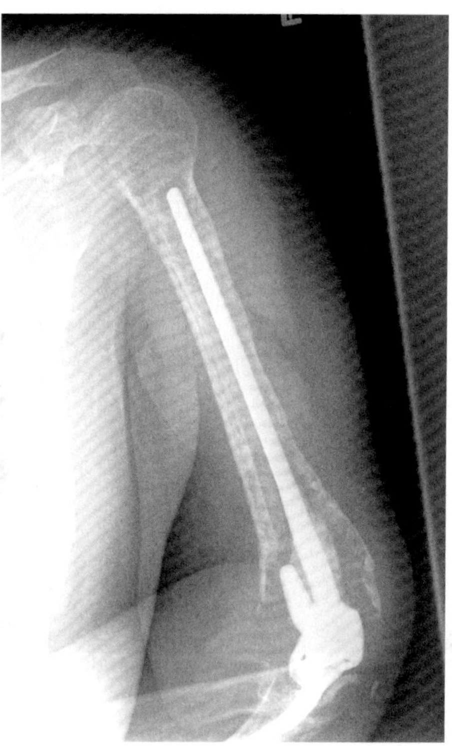
B

FIGURE 28-17 Total elbow arthroplasty can provide very good early functional results in the treatment of fractures of the distal humerus, but there are several problems that limit the enthusiasm for their use. **A.** Wound problems and infections are very difficult to salvage and can be a major problem. **B.** This young patient developed massive osteolysis after revision total elbow arthroplasty. Future treatment options are limited.

fragmentation of the articular surface and therefore an interfragmentary compression screw between the major medial and lateral fragments—as is often described—can rarely be used.

Metaphyseal comminution can be addressed by either bridging the fragments with stable internal fixation or by resecting comminution and shortening the distal humerus. Bridging the fragments preserves the olecranon and coronoid fossas, avoids the need for shortening of a relatively intact column given that metaphyseal comminution often involves only one column, and usually does not impede healing, provided that stable internal fixation is achieved (this is a metaphyseal region with an excellent blood supply). On the other hand, resecting the comminution in order to obtain stable apposition of major fracture fragments increases the initial stability of the fixation. In practice, I balance these two rationales and make the decision intraoperatively. In my experience, the need to shorten the bone is uncommon.

Operative Technique: Olecranon Osteotomy. The patient is placed in a lateral decubitus position with the arm supported over a bolster. Either the prior incision or a straight posterior incision is used. Medial and lateral skin flaps are elevated with care taken to protect cutaneous nerve branches and keep them within the skin flaps. The ulnar nerve is identified along the medial border of the triceps, dissected at least 6 cm proximally and distally, and left in an anteriorly transposed position in the subcutaneous tissues.

The insertion of the anconeus onto the proximal ulna is partially elevated to directly view the arc of the trochlear notch. Alternatively, if the ulnar nerve has been transposed, the medial elbow capsule can be incised in the bed where the ulnar nerve originally lay. If the fracture is simple enough that reduction of the metaphyseal fracture lines can be relied upon to achieve a good articular reduction, the triceps can be elevated from the posterior aspect of the distal humerus on both the medial and lateral sides and the osteotomy made only if necessary. In most patients, however, an osteotomy is necessary for adequate reduction and fixation.

An apex distal chevron-shaped osteotomy is planned so that it enters the joint at the depths of the trochlear notch. An oscillating saw is used to start the osteotomy (Fig. 28-18A). A small, straight osteotome is then used to complete it, by levering the osteotome proximally and cracking the subchondral bone (Fig. 28-18B). This maneuver creates an uneven surface that facilitates repositioning and may enhance stability. The posterior elbow capsule is then incised and the olecranon fragment and triceps are elevated from the posterior aspect of the humerus (Fig. 28-18C).

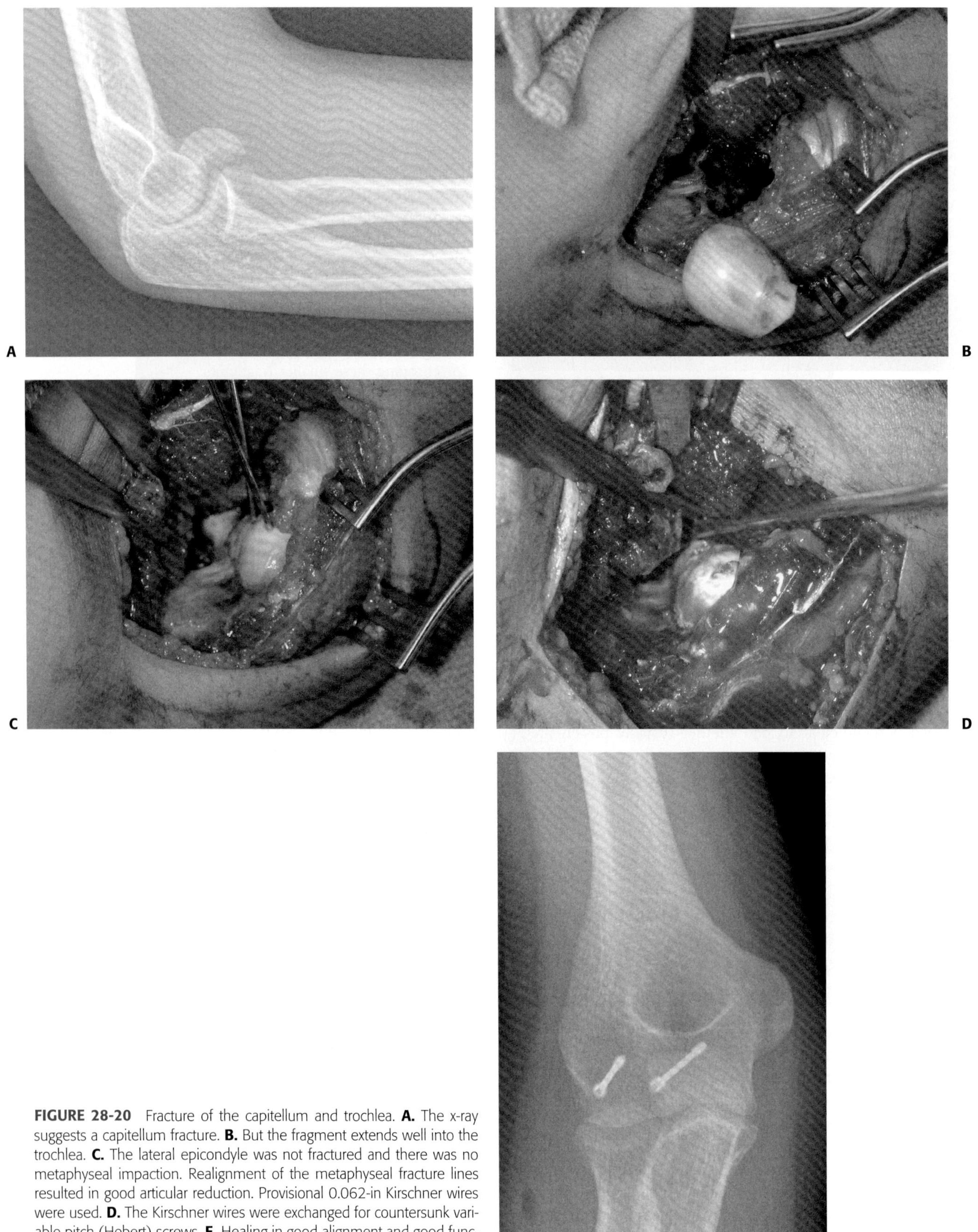

FIGURE 28-20 Fracture of the capitellum and trochlea. **A.** The x-ray suggests a capitellum fracture. **B.** But the fragment extends well into the trochlea. **C.** The lateral epicondyle was not fractured and there was no metaphyseal impaction. Realignment of the metaphyseal fracture lines resulted in good articular reduction. Provisional 0.062-in Kirschner wires were used. **D.** The Kirschner wires were exchanged for countersunk variable pitch (Hebert) screws. **E.** Healing in good alignment and good function were obtained.

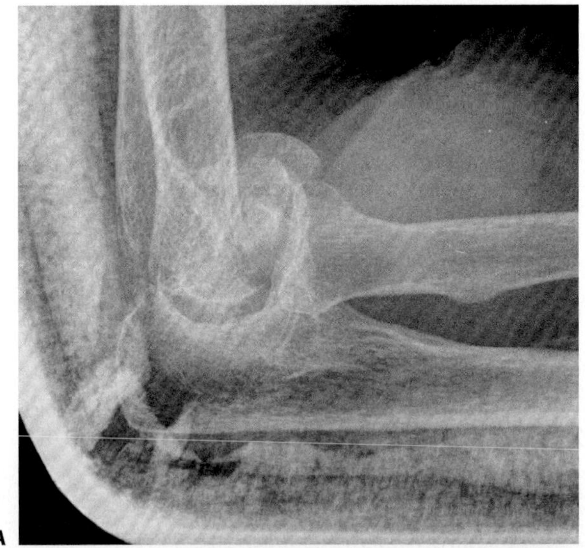

FIGURE 28-21 **A.** At first glance this fracture may look like a capitellar fracture. A closer look suggests a much more complex articular fracture. **B.** The quality of these three-dimensional CT image is limited by the technique used to make the original CT, but it can be seen that the entire anterior articular surface is fractured and displaced anteriorly. **C.** Through an olecranon osteotomy, the multifragmented fracture was pieced together with small threaded Kirschner wires and then additional stabilization was provided by a plate with small (2.7 mm) distal screws.

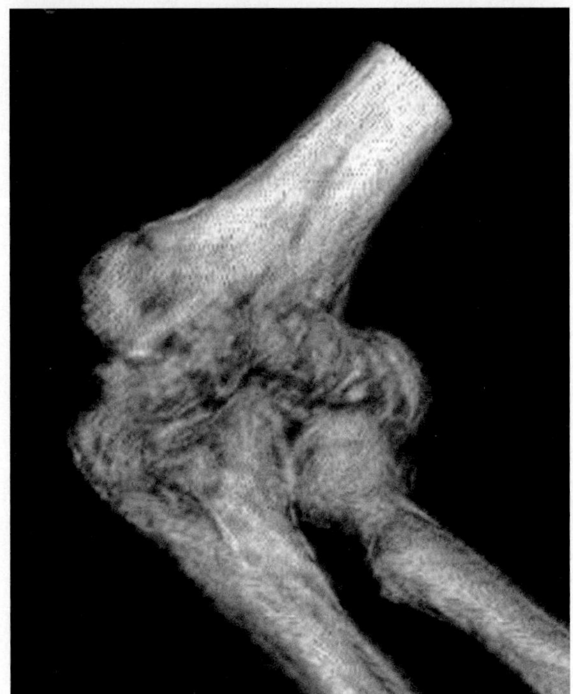

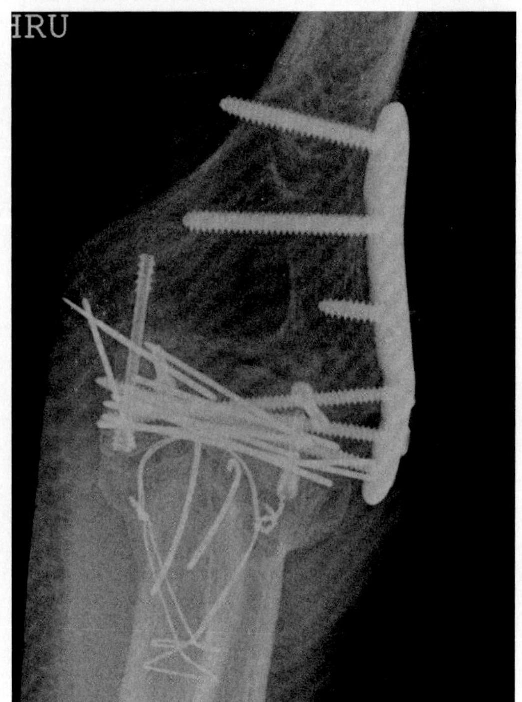

excised and the triceps is elevated from the posterior aspect of the humerus. The triceps is elevated slightly from the olecranon tip that will be excised in order to facilitate passage of the ulnar component of the prosthesis, but there is no need for an extensive elevation of the triceps from the ulna in the treatment of a distal humerus fracture with total elbow arthroplasty—a sufficient working space is created by removing the fracture fragments (Fig. 28-22).

A semi-constrained (linked) total elbow arthroplasty is inserted according to the specific technique for the implant used. Repair of the common extensor and flexor muscles can improve coverage of the implant, but is not necessary for good arm function. The elbow is splinted for comfort only and the patient is allowed to begin active use of and exercise the arm as soon as possible.

Complications

Ulnar Neuropathy

Management of the ulnar nerve is debated. Some surgeons always transpose the nerve (98), some never (106), and most fall somewhere in between.

Ulnar nerve dysfunction can result from entrapment by normal anatomic structures or scar, but can also result from handling and transposition of the nerve. It can be difficult to predict when the nerve will have dysfunction after transposition, but vigorous retraction seems to be the most preventable aspect of treatment—for this reason I use a small vessel loop rather than a Penrose drain to isolate the nerve and assist with dissection and I never attach a clamp to the loop. It is also useful to have an oscillating drill to avoid wrapping the nerve up on the drill.

In practice, the ulnar nerve must be at least partially released and mobilized in order to achieve secure fixation and to keep the nerve safe. Given the many potential areas of constriction in the normal anatomical course of the ulnar nerve, it is inadvisable to perform a partial release. In our practice ulnar nerve dysfunction after treatment of a fracture of the distal humerus is frequently encountered and often seems related to incomplete release of the nerve with resultant nerve compression. Consequently, it is my practice to perform a complete release of the ulnar nerve for the vast majority of fractures (from the passage of the nerve through the medial intermuscular septum through Osbourne's fascia), and to leave the nerve in an anteriorly transposed, subcutaneous position at the end of the case.

Stiffness and Heterotopic Ossification

Failure to restore the anterior translation of the trochlea with respect to the humeral shaft will lead to limitation of flexion that cannot be improved with capsular release (Fig. 28-23). Articular incongruities and arthrosis can also result in unsalvageable stiffness. Heterotopic ossification that blocks motion usually occurs on the anterior aspect of the distal humerus after distal humerus fracture, causing limitation of flexion. Resection of this bone is straightforward, restores flexion, and does not required prophylaxis against recurrence because recurrence after resection of this anterior heterotopic bone is unusual.

Nonunion

Nonunion is nearly always related to inadequate fixation (107–109), but can also be related to infection, avascular necrosis, or excessively forceful use or manipulation of the arm prior to healing. The weakest point is fixation of the distal, articular fragments to the shaft and nonunion tends to occur at the supracondylar region, and only occasionally involves the articular fragments. A sufficient number of screws in the distal fragments, good contact between the shaft and the distal fragments, and strong plates will help limit the risk of nonunion.

Nonunion can nearly always be salvaged with repeat open reduction, internal plate fixation, and autogenous cancellous bone grafting. The addition of capsulectomy of the elbow joint and neurolysis and transposition of the ulnar nerve seem to have improved the success of surgery for nonunion (60).

Total elbow arthroplasty can also be used to salvage nonunion of the distal humerus, but is most appropriate in older, low-demand patients (110,111). In addition, total elbow arthroplasty for post-traumatic reconstruction may have an increased rate of complications (92).

Implant-Related Complications

The frequent need for a second surgery to remove the wires used to repair an olecranon osteotomy has been viewed by some as representing a complication. This may be a biased view as it is also appropriate to say that the need for two surgeries (the second being relatively straightforward) to restore elbow function after such a complex injury is reasonable. It could be detrimental to the patient for the surgeon to compromise his or her exposure of and access to the fracture in the attempt to avoid a relatively simple second surgery for implant removal. Furthermore, with careful attention to the technique of creation and fixation of the osteotomy, the need for a second surgery to remove the screw or wires does not arise routinely.

Controversies and Future Directions

Current areas of debate and innovation in the treatment of distal humerus fractures include: (a) Which technique of exposure best balances visualization and access to the fragments with complications related to the exposure? (b) Are parallel plating techniques and the associated concepts superior to orthogonal plating techniques? (c) How will plates with angular stable (locked) screws influence the treatment of fractures of the distal humerus? and (d) What is the role of total elbow arthroplasty in the treatment of fractures of the distal humerus?

RADIAL HEAD FRACTURES

Mechanism of Injury

The radial head fractures when it collides with the capitellum. This can occur with a pure axial load [the most extreme example

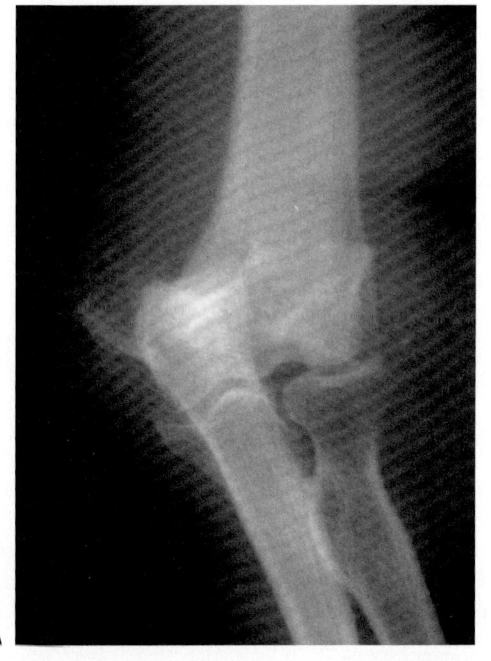

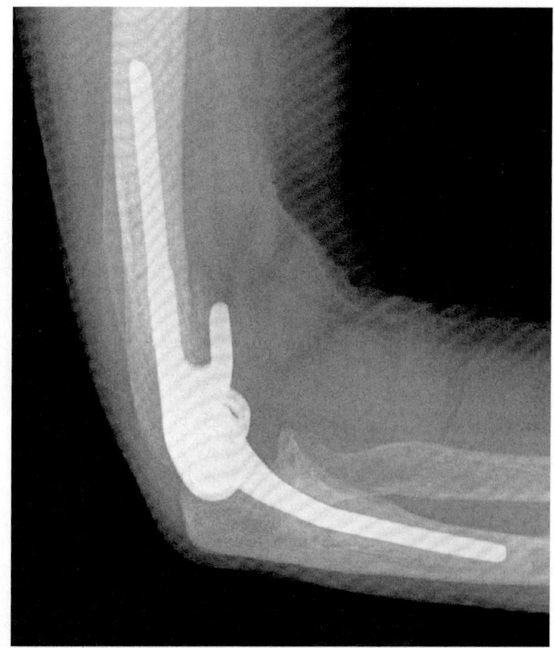

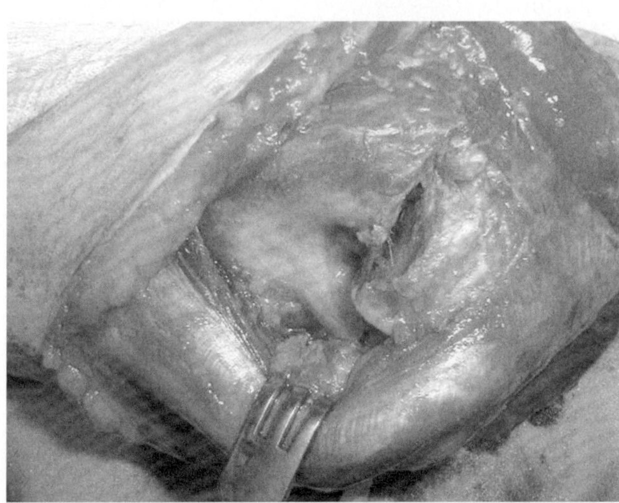

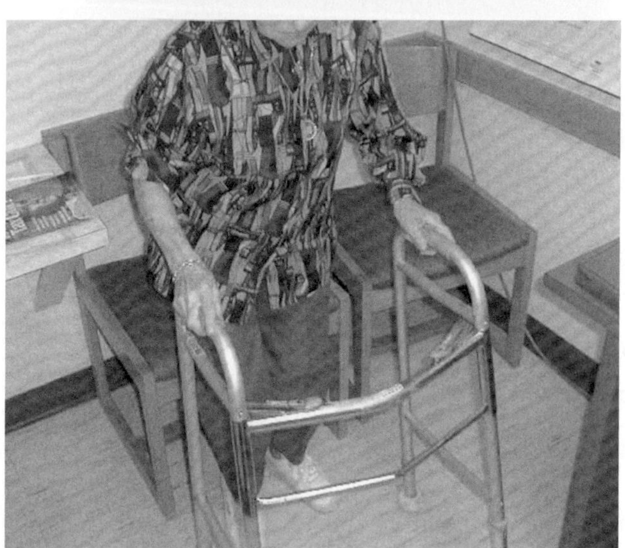

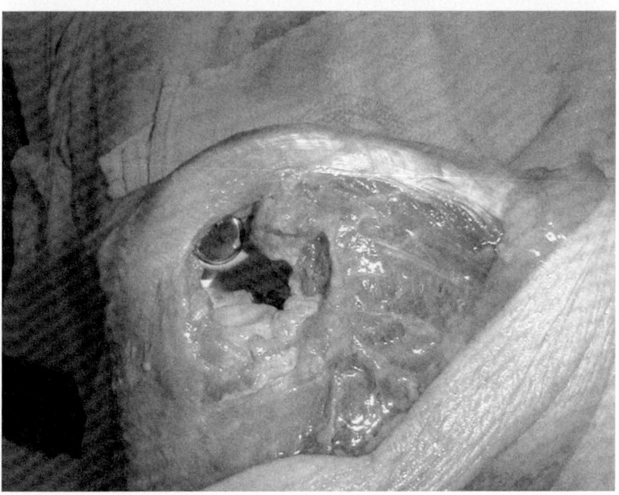

FIGURE 28-22 The early results of total elbow arthroplasty for fracture of the distal humerus can be quite gratifying. **A.** This fracture occurred in an elderly woman who needed to use a walker to ambulate. **B.** Excision of the distal fracture fragments creates a working space. **C.** The prosthesis can be inserted without detaching the triceps insertion. **D.** Semiconstrained total elbow arthroplasty provides immediate stability. **E.** This allowed the patient to use her walker and avoid being bed and wheelchair bound.

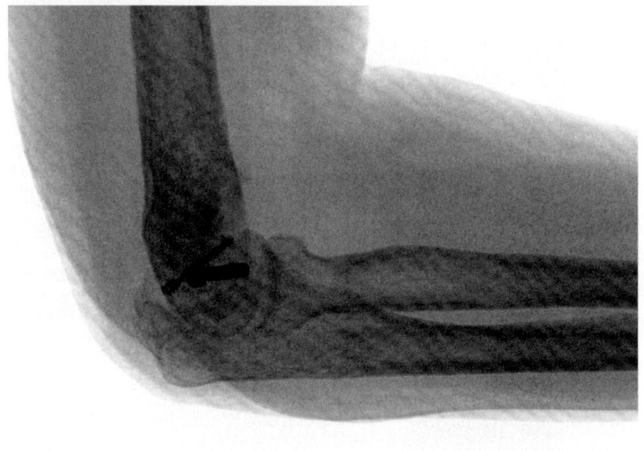

FIGURE 28-23 Loss of the anterior translation of the distal humerus makes it impossible for this patient to regain more than about 95 degrees of flexion in spite of removing most of the implants and excision of contracted capsule.

of which is the Essex-Lopresti injury, a valgus load (12)], with a posterolateral rotatory (elbow dislocation) type of load, or as the radial head dislocates posteriorly as part of a posterior Monteggia fracture or posterior olecranon fracture-dislocation. The vast majority of these injuries are the result of a fall onto the outstretched hand, the higher energy injuries representing falls from a height or during sports.

Signs and Symptoms

Even relatively minor fractures of the radial head (radiographically occult fractures, for instance) can be quite painful because the elbow joint is usually distended with blood. There is a variable amount of swelling and ecchymosis, which may correspond with the degree of associated ligament injury. The distal radioulnar joint, interosseous space, and medial side of the elbow should be examined for signs of associated ligament injury. There is often crepitation of the radial head with forearm rotation and occasionally a fracture fragment will block forearm rotation.

Associated Injuries

Isolated radial head fractures are straightforward to treat. One of the keys to successful management of a fracture of the radial head is to identify and address associated injuries. This is particularly important for very displaced fractures and fractures that involve the entire head of the radius. In the study of Davidson and colleagues, all 11 patients with a fracture involving the entire radial head had associated injury to the elbow or forearm (113). In my experience, complex fractures of the entire head do occur without associated ligament damage on occasion—particularly in older patients—but I agree with Davidson and colleagues that one should assume there is an associated injury until it has been proved otherwise. In fact, a markedly displaced partial head fracture should raise similar concerns.

There are several patterns of complex injury that include a fracture of the radial head. Identification of these injury patterns can help guide treatment. These patterns include: (a) fracture of the radial head associated with rupture of the MCL; (b) concomitant fracture of the radial head and capitellum; (c) posterior dislocation of the elbow with fracture of the radial head; (d) posterior dislocation of the elbow with fracture of the radial head and the coronoid process (the so-called terrible triad of the elbow); (e) posterior Monteggia fractures including posterior olecranon fracture-dislocations; and (f) Essex-Lopresti lesions and variants.

The x-ray evaluation alone may not disclose associated ligament injury. In particular, intraoperative examination after removal of the radial head is important to avoid missing injury to the interosseous ligament of the forearm. After removing the radial head fragments, the surgeon should push and pull on the radius. If the radial neck is very mobile and collides with the capitellum, the surgeon should assume that the interosseous ligament of the forearm is injured (114).

Rationale

The goals of treatment of fracture of the radial head include: (a) correction of any hindrance of forearm rotation by the fracture; (b) restoration of elbow and forearm motion by early initiation of an adequate exercise program; (c) stability of the forearm and elbow; (d) limitation of the potential for ulnohumeral and radiocapitellar arthrosis, although the latter seems to be an uncommon problem; and (e) avoidance of injury-related complications and complications related to operative intervention including nonunion, avascular necrosis, an expanded or incongruous radial head that restricts motion, restriction of motion by plates and screws, radioulnar synostosis, posterolateral rotatory instability, and a prominent radial head prosthesis leading to capitellar wear.

Diagnosis and Classification

In combination with the evaluation of the signs and symptoms previously described, x-rays of the elbow and wrist will disclose most associated injuries. For isolated partial fractures of the radial head, the ability of the patient to fully pronate and supinate the forearm will influence treatment. Pain can make this very difficult to evaluate during the first few days after injury. If the x-rays reveal a fracture that may restrict forearm rotation and operative treatment is being considered, it may be useful to aspirate some of the blood from the elbow joint and instill some local anesthetic (usually lidocaine). This can be done at the anatomic soft-spot (roughly at the center of a triangle formed by the dorsal point of the olecranon, the radial head, and the lateral epicondyle) on the lateral side of the elbow. Alternatively, if the patient returns to the office a few days to a week after injury, they are likely to feel much better and be capable of demonstrating forearm rotation. A true block to forearm rotation is uncommon, so either injection or delayed serial examination, or both are important steps in decision making.

Operative treatment of widely displaced fractures of the radial head typically reveals a more complex fracture than was apparent on x-rays. Although two-dimensional and three-dimensional CT will depict these aspects in greater detail and thereby facilitate planning of the operation, it is not necessary to obtain these studies provided that the surgeon is prepared for all possible treatment options including repair with plates and/or screws or excision of the fractured radial head with insertion of a metal prosthesis if there is an associated forearm or elbow injury.

Mason classified fractures of the radial head at a time when fractures were either excised or treated nonoperatively (115). He distinguished nondisplaced fractures that did well with nonoperative treatment (Type 1), comminuted fractures of the entire head of the radius (Type 3) that were best treated by excision, and displaced fractures involving part of the radial head (Type 2), which presented a treatment dilemma in that the majority of the head was intact, but some fractures had poor results. His classification did not include radial neck fractures, did not account for associated injuries, and did not quantify displacement.

Morrey (116) modified Mason's classification to (a) include fractures of the radial neck, (b) provide a quantitative definition of displacement (a fragment involving 30% or more of the articular surface that is displaced more than 2 mm), and (c) incorporate fracture-dislocations of the elbow as suggested by Johnston (117) as a Mason Type 4 fracture. The inclusion of radial neck fractures is not useful because these fractures have different management issues and should be considered separately. The inclusion of dislocations is also not useful because fractures of the radial head are associated with a variety of complex injury patterns and, regardless of which injury pattern is present, it is still important to characterize the fracture of the radial head. Finally, there are few data to support the quantitative definition of displacement that is offered in this system.

Hotchkiss' modification of Mason's classification directly reflects current treatment options: Type 1 fractures are minimally displaced fractures that do well with nonoperative treatment; Type 2 fractures are displaced partial head fractures that block forearm rotation and fractures involving the entire head that are repairable; and Type 3 fractures are irreparable fractures that require excision with or without prosthetic replacement (26). This classification is useful conceptually, but the means for distinguishing repairable from unrepairable fractures are incompletely defined.

The Comprehensive Classification of Fractures (118) mixes fractures of the proximal radius and ulna in a way that is not useful for patient management; however, one useful aspect of this system is a modifier that distinguished fractures with greater than three fragments from those with two or three major fragments. The presence of greater than three fragments has been associated with a much higher risk of early failure of internal fixation, nonunion, and loss of forearm rotation (59).

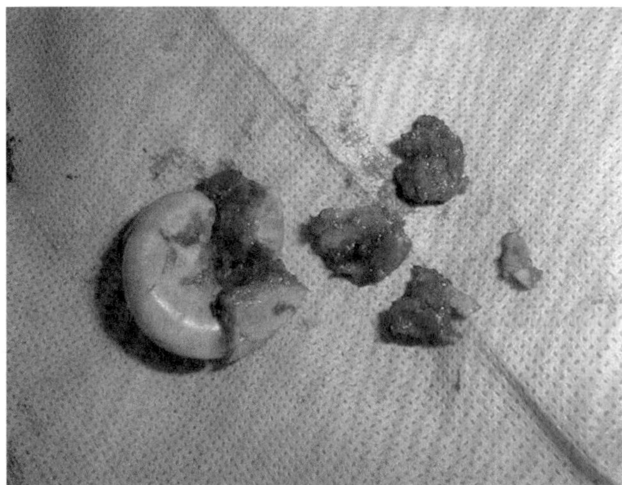

FIGURE 28-24 These fracture fragments demonstrate impaction and deformation of the head in the largest fragment (*left*), metaphyseal fragmentation and small unrepairable articular fragments (*right*).

Other factors that may have an important influence on treatment, but are not well accounted for in current classification systems include: (a) lost fragments—a very common occurrence with displaced fractures, (b) fragments that are too small to be repaired and must be discarded, (c) fragments with little or no subchondral bone, (d) fragments with osteoporotic bone, (e) impaction and deformation of the fracture fragments, and (f) metaphyseal bone loss (Fig. 28-24). Partial resection of the radial head has long been associated with inferior results (119) and was one factor associated with problems in our study of operative treatment (11). Therefore, when fragments are lost, too small to fix, or have inadequate or poor quality bone and must be discarded, the surgeon probably ought to err toward resection of the radial head with or without prosthetic replacement depending upon the presence or absence of associated injuries. Impacted fractures may be less suitable for operative fixation because enlargement and deformation of the radial head have been observed in long-term follow-up and seem to hinder forearm rotation. Metaphyseal bone loss and impaction are observed even with partial radial head fractures and a plate may be superior to screws alone in this circumstance (Fig. 28-25).

Current Treatment Options

Nonoperative Treatment

The vast majority of isolated fractures of the radial head are treated nonoperatively. The major problem patients encounter after an isolated fracture of the radial head is elbow stiffness. Only one study has noted fracture displacement with immediate active motion (120) and it would seem to be a very unusual problem. Nonunion occurs on occasion, but is usually asymptomatic (57,58).

There are no radiographic criteria that have been consistently associated with a poor result with nonoperative treatment

TABLE 28-2 Pearls and Pitfalls for Fractures of the Radial Head

Pitfalls	Pearls
• Resection of the radial head contributing to elbow or forearm instability	• Beware of complex injury patterns associated with fracture of the radial head • Do not use radial head resection for terrible triad and Essex-Lopresti injuries • Only use resection when radius pull test is normal
• Early failure of radial head fixation	• Do not repair the radial head if the fracture is too complex. More than 3 articular fragments, loss fragments, metaphyseal comminution, and impaction/deformation of radial head fragments should make the surgeon less enthusiastic about operative fixation. • Do not accept tenuous fixation for injury patterns with a high potential for instability (e.g., terrible triad and Essex-Lopresti)
• Impingement of implants in proximal radioulnar joint blocking motion	• Respect the safe zones for internal fixation • Countersink all implants outside the safe zone
• Overstuffing of the radio-capitellar joint with a metal prosthesis leading to malalignment of the ulnohumeral joint and painful capitellar erosions	• The proximal articular surface of the radial head should protrude no more than 1 to 2 mm from the lateral edge of the coronoid process.

this area has been suggested to increase the risk of proximal radioulnar synostosis (136,137).

When treating a complex fracture of the radial head with the LCL complex intact (for instance an Essex-Lopresti injury), it may be difficult to gain adequate exposure without releasing the LCL complex from the lateral epicondyle. This can be done either by directly incising the origin of the LCL complex from bone or by performing an osteotomy of the lateral epicondyle (22,29–31,138). In either case a secure repair and avoidance of varus stress in the early postoperative period are important.

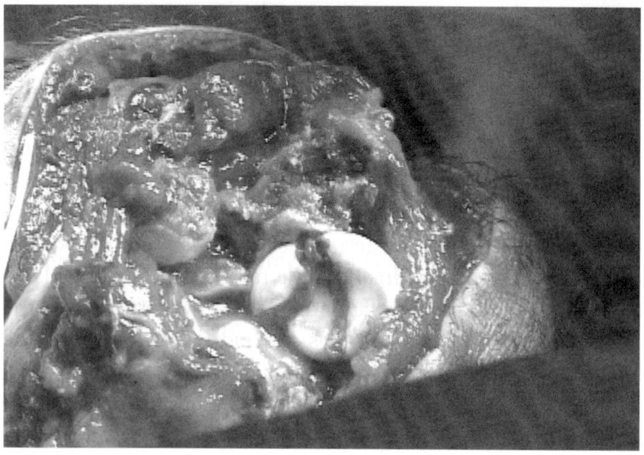

FIGURE 28-30 When treating a posterior olecranon fracture-dislocation or posterior Monteggia injury the radial head can often be addressed through the posterior traumatic interval.

Excision

The fragments are excised and the neck smoothed off. In the setting of an olecranon fracture-dislocation or posterior Monteggia injury, it may be useful to seal the end of the radius with bone wax. The LCL complex should be repaired if injured.

Open Reduction and Internal Fixation

Increased enthusiasm for open reduction and internal fixation of the radial head paralleled the development of small screws (2.7 mm, 2.0 mm, and 1.5 mm) and the techniques for using them (31). At the same time small, headless, variable pitch compression screws (such as the Herbert screw) were developed, allowing for fixation of entirely articular fragments (139–141). Standard screws can be used in this way as well, countersinking the head below the articular surface, although they are prone to backing out into the joint with the slightest amount of settling at the fracture site.

Some small fragments can only be repaired with small Kirschner wires. Threaded wires are usually used because of the tendency for smooth wires to migrate and potentially travel to various parts of the body (142). Absorbable pins and screws are being developed for similar uses (143,144), but are still somewhat brittle and sometimes associated with an inflammatory response.

Small plates are available for fractures that involve the entire head. Plate types include T- and L-shaped plates with standard screws, small (condylar) blade plates, and new plates designed specifically for the radial head (many of which incorporate angular stable screws—screws that thread directly into the plate). The use of plates that are placed within the radial head or countersunk into the articular surface has also been described (138).

Prosthetic Replacement

When preparing for prosthetic replacement, if some of the radial head is still attached to the neck, it is separated at the point on the radial neck where the flare of the head begins. I prefer to use a prosthesis with a smooth neck that serves as a loose spacer. The laxity in the neck facilitates insertion and removal of the prosthesis and accommodates for some of the nonanatomic features of the prosthesis as compared to the native radial head. I use a neck diameter one size less than the reamer that can be passed with slight effort. I use a head size of slightly smaller diameter than the native head. I almost never add more length through the head. It is important to realize that the prosthesis will sit on the most prominent portion of the radial neck; therefore, one should be careful to choose a head thickness based upon the thinnest portion of the radial head. I smooth off, but do not evenly plane the remaining radial neck. It is important to check the level of the radial head with respect to the lateral edge of the coronoid process—it should be no more than 1 mm more proximal.

In the unusual patient in whom the comminution extends into the neck, a prosthetic head of greater thickness can be used. In cases of extreme neck comminution the prosthesis can be cemented in the neck.

Complications

Laceration or permanent injury to the posterior interosseous nerve during open reduction and internal fixation of a radial head fracture is unusual. Most commonly this complication is experienced as a palsy related to retraction or exposure that resolves over weeks to months. To limit the potential for this complication, retractors should not be placed around the radial neck, the forearm should be pronated during exposure of the radial neck, and consideration should be given to identifying and protecting the nerve when more distal dissection and internal fixation are needed, particularly when a more anterior muscle interval is used for exposure.

Early failure of fixation and later nonunion are not infrequent, particularly after open reduction and internal fixation of complex fractures involving the entire head. In a recent series, 3 of 14 fractures involving the entire radial head and creating more than 3 articular fragments had failure of fixation within the first month (59). Because this situation can contribute to instability of the forearm or elbow, unstable or unpredictable fixation is undesirable and such fractures should probably be treated with prosthetic replacement. Among fractures of the entire radial head 6 of 11 in one series (30) and 8 of 26 fractures in another series (59) (including 2 of 12 fractures with three or fewer fragments and 6 of 14 fractures with more than three articular fragments) had nonunion.

Delayed resection of the radial head has usually been performed to improved forearm rotation, and not for painful arthrosis of the radiocapitellar joint (145,146). Incongruity of the proximal radioulnar joint presents as stiffness rather than pain or arthrosis and incongruity of the radiocapitellar joint inconsistently and unpredictably leads to radiocapitellar arthrosis, which seems to be an uncommon problem.

A radial head prosthesis that is too large can cause malalignment of the elbow, capitellar wear, and synovitis and usually needs to be removed. Removal of a metal radial head prosthesis can be very difficult. Given the alternative of releasing the origin of the LCL complex in order to subluxate the elbow, in most patients, I prefer to excise a portion of the radial neck so that I can pry the prosthesis out. The difficulty encountered in removing these prostheses is one reason I prefer to use a slightly loose prosthetic stem.

Controversies and Future Directions

Several new plates are in development, including plates with screws that lock to the plate. Prostheses also continue to evolve. It remains unclear how appropriately sized prostheses will function over the long term. If they continue to perform as well as they have in published studies, surgeons will likely gradually become more confident with prosthetic replacement and less accepting of tenuous internal fixation.

TRAUMATIC ELBOW INSTABILITY

Traumatic elbow instability occurs in three basic forms: posterolateral rotatory instability (elbow dislocations with or without associated fractures), varus posteromedial rotational instability (anteromedial coronoid facet fractures), and olecranon fracture-dislocations. Identification of the specific pattern of traumatic elbow instability will indicate which structures are likely to be injured, the morphology of the injuries, and the prognosis, all of which will help to guide management.

Mechanism

Posterolateral rotatory instability results in dislocation of the elbow with or without fractures of the radial head and coronoid. Posterolateral rotatory injuries occur during a fall onto the outstretched arm that creates a valgus, axial, and posterolateral rotatory force. The ulna and the forearm supinate away from the humerus and dislocate posteriorly. Sometimes this results in injury to the radial head or coronoid. The soft tissue injury proceeds from lateral to medial, with the anterior band of the MCL being the last structure injured (Fig. 28-3) (15). It is possible to dislocate the elbow with the anterior band of the MCL remaining intact.

Varus, posteromedial rotational instability occurs with a fall onto the outstretched arm that creates a varus stress, axial load, and posteromedial rotational force to the elbow (1). This results in fracture of the anteromedial facet of the coronoid process and (a) injury to the LCL, or (b) fracture of the olecranon, or (c) an additional fracture of the coronoid at its base.

Anterior olecranon fracture-dislocations are the result of a direct blow to the flexed elbow, but the mechanism of posterior olecranon fracture dislocations is more speculative, with some authors suggesting they may result from the same mechanism that usually creates elbow dislocations, particularly in older osteopenic individuals (147,148).

Signs and Symptoms

In the majority of patients with traumatic elbow instability, the problem is evident. In some patients the dislocation has reduced, either spontaneously or with assistance. Pain, ecchymosis, and swelling are present along with deformity if the elbow is still dislocated. The point of the olecranon process and the medial and lateral epicondyles should form a triangle in the coronal plane with the elbow flexed 90 degrees. If the point of the olecranon is well posterior to the epicondyles, the elbow is likely dislocated.

Associated Injuries

Acute neurovascular injuries are uncommon, but the ulnar and median nerves are most commonly involved. The brachial artery may also be injured, particularly with an open dislocation, which is also unusual.

Rationale

The treatment of fracture-dislocations of the elbow is intended to restore the inherent bony stability of the elbow that allows us to treat most simple elbow dislocations with immediate active motion with a high degree of success. Critical to achieving this is restoration of the trochlear notch of the ulna, particularly the coronoid process. Anatomic alignment of anteromedial and basal coronoid fractures is necessary for elbow stability and function. Radiocapitellar contact is also very important to the stability of the injured elbow. The LCL is far more important than the MCL in the setting of most cases of traumatic elbow instability. The trochlear notch (coronoid and olecranon), radial head, and LCL are repaired or reconstructed, but the MCL rarely needs to be repaired. Some surgeons are still becoming comfortable with the idea that MCL repair is not necessary for most fracture-dislocations (149). If the elbow is stable, or can be made stable with surgery on the lateral side, the MCL will heal properly with active motion and its repair is not necessary for stability (18).

Diagnosis and Classification

The majority of elbow dislocations and fracture-dislocations result in injury to all of the capsuloligamentous stabilizers of the elbow joint (15,125,134,135). The exceptions include fracture-dislocations of the olecranon and other injuries with fractures of the coronoid involving nearly the entire coronoid process (1,12,55,56).

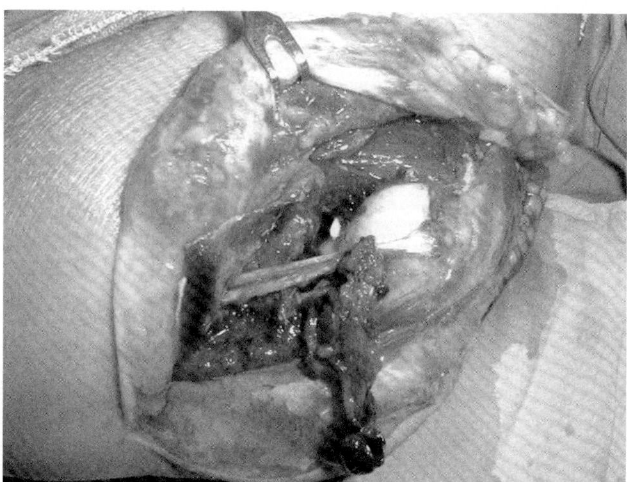

FIGURE 28-31 The LCL nearly always fails via avulsion of its lateral epicondylar origin. The remaining tissue attached to the epicondyle is the remnant of the common extensor musculature, much of which has been torn more distally.

The capsuloligamentous injury progresses from lateral to medial and the elbow can completely dislocate with the anterior band of the MCL remaining intact (15). There is also a variable degree of injury to the common flexor and extensor musculature (43,134,135,150).

One recent study notes that the LCL complex fails by avulsion from the lateral epicondyle in more than 75% of patients with elbow dislocations (16). In my personal observations treating more than 60 fracture-dislocations of the elbow, I have found that the LCL is always avulsed from the lateral epicondyle. In many patients there are small pieces of the ligament or other long strands of musculotendinous tissue, which may lead the surgeon to misinterpret the situation (Fig. 28-31). Defined practically, reattachment of the soft tissue sleeve to the lateral epicondyle is nearly always sufficient.

O'Driscoll has described several stages of elbow instability (Fig. 28-32) (15). Stage 1 involves partial or complete disruption of the LCL, which may result in slight posterior subluxation of the radial head with respect to the capitellum. Stage 2 involves an incomplete posterior dislocation with disruption of the lateral ligamentous complex and further injury to the osseous or ligamentous supporting structures anteriorly and/or posteriorly. The medial edge of the ulna may be found to rest on the trochlea. This gives the appearance of the coronoid being perched on the trochlea on a lateral x-ray (15). Stage 3 is divided into three subgroups (A–C). Stage 3A involves injury to all the soft tissue support except the anterior band of the MCL. The elbow dislocates in a posterolateral direction rotating about the intact anterior MCL. Stage 3B involves injury to the entire medial ligamen-

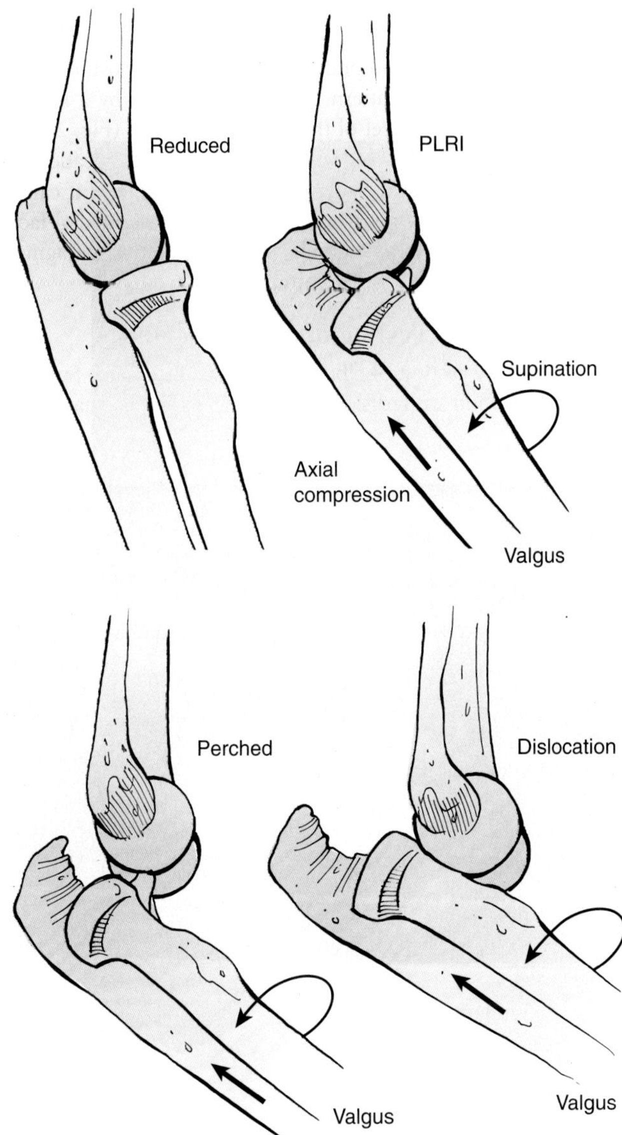

FIGURE 28-32 Posterolateral rotatory instability (PLRI) occurs in several stages. Elbow dislocation is the final stage.

tous complex resulting in varus, valgus, and rotary instability. Stage 3C injuries are very unstable due to complete soft tissue disruption from the distal humerus with the elbow having the ability to dislocate even when immobilized in a cast (1).

Elbow dislocations that are associated with one or more intraarticular fractures are at greater risk for recurrent or chronic instability (12,125,151). Fracture-dislocations of the elbow usually occur in one of several distinct, recognizable injury patterns: (a) posterior dislocation with fracture of the radial head; (b) posterior dislocation with fractures of the radial head and coronoid process—the so-called terrible triad injury (Fig. 28-33); (c) varus posteromedial rotational instability pattern injuries (Fig. 28-34); (d) anterior olecranon fracture-dislocations (Fig. 28-35); and (e) posterior olecranon fracture-dislocations (Fig. 28-36). Each of these patterns is associated with characteristic injury components and fracture morphologies, the knowledge of which can help guide effective management.

Varus posteromedial rotational instability pattern injuries and olecranon fracture-dislocations are not true dislocations in that apposition of the articular surfaces is not lost (see Fig. 28-34). Rather, they are usually fracture-subluxation injuries where the major problem is disruption of the trochlear notch

Recent reports on elbow instability have emphasized the importance of the coronoid process (1,12,20). The injuries that give surgeons the most trouble are the terrible triad, varus posteromedial, and olecranon fracture-dislocations with associated coronoid fractures (1). In each case, the fracture of the coronoid is the most important and challenging part of the injury.

Regan and Morrey (152) classified coronoid fractures based on the size of the fragment: Type I, avulsion of the tip of the coronoid process; Type II, a single or comminuted fragment involving 50% of the process or less; and Type III, a single or comminuted fragment involving more than 50% of the process (152). They also included a modifier to indicate the presence (Type B) or absence (Type A) of an elbow dislocation. However, it has become clear that the pattern of the overall injury and morphology of the fracture may be equally or more important than the size of the fragment and the presence or absence of dislocation.

O'Driscoll proposed a new classification system for coronoid fractures based on the anatomic location of the fracture. Fractures may involve the tip, the anteromedial facet, or the basal aspect of the coronoid. The three groups are further divided into subtypes based on the severity of coronoid involvement. His system considers the mechanism of injury along with the associated fractures and soft-tissue injuries and helps to dictate treatment (Fig. 28-37) (1).

The first group of coronoid fractures involves the tip but does not extend medially past the sublime tubercle or into the body. Tip, subtype 1 fractures involve less than 2 mm of the coronoid and may be found in isolation or with a fracture dislocation. Tip, subtype 2 fractures involve more than 2 mm and are largely associated with terrible triad injuries. In my experience all of these fracture fragments contain the insertion of the anterior capsule and the 2-mm distinction between subtypes 1 and 2 is arbitrary and does not influence treatment.

The second group of coronoid fractures involves the anteromedial aspect of the coronoid. Anteromedial subtype 1 fractures extend from just medial to the tip of the coronoid to the anterior half of the sublime tubercle (insertion of the anterior band of the MCL). Anteromedial subtype 2 fractures are subtype 1 injuries with extension of the fracture line into the tip. Anteromedial subtype 3 fractures involve the anteromedial rim and the entire sublime tubercle with or without involvement of the tip of the coronoid. The mechanism of injury is usually a varus/posteromedial rotation injury with axial loading. The LCL com-

a cast brace that allows elbow motion with the forearm held in this position. It is interesting to check varus and valgus stability in order to note that in some patients valgus stability is preserved, but this examination does not usually alter treatment.

A posterior splint immobilizing the elbow in 90 degrees of flexion and the forearm in neutral rotation is applied for comfort and discarded within 2 weeks of injury. Active elbow motion is encouraged as soon as the patient can tolerate it. Specific exercises to regain terminal elbow extension and flexion are often helpful and can be taught by the physician or a therapist.

Treatment of Persistent Subluxation

Patients with persistent subluxation have been treated with a cast brace with the forearm held in pronation (157). An alternative is to forego the brace or cast and encourage confident active motion of the elbow (9). Patients with persistent subluxation of the elbow resemble patients with so-called pseudosubluxation of the shoulder related to pain-related inhibition of the shoulder muscles. Active elbow mobilization adds an additional dynamic muscular contribution to elbow stability. This should only be attempted in patients with slight subluxation or opening of the joint and not in patients with so-called perched dislocations in which the trochlea is resting on and scraping against the coronoid process (Fig. 28-39).

Treatment of Unstable Dislocations

When the elbow cannot be held in a concentrically reduced position, redislocates before getting a postreduction x-ray, or dislocates later in spite of splint immobilization, the dislocation is deemed unstable and operative treatment is required. There are three general approaches to this problem: (a) open relocation and repair of soft tissues back to the distal humerus (Fig. 28-40); (b) hinged external fixation (Fig. 28-41); and (c) cross-pinning of the joint (Fig. 28-42).

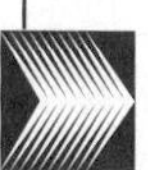

AUTHOR'S PREFERRED TREATMENT

After closed manipulative reduction, I prefer to avoid a splint if possible and start immediate active mobilization of the elbow. I do not immobilize the elbow longer than 1 week. Slight subluxations nearly always recover with confident elbow exercises and I have used this technique following reduction as late as 6 weeks after a simple elbow dislocation (Table 28-3).

In my opinion neither persistent subluxation nor an unstable elbow dislocation benefits from cast immobilization. Persistent subluxation may be exacerbated by additional weight on a relaxed elbow and the elbow also becomes very stiff. Unstable elbows can dislocate in spite of cast or brace immobilization and the patient may not be aware (20).

I believe that persistent subluxation or dislocation of the elbow after manipulative reduction and active elbow exercises requires operative treatment. In older patients, it is often sufficient to repair the lateral soft tissues back to the lateral epicondyle. In younger patients with high-energy injuries, I have found that repair of both the medial and lateral soft tissue structures back to the distal humerus does not completely stabilize the elbow, but this might be enhanced by reattachment of the anterior capsule to the coronoid process. Instead of this extensive dissection, which I fear might enhance the potential for heterotopic ossification, I prefer to apply a hinged external fixator to maintain reduction while allowing active exercises for the first 4 weeks after injury.

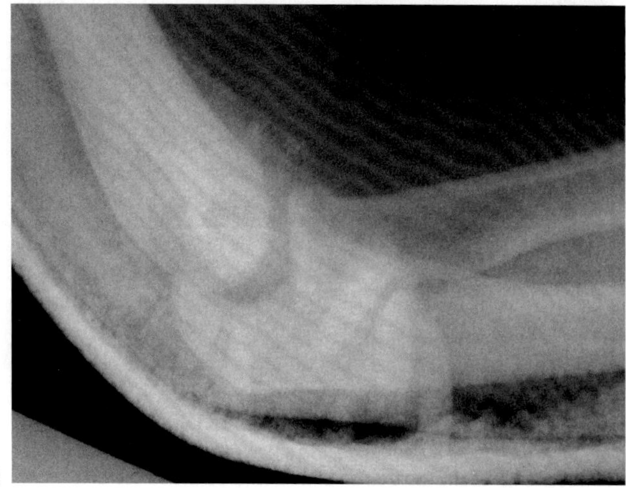

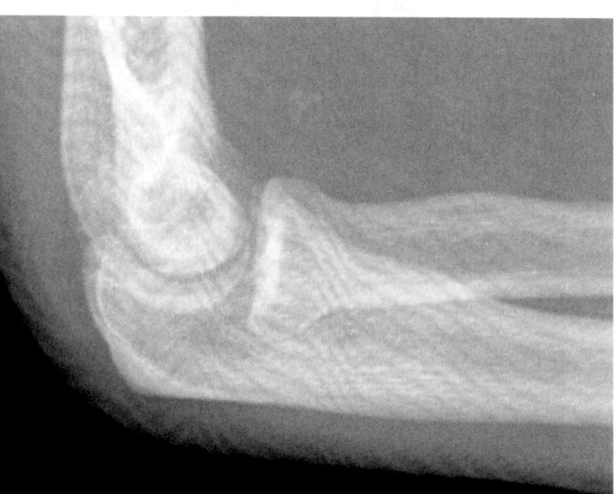

FIGURE 28-39 Residual subluxation of the elbow after a simple elbow dislocation can be effectively treated with active elbow exercises in most patients. **A.** This is attempted when the subluxation is more of a pseudosubluxation, as seen here, and not when the trochlea is perched on the coronoid. **B.** An x-ray taken after confident active mobilization of the elbow shows a concentric reduction.

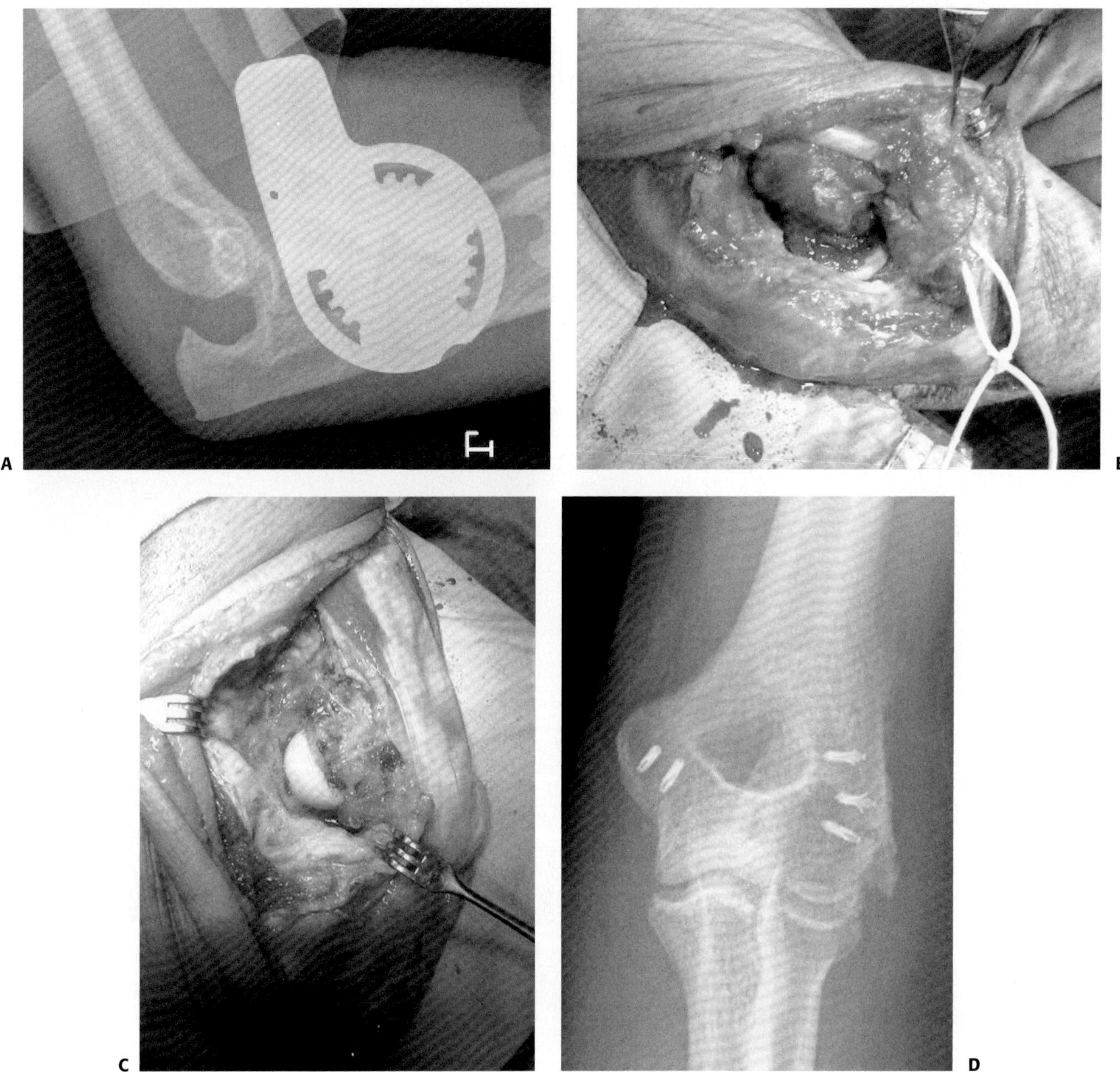

FIGURE 28-40 A 35-year-old man who fell from four stories had an unstable simple elbow dislocation. **A.** In spite of a hinged brace, the trochlea is perched on the coronoid process. **B.** The MCL and common flexor muscles were avulsed from the medial epicondyle. **C.** The LCL and common extensor muscles were stripped off of the lateral epicondyle. **D.** Anteroposterior x-ray after reattachment of the soft tissues to the epicondyles shows concentric reduction.

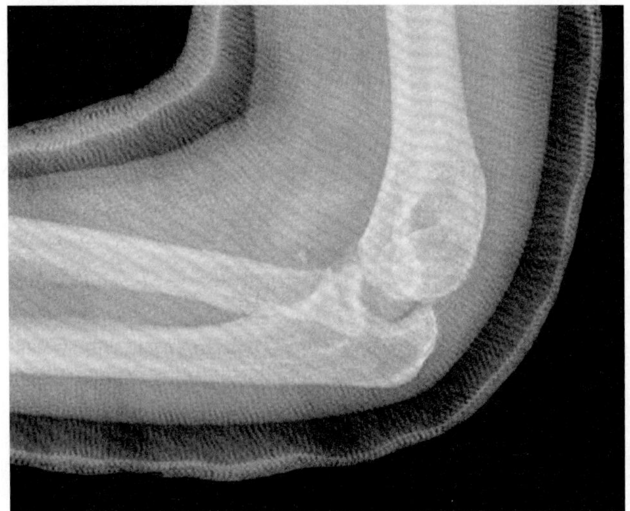

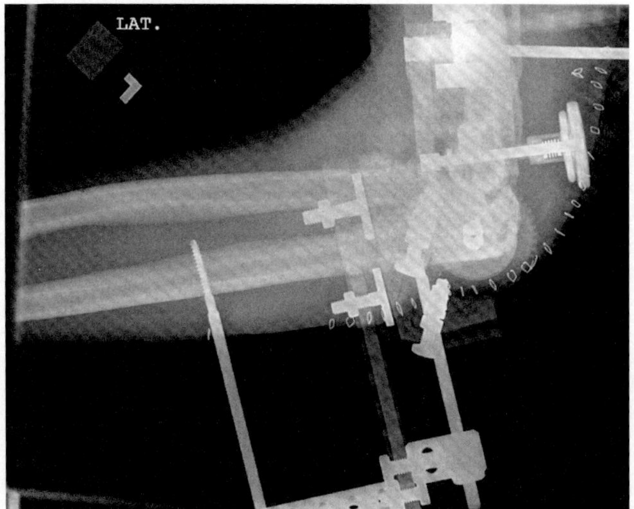

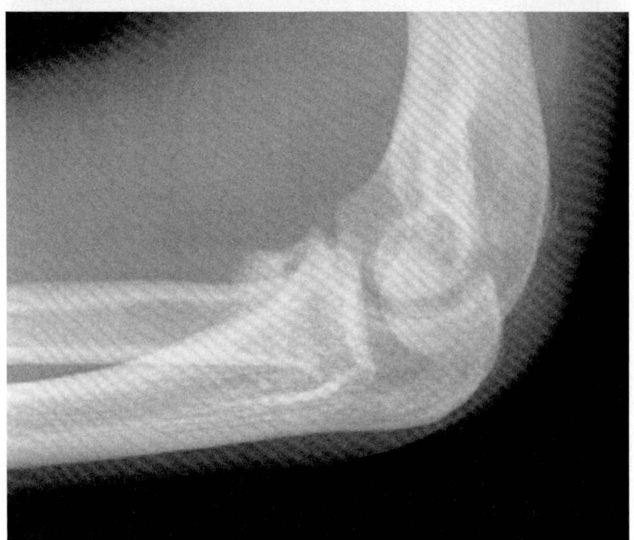

FIGURE 28-41 A 30-year-old man injured in a fall from a height had an unstable simple elbow dislocation. **A.** The trochlea remains perched on the coronoid process in spite of cast immobilization. **B.** An open reduction, reattachment of the lateral collateral ligament to the lateral epicondyle and application of hinged external fixation were performed. **C.** A second procedure to remove anterior heterotopic bone was performed and a stable elbow with near-normal elbow motion was obtained.

Hinged external fixation is usually used in addition to open relocation of the elbow and reattachment of the origin of the LCL to the lateral epicondyle. In older, infirm patients, cross-pinning of the ulnohumeral joint is adequate and can be accomplished with sedation and local anesthesia.

Surgical Procedure: Soft Tissue Repair

A midline posterior incision is created and a lateral skin flap elevated. The extent of the soft tissue injury may not be apparent until the overlying fascia is incised. The avulsed LCL origin and common extensor musculature are reattached to the lateral epicondyle with suture anchors or sutures passed through drill holes in bone. I place one anchor or drill hole at the origin of the LCL and one more proximally if necessary for repair of the avulsed or detached radial wrist extensor muscle origins (Fig. 28-43). This lateral soft tissue repair is often sufficient in older patients, but a medial sided repair will be necessary in most young patients with high-energy injuries (Fig. 28-40).

If the elbow redislocates with gravity extension, a medial flap is elevated and the ulnar nerve is released from where it passes through the medial intermuscular septum proximally through Osbourne's fascia distally and transposed into the subcutaneous tissues anteriorly. The anterior capsule is reattached to the coronoid using sutures passed through drill holes in the coronoid (entering from the dorsal surface of the ulna) and the MCL and common flexor origins are then repaired back to the medial epicondyle using suture anchors or sutures passed through drill holes in bone. If the elbow dislocates in gravity extension, hinged external fixation or cross-pinning of the elbow should be considered. If stability is restored with soft tissue repair alone, the elbow can be mobilized within a few days of surgery, but I usually splint the elbow until suture removal about 10 days later and then initiate active elbow exercises.

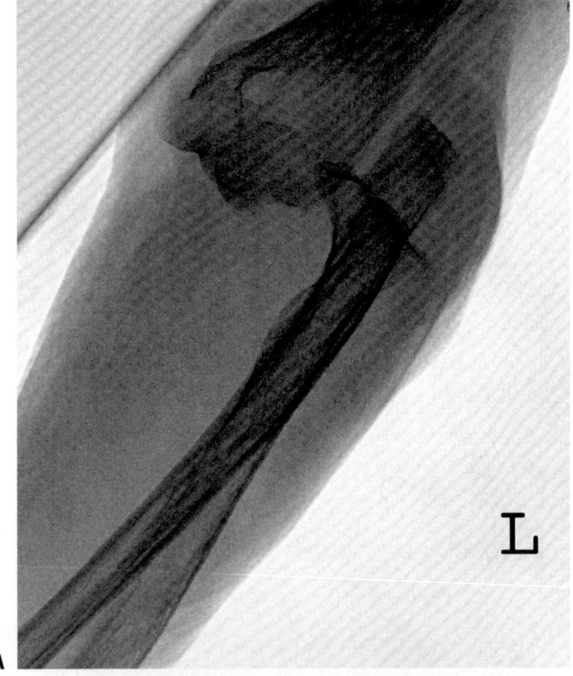

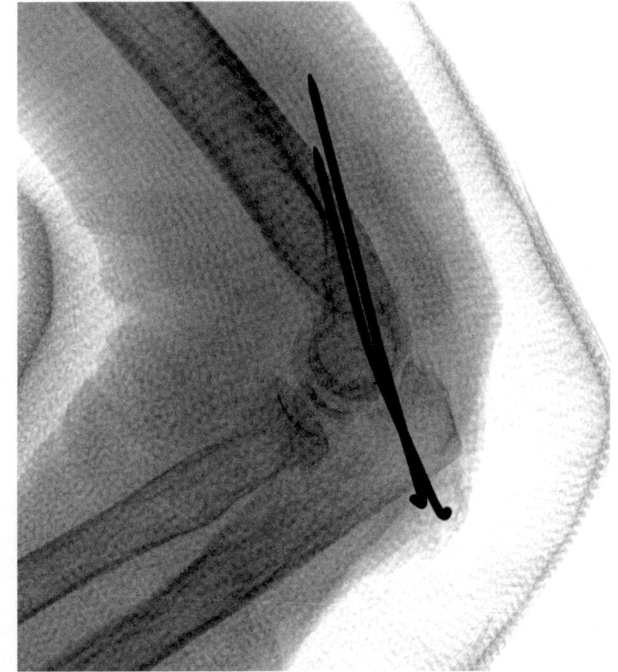

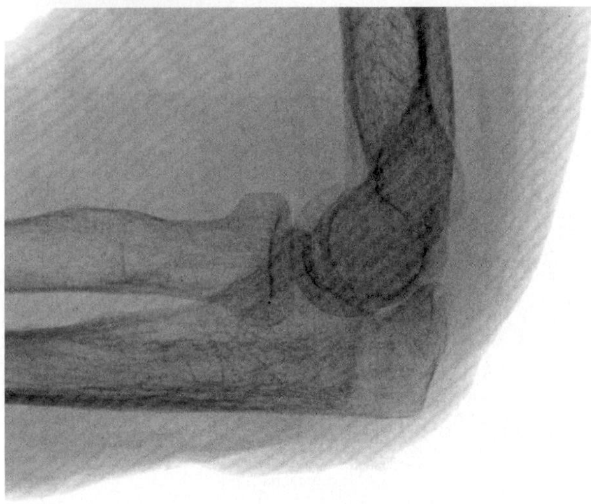

FIGURE 28-42 An 80-year-old woman had an unstable simple elbow dislocation after a fall. **A.** The x-ray of the initial injury. **B.** The elbow was stabilized with two smooth Kirschner wires under sedation and local anesthesia and a long arm cast was applied. The pins and cast were removed 4 weeks later. **C.** A stable concentric reduction with near-normal motion was obtained.

TABLE 28-3 Pitfalls and Pearls for Simple Elbow Dislocations

Pitfalls	Pearls
• Stiffness of the elbow	• Immobilize the elbow for comfort only. Initiate active exercises within 2 weeks of injury.
• Continued casting or operative treatment to treat slight subluxation after elbow relocation	• The majority of patients with slight subluxation (or pseudosubluxation) of the elbow after an elbow dislocation will improve with active elbow motion.
• Unrecognized redislocation	• Beware of the potential for a simple elbow dislocation to be unstable in (a) elderly patients, and (b) younger patients after high-energy injuries.

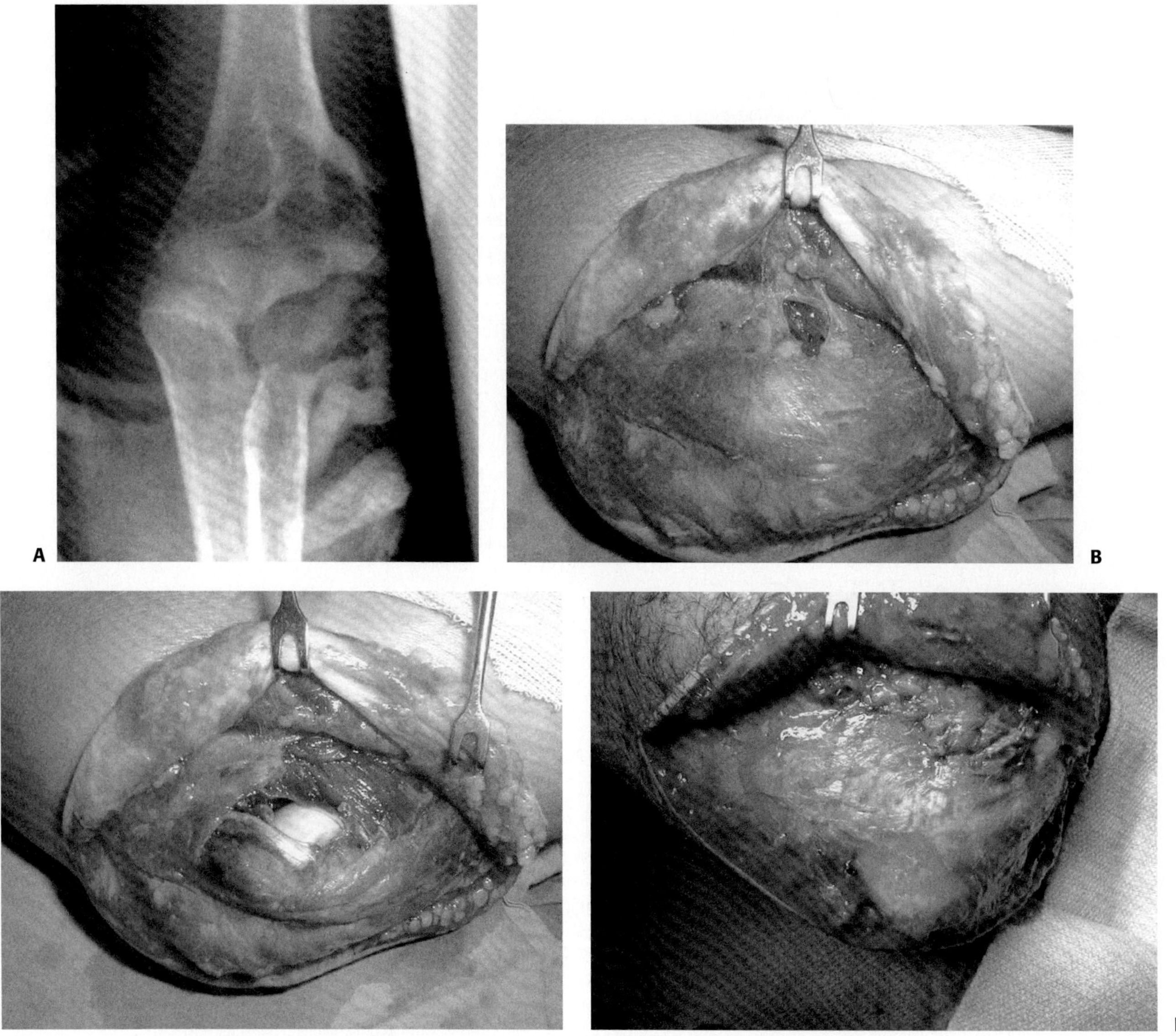

FIGURE 28-43 A 65-year-old woman had an unstable simple elbow dislocation. **A.** The elbow seems to be hinging open on some intact medial soft tissues. **B.** After elevating a lateral skin flap, there is very little damage evident. **C.** After incision of the overlying fascia, the injury to the lateral collateral ligament and common extensors is apparent. The remaining tissue on the lateral epicondyle is tendon and not ligament. **D.** Repair of the lateral sided soft tissue injury restored stability.

Surgical Procedure: Hinged External Fixation

The elbow joint is reduced and held in a reduced position with temporary cross-pinning of the joint using smooth 0.078 inch Kirschner wires and a hinged external fixator is applied. There are several varieties of hinged external fixators including unilateral (lateral) fixators, fixators with transfixation pins, and fixators based on an Ilizarov-type frame—the specific instructions for application should be followed (Fig. 28-41).

Active mobilization is allowed the morning after surgery. Some fixators include a mechanism for applying a static progressive stretch to the elbow and this can be instituted immediately. The fixator is removed 4 weeks after surgery and the exercises are continued.

Surgical Procedure: Cross-Pinning

Under sedation, the skin over the olecranon is infiltrated with local anesthesia. The elbow is manipulated and two 0.078-inch Kirschner wires are drilled across the ulnohumeral joint. Usually one axially directed wire and one obliquely directed wire (starting lateral to avoid the ulnar nerve) are adequate (Fig. 28-42). The wires are aimed somewhat posteriorly in order to account for the anterior translation of the trochlea with respect to the humeral shaft. The adequacy of the reduction is confirmed by x-ray, the wires are trimmed and bent above the skin and a well-padded cast is applied. The cast and pins are removed 3 or 4 weeks later and active exercises are initiated. Some surgeons who use cross-pinning prefer to use screws because they are worried about breakage of the pins, but I have not found this desirable or necessary.

Complications

Varus, valgus, and posterolateral rotatory instability are very uncommon after elbow dislocation. Persistent subluxation and dislocation can destroy the ulnohumeral articulation if not promptly identified and treated as the joint surfaces scrape against one another. Slight subluxation with relative congruence of the articular surfaces can be treated with active exercises as previously described. Wide dislocation is actually preferred over subluxation with abnormal contact of the articular surfaces, because the articular surfaces are less likely to be damaged. We have had substantial success treating a chronic simple elbow dislocation with relocation and 6 weeks of hinged external fixation without ligament repair or reconstruction, likely because the articular surfaces have been relatively well preserved (158).

ELBOW FRACTURE-DISLOCATIONS AND CORONOID FRACTURES

Posterior Dislocation and Fracture of the Radial Head

The simplest pattern of elbow fracture-dislocation is posterior dislocation of the elbow with fracture of the radial head. This injury is identical to a simple elbow dislocation with the addition of a fracture of the radial head as it collides with the capitellum during dislocation.

Rationale

Loss of support between the radial head and capitellum via fracture of the radial head creates an additional measure of instability, but this injury pattern is not as problematic as when the coronoid process is fractured as well. Broberg and Morrey (124) and Josefsson and colleagues (125) documented good results treating these injuries with or without radial head resection and a month of cast immobilization with two caveats: (a) patients with associated coronoid fractures redislocated in the cast, and (b) patients treated nonoperatively often needed secondary procedures to address restriction of forearm rotation due to the fracture of the radial head. Although the radial head may not be necessary to keep the elbow concentrically reduced in this injury pattern, some authors have suggested that preservation of the stabilizing influence of radiocapitellar contact may delay the onset of ulnohumeral arthrosis (159).

Current Treatment Options

Nonoperative Treatment. Some patients are wary of operative treatment. Whereas avoidance of operative treatment might be unwise when the elbow dislocation is associated with both coronoid and radial head fractures, it is a reasonable treatment option in patients with dislocation and fracture of the radial head only. A CT scan may be necessary to be certain that the coronoid is not fractured. Patients who elect nonoperative treatment need to be aware of the slight potential for instability and the substantial potential for restriction of motion or arthrosis from the radial head fracture. The literature documents the results after 1 month of cast immobilization (124,125), but under close supervision, it is reasonable to remove the splint and begin active motion at the patient's first visit to the office, typically about a week after injury.

Operative Treatment: Radial Head Resection, Repair or Replacement and Lateral Collateral Ligament Repair. When the fracture of the radial head cannot be repaired with confidence, it is reasonable to resect it (without prosthetic replacement). Good results with this treatment have been reported, provided that there is no coronoid fracture (124,125). The experience reported in the literature does not include collateral ligament repair. We now understand the importance of the LCL to elbow stability, and it is helpful to reattach this ligament to the lateral epicondyle (18).

When feasible, repair of the radial head restores the native anatomy and contributes to the immediate and long-term stability of the elbow. The injured LCL facilitates exposure of the radial head.

If the radial head cannot be repaired, resection, and replacement with a metal prosthesis will enhance immediate and long-term stability, but also exposes the patient to its potential complications.

When the LCL is repaired, immediate active motion is usually possible (particularly if radiocapitellar contact has also been restored), but up to 10 days of immobilization is reasonable (132).

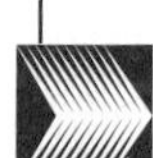

AUTHOR'S PREFERRED TREATMENT

I usually recommend operative treatment, but I have treated a few very motivated and informed patients nonoperatively and been delightfully surprised with the results (Fig. 28-44). Most patients will benefit from treatment of the radial head fracture. I repair the radial head only when all the fragments are present, the bone quality is adequate, and secure fixation can be accomplished. Otherwise, I resect the radial head and replace it with a metal prosthesis. I have treated a few lower-demand patients who did not want a prosthesis (again well-informed and motivated) with resection and LCL repair alone, also with good results. Operative treatment of the radial head fracture and collateral ligament injury are described above.

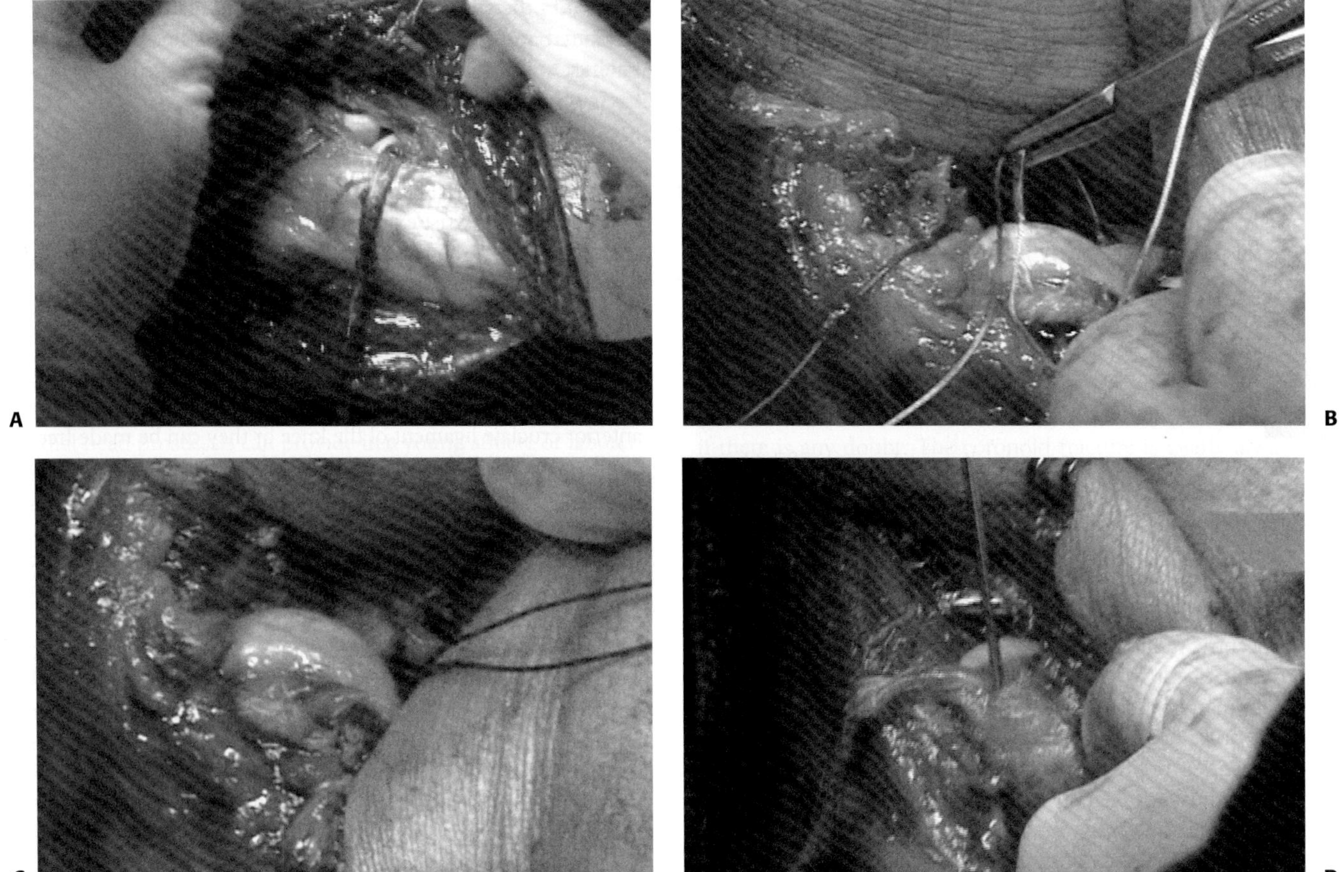

FIGURE 28-45 Operative treatment of a terrible triad elbow fracture-dislocation. **A.** A traumatic rent in the common extensors was developed distally. The strand of tissue still attached to the lateral epicondyle is musculotendinous, not ligament. **B.** Sutures passed through drill holes in the ulna are passed through drill holes in the large coronoid fragment. **C.** The coronoid is reduced, restoring an anterior buttress and the function of the anterior capsule. **D.** The lateral collateral ligament complex is reattached to the lateral epicondyle using a suture anchor. The radial head has been replaced with a prosthesis.

treatment and radial head resection without prosthetic replacement risks redislocation (20), and data that fixation of the coronoid can restore stability in most cases (18), but we do not have data regarding the efficacy of treatment of the radial head and collateral ligaments alone.

The role of MCL repair is debatable. I, and others, find that it is rarely necessary when all of the lateral structures and the coronoid have been repaired (18). In fact, it is my impression that in the rare patient in whom treatment of the coronoid, radial head, and LCL do not restore stability, then repair of the MCL will not add much and one should be prepared to proceed to hinged external fixation or cross-pinning of the joint.

The use of cross-pinning of the joint is very controversial. I would point out that a stiff elbow with preserved articular surface is easier to treat than an elbow with a damaged articular surface due to chronic subluxation and abnormal wear. Recognizing the expense, skill, and resources needed to apply a hinged fixator successfully, I think cross-pinning has a useful role for the very unstable elbow.

Varus Posteromedial Rotational Instability Injuries

Signs and Symptoms

With this injury the elbow is swollen and painful as expected, but the patient is often capable of substantial active motion. In fact, given the small size of the associated coronoid fracture in most cases, the surgeon may be tempted to treat the injury with early active motion to avoid instability (Table 28-4). Patients will often report clunking or giving way of the elbow when this is attempted—evidence of the underlying instability.

TABLE 28-4 Pitfalls and Pearls for Elbow Fracture-Dislocations and Coronoid Fractures

Pitfalls	Pearls
• Failure to recognize a complex injury pattern	• The majority of small coronoid fractures are part of a potentially troublesome complex injury pattern. • In the setting of a dislocation with fracture of the radial head, a small triangular fragment in front of the trochlea or in the coronoid fossa is the coronoid. When in doubt use CT. • Anteromedial coronoid facet fractures are associated with varus instability—beware of associated LCL or olecranon injury.
• Recurrent instability	• Never resect the radial head without replacing it with a prosthesis in the setting of a terrible triad injury. • Identify the injury pattern and treat each of the components of the injury. • Do not trust a cast to maintain reduction.
• Arthrosis due to persistent subluxation	• Check the elbow frequently for the first 6 weeks after injury and surgery. • When substantial subluxation (perching of the trochlea on the coronoid) is identified, the surgeon should intervene before articular damage occurs.
• Underestimation of the importance of a small coronoid fracture with resultant instability	• Become comfortable with operative fixation of coronoid fractures or refer patients to surgeons who are comfortable with these techniques.

Rationale

This is an unstable injury that can lead to chronic subluxation and arthrosis of the elbow. It has only recently been recognized and it is relatively uncommon, so our knowledge of the results of nonoperative treatment is limited. Early experience would suggest that these injuries benefit from operative treatment (1).

Diagnosis and Classification

This injury is under-recognized. The key element of this injury is a displaced fracture of the anteromedial facet of the coronoid process (Fig. 28-46A), reflecting the varus injury mechanism. Associated injuries include one of the following: (a) injury to the LCL (Fig. 28-46B), (b) fracture of the olecranon (Fig. 28-46C), or (c) an additional fracture of the coronoid at its base (Fig. 28-46D–F). It is uncommon to have more than one of these associated injuries.

When the olecranon is not fractured, a varus stress x-ray may be necessary to appreciate the LCL injury (Fig. 28-46A,B). Computed tomography, particularly three-dimensional reconstructions, are useful to plan treatment of the coronoid fracture. The coronoid fracture usually involves anteromedial facet and tip fragments and occasionally extends to the base of the coronoid process.

Current Treatment Options/Author's Preferred Treatment

This injury is treated with operative repair of all injured structures. The LCL and/or olecranon fracture are repaired, the coronoid is repaired through a medial exposure using some combination of wires, plates, and screws. A buttress plate is particularly useful.

Surgical Procedure: Anteromedial Coronoid Facet Fracture. A medial skin flap is elevated with care taken to protect the medial antebrachial cutaneous nerve and the ulnar nerve. We prefer to mobilize the ulnar nerve from the cubital tunnel allowing it to remain anteriorly transposed in the subcutaneous tissues at the end of the procedure (Fig. 28-34E). From the medial side, the coronoid can be exposed directly medially—between the heads of the flexor carpi ulnaris where the ulnar nerve usually lies—or superiorly through the over-the-top approach described by Hotchkiss (24) for contracture release (Fig. 28-5). Taylor and Scham (25) described elevation of the entire flexor-pronator mass, but this requires far more dissection than elevation from within the split in the flexor carpi ulnaris. It is useful for very large fragments.

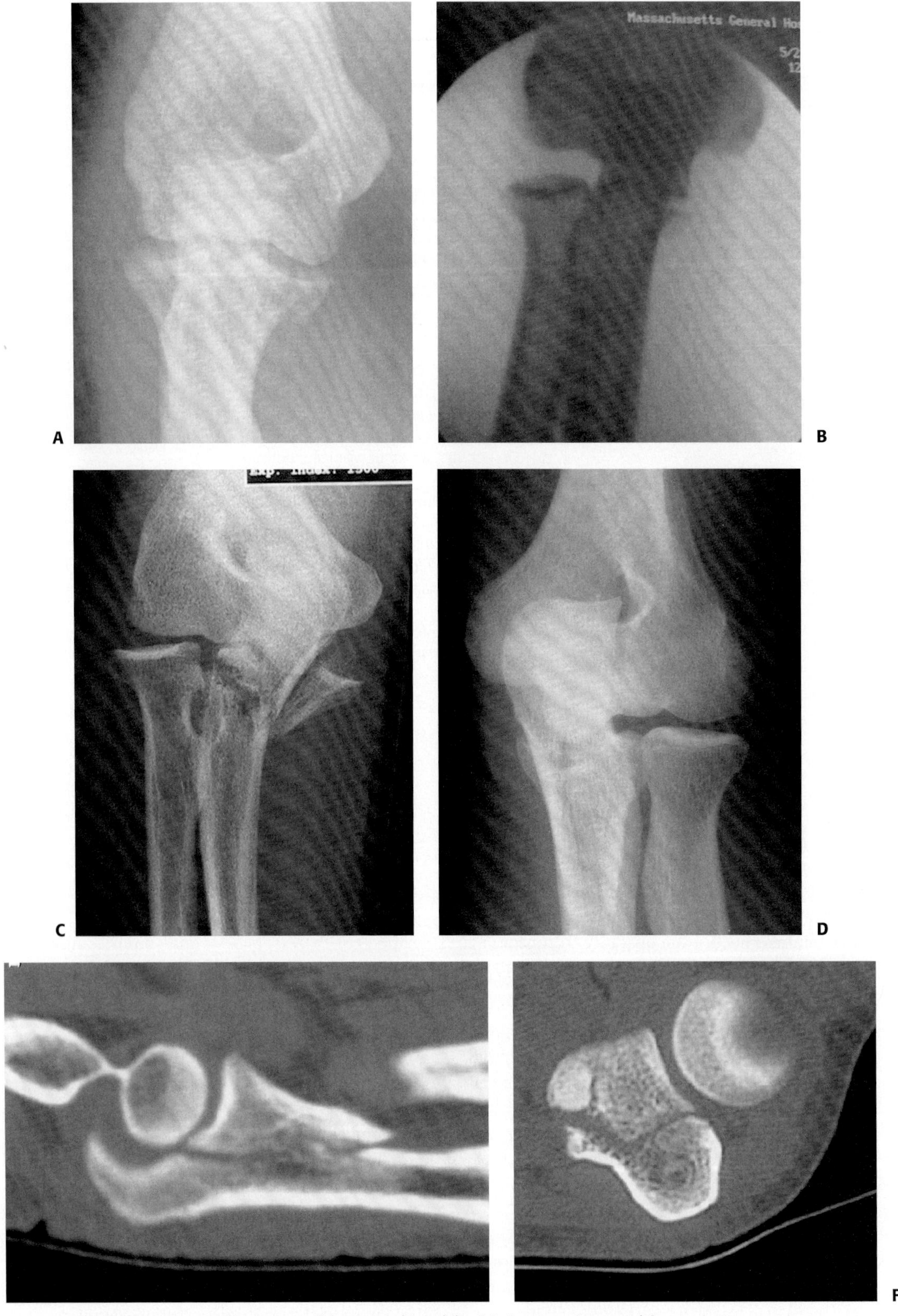

FIGURE 28-46 Varus posteromedial rotational instability injuries occur in several forms. **A.** Some patients present with small isolated anteromedial facet coronoid fractures. **B.** Stress x-rays reveal injury to the lateral collateral ligament. **C.** Alternatively, there may be a fracture of the olecranon, in which case there is usually not a lateral collateral ligament injury. **D–F.** Finally, some patients with anteromedial coronoid facet fractures may have a fracture of the coronoid at its base.

The dissection on the medial side should remain superficial to the anterior band of the MCL. In addition, capsular attachments to the tip of the coronoid should be preserved. Through this exposure a small T-plate or a plate designed specifically for internal fixation of the coronoid can be applied.

Complications

An extensive dissection, transposition, and retraction of the ulnar nerve is needed to perform a medial repair and ulnar nerve palsies sometimes occur. Large tapes and tapes with hemostats should not be used as they may lead to excessive traction. A means for providing adequate retraction of the nerve without prolonged pressure needs to be devised. I have sutured the skin to the forearm fascia to hold the nerve anteriorly as I work on the coronoid.

Subluxation of the elbow can occur with rotation of the humerus into the coronoid defect leading to arthrosis (1). Heterotopic bone formation is uncommon after this injury.

Controversies and Future Directions

This injury has only recently been recognized and our understanding of it and the best treatment methods are evolving. Improved exposure and plating techniques for the medial coronoid will most likely be developed with increasing experience with this injury pattern.

OLECRANON AND PROXIMAL ULNA FRACTURES

Rationale

The key element in the treatment of a fracture of the proximal ulna, no matter how complex, is to restore the contour and dimensions of the trochlear notch of the ulna. Small articular incongruities and comminution in the relatively nonarticular transverse groove will be of little consequence provided that stable realignment of the coronoid and olecranon facets is achieved (1,55,56). These fractures often occur in patients with poor bone quality (55). Careful technique and an understanding of how to achieve reliable internal fixation are important. Restoration of the trochlear notch is the key to restoring elbow stability. Also important are repair or replacement of the radial head and repair of the LCL complex when they are injured. Stable fixation will allow immediate mobilization, thereby diminishing the risk of stiffness and heterotopic ossification (Table 28-5).

Diagnosis and Classification

The initial x-rays obtained after the injury are often of limited quality due to the deformity and pain in the limb. Nevertheless, it is usually possible to discern the overall pattern of the injury, which in turn leads one to suspect other injury components that may not be immediately obvious. For example, a posterior olecranon fracture-dislocation is often associated with fractures of the radial head and coronoid process as well as injury to the LCL complex (55), whereas an anterior fracture-dislocation rarely involves injury to the radial head or collateral ligaments (56).

X-rays obtained after manipulative reduction and splint immobilization of the limb (when appropriate) may provide better views of the elbow and additional information about the injury. When additional information about fractures of the radial head or coronoid may influence decision making, CT is useful. In particular, three-dimensional reconstructions with the distal humerus removed can provide a very accurate characterization of the injury. Using such images, the preoperative planning will be more accurate.

Additional information regarding the character of the injury can be obtained by viewing the elbow under the image intensifier once the patient is anesthetized. For some complex injuries, complete characterization of the injury pattern—and therefore a final treatment plan—can only be made based upon operative exposure. The surgeon must therefore be comfortable with extensile exposures providing adequate access to the injury components.

Monteggia Fractures

Fractures of the proximal ulna that do not involve the trochlear notch often have an associated dislocation of the proximal radioulnar joint—the so-called Monteggia lesion (55,161,162). The most commonly used classification of these injuries is that by Bado who distinguished four lesions based upon the direction of dislocation of the radial head: Type 1, anterior; Type 2, posterior; Type 3, lateral; Type 4, any direction, associated with a diaphyseal fracture of the radius (163). In practice the most useful distinction is between fractures with anterior or lateral displacement of the radial head and those with posterior displacement. The management of injuries with anterior or lateral displacement centers upon stable restoration of the ulnar alignment, which nearly always restores alignment and function of the proximal radioulnar joint (55,120,162).

The Bado Type 2 or posterior Monteggia lesion has long been recognized as a distinct injury that is usually associated with fracture of the radial head and often occurs in the setting of osteoporosis (147,148,164). There is a spectrum of posterior Monteggia injuries with similar features that vary according to the location of the ulnar fracture (164). These have been subclassified as Type A when the fracture is at the level of the trochlear notch (involving the olecranon and often the coronoid processes); Type B, in the metaphysis just distal to the trochlear notch; and Type C, in the diaphysis. Type D fractures are multifragmented fractures that involve more than one region (164). These fractures are inherently unstable by virtue of the associated capsuloligamentous damage, fracture and dislocation of the radial head, and the morphology of the ulnar fracture, which often involves a triangular or quadrangular fragment of the ulna that includes the anterior ulnar cortex and sometimes the coronoid process.

TABLE 28-5 Pitfalls and Pearls for Olecranon and Proximal Ulna Fractures

Pitfalls	Pearls
• Use of tension band wiring for complex injury patterns	• Recognize anterior and posterior olecranon fracture-dislocations and use plate and screw fixation.
• Failure to restore alignment of a large coronoid fracture	• Recognize complex injury patterns. • Be prepared for large coronoid fractures. • Be prepared for complex comminution. • Become familiar with the techniques of exposure and internal fixation of large coronoid fractures as part of an olecranon fracture-dislocation or refer to a surgeon who is.
• Postoperative dislocation of the ulnohumeral joint	• Be aware of the potential for ulnohumeral instability with posterior olecranon fracture-dislocations. • Restore radiocapitellar contact, realign the ulna including the coronoid, repair the LCL.
• Early loss of fixation and nonunion	• Use a long plate that follows the contour of the olecranon, preferably on the dorsal surface. This provides for a greater number of screws and screws in orthogonal directions. • Be aware of the likelihood of osteoporosis, particularly with posterior olecranon fracture-dislocations after low-energy injuries.

Olecranon Fractures

The Mayo classification of olecranon fractures distinguishes three factors that have a direct influence on treatment: (a) fracture displacement, (b) comminution, and (c) ulnohumeral instability (Fig. 28-47) (161). Type I fractures that are nondisplaced or minimally displaced, are either noncomminuted (Type IA) or comminuted (Type IB) and are treated nonoperatively. Type II fractures feature displacement of the proximal fragment without elbow instability—these fractures require operative treatment. Type IIA fractures, which are noncomminuted, are well treated by tension band wire fixation. When the fracture is oblique, an ancillary interfragmentary compression screw can be added. Type IIB fractures are comminuted and require plate fixation. Type III fractures feature instability of the ulnohumeral joint and require surgical treatment.

Olecranon Fracture-Dislocations

Fractures of the proximal ulna can appear extremely complex. The identification of basic injury patterns can facilitate management. Even a simple fracture pattern of the olecranon can have associated injuries, which the surgeon must be careful not to miss.

Varus posteromedial rotational instability pattern injuries have only recently been recognized and described. The central element of this injury is a fracture of the anteromedial facet of the coronoid process, resulting in varus instability (14). There is an associated injury, either an avulsion of the LCL complex from the lateral epicondyle or a fracture of the olecranon—but rarely both. The radial head is rarely fractured.

The majority of olecranon fracture-dislocations occur in either an anterior or a posterior direction (55,56). Anterior olecranon fracture-dislocations have been described as trans-olecranon fracture dislocations because the trochlea of the distal humerus implodes through the trochlear notch of the ulna as the forearm translates anteriorly (Fig. 28-35) (56,165). This pattern can be confused with posterior fracture-dislocations with a similar appearance, so the term anterior olecranon fracture-dislocation may be preferable. Anterior fracture dislocations are injuries to the ulnohumeral articulation with the radioulnar relationship being relatively preserved and the radial head rarely injured. The fracture of the proximal ulna can be a simple oblique fracture, but is often very complex including fragmentation of the olecranon, fragmentation extending into the ulnar diaphysis, and fracture of the coronoid. Associated collateral ligament injury is unusual (56,165).

It is useful to consider posterior fracture-dislocations of the olecranon as the most proximal type of posterior Monteggia injury (164). Common factors of posterior Monteggia injuries include an apex posterior fracture of the ulna, posterior translation of the radial head with respect to the capitellum, fracture of the radial head, and frequent injury to the LCL complex. With posterior olecranon fracture-dislocations [or Type A posterior Monteggia fractures according to Jupiter and colleagues (164)] the fracture of the ulna occurs at the level of the olecranon and is nearly always associated with a fracture of the coronoid process. When a complex olecranon fracture-dislocation is identified as being posterior in direction, fractures of the radial

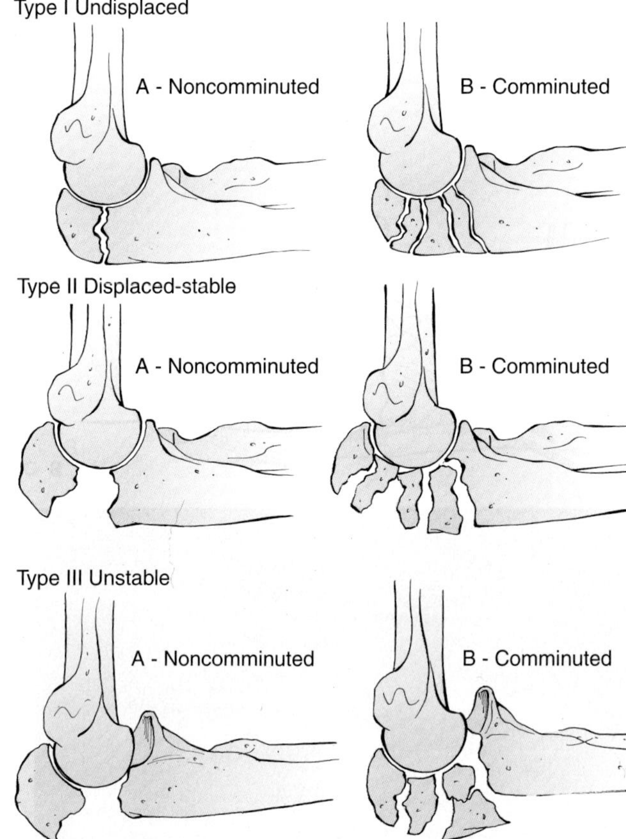

FIGURE 28-47 The Mayo classification of olecranon fractures divides fractures according to displacement, comminution, and sub-luxation/dislocation.

head and coronoid and injury to the LCL should be suspected (Fig. 28-36).

The fracture of the coronoid varies somewhat with each specific type of olecranon fracture-dislocation. Those associated with a varus posteromedial mechanism will involve the anteromedial facet and the tip and the radial head will not be fractured. The fracture of the coronoid that occurs with an anterior olecranon fracture-dislocation is usually a single, large fragment involving nearly the entire coronoid, but it is occasionally split once or twice in the sagittal plane. The fractures of the coronoid associated with posterior olecranon fracture-dislocations are more variable including the occasional fracture of the tip, a single large fragment, comminution into three fragments (anteromedial, central, and sigmoid notch), and more extensive comminution (Fig. 28-35).

Current Treatment Options

Nonoperative Treatment

The unusual fracture of the olecranon that is minimally displaced and does not displace further with the arm placed in 90 degrees of flexion can be treated nonoperatively. The elbow is splinted for 3 to 4 weeks in 90 degrees of flexion and then gentle active motion is started progressing gradually to active assisted motion.

Excision and Triceps Advancement

The olecranon process is rarely so fragmented that it cannot be repaired. Tension band wiring techniques can gain fixation of the soft tissue attachments until healing occurs. As a result, excision of the olecranon and triceps advancement is used sparingly for primary treatment of fractures of the olecranon and occasionally for treatment of secondary complications. As primary treatment, excision of the olecranon is best suited to infirmed older patients with limited functional demands (166,167). The surgeon must be certain that the collateral ligaments, radial head, and coronoid process are intact.

Tension Band Wiring

Tension band wiring is appropriate for relatively simple fractures at the level of the transverse groove of the trochlear notch, without associated ligament injuries or fracture of the coronoid or radial head (Fig. 28-48). Tension band wire techniques have been described using screws or Kirschner wires.

Plate and Screw Fixation

A plate and screw fixation is used for comminuted olecranon fractures, Monteggia fractures, and olecranon fracture-dislocations (Fig. 28-49). In addition to standard plates, there are several precontoured plates for the proximal ulna now available.

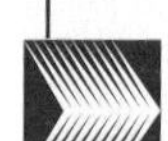

AUTHOR'S PREFERRED TREATMENT

I use cast immobilization on occasion for a stable, nondisplaced fracture of the olecranon, but prefer to repair the majority of these fractures in order to start confident active motion exercises and functional use of the limb.

For simple, noncomminuted fractures without associated ligament injuries, I use tension band wiring with Kirschner wires rather than a screw. For comminuted fractures and fracture dislocations I use a dorsal plate and screws contoured to wrap around the proximal ulna (12,55,56). For some complex fractures I place the proximal aspect of the plate over the triceps insertion and otherwise I elevate the triceps insertion and place the plate directly on bone. When the proximal olecranon fragment is small, fragmented, or osteopenic, I also use a tension wire that engages the triceps insertion (Fig. 28-49).

For fractures of the coronoid that involve the anteromedial facet I use a medial plate unless the fragments are large enough to be reliably repaired with screws (14). For unreconstructable or very complex fractures of the coronoid I use 4 to 8 weeks of hinged external fixation to maintain a concentric ulnohumeral reduction and protect the healing coronoid.

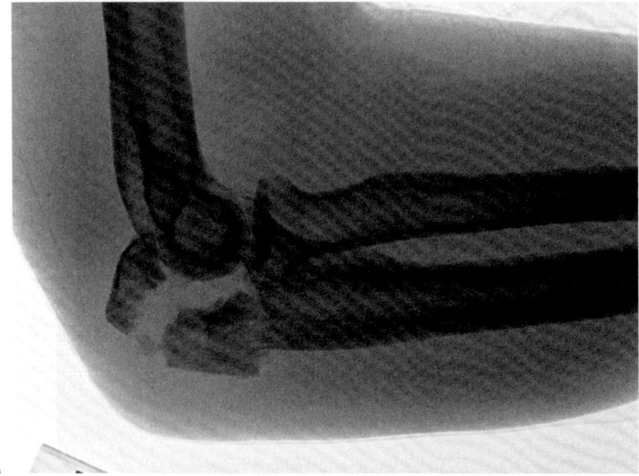

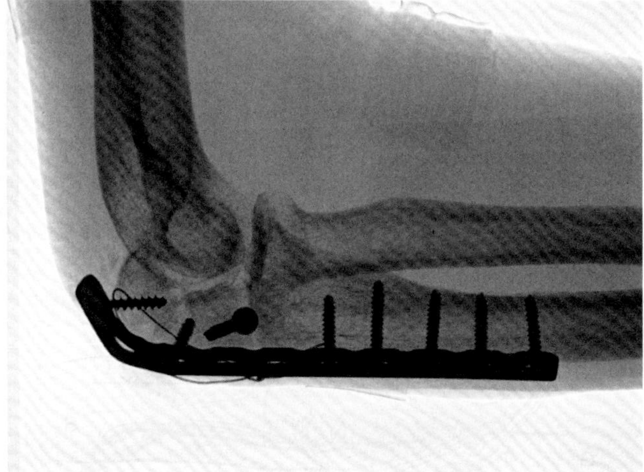

FIGURE 28-49 Comminuted olecranon fractures require plate and screw fixation. **A.** This injury created a small olecranon fragment. **B.** In addition to the plate and screws used to maintain alignment of the trochlear notch, a tension wire is used to gain hold of the small proximal fragment.

clamp can be used to maintain reduction of the olecranon. A drill hole made in the dorsal surface of the ulna can provide a good anchor point for the distal tine of the clamp.

Kirschner Wire Technique

Two parallel Kirschner wires are drilled across the osteotomy site. The majority of surgeons use 0.062-in wires, but we use 0.045-in wires with few problems. The wires are often drilled parallel to the ulnar diaphysis, but we and others favor drilling the wires obliquely so that they pass through the anterior ulnar cortex, just distal to the coronoid process (168,169). This is intended to limit the potential for wire migration. After exiting the anterior cortex, the wires are retracted between 5 and 10 mm anticipating subsequent impaction of the wires into the olecranon process proximally.

The extensor carpi ulnaris and flexor carpi ulnaris muscles are partly elevated from the apex of the ulna distal to the osteotomy site to expose the cortex. The appropriate distance between the fracture and this drill hole has been commented on based upon mechanical calculations, but the placement of these holes is determined more practically by the transition from the flat proximal ulna to the apex posterior triangular shape of the diaphysis. Likewise, the placement of the drill holes in the anteroposterior plane is not critical except that they should not be so dorsal as to risk breaking out of the ulna. Large drill holes (2.5 mm) facilitate wire passage.

Many surgeons use a single 18-gauge stainless-steel wire for the tension wire, but we prefer to use two 22-gauge stainless-steel wires, each passed through its own drill hole distally (Fig. 28-48). The smaller wires are less prominent.

The tension wires are placed in a figure-eight over the dorsal ulna. The proximal end of the wire is passed deep to the Kirschner wires, through the insertion of the triceps using a large gauge needle. The tension wires are then tensioned on both the medial and lateral sides of the ulna until the wire rests flush with the ulna. Some surgeons prefer to twist the wires until they are very tight, but this cannot be done with smaller gauge wires—they will break. The wire does not need to be tight, it is only important to take up all of the slack in the wires. This is done by twisting the wire until it starts to bend over itself. The twisted ends are trimmed and bent into adjacent soft tissues to limit prominence.

The proximal ends of the Kirschner wires are bent 180° and trimmed. The triceps insertion is then incised and these bent ends are impacted into the proximal olecranon with a bone tamp. The strength of the fixation can be tested by completely flexing the elbow—the fracture should not separate.

Screw Technique

Some surgeons prefer to use screws instead of Kirschner wires. Some recommend using a very long screw that engages the medullary canal of the ulnar diaphysis distally (170). Others recommend aiming the screw anteriorly to engage the anterior ulnar cortex. An oblique screw is particularly well suited to an oblique fracture. The remaining portion of the technique is as described for the Kirschner wire technique.

Operative Technique: Plate and Screw Fixation. When a plate is applied to the proximal ulna, it should be contoured to wrap around the proximal aspect of the ulna (Fig. 28-49). A straight plate will only have two or three screws in metaphyseal bone proximal to the fracture. Many patients with complex proximal ulna fractures have osteopenic bone, which further compromises the strength of plate and screw fixation. Bending the plate around the proximal aspect of the olecranon provides additional screws in the proximal fragment. In addition, the most proximal screws are oriented orthogonal to the more distal screws. Finally, the most proximal screws can be very long, crossing the fracture line into the distal fragment. In some cases, these screws can be directed to engage one of the cortices of the distal fragment, such as the anterior ulnar cortex.

A plate applied to the dorsal surface of the proximal ulna also has several advantages over plates applied to the medial or lateral aspects of the ulna. Placing the plate along the flat dorsal surface can assist in obtaining and maintaining reduction. The dorsal surface is in the plane of the forces generated by active elbow motion so that the plate functions to a certain extent as a tension band. Finally, dorsal plate placement requires very limited soft-tissue stripping.

Exposure of the ulna should preserve periosteal and muscle attachments. A plate contoured to wrap around the proximal ulna can be placed on top of the triceps insertion with few problems. This is particularly useful when the olecranon fragment is small or fragmented. Alternatively, the triceps insertion can be incised longitudinally and partially elevated medially and laterally sufficiently to allow direct plate contact with bone.

Distally, a dorsal plate will lie directly on the apex of the ulnar diaphysis. This might seem unsettling to some surgeons, but has not been a problem in our hands. One advantage of this situation is that the muscle need only be split sufficiently to gain access to this apex—there is no need to elevate the muscle or periosteum off either the medial or lateral flat aspect of the ulna. No attempt is made to precisely realign intervening fragmentation—once the relationship of the coronoid and olecranon facets is restored and the overall alignment is restored, the remaining fragments are bridged, leaving their soft tissue attachments intact. In spite of extensive fragmentation, bone grafts (171) are rarely necessary if the soft tissue attachments are preserved (55,56).

Operative Technique: Monteggia Fractures. The majority of anterior and lateral Monteggia lesions feature diaphyseal fractures of the ulna. Standard plating techniques with the plate applied to one of the flat surfaces of the ulna should restore forearm alignment (55). Residual radiocapitellar or proximal radioulnar subluxation usually indicates inadequate alignment of the ulna. On rare occasions, open reduction of the radial head is necessary.

Posterior Monteggia injuries that do not involve the ulnohumeral joint, most frequently occur at the level of the proximal ulnar metaphysis. In this location a dorsally applied plate is preferred (162). Posterior Monteggia injuries are also associated with radial head fractures and LCL injuries that may need to be addressed.

Operative Technique: Fracture-Dislocations. Fractures of the radial head and coronoid process can be evaluated and often definitively treated through the exposure provided by the fracture of the olecranon process. With little additional dissection, the olecranon fragment can be mobilized proximally, providing exposure of the coronoid through the ulnohumeral joint. If the exposure of the radial head through the posterior injury is inadequate, a separate muscle interval [e.g., Kocher's or Kaplan's intervals (27)], accessed by the elevation of a broad lateral skin flap, can be used.

If the exposure of the coronoid is inadequate through the straight dorsal skin incision, a separate medial or lateral exposure can be developed. Posterior olecranon fracture-dislocations often require a lateral exposure to address a fracture of the radial head or coronoid, or to repair the LCL. When the LCL is injured it is usually avulsed from the lateral epicondyle. This facilitates both exposure and repair. The LCL origin and common extensor musculature can be included in an anterior or posterior flap, or mobilized distally.

Improved exposure of the coronoid can be obtained by releasing the origins of the radial wrist extensors from the lateral supracondylar ridge and elevating the brachialis from the anterior humerus, and by excising the fractured radial head (14,19). A medial exposure, between the two heads of the flexor carpi ulnaris, or by splitting the flexor-pronator mass more anteriorly may be needed to address a complex fracture of the coronoid, particularly one that involves the anteromedial facet of the coronoid process.

The fracture of the coronoid can often be reduced directly through the elbow joint using the limited access provided by the olecranon fracture (151,172,173). Provisional fixation can be obtained using Kirschner wires to attach the fragments either to the metaphyseal or diaphyseal fragments of the ulna, or to the trochlea of the distal humerus when there is extensive fragmentation of the proximal ulna (174,175). An alternative to keep in mind when there is extensive fragmentation of the proximal ulna is the use of a skeletal distractor (a temporary external fixator) (56,175). External fixation applied between a wire driven through the olecranon fragment and up into the trochlea and a second wire in the distal ulnar diaphysis can often obtain reduction indirectly when distraction is applied between the pins. Definitive fixation can usually be obtained with screws applied under image intensifier guidance. The screws are placed through the plate when there is extensive fragmentation of the proximal ulna. If the coronoid fracture is very comminuted and cannot be securely repaired, the ulnohumeral joint should be protected with temporary hinged or static external fixation, or temporary pin fixation of the ulnohumeral joint depending on the equipment and expertise available.

A long plate is contoured to wrap around the proximal olecranon. A very long plate should be considered (between 12 and 16 holes), particularly when there is extensive fragmentation or the bone quality is poor. When the olecranon is fragmented or osteoporotic, a plate and screws alone may not provide reliable fixation. In this situation, it has proved useful to use ancillary tension wire fixation to control the olecranon fragments through the triceps insertion.

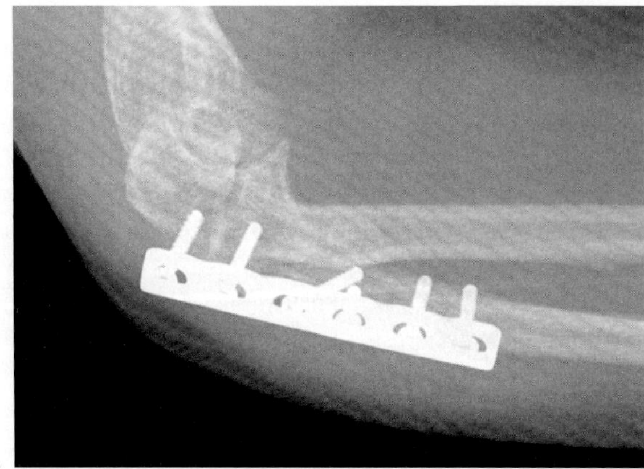

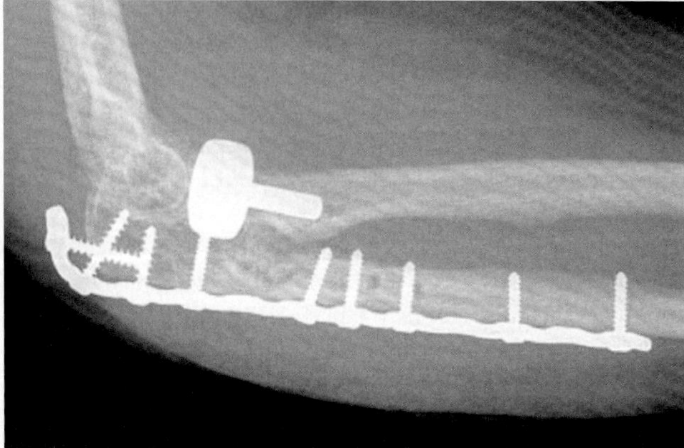

FIGURE 28-50 Medial and lateral plates seem prone to failure when treating posterior Monteggia injuries. **A.** This plate only has two screws in the proximal, osteoporotic metaphyseal fragment and it is therefore not surprising that it loosened. **B.** A much more secure plate applied to the dorsal surface and contoured to wrap around the olecranon process has four screws in the proximal fragment with orthogonal interlocking of the most proximal screws.

Complications

Tension band wire constructs can fail when used for complex fractures or fracture-dislocations, but rarely fail when used for simple fractures unless the patient returns to forceful activity too soon. Plate loosening is most common in older patients with fracture-dislocations when a noncontoured plate has been placed on either the medial or lateral side of the proximal ulna (Fig. 28-50) Failed internal fixation can be salvaged with realignment and repeat internal fixation using a dorsal contoured plate and screws. If there is a bone defect or delayed union, autogenous cancellous bone graft can be applied to the fracture site.

Nonunion after simple olecranon fractures is very unusual (53). Proximal ulnar nonunion usually occurs after a fracture-dislocation of the proximal ulna. Union can usually be achieved with contoured dorsal plate fixation and autogenous bone grafting (53,54).

Ulnohumeral instability is sometimes a surprise to the surgeon treating a complex proximal ulna fracture. It is usually the result of some combination of fixation of the proximal ulna with apex dorsal deformity, as well as inadequate treatment of the coronoid, radial head and LCL complex. These can often be salvaged by secondary surgery, often including the use of hinged external fixation (13,38,52,150).

Both the elbow and the forearm can become stiff with these injuries, particularly posterior olecranon-fracture dislocations. Proximal radioulnar synostosis occurs fairly frequently with these injuries.

Controversies and Future Directions

Many surgeons are starting to use plate and screw fixation for even relatively simple fractures of the olecranon. In some ways, the tension wire is a more reliable way to fix these relatively small fracture fragments. Additional data is needed to understand the relative advantages and disadvantages of each technique.

Our understanding of complex fractures of the proximal ulna and olecranon fracture-dislocations continues to evolve and improve. In particular, the handling of a complex comminuted basal coronoid fracture still represents a substantial challenge.

REFERENCES

1. O'Driscoll SW, Jupiter JB, Cohen M, et al. Difficult Elbow Fractures: Pearls and Pitfalls. Instructional Course Lectures 2003;52:113–134.
2. Morrey BF, An KN. Articular and ligamentous contributions to the stability of the elbow joint. *Am J Sports Med* 1983;11:315–320.
3. Morrey BF, Tanaka S, An KN. Valgus stability of the elbow. A definition of primary and secondary constraints. *Clin Orthop* 1991;265:187–195.
4. Jobe FW, Stark H, Lombardo SJ. Reconstruction of the ulnar collateral ligament in athletes. *J Bone Joint Surg* 1986;68A:1158–1163.
5. Cohen MS, Hastings H. Rotatory instability of the elbow: the anatomy and role of the lateral stabilizers. *J Bone Joint Surg* 1997;79A:225–233.
6. Nestor BJ, O'Driscoll SW, Morrey BF. Ligamentous reconstruction for posterolateral rotatory instability of the elbow. *J Bone Joint Surg* 1992;74A:1235–1241.
7. O'Driscoll SW, Bell DF, Morrey BF. Posterolateral rotatory instability of the elbow. *J Bone Joint Surg* 1991;73A:440–446.
8. Osbourne G, Cotterill P. Recurrent dislocations of the elbow. *J Bone Joint Surg* 1966; 48B:340–346.
9. Dunning CE, Zarzour ZD, Patterson SD, et al. Muscle forces and pronation stabilize the lateral ligament deficient elbow. *Clin Orthop* 2001;388:118–124.
10. Kapandji IA. The physiology of the joints. 5th ed. Edinburgh: Churchill Livingstone, 1982.
11. Ring D, Gulotta L, Jupiter J. Articular fractures of the distal part of the humerus. *J Bone Joint Surg* 2003;85A:232–238.
12. Ring D, Jupiter JB. Fracture-dislocation of the elbow. *J Bone Joint Surg* 1998;80A: 566–580.
13. Ring D, Jupiter JB. Reconstruction of post-traumatic elbow instability. *Clin Orthop* 2000; 370:44–56.
14. Ring D, Jupiter JB. Surgical exposure of coronoid fractures. *Tech Should Elbow Surg* 2002;3:48–56.
15. O'Driscoll SW, Morrey BF, Korinek S, et al. Elbow subluxation and dislocation. a spectrum of instability. *Clin Orthop* 1992;280:186–197.

16. McKee MD, Schemitsch EH, Sala MJ, et al. The pathoanatomy of lateral ligamentous disruption in complex elbow instability. *J Should Elbow Surg* 2003;12:391–396.
17. Cage DJN, Abrams RA, Callahan JJ, et al. Soft tissue attachments of the ulnar coronoid process. *Clin Orthop* 1995;320:154–158.
18. Pugh DM, Wild LM, Schemitsch EH, et al. Standard surgical protocol to treat elbow dislocations with radial head and coronoid fractures. *J Bone Joint Surg* 2004;86A: 1122–1130.
19. Ring D, Jupiter JB. Operative fixation and reconstruction of the coronoid. *Tech Orthop* 2000;15(2).
20. Ring D, Jupiter JB, Zilberfarb J. Posterior dislocation of the elbow with fractures of the coronoid and radial head. *J Bone Joint Surg* 2002;84A:547–551.
21. Morrey BF. Anatomy of the elbow joint. In: Morrey BF, ed. *The elbow and its disorders.* 2nd ed. Philadelphia: W.B. Saunders, 1995:16–52.
22. Patterson SD, Bain GI, Mehta JA. Surgical approaches to the elbow. *Clin Orthop* 2000; 370:19–33.
23. Dowdy PA, Bain GI, King GJW, et al. The midline posterior elbow incision. *J Bone Joint Surg* 1995;77B:696–699.
24. Hotchkiss RN. Elbow contracture. In: Green DP, Hotchkiss RN, Pederson WC, eds. *Green's operative hand surgery.* Philadelphia: Churchill-Livingstone, 1999:667–682.
25. Taylor TKF, Scham SM. A posteromedial approach to the proximal end of the ulna for the internal fixation of olecranon fractures. *J Trauma* 1969;9:594–602.
26. Hotchkiss RN. Displaced fractures of the radial head: Internal fixation or excision. *J Amer Acad Orthop Surg* 1997;5:1–10.
27. Morrey BF. Surgical exposures of the elbow. In: Morrey BF, ed. *The elbow and its disorders.* 2nd ed. Philadelphia: WB Saunders, 1993:139–166.
28. Kocher T. *Textbook of operative surgery.* 3rd ed. London: Adam and Charles Black, 1911.
29. Geel CW, Palmer AK, Rüedi T, et al. Internal fixation of proximal radial head fractures. *J Orthop Trauma* 1990;4:270–274.
30. Heim U. Surgical treatment of radial head fracture. *Z Unfallchir Versicherungsmed* 1992; 85:3–11.
31. Heim U, Pfeiffer KM. *Internal fixation of small fractures.* 3rd ed. Berlin: Springer-Verlag, 1988.
32. Diliberti T, Botte MJ, Abrams RA. Anatomical considerations regarding the posterior interosseous nerve during posterolateral approaches to the proximal part of the radius. *J Bone Joint Surg* 2000;82A:809–813.
33. Henry AK. *Extensile exposure.* 2nd ed. Edinburgh: Churchill Livingstone; 1973.
34. Smith GR, Hotchkiss RN. Radial head and neck fractures: anatomic guidelines for proper placement of internal fixation. *J Should Elbow Surg* 1996;5:113–117.
35. Soyer AD, Nowotarski PJ, Kelso TB, et al. Optimal position for plate fixation of complex fractures of the proximal radius: a cadaver study. *J Orthop Trauma* 1998;12:291–293.
36. Caputo AE, Mazzocca AD, Santoro VM. The nonarticulating portion of the radial head: anatomic and clinical correlations for internal fixation. *J Hand Surg* 1998;23A: 1082–1090.
37. van Riet R, Glabbeek FV, Neale PG, et al. The noncircular shape of the radial head. *J Hand Surg [Am]* 2003;28:972–978.
38. Ring D, Kloen P, Tavakolian J, et al. Loss of alignment after operative treatment of posterior Monteggia fractures: salvage with dorsal contoured plate fixation. *J Hand Surg [Am]* 2004;29:694–702.
39. Cohen MS, Hastings H. Post-traumatic contracture of the elbow: operative release using a lateral collateral ligament sparing approach. *J Bone Joint Surg* 1998;80B:805–812.
40. Jupiter JB, Ring D. Operative treatment of post-traumatic proximal radioulnar synostosis. *J Bone Joint Surg* 1998;80A:248–257.
41. Mansat P, Morrey BF. The column procedure: a limited lateral approach for extrinsic contracture of the elbow. *J Bone Joint Surg* 1998;80A:1603–1615.
42. Ring D, Jupiter J. The operative release of complete ankylosis of the elbow due to heterotopic bone in patients without severe injury of the central nervous system. *J Bone Joint Surg* 2003;85A:849–857.
43. Josefsson PO, Gentz CF, Johnell O, et al. Surgical versus non-surgical treatment of ligamentous injuries following dislocation of the elbow joint. *J Bone Joint Surg* 1987; 69A:605–608.
44. Ring D, Jupiter JB. Fractures of the distal humerus. *Orthop Clin N Amer* 2000;31: 103–113.
45. Gelinas JJ, Faber KJ, Patterson SD, et al. The effectiveness of turnbuckle splinting for elbow contractures. *J Bone Joint Surg* 2000;82B:74–78.
46. Green DP, McCoy H. Turnbuckle orthotic correction of elbow-flexion contractures after acute injuries. *J Bone Joint Surg* 1979;61A:1092–1095.
47. McAuliffe JA, Wolfson AH. Early excision of heterotopic ossification about the elbow followed by radiation therapy. *Orthop Trans* 1995;19:827.
48. Viola RW, Hanel DP. Early "simple" release of posttraumatic elbow contracture associated with heterotopic ossification. *J Hand Surg* 1999;24:370–380.
49. McKee MD, Jupiter JB, Bosse G, Hinds L, et al. The results of ulnar neurolysis for ulnar neuropathy during post-traumatic elbow reconstruction. *Orthop Trans* 1995;19: 162–163.
50. Faierman E, Wang J, Jupiter JB. Secondary ulnar nerve palsy in adults after elbow trauma: a report of two cases. *J Hand Surg* 2001;26A:675–678.
51. Ring D, Jupiter JB, Gulotta L. Unstable nonunions of the distal humerus. *J Bone Joint Surg* 2003;85A:1040–1046.
52. Ring D, Hannouche D, Jupiter JB. Surgical treatment of persistent dislocation or subluxation of the ulnohumeral joint after fracture-dislocation of the elbow. *J Hand Surg [Am]* 2004;29A:470–480.
53. Papagelopoulos PJ, Morrey BF. Treatment of nonunion of olecranon fractures. *J Bone Joint Surg* 1994;76B:627–635.
54. Ring D, Jupiter JB, Gulotta L. Atrophic nonunions of the proximal ulna. *Clin Orthop* 2003;409:268–274.
55. Ring D, Jupiter JB, Simpson NS. Monteggia fractures in adults. *J Bone Joint Surg* 1998; 80A:1733–1744.
56. Ring D, Jupiter JB, Sanders RW, et al. Trans-olecranon fracture-dislocation of the elbow. *J Orthop Trauma* 1997;11:545–550.
57. Cobb TK, Beckenbaugh RD. Nonunion of the radial head and neck. *Orthopaedics* 1998; 21:364–368.
58. Ring D, Chin K, Jupiter JB. Nonunion of nonoperatively treated fractures of the radial head. *Clin Orthop* 2002;398:235–238.
59. Ring D, Quintero J, Jupiter JB. Open reduction and internal fixation of fractures of the radial head. *J Bone Joint Surg* 2002;84A:1811–1815.
60. Helfet DL, Kloen P, Anand N, et al. Open reduction and internal fixation of delayed unions and nonunions of fractures of the distal part of the humerus. *J Bone Joint Surg* 2003;85A:33–40.
61. Sherman R. Soft-tissue coverage for the elbow. *Hand Clinics* 1997;13(2):291–302.
62. Stevanovic M, Sharpe F, Itamura J. Treatment of soft tissue problems about the elbow. *Clin Orthop* 2000;370:127–137.
63. Antuna SA, Morrey BF, Adams RA, et al. Ulnohumeral arthroplasty for primary degenerative arthritis of the elbow: long-term outcome and complications. *J Bone Joint Surg* 2002;84A:2168–2173.
64. Cheng SL, Morrey BF. Treatment of the mobile, painful arthritic elbow by distraction interposition arthroplasty. *J Bone Joint Surg* 2000;82B:233–238.
65. Froimson AI, Silva JE, Richey DG. Cutis arthroplasty of the elbow joint. *J Bone Joint Surg* 1976;58A:863–865.
66. Morrey BF, Adams RA, Bryan RS. Total elbow replacement for post-traumatic arthritis of the elbow. *J Bone Joint Surg* 1991;73B:607–612.
67. Cobb TK, Morrey BF. Total elbow arthroplasty as primary treatment for distal humeral fractures in elderly patients. *J Bone Joint Surg* 1997;79A:826–832.
68. Frankle MA, Herscovici D, Pasquale TF, et al. A comparison of open reduction and internal fixation and primary total elbow arthroplasty in the treatment of intraarticular distal humerus fractures in women older than age 65. *J Orthop Trauma* 2003;17: 473–480.
69. Riseborough EJ, Radin EL. Intercondylar T fractures of the humerus in the adult. *J Bone Joint Surg* 1969;51A:130–141.
70. Mehne DK, Jupiter JB. Fractures of the distal humerus. In: Browner B, Jupiter JB, Levine A, Trafton P, eds. *Skeletal trauma.* Philadelphia: WB Saunders, 1991:1146–1176.
71. Jupiter JB, Barnes KA, Goodman LJ, et al. Multiplane fracture of the distal humerus. *J Orthop Trauma* 1993;7:216–220.
72. Bryan RS, Morrey BF. Fractures of the distal humerus. In: Morrey BF, ed. *The elbow and its disorders.* Philadelphia: WB Saunders, 1985:302–339.
73. McKee MD, Jupiter JB, Bamberger HB. Coronal shear fractures of the distal end of the humerus. *J Bone Joint Surg* 1996;78A:49–54.
74. Collert S. Surgical management of fracture of the capitulum humeri. *Arch Orthop Scan* 1977;48:603–606.
75. Darrach W. Fracture of lower articular surface of humerus. *Ann Surg* 1916;64:724–725.
76. Fowles JV, Kassab MT. Fracture of the capitulum humeri: treatment by excision. *J Bone Joint Surg* 1974;56A:794–798.
77. Gejrot W. On intra-articular fractures of the capitellum and trochlea of the humerus with special reference to the treatment. *Acta Chir Scand* 1932;71:253–270.
78. Grantham SA, Norris TR, Bush DC. Isolated fracture of the humeral capitellum. *Clin Orthop* 1981;161:262–269.
79. Lee WE, Summey TJ. Fracture of the capitellum of the humerus. *Ann Surg* 1934;99: 497–509.
80. Lindem MC. Fractures of the capitellum and trochlea. *Ann Surg* 1922;76:78–82.
81. Mazel MS. Fracture of the capitellum: a report of a case. *J Bone Joint Surg* 1935;17: 483–488.
82. Oppenheim W, Davlin LB, Leipzig JM, et al. Concomitant fractures of the capitellum and trochlea. *J Orthop Trauma* 1989;3:260–262.
83. Rhodin R. On the treatment of fracture of the capitellum. *Acta Chir Scand* 1942;86: 475–486.
84. Robertson RC, Bogart RB. Fracture of the capitellum and trochlea, combined with fracture of the external humeral condyle. *J Bone Joint Surg* 1933;15:206–213.
85. Brown RF, Morgan RG. Intercondylar T-shaped fractures of the humerus: results in ten cases treated by early mobilization. *J Bone Joint Surg* 1971;53B:425–428.
86. Wilkinson JM, Stanley D. Posterior surgical approaches to the elbow: a comparative anatomic study. *J Should Elbow Surg* 2001;10:380–382.
87. Alonso-Llames M. Bilaterotricipital approach to the elbow. *Acta Orthop Scand* 1972; 43:479–490.
88. McKee MD, Kim J, Kebaish K, et al. Functional outcome after open supracondylar fractures of the humerus. The effect of the surgical approach. *J Bone Joint Surg* 2000; 82B:646–651.
89. McKee MD, Wilson TL, Winston L, et al. Functional outcome following surgical treatment of intraarticular distal humerus fractures through a posterior approach. *J Bone Joint Surg* 2000;82A:1701–1707.
90. Bryan RS, Morrey BF. Extensive posterior exposure of the elbow: a triceps sparing approach. *Clin Orthop* 1982;166:188–193.
91. O'Driscoll SW. The triceps-reflecting anconeus pedicle (TRAP) approach for distal humerus fractures and nonunions. *Orthop Clin N Amer* 2000;31(1):91–101.

92. Hildebrand KA, Patterson SD, Regan WD, et al. Functional outcome of semiconstrained total elbow arthroplasty. *J Bone Joint Surg* 2000;82A:1379–1386.
93. Pierce TD, Herndon JH. The triceps preserving approach to total elbow arthroplasty. *Clin Orthop* 1998;354:144–152.
94. Helfet DL, Hotchkiss RN. Internal fixation of the distal humerus: a biomechanical comparison of methods. *J Orthop Trauma* 1990;4:260–264.
95. Kirk P, Goulet JA, Freiberg A, et al. A biomechanical evaluation of fixation methods for fractures of the distal humerus. *Orthop Trans* 1990;14:674.
96. Schemitsch EH, Tencer AF, Henley MB. Biomechanical evaluation of methods of internal fixation of the distal humerus. *J Orthop Trauma* 1994;8:468–475.
97. Müller ME, Allgower M, Schneider R, et al. *Manual of internal fixation. Techniques recommended by the AO-ASIF Group*. 3rd ed. Berlin: Springer–Verlag; 1991.
98. Jupiter JB. Complex fractures of the distal part of the humerus and associated complications. *J Bone Joint Surg* 1994;76A:1252–1264.
99. Jupiter JB, Goodman LJ. The management of complex distal humerus nonunion in the elderly by elbow capsulectomy, triple plating, and ulnar nerve neurolysis. *J Should Elbow Surg* 1992;1:37–46.
100. Self J, Viegas SF, Buford WL, et al. A comparison of double-plate fixation methods for complex distal humeral fractures. *J Should Elbow Surg* 1995;4:11–16.
101. Houben PF, Bongers KJ, Wildenberg FA. Double tension band osteosynthesis in supra- and transcondylar humeral fractures. *Injury* 1994;25:305–309.
102. Zhao J, Wang X, Zhang O. Surgical treatment of comminuted intra-articular fractures of the distal humerus with double tension band osteosynthesis. *Orthopaedics* 2000;23: 449–452.
103. Cobb TK, Morrey BF. Total elbow arthroplasty as primary treatment for distal humerus fractures in elderly patients. *J Bone Joint Surg* 1997;79A:826–832.
104. Garcia JA, Mykula R, Stanley D. Complex fractures of the distal humerus in the elderly. *J Bone Joint Surg* 2001;84B:812–816.
105. Ray PS, Kakarlapudi K, Rajsekhar C, et al. Total elbow arthroplasty as primary treatment for distal humeral fractures in elderly patients. *Injury* 2000;31:687–692.
106. Gupta R, Khanchandani P. Intercondylar fractures of the distal humerus in adults: a critical analysis of 55 cases. *Injury* 2002;33:511–515.
107. Papaioannou N, Babis GC, Kalavritinos J, et al. Operative treatment of type C intra-articular fractures of the distal humerus: the role of stability achieved at surgery on final outcome. *Injury* 1995;26:169–173.
108. Södergård J, Sandelin J, Böstman O. Mechanical failures of internal fixation in T and Y fractures of the distal humerus. *J Trauma* 1992;33:687–690.
109. Södergård J, Sandelin J, Böstman O. Postoperative complications of distal humeral fractures: 27 of 96 adults followed up for 6 (2–10) years. *Acta Orthop Scand* 1992;63: 85–89.
110. Figgie MP, Inglis AE, Mow CS, et al. Salvage of non-union of supracondylar fracture of the humerus by total elbow arthroplasty. *J Bone Joint Surg* 1989;71A:1058–1065.
111. Morrey BF, Adams RA. Semiconstrained elbow replacement for distal humeral non-union. *J Bone Joint Surg* 1995;77B:67–72.
112. Essex-Lopresti P. Fractures of the radial head with distal radioulnar dislocation. *J Bone Joint Surg* 1951;33B:244–247.
113. Davidson PA, Moseley JB, Tullos HS. Radial head fracture. A potentially complex injury. *Clin Orthop* 1993;297:224–230.
114. Smith AM, Urbanosky LR, Castle JA, et al. Radius pull test: predictor of longitudinal forearm instability. *J Bone Joint Surg Am* 2002;84A:1970–1976.
115. Mason ML. Some observations on fractures of the head of the radius with a review of one hundred cases. *Br J Surg* 1959;42:123–132.
116. Morrey BF. Radial head fractures. In: Morrey BF, ed. *The elbow and its disorders*. Philadelphia: WB Saunders, 1985:355.
117. Johnston GW. A follow-up of one hundred cases of fracture of the head of the radius. *Ulster Med J* 1952;31:51–56.
118. Muller ME, Nazarian S, Koch P, et al. *The comprehensive classification of fractures of long bones*. Berlin: Springer-Verlag; 1990.
119. Carstam N. Operative treatment of fractures of the upper end of the radius. *Acta Orthop Scan* 1950;19:502–526.
120. Radin EL, Riseborough EJ. Fractures of the radial head. *J Bone Joint Surg* 1966;48A: 1055–1065.
121. Herbertsson P, Josefsson PO, Hasserius R, et al. Uncomplicated Mason type II and III fractures of the radial head and neck in adults. A long-term follow-up study. *J Bone Joint Surg* 2004;86A:569–574.
122. Miller GK, Drennan DB, Maylahn DJ. Treatment of displaced segmental radial head fractures: Long-term follow-up. *J Bone Joint Surg* 1981;63A:712–717.
123. Weseley MS, Barenfeld PA, Eisenstein AL. Closed treatment of isolated radial head fractures. *J Trauma* 1983;23:36–39.
124. Broberg MA, Morrey BF. Results of treatment of fracture-dislocations of the elbow. *Clin Orthop* 1987;216:109–119.
125. Josefsson PO, Gentz CF, Johnell O, et al. Dislocations of the elbow and intraarticular fractures. *Clin Orthop* 1989;246:126–130.
126. Beingessner DM, Dunning CE, Beingessner CJ, et al. The effect of radial head fracture size on radiocapitellar joint stability. *Clin Biomech* 2003;18:677–681.
127. Carn RM, Medige J, Curtain D, et al. Silicone rubber replacement of the severely fractured radial head. *Clin Orthop* 1986;209:259–269.
128. Gordon M, Bullough PG. Synovial and osseous inflammation in failed silicone-rubber prosthesis. *J Bone Joint Surg* 1982;64A:574–580.
129. Vanderwilde RS, Morrey BF, Melberg MW, et al. Inflammatory arthritis after failure of silicone rubber replacement of the radial head. *J Bone Joint Surg* 1994;76B:78–81.
130. Harrington IJ, Tountas AA. Replacement of the radial head in the treatment of unstable elbow fractures. *Injury* 1980;12:405–412.
131. Moro JK, Werier J, MacDermid JC, et al. Arthroplasty with a metal radial head for unreconstructable fractures of the radial head. *J Bone Joint Surg* 2001;83A:1201–1211.
132. Judet T, de Loubresse CG, Piriou P, et al. A floating prosthesis for radial head fractures. *J Bone Joint Surg* 1996;78B:244–249.
133. van Riet RP, Glabbeek FV, Verborgt O, et al. Capitellar erosion caused by a metal radial head prosthesis. A case report. *J Bone Joint Surg* 2004;86A:1061–1064.
134. Dürig M, Müller W, Rüedi TP, et al. The operative treatment of elbow dislocation in the adult. *J Bone Joint Surg* 1979;61A:239–244.
135. Josefsson PO, Johnell O, Wendeberg B. Ligamentous injuries in dislocations of the elbow joint. *Clin Orthop* 1987;221:221–225.
136. Bauer G, Worsdorfer O, Braun K. Radio-ulnar bridge callus following osteosynthesis of forearm fractures. *Aktuelle Traumatol* 1990;20:194–198.
137. Vince KG, Miller JE. Cross union complicating fracture of the forearm. Part I. 1987; 69A:640–653.
138. Geel C. Fractures of the radial head. In: McQueen MM, Jupiter JB, ed. *Radius and ulna*. Oxford: Butterworth-Heinemann, 1999:159–168.
139. Bunker TD, Newman LH. The Herbert differential pitch bone screw in displaced radial head fractures. *Injury* 1987;16:621–624.
140. McArthur RA. Herbert screw fixation of the head of the radius. *Clin Orthop* 1987;224: 79–87.
141. Pearce MS, Gallannaugh SC. Mason type II radial head fractures fixed with Herbert bone screws. *J R Soc Med* 1996;89:340–344.
142. Lyons FA, Rockwood CA. Migration of pins used in operations on the shoulder. *J Bone Joint Surg* 1990;72A:1262–1267.
143. Hirvensalo E, Böstman O, Rokkanen P. Absorbable polyglycolide pins in fixation of displaced fractures of the radial head. *Arch Orthop Trauma Surg* 1990;109:258–261.
144. Pelto K, Hirvensalo E, Bostman O, et al. Treatment of radial head fractures with absorbable polyglycolide pins: a study on the security of fixation in 38 cases. *J Orthop Trauma* 1994;8:94–98.
145. Broberg MA, Morrey BF. Results of delayed excision of the radial head after fracture. *J Bone Joint Surg* 1986;68A:669–674.
146. Goldberg I, Peylan J, Yosipovitch Z, et al. Late results of excision of the radial head for an isolated closed fracture. *J Bone Joint Surg* 1986;68A:675–679.
147. Pavel A, Pittman JM, Lance EM, et al. The posterior Monteggia fracture. A clinical study. *J Trauma* 1965;5:185–199.
148. Penrose JH. The Monteggia fracture with posterior dislocation of the radial head. *J Bone Joint Surg* 1951;33B:65–73.
149. Ring D, Jupiter JB, Zilberfarb J. Roles of the medial collateral ligament and the coronoid in elbow stability. Reply to letter to the editor. *J Bone Joint Surg* 2003;85A:568–569.
150. McKee MD, Bowden SH, King GJ, et al. Management of recurrent, complex instability of the elbow with a hinged external fixator. *J Bone Joint Surg* 1998;80B:1031–1036.
151. Heim U. Combined fractures of the upper end of the ulna and the radius in adults: a series of 120 cases. *Rev Chir Orthop* 1998;84:142–153.
152. Regan W, Morrey BF. Fractures of the coronoid process of the ulna. *J Bone Joint Surg* 1990;71A:1348–1354.
153. Morrey BF. Complex instability of the elbow. *J Bone Joint Surg* 1997;79A:460–469.
154. Melhoff TL, Noble PC, Bennet JB, et al. Simple dislocation of the elbow in the adult: results after closed treatment. *J Bone Joint Surg* 1988;70A:244–249.
155. Protzman RR. Dislocation of the elbow joint. *J Bone Joint Surg* 1978;60A:539–541.
156. O'Driscoll SW. Classification and spectrum of elbow instability: recurrent instability. In: Morrey BF, ed. *The elbow and its disorders*. 2nd ed. Philadelphia: WB Saunders, 1993:453–463.
157. Linsheid RL, O'Driscoll SW. Elbow dislocations. In: Morrey BF, ed. *The elbow and its disorders*. 2nd ed. Philadelphia: WB Saunders, 1993:441–452.
158. Jupiter JB, Ring D. Treatment of unreduced elbow dislocations with hinged external fixation. *J Bone Joint Surg* 2002;84A:1630–1635.
159. Sanchez-Sotelo J, Romanillos O, Garay EG. Results of acute excision of the radial head in elbow radial head fracture-dislocations. *J Orthop Trauma* 2000;14:354–358.
160. Hotchkiss RN. Fractures and dislocations of the elbow. In: Rockwood CA, Green DP, Bucholz RW, Heckman JD, eds. *Rockwood and Green's fractures in adults*. 4th ed. Philadelphia: Lippincott-Raven, 1996:929–1024.
161. Morrey BF. Current concepts in the treatment of fractures of the radial head, the olecranon, and the coronoid. *J Bone Joint Surg* 1995;77A:316–327.
162. Ring D, Jupiter JB, Waters PM. Monteggia fractures in children and adults. *J Am Acad Orthop Surg* 1998;6:215–224.
163. Bado JL. The Monteggia lesion. *Clin Orthop* 1967;50:71–76.
164. Jupiter JB, Leibovic SJ, Ribbans W, et al. The posterior Monteggia lesion. *J Orthop Trauma* 1991;5:395–402.

165. Biga N, Thomine JM. La luxation trans-olecranienne du coude. *Rev Chir Orthop* 1974; 60:557–567.
166. Didonna ML, Fernandez JJ, Lim TH, et al. Partial olecranon excision: the relationship between triceps insertion site and extension strength of the elbow. *J Hand Surg Am* 2003;28A:117–122.
167. Gartsman GM, Scales JC, Otis JC. Operative treatment of olecranon fractures. *J Bone Joint Surg* 1981;63A:718–721.
168. Chin KR, Ring D, Jupiter JB. Double tension-band fixation of the olecranon. *Tech Should Elbow Surg* 2000;1:61–66.
169. Prayson MJ, Williams JL, Marshall MP, et al. Biomechanical comparison of fixation methods in transverse olecranon fractures: a cadaveric study. *J Orthop Trauma* 1997; 11:565–572.
170. Hutchinson DT, Horowitz DS, Ha G, et al. Cyclic loading of olecranon fracture fixation constructs. *J Bone Joint Surg* 2003;85A:831–837.
171. Ikeda M, Fukushima Y, Kobayashi Y, Oka Y. Comminuted fractures of the olecranon. *J Bone Joint Surg* 2001;83B:805–808.
172. Heim U. Kombinierte Verletzungen von Radius und Ulna im proximalen Unterarmsegment. *Hefte Unfallchir* 1994;241:61–79.
173. O'Driscoll SW. Technique for unstable olecranon fracture-subluxations. *Oper Tech Orthop* 1994;4:49–53.
174. Hastings H, Engles DR. Fixation of complex elbow fractures, part II: proximal ulna and radius fractures. *Hand Clinics* 1997;13(4):721–735.
175. Mast J, Jakob RP, Ganz R. *Planning and reduction techniques in fracture surgery*. Heidelberg: Springer-Verlag, 1979.

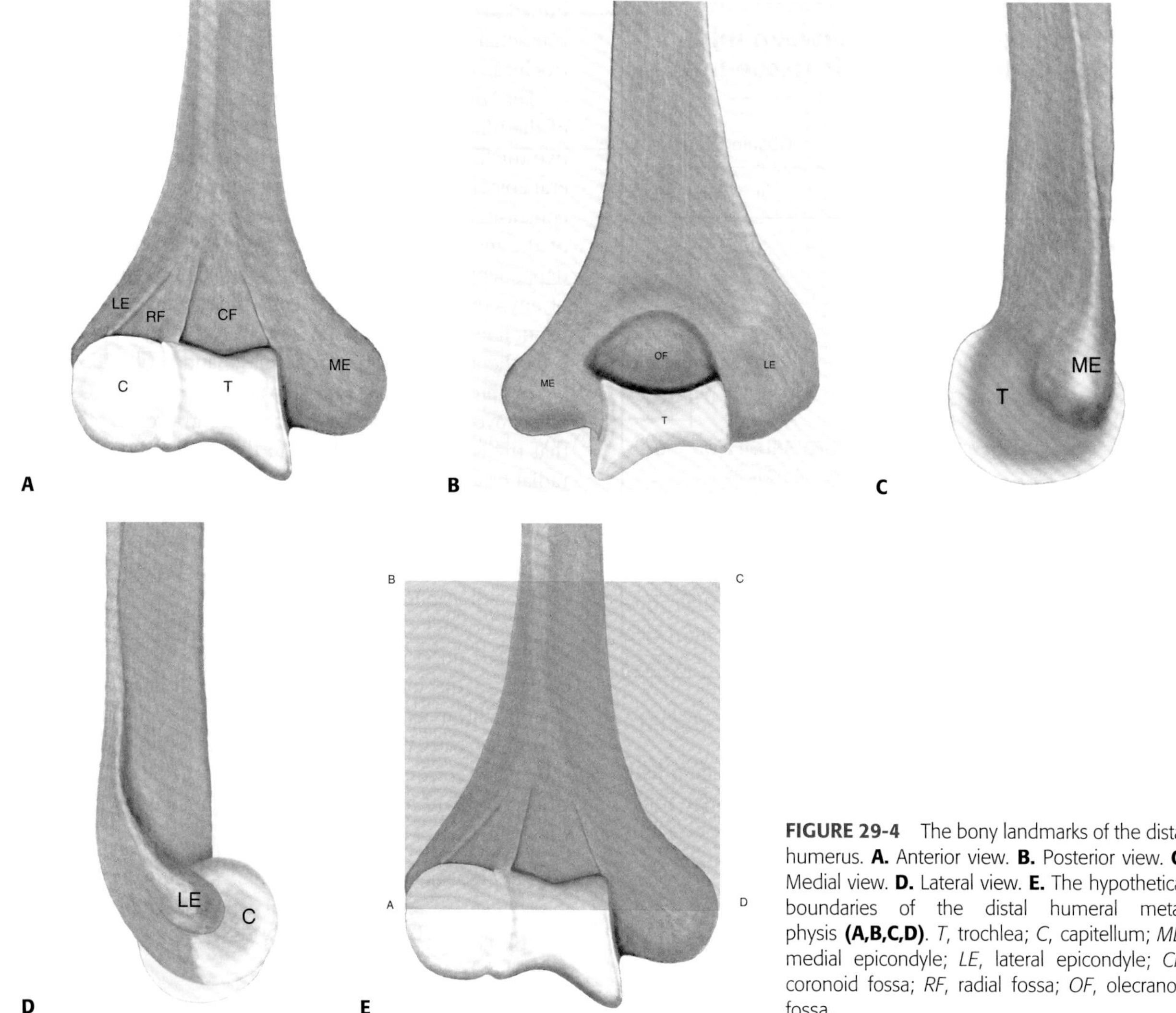

FIGURE 29-4 The bony landmarks of the distal humerus. **A.** Anterior view. **B.** Posterior view. **C.** Medial view. **D.** Lateral view. **E.** The hypothetical boundaries of the distal humeral metaphysis **(A,B,C,D)**. *T*, trochlea; *C*, capitellum; *ME*, medial epicondyle; *LE*, lateral epicondyle; *CF*, coronoid fossa; *RF*, radial fossa; *OF*, olecranon fossa.

extends to the distal and lateral aspect of the trochlea, where its cartilage-covered anterior surface forms the capitellum. The medial epicondyle and distal aspect of the lateral column are frequently difficult to visualize due to their soft-tissue attachments.

The posterior fossa, which accommodates the olecranon during elbow extension, is located within the triangle formed by the medial and lateral columns and the trochlea. The intramedullary canal of the humerus becomes narrow distally as it converges on the olecranon fossa. Approximately one in 20 individuals has a bony defect (or "septal aperture") between the two columns where the olecranon fossa is deficient.

A posterior approach to the elbow can be made either with the patient in the lateral decubitus position, with the arm suspended over a bolster (Fig. 29-7A), or supine, with the arm draped across the chest (Fig. 29-7B). The former provides greater stability for the arm during the surgery, whereas the latter is easier to set up and is more convenient for the anesthetist. All posterior approaches use a longitudinal midline incision over the posterior aspect of the elbow, beginning well proximal to the tip of the olecranon, curving slightly medially at its distal extent, then returning to the midline and extending approximately 5 cm distal to the tip of the olecranon.

The ulnar nerve should be routinely identified behind the medial epicondyle, and protected in all posterior approaches to the elbow. Extensive dissection of the nerve is inadvisable, as this increases the risk of tethering and damage to its vascularity. However, adequate exposure of the nerve is required to reduce the risk of its injury if olecranon osteotomy or insertion of hardware is required. The nerve should be transposed anterior to the medial epicondyle, either subcutaneously or using a fasciodermal sling (14,15), if it is in proximity to hardware at the end of the procedure.

There are several variations of approach to gain access to the posterior aspect of the distal humerus, which have different advantages, disadvantages, and indications. Although many nu-

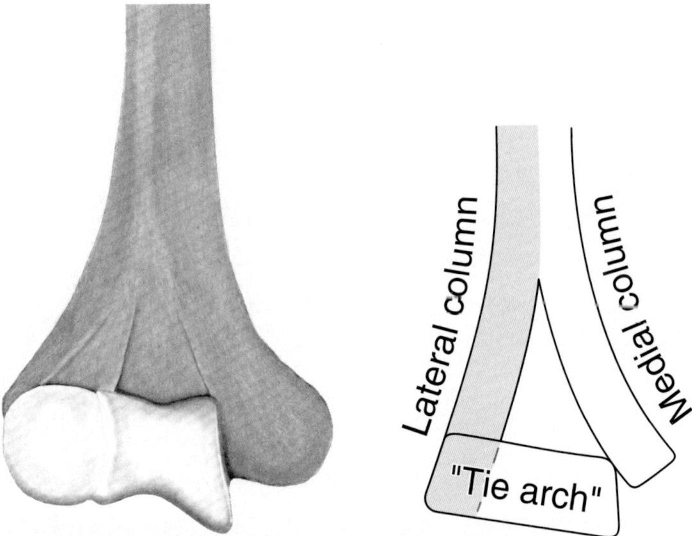

FIGURE 29-5 The distalmost part of the lateral column is the capitellum, and the distalmost part of the medial column is the nonarticular medial epicondyle. The trochlea is the medialmost part of the articular segment and is intermediate in position between the medial epicondyle and capitellum. The articular segment functions architecturally as a "tie arch."

ances and variations exist, there are four main types of posterior approach, which have been described as follows.

Olecranon Osteotomy

Reflection of the triceps tendon and its bony insertion, by use of an olecranon osteotomy, has been the most widely used approach to the elbow, since operative treatment of these injuries was popularized (Fig. 29-8A). It remains the approach of choice for most bicolumn and transcolumn fractures that are amenable to dual plating.

The triceps insertion is isolated and the joint surfaces on either side of the trochlear notch are identified by opening the

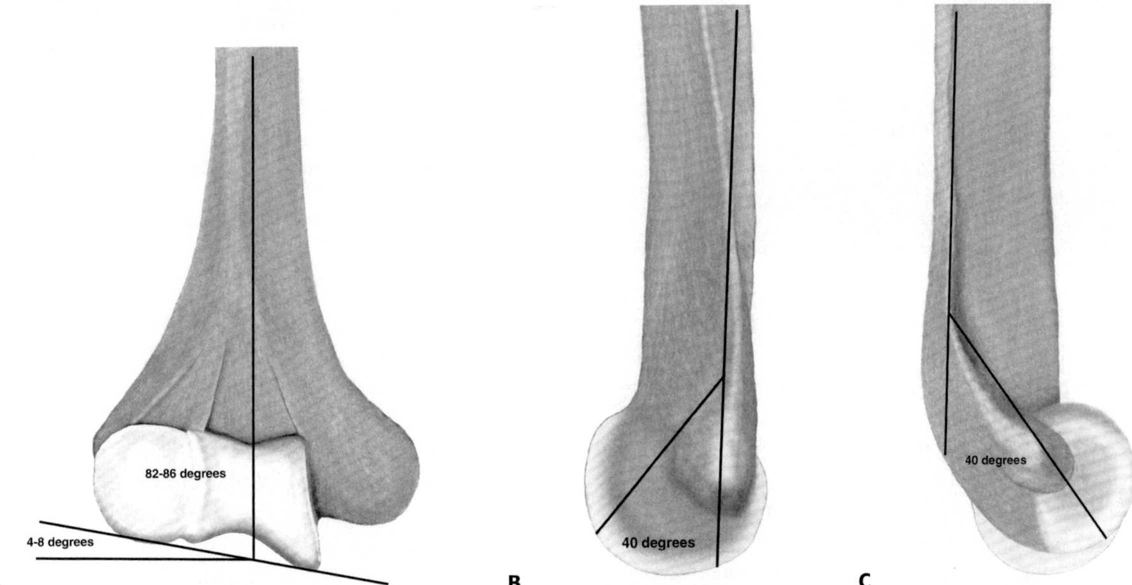

FIGURE 29-6 The joint surface to shaft axis is 4° to 8° of valgus—the A-carrying angle **(A)**. The articular segment juts forward from the line of the shaft at 40° and functions architecturally as the tie arch at the point of maximum column divergence distally. It is important to note that the medial epicondyle is on the projected axis of the shaft, whereas the lateral epicondyle is projected slightly forward from the axis **(B,C)**.

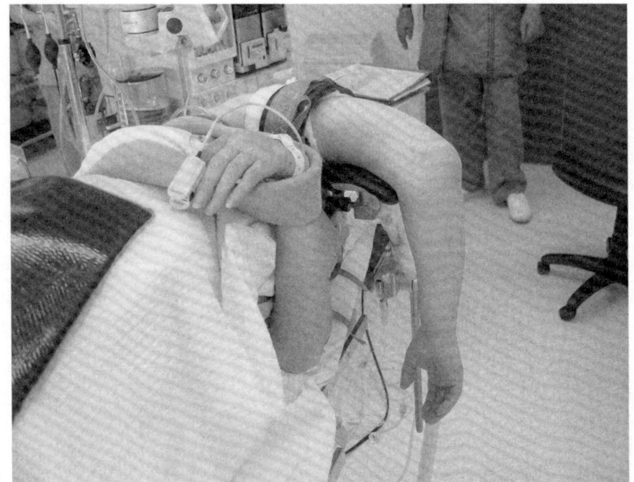

A

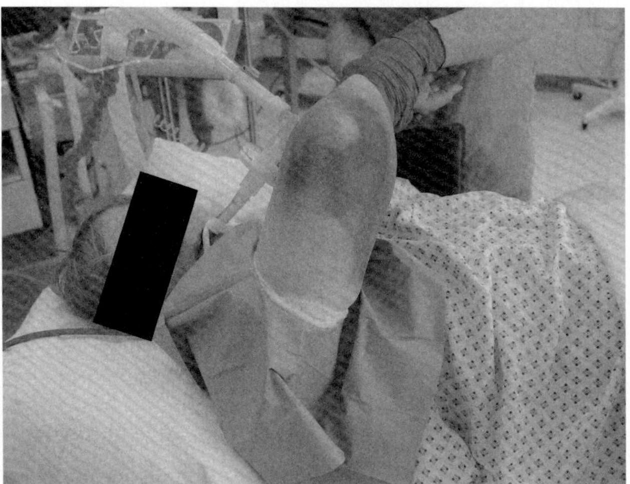

B

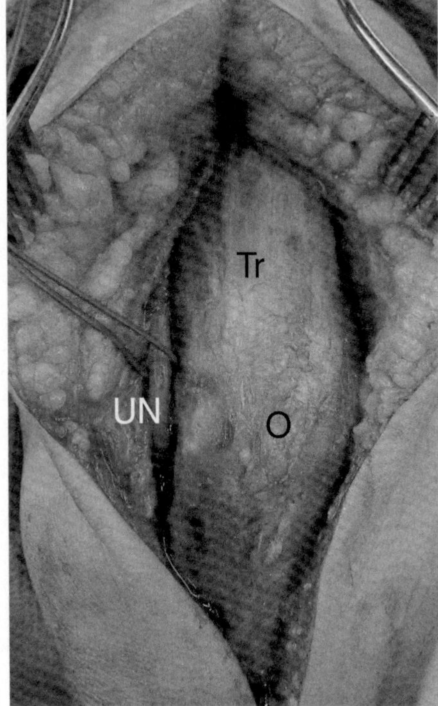

C

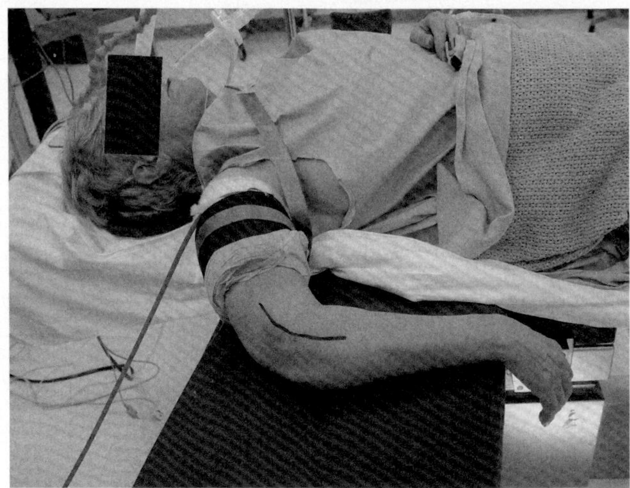

D

FIGURE 29-7 The commonly used intraoperative patient positions. **A.** The lateral decubitus position for a posterior approach. **B.** The supine position, with the arm across the chest for a posterior approach. **C.** Intraoperative view of the posterior approach to the right elbow. *O*, olecranon; *Tr*, triceps; *UN*, ulnar nerve. **D.** The supine position using an arm board extension for the direct lateral approach.

joint capsule. An elevator or gauze swab is then inserted from medial to lateral through the joint across the notch. This serves to protect the articular surfaces during the subsequent osteotomy, and also facilitates the accurate placement of the osteotomy (Fig. 29-8B). The approach initially recommended by the AO group was an extra-articular oblique osteotomy of the olecranon (16), although the approach more commonly used is an intra-articular osteotomy, through the mid-portion of the greater sigmoid notch (17). The osteotomy must be proximal to the coronoid process, to provide a balance between an osteotomy that is too small, which may compromise the exposure of the articular surfaces, and one that is too large, which may cause an inadvertent osteotomy at the level of the coronoid and destabilize the elbow.

Predrilling and tapping of the olecranon should be performed if screw fixation of the osteotomy is planned. The screw can then be partially inserted through the olecranon and used as a surgical retractor for the olecranon and its attached triceps after completion of the osteotomy. The osteotomy should be performed as a chevron, with its apex directed distally, perpendicular to the long axis of the shaft of the ulna. The chevron facilitates reduction and fixation of the osteotomy and also pro-

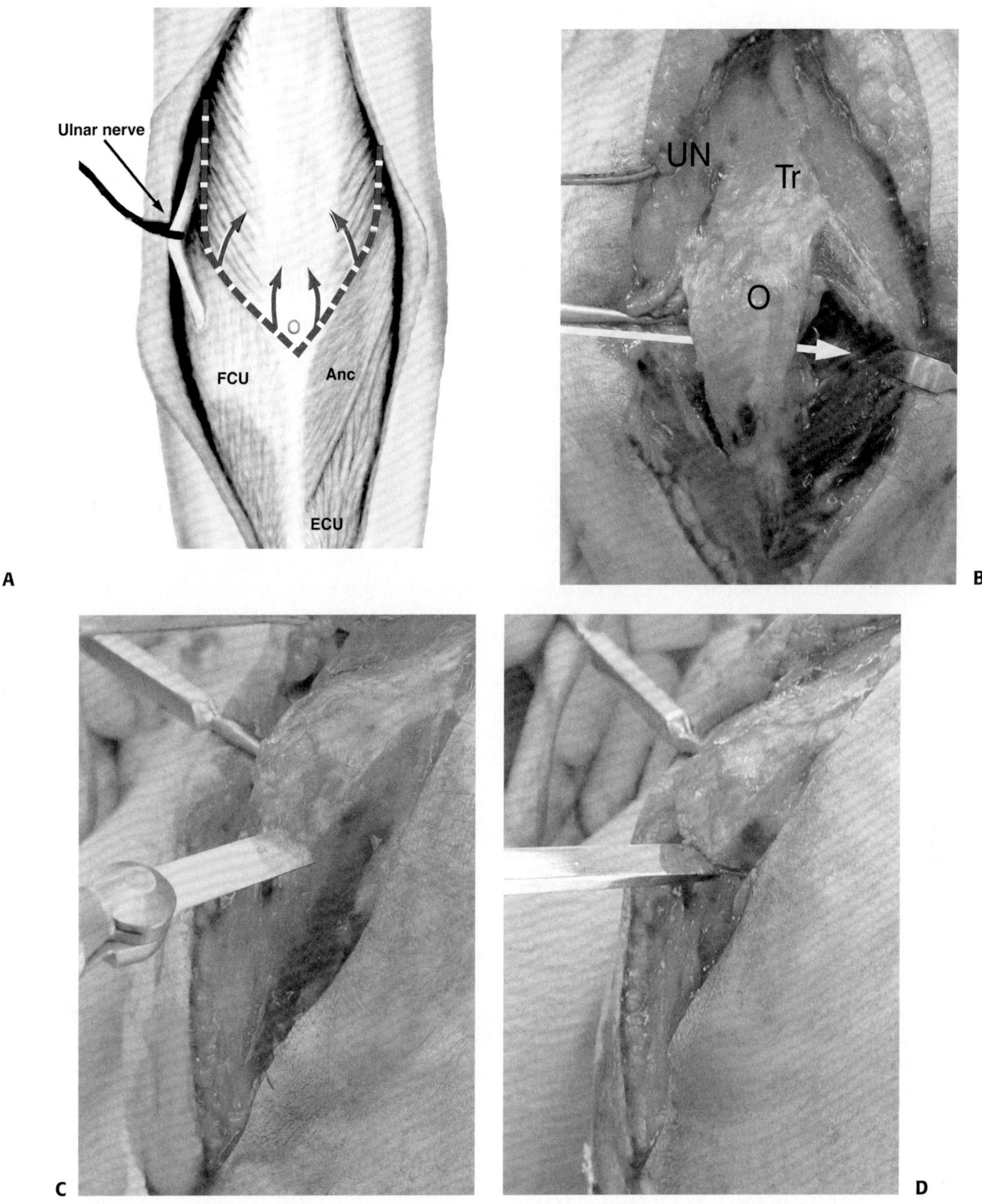

FIGURE 29-8 The olecranon osteotomy approach. **A.** Schematic diagram of the surgical approach for the osteotomy in a right elbow with the patient in a lateral decubitus position (*FCU*, flexor carpi ulnaris; *ECU*, extensor carpi ulnaris; *Anc*, anconeus). **B.** Preparation of site for osteotomy. An elevator (*white arrow*) is introduced across the greater sigmoid notch to facilitate optimal placement of the osteotomy (*Tr*, triceps; *UN*, ulnar nerve; *O*, olecranon). **C.** Performing the chevron osteotomy with an oscillating saw. **D.** Completion of the osteotomy with an osteotome. (*continues*)

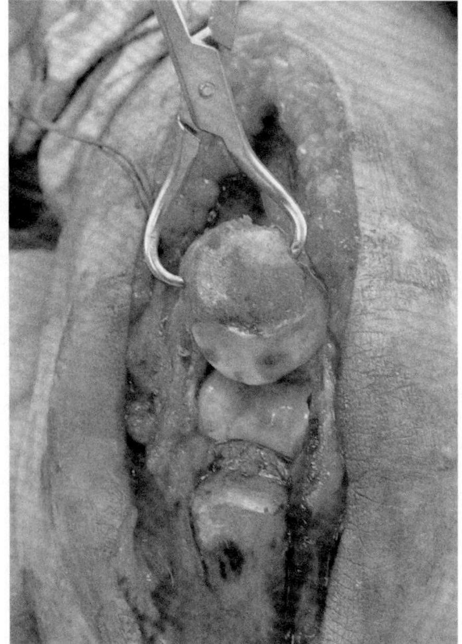

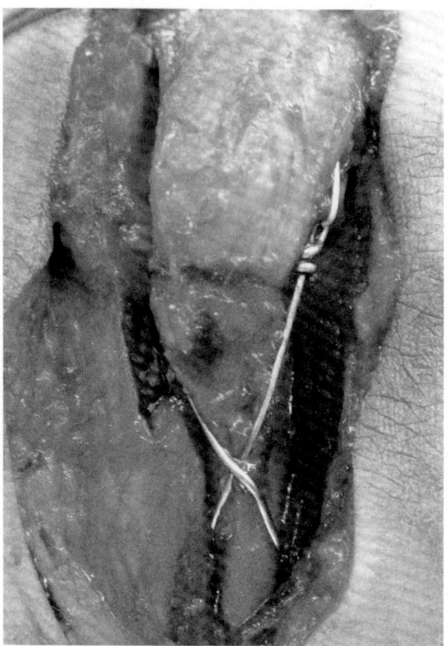

FIGURE 29-8 *(continued)* **E.** Retraction of the olecranon with a towel forceps to expose the distal humeral articular surface. **F.** Fixation of the osteotomy using a tension band wiring technique after the fixation procedure.

vides a greater surface area of cancellous bone over which healing can occur. The osteotomy is performed using a narrow saw (Fig. 29-8C) and completed using an osteotome, to "crack" through the articular surface (Fig. 29-8D). This maneuver facilitates subsequent anatomic reconstruction of the osteotomy fragments (14).

At the completion of surgery, the osteotomy can be secured either with an intramedullary 6.5-mm, partially threaded cancellous screw, or using two K-wires and a tension-banding technique (Fig. 29-8E). Screw fixation may be less secure in osteoporotic bone, but the hardware is less obtrusive over the subcutaneous border of the elbow, when compared with the K-wire and tension-banding technique.

The approach has the advantage of providing excellent access to the whole of the distal humerus, especially to view the distal posterior articular surfaces. It provides only limited exposure of the capitellum, but its major drawback is the postoperative morbidity, which is associated with the internal fixation of the osteotomy.

Triceps-Splitting Approaches

The triceps-splitting approach has been developed to attempt to overcome the morbidity associated with the use of olecranon osteotomy. It is made by fashioning a direct midline posterior split in the triceps (18–22). Distally sharp dissection is used to reflect the triceps insertion off the olecranon and proximal ulna medially and laterally (Fig. 29-9A,B). A thin wafer of bone may be detached from the olecranon at the level of the triceps insertion (21). The triceps may also be detached as a distally based "tongue" or "V" muscle flap with splitting of only its deeper portion, though this has been less commonly used for fracture surgery (23–25).

The limited access to the joint surfaces can be improved by flexing the elbow and grasping and posteriorly retracting the olecranon with reduction forceps. Meticulous repair of the tendon through drill holes in the olecranon must be performed at the conclusion of surgery, to minimize the risk of triceps tendon pull-off. This approach does not appear to be detrimental to elbow function (26) and reduces the risk of later hardware complications, encountered with the use of an olecranon osteotomy (26,27). Although some authors have reported a better functional outcome following the use of a triceps-splitting approach compared with olecranon osteotomy (26,27), others have reported the converse (28).

Although the access to the elbow joint is more restricted than with an olecranon osteotomy, the intact trochlear notch may be used as a template, against which the reduction of the trochlea can be assessed, when treating bicolumn and transcolumn fractures. Another major advantage of this approach is that it allows greater intraoperative flexibility, because either internal fixation or total elbow arthroplasty (TER) can be performed. This is particularly useful if there is uncertainty as to whether reduction and internal fixation of the fracture will be technically feasible, and TER might be required. In these circumstances, the use of an olecranon osteotomy would prohibit the use of a TER, whereas a triceps-reflecting approach would make internal fixation technically difficult.

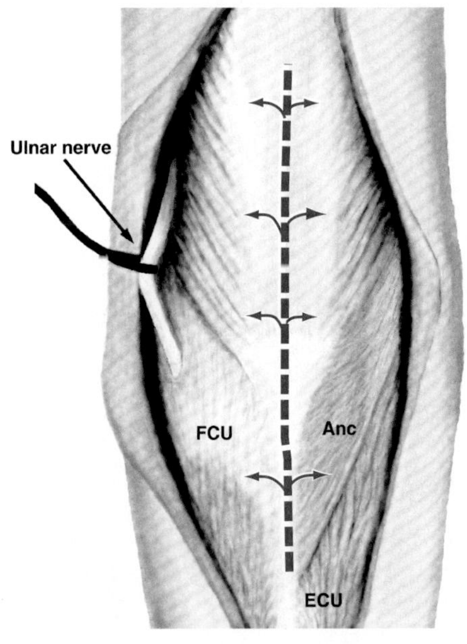

A

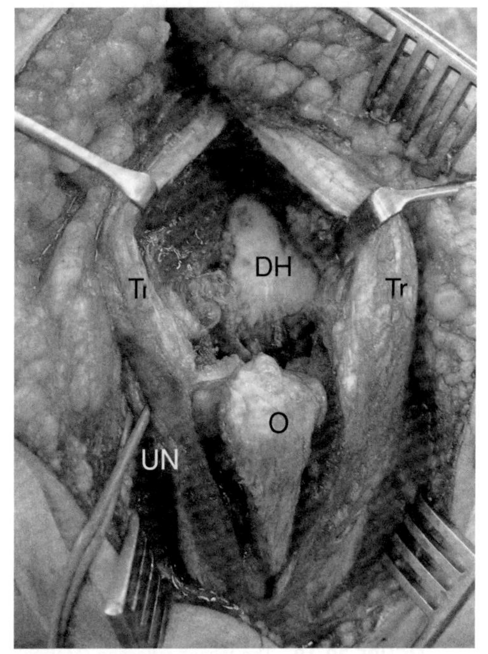

B

FIGURE 29-9 The triceps-splitting approach. **A.** Schematic diagram of the approach in a right elbow with the patient in a lateral decubitus position (*FCU*, flexor carpi ulnaris; *ECU*, extensor carpi ulnaris; *Anc*, anconeus). **B.** Intraoperative view of the approach (*Tr*, triceps; *UN*, ulnar nerve; *O*, olecranon; *DH*, distal humerus).

The major drawback of the triceps-splitting approach is the theoretical risk of postoperative detachment of the tendon from the proximal ulna, though this has not been reported to date. In addition, the radial nerve may be at risk if the split is continued too far proximally, and care must be taken to avoid this (27).

Triceps-Reflecting Approaches

The triceps-reflecting approach was developed for insertion of a TER, without the requirement to fully detach the triceps insertion, in patients with degenerative joint disease (29,30). It can also be used to treat a distal humerus fracture because the distal portions of both columns and the articular surfaces are excised, creating a sloppy "working space," in which the components of the elbow replacement can be inserted. The approach has been used less frequently for open reduction with internal fixation (ORIF), because of the limited exposure of the lateral column that it provides, and it should only be used if the surgeon is convinced that a TER will be required.

The whole of the triceps is reflected as a continuous cuff of tissue, from medial to lateral (Fig. 29-10A,B). The medial aspect of the triceps is sharply reflected off the proximal ulna at its insertion, taking care to only continue dissection until adequate exposure of the joint has been obtained. As with the triceps-splitting approach, careful repair of the triceps tendon through drill holes is required to reduce the risk of postoperative tendon pull-off (Table 29-3).

Several variations of this approach have been described:

1. As originally described there is a risk of ulnar nerve palsy from retraction during surgery (29). To protect against this the triceps may be split so that 75% of the muscle lies laterally and 25% medially (31). The triceps is then reflected laterally as for the standard technique. The ulnar nerve and its blood supply are protected from traction injury by the medial triceps during surgery.
2. A wafer of bone carrying the triceps insertion may be detached, to facilitate later closure. The triceps is then reflected laterally as an "osteo-anconeus flap" to provide exposure of the lateral column (32).
3. The paratricipital approach, originally described by Alonso-Llames (33) has been adapted for use in transcolumn and simple bicolumn fractures (34). Through a single posterior incision, exposure of the medial and lateral columns is made by separate medial and lateral paratricipital incisions, with minimal retraction of the triceps.
4. The triceps may be reflected from lateral to medial (extended Kocher approach). This approach has seldom been used for fractures of the distal humerus.
5. Morrey has further modified his original approach for nonunion surgery, where the distal humeral articular surface is to be excised to insert a hinged TER (35). If the patient has undergone previous surgery, detachment of the triceps

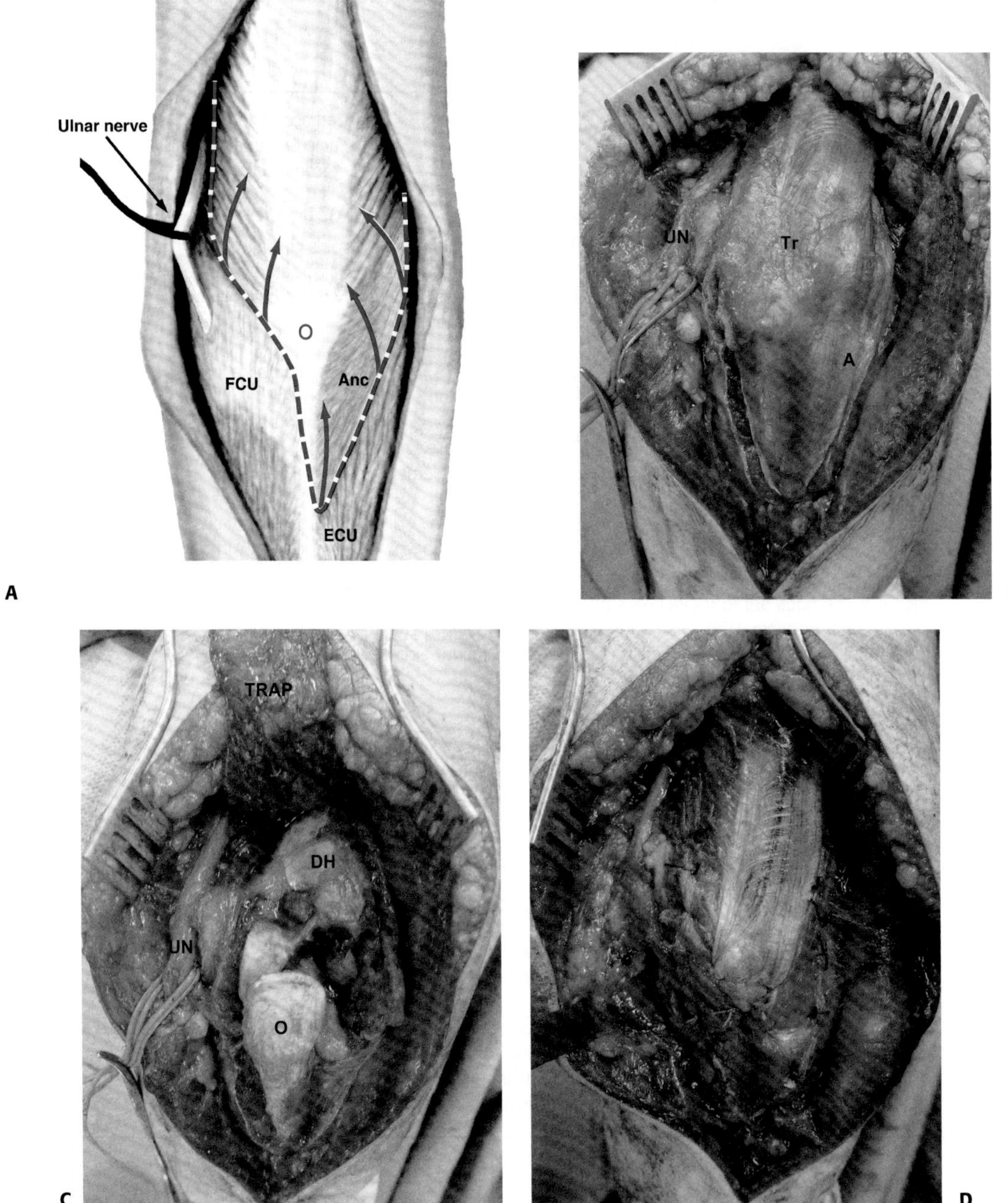

FIGURE 29-11 Diagrams and operative photos of the triceps-reflecting anconeus pedicle approach. **A.** Schematic diagram of the approach in a right elbow with the patient in a lateral decubitus position (*FCU*, flexor carpi ulnaris; *ECU*, extensor carpi ulnaris; *Anc*, anconeus). **B.** Intraoperative view of the approach (*Tr*, triceps; *UN*, ulnar nerve; *A*, anconeus). **C.** Elevation of the flap (*TRAP*, triceps-reflecting anconeus pedicle; *DH*, distal humerus; *UN*, ulnar nerve; *O*, olecranon). **D.** Closure of the flap following reconstruction, using a figure-of-eight suture.

can be detached from the lateral epicondyle to provide exposure of the lateral aspect of the elbow joint. Exposure of the posterior aspect of the posterior column can also be gained to internally fix capitellar fractures.

If more distal access to perform an arthrotomy is required, this is achieved by entering the interval between the extensor carpi radialis longus and extensor digitorum tendons, or more posteriorly between the extensor carpi ulnaris and anconeus. The latter approach is preferred, because it provides greater protection to the radial nerve. The lateral epicondyle may be osteotomized or fractured as a result of injury, providing an improved portal of access to the lateral side of the joint for reconstruction (39).

The lateral epicondyle is smaller than its medial counterpart (Fig. 29-4) and serves as origin for the lateral collateral ligament, which blends with the common extensor origin and the annular ligament. The anterior fibers of the lateral collateral ligament insert on the supinator crest of the proximal ulna. The common extensor muscle mass takes its origin from the lateral epicondyle, posterior to the radial part of the lateral collateral ligament. The lateral column diverges from the humeral shaft at the same level as the medial column (Fig. 29-6). The proximal part of this column is hard and predominantly cortical bone, whereas the distal half of the lateral column is largely cancellous. The capitellum consists of a 180 degrees hemisphere of cartilage, which faces directly anteriorly. Its rotational center is displaced between 1 and 2 cm anterior to the axis of the humeral shaft axis, to align it with the trochlea, and allow the radius and ulna to flex and extend coaxially.

Anterior Approach

Anterior approaches to the elbow are infrequently used in adult distal humeral fracture treatment (40,41). Occasionally, this approach will be required for vascular access if there is a significant injury to the brachial artery at the level of the fracture. It is never used for reconstruction because of the poor access it provides to the medial and lateral columns. This is due to the intervening flexor muscles and neurovascular structures, which are at risk of injury.

The columns are less apparent from an anterior perspective because there is no anterior counterpart of the deep olecranon fossa, which emphasizes them posteriorly. The two corresponding anterior recesses are the coronoid and radial fossae, which accommodate the coronoid process and radial head during elbow flexion. The fossae are separated by a longitudinal ridge of bone that continues distally as the lateral eminence of the trochlea (Fig. 29-4A).

Blood Supply

The extraosseous circulation receives a rich blood supply, which is organized into three arcades situated medially, laterally, and posteriorly (42). The medial arcade is formed from the superior collateral, inferior collateral, and posterior recurrent ulnar arteries; the lateral arcade from radial and middle collateral, interosseous and radial recurrent arteries; and the posterior arcade receives contributions from both medial and lateral arcades, as well as the middle collateral artery (Fig. 29-12A,B).

The interosseous blood supply is segmental in organization, and derived from feeding perforating vessels derived from the

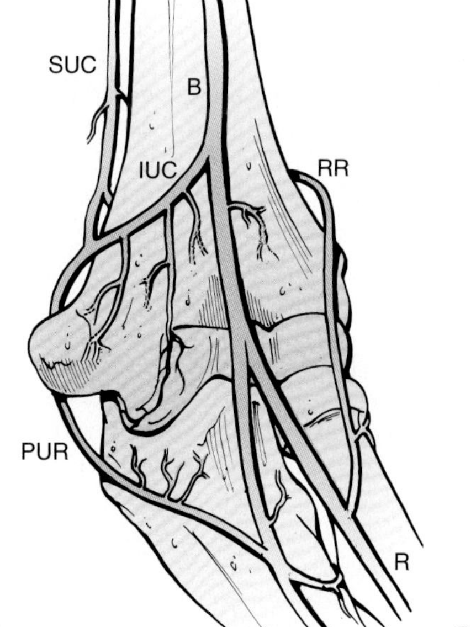

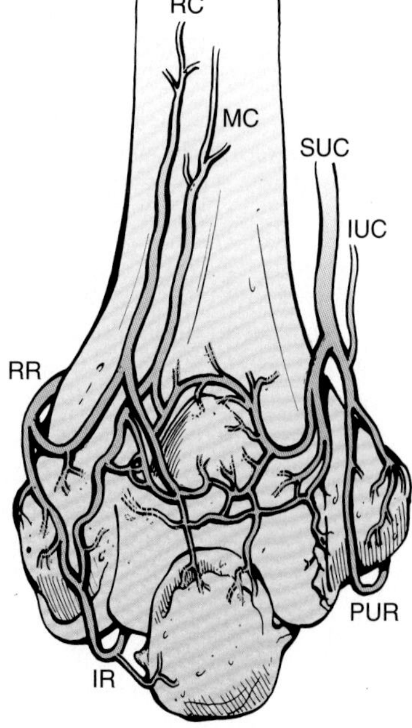

FIGURE 29-12 The blood supply of the distal humerus. **A.** Anterior view. **B.** Posterior view. *SUC*, superior ulnar collateral artery; *B*, brachial artery; *IUC*, inferior ulnar collateral artery; *RR*, radial recurrent artery; *PUR*, posterior ulnar recurrent artery; *R*, radial artery; *RC*, radial collateral artery; *MC*, middle collateral artery; *IR*, interosseous recurrent artery. (Redrawn after Yamaguchi K, Sweet FA, Bindra R, et al. The extraosseous and intraosseous arterial anatomy of the adult elbow. *J Bone Joint Surg Am* 1997;79:1653–1662, with permission.)

three arcades. The capitellum and lateral aspect of the trochlea are supplied by posterior perforating vessels derived from the radial recurrent, radial collateral, and interosseous recurrent arteries, whereas the medial aspect of the trochlea is supplied by a circumferential vascular ring originating from the inferior ulnar recurrent artery. Watershed areas are apparent between the blood supplies to the medial and lateral aspects of the distal humerus.

The distal humerus thus has a rich anastomotic blood supply and problems with healing and osteonecrosis (ON) are therefore relatively uncommon. During reduction and internal fixation of complex closed distal humeral fractures, retention of even completely devascularized fragments is appropriate if they are large and contributing to the stability of the reconstruction. Revascularization of these fragments may subsequently occur by creeping substitution.

CLASSIFICATION

The change in treatment of distal humeral fractures over the last 30 years, from largely nonoperative to mostly operative treatment, has resulted in a greater requirement for a classification system that can be used to guide treatment and predict the outcome. Before 1970, these fractures were classified by anatomical regions, using terms such as condylar, epicondylar, supracondylar, and by displacement (43,44).

The first comprehensive classification was produced by the AO Group (45) and the original OTA classification (46) has now been modified, so that it is identical (47). Both use an alphanumeric system, with subclassification according to the degree of articular involvement. Type A fractures are extra-articular, Type B fractures are partial articular, and Type C are complete articular. Further classification into subgroups produces 27 main fracture types (Fig. 29-13), and 61 types, if all qualifications are considered. Although still widely used, the classification has been criticized for being too rigid, overcomplex in some areas and too simple in others (48).

The other recent classification system has been produced by Jupiter et al (49–51). This uses the modern understanding of the stability of the elbow, based upon the concept of the "two column and tie-arch elbow" (Fig. 29-14). The columns of the elbow correspond closely to the condyles described in the AO system. The classification also allows distinction of the level of the fracture, which is a major determinant of the complexity of any reconstructive procedure.

There are many similarities between the two classifications; the AO system has the advantage that through its ubiquity, the major subdivisions can be easily remembered and understood. The Jupiter classification is less intuitive, and does not distinguish the different types of articular surface fractures, which should be identified for treatment purposes. Both have the drawbacks of observer error (52,53), lack of validation, and neither considers the extent of displacement of fracture fragments as a factor. Overall, it is the author's opinion that the Jupiter classification provides a better guide to the problems of reconstruction. For this reason we have used this classification in this chapter, although the corresponding AO classification is given for comparison.

CLINICAL ASSESSMENT

Fractures of the distal humerus present with pain, swelling, bruising, and the elbow may appear deformed and shortened. If there is a fracture of the capitellum there may be more specific pain on rotational movements of the forearm. The degree of swelling is often a poor marker of the severity of the underlying bony injury.

Excessive pain in a patient with a history of a high-energy injury should raise the suspicion of a concomitant compartment syndrome of the forearm. Direct measurement of tissue pressures should be undertaken, if there is suspicion on clinical grounds (54). Urgent fasciotomies are indicated if the tissue pressures are elevated (4).

Open fractures of the distal humerus are relatively common (see Tables 29-2 and 29-9), and careful circumferential inspection of the elbow is required, prior to application of a temporary, well-padded plaster back-shell. This will detect any open wounds, or areas of bone extrusion from the soft-tissue envelope, which may cause skin tenting and necrosis.

Although vascular injuries are rarely associated with distal humeral fracture in adults (4), assessment of the circulation distal to the fracture is mandatory. These are particularly associated with the extension transcolumn fracture subtypes, where the distal humerus projects forward and comes into close proximity to the brachial artery. Any patient with ongoing signs of vascular compromise should be referred for specialist vascular surgical advice. An arteriogram should also be performed if there is a history of transient ischemia of the extremity. This may be caused by flap-like intimal tears, which can re-occlude and cause vascular compromise during surgery

A careful assessment of the neurological status of the hand must also be made. Specific assessment of the ulnar, median and radial nerve is difficult immediately after trauma because hand movements may be inhibited by pain, or the elbow may have been placed in a plaster back-shell. However, it is mandatory to exclude injury to these structures prior to any therapeutic intervention. The radial and median nerve palsies are more commonly associated with extension-type transcolumn or bicolumn fractures, whereas injury to the ulnar nerve is more commonly associated with flexion injuries and medial epicondyle fractures.

Patients with distal humeral fractures often have multiple injuries (55) and the initial treatment of life-threatening injuries takes precedence over the reconstruction of the elbow. In closed injuries the articular reconstruction can often be delayed for several days, until the patient is stable enough to undergo definitive treatment.

Concomitant fractures of the distal radius, olecranon, radial head, or proximal humerus, may occur in association with

Extra-articular fractures (Type A)

Apophyseal avulsion fractures (A1)

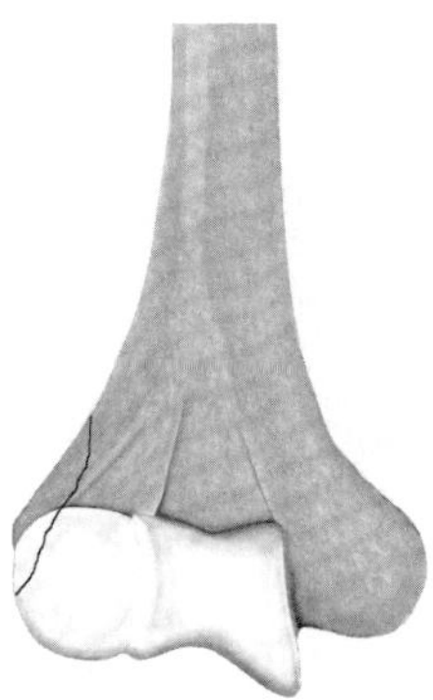

A. A1.1 fracture (lateral epicondylar avulsion)

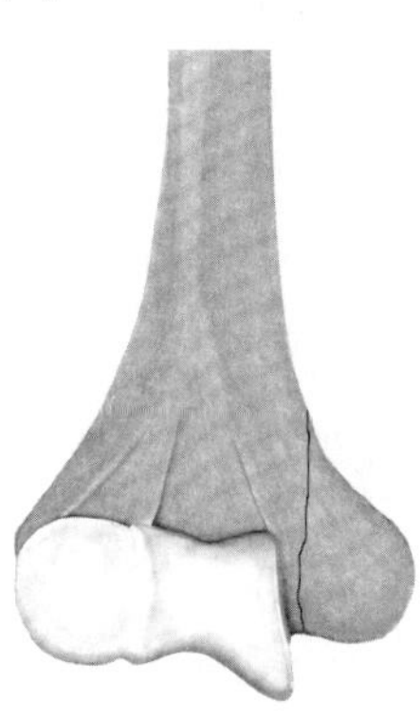

B. A1.2 fracture (medial epicondyle, nonincarcerated)

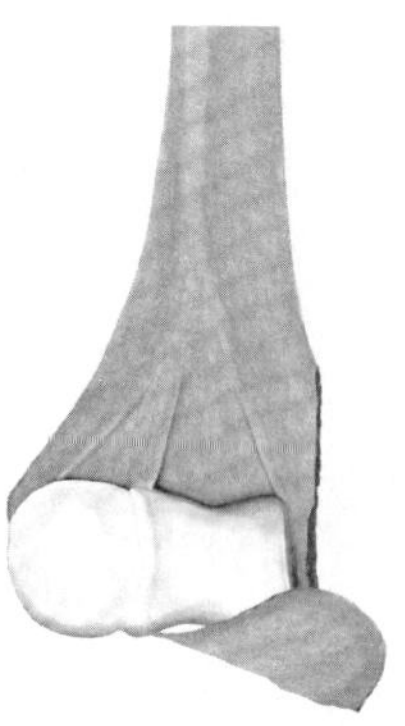

C. A1.3 fracture (medial epicondyle, incarcerated)

Simple metaphyseal transcolumn fractures (A2)

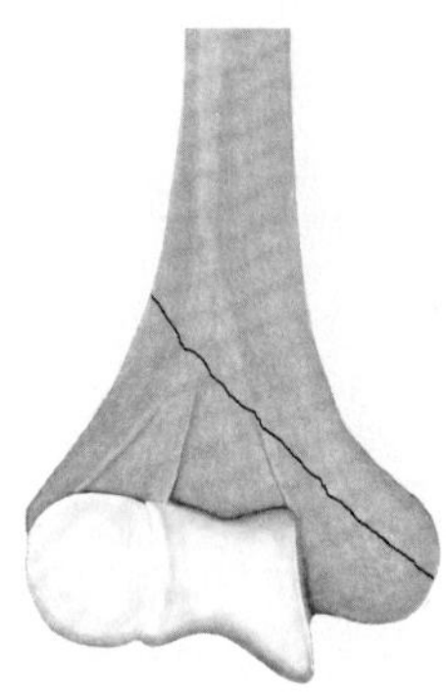

D. A2.1 fracture (oblique downward and inward)

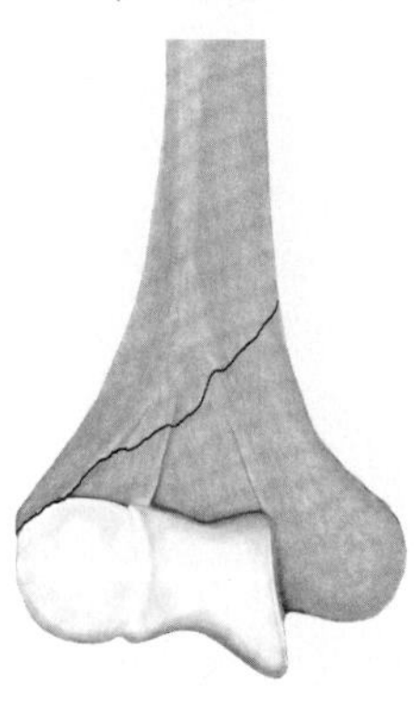

E. A2.2 fracture (oblique downward and outward)

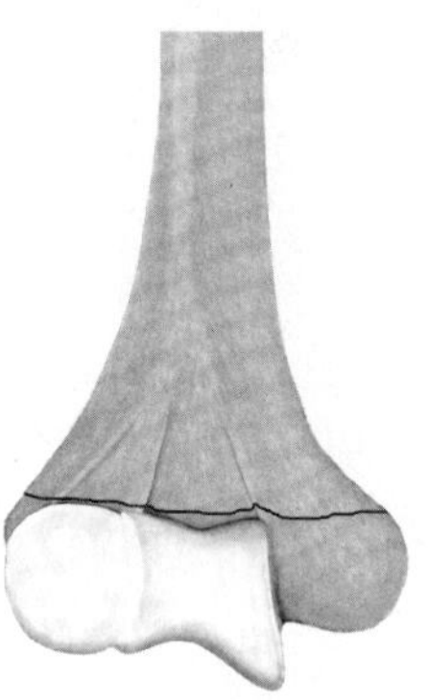

F. A2.3 fracture (transverse)

Complex multifragmentary metaphyseal transcolumn fractures (A3)

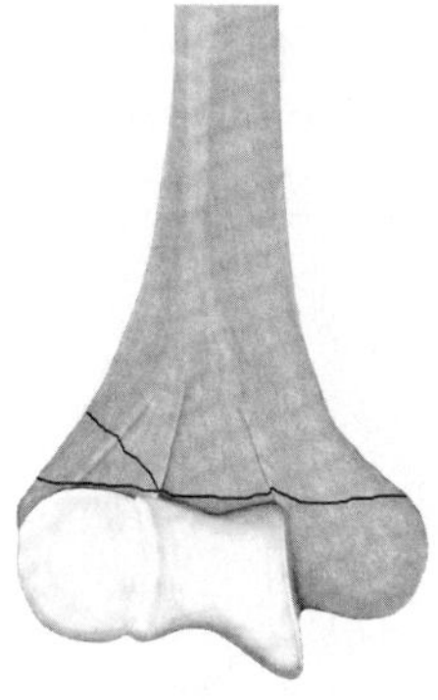

G. A3.1 fracture (with an intact wedge)

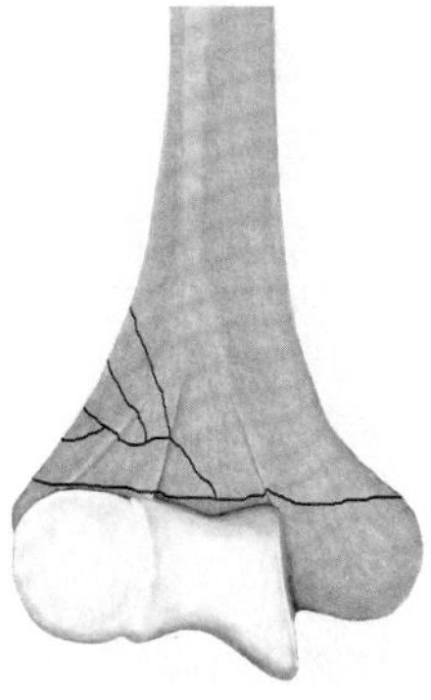

H. A3.2 fracture (with a fragmented wedge)

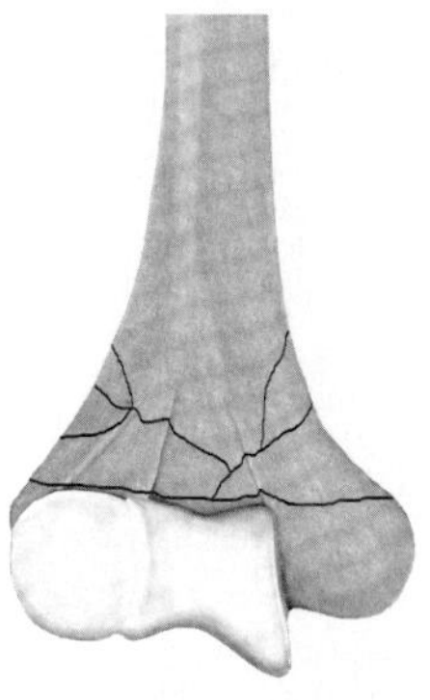

I. A3.3 fracture (complex)

FIGURE 29-13 The AO classification of distal humeral fractures. (*continues*)

Partial articular fractures (Type B)

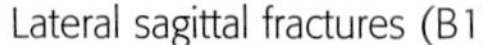
Lateral sagittal fractures (B1)

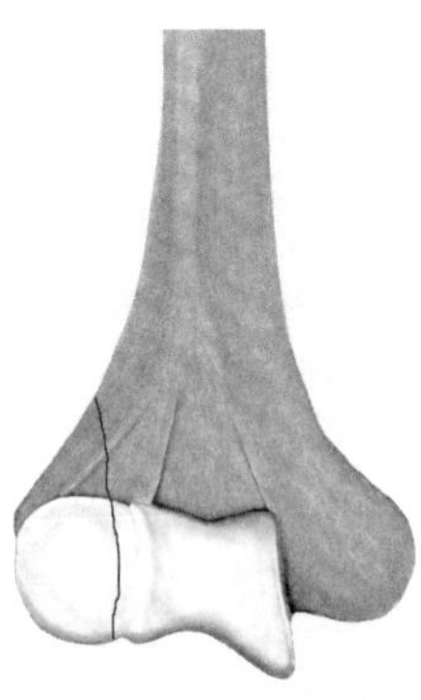

J. B1.1 fracture (transcapitellar, Milch Type I)

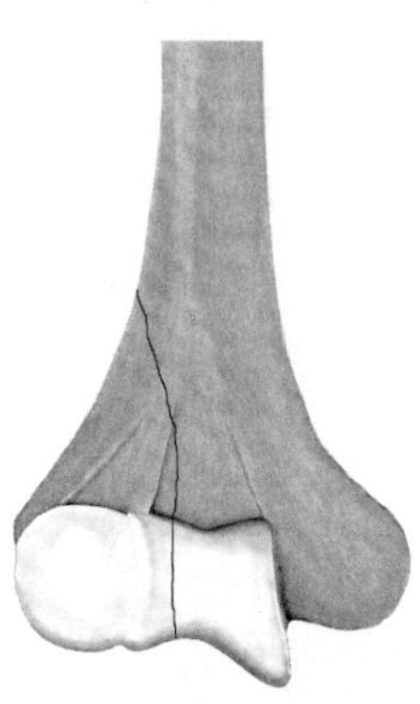

K. B1.2 fracture (transtrochlear, Milch Type II)

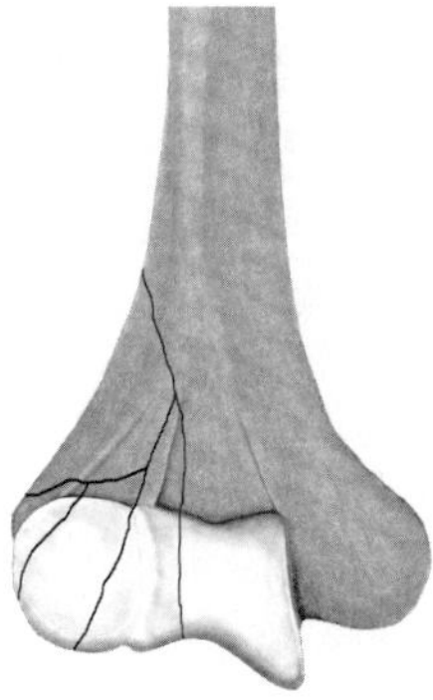

L. B1.3 fracture (transtrochlear, Milch Type II, multifragmentary)

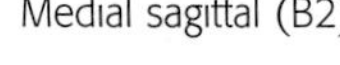
Medial sagittal (B2)

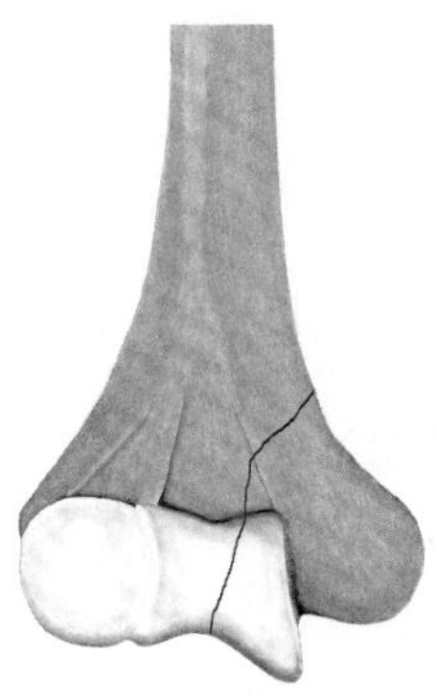

M. B2.1 fracture (transtrochlear simple, through the medial side, Milch Type I)

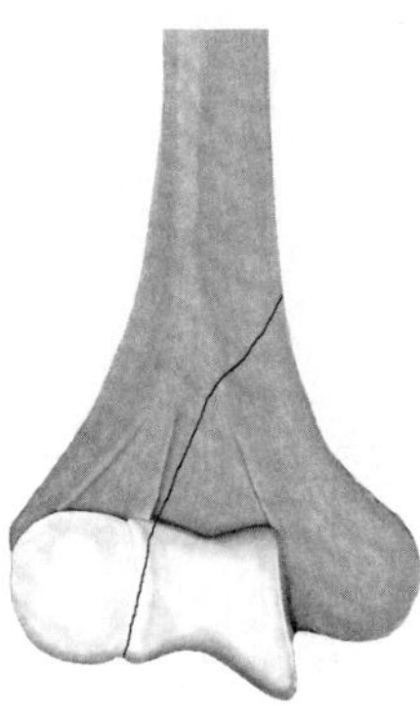

N. B2.2 fracture (transtrochlear, through the groove, Milch Type II)

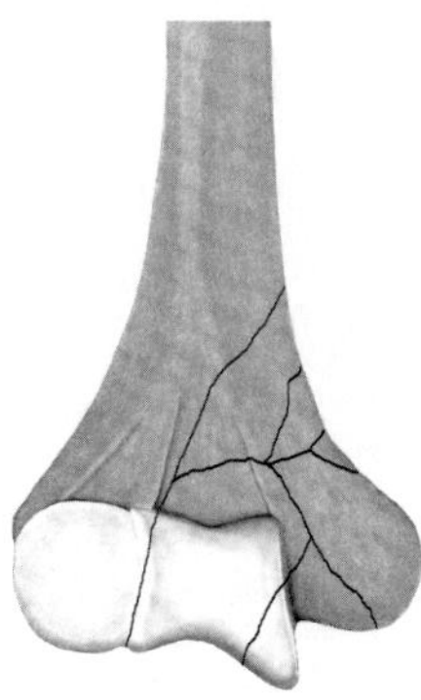

O. B2.3 fracture (transtrochlear, Milch Type II, multifragmentary)

Frontal (B3)

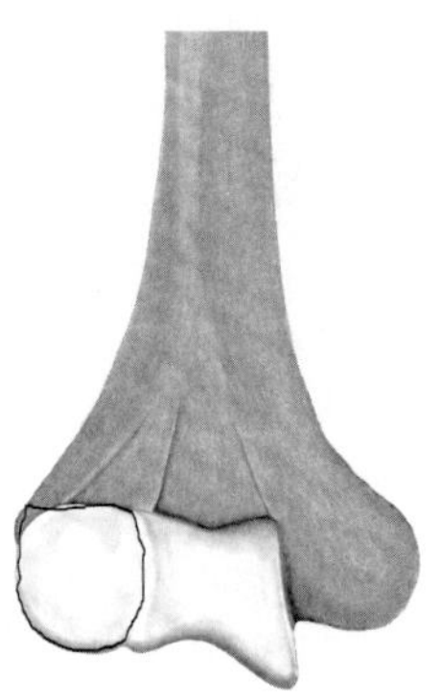

P. B3.1 fracture (capitellum)

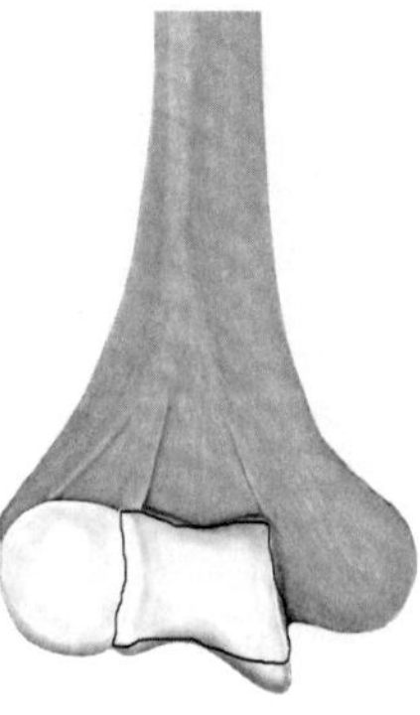

Q. B3.2 fracture (transtrochlear simple)

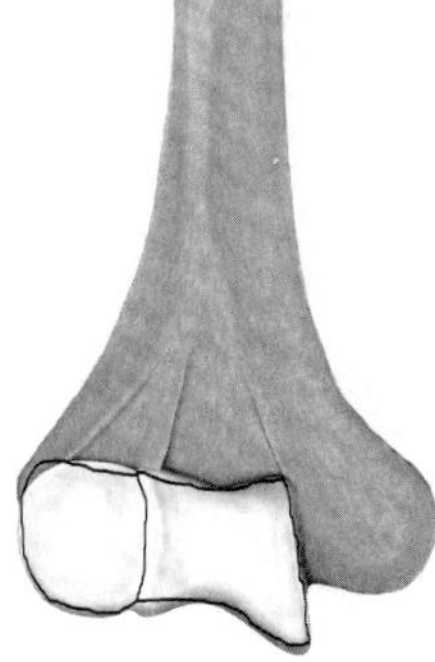

R. B3.3 fracture (capitellum and trochlea)

FIGURE 29-13 *(continued)*

Complete articular fractures (Type C)

Articular and metaphyseal simple (C1)

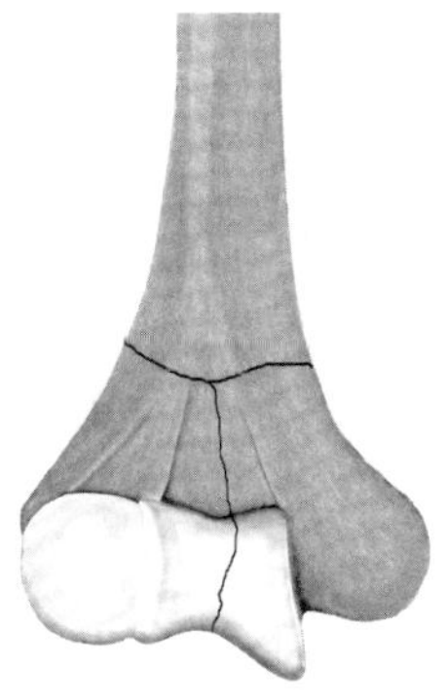

S. C1.1 fracture (slight displacement)

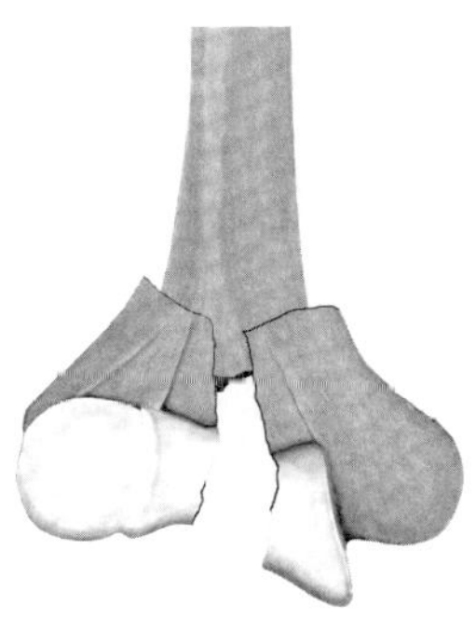

T. C1.2 fracture (marked displacement)

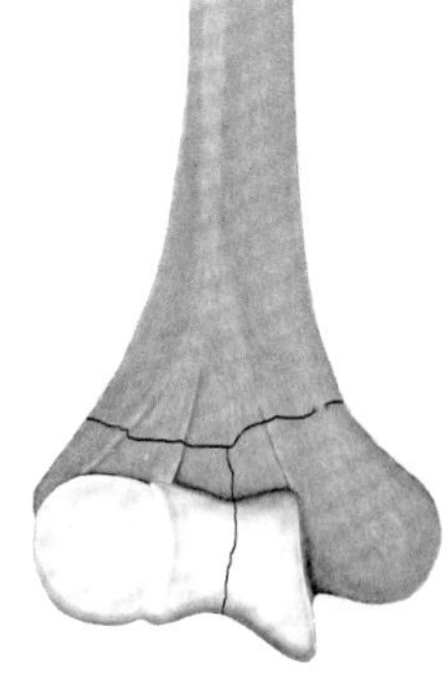

U. C1.3 fracture (T-shaped epiphyseal)

Articular simple, metaphyseal complex (C2)

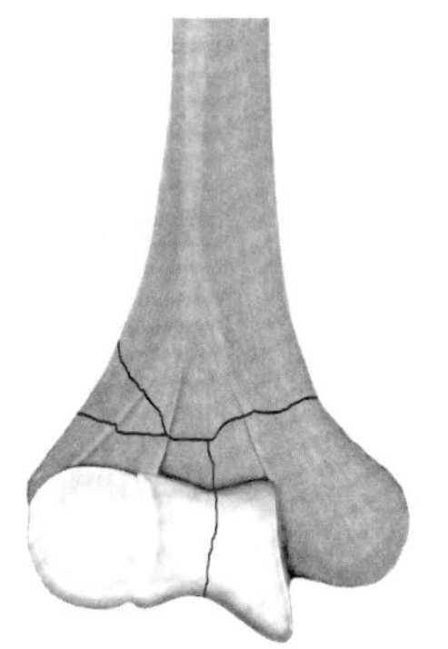

V. C2.1 fracture (with an intact wedge)

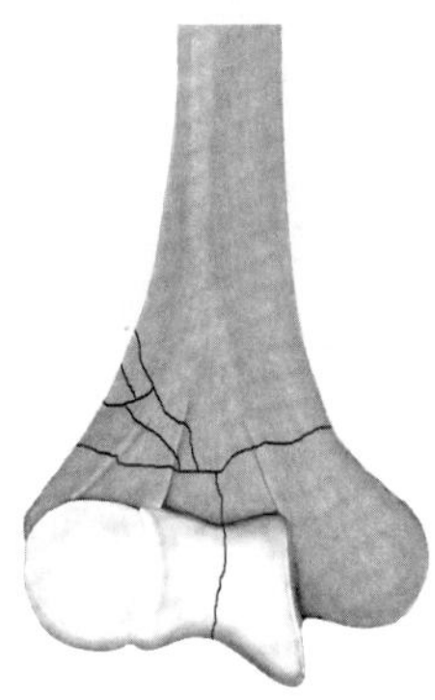

W. C2.2 fracture (with fragmented wedge)

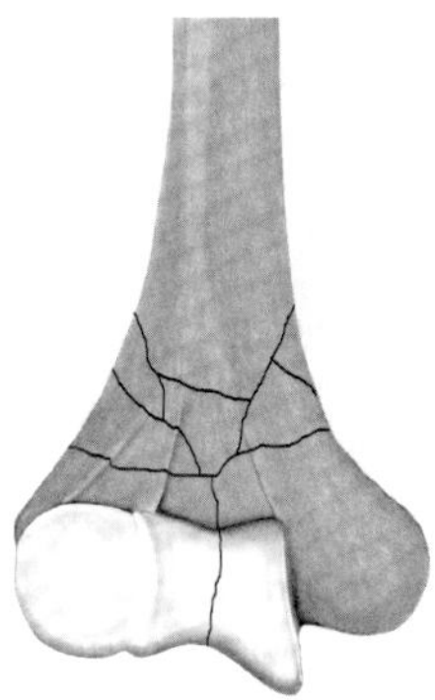

X. C2.3 fracture (complex)

Multifragmentary (C3)

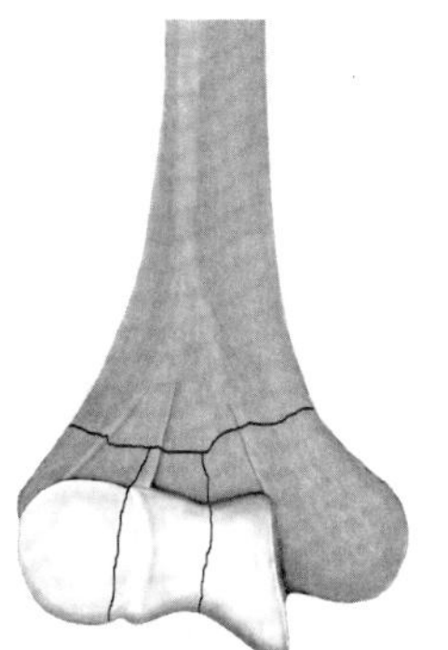

Y. C3.1 fracture (metaphyseal simple)

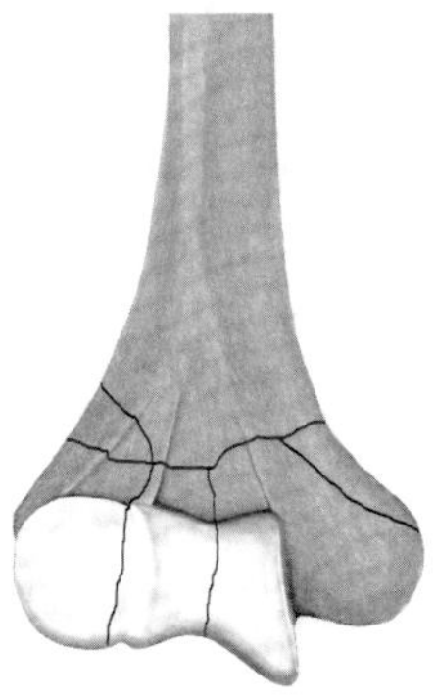

Z. C3.2 fracture (metaphyseal wedge)

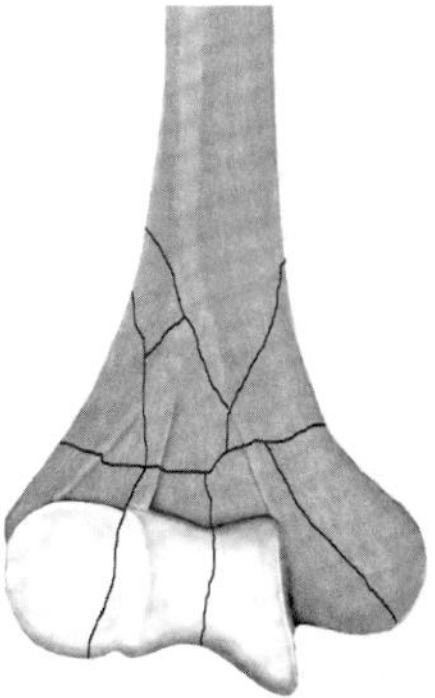

AA. C3.3 fracture (metaphyseal complex)

FIGURE 29-13 *(continued)*

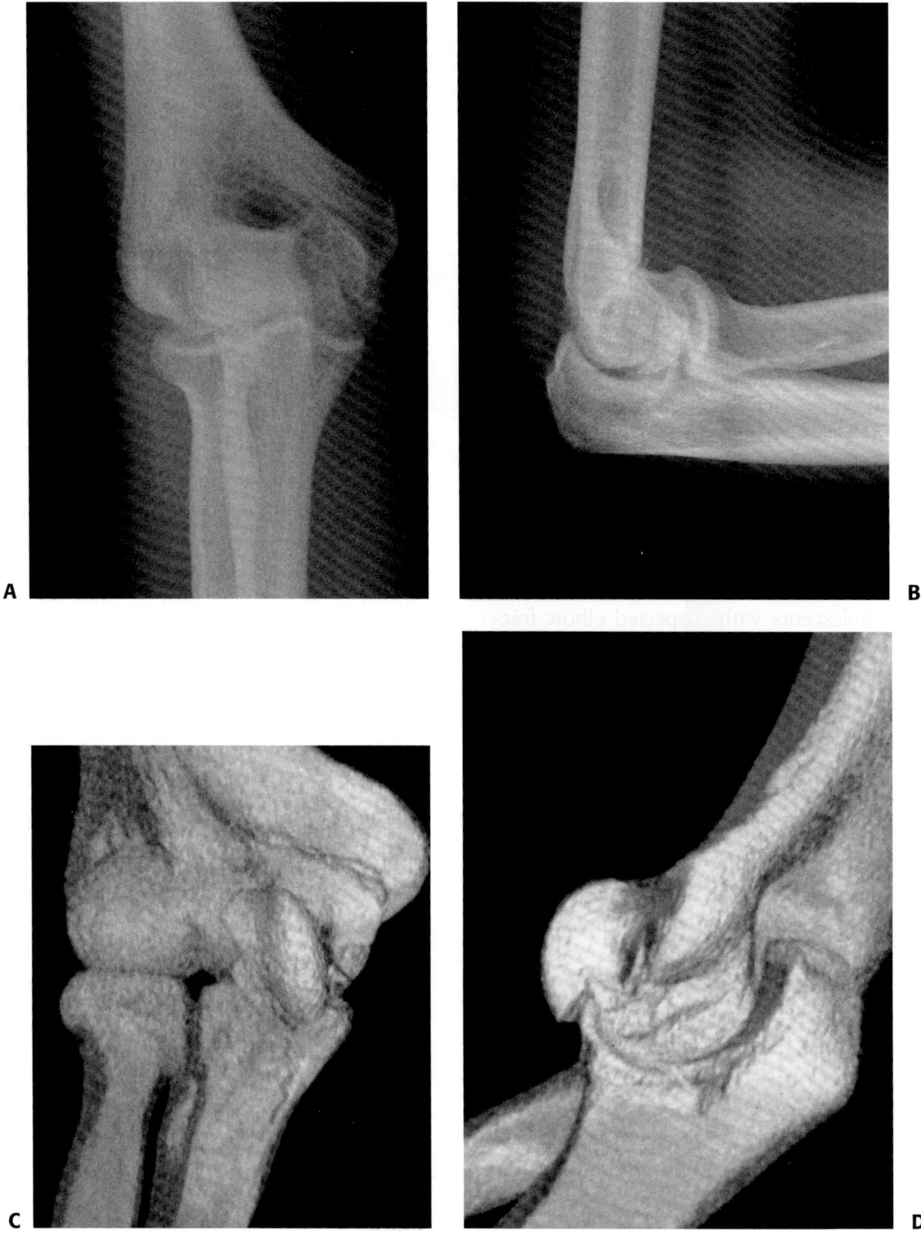

FIGURE 29-15 X-rays of a 23-year-old male who sustained a trochlear fracture during a high-speed fall off a motorbike. The severity and displacement of the fracture is poorly appreciated with conventional anteroposterior and lateral x-rays **(A,B)**. The use of three-dimensional CT reconstruction provides a better appreciation of the complex geometry of the fracture **(C,D)**.

Level IV (case series) and Level V (expert opinion) studies. Although there are several key areas of controversy in the treatment of these injuries, there are few randomized controlled trials, prospective cohort studies, or case-control studies (Level I to III) to help formulate evidence-based treatment protocols. Furthermore, the bulk of the published results emanate from centers of excellence, where the patterns of injury encountered may be different from everyday practice. The excellent results reported by elbow specialists working with modern facilities in tertiary referral centers, may be not be reproducible in centers where expertise and resources are more limited.

Most of the published results of treatment include an assessment of pain, range of movement, and ability to perform normal activities, which are usually collectively amalgamated to produce a functional score (Table 29-5). This score is then used to grade the outcome, usually into the four categories of "excellent," "good," "fair," and "poor." The other surrogate outcome measure, which has been used historically, is to assess the inci-

TABLE 29-4 Summary of the Medical Co-Morbidities Commonly Associated with Increased Risk of Surgical Complications

Co-morbidity	Operative Risk
Dementia/mental impairment	Poor compliance with rehabilitation
Diabetes mellitus	Deep infection
Immunocompromise	Nonunion/infection
Parkinson's disease	Fixation failure
Rheumatoid arthritis	Nonunion/infection
Disseminated malignancy	Nonunion/infection
Steroid medication	Nonunion/infection
Heavy tobacco usage	Nonunion
Alcohol abuse	Nonunion, poor compliance with rehabilitation

dence of complications associated with a specific form of treatment.

Assessment of Functional Outcome

The deficiency of many of the functional scores that have traditionally been used is that they are not sufficiently flexible to accommodate the variability in patients' own expectations from treatment. This may vary widely dependent upon their age and level of activity. More recently, newer audit tools have been produced, which attempt to address this deficiency, by assessing the patient's own aspirations and feelings about their injury and its treatment. The newer tools are administered as questionnaires, which either selectively assess limb function (the DASH score and the ASES-e), or assess the patient's general health status in response to injury (the SF-36, Musculoskeletal Function Assessment, Nottingham Health Profile). The chief drawback of these is their inability to assess the patient's functional status prior to their injury, in order to evaluate the efficacy of the treatment used. Although normative "control" values are available for the general population, the patients who sustain distal humeral fractures may not be strictly comparable.

More objective measurement instruments are now available that more accurately and reproducibly assess the key components of elbow function. Assessment of muscle strength and range of movement can be made using commercially available muscle testing machines, which can selectively "isolate" muscle groups, and produce computer-generated simulations of normal daily activities. The strength in the injured elbow in flexion, extension, forearm pronation and supination, and grip strength are assessed and compared with the normal uninjured side, thereby "controlling" for the effect of age and individual variation in muscle strength. These systems have the advantage of providing a quantitative evaluation of function, and repeated testing allows appraisal of the recovery of function over time. Their major drawback is that objective evidence of weakness may not correlate well with the patient's overall level of function, and degree of satisfaction with their outcome (26,27,60).

The Expected Functional Outcome after Distal Humeral Fracture

Functional normality is seldom restored after a significantly displaced distal humeral fracture. Minor complaints of activity-related ache and sensitivity to cold or damp weather ("barometric elbow"), together with a sensation of stiffness, particularly after unaccustomed heavy activity are common, even in patients who have near-normal functional outcome scores (61). There is evidence to suggest that continued functional recovery may take place during the first 2 years after the injury. However, the rate of recovery is rapid in the first 6 months, slows exponentially during the subsequent 6 months and is minimal in the second year (24).

Recovery of flexion is usually rapid, whereas extension recovers more slowly and is more often incomplete, with a residual lag of 20 to 30 degrees after more severe injuries. With early mobilization of the elbow, the range of supination and pronation movements are usually unaffected. Most activities of daily living can be performed with a pain-free functional arc of 100° of elbow movement or a range of 30 to 130 degrees (62). Lesser degrees of movement may be well-tolerated in low-demand elderly individuals, whereas more movement is often required for function in younger, active patients. Formal measurements of muscle strength frequently reveal continued long-term weakness in the elbow, which may be clinically undetectable by standard means of testing. This weakness may be a cause of the minor complaints, which patients describe long after their fracture has healed and movement has been restored. A wide range of intrinsic and extrinsic factors have been associated with poorer functional outcomes from treatment (Table 29-6).

Assessment of Complications

Although it is widely accepted that most distal humeral fractures are best treated operatively, it is also acknowledged that this is a high-risk strategy. Complications of treatment frequently occur during treatment and vary from the relatively benign superficial wound infection, to the difficult infected nonunion. More than one-fourth of patients can expect to develop one or more significant complications during treatment, with one-eighth requiring further surgery (4).

Complications of treatment may be incompletely or inaccurately reported in many of the retrospective studies that have reported results of treatment, owing to incomplete documentation in case records. Prospective cohort studies usually report

TABLE 29-5 Summary of the Outcome Assessment Tools Which Have Been Used to Evaluate the Results Following the Treatment of Distal Humeral Fractures

			Range of Movement				Pain/ADL Assessment			
Author	Type	Other Components	Excellent	Good	Fair or Satisfactory	Poor	Excellent	Good	Fair or Satisfactory	Poor
Riseborough[44]	Nominal categorical			30 to 115°	30–60 to 115°	>60 to <115°	N/A	"Minor" symptoms	"Minor" symptoms	"Major" symptoms
Cassebaum[90]	Nominal categorical		15 to 130°	30 to 120°	40 to 90–120°	>40° to <90°	N/A			
Burri[250,251]	Nominal categorical	PS, AR	<10% arc	<33% loss	<50% loss	>50% loss	Preinjury levels	Preinjury levels	Reduced ability to work	Unable to work
Horne[76]	Nominal categorical		10 to 120°	30 to 90°		>30° and <90°	No pain	Minimal/ occassional		Severe/ persistent
Jupiter[64]	Nominal categorical		15 to 130°	30 to 120°	40 to 90–120°	>40° and <90°	No pain	Minimal/ occassional	Moderate/with activity	Severe
MEPI[252a]	Ordinal categorical	S	Point scoring system				Point scoring system			
Browne[56]	Nominal categorical	AR	<10 to >120°	<30 to >90°		>30 to <90°	N/A			
Aitken[95]	Nominal categorical		>100° arc	>75° arc	>60° arc	<60° arc	No pain/ unlimited ADL	Minimal/normal ADL	Mild/normal ADL	Severe/no ADL
Gabel[92]	Nominal categorical		<30 to >130°	30 to >130°	<30 to 130°	>30 to <130°	N/A			
Caja[146]	Ordinal categorical	AR	Point scoring system				Point scoring system			
DASH[26]	Ordinal categorical		N/A				30 item questionnaire for upper limb disorders			
OTA[28]	Nominal categorical	AR, PS	>125° arc	>95° arc	>70° arc	<70° arc	Preinjury levels	Preinjury levels	Reduced ability to work	Unable to work
ASES-e[60]	Ordinal categorical		N/A				N/A			
IMST[60]	Continuous numeric		N/A				N/A			
SF-36[26,60]	Ordinal categorical		N/A				Patient orientated general health questionnaire			

[a] The Mayo elbow performance index (MEPI) has been evolved by Morrey and is based upon three slightly different elbow rating systems, which he described previously. ROM = goniometer assessment of range of movement, PS = patients subjective assessment of outcome, AR = degree of clinical/radiological malunion, ADL = assessment of ability to perform specific normal daily activities, S = stability and/or strength of elbow function,, ASES-e = American Shoulder and Elbow Surgeons elbow form, IMST = isometric muscle strength testing, N/A = not assessed or applicable.

TABLE 29-6 Factors Associated with a Poorer Functional Outcome and Increased Risk of Complications After a Distal Humeral Fracture

Category	Factor	Adverse Factors	References
Patient-related factors	Patient motivation/compliance[a]	Poor compliance/motivation	
	Worker's compensation claim[a]	Claim pending	
	Age	Advanced age	28,72,146,147
	Osteoporosis		28,175
	Medical co-morbidity	See Table 29-4	175
	Joint disease prior to injury	Degenerative joint disease Inflammatory joint disease	175
Injury-related factors	Fracture configuration	Bicolumn/transcolumn fracture Higher AO/Jupiter grade of Type C fracture "Low" bicolumn and trans-column fracture configurations	4,14,55,60,72,253
	Injury mechanism/injuries sustained	High-energy injury Multiple injuries Head injury Ipsilateral upper limb injury	4,55
	Soft-tissue injury	Open fracture Skin/muscle loss Neurovascular injury	4,28,55,147
Surgery-related factors	Internal fixation	Nonrigid fixation Technical error	55,61,76,147,254
	Immobilization	Prolonged immobilization	28
	Recovery	Postsurgical complications Reoperations	117,122
	Type of intervention	Nonoperative treatment	4,95,97,255
	Timing of surgery	Late surgery	55,254

[a] Although these factors adversely affect functional outcome, they probably do not increase the risk of complications after surgery.

higher incidences, and this may explain the wide variation in the literature (see Table 29-11).

Although some postsurgical complications are ubiquitous, many are unique to specific fracture patterns. There are identifiable risk factors associated with an increased risk of specific complications, and many of these are similar to those associated with a poorer functional outcome (Table 29-6).

Treatment of Single Column Fractures (AO/OTA Type B1 and B2 Fractures)

Epidemiology and Subclassification of Single Column Fractures

Single column fractures are rare, comprising approximately 15% of all distal humeral fractures (4). The system devised by Milch has been traditionally used to subclassify these fractures (43,63,64). Both medial and lateral single column fractures are subclassified into two types, dependent upon whether the lateral eminence of the trochlea remains attached to the main mass of the humerus (Type I fracture) or is part of the fractured segment (Type II fracture). Type I fractures extend for a shorter distance on their respective column than Type II fractures, often exiting at the level of the olecranon fossa (Fig. 29-16). For this reason Type I and II fractures are also referred to as "low" and "high" fractures (Fig. 29-16). Both the AO/OTA and the Jupiter classifications (Figs. 29-13 and 29-14) use a similar system of subclassification, though the AO/OTA classification includes subcategories for fractures that are significantly comminuted (Types B1.3 and B2.3).

Most single column fractures are displaced, although Type I ("low") injuries are more stable fractures than the Type II subtype, because the lateral trochlear eminence remains intact (43). In Type II injuries the eminence forms part of the fracture and in the presence of a concomitant collateral ligament injury a dislocation of the elbow can occur (Fig. 29-16).

A rare third type of "divergent" single column fracture has been described (65), which occurs in adolescents who are predisposed to this injury because they have a septal aperture in the olecranon fossa (66). Following an axial loading injury, the olecranon is driven proximally, and produces a divergent split between the medial and lateral columns, with the fracture exiting high up on a single column.

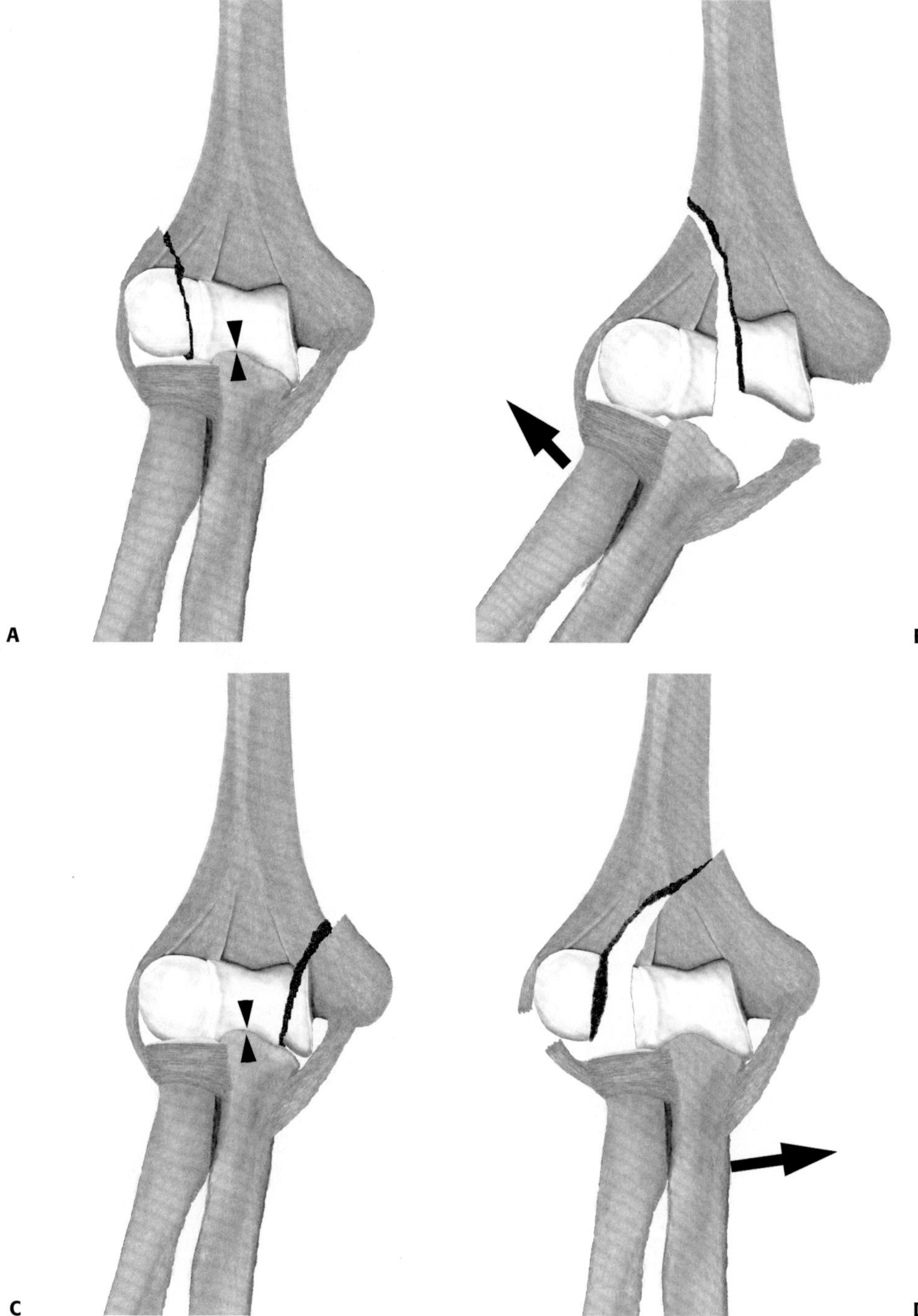

FIGURE 29-16 The lateral trochlear eminence is the key to analyzing single column distal humeral fractures. In low lateral column (Milch Type I) fractures the lateral trochlear eminence is intact and provides medial to lateral elbow stability **(A)**. In high lateral column (Milch Type II) fractures the eminence is a part of the fractured column, which may allow the elbow to dislocate laterally, if the medial ligament complex is disrupted **(B)**. In low medial column (Milch Type I) fractures the lateral ridge is intact and provides medial to lateral stability **(C)**. In high medial column (Milch Type II) fractures, the lateral trochlear ridge is again part of the fractures column and the elbow can potentially dislocate in a medial direction, if the lateral ligamentous complex is disrupted **(D)**.

Lateral column fractures (Type B1) outnumber medial column fractures (Type B2) by almost four-fold (4,43,63), and two-thirds of fractures in both medial and lateral columns are the "high" type, which involve the lateral wall of the trochlea. Fifteen percent of lateral column fractures are comminuted (AO/OTA Type B1.3), whereas significant fragmentation of a medial column fracture (Type B2.3) is uncommon (4).

Single column fractures tend to occur in a relatively young age group of patients, and there is an almost equal gender distribution (Tables 29-7 and 29-8). They are most commonly produced either from falls onto the outstretched hand or directly onto the elbow, although a significant proportion of high-energy injuries also occur.

Treatment of Single Column Fractures

Completely undisplaced fractures should be immobilized for 4 to 6 weeks, with careful x-ray monitoring to ensure secondary displacement does not occur. Early open reduction and internal fixation (ORIF) is now recommended for any fracture that is displaced, irrespective of their classification.

A lateral Kocher approach will often be sufficient to gain access to the lateral column to allow adequate fixation. A medial approach, posterior triceps reflecting, or transolecranon approach may be required to provide adequate exposure to treat a medial column fracture or a more comminuted low medial or lateral column fracture. High fractures are more unstable, but easier to reconstruct, because of the larger fracture fragment, which will more easily accommodate internal fixation (Fig. 29-17).

Reduction of the fracture is carried out and a formal arthrotomy is usually required to assess the adequacy of the articular reduction. After provisional stabilization of the fracture, multiple interfragmentary lag screws may be sufficient to stabilize the fracture in younger individuals. The use of bioabsorbable fixation has been explored to treat these fractures, but is not widely practiced (67). In the elderly, and in fractures that are significantly comminuted, a single small fragment dynamic compression plate, reconstruction plate, or locking compression plate secured to the fractured column is preferable. The postoperative rehabilitation following surgical reconstruction is essentially the same as for bicolumn fractures.

Occasionally with high-energy trauma or with severe osteoporosis, the fracture may be so badly comminuted that it is unreconstructable. Excision of the lateral column has been successfully used for low (Type I) fractures in these circumstances, when the elbow is not unstable (the MCL and forearm interosseous are intact) (68). In some elderly individuals, TER has also been used to treat osteoporotic high (Type II) fractures, where excision of the fracture would cause instability (69–71).

Outcome of Single Column Fractures

Few studies have examined the results of treatment of single column fractures in isolation, and most are included in series reviewing the outcome after operative treatment of bicolumn fractures (55,72–76). Of the three studies that have specifically examined these fractures, good or excellent functional results are reported in 55 of 64 patients (86%) treated by ORIF (64,65,77).

Complications of Single Column Fractures

Nonunion of a unicolumn fracture may rarely occur following ORIF (4,64). However, nonunion and malunion are more frequently encountered following nonoperative treatment, typically of lateral condylar fractures in childhood (78–82). The typical presenting features are pain, stiffness, and deformity, which is more severe following low (Milch Type I) injuries. Severe ulnar neuritis may be present following malunion or nonunion of a lateral condylar fracture. Satisfactory results may be achieved following ORIF with bone grafting, combined with neurolysis and transposition of the ulnar nerve (79,83,84). An intra-articular osteotomy is often required, when there is significant malunion of the fracture.

Early osteoarthrosis may develop following nonoperative treatment or as a delayed complication of operative treatment (64,77). Jupiter (64) encountered four patients with extensive posttraumatic osteoarthrosis following internal fixation on medium-term follow-up, which was associated with a poorer functional outcome. The overall rate of decline of these joints over time is unknown, as long-term follow-up studies have not been performed. Severe symptomatic osteoarthrosis in more elderly individuals may require an elbow arthroplasty. The other complications described after open reconstruction of single column fractures are similar to those seen after the treatment of bicolumn fractures.

Treatment of Bicolumn Fractures (AO/OTA Type C Fractures)

Subclassification

Subclassification of these fractures aims to predict the likely technical difficulty of surgery and the feasibility of reconstruction. In the AO/OTA system, bicolumn fractures are classified as Type C fractures. They become more comminuted, both in the metaphysis and in the articular segment, proceeding from the C1.1 to the C3.3 fracture (Fig. 29-13). The Jupiter system (Fig. 29-14) attempts to describe the commonly encountered articular fracture configurations, and places particular emphasis on the level of the transverse fracture line across the condyles, distinguishing "high" (transverse fracture line above the olecranon fossa) from the "low" (transverse fracture line below the olecranon fossa, usually just proximal to the trochlea) subtypes.

In reality, the severity of comminution, the quality of the bone, and the level of the fracture are a continuum, which may defy finite classification. Neither system takes into account the separation of the fragments and severely comminuted fractures may be unclassifiable. Radiologically occult fracture lines are frequently encountered at surgery, and it is important to adopt a flexible approach to the operative reconstruction of these injuries.

Epidemiology

Fractures involving both columns are the most common type of distal humeral fracture, accounting for more than one-third

TABLE 29-7 Demographic Details of Distal Humeral Fractures, Classified Using the Two Most Commonly Used Systems

Classification System	Categories	Fracture Subtypes	Number of Fractures *(number open)*	Percentage of Total	Average Age in Years (range)	Males	Females	M:F Ratio
AO classification	Extra-articular	A1	47	15	24.6 (12–81)	34	13	2.6 : 1
		A2	54	17	59.6 (12–93)	28	26	0.6 : 1
		A3	23 *(1)*	7	45.1 (12–89)	12	11	1.1 : 1
		All type A	124 (1)	39	44.6 (12–93)	74	50	1.5 : 1
	Partial articular	B1	38 *(2)*	12	43.1 (13–93)	21	17	1.2 : 1
		B2	10 *(2)*	3	34.4 (13–64)	5	5	1.0 : 1
		B3	29	9	39.9 (13–84)	11	18	0.6 : 1
		All type B	77 (4)	24	40.7 (13–93)	37	40	0.9 : 1
	Complete articular	C1	39 (5)	12	55.5 (13–97)	12	27	0.4 : 1
		C2	42 *(7)*	13	53.4 (14–89)	21	21	1.0 : 1
		C3	38 *(6)*	12	68.9 (29–99)	15	23	0.7 : 1
		All type C	119 (18)	37	62.7 (13–99)	48	71	0.7 : 1
Jupiter classification	Single-column	Medial high	7 *(2)*	2	38.1 (14–64)	3	4	0.8 : 1
		Medial low	3	1	25.7 (13–39)	2	1	2.0 : 1
		Lateral high	27 *(1)*	8	45.1 (13–93)	12	15	0.8 : 1
		Lateral low	11 *(1)*	3	39.3 (13–84)	9	2	4.5 : 1
		Divergent	0	0	N/A	N/A	N/A	N/A
		All single column	48 (4)	15	39.8 (13–93)	26	22	1.2 : 1
	Bicolumn	High T type	19 *(2)*	6	50.1 (14–87)	6	13	0.5 : 1
		Low T type	24 *(2)*	8	63.4 (14–97)	9	15	0.6 : 1
		Y type	15 *(1)*	5	53.3 (16–89)	6	9	0.7 : 1
		H type	19 *(5)*	6	61.4 (18–91)	7	12	0.6 : 1
		Medial lamba	12 *(2)*	4	58.4 (17–97)	6	6	1.0 : 1
		Lateral lambda	11 *(1)*	3	62.1 (17–90)	5	6	0.8 : 1
		Multiplanar	19 *(5)*	6	68.2 (29–96)	9	10	0.9 : 1
		All bicolumn	119 (18)	37	62.7 (13–99)	48	71	0.7 : 1
	Articular surface		29	9	39.9 (13–84)	11	18	0.6 : 1
	Transcolumn	High extension	29 *(1)*	9	44.2 (12–99)	16	13	1.2 : 1
		High flexion	0	0	N/A	N/A	N/A	N/A
		High abduction	10	3	59.3 (18–80)	5	5	1.0 : 1
		High adduction	14	4	58.7 (17–77)	7	7	1.0 : 1
		Low flexion	3	1	56.4 (47–90)	2	1	2.0 : 1
		Low extension	21[a]	7	60.6 (14–94)	10	11	0.9 : 1
		All transcolumn	77 (1)	24	56.3 (12–93)	40	37	1.1 : 1
	Extracapsular	Medial epicondyle	38	12	18.6 (12–81)	17	6	2.8 : 1
		Lateral epicondyle	9	3	32.7 (18–68)	17	7	2.4 : 1
Total			320		48.4 (12–99)	159	161	1.0 : 1

[a]Six fractures in this group were minimally displaced, but of extension pattern. N/A = not applicable, M:F ratio = male:female ratio.

Some data from Robinson et al, 2003.[4]

TABLE 29-8 Mechanism of Injury in Fracture Subtypes

Classification System	Categories	Fracture Subtype	Mechanism of Injury: Simple Falls	Falls from Height	RTA	Sport	Other	Total
AO classification	Extra-articular	A1	18 (*38.3*)	2 (*4.3*)	5 (*10.6*)	16 (*34.0*)	6 (*12.8*)	47
		A2	44 (*81.5*)	0	3 (5.5)	5 (*6.0*)	2 (*3.7*)	54
		A3	11 (*47.8*)	0	6 (*26.1*)	6 (*26.1*)	0	23
		All type A	73 (58.9)	2 (*1.3*)	14 (11.4)	27 (21.8)	8 (6.6)	154
	Partial articular	B1	28 (*73.7*)	0	5 (*13.2*)	3 (*7.9*)	2 (*5.3*)	38
		B2	6 (*60.0*)	1 (*10.0*)	3 (*30.0*)	0	0	10
		B3	21 (*72.4*)	0	5 (*17.2*)	3 (*10.3*)	0	29
		All type B	55 (*71.4*)	1 (*1.3*)	13 (*16.9*)	6 (*7.8*)	2 (*2.6*)	77
	Complete articular	C1	34 (*87.2*)	0	2 (*5.1*)	3 (*7.7*)	0	39
		C2	26 (61.9)	1 (2.4)	9 (*21.4*)	5 (*11.9*)	1 (*3.7*)	42
		C3	31 (*76.5*)	1 (2.6)	4 (*10.5*)	0	2 (*5.3*)	38
		All type C	91 (*76.5*)	2 (1.7)	15 (*12.6*)	8 (*6.7*)	3 (*2.5*)	119
Jupiter classification	Single-column	Medial high	4 (*57.1*)	1 (*14.3*)	2 (*28.6*)	0	0	7
		Medial low	2 (*66.7*)	0	1 (*33.3*)	0	0	3
		Lateral high	20 (*74.1*)	0	3 (*11.1*)	2 (*7.4*)	2 (*7.4*)	27
		Lateral low	8 (*72.7*)	0	2 (*18.2*)	1 (*9.1*)	0	11
	Bicolumn	High T type	14 (*73.7*)	0	2 (*10.5*)	3 (*15.8*)	0	19
		Low T type	19 (*79.2*)	0	3 (*12.5*)	1 (*4.2*)	1 (*4.2*)	24
		Y type	13 (*86.7*)	0	0	2 (*13.3*)	0	15
		H type	13 (*68.4*)	1 (*5.3*)	4 (*21.1*)	0	1 (*5.3*)	19
		Medial lamba	10 (*83.3*)	0	1 (*8.3*)	1 (*8.3*)	0	12
		Lateral lambda	9 (*81.2*)	0	1 (*9.1*)	1 (*9.1*)	0	11
		Multiplanar	13 (*68.4*)	1 (*5.3*)	4 (*21.1*)	0	1 (*5.3*)	19
	Articular surface		21 (*72.4*)	0	5 (*17.2*)	3 (*10.3*)	0	29
	Transcolumn	High extension	21 (*72.4*)	0	4 (*13.8*)	4 (*13.8*)	0	29
		High flexion	0	0	0	0	0	0
		High abduction	9 (*90*)	0	0	1 (*10*)	0	10
		High adduction	10 (*71.4*)	0	1 (*7.1*)	1 (*7.1*)	2 (*14.3*)	14
		Low flexion	1 (*33.3*)	0	1 (*33.3*)	1 (*33.3*)	0	3
		Low extension	14 (*66.7*)	0	3 (*14.3*)	4 (*19.0*)	0	21
	Extracapsular	Medial epicondyle	15 (*39.5*)	2 (*5.3*)	5 (*13.2*)	13 (*34.2*)	3 (*7.9*)	38
		Lateral epicondyle	3 (*33.3*)	0	0	3 (*33.3*)	3 (*33.3*)	9
Total population			219 (*68.4*)	5 (*1.6*)	42 (*13.1*)	41 (*12.8*)	13 (*4.1*)	320

Percentage indices are in parentheses.
RTA = road traffic accident.
Some data from Robinson et al, 2003.

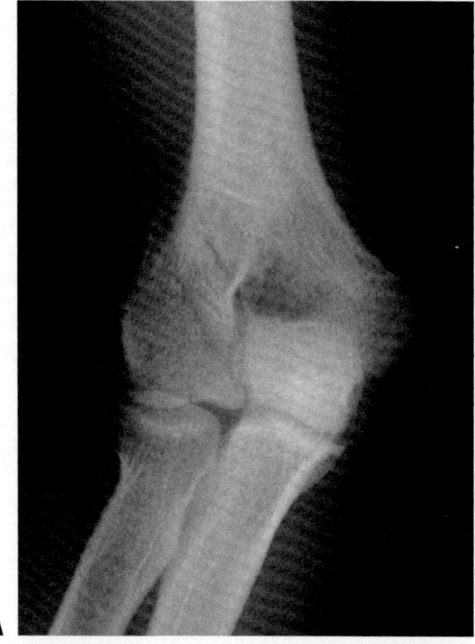

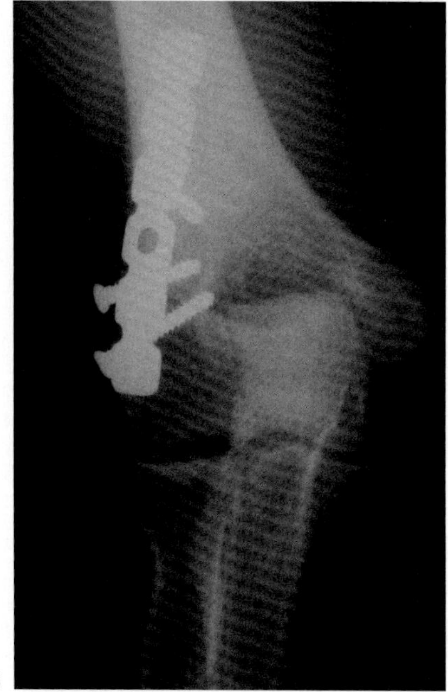

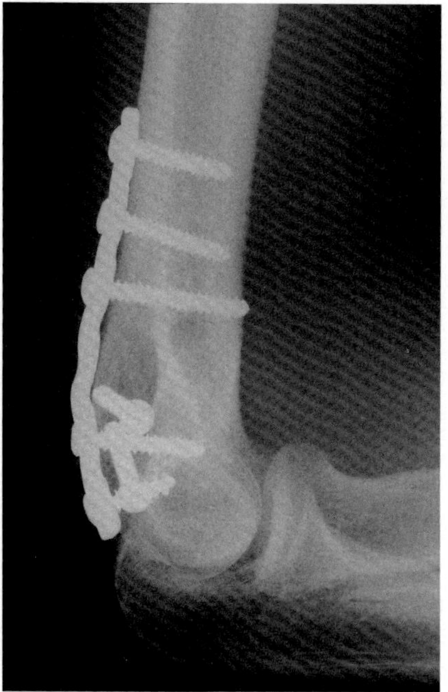

FIGURE 29-17 Reconstruction of a Milch Type II lateral column fracture in an 18-year-old who sustained the injury while playing rugby **(A)**. The fracture healed uneventfully after internal fixation with a lateral column reconstruction plate **(B,C)**, inserted through an extended Kocher approach.

of all injuries seen in this area (Tables 29-7 and 29-8). These fractures occur in the middle-aged and elderly females during simple falls, and in younger individuals during high-energy sporting injuries or road traffic accidents (Table 29-8). There is evidence that these fractures are sustained when the arm is axially loaded when the elbow is flexed beyond 90° (51,85).

Comminuted fractures of "low" configuration, according to the Jupiter classification are more commonly encountered than high fractures (Table 29-7). Although the more simple (Jupiter high "T" and "Y" or AO Type C1) subtypes occur in younger individuals, it is more common for the patient to be elderly, osteoporotic, and have significant articular or metaphyseal comminution, or both. The vast majority of bicolumn fractures are displaced (4) and nearly one-fourth are open (Table 29-9).

Overview of Treatment of Bicolumn Fractures

Although some pioneering studies successfully treated patients with bicolumnar fractures by internal fixation (23,86), prior to the 1980s most complete articular fractures of the distal humerus fractures were treated nonoperatively (44). This was because surgical treatment with limited access and minimal, nonrigid methods of internal fixation produced poor results, which were often worse than nonoperative treatment (44,76). Most patients with these fractures were consequently treated using overhead

TABLE 29-9 Summary of the Published Results of the Primary Treatment of Bicolumn Fractures by Modern Double Plating Techniques

Author	Year	Number of Fractures	Average Age of Patients (range)	Percentage of Open Fractures	Surgical Approach	Average Follow-up (range)	Outcome Assessment Used	Percentage with Excellent or Good Outcomes	Percentage with Satisfactory or Poor Outcomes
Jupiter[64]	1985	34	57 (17–79)	41	TOO[d]	70 (24–144)	Jupiter	79	21
Browne[56]	1986	24	36 (N/R)	25	6TOO, 18TS	12 (N/R)	Browne	88	12
Henley[46]	1987	33	32 (15–61)	42	TOO	18 (N/R)	Jupiter and Cassebaum	92	8
Gabel[92]	1987	10	45 (17–75)	30	TOO	26 (13–36)	Author's system	90	10
Waddell[93]	1988	34	49 (17–83)	26	TOO	29 (6–120)	Home	77	23
Luppino[25]	1989	12	56 (14–81)	17	TS	24 (6–60)	N/A	N/A	N/A
Holdsworth[72]	1990	38	36 (13–72)	34	TOO	37 (6–85)	Jupiter	76	24
Wildburger[61]	1991	29	56 (N/R)	45	TOO	47 (12–170)	Burri	72	28
John[73b]	1994	28	80 (75–90)	0	TOO/TS	18 (5–132)	Cassebaum	79	21
Wang[14]	1994	20	47 (20–68)	25	TOO	N/R (15–35)	Cassebaum	75	25
Kaushal[253]	1994	75	47 (18–76)	36	TOO[d]	N/R (18–144)	Burri	77	23
Caja[146]	1994	22	39 (13–70)	9	TOO	43 (24–72)	Author's system	50	50
Papaioannou[254]	1995	54	51 (17–83)	17	TOO	48 (12–144)	Cassebaum	78	22
Kundel[55a]	1996	99	54 (14–87)	37	TOO[d]	40 (12–89)	Cassebaum	52	48
Pereles[57b]	1997	9	71 (63–85)	11	TOO	39 (13–96)	Morrey/Chao, SF-36	100	0
Kinik[74]	1999	30	49 (17–67)	3	TOO	32 (4–69)	N/A	N/A	N/A
McKee[27c]	2000	25	47 (18–75)		11TOO, 14TS	37 (18–75)	DASH, IMST, SF-36	N/A	N/A
Eralp[256]	2001	17	31 (19–77)	0	TOO	35 (14–107)	Jupiter	88	12

(Continues)

TABLE 29-9 Continued

Author	Year	Number of Fractures	Average Age of Patients (range)	Percentage of Open Fractures	Surgical Approach	Average Follow-up (range)	Outcome Assessment Used	Percentage with Excellent or Good Outcomes	Percentage with Satisfactory or Poor Outcomes
Pajarinen[28]	2002	18	44 (16–81)	28	TOO[d]	25 (10–41)	OTA	56	44
Ozdemir[147]	2002	34	38 (20–78)	15	TOO	82 (24–141)	Jupiter	62	38
Gupta[24]	2002	55	39 (18–65)	11	13TOO, 42TS	48 (24–108)	Aitken	93	7
Robinson[4]	2003	119	53 (13–99)	15	TOO	19 (5–32)	N/A	N/A	N/A
Gofton[60]	2003	23	45 (14–89)	30	TOO[d]	45 (14–89)	DASH, PRUNE, ASES-e, IMST, SF-36	N/A	N/A
Yang[106]	2003	17	41 (16–69)	29	TOO	17 (13–38)	MEPI	88	12
Frankle[175b]	2003	12	74 (65–86)	0	10TOO, 2TS	57 (24–78)	MEPI	67	33
Allende[113]	2004	40	42 (16–77)	25	31TOO, 9TR	47 (13–94)	Jupiter and OTA	85	15
Aslam[257]	2004	26	56 (18–82)	12	TOO	35 (24–48)	Broberg/Morrey, Grip strength	70	30
Soon[116]	2004	12	43 (21–80)	0	5TOO, 7TS	11 (2–21)	MEPI	92	8
Total		949	45 (13–99)	23		36 (2–170)		78	22

[a] Includes 16 patients with unicondylar fractures, [b]study confined to elderly patients, [c]study confined to closed fractures, [d]transolecranon osteotomy performed in the majority of cases. N/A 5 not applicable, N/R 5 not recorded, TOO 5 transolecranon osteotomy, TS 5 triceps-splitting approach, TR 5 triceps-reflecting approach, MEPI 5 Mayo elbow performance index, IMST 5 isometric muscle strength testing.
Only English-language studies, or studies with an English-language translation, appearing in peer-reviewed journals during the last 20 years are shown.

transolecranon traction or "bag of bones" treatment (44, 87–89). If the fractures united, the endresult was usually a stiff, functional elbow (44,90), although when nonunion occurred, the elbow was often flail, functionally useless, and difficult to reconstruct.

In the mid 1980s the critical concepts required to successfully treat these fractures operatively were defined in AO centers and elsewhere (Table 29-10) (91–94). Since this time, the results of operative treatment have been shown to be superior to nonoperative methods (89,95–97), although the rate of complications is high for both. Many publications have now documented satisfactory results using these methods, when the standard technique is followed (Tables 29-9 and 29-11).

Although some studies report satisfactory results following internal fixation in elderly patients (57,73,98,99), in many the results are poorer in these individuals (Tables 29-6 and 29-11). This is because the internal fixation is often unstable, predisposing to fixation failure and nonunion (67,100). Noncustom total elbow arthroplasty (TER), incorporating a semiconstrained hinge, has been used successfully as a primary treatment in these patients. TER has the advantage that immediate motion may be started for an injury in which stable fixation cannot be achieved and a period of immobilization would be required after ORIF. The use of TER removes the risk of several fracture related complications, such as nonunion, malunion, and ON, but increases the risk of late prosthesis-related complications. The technique is particularly applicable to patients with short life expectancy and those with preexisting elbow pathology, especially those with rheumatoid arthritis, who have poor results from ORIF.

Open Reduction and Internal Fixation to Treat Acute Bicolumn Fractures

Preoperative Planning and Surgical Approach. Surgery should ideally be performed as soon as other medical conditions permit. Access to the distal humerus can be gained using either the olecranon osteotomy, triceps-splitting, or TRAP approaches. The former is most commonly used and remains the "gold standard" against which others must be validated in clinical trials. The latter two approaches are more commonly considered if there are doubts about whether the fracture will be reconstructable by internal fixation. Careful preoperative planning is essential and this should extend to all aspects of the patient's treatment: a preoperative "checklist" is invaluable (Table 29-12).

The fracture hematoma is gently irrigated away, and the raw cancellous surfaces are cleaned of loose debris. All attempts are made to minimize further soft-tissue detachment. The usual protocol is to reconstruct the articular surface tie-arch first, and then reconstruct the two columns.

Reconstruction of the Articular Surface. The articular fracture is reduced and internally fixed, normally using one or two partially threaded cancellous screws inserted across the capitellar-trochlear axis. It is important to ensure central placement of the screws, to avoid inadvertent anterior joint penetration. The use of 3.5-mm cannulated screws make this part of the procedure technically easier as the guide wire can be inserted across one condyle, and can then be used as a reduction aid to transfix the other articular fragment. The self-tapping screw is then inserted over the guide wire. If there is significant articular comminution, it is preferable to use a fully threaded screw, rather than a partially threaded lag screw, to avoid compressing the joint surface in the area of comminution. Whichever approach is used, the ulnar nerve must be clearly identified, to avoid inadvertent injury by reduction forceps, screws, or guide wires.

If the articular surface is comminuted, as occurs in "H," lambda, and multiplanar fractures (see following text), it may be reconstructed using countersunk standard small fragment screws or Herbert or Acutrak screws, which are self-countersinking and low-profile.

Reconstruction of the Columns. The distal portions of the medial and lateral columns attached to the reconstructed articular surface are now reduced and fixed to their respective columns. The use of two orthogonal plates is the most stable method of treating these fractures (94,101), although this requires further dissection along the medial supracondylar crest, which may further devascularize a comminuted fracture. For this reason, some authors now advocate the use of two plates applied posteriorly, but with eccentrically located screws (24,51,102,103). Three-dimensional contouring is required to make plates conform to the complex shape of the two columns and reconstruction plates are therefore preferable to dynamic compression plates. One-third tubular plates should not be used, as they are too weak and prone to breakage (46,104).

Screw insertion through the plates should proceed in a distal to proximal direction. Consecutive screws should be inserted eccentrically to each other, to improve the rigidity of fixation. The internal fixation is always weakest distal to the fracture and failure usually occurs in this area. This is due to the poor purchase of screws in the cancellous bone of the distal metaphysis, and the small number of screws that can be inserted distal to the fracture, especially with "low" fracture configurations.

On the medial side, the distal part of the plate may be bent through 90° to allow it to cradle the medial epicondyle to facilitate screw placement, such that a "column screw" can sometimes

TABLE 29-10 The Three Key Concepts for Successful Internal Fixation of Closed Distal Humeral Fractures

Anatomic and stable reconstruction of the articular surface

Stable reconstruction of both distal humeral columns using two orthogonal plates

Early postoperative motion to reduce elbow stiffness

TABLE 29-11 **Summary of the Complications of Treatment of Bicolumn Fractures by Modern Double Plating Techniques**

Author	Year	Number of Fractures	Number of Deep Infections	(%)	Number of Implant Failures or Nonunions	(%)	Number of Operative Nerve Palsies	(%)	Ulnar Nerve Transposition Performed?	Number of Postoperative Nerve Palsies	(%)	Surgical Approach	Number of Olecranon Osteotomy Complications	(%)	Other Complications Requiring Intervention
Jupiter[64]	1985	34	1	*3*	2	*6*	0	*0*	In 9	5 (1 MN, 4UN)	*15*	TOO[d]	1 (1NU)	*4*	1HO, 1RF, 24HR
Browne[56]	1986	24	0	*0*	1 (FF)	*4*	1 (N/S)	*4*	N/S	0	*0*	6TOO, 18TS	N/A	*0*	
Henley[46]	1987	33	1	*3*	5 (2FF+NU, 3FF)	*15*	0	*0*	No	0	*0*	TOO	8 (6FF, 2NU)	*28*	2HO
Gabel[92]	1987	10	0	*0*	0	*0*	0	*0*	No	0	*0*	TOO	0	*0*	2HR
Waddell[93]	1988	34	1	*3*	1 (1NU)	*3*	0	*0*	N/S	3 (2RN, 1UN)	*9*	TOO	0	*0*	
Luppino[25]	1989	12	0	*0*	0	*0*	2 (2RN)	*17*	N/S	2 (1RN, 1UN)	*17*	TS	N/A	*N/A*	
Holdsworth[72]	1990	38	1	*3*	4 (3FF, 1NU)	*11*	2 (2UN[d])	*5*	N/S	0	*0*	TOO	2 (2NU)	*5*	
Wildburger[61]	1991	29	1	*3*	3 (3FF)	*10*	0	*0*	N/S	0	*0*	TOO	1 (1FF)	*3*	4STR for HO
John[73b]	1994	28	1	*4*	3 (1FF+NU, 2FF)	*11*	6 (6UN[d])	*21*	N/S	0	*0*	TOO/TS	2 (2NU)	*13*	
Wang[14]	1994	20	1	*5*	1 (FF+NU)	*5*	0	*0*	Yes	0	*0*	TOO	0	*0*	
Kaushal[253]	1994	75	0	*0*	1 (1FF)	*1*	0	*0*	N/S	0	*0*	TOO[e]	3 (3NU)	*4*	
Caja[145]	1994	22	0	*0*	2 (2FF+NU)	*9*	0	*0*	N/S	0	*0*	TOO	1 (1NU)	*5*	
Papaioannou[254]	1995	54	2	*4*	5 (2FF, 3NU)	*9*	5 (2RN, 3UN[d])	*9*	N/S	0	*0*	TOO	1 (1NU)	*2*	6HO
Kundel[55a]	1996	99	10	*10*	10 (4FF, 6NU)	*10*	13	*13*	In 13	13 (N/S)	*13*	TOO[e]	4 (4NU)	*7*	1 AVN, 47HR, 22STR
Pereles[57b]	1997	9	0	*0*	0	*0*	1 (1UN)	*11*	Yes	0	*0*	TOO	0	*0*	2HR, 2HO
Kinik[74]	1999	30	0	*0*	1 (1FF)	*3*	3 (3UN)	*10*	Yes	2 (2UN)	*7*	TOO	0	*0*	4HO
McKee[27c]	2000	25	0	*0*	1 (FF+NU)	*4*	3 (3UN)	*12*	Yes	1 (1RN)	*4*	11TOO, 14TS	3 (3FF)	*27*	2STR

(*continues*)

TABLE 29-11 Continued

Author	Year	Number of Fractures	Number of Deep Infections	(%)	Number of Implant Failures or Nonunions	(%)	Number of Operative Nerve Palsies	(%)	Ulnar Nerve Transposition Performed?	Number of Postoperative Nerve Palsies	(%)	Surgical Approach	Number of Olecranon Osteotomy Complications	(%)	Other Complications Requiring Intervention
Eralp[256]	2001	17	0	*0*	0	*0*	2 (1RN+UN, 1UN)	*12*	Yes	1 (1UN)	*6*	TOO	1 (1NU)	*6*	
Pajarinen[28]	2002	18	1	*6*	2	*11*	3 (1MN, 1UN, 1RN)	*17*	N/S	0	*0*	TOO[d]	1 (1NU)	*6*	
Ozdemir[147]	2002	34	4	*12*	1 (FF)	*3*	0	*0*	N/S	4	*12*	TOO	1 (1NU)	*3*	
Gupta[24]	2002	55	2	*4*	1 (FF)	*2*	0	*0*	No	3 (3UN)	*5*	13TOO, 42TS	4 (4FF)	*31*	1HO
Robinson[4]	2003	119	4	*3*	9 (4FF, 5NU)	*8*	5 (2MN, 1RN, 2UN)	*4*	No	6 (1MU, 3TP, 2UN)	*5*	TOO	2 (2NU)	*2*	4MO, 1CS, 4PM
Gofton[60]	2003	23	1	*4*	1 (NU)	*4*	6 (6UN)	*26*	Yes	1 (1UN)	*4*	TOO[d]	2 (2NU)	*9*	1RSD, 3HO
Yang[105]	2003	17	0	*0*	0	*0*	0	*0*	N/S	0	*0*	TOO	1	*6*	5STR
Frankle[175b]	2003	12	1	*8*	3	*25*	0	*0*	N/S	0	*0*	10TOO, 2TS	0	*0*	
Allende[113]	2004	40	0	*0*	4 (2FF, 2NU)	*10*	4 (4UN)	*10*	In 12	3 (3NU)	*8*	31TOO, 9TR	1 (1NU)	*3*	2HO
Aslam[257]	2004	26	0	*0*	0	*0*	1 (1UN)	*4*	No	0	*0*	TOO	3 (HR)	*12*	2HO
Soon[116]	2004	12	0	*0*	3 (3FF)	*25*	0	*0*	In 2	2 (2UN)	*17*	5TOO, 7TS	0	*0*	3STR
Total		949	32	*3*	64	*6*	56	*6*		46	*5*		35	*6*	

[a] Includes 16 patients with unicondylar fractures, [b]study confined to elderly patients, [c]study confined to closed fractures, [d]not specified if nerve palsy occurred pre- or postoperatively, [e]transolecranon osteotomy performed in the majority of cases, N/S = not specified, FF = fixation failure, NU = nonunion, MN = median nerve palsy, RN = radial nerve palsy, UN = ulnar nerve palsy, TP = tourniquet palsy, TOO = transolecranon osteotomy, TS = triceps-splitting approach, TR = triceps-reflecting approach, HO = clinically significant heterotopic ossification, producing restriction of movement or requiring excision, HR = hardware removal for prominence, RP = refracture, AVN = avascular necrosis, STR = soft-tissue release procedure for persistent elbow stiffness.

Only English-language studies, or studies with an English-language translation, appearing in peer-reviewed journals during the last 20 years are shown.

TABLE 29-12 Surgical Pearls: "Checklist" for the Reconstruction of a Bicolumn Fractures

Admission checklist	Ensure no open wounds, skin tenting or areas of skin necrosis around the elbow Document any neurological deficit Ensure routine hematological, biochemical and cardiorespiratory work-up is performed Optimize any co-morbidities with medical treatment Explain risks of surgery to patient and likely prognosis Obtain informed consent Draw up a fracture plan based upon radiographs CT scan with 3D reconstruction for complex fractures Antithrombotic prophylaxis Heterotopic ossification prophylaxis in head-injured patients
Preoperatively	Discuss postoperative analgesia with anaesthetist (regional anesthesia if early postoperative passive movement is planned) Confirm availability of an assistant (preferrably "skilled") Antibiotic prophylaxis before tourniquet inflation Radiographer available for preoperative traction film and intraoperative radiographs Upper arm tourniquet Position patient—check supports Ensure free access to airway for the anesthetist before draping Drape iliac crest if bone grafting may be required
Equipment to be available in theater	Small and large fragment screw sets Small fragment plates and reconstruction plates Bending pliers and press for plate contouring K-wiring and tension band wire equipment Nerve slings Small oscillating saw Osteotomes Small and large reduction clamps Small cannulated screw set (if available) Hinged total elbow arthroplasty trays (if fracture may not be reconstructable)
Postoperatively	Liase with physiotherapist regarding rehabilitation protocol Update patient regarding surgical reconstruction obtained Wound check before discharge

be placed through the most distal hole (Fig. 29-18A). The remainder of the distal screws can be inserted through the medial epicondyle, and may penetrate anteriorly, as it does not carry any articular surface. The lateral plate should be applied as close as possible to the capitellar articular surface, without causing impingement. This is so that it can gain the best possible purchase of its screws in the distal fragment (Fig. 29-18B).

Several recent innovations have further refined the technique, although evidence of their clinical benefit is as yet unavailable:

1. Many implant manufacturers are now producing specially precontoured distal humeral plates (51,93,105,106), which may reduce the risk of implant breakage (Fig. 29-20).
2. A third posterolateral plate may be used to increase the rigidity of fixation (107), if extra stability is required (see Fig. 29-20A). It may be possible to insert "column" screws through the most distal holes in two of the plates to further improve stability.
3. Polymethyl-methacrylate bone cement or bone substitutes may augment distal fixation in osteoporotic bone (108). In addition, cancellous autograft has sometimes been used to improve the prospects of primary healing in elderly osteoporotic individuals (55,57,73).
4. Double-column tension-band osteosynthesis has been advocated for elderly patients with distal fractures (109–111). However, equivalent or superior results have been achieved using the standard double-plating techniques (57,73,98,99), and this remains the more generally accepted method for these patients.
5. Locking compression plates are now generally available (112), although there are no clinical series reporting their use. However, these plates may prove to be a major advance in treatment, because of the greater stability of fixation they obtain in osteoporotic fractures.
6. With severe comminution, a temporary hinged external fixa-

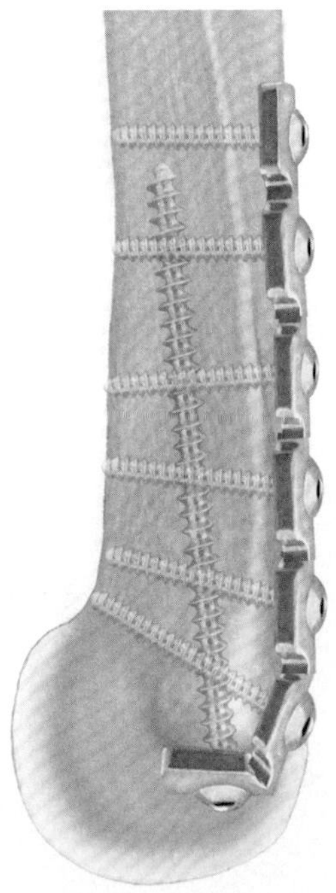

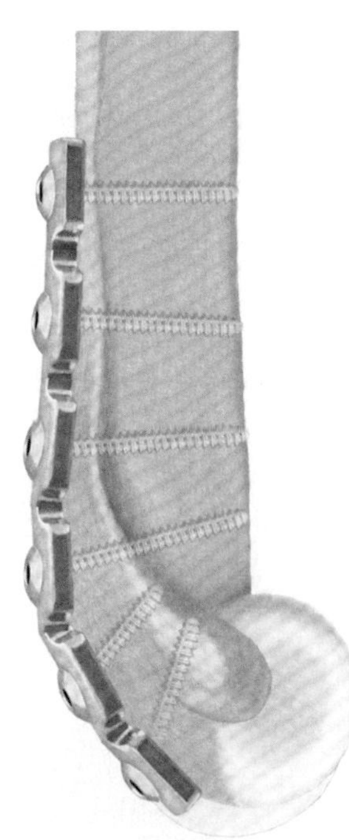

FIGURE 29-18 Schematic diagrams of the optimal placement of the lateral **(A)** and medial **(B)** column plates. The medial column plate can also be applied to the medial supracondylar ridge.

tor may be used to confer extra stability to the ORIF in the first few weeks postsurgery (113).

Reconstruction by Internal Fixation of Specific Fracture Types.

T Pattern. In a high fracture, the transverse component of the fracture crosses both columns proximal to or at the upper extent of the olecranon fossa. The large fracture fragments make this configuration relatively easy to reconstruct with standard fixation protocol (Fig. 29-19).

A low fracture is the most complex to reconstruct. The transverse component crosses the olecranon fossa just proximal to the trochlea, producing small distal fragments, which are difficult to stabilize. Both plates must be applied as distally as possible to maximize the number of screw holes available for fixation

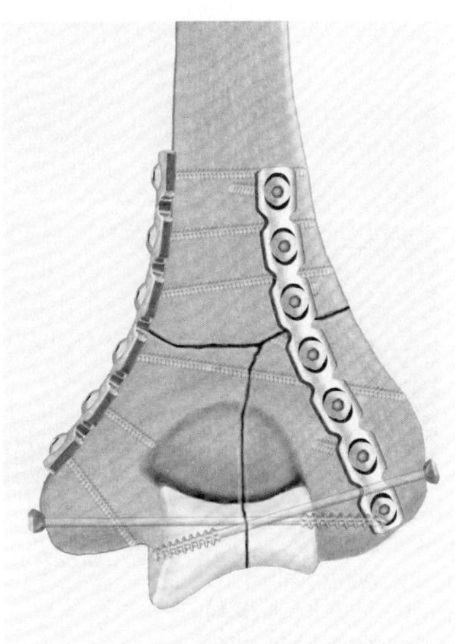

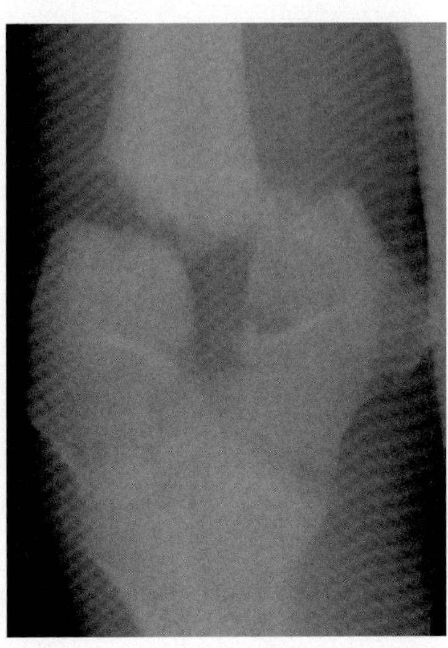

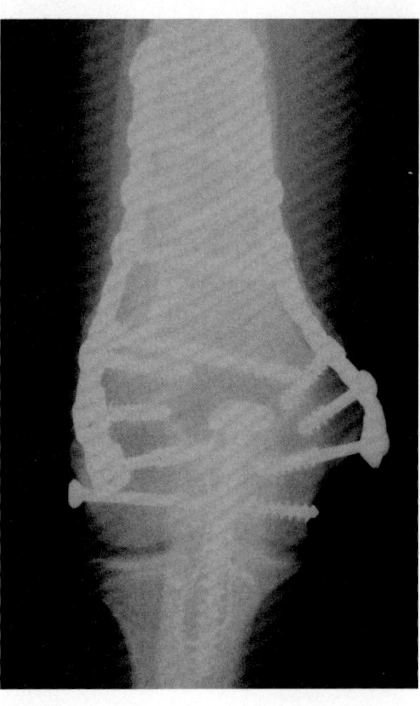

FIGURE 29-19 Schematic picture of a reconstruction of a high T or Y fracture **(A)**. X-rays of a reconstruction of a T fracture using traditional bicolumn fixation **(B,C)**.

of the distal fragment. The lateral fragment is often particularly small and difficult to stabilize, although the lateral plate can sometimes be twisted sagittally around the lateral column. A lateral "column" screw inserted through the most distal hole in the plate may then be feasible to enhance the fixation. Alternatively, if more modern precontoured plates are available these may provide enhanced distal fixation options (Fig. 29-20).

Y Fracture. A vertical split though the centre of the articular surface exits obliquely out into each column. The large fracture fragments make this a technically easy fracture to reconstruct with the standard protocol.

H Fracture. The medial epicondyle and lateral condyle are both fractured away from their respective columns and there is a transverse fracture line across the columns, which potentially renders the trochlea free of soft-tissue attachments and at risk for ON. Several variants, with different degrees of comminution, may be encountered but this fracture is usually technically difficult to treat.

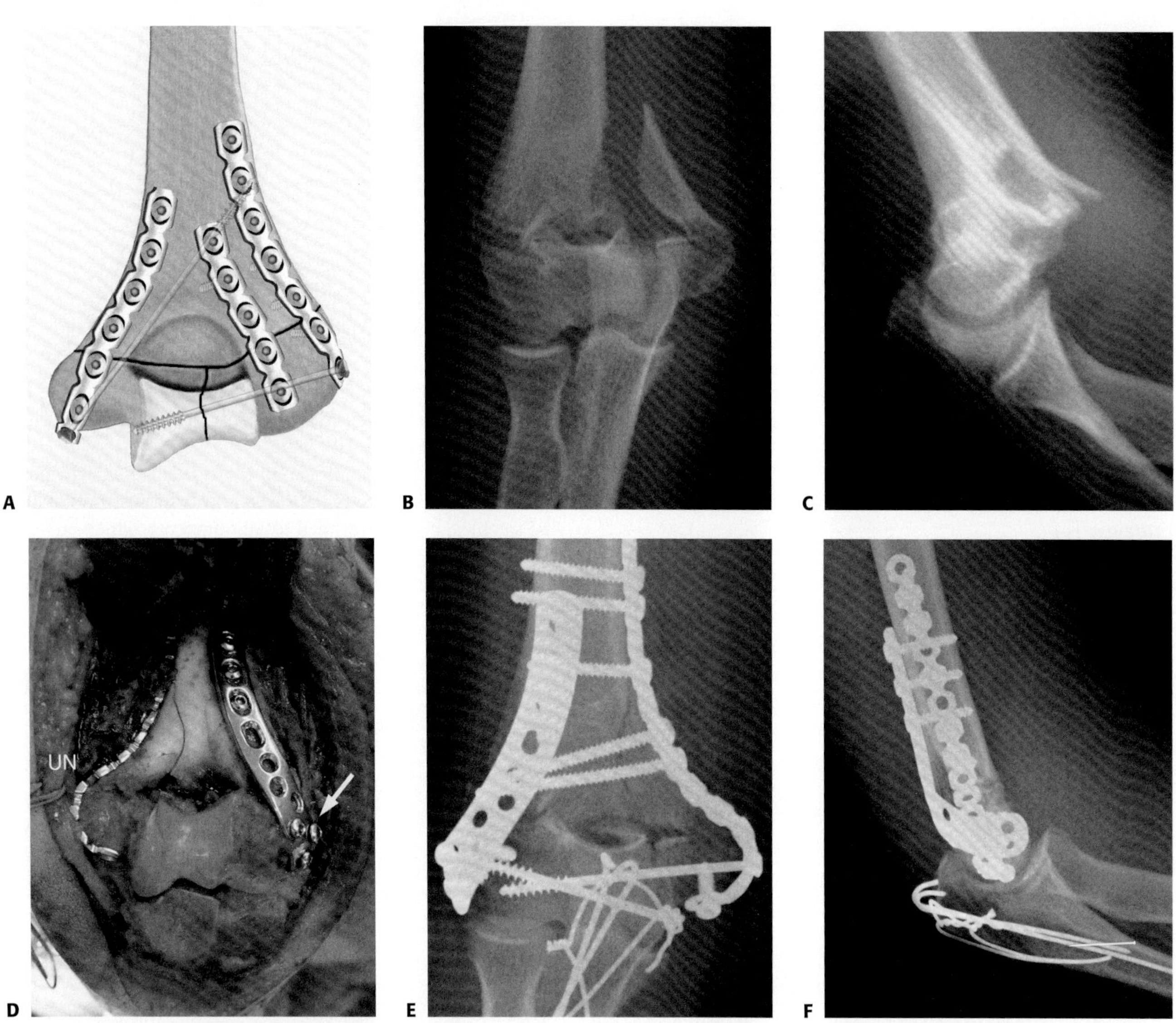

FIGURE 29-20 Schematic picture of a reconstruction of a low T fracture using standard plate fixation **(A)**. The intermediate third plate is optional if the bone quality is good and the reconstruction with two plates is stable. Preoperative x-rays of a 17-year-old girl who sustained a low bicondylar fracture, with comminuted wedge extension into the medial epicondyle and considerable comminution in the olecranon fossa **(B,C)**. Reconstruction through an olecranon osteotomy, using precontoured plate fixation was useful, as enhanced fixation using three screws below the fracture on the lateral column *(arrow)* and two screws below the fracture of the medial epicondyle was possible **(D)**. UN, ulnar nerve. Solid internal fixation permitted mobilization of the elbow in the early postoperative period. Postoperative x-rays **(E,F)**.

Reconstruction of the articular surface may be initially attempted using a 3.5-mm cannulated screw guide wire, but with severe comminution this may not be feasible. Instead, temporary reduction of the epicondylar fragments onto their respective columns using temporary K-wires may be preferable to provide a "template" to which the articular surface can be reduced. Following reconstruction of the articular surface using cannulated screws, column fixation is performed in a standard manner (Fig. 29-21).

Lambda Fracture

Medial Lambda. The transcolumn fracture line extends from the tip of the lateral epicondyle distally, exiting high on the medial column proximally. An intra-articular split extends from this fracture line through the trochlea to produce a lateral capitellar-trochlear fragment, while the medial part of the trochlea remains attached to the medial column. Technical difficulty may be encountered with internal fixation of the lateral column due to the distal extension of the fracture line on this side, which leaves a small zone for internal fixation. In addition, the medial trochlear fragment may be too small to gain adequate internal fixation.

The solution to these problems is usually provided by initial reconstruction of the trochlea by reduction and screw fixation of the capitellar-trochlear fragment onto the medial column, bearing the medial part of the trochlea. The lateral column is then secured to the reconstituted articular surface using further interfragmentary screws, placed through the lateral column plate. A medial column plate is then inserted to complete the reconstruction (Fig. 29-22).

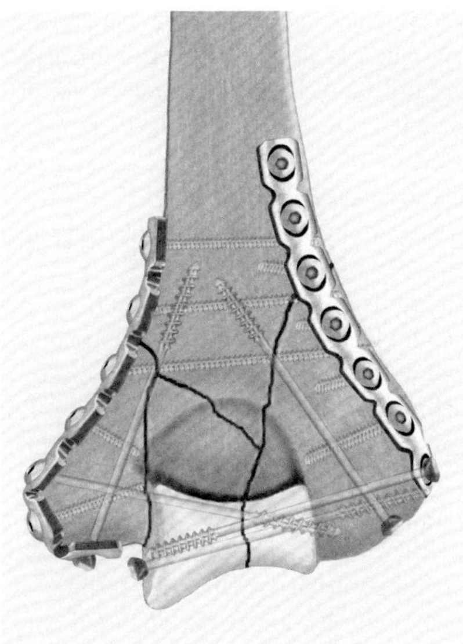

FIGURE 29-21 Schematic picture of a reconstruction of an H fracture.

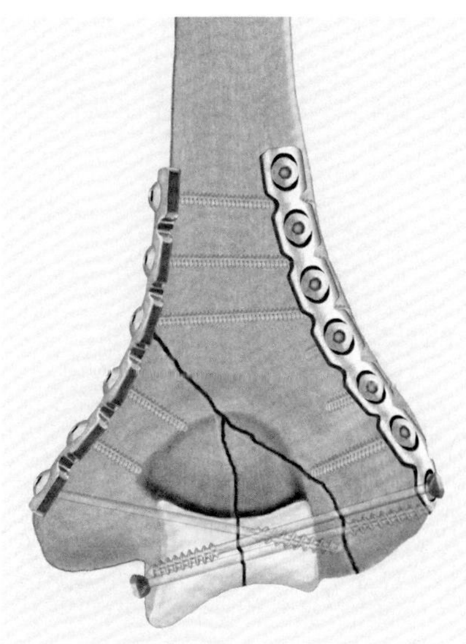

FIGURE 29-22 Schematic picture of a reconstruction of a medial lambda fracture.

Lateral Lambda. The transcolumn fracture extends from low on the medial column (normally below or through the medial epicondyle) to exit higher on the lateral column. The intercondylar split extends distally from this fracture line, to produce a capitellar-trochlear fragment, with a variable amount of the articular surface remaining attached to the lateral column. The capitellar-trochlear fragment may be relatively free of soft-tissue attachments and therefore at risk of ON. Technical difficulty is encountered due to the lack of distal fixation on the medial side.

As with the medial lambda fracture, reduction and fixation of the articular surface may be accomplished by reduction of the free fragment of articular surface onto the lateral column fragment. However, the free articular fragment is often small and it may be preferable to stabilize this to the intact medial column first. This is accomplished using a medial plate, which is twisted around the medial column to allow the lower two screw holes to pass screws transversely across the free articular fragment and into the lateral column fragment to lag the articular fragments together. This may again be facilitated by the use of a 3.5-mm cannulated screw guide pin inserted through the lower hole, which is then replaced with a 3.5-mm cannulated screw once reduction has been achieved. The proximal part of the plate is secured to the medial column and a lateral column plate is then applied to complete the reconstruction (Fig. 29-23).

Multiplane Fracture. This fracture consists of the standard T-type distal humeral fracture with the added complexity of an additional coronal plane fracture of the trochlea and/or capitellum, which may be free of soft-tissue attachments. This fracture is a true triplane fracture, due to the separate fracture lines traversing the transverse, coronal, and sagittal planes (114). In addition to the standard bicolumnar fixation, Herbert

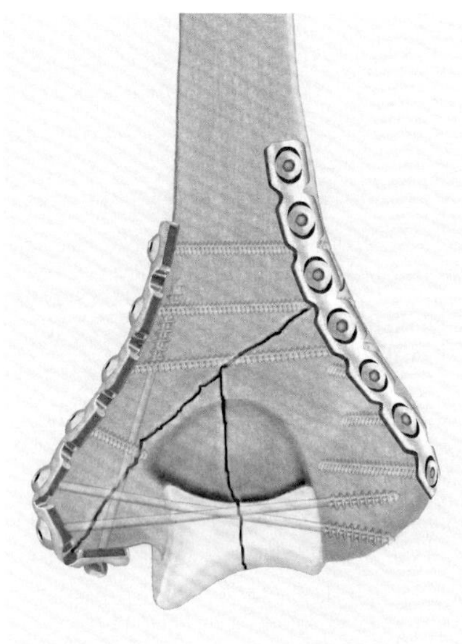

FIGURE 29-23 Schematic picture of a reconstruction of a lateral lambda fracture.

or Acutrak screws may be required to fix the coronal plane fracture.

These sagittally orientated screws may block the subsequent placement of interfragmentary screws to stabilize the sagittal split in the articular surface. Careful planning of the articular reconstruction is therefore required in these cases. Subsequent bicolumnar fixation should proceed according to the standard protocol.

Closure and Postoperative Regime. The stability of the reconstruction, and lack of impingement from the inserted metal work should be tested by moving the elbow through a full range of movement. If instability is detected at the fracture, consideration should be given to revision of the fixation, using one of the modifications previously described.

After thorough irrigation of the wound, the tourniquet is deflated and hemostasis is secured. A meticulous layered closure of the wound is affected, and a plaster back-shell is applied. Alternatively, a continuous passive movement machine may be used to facilitate early movement, under regional anesthesia (115,116).

Following stable fixation, passive range of movement exercises, under physiotherapy supervision, should be commenced in the early postoperative period. The elbow should be rested in a splint and sling during the intervening periods. If absolute stability has not been restored, the elbow should be immobilized in the first 4 weeks after surgery.

Patients are normally able to be discharged from hospital after 48 hours, if social circumstances permit. Regular clinical and x-ray review should continue for the first year after surgery, with review appointments at 1 week, 6 weeks, 3 months, 6 months, and 1 year. Active range of movement and strengthening exercises are commenced at 6 weeks, if there is evidence of early fracture consolidation on x-rays.

Functional Outcome after Internal Fixation of Bicolumn Fractures

The functional outcome following reconstruction of bicolumn fractures, using modern fixation methods, has been shown to be reproducibly good, with an overall average of 78% (range 50% to 100%) good or excellent results (Table 29-9). Three recent studies (27,57,60), using modern functional assessment tools have confirmed that the outcome following these injuries is generally good.

However, patients often have continued aching in their elbow associated with activity and frequently complain of "weather-sensitivity." Although most patients regain a functional arc of movement of 100° or more, restoration of full range of movement, in either flexion or extension is unusual. Patients often have objective evidence of residual muscle weakness in the long-term (27,57,60). This may explain the mild degrees of physical impairment, detected by patient-oriented, limb-specific outcome measures and physical function components of general health-status measures (27,57,60).

Complications of ORIF of Bicolumn Fractures

Nonunion/Fixation Failure. Historically, nonunions were common following nonoperative treatment of distal humeral fractures. These were frequently unsalvageable by internal fixation and were treated either nonoperatively by excision, or by arthroplasty. Despite the advances in fixation techniques, fixation failure and nonunion continue to occur, and pose their own set of challenges to reconstruction.

Definition and Classification. The terms fixation failure and nonunion have often been used interchangeably in the literature, and the two frequently coexist. The former is typically used to refer to implant failure occurring at an early stage after surgery (117), whereas the latter is used to describe a more delayed failure of union. Both commonly occur at the level of the transcolumn fracture. Nonunions have been classified, using Weber and Cech (118) guidelines, into hypervascular (hypertrophic) and avascular (atrophic) types (119), whereas Mitsunaga (80) classified nonunions according to their anatomic locations.

Fixation failure is usually clearly apparent on postoperative x-rays as implant breakage, migration, or loosening. Nonunion following nonoperative treatment, or technically inadequate ORIF, is usually easily detected by pain, loss of function, and abnormal movement at the fracture, at more than 6 months after the injury. In x-rays, there are signs of early failure of fixation and lack of healing across fracture gaps. Following a satisfactory ORIF, it may be difficult to establish by x-ray whether the fracture is healed. Nonunion in these circumstances usually presents with pain and x-ray-apparent widening of the fracture gaps, and/or delayed loosening or breakage of internal fixation.

Incidence and Specific Risk Factors. The risk of nonunion using modern treatment methods is 6% (range 0% to 25%) (Table 29-11), and most series that have specifically examined the treatment of nonunions include a substantial number of bicolumn fractures (80,119–121). "Low" fracture configurations, particularly associated with extreme porosity of the distal fragment, and inadequate internal fixation, using K-wires or screws to fix the columns (117,122), have been specifically associated with higher risk of nonunion (Fig. 29-24).

Clinical Features. Fixation failure or nonunion are associated with pain, stiffness, and loss of function. Pain may be from instability at the fracture, from ulnar neuritis (119,120,123), or from posttraumatic osteoarthritis. Stiffness may be articular deformity or necrosis or from posttraumatic adhesions. The level of interference with normal daily activities is dependent on the age and level of physical activity of the patient. If there is concomitant fixation failure, the elbow will frequently be unstable due to gross movement at the site of the fracture. This feature may not be present if there is fibrous union, or if the implants are still conferring a degree of stability.

Treatment. The symptoms from a nonunion or fixation failure are usually severe enough to warrant further intervention. However, symptomatic treatment may be more appropriate in frail, elderly patients and those with high risk of failure of revision surgery.

If fixation failure with separation of fragments is recognized at an early stage, immediate reoperation should be considered, especially if the original surgery was technically inadequate. On

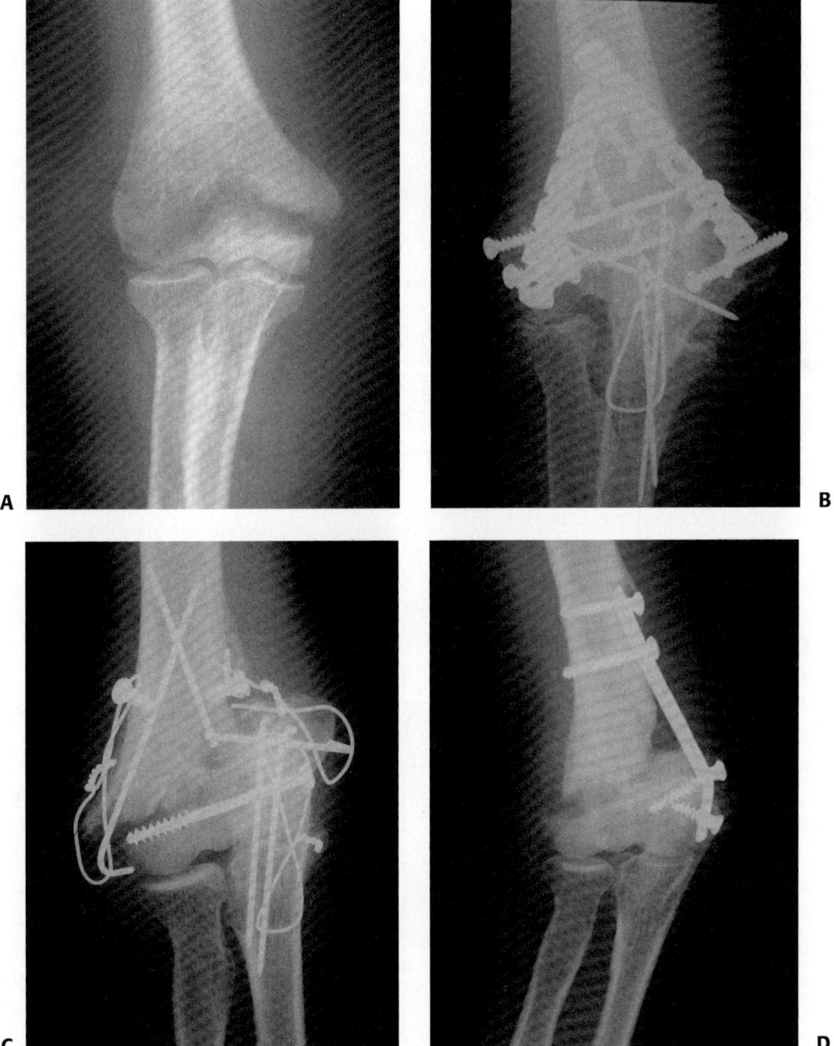

FIGURE 29-24 Nonunion may be associated with low fracture configurations **(A)** and with fixation failure which is usually caused by inadequate stabilization of the intra-articular component of the fracture **(B)** or inadequate restoration of stability to both columns of the distal humerus **(C,D)**.

occasion, fixation failure is a more insidious process due to loss of absolute stability with more minor displacement of the fixation. The choice of treatment in this situation rests between cast immobilization, which offers the possibility of obtaining union without further surgery, and early revision, which offers the possibility of restoring stability, but risks introducing infection or further postoperative complications. The former option is most commonly used in the elderly patient, whereas the latter option is more commonly preferred in younger individuals.

Nonunion after nonoperative treatment is difficult to treat by internal fixation, owing to the complex malorientation of osteoporotic fracture fragments. Although rigid internal fixation with bone grafting may be appropriate in selected cases, most will be treated by a semiconstrained TER replacement.

The degree of deformity and bone loss is often less severe if nonunion develops after ORIF, and revision osteosynthesis is often feasible. However, this is not without risks, and there may be particular technical problems encountered due to scarring from previous surgical approaches, broken implants, infection, gross osteopenia from previous fixation, and the viability of articular surface fragments. These problems will often be deemed to be insurmountable, and revision to a TER may be preferred. Revision to an arthroplasty is also the procedure of choice in elderly patients with limited functional expectations, and in patients with advanced arthritic change in their elbow.

Before any further reconstructive procedure, it is important to establish the cause of failure of union. In many instances, this will be from inadequate fixation, from devascularization of bone fragments, or from inadequate bone stock. However, it is mandatory to exclude infection as a contributory factor to nonunion before any further attempts at reconstruction, especially if the original fracture was open, or there was delayed wound healing after the original surgery. Revision fixation or elbow arthroplasty is doomed in the presence of active infection and initial attempts must be made to eradicate infection by metalwork removal, surgical debridement, and antibiotic therapy before revision is undertaken.

Revision ORIF. Olecranon osteotomy is the preferred surgical approach to allow sufficient access for the complex surgery (120,124,125). The goals of surgery are restoration of congruity of the articular surface, using an articular osteotomy if necessary, restoration of stability by rigid internal fixation of both columns, and stimulation of the healing process by autologous bone grafting. Essential adjuvant treatment includes ulnar neurolysis and transposition, and radical soft-tissue release with capsulectomy to increase the arc of movement (120,124,125). Postoperatively, aggressive early mobilization of the elbow is important to retain the movement regained intraoperatively.

Although the risk of complications from revision ORIF is high (Table 29-13) and the functional outcome is frequently imperfect, most patients report subjective improvement of their debilitating preoperative symptoms. Medium-term follow-up has not demonstrated significant deterioration in these results or progression to osteoarthrosis of the joint (119).

Total Elbow Arthroplasty. Total elbow arthroplasty, using a noncustom semiconstrained hinge design, is used to treat unsalvageable nonunions. If the patient has had a well-healed olecranon osteotomy following previous surgery, simple hardware removal is performed and either a triceps-reflecting or triceps-splitting approach can be used. If there is a nonunion of an olecranon osteotomy, the elbow is approached through the nonunion. This is then repaired with either tension band wiring or nonabsorbable sutures (126,127), after prosthetic insertion,

All metalwork is removed prior to excision of the nonunion and insertion of the cemented arthroplasty. Prosthetic insertion follows the same principles adopted for primary arthroplasty, although transposition of the ulnar nerve should always be performed, and both anterior and posterior capsular releases are required to restore an adequate range of elbow movement.

Revision to a TER of noncustom semiconstrained hinge design has been used successfully to treat unsalvageable nonunions, which have initially been treated either nonoperatively or operatively (Fig. 29-25). The results of treatment in these series cannot be directly compared with the results of revision internal fixation, as the group demographics and indications for surgery are different (Table 29-13) (128). However, as with revision internal fixation, the results appear to be improving with refinements to the technique over time. Despite the suboptimal functional results, most patients appear to have subjective improvement of their symptoms from the surgery.

Other Techniques. Several other methods of treatment for nonunions have been described, including intramedullary nailing and transcondylar rod techniques (129,130), osteochondral allograft replacement of the distal humerus (119,131–133), joint distraction, or interposition arthroplasty (134). However, most of these techniques have significant drawbacks and are not widely used. Arthrodesis has a limited role to play in the treatment of the patient who has had multiple failed attempts at reconstruction, or in whom deep sepsis cannot be eradicated (135).

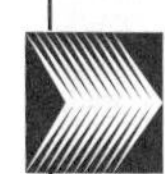

AUTHOR'S PREFERRED TREATMENT

It is the author's policy to attempt revision internal fixation and bone grafting, combined with soft-tissue release and ulnar nerve decompression, wherever possible in younger individuals, aged 60 or under. This is because of concerns regarding the longevity of hinged TER in patients with prolonged life expectancy. The author reserves the use of TER for elderly symptomatic patients who are intolerant of an orthosis, and for the rare instances in younger patients where excessive bone loss or osteoarthrosis dictate that revision internal fixation is unlikely to produce a satisfactory outcome.

TABLE 29-13 Comparison of the Results of Revision ORIF with Bone Grafting and TER to Treat Distal Humeral Nonunion

Technique	Author	Year	Number of Fractures (with Mitsunaga subclassification)	Average Age of Patients (range)	Adjuvant Treatment	Follow-up in Months (range)	Percentage United after Treatment	Complications	Functional Assessment	Percentage Good or Excellent Results	Percentage Fair or Poor Results
Internal fixation and bone grafting	Mitsunaga[80a]	1982	25 (N/S)	46 (21–77)		29 (12–72)	88	6FF,1 NU, 2DI+NU	N/A	N/A	N/A
	McKee[120]	1984	7 (All BC)	43 (25–62)	APC, UN	23 (12–48)	100		Morrey	71	29
	Ackerman[119]	1988	20 (7BC, 13HT or LT)[b]	40 (20–70)		42 (13–108)	94	1RNP, 1DI, 50A	Jupiter	35	65
	Sanders[258]	1990	5 (All BC)	56 (22–81)		40 (24–65)	100		Cassebaum	40	60
	Jupiter[107]	1992	6 (All BC)	68 (55–85)	APC, UN	18 (12–30)	100	20A	Morrey	83	17
	Helfet[124]	2003	52 (27HT, 13BC, 2LC, 6LT, 4MC)[c]	47 (16–88)	APC, UN	33 (3–198)	98	2DI, 5UNP, 2RNP, 13ROM, 1CF	N/A	N/A	N/A
	Ring[125]	2003	15 (N/A)	60 (26–84)	APC, UN, 2FG	51 (24–130)	80	3NU+FF, 2UN, 4ER, 80A	MEPI	73	27
Total elbow arthroplasty	Mitsunaga[80a]	1982	7 (N/S)	46 (21–77)		29 (12–72)	N/A	2EL	N/A	N/A	N/A
	Figgie[259]	1989	14 (N/S)	65 (31–77)		16 (N/A)	N/A	2DI, 1LH, 1LU, 1DP, 1UNP	HSS	57	43
	Morrey[260]	1995	36 (4MC or LC, 10BC, 21HT, 4LT)	67 (40–89)		50 (24–127)	N/A	2DI, 2PS, 2UN, 1WB	MEPI	86	14
	Ramsey[261]	1999	19 (8BC, 11HT or LT)	61 (22–81)		72 (25–128)	N/A	2UP, 10F, 1LH	MEPI	84	16

[a] Mixed series of patients treated by internal fixation and total elbow arthroplasty, [b]2 patients underwent allograft replacement of the distal humerus, [c]13 delayed unions and 39 nonunions. N/A = not assessed or applicable, N/S = not specified, MC = medial single column nonunion, LC = lateral single column nonunion, BC = bicolumn nonunion, HT = high transcolumn nonunion, LT = low transcolumn nonunion, MEPI = Mayo elbow performance index, HSS = Hospital for Special Surgery scoring system, APC = anterior and posterior capsulectomy, UN = ulnar neurolysis, EL = early loosening, FF = fixation failure, NU = nonunion, DI = deep infection, FG = vascularized fibular graft, RNP = radial nerve palsy, UNP = ulnar nerve palsy, ROM = removal of prominent metalwork, +/− ulnar neurolysis and manipulation under anesthesia, IF = fracture of lateral column of distal humerus during manipulation under anesthesia, CF = forearm fasciotomies for compartment syndrome, OA = posttraumatic osteoarthrosis on follow-up radiographs, ER = elbow soft-tissue release for recurrent contracture, UP = fracture of prosthetic ulnar component, OF = intraoperative olecranon fracture, LH = loose humeral prosthetic component, LU = lucency around ulnar component, DP = dislocation of prosthesis, PS = particulate synovitis, WB = worn prosthetic bushings.

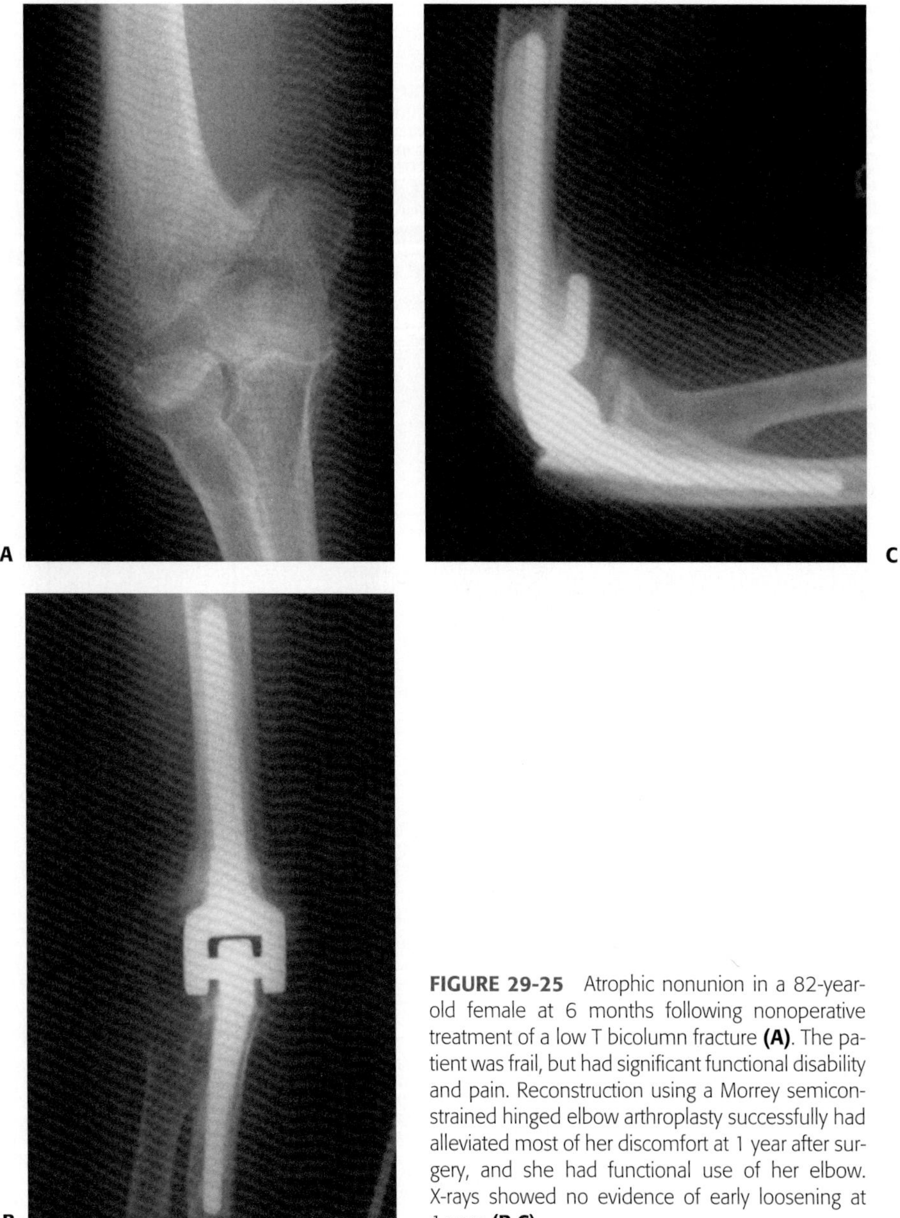

FIGURE 29-25 Atrophic nonunion in a 82-year-old female at 6 months following nonoperative treatment of a low T bicolumn fracture **(A)**. The patient was frail, but had significant functional disability and pain. Reconstruction using a Morrey semiconstrained hinged elbow arthroplasty successfully had alleviated most of her discomfort at 1 year after surgery, and she had functional use of her elbow. X-rays showed no evidence of early loosening at 1 year **(B,C)**.

Malunion. Malunion following bicolumn fracture may occur either in the metaphysis of the distal humerus from malreduction of the transcolumn fracture, or in the joint surface from malreduction of the articular fracture (121,136).

In theory, deformity from malreduction of the transcolumn fracture may occur in any one or a combination of all three dimensions. It is likely that minor degrees of subclinical rotational deformity, procurvatum/recurvatum, and varus/valgus deformity commonly occur following the reconstruction of complex comminuted bicolumnar fractures.

Extensive procurvatum or recurvatum may cause loss of flexion or extension movement, whereas cubitus varus and valgus deformity may cause significant cosmetic deformity, instability, or may be associated with ulnar neuritis (24,120). In patients with no signs of degenerative change within the elbow joint, osteotomy and correction of the metaphyseal deformity, combined with intra-articular opening wedge osteotomy to correct the articular malunion, has been shown to be effective in the medium-term in small numbers of patients (120,121,136). As with nonunion surgery, anterior and posterior capsular releases, and ulnar nerve transposition are important adjunctive components of this procedure.

Wound Complications and Infection. Superficial infection (defined as a bacteriologically proven growth of pathogenic organisms on culture, which is confined to the wound, without a collection) is common following operative treatment, but is sporadically reported in the literature (4). Often it is difficult to distinguish between a superficial infection, and mild wound hematoma or erythema, especially if cultures are equivocal. Broad-spectrum antibiotic therapy and topical dressings are often given empirically following discharge from hospital, and most superficial infections resolve on this regime.

In the presence of more severe superficial infection, parenteral antibiotics should be administered, guided by wound cultures. A severe wound infection raises the suspicion of deep infection and an ultrasound scan must be performed to diagnose any collection. An ultrasound guided aspirate is useful in distinguishing a deep purulent infection from a sterile wound hematoma. Large sterile wound hematomas require surgical drainage, as wound dehiscence may otherwise occur, with risk of subsequent bacterial colonization and deep infection.

Deep infection (defined as a bacteriologically proven growth of known pathogenic organisms on culture, associated with a purulent collection or discharge, implant failure or bony changes) is uncommon, occurring in 3% (range 0% to 12%) of operatively treated bicolumn fractures (Table 29-11). The risk of deep infection is higher with open fractures, particularly when there is gross contamination, or soft-tissue and bone loss (4,55).

Early deep infection with stable internal fixation should be treated with a protocol of repeated surgical irrigation and debridement, and parenteral and topical antibiotic therapy (137). Most series report satisfactory outcome following this protocol, although subsequent nonunion frequently occurs and requires bone grafting once the infection has been eradicated.

Deep infection may be refractory to this treatment protocol, and failure of the internal fixation usually occurs in these circumstances (122). In older patients, radical debridement, metalwork removal, and excision of the distal humerus may sometimes be effective in controlling infection, to allow later insertion of a hinged TER or arthrodesis (93). In younger patients, salvage of the articular surface may be achieved after metalwork removal by the use of a fine-wire external fixator to provide skeletal stabilization, while infection is brought under control. Subsequent, internal fixation and bone grafting procedures have been successful in promoting aseptic healing in small numbers of patients with resistant infections (138).

Late infection of the metalwork, or septic arthritis of the elbow, may occur several years after the original surgery in elderly debilitated or immunocompromised patients. The infection may occur following a bacteremia and the organism may be of low-virulence or antibiotic-resistant. Debridement, metalwork removal, and long-term antibiotic therapy may help to suppress or eradicate infection in these patients.

Nerve Injury. Neural injuries are commonly associated with bicolumn fractures and are classified according to when they occur, the nerves involved, and the severity of the neural injury. Nerve palsies occur following injury in 6% (range 0% to 26%) of patients, with a further 5% (range 0% to 17%) being apparent after operative treatment (Table 29-11). Intraoperative nerve division, manipulation and devascularization, inadequate release, impingement, or injury by bony fragments or hardware, and postoperative fibrosis may all contribute to the development of neural problems after surgery. Ulnar neuritis may develop at a later stage of treatment, and may be associated either with nonunion or a cubitus valgus deformity (139,140).

Although injury to any of the three major nerves that cross the elbow can occur (4), the ulnar nerve is the most commonly involved, both at the time of injury and intraoperatively. This is unsurprising given its close anatomic relationship with the medial epicondyle, and the nerve is particularly at risk if there is wide displacement of the columns. During ORIF, the ulnar nerve is more at risk in triceps-reflecting approaches (29), or if it is not transposed (60). The radial nerve is at risk with triceps-splitting approaches, if the split is continued too far proximally (27). Tourniquet palsy may occur with prolonged surgical procedures and routine deflation should be performed for procedures that continue for longer than 90 minutes.

Nerve injury may vary in severity from minor dysesthesia, to complete sensory loss and paralysis. A satisfactory method of assessing the severity of motor injury is provided by the commonly used Medical Research Council (MRC) scale (141). More specialist evaluation of ulnar nerve palsy may be undertaken using the McGowan classification (142), the Gabel score (143), or the PRUNE score (60). These scores may be useful clinically in quantifying the degree of recovery of function during follow-up.

Nerve exploration is mandatory if dysfunction is detected prior to surgical intervention, particularly with penetrating trauma. If the nerve is found to be intact, it must be fully decompressed, whereas if the nerve is transected, an immediate repair is undertaken.

Ulnar nerve lesions that occur following surgery can be managed expectantly if the nerve was transposed at surgery, whereas reexploration decompression and transposition is indicated if this was not initially performed. It is important that decompression is performed at all possible levels of compression, including the arcade of Struthers (5 cm above the medial epicondyle), the medial intermuscular septum, the cubital tunnel, the flexor carpi ulnaris (Osborne) arcade, and the deep aponeurosis of the common flexor mass (143). A radial or median nerve palsy detected postoperatively requires early reexploration, as these nerves are not routinely identified and surgical injury must be excluded.

The prognosis for most nerve injuries in continuity is good, but the recovery is much more variable following transection or avulsion. Ulnar nerve symptoms should be treated by neurolysis and transposition, combined with surgery to address any deformity or nonunion. Although this produces reproducibly good results (120,123), most patients do not achieve functional normality. This emphasizes the importance of adequate protection and anterior transposition of the ulnar nerve away from implanted hardware and bony fragments at time of the primary surgery.

Elbow Stiffness and Heterotopic Ossification. The elbow is prone to stiffness after trauma because of the high degree of congruency of the joint and the proximity of the brachialis anteriorly to the capsule, which forms scar tissue and heterotopic bone after injury. Restoration of a full range of movement is uncommon, although the degree of posttraumatic elbow stiffness is a continuum, the significance of which varies according to the patient's functional expectations. Furthermore the degree of stiffness often improves gradually with time, and it is important to have objective evidence that improvement in range of movement has reached a plateau before deciding whether intervention is required. Most active individuals complain of functional disability and require treatment when their steady-state extension deficit is more than 40 degrees, or they are unable to flex beyond 120 degrees (144). More minor restriction of movement may require treatment for younger patients who are in manual work, or who are keen to return to playing sport.

It is difficult to quantify the exact incidence of this problem, although many series report individuals who require secondary soft-tissue release (27,55,61,106,116). In a large series of elbow contractures, it was estimated that one-third were due to fractures (145). Risk factors for postsurgical stiffness include more severe soft-tissue or bone injury, particularly of the articular surface, delayed surgery, advanced age, and prolonged immobilization after surgery (28,55,72,146,147).

Clinical evaluation of the patient with a post-traumatic elbow contracture should attempt to define all of the contributory factors to stiffness. Morrey (134) has classified these into extrinsic, intrinsic, or mixed. Extrinsic causes of stiffness include heterotopic ossification, and contractures of the anterior and posterior capsule, collateral ligaments, and muscles. The severity of postsurgical heterotopic ossification is variable and can be classified according to the system of Hastings (Table 29-14) (148). Lesser degrees of ossification (Class I) are frequently encountered and are usually asymptomatic. More severe and clinically significant heterotopic bone formation (Class II and III) is rare (149): risk factors include head injury (150), severe soft-tissue and bony trauma, and delayed surgical intervention. Prophylactic diphosphonates, nonsteroidal anti-inflammatory medication, or radiation may help to reduce the formation of heterotopic bone, but may retard bone healing. The use of these agents varies widely and there is little evidence to support their routine use (151).

TABLE 29-14 The Hastings[148] Classification of Heterotopic Ossification

Class	Subtype	Description
I		Radiographic heterotopic ossification without functional limitation
II	A	Limitation of flexion/extension
	B	Limitation of forearm pronation/supination
	C	Limitation in both planes
III		Bony ankylosis of either the elbow or forearm

Intrinsic stiffness is produced by joint incongruity or osteoarthrosis. Common causes include intra-articular nonunion or malunion of the fracture, osteophytes, and loose fracture fragments causing third-body wear. Implant impingement, due to intra-articular screw placement, screws violating the olecranon fossa, and excessively low placement of column plates may also cause restriction of movement. In most instances, both intrinsic and extrinsic causes are contributory to stiffness, and each component should be addressed if surgical release is performed.

Sustained nonoperative physical therapy may be useful in further improving range of movement without recourse to surgery, especially if there is still a "springy" end-point to movement. Nonoperative treatment should attempt to regain movement gradually, without precipitating inflammation. Oral nonsteroidal anti-inflammatory medication and serial splinting may be useful in helping to regain movement. Closed manipulation under anesthesia is not recommended due to the risk of iatrogenic fracture.

Soft-tissue release is usually indicated for refractory stiffness in symptomatic patients beyond 6 months postinjury. Radiologically, any heterotopic ossification must be corticated and quiescent. Open contracture release is most commonly performed, although arthroscopic capsular release is gaining in popularity. The surgery should be lesion-specific to address all components of the contracture. A posterior skin incision, raising skin flaps to allow medial and lateral approaches to be made through the same skin incision, is recommended. The lateral approach alone may be sufficient for lesser degrees of contracture, although an additional medial approach is usually required for more complex releases.

Lesion-specific surgery may include anterior and posterior capsulectomy for capsular contracture, subperiosteal elevation of the brachialis and triceps muscles, subtotal collateral ligament release and excision of all heterotopic bone (49,144,152–154). Rarely, more severe contractures may require fractional lengthening of muscles, excision of the tip of the olecranon, and fenestration of the olecranon fossa to regain satisfactory movement. Only gentle manipulation is used to regain movement, to reduce the risk of fracture or subchondral impression lesions from forceful manipulation. All previous internal fixation should be removed at the end of surgery. If there is less than half of the articular surface covered with hyaline cartilage, or severe malunion, interposition or joint distraction may be considered in younger individuals (134).

Postoperatively, adjuvant radiation, and medical therapy to

prevent the re-formation of heterotopic bone have been recommended. However, guidelines for their usage are lacking and evidence of their benefit is much less clear than for the hip joint (151). It is important that movement is sustained in the early postoperative period, ideally using a continuous passive motion machine, with regional anesthesia (155,156).

Soft-tissue releases have been more commonly performed in recent times, as experience has grown in the use of these techniques. Most studies report good results in terms of return of movement and levels of patient satisfaction. More than three-fourths of patients will regain a functional arc of motion from 30 to 130 degrees or more, and most will regain at least 50% of the movement which was absent preoperatively (106,134, 155–157). Patients with more severe deformities have a proportionately greater degree of improvement than those with more minor contractures.

Osteoarthritis. Early rapid progression to symptomatic osteoarthrosis is more likely if the fracture is initially treated nonoperatively or restoration of articular congruity has not been achieved following surgical reconstruction. Early collapse of the articular surface despite a technically adequate ORIF raises the suspicion of ON, which may involve the whole articular surface (55), or occur segmentally, affecting either the trochlea (60,61) or the lateral joint surface (113). Other causes of rapid postsurgical articular cartilage deterioration include loose bodies producing third-body wear and inadvertent intra-articular placement of metalwork.

The radiological severity of osteoarthrosis may be classified using the scale of Knirk and Jupiter (Table 29-15) (158). Minor degrees of posttraumatic arthrosis are inevitable in later life following reconstruction of severe bicolumn fractures in younger individuals (91,159). Exact quantification of the lifetime risk is not possible, because long-term follow-up studies have not been performed.

Older patients with symptomatic osteoarthrosis following reconstruction are usually treated by TER of hinged design. Similar technical problems may be encountered to those seen during elbow replacement for nonunion. In addition, there may be marked bone loss either from the original injury or from prior surgery. Morrey classified the severity of bone loss that may be encountered at surgery (Table 29-16) (160).

TABLE 29-15 The Knirk and Jupiter[158] Classification of Elbow Osteoarthrosis

Grade	Description
0	No degenerative change
1	Slight narrowing of joint space
2	Marked narrowing of joint space
3	Total loss of joint space

TABLE 29-16 The Morrey[160] Classification of Bone Loss in Arthritic Elbows Treated by Elbow Replacement

Grade	Description
1	Trochlea and capitellum present
2	Trochlea/capitellum absent, columns intact
3	Either of the columns are absent
4	Both columns absent/loss of bone up to or above the olecranon fossa

The initial results of elbow replacement for osteoarthrosis were disappointing (29,161–164). However, satisfactory medium-term results have been reported more recently following refinements to prosthetic design, and restriction of the use of arthroplasty to older patients with low physical demands on their elbow (160,165,166).

The problem patient remains the younger active individual who develops early symptomatic posttraumatic osteoarthritis after a bicolumn fracture. Currently the results of elbow replacements in these individuals are poor, with high rates of early loosening. The choice of treatment rests between nonoperative treatment with orthotic and medical management, or nonprosthetic arthroplasty (either by resection, interposition, or distraction).

Instability. Instability is uncommon after these injuries because the collateral ligaments are intact and anatomic healing of the bicolumn fracture will normally restore bony congruity. The elbow is therefore more at risk of stiffness from capsular scarring and fibrosis, than instability. In severely comminuted fractures, anatomical reconstruction may not be possible and malreduction may be associated with instability (167). If this is recognized early, a temporary external fixator (113,168), ideally of hinged design (167), should be used to augment the internal fixation for the first four weeks after surgery.

Olecranon Osteotomy Complications. Prominence of the implants used to repair the olecranon osteotomy is common, and may lead to painful local symptoms or recurrent olecranon bursitis. These problems will usually be alleviated with metalwork removal, although this must be deferred until the osteotomy has healed.

Fixation failure, delayed union and nonunion are not uncommon following olecranon osteotomy and 6% of patients (range 0% to 31%) will require treatment for this (Table 29-

11). It is not uncommon for the olecranon osteotomy to require longer to heal than the distal humeral fracture (169). Some studies have suggested that this nonunion of the osteotomy is more commonly associated with use of the tension band wiring technique (46), whereas others have shown higher rates with solitary screw techniques (169). It is unclear whether refinements to the technique, such as using a chevron osteotomy, will reduce the risk of these problems.

Nonunion and early fixation failure of the osteotomy should be treated by revision internal fixation using a contoured ulnar plate, and bone grafting. If the olecranon fragment is small this may not be feasible and excision of the fragment, with reattachment of the triceps tendon, using suture anchors may be preferable.

Total Elbow Replacement to Treat Acute Bicolumn Fractures

Currently the use of TER has been confined largely to elderly, low-demand patients with bicolumn fractures that are not amenable to reconstruction by ORIF (typically low "T" fractures, and some comminuted multiplane, H and lambda fractures), or who have preexisting conditions of the elbow, most notably rheumatoid arthritis (69–71,170–172).

Technical Considerations. There are considerable technical problems which may be encountered in performing this technique, and a surgeon experienced in elbow arthroplasty techniques should ideally perform the surgery. A posterior triceps-reflecting, triceps-splitting, or triceps-detaching approach may be used. The latter two approaches are preferable if it is uncertain preoperatively as to whether the fracture might be reconstructable by internal fixation. The olecranon osteotomy approach should never be used if elbow arthroplasty is contemplated, as this will destabilize the ulnar component.

The articular fragments and condyles are excised and the medullary canals of the distal humerus and ulna are prepared in the working space that is created. Condylar resection does not appear to adversely affect subsequent elbow function (173).

Although a resurfacing arthroplasty may be used if both epicondyles are intact, and may be associated with lower rates of loosening, the use of a noncustom semi-constrained hinge is usually preferred, as it removes the risk of dislocation in patients with limited life expectancy. The Coonrad-Morrey implant has been most commonly used. This is a linked device with seven degrees of varus/valgus laxity and is less reliant on soft tissue or bony support than unconstrained or resurfacing arthroplasties. It can therefore be used in patients with greater degrees of bone loss or deformity, without the risk of subsequent instability. Long-stemmed components are usually not required unless the patient is very osteoporotic. It is important to place the hinge of the components at the center of the axis of rotation of the elbow, to minimize the risk of early loosening. Trial reduction of components is therefore important. The center of the ulnar component should be inserted initially to align with the center of the greater sigmoid notch, while the base of the flange of the humeral component will usually be flush with the anterior bone of the coronoid fossa (Fig. 29-26). If the central axis of the prosthesis is located at the correct level and adequately tensioned, the elbow should be able to be brought into full extension and flexed well beyond 90 degrees.

Both components should be cemented with the same mix of cement, and the hinge secured with the central axis pin before cement hardening, to ensure adequate alignment of the prosthetic components. The elbow is brought into full extension while the cement sets, to secure adequate tensioning of the prosthesis. The postoperative regime following TER is identical to that for ORIF.

Functional Outcome of TER. The functional outcome following reconstruction of bicolumn fractures with a TER of hinged design have been shown to be reproducibly good, with the large majority of patients achieving good or excellent results on medium-term follow-up (Table 29-17). These results should not be directly compared with those of ORIF, because of the different indications for the two procedures, and more limited functional expectations of patients who are treated by arthroplasty. There are some concerns regarding the longer-term functional outcome of TER, although many patients have a limited life expectancy and may not survive long enough to develop problems from wear or loosening of the components.

Studies using more modern general health measures have shown generally favorable outcomes, though the levels of patient satisfaction are poorer than when the procedure is performed electively for inflammatory arthritis (174).

Complications of TER. Postoperative cardiorespiratory and cerebrovascular complications have been commonly reported after surgery, which is unsurprising given the elderly population treated. It is difficult to accurately estimate the incidence of surgery-related complications following TER, owing to the paucity of large clinical reviews. Intraoperative complications described include fracture of both the humerus and ulna during the preparation of the medullary canal or during prosthetic insertion (174) and failure to adequately insert the central axis pin, which causes later prosthetic uncoupling (175). Early postoperative complications that have been described include wound hematoma or dehiscence, deep sepsis, and triceps rupture (Table 29-17). These complications usually require early reoperation. Deep sepsis is usually initially managed by repeated debridements, and parenteral antibiotic therapy with the prosthesis left in situ (69,174); acute triceps ruptures should be repaired.

Ulnar nerve palsy, heterotopic ossification, and reflex sympathetic dystrophy have also been described in the rehabilitative phase of treatment (Table 29-17), and are usually managed expectantly. Periprosthetic fractures, as well as fractures of the components themselves have both been described. The former

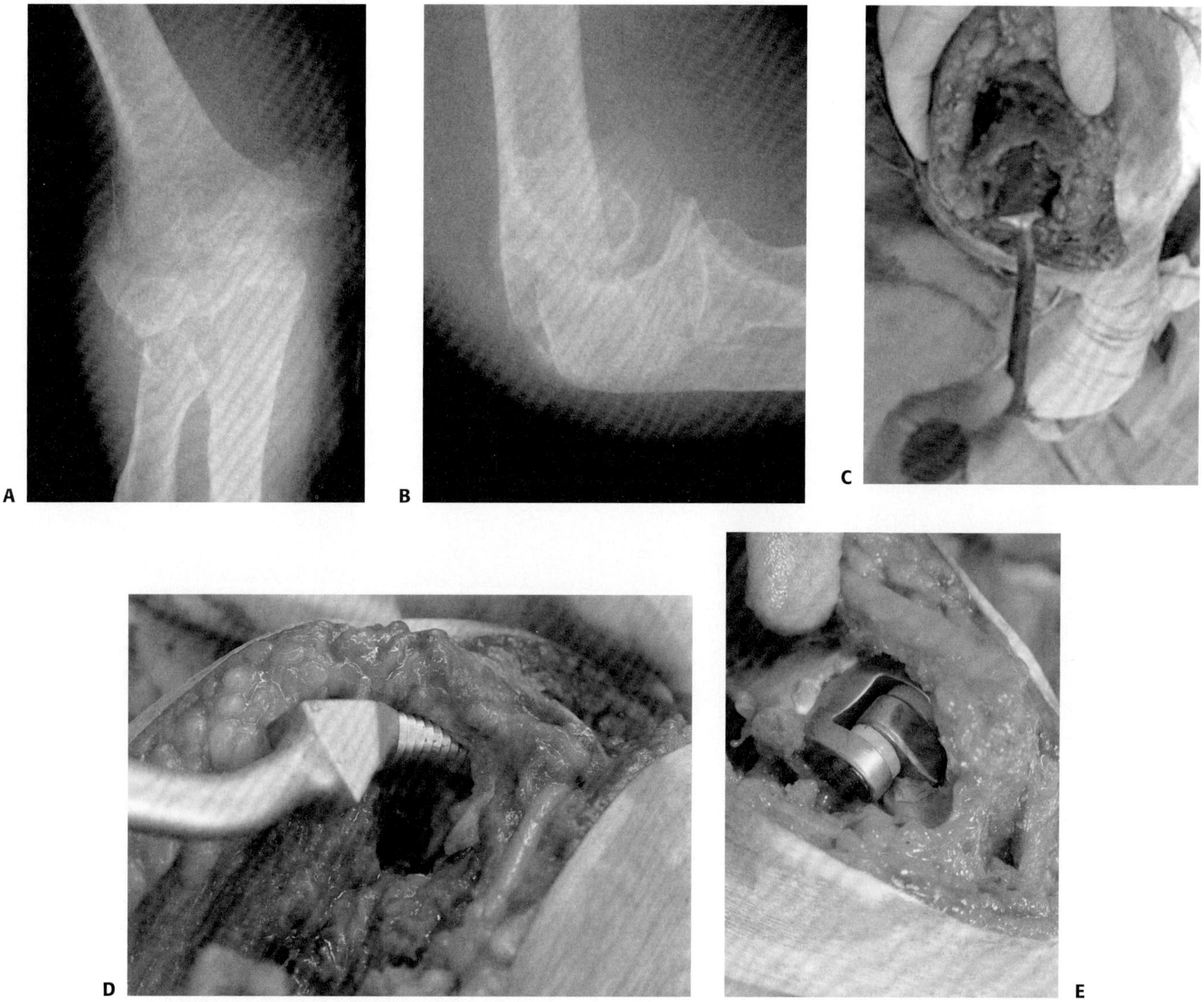

FIGURE 29-26 Preoperative x-rays of a 79-year-old female who sustained a low transcolumn fracture in a simple fall **(A,B)**. The fracture was deemed to be unreconstructable and a Coonrad-Morrey hinged elbow arthroplasty was performed as a primary procedure, using a Morrey approach. Operative detail of preparation of the medullary canals of the humerus and ulna **(C,D)** and the completed assembly **(E)**.

usually requires revision, whereas the latter may heal with immobilization, if the prosthesis is stable.

Late complications include wear of the prosthetic bushings, and loosening of the cement mantle around either the ulnar or humeral prosthetic components. These complications may require revision of the prosthesis if the patient is active and symptomatic, whereas frailer patients with more minor complaints may be treated nonoperatively.

Prolonged follow-up of patients who receive an arthroplasty is difficult because of their limited life-expectancy, and the incidence of complications in the long term has not yet been evaluated.

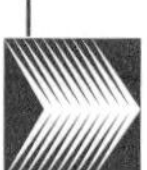

AUTHOR'S PREFERRED TREATMENT

Although, it is generally accepted that patients under the age of 60 merit attempted ORIF of their fracture, there is considerable debate over whether this technique or TER is better in more elderly patients, with limited functional need. At present only one small retrospective review exists that has compared the two techniques (175). This found that the functional results were better, and the revision rates were lower, following elbow replacement on medium-term follow-up (175). Currently, there is a need for further prospec-

TABLE 29-17 Summary of the Published Results of the Primary Treatment of Bicolumn Fractures by Total Elbow Arthroplasty

Author	Year	Number of Fractures (no. with rheumatoid arthritis)	Average Age of Patients (range)	Surgical Approach	Follow-up in Months (range)	Outcome Assessment Used	Percentage with Excellent or Good Outcomes	Percentage with Satisfactory or Poor Outcomes	Complications	Radiological Follow-up
Cobb[71b]	1997	21 (10)	77 (48–92)	Bryan/Morrey	36 (3–126)	MEPI	100	0	3UN, 1UCF, 1RSD	3UNP
Ray[170]	2000	7 (3)	82 (74–88)	Bryan/Morrey	32 (24–48)	MEPI	100	0	1TR	Not assessed
Hildebrand[174]	2000	7 (0)	74 (64–87)	Bryan/Morrey	50 (24–97)	Muscle strength, MEPI, SF-36 and DASH	N/A	N/A	UN, DS, UF, HF, UPF, TR[c]	UP[c]
Gambirasio[70b]	2001	10 (N/R)	85 (57–95)	Bryan/Morrey	18 (12–34)	MEPI	100	0	1HO, 1RSD	2HNP
Ikavalko[171a]	2001	26 (26)	57 (20–81)	Triceps split	30 (6–96)	N/A	N/A	N/A	1DS, 2TR	3HP
Garcia[172b]	2002	16 (0)	73 (61–95)	Triceps split	36 (12–66)	MEPI, DASH	100	0	1UN, 1HO	1UNP
Frankie[175]	2003	12 (8)	72 (65–88)	Bryan/Morrey	57 (24–78)	MEPI	100	0	2UN, 1UP, 1H, 1DS	1UP
Kamineni[69b]	2004	43 (19)	69 (34–92)	Bryan/Morrey	84 (24–180)	MEPI	93	7	7HO, 4BW, 3UPF, 1HPF, 5H, 1DS	2UNP, 1HNP
Total		142	74 (20–95)		43 (3–180)		98	2		

[a] Open reduction and internal fixation of the epicondylar fractures around a Souter prosthesis used, [b]Some transcolumn and/or single column fractures included in the series, [c]Complications described but not specified how many occurred in the fracture group. N/A = not applicable, N/R = not recorded, MERI, = Mayo elbow performance index, UN = ulnar nerve palsy, UCF = ulnar component fracture, RSD = reflex sympathetic dystrophy, TR = triceps rupture, UPF = ulnar prosthetic fracture, HPF = humeral prosthetic fracture, UF = intraoperative ulnar fracture, HF = intraoperative humeral fracture, HO = heterotopic ossification, DS = deep infection, UP = uncoupled prosthesis, H = wound hematoma or dehiscence, BW = bushing wear, UNP = ulnar component nonprogressive cement line, UP = ulnar component progressive cement line, HNP = humeral component nonprogressive cement line, HP = humeral component progressive cement line.

Only English-language studies, or studies with an English-language translation, appearing in peer-reviewed journals are shown.

tive, randomized, multicenter controlled trials to evaluate the results of the two techniques in elderly patients, in order to resolve this controversy.

Currently it is the author's belief that preoperative planning should attempt to place the patient into one of three groups, which determines the surgical approach and implants used.

The Fracture Is Definitely Reconstructable by Internal Fixation. This scenario applies to all age groups of patients, and fractures configurations that are usually amenable to fixation include "high T," "Y," and minimally comminuted "H" and lambda patterns. In these circumstances, an olecranon osteotomy or triceps-splitting approach is used to gain access. Standard reconstruction of the articular fragments and stabilization of both columns should be accomplished using two orthogonal plates, following the protocol described previously. The author routinely transposes the ulnar nerve.

The Fracture Is Unreconstructable by Internal Fixation, or the Patient Has Rheumatoid Arthritis. Most of the patients in this category are elderly or have preexisting joint diseases. Fracture configurations which are frequently difficult to reconstruct include "low T" fractures and some comminuted multiplane, "H," and lambda fractures. In these patients, the author uses a triceps-reflecting approach to gain access to perform a hinged, semiconstrained TER.

The Fracture May Be Unreconstructable by Internal Fixation. This scenario usually applies to older patients and common fracture configurations in which there is uncertainty about the feasibility of reconstruction by internal fixation include "H" fractures, multiplane fracture, lambda fractures, and low transcolumn fractures. A triceps-splitting or triceps-detaching approach is used to keep options open for internal fixation or joint replacement, dependent on the findings at surgery. In younger patients, all attempts are made to salvage the joint if possible by reduction and internal fixation, even if absolute stability cannot be restored. The author has found 3.5-mm cannulated screws to reduce the articular surface and locking compression plates to reconstruct the two columns to be particularly useful. In more elderly patients, a hinged TER is performed, if the fracture is found to be unreconstructable by internal fixation.

ARTICULAR SURFACE FRACTURES (AO/OTA TYPE B3 FRACTURES)

Subclassification

Fractures of the articular surface of the capitellum or trochlea of the distal humerus are a distinct and complex subgroup of injuries. They are distinguished from single and bicolumn fractures by the lack of any metaphyseal extension of fracture lines into either column above the olecranon fossa.

Most articular surface fractures involve the capitellum, with variable additional components of the trochlea and/or epicondyles. Isolated fractures of the trochlea are extremely rare (176,177), and more commonly a portion of the trochlea is fractured with the capitellum (39,178,179). Isolated osteochondral injury to the trochlea may occur in association with elbow dislocation (176).

Three "simple" subtypes of fracture have been recognized: The first is a "complete" fracture of the capitellum, comprising the hemisphere of the articular surface and the underlying cancellous bone. This fracture is usually referred to as the Hahn-Steinthal or Type I fracture (Fig. 29-27). The second and more uncommon type consists of an osteochondral shell of the anterior cartilage and is referred to as the Kocher-Lorenz fracture or Type II fracture. An uncommon third type of injury (Type III) has been described, where there is significant comminution of the fragment (180). It is increasingly appreciated that these fractures are often more "complex" than is initially apparent with plain x-rays, and frequently involve a significant portion of either the trochlea, or one or both epicondyles (Fig. 29-27) (39,181).

Preoperative radiological distinction of these subtypes, ideally using three-dimensional reconstruction of CT scaning of the elbow is of considerable importance if surgical reconstruction is planned. A poorly chosen surgical approach may provide restricted access and result in suboptimal reconstruction.

Epidemiology

Articular surface fractures are uncommon, but account for approximately 10% of all distal humeral fractures (Table 29-7). The large majority of these are usually considered to be Type I "simple" capitellar fractures, although the increasing use of CT in the future may result in increased recognition of the more "complex" subtypes. Most patients who sustain these injuries are middle-aged (Table 29-7), with a slight male predominance. Most injuries are produced in simple falls, although one-third are sustained in motor vehicle accidents or sporting injuries (Table 29-8).

These fractures are produced by coronal shearing forces, which displace the capitellum from the lateral column. Other associated elbow injuries may be present in up to 20% of cases, including MCL avulsion, dislocation of the elbow, or radial head fractures (181–186). It has been suggested that radiologically occult osteochondral fractures of the capitellum may often be associated with fracture of the radial head, and account for the occasional, unexpectedly poor outcome following this injury (184). Combined injuries can be associated with postero-lateral instability, which will usually be clinically inapparent until the fractures have united (181,187).

Treatment

"Simple" Fractures

Completely undisplaced fractures may be treated nonoperatively, though careful monitoring is required to ensure that sec-

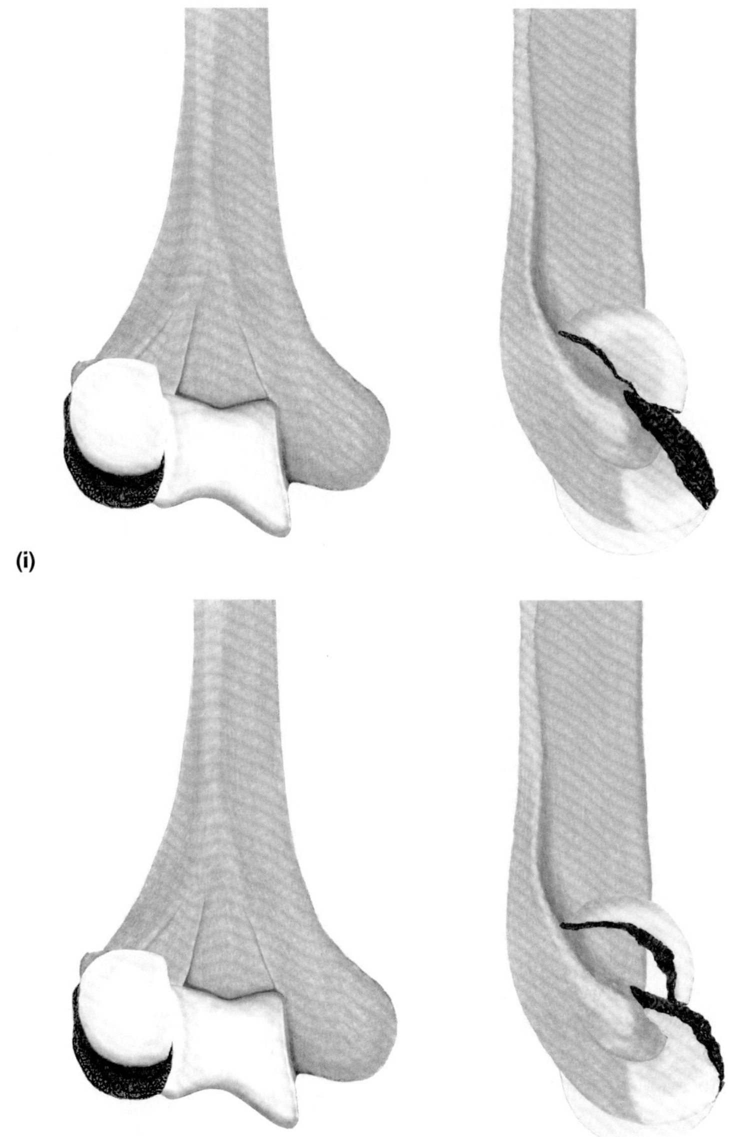

FIGURE 29-27 Classification of articular surface fractures, according to the traditionally used system and the newer classification of Ring and Jupiter (i). **A.** The type I (Hahn-Steinthal) capitellar fracture. A portion of the trochlea may be involved in this fracture. In the type II (Kocher-Lorenz) capitellar fracture (ii), very little subchondral bone is attached to the capitellar fragment. There is no fracture through the lateral condyle in the sagittal plane in either the Type I or II capitellar fracture. *(continues)*

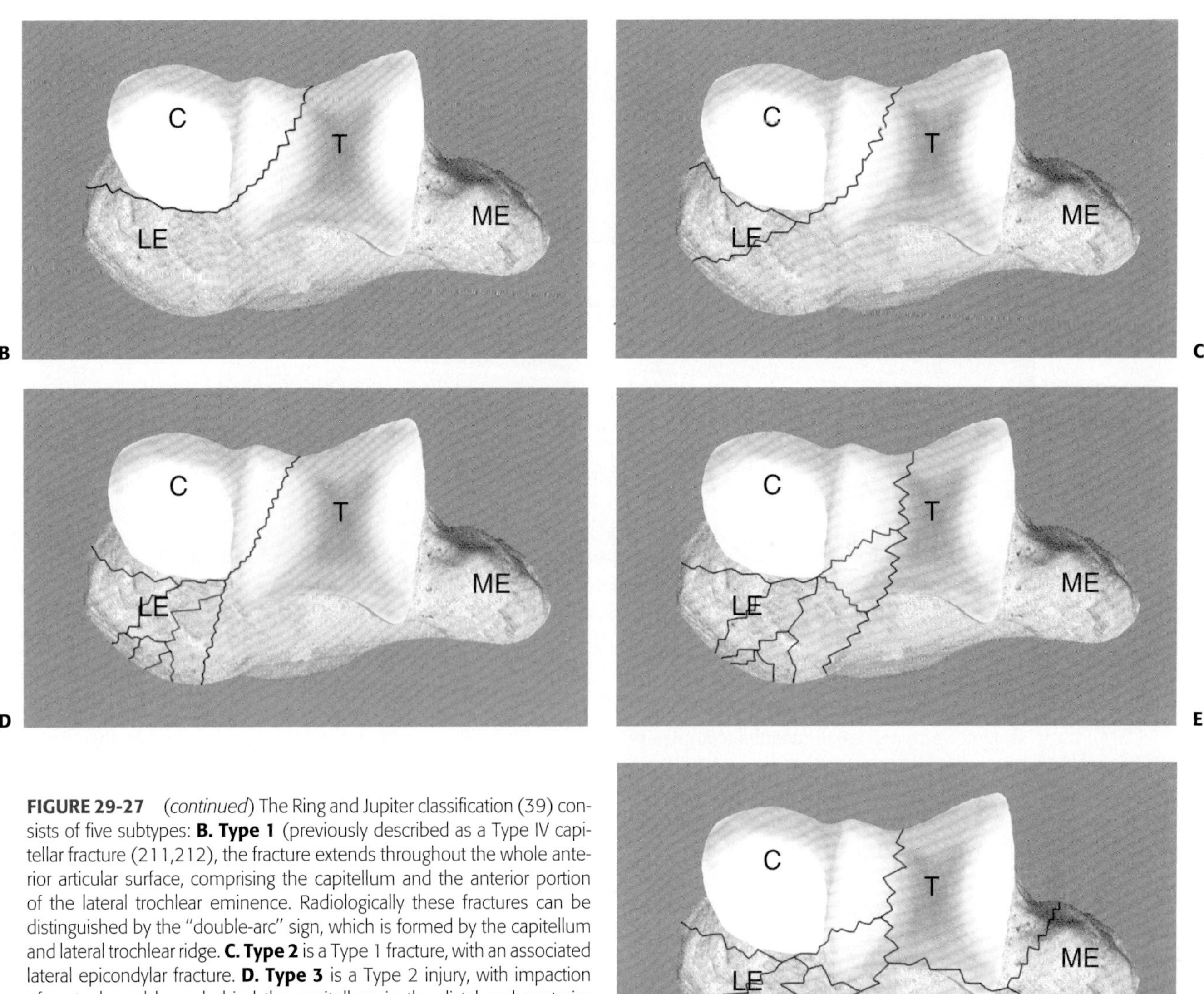

FIGURE 29-27 (*continued*) The Ring and Jupiter classification (39) consists of five subtypes: **B. Type 1** (previously described as a Type IV capitellar fracture (211,212), the fracture extends throughout the whole anterior articular surface, comprising the capitellum and the anterior portion of the lateral trochlear eminence. Radiologically these fractures can be distinguished by the "double-arc" sign, which is formed by the capitellum and lateral trochlear ridge. **C. Type 2** is a Type 1 fracture, with an associated lateral epicondylar fracture. **D. Type 3** is a Type 2 injury, with impaction of metaphyseal bone behind the capitellum in the distal and posterior aspect of the lateral column. **E. Type 4** is a Type 3 injury in which there is an additional fracture of whole of the posterior aspect of the trochlea. **F. Type 5** is a Type 4 fracture with an additional fracture of the medial epicondyle.

ondary displacement does not occur during the first 2 weeks postinjury. The contemporary treatment for most displaced fractures is surgical, unless there are medical contraindications or the patient is very frail and elderly. This is because closed reduction is difficult to achieve and maintain (187–190) and operative treatment is the most reliable way of restoring stability, to allow early mobilization of the elbow (51).

The preferred approach to all of these fractures is the direct lateral (Kocher) approach. Following arthrotomy, the capitellar fragment is initially reduced, and temporarily stabilized with either a reduction forceps or with K-wires. Permanent internal fixation can be carried out either using countersunk cancellous screws placed from anterior to posterior through the articular cartilage, or from posterior to anterior (Fig. 29-28). Although dissection has to be continued posteriorly in the latter technique, it has the advantage that the joint surface is not further damaged by placement of hardware through it.

The Herbert or Acutrak screw can also be used for internal fixation through the articular cartilage in an anteroposterior direction (191–193). Both of these implants have been shown to be more stable than more traditional methods of screw or K-wire fixation (194,195). Other implants which have been

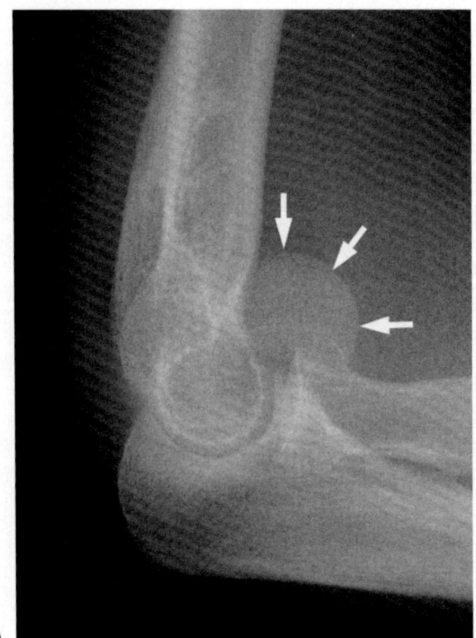

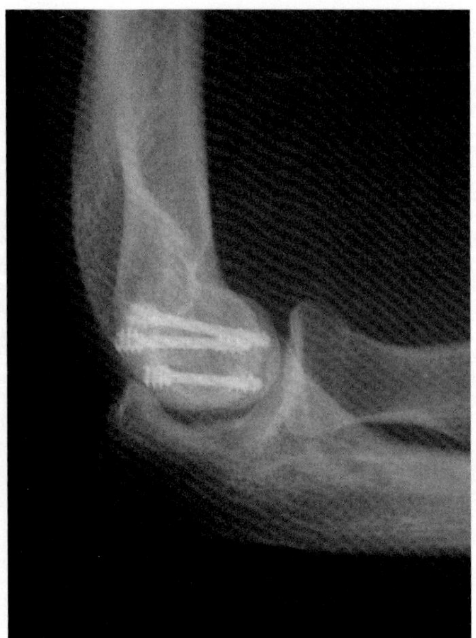

FIGURE 29-28 A "simple" Type I (Hahn-Steinthal) capitellar fracture (*arrows*) in a 42-year-old female (**A**), treated by multiple Herbert screw fixation through a Kocher approach (**B**).

used with success include bioabsorbable pins (67,196,197), K-wires (194), fibrin sealants (65), and small maxillofacial plates (198).

When solid fixation has been achieved, early postoperative range of movement exercises can be commenced as comfort permits. If there is significant osteoporosis, which potentially compromises the stability of the reconstruction, a period of 4 weeks' immobilization in a plaster cast or splint, which restricts pronation and supination, is advisable, to reduce the risk of early fixation failure.

Stable internal fixation of Type II and III fractures is not easily accomplished, due to the small size of the fracture fragment or the comminution. Although prosthetic replacement of the capitellum has been described (199), this has not been widely used and excision of the fragment is the preferred option in most cases (200). Although excision has been achieved arthroscopically (201), an open lateral approach is more commonly adopted. Excision is also the preferred option for most isolated capitellar fractures that present late, at more than 3 weeks post-injury (200,202).

There are only a few small reports of the treatment of combined radial head and capitellar fractures (182,184–186). Most suggest that internal fixation of both fractures is advisable, if this is possible. In the presence of severe comminution of both fractures, attempts should be made toward preferential salvage of the capitellum. This is because there is frequently an associated MCL injury, and excision of the capitellum may predispose to subsequent posterolateral instability. A metallic radial head spacer should be inserted if the head fracture cannot be reconstructed.

The rare isolated trochlea fracture should be treated by ORIF, using multiple Herbert or Acutrak screw fixation through a posterior approach. It is important to restore the spool shape of the trochlea to recreate a congruous articulation, and minimize the risk of later osteoarthrosis.

"Complex" Articular Surface Fractures

In young individuals, reconstruction of these fractures should be attempted wherever possible. For the simpler Type I-4, fracture configurations ORIF using Herbert or Acutrak screws can be accomplished through a lateral approach. As all of these fractures involve the lateral trochlear eminence, excision of the fracture is contraindicated, as this may de-stabilize the elbow.

In Type 2-4 injuries, the lateral epicondyle can be reflected distally, with its attached common extensor origin and lateral ligamentous complex, to allow the elbow to be hinged open laterally. Exposure of most of the anterior and posterior aspects of the articular surfaces should be possible after further elevation of the lateral triceps from the distal humerus and proximal part of the olecranon. The lateral epicondyle should be reattached after the articular reconstruction using either a lateral plate if the fragment is large (Fig. 29-29) or interosseous sutures if the fragment is too small to accept screw fixation. In Type 5 injuries, a posterior approach with olecranon osteotomy should be carried out to allow better access to the whole of the distal humerus. Following articular reconstruction, both epicondyles should be reattached using either plates or interosseous suturing, dependent on their size.

In elderly patients, severe comminution and destruction of the articular surface may preclude ORIF, and a TER should be

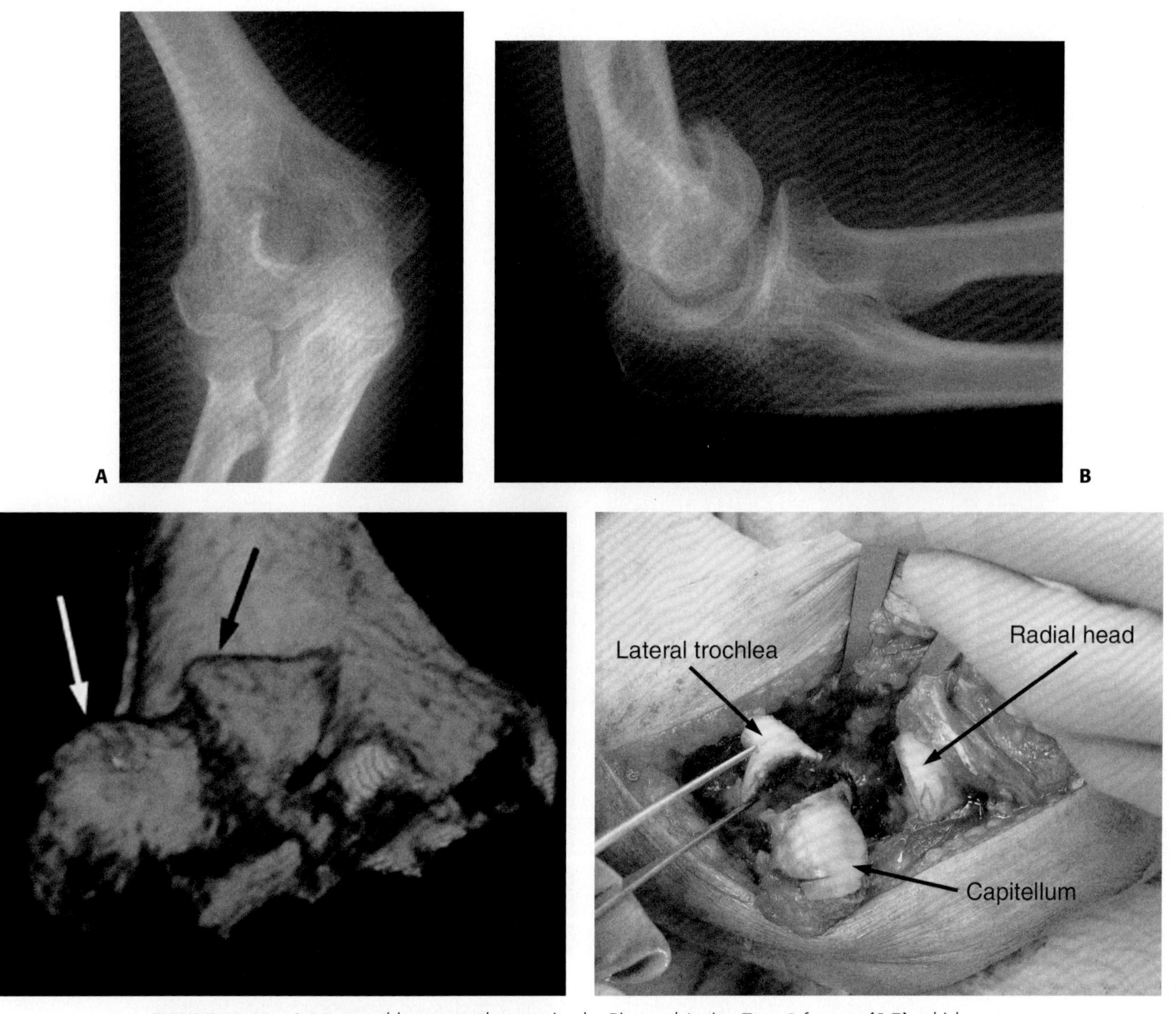

FIGURE 29-29 A 32-year-old woman who sustained a Ring and Jupiter Type 2 fracture **(A,B)**, which was confirmed on three-dimensional CT reconstructions. The white arrow indicates the capitellar fracture and the black arrow indicates the fracture of the lateral trochlea eminence **(C)**. The fracture was reconstructed through an extended lateral approach **(D)** (*continues*)

used (Fig. 29-30) (172). The postoperative management and rehabilitation protocols for these injuries are identical to those for bicolumn fractures.

Functional Outcome after Articular Surface Fractures

"Simple" Capitellar Fractures

Although satisfactory results have been reported following closed manipulation (181,188,189,203), redisplacement of the fracture may occur and the requirement for immobilization of the elbow often produces unpredictable results. Although many of the clinical series of the results of ORIF of Type I (Hahn-Steinthal) are small, most have shown predictably good functional outcomes, irrespective of the method of internal fixation used (4,181,183,193,194,196,198,203–209).

The results achieved after excision, usually for Type II (Kocher-Lorenz) fractures have been shown to be satisfactory in the short term (187,200,201,210), although frequently deterioration subsequently occurs, with stiffness and instability being frequently encountered (181,187,203). The results of treatment of combined capitellar and radial head fractures are unsurprisingly poorer than when either injury occurs in isolation (182,184,186).

"Complex" Articular Surface Fractures

Fractures involving the capitellum and the anterior trochlea (Ring and Jupiter Type 1 fracture) have been shown to have a

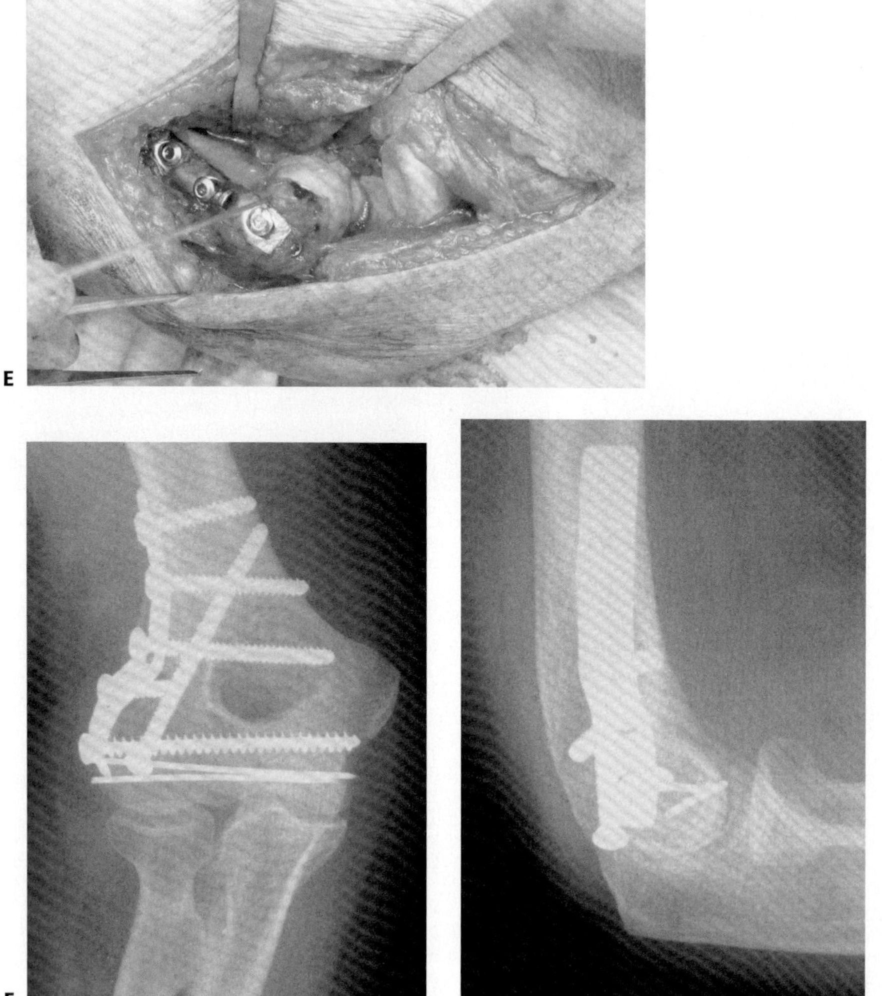

FIGURE 29-29 *(continued)* using a plate to secure the lateral epicondylar fracture and threaded K-wires to fix the flimsy capitellar fragment **(E)**. The fracture united at 3 months and the patient had an excellent functional outcome. Postoperative x-rays showed uneventful healing **(F,G)**.

favorable prognosis following ORIF on medium-term follow-up (39,178,211,212). Satisfactory early results have also been reported after internal fixation of the more complex articular surface injuries (39). However, longer-term follow-up studies have not been performed, and it is uncertain whether these joints will deteriorate over time.

Complications of Capitellar Fractures

The principal complication of a capitellar fracture is loss of elbow movement (181,203). Restriction does not tend to be confined to pronation and supination movements, and frequently there is also a loss of the full arc of elbow flexion and extension. Loss of movement has been frequently reported after excision of Type II fractures, but may occur despite technically adequate ORIF of Type I fractures. Intra-articular metalwork, nonunion, and ON may all cause severe stiffness and require treatment. However, the cause of stiffness is frequently obscure, and in refractory cases a soft-tissue release may be required to regain movement. Elbow contracture is more frequently encountered after treatment of the more complex articular surface fractures (39), but satisfactory movement may be regained after a soft-tissue release.

Malunion or nonunion may occur if there is a delay in diagnosis, through late presentation or failure to diagnose the injury. The patient usually presents with a severe block to flexion, pronation, and supination movements at the elbow. More rarely nonunion may occur despite early adequate treatment with internal fixation. This complication is more likely with more severe initial displacement and devascularization of the capitellar

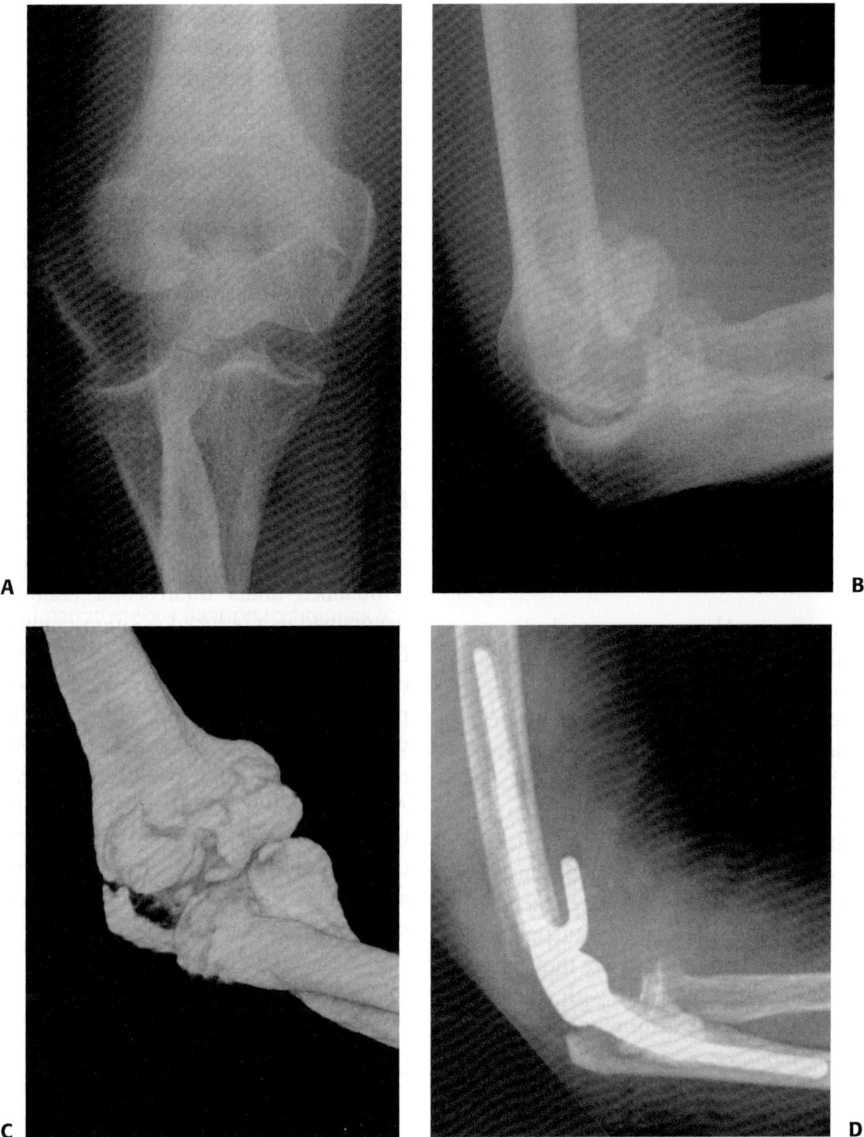

FIGURE 29-30 Standard x-rays and three-dimensional reconstructions of a complex Ring and Jupiter Type IV fracture of the lateral epicondyle, capitellum, and the lateral half of the trochlea **(A–C)**. The patient was a 78-year-old female and significant articular comminution dictated that total elbow arthroplasty was the only reconstructive option **(D)**.

fragment, which causes ON. Excision of the fragment is usually performed to treat malunion and nonunion (200,202). Although some degree of improvement usually occurs following this procedure, the final clinical outcome is often imperfect. A persistent block to flexion after excision may require further treatment with an anterior soft-tissue release.

Collapse and ON of the fractures of the capitellum and trochlea have been described (39,64,183,210,213). This complication may be relatively common but clinically occult because of revascularization of the small fractured fragment following internal fixation. Delayed excision is usually indicated for patients who develop symptomatic ON.

Valgus instability has been described following this injury, but given the mechanism of injury this complication is surprisingly uncommon. This may be due to the soft-tissue scarring that occurs in these severe injuries (181) or the comparative rarity of associated MCL injuries (187). Elbow osteoarthrosis has been described after these injuries (181,183,211,212), although this is frequently low-grade, producing few or no symptoms. The long-term risk of this complication is difficult to estimate as prolonged follow-up studies have not been performed. Late ulnar neuritis has also been described following articular surface fractures (39), which is usually successfully treated by nerve decompression and transposition.

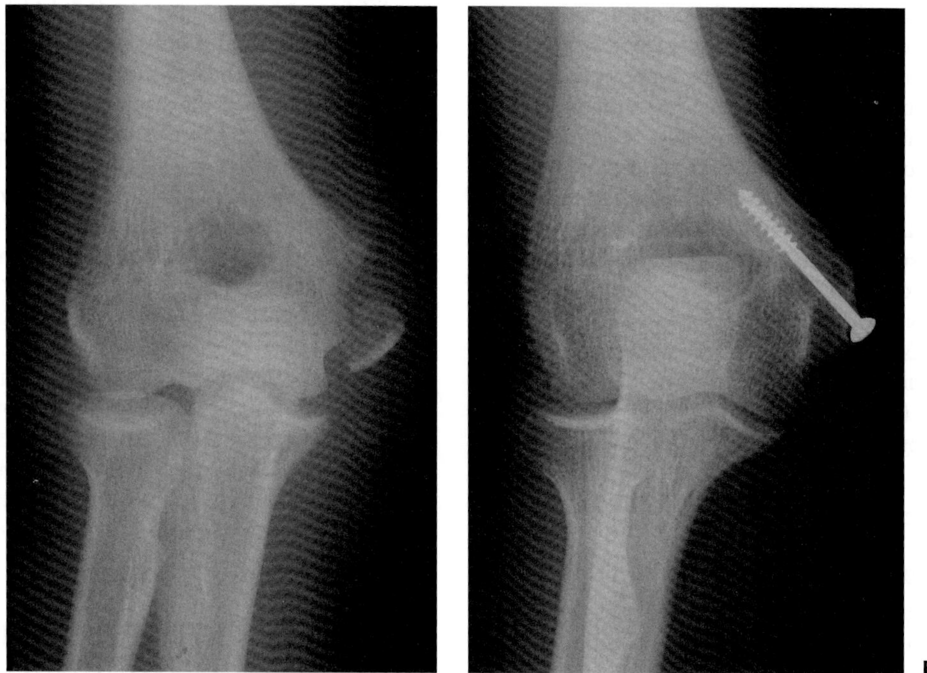

FIGURE 29-31 X-rays of a 16-year-old with a medial epicondylar avulsion fracture-dislocation. Following relocation of the elbow the fracture remained displaced **(A)**, and was treated by open reduction and internal fixation. The fracture healed uneventfully **(B)** and he had full function at 1 year postinjury.

should be treated by ORIF (226,233) to reduce the potential problems of weakness of grip, ulnar nerve dysfunction, or elbow instability (Fig. 29-31). For large fragments, lag screw fixation is most appropriate, whereas smaller fragments are best secured using interosseous wires, or using bone suture anchors with nonabsorbable sutures. Careful identification and protection of the ulnar nerve is mandatory throughout, and it should be decompressed and transposed, if the patient had preoperative symptoms of ulnar nerve dysfunction.

For fractures associated with dislocations of the elbow, initial closed reduction should be undertaken under general anesthesia. A check x-ray of the position of bony fragments should be taken in the operating room, and the elbow carefully examined for residual instability. Operative intervention is indicated in the presence of residual instability and/or continued displacement of the epicondyle. A soft-tissue elbow reconstruction may be required in addition to repair of the epicondylar fracture in more complex instability patterns.

Outcome after Epicondylar Fractures

Owing to the rarity of these injuries in the adult, there is little information on their functional outcome following treatment. Minimally displaced avulsion fractures have been shown to have good outcome, irrespective of the method of treatment adopted (227,233). Satisfactory outcomes have also been reported in the subgroup of adolescent patients who sustain medial epicondylar avulsion injuries while arm-wrestling (229–231).

Nonunion following treatment of medical epicondylar fractures may occur (4) and these may present in adult life as a sequel of an injury in childhood. Nonunion of the medial epicondyle may often be asymptomatic (234), although symptoms of local pain, valgus instability, stiffness and ulnar neuritis have been described (231,234,235). Bony union may be difficult to achieve and excision of the medial epicondylar fragment and MCL advancement and repair has been recommended as a treatment for this complication (235). Varus instability associated with nonunion of lateral epicondylar fractures has also been described, although this is rare (236).

FRACTURES IN SPECIAL SITUATIONS

Open Fractures

Only 7% of all fractures of the distal humerus are open (4), although bicolumn fractures tend to be at much higher risk, with up to one-fourth of these injuries being open (Table 29-9). Open fractures of the distal humerus are usually classified according to the classification of Gustilo and Anderson (237). The injuries tend to be either Type I puncture wounds, or larger Grade IIIB wounds, which are commonly caused by blunt high-energy trauma, or penetrating blast and gunshot injuries (4,7). Following blunt trauma, the open wound tends to be situated posteriorly through a tear in the triceps mechanism (26), where the distal end of the humerus has pierced the soft-tissue envelope. In contrast, blast and gunshot entry wounds are more often situated anteriorly or laterally, and usually have separate exit wounds.

These injuries should be treated with a protocol of early prophylactic broad-spectrum antibiotic cover in the first 48 hours postinjury, tetanus cover, immediate debridement, and removal of any devitalized soft-tissue. It is customary to irrigate the wound using at least 3 L of warmed saline solution. Pulsed lavage is particularly useful and allows the rapid delivery of higher fluid volumes through the soft tissues. Particular attention must be paid to the distal end of the humerus that has penetrated the soft-tissue envelope and is often heavily contaminated. ORIF should then be carried out as for a standard closed fracture. If the posterior triceps has been torn, it is preferable to use a triceps-splitting approach, rather than disrupting the extensor mechanism again by performing an olecranon-osteotomy. Delayed primary closure of the wound should be performed for higher-grade, open fractures. We have found the use of an antibiotic bead pouch technique to be useful following the primary surgery (137).

Large, potentially contaminated, devascularized segments of articular surface encountered during debridement, may pose a dilemma as to whether they should be retained, with the attendant risk of infection, or discarded, thereby increasing the risk of elbow stiffness, instability, and secondary osteoarthritis. It is the authors practice to attempt to retain these fragments whenever possible after thorough debridement, unless gross contamination precludes this. If a large area of articular surface has to be discarded, it can subsequently be reconstructed using either bicortical autograft (238), or an osteochondral allograft (103). Soft-tissue cover is usually not a problem unless there is tissue loss either from the triceps or the integument, when a plastic surgical reconstructive procedure may be required.

Although most studies of bicolumn fractures include patients with open fractures, there are few studies that have specifically examined the results of treatment of these injuries (26,239). One such study suggested a generally satisfactory outcome of treatment, following the protocol previously described. A better outcome followed the use of a triceps-splitting approach, when compared with olecranon osteotomy (26).

Most studies suggest that the rate of complications following treatment of open injuries is higher. This is unsurprising given that many are caused by high-energy injuries, and there is a correspondingly greater severity of both soft-tissue injury and fracture grade (239). High rates of nonunion and implant failure are reported after open fractures, although deep infection is the most serious complication. This occurred in 14% of open fractures treated in three series using modern treatment methods (4,26,239). Infection is treated by repeated surgical debridements in the manner described previously for bicolumn fractures. It is mandatory that any devitalized soft-tissue or bone that may harbor infection is radically excised. Delayed or nonunion is almost inevitable after open fracture complicated by deep infection, which frequently requires bone grafting, once the infection has been eradicated.

The "Smashed" Distal Humerus

Although this type of injury defies rigid definition, most trauma surgeons are familiar with the severe injuries, where there are more extensive, comminuted fractures of the articular surfaces and metaphysis of the distal humerus (103,240). These rare, but catastrophic injuries are caused by high-energy blunt trauma, crush injuries, and penetrating blast or gunshot injuries. A common mechanism is a motor vehicle "side-swipe" injury, caused by an oncoming car hitting the elbow while it is resting on the ledge of the rolled-down car window (241).

These injuries are often associated with either primary bone loss through open wounds, or with contaminated, devascularized segments of bone, extending into the diaphysis of the humerus that must be discarded during the initial debridement (7,49,103,114,167,168,242). Often there are associated injuries of the proximal radius and ulna ("floating elbow") (7,243–247), or there may be extension of the distal humeral fracture into the diaphysis. In addition, there is frequently neurovascular injury and skin or muscle loss (5).

Revascularization of an ischemic limb should take priority in these instances (5). With arteriographic confirmation of injury, immediate exploration and revascularization are performed. If there is a prolonged ischemic time, revascularization may produce a compartment syndrome of the forearm (4,113), and generous flexor and extensor compartment releases should be performed routinely.

Successful revascularization should be followed by wound debridement, irrigation, and skeletal stabilization. Heavily contaminated wounds and those with tissue loss should be left open primarily and reexplored at 48 hours (Fig. 29-32). If the fracture is technically reconstructable, this will usually be performed using standard techniques (5). Any concomitant fractures in the same limb should also be treated by internal fixation, particularly if there is a "floating elbow." Frequently, the extensive comminution and bone loss preclude standard internal fixation. Modifications to the standard treatment protocol are often required to treat these injuries. These may include the use of standard (248), fine-wire (242), or hybrid (7,168) external fixation systems, applied rigidly across the elbow (248) or in hinged mode (7); plastic surgical interventions in the presence of integumental or muscle loss; supracondylar shortening, if there is extensive metaphyseal bone loss (103); and delayed tricortical bone grafting if there are significant articular surface defects (238,249). Occasionally, in the presence of a devastating injury with bone or soft-tissue loss and vascular compromise, the limb may be deemed to be unsalvageable, and a primary amputation is performed (244).

Even with limb salvage the functional outcome following these injuries is unsurprisingly poor (247). There is usually a high rate of complications and requirement for multiple secondary surgical procedures, including bone grafting procedures, debridements to treat infection, and soft-tissue releases to regain movement.

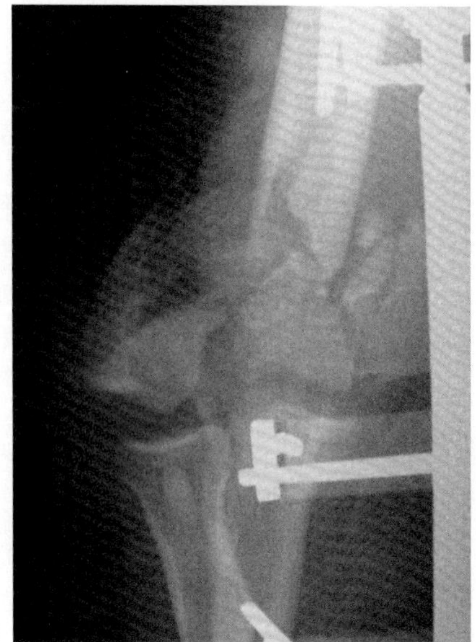
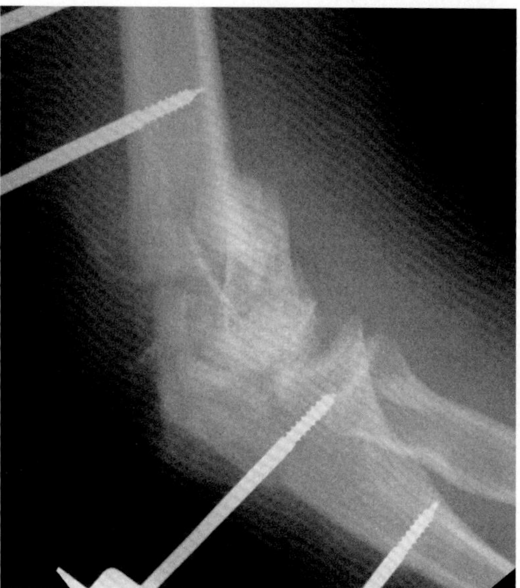

FIGURE 29-32 A "smashed" distal humeral fracture sustained in a motor vehicle accident by a 17-year-old female. There was extensive skin loss and metaphyseal bone loss, and an associated olecranon fracture. After the initial debridement, a temporary external fixator was applied **(A,B)**, until a delayed plastic surgical reconstructive procedure and definitive skeletal stabilization could be performed at 48 hours.

Fractures of the Supracondylar Process

The supracondylar process is a congenital anomaly, which is present in approximately 1% of individuals. It is a bony or cartilaginous projection that arises from the anteromedial surface of the distal humerus, approximately 5 cm above the medial epicondyle. The ligament of Struthers projects forward for the tip of the process to the medial epicondyle, and the median nerve and brachial artery pass beneath this arcade.

When present, the process is susceptible to fracture, and this may cause compression of the neurovascular structures passing beneath it. Most fractures of the process will heal with nonoperative treatment, though late excision may be required if symptoms of median nerve compression ensue. The process must be removed in its entirety, with its periosteum and the fibers of the pronator teres origin, to prevent reformation.

CONCLUSIONS

It is now more than 25 years since surgical treatment by internal fixation became the "gold standard" of treatment for most distal humeral fractures. It is clear that the outcome following the treatment of these "problem" fractures is good in the majority of patients. Although surgical treatment is complex and time-consuming, with a substantial risk of complications, most patients can expect a functional elbow at the conclusion of treatment.

The changing population demographic has produced an ever increasing elderly population of dependent patients who sustain these fractures. Poor bone quality, fracture comminution, and reduced rehabilitative capacity pose yet further challenges to the successful treatment of these injuries. Currently, the commonly encountered "unsolved" fractures remain the "low" complex articular surface, transcolumn and bicolumn fractures with their higher risk of complications, whichever form of surgical treatment is used. The challenge for the next 25 years will be to properly define the complementary roles of internal fixation and arthroplasty in their treatment.

REFERENCES

1. Nicholson JT. Compound comminuted fractures involving the elbow joint. Treatment by resection of the fragments. *J Bone Joint Surg Am* 1946;28:565–575.
2. Jupiter JB, Morrey BF. Fractures of the distal humerus in the adult. In: Morrey BF, ed. *The elbow and its disorders,* 2nd ed. Philadelphia: WB Saunders, 1993:328–366.
3. Rose SH, Melton LJ III, Morrey BF, et al. Epidemiologic features of humeral fractures. *Clin Orthop* 1982;24–30.
4. Robinson CM, Hill RM, Jacobs N, et al. Adult distal humeral metaphyseal fractures: epidemiology and results of treatment. *J Orthop Trauma* 2003;17:38–47.
5. Brannon JK, Woods C, Chandran RE, et al. Gunshot wounds to the elbow. *Orthop Clin North Am* 1995;26:75–84.
6. Zinman C, Norman D, Hamoud K, et al. External fixation for severe open fractures of the humerus caused by missiles. *Ortho Trauma* 1997;11:536–539.
7. Lerner A, Stahl S, Stein H. Hybrid external fixation in high-energy elbow fractures: a modular system with a promising future. *J Trauma* 2000;49:1017–1022.
8. Palvanen M, Niemi S, Parkkari J, et al. Osteoporotic fractures of the distal humerus in elderly women. *Ann Intern Med* 2003;139:W–W61.
9. Palvanen M, Kannus P, Niemi S, et al. Secular trends in the osteoporotic fractures of the distal humerus in elderly women. *Eur J Epidemiol* 1998;14:159–164.
10. Kannus P, Niemi S, Parkkari J, et al. Why is the age-standardized incidence of low-trauma fractures rising in many elderly populations? *J Bone Miner Res* 2002;17:1363–1367.
11. Palvanen M, Kannus P, Parkkari J, et al. The injury mechanisms of osteoporotic upper extremity fractures among older adults: a controlled study of 287 consecutive patients and their 108 controls. *Osteoporos Int* 2000;11:822–831.
12. An K-N, Morrey BF. Biomechanics of the elbow. In: Morrey BF, ed. *The elbow and its disorders,* 1st ed. Philadelphia: WB Saunders, 1993:53–72.

13. O'Driscoll SW, An KN, Korinek S, et al. Kinematics of semi-constrained total elbow arthroplasty. *J Bone Joint Surg Br* 1992;74:297–299.
14. Wang KC, Shih HN, Hsu KY, et al. Intercondylar fractures of the distal humerus: routine anterior subcutaneous transposition of the ulnar nerve in a posterior operative approach. *J Trauma* 1994;36:770–773.
15. Glousman RE. Ulnar nerve problems in the athlete's elbow. *Clin Sports Med* 1990;9: 365–377.
16. Muller ME, Allgower M, Willenegger H. In: *Manual of internal fixation: techniques recommended by the AO Group.* New York: Springer-Verlag, 1970.
17. MacAusland WR. Ankylosis of the elbow: with report of 4 cases treated by arthroplasty. *JAMA* 1915;64:312–319.
18. Campbell WC. Incision for exposure of the elbow joint. *Am J Surg* 1932;15:65–70.
19. Gschwend N, Loehr J, Ivosevic-Radovanovic D, et al. Semiconstrained elbow prostheses with special reference to the GSB III prosthesis. *Clin Orthop* 1988;104–111.
20. Gschwend N, Loehr J. [Elbow arthroplasty] *Orthopade* 1980;9:158–168.
21. Olson SA, Hertel R, Jakob RP. The trans-tricipital approach for intra-articular fractures of the distal humerus: a report of two cases. *Injury* 1994;25:193–198.
22. Kasser JR, Richards K, Millis M. The triceps-dividing approach to open reduction of complex distal humeral fractures in adolescents: a Cybex evaluation of triceps function and motion. *J Pediatr Orthop* 1990;10:93–96.
23. Vangorder GW. Surgical approach in supracondylar "T" fractures of the humerus requiring open reduction. *J Bone Joint Surg Am* 1940;22:278–292.
24. Gupta R, Khanchandani P. Intercondylar fractures of the distal humerus in adults: a critical analysis of 55 cases. *Injury* 2002;33:511–515.
25. Luppino T, Fiocchi R, Salsi A, et al. Stable osteosynthesis by the AO method in comminuted intra-articular fractures of the distal humerus. *Ital J Orthop Traumatol* 1989;15: 165–170.
26. McKee MD, Kim J, Kebaish K, et al. Functional outcome after open supracondylar fractures of the humerus. The effect of the surgical approach. *J Bone Joint Surg Br* 2000; 82:646–651.
27. McKee MD, Wilson TL, Winston L, et al. Functional outcome following surgical treatment of intra-articular distal humeral fractures through a posterior approach. *J Bone Joint Surg Am* 2000;82-A:1701–1707.
28. Pajarinen J, Bjorkenheim JM. Operative treatment of type C intercondylar fractures of the distal humerus: results after a mean follow-up of 2 years in a series of 18 patients. *J Shoulder Elbow Surg* 2002;11:48–52.
29. Morrey BF, Bryan RS, Dobyns JH, et al. Total elbow arthroplasty. a five-year experience at the Mayo Clinic. *J Bone Joint Surg Am* 1981;63:1050–1063.
30. Bryan RS, Morrey BF. Extensive posterior exposure of the elbow: a triceps-sparing approach. *Clin Orthop* 1982;188–192.
31. Shahane SA, Stanley D. A posterior approach to the elbow joint. *J Bone Joint Surg Br* 1999;81:1020–1022.
32. Wolfe SW, Ranawat CS. The osteo-anconeus flap. An approach for total elbow arthroplasty. *J Bone Joint Surg Am* 1990;72:684–688.
33. Alonso-Llames M. Bilaterotricipital approach to the elbow. *Acta Orthop Scand* 1972; 43:479–490.
34. Schildhauer TA, Nork SE, Mills WJ, et al. Extensor mechanism-sparing paratricipital posterior approach to the distal humerus. *J Orthop Trauma* 2003;17:374–378.
35. Morrey BF. Revision total elbow arthroplasty. In: Morey BF, ed. *Joint replacement arthroplasty.* New York: Churchill-Livingstone, 1991.
36. O'Driscoll SW. The triceps-reflecting anconeus pedicle (TRAP) approach for distal humeral fractures and nonunions. *Orthop Clin North Am* 2000;31:91–101.
37. Kocher T. *Textbook of operative surgery*, 3rd ed. London: A and C Black, 1911.
38. Moran MC. Modified lateral approach to the distal humerus for internal fixation. *Clin Orthop* 1997;190–197.
39. Ring D, Jupiter JB, Gulotta L. Articular fractures of the distal part of the humerus. *J Bone Joint Surg Am* 2003;85-A:232–238.
40. Henry AK. *Extensile exposure*, 2nd ed. Baltimore: Williams & Wilkins, 1957.
41. Kelly RP, Griffin TW. Open reduction of T-condylar fractures of the humerus through an anterior approach. *J Trauma* 1969;9:901–914.
42. Yamaguchi K, Sweet FA, Bindra R, et al. The extraosseous and intraosseous arterial anatomy of the adult elbow. *J Bone Joint Surg Am* 1997;79:1653–1662.
43. Milch H. Fractures and fracture dislocations of the humeral condyles. *J Trauma* 1964; 15:592–607.
44. Riseborough EJ, Radin EL. Intercondylar T fractures of the humerus in the adult. A comparison of operative and non-operative treatment in twenty-nine cases. *J Bone Joint Surg Am* 1969;51:130–141.
45. Muller ME. The comprehensive classification of fractures of long bones. In: Muller ME, Allgower M, Schneider R, et al, eds. *Manual of internal fixation,* 3rd ed. Berlin: Springer-Verlag, 1991:118–150.
46. Henley MB, Bone LB, Parker, B. Operative management of intra-articular fractures of the distal humerus. *J Orthop Trauma* 1987;1:24–35.
47. Orthopaedic Trauma Association Committee for Coding and Classification. OTA Coding and Classification Committee. Fracture and dislocation compendium. *J Orthop Trauma* 1996;10[Suppl 1]:154.
48. Schatzker J. Fractures of the distal end of the humerus. In: Schatzker J, Tile M, eds. *Rationale of operative fracture care.* Berlin: Springer-Verlag, 1987;70–87.
49. Jupiter JB. Complex fractures of the distal part of the humerus and associated complications. *Instructional Course Lecture* 1995;44:187–198.
50. Jupiter JB, Mehne DK. Fractures of the distal humerus. *Orthopedics* 1992;15:825–833.
51. McKee MD, Jupiter JB. Fractures of the distal humerus. In: Browner B, Jupiter J, Levine A, et al, eds. *Skeletal trauma,* 3rd ed. Philadelphia, WB Saunders, 2003;1436–1480.
52. Wainwright AM, Williams JR, Carr AJ. Interobserver and intraobserver variation in classification systems for fractures of the distal humerus. *J Bone Joint Surg Br* 2000;82: 636–642.
53. Smith RM. The classification of fractures. *J Bone Joint Surg Br* 2000;82:625–626.
54. McQueen MM, Gaston P, Court-Brown CM. Acute compartment syndrome. Who is at risk? *J Bone Joint Surg Br* 2000;82:200–203.
55. Kundel K, Braun W, Wieberneit J, et al. A. Intraarticular distal humerus fractures. Factors affecting functional outcome. *Clin Orthop* 1996;200–208.
56. Browne AO, O'Riordan M, Quinlan W. Supracondylar fractures of the humerus in adults. *Injury* 1986;17:184–186.
57. Pereles TR, Koval KJ, Gallagher M, et al. Open reduction and internal fixation of the distal humerus: functional outcome in the elderly. *J Trauma* 1997;43:578–584.
58. Corbett RH. Displaced fat pads in trauma to the elbow. *Injury* 1978;9:297–298.
59. O'Dwyer H, O'Sullivan P, Fitzgerald D, et al. The fat pad sign following elbow trauma in adults: its usefulness and reliability in suspecting occult fracture. *J Comput Assist Tomogr* 2004;28:562–565.
60. Gofton WT, Macdermid JC, Patterson SD, et al. Functional outcome of AO type C distal humeral fractures. *J Hand Surg Am* 2003;28:294–308
61. Wildburger R, Mahring M, Hofer HP. Supraintercondylar fractures of the distal humerus: results of internal fixation. *J Orthop Trauma* 1991;5:301–307.
62. Morrey BF, Askew LJ, Chao EY. A biomechanical study of normal functional elbow motion. *J Bone Joint Surg Am* 1981;63:872–877.
63. Niemann KM. Condylar fractures of the distal humerus in adults. *South Med J* 1977; 70:915–918.
64. Jupiter JB, Neff U, Regazzoni P, et al. Unicondylar fractures of the distal humerus: an operative approach. *J Orthop Trauma* 1988;2:102–109.
65. Kuhn JE, Louis DS, Loder RT. Divergent single-column fractures of the distal part of the humerus. *J Bone Joint Surg Am* 1995;77:538–542.
66. Glanville EV. Perforation of the coronoid-olecranon septum. Humero-ulnar relationships in Netherlands and African populations. *Am J Phys Anthropol* 1967;26:85–92.
67. Pelto-Vasenius K, Hirvensalo E, Rokkanen P. Absorbable implants in the treatment of distal humeral fractures in adolescents and adults. *Acta Orthop Belg* 1996;62[Suppl 1]: 93–102.
68. Ferlic RJ, Lee DH. Excision of comminuted distal humeral lateral condyle fractures: a report of two cases. *J Shoulder Elbow Surg* 2003;12:188–192.
69. Kamineni S, Morrey BF. Distal humeral fractures treated with noncustom total elbow replacement. *J Bone Joint Surg Am* 2004;86-A:940–947.
70. Gambirasio R, Riand N, Stern, R, et al. Total elbow replacement for complex fractures of the distal humerus. An option for the elderly patient. *J Bone Joint Surg Br* 2001;83: 974–978.
71. Cobb TK, Morrey BF. Total elbow arthroplasty as primary treatment for distal humeral fractures in elderly patients. *J Bone Joint Surg Am* 1997;79:826–832.
72. Holdsworth BJ, Mossad MM. Fractures of the adult distal humerus. Elbow function after internal fixation. *J Bone Joint Surg Br* 1990;72:362–365.
73. John H, Rosso R, Neff U, et al. Operative treatment of distal humeral fractures in the elderly. *J Bone Joint Surg Br* 1994;76:793–796.
74. Kinik H, Atalar H, Mergen E. Management of distal humerus fractures in adults. *Arch Orthop Trauma Surg* 1999;119:467–469.
75. Letsch R, Schmit-Neuerburg KP, Sturmer KM, et al. Intraarticular fractures of the distal humerus. Surgical treatment and results. *Clin Orthop* 1989;238–244.
76. Horne G. Supracondylar fractures of the humerus in adults. *J Trauma* 1980;20:71–74.
77. Bodoky A, Neff U, Regazzoni P. [Intra-articular unicondylar humerus fractures. Late results following stable osteosynthesis]. *Orthopade* 1988;17:257–261.
78. Toh S, Tsubo K, Nishikawa S, et al. Long-standing nonunion of fractures of the lateral humeral condyle. *J Bone Joint Surg Am* 2002;84-A:593–598.
79. Masada K, Kawai H, Kawabata H, et al. Osteosynthesis for old, established non-union of the lateral condyle of the humerus. *J Bone Joint Surg Am* 1990;72:32–40.
80. Mitsunaga MM, Bryan RS, Linscheid RL. Condylar nonunions of the elbow. *J Trauma* 1982;22:787–791.
81. Flynn JC. Nonunion of slightly displaced fractures of the lateral humeral condyle in children: an update. *J Pediatr Orthop* 1989;9:691–696.
82. Flynn JC, Richards JF Jr, Saltzman RI. Prevention and treatment of non-union of slightly displaced fractures of the lateral humeral condyle in children. An end-result study. *J Bone Joint Surg Am* 1975;57:1087–1092.
83. Toh S, Tsubo K, Nishikawa S, et al. Osteosynthesis for nonunion of the lateral humeral condyle. *Clin Orthop* 2002;Dec:230–241.
84. Inoue G, Tamura Y. Osteosynthesis for longstanding nonunion of the lateral humeral condyle. *Arch Orthop Trauma Surg* 1993;112:236–238.
85. Amis AA, Miller JH. The mechanisms of elbow fractures: an investigation using impact tests in vitro. *Injury* 1995;26:163–168.
86. Bryan RS, Bickel WH. "T" condylar fractures of distal humerus. *J Trauma* 1971;11: 830–835.
87. Brown RF, Morgan RG. Intercondylar T-shaped fractures of the humerus. Results in ten cases treated by early mobilisation. *J Bone Joint Surg Br* 1971;53:425–428.
88. Keon-Cohen BT. Fractures at the elbow. *J Bone Joint Surg Am* 1966;48-A:1623–1639.
89. Miller WE. Comminuted fractures of the distal end of the humerus in the adult. *J Bone Joint Surg Am* 1964;46:644–657.
90. Cassebaum WH. Open reduction of T & Y fractures of the lower end of the humerus. *J Trauma* 1969;9:915–925.
91. Jupiter JB, Neff U, Holzach P, et al. Intercondylar fractures of the humerus. An operative approach. *J Bone Joint Surg Am* 1985;67:226–239.
92. Gabel GT, Hanson G, Bennett JB, et al. Intraarticular fractures of the distal humerus in the adult. *Clin Orthop* 1987;99–108.

93. Waddell JP, Hatch J, Richards R. Supracondylar fractures of the humerus—results of surgical treatment. *J Trauma* 1988;28:1615–1621.
94. Helfet DL, Hotchkiss RN. Internal fixation of the distal humerus: a biomechanical comparison of methods. *J Orthop Trauma* 1990;4:260–264.
95. Aitken GK, Rorabeck CH. Distal humeral fractures in the adult. *Clin Orthop* 1986; 191–197.
96. Lansinger O, Mare K. Intercondylar T-fractures of the humerus in adults. *Arch Orthop Trauma Surg* 1982;100:37–42.
97. Zagorski JB, Jennings JJ, Burkhalter WE, et al. Comminuted intraarticular fractures of the distal humeral condyles. Surgical vs. nonsurgical treatment. *Clin Orthop* 1986; 197–204.
98. John H, Rosso R, Neff U, et al. [Distal humerus fractures in patients over 75 years of age. Long-term results of osteosynthesis]. *Helv Chir Acta* 1993;60:219–224.
99. Noack W, Kreusch-Brinker R, Trepte CT. [Indications and results of the surgical treatment of distal intra-articular humeral fractures in the elderly]. *Z Orthop Ihre Grenzgeb* 1987;125:233–242.
100. Seiler H, Trentz O. [Bicondylar fractures]. *Orthopade* 1988;17:262–271.
101. Jacobson SR, Glisson RR, Urbaniak JR. Comparison of distal humerus fracture fixation: a biomechanical study. *J South Orthop Assoc* 1997;6:241–249.
102. Schemitsch EH, Tencer AF, Henley MB. Biomechanical evaluation of methods of internal fixation of the distal humerus. *J Orthop Trauma* 1994;8:468–475.
103. O'Driscoll SW, Sanchez-Sotelo J, Torchia ME. Management of the smashed distal humerus. *Orthop Clin North Am* 2002;33:19–33, vii.
104. Henley MB. Intra-articular distal humeral fractures in adults. *Orthop Clin North Am* 1987;18:11–23.
105. Lortat-Jacob A, Hardy P. [An internal premoulded plate for complex fractures of the lower end of the humerus. A complement of the external premoulded plate]. *Rev Chir Orthop Reparatrice Appar Mot* 1989;5:347–349.
106. Yang KH, Park HW, Park SJ, et al. Lateral J-plate fixation in comminuted intercondylar fracture of the humerus. *Arch Orthop Trauma Surg* 2003;123:234–238.
107. Jupiter JB, Goodman LJ. The management of complex distal humerus nonunion in the elderly by elbow capsulectomy, triple plating and ulnar nerve neurolysis. *J Shoulder Elbow Surg* 1992;1:37–46.
108. Ring D, Jupiter JB. Fractures of the distal humerus. *Orthop Clin North Am* 2000;31: 103–113.
109. Houben PF, Bongers KJ, Wildenberg FA. Double tension band osteosynthesis in supra- and transcondylar humeral fractures. *Injury* 1994;25:305–309.
110. Fama G. Supraintercondylar fractures of the humerus—treatment by the Vigliani osteosynthesis. *Ital J Orthop Traumatol* 1987;13:55–65.
111. Zhao J, Wang X, Zhang Q. Surgical treatment of comminuted intra-articular fractures of the distal humerus with double tension band osteosynthesis. *Orthopedics* 2000;23: 449–452.
112. Korner J, Lill H, Muller LP, et al. The LCP-concept in the operative treatment of distal humerus fractures—biological, biomechanical and surgical aspects. *Injury* 2003; 34[Suppl 2]:B20–B30.
113. Allende CA, Allende BT, Allende BL, et al. Intercondylar distal humerus fractures—surgical treatment and results. *Chir Main* 2004;23:85–95.
114. Jupiter JB, Barnes KA, Goodman LJ, et al. Multiplane fracture of the distal humerus. *J Orthop Trauma* 1993;7:216–220.
115. Soffer SR, Yahiro MA. Continuous passive motion after internal fixation of distal humerus fractures. *Orthop Rev* 1990;19:88–93.
116. Soon JL, Chan BK, Low CO. Surgical fixation of intra-articular fractures of the distal humerus in adults. *Injury* 2004;35:44–54.
117. Sodergard J, Sandelin J, Bostman O. Mechanical failures of internal fixation in T and Y fractures of the distal humerus. *J Trauma* 1992;33:687–690.
118. Weber BG, Cech O. Pseudarthrosen. In: *Pseudarthrosen.* Bern, Stuttgart-Wien: Huber, 1973.
119. Ackerman G, Jupiter JB. Non-union of fractures of the distal end of the humerus. *J Bone Joint Surg Am* 1988;70:75–83.
120. McKee M, Jupiter J, Toh CL, et al. Reconstruction after malunion and nonunion of intra-articular fractures of the distal humerus. Methods and results in 13 adults. *J Bone Joint Surg Br* 1994;76:614–621.
121. Cobb TK, Linscheid RL. Late correction of malunited intercondylar humeral fractures. Intra-articular osteotomy and tricortical bone grafting. *J Bone Joint Surg Br* 1994;76: 622–626.
122. Sodergard J, Sandelin J, Bostman O. Postoperative complications of distal humeral fractures. 27/96 adults followed up for 6 (2–10) years. *Acta Orthop Scand* 1992;63: 85–89.
123. McKee MD, Jupiter JB, Bosse G, et al. Outcome of ulnar neurolysis during post-traumatic reconstruction of the elbow. *J Bone Joint Surg Br* 1998;80:100–105.
124. Helfet DL, Kloen P, Anand N, et al. Open reduction and internal fixation of delayed unions and nonunions of fractures of the distal part of the humerus. *J Bone Joint Surg Am* 2003;85-A:33–40.
125. Ring D, Gulotta L, Jupiter JB. Unstable nonunions of the distal part of the humerus. *J Bone Joint Surg Am* 2003;85-A:1040–1046.
126. Gallay SH, McKee MD. Operative treatment of nonunions about the elbow. *Clin Orthop* 2000;(Jan):87–101.
127. Papagelopoulos PJ, Morrey BF. Treatment of nonunion of olecranon fractures. *J Bone Joint Surg Br* 1994;76:627–635.
128. McKee MD, Jupiter JB. Semiconstrained elbow replacement for distal humeral nonunion. *J Bone Joint Surg Br* 1995;77:665–666.
129. Paramasivan ON, Younge DA, Pant R. Treatment of nonunion around the olecranon fossa of the humerus by intramedullary locked nailing. *J Bone Joint Surg Br* 2000;82: 332–335.
130. Chadwick CJ. The treatment of nonunion of the distal humerus by means of a transcondylar rod: a report of 3 cases. *J Shoulder Elbow Surg* 2000;9:244–247.
131. Dean GS, Holliger EH, Urbaniak JR. Elbow allograft for reconstruction of the elbow with massive bone loss. Long term results. *Clin Orthop* 1997;(Aug):12–22.
132. Urbaniak JR, Aitken M. Clinical use of bone allografts in the elbow. *Orthop Clin North Am* 1987;18:311–321.
133. Urbaniak JR, Black KE, Jr. Cadaveric elbow allografts. A six-year experience. *Clin Orthop* 1985;197:131–140.
134. Morrey BF. Post-traumatic contracture of the elbow. Operative treatment, including distraction arthroplasty. *J Bone Joint Surg Am* 1990;72:601–618.
135. Rashkoff E, Burkhalter WE. Arthrodesis of the salvage elbow. *Orthopedics* 1986;9: 733–738.
136. Kazuki K, Miyamoto T, Ohzono K. Intra-articular corrective osteotomy for the malunited intercondylar humeral fracture: a case report. *Osaka City Med J* 2002;48:95–100.
137. Henry SL, Ostermann PA, Seligson D. The antibiotic bead pouch technique. The management of severe compound fractures. *Clin Orthop* 1993;295:54–62.
138. Ring D, Jupiter JB, Toh S. Salvage of contaminated fractures of the distal humerus with thin wire external fixation. *Clin Orthop* 1999;359:203–208.
139. Uchida Y, Sugioka Y. Ulnar nerve palsy after supracondylar humerus fracture. *Acta Orthop Scand* 1990;61:118–119.
140. Schwarz B, Schmitt O, Mittelmeier H. [Late damage to the ulnar nerve following trauma to the elbow joint]. *Unfallchirurg* 1985;88:208–213.
141. Medical Research Council. *Aids to the examination of the peripheral nervous system. Memorandum no. 45.* London: HMSO, 1976.
142. McGowan AJ. The results of transposition of the ulnar nerve for traumatic ulnar neuritis. *J Bone Joint Surg Br* 1950;32-B:293–301.
143. Gabel GT, Amadio PC. Reoperation for failed decompression of the ulnar nerve in the region of the elbow. *J Bone Joint Surg Am* 1990;72:213–219.
144. King GJ, Faber KJ. Posttraumatic elbow stiffness. *Orthop Clin North Am* 2000;31: 129–143.
145. Mohan K. Myositis ossificans traumatica of the elbow. *Int Surg* 1972;57:475–478.
146. Caja VL, Moroni A, Vendemia V, et al. Surgical treatment of bicondylar fractures of the distal humerus. *Injury* 1994;25:433–438.
147. Ozdemir H, Urguden M, Soyuncu Y, et al. [Long-term functional results of adult intra-articular distal humeral fractures treated by open reduction and plate osteosynthesis]. *Acta Orthop Traumatol Turc* 2002;36:328–335.
148. Hastings H, Graham TJ. The classification and treatment of heterotopic ossification about the elbow and forearm. *Hand Clin* 1994;10:417–437.
149. Thompson HC III, Garcia A. Myositis ossificans: aftermath of elbow injuries. *Clin Orthop* 1967;50:129–134.
150. Garland DE, O'Hollaren RM. Fractures and dislocations about the elbow in the head-injured adult. *Clin Orthop* 1982;38–41.
151. Ellerin BE, Helfet D, Parikh S, et al. Current therapy in the management of heterotopic ossification of the elbow: a review with case studies. *Am J Phys Med Rehabil* 1999;78: 259–271.
152. Ring D, Jupiter JB. Operative release of complete ankylosis of the elbow due to heterotopic bone in patients without severe injury of the central nervous system. *J Bone Joint Surg Am* 2003;85-A:849–857.
153. Ring D, Jupiter JB. Operative release of ankylosis of the elbow due to heterotopic ossification. Surgical technique. *J Bone Joint Surg Am* 2004;86-A[Suppl 1]:2–10.
154. Modabber MR, Jupiter JB. Reconstruction for post-traumatic conditions of the elbow joint. *J Bone Joint Surg Am* 1995;77:1431–1446.
155. Rymaszewski L, Glass K, Parikh R. Post-traumatic elbow contracture treated by arthrolysis and continual passive motion under brachial plexus anaesthesia. *J Bone Joint Surg Br* 1996;76-B[Suppl]:30.
156. Parikh RK, Rymaszewski LR, Scott NB. Prolonged postoperative analgesia for arthrolysis of the elbow joint. *Br J Anaesth* 1995;74:469–471.
157. Urbaniak JR, Hansen PE, Beissinger SF, et al. Correction of post-traumatic flexion contracture of the elbow by anterior capsulotomy. *J Bone Joint Surg Am* 1985;67: 1160–1164.
158. Knirk JL, Jupiter JB. Intra-articular fractures of the distal end of the radius in young adults. *J Bone Joint Surg Am* 1986;68:647–659.
159. Perry CR, Gibson CT, Kowalski MF. Transcondylar fractures of the distal humerus. *J Orthop Trauma* 1989;3:98–106.
160. Morrey BF, Adams RA, Bryan RS. Total replacement for post-traumatic arthritis of the elbow. *J Bone Joint Surg Br* 1991;73:607–612.
161. Inglis AE, Pellicci PM. Total elbow replacement. *J Bone Joint Surg Am* 1980;62: 1252–1258.
162. Kasten MD, Skinner HB. Total elbow arthroplasty. An 18-year experience. *Clin Orthop* 1993;290:177–188.
163. Soni RK, Cavendish ME. A review of the Liverpool elbow prosthesis from 1974 to 1982. *J Bone Joint Surg Br* 1984;66:248–253.
164. Lowe LW, Miller AJ, Allum RL, et al. The development of an unconstrained elbow arthroplasty. A clinical review. *J Bone Joint Surg Br* 1984;66:243–247.
165. Schneeberger AG, Adams R, Morrey BF. Semiconstrained total elbow replacement for the treatment of post-traumatic osteoarthrosis. *J Bone Joint Surg Am* 1997;79: 1211–1222.
166. Kraay MJ, Figgie MP, Inglis AE, et al. Primary semiconstrained total elbow arthroplasty. Survival analysis of 113 consecutive cases. *J Bone Joint Surg Br* 1994;76:636–640.
167. Hall J, Schemitsch EH, McKee MD. Use of a hinged external fixator for elbow instability after severe distal humeral fracture. *J Orthop Trauma* 2000;14:442–445.
168. Skaggs DL, Hale JM, Buggay S, et al. Use of a hybrid external fixator for a severely comminuted juxta-articular fracture of the distal humerus. *J Orthop Trauma* 1998;12: 439–442.

169. Gainor BJ, Moussa F, Schott T. Healing rate of transverse osteotomies of the olecranon used in reconstruction of distal humerus fractures. *J South Orthop Assoc* 1995;4: 263–268.
170. Ray PS, Kakarlapudi K, Rajsekhar C, et al. Total elbow arthroplasty as primary treatment for distal humeral fractures in elderly patients. *Injury* 2000;31:687–692.
171. Ikavalko M, Lehto MU. Fractured rheumatoid elbow: treatment with Souter elbow arthroplasty—a clinical and radiologic midterm follow-up study. *J Shoulder Elbow Surg* 2001;10:256–259.
172. Garcia JA, Mykula R, Stanley D. Complex fractures of the distal humerus in the elderly. The role of total elbow replacement as primary treatment. *J Bone Joint Surg Br* 2002; 84:812–816.
173. McKee MD, Pugh DM, Richards RR, et al. Effect of humeral condylar resection on strength and functional outcome after semiconstrained total elbow arthroplasty. *J Bone Joint Surg Am* 2003;85-A:802–807.
174. Hildebrand KA, Patterson SD, Regan WD, et al. Functional outcome of semiconstrained total elbow arthroplasty. *J Bone Joint Surg Am* 2000;82-A:1379–1386.
175. Frankle MA, Herscovici D Jr, DiPasquale TG, et al. A comparison of open reduction and internal fixation and primary total elbow arthroplasty in the treatment of intraarticular distal humerus fractures in women older than age 65. *J Orthop Trauma* 2003;17: 473–480.
176. Grant IR, Miller JH. Osteochondral fracture of the trochlea associated with fracture-dislocation of the elbow. *Injury* 1975;6:257–260.
177. Foulk DA, Robertson PA, Timmerman LA. Fracture of the trochlea. *J Orthop Trauma* 1995;9:530–532.
178. Oppenheim W, Davlin LB, Leipzig JM, et al. Concomitant fractures of the capitellum and trochlea. *J Orthop Trauma* 1989;3:260–262.
179. Mehdian H, McKee MD. Fractures of capitellum and trochlea. *Orthop Clin North Am* 2000;31:115–127.
180. Bryan RS, Morrey BF. Fractures of the distal humerus. In: Morrey BF, ed. *The elbow and its disorders,* 1st ed. Philadelphia: WB Saunders, 1985:302–339.
181. Grantham SA, Norris TR, Bush DC. Isolated fracture of the humeral capitellum. *Clin Orthop* 1981;262–269.
182. Hendel D, Halperin N. Fracture of the radial head and capitulum humeri with rupture of the medial collateral ligament of the elbow. *Injury* 1982;14:98–99.
183. Lansinger O, Mare K. Fracture of the capitulum humeri. *Acta Orthop Scand* 1981;52: 39–44.
184. Newman JH. Radius fractures and damage to the capitulum humeri. *Injury* 1983;14: 477.
185. Hendel D, Aghasi M, Halperin N. Unusual fracture dislocation of the elbow joint. *Arch Orthop Trauma Surg* 1985;104:187–188.
186. Ward WG, Nunley JA. Concomitant fractures of the capitellum and radial head. *J Orthop Trauma* 1988;2:110–116.
187. Dushuttle RP, Coyle MP, Zawadsky JP, et al. Fractures of the capitellum. *J Trauma* 1985;25:317–321.
188. Ma YZ, Zheng CB, Zhou TL, et al. Percutaneous probe reduction of frontal fractures of the humeral capitellum. *Clin Orthop* 1984;17–21.
189. Ochner RS, Bloom H, Palumbo RC, et al. Closed reduction of coronal fractures of the capitellum. *J Trauma* 1996;40:199–203.
190. Christopher F, Bushnell L. Conservative treatment of fractures of the capitellum. *J Bone Joint Surg Am* 1935;17:489–492.
191. Silveri CP, Corso SJ, Roofeh J. Herbert screw fixation of a capitellum fracture. A case report and review. *Clin Orthop* 1994;30:123–126.
192. Simpson LA, Richards RR. Internal fixation of a capitellar fracture using Herbert screws. A case report. *Clin Orthop* 1986;209:166–168.
193. Lambert SM, Pike J, Railton GT. Fractures of the humeral capitellum: Herbert screw fixation. *J R Coll Surg Edinb* 1994;39:321–323.
194. Poynton AR, Kelly IP, O'Rourke SK. Fractures of the capitellum—a comparison of two fixation methods. *Injury* 1998;29:341–343.
195. Elkowitz SJ, Polatsch DB, Egol KA, et al. Capitellum fractures: a biomechanical evaluation of three fixation methods. *J Orthop Trauma* 2002;16:503–506.
196. Hirvensalo E, Bostman O, Partio E, et al. Fracture of the humeral capitellum fixed with absorbable polyglycolide pins. 1-year follow-up of 8 adults. *Acta Orthop Scand* 1993; 64:85–86.
197. Kramer M, Pamnani A, Strauch RJ. Internal fixation of a capitellum fracture using a biodegradable screw. *Orthopedics* 2002;25:765–766.
198. Clough TM, Jago ER, Sidhu DP, et al. Fractures of the capitellum: a new method of fixation using a maxillofacial plate. *Clin Orthop* 2001;384:232–236.
199. Jackobsson A. Fracture of the capitellum of the humerus in adults: treatment with intra-articular chrome-cobalt-molybdenum prosthesis. *Acta Orthop Scand* 1957;26:184–190.
200. Fowles JV, Kassab MT. Fracture of the capitulum humeri. Treatment by excision. *J Bone Joint Surg Am* 1974;56:794–798.
201. Feldman MD. Arthroscopic excision of type II capitellar fractures. *Arthroscopy* 1997; 13:743–748.
202. Di Schino M, Allizard M, Dran G, et al. [Fractures of the capitellum humeri with late discovery]. *Rev Chir Orthop Reparatrice Appar Mot* 1991;77:432–434.
203. Collert S. Surgical management of fracture of the captulum humeri. *Acta Orthop Scand* 1977;48:603–606.
204. Liberman N, Katz T, Howard CB, et al. Fixation of capitellar fractures with the Herbert screw. *Arch Orthop Trauma Surg* 1991;110:155–157.
205. Richards RR, Khoury GW, Burke FD, et al. Internal fixation of capitellar fractures using Herbert screws: a report of four cases. *Can J Surg* 1987;30:188–191.
206. Imatani J, Morito Y, Hashizume H, et al. Internal fixation for coronal shear fracture of the distal end of the humerus by the anterolateral approach. *J Shoulder Elbow Surg* 2001;10:554–556.
207. Malki AA, Salloom FM, Wong-Chung J, et al. Cannulated screw fixation of fractured capitellum: surgical technique through a limited approach. *Injury* 2000;31:204–206.
208. Fioretta G, Rotolo F, Zanasi L. The treatment of fractures of the capitulum of the humerus. *Ital J Orthop Traumatol* 1984;10:81–84.
209. Mosheiff R, Liebergall M, Elyashuv O, et al. Surgical treatment of fractures of the capitellum in adults: a modified technique. *J Orthop Trauma* 1991;5:297–300.
210. Alvarez E, Patel MR, Nimberg G, et al. Fracture of the capitulum humeri. *J Bone Joint Surg Am* 1975;57:1093–1096.
211. Stamatis E, Paxinos O. The treatment and functional outcome of type IV coronal shear fractures of the distal humerus: a retrospective review of five cases. *J Orthop Trauma* 2003;17:279–284.
212. McKee MD, Jupiter JB, Bamberger HB. Coronal shear fractures of the distal end of the humerus. *J Bone Joint Surg Am* 1996;78:49–54.
213. Scapinelli R. Treatment of fractures of the humeral capitulum using fibrin sealant. *Arch Orthop Trauma Surg* 1990;109:235–237.
214. Soltanpur A. Anterior supracondylar fracture of the humerus (flexion type). A simple technique for closed reduction and fixation in adults and the aged. *J Bone Joint Surg Br* 1978;60-B:383–386.
215. Bryan RS. Fractures about the elbow in adults. *Instruct Course Lecture* 1981;30: 200–223.
216. Charnley J. Supracondylar fractures of the humerus in children. In: *The closed treatment of common fractures.* Charnley J, ed. Cambridge, UK: Colt Books Ltd, 1999:105–115.
217. Fowles JV, Kassab MT. Displaced supracondylar fractures of the elbow in children. A report on the fixation of extension and flexion fractures by two lateral percutaneous pins. *J Bone Joint Surg Br* 1974;56B:490–500.
218. Merle d'aubigne R, Carlioz J, Meary R. Fractures sus et intercondyliennes recentes de l'adulte. *Rev Chir Orthop Reparatrice Appar Mot* 1964;50:279–288.
219. Swenson AL. The treatment of supracondylar fractures of the humerus by Kirschner wire transfixation. *J Bone Joint Surg Am* 1948;30-A:993–997.
220. Jones, KG. Percutaneous pin fixation of fractures of the lower end of the humerus. *Clin Orthop* 1967;50:53–69.
221. Lecestre P, Dupont JY, Lortat JA, et al. [Severe fractures of the lower end of the humerus in adults (author's transl)]. *Rev Chir Orthop Reparatrice Appar Mot* 1979;65:11–23.
222. Song HR, Cho SH, Jeong ST, et al. Supracondylar osteotomy with Ilizarov fixation for elbow deformities in adults. *J Bone Joint Surg Br* 1997;79:748–752.
223. Chung MS, Baek GH. Three-dimensional corrective osteotomy for cubitus varus in adults. *J Shoulder Elbow Surg* 2003;12:472–475.
224. Purser DW. Dislocation of the elbow and inclusion of the medial epicondyle in the adult. *J Bone Joint Surg Br* 1954;36-B:247–249.
225. Smith FM. Displacement of the medial epicondyle of the humerus into the elbow joint. *Ann Surg* 1946;124:410–425.
226. Patrick J. Fracture of the medial epicondyle with displacement into the elbow joint. *J Bone Joint Surg Am* 1946;28:143–147.
227. Smith FM. Medial epicondyle injuries. *JAMA* 1950;142:396–402.
228. Durig M, Muller W, Ruedi TP, et al. The operative treatment of elbow dislocation in the adult. *J Bone Joint Surg Am* 1979;61:239–244.
229. Moon MS, Kim I, Han IH, et al. Arm wrestler's injury: report of seven cases. *Clin Orthop* 1980;219–221.
230. Lokiec F, Velkes S, Engel J. Avulsion of the medial epicondyle of the humerus in arm wrestlers: a report of five cases and a review of the literature. *Injury* 1991;22:69–70.
231. Ogawa K, Ui M. Fracture-separation of the medial humeral epicondyle caused by arm wrestling. *J Trauma* 1996;41:494–497.
232. Nyska M, Peiser J, Lukiec F, et al. Avulsion fracture of the medial epicondyle caused by arm wrestling. *Am J Sports Med* 1992;20:347–350.
233. Kobayashi Y, Oka Y, Ikeda M, et al. Avulsion fracture of the medial and lateral epicondyles of the humerus. *J Shoulder Elbow Surg* 2000;9:59–64.
234. Wilson JN. The treatment of fractures of the medial epicondyle of the humerus. *J Bone Joint Surg Br* 1960;42-B:778–781.
235. Gilchrist AD, McKee MD. Valgus instability of the elbow due to medial epicondyle nonunion: treatment by fragment excision and ligament repair—a report of 5 cases. *J Shoulder Elbow Surg* 2002;11:493–497.
236. Li YH, Leong JC. Fractured lateral epicondyle associated with lateral elbow instability. *Injury* 1995;26:267–268.
237. Gustilo RB, Anderson JT. Prevention of infection in the treatment of 1025 open fractures of long bones. *J Bone Joint Surg Am* 1976;58-A:453–458.
238. Perry CR, Court-Brown CM. Masterclasses: orthopaedic trauma. In: Perry CR, Court-Brown CM, eds. *Masterclasses: orthopaedic trauma.* New York: Thieme, 1999:79–86.
239. Feil J, Burri C, Kiefer, H. [Open fractures of the elbow joint]. *Orthopade* 1988;17: 272–278.
240. Perry CR, Court-Brown CM. Masterclasses: orthopaedic trauma. In: Perry CR, Court-Brown CM, eds. *Masterclasses: orthopaedic trauma.* New York: Thieme, 1999:59–65.
241. Raab MG, Lapid MA, Adair D. Sideswipe elbow fractures. *Contemp Orthop* 1995;30: 199–205.
242. Komurcu M, Yanmis I, Atesalp AS, et al. Treatment results for open comminuted distal humerus intra-articular fractures with Ilizarov circular external fixator. *Mil Med* 2003; 168:694–697.
243. Solomon HB, Zadnik M, Eglseder WA. A review of outcomes in 18 patients with floating elbow. *J Orthop Trauma* 2003;17:563–570.
244. Lange RH, Foster RJ. Skeletal management of humeral shaft fractures associated with forearm fractures. *Clin Orthop* 1985;195:173–177.
245. Yokoyama K, Itoman M, Kobayashi A, et al. Functional outcomes of "floating elbow" injuries in adult patients. *J Orthop Trauma* 1998;12:284–290.
246. Dorow C, Markgraf E. [Fractures of the distal humerus and proximal forearm]. *Unfallchirurg* 1996;99:440–449.

247. Pierce RO Jr, Hodurski DF. Fractures of the humerus, radius, and ulna in the same extremity. *J Trauma* 1979;19:182–185.
248. Mostafavi HR, Tornetta P III. Open fractures of the humerus treated with external fixation. *Clin Orthop* 1997;337:187–197.
249. Moritomo H. Tricortical bone-block grafting for comminuted supracondylar and intercondylar fracture of the elbow in an elderly woman: case report. *J Trauma* 2001;51:784–787.
250. Burri C, Henkemeyer H, Spier W. Results of operative treatment of intraarticular fractures of the distal humerus. *Acta Orthop Belg* 1975;41:227–234.
251. Burri C, Kinzl L, Pusterla C, et al. [Therapeutic results following surgical management of distal intra-articular humerus fractures]. *Chirurg* 1973;44:78–82.
252. Morrey BF. Functional assessment of the elbow. In: Morrey BF, ed. *The elbow and its disorders*, 2nd ed. Philadelphia: WB Saunders, 1993.
253. Kaushal L, Rai J, Singh SP. Comminuted intra-articular fractures of the distal humerus. *Int Orthop* 1994;18:276–279.
254. Papaioannou N, Babis GC, Kalavritinos J, et al. Operative treatment of type C intra-articular fractures of the distal humerus: the role of stability achieved at surgery on final outcome. *Injury* 1995;26:169–173.
255. Zagorski JB. Complex fractures about the elbow. *Instrucional Course Lecture* 1990;39:265–270.
256. Eralp L, Kocaoglu M, Sar C, et al. Surgical treatment of distal intraarticular humeral fractures in adults. *Int Orthop* 2001;25:46–50.
257. Aslam N, Willett K. Functional outcome following internal fixation of intraarticular fractures of the distal humerus (AO type C). *Acta Orthop Belg* 2004;70:118–122.
258. Sanders RA, Sackett JR. Open reduction and internal fixation of delayed union and nonunion of the distal humerus. *J Orthop Trauma* 1990;4:254–259.
259. Figgie MP, Inglis AE, Mow CS, et al. Salvage of non-union of supracondylar fracture of the humerus by total elbow arthroplasty. *J Bone Joint Surg Am* 1989;71:1058–1065.
260. Morrey BF, Adams RA. Semiconstrained elbow replacement for distal humeral nonunion. *J Bone Joint Surg Br* 1995;77:67–72.
261. Ramsey ML, Adams RA, Morrey BF. Instability of the elbow treated with semiconstrained total elbow arthroplasty. *J Bone Joint Surg Am* 1999;81:38–47.

30

FRACTURES OF THE SHAFT OF THE HUMERUS

Michael D. McKee

GENERAL CONSIDERATIONS

A fracture of the humeral shaft is a common event, occurring over 70,000 times a year in North America, and representing between 3% and 5% of all fractures (1–3). Most will heal with appropriate conservative care, although a small but consistent number will require surgery for optimal outcome (1,4,5). Given the extensive range of motion of the shoulder and elbow, and the minimal effect from minor degrees of shortening, a wide range of radiographic malunion can be accepted with little functional deficit (6). Current research in this area focuses on defining the incidence and health care resources required to treat this injury, refining the indications for surgical intervention, decreasing the surgical failure rate through new implants and techniques, and minimizing the duration and magnitude of disability postinjury (3,7–9). The successful treatment of a humeral shaft fracture may not end with bony union: in the current emphasis on a "holistic" approach to patient care the treating orthopaedic surgeon may be in an ideal position to intervene and improve a patients life beyond what is traditionally recognized as the surgeons' role. Recognition of the injury as an osteoporotic fragility fracture in an elderly patient should prompt a referral for diagnostic investigations of, and potentially treatment for, an underlying osteoporotic condition. Similarly, fractures resulting from abusive domestic relationships or drug/alcohol addiction may represent opportunities to intervene. As with most orthopaedic injuries, the successful treatment of a humeral shaft fracture demands a knowledge of anatomy, surgical indications, techniques and implants, and patient function and expectations.

EPIDEMIOLOGY

The advent of comprehensive fracture databases at dedicated trauma units and the proliferation of capitated insurance contract populations (where one single orthopaedic provider group has the responsibility of caring for a set number of patients under a specific insurance contract) has dramatically improved the information available regarding the epidemiology of fractures and dislocations. While in the past (in the typical doctor–patient relationship) this was of little importance, orthopaedic surgeons around the globe are increasingly aware that the complexity of economics and politics involved in the delivery of sound orthopaedic care is increasing exponentially. As the persons who know the most about the practical aspects and human side of this topic, it is important that orthopaedic surgeons take a leading role in this type of research.

A review by Tytherleigh-Strong et al provided an excellent picture of the epidemiology of humeral shaft fractures in the United Kingdom (8). This research was based at a single orthopaedic trauma center solely responsible for the fracture care of 600,000 people, thus providing a defined population for study. They found that there was a bimodal distribution of fractures (Fig. 30-1), with a peak (25 per 100,000-population per year), in young, primarily male patients in the 21 to 30 age bracket and a larger peak (100 per 100,000 per year) primarily in older

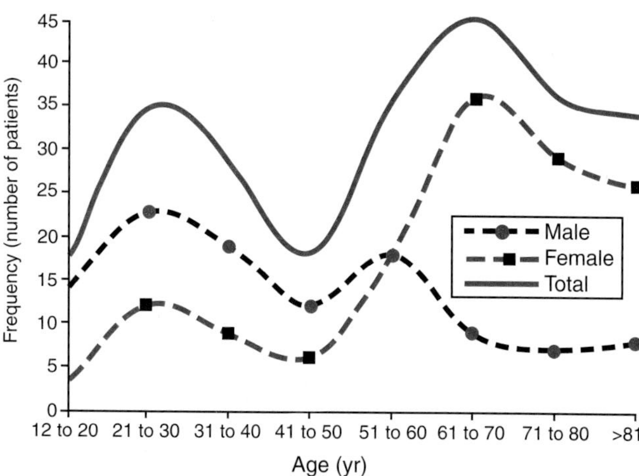

FIGURE 30-1 Age and gender distribution of fractures of the humeral shaft in 249 patients from Edinburgh: (From Tytherleigh-Strong G, Walls N, McQueen MM. The epidemiology of humeral shaft fractures. *J Bone Joint Surg Br* 1998;80:249–253; with permission).

females 60 to 80 years old. They point out that high energy trauma was responsible for the majority of injuries in young patients, and that this is the population that most of the orthopaedic literature focuses on. The fractures caused primarily by simple falls in older women (the second peak) thus represent a population intrinsically different from that described in reports on surgical intervention for these fractures. Only 5% of the injuries were associated with an open wound and 63% were "simple" fracture patterns (AO/OTA type "A", Table 30-1). Again, this represents a fracture population different from most reports that concentrate on higher energy, open fractures (10). This type of information that has implications for resident training (relatively few "operative" fractures per center per year), resource management (the largest single group is elderly females with simple humeral fractures after falls), and research (to ensure comparisons of equivalent groups) (8).

Brinker et al examined prospectively gathered data from a capitated insurance contract where orthopaedic services for 135,000 (average annual enrollment) young (mean age 28.9 years) people were provided by a single physician group of 62 orthopaedic surgeons (3). The overall incidence of fractures was 847 per 100,000 persons per year, with the incidence of humeral fractures being 13.1 per 100,000 persons per year. As would be expected in a young population, males predominated in all fracture groups. This data is useful in estimating the orthopaedic resources (and costs) required to service a young, active North American population.

ANATOMY

It is generally accepted that a humeral shaft fracture is one in which the main fracture line is distal to the surgical neck of the proximal humerus and proximal to the supracondylar ridge distally (1,4,6). Proximally the humerus is roughly cylindrical

TABLE 30-1 Fracture Pattern of 249 Fractures of the Humeral Shaft as Classified by the AO System

Type	Percentage	Average Age (yr)
A1	29.2	
A2	10.8	
A3	23.3	
Total	63.3	56.5
B1	17.1	
B2	8.3	
B3	0.8	
Total	26.2	47.5
C1	5.4	
C2	3.3	
C3	1.7	
Total	10.4	56.2

From Tytherleigh-Strong G, Walls N, McQueen MM. The epidemiology of humeral shaft fractures. *J Bone Joint Surg Br* 1998;80:249–253.

in cross section, tapering to a triangular shape distally (11). The medullary canal of the humerus tapers to an end above the supracondylar expansion. This is different from the wide metaphyseal flares of the distal tibia and distal femur and has implications in intramedullary nailing of humeral shaft fractures. The humerus is well enveloped in muscle and soft tissue, hence its good prognosis for healing in the majority of uncomplicated fractures. The medial and lateral intermuscular septa are tough fibrous bands that divide the arm into anterior and posterior compartments. The brachial artery, median nerve, and musculocutaneous nerve all remain in the anterior compartment for their entire course, while the ulnar nerve begins in the anterior compartment and passes through to the posterior compartment at the elbow. The radial nerve begins in the posterior compartment and passes through into the anterior compartment (Fig. 30-2). A thorough knowledge of anatomy is important for the successful treatment of humeral shaft fractures.

DIAGNOSIS

History

As with most fractures, a careful and detailed history and physical examination provide critical information that serves as a starting point for treatment. The predominant causes of humeral shaft fractures include simple falls or rotational injuries in the older population and higher-energy mechanisms in the younger patient including motor vehicle accidents, assaults, falls from a height, and throwing injuries. A history of minimal trauma causing fracture in the older patient may be the first point to alert the surgeon that the fracture may involve pathologic bone (be it from metastatic disease or severe osteoporosis) and prompt a thorough history (e.g., for prior cancer) and possibly a systemic work-up. In this situation, the treating surgeon has the potential to help the patient both in terms of the presenting fracture and the prevention of further fractures. Comorbidities, especially as they relate to the patient's suitability for a potential anesthetic, should be elucidated. These may also be relevant with regards to the etiology of the fall that resulted in fracture: an unrecognized arrhythmia can cause recurrent falls and injuries. Thus, a clear description of the actual mechanism of the injury is important.

The described mechanism of injury should match the fracture type: while exceptions do occur, the presence of a spiral fracture indicates a rotational force (such as that which occurs when the arm is forcibly wrenched behind the back) that is not consistent with, for example, striking the arm against a door. Discordance between history and fracture type is a hallmark of domestic abuse, and again this may represent an opportunity to intervene in a potentially lethal situation (12). Alcohol abuse, smoking, and/or illicit drug use are all potential risk factors for negative fracture outcome through repeat injury, noncompliance, or poor biology at the fracture site, and represent an opportunity to improve outcome. For example, while it is unrealistic to expect uniform compliance, modern smoking cessation strategies have a success rate from 20% to 60%. It is also becoming apparent that the use of nonsteroidal anti-inflammatory drugs (NSAIDs), for years a standard treatment for pain and swelling after acute injury, is associated with prolonged fracture healing times (13). Burd et al, in a randomized clinical trial, investigated the effect of indomethacin on the prevention of heterotopic ossification in a group of polytrauma patients with acetabular fractures (14). One group received indomethacin, one group local irradiation, and the control group nothing. These patients also had a number of associated long bone fractures: the incidence of delayed and nonunion in the indomethacin-treated group was 26% versus 7% in the other two groups, a significantly higher rate ($p = 0.004$). We strongly discourage the use of NSAIDs in patients with humeral shaft fractures (14,15).

Physical Examination

In the multiple trauma situation, history from the patient may be unobtainable, but any available information from the accident scene, paramedical personnel, or family members is important. In general, the treatment of a humeral fracture is a relatively low priority in the resuscitation of a severely injured patient, which should proceed according to the guidelines of the Advanced Trauma Life Support (ATLS) protocol (16). Following stabilization of the patient, attention is turned to the affected

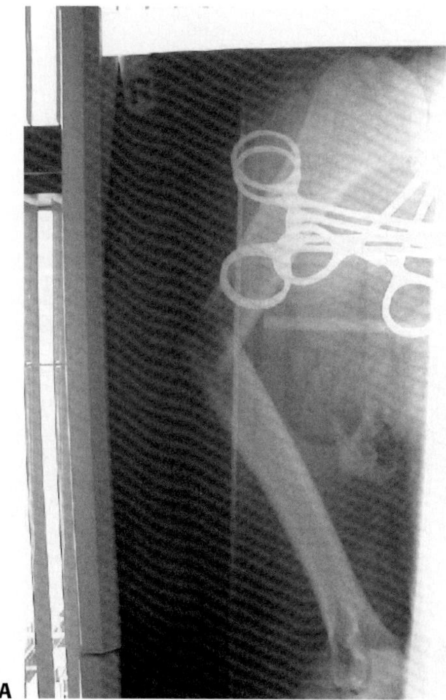

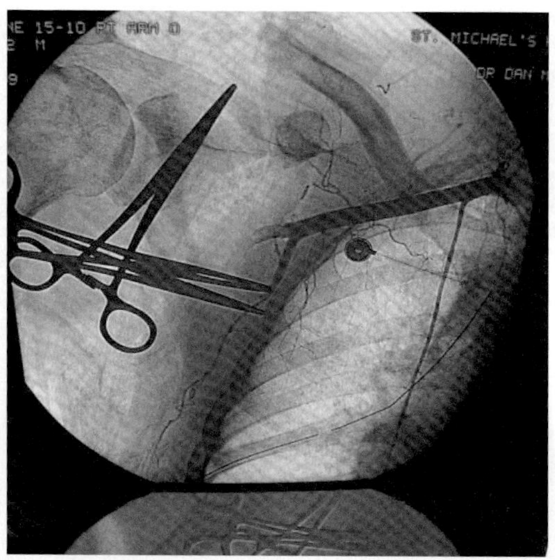

FIGURE 30-4 **A.** An angulated, open fracture of the humeral shaft in a patient from a rollover motor vehicle accident. **B.** Angiogram demonstrates axillary artery injury with associated scapulothoracic dissociation (note the wide separation of the distal clavicle and acromion process).

A careful search for open wounds is very important, as the presence of an open fracture accelerates the urgency of the situation. Examination of the shoulder and elbow joint is mandatory: associated injuries or preexisting joint pathology may be an indication for operative management as stiffness may transfer physiologic stress to the fracture site and increase healing time (Fig. 30-5) (25). This will have implications for treatment and counseling of the patient with regards to prognosis.

Imaging

Standard imaging for any humeral shaft fracture includes two radiographs at 90 degrees to each other that include the shoulder and elbow joints in each view. Further views can be ordered depending on the clinical examination and any abnormalities noticed on the initial films. For the typical humeral shaft fracture it is rarely necessary to obtain further imaging. Exceptions to this would include shaft fractures with associated vascular injuries that should be investigated further with an angiogram (Fig. 30-4) or computed tomographic (CT) scans of associated intra-articular injuries proximally or distally (1,4,25). CT scanning may also be indicated in the rare situation where a significant rotational abnormality exists: rotational alignment is difficult to judge from plain radiographs of a diaphyseal long bone fracture and a CT scan through the humeral condyles distally and the humeral head proximally can provide exact rotational alignment, especially when compared to the normal side. Given the broad rotational range of the shoulder, fairly large degrees of rotational malalignment can be (and probably routinely are) accepted (6). However, severe degrees of rotational malalignment (>30 degrees) should be avoided as they have a deleterious effect on the functional "sphere of action" of the upper extremity. Bae et al reported an extreme case of a 270-degree rotational malunion following humeral shaft fracture with obvious functional impairment that required corrective osteotomy, and we have had experience with a similar case in an adult male (27).

In developing countries ultrasound may provide an attractive alternative to the expense, maintenance, safety issues and space required for conventional radiography. The diagnostic accuracy of ultrasound for long bone fractures is excellent: Hubner et al reported a sensitivity of 100%, indicating that a negative ultrasound study essentially rules out a fracture (28). While this technique is unlikely to become routine in North America or Europe, it has potential in other areas where social circumstances or economics make medical resources scarce.

CLASSIFICATION

Bone

A number of factors are important when describing humeral shaft fracture classification. These include the mechanism of injury (low energy, high energy, gunshot associated), the location of the fracture (proximal, mid-shaft, distal) along with any potential peri- or intra-articular extension, concomitant soft-tissue wounds or lesions, associated nerve or vessel injury (radial nerve most commonly), the nature of the underlying bone (normal, osteopenic, pathologic), and the presence of any asso-

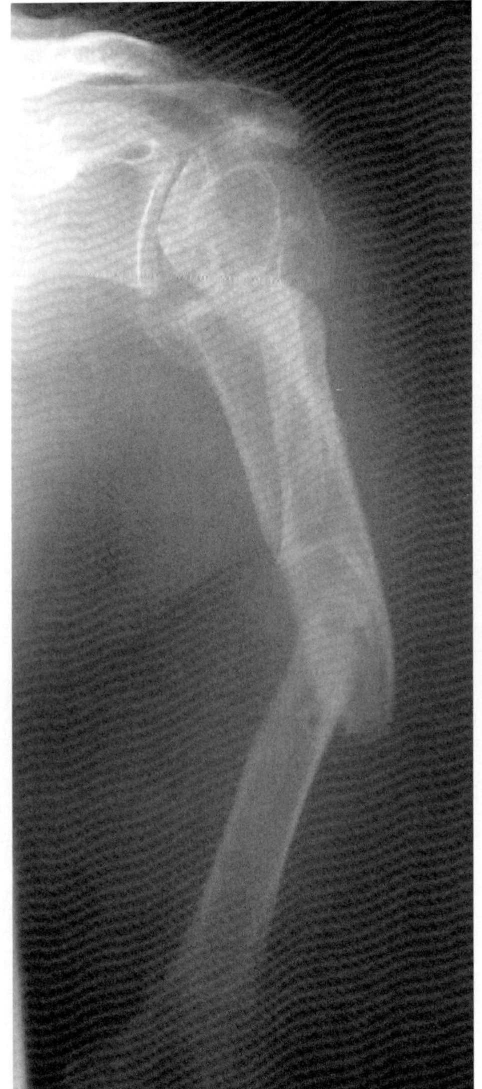

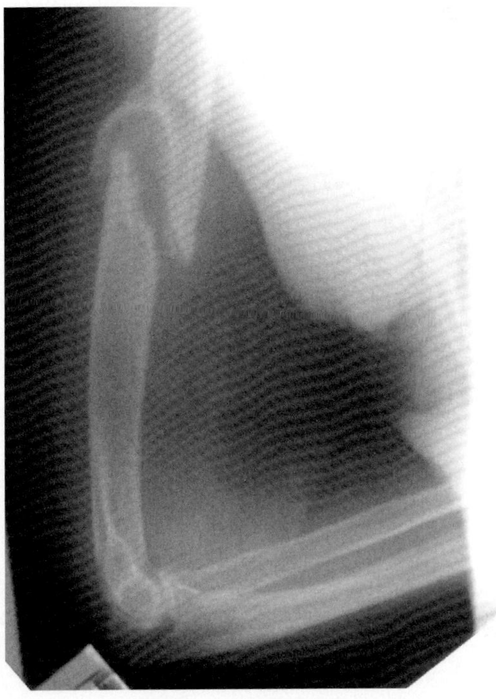

FIGURE 30-5 This elderly osteoporotic woman had previously sustained a humeral head and neck fracture treated conservatively that had resulted in a very stiff shoulder. She fell 4 years later and fractured the shaft of the humerus distal to the prior injury. **A.** Despite appropriate splinting, she developed a painful pseudarthrosis, as seen on the lateral radiograph **(B)**. Adjacent joint stiffness transfers much of the motion and stress of the limb to an ipsilateral fracture and increases the rate of delayed union and nonunion. This factor should be considered when deciding on treatment options.

ciated prosthesis. Descriptive terms such as these are useful in providing an overall picture of a particular humeral shaft fracture, although they may not lend themselves well to categorizing injuries for research or clinical trials. For this reason, more "objective" classification schemes have been developed to aid in such endeavors.

A popular and useful scheme is the Orthopaedic Trauma Association's Fracture and Dislocation Compendium, first published in 1996 (29). This system is based on the AO/ASIF Comprehensive Long Bone Classification, adds previously unclassified fractures and reorders them in an alpha-numeric system. The humerus is designated bone "1" and is divided into proximal (11), diaphyseal (12), and distal (13) segments (Fig. 30-6). Fractures are divided into three types: "A" or "Simple" fractures of two main fragments, proximal and distal (cortical fragments of less than 10% of the circumference are ignored); "B" or "Wedge" fractures where there are one or more intermediate fracture fragments but, after reduction, there is contact between the main proximal and distal fragments; and "C" or "Complex" fractures, where there are one or more intermediate fragments such that, after reduction, there is no contact between the main fragments. These main types are then subdivided into groups based on fracture pattern (spiral, oblique, transverse) and subgroups based on proximal, middle, or distal zones of the diaphysis. The system is designed to reflect increasing fracture severity as one progresses from A to C types, and to help aid in treatment, prognosis, and research. The reliability and reproducibility of this type of scheme has not been critically assessed for the humeral shaft but has been looked at for both the proximal and distal segments of the bone. These investigators found that while there was poor inter- and intraobserver agreement for subgroup classification, there was "substantial" (kappa value

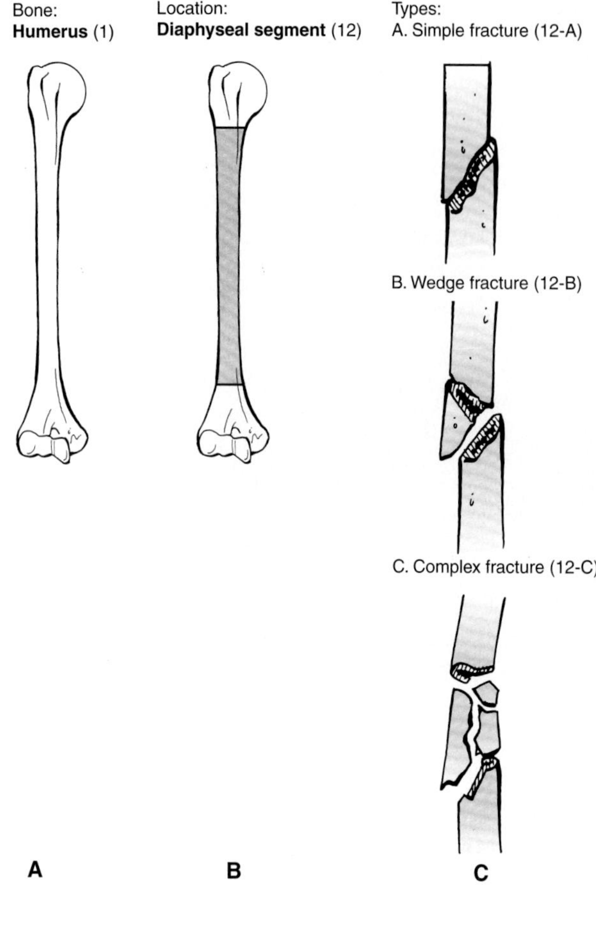

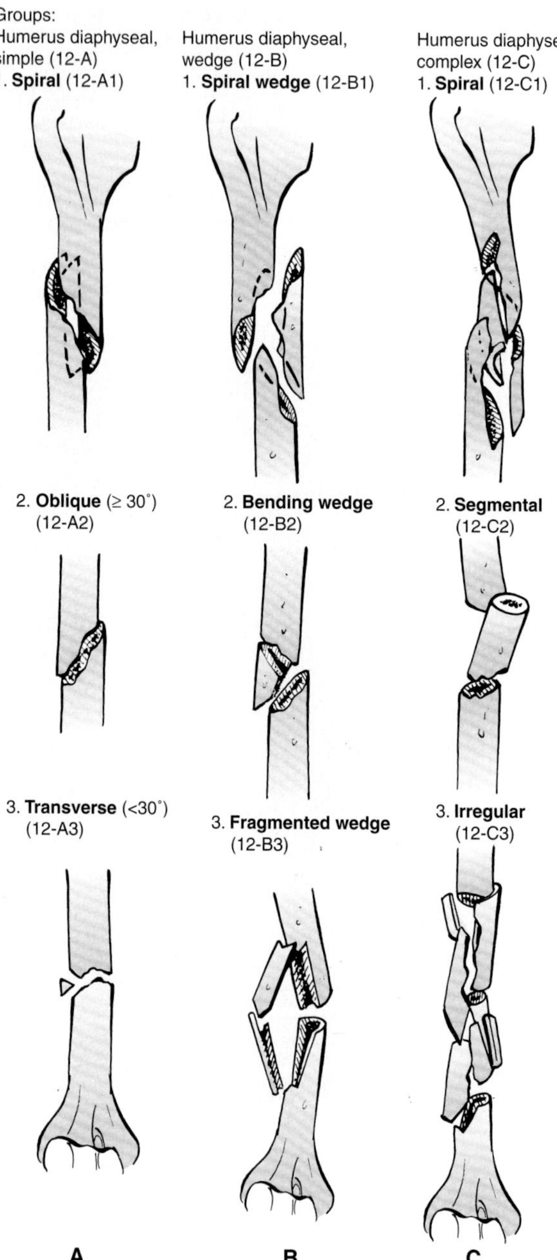

FIGURE 30-6 The OTA classification of humeral shaft fractures.

0.66) agreement for type (A, B, C) and "moderate" (kappa value 0.52) agreement for group designation (30,31). Thus, it seems reasonable to assume that (the anatomically simpler) humeral shaft fractures can reliably be classified at least as to type (simple, wedge, complex) and group (spiral, oblique, transverse) by the typical orthopaedic surgeon.

Soft Tissue

Soft-tissue lesions are classified by one of two schemes. The Gustilio classification (popular in North America) divides wounds into three grades (32). Grade I is a wound less then 1 cm (typically low-energy wounds caused by an inside-out puncture of the fragment end). A grade II wound is greater than 1 cm and of higher energy. A grade III wound is produced by high energy, is 10 cm or greater and often has extensive soft-tissue and/or periosteal stripping. Depending on the severity of the stripping, grade III lesions are subclassified into A, B, and C types, with C depicting an associated arterial injury that requires surgical repair for viability of the limb. The scheme of Tscherne (popular in Europe) has the advantage of including various degrees of closed soft-tissue contusions and compartment syndromes (33) as well. Type O fractures are from indirect violence (e.g., torsion) and have minimal soft-tissue injury. Type I injuries have superficial abrasions or contusions caused by pressure from within. Type II injuries have deep abrasions with contused skin and/or muscle, and may have an impending compartment syndrome. Type III injuries have extensive contusions or crushed muscle, subcutaneous avulsions, vascular injuries and compartment syndromes. The reproducibility of soft-tissue injury grading schemes has also been called into question (34).

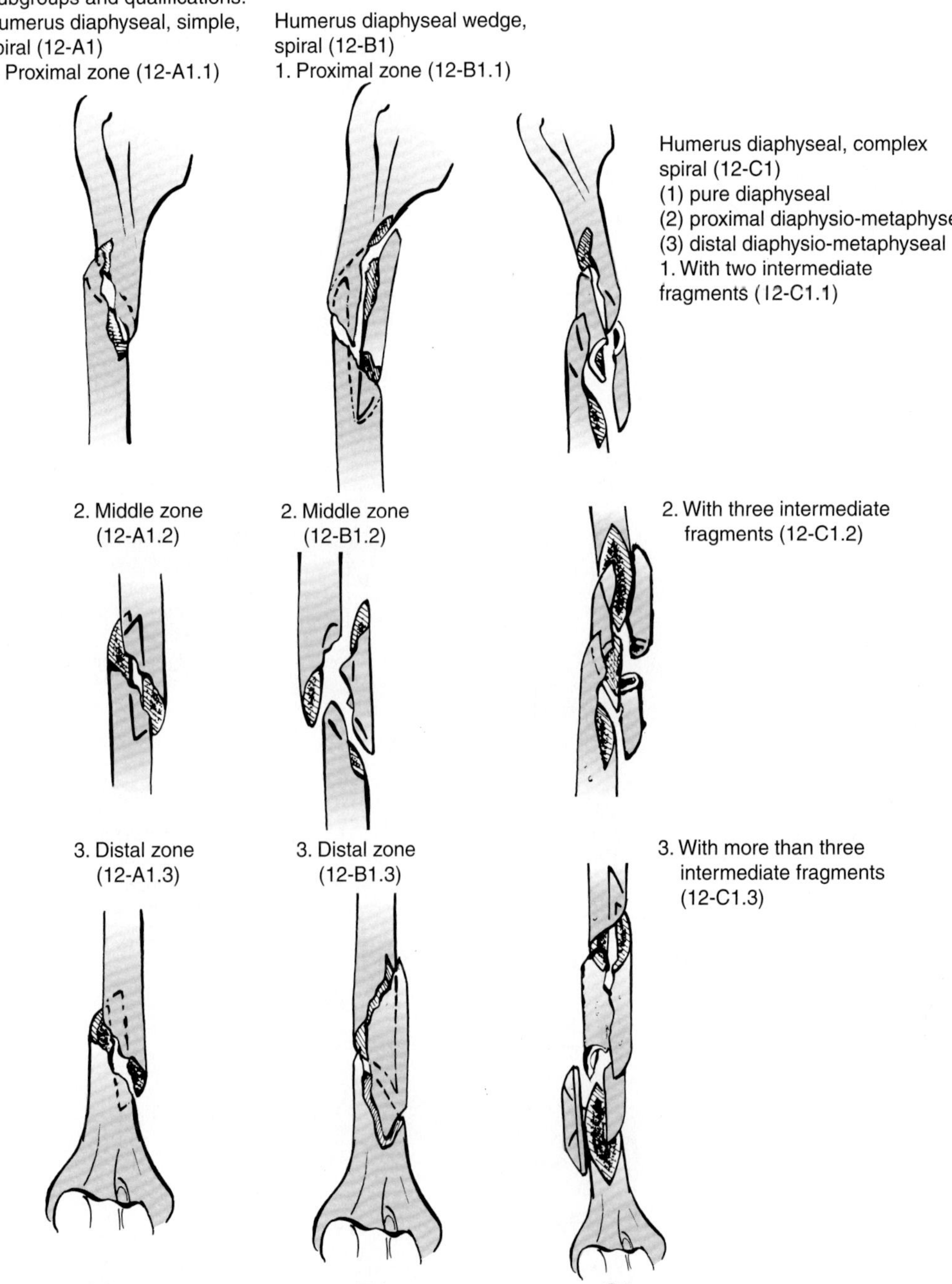

FIGURE 30-6 (*continued*) The OTA classification of humeral shaft fractures. (*continues*)

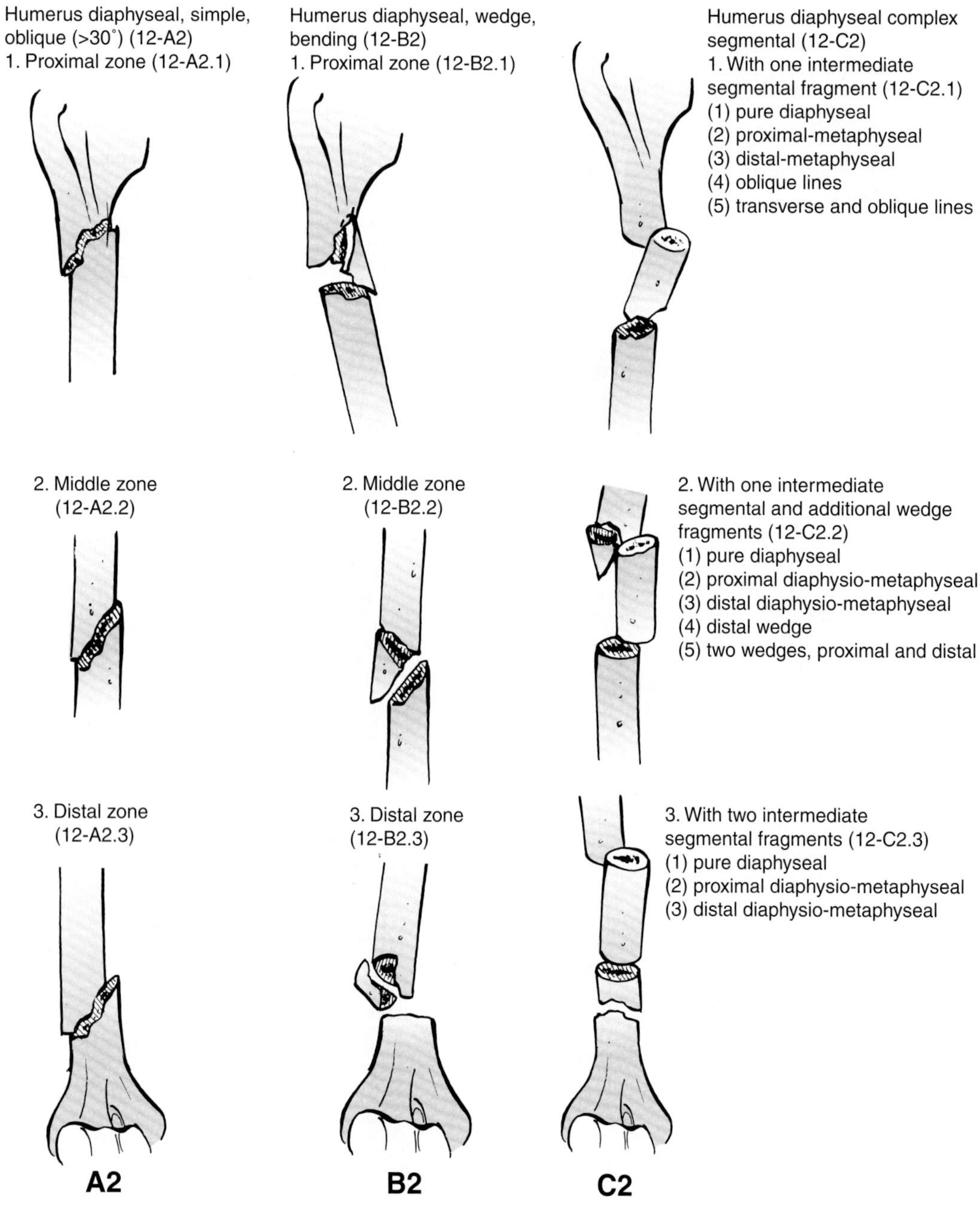

Humerus diaphyseal, simple, oblique (>30°) (12-A2)
1. Proximal zone (12-A2.1)

Humerus diaphyseal, wedge, bending (12-B2)
1. Proximal zone (12-B2.1)

Humerus diaphyseal complex segmental (12-C2)
1. With one intermediate segmental fragment (12-C2.1)
(1) pure diaphyseal
(2) proximal-metaphyseal
(3) distal-metaphyseal
(4) oblique lines
(5) transverse and oblique lines

2. Middle zone (12-A2.2)

2. Middle zone (12-B2.2)

2. With one intermediate segmental and additional wedge fragments (12-C2.2)
(1) pure diaphyseal
(2) proximal diaphysio-metaphyseal
(3) distal diaphysio-metaphyseal
(4) distal wedge
(5) two wedges, proximal and distal

3. Distal zone (12-A2.3)

3. Distal zone (12-B2.3)

3. With two intermediate segmental fragments (12-C2.3)
(1) pure diaphyseal
(2) proximal diaphysio-metaphyseal
(3) distal diaphysio-metaphyseal

A2 B2 C2

FIGURE 30-6 (*continued*) The OTA classification of humeral shaft fractures. (*continues*)

Humerus diaphyseal, simple, transverse (<30°) (12-A3)
1. Proximal zone (12-A3.1)

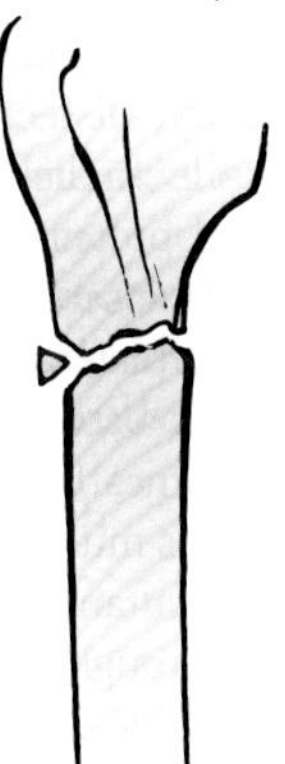

Humerus diaphyseal, wedge, fragmented (12-B3)
1. Proximal zone (12-B3.1)

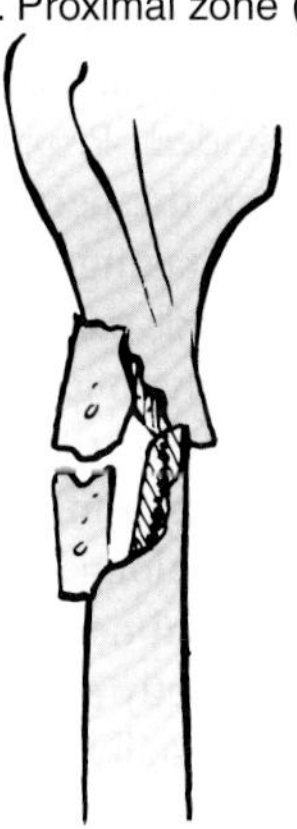

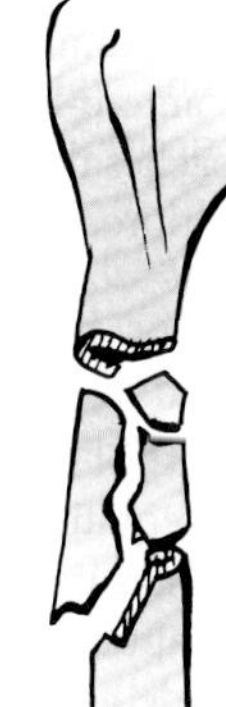

Humerus diaphyseal, complex irregular (12-C3)
1. With two or three intermediate fragments (12-C3.1)
(1) two main intermediate fragments
(2) three main intermediate fragments

2. Middle zone (12-A3.2)

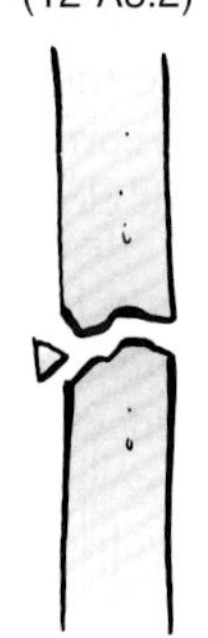

2. Middle zone (12-B3.2)

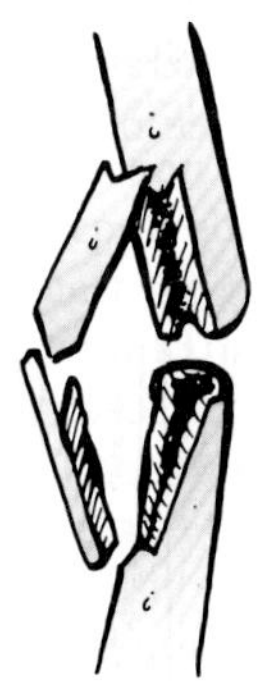

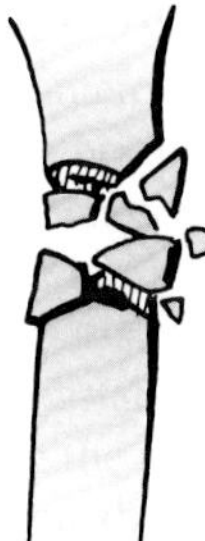

2. With limited shattering (<4 cm) (12-C3.2)
(1) proximal zone
(2) middle zone
(3) distal zone

3. Distal zone (12-A3.3)

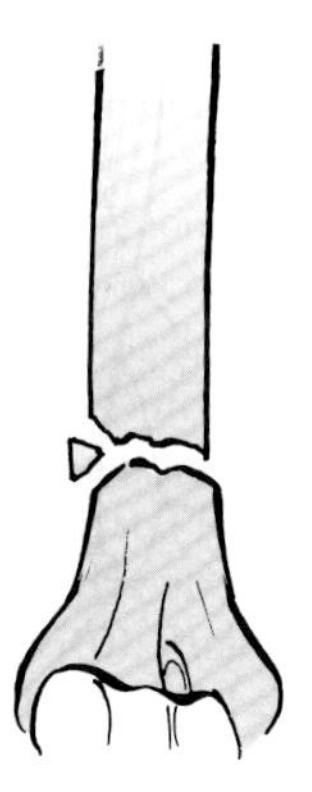

3. Distal zone (12-B3.3)

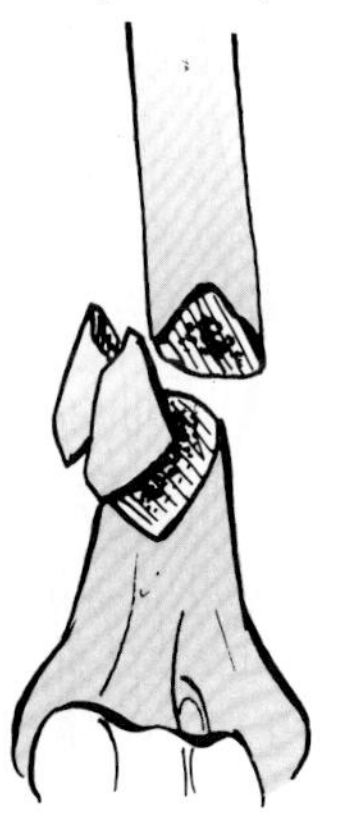

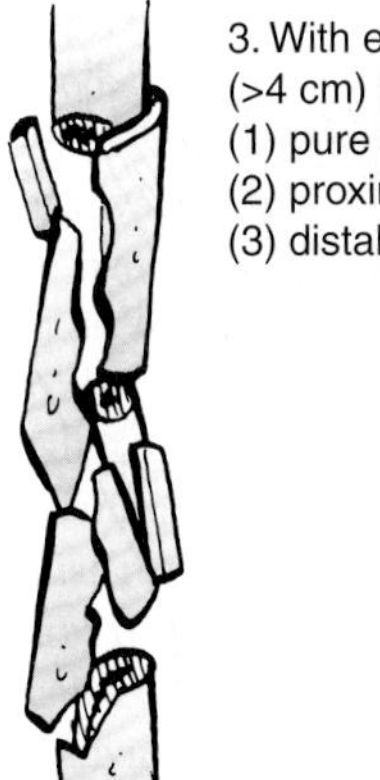

3. With extensive shattering (>4 cm) (12-C3.3)
(1) pure diaphyseal
(2) proximal diaphysio-metaphyseal
(3) distal diaphysio-metaphyseal

A3 **B3** **C3**

FIGURE 30-6 (*continued*) The OTA classification of humeral shaft fractures.

tion is rarely achieved with nonoperative treatment of these injuries, it is rarely necessary due to the wide range of motion of the shoulder and elbow, such that angulatory, axial, or rotational malunion is easily accommodated and functional limitation is minimal. The humeral shaft is well enveloped in muscle, has a robust blood supply (43), does not bear weight, and is easily splinted, leading Sir John Charnley to state, "It is perhaps the easiest of the major long bones to treat by conservative methods" (49). Described techniques include hanging casts, "sugar tong" or coaptation splints, sling and swathes, long-arm casts, shoulder spica casts, and olecranon pin traction. However, while good results have been described with most of these methods, functional bracing has become the gold standard for nonoperative treatment due to its ease of application, adjustability, low cost, allowance of shoulder and elbow motion, and reproducible record of success (6,45). While a detailed description of nonoperative care is beyond the scope of this chapter, a review of functional bracing is an integral part of any description of humeral shaft fracture treatment.

Functional bracing was first described by Sarmiento et al in 1977, and consisted of a custom-made, circumferential orthosis that allowed elbow and shoulder motion and was worn for a mean of 10 weeks in 51 patients, with one nonunion (45). The device has been modified since and now is a prefabricated device with plastic supports and adjustable Velcro straps that can be tightened as the swelling associated with the fracture recedes (6). The device works on the principles of active muscle contraction correcting rotation and angulation, the "hydraulic" effect of soft-tissue compression aligning the fracture fragments, and the beneficial effect of gravity on alignment. In the largest series to date of 922 patients (620 were followed to definitive outcome) with humeral shaft fractures treated with functional bracing, Sarmiento reported union in 98% of 465 closed fractures and 94% of 155 low-grade open fractures. Open fractures took longer to heal than closed fractures (14 weeks versus 9.5 weeks). These results are consistent with those reported by Ostermann et al (4 nonunions of 191 fractures), Zagorski et al (3 nonunions of 170 fractures), and Ricciardi-Pollini (2 nonunions of 36 fractures) (50–52). It is clear that, for properly selected patients, this technique results in a high rate of union. Given the early motion that is encouraged with this method, functional outcome of the elbow and shoulder is well maintained with 89% of patients losing 10 degrees of motion or less of the shoulder and 93% of patients losing 10 degrees of motion or less of the elbow in Sarmiento's series. It should be noted however that many of the patients in this series were indigent and functional outcome data was rudimentary. For instance, elbow range of motion was recorded for only 301 of the original 922 patients.

Significant degrees of initial deformity are often surprisingly well corrected with this method under the influence of gravity, time and the brace (Fig. 30-11). Sarmiento et al reported that 55% of patients healed within 5 degrees of anatomic alignment following functional bracing of humeral shaft fractures, with varus being the commonest deformity: 42% of patients healed with 6 to 25 degrees of varus deformity (6). Eighty-six percent of patients healed within 10 degrees of anatomic alignment in the anteroposterior plane. These deformities did not seem to influence functional results. However, as mentioned functional outcome data was minimal, and it is quite possible subtle or delayed complications would not be detected. For example, recently the negative biomechanical and clinical effects of distal humeral varus malunion have been elucidated. Twenty patients with a mean varus malunion of 19 degrees developed posterolateral rotatory instability (PLRI) of the elbow a mean of 15 years after their initial distal humeral fracture (53). It is unlikely this type of problem would have been elucidated in Sarmiento's study.

OPERATIVE TREATMENT

Operative Indications

The majority of isolated, simple humeral shaft fractures can be managed nonoperatively; however, there are specific operative indications that have been shown to enhance the outcome of the fracture or patient. These indications can be divided into three groups: fracture indications, associated injuries, and patient indications (Table 30-2). While some of these indications are absolute, such as an associated vascular injury or an associated higher grade open wound, many are relative indications where both patient and fracture features must be taken into consideration prior to deciding on treatment. For instance, although most segmental fractures are high-energy injuries with significant deformity, a segmental fracture in which both fracture lines are minimally displaced and the overall alignment is acceptable is a good candidate for a trial of conservative care with functional bracing. It is important to note that fracture comminution, in isolation, is *not* an indication for operative intervention. Although intuitively it would seem that such fractures are more likely to develop delayed or nonunion, this is not the case. In his large series of functional bracing, Sarmiento found the median healing time of the humeral shaft was 11 weeks for the comminuted fractures and *12* weeks for the transverse fractures: others have reported similar findings (6). In fact, some authorities have noted the "relative propensity for delayed union in transverse or short oblique fractures managed nonoperatively in an active individual" (1,25), and considered such injuries a relative indication for operative repair. Also, operative fixation of comminuted fractures is associated with a higher complication and mechanical failure rate, and thus is best avoided if conservative treatment is feasible.

Plate Osteosynthesis

Plate osteosynthesis remains the gold standard of fixation of humeral shaft fractures against which other methods must be compared (1,4,17,25,55–59). It is associated with a high union rate, low complication rate, and a rapid return to function. It can be used for fractures with both proximal and distal extension, is safe and effective in open fractures (see below), has essentially

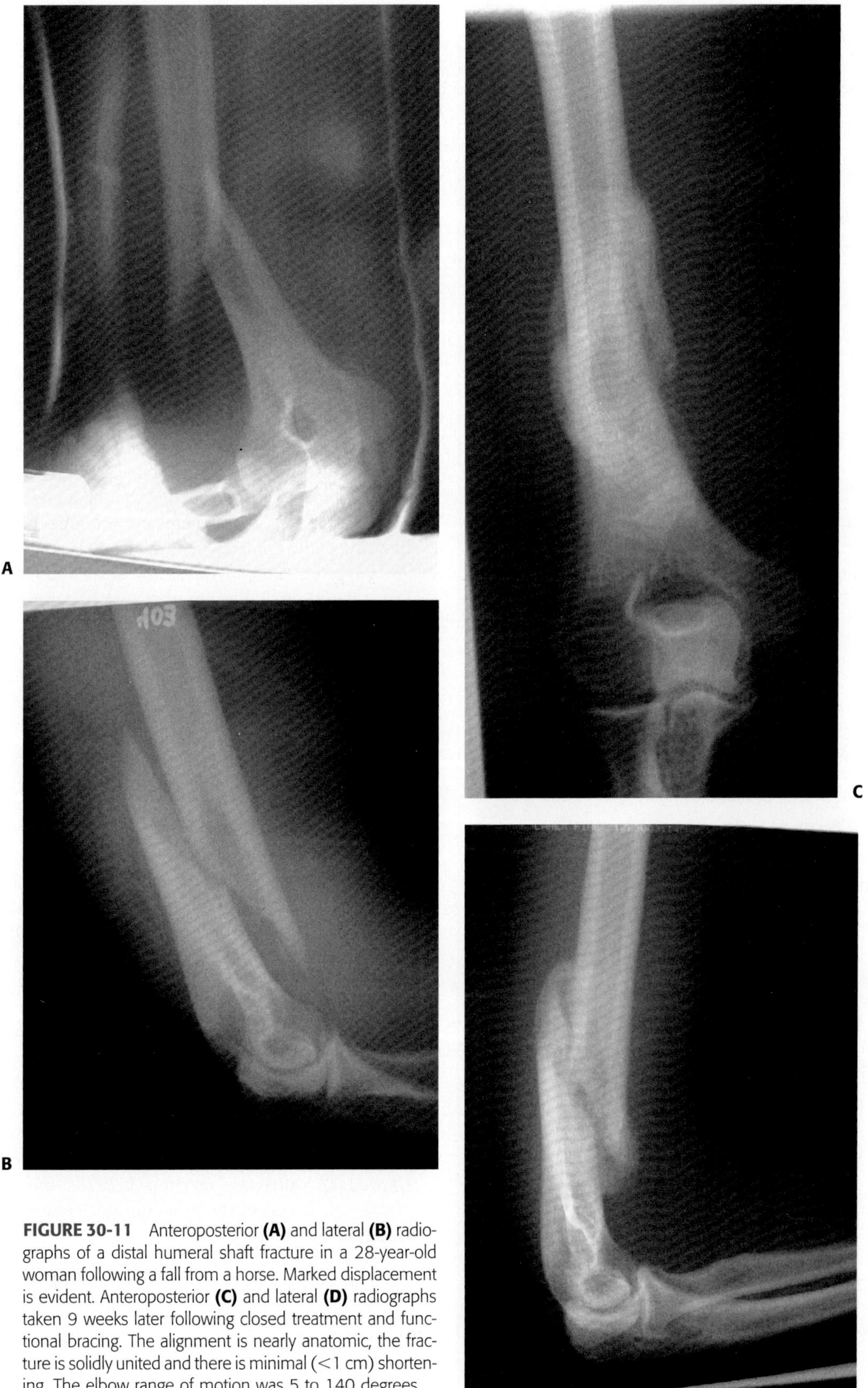

FIGURE 30-11 Anteroposterior **(A)** and lateral **(B)** radiographs of a distal humeral shaft fracture in a 28-year-old woman following a fall from a horse. Marked displacement is evident. Anteroposterior **(C)** and lateral **(D)** radiographs taken 9 weeks later following closed treatment and functional bracing. The alignment is nearly anatomic, the fracture is solidly united and there is minimal (<1 cm) shortening. The elbow range of motion was 5 to 140 degrees.

TABLE 30-2 Indications for Primary Operative Treatment of Humeral Shaft Fractures

Fracture Indications
Failure to obtain and maintain adequate closed reduction:
Shortening >3 cm
Rotation >30°
Angulation >20°
Segmental fractures
Pathologic fractures
Intra-articular extension:
Shoulder joint
Elbow joint
Associated Injuries
Open wound
Vascular injury
Brachial plexus injury
Ipsilateral forearm fractures
Ipsilateral shoulder or elbow fractures
Bilateral humeral fractures
Lower extremity fractures requiring upper extremity weight-bearing
Burns
High-velocity gun shot injury
Chronic associated joint stiffness—elbow, shoulder
Patient Indications
Multiple injuries—polytrauma
Head injury (Glasgow Coma Scale ≤8)
Chest trauma
Poor patient tolerance, compliance
Unfavorable body habitus:
Morbid obesity
Large breasts

no elbow or shoulder morbidity, and is stable enough to allow early upper extremity weight-bearing in the multiply injured patient (60). The surgical approaches, implants, and techniques are familiar to most orthopaedic surgeons, and it remains the procedure of choice at our institution for humeral shaft fractures that require operative fixation (Fig. 30-12). Vander Griend et al reported union in 35 of 36 plated humeral shaft fractures with no shoulder or elbow morbidity and one temporary radial nerve palsy (58). Bell et al had similar results (union in 37 of 39 fractures) as did Tingstad et al (union in 78 of 83 fractures) (59,60). The union rate following open reduction and internal fixation of humeral shaft fractures averages 96% in a number of large series (55–60). Complications are infrequent, and include radial nerve palsy (2% to 5%, usually neuropraxic injuries which recover), infection (1% to 2% for closed fractures, 2% to 5% for open fractures) and refracture (1%).

Fractures in the middle or proximal third are best approached through an anterolateral incision. Fractures that extend into the distal third of the bone are best approached posteriorly. A broad 4.5-mm dynamic compression or limited contact compression (LCC) plate helps prevent longitudinal fracture or fissuring of the humerus because the screw holes in these plates are staggered (25). In physically small individuals with thin humerii, a narrow 4.5-mm plate may be used. Inserted screws can be angled medially and laterally so they exit staggered on the opposite cortex, minimizing longitudinal stress. Other plates are not strong enough, especially in active individuals (Fig. 30-13). In the transition zone distally between the shaft and the supracondylar ridges, as the medial and lateral columns diverge, fixation can be achieved with two 3.5-mm compression plates along each column, avoiding plate impingement in the olecranon fossa (Fig. 30-10). A lag screw placed across the main fracture line (either outside or through the plate) can increase construct strength by 30% to 40%, and if fracture or nonunion geometry permits, should be inserted (Fig. 30-14) (25). With a solid lag screw, three screws (six cortices) proximal and three screws (six cortices) distal constitute the minimum fixation: without a lag screw, at least four screws (eight cortices) proximally and distally are required. Fracture comminution, poor screw purchase, poor bone quality, or other negative factors should prompt longer plate application with more screws. Previously, it was recommended that a unicortical screw be placed in the last hole of the plate to minimize the stress-riser effect of the plate, provide a smoother transition of stress from plate to bone and decrease the potential risk of fracture at the end of the implant. However, a biomechanical study by Davenport showed no difference in stress between uni- and bicortical screws in the end of the plate and this technique is no longer recommended (61).

There are several practical advantages to the use of the limited contact dynamic (LCD) plates over standard compression plates: they are easier to contour, allow for wider angle of screw insertion, and have bidirectional compression holes. Theoretical advantages include decreased stress shielding and improved bone blood flow due to limited plate–bone contact (62). One

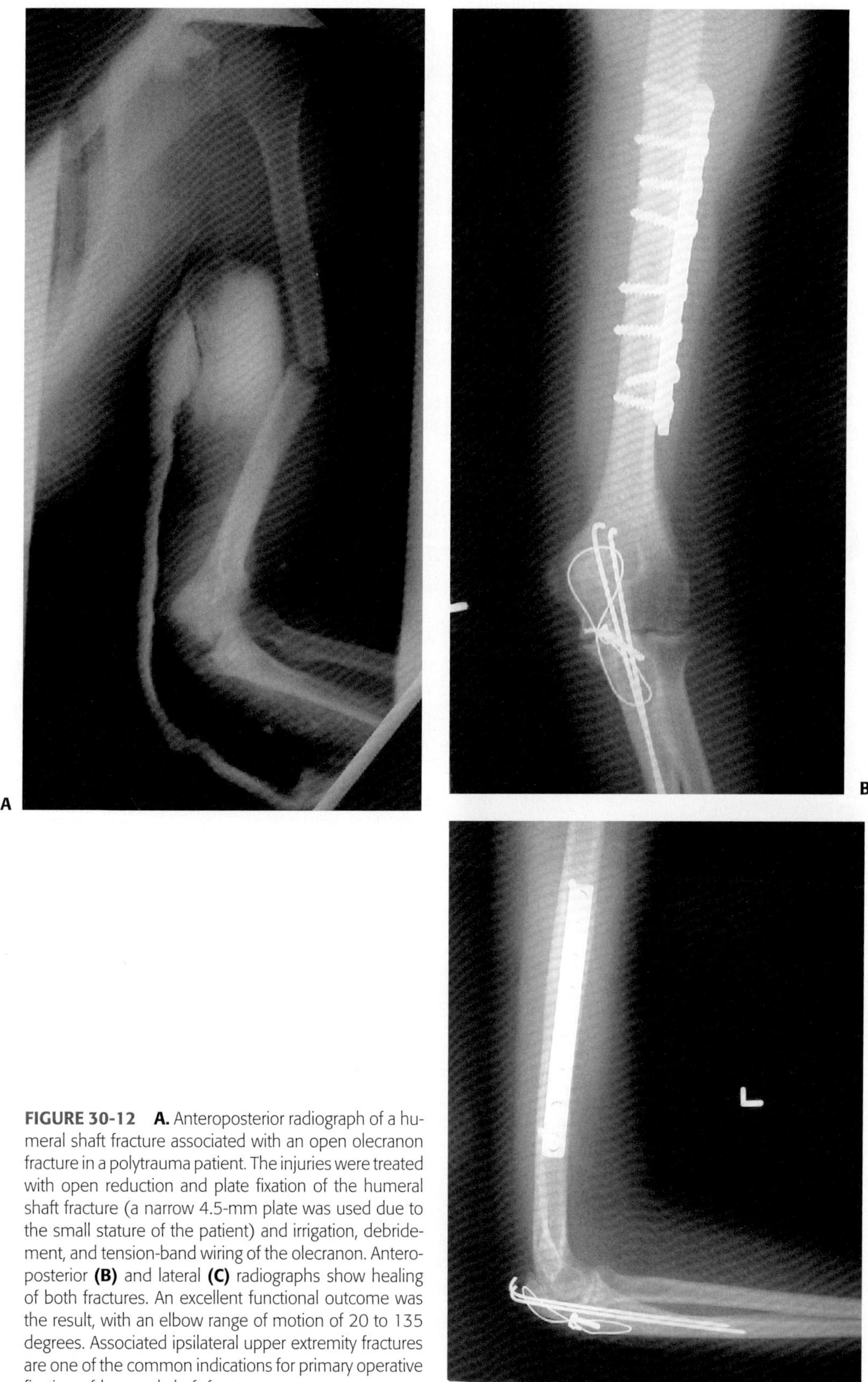

FIGURE 30-12 **A.** Anteroposterior radiograph of a humeral shaft fracture associated with an open olecranon fracture in a polytrauma patient. The injuries were treated with open reduction and plate fixation of the humeral shaft fracture (a narrow 4.5-mm plate was used due to the small stature of the patient) and irrigation, debridement, and tension-band wiring of the olecranon. Anteroposterior **(B)** and lateral **(C)** radiographs show healing of both fractures. An excellent functional outcome was the result, with an elbow range of motion of 20 to 135 degrees. Associated ipsilateral upper extremity fractures are one of the common indications for primary operative fixation of humeral shaft fractures.

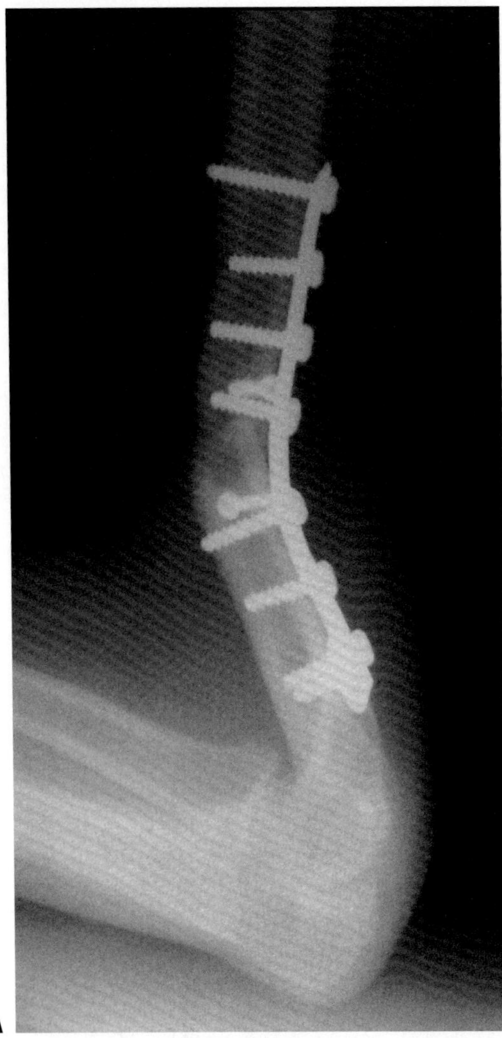

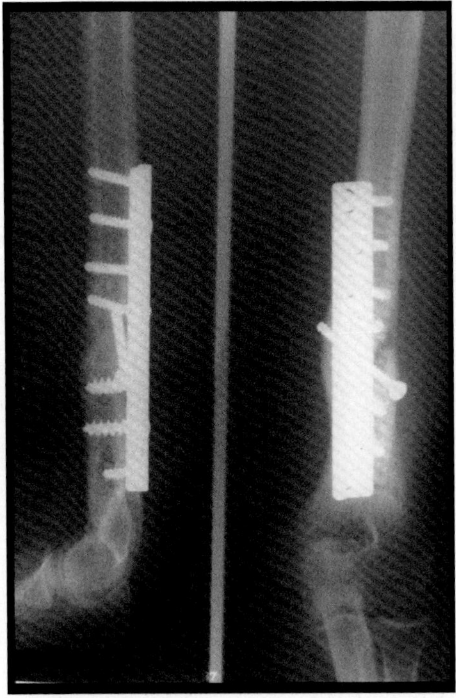

FIGURE 30-13 **A.** Proper plate selection is important in the fixation of humeral shaft fractures. This 18-year-old man had a displaced distal humeral shaft fracture fixed with a thin "T" plate placed directly posteriorly. This plate, with its thinnest dimension directly in the plane of motion of the elbow, was insufficient to withstand the forces applied to it in this muscular, active young man. An unacceptable 30 degrees recurvatum deformity soon developed, with pain and instability at the fracture site. **B.** Revision with a lag screw and broad 4.5-mm compression plate restored local anatomy and resulted in rapid union. Compression plates are the implants of choice for humeral shaft fractures, especially in active young individuals.

study showed a 97% union rate in upper extremity injuries in which plate fixation was accomplished with LCD plates (57).

Locking plates represent the newest advance in plate technology. Screws are inserted into combination holes that can act in a conventional compression fashion or a locking mode. This is made possible by specially designed screws with threaded heads that lock into corresponding threads in the locking part of the screw hole, providing fixed-angle stability from multiple screws. At the present time, there is some preliminary evidence that the improved fixation seen with this device may be advantageous in the humeral shaft, especially when dealing with osteopenic bone (9,63).

Pearls and Pitfalls

Compression Plating

- Use an anterolateral approach for midshaft or proximal fractures, and a posterior approach for distal fractures
- Use a broad 4.5-mm compression plate in most patients, with a minimum of three (and preferably four) screws proximal and distal. A 4.5-mm narrow plate is acceptable for smaller individuals
- Insert a lag screw between major fracture fragments, if possible
- Check the distal corner of the plate for radial nerve entrapment prior to closure following the anterolateral approach
- The intraoperative goal is to obtain sufficient stability to allow immediate postoperative shoulder and elbow motion

Intramedullary Nailing

Locking, large-diameter humeral nails were introduced with the hope that the results from their use would parallel the clinical success seen with similar devices used for femoral and tibial fractures (7,64–69). Previously available intramedullary implants for the humerus such as Rush pins or Enders nails, while effective in many cases with simple fracture patterns, had significant drawbacks such as poor or nonexistent axial or rotational stability (70–73). Henley reported a series of 49 patients with

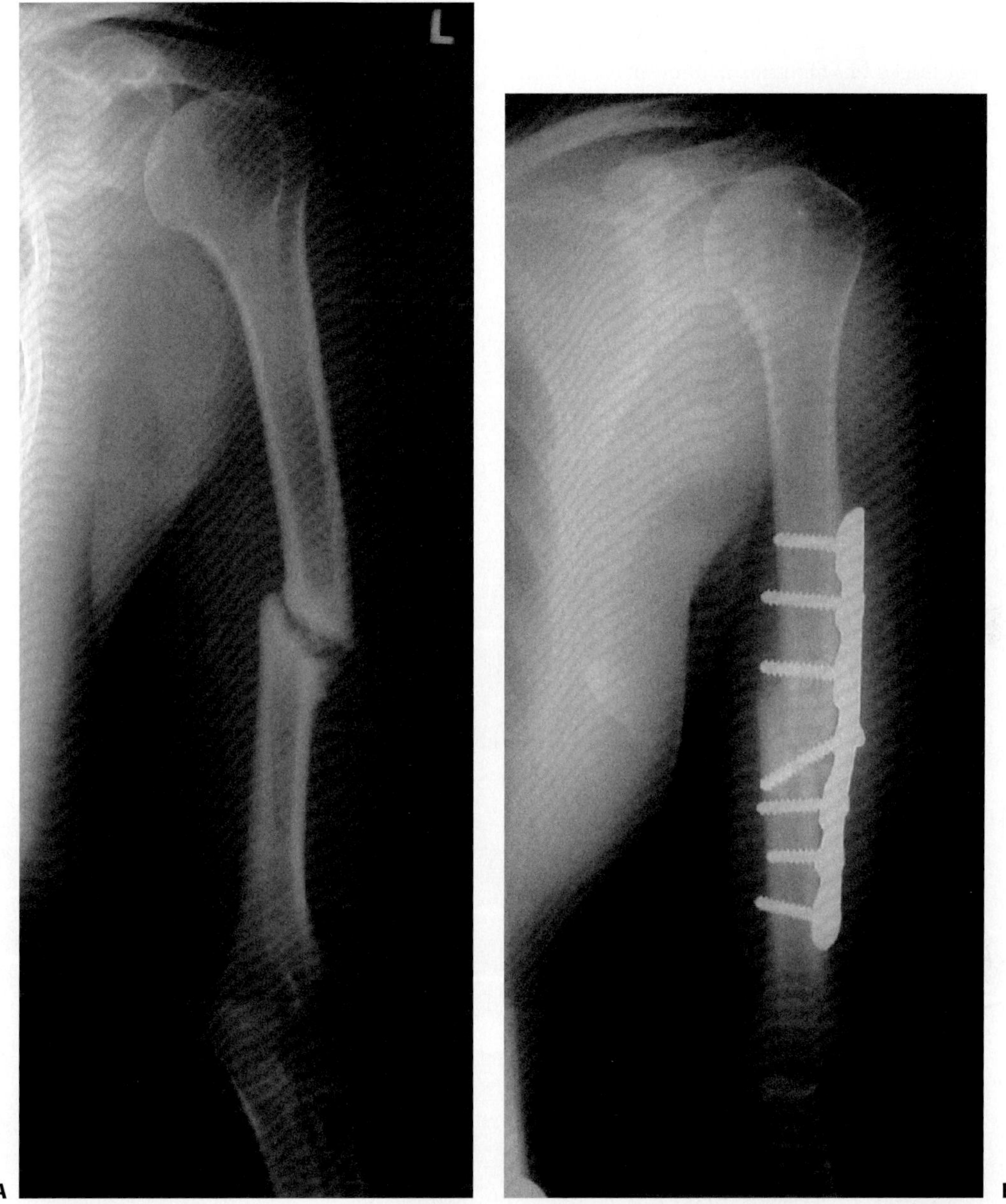

FIGURE 30-14 **A.** Humeral shaft nonunion in a 37-year-old woman 14 months following conservative treatment with functional bracing. **B.** Solid bony union after compression plate fixation (with a lag screw through the plate). The limited contact dynamic (LCD) plate allows greater angulation of screw placement through the plate compared to a conventional plate. The nonunion was not formally "taken down" or bone grafted since the alignment were reasonable and there were some intrinsic signs of bony healing. In this situation, where alignment and biology are favorable, rigid fixation and nonunion site compression alone are usually successful. (From Pugh DMW, McKee MD. Advances in the management of humeral nonunion. *J Am Acad Orthop Surg* 2003;11:48–59.)

humeral shaft fractures treated with Ender nailing and had only one nonunion, and Brumback reported a 94% union rate with Rush pins and Enders nails, although there was a significant rate of insertion site morbidity and backing out of the nails such that the "excellent" clinical success rate was much lower (62%) (18,74). However, especially when used for comminuted or unstable fracture patterns, some form of additional stabilization was required, either internal (cerclage wire at the fracture site) or external (prolonged splinting). The construct that resulted was often not stable enough to allow early motion or upper extremity weight-bearing in the case of the multiply injured patient with concomitant lower extremity injuries.

With the newer generation of nails came a number of locking mechanisms distally including interference fits from expandable bolts (Seidel nail) or ridged fins (Trueflex nail) or interlocking screws (Russell-Taylor nail, Synthes nail, Biomet nail). Unfortunately, despite favorable initial reports, these devices have not enjoyed the unparalled success of lower extremity locking nails. Problems such as insertion site morbidity, iatrogenic fracture comminution (especially in small diameter canals), and nonunion (and significant difficulty in its salvage) have been reported (Fig. 30-15) (75–79). In addition, some of the perceived advantages of nailing over compression plating (such as earlier upper extremity ambulation and avoiding peri-implant fracture) have proven to be illusory (66,76). A number of randomized clinical trials comparing these intramedullary implants to compression plating have been performed (73,80–82). They have shown a higher reoperation rate and greater shoulder morbidity with the use of nails. At the present time, in our institution, the use of locking nails is restricted to widely separate segmental fractures, pathological fractures, fractures in patients with morbid obesity, and fractures with poor soft tissue over the fracture site (such as burns). A number of newer nails, designed to eliminate insertion site morbidity through an extra-articular start point, have been introduced (see below); it remains to be seen whether prospective, randomized trials will prove their advantages.

Original nail sizes were limited; thus, most locking humeral nails required reaming prior to insertion. While the reamings produced may improve fracture union, there are some drawbacks. The fracture site must be kept closely apposed during reaming to prevent radial nerve damage. Also, the distal humeral canal tapers to a blind end above the olecranon fossa: it does not have a wide metaphyseal flare to vent debris or heat in front of an advancing reamer as does the femur or tibia. There is evidence that excessive reaming of the medullary canal can be detrimental. Reimer et al reported a 58% complication rate in patients undergoing Seidel humeral nailing when the humeral canal size was 9 mm or less, and postulated extensive reaming was one of the contributing factors (83). Others have reported extensive heat necrosis from excessive reaming, and we have experience with similar cases (84,85). If there is not sufficient

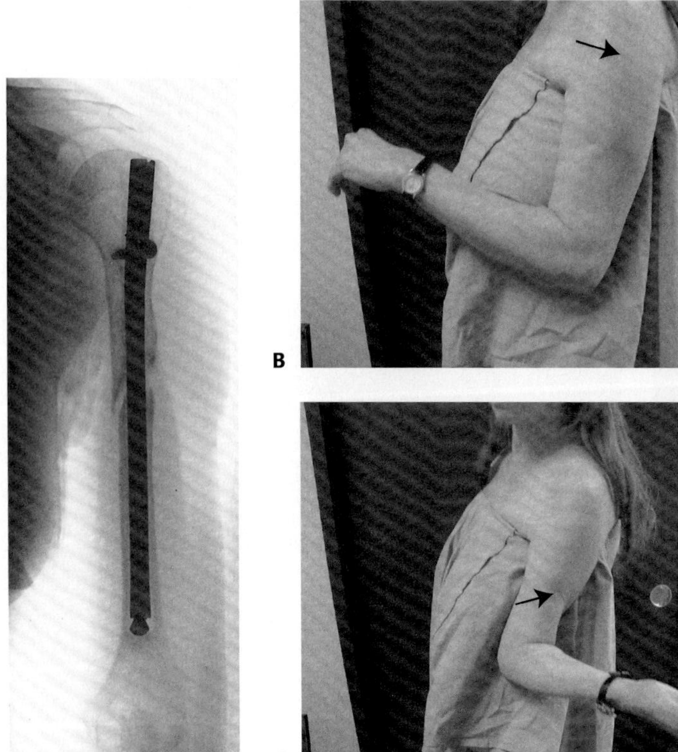

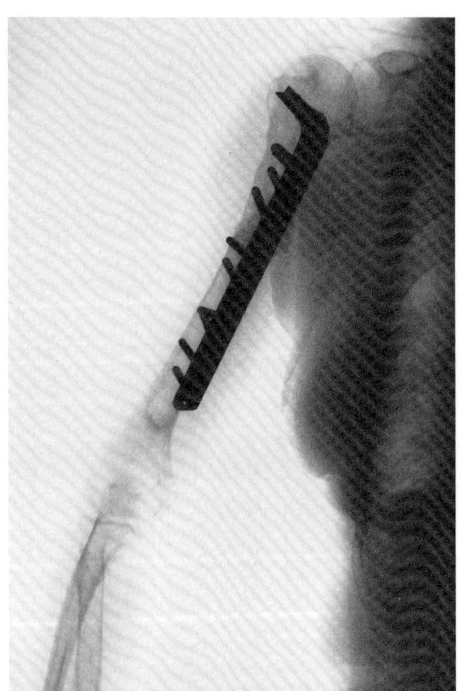

FIGURE 30-15 **A.** Gross rotational instability was present in a 41-year-old woman 7 months after having undergone reamed antegrade intramedullary nailing of a humeral shaft fracture. The distal interference fit of the nail failed. **B.** Clinical photographs of a similar patient. The incisional scar can be seen on the anterior aspect of her shoulder (*arrow*). The patient is facing straight ahead. **C.** It is possible for the patient to externally rotate her lower arm over 90 degrees without changing the orientation of her shoulder at all: the rotation occurs completely through the rotationally unstable nonunion. The skin and soft tissue can be seen bunching up at the mid-humeral level of the nonunion (*arrows*). **D.** Union following nail removal, bone grafting, judicious humeral shortening and blade plate fixation. (**A,D** from McKee MD, Miranda MA, Riemer BL, et al. Management of humeral nonunion after the failure of locking intramedullary nails. *J Orthop Trauma* 1996;10(7)492–499.)

space, one risks distracting the fracture site as the nail wedges in the distal fragment during insertion (Fig. 30-16). One point emphasized in most series of large-diameter nails is that the humerus does not tolerate distraction. This is a risk factor for delayed and nonunion. Newer nail designs have smaller (7, 8, or 9 mm) diameter implants that are better suited to small canal diameters.

Antegrade Technique

The patient is placed in the beach-chair, semisitting position, with the affected arm draped free. The image intensifier is brought in directly laterally on the injured side, and the patient brought to the edge of the table. The head is taped in place on a pad. Before proceeding, it is important to check and ensure a good x-ray of the entire humerus is possible. It may be necessary to have the patient lying partially off the table on a radiolucent support. The surgeon stands at the top of the bed looking down on the shoulder and the assistant stands below on the other side of the image holding the arm. A small incision is made at the antero-lateral corner of the acromion, the deltoid is split, and any visible subdeltoid bursa is excised. The supraspinatus tendon is identified, and split for 1 to 2 cm in line with its fibers. The entry point for a standard antegrade nail is in the greater tuberosity, just lateral to the articular margin. The canal is broached with either an awl or a starter reamer placed over a guide wire. A long guide wire is then passed to the fracture site, and it should be colinear with the medullary canal. If the start point is too lateral, iatrogenic fracture of the proximal lateral cortex is a risk when the nail is inserted. The fracture is reduced with gentle longitudinal traction and manipulation, and the guide wire is passed across the fracture site. Extreme difficulty in reducing the fracture and passing the guide wire, especially in isthmal fractures, should alert the surgeon to the possibility of soft tissue (radial nerve) entrapment. In technology similar to that used for sciatic nerve monitoring during acetabular fracture fixation, Mills et al described using somatosensory evoked potentials (SSEP) during closed humeral nailing to detect nerve injury. They found that they could detect signal change with impending nerve injury and in at least one case this prompted an open procedure with the finding of radial nerve entrapment in the fracture site (86). However, this technology is not widely used at this time and the incidence of permanent radial nerve injury, despite its proximity to the humeral shaft, is surprisingly low during closed nailing. If the fracture is open, the fracture site should be inspected visually to be sure it is free of soft-tissue entrapment as the guide wire is passed. Using a combination of fluoroscopy and arm rotation, the guide wire is checked in two planes to ensure accurate placement.

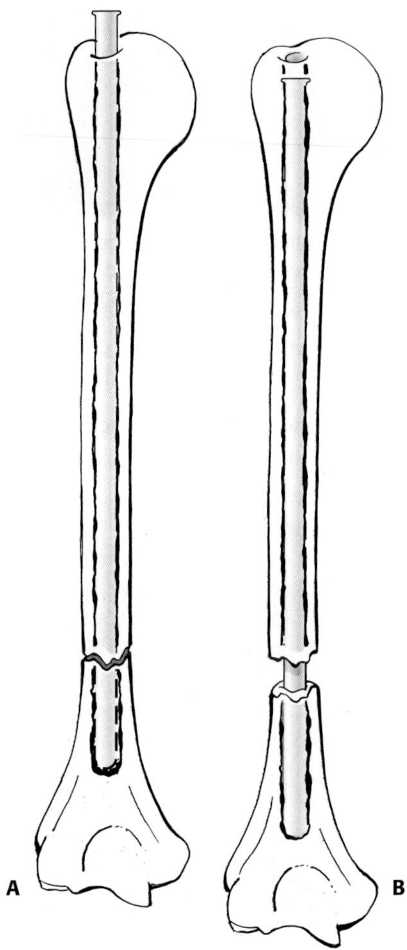

FIGURE 30-16 Fracture site distraction during intramedullary nailing. Since the humeral canal tapers to a blind end, if the nail is too long as it is impacted to avoid impingement in the shoulder **(A)**, it abuts the end of the canal and distracts the fracture site **(B)**. Fracture site distraction following humeral nailing is poorly tolerated and is a common finding in delayed unions and nonunions.

We usually ream minimally, until the sound of cortical chatter is heard, and then insert a nail 1 mm smaller in diameter than the last reamer used. Care is taken to keep the fracture well reduced during the reaming process. The length of nail is carefully chosen and checked twice: if a nail too long is picked, one risks distracting the fracture site as the nail impacts the tapered end of the humeral canal as it is advanced in an attempt to seat it below the tuberosity proximally. Leaving the nail proud proximally will result in an increased incidence and severity of impingement (Fig. 30-17). Biomechanical studies have shown that nails locked with screws are axially and torsionally superior to so-called interference fit nail designs (Fig. 30-18) (87). The nail is then locked with screws using a jig proximally and a freehand technique distally. Distal anteroposterior locking is done through a small open incision; risk to the brachial artery, median nerve, and musculocutaneous nerve is minimized by the open approach and by staying lateral to the biceps muscle and tendon. The radial nerve is at risk during lateral to medial locking (88). While the nerve does not necessarily need to be seen and isolated, a incision with blunt dissection to bone, clear visualization of the tract and bony drill site, and use of a protec-

ment for pin tract infections. Although Mostafavi and Tornetta had good or excellent results in 12 of 18 of their patients treated with external fixation the complication rate was high: three malunions, one delayed union, eight pin tract infections (two with a sequestrum), and two refractures following fixator removal (101). While these results may indicate a selection bias, where only the worst injuries with the most extensive soft-tissue damage were treated with this technique, in general external fixation is cumbersome for the humerus and the complication rate is high. This is especially true for the pin sites, where a thick envelope of muscle and soft tissue between the bone and the skin and constant motion of the elbow and shoulder accentuate the risk of delayed union and malunion, resulting in significant rates of pin tract irritation, infection, and pin breakage.

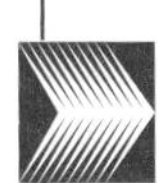

AUTHOR'S PREFERRED TREATMENT

Compression plate fixation is my treatment of choice for those humeral shaft fractures that have an operative indication. I prefer the anterolateral approach unless the fracture is so distal that preoperative planning suggests it will not be possible to place four screws distally: if this is the case, a posterior approach is performed (102). When dealing with open humeral shaft fractures it is important to adhere to the principles of open fracture treatment. The open wound is inspected, any obvious debris (e.g., grass, clothing, dirt) is removed, and a sterile dressing is applied. The arm is splinted and prophylactic antibiotics started intravenously. Penicillin is added for injuries that occur in barnyard or sewer environments. Tetanus prophylaxis is given if required. The patient should be transferred emergently to the operating room where any associated life-threatening injuries take priority. Once these (or other orthopaedic injuries of greater urgency) are dealt with, attention is focused on the (open) humeral shaft fracture. Grossly contaminated wounds are subjected to a nonsterile scrub with copious sterile saline and a chlorhexidine scrub brush. For the anterolateral approach, the patient is positioned sitting up 30 to 45 degrees (favorable for polytrauma patients with abdominal, chest, or head injuries) and the arm is prepared in sterile fashion and draped free. An anterolateral approach is then performed (see Surgical Approach): any open wounds are debrided, and if possible, included in the incision. The bone ends are exposed and thoroughly cleaned of debris and hematoma, taking care to preserve any soft-tissue attachments to bony fragments. In open fractures, the medullary canal is carefully inspected as occasionally ground debris can be impacted far up the canal of the proximal fragment, especially in falls from a height, and this material must be removed. Completely devitalized cortical fragments are removed. For open fractures, the wound and incision are then copiously irrigated with a minimum of nine liters of sterile saline with added bacitracin (50,000 IU/L). The radial nerve is identified distally between the brachialis and the brachioradialis, and protected throughout the case. Care is taken not to pinch the nerve under the distal lateral corner of the plate (Fig. 30-8). If radial nerve function is impaired or absent preoperatively, it is explored. This protects the nerve from further damage and adds useful prognostic information. If the nerve is found to be completely avulsed, the epineurium at the ends is tagged with a nonabsorbable, colored suture, for easier identification later, but primary repair (in blunt trauma cases) is usually not indicated (21–24).

The fracture is then reduced and temporarily fixed with a 2-mm Kirschner wire. If possible a lag screw is inserted across the main fracture line. For most individuals, a broad 4.5-mm compression plate will be the implant of choice. The occasional small-boned patient may require a narrow 4.5-mm plate. A minimum six hole (with a lag screw) or eight hole (no lag screw) plate is contoured and applied. The fixation and radial nerve are checked, and an intraoperative radiograph is taken. Adjacent muscle is loosely approximated to obtain complete coverage of the plate, and a standard closure performed: drains are not typically necessary. Any open wounds are left open, and only the surgical extensions are closed. A sterile dressing and well-padded posterior splint are applied. The dressing and splint are removed at 48 hours postinjury. Wounds that have residual necrotic tissue, appear infected, have exposed bone or require repeat debridement due to a high probability of residual contaminated material are returned to the operating room for repeat debridement and irrigation. The wound can then be closed in a delayed primary fashion, if possible, or allowed to granulate in and heal by secondary intention. Larger defects may require a split-thickness skin graft to accelerate rehabilitation. More extensive soft-tissue defects can be dealt with by a variety of local rotational (biceps) or pedicled (latissimus) flaps. Patients are encouraged to begin early, active motion of the shoulder and elbow under the supervision of a physiotherapist. If upper extremity weight-bearing is required, an elbow gutter crutch is prescribed.

I reserve intramedullary nailing for patients with pathological fractures, widely separate segmental fractures, or fractures with soft-tissue conditions that would preclude or complicate plating, such as morbid obesity or local burns. While either plating or nailing is acceptable for most patients with humeral shaft fractures, I specifically avoid nailing in patients with preexisting shoulder pathology, those with narrow diameter humeral canals (<9 mm), those who will be permanent upper extremity weight-bearers and those with recognized radial nerve palsies. An antegrade approach is used for midshaft or proximal fractures, and a retrograde approach for distal fractures is ideal. I use a reamed nail locked with screws proximally and distally. I ream sparingly, stopping at the sound or feel of cortical "chatter," and insert a nail 1 mm narrower than the last reamer. Great care is taken not to distract the fracture site with nail insertion. I usually err on the side of choosing a shorter, rather than longer, nail for this reason (Fig. 30-16). It is important to use a mini-open approach for the distal locking screws to avoid damage to neurovascular structures (88–90).

I no longer use small-diameter flexible nails for humeral shaft fractures.

External fixation is useful in two situations. One is when rapid stabilization of the humerus is required, as in a critically ill patient with multiple injuries, or in a fracture associated with a vascular injury where rapid stabilization can provide a stable platform for emergent vascular repair (98–101). The other is when the associated soft tissue injuries or contamination (Gustilo type III) are so severe that plate fixation would result in exposed hardware or residual contamination. Using a large external fixator set, I insert two pins from an anterolateral direction proximally and two pins distally (using a mini-open technique) and connect them with two straight bars. However, our recent experience with compression plating in these situations has been so favorable that the indications for external fixation in my practice have become very limited.

CLINICAL TRIALS OF PLATE FIXATION VERSUS INTRAMEDULLARY NAILING

There are numerous retrospective reviews of antegrade-locked intramedullary nailing and compression plating in the literature (17,55–60,64–67). Overall, they would suggest that the risk of shoulder pain is much less in patients treated with plates (essentially zero versus 5% to 42% with antegrade nailing) and there is a trend toward a decreased nonunion rate with plating. However, these studies, like all retrospective studies, have inherent biases, including patient selection, a high lost to follow-up rate, incomplete outcome data, and surgeon bias. Randomized clinical trials (RCTs) have been designed to overcome the biases inherent in prior observational studies, and are now considered the gold standard for evaluating fracture treatment. There have been three RCTs that have compared locked intramedullary nailing to compression plating (80–82). Although they are small in numbers, their design is solid and represents the best information on this topic. A recent meta-analysis conducted on these studies revealed that patients in the plated group had a lower rate of reoperation (6% vs. 18%, $p = 0.03$), and a lower rate of shoulder pain (1% vs. 21%, $p = 0.002$) (54). There were also more nonunions in the nail group (8/73, 11%) than in the plate group (5/83, 6%), although this difference did not reach statistical significance with the numbers available. These studies certainly did not confirm the theoretical advantages of locked intramedullary nailing of humeral shaft fractures and have re-established compression plating as the treatment of choice for the majority of these injuries (Table 30-3).

HUMERAL FRACTURES ASSOCIATIONS

Radial Nerve Palsy

There is an intimate anatomic relationship between the radial nerve and the humeral shaft (11,21,88). Thus, it is not surprising that the commonest nerve palsy following a humeral shaft fracture is a radial nerve palsy. This is typically due to contusion and/or stretching of the nerve in the spiral groove at the moment of fracture. There is limited "give" in the nerve as it is tethered proximally as a terminal branch of the brachial plexus and distally as it exits through the lateral intermuscular septum. The incidence of radial nerve palsy is directly proportional to the degree of violence of the initial trauma. It ranges from 3% to 34% and increases with open fractures, polytrauma, vascular injury, and multiple ipsilateral fractures (1,4,20–24). Tingstad et al reported an incidence of radial nerve palsy of 34% in 111 fractures predominantly in polytrauma patients (60), and Connolly et al reported an incidence of 14 radial nerve injuries in 53 open fractures (26%) (103). Fortunately most of these lesions are neuropraxic injuries of the nerve: spontaneous recovery is the rule. Ogawa and Ui reported 100% recovery in one large series (104), Pollock et al reported a recovery rate of 90% in closed fractures (23), and Sarmiento et al reported a 100% recovery rate in 85 patients with distal humeral shaft fractures (105). However, there is some evidence that the prognosis for recovery with high-energy or open fractures is not as good. Sanders et al presented 12 cases of open humeral shaft fractures associated with radial nerve injury; only four recovered function (106). Ring et al described six radial nerve transections in 24 patients with high-energy humeral shaft fractures with an associated radial nerve palsy (24). Connolly reported that 4 of 14 radial nerve injuries in patients with open fractures did not recover and required nerve grafting (103).

Given the propensity for spontaneous recovery (and the lack of any evidence that early exploration improves outcome), it is clear that, in general, the presence of a radial nerve injury in isolation is not an indication for operative management of a humeral shaft fracture (Fig. 30-21). However, there are accepted indications for exploration of the radial nerve in the setting of a humeral shaft fracture. If there is another indication for operative repair, such as an open wound or an associated ipsilateral injury, then the injured nerve should be explored for a number of reasons. First, it is of prognostic value. While a contused or stretched nerve is the most likely finding, if a completely severed nerve is found then this helps guide early nerve reconstruction or tendon transfer after fracture healing (24,106). Secondly, the nerve may be injured due to entrapment in the fracture site, compression by bony fragments or other physical obstruction and thus it is prudent to release and protect the nerve during fracture fixation. Third, in rare instances, primary repair of a completely lacerated nerve may be indicated. In most cases, extensive contusion and stretching make such an endeavor unrewarding, as the zone of injury of the nerve is often indistinct and the chance of recovery slim. For example, Ring et al reported that none of the five transected radial nerves repaired

TABLE 30-3 Advantages and Disadvantages of Plate Fixation, Intramedullary Fixation, and External Fixation of Humeral Shaft Fractures

Parameter	Plate Fixation	Intramedullary Nails	External Fixators
Fracture around implant	–	–	+
Shoulder morbidity	+	–	+
Difficulty of reconstruction if primary treatment fails	+/–	–	+
Nonunion rate	+	–	–
Reoperation rate	+	–	–
Radial nerve injury	+/–	+/–	+/–
Small canal	+	–	+
Radiation exposure	+	–	–
Complex fractures	–	+	–
Intra-articular fracture extension	+	–	–

+, advantage; –, disadvantage.

primarily in a series of high-energy humeral shaft fractures recovered (24). However, in instances where there is a clean laceration of the nerve from a bone fragment or sharp instrument (such as a machete) then primary repair may be successful and Foster et al reported good results with primary nerve repair (four of five repaired nerves recovered) (55).

Radial nerve palsies associated with low-velocity gunshot wounds may also recover spontaneously. Rather than being transected by the projectile, in most cases the nerve has been damaged by the concussive blast or shock-wave associated with the path of the bullet, or contused by bony fragments, and is structurally intact (6).

Following a radial nerve injury, the patient should be given a cock-up wrist splint and instructed to perform daily passive wrist, finger, and thumb range of motion exercises to prevent the development of a flexion contracture. Some authorities recommend that baseline electromyography and nerve conduction studies be performed at 3 weeks postinjury so that later studies can be compared to them (107,108). The patient is observed clinically for any sign of recovery of the nerve, which is typically seen in the first muscles innervated distal to the injury: the brachioradialis and extensor carpi radialis brevis and longus. The electrical equivalent is the development of action potentials where complete denervation or fibrillation was noted before. One should expect to see nerve regeneration proceed at a rate of 1 inch per month. If no electrical or clinical activity can be identified by 3 to 4 months postinjury (depending on the site of the fracture), then surgical exploration of the nerve is indicated. Resection of the damaged portion of the nerve followed by cable graft reconstruction is usually required. If nerve reconstruction is unsuccessful or not indicated, tendon transfers are an ideal procedure to restore function, since the major contribution of the radial nerve to the hand is motor function.

Brachial Plexus Palsy

The successful outcome of functional bracing for humeral shaft fractures depends on a number of factors, including a compliant patient, an upright position, the "hydraulic" effect of a well-fitted splint, and the contraction of the associated muscles. Sarmiento et al point out that the muscle contraction during activity when the patient is in a splint helps to "align the fragments in a parallel direction, correcting the malrotation" (6). In patients with a significant brachial plexus palsy this intrinsic muscle tone and contraction may be lost, resulting in a much higher incidence of malunion and/or nonunion (Fig. 30-22). Also, the associated sensory loss may lead to ulceration of insensate skin under a tight splint or cast. There is relatively little in the literature regarding this topic, but Brien et al reported on 21 cases of humeral shaft fracture with associated brachial plexus palsy and reported superior results with plate fixation (three of three united) (109). Of the 11 fractures treated nonoperatively, there were five nonunions, two delayed unions, and two malunions. The flail extremity interfered with rehabilitation and led to pro-

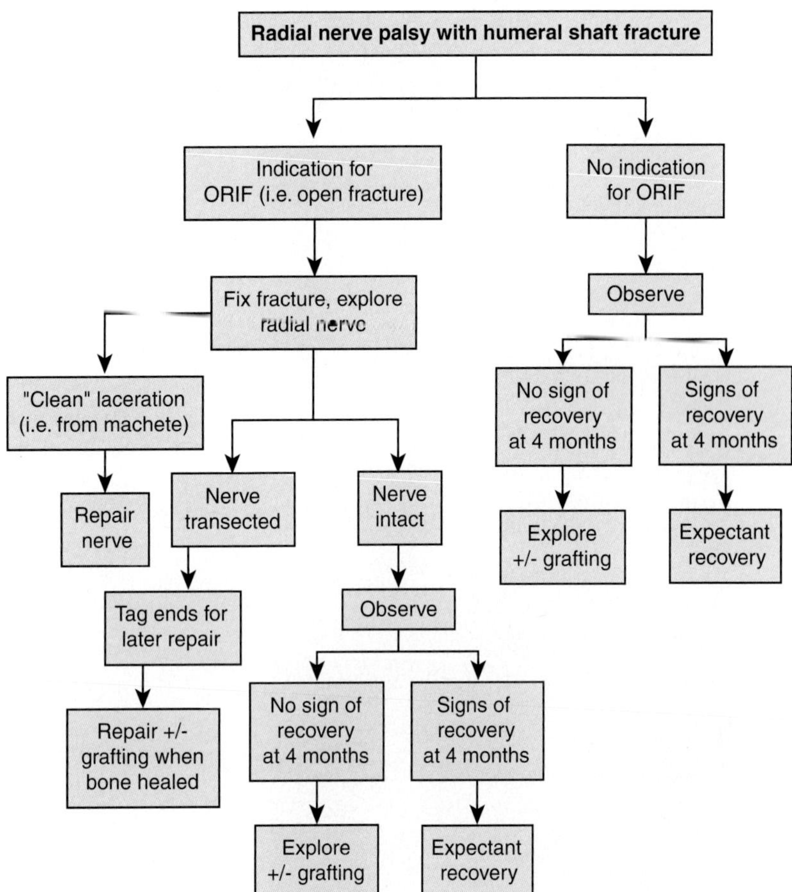

FIGURE 30-21 An algorithm for the management of radial nerve palsy in association with a humeral shaft fracture.

longed hospital stays. Additionally, only 2 of 21 patients showed any neurologic recovery. The authors described a much higher incidence of associated injuries in this patient population (11 traumatic brain injuries), which often represent independent indications for operative intervention. Thus, an ipsilateral brachial plexus injury represents a strong relative indication for primary plate fixation of an associated humeral shaft fracture.

Pathological Bone

A metastatic deposit from a malignant neoplasm is the commonest cause of a pathologic fracture of the shaft of a long bone in an adult (110,111). The long bone most affected is the femur, followed by the humerus, which accounted for 96 of 588 pathological fractures (16%) in one large series (112). These fractures usually occur late in the clinical course of the illness and are often a significant source of pain. The associated functional loss can be critically important in the typical older, debilitated patient and can result in a decreased quality of life, dependency on others, possible hospitalization or institutionalization, and increased medical costs. While aggressive surgical treatment is not usually indicated in the moribund, cachetic patient, judicious intervention in a patient with a life expectancy measured in months or greater is often beneficial from both a patient-oriented and societal perspective.

Unfortunately, when dealing with pathological humeral shaft fractures from malignant lesions, conservative care (consisting mainly of splinting and/or radiation) provides some symptomatic relief but rarely provides fracture healing or stability. Douglass et al reported dismal results in a series of patients with pathological humeral shaft fractures treated with radiation and immobilization (113). Pain relief was evident in 5 of 9 treated with radiotherapy and only 3 of 12 treated with immobilization. Flemming and Beals reported on eight such patients treated conservatively and described poor pain relief with half having poor function (114). These unsatisfactory results have led other investigators to pursue operative avenues of treatment. For patients with a finite life expectancy, the ideal treatment would stabilize the entire shaft of the humerus, be performed through a small incision away from the metastatic disease (to allow radiotherapy without affecting incisional healing), minimize bleeding by not exposing the fracture site and tumor, and allow early motion and rapid return of function. Fracture healing per se is not as important as it is in a routine patient, and a stable mechanical construct that will last a finite period of time is the main goal. This discussion pertains to patients with established

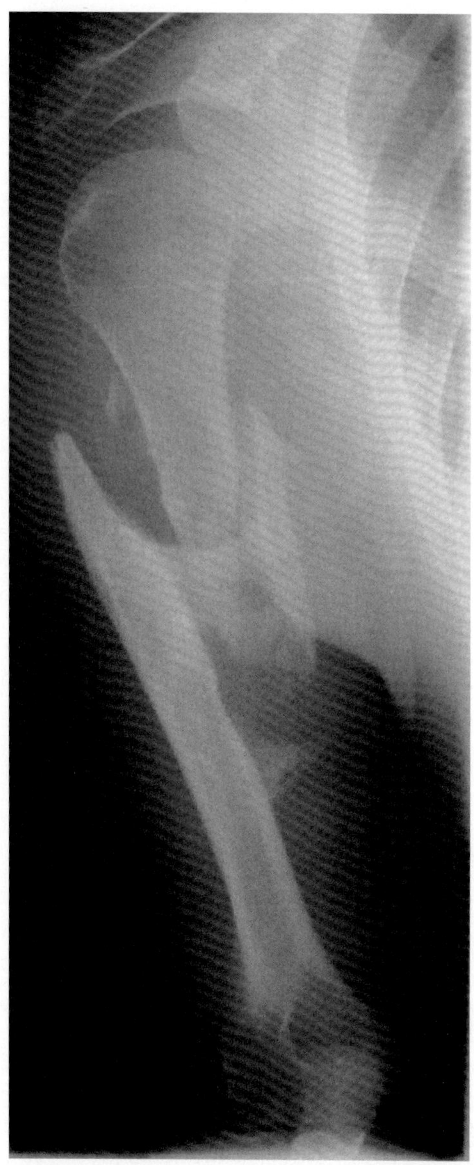

FIGURE 30-22 A humeral pseudarthrosis 14 months following a fracture complicated by a severe brachial plexus injury. Lacking normal muscle tension and tone, these injuries have a high rate of delay and nonunion.

metastatic disease from an incurable systemic cancer; resection and reconstruction of primary malignant disease or an isolated metastasis with the potential for long-term survival (such as renal cell carcinoma) is beyond the scope of this chapter.

Harrington et al reported one of the first surgical experiences with a large number of patients with pathological humeral fractures, and reported good results in 68 cases treated with Rush pinning and, in most cases, polymethlymethacrylate cement augmentation (115). In a series that originated from the Mayo Clinic, Lewallen et al (and later Yazawa et al) described a similar technique with good results: 48 of 55 patients in Lewallen's paper had good relief of pain (116,117). Lancaster used a larger diameter Kuntscher nail and reported pain relief in 26 of 29 patients (118). However, they also had to open the fracture site and add polymethylmethacrylate cement to obtain rotational and axial stability. This is undesirable from a number of standpoints including increased blood loss, increased operative time, higher morbidity (from infection), and, if radiation is to be used, wound healing complications. The advent of larger diameter locking humeral nails has dramatically improved the care of patients with pathological humeral shaft fractures. In a definitive article on the subject, Redmond et al performed closed, locked humeral nailing on 16 patients and reported good to excellent pain relief in all but one patient, with 14 extremities returning to "near normal" function within 3 weeks (119). Radiation was initiated at a mean of 7 days postoperatively in 14 humeri, with no infections, nerve palsies, or implant failures; and only one reoperation for the removal of a locking screw was required (Fig. 30-23). The rotational and axial control obtained by the locking screws eliminates the need to address stability at the fracture site directly. Thus, radiotherapy can be initiated earlier because there is no incision there. In this specific situation, closed locked humeral nailing has significant advantages over compression plating, and should be considered the treatment of choice for affected individuals.

An open approach to the tumor site is best reserved for patients where tissue is required for diagnosis, or a definitive resection of the tumor mass is planned to gain sufficient local control to allow anticipated long-term survival (such as in isolated metastasis from renal cell carcinoma). In this situation, the technique of Chin et al, with segmental resection followed by metallic, cement, or allograft replacement and plating is recommended (120). Fractures in the metaphyseal region that are not amenable to stabilization with an intramedullary nail are best treated with prosthetic reconstruction.

Benign tumors or conditions (such as aneurysmal bone cysts or fibrous dysplasia) may weaken the bone sufficiently to result in a fracture from minimal force or trauma. In most cases, despite what may appear to be an unfavorable radiographic picture, closed treatment will result in healing. Often, the healing osseous response will obliterate or at least attenuate the lesion. Thus, the initial approach for the majority of pathological fractures from benign tumors is nonoperative.

Open Wounds

Although present in less than 10% of humeral shaft fractures, an open wound complicates treatment, and there is relatively little specific information in the literature to aid in decision making. The patient with an open humeral shaft fracture has often sustained high-energy trauma and has an increased incidence of radial nerve palsy, fracture comminution, ipsilateral upper extremity fractures, and systemic injuries. Most available information is contained in larger series on the treatment of humeral shaft fractures that include a small percentage of fractures with associated open wounds, and a variety of treatment techniques have been described (55–60).

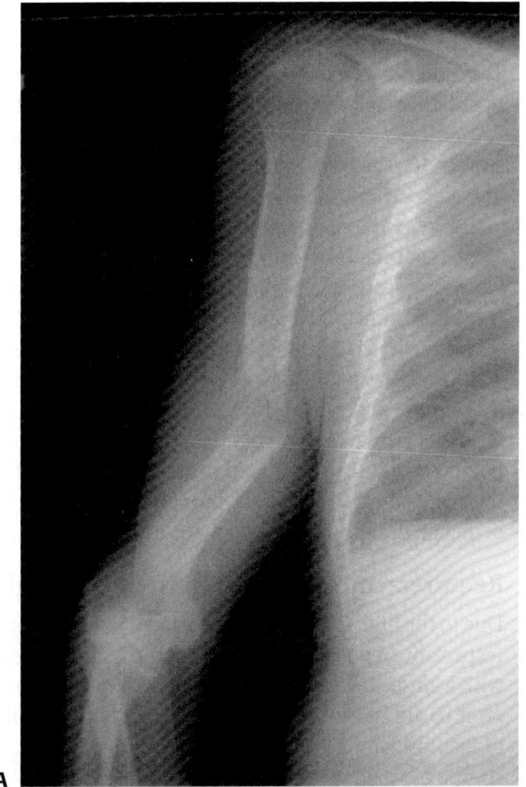

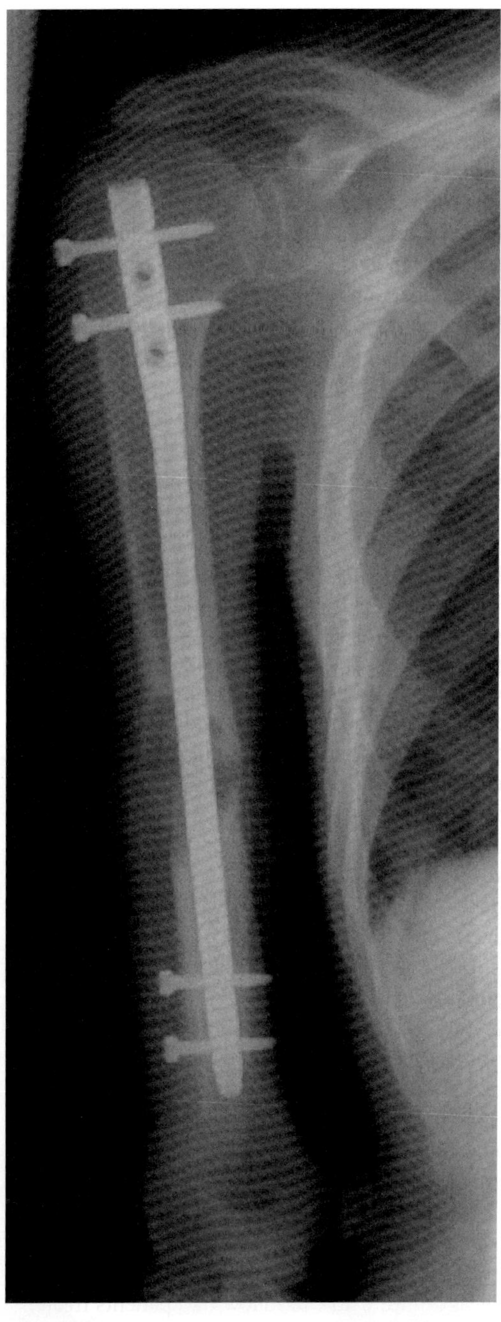

FIGURE 30-23 **A.** Pathological humeral shaft fracture through a lytic defect caused by a deposit of metastatic carcinoma. **B.** Treatment with a statically locked closed humeral nail resulted in immediate stability and good pain relief: since there was no incision over the fracture site, early radiation therapy could be initiated (courtesy of Ralph B. Blasier, MD).

Open Reduction and Internal Fixation

Vander Griend and colleagues reported on open reduction and internal fixation of 34 humeral shaft fractures, 13 of which were open (58). Although all 13 were plated and eventually healed without infection, only five had immediate plate osteosynthesis. The remaining eight were plated secondarily after temporizing methods were used initially. In the only series dealing exclusively with the issue, Connolly et al reviewed 53 consecutive patients from our level 1 trauma center managed with immediate plating of open humeral shaft fractures (103). Three patients underwent early amputation due to associated vascular injuries with mangled extremities, three were lost to follow-up, and one died. Forty-six patients were followed to definitive outcome, and they reported excellent results with no deep infections, no malunions and nonunions. Forty fractures healed at an average of 18.6 weeks postinjury. There were six delayed unions that healed on average at 10.1 months postinjury, but none of these patients required other operative procedures to obtain union. The authors stressed the importance of a standard surgical protocol including thorough irrigation and debridement, stable fix-

Total Shoulder Arthroplasty

There are a number of reports describing periprosthetic fractures following total shoulder arthroplasty, and the prevalence of such injuries has ranged from 1.6% to 2.4% (124–127). As with other periprosthetic fractures, the quality of the bone, location of the fracture and implant fixation are the main determinants of treatment and outcome. These fractures are classified as type A—at the tip of the stem extending proximally, type B—at the tip of the stem plus or minus some distal extension, and type C—distal to the tip of the stem (127). The conservative treatment of type C fractures is associated with a high success rate. Campbell reported healing in four of four such fractures (125), and the high union rate (five of six) of these fractures treated in a splint in the series by Kumar et al led the authors to state that for type C fractures "a trial of nonoperative treatment is recommended" (126). Type B fractures have a worse prognosis with conservative care. Six of seven did not heal in a series by Boyd et al, and four of five did not heal in the series of Kumar et al (124,126). While a trial of conservative care in a well-aligned type B fracture with a stable component may be reasonable, a lack of clear progression toward union should prompt operative intervention. Newer plates with the ability to enhance fixation proximally with cerclage wire mounts are useful in this regard. A fracture around a loose prosthesis should be treated with a long-stem revision, with autogenous bone grafting of the fracture site. Type A fractures are usually associated with a loose stem, and if this is the case, require operative intervention similar to type B fractures. In the unlikely event that the humeral component is stable, a trial of splinting is indicated.

COMPLICATIONS

Complications after Intramedullary Nailing

Insertion Site Morbidity

Insertion site pain and discomfort is a feature of many intramedullary nails, be it anterior knee pain following tibial nailing or shoulder pain after antegrade humeral nailing. Despite variations in insertion technique and implant design, persistent shoulder pain remains a problem following antegrade humeral nailing. Modifications of the insertion technique have ranged from "mini" incisions at the edge of the rotator cuff in an attempt to avoid cuff damage altogether to formal open approaches with partial anterior acromioplasty, division of the rotator cuff, insertion of the nail, and subsequent cuff repair (64–68). The basic problem lies in the fact that the medullary canal is in line with the articular surface of the humeral head and the rotator cuff, and the insertion area is an anatomically limited one where any soft-tissue swelling, nail protrusion, or other perturbation can result in painful impingement-like symptoms (Fig. 30-17). In the initial enthusiasm for this technique the incidence of shoulder problems was extremely variable, and, in general, underreported. Reimer reported excellent shoulder function in 17 of 18 patients who underwent antegrade Seidel nailing (67). In 1991 Habernek and Ortner (in their original series on Seidel nailing of humeral shaft fractures) reported that "all cases regained full shoulder movement with no functional impairment by an average of six weeks" (130). However, to their credit, the same authors later stated in a letter to the editor of the journal in which their work was published, regarding antegrade humeral nailing through a standard portal, that "this inevitably leads to damage of the cuff. . . .When we reviewed the 19 active patients in 1991, we did not address their shoulders and this should have been addressed" (131). Subsequently, other authors reported much higher rates of shoulder pain and dysfunction following antegrade nailing including Robinson et al (12 of 17 patients) and Ingman and Waters (100%) causing a change to the retrograde technique (64,66).

With proper technique, the shoulder pain that is associated with the insertion of humeral nails is usually self-limited and temporary. Proper technique includes minimizing damage to the cuff by protecting the edges during reaming, seating the nail well below the osseous surface, removing all reaming debris, carefully repairing the cuff on completion of the procedure and instituting early shoulder motion. However, despite all precautions shoulder pain may be severe enough to warrant further surgical intervention, up to and including acromioplasty, subacromial bursectomy, nail removal, and cuff repair. Patients who will be permanent upper extremity ambulators (such as those who are rendered para- or quadriplegic in the accident that causes their concomitant humeral shaft fracture) seem to be particularly vulnerable to violations of their subacromial space and rotator cuff. Intractable pain and impingement can be the result. Antegrade humeral nailing is relatively contraindicated in such individuals, and in those with a prior history of impingement, and a humeral shaft fracture should be plated if an indication for operative intervention exists in these patients.

There have been two separate approaches to eliminating the insertion site morbidity seen with antegrade humeral nailing. One was to adopt a retrograde technique, where the nail is inserted through the olecranon fossa. There are several series that describe this technique (66,92–94). However, complications include supracondylar fracture, elbow pain, triceps weakness, or elbow stiffness/ankylosis (Fig. 30-19).

The other approach was to design humeral nails that avoid the articular surface and rotator cuff by having alterations in the proximal portion of the nail that allow an extra-articular start point, analogous to the proximal bend in a tibial nail. A report in 2003 by Stannard et al describes a titanium, flexible, locking nail with a unique mechanism (7). Inserted in a flexible format, it allows an extra-articular starting point (1.5 cm distal to the greater tuberosity for antegrade insertion) and is tensioned by a screw in the end of the nail which stiffens the intercalated segments, producing a rigid construct. This is then locked in standard fashion. The Birmingham group reported on 42 fractures treated with this device, and reported an excellent union rate. Thirty-eight of 42 had no shoulder pain (mean Constant score of 90 points, range 50 to 100). There were however, five major complications requiring reoperation (nonunion, hardware failure, deep infection), all associated with the smaller

7.5-mm version of the implant. The authors cautioned that, considering these complications, "options other than intramedullary fixation should be considered" in patients with canals 8 mm or less in diameter (7). Analogous to previous reports of humeral nails, however, these results need further confirmation before the device can be recommended for general use.

Fractures at the End of the Nail

A well-recognized complication of plating of humeral shaft fractures is the potential for fracture at the end of the plate due to the stress-concentrating effect of the screws, or refracture following plate removal (Fig. 30-25) (25). It was thought that the introduction of locking humeral nails would lead to the elimination of this problem, as it has in the lower extremity with locked femoral and tibial nails. However, the anatomy of the distal humerus is fundamentally different from the tibia or femur: these lower extremity bones have a wide metaphyseal flare. The medullary canal of the distal humerus tapers rapidly to a narrow end above the olecranon fossa (11,36). Thus, the tip of the nail ends in diaphyseal, rather than metaphyseal, bone.

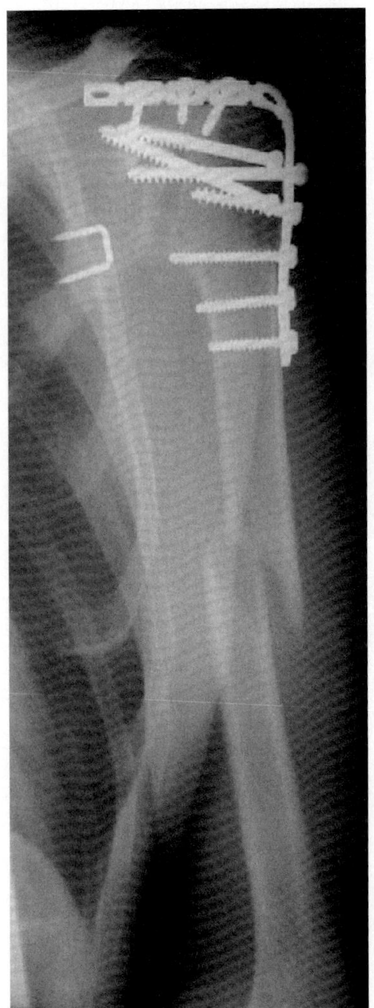

A

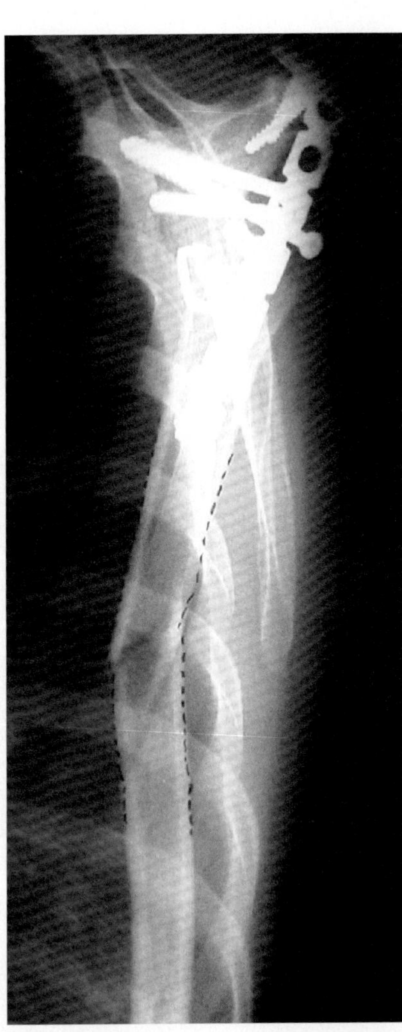

B

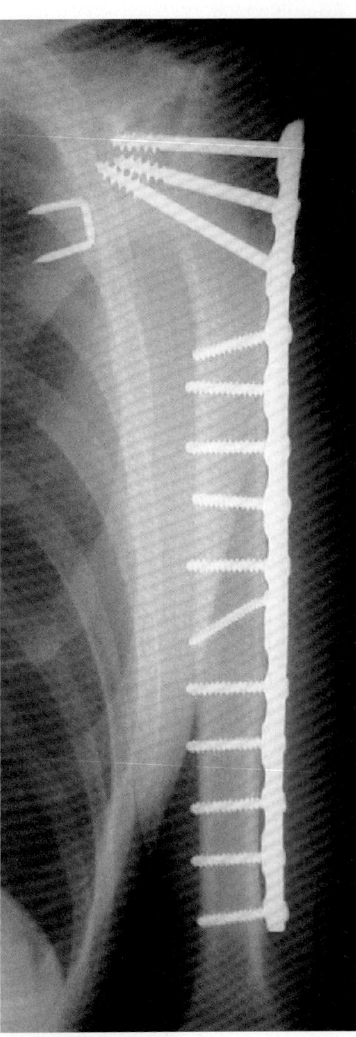

C

FIGURE 30-25 **A.** A 43-year-old man had a successful glenohumeral fusion following multiple failed surgical procedures for shoulder instability with subsequent arthritic change. He fell approximately 9 months postoperatively and sustained a humeral shaft fracture below the fusion plate. **B.** The lateral radiograph demonstrates the extension deformity at the fracture site (*dotted outline*). Operative intervention was recommended for two reasons: the long lever arm and shoulder fusion meant that there would be excessive force and motion at the fracture site, making a delayed or nonunion more likely. Second, the fracture would be very difficult to control in a splint, and the extension deformity would result in significant loss of function since compensatory motion through the shoulder was not available. **C.** Anteroposterior radiograph following open reduction and internal fixation. The old plate was removed and a long, broad large fragment plate was used for fixation. Extra screws were placed distally due to the increased stress anticipated, and fixation extended proximally to protect the arthrodesis.

The juxtaposition of a long rigid implant with locking screws at the tip in diaphyseal bone leads to a significant stress-riser effect, especially if there is a transcortical hole drilled for a missed distal locking screw. This is analogous clinically to the introduction of short-locking nails for intertrochanteric and subtrochanteric fractures in the femur that were associated with a low but persistent incidence of femoral shaft fracture at the tip of the implant (132,133). Similar fractures have been reported following locked humeral nailing (76). These fractures were reported eight to 26 weeks after the humeral shaft fracture had been treated. A sudden rotational motion was accompanied by an audible crack associated with an oblique or spiral distal humeral fracture at the distal end of the nail (Fig. 30-26). A number of factors result in delayed healing in this situation including the distal locking screw(s) and nail tip in the fracture site, the "Holstein-Lewis" pattern of fracture and the poor natural history of fractures at the end of long, rigid implants (20,124,125,134). The limited numbers of reported cases make treatment recommendations difficult. It would appear that these fractures are best treated with repeat operative intervention where the distal locking screws (and nail, if the shaft fracture is solidly healed) are removed and the fracture site reduced and then internally fixed. If the nail is left in place then transcortical screws and/or cerclage wires will be required to augment proximal fixation.

Nonunion

Nonunion can occur following closed or operative treatment. Nonunion following operative repair is often the result of technical error, including inadequate plate size (Fig. 30-13), fracture site distraction (Figs. 30-15 and 30-16), inadequate screw purchase (Fig. 30-27), or mechanical failure from osteopenic bone (Fig. 30-28) (25,55,56,102,103). Thus, careful attention to surgical technique and proper implant choice can reduce the incidence of nonunion. The treatment of nonunion is based on establishing mechanical stability and stimulating nonunion site biology (135–147). Open reduction and internal fixation with iliac crest bone grafting has had consistently good results in the treatment of humeral shaft nonunion, regardless of the cause. Ring et al reported union in 24 of 25 humeral shaft nonunions treated in this fashion (146), and Otsuka et al reported union in all 25 patients from a similar series (135). Proper technique is essential and includes removal of all preexisting implants, debridement to bleeding healthy bone, reestablishing the medullary canals of the fragments, correction of deformity, stable fixation with compression and bone grafting. Bone grafting is typically required for atrophic nonunions, as hypertrohic nonunions have favorable biology and will generally heal with mechanical stabilization alone. More recently, there has been increasing interest in the use of bone graft substitutes in an attempt

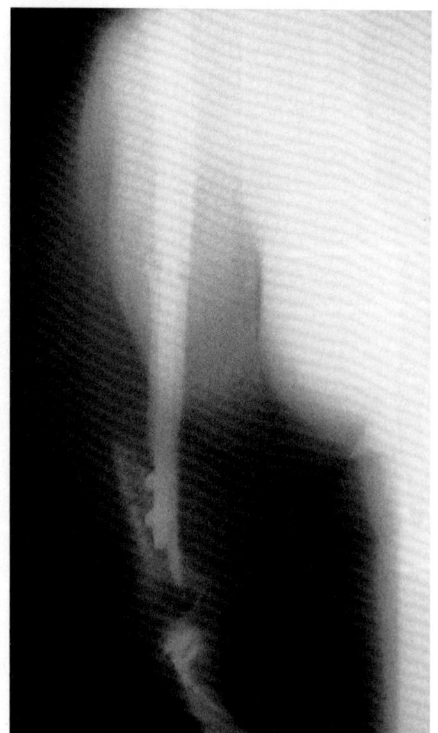

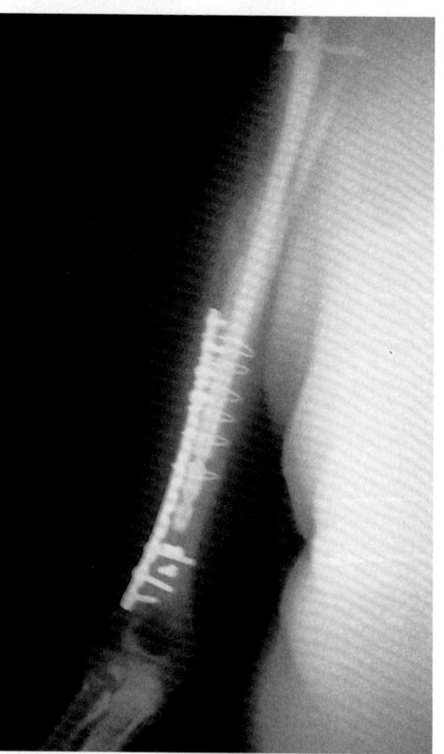

FIGURE 30-26 **A.** A fracture occurred at the distal tip of this interlocking humeral nail following a rotational injury 8 weeks after intramedullary nailing for a humeral shaft fracture. **B.** The fracture was repaired by removal of the interlocking screws from the fracture site, reduction of the fracture and plate fixation with a combination of screws and cerclage wires. (From McKee MD, Pedlow FX, Cheney PJ, et al. Fractures below the end of locking humeral nails: a report of three cases. *J Orthop Trauma* 1996;10(7)500–504.)

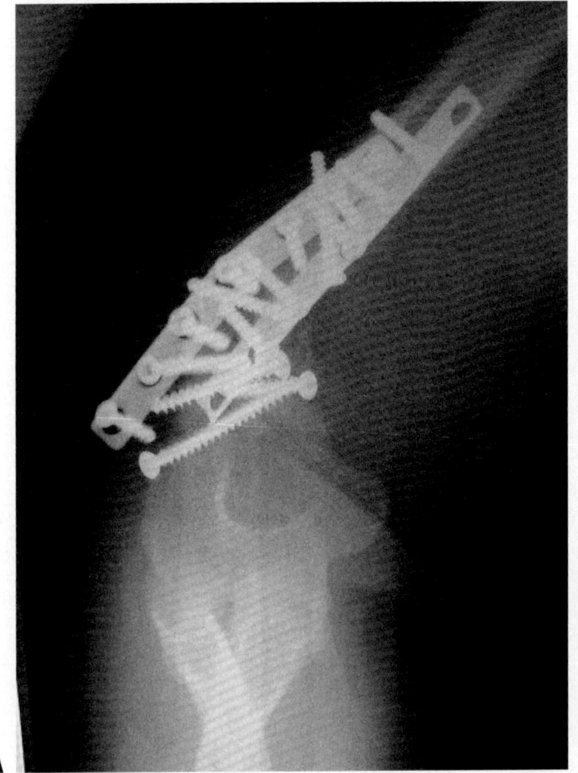

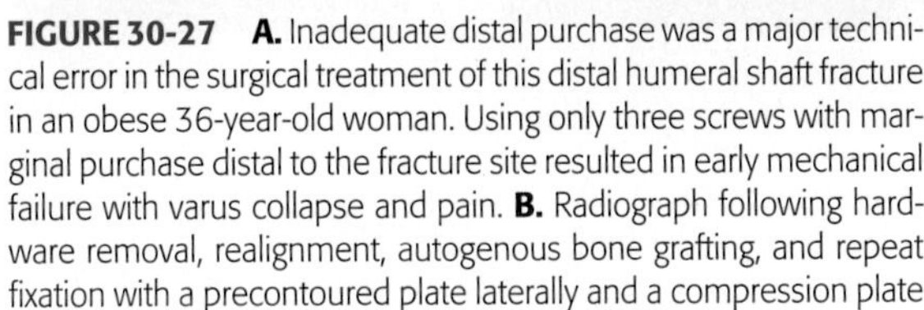

FIGURE 30-27 **A.** Inadequate distal purchase was a major technical error in the surgical treatment of this distal humeral shaft fracture in an obese 36-year-old woman. Using only three screws with marginal purchase distal to the fracture site resulted in early mechanical failure with varus collapse and pain. **B.** Radiograph following hardware removal, realignment, autogenous bone grafting, and repeat fixation with a precontoured plate laterally and a compression plate medially. The fracture healed promptly but the patient had an iatrogenic radial nerve palsy postoperatively that lasted 4 months. Revision surgery for humeral fractures carries with it a higher rate of complications, especially nerve injury.

to eliminate the morbidity of autogenous bone grafting. While there is some preliminary evidence that materials such as bone morphogenetic proteins (BMP, e.g., BMP-7 or BMP-2) will provide sufficient biologic stimulus to produce union, it is important to use them properly (148). They should form an integral part of a standard orthopaedic procedure. For patients with bone loss of more than 5 to 6 cm, or those who have failed conventional care, vascularized fibular grafting is a good option; Jupiter reported healing in four patients treated in this fashion (40).

Often nonunion is associated with severe osteopenia, be it as a cause of prior mechanical failure or as a result of prolonged disuse. There are several options for dealing with this situation: longer plates with more screws, cement augmentation of screw fixation, blade plate fixation, and the use of Schuli nuts for plate fixation (136,137,144,149). Allograft can be used as intramedullary fixation or as cortical struts to aid in mechanical fixation (Fig. 30-28). Wright reported success in 17 of 19 patients augmented with intramedullary allograft fibular fixation (145); Van Houwelingen and McKee had union in all of six recalcitrant nonunions treated with onlay strut allografts to augment screw fixation (148). More recently, Ring et al reported on the use of a locking plate to enhance fixation in severely osteoporotic elderly patients (mean age 72 years), and had success with their primary procedure in 22 of 24 patients (63). This new technology has great promise in the treatment of fractures or nonunions with poor bone quality.

Nonunion following intramedullary nailing represents a unique problem. Originally, it was thought that exchange nailing would be routinely successful in this situation, just as it has been in the lower extremity. However, McKee et al found that exchange nailing was successful in only four of ten such cases, and then had better success with nail removal, compression plating and bone grafting (union in nine of nine cases) (75). Similarly, Robinson et al had success with exchange nailing in only two of five cases (64). Nonunion associated with a loose nail is a difficult reconstructive problem and requires longer plates, liberal bone grafting, and extensive dissection to remove

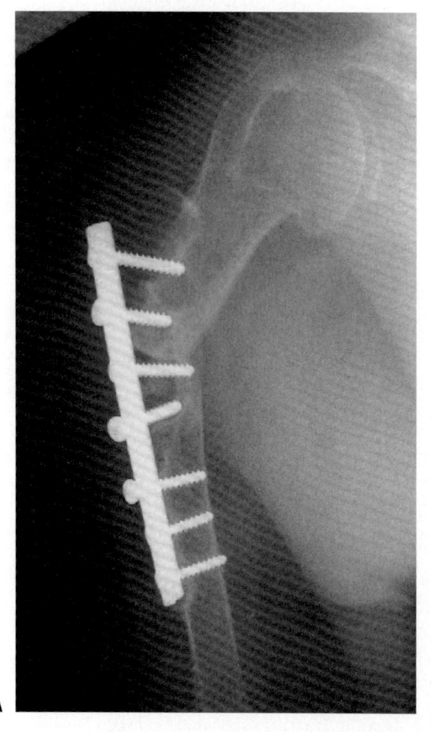

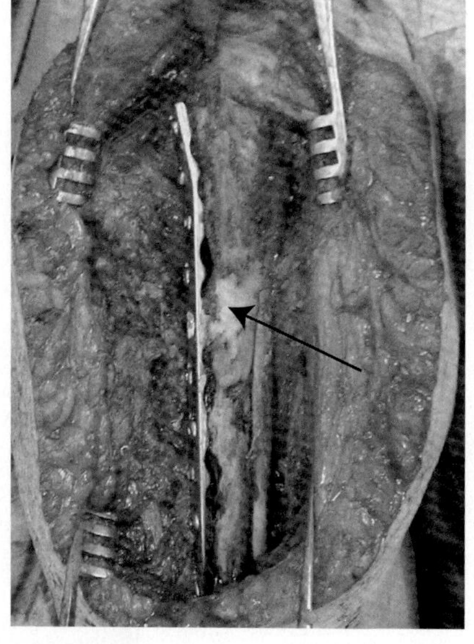

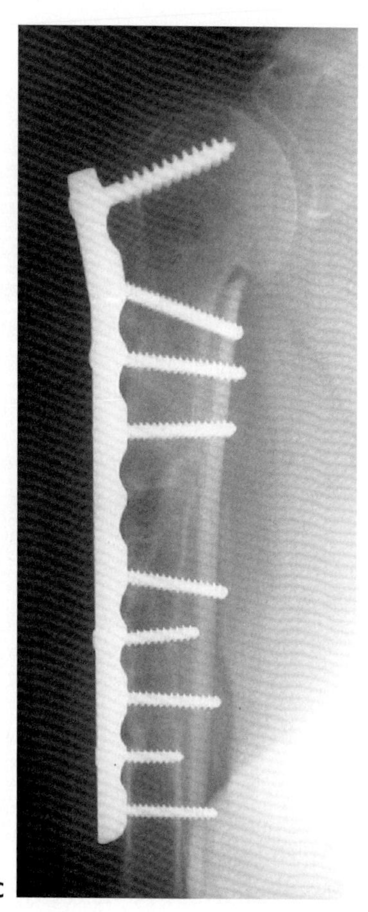

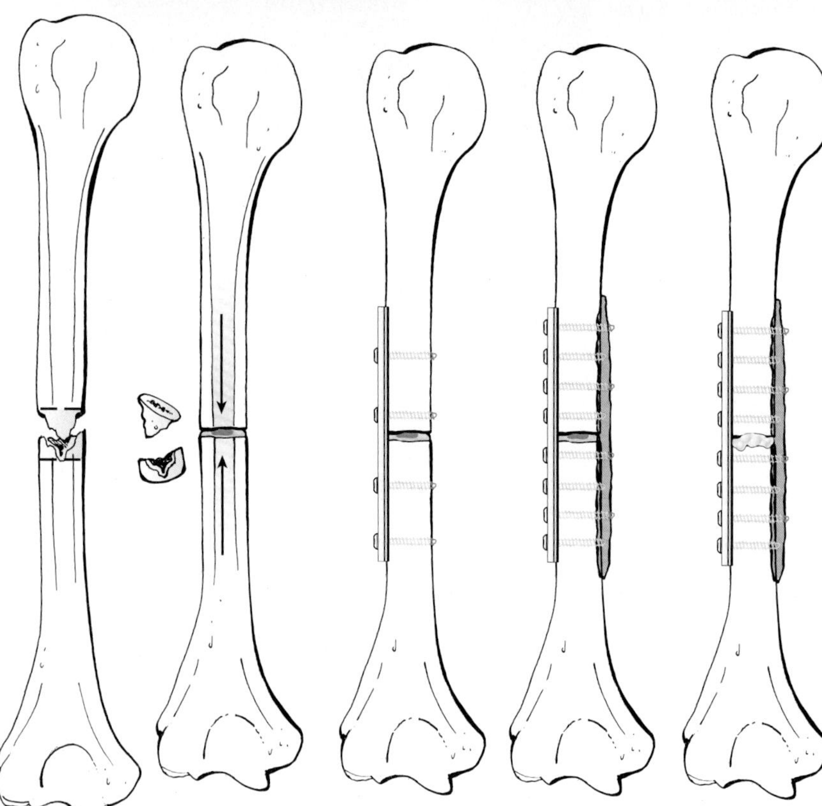

FIGURE 30-28 This 77-year-old patient had had two attempts at fixation of a nonunion following conservative treatment of a humeral shaft fracture. **A.** There are two main problems: one is mechanical, with obvious loss of fixation in very osteopenic bone, and the second is biologic, with no evidence of callous formation or healing, an atrophic nonunion. **B.** Intraoperative photograph after realignment, debridement of the nonunion, reestablishment of the medullary canals, and plate fixation with a broad 4.5-mm compression plate. Following provisional fixation of the plate with one screw proximally and distally, a cortical strut allograft was applied medially and the remaining screws were inserted into it, dramatically enhancing fixation. rhBMP-7 was applied to the nonunion site (*arrow*) instead of autogenous bone (both anterior iliac crests had been harvested previously). With a stable arm and no bone graft donor site, the patient left the hospital the day after surgery. **C.** A follow-up radiograph taken at 4 months postoperatively revealing solid bony union. **D.** The steps in the procedure are depicted. (**A–C** from Van Hounelingen AP, McKee MD. Treatment of osteopenic humeral shaft nonunion with compression plating, humeral cortical allograft struts, and bone grafting. *J Orthop Trauma* 2005; 19(1):36–42.)

the implanted nail. Wu and Shih presented a comparative study on the use of intramedullary nails versus plates in the primary treatment of humeral nonunion, and found similar results in both groups (89.5% union in the plate group, 87.5% union in the nail group) (150). However, if nailing is chosen as a treatment, bone grafting seems advisable.

Delayed union or nonunion following nonoperative treatment can be due to soft-tissue interposition, displaced transverse fracture patterns, noncompliance with bracing (Fig. 30-29), unfavorable body habitus (e.g., morbid obesity), or severe fracture angulation (Fig. 30-30). A true synovial pseudarthrosis can result (Fig. 30-29), which requires extensive debridement at the time of surgical repair.

Some authorities have reported that nonunion of the upper extremity is relatively well-tolerated, compared to lower extremity nonunion, especially in elderly patients or those with multiple medical comorbidities whose functional demands are limited. However, Ring et al showed that a humeral pseudarthrosis can be very debilitating in elderly patients whose independent functioning is often marginal, and can often be the difference

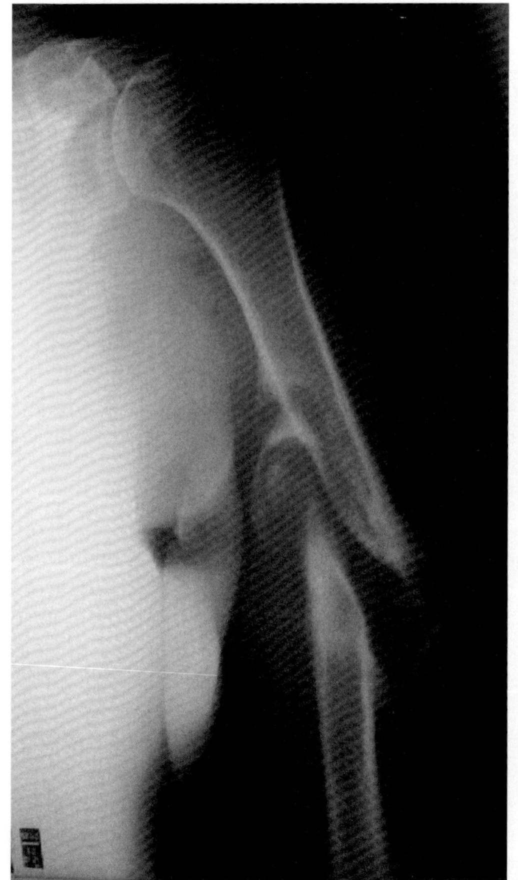
A

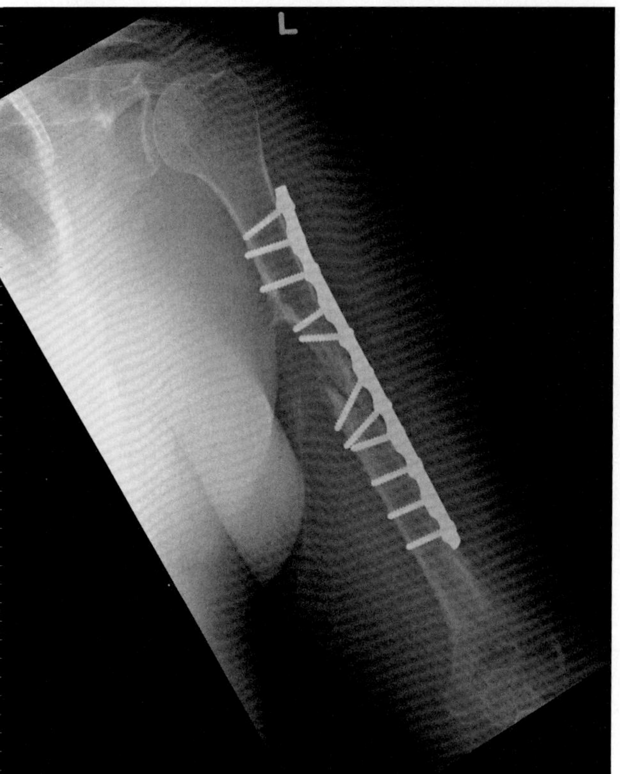

C

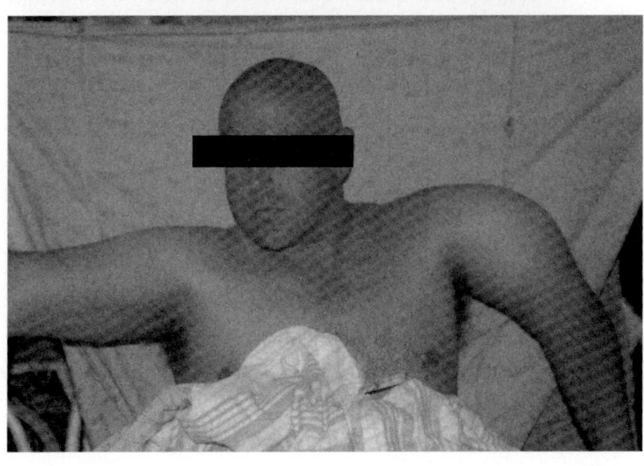
B

FIGURE 30-29 **A.** A synovial pseudarthrosis followed conservative treatment of a mid-shaft humeral fracture in a 38-year-old who was noncompliant with treatment and did not wear his functional brace. Note the pseudoarticulation between the distal fragment and the reactive bone on the medial aspect of the proximal fragment. **B.** There was gross mobility at the nonunion site. This photograph also demonstrates why varus malalignment is common with these injuries. The intrinsic pull of the deltoid on the proximal fragment produces the typical deformity. Surgical tactics included excision of the interposed soft tissue and pseudo-capsule, debridement of the bone ends to bleeding bone, reestablishment of the medullary canals with a drill, shortening, and re-approximation of the bony fragments. A broad 4.5-mm plate was applied following lag screw fixation of the nonunion and rhBMP-7 was applied to the nonunion site to stimulate healing. **C.** Postoperative radiograph revealing excellent alignment and stable fixation. Early motion of the elbow and shoulder was allowed and union occurred.

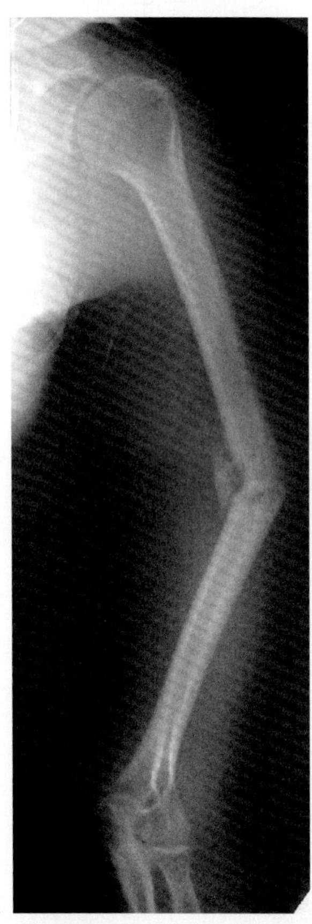

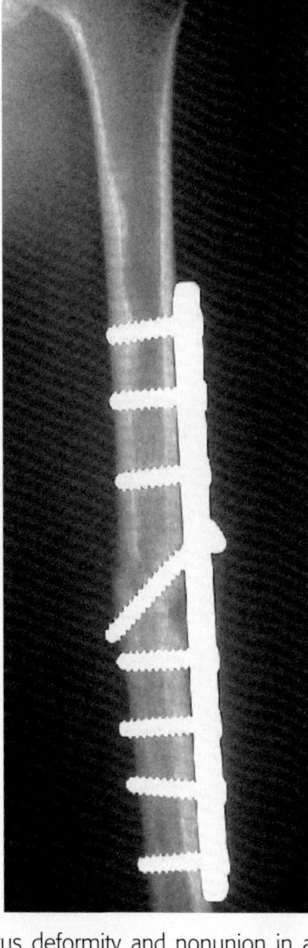

FIGURE 30-30 **A.** Unacceptable varus deformity and nonunion in a 22-year-old female student 6 months following a humeral shaft fracture treated conservatively. While a fairly broad range of angulatory, translational and rotational malunion can be accepted in the humeral shaft due to the compensatory motion of the shoulder and elbow, this degree of deformity has functional and cosmetic consequences. The lack of osseous union caused ongoing pain at the nonunion site. **B.** Uneventful union following open reduction, correction of deformity, compression plating and addition of bone morphogenetic protein.

between independent living and institutionalization (151). They used the Enforced Social Dependency Scale to evaluate 22 elderly patients (mean age 72 years) with humeral nonunion and found a mean value of 39 points (0 = complete independence, 100 = complete dependency). The authors stated that eight patients had been told there was nothing that could be done surgically for their problem. Following successful operative repair of the nonunion, the Enforced Social Dependency Score decreased to a mean of 9 points, reflecting a dramatic improvement in independent functioning. Recognition of the associated impairment and knowing about the improved implants and techniques for the operative repair of humeral nonunion in the elderly population can lead to a more aggressive surgical approach to this problem; age alone should not be used as a contraindication to fixation (151).

Pearls and Pitfalls

Nonunion Treatment

- Investigate for infection prior to initiating treatment
- Some bone shortening (<3 cm), in order to have apposition of healthy, viable bone ends, is acceptable in treatment of nonunion of the humeral shaft
- Correction of deformity and compression plating is the treatment of choice
- Add a bone graft or osteoinductive bone graft substitute to atrophic nonunions
- A variety of techniques are available to deal with osteoporotic bone

Infection

Fortunately, due to its excellent blood supply and thick soft-tissue and muscle coverage, deep infection of the humerus is relatively rare, even in open fractures treated aggressively with immediate internal fixation. In our experience, infection in this setting is usually related to underlying medical comorbidities, especially diabetes, or severe, mutilating injuries that are often near-amputations.

Where deep infection develops following fracture fixation, general principles of treatment are adhered to. Cultures are taken to establish the causative bacteria, appropriate antibiotics are administered intravenously, the patient's medical condition is optimized, and the infected fracture is debrided and irrigated. If the implanted fixation is solid, it is left in place; if not, it is removed and a spanning external fixator is applied (two pins proximal, two distal). We have had excellent success in augmenting standard techniques through the addition of an antibiotic impregnated, osteoconductive bone substitute at the fracture or infection site. It provided a very high local concentration of antibiotics and it then contributed to eradicating infection in 23 of 25 patients (152). If necessary, serial debridements are performed. If the original plate or nail has been left in place, the hardware can be removed following union, if necessary. If an external fixator is used, repeat fixation with bone grafting can be performed when the wound is clean and the infection eradicated as evidenced clinically and hematologically. In recalcitrant cases, the Ilizarov technique has been described as a useful salvage option (142,143). However, in the humerus it is associated with a high complication rate, a prolonged period of time in the frame, and a significant risk of re-fracture.

CONCLUSION

Humeral shaft fractures are common. While most of these fractures can be treated nonoperatively with the expectation of a high degree of success, the alert orthopaedic surgeon can also use the interaction as an opportunity to intervene in other related health areas, such as the recognition, diagnosis, and referral for treatment of osteoporosis. There remains a consistent subset of these fractures that will have improved outcomes with operative intervention. Open reduction and compression plating has a consistent record of high union rates, low complication rates and rapid functional restoration that makes it the standard against which other methods are compared. Locked intramedullary nailing is an attractive option in select fracture types or clinical situations. Future innovations, be they technique or implant related, should be subjected to rigorous, prospective randomized studies prior to universal acceptance or recommendation.

REFERENCES

1. Schemitsch EH, Bhandari M. Fractures of the diaphyseal humerus. In: Browner BD, Jupiter JB, Levine AM, Trafton PG, eds. *Skeletal trauma*, 3rd ed. Toronto: WB Saunders; 2001:1481–1511.
2. Praemer A, Furner S, Rice DP. *Musculoskeletal conditions in the United States*. Rosemont, IL: American Academy of Orthopaedic Surgeons; 1999.
3. Brinker MR, O'Connor DP. The incidence of fractures and dislocations referred for orthopaedic services in a capitated population. *J Bone Joint Surg Am* 2004;86:290–297.
4. Gregory PR. Fractures of the humeral shaft. In: Bucholz RW, Heckman JD, eds. *Rockwood and Green's fractures in adults*, 5th ed. Philadelphia: Lippincott Williams & Wilkins; 2001:973–996.
5. Fears RL, Gleis GE, Seligson D. Diagnosis and treatment of complications: Fractures of the diaphyseal humerus. In: Browner BD, Jupiter JB, Levine AM, Trafton PG, eds. *Skeletal Trauma*, 2nd ed. Toronto: WB Saunders; 1998:567–578.
6. Sarmiento A, Zagorski JB, Zych G, et al. Functional bracing for the treatment of fractures of the humeral diaphysis. *J Bone Joint Surg Am* 2000;82:478–486.
7. Stannard JP, Harris HW, McGwin G Jr, et al. Intramedullary nailing of humeral shaft fractures with a locking, flexible nail. *J Bone Joint Surg Am* 2003;85:2103–2110.
8. Tytherleigh-Strong G, Walls N, McQueen MM. The epidemiology of humeral shaft fractures. *J Bone Joint Surg Br* 1998;80:249–253.
9. Sommer C, Gautier E, Muller M, et al. First clinical results of the Locking Compression Plate (LCP). *Injury* 2003;34(suppl 2):B43–54.
10. Rose SH, Melton LJ, Morrey BF, et al. Epidemiolgic features of humeral fractures. *Clin Orthop Relat Res* 1982;168:24–30.
11. Goss CM, ed. *Gray's anatomy*, 25th ed. Philadelphia: Lea & Febiger; 1950.
12. Worlock P, Stower M, Barbor P. Patterns of fractures in accidental and non-accidental injury in children: A comparative study. *British Med J* 1986;293:100–102.
13. Lancaster T, Stead L. Physician advice for smoking cessation. *Cochrane Database Syst Rev* 2004, Oct 18(4), CD000165.
14. Burd TA, Hughes MS, Anglen JO. Heterotopic ossification prophylaxis with indomethacin increases the risk of long-bone nonunion. *J Bone Joint Surg Br* 2003;85:700–705.
15. Giannoudis PV, MacDonald DA, Matthews SJ, et al. Nonunion of the femoral diaphysis: The influence of reaming and non-steroidal anti-inflammatory drugs. *J Bone Joint Surg Br* 2000;5:655–658.
16. American College of Surgeons. *Advanced Trauma Life Support (ATLS) manual*. Chicago: American College of Surgeons; 1993:17–46.
17. Bone L. Fractures of the shaft of the humerus. In: Chapman MW, ed. *Operative orthopedics*, Vol. 1. Philadelphia: JB Lippincott; 1988:221–234.
18. Brumback RJ, Bosse MJ, Poka A, et al. Intramedullary stabilization of humeral shaft fractures in patients with multiple trauma. *J Bone Joint Surg Am* 1986;68:960–969.
19. Ring D, Waters PM, Hotchkiss RN, et al. Pediatric floating elbow. *J Pediatr Orthop* 2001;21(4):456–459.
20. Holstein A, Lewis GB. Fractures of the humerus with radial nerve paralysis. *J Bone Joint Surg Am* 1963;45:1382–1388.
21. Garcia A Jr, Maeck BH. Radial nerve injuries of fractures of the shaft of the humerus. *Am J Surg* 1960;99:625–627.
22. Kettlekamp DB, Alexander H. Clinical review of radial nerve injury. *J Trauma* 1967; 7:424.
23. Pollock FH, Drake D, Bovill EG, et al. Treatment of radial neuropathy associated with fractures of the humerus. *J Bone Joint Surg Am* 1981;63:239–243.
24. Ring D, Chin K, Jupiter JB. Radial nerve palsy associated with high-energy humeral shaft fractures. *J Hand Surg* 2004;29:144–147.
25. Schatzker J. Fractures of the humerus. In: Schatzer J, Tile M, eds. *The rationale for operative fracture care*, 2nd ed. Berlin: Springer Verlag; 1996:83–94
26. McNamara JJ, Brief DK, Stremple JF, et al. Management of fractures with associated arterial injury in combat casualties. *J Trauma* 1973;13:17–19.
27. Bae H, Widmann RF, Hotchkiss RN. Extreme rotational malunion of the humerus. *J Bone Joint Surg Am* 2001;83(3):424–427.
28. Hubner U, Schlicht W, Outzen S, et al. Ultrasound in the diagnosis of fractures in children. *J Bone Joint Surg Br* 2000;82:1170–1173.
29. Orthopaedic Trauma Association Committee for Coding and Classification. Fracture and dislocation compendium. *J Orthop Trauma* 1996;10(suppl 1):v–ix, 1–154.
30. Wainwright AM, Williams JR, Carr AJ. Interobserver and intraobserver variation in classification systems for fractures of the distal humerus. *J Bone Join Surg Br* 2000;82: 636–642.
31. Siebenrock KA, Gerber C. The reproducibility of classification of fractures of the proximal end of the humerus. *J Bone Joint Surg Am* 1993;75(12):1751–1755.
32. Gustilo RB, Anderson JT. Prevention of infection in the treatment of 1025 open fractures of the long bones. Retrospective and prospective analysis. *J Bone Joint Surg Am* 1976; 58:453–458.
33. Schandelmaier P, Krettek C, Rudolf J, et al. Outcome of tibial shaft fractures with severe soft tissue injury treated by unreamed nailing versus external fixation. *J Trauma* 1995; 39:707–711.
34. Brumback RJ, Jones AL. Interobserver agreement in the classification of open fractures of the tibia. The results of a survey of two hundred and forty-five orthopedic surgeons. *J Bone Joint Surg Am* 1994;76:1162–1166.
35. DePalma AF. *The management of fractures and dislocations*. Philadelphia: W.B. Saunders; 1970.
36. Hollinshead WH. *Anatomy for surgeons*, Vol. 3. New York: Hoeber-Harper; 1958.
37. Hoppenfeld S, De Boer P. *Exposures in orthopedics*. Philadelphia: JB Lippincott; 1984: 47–75.
38. Mills WJ, Hanel DP, Smith DG. Lateral approach to the humeral shaft: An alternative approach for fracture treatment. *J Orthop Trauma* 1996;10:81–86.
39. Kellar A. The management of gunshot fractures of the humerus. *Injury* 1995;26:93–95.
40. Jupiter JB. Complex nonunion of the humeral diaphysis: treatment with a medial approach, an anterior plate, and a vascularized fibular graft. *J Bone Joint Surg Am* 1990; 72:701–707.
41. Chesser TJ, Leslie IJ. Radial nerve entrapment by the lateral intermuscular septum in trauma. *J Orthop Trauma* 2000;14:65–66.
42. Baker DM. Fracture of the humeral shaft associated with ipsilateral fracture dislocation of the shoulder: Report of a case. *J Trauma* 1971;11:532–534.
43. Laing PG. The arterial supply of the adult humerus. *J Bone Joint Surg Am* 1956;38: 1–105.
44. Connolly J. Management of fractures associated with arterial injuries. *Am J Surg* 1970; 120:331.
45. Sarmiento A, Kinman PB, Calvin EG, et al. Functional bracing of fractures of the shaft of the humerus. *J Bone Joint Surg Am* 1977;59:596–601.
46. Holm CL. Management of humeral shaft fractures. Fundamental nonoperative techniques. *Clin Orthop Relat Res* 1970;91:132–139.
47. Christensen S. Humeral shaft fractures: Operative and conservative treatment. *Acta Chir Scand* 1967;133:455.
48. Caldwell JA. Treatment of fracture of the shaft of the humerus by hanging cast. *Surg Gynecol Obstet* 1940;70:421.
49. Charnley J. *The closed treatment of common fractures*. Baltimore: Williams & Wilkins; 1961.
50. Ostermann PA, Ekkernkamp A, Muhr G. Functional bracing of shaft fractures of the humerus—an analysis of 195 cases. *Orthop Trans* 1993–1994;17:937.
51. Zagorski JB, Latta LL, Zych GA, et al. Diaphyseal fractures of the humerus. Treatment with prefabricated braces. *J Bone Joint Surg Am* 1988;70:607–610.
52. Ricciardi-Pollini PT, Falez F. The treatment of diaphyseal fractures by functional bracing. *Ital J Orthop Traumatol* 1985;11:199–205.
53. O'Driscoll SW, Spinner RJ, McKee MD, et al. Tardy posterolateral instability of the elbow due to cubitus varus. *J Bone Joint Surg Am* 2001;83:1358–1369.
54. Bhandari M, McKee MD, Schemitsch EH. Compression plating versus intramedullary nailing of humeral shaft fractures: a meta-analysis. *Acta Orthop Scand*. In press.
55. Foster RJ, Dixon JL, Bach AW, et al. Internal fixations of fractures and nonunions of the humeral shaft. *J Bone Joint Surg Am* 1985;67:857–864.
56. Mast JW, Spiegal PG, Harvey JP, et al. Fractures of the humeral shaft. *Clin Orthop Relat Res* 1975;12:254–262.
57. McKee MD, Seiler J, Jupiter JB. The application of the limited contact dynamic compression plate in the upper extremity: an analysis of 114 cases. *Injury* 1995;26:661–666.
58. Vander Griend RA, Tomasin J, et al. Open reduction and internal fixation of humeral shaft fractures. *J Bone Joint Surg Am* 1986;68:430–433.
59. Bell MJ, Beauchamp CG, Kellam JK, et al. The results of plating humeral shaft factures in patients with multiple injuries. *J Bone Joint Surg Br* 1985;67:293–296.
60. Tingstad EM, Wolinsky PR, Shyr Y, et al. Effect of immediate weight-bearing on plated fractures of the humeral shaft. *J Trauma* 2000;49:278–280.
61. Davenport SR, Lindsey R, Leggon R, et al. Dynamic compression plate fixation: a biomechanical comparison of unicortical and biocortical distal screw fixation. *J Orthop Trauma* 1988;2:146–150.
62. Jain R, Podworthy N, Hupel TM, et al. Influence of plate design on cortical bone perfusion and fracture healing in segmental tibia fractures. *J Orthop Trauma* 1999;13: 178–186.
63. Ring D, Kloen P, Kadzielski J, et al. Locking compression plates for osteoporotic nonunions of the diaphyseal humerus. *Clin Orthop Relat Res* 2004;425:50–54.
64. Robinson CM, Bell KM, Court-Brown CM, et al. Locked nailing of humeral shaft fractures. *J Bone Joint Surg Br* 1992;74:558–561.
65. Crolla KMP, de Varis LS, Clevers GJ. Locked intramedullary nailing of humeral fractures. *Injury* 1993;24:403–406.
66. Ingman AM, Waters DA. Locked intramedullary nailing of the humeral shaft fractures. *J Bone Joint Surg Br* 1994;76:23–29.
67. Reimer B. Humeral shaft fractures—intramedullary nailing. In: Wiss D, ed. *Master techniques in orthopedic surgery: fractures*. Philadelphia: Lippincott-Raven; 1998:81–94.
68. Reimer BL, D'Ambrosia R, Kellman JF, et al. The anterior acromial approach for antegrade intramedullary nailing of the humeral diaphysis. *Orthopedics* 1993;16: 1219–1223.

69. Kuntscher G. *Practice of intramedullary nailing*. Springfield, IL: Charles C Thomas; 1967.
70. Allen WC, Piotrowski G, Burstein AH, et al. Biomechanical principles of intramedullary fixation. *Clin Orthop Relat Res* 1968;60:1320.
71. Hall RF, Pankovich AM. Ender nailing of acute fractures of the humerus. *J Bone Joint Surg Am* 1987;69:558–567.
72. Pritchett JW. Delayed union of humeral shaft fractures treated by closed flexible intramedullary nailing. *J Bone Joint Surg Br* 1985;67:715–718.
73. Rodrigues-Merchan EC. Compression plating versus Hackethal nailing in closed humeral shaft fractures failing nonoperative reduction. *J Orthop Trauma* 1995;9(3): 194–197.
74. Henley MB, Chapman JR, Claudi BF. Closed retrograde Hackethal nail stabilization of humeral shaft fractures. *J Orthop Trauma* 1992;6:18–24.
75. McKee MD, Miranda MA, Reimer BL, et al. Management of humeral nonunion after the failure of locking intramedullary nails. *J Orthop Trauma* 1996;10:492–499.
76. McKee MD, Pedlow FX, Cheney PJ, et al. Fracture below the end of locking humeral nails: A report of three cases. *J Orthop Trauma* 1996;10:500–551.
77. Farragos AF, Schemitsch ED, McKee MD. Complications of intramedullary nailing for fractures of the humeral shaft: A review. *J Orthop Trauma* 1999;13:258–267.
78. Rupp RE, Chrissos MG, Ebraheim N. The risk of neurovascular injury with distal locking screws of humeral intramedullary nails. *Orthopedics* 1996;19:593–595.
79. Simon P, Jobard D, Bistour L, et al. Complications of Marchetti locked nailing for humeral shaft fractures. *Int Orthop* 1999;23:320–324.
80. McCormack RG, Brien D, Buckley RE, et al. Fixation of fractures of the shaft of the humerus by dynamic compression plate or intramedullary nail: a prospective randomized trial. *J Bone Joint Surg Br* 2000;82:336–339.
81. Chapman JR, Henley MB, Agel J, et al. Randomized prospective study of humeral shaft fracture fixation: intramedullary nails versus plates. *J Orthop Trauma* 2000;14:162–166.
82. Bolano LE, Iaquinto JA, Vasicek V. Operative treatment of humerus shaft fractures: a prospective randomized study comparing intramedullary nailing with dynamic compression plating. Presented at the 62nd Annual Meeting of the American Academy of Orthopaedic Surgeons. Orlando, FL; February 1995.
83. Reimer BL, Foglesong ME, Burke CJ, et al. Complications of Seidel nailing of narrow diameter humeral diaphyseal fractures. *Orthopaedics* 1994;17:19–29.
84. Utvag SE, Grundnes O, Reikeras O. Effects of degrees of remaining on healing of segmental fractures. *J Bone Joint Surg Am* 1998;12:192–199.
85. Leung M, Hertel R. Thermal necrosis after tibial reaming for intramedullary nail fixation. *J Bone Joint Surg Br* 1996;78:584–587.
86. Mills WJ, Chapman JR, Robinson LR, et al. Somatosensory evoked potential monitoring during closed humeral nailing: a preliminary report. *J Orthop Trauma* 2000;14: 167–170.
87. Zimmerman MC, Waite AM, Deehan M, et al. A biomechanical analysis of four humeral fracture fixation systems. *J Orthop Trauma* 1994;8:233–239.
88. Bono CM, Grossman MG, Hochwald N, et al. Radial and axillary nerves. Anatomic considerations for humeral fixation. *Clin Orthop Relat Res* 2000;373:259–264.
89. Port AM, Nanu AM, Cross AT. Windows for humeral interlocking nails—an anatomical study. *J Bone Joint Surg Br* 1997;79(suppl 1):102.
90. Faruqui NA, Hutchins PM. Humeral nailing—an anatomical study. *J Bone Joint Surg Br* 1997;79(suppl 1):102.
91. Strothman D, Templeman DC, Varecka T, et al. Retrograde nailing of humeral shaft fractures: a biomechanical study of its effects on the strength of the distal humerus. *J Orthop Trauma* 2000;14:101–104.
92. Lin J, Inoue N, Valdevit A, et al. Biomechanical comparison of antegrade and retrograde nailing of humeral shaft fracture. *Clin Orthop Relat Res* 1998;351:203–213.
93. Rommens PM, Verbruggen J, Broos PL. Retrograde locked nailing of the humeral shaft fractures. *J Bone Joint Surg Br* 1995;77:84–89.
94. Blum J, Machemer H, Baumgart F, et al. Biomechanical comparison of bending and torsional properties in retrograde intramedullary nailing of humeral shaft fractures. *J Orthop Trauma* 1999;13:344–350.
95. Kamhin M, Michaelson M, Waisbrod H. The use of external skeletal fixation in the treatment of fractures of the humeral shaft. *Injury* 1977;9:245–248.
96. Rich NM, Metz CW, Hutton JE, et al. Internal versus external fixation of fractures with concomitant vascular injuries in Vietnam. *J Trauma* 1971;11:463–473.
97. Choong PF, Griffiths JD. External fixation of complex open humeral fractures. *Aust NZ J Surg* 1988;2:137–142.
98. Modabber MR, Jupiter JB. Operative management of diaphyseal fractures of the humerus. *Clin Orthop Relat Res* 1998;347:93–104.
99. Ruland WO. Is there a place for external fixation in humeral shaft fracture? *Injury* 2000;31(suppl 1):27–34.
100. Marsh JL, Mahoney CR, Steinbronn D. External fixation of open humerus fractures. *Iowa Orthop J* 1999;19:35–42.
101. Mostafavi HR, Tornetta P. Open fractures of the humerus treated with external fixation. *Clin Orthop Relat Res* 1997;337:187–197.
102. O'Brien PJ, Guy P, Blachut P. Humeral shaft fractures-open reduction internal fixation. In: Wiss D, ed. *Master techniques in orthopedic surgery: fractures*. Philadelphia: Lippincott-Raven; 1998:63–80.
103. Connolly S, Nair R, Waddell JP, et al. Immediate plate osteosynthesis of open fractures of the humeral shaft. Proceedings of the 55th Canadian Orthopaedic Association Annual Meeting. Edmonton, Alberta; June 3–6, 2000.
104. Ogawa K, Ui M. Humeral shaft fracture sustained during arm wrestling: report on 30 cases and review of the literature. *J Trauma* 1997;42(2):243–246.
105. Sarmiento A, Horowitch A, Aboulafia A, et al. Functional bracing for comminuted extra-articular fractures of the distal third of the humerus. *J Bone Joint Surg Br* 1990; 72(2):283–287.
106. Sanders R, Yach J, Dipasquale T, et al. Radial nerve palsy associated with humeral fractures. Presented at the 16th Annual Meeting of the Orthopaedic Trauma Association. San Antonio, TX; Oct. 12, 2000.
107. Swenson MR, Villasana DR. Neurologic evaluation of the upper extremity. In: Kasdan ML, ed. *Occupational hand and upper extremity injuries and diseases*. Philadelphia: Hanley and Belfus; 1991:115–130.
108. Bodine SC, Lieber RL, Peripheral nerve physiology, anatomy, and pathology. In: Simon SR, ed. *Orthopaedic basic science*. Rosemont, IL: American Academy of Orthopaedic Surgeons; 1994:325–396.
109. Brien WW, Gellman H, Becker V, et al. Management of fractures of the humerus in patients who have an injury of the ipsilateral brachial plexus. *J Bone Joint Surg Am* 1990;72:1208–1210.
110. Kunec JR, Lewis RJ. Closed intramedullary rodding of pathological fractures with supplemental cement. *Clin Orthop Relat Res* 1984;188:183–186.
111. Lancaster JM, Koman AL, Gristina AG, et al. Treatment of pathologic fractures of the humerus. *South Med J* 1988;81:52–55.
112. Habermann ET, Lopez RA. Metastatic disease of bone and treatment of pathological fractures. *Orthop Clin North Am* 1989;20:469–486.
113. Douglass HO, Shukla SK, Mindell E. Treatment of pathological fractures of long bones excluding those due to breast cancer. *J Bone Joint Surg Am* 1976;76:839–847.
114. Flemming JE, Beals RK. Pathologic fracture of the humerus. *Clin Orthop Relat Res* 1986; 203:258–260.
115. Harrington KD, Sim FH, Enis JE, et al. Methylmethacrylate as an adjunct in internal fixation of pathological fractures. Experience with three hundred and seventy five cases. *J Bone Joint Surg Am* 1976;58:1047–1055.
116. Lewallen RP, Pritchard DJ, Sim FH. Treatment of pathologic fractures or impending fractures of the humerus with Rush rods and methylmethacrylate. Experience with 55 cases in 54 patients 1968–1977. *Clin Orthop Relat Res* 1982;166:193–198.
117. Yazawa Y, Frassica FJ, Chao EYS, et al. Metastatic bone disease. A study of the surgical treatment of 166 pathologic humeral and femoral fractures. *Clin Orthop Relat Res* 1990; 251:213–219.
118. Lancaster JM, Koman LA, Gristina AG, et al. Pathologic fractures of the humerus. *South Med J* 1988;81:52–55.
119. Redmond BJ, Biermann JS, Blasier RB. Interlocking intramedullary nailing of pathological fractures of the shaft of the humerus. *J Bone Joint Surg Am* 1996;78:891–896.
120. Chin HC, Frassica FJ, Hein TJ, et al. Metastatic diaphyseal fractures of the shaft of the humerus. The structural strength evaluation of a new method of treatment with a segmental defect prosthesis. *Clin Orthop Relat Res* 1989;248:231–239.
121. Crates J, Whittle AP. Antegrade interlocking nailing of acute humeral shaft fractures. *Clin Orthop Relat Res* 1998;350:40–50.
122. Sims SH, Smith SE. Intramedullary nailing of humeral shaft fractures. *J South Orthop Assoc* 1995;(1):24–31.
123. Henley MB, Monroe M, Tencer AF. Biomechanical comparison of methods of fixation of a midshaft osteotomy of the humerus. *J Orthop Trauma* 1991;5:14–20.
124. Boyd AD, Thornhill TS, Barnes CL. Fractures adjacent to humeral prostheses. *J Bone Joint Surg Am* 1992;74:1498–1504.
125. Campbell JT, Moore RS, Iannotti JP, et al. Periprosthetic humeral fractures: mechanisms of fracture and treatment options. *J Shoulder Elbow Surg* 1998;7:406–413.
126. Kumar S, Sperling JW, Haidukewych GH, et al. Periprosthetic humeral fractures after shoulder arthroplasty. *J Bone Joint Surg Am* 2004;86:680–689.
127. Worland RL, Kim DY, Arrendondo J. Periprosthetic humeral fractures: management and classification. *J Shoulder Elbow Surg* 1999;8:590–594.
128. O'Driscoll SW, Morrey BF. Periprosthetic fractures about the elbow. *Orthop Clin North Am* 1999;30:319–325.
129. Sanchez-Sotelo J, O'Driscoll S, Morrey BF. Periprosthetic humeral fractures after total elbow arthroplasty: treatment with implant revision and strut allograft augmentation. *J Bone Joint Surg Am* 2004;9;1642–1650.
130. Habernek H, Ortner E. A locking nail for fractures of the humerus. *J Bone Joint Surg Br* 1991;73:651–653.
131. Habernek H. A locking nail for fractures of the humerus [Letter to the editor]. *J Bone Joint Surg Br* 1998;80:557.
132. Halder SC. The Gamma nail for peritrochanteric fractures. *J Bone Joint Surg Br* 1992; 74:340–344.
133. Leung KS, So WS, Shen WY, et al. Gamma nails and dynamic hip screws for peritrochanteric fractures: a randomized prospective study in elderly patients. *J Bone Joint Surg Br* 1992;74:345–351.
134. Lewallen DG, Berry DJ. Periprosthetic fracture of the femur after total hip arthroplasty: treatment and results to date. *Instr Course Lect* 1998;47:2443–2449.
135. Otsuka NY, McKee MD, Liew A, et al. The effect of comorbidity and duration of nonunion on outcome after surgical treatment for nonunion of the humerus. *J Shoulder Elbow Surg* 1998;7:127–133.
136. Ring D, McKee MD, Perey BH, et al. The use of a blade plate and autogenous cancellous bone graft in the treatment of ununited fractures of the proximal humerus. *J Shoulder Elbow Surg* 2001;10:501–507.
137. Palmer SH, Handley R, Willett K. The use of interlocked 'customized' blade plates in the treatment of metaphyseal fractures in patients with poor bone stock. *Injury* 2000; 31;187–191.
138. Rosen H. The treatment of nonunions and pseudarthroses of the humeral shaft. *Orthop Clin North Am* 1990;21:725–742.
139. Jupiter JB, von Deck M. Ununited humeral diaphyses. *J Shoulder Elbow Surg* 1998;7: 644–652.

140. Valchanou VD, Michailov P. High-energy shock waves in the treatment of delayed and nonunion of fractures. *Int Orthop* 1991;15:181–184.
141. Gill DRJ, Torchia ME. The spiral compression plate for proximal humeral shaft nonunion: A case report and description of a new technique. *J Orthop Trauma* 1999;13:141–144.
142. Patel VR, Menon DK, Pool RD, et al. Nonunion of the humerus after failure of surgical treatment: Management using the Ilizarov circular fixator. *J Bone Joint Surg Br* 2000;82:977–983.
143. Lammens J, Bauduin G, Dreisen R, et al. Treatment of nonunion of the humerus using the Ilizarov external fixator. *Clin Orthop Relat Res* 1998;353:223–230.
144. Jupiter JB. Complex non-union of the humeral diaphysis. *J Bone Joint Surg Am* 1990;72:701–707.
145. Wright TW, Miller GJ, Vander Griend RA, et al. Reconstruction of the humerus with an intramedullary fibular graft. *J Bone Joint Surg Br* 1993;75:801–807.
146. Ring D, Jupiter JB, Quintero J, et al. Atrophic ununited diaphyseal fractures of the humerus with a bony defect. *J Bone Joint Surg Am* 2000;82:867–871.
147. Hornicek FJ, Zych GA, Hutson JJ, et al. Salvage of humeral nonunions with onlay bone plate allograft augmentation. *Clin Orthop Relat Res* 2001;386:203–209.
148. Van Houwelingen A, McKee MD. Treatment of osteopenic humeral shaft nonunion with compression plating, humeral cortical allograft struts and bone grafting. *J Orthop Trauma* 2005;19(1):36–42.
149. Cameron HU, Jacob R, Macnab I, et al. Use of polymethyl methacrylate to enhance screw fixation in bone. *J Bone Joint Surg Am* 1975;57:655–656.
150. Wu CC, Shih CH. Treatment for nonunion of the shaft of the humerus: comparison of plates and Seidel interlocking nails. *Can J Surg* 1992;35:661–665.
151. Ring D, Perey B, Jupiter J. The functional outcome of operative treatment of ununited fractures of the humeral diaphysis in older patients. *J Bone Joint Surg Am* 1999;81:177–190.
152. McKee MD, Wild LM, Schemitsch EH, et al. The use of an antibiotic-impregnated, osteoconductive, bioabsorbable bone substitute in the treatment of infected long bone defects. *J Orthop Trauma* 2002;16:622–627.

FRACTURES OF THE PROXIMAL HUMERUS

Jon J. P. Warner, John G. Costouros, and Christian Gerber

INCIDENCE

One of the most detailed accounts on fractures about the shoulder was published by Cave, who reported on the Massachusetts General Hospital experience of 1,603 shoulder traumas (1). Clavicle fractures were by far the most common fracture type, with an incidence of 700 (44%), compared to 273 (17%) proximal humerus fractures. Fractures of the proximal humerus are thus relatively rare and represent no more than 3% of all upper extremity fractures (2). Their overall incidence has been reported to be 73 cases per 100,000 individuals per year (3–8). Most of these fractures occur in women over the age of 50, with the exception of isolated greater tuberosity fractures, which occur with greater frequency in younger individuals (5). More than 85% of these fractures are only minimally displaced. The more complex displaced fracture patterns, which are difficult to classify in reproducible fashion, are thus relatively infrequent (9,10). Significant controversy continues regarding the best methods of treating displaced proximal humerus fractures. Classification of fracture types has been inconsistent, and thus selection of surgical approaches has been variable. Most published series are retrospective reviews of small numbers of cases, often with mixed approaches and techniques used by different surgeons. Furthermore, surgeons coming from different disciplines often have a different approach to the treatment of proximal humerus fractures. For example, traumatologists favor rigid fixation and implants that are typically used for lower extremity fractures (11–14). On the other hand, upper extremity surgeons with specialty training in shoulder surgery tend to favor less invasive approaches and less rigid methods of fixation.

HISTORICAL APPROACHES TO TREATMENT

Ancient physicians advocated bandaging and rest for closed proximal humerus fractures, while open fractures were usually fatal (15,16). In medieval Europe, "bonesetters" performed some manipulations and operations, but little detail of these treatment methods is available in written documentation (16).

In the past century, nonoperative treatment of proximal humerus fractures has been documented as an acceptable approach (17–21). Treatment modalities have included traction (22–27), manipulation (28–30), and casting (31), with an emphasis on early functional range of motion. It has generally been considered that results could be good even with malunion (9,32–41). However, some surgeons did recognize that significant displacement, especially in comminuted proximal humerus fractures, was associated with a poor functional outcome (42–44). That said, in a recent study, Zyto (45) reported on a series of elderly patients with four-part fractures who were randomized into nonoperative treatment or open reduction and internal fixation. They observed no difference in the functional outcome between the two groups, although they did not report on whether displacement was corrected with their operative management.

The first systematic approach to surgical fixation of proximal humerus fractures was described by Lambotte in Belgium and Lane in Great Britain (46,47). Subsequently, other surgeons described many methods of surgical repair and fixation of proximal humerus fractures, including staples (48), plates and screws (49–54), blade plates (55,56), intramedullary (IM) nails (57–68), retrograde nails and pins (69–77), external fixation (78–80), and tension-band fixation (58,81–88).

In 1970 the AO Group published its *Manual of Internal Fixation*, the first practical guide to fracture fixation using combinations of plates and screws (89). The concept of minimal fixation to preserve "the blood supply to the head and the anterolateral artery" was first described by Neer (90). This set the stage for an ongoing controversy between proponents of rigid fixation of fractures and those advocating "minimal fixation" (50,91). This controversy is discussed further in this chapter as it pertains to current approaches in the treatment of specific fracture types.

PRINCIPLES OF TREATMENT

Anatomy of the Humerus, Rotator Cuff, and Neurovascular Anatomy

The proximal humerus is uniquely adapted to allow for the large range of motion of the shoulder joint. The diaphysis expands into the surgical neck, which is just below the greater and lesser tuberosities of the metaphyseal flare (Fig. 31-1). The anatomic neck is just above the tuberosities, and it is the region just below the humeral articular surface. The humeral articular segment is almost spherical, with a diameter of curvature averaging 46 mm (ranging from 37 to 57 mm) (92). The inclination of the humeral head relative to the shaft averages 130 degrees, and the geometric center of the humeral head is offset an average of 3 mm posteriorly and 7 mm medially from the axis of the humeral shaft (92).

Humeral retroversion, as measured with respect to the epicondyles of the distal humerus, averages about 20 degrees. However, it can be significantly variable among individuals, and the range has been reported to be between 10 degrees of anteversion and 60 degrees of retroversion (see Fig. 31-1) (92–99).

The bone density of the proximal humerus is relevant to fracture fixation, and generally the bone density of the subchondral bone just underneath the articular surface is strongest, while the bone of the central humeral head and neck is more porous (Fig. 31-2) (100–105).

Rotator Cuff

The greater tuberosity has three regions into which the supraspinatus, infraspinatus, and teres minor insert. Recognition of these three prominences may aid in determining which tendons are involved in the fracture. The subscapularis tendon inserts into the lesser tuberosity, which is separated from the greater tuberosity by the bicipital groove. This groove in which courses the

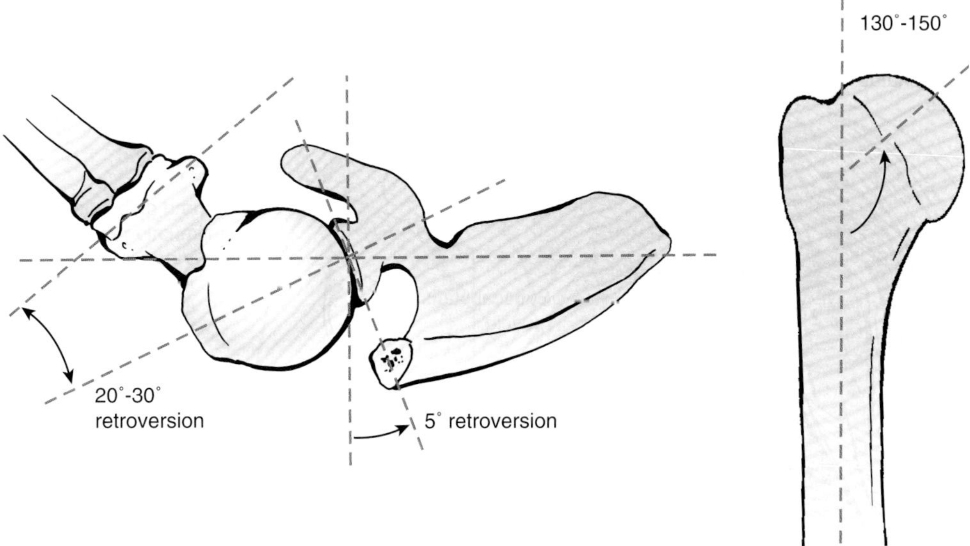

FIGURE 31-1 Proximal humerus anatomy.

biceps tendon is a useful landmark for fixation of the tuberosities during fracture repair.

The orientation of the rotator cuff attachments onto the humerus is important to understanding displacement of the tuberosities in proximal humerus fractures (Fig. 31-3). This can also aid in closed or open reduction of fracture fragments. Typically the tendon structure is stronger than the adjacent bone of the tuberosities, and this is the basis for a variety of suture fixation methods for proximal humerus fracture repairs.

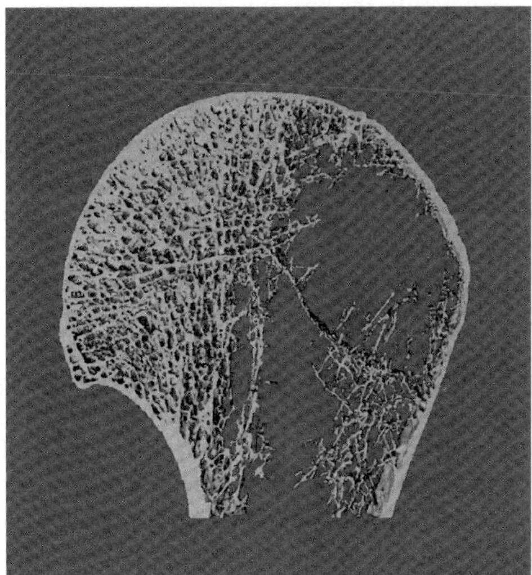

FIGURE 31-2 Micro-CT study of cancellous trabeculae in humeral head shows marked porosity in greater tuberosity region and densest bone just underneath humeral head. (Reprinted with permission from Meyer DC, Fucentese SF, Koller B, Gerber C. Association of osteopenia of the humeral head with full-thickness rotator cuff tears. *J Shoulder Elbow Surg* 2004; 13(3):333–337.)

Vascular Anatomy

The vascular anatomy of the proximal arm is relevant to proximal humerus fractures due to implications for vascular supply to the articular segment and also due to the risk of vascular injury with certain fracture configurations. The axillary artery and vein and the branches of the anterior and posterior humeral circumflex vessels are important to consider (Fig. 31-4A).

The anterior humeral circumflex artery originates from the axillary artery at the inferior border of the subscapularis muscle. The anterior humeral circumflex artery courses around the humeral shaft and anastomoses with the posterior humeral circumflex artery, which accompanies the axillary nerve through the quadrilateral space.

The ascending branch of the anterior humeral circumflex artery courses immediately lateral to the bicipital groove and is paramount in maintaining vascularity of the articular segment (see Fig. 31-4B) (106–110). This vessel enters the humeral head just below the articular surface to form the arcuate artery, which perfuses the majority of the humeral head. Loss of vascularity to the humeral head can occur if this vessel is disrupted in the setting of a fracture that involves the articular segment of the humerus at the anatomic neck level (107,111). This anatomy is relevant to fracture fixation, since excessive soft tissue stripping may damage the residual vascular supply to the humeral articular segment and increase the risk of osteonecrosis. This is considered in further detail under specific fracture types below.

Rarely, proximal humerus fractures with significant displacement of the humeral shaft can injure the axillary artery near the take-off of the circumflex vessels. The reason for this is that a sharp edge of bone may occur with a fracture at the surgical neck, and the pectoralis major tends to pull the shaft of the humerus medially toward the axillary artery. Furthermore, the circumflex vessels act as a tether, preventing the axillary vessels

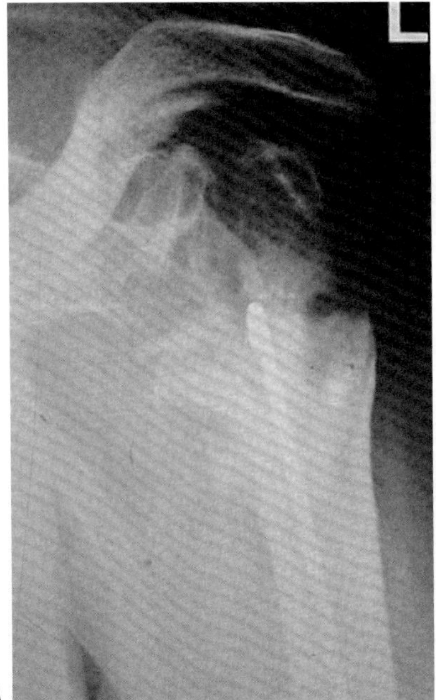

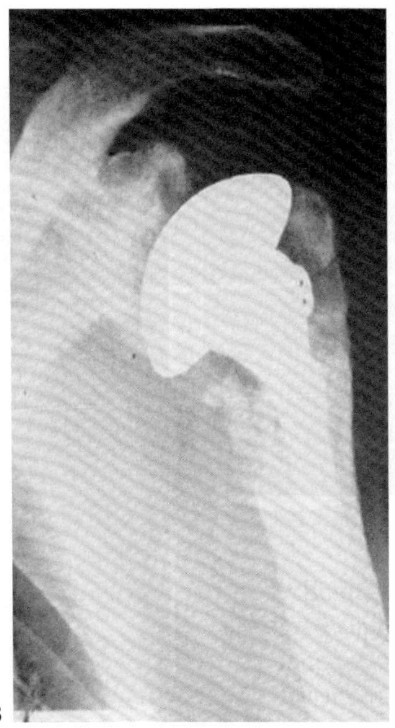

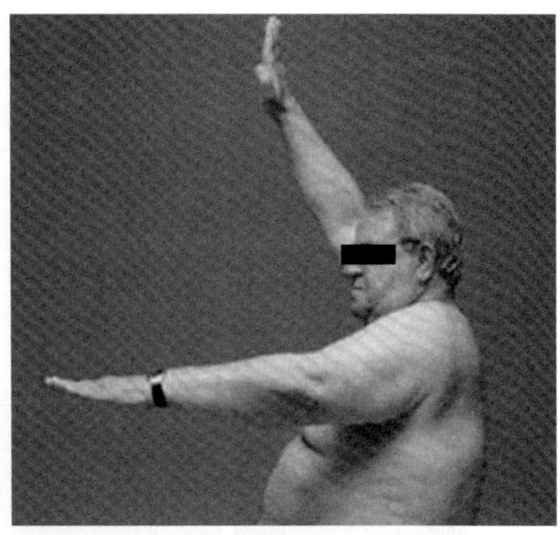

FIGURE 31-8 A. Fracture malunion with osteonecrosis. **B.** Hemiarthroplasty. **C.** Poor clinical outcome.

The currently used classification systems for proximal humerus fractures are the basis for deciding about the need for surgical fixation, since the degree of displacement is an index of fracture severity. McLaughlin (152) first proposed in 1963 that displacement of the greater tuberosity beyond 5 mm was likely to be associated with a poor functional outcome. Neer's landmark four-part classification system (153) was based on the selection of 1 cm of displacement or 45 degrees of angulation as criteria for operative intervention. Although somewhat arbitrary, it has nonetheless stood the test of time as a useful clinical decision-making tool and a gauge of the degree of fracture fragment separation that may warrant surgical treatment. In practice, though, the reproducibility and reliability of this method of radiographic measurement have come under question (see the following section).

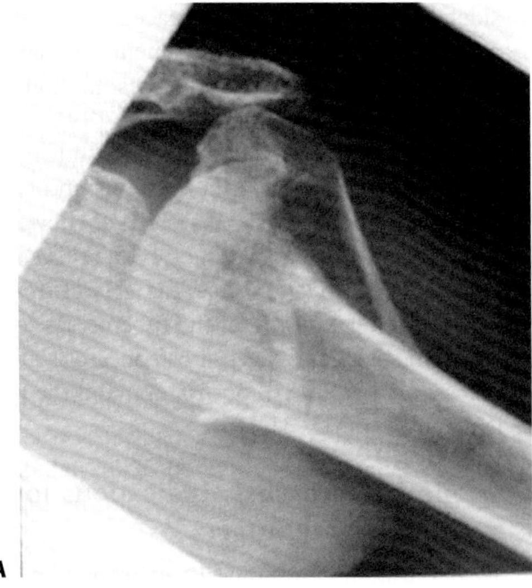

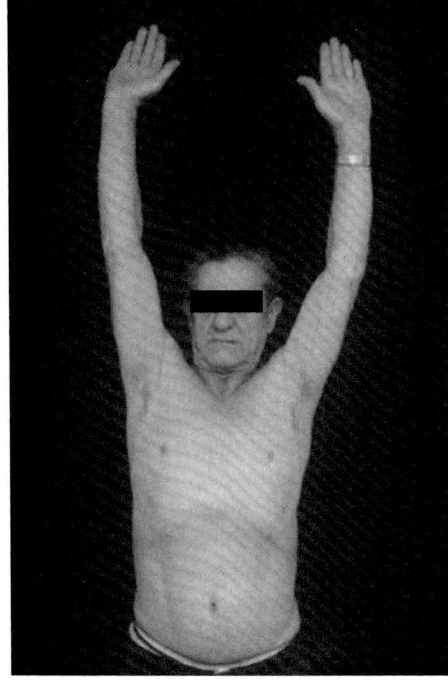

FIGURE 31-9 A. Malunited greater tuberosity fracture. **B.** Good function in patient with malunited greater tuberosity fracture.

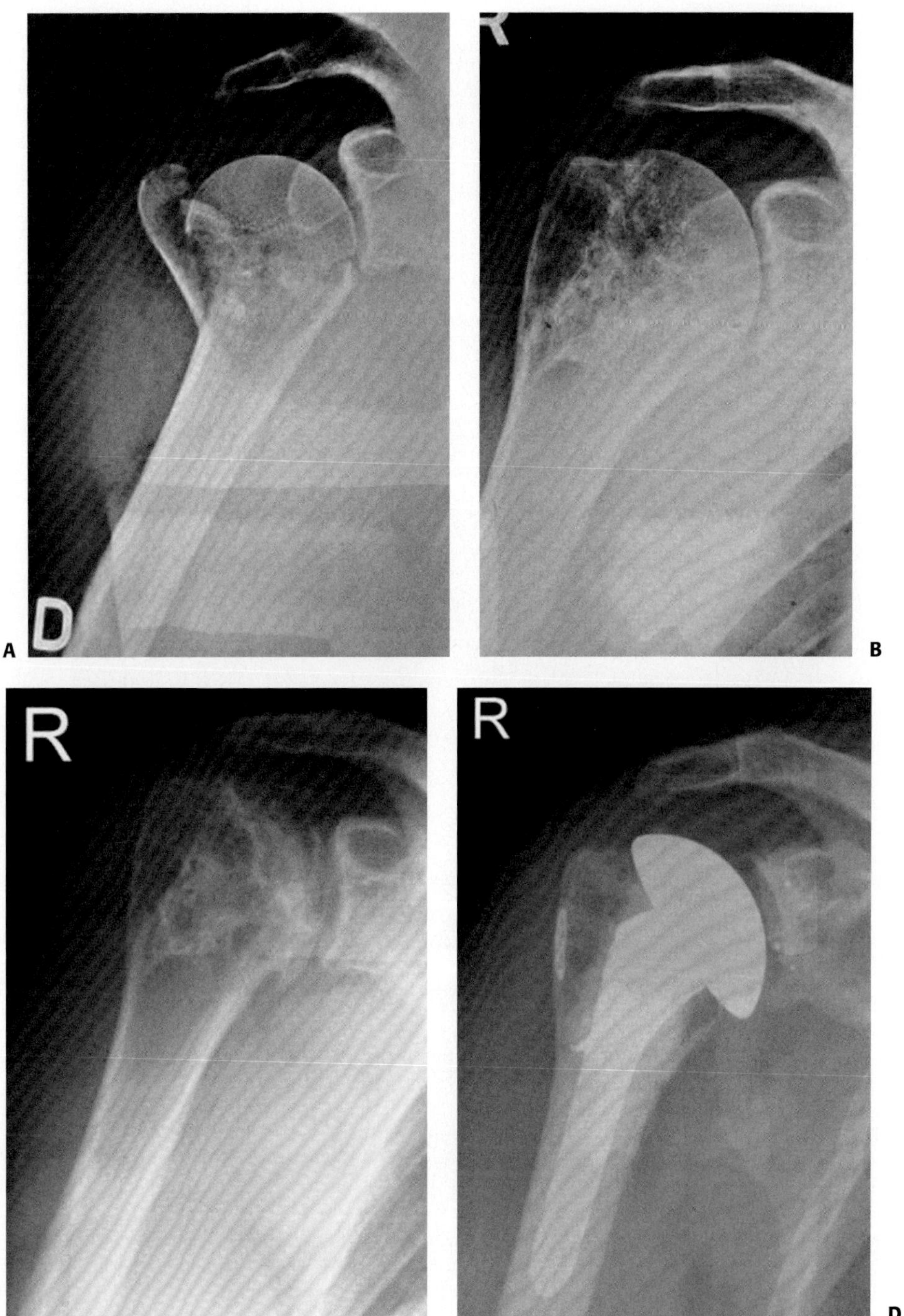

FIGURE 31-10 **A.** Valgus-impacted three-part fracture in a 42-year-old patient. **B.** One year after anatomic reconstruction and removal of hardware. This is a normal joint. **C.** Osteonecrosis develops 3 years after stabilization of fracture, resulting in poor function and the need for arthroplasty **(D)**. (Reprinted with permission from Gerber C, Werner CML, Vienne P. Internal fixation of complex fractures of the proximal humerus. *J Bone Joint Surg Br* 2004;86:848–855.)

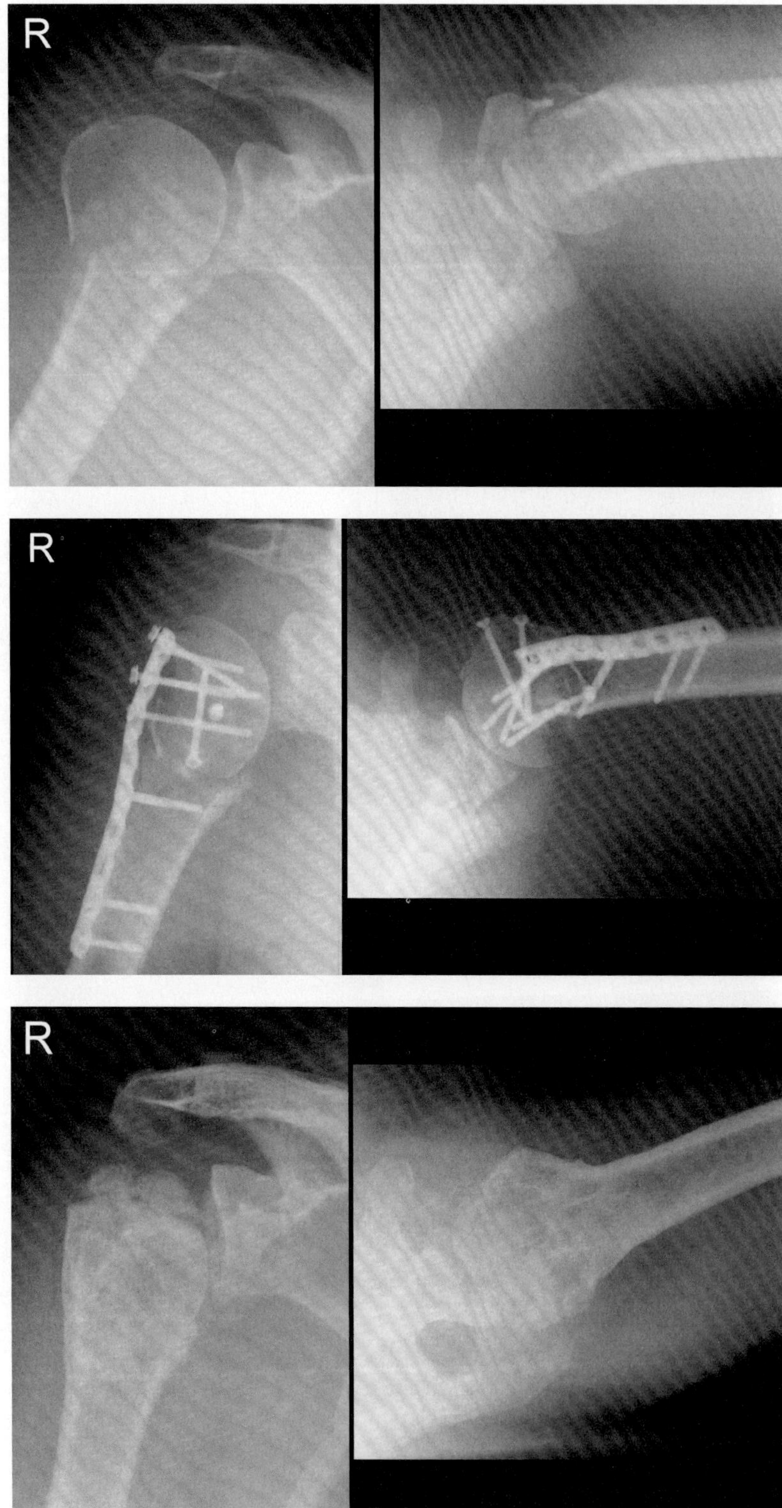

FIGURE 31-11 Rigid fixation of a fracture resulting in osteonecrosis due to disruption of residual vascularity to the articular segment.

Once the surgeon decides that a fracture must be treated surgically, the goal is restoring articular anatomy and its relationship to the tuberosities while at the same time maintaining the vascular integrity of the anatomic head. The problem with rigid internal fixation using plates has been the relative risk of disruption of the residual vascularity to the articular segment (Fig. 31-11). An alternative method of treatment that has been developed over the past few decades is percutaneous fixation with indirect reduction using closed methods (154–159). This method has been shown to be useful in certain fracture configurations, such as valgus-impacted three- and four-part fractures, which carry a relatively low rate of osteonecrosis (160,161). It is believed that this is because the ascending branch of the anterior humeral circumflex artery is not disrupted, since there is no surgical dissection in this region (see Fig. 31-4) (83,156,157,162). Despite these advantages, this is a demanding technique with complications such as loss of fixation and pin tract infection, which have been variably reported in the literature (155,163,164). This method and its applications are discussed in a later section.

EVALUATION AND CLASSIFICATION

Signs and Symptoms

In most cases of proximal humerus fracture, there is significant swelling and pain; they may worsen over several days after the injury and are usually associated with ecchymosis. As the swelling subsides over the first 2 to 4 weeks, the ecchymosis changes from the classic blue bruising to green and then yellow and may move distally down the arm. Patients should be instructed initially to remove any constricting jewelry such as rings and bracelets. Bony deformity is not usually very apparent due to the marked swelling. Patients may occasionally note tingling or numbness in the extremity, which may be related to brachial plexus stretch or, rarely, more serious injury. A careful physical examination must be performed to rule out neurovascular injury.

Physical Findings

Initially, other injuries of the neck or chest wall must be excluded, since this association is not uncommon, especially if high-energy trauma such as a motor vehicle accident has occurred. Neurovascular evaluation is the next step, and this may be difficult in the setting of acute swelling and pain, as pseudoparalysis (inability to move the arm due to pain from the fracture) makes motor examination unreliable. Light touch sensation should be documented, although preserved sensation over the deltoid does not necessarily rule out an axillary nerve injury (165). Function of the distal upper extremity (including biceps, triceps, wrist extensors, and hand intrinsics) can help rule out brachial plexus injury, and careful documentation of extremity perfusion is also necessary, since rare injuries to the vessels of the brachial plexus can occur with marked fracture displacement.

If the patient has had loss of consciousness, bilateral injuries, and especially a posterior fracture–dislocation, a seizure disorder or electric shock should be considered and ruled out through appropriate neurologic evaluation.

X-Rays and CT Scans

Adequate radiographic evaluation is essential for accurate fracture classification and treatment decisions. Not uncommonly, oblique x-rays or an inadequate number of views results in an inaccurate fracture classification or missed fractures and dislocations, which can lead to errors in treatment (Fig. 31-12).

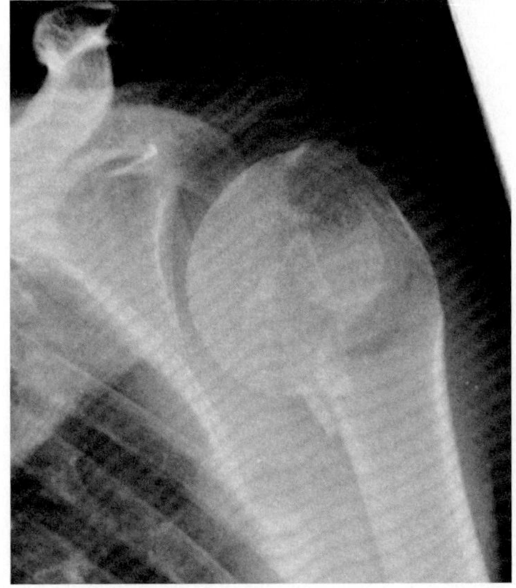

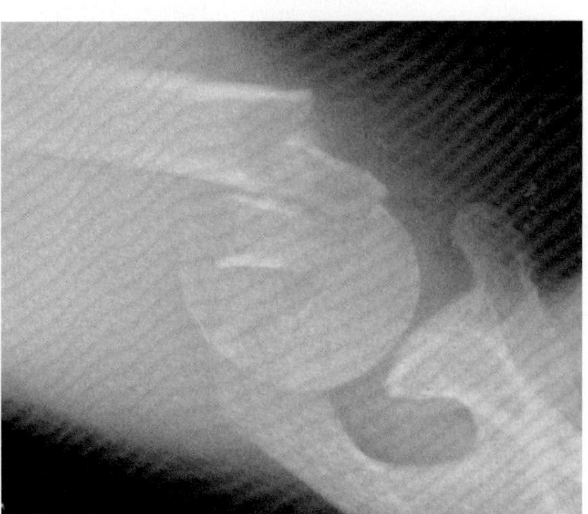

FIGURE 31-12 **A.** True AP view gives the impression of a one-part fracture. **B.** Axillary image shows that this is a two-part surgical neck fracture.

A trauma series is mandatory, and this consists of an anteroposterior (AP) view of the scapula, which is a true AP view of the shoulder joint, an axillary view, and a lateral Y-view of the scapula (Fig. 31-13). If abduction of the shoulder for an axillary view cannot be performed due to pain, a Velpeau axillary view can be substituted while the patient's arm remains in the sling. However, the physician should be willing to assist with positioning the patient's arm to obtain an accurate axillary image, as this is the most commonly omitted x-ray and a reason for missing dislocations and fractures. If the physician carefully brings the arm into abduction, inability to obtain an axillary view is quite rare.

A CT scan may be helpful when plain x-rays fail to clearly show the fracture or if there is concern for concomitant glenoid or scapular injury (Fig. 31-14). MRI studies are rarely needed and do not usually give the osseous detail of a CT scan.

Classification

Historically, proximal humerus fracture classification evolved based on the location of the fracture lines or the supposed mech-

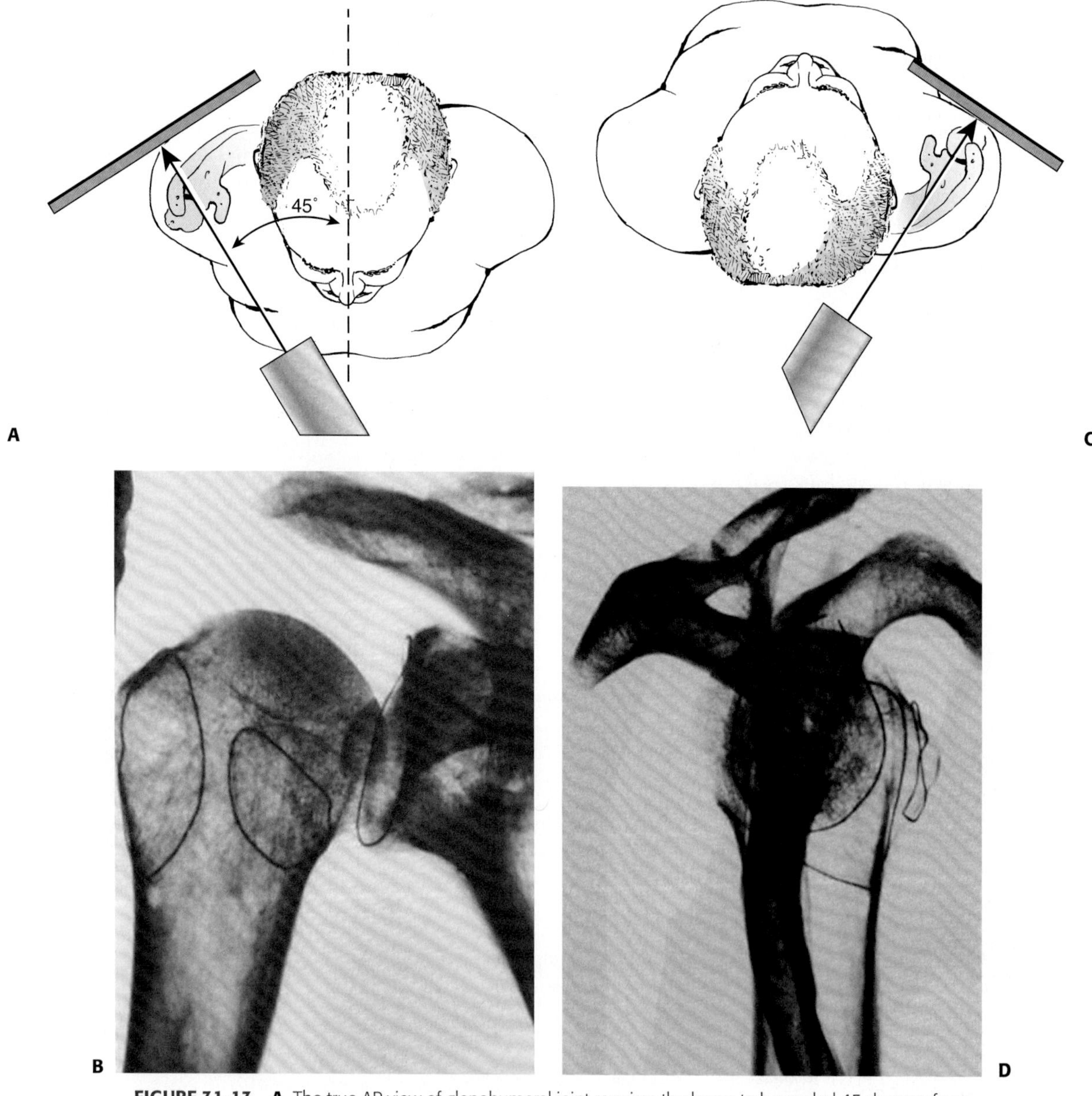

FIGURE 31-13 **A.** The true AP view of glenohumeral joint requires the beam to be angled 45 degrees from the sagittal plane. **B.** True AP view shows the joint in profile and the tuberosities are outlined. **C.** The Y-lateral view orientation of x-ray beam. **D.** The Y-lateral view shows the humeral head centered in the glenoid. (*continues*)

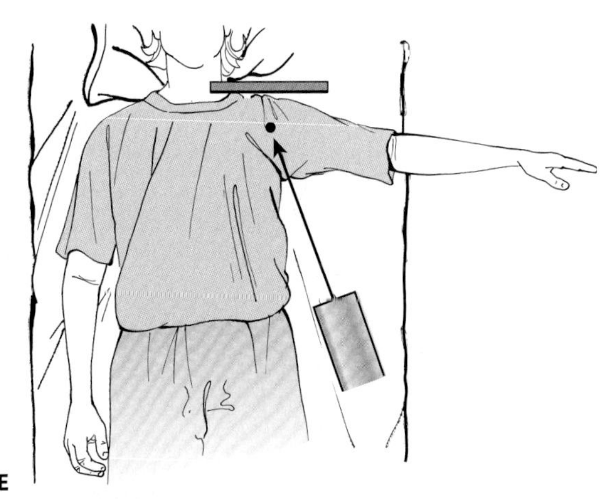
E

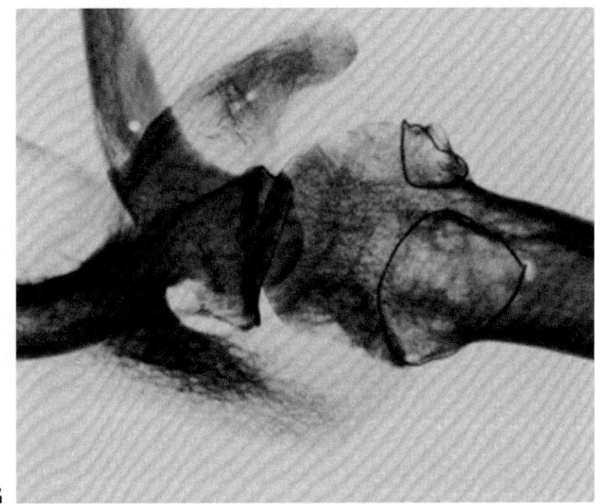
G

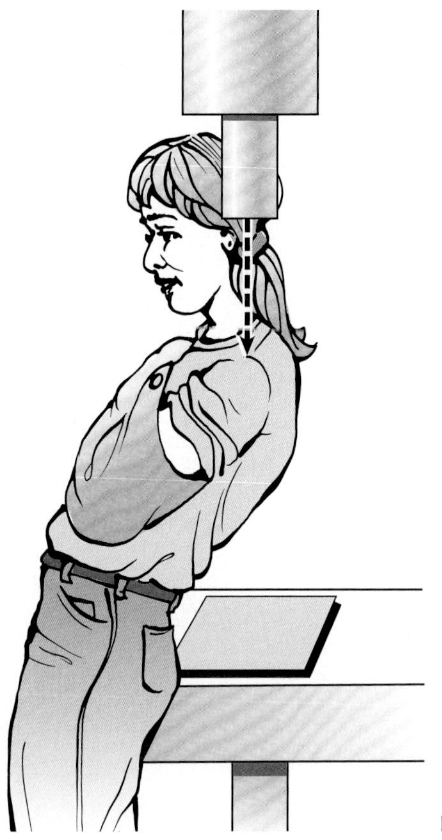
F

FIGURE 31-13 (*continued*) **E.** The axillary lateral view requires the shoulder to be abducted. **F.** A Velpeau axillary view can be obtained without abducting the shoulder. **G.** Axillary lateral x-ray shows the humeral head centered in the glenoid.

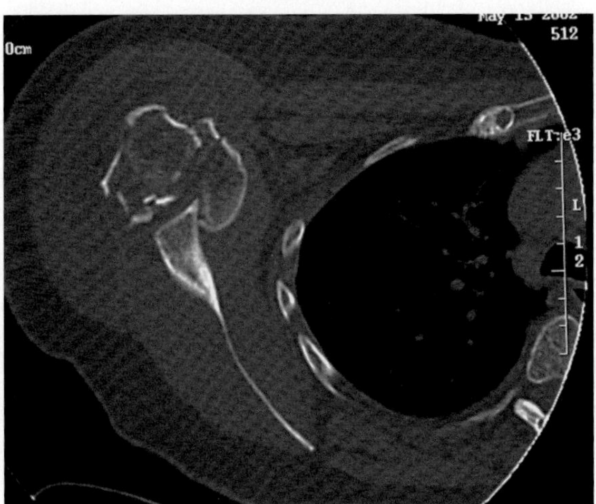

FIGURE 31-14 Locked fracture–dislocation of anatomic neck shown on a CT scan.

anism of injury (29,118,166–169). Consideration of fracture classification based on regions of the proximal humerus including the tuberosities, articular segment, and shaft was separately proposed by DeAnquin (170) and Neer (171). DePalma and Cautilli (35) first emphasized the difference between fractures with and without dislocation of the joint surfaces. Neer subsequently modified and emphasized this fracture type in his classic four-part classification scheme (171,172).

Codman was the first to observe that there were four major fracture fragments when a proximal humerus fracture occurred, and that these occurred in varying combinations depending on the mechanism of injury (Fig. 31-15) (115). These fragments were the articular head, the greater and lesser tuberosities, and the humeral shaft.

Neer's classification scheme was first published in 1975 after more than 15 years of experience and analysis of 300 displaced proximal humerus fractures. He modified and improved on Codman's classification by emphasizing patterns and degree of displacement rather than the location of fracture lines. He believed this gave important insight into humeral articular seg-

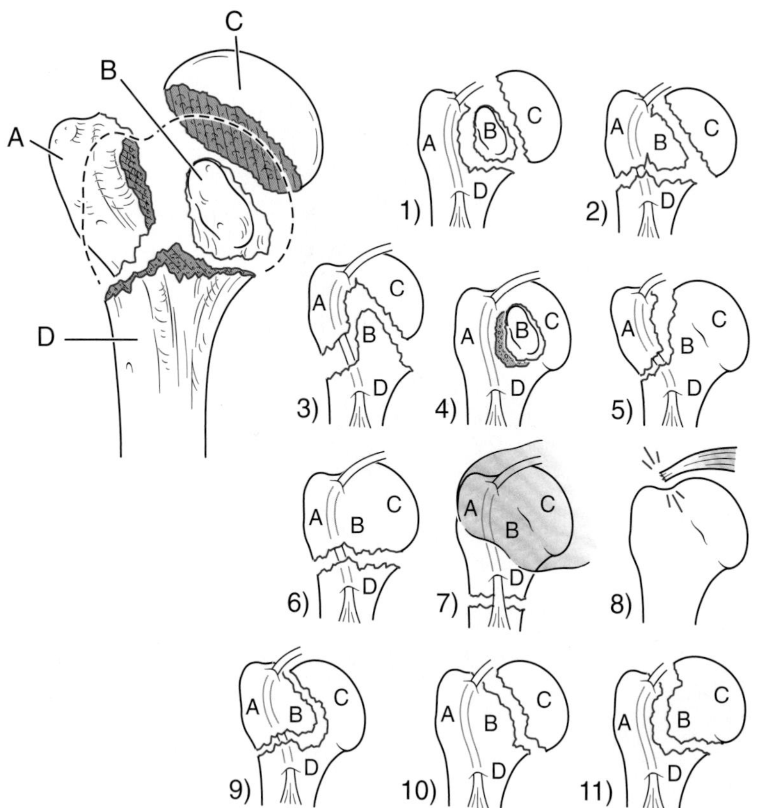

FIGURE 31-15 Codman's drawing of patterns of fracture of the proximal humerus. (Adapted from Codman EA. *The shoulder: rupture of the supraspinatus tendon and other lesions in or about the subacromial bursa*. Boston: Thomas Todd, 1934; with permission.)

ment viability by providing evidence of the likelihood of disruption of soft tissue and vascular integrity to the head. He emphasized the prognostic importance of fracture–dislocations, which he felt had a high likelihood of osteonecrosis due to loss of soft tissue attachments to the humeral head, and this led to the development of proximal humeral replacements as early as 1953 (97).

Neer's classification scheme is the system most widely used by orthopaedic surgeons today (Fig. 31-16) (171). It groups fractures based on the number of parts and their displacement from each other. In this system, the criteria for displacement are 45 degrees of angulation or more than 1 cm of displacement between fracture parts. If displacement is less than this, then the fracture is considered to be "minimally displaced" regardless of the number of fracture lines.

A two-part fracture means that only one segment is displaced, and the most common type is a surgical neck fracture. Greater tuberosity displacement is another not uncommon form of two-part fracture. Two-part fractures that involve the lesser tuberosity or the anatomic neck are rare. A three-part fracture involves displacement of the shaft and humeral head from either the greater tuberosity (more common) or the lesser tuberosity. The pattern of deformity is then based on the pull upon each segment, as previously described.

A four-part fracture isolates the humeral articular segment from the tuberosities and the shaft. The typical scenario is dislocation of the humeral segment out of the glenoid with no remaining soft tissue attachments. The so-called valgus-impacted four-part fracture was described after Neer's original classification and is an important variant, since it may have a better prognosis than the classic four-part fracture (Fig. 31-17) (83,156,159,173). In this fracture, residual vascularity may be maintained through an intact medial soft tissue sleeve despite more than 45 degrees of angulation of the humeral head segment as well as greater and lesser tuberosity displacement. Thus, the risk for osteonecrosis is less than in the case of a classic four-part fracture (83,156,159,162,174).

Jakob et al proposed the AO Group classification of proximal humerus fractures based on a study of 730 cases. This system creates subgroups of fractures according to the degree of displacement, resulting in 27 subgroups (157,175). Its complexity has resulted in limited use (176).

Recently, Hertel et al (162) analyzed factors associated with the development of osteonecrosis and found that the number of "parts" and degree of displacement were not as important as the length of the dorsomedial metaphyseal extension of the fracture and integrity of the medial soft tissue. Despite this new insight, the Neer classification system remains the most widely used, and it will be the basis for presentation of fracture management in this chapter.

Concerns for reliability of these classification schemes have been raised, and several studies have documented poor interob-

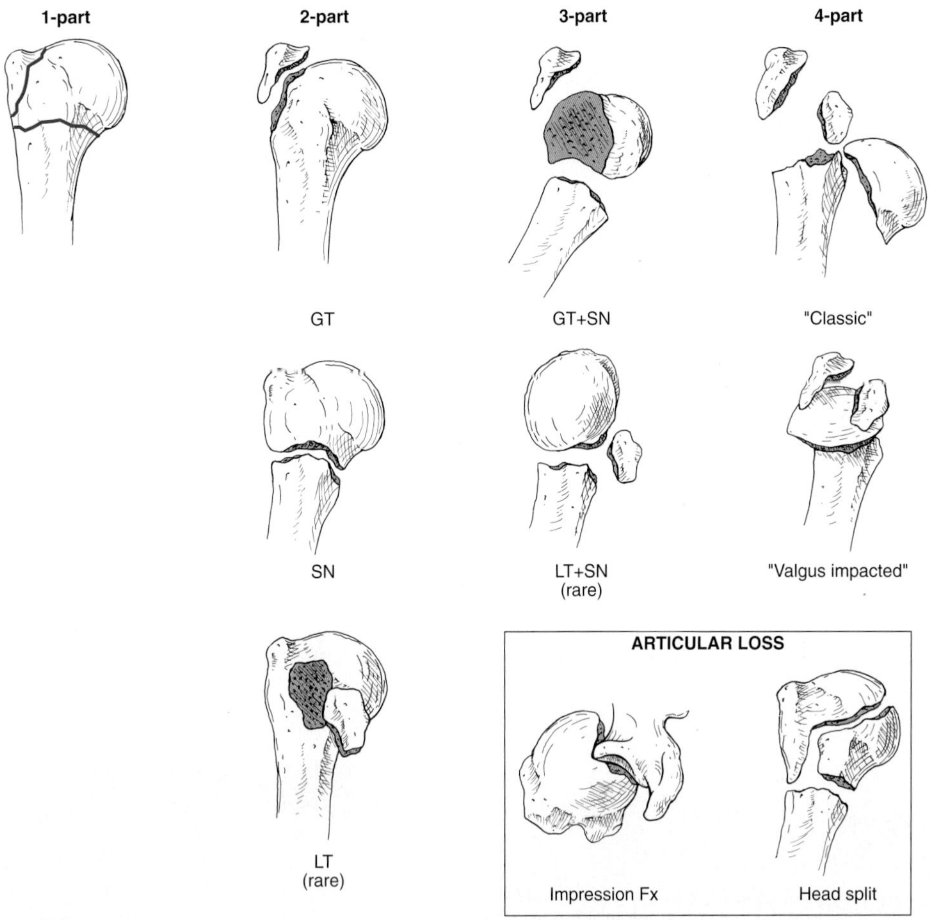

FIGURE 31-16 Neer's classification of proximal humerus fractures. (Reprinted with permission from Neer CS. Displaced proximal humeral fractures: I. Classification and evaluation. *J Bone Joint Surg Am* 1970;52: 1077–1089.)

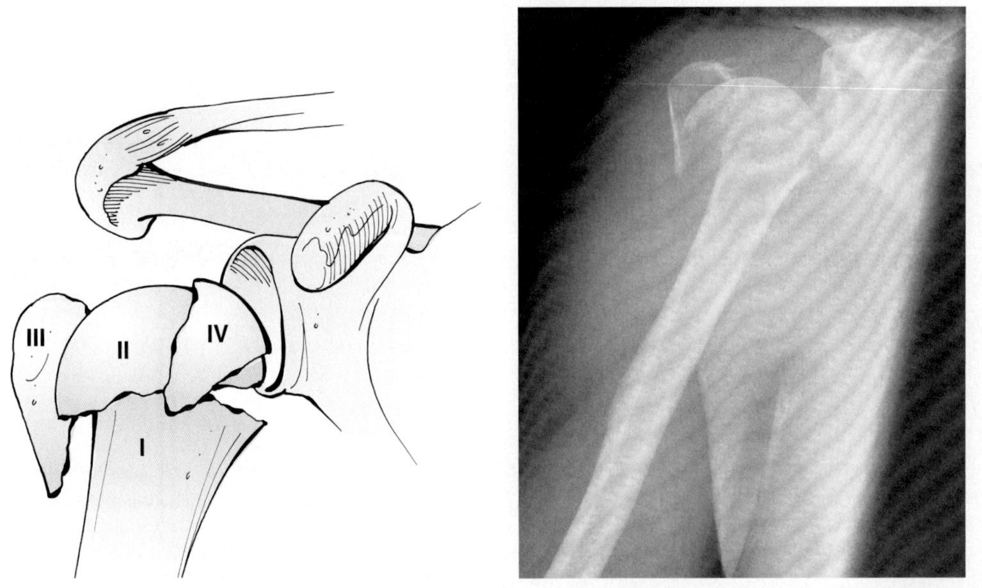

FIGURE 31-17 **A.** Drawing showing anatomy of a valgus-impacted four-part fracture. **B.** A valgus-impacted four-part fracture. (**A** adapted from Jakob RP, Miniaci A, Anson PS, et al. Four-part valgus-impacted fractures of the proximal humerus. *J Bone Joint Surg Br* 1991;73:295–298.)

server reliability (different observers classify the same fracture differently based on the same x-rays) and intraobserver repeatability (the same observer classifies the same fracture differently) (176–179). However, the experience of the physician in treating proximal humerus fractures has correlated with the reliability of the classification (180,181). Recently, Parsons et al (149) showed that multiple radiographic views may be necessary to accurately classify the degree of greater tuberosity displacement, and that a true AP of the shoulder joint with the arm in external rotation is the best method to detect small degrees of greater tuberosity displacement. It is likely that the degree of variability between examiners may reflect differences in radiographic views as well as the observation that fracture configuration may change when the arm is placed into different positions for an x-ray.

CT scans may help with classification in certain situations, such as unrecognized displacement of the lesser tuberosity or greater tuberosity, as well as providing a more accurate determination of proximal humeral angulation in the axial plane. The reproducibility of classification, however, does not increase (151,176,182,183).

SURGICAL TREATMENT OF SPECIFIC FRACTURE TYPES

Two-Part (Displaced Greater Tuberosity)

Isolated greater tuberosity fracture is not uncommon, but unfortunately the extent of tuberosity displacement is not always appreciated (81,149,184). Careful attention to obtaining proper x-rays in biplanar orientation and CT scans when needed is the only way to ensure accurate detection of significant tuberosity displacement.

The consequences of an untreated malunited greater tuberosity fracture may be limited motion and/or pain (see Fig. 31-9) (81). Typically this fracture occurs when there is an anterior dislocation as the posterior rotator cuff bony insertion is avulsed (185). About 7% to 15% of anterior shoulder dislocations are associated with a greater tuberosity fracture (1,52,138,186). As with all dislocations, careful attention to radiographic analysis is important to make sure no other fractures are present in the proximal humerus, as displacement of an otherwise minimally displaced fracture of the anatomic neck has been described, and the consequences of this can be dire (150,187,188). If there is any

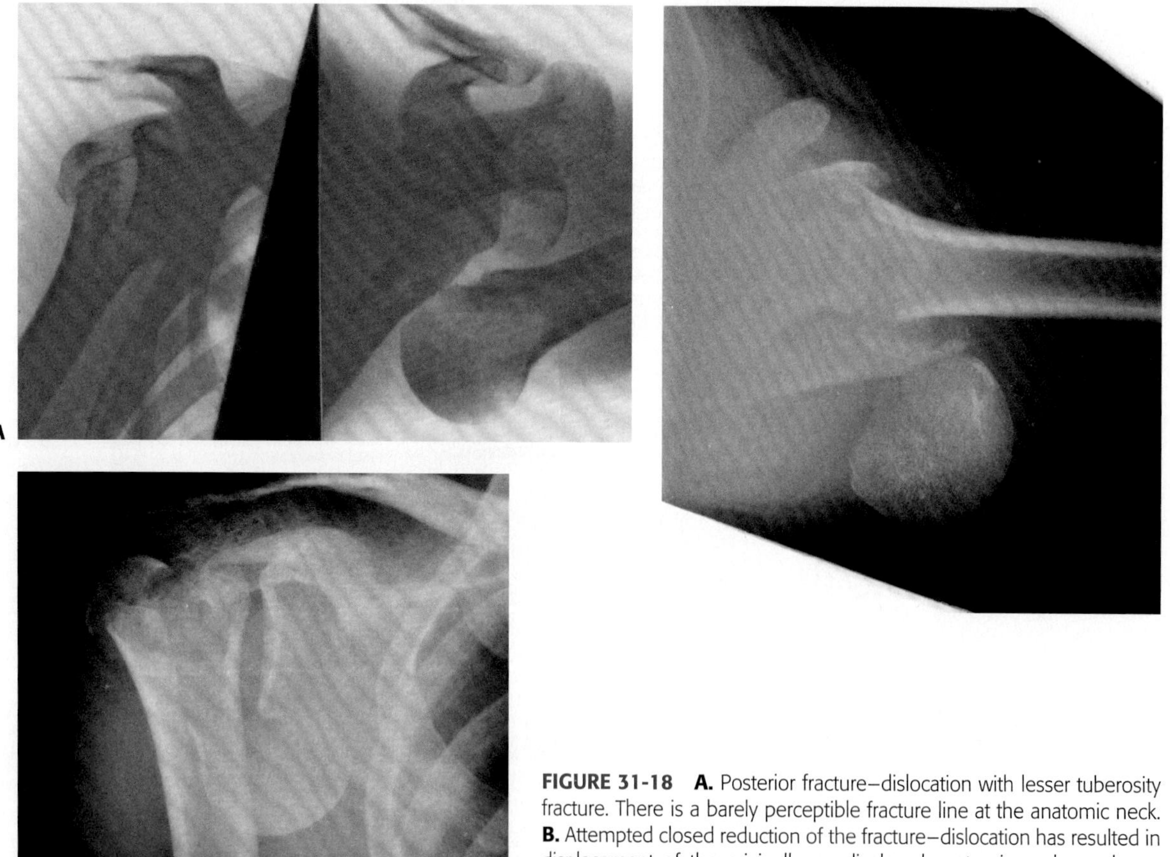

FIGURE 31-18 A. Posterior fracture–dislocation with lesser tuberosity fracture. There is a barely perceptible fracture line at the anatomic neck. **B.** Attempted closed reduction of the fracture–dislocation has resulted in displacement of the originally nondisplaced anatomic neck, as shown on the anteroposterior radiograph **(B)** and the axillary radiograph **(C)**. (Reprinted with permission from Hersche O, Gerber C. Iatrogenic displacement of fracture–dislocations of the shoulder. A report of seven cases. *J Bone Joint Surg Br* 1994;76(1):30–33.)

possibility of a minimally displaced anatomic or surgical neck fracture component in an otherwise unreduced anterior dislocation with avulsion of the greater tuberosity, reduction under general anesthesia using open methods is preferred (Fig. 31-18). Stabilizing the neck fracture with a short plate and screws before reduction, then reduction and removal of the protective plate, seems to be the most prudent way of treating this situation.

During closed reduction, the greater tuberosity is usually reduced into an acceptable position, as the remaining intact rotator cuff tethers the bony fragment back into its bed (Fig. 31-19). This kind of fracture–dislocation has been shown to be associated with a lower recurrence of anterior instability, presumably due to healing of the greater tuberosity (152). In some cases, however, the tuberosity fragment may be displaced superiorly or posteriorly, and while there is no absolute consensus as to the acceptable degree of displacement, generally less than 5 mm of displacement is the criterion for nonoperative treatment (189,190). There are, however, individual exceptions to this rule (see Fig. 31-9). When this occurs, it is usually advisable to reduce and repair the greater tuberosity acutely. In some cases, soft tissue interposition may be the reason for continued displacement (Fig. 31-20).

Historically, treatment has consisted of traction, spica casting, and even excision of the fragment and repair of the tendon (25,191–194). None of these methods resulted in consistent restoration of function. Most surgeons now advocate surgical repair when there is displacement, with options including open reduc-

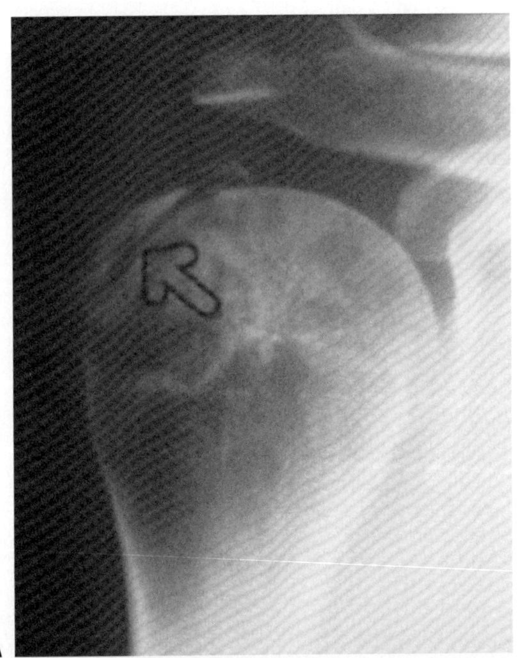

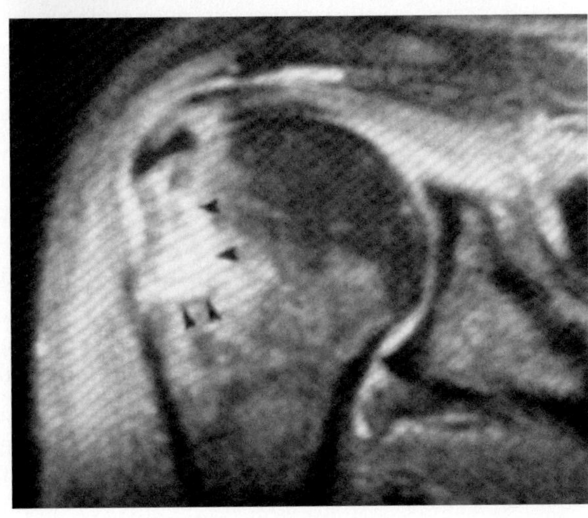

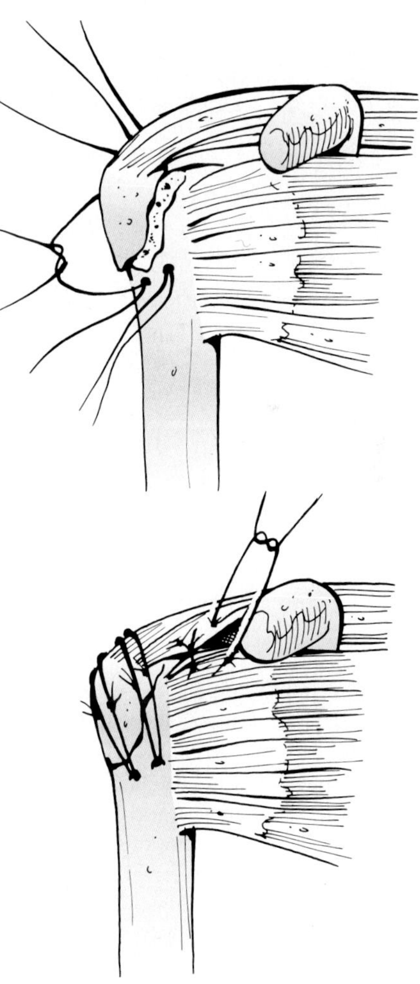

FIGURE 31-19 A. Displaced greater tuberosity (*arrow*) after reduction of humerus. **B.** MRI of displaced greater tuberosity fracture. **C.** Open reduction and repair of greater tuberosity fracture.

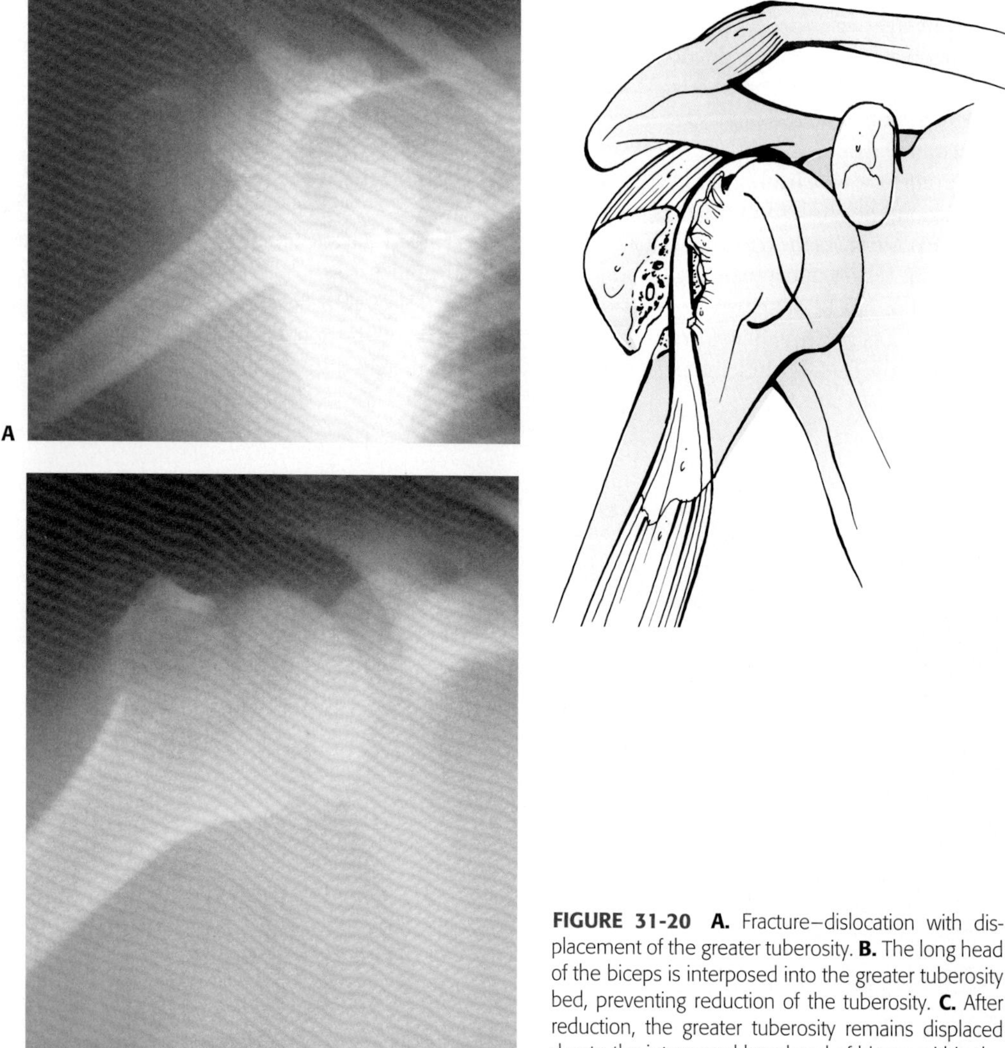

FIGURE 31-20 A. Fracture–dislocation with displacement of the greater tuberosity. **B.** The long head of the biceps is interposed into the greater tuberosity bed, preventing reduction of the tuberosity. **C.** After reduction, the greater tuberosity remains displaced due to the interposed long head of biceps within the fracture site.

tion and screw fixation (in the case of a large fragment of good bone in a younger patient) or suture fixation. In practice, many of these cases are associated with soft bone, which may be fragmented, and most surgeons prefer to use heavy sutures placed through the adjacent rotator cuff tendon and then through holes placed in the adjacent proximal humerus (81,195–197). One study recently showed good results with arthroscopically guided percutaneous repair of the greater tuberosity (198).

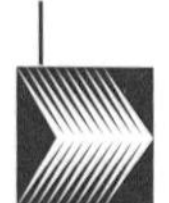

AUTHORS' PREFERRED TREATMENT

A superior open approach, similar to that used for rotator cuff repair, provides good access for reduction and repair of a displaced greater tuberosity. On rare occasions, if there is a long spiral extension into the metaphysis, or if there is an associated subscapularis disruption, a deltopectoral approach is used.

An incision is made over the top of the shoulder in the skin crease lines, and the skin is undermined to facilitate adequate exposure. The deltoid is then split in line with its fibers at the lateral edge of the mid-acromion. Some surgeons prefer to split the deltoid in its anterior raphe; however, we have found that splitting it at the mid-acromion and then elevating it off the acromion as a sleeve with electrocautery allows for extensive posterior exposure, which facilitates mobilization and repair of even a posteriorly retracted greater tuberosity. If there is a large bony fragment, it may be fixed with AO screws. We prefer 4.0 cannulated cancellousscrews, usually without washers. More frequently the quality of the bone is soft; in these cases, No. 5 braided, nonabsorb-

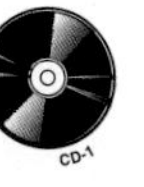

able suture (Fiberwire, Arthrex, Naples, Florida) is placed through the tendon at its junction with the tuberosity and then through drill holes in the humerus to reduce the fragment anatomically (see Fig. 31-19). Several additional sutures are placed to close the lateral portion of the rotator interval, between the supraspinatus and subscapularis tendons. The deltoid is then closed with the same sutures through drill holes in the acromion, and skin closure is usually achieved using subcuticular absorbable suture.

Postoperative Rehabilitation. In most cases, secure fixation is achieved and immediate passive range of motion is instituted to avoid formation of adhesions and adhesive capsulitis. Passive motion is performed by a therapist, and patient self-assisted exercises with a pulley and stick are delayed until 4 to 6 weeks after surgery. A sling is worn for 4 to 6 weeks as well. If a water therapy program is available, we ask the patient to go into a warm pool and gently let the shoulder float on postoperative day 1. The incision remains covered with a sterile, watertight adhesive dressing that is placed at the completion of the surgical procedure. This zero-gravity situation allows for some muscle activation without loading the fracture and also seems to restore motion more quickly (199). While active motion and discontinuation of the sling can usually commence after 6 weeks, strengthening and stretching into internal rotation are usually avoided until 3 months after surgery.

Results. Early repair using this method has been shown in one series to give consistently excellent results with near-normal range of motion (81). This has also been our experience, though unfortunately we are seeing more cases of malunited or nonunited greater tuberosity fractures, and the consequences of these conditions are discussed in a later section of this chapter.

Two-Part (Displaced Lesser Tuberosity)

The isolated lesser tuberosity fracture is rare (81,195–197). In the series used as a basis for the AO classification, these fractures represented only 2 of the 730 cases analyzed (175). Just as with greater tuberosity fractures, where anterior dislocation may be a concurrent event, posterior dislocation should be suspected with a lesser tuberosity fracture that is displaced. Our experience is that this is often associated with a severe trauma, so nondisplaced anatomic or surgical neck fractures should also be ruled out. When initially treating a posterior dislocation with a displaced lesser tuberosity, care should be taken not to create a displaced fracture of the anatomic neck. If there is any question about the presence of a nondisplaced anatomic neck fracture, a CT scan should be obtained and the reduction maneuver performed after preliminary fixation either by percutaneous pins for a closed reduction or with plate and screw fixation of the neck fracture for the preferred open reduction.

Since these fractures are so rare, in cases where the posterior dislocation reduces, the displacement of the lesser tuberosity may be missed. This can lead to chronic subscapularis insufficiency, which is demonstrated clinically with a classic lift-off or belly-press sign (Fig. 31-21) (200–202). Few reports of treatment are available in the literature; however, excision with repair of the subscapularis or internal fixation with a screw has been described in a few cases (202,203).

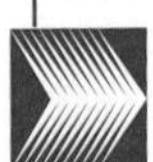

AUTHORS' PREFERRED TREATMENT

Axillary x-rays are helpful to detect the degree of medial displacement, and we often obtain a CT scan as well, since this more accurately defines the degree of displacement. The surgical approach for repair is an extended deltopectoral ap-

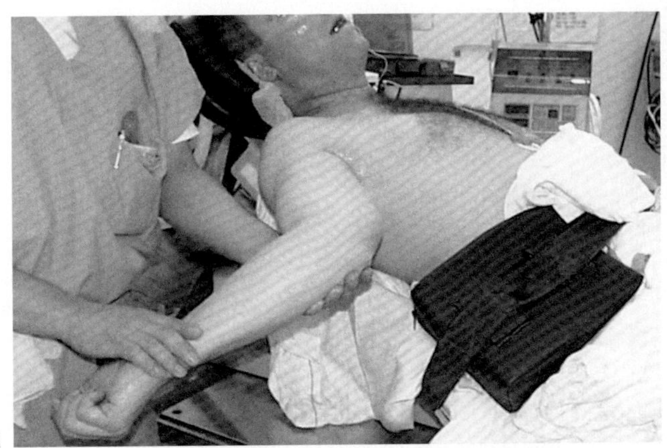

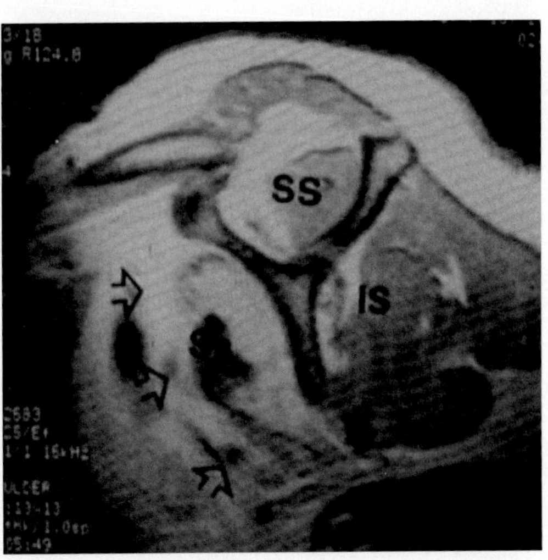

FIGURE 31-21 **A.** Increased external rotation in a 27-year-old physician with a chronic nonunion of a lesser tuberosity fracture and subscapularis insufficiency. **B.** Oblique sagittal MRI image showing marked fatty replacement of the subscapularis muscle (*arrows*) 10 years after a nonunion of the lesser tuberosity.

proach similar to that used for a shoulder arthroplasty. The long head of the biceps should be assessed to make sure it is not displaced medially into the joint. If it is displaced out of the bicipital groove, it should be tenodesed in situ at the lower portion of the metaphysis. The subscapularis, in the case of an acute lesser tuberosity fracture, is freely mobile and if the bony fragment is large it is fixed with two 4.0 cannulated AO cancellous screws into the humeral bed from which it was avulsed. If it is small and soft, then repair is performed with heavy transosseous, nonabsorbable, braided sutures using a similar technique as used for lesser tuberosity osteotomy repair in total shoulder replacement (204,205). We do not hesitate to expose and mobilize the axillary nerve if needed to restore mobility to the subscapularis, since a delay of only several weeks can lead to medial retraction of the tendon and the need for its mobilization. This step cannot be safely performed without visualizing and dissecting the axillary nerve.

Results. There are few reports of repair of isolated lesser tuberosity fractures (202,206–212). Our experience has been identical to repair of an acute subscapularis rupture in that repair without a delay of greater than 6 months uniformly leads to an excellent result, even though rehabilitation may last up to 6 months. Late repair is usually difficult due to the scarring and retraction that accompany the chronic tendon tear as well as fatty replacement of the muscle (see Fig. 31-21) (213–217). Loss of external rotation after repair must be anticipated in these cases.

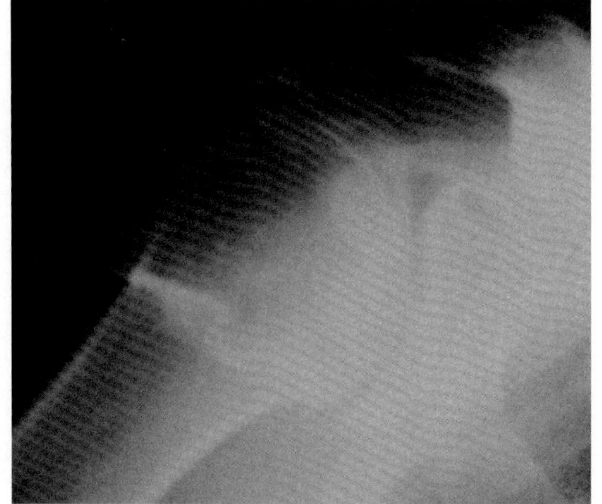
A

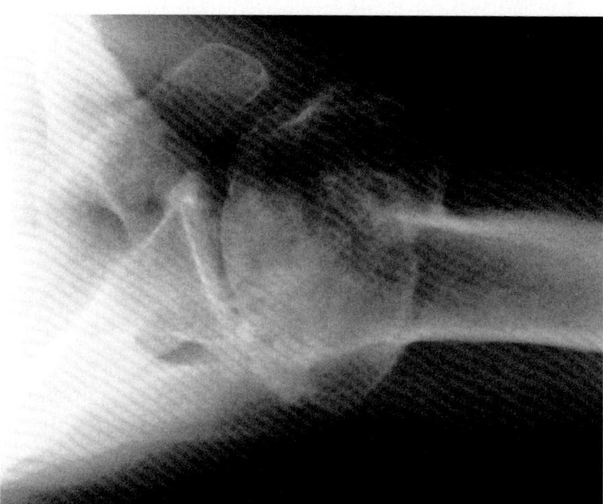
B

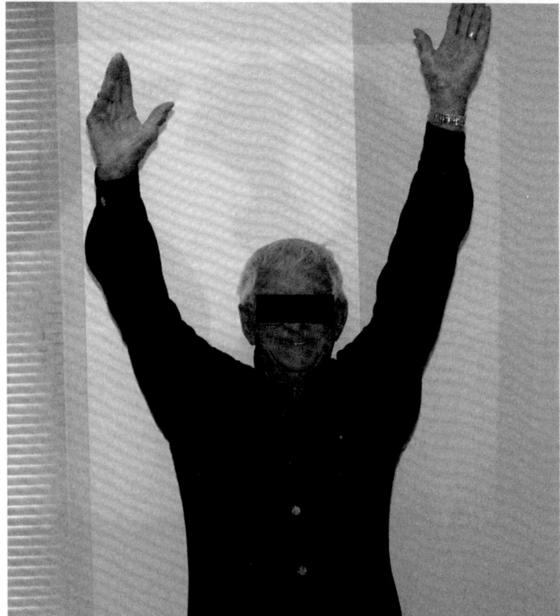
C

FIGURE 31-22 A. AP x-ray of a malunited proximal humerus fracture. **B.** Axillary x-ray of malunited proximal humerus fracture. **C.** The patient had good clinical function and no pain despite the chronic malunited fracture.

Two-Part (Displaced Surgical Neck)

Unlike displacement between the articular surface and the tuberosities, displacement and angulation between the articular surface and the humeral shaft can be relatively well tolerated due to the large range of motion available to the shoulder. In elderly individuals, it is thus acceptable to opt for conservative treatment if union is likely to occur even with angulation (Fig. 31-22). Surgical neck fractures are at risk for nonunion if the bone is very osteopenic, the fracture line is very proximal, or the degree of displacement between the humeral shaft and proximal humerus is substantial (218–221). Complete displacement of the proximal segment from the shaft is an indication for surgery in most cases (Fig. 31-23). Options for treatment include closed reduction with or without percutaneous pinning and open reduction with minimal or rigid fixation using plates, IM fixation, and fixation with heavy sutures. These options are briefly presented and the technique of closed reduction and percutaneous pinning (CRPP) is discussed in the context of even more complex fractures in greater detail.

Closed Reduction

This technique should be performed only after adequate biplanar x-rays are available. It is usually indicated in an elderly individual without significant comminution at the calcar level and if there is no substantial extension of the fracture into the (medial) metaphysis. Complete muscle paralysis is necessary either with general anesthesia or with regional anesthetic blockade. Biplanar fluoroscopic guidance is mandatory. Before draping, the surgeon must ascertain that AP and axillary views can be obtained with the selected positioning of the patient at the table. Typically, the deformity is one in which the apex of the fracture is angulated anteriorly or the shaft is displaced anteriorly while the humeral head remains in the glenoid. The pull of the pectoralis major on the distal segment causes this deformity (Fig. 31-24). The reduction maneuver involves holding one hand anteriorly on the fracture site and then forceful flexion of the arm combined with adduction to disimpact the posterior impaction and to relax the pectoralis major muscle. The proximal shaft next to the fracture site is thereby manipulated posteriorly and laterally (Fig. 31-25). A reduction may be felt, and fluoroscopy should confirm if alignment is acceptable and if the reduction is stable. If this is not the case, then percutaneous fixation is performed as described below. If the reduction is stable, the shoulder is immobilized in a sling and swathe for 4 weeks, after which active motion may begin as long as radiographic control demonstrates a stable reduction.

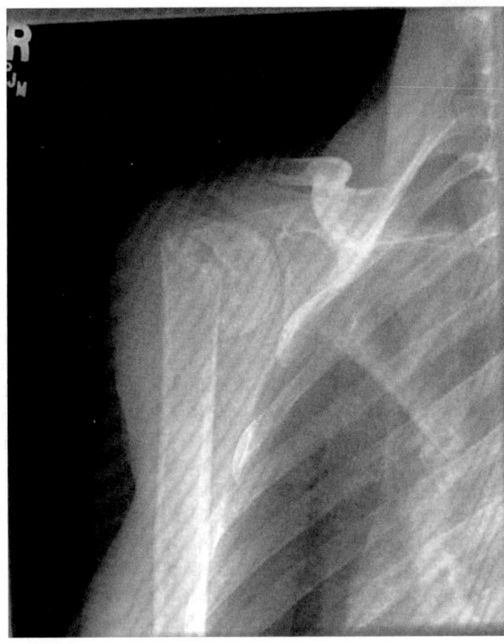

FIGURE 31-23 AP x-ray of a nonunion of a proximal humerus fracture.

Open Reduction and Internal Fixation (ORIF) with Plates

In the case of an unstable fracture that cannot be reduced closed, and if there is significant comminution of the fracture fragments, ORIF is indicated. Several options currently exist. The small blade plate from the AO Group (AO, Synthes, Paoli, Pennsylvania) has been a reliable construct to maintain fixation (Fig. 31-26) (222–224). More recently, special proximal humeral locking plates allow multiple screw fixation through the plate if rigid fixation is required (222). Advantages include better purchase in osteoporotic bone and potentially easier application than a blade plate (Fig. 31-27). These plates do not easily allow for indirect reduction using the plate-shaft or plate-head construct but require that the fracture be reduced before definitive fixation.

IM Fixation

A variety of IM devices have been advocated for ORIF of surgical neck fractures. Their advantages include a limited need for dissection around the fracture. Disadvantages include the need to penetrate the greater tuberosity and rotator cuff for insertion of some of them, and the suggestion of reduced torsional stability compared to rigid fixation with a plate and screws (11,13,14,225). A technique using modified Enders nails and tension-band fixation with heavy sutures has been described with excellent results in surgical neck fractures (Fig. 31-28) (226).

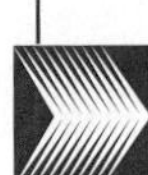

AUTHORS' PREFERRED TREATMENT

Displaced Surgical Neck Fracture (No Comminution). Our preference in this setting is to perform a CRPP. This technique has been used by many surgeons and recently has been extended to more complex three-part and even selected four-part fractures (83,156,159).

Technique of CRPP. This technique requires a team approach on the part of anesthesia, surgeons, and radiology

(text continues on page 1185)

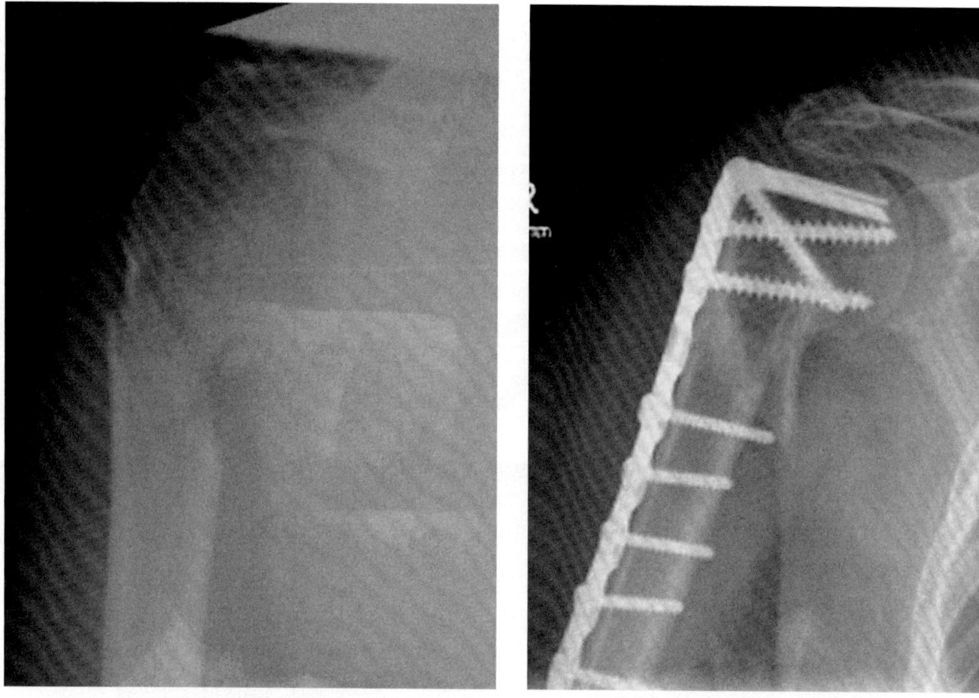

FIGURE 31-26 **A.** Comminuted proximal humerus fracture. **B.** Fixation of comminuted fracture with blade plate and indirect reduction. (**B** Courtesy of David Ring, MD.)

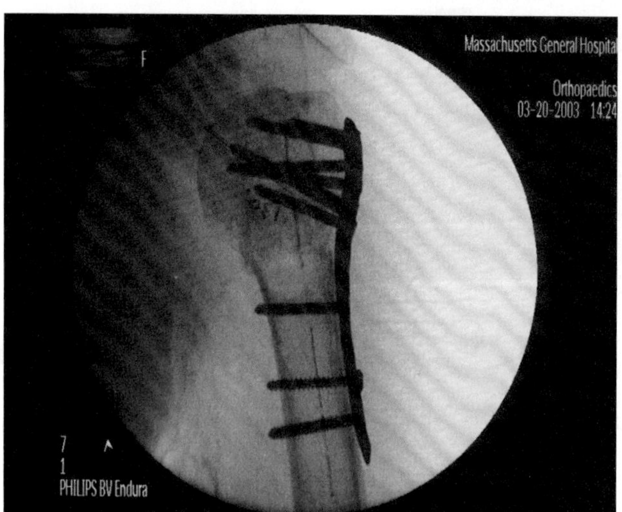

FIGURE 31-27 Proximal humeral locking plate used to treat a two-part surgical neck fracture.

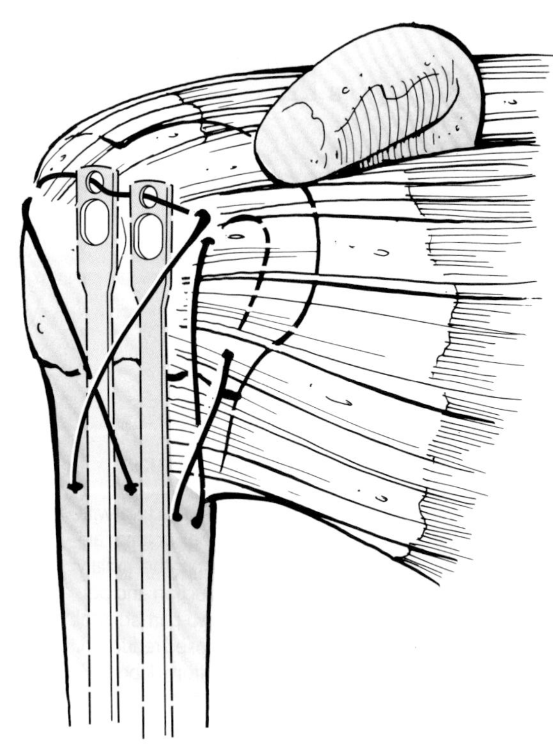

FIGURE 31-28 Technique of modified Enders nails and figure-of-eight sutures for two-part surgical neck fracture repair.

technicians. Careful positioning of the patient and the C-arm is essential for the success of the procedure. Complete muscle paralysis either by general anesthesia or regional anesthetic block is essential to allow for a safe reduction maneuver.

The patient is positioned supine on the operating table and the head of the bed is elevated to about 30 degrees. We prefer to use a special beach chair device (Tmax Beach Chair, Tenet Medical Engineering, Calgary, Canada), which permits the back of the shoulder to be freely exposed for fluoroscopic imaging; however, a long bean-bag can be used on a regular operating room table; once it is contoured so that the patient's shoulder is free, the patient can be moved laterally sufficient for a good fluoroscopic image (Fig. 31-29). We also prefer to use a mechanical arm holder, as this eliminates the need for an assistant (Spider arm holder, Tenet Medical Engineering). The patient's arm can simply be rotated during the procedure to see the proximal humerus in an AP and an axillary projection. The C-arm unit is positioned parallel to the patient from the head of the bed so that it does not interfere with movement of the arm, and prior to preparing and draping the shoulder a trial closed reduction is performed with fluoroscopic guidance. It is important to accomplish the reduction in this stage, as failure to do so will then mandate an open approach. After marking its position on the floor with tape for future correct placement, the C-arm is then moved out of the way and the patient's arm is prepared and draped.

The reduction maneuver is then repeated if necessary, and the reduction can be held in place by the assistant while the fracture is pinned with 2.5-mm terminally threaded Schanz pins. We begin by holding one pin over the front of the shoulder and obtaining an AP image. The location for the pin is chosen so that it will enter the shaft of the humerus and then be placed up into the articular fragment. This orientation is marked on the skin with a skin marker. A small incision is then made over the humerus and a straight clamp is used to spread down to the humeral shaft. This maneuver will push aside any neurovascular elements; however, the entrance of the pin is usually below the course of the axillary nerve (Fig. 31-30) (227,228). The pin is then introduced so that it is against the lateral shaft of the humerus. A drill guide can be used for this step. The pin is then directed up into the humeral head, as visualized under fluoroscopy in two planes. We usually place a second pin parallel to the first. A third pin is placed from a more anterior position so that it enters the humeral head almost perpendicular to the first two. A fourth pin directed downward from the greater tuberosity is usually optional in two-part fractures but is a requirement in three- and four-part fractures. The goal is to place three or four pins with as wide a separation in the humeral head as possible.

The pins are then cut off so that they are below the skin, and the small incisions are closed with monofilament suture and sterilely dressed.

Aftercare. The shoulder is placed into a sling and swathe or shoulder immobilizer, and no motion is permitted for 3 weeks. Radiographic control on a weekly basis is preferred to make sure no pin migration occurs and the reduction is maintained. After 3 to 4 weeks the pins can be removed with local anesthesia, and we usually perform this step in an outpatient facility. Fluoroscopy can then confirm stable union. Gentle active and passive range of motion under the supervision of a therapist is then begun.

Displaced Surgical Neck Fracture (Comminution). In these cases we prefer rigid fixation. Our current implant of choice is the proximal humeral locking plate. A standard deltopectoral approach is used after the patient is positioned as described above for CRPP. We use fluoroscopic guidance if anatomic reduction is not certain intraoperatively. Surgical dissection remains lateral to the bicipital groove so as not to risk disruption of the vascular supply to the humeral head. The fracture is reduced after removing any interposed soft tissue. In some cases with marked comminution or segmental bone loss, an AO distractor can be used to keep the humerus at the correct length while the plate is applied. Intercalated autogenous or allograft bone grafting can then be performed, although one of us (C.G.) never performs primary bone grafting.

Aftercare. If rigid fixation is achieved, immediate passive range of motion is begun and active motion can commence after 3 to 4 weeks, once the sling is removed.

Two-Part Surgical Neck Fracture with Very Osteoporotic Bone. In rare cases, the bone may be so soft that internal fixation is almost impossible with pins or rigid implants. This is especially the case in elderly women. In this situation fixation of the humeral shaft by impacting it into the humeral head and using heavy sutures as tension bands through the rotator cuff and a hole in the humeral shaft is a good alternative (132). The tendon quality is usually better than the osteoporotic bone, so heavy sutures are placed in the supraspinatus, infraspinatus, and subscapularis and then through one or two holes in the humeral shaft just distal to the metaphysis. When these sutures are tied down, the humeral shaft is compressed into the softer metaphyseal bone. It may be necessary to accept some valgus angulation and humeral shortening with this approach (Fig. 31-31).

Results and Complications. While technically challenging, the method of CRPP has been shown to have excellent results (83,156,159,229). However, complications have included loss of fixation, pin migration and infection, and malunion (156,159,230). Migration of the pins can be prevented by a fixation clamp positioned on the humerus to hold the Kirschner wires in place (159). General guidelines for pin

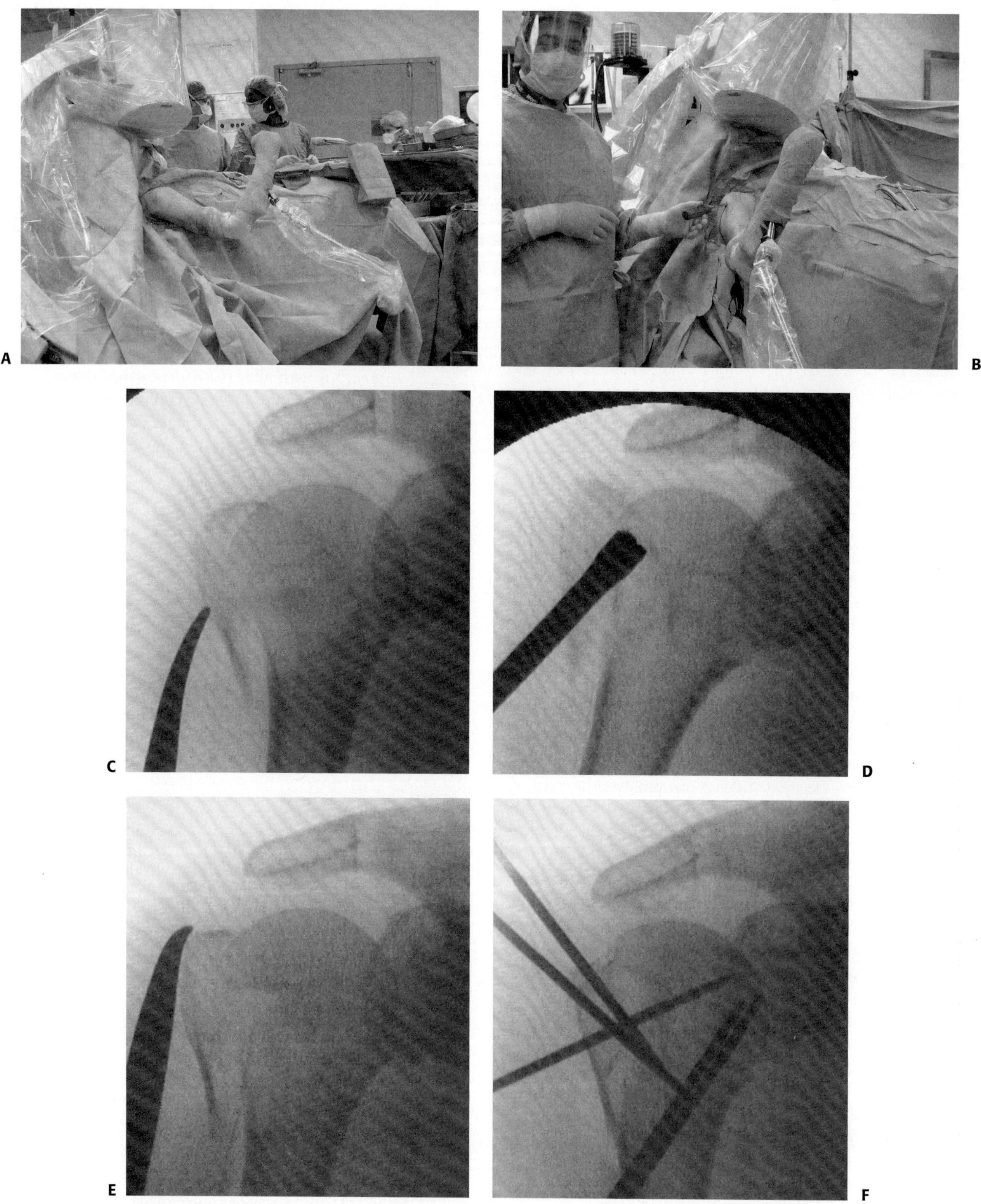

FIGURE 31-29 **A.** Positioning for closed reduction and percutaneous pinning. An articulated arm holder is used and the C-arm is positioned over the shoulder with its base at the top of the table. **B.** The arm can be maintained in any position of abduction and rotation with the arm holder to facilitate imaging with the C-arm and reduction of the fracture. **C.** Orientation of the clamp to reduce valgus angulation of the humeral head. **D.** Elevation of humeral head fracture out of valgus with a bone tamp. **E.** The greater tuberosity is pulled inferiorly with a clamp or a hook. **F.** Maintenance of fracture reduction with percutaneous pins.

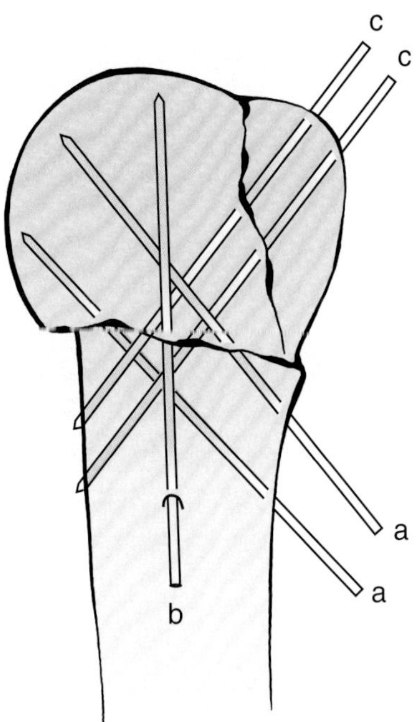

FIGURE 31-30 Pinning technique. (Reprinted with permission from Jaberg H, Warner JJP, Jakob RP. Percutaneous stabilization of unstable fractures of the humerus. *J Bone Joint Surg Am* 1992;74:508–515.)

placement are to place multiple parallel pins spread widely apart in the proximal fragment. These pins should be terminally threaded to prevent migration. Unrecognized comminution and failure to trim the pins beneath the skin are common causes for complication and failure of the technique, although surgeon error in pin placement can also be a cause of failure and complications (Fig. 31-32).

ORIF with plates and screws has also given excellent results (49–56,89,108). Loss of fixation due to osteopenic bone, however, has been a common complication.

Two-Part (Anatomic Neck)

There are no reported series of open reduction and fixation of isolated anatomic neck fractures; however, Gerber (187) has described iatrogenic anatomic neck fracture with closed reduction of shoulder dislocation where there was a nondisplaced fracture that was unrecognized. In these cases open fixation of the humeral articular segment was performed, as many of these patients were very young. While osteonecrosis can ensue, it is not immediately symptomatic in all patients (Fig. 31-33).

Three-Part Fractures

The classic three-part fracture as described by Neer (90, 153,171,172,196,231,232) involves either the greater or lesser tuberosity. Consequently, the direction of displacement and

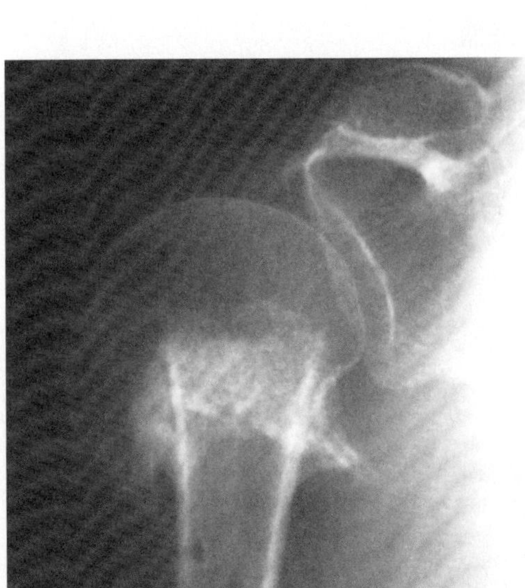

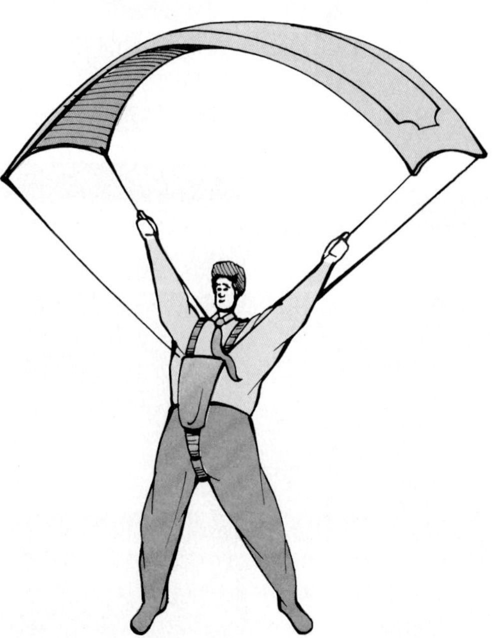

FIGURE 31-31 Parachute method of Fenlin. Union with impaction of fragments using repair with heavy sutures through the rotator cuff and humeral shaft in the case of osteoporotic bone and a two-part fracture.

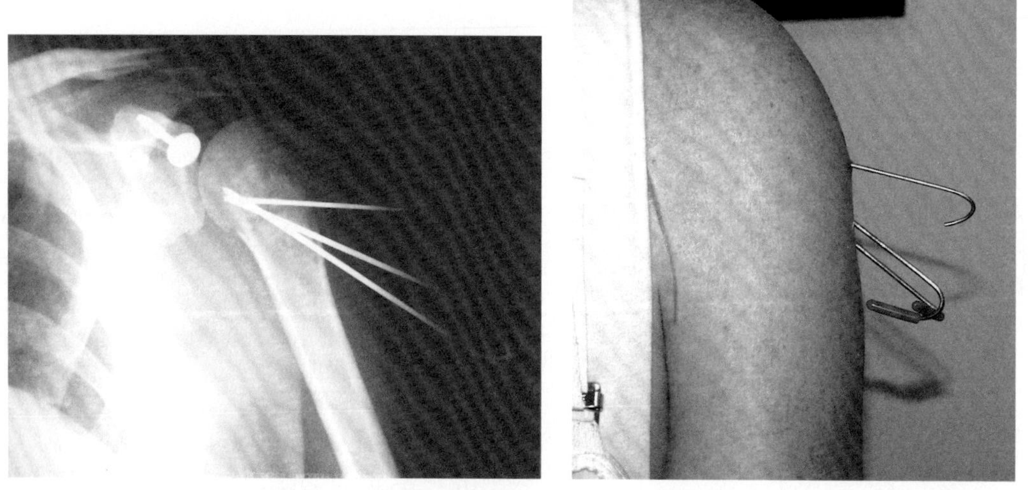

FIGURE 31-32 **A.** Smooth pins placed in convergent orientation during CRPP with a resultant nonunion. **B.** Pins have been bent and cut out over the skin.

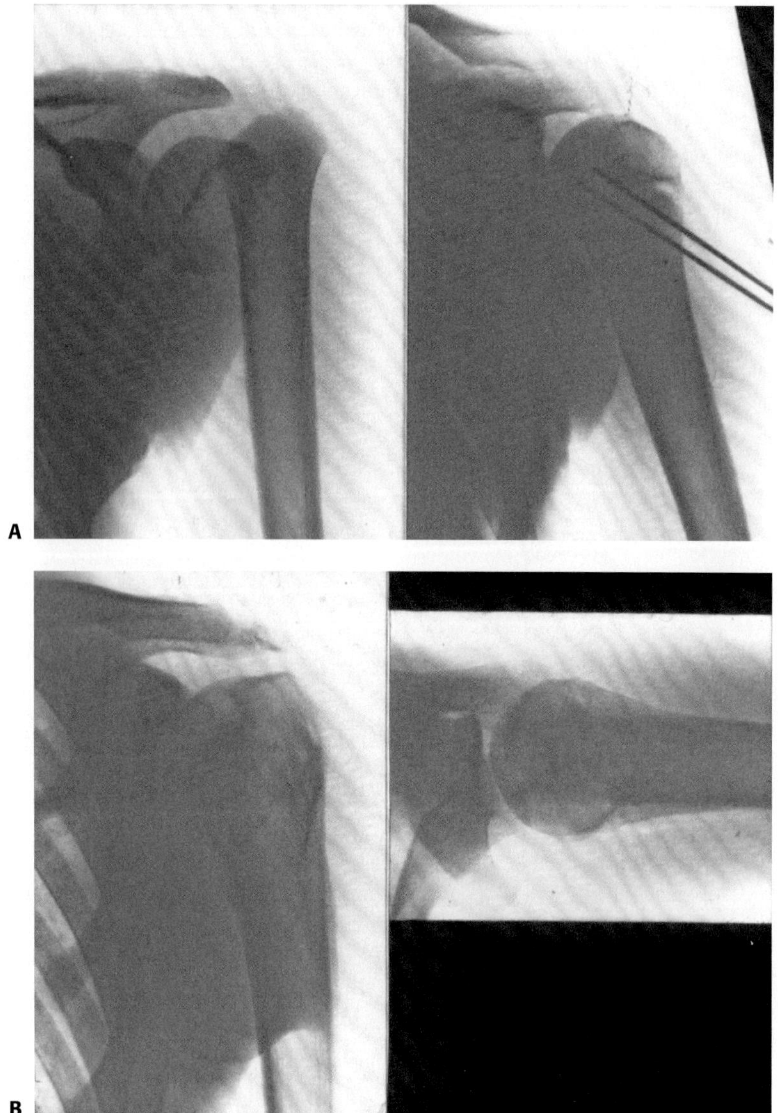

FIGURE 31-33 **A.** Young patient with an anatomic neck fracture treated with CRPP. **B.** One year after surgery, there is maintenance of the joint space and the humeral head has not collapsed.

fracture deformity will be determined by the remaining muscle forces across the head segment to which the tuberosity remains attached. If the greater tuberosity is displaced, the subscapularis rotates the humeral head into internal rotation through its attachment to the lesser tuberosity. Thus, the articular surface faces posteriorly (see Fig. 31-5). In the rare three-part fracture that involves the lesser tuberosity, the pull of the supraspinatus and infraspinatus on the greater tuberosity rotates the humeral head externally so that the articular surface faces anteriorly (see Fig. 31-5).

Radiographic classification can be very challenging in these cases, and what initially appears as a three-part fracture in one radiographic plane may appear to be a four-part fracture in another plane (176,179,182,233–237). Tuberosity displacement may be quite subtle and difficult to judge due to rotatory deformities. CT may be helpful in these cases.

The surgical approach to these fractures depends not only on the fracture configuration but also on the quality of bone. In rare cases involving elderly patients with very osteopenic bone and comminution, hemiarthroplasty may be the preferable treatment. In most cases, however, it is preferable to perform a reduction and fixation to restore the relationship of the articular segment to the shaft and, more importantly, to the tuberosities. In all cases, careful preservation of the medial soft tissue in the region of the bicipital groove is preferred so as not to jeopardize the vascularity to the humeral head segment. Due to the rotational component of this fracture, it is difficult to reduce these fractures through closed means. Thus, an open deltopectoral approach is usually preferred. Options for fixation include open reduction and stabilization with heavy sutures around the tuberosities and to the humeral shaft, with or without an intramedullary device (150,238), plate fixation with either a blade plate or fixation with a proximal humeral locking plate (see Figs. 31-26 and 31-27). The latter is our preferred method of treatment.

A valuable alternative is open reduction and minimal internal fixation. The fracture site is exposed through a deltopectoral approach. If the head is impacted, it is elevated using a rasp, which is introduced through the fracture and brought underneath the proximal fragment. If the bone is severely osteoporotic, bone graft (either allograft or autograft) is then used as a buttress material. To ascertain length and orientation, the greater and/or the lesser tuberosity are then reduced to the shaft, where their proper location can usually be identified easily by the triangular shape of the fracture. The greater tuberosity and/ or lesser tuberosity are then stabilized with sutures only (Fig. 31-34).

The fracture pattern known as valgus-impacted is usually associated with a four-part fracture, although it is a matter of debate as to whether there is always significant displacement of the lesser tuberosity to qualify as such. To determine the answer to this question, a Y radiographic view is often helpful. If the anterior contour of the head is followed, it can be determined whether the head is separated from the lesser tuberosity. It may in some circumstances be a three-part fracture. This fracture configuration represents a separate consideration due to its potential for excellent reduction with preservation of humeral head vascularity, either by closed or open means (159,239,240). This is discussed in the following section on four-part fractures.

Results

In general, different methods of open reduction and fixation result in good to excellent outcomes in about 60% to 80% of cases (11,127), whereas acute hemiarthroplasty generally leads to excellent to good results in less than 50% of cases (97,144, 172,196,241–251).

Four-Part Fractures

By definition, a four-part fracture is one in which the articular segment is isolated from both tuberosities and the humeral shaft. Historically, these fractures were treated by resection of the articular segment (29,69,252–257), which yielded uniformly poor results. Nonoperative treatment has also often been reported to lead to poor results in terms of pain and function, although some studies have been less disappointing (45,258).

The typical fracture pattern is one in which the articular segment is dislocated anteriorly into the axillary pouch while the shaft of the humerus sits laterally and the lesser and greater tuberosities are displaced anteriorly and posteriorly, respectively (Fig. 31-35). In most cases an immediate hemiarthroplasty is indicated. Our approach to this is presented in the following text. In some rare cases of a young individual with a four-part fracture, we perform an immediate open reduction and fixation with a combination of plates, screws, and sometimes heavy sutures. The key is to restore an anatomic relationship to the humeral head and tuberosities, since osteonecrosis may be well tolerated in this situation and future conversion to an arthroplasty is much more successful following an anatomic reduction (Fig. 31-36) (107).

Results

Open reduction and fixation usually leads to a poor outcome as a result of osteonecrosis, loss of fixation, posttraumatic arthritis, and stiffness (11,45,162,196,235,238,259–263). However, some authors have reported good results in selected patients (155,264–266) and continue to use open reduction and minimal internal fixation if possible. These fractures often require solutions on a case-by-case basis, with the common goal being the use of as few implants as possible to achieve stability to allow healing of the immobilized arm. In these cases, which usually do not involve full exposure of the joint, immobilization for 3 or 4 weeks is mandatory and not usually associated with stiffness (Fig. 31-37).

The Valgus-Impacted Four-Part Fracture

This fracture configuration should be considered separately due to the preserved medial soft tissue hinge, which preserves vascularity to the articular segment (Fig. 31-38). Thus, the risk for osteonecrosis is lower than for a typical four-part fracture, pro-

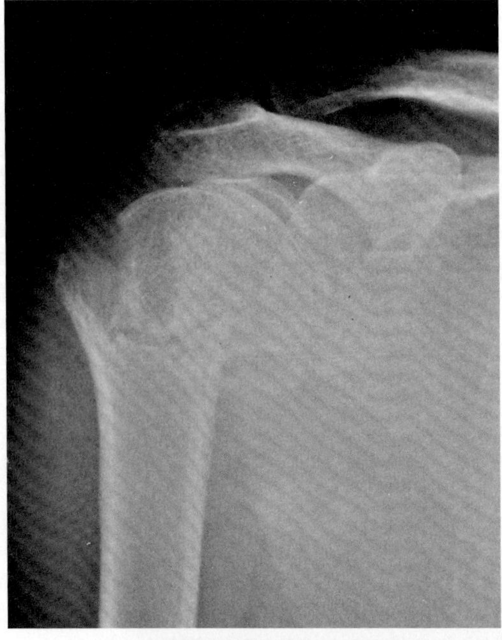

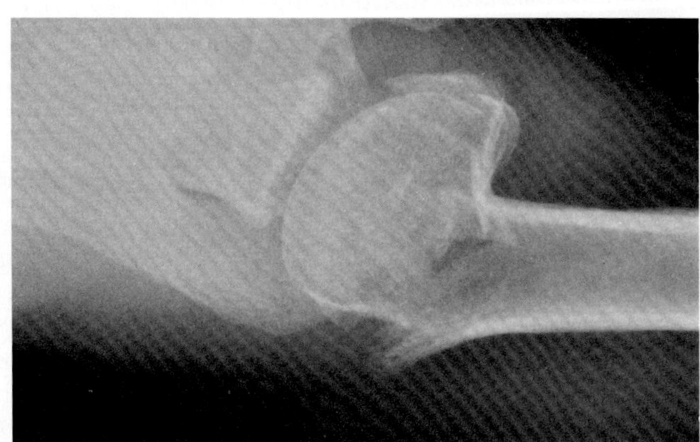

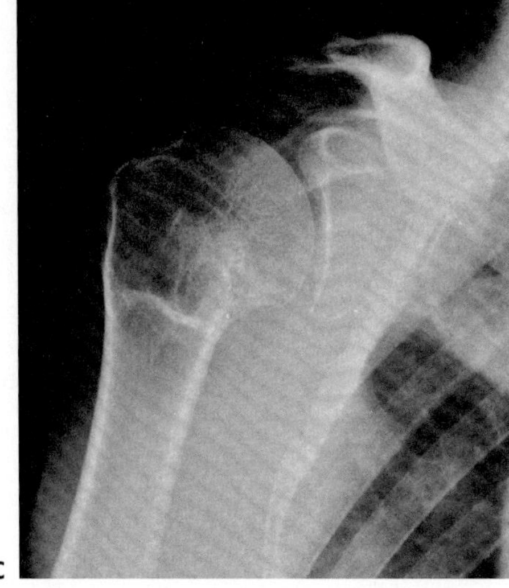

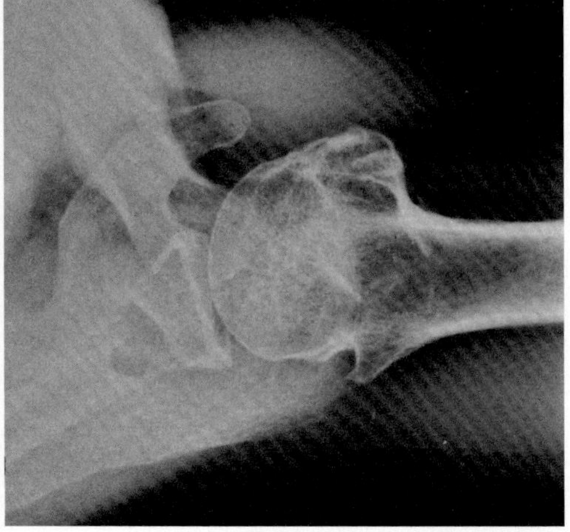

FIGURE 31-34 **A,B.** Three-part proximal humerus fracture treated with open reduction and suture fixation of the greater to the lesser tuberosity. **C.** The postoperative x-ray indicates successful fracture union. The patient had excellent function.

vided that iatrogenic disruption of the vessels is not a consequence of treatment. Both open reduction and internal fixation and closed reduction and internal fixation are well suited to this fracture configuration. Both methods are described below according to our treatment approaches.

Closed Reduction and Percutaneous Pinning. This method is described for a four-part valgus-impacted fracture, but the steps are the same in the case of a two-part or three-part fracture.

The patient is positioned supine in a fashion that allows for free mobility of the shoulder girdle and adequate image intensification. Two of us (JJPW, JGC) prefer to use a special beach chair device with the shoulder completely free and the head of the bed elevated to about a 30-degree angle. Complete muscle relaxation is necessary for the reduction maneuver. The C-arm is moved into position at the top of the bed and brought over the shoulder (see Fig. 31-29). Radiographic images are then obtained in both the AP and axillary planes before preparing the patient's shoulder using sterile technique. The patient then receives an intravenous cephalosporin as infection prophylaxis.

The first step is to reduce the humeral head segment from its valgus position. A special bone punch or elevator is inserted through a small lateral incision while visualizing with the C-arm in the AP plane. The head fragment is then levered upward from laterally, so that the proper humeral neck angle is restored (see Fig. 31-38). One may sometimes feel the head shift back into position as it falls into contact with the glenoid. The medial soft tissue sleeve will facilitate this indirect reduction

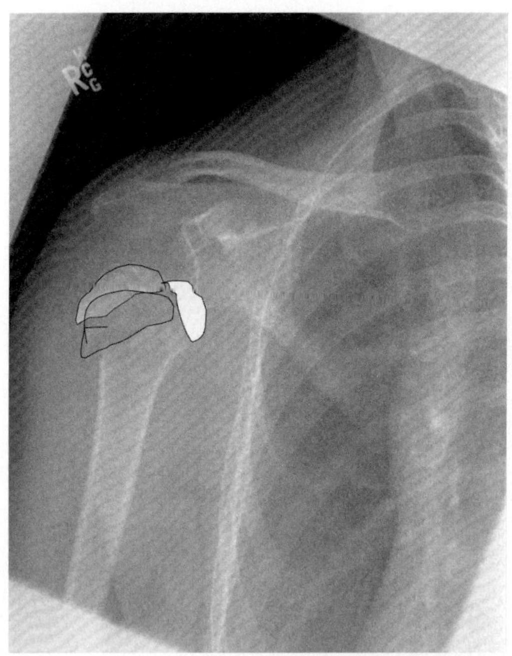

FIGURE 31-35 Classic four-part fracture. The segments have been shaded on the x-ray.

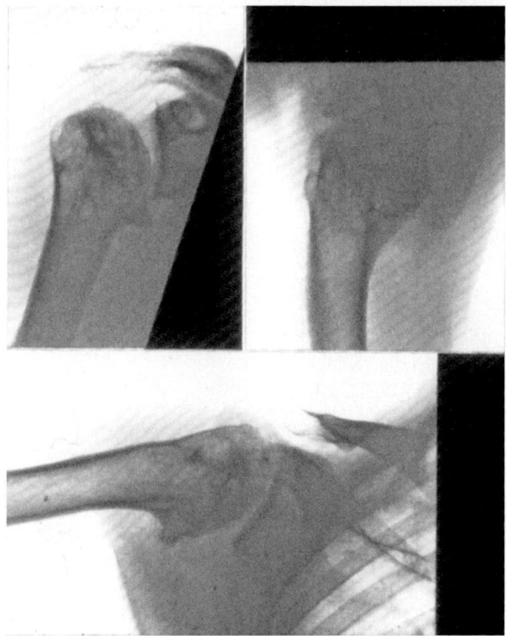

FIGURE 31-36 This patient with osteonecrosis 6 years after anatomic reconstruction of a four-part fracture had excellent function with only mild shoulder pain.

as it will prevent the head from moving medially on the shaft of the humerus, since it will act as a hinge. This reduction is then held in position while a 2.5-mm Shantz pin is drilled from inferior and lateral through the shaft and up into the humeral head. A second pin may be place to ensure stable fixation.

The greater tuberosity may then be more closely reduced to its proper position once the humeral head is elevated to its correct position. The tuberosity can be reduced into the lateral defect underneath the humeral head using a 2.5-mm Shantz pin from superiorly so that the bone fragment can be moved as with a "joystick."

If the lesser tuberosity is displaced medially, an axillary view is obtained and a small bone hook is inserted percutaneously and the tuberosity is pulled laterally to its correct position underneath the humeral head. This fragment is then fixed with one or two percutaneous pins as above.

Resch has recently demonstrated a technique similar to the one described above, except that he uses cannulated screws so that later removal of wires is not required (Fig. 31-39) (159).

Open Reduction and Fixation. This method may be used if reduction cannot be obtained by closed and percutaneous means. The setup is the same as that described above and includes fluoroscopic guidance. A deltopectoral approach is performed without dissection in the area of the bicipital groove or medially. The head fragment is then elevated with a bone elevator and the greater tuberosity is reduced underneath the humeral head. In some cases of comminution, bone grafting may be performed between the greater tuberosity and the humeral head; however, we do not usually find this to be necessary. There are then several ways to fix the fragments. If there is good bone with large pieces, a simple lateral plate will fix the tuberosity against the humeral head and the humeral head to the shaft. The medial soft tissue hinge allows restoration of height through the lateral plate (Fig. 31-40). Screw fixation to the humeral head and shaft or suture fixation are also possible (Fig. 31-41).

Aftercare. This is essentially the same as the methods described above, with minimal or no motion permitted for 4 weeks, after which gentle range of motion is permitted if stable fixation is confirmed by radiographic control. If percutaneous pins have been placed, they are trimmed underneath the skin and removed at 4 to 6 weeks.

Results. Both percutaneous and open methods have led to excellent results (150,226,267–272). Jakob described 74% good to excellent results, with only a 26% incidence of osteonecrosis (175), using the open method. Recently, Resch et al reported a postoperative Constant Score of 91% out of 100% in 27 patients with three- and four-part fractures using percutaneous pinning and screw fixation (159,173). Of these, 13 were valgus-impacted four-part fractures. The overall incidence of osteonecrosis was only 11%, and some of these were only partial

(text continues on page 1195)

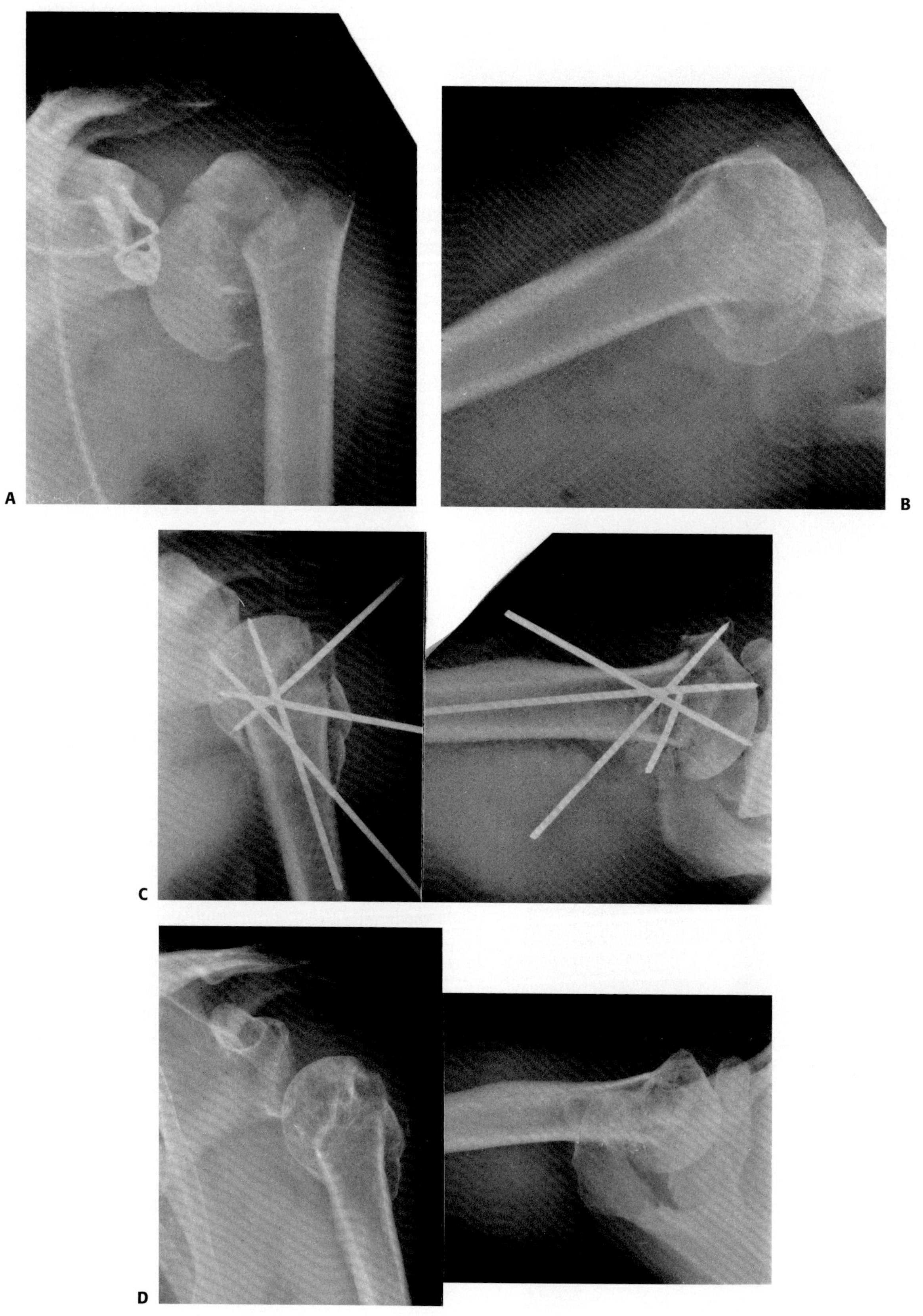

FIGURE 31-37 A–C. Four-part proximal humerus fracture treated with closed reduction and percutaneous pinning. **D.** The postoperative x-ray shows satisfactory fracture union. The patient had excellent function 1 year after surgery.

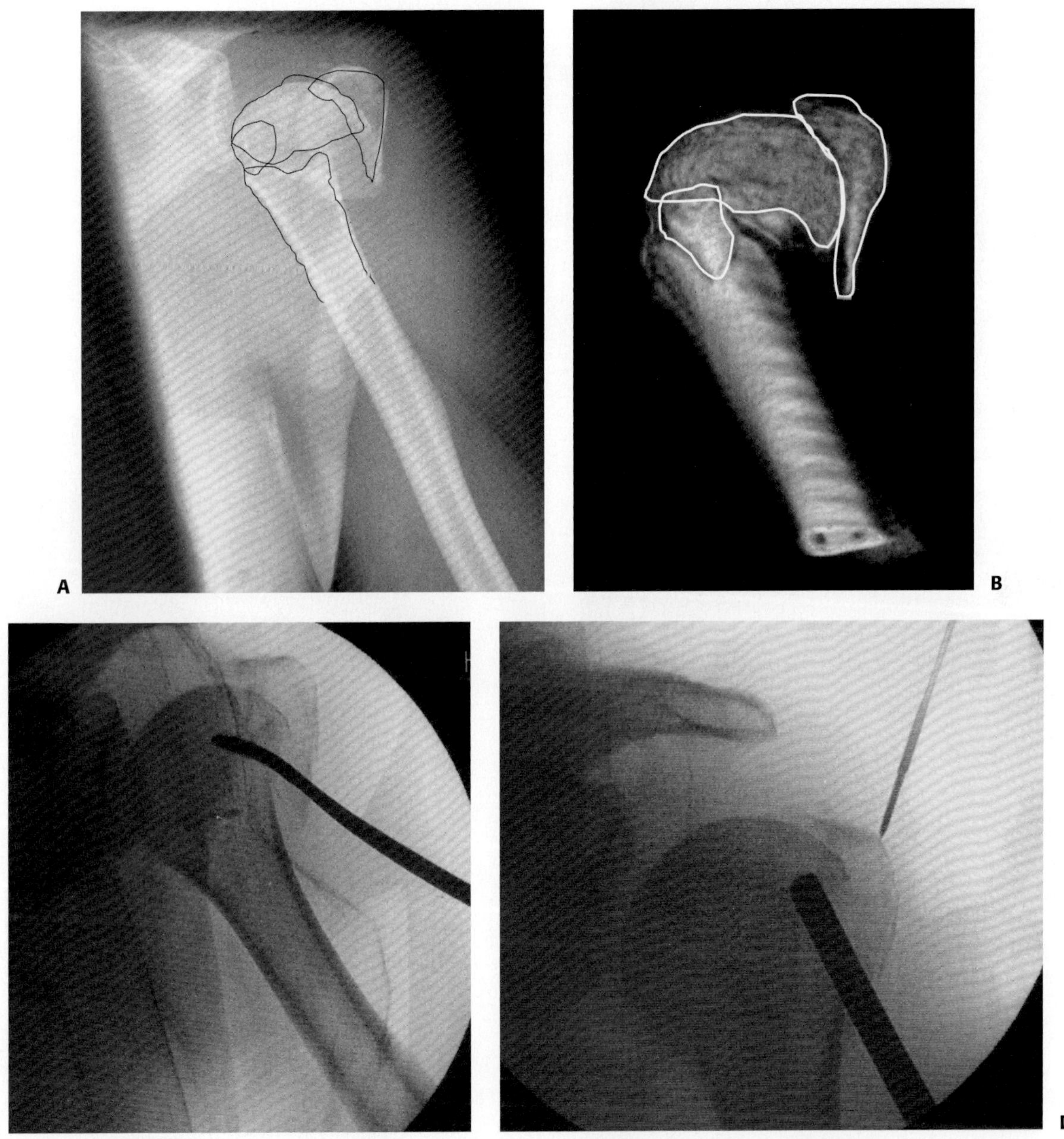

FIGURE 31-38 **A.** Valgus-impacted four-part fracture. The segments of the fracture are outlined. **B.** CT scan confirms fracture configuration. **C.** Elevation of head segment percutaneously. **D.** Reduction of greater tuberosity using a pin as a joystick. (*continues*)

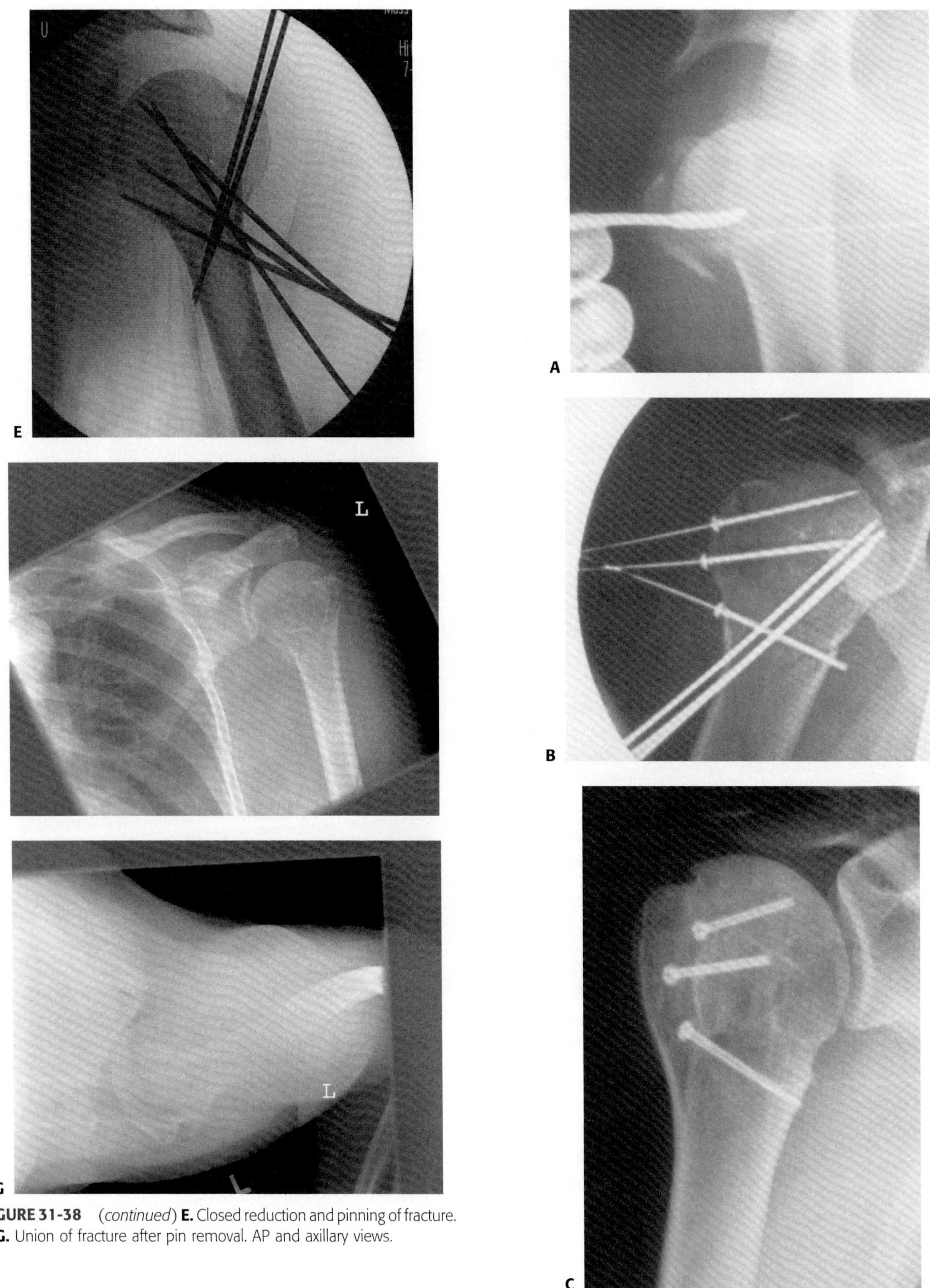

FIGURE 31-38 (*continued*) **E.** Closed reduction and pinning of fracture. **F,G.** Union of fracture after pin removal. AP and axillary views.

FIGURE 31-39 Closed reduction and percutaneous screw fixation. **A.** Four-part fracture. **B.** Initial reduction. **C.** Final radiographic result. (Courtesy of Herbert Resch, MD.)

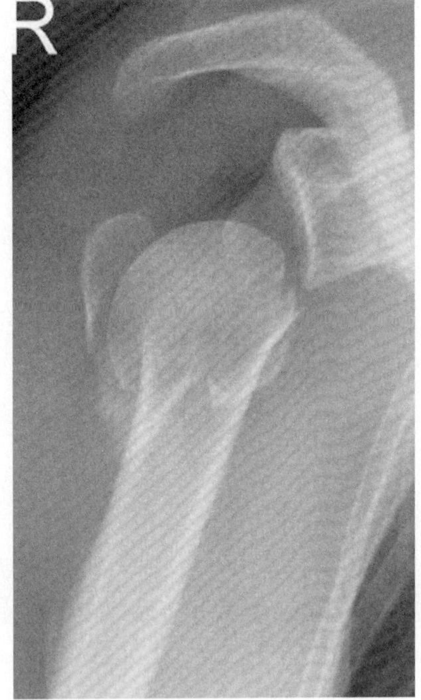

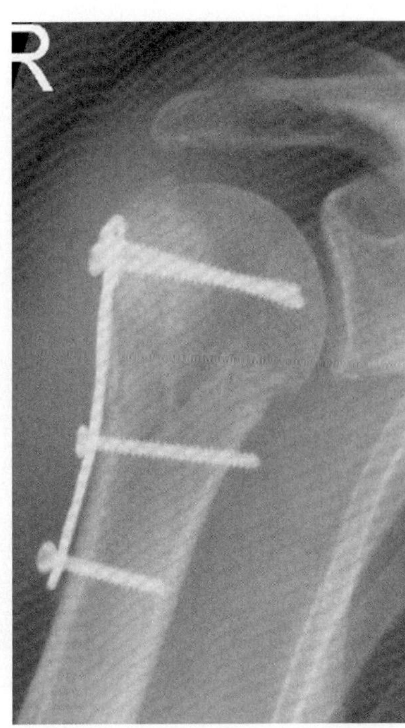

FIGURE 31-40 **A.** Valgus-impacted four-part fracture. **B.** Anatomic reduction and maintenance of position with lateral plate. (Reprinted with permission from Gerber C, Werner CML, Vienne P. Internal fixation of complex fractures of the proximal humerus. *J Bone Joint Surg Br* 2004;86:848–855.)

osteonecrosis. In only one case was conversion to hemiarthroplasty required.

One study (273) reported a complete osteonecrosis rate of 0%, but evidence of partial osteonecrosis and humeral head collapse was found in 30% of 85 patients. Another study (274) reported only that 1 of 12 cases developed osteonecrosis after open reduction and fixation of a valgus-impacted four-part fracture.

These studies support the experience of the senior author (CG) that osteonecrosis can be well tolerated as long as anatomic tuberosity fixation can be obtained (275).

Head-Splitting and Impression Fractures

Head-splitting and impression fractures are usually the result of a severe impaction of the humeral head into the glenoid,

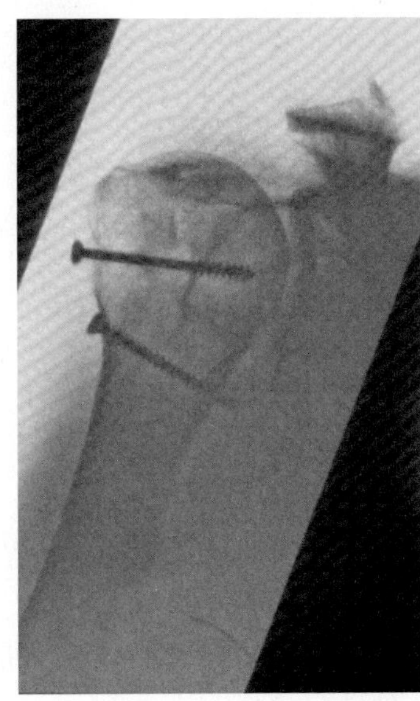

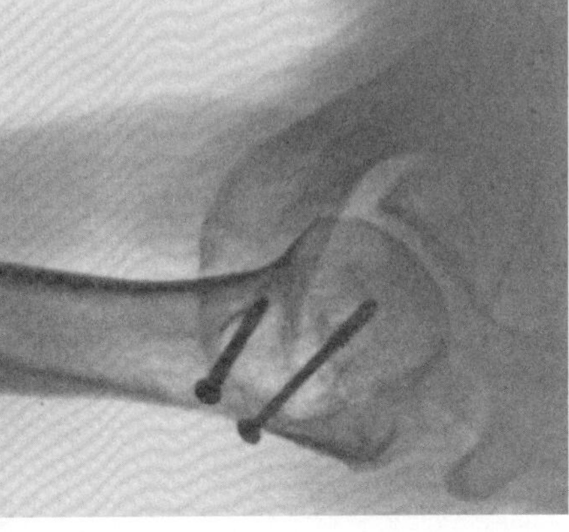

FIGURE 31-41 Open reduction and screw fixation of valgus-impacted four-part fracture.

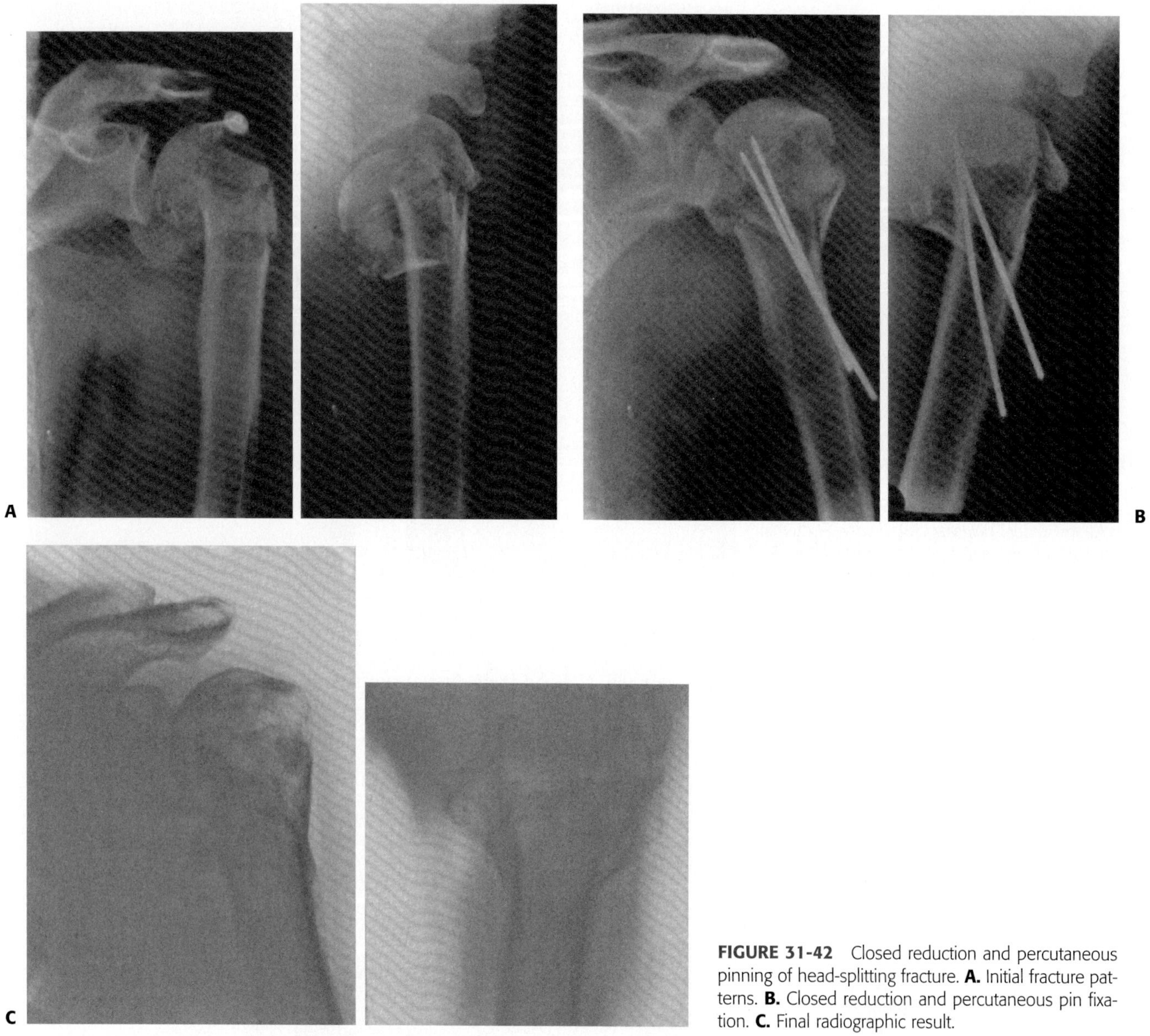

A B C

FIGURE 31-42 Closed reduction and percutaneous pinning of head-splitting fracture. **A.** Initial fracture patterns. **B.** Closed reduction and percutaneous pin fixation. **C.** Final radiographic result.

with or without a dislocation (Fig. 31-42) (166,167,276). In the case of a head-splitting fracture, there are few isolated reports of open reduction and fixation (277). A number of reports exist about severe impression fractures of the humeral head (134,278,279). In most cases the defect is anterior and represents a reverse Hill-Sachs lesion that occurs with a traumatic posterior dislocation. In these cases we always obtain a CT scan to quantitate the extent of humeral head involvement. In general, with a chronic locked posterior dislocation, the defect may be very large. When the defect is small (less than 20% of the humeral head), transfer of the subscapularis with the lesser tuberosity into the defect through a deltopectoral approach is the preferred method of treatment. When the defect involves up to 40% of the humeral head, reconstruction with a matched osteochondral allograft has been a very successful method of treatment (200). When the humeral head defect is more than 40% or if the bone is soft and of poor quality, an acute hemiarthroplasty is performed.

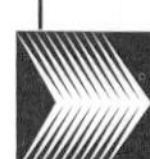

AUTHORS' PREFERRED TREATMENT

When a young patient has a head-splitting fracture, we prefer to perform ORIF according to standard fracture repair principles to restore articular congruity. Usually a deltopectoral approach is needed, and we try to leave as much of the subscapularis in place as possible, opening only the superior rotator interval and detaching the upper portion of the subscapularis. The fracture fragments are then reduced and fixed with a variety of screws, which may be cannulated, or with pins from an extra-articular approach (Fig. 31-43). If the fracture is so comminuted that reconstruction is impossible, or if the patient is of advanced age, an acute hemiarthroplasty is performed.

Results

To our knowledge there is no report in the literature describing the outcome with this type of fracture. Our experience with the occasional case of ORIF in young patients has been very favorable.

Special Situations: Fracture–Dislocation, Extensive Comminution

A fracture–dislocation has occurred when the articular surface is out of contact with the glenoid and there is a displaced fracture of one of the segments of the proximal humerus. Typically, this involves a greater tuberosity fracture with an anterior dislocation.

Even more challenging is a fracture in which the anatomic head is dislocated from the humeral shaft and the displaced tuberosities. As previously discussed, such a fracture may be created iatrogenically by displacing a nondisplaced proximal humerus fracture when attempting closed reduction of a dislocation in the presence of a subcapital fracture line (see Fig. 31-18). This by definition is a four-part fracture–dislocation, and the appropriate treatment appears to be hemiarthroplasty reconstruction. The surgical dissection can, however, be challenging, with chronic displacement of the articular segment into the axillary pouch. Extensive scarring may make surgical mobilization and removal of the articular segment difficult, as the brachial plexus may lie over the displaced humeral head.

Extensive comminution from the articular head and tuberosities into the diaphysis is rare and usually associated with severe trauma. This kind of severe comminution may be very challenging to manage due to the need to stabilize the diaphyseal component as well as the properly oriented articular component and tuberosities. The first priority is usually reconstruction of the proximal humeral component, after which the diaphyseal component may be addressed with one of a variety of rigid fixation techniques (Fig. 31-44).

Hemiarthroplasty: Indications and Authors' Technique

The technique of hemiarthroplasty and its results are discussed in detail in other publications (90,122,141,144,153,204,242–251,280–282). Hemiarthroplasty is reserved for fractures in which severe comminution, articular segment separation or destruction, and poor-quality bone preclude osteosynthesis due to the risk of osteonecrosis, malunion, or nonunion. While in general pain relief is usually expected, functional recovery is less predictable. This is mainly due to the technical challenge of achieving anatomic restoration of the humeral head as well as the biologic and surgical problems of obtaining anatomic healing of the greater tuberosity and the associated rotator cuff. Common errors include placement of the prosthetic implant too low, too high, with too large a head, and/or in too much retroversion (144,145,283–285). One reason for this high complication rate is the lack of anatomic reference points due to fracture comminution. Furthermore, most surgeons are faced with treating these complex fractures only on rare occasions, so the method of treatment and the steps for successful reconstruction may not be clear or apparent (286,287).

The goal of hemiarthroplasty reconstruction for proximal humerus fracture is to restore the anatomic relationship of the humeral head to the tuberosities and to the shaft by achieving proper component height, offset, and version. It is believed that this will not only ensure healing of the tuberosities and thus improved function, but also may avoid the late complication of glenoid arthrosis (122,144,145,284,288). Currently, it is accepted that the key determinant of success is obtaining healing of the greater tuberosity to the shaft and to the lesser tuberosity. Anatomic healing of the greater tuberosity is associated with good functional outcome, while absence of healing or secondary displacement of the greater tuberosity is associated with functional failure. It is therefore critical not only to ensure optimal surgical fixation of the greater tuberosity, but also to prevent its secondary displacement by strict postoperative protection of the shoulder. We have found that partial stiffness in the presence of tuberosity healing is an easily manageable problem. In contrast, secondary displacement of the greater tuberosity remains an unmanageable problem.

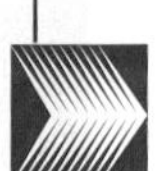

AUTHORS' PREFERRED TREATMENT

Preoperative Planning. Our current approach to preoperative imaging includes a true AP and axillary x-ray. Two of us (JJPW, JGC) prefer to obtain bilateral long-arm films that include the entire length of the humerus from the humeral head to the elbow. Magnification markers are used so that an accurate comparison of length can be made. The normal side then serves as a basis for templating the fractured side for selection of the articular head size and the length of the reconstruction (Fig. 31-45). CT scans are not usually necessary unless there is concern for an associated glenoid fracture or an anterior or posterior dislocation of the humeral head. They may, however, yield valuable information concerning

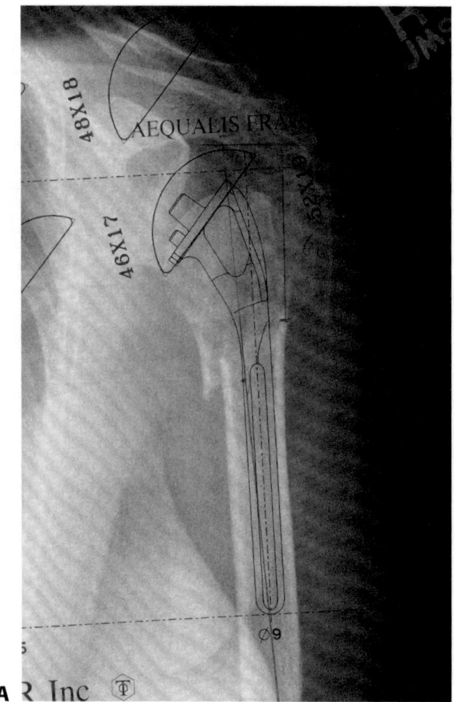

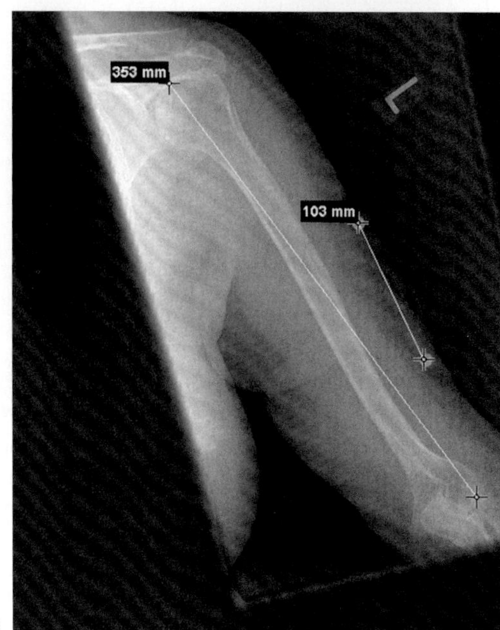

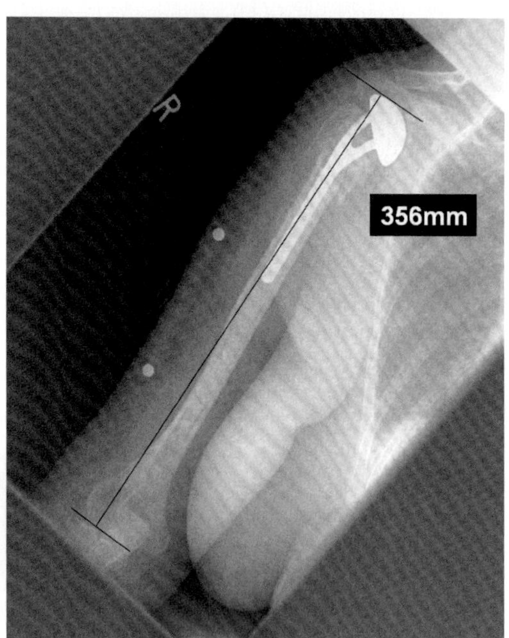

FIGURE 31-45 **A.** Preoperative templating of the fracture prior to hemiarthroplasty. **B.** Long-arm x-ray of the contralateral shoulder is performed to ensure restoration of proper length prior to hemiarthroplasty. **C.** The postoperative long-arm x-ray shows satisfactory length restoration compared to the normal contralateral side.

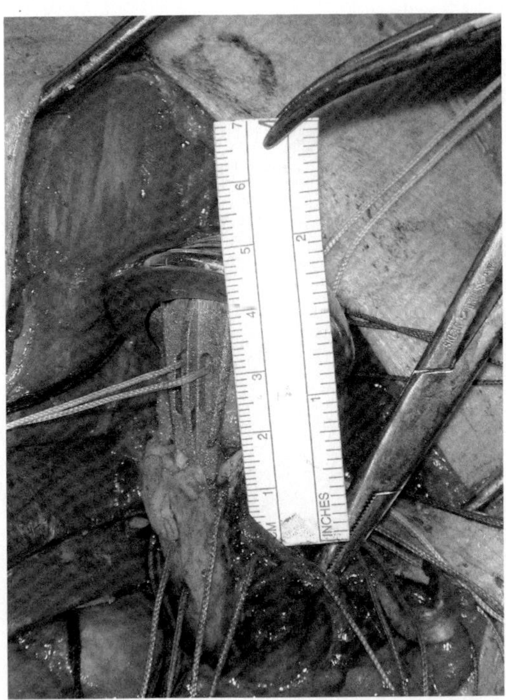

FIGURE 31-46 Measuring the distance from the superior border of the pectoralis major tendon to the top of the humeral head (average 5.3 cm) as an intraoperative reference for restoration of proper height of the humeral component.

begun no earlier than 6 weeks postoperatively. The brace or sling can be discontinued at this time as well. Strengthening can commence at 3 months.

Expected Results. Usually the patient can reach to the top of the head. If proper prosthesis placement is combined with secure tuberosity fixation and a compliant physical therapy program, overhead use can be expected.

COMPLICATIONS

Complications are not uncommon after surgical treatment of proximal humerus fractures. This is usually due to errors in procedure selection and in surgical technique (45,258). Furthermore, many complications such as greater tuberosity displacement are typically missed on postoperative follow-up. This makes revision surgery more difficult.

Instability

True instability is rare after treatment of fractures, and subluxation of the humeral head out of the glenoid is usually the consequence of hemarthrosis, deltoid atony, or rotator cuff dysfunction (166,289–292). This is usually transient as muscle tone returns and hemarthrosis is resorbed; however, axillary nerve dysfunction should be considered when inferior subluxation persists.

In the setting of hemiarthroplasty, inferior subluxation can also be due to incorrect placement of the prosthesis at a level that is too low, so that the deltoid tension is insufficient to maintain the humeral head in the glenoid (Fig. 31-48).

Hardware Problems

Problems with hardware are usually associated with other complications such as nonunion and sometimes neurovascular problems. These problems are sometimes related to inappropriate use of rigid devices in poor bone (see Fig. 31-7) or placement of metallic implants with a poor construct that cannot withstand the forces across the fracture. A thorough understanding of fracture geometry and bone quality is essential to avoid such problems.

Delayed Treatment and Missed Fractures

Delay in treatment, especially in the setting of missed fractures, can lead to a poor outcome because heterotopic bone formation may ensue and soft tissue contractures may prevent the restoration of normal anatomy. In some cases the reconstruction option that remains will not have been the option available in the acute case (see Figs. 31-8 and 31-21).

Neurovascular Problems

Although rare, neurovascular problems are unfortunately usually due to iatrogenic causes (293). Misplaced pins and excessive dissection and mobilization may be involved. Vascular injury in the case of marked fracture displacement has been reported (294–300), and careful neurovascular examination is required in all patients with a fracture.

Malunion

Malunion in the case of proximal humerus fracture is not rare, but often it does not result in significant functional disability. Rotational deformities as well as angular deformities in the plane of motion of the joint are relatively well tolerated (156), but malunions of the tuberosity relative to the articular segment are less well tolerated (92,107,127,142,143,145,147,148,301–304). Furthermore, some degree of soft tissue contracture accompanies all chronic malunions.

In cases of varus malunion, an angular osteotomy usually leads to an excellent outcome, whereas osteotomy of displaced tuberosity fragments, with or without arthroplasty, usually leads to weakness and a poor overall functional outcome (see Fig. 31-8) (143–145,305).

Nonunion

Surgical neck nonunion is much more common than tuberosity nonunion (see Fig. 31-23) (218,219,306,307). The inci-

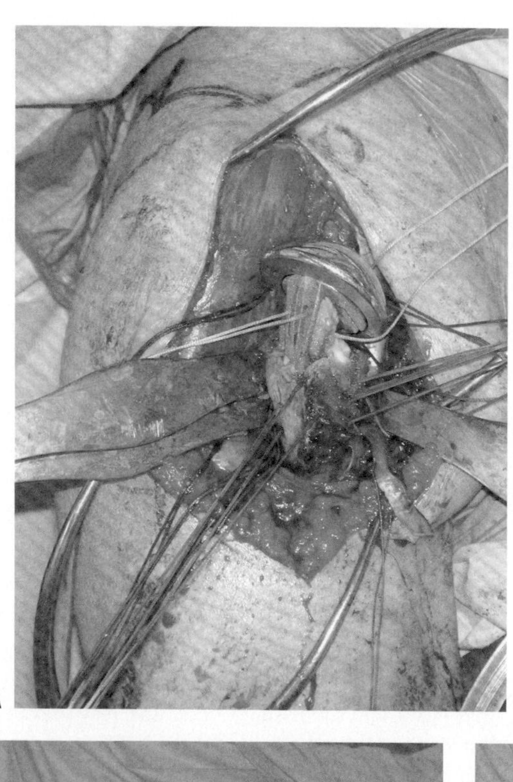

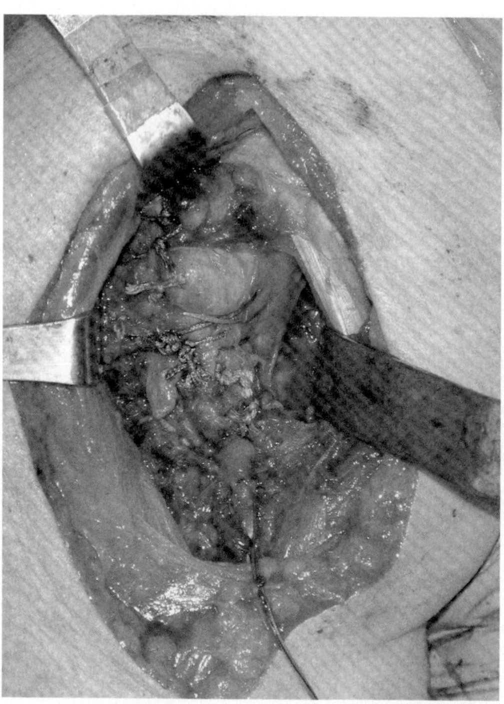

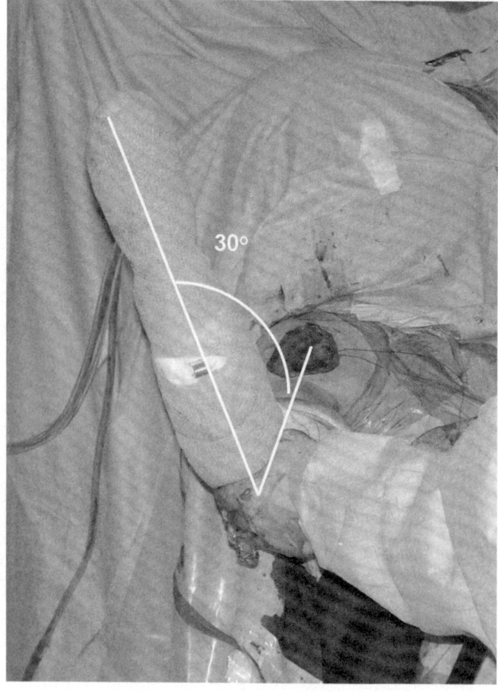

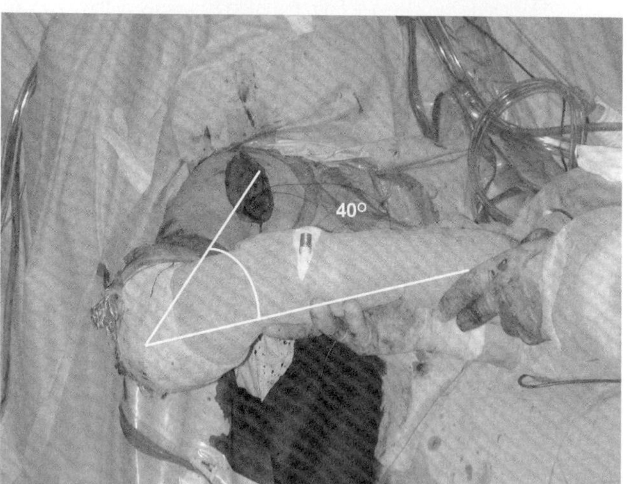

FIGURE 31-47 **A.** Placement of heavy sutures through the humeral shaft and around the stem of the prosthesis for reconstruction of the tuberosities. **B.** Reconstruction of the tuberosities. Determination of safe range of external rotation **(C)** and internal rotation **(D)** after repair of the tuberosities.

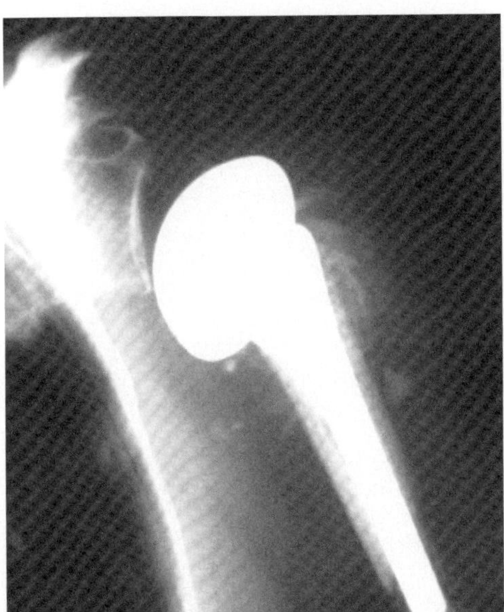

FIGURE 31-48 Inferior subluxation as a result of the hemiarthroplasty being placed too low and deltoid tension being insufficient.

dence of surgical neck nonunion in the setting of conservative treatment has actually been reported to be as high as 20%. Surgical neck nonunion usually occurs in conjunction with tuberosity displacement, and reconstruction with hemiarthroplasty when performed in this setting usually leads to poor function (107,143–145,220,308). Isolated surgical neck nonunion has been successfully treated with blade plate or proximal humeral locking plate fixation. Bone graft can be either used as an intramedullary plug or placed along the nonunion (309,310).

Osteonecrosis

Osteonecrosis can occur either as complete humeral head collapse or as a partial involvement of the humeral head either with or without articular collapse (107,147,159,276,311). The extent of osteonecrosis depends on the fracture configuration and the associated fracture treatment, as iatrogenic osteonecrosis is associated with excessive stripping of the medial soft tissues that contain the residual vascularity to the articular segment (see Fig. 31-11) (86,196,251,257,259,267,312–315).

When it occurs, osteonecrosis is often associated with progressive humeral head collapse and painful arthritis; however, this is not always the case (70,157,161,275,316–319). Gerber et al (107) observed that osteonecrosis in the setting of anatomic tuberosity reconstruction relative to the articular segment can result in less pain and far superior function than when there is an associated tuberosity malunion.

In symptomatic osteonecrosis, hemiarthroplasty is usually indicated, as other joint-preserving techniques such as core decompression remain unproven (320,321). In such cases, humeral reconstruction with an arthroplasty is much more successful if there is no associated malunion that requires treatment (see Fig. 31-10). If the malunion is associated with marked stiffness, total joint arthroplasty may be more successful in relieving pain and restoring motion. Conversely, hemiarthroplasty may be associated with relatively early glenoid erosion.

Stiffness and Arthritis

Stiffness may occur with or without operative treatment of a fracture, and it is usually due to prolonged immobilization that leads to scarring between tissue planes. In general, this complication is less common with closed reduction and percutaneous fixation than with open reduction and percutaneous fixation (156,159).

Posttraumatic arthritis is usually associated with loss of motion as well and may or may not occur in the setting of joint incongruity with fracture malunion (231,251). In associated malunions, the result of arthroplasty is less satisfactory than when there is an anatomic relationship between the tuberosity fragments.

Infection

Infection is relatively rare in the shoulder, even after surgical repair using open methods. This is due to the rich vascularity to this region and the good soft tissue coverage (195). Pin tract infections have been implicated as a common complication in the setting of percutaneous pinning of fractures (156,226). Pins that protrude from the skin create an increased risk for pin tract infection (see Fig. 31-32).

In the setting of arthroplasty, *Propionibacterium* infections appear to be much more frequent than previously believed (322), although the diagnosis may be difficult to make in the setting of a normal sedimentation rate, equivocal C-reactive protein tests, and no radiographic evidence of loosening. Persistent pain with stiffness under these circumstances should raise concern of a possible indolent *Propionibacterium* infection.

CONTROVERSIES AND FUTURE DIRECTIONS

Four-Part Fractures in the Elderly: Hemiarthroplasty versus Immediate Reverse Prosthesis

In elderly individuals, the results after hemiarthroplasty are often poor due to tuberosity nonunion and thus rotator cuff insufficiency. Recent experience in some European centers has demonstrated that immediate reconstruction with a reverse ball-in-socket prosthesis may be an option to restore better motion in some patients (Fig. 31-49). Surgical series are only just being presented, and the peer-reviewed literature has not yet validated this concept.

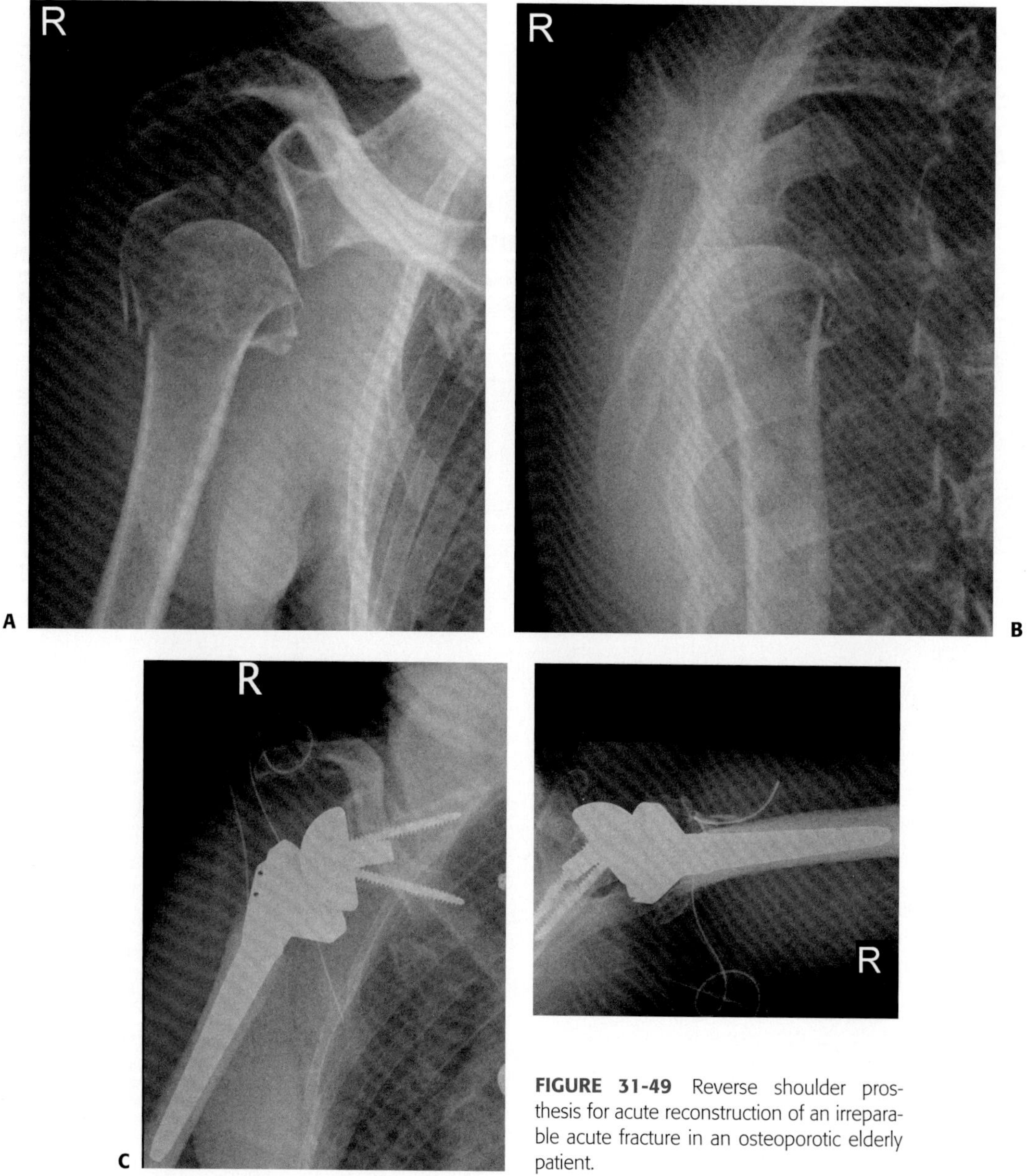

FIGURE 31-49 Reverse shoulder prosthesis for acute reconstruction of an irreparable acute fracture in an osteoporotic elderly patient.

CONCLUSIONS

Optimal proximal humerus fracture management requires a clear appreciation of the fracture configuration and fracture classification, as well as the quality of the bone in which the fracture occurs. Advanced age is an important risk factor and affects the prognosis. The best method of treatment must be selected with an appreciation of the natural history of these fractures. Postoperative physical therapy should be tailored to each patient, and a realistic approach should also set the surgeon and the patient up for a logical next step if additional surgical treatment becomes necessary.

REFERENCES

1. Cave EF. Shoulder girdle injuries. In: *Fractures and other injuries*. Chicago: Year Book, 1958.
2. Hulke JW. *Injuries of the upper extremity*. New York: William Wood, 1879.
3. Buhr AJ, Cooke AM. Fracture patterns. *Lancet* 1959;1:531–536.
4. Garraway WM, Stauffer RN, Kurland LT, et al. Limb fractures in a defined population. Frequency and distribution. *Mayo Clin Proc* 1979;54:701–707.
5. Horak J, Nilsson B. Epidemiology of fractures of the upper end of the humerus. *Clin Orthop* 1975;112:250–253.
6. Lind T, Kroner K, Jensen J. The epidemiology of fractures of the proximal humerus. *Arch Orthop Trauma Surg* 1989;108:285–287.
7. Razemon JP, Baux S. Fractures and fracture-dislocations of the upper extremity of the humerus. *Rev Chir Orthop Reparatrice Appar Mot* 1969;55:387–496.
8. Rose SH, Melton LJ, Morrey BF, et al. Epidemiologic features of humeral fractures. *Clin Orthop* 1982;64:24–30.

9. Koval KJ, Gallagher MA, Marsicano JG, et al. Functional outcome after minimally displaced fractures of the proximal part of the humerus. *J Bone Joint Surg Am* 1997;79:203–207.
10. Meyerding HW. Fracture-dislocation of the shoulder. *Minn Med* 1937;20:717–726.
11. Adedapo AO, Ikpeme JO. The results of internal fixation of three- and four-part proximal humerus fractures with the Polaris Nail. *Injury* 2001;32:115–121.
12. Hessmann M, Baumgaertel F, Gehling H, et al. Plate fixation of proximal humerus fractures with indirect reduction: surgical technique and results utilizing three shoulder scores. *Injury* 1999;30(7):453–462.
13. Ruch DS, Glisson RR, Marr AW, et al. Fixation of three-part proximal humerus fractures: a biomechanical evaluation. *J Orthop Trauma* 2000;14(1):36–40.
14. Wachtl SW, Marti CB, Hoogewoud HM, et al. Treatment of proximal humerus fracture using multiple intramedullary flexible nails. *Arch Orthop Trauma Surg* 2000;120(3–4):171–175.
15. Breasted JH. *The Edwin Smith surgical papyrus*. Chicago: University of Chicago Press, 1930.
16. Peltier LF. *Fractures: a history and iconography of their treatment*. San Francisco: Norman Publishing, 1990.
17. Bertoft ES, Lundh I, Ringqvist I. Physiotherapy after fracture of the proximal end of the humerus. *Scand J Rehabil Med* 1984;16:11–16.
18. Gordon D. Fractures of the upper end of the humerus. *JAMA* 1931;96:332–336.
19. Gurd FB. A simple effective method for the treatment of fractures of the upper part of the humerus. *Am J Surg* 1940;47:433–453.
20. Lucas-Championnière J. *Traitement des fractures par le massage et la mobilization*. Paris: Rueff, 1895.
21. Young TB, Wallace WA. Conservative treatment of fractures and fracture-dislocations of the upper end of the humerus. *J Bone Joint Surg Br* 1985;67:373–377.
22. Caldwell JA, Smith J. Treatment of unimpacted fractures of the surgical neck of the humerus. *Am J Surg* 1936;31:141–144.
23. Coonse GK. An improved humerus splint for hospital use. *J Bone Joint Surg* 1931;13:374–375.
24. Coonse GK, Moore H. Treatment of fractures of the humerus by mobilization and traction. *N Engl J Med* 1930;203:829–832.
25. Jones R. On certain fractures about the shoulder. *Ir J Med Sci* 1932;78:282–291.
26. Santee HE. Fractures about the upper end of the humerus. *Ann Surg* 1924;80:103–114.
27. Stevens JH. Fracture of the upper end of the humerus. *Ann Surg* 1919;69:147–160.
28. Callahan DJ. Anatomic considerations: closed reduction of proximal humeral fractures. *Orthop Rev* 1984;13:79–85.
29. de Mourgues G, Razemon JP, Leclaire HP, et al. Les fractures-luxations de l'épaule. *Rev Chir Orthop Reparatrice Appar Mot* 1965;51:151–165.
30. Frankau C. A manipulative method for the reduction of fractures of the surgical neck of the humerus. *Lancet* 1933;2:755.
31. Griswold RA, Hucherson DC, Strode EC. Fractures of the humerus treated with hanging cast. *South Med J* 1941;34:777–778.
32. Aldredge RH, Knight MP. Fractures of the upper end of the humerus treated by early relaxed motion and massage. *New Orleans Med Surg J* 1940;92:519–524.
33. Basti JJ, Dionysian E, Sherman PW, et al. Management of proximal humeral fractures. *J Hand Ther* 1994;7(2):111–121.
34. Brostrom F. Early mobilization of fractures of the upper end of the humerus. *Arch Surg* 1943;46:614–615.
35. DePalma AF, Cautilli RA. Fractures of the upper end of the humerus. *Clin Orthop* 1961;20:73–93.
36. Drapanas T, McDonald J, Hale HW. A rational approach to classification and treatment of fractures of the surgical neck of the humerus. *Am J Surg* 1960;99:617–624.
37. Ekstrom T, Lagergren C, von Schreeb T. Procaine injections and early mobilization for fractures of the neck of the humerus. *Acta Chir Scand* 1965;130:18–24.
38. Hermann OJ. Fractures of the shoulder joint with special reference to correction of defects. *AAOS Instr Course Lect* 1944;2:359–370.
39. Lundberg BJ, Svenungson-Hartwig E, Vikmark R. Independent exercises versus physiotherapy in non-displaced proximal humeral fractures. *Scand J Rehabil Med*. 1979;11:133–136.
40. Mills KL. Severe injuries of the upper end of the humerus. *Injury* 1974;6:13–21.
41. Roberts SM. Fractures of the upper end of the humerus: an end-result study which shows the advantage of early active motion. *JAMA* 1932;98:367–373.
42. Clifford PC. Fractures of the neck of the humerus: a review of the late results. *Injury* 1980;12:91–95.
43. Keene JS, Huizenga RE, Engber WD, et al. Proximal humeral fractures: a correction of residual deformity with long-term function. *Orthopedics* 1983;6:173–178.
44. Leyshon RL, Rehn J, Decker S, et al. Closed treatment of fractures of the proximal humerus (results of rotation osteotomy in habitual shoulder dislocation): radiology of the humeral head in recurrent anterior shoulder dislocations: brief report. *Acta Orthop Scand* 1984;55:48–51.
45. Zyto K, Ahrengart L, Sperber A, et al. Treatment of displaced proximal humeral fractures in elderly patients. *J Bone Joint Surg Br* 1997;79:412–417.
46. Colton CL. *The history of fracture treatment*. Philadelphia: WB Saunders, 1992.
47. Van Der Ghinst M, Houssa P. Acrylic prosthesis in fractures of the head of the humerus. *Acta Chir Belg* 1951;50:31–40.
48. Lorenzo FT. Osteosynthesis with Blount staples in fracture of the proximal end of the humerus: a preliminary report. *J Bone Joint Surg Am* 1955;37:45–48.
49. Krakovic M, Schmidt A, El Sigai A. Indication for surgery in shoulder-joint proximal fractures of the humerus and results. *Monatsschr Unfallheilkd* 1975;78:326–332.
50. Kristiansen B, Christensen SW. Plate fixation of proximal humeral fractures. *Acta Orthop Scand* 1986;57:320–323.
51. Moda SK, Chadha NS, Sangwan SS, et al. Open reduction and fixation of proximal humeral fractures and fracture-dislocations. *J Bone Joint Surg Br* 1990;72:1050–1052.
52. Savoie FH, Geissler WB, Vander Griend RA. Open reduction and internal fixation of three-part fractures of the proximal humerus. *Orthopedics* 1989;12:65–70.
53. Weise K, Meeder PJ, Wentzensen A. Indications and operative technique in osteosynthesis of fracture-dislocations of the shoulder joint in adults. *Langenbecks Arch Chir* 1980;351:91–98.
54. Yamano Y. Comminuted fractures of the proximal humerus treated with hook plate. *Arch Orthop Trauma Surg* 1986;105:359–363.
55. Neviaser JS. Complicated fractures and dislocations about the shoulder joint. *J Bone Joint Surg Am* 1962;44:984–998.
56. Sehr JR, Szabo RM. Semitubular blade plate for fixation in the proximal humerus. *J Orthop Trauma* 1988;2:327–332.
57. Chandler RW. Displaced proximal humeral fractures treated with a locked intramedullary device. *Tech Orthop* 1994;8:192–198.
58. Cuomo F, Flatow EL, Maday M, et al. Open reduction and internal fixation of two- and three-part displaced surgical neck fractures of the proximal humerus. *J Shoulder Elbow Surg* 1992;1:287–295.
59. Doursounian L, Grimberg J, Touzard RC. A new method of internal fixation for fractures of the upper end of the humerus: the Bilboquet implant. A study of 27 cases reviewed after more than 2 years. *Orthop Trans* 1996;20:457–458.
60. Haas K. Displaced proximal humeral fractures operated by Rush pin technique. *Opuscula Med* 1978;23:100–102.
61. Habernek H, Orthner E. A locking nail for fractures of the humerus. *J Bone Joint Surg Br* 1991;73:651–653.
62. Lentz W, Meuser P. The treatment of fractures of the proximal humerus. *Arch Orthop Trauma Surg* 1980;96:283–285.
63. Mazet R. Intramedullary fixation in the arm and the forearm. *Clin Orthop* 1953;2:75–92.
64. Mouradian WH. Displaced proximal humeral fractures: seven years' experience with a modified Zickel supracondylar device. *Clin Orthop* 1986;212:209–218.
65. Seidel H. Humeral locking nail: a preliminary report. *Orthopedics* 1989;12:219–226.
66. Weseley MS, Barenfeld PA, Eisenstein AL. Rush pin intramedullary fixation for fractures of the proximal humerus. *J Trauma* 1977;17:29–37.
67. Widen A. Fractures of the upper end of humerus with great displacement treated by marrow nailing. *Acta Chir Scand* 1959;97:439–441.
68. Zuipp H, Thermann H, Tscherne H. Interlocking screw-nail: a new device for unstable 2- and 3-part fractures of the proximal humerus. *Orthop Trans* 1992;16:231.
69. Checchia SL, Miranda DL, Carneiro MU, et al. Tratamento das fracturas do colo cirúrgico do úmero pela técnica de Kapandji. *Rev Bras Ortop* 1993;28:43–49.
70. Geneste R, Durandeau A, Gauzere JM, et al. The treatment of fracture-dislocation of the humeral head by blind pinning. *Rev Chir Orthop Reparatrice Appar Mot* 1980;66:383–386.
71. Halder SC, Chapman JA. Proximal humeral fractures: a new internal fixation device. *J Bone Joint Surg Br* 1997;79[Suppl 4]:408–409.
72. Henley MB, Chapman JR, Claudi BF. Closed retrograde Hackethal nail stabilization of humeral shaft fractures. *J Orthop Trauma* 1992;6:18–24.
73. Ingman AM, Waters DA. Locked intramedullary nailing of humeral shaft fractures: implant design, surgical technique, clinical results. *J Bone Joint Surg Br* 1994;76:23–29.
74. Kapandji A. L'ostéosynthèse par la technique des broches "en palmier" des fractures du col chirurgical de l'humérus. *Ann Chir Main* 1989;8:39–52.
75. Markel DC, Donley BG, Blasier RB. Percutaneous intramedullary pinning of proximal humeral fractures. *Orthop Rev* 1994;23:667–671.
76. Yano S, Takamura S, Kobayashi I, et al. Use of the spiral pin for fracture of the humeral neck: case report 165:BCG-osteomyelitis of the proximal end of the humerus with an abscess dissecting into the deltoid muscle. *Nippon Seikeigeka Gakkai Zasshi* 1981;55:1607–1619.
77. Zifko B, Poigenfürst J, Pezzei C, et al. Flexible intramedullary pins in the treatment of unstable proximal humeral fractures. *Injury* 1991;22:60–62.
78. Kristiansen B. External fixation of proximal humerus fracture: clinical and cadaver study of pinning technique. *Acta Orthop Scand* 1987;58:645–648.
79. Kristiansen B, Kofoed H. External fixation of displaced fractures of the proximal humerus: technique and preliminary results. *J Bone Joint Surg Br* 1987;69:643–646.
80. Kristiansen B, Kofoed H. Transcutaneous reduction and external fixation of displaced fractures of the proximal humerus: a controlled clinical trial. *J Bone Joint Surg Br* 1988;70:821–824.
81. Flatow EL, Cuomo F, Madey MG, et al. Open reduction and internal fixation of two-part displaced fractures of the greater tuberosity of the proximal part of the humerus. *J Bone Joint Surg Am* 1991;73:1213–1218.
82. Hawkins RJ, Switlyk P. Acute prosthetic replacement for severe fractures of the proximal humerus. *Clin Orthop* 1993;289:156–160.
83. Jakob RP, Miniaci A, Anson PS, et al. Four-part valgus-impacted fractures of the proximal humerus. *J Bone Joint Surg Br* 1991;73:295–298.
84. Koval KJ, Sanders R, Zuckerman JD, et al. Modified-tension band wiring of displaced surgical neck fractures of the humerus. *J Shoulder Elbow Surg* 1993;2:85–92.
85. Magerl F. Osteosyntheses in the shoulder region: pertubercular humeral fractures, scapular neck fractures. *Helv Chir Acta* 1974;41:225–232.
86. Meeder PJ, Wiese K, Wentzensen A. Results of an operative therapy of dislocated fractures of the humeral head in adults. *Aktuel Traumatol* 1980;10:201.
87. Stewart MJ, Hundley JM. Fractures of the humerus: a comparative study in methods of treatment. *J Bone Joint Surg Am* 1955;37:681–692.
88. Wörsdörfer O, Magerl F. Operative Behandlung der proximalen Humerusfrakturen. *Hefte Unfallheilkd* 1982;160:136–154.

89. Muller ME, Allgower M, Willeneger H. *Manual of internal fixation.* New York: Springer-Verlag, 1970.
90. Neer CS. I. Displaced proximal humeral fractures. II. Treatment of three-part and four-part displacement. *J Bone Joint Surg Am* 1970;52:1090–1103.
91. Paavolainen P, Bjorkenheim JM, Slatis P, et al. Operative treatment of severe proximal humeral fractures. *Acta Orthop Scand* 1983;54:374–379.
92. Boileau P, Huten D, Pietu G, et al. *L'arthroplastie prosthétique dans les fractures récentes complexes de l'extrémité supérieure de l'humérus: technique et indications.* Paris: Expansion Scientifique Publications, 1999.
93. Debevoise NT, Hyatt GW, Townsend GB. Humeral torsion in recurrent shoulder dislocations: a technic of determination by X-ray. *Clin Orthop* 1971;76:87–93.
94. Hill JA, Tkach L, Hendrix RW. A study of glenohumeral orientation in patients with anterior recurrent shoulder dislocations using computerized axial tomography. *Orthop Rev* 1989;18:84–91.
95. Krahl V. The torsion of the humerus: its localization, cause, duration in man. *Am J Anat* 1947;80:275–319.
96. Kronberg M, Brostrom LA, Soderlund V. Retroversion of the humeral head in the normal shoulder and its relationship to the normal range of motion. *Clin Orthop* 1990; 253:113–117.
97. Neer CS. Articular replacement for the humeral head. *J Bone Joint Surg Am* 1955;37: 215–228.
98. Pieper HG. Shoulder dislocation in skiing: choice of surgical method depending on the degree of humeral retrotorsion. *Int J Sports Med* 1985;6:155–160.
99. Randelli M, Gambrioli PL. Glenohumeral osteometry by computed tomography in normal and unstable shoulders. *Clin Orthop* 1986;208:151–156.
100. Hall MC, Rosser M. The structure of the upper end of the humerus, with reference to osteoporotic changes in senescence leading to fractures. *Can Med Assoc J* 1963;88: 290–294.
101. Hepp P, Lill H, Bail H, et al. Where should implants be anchored in the humeral head? *Clin Orthop* 2003;415:139–147.
102. Saitoh S, Nakatsuchi Y. Osteoporosis of the proximal humerus: comparison of bone mineral density and mechanical strength with the proximal femur. *J Shoulder Elbow Surg* 1993;2:78–84.
103. Saitoh S, Nakatsuchi Y, Latta L, et al. Distribution of bone mineral density and bone strength of the proximal humerus. *J Shoulder Elbow Surg* 1994;3:234–242.
104. Tingart M, Apreleva M, von Stechow D, et al. Cortical thickness of the proximal humeral diaphysis predicts bone mineral density of the proximal humerus. *J Bone Joint Surg Br* 2003;85(4):611–617.
105. Tingart M, Lehtinen J, Zurakowski D, et al. Proximal humeral fractures: regional differences in bone mineral density affect the fixation strength of cancellous screws. *J Shoulder Elbow Surg (submitted)*, 2005.
106. Galle P, Munk P, Passl R, et al. Zur Gefassversorgung des Oberarmkopfes. *Hefte Unfallheilkd* 1975;126:19–20.
107. Gerber C, Hersche O, Berberat C. The clinical relevance of posttraumatic avascular necrosis of the humeral head. *J Shoulder Elbow Surg* 1998;7:586–590.
108. Laing PG. The arterial supply of the adult humerus. *J Bone Joint Surg Am* 1956;38: 1105–1116.
109. Moseley HF, Goldie I. The arterial pattern of the rotator cuff and the shoulder. *J Bone Joint Surg Br* 1963;45:780–789.
110. Rothman RH, Parke WW. The vascular anatomy of the rotator cuff. *Clin Orthop* 1965; 41:176–186.
111. Brooks CH, Revell WJ, Heatley FW. Vascularity of the humeral head after proximal humeral fractures: an anatomical cadaver study. *J Bone Joint Surg Br* 1993;75:132–136.
112. Decq P, Filipetti P, Feve A, et al. Peripheral selective neurotomy of the brachial plexus collateral branches for the treatment of spastic shoulder: anatomical study and clinical results in five patients. *J Neurosurg* 1997;86(4):648–653.
113. Fischer L, Neidhardt JH, Tissot E, et al. Anatomical variations of scalenus muscle and brachial plexus relationships. *Lyon Med* 1971;225(8):750–752.
114. Gardener E. Innervation of the shoulder joint. *Anat Rec* 1948;102:1–18.
115. Codman EA. *The shoulder: rupture of the supraspinatus tendon and other lesions in or about the subacromial bursa.* Boston: Thomas Todd, 1934.
116. Gold AM. Fractured neck of the humerus with separation and dislocation of the humeral head (fracture-dislocation of the shoulder, severe type). *Bull Hosp Jt Dis* 1971; 32:87–99.
117. Kocher MS, Feagin JAJ. Shoulder injuries during Alpine skiing. *Am J Sports Med* 1996; 24:665–669.
118. Kocher T. *Beiträge zur Kenntnis Einiger Praktisch Wichtiger Fracturformen.* Basel: Carl Sallmann, 1896.
119. Howard NJ, Eloesser L. Treatment of fractures of the upper end of the humerus: an experimental and clinical study. *J Bone Joint Surg* 1934;32:1–29.
120. Garceau GJ, Cogland S. Early physical therapy in the treatment of fractures of the surgical neck of the humerus. *Indiana Med* 1941;34:293–295.
121. Ehlinger M, Gicquel P, Clavert P, et al. A new implant for proximal humeral fracture: experimental study of the basket plate. *Rev Chir Orthop Reparatrice Appar Mot* 2004; 90(1):16–25.
122. Frankle MA, Greenwald DP, Markee BA, et al. Biomechanical effects of malposition of tuberosity fragments on the humeral prosthetic reconstruction for four-part proximal humerus fractures. *J Shoulder Elbow Surg* 2001;10:321–326.
123. Gicquel P, Bonnomet F, Boutemy P, et al. Experimental comparative study of 3 systems of osteosynthesis for proximal humeral fractures. Preliminary study of the mechanical properties of conserved trabecular bone. *Rev Chir Orthop Reparatrice Appar Mot* 1999; 85(8):811–820.
124. Marchetti PG, Vicenzi G, Impallomeni C, et al. The use of elastic nails for intramedullary fixation of humeral fractures and nonunions. *Orthopedics* 2000;23(4):343–347.
125. Clare DJ, Hersh CK, Athanasiou K, et al. Biomechanical fixation strength in surgical neck fractures of the proximal humerus. *Orthop Trans* 1998;22:339.
126. Ruch DS, Kuzma GR. Biomechanical rigidity following fixation of proximal humerus fractures. *Orthop Trans* 1998;22:599.
127. Chu SP, Kelsey JL, Keegan TH, et al. Risk factors for proximal humerus fracture. *Am J Epidemiol* 2004;160(4):360–367.
128. Gaebler C, McQueen MM, Court-Brown CM. Minimally displaced proximal humerus fractures: epidemiology and outcome in 507 cases. *Acta Orthop Scand* 2003;74(5): 580–585.
129. Gerber C, Werner CM, Vienne P. Internal fixation of complex fractures of the proximal humerus. *J Bone Joint Surg Br* 2004;86(6):848–855.
130. Tingart MJ, Bouxsein ML, Zurakowski D, et al. Three-dimensional distribution of bone density in the proximal humerus. *Calcif Tissue Int* 2003;73(6):531–536.
131. Liew AS, Johnson JA, Patterson SD, et al. Effect of screw placement on fixation in the humeral head. *J Shoulder Elbow Surg* 2000;9:423–426.
132. Banco SP, Andrisani D, Ramsey M, et al. The parachute technique: valgus impaction osteotomy for two-part fractures of the surgical neck of the humerus. *J Bone Joint Surg Am* 2001;83(Suppl 2[Pt 1]):38–42.
133. Hawkins RJ, Bell RH, Gurr K. The three-part fracture of the proximal part of the humerus. Operative treatment. *J Bone Joint Surg Am* 1986;68(9):1410–1414.
134. Hawkins RJ, Kiefer GN. Internal fixation techniques for proximal humeral fractures. *Clin Orthop* 1987;223:77–85.
135. Schlegel TF, Hawkins RJ. Displaced proximal humeral fractures: evaluation and treatment. *J Am Acad Orthop Surg* 1994;2(1):54–78.
136. Einarsson F. Fracture of the upper end of the humerus: discussion based on the follow-up of 302 cases. *Acta Orthop Scand* 1958;27(Suppl 32):1–215.
137. Rasmussen S, Hvass I, Dalsgaard J, et al. Displaced proximal humeral fractures: results of conservative treatment. *Injury* 1992;23(1):41–43.
138. Wentworth ET. Fractures involving the shoulder joint. *NY State J Med* 1940;40: 1282–1288.
139. Hodgson SA, Mawson SJ, Stanley D. Rehabilitation after two-part fractures of the neck of the humerus. *J Bone Joint Surg Br* 2003;85:419–422.
140. Levin LS, Goldner RD, Urbaniak JR, et al. Management of severe musculoskeletal injuries of the upper extremity. *J Orthop Trauma* 1990;4(4):432–440.
141. O'Brien PJ. Fracture fixation in patients having multiple injuries. *Can J Surg* 2003; 46(2):124–128.
142. Beredjiklian PK, Iannotti JP. Treatment of proximal humerus fracture malunion with prosthetic arthroplasty. *AAOS Instr Course Lect* 1998;47:135–140.
143. Beredjiklian PK, Iannotti JP, Norris TR, et al. Operative treatment of malunion of a fracture of the proximal aspect of the humerus. *J Bone Joint Surg Am* 1998;80: 1484–1497.
144. Boileau P, Krishnan SG, Tinsi L, et al. Tuberosity malposition and migration: reasons for poor outcomes after hemiarthroplasty for displaced fractures of the proximal humerus. *J Shoulder Elbow Surg* 2002;11(5):401–412.
145. Boileau P, Trojani C, Walch G, et al. Shoulder arthroplasty for the treatment of the sequelae of fractures of the proximal humerus. *J Shoulder Elbow Surg* 2001;10(4): 299–308.
146. Demirhan M, Kilicoglu O, Altinel L, et al. Prognostic factors in prosthetic replacement for acute proximal humerus fractures. *J Orthop Trauma* 2003;17(3):181–188.
147. Gerber C. Reconstructive surgery following malunion of fractures of the proximal humerus in adults. *Orthopade* 1990;19:316–323.
148. Siegel JA, Dines DM. Proximal humerus malunions. *Orthop Clin North Am* 2000;31(1): 35–50.
149. Parsons BO, Klepps SJ, Miller SR, et al. Reliability and reproducibility of radiographs of greater tuberosity displacement. Cadaver study. *J Bone Joint Surg Am* 2005;87:58–65.
150. Gerber C, Werner CM, Vienne P. Internal fixation of complex fractures of the proximal humerus. *J Bone Joint Surg Br* 2004;86(6):848–855.
151. Bernstein J, Adler LM, Blank JE, et al. Evaluation of the Neer system of classification of proximal humeral fractures with computerized tomographic scans and plain radiographs. *J Bone Joint Surg Am* 1996;78:1371–1375.
152. McLaughlin HL. Dislocation of the shoulder with tuberosity fracture. *Surg Clin North Am* 1963;43:1615–1620.
153. Neer CS. Displaced proximal humeral fractures. I. Classification and evaluation. *J Bone J Surg Am* 1970;52:1077–1089.
154. Benirschke SK, West GG, Henley MD, et al. Percutaneous pin fixation of surgical neck fractures of the humerus. *Orthop Trans* 1992;16:231.
155. Herscovici DJ, Saunders D, Sanders R, et al. The use of percutaneous fixation for the operative management of proximal humerus fractures. *Orthop Trans* 1996;21:624.
156. Jaberg H, Warner JJ, Jakob RP. Percutaneous stabilization of unstable fractures of the humerus. *J Bone Joint Surg Am* 1992;74:508–515.
157. Jakob RP, Ganz R. Proximale Humerusfrakturen. *Helv Chir Acta* 1981;48:595–610.
158. Mestdagh H, Butruille Y, Tillie B, et al. Résultats du traitement des fractures de l'extrémité supérieure de l'huméus par embrochage percutane: à propos de cent quarante deux cas. *Ann Chir* 1984;38:5–13.
159. Resch H, Povacz P, Frohlich R, et al. Percutaneous fixation of three- and four-part fractures of the proximal humerus. *J Bone Joint Surg Br* 1997;79(2):295–300.
160. Lavender A, Srinivasan M, Henderson AA. Percutaneous reduction and fixation of the valgus impacted fracture of the proximal humerus: a new method. *J Bone Joint Surg Br* 1998;80[Suppl 1]:105.

161. Molé D, Roche O. Impacted fractures of the upper end of the humerus: comparison between conservative and closed surgical treatment. *J Bone Joint Surg Br* 1997;79[Suppl 1]:46.
162. Hertel R, Hempfing A, Stiehler M, et al. Predictors of humeral head ischemia after intracapsular fracture of the proximal humerus. *J Shoulder Elbow Surg* 2004;13(4): 427–433.
163. Kocialkowski A, Wallace WA. Closed percutaneous K-wire stabilization for displaced fractures of the surgical neck of the humerus. *Injury* 1990;21:209–212.
164. Stoller C, Gerber C. Secondary fracture of the humerus after closed reduction and percutaneous stabilization of a subcapital fracture. *J Shoulder Elbow Surg* 1994;3: 100–106.
165. Blom S, Dahlback LO. Nerve injuries in dislocations of the shoulder joint and fracture of the neck of the humerus. *Acta Chir Scand* 1970;136:461–466.
166. Dehne E. *Arch Orthop Unfallchir* 1939;39:477–485.
167. Dehne E. Fractures at the upper end of the humerus. *Surg Clin North Am* 1945;25: 28–47.
168. Watson-Jones R. *Fracture of the neck of the humerus*. Baltimore: Williams & Wilkins, 1955.
169. Watson-Jones R. *Fracture of the neck of the humerus*. Baltimore: Williams & Wilkins, 1940.
170. De Anquin CE, De Anquin CA. *Prosthetic replacement in the treatment of serious fractures of the proximal humerus*. Berlin: Springer-Verlag, 1982.
171. Neer CS. Four-segment classification of displaced proximal humeral fractures. *AAOS Instr Course Lect* 1975;24:160–168.
172. Neer CS. *Shoulder reconstruction*. Philadelphia: WB Saunders, 1990.
173. Resch H, Hubner C, Schwaiger R. Minimally invasive reduction and osteosynthesis of articular fractures of the humeral head. *Injury* 2001;32(Suppl 1):25–32.
174. Seggl W, Weiglein A. Die arterielle Blutversorgung des Oberarmkopfes und ihre prognostische Bedeutung bei Luxationen, Frakturen, und Luxationsfrakturen des Oberarmkopfes. *Acta Chir Austriaca* 1991;23:1–19.
175. Jakob RP, Kristiansen T, Mayo K, et al. *Classification and aspects of treatment of fractures of the proximal humerus*. Philadelphia: BC Decker, 1984.
176. Siebenrock KA, Gerber C. The reproducibility of classification of fractures of the proximal end of the humerus. *J Bone Joint Surg Am* 1993;75:1751–1755.
177. Bigliani LU, Flatow EL, Pollock RG. Fracture classification systems: do they work and are they useful? *J Bone Joint Surg Am* 1994;76:790–792.
178. Burstein AH. Fracture classification systems: do they work and are they useful? *J Bone Joint Surg Am* 1993;75:1743–1744.
179. Sidor ML, Zuckerman JD, Lyon T, et al. The Neer classification system for proximal humeral fractures: an assessment of interobserver reliability and intraobserver reproducibility. *J Bone Joint Surg Am* 1993;75:1745–1750.
180. Kristiansen B, Anderson UL, Olsen CA, et al. The Neer classification of fractures of the proximal humerus: an assessment of interobserver variation. *Skeletal Radiol* 1988;17: 420–422.
181. Landis JR, Koch GG. The measurement of observer agreement for categorical data. *Biometrics* 1977;33:159–174.
182. Edelson G, Kelly I, Vigder F, et al. A three-dimensional classification for fractures of the proximal humerus. *J Bone Joint Surg Br* 2004;86:413–425.
183. Simon JA, Puopolo SM, Capla EL, et al. Accuracy of the axillary projection to determine fracture angulation of the proximal humerus. *Orthopedics* 2004;27(2):205–207.
184. Green A, Izzi JJ. Isolated fractures of the greater tuberosity of the proximal humerus. *J Shoulder Elbow Surg* 2003;12(6):641–649.
185. Stevens JH. Dislocation of the shoulder. *Ann Surg* 1926;83:84–103.
186. Marke DC, Blasier RB. Bilateral anterior dislocation of the shoulders with greater tuberosity fractures. *Orthopedics* 1994;17:945–949.
187. Hersche O, Gerber C. Iatrogenic displacement of fracture-dislocations of the shoulder. A report of seven cases. *J Bone Joint Surg Br* 1994;76(1):30–33.
188. Ogawa K, Yoshida A, Inokuchi W. Posterior shoulder dislocation associated with fracture of the humeral anatomic neck: treatment guidelines and long-term outcome. *J Trauma* 1999;46(2):318–323.
189. Bono CM, Renard R, Levine RG, et al. Effect of displacement of fractures of the greater tuberosity on the mechanics of the shoulder. *J Bone Joint Surg Br* 2001;83(7): 1056–1062.
190. Green A, Izzi JJ. Isolated fractures of the greater tuberosity of the proximal humerus. *J Shoulder Elbow Surg* 2003;12(6):641–649.
191. McWhorter GL. Fractures of the greater tuberosity of the humerus with displacement. *Surg Clin North Am* 1925;5:1005–1017.
192. Miller SR. Practical points in the diagnosis and treatment of fractures of the upper fourth of the humerus. *Indust Med* 1940;9:458–460.
193. Sever JW. Fracture of the head of the humerus: treatment and results. *N Engl J Med* 1937;216:1100–1107.
194. Taylor HL. Isolated fracture of the greater tuberosity of the humerus. *Ann Surg* 1908; 54:10–12.
195. Johansson O. Complications and failures of surgery in various fractures of the humerus. *Acta Chir Scand* 1961;120:469–478.
196. Neer CSI, McIlveen SJ. Remplacement de la tète humérale avec reconstruction des tubérosités et de la coiffe dans les fractures déplacées à 4 fragments. *Rev Chir Orthop Reparatrice Appar Mot* 1988;74[Suppl 2]:31–40.
197. Olivier H, Dufour G, Duparc J. Fracture of the trochiter. *Rev Chir Orthop Reparatrice Appar Mot* 1976;62:113–118.
198. Levy AS. Greater tuberosity fractures of the humerus. *Orthop Trans* 1998;22:594.
199. Fujisawa H, Suenaga N, Minami A. Electromyographic study during isometric exercise of the shoulder in head-out water immersion. *J Shoulder Elbow Surg* 1998;7:491–494.
200. Gerber C, Hersche O, Farron A. Isolated rupture of the subscapularis tendon. *J Bone Joint Surg Am* 1996;78(7):1015–1023.
201. Hertel R, Ballmer FT, Lombert SM, et al. Lag signs in the diagnosis of rotator cuff rupture. *J Shoulder Elbow Surg* 1996;5(4):307–313.
202. Paschal SO, Hutton KS, Weatherall PT. Isolated avulsion fracture of the lesser tuberosity of the humerus in adolescents. *J Bone Joint Surg Am* 1995;77:1427–1429.
203. Haas SL. Fracture of the lesser tuberosity of the humerus. *Am J Surg* 1944;63:253–256.
204. Gerber A, Warner JJP. *Hemiarthroplasty for management of complex proximal humerus fractures: preoperative planning and surgical solution*. Philadelphia: Lippincott-Raven, 2005.
205. Gerber C, Yian E, Pfirrmann CAW, et al. Evaluation of subscapularis muscle function and structure after total shoulder replacement using lesser tuberosity osteotomy and repair. *J Bone Joint Surg Am* 2005 (*in press*).
206. Caniggia M, Maniscalco P, Picinotti A. Isolated avulsion fracture of the lesser tuberosity of the humerus. Report of two cases. *Panminerva Med* 1996;38(1):56–60.
207. Coates MH, Breidahl W. Humeral avulsion of the anterior band of the inferior glenohumeral ligament with associated subscapularis bony avulsion in skeletally immature patients. *Skeletal Radiol* 2001;30(12):661–666.
208. Kanso I, Bricout JM. Isolated avulsion fracture of the lesser tuberosity of the humerus. Apropos of a case. *Rev Chir Orthop Reparatrice Appar Mot* 1998;84(6):554–557.
209. Leslie A, Cassar-Pullicino VN. Avulsion of the lesser tuberosity with intra-articular injury of the glenohumeral joint. *Injury* 1996;27(10):742–745.
210. Ogawa K, Takahashi M. Long-term outcome of isolated lesser tuberosity fractures of the humerus. *J Trauma* 1997;42(5):955–999.
211. Sugalski MT, Hyman JE, Ahmad CS. Avulsion fracture of the lesser tuberosity in an adolescent baseball pitcher: a case report. *Am J Sports Med* 2004;32(3):793–796.
212. van Laarhoven HA, te Slaa RL, van Laarhoven EW. Isolated avulsion fracture of the lesser tuberosity of the humerus. *J Trauma* 1995;39(5):997–999.
213. Fuchs B, Weishaupt D, Zanetti M, et al. Fatty degeneration of the muscles of the rotator cuff: assessment by computed tomography versus magnetic resonance imaging. *J Shoulder Elbow Surg* 1999;8(6):599–605.
214. Gerber C, Meyer DC, Schneeberger AG, et al. Effect of tendon release and delayed repair on the structure of the muscles of the rotator cuff: an experimental study in sheep. *J Bone Joint Surg Am* 2004;86(9):1973–1982.
215. Hersche O, Gerber C. Passive tension in the supraspinatus musculotendinous unit after long-standing rupture of its tendon: a preliminary report. *J Shoulder Elbow Surg* 1998; 7(4):393–396.
216. Meyer DC, Hoppeler H, von Rechenberg B, et al. A pathomechanical concept explains muscle loss and fatty muscular changes following surgical tendon release. *J Orthop Res* 2004;22(5):1004–1007.
217. Pfirrmann CW, Zanetti M, Weishaupt D, et al. Subscapularis tendon tears: detection and grading at MR arthrography. *Radiology* 1999;213(3):709–714.
218. Galatz LM, Iannotti JP. Management of surgical neck nonunions. *Orthop Clin North Am* 2000;31(1):51–61.
219. Healy WL, Jupiter JB, Kristiansen TK, et al. Nonunion of the proximal humerus. A review of 25 cases. *J Orthop Trauma* 1990;4(4):424–431.
220. Nayak NK, Schickendantz MS, Regan WD, et al. Operative treatment of nonunion of surgical neck fractures of the humerus. *Clin Orthop* 1995;313:200–205.
221. Wirth MA. Late sequelae of proximal humerus fractures. *AAOS Instr Course Lect* 2003; 52:13–16.
222. Fankhauser F, Boldin C, Schippinger G, et al. A new locking plate for unstable fractures of the proximal humerus. *Clin Orthop* 2005;430:176–181.
223. Ring D, McKee BH, Perey BH, Jupiter JB. The use of a blade plate and autogenous cancellous bone graft in the treatment of ununited fractures of the proximal humerus. *J Shoulder Elbow Surg* 2001;10:501–507.
224. Thompson NW, Sloan SC, Adair A, et al. The limited-contact dynamic compression plate in the management of proximal humeral non-union. *Injury* 2004;35(11): 1137–1139.
225. Qidwai SA. Treatment of proximal humerus fractures by intramedullary Kirschner wires. *J Trauma* 2001;50(6):1090–1095.
226. Dander AJ, Dander A, Gomar F. Complications in operative treatment for displaced proximal humeral fractures. *J Bone Joint Surg Br* 1995;77[Suppl 2]:146.
227. Kamineni S, Ankem H, Sanghavi S. Anatomical considerations for percutaneous proximal humeral fracture fixation. *Injury* 2004;35(11):1133–1136.
228. Rowles DJ, McGrory JE. Percutaneous pinning of the proximal part of the humerus. An anatomic study. *J Bone Joint Surg Am* 2001;83:1695–1699.
229. Chen CY, Chao EK, Tu YK, et al. Closed management and percutaneous fixation of unstable proximal humerus fractures. *J Trauma* 1998;45(6):1039–1045.
230. Mellado JM, Calmet J, Garcia Forcada IL, et al. Early intrathoracic migration of Kirschner wires used for percutaneous osteosynthesis of a two-part humeral neck fracture: a case report. *Emerg Radiol* 2004;11(1):49–52.
231. Neer CS, Borwn TH, McLaughlin HL. Fracture of the neck of the humerus with dislocation of the head fragment. *Am J Surg* 1953;85:252–258.
232. Neer CS. Displaced proximal humeral fractures. Part I. Classification and evaluation. *Clin Orthop* 1987;223:3–10.
233. Brorson S, Bagger J, Sylvest A, et al. Improved interobserver variation after training of doctors in the Neer system. A randomised trial. *J Bone Joint Surg Br* 2002;84(7): 950–954.
234. Brorson S, Bagger J, Sylvest A, et al. Low agreement among 24 doctors using the Neer classification; only moderate agreement on displacement, even between specialists. *Int Orthop* 2002;26(5):271–273.
235. Rees J, Hicks J, Ribbans W. Assessment and management of three- and four-part proximal humeral fractures. *Clin Orthop* 1998;353:18–29.
236. Sallay PL, Pedowitz RA, Mallon WJ, et al. Reliability and reproducibility of radiographic

interpretation of proximal humeral fracture pathoanatomy. *J Shoulder Elbow Surg* 1997; 6(1):60–69.

237. Sjoden GO, Movin T, Guntner P, et al. Poor reproducibility of classification of proximal humeral fractures. Additional CT of minor value. *Acta Orthop Scand* 1997;68(3): 239–242.
238. Naranja RJJ, Iannott IJP. Displaced three- and four-part proximal humerus fractures: evaluation and management. *J Am Acad Orthop Surg* 2000;8(6):373–382.
239. Panagopoulos AM, Dimakopoulos P, Tyllianakis M, et al. Valgus-impacted proximal humerus fractures and their blood supply after transosseous suturing. *Int Orthop* 2004; 28:333–337.
240. Williams GRJ, Wong KL. Two-part and three-part fractures: open reduction and internal fixation versus closed reduction and percutaneous pinning. *Orthop Clin North [Am]* 2000;31(1):1–21.
241. Bosch U, Skutek M, Fremerey RW, et al. Outcome after primary and secondary hemiarthroplasty in elderly patients with fractures of the proximal humerus. *J Shoulder Elbow Surg* 1998;7(5):479–484.
242. Dimakopoulos P, Potamitis N, Lambiris E. Hemiarthroplasty in the treatment of comminuted intraarticular fractures of the proximal humerus. *Clin Orthop* 1997;341:7–11.
243. Frankle MA, Ondrovic LE, Markee BA, et al. Stability of tuberosity reattachment in proximal humeral hemiarthroplasty. *J Shoulder Elbow Surg* 2002;11(5):413–420.
244. Goldman RT, Koval KJ, Cuomo F, et al. Functional outcome after humeral head replacement for acute three- and four-part proximal humeral fractures. *J Shoulder Elbow Surg* 1995;4(2):81–86.
245. Lervick GN, Carroll RM, Levine WN. Complications after hemiarthroplasty for fractures of the proximal humerus. *AAOS Instr Course Lect* 2003;52:3–12.
246. Mighell MA, Kolm GP, Collinge CA, et al. Outcomes of hemiarthroplasty for fractures of the proximal humerus. *J Shoulder Elbow Surg* 2003;12(6):569–577.
247. Moeckel BH, Dines DM, Warren RF, et al. Modular hemiarthroplasty for fractures of the proximal part of the humerus. *J Bone Joint Surg [Am]* 1992;74(6):884–889.
248. Prakash U, McGurty DW, Dent JA. Hemiarthroplasty for severe fractures of the proximal humerus. *J Shoulder Elbow Surg* 2002;11(5):428–430.
249. Skutek M, Fremerey RW, Bosch U. Level of physical activity in elderly patients after hemiarthroplasty for three- and four-part fractures of the proximal humerus. *Arch Orthop Trauma Surg* 1998;117(4–5):252–255.
250. Wretenberg P, Ekelund A. Acute hemiarthroplasty after proximal humerus fracture in old patients. A retrospective evaluation of 18 patients followed for 2–7 years. *Acta Orthop Scand* 1997;68(2):121–123.
251. Zyto K, Wallace WA, Frostick SP, et al. Outcome after hemiarthroplasty for three- and four-part fractures of the proximal humerus. *J Shoulder Elbow Surg* 1998;7:85–89.
252. Jones L. Reconstructive operation for non-reducible fractures of the head of the humerus. *Ann Surg* 1933;97:217–225.
253. Luppino D, Santangelo G, Vicenzi G, et al. Le fratture dell'estremità prossimale dell'omero de interesse chirurgico (studio de 40 casi). *Chir Organi Mov* 1982;67:373–381.
254. Michaelis LS. Comminuted fracture-dislocation of the shoulder. *J Bone Joint Surg Am* 1944;26:363–365.
255. Prahinski JR, Schaefer RA, McHale KA. New York-Tidewater Chapters History of Military Medicine Essay Award: surgical resection of the proximal humerus in the American Civil War. *Mil Med* 1998;163:257–264.
256. Skruodies B, Wening JV, Jungbluth KH. Humeruskopfresektion als Therapie bei Oberarmkopftrümmerfrakturen-Ergebnisse. *Langenbecks Arch Chir* 1990;375:225–230.
257. Svend-Hansen H. Displaced proximal humeral fractures: a review of 49 patients. *Acta Orthop Scand* 1974;45:359–364.
258. Tornkvist H, Ahrengart L, Sperber A. Tension band wiring vs. non-operative treatment of displaced proximal humerus fractures: a prospective randomized study. *Orthop Trans* 1997;21:592.
259. Knight RA, Mayne JA. Comminuted fractures and fracture-dislocations involving the articular surface of the humeral head. *J Bone Joint Surg Am* 1957;39:1343–1355.
260. Lasher WW. Fracture dislocation of the head of the humerus. *JAMA* 1925;84:356–358.
261. Silverskoild N. On the treatment of fracture-dislocations of the shoulder-joint with special reference to the capability of the head-fragment, disconnected from capsule and periosteum to enter into bony union. *Acta Chir Scand* 1928;64:227–293.
262. Szyszkowitz R, Seggl W, Schleifer P, et al. Proximal humeral fractures: management techniques and expected results. *Clin Orthop* 1993;292:13–25.
263. Wijgman AJ, Roolker W, Patt TW, et al. Open reduction and internal fixation of three- and four-part fractures of the proximal part of the humerus. *J Bone Joint Surg Am* 2002; 84(11):1919–1925.
264. Dewar FP, Yabsley RH. Fracture-dislocation of the shoulder: report of a case. *J Bone Joint Surg Br* 1967;49:540–543.
265. Ilchmann T, Ochsner PE, Wingstrand H, et al. Non-operative treatment versus tension-band osteosynthesis in three- and four-part proximal humeral fractures. *Int Orthop* 1998;22:316–320.
266. Imhoff VM, Sadr I, Tassler H, et al. Die konservative und operative Therapie der Humerusfrakturen des Collum chirurgicum. *Zentralbl Chir* 1989;114:228–237.
267. Esser RD. Treatment of three- and four-part fractures of the proximal humerus with a modified cloverleaf plate. *J Orthop Trauma* 1994;8:15–22.
268. Ko JY, Yamamoto R. Surgical treatment of complex fracture of the proximal humerus. *Clin Orthop* 1996;327:225–237.
269. Resch H, Benedetto KP, Kadletz R, et al. Roentgen examination in recurrent shoulder luxation: value of different exposure technics: simultaneous bilateral anterior and posterior shoulder dislocations. *Unfallchirurgie* 1985;11:65–69.
270. Ruedi T. Treatment of displaced metaphyseal fractures with screw and wiring systems. *Orthopedics* 1989;12:55–59.
271. Siebler G, Walz H, Kuner EH. Minimal osteosynthesis of fractures of the head of the humerus. Indications, technic, results. *Unfallchirurg* 1989;92:169–174.
272. Van Der Elst E. *Early stages of internal fixation of fractured bones (osteosynthesis) in Belgium*. Brussels, 1971.
273. Kasperczyk WJ, Tscherne H. Avascular necrosis after four-part fractures and fracture-dislocations of the proximal humerus: is reconstruction really advisable? *Orthop Trans* 1997;21:592–593.
274. Bellumore Y, Determe P, Bonnevialle M, et al. Preliminary results of internal fixation combined with disto-proximal Kapandji nailing in fractures of the head and tuberosities of the humerus. *J Bone Joint Surg Br* 1997;79:45.
275. Gerber C, Schneeberger AG, Vinh TS. The arterial vascularization of the humeral head: an anatomical study. *J Bone Joint Surg Am* 1990;72:1486–1494.
276. Murphy JB. Fracture and luxation of the neck of the humerus. *Surg Clin Chicago* 1913; 2:137–148.
277. Collopy D, Skirving A. Transchondral fracture dislocation of the shoulder. *J Bone Joint Surg Br* 1995;77:975–976.
278. Hartsock LA, Estes WJ, Murray CA, et al. Shoulder hemiarthroplasty for proximal humeral fractures. *Orthop Clin North Am* 1998;29(3):467–475.
279. Heers G, Torchia ME. Shoulder hemi-arthroplasty in proximal humeral fractures. *Orthopade* 2001;30(6):386–394.
280. Kralinger F, Schwaiger R, Wambacher M, et al. Outcome after primary hemiarthroplasty for fracture of the humeral head. A retrospective multicenter study of 167 patients. *J Bone Joint Surg Br* 2004;86:217.
281. Robinson CM, Page RS, Hill RMF, et al. Primary hemiarthroplasty for treatment of proximal humerus fractures. *J Bone Joint Surg Am* 2003;85(7):1215–1223.
282. Tanner RW, Cofield RH. Prosthetic arthroplasty for fracture and fracture-dislocation of the proximal humerus. *Clin Orthop* 1983;179:116.
283. Boileau P, Tinsi P, Le Huec J, et al. Results of shoulder arthroplasty in acute fractures of the proximal humerus. In Walch G, Boileau P, eds. *Shoulder arthroplasty*. Berlin/Heidelberg/New York: Springer, 1999.
284. Frankle MA, Mighell MA. Techniques and principles of tuberosity fixation for proximal humeral fractures treated with hemiarthroplasty. *J Shoulder Elbow Surg*. 2004;13:239.
285. Norris TR, Green A, McGuigan FX. Late prosthetic shoulder arthroplasty for displaced proximal humerus fractures. *J Shoulder Elbow Surg* 1995;4(4):271.
286. Hammon JW, Queale WS, Kim TK, et al. Surgeon experience and clinical and economic outcomes of shoulder arthroplasty. *J Bone Joint Surg Am* 2003;12:164.
287. Hasan SS, Leith JM, Smith KL, et al. The distribution of shoulder replacement among surgeons and hospitals is significantly different than that of hip or knee replacement. *J Shoulder Elbow Surg* 2003;12:164.
288. Parsons IM, Millett PJ, Warner JJP. Glenoid erosion after hemiarthroplasty. *Clin Orthop* 2004;421:120.
289. Cotton FJ. Subluxation of the shoulder downward. *Boston Med Surg J* 1921;185: 405–407.
290. Fairbank TJ. Fracture-subluxations of the shoulder. *J Bone Joint Surg Br* 1948;30: 454–460.
291. Thompson FR, Winant EM. Comminuted fracture of the humeral head with subluxation. *Clin Orthop* 1961;20:94–96.
292. Thompson FR, Winant EM. Unusual fracture subluxations of the shoulder joint. *J Bone Joint Surg Am* 1950;32:575–582.
293. de Laat EA, Visser CP, Coene LN, et al. Nerve lesions in primary shoulder dislocations and humeral neck fractures: a prospective clinical and EMG study. *J Bone Joint Surg Br* 1994;76:381–383.
294. Hayes JM, Van Winkle GN. Axillary artery injury with minimally displaced fracture of the neck of the humerus. *J Trauma* 1983;23:431–433.
295. Henson GF. Vascular complications of shoulder injuries: a report of two cases. *J Bone Joint Surg Br* 1956;38:528–531.
296. Laverick MD, D'Sa AA, Kirk SJ, et al. Management of blunt injuries of the axillary artery and the neck of the humerus: case report. *J Trauma* 1990;30:360–361.
297. Lim EVA, Day LJ. Thrombosis of the axillary artery complicating proximal humeral fractures. *J Bone Joint Surg Am* 1987;69:778–780.
298. Linson MA. Axillary artery thrombosis after fracture of the humerus: a case report. *J Bone Joint Surg Am* 1980;62:1214–1215.
299. Sathyarup D, Huilgol AK, Iyer KM. Axillary artery thrombosis following a fracture of the neck of the humerus. *Injury* 1988;19:45–47.
300. Zuckerman JD, Flugstad DL, Teitz CC, et al. Axillary artery injury as a complication of proximal humeral fractures: two case reports and a review of the literature. *Clin Orthop* 1984;189:234–237.
301. Boileau P, Walch G. The three-dimensional geometry of the proximal humerus. *J Bone Joint Surg Br* 1997;79:857–865.
302. Mansat P, Guity MR, Bellumore Y, et al. Shoulder arthroplasty for late sequelae of proximal humeral fractures. *J Shoulder Elbow Surg* 2004;13(3):305–312.
303. Rodosky MW, Duralde XA, Connor PM, et al. Operative treatment of malunions of proximal humerus fractures. *Orthop Trans* 1997;21:624–625.
304. Solonen KA, Vastamaki M. Osteotomy of the neck of the humerus for traumatic varus deformity. *Acta Orthop Scand* 1985;56:79–80.
305. Dines DM, Warren RF, Altchek DW, et al. Posttraumatic changes of the proximal humerus: malunion, nonunion, osteonecrosis: treatment with modular hemiarthroplasty or total shoulder arthroplasty. *J Shoulder Elbow Surg* 1993;2:11–21.
306. Checchia SL, Doneux P, Miyazaki AN, et al. Classification of non-unions of the proximal humerus. *Int Orthop* 2000;24(4):217–220.
307. Rooney PJ, Cockshott WP. Pseudarthrosis following proximal humerus fractures: a possible mechanism. *Skeletal Radiol* 1986;15:21–24.
308. Duralde XA, Flatow EL, Pollock RG, et al. Operative treatment of nonunions of the surgical neck of the humerus. *J Shoulder Elbow Surg* 1996;5:169–180.

309. Simpson NS, Jupiter JB. Reconstruction of nonunion of the proximal humerus with a custom blade plate. *Orthop Trans* 1996;20:11–12.
310. Walch G, Badet R, Nove-Josserand L, et al. Nonunions of the surgical neck of the humerus: surgical treatment with an intramedullary bone peg, internal fixation, cancellous bone grafting. *J Shoulder Elbow Surg* 1996;5:161–168.
311. Lee CK, Hansen HR, DeGiorgi G, et al. Post-traumatic avascular necrosis of the humeral head in displaced proximal humeral fractures: malformations of the shoulder girdle. *J Trauma* 1981;21:788–791.
312. Bohler J. Les fractures récentes de l'épaule. *Acta Orthop Belg* 1964;30:235–242.
313. Hagg O, Lundberg B. *Aspects of prognostic factors in comminuted and dislocated proximal humeral fractures*. Philadelphia: BC Decker, 1984.
314. Schai P, Imhoff A, Preiss S. Comminuted humeral head fractures: a multicenter analysis. *J Shoulder Elbow Surg* 1995;4:319–330.
315. Sturzenegger M, Fornaro E, Jakob RP. Results of surgical treatment of multifragmented fractures of the humeral head. *Arch Orthop Trauma Surg* 1982;100:249–259.
316. Fourrier P, Martini M. Post-traumatic avascular necrosis of the humeral head. *Int Orthop* 1977;1:187–190.
317. Kofoed H. Revascularization of the humeral head: a report of two cases of fracture-dislocation of the shoulder. *Clin Orthop* 1983;179:175–178.
318. Lim TE, Ochsner PE, Marti RK, et al. The results of treatment of comminuted fractures and fracture dislocations of the proximal humerus. *Neth J Surg* 1983;35:139–143.
319. Rechtman AM. Open reduction of fracture dislocation of the humerus. *JAMA* 1930; 94:1656–1657.
320. Mohan V, Mont MA, Pierre-Jacques H, et al. Osteonecrosis of the humeral head treated by core decompression. *Orthop Trans* 1997;21:279.
321. Mont MA, Maar DC, Urquhart MW, et al. Avascular necrosis of the humeral head treated by core decompression: a retrospective review. *J Bone Joint Surg Br* 1993;75: 785–788.
322. Sperling JW, Kozak TK, Hanssen AD, et al. Infection after shoulder arthroplasty. *Clin Orthop Rel Res* 2001;382:206–216.

FRACTURES OF THE CLAVICLE

Mark D. Lazarus and Carl Seon

Let us imagine a game of word association. The initial phrase is "clavicle fracture." Close your eyes and picture your response. Likely, free association will bring images of simple injuries, simple treatments, and favorable outcomes. Yet, there is still a great degree of controversy to the management of these injuries.

From the earliest recorded mention of clavicle fractures, the treatment has been considered supportive, the results considered excellent. Hippocrates wrote that the patient with a fractured clavicle could be treated with observation and that the treating physician would not be "sorry at the neglect of the patients," for, although deformity was universal, healing and return to normal function were equally expected (1). Although various types of immobilization and treatment were later advocated, most subsequent writings similarly discussed the excellent rate of healing and recovery that was expected after clavicular fracture.

As anyone who has treated this injury is aware, discussion of universal healing rates after clavicular fracture is overly optimistic. Recently, investigators have discovered that union after midshaft clavicle fracture is not as universal as once thought. Moreover, certain types of clavicular fractures have declared themselves to be problematic. Finally, there has been newfound interest in the treatment of problem fractures and nonunions.

SURGICAL/APPLIED ANATOMY

Osteology

As viewed in the coronal plane, the clavicle is a slender bone, wider medially at its sternal articulation and noticeably thinner at its lateral third. Viewed axially, however, the three-dimensional structure becomes more apparent. The clavicle assumes a gentle s-shape, the medial end convex forward and the lateral end concave forward. This shape has been likened to the musical symbol the clavicula, thus the name (2). In the axial projection, the clavicle is also noted to have both medial and lateral flat expanses, linked by a thin, tubular middle. This central transitional area represents a weak link in clavicular structure. The midclavicle, therefore, is the most common site of fracture (3). Finally, when viewed in the sagittal plane, the extent of anterior to posterior transition is clearly identified.

Medial Ligamentous Anatomy

The bulbous medial clavicular end serves as the lateral contribution to the sternoclavicular joint. There are several layers of ligamentous support to this articulation, some extremely important to fracture anatomy and displacement (Fig. 32-1).

Capsular Ligaments

Specific thickenings of the sternoclavicular joint capsule are referred to as the capsular ligaments. These thickenings are the anterosuperior and posterior aspects of the capsule. These ligaments may be the strongest of the sternoclavicular articulation and are responsible for limiting superior displacement of the medial clavicular or, through the clavicular moment arm, inferior displacement of the lateral end of an intact clavicle (4).

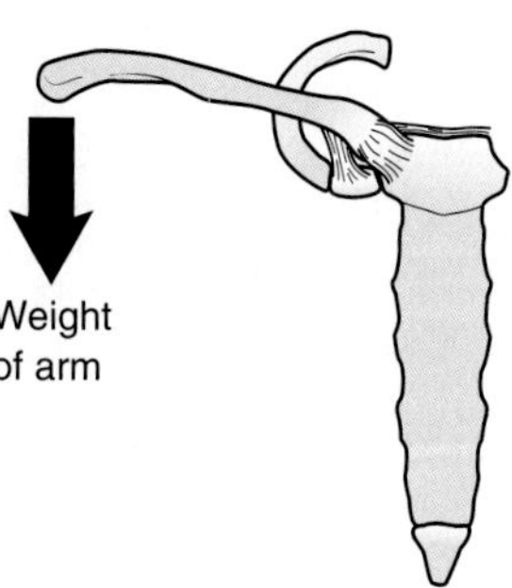

FIGURE 32-1 Strong sternoclavicular ligaments serve to hold the clavicle in appropriate position, countering muscular forces and the weight of the arm.

The posterior capsule has recently been determined to be the most important structure in resisting both anterior and posterior translation at the sternoclavicular joint (5).

Interclavicular Ligament

This strong ligamentous band spans from the medial clavicle to the superior sternum to the contralateral clavicle. The ligament loosens with shoulder elevation but serves as a support to prevent downward displacement of the lateral end of the clavicle.

Costoclavicular Ligament

These strong ligaments run from the upper aspect of the first rib and adjacent aspects of the sternum to the inferior clavicle. Occasionally, a depression exists in the medial clavicle that serves as a ligamentous attachment site, the rhomboid fossa (6). For the purposes of studying clavicular fracture anatomy, the anterior and posterior fibers of the costoclavicular ligament stabilize the medial clavicle against both upward and downward rotation, respectively (4).

Lateral Ligamentous Anatomy

Coracoclavicular Ligaments

The trapezoid and conoid are thick, strong ligaments traveling from the base of the coracoid process of the scapula to the inferior aspect of the lateral clavicle. The more lateral trapezoid attaches on a specific osseous ridge, whereas the more medial conoid inserts at the conoid tubercle. These ligaments serve the important function of suspension of the shoulder girdle from the clavicle.

Acromioclavicular Ligaments

The capsule of the acromioclavicular joint forms the acromioclavicular ligaments. Superiorly, and more specifically posterosuperiorly, the ligament serves to resist anteroposterior (AP) displacement of the distal clavicle (7). A recent biomechanical study confirmed that the acromioclavicular capsule mainly resists anterior-posterior translation (8). Furthermore, differential loading occurred in the coracoclavicular ligaments when the acromioclavicular ligaments were disrupted. The conoid served to resist anterior and superior loading, whereas the trapezoid predominantly resisted posterior loading.

Muscular Anatomy

Several important muscles originate or insert on the clavicle. Medially, the clavicle serves as origin of the pectoralis major and sternohyoid muscles. Of great importance from a fracture standpoint, the superomedial clavicle serves as an origin of the sternocleidomastoid. In a midshaft clavicle fracture, this origin is converted to an insertion, the sternocleidomastoid becoming a medial clavicle elevator. The undersurface of the middle clavicle serves as an insertion point for the subclavius muscle. Laterally, the anterior clavicle is the site of origin for the anterior deltoid with the posterosuperior clavicle serving as an accessory insertion for the trapezius.

The other important muscle related to clavicular anatomy is the platysma. Located in the subcutaneous tissue superficial to the cervical fascia, the platysma originates over the deltoid and pectoralis major and crosses the superficial anterior surface of the clavicle before inserting on the mandible and skin and muscles of the mouth. Because of its location, division of the platysma is necessary for surgical approach to the midclavicle.

Neurovascular Anatomy

From a surgical standpoint, the important neurovascular relationships to the clavicle can be divided into anterior and posterior. Anteriorly, the main structures are the supraclavicular nerves. Branches of the cervical plexus, these nerves originate as a common trunk at the level of the posterior border of the sternocleidomastoid. This trunk then divides into anterior, middle, and posterior nerves that cross the superficial surface of the clavicle deep to the platysma. Jupiter and Ring have recommended locating and preserving these nerves during surgical approach to the midclavicle (9).

More important than its own neurovascular anatomy is the clavicle's relational neurovascular anatomy. The clavicle has an important function as an osseous protector of the brachial plexus and jugular and subclavian vessels. Specifically, the superior surface of the middle third of the clavicle forms the inferior border of the posterior triangle of the neck. The important contents of that triangle include the brachial plexus and subclavian artery. The fracture and surgical implications of the proximity of these structures are clear.

BIOMECHANICS

The functional role of the clavicle has long been debated. There are several facts that would support the concept of minimal function. Children with cleidocranial dysostosis (congenital absence of the clavicle) often function well. Patients with nonunion of a clavicle fracture often have minimal to no symptoms (10,11). Moreover, surgical excision of the clavicle can result in a fairly good functional result (12–14). In fact, older vascular surgical references recommended excisional clavicular osteotomy as an approach to the subclavian vessels (15). Because some patients were noted to function well even after complete claviculectomy, Gurd stated that "apart from its function in serving for the attachment of muscles, this bone serves no useful purpose" (16). Yet, there are some important biomechanical functions of the clavicle, particularly in reference to fractures.

Normal Clavicular Functions

Strut Function

Like the strut of an awning, the clavicle is responsible for bracing the shoulder girdle and propping it away from the sternum and thoracic cage (Fig. 32-2). Having this strut allows the shoulder to reach into cross-body and internal rotation positions without medial collapse. Similar to the way that wrist extension permits optimal muscle-tendon unit length for power grip, the strut or prop function of the clavicle allows the thoracohumeral muscles to maintain their optimal working distance. Therefore, the clavicle increases the strength of shoulder girdle movements (17). Finally, this strut function affords cosmesis and posture to the shoulder girdle. In a displaced midshaft fracture, the strut function of the clavicle is lost and clavicular shortening may result.

Suspensory Function

The shoulder girdle is stabilized against inferior displacement by two mechanisms, one dynamic and one static. Posteriorly, the trapezius acts as a dynamic scapular elevator. Anteriorly, the shoulder girdle hangs from the clavicle by the coracoclavicular ligaments, similar to a sign hanging from a signpost. The sturdy sternoclavicular ligaments allow the clavicle to remain in position to withstand this downward load (Fig. 32-3).

As with the strut function, loss of suspensory function in a fracture model has important displacement implications. The sternoclavicular ligaments and sternocleidomastoid muscle hold the medial clavicular segment in an elevated position. The lateral segment can be expected to succumb to the weight of the arm

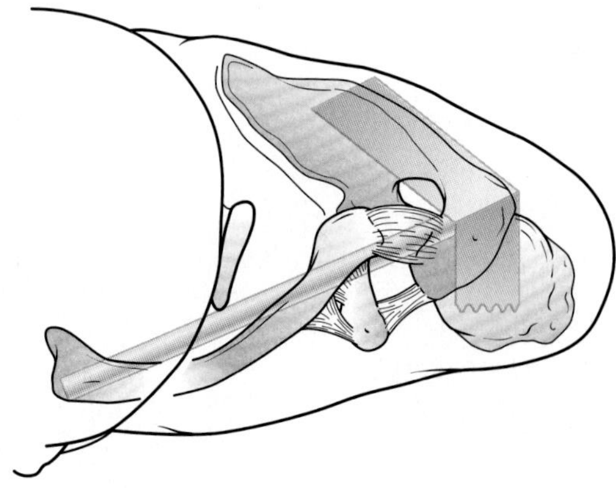

FIGURE 32-2 Strut function of the clavicle.

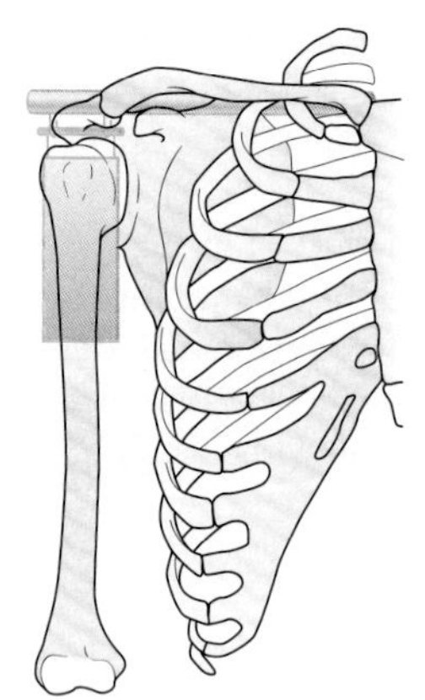

FIGURE 32-3 Suspension function of the clavicle.

and be displaced inferiorly through the pull of the coracoclavicular ligaments. Thus, fracture displacement will follow.

Fracture Biomechanics

Just as the articulations and muscular attachments support the normal functions of the clavicle, these same structures may serve as displacing forces in a fracture. For a midshaft fracture, the displacing forces are as follows (Fig. 32-4):

1. stabilizing on the medial segment by the sternoclavicular ligaments
2. superior on the medial segment through the sternocleidomastoid
3. inferior and medial on the lateral segment through the pectoralis major
4. inferior on the lateral segment through the weight of the arm pulling through the coracoclavicular ligaments

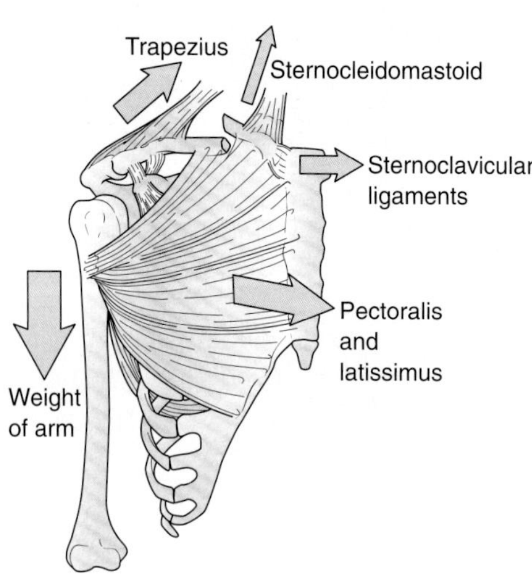

FIGURE 32-4 Displacing forces on a midshaft clavicle fracture.

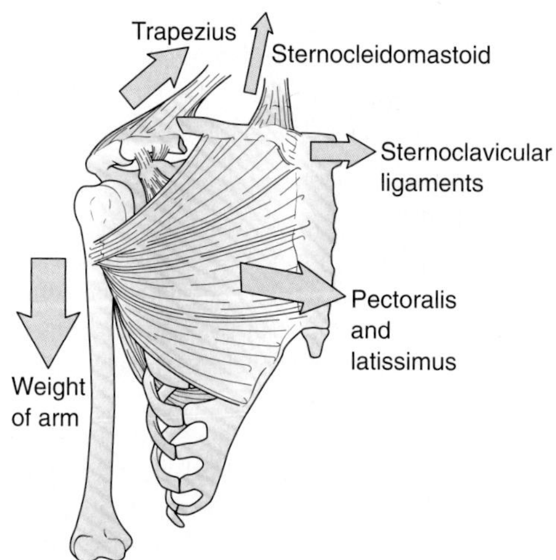

FIGURE 32-5 Displacing forces on a lateral clavicle fracture.

The trapezius provides a stabilizing force against inferior displacement of the lateral segment.

For more lateral fractures, the displacing forces are as follows (Fig. 32-5):

1. superior on the medial segment through the sternocleidomastoid and trapezius
2. medial on the distal segment through the pull of the pectoralis major, pectoralis minor, and latissimus dorsi
3. inferior on the distal segment through the weight of the arm

Because the trapezius is the main stabilizer of midshaft fractures, reasonable function after total claviculectomy or clavicular nonunion is likely because of the enhanced trapezius function (14). In patients without intact trapezius function, such as those who have injury to the spinal accessory nerve, loss of clavicular stability with a fracture is extremely disabling. Although an uncommon scenario, given the combination of radical neck dissection plus postoperative irradiation as a treatment for head and neck carcinomas, the risk of pathologic clavicular fracture in a patient with spinal accessory palsy is present (18). In this scenario, loss of clavicular function can result in inferior and medial collapse of the shoulder girdle secondary to loss of normal strut and suspensory function (Fig. 32-6).

MECHANISM OF INJURY

Indirect Trauma

In his initial description of clavicle fracture classification, Allman described the mechanism of injury as either a fall onto an outstretched hand or a fall onto the point of the shoulder (19). More recent data, however, indicate direct trauma as the predominant cause of clavicle fractures. Stanley et al (20) questioned 122 patients who had a clavicle fracture and asked them to group their mechanism of injury as a fall onto an outstretched

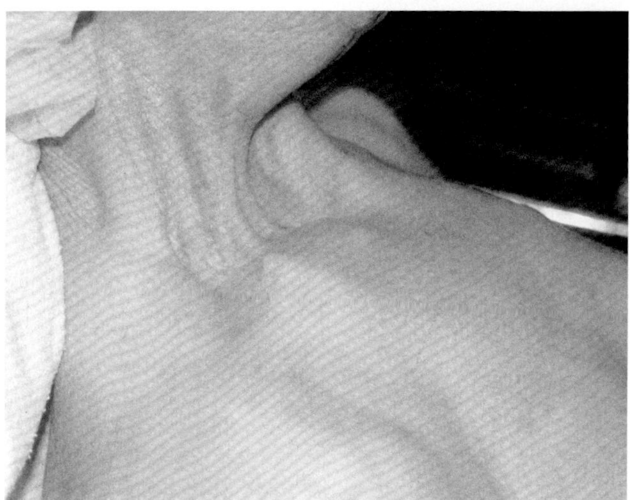

FIGURE 32-6 This patient had a pathologic medial clavicle fracture and loss of trapezius function. The result was loss of clavicular strut function and medial collapse of the shoulder girdle.

hand, fall onto the shoulder, direct blow to the shoulder, or other. In 87% of patients, the described mechanism was a fall onto the shoulder. Seven percent of patients described a direct blow to the shoulder with only 6% describing a fall onto an outstretched hand. There was no correlation between fracture location and mechanism of injury. These data confirm the postulates of other authors that direct trauma is the main mode of clavicular failure (21,22).

The primary mechanism of clavicular failure is compression (20–22,). For most injury types, this requires a fall or blow directly to the lateral aspect of the shoulder. Unless the arm is significantly outstretched relative to the shoulder, a fall on an outstretched hand will result in tension and not compression loading of the clavicle (Fig. 32-7).

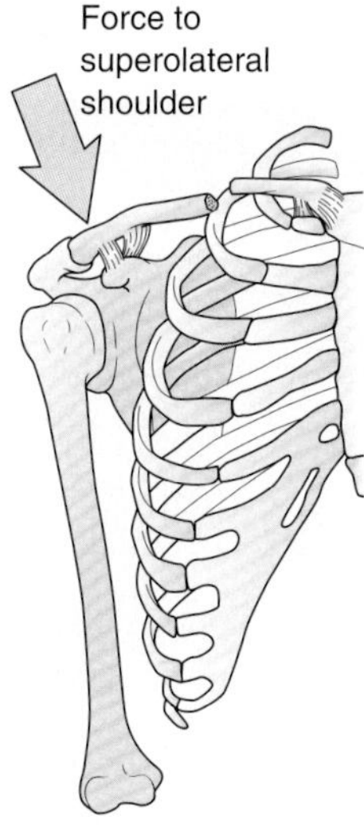

FIGURE 32-7 The most common mechanism of clavicle fracture is a fall on the superolateral shoulder. Because the sternoclavicular ligaments are extremely strong, the force exits the clavicle in the midshaft.

Direct Trauma

Given the subcutaneous position of the clavicle, there is an inherent susceptibility to direct injury, similar to a tibia or ulna. This mechanism can occur with either blunt or penetrating trauma. Because direct trauma is independent of muscular forces or arm position, all regions of the clavicle are vulnerable (Fig. 32-8A,B).

Sporting activities that may result in direct trauma to the clavicle include bicycling and skiing. A recent Swedish study cites that bicycling accidents were the most common cause of clavicle fractures in both sexes. The authors confirmed that clavicle fractures resulting from a fall on an outstretched hand was uncommon (23).

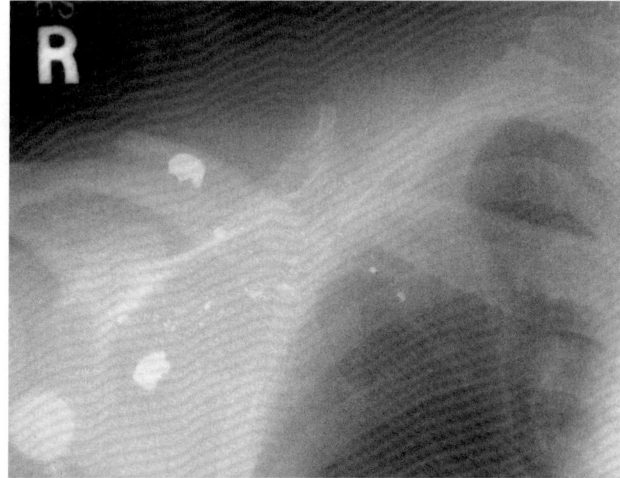

A

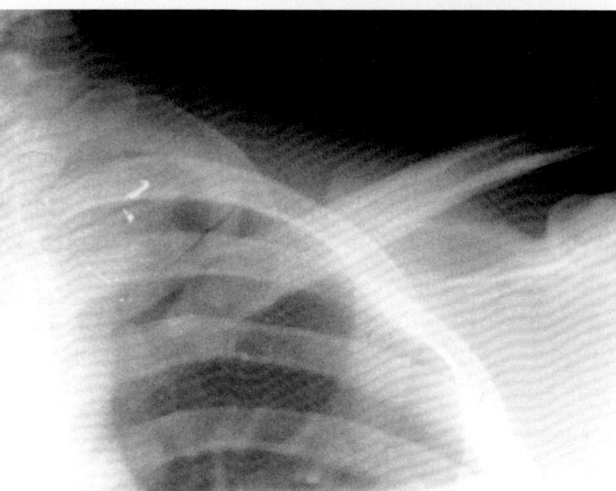

B

FIGURE 32-8 A,B. Fracture from direct trauma, as in gunshot wounds, can occur anywhere along the clavicular length.

A group of Japanese physicians recently examined 3103 upper extremity fractures or dislocations in snowboarders and skiers (24). The clavicle was the most frequently fractured bone in skiers (32% of all fractures) in contrast with the wrist in snowboarders (62% of all fractures). The difference was attributed to snowboarders having a tendency to fall in the anterior-posterior direction. This allowed the outstretched arms to have more of a chance to absorb the impact of the fall. This supports the notion that most clavicle fractures are the result of a direct trauma rather than a fall onto an outstretched upper extremity.

Pathologic

The clavicle is vulnerable to pathologic fracture from several causes. Although uncommon, the clavicle can be a site of primary or metastatic neoplasm (Fig. 32-9A) (25). More commonly, given the use of adjunctive radiation treatment for carcinomas of the neck and breast, clavicular weakening from post-irradiation osteitis can occur (Fig. 32-9B) (18). Stress fractures of the clavicle have been reported after radical neck dissection for carcinoma (26–29). This may be secondary to an imbalance of stabilizing forces on the clavicle as the sternocleidomastoid muscle is resected.

Stress

Although stress fractures of the clavicle are considered a rarity without medical history, case reports continue to appear (30,31). Recent case reports of a stress fracture involving a young female lightweight rower and middle-aged male cablemaker highlight the importance of taking a detailed history (32,33). Both were involved in repetitive upper extremity activity, and both stress fractures involved the medial third near the sternoclavicular joint. This is consistent with previous case reports that the majority of athletic-related stress fractures occur in the medial third (34,35).

CLASSIFICATION

There are several classification schemes for fractures of the clavicle, ranging from the simple to complex. Although somewhat helpful for description, the benefit of each system in determining a treatment choice or outcome potential is limited.

Possibly the most commonly used system is that of Allman (19). He separated clavicle fractures into three groups:

Group I: middle third fractures

Group II: lateral third fractures

Group III: medial third fractures

Although helpful in terms of localizing the injury, the system does not describe displacement, comminution, or shortening, all potentially important prognostic and treatment variables.

Neer recognized the unique behavior of distal clavicle fractures and proposed a separate classification system for this group (36,37). He recommended dividing Allman's Group II into three distinct types:

Type I: coracoclavicular ligaments intact (Fig. 32-10A)

Type II: coracoclavicular ligaments detached from the medial segment but trapezoid intact to distal segment (Fig. 32-10B)

Type III: intra-articular extension into the acromioclavicular joint

Later, Rockwood created two distinct subsets of Neer's Type II fracture of the distal clavicle, Type IIA, in which both the conoid and trapezoid remain attached to the distal segment, and Type IIB, in which the medial segment is unstable with the conoid torn (38).

Craig advanced a classification scheme that combines the Allman and Neer classes while also providing more detail (Table 32-1) (39). The system gives more descriptive and functional information than the Allman scheme and has the advantage of

A

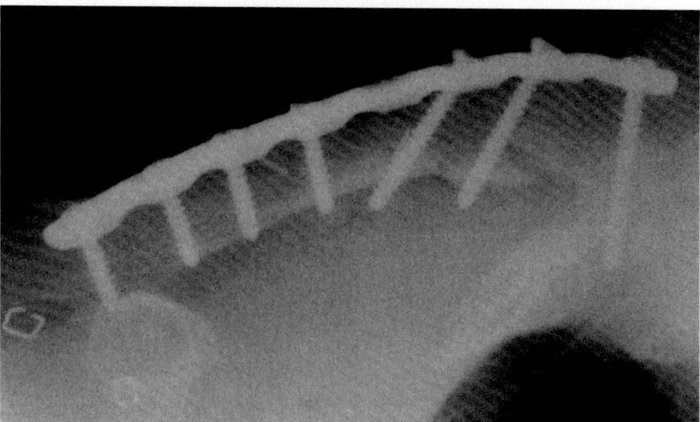

B

FIGURE 32-9 **A.** Pathologic midshaft clavicle fracture secondary to metastatic prostatic carcinoma. **B.** Pathologic medial clavicle fracture resulting from post-irradiation osteonecrosis. This fracture required operative fixation.

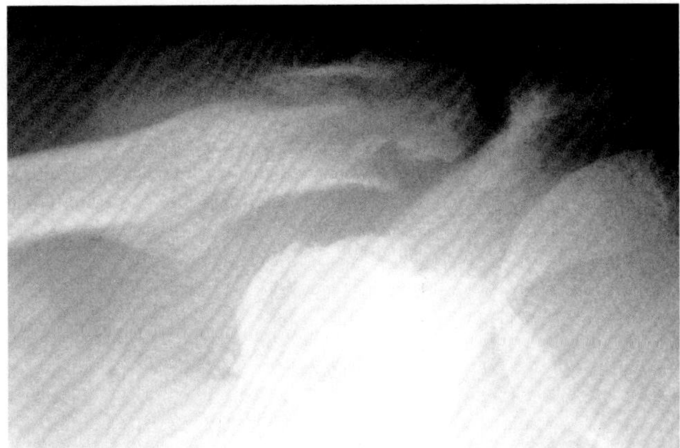
A

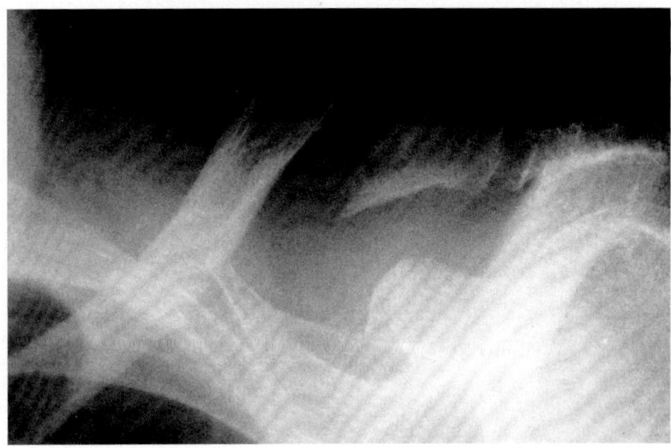
B

FIGURE 32-10 **A.** Type I distal clavicle fracture. **B.** Type II distal clavicle fracture.

including more unusual injuries, such as epiphyseal separations and periosteal sleeve fractures. Although more descriptive and filled with important treatment applications, this system still leaves the majority of fractures, those of the middle third, without any subclassification.

Nordqvist and Petersson (40) studied the incidence of clavicle fractures in 2035 cases occurring in the population of Malmo, Sweden. This impressive undertaking included all clavicular fractures seen over a 10-year period. The authors also proposed a simple classification tightly based on the Allman grading system (40). In this scheme, Allman Types I to III are maintained. Each type is then given a subtype of displaced or nondisplaced. Finally, for the important Type I group (middle), a final subgroup of comminution is given. This system has the advantage of providing more description to the important midshaft fracture group.

Robinson analyzed 1000 consecutive clavicle fractures seen at the Orthopaedic Trauma Unit of the Royal Infirmary of Edinburgh over a 6-year period (41). Because of the lack of a single system that would have prognostic and therapeutic value, he proposed his own classification (Table 32-2 and Fig. 32-11). This system has several advantages:

1. It continues the traditionally accepted practice of analyzing the clavicle in thirds.

TABLE 32-1 Craig Classification of Clavicular Fractures

Group I—fracture of the middle third

Group II—fracture of the distal third
- Type I—minimal displacement (interligamentous)
- Type II—displaced secondary to fracture line medial to the coracoclavicular ligaments
  - (A) conoid and trapezoid attached
  - (B) conoid torn, trapezoid attached
- Type III—fractures of the articular surface
- Type IV—periosteal sleeve fracture (children)
- Type V—comminuted with ligaments attached neither proximally nor distally, but to an inferior comminuted fragment

Group III—fractures of the proximal third
- Type I—minimal displacement
- Type II—displaced (ligaments ruptured)
- Type III—intraarticular
- Type IV—epiphyseal separation (children and young adults)
- Type V—comminuted

TABLE 32-2 Robinson Classification of Clavicular Fractures

Type 1—medial
- A—nondisplaced
  - A1—extraarticular
  - A2—intraarticular
- B—displaced
  - B1—extraarticular
  - B2—intraarticular

Type 2—middle
- A—cortical alignment
  - A1—nondisplaced
  - A2—angulated
- B—displaced
  - B1—simple or single butterfly fragment
  - B2—comminuted or segmental

Type 3—distal
- A—nondisplaced
  - A1—extraarticular
  - A2—intraarticular
- B—displaced
  - B1—extraarticular
  - B2—intraarticular

Robinson Cortical Alignment Fracture (Type 2A)

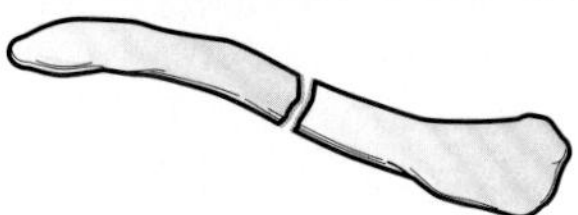

Undisplaced (Type 2A1)

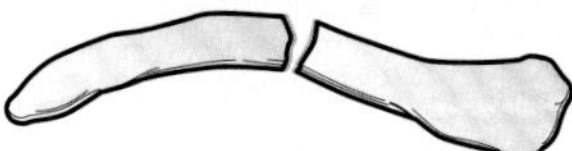

Angulated (Type 2A2)

Robinson Displaced Fractures (Type 2B)

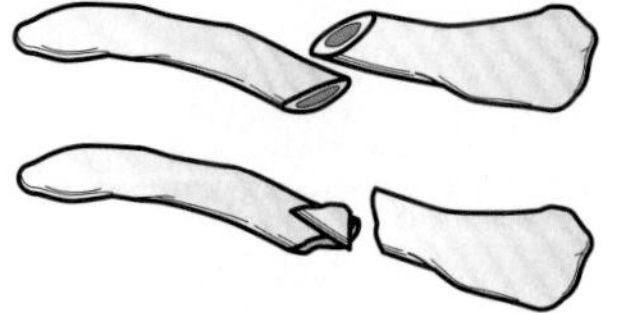

Simple or single butterfly (Type 2B1)

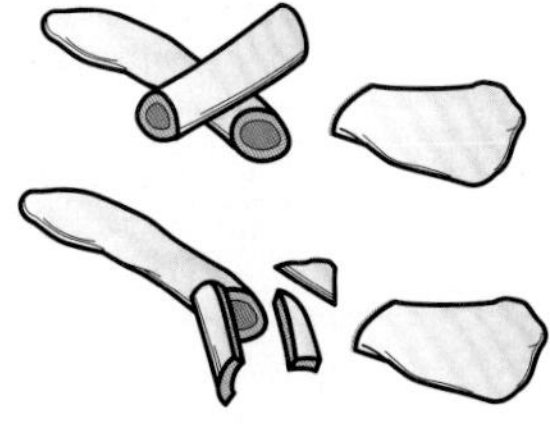

Segmental or comminuted (Type 2B2)

Allman Group I
Craig Group I

Robinson Cortical Alignment Fracture (Type 3A)

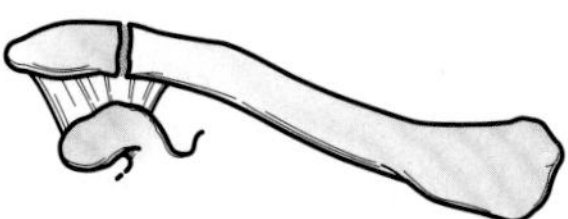

Extra-articular (Type 3A1)
Neer Type I
Craig Type I

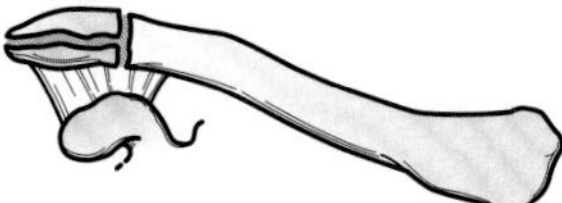

Intra-articular (Type 3A2)
Neer Type III
Craig Type III

Robinson Displaced Fractures (Type 3B)

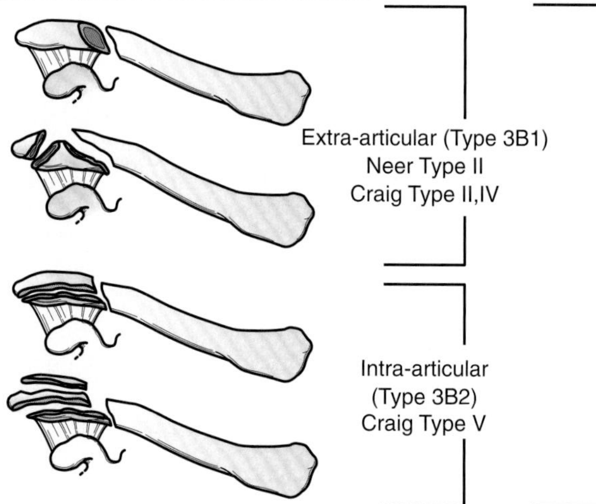

Robinson Undisplaced Fractures (Type 1A)

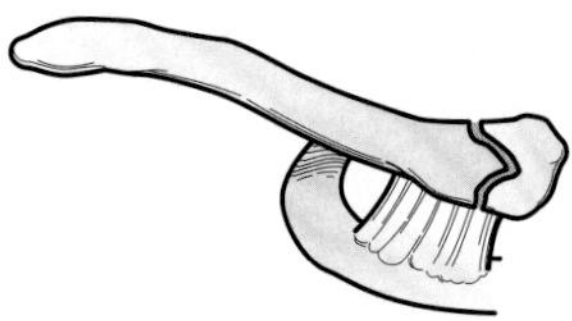

Extra-articular (Type 1A1)
Craig Type I

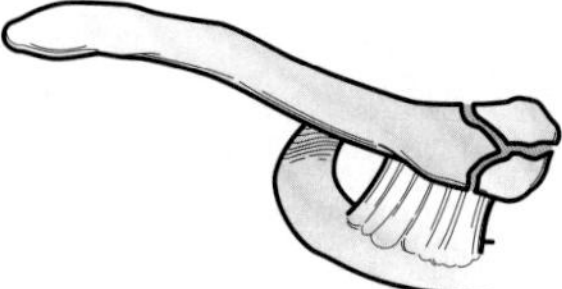

Intra-articular (Type 1A2)
Craig Type III

Robinson Displaced Fractures (Type 1B)

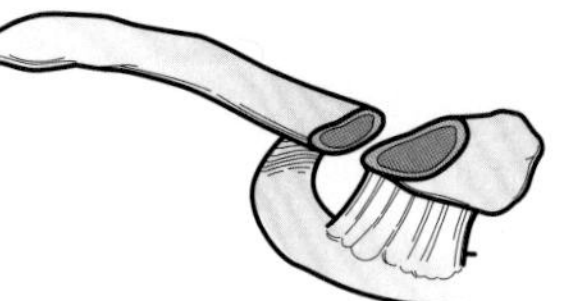

Extra-articular (Type 1B1)
Craig Type II

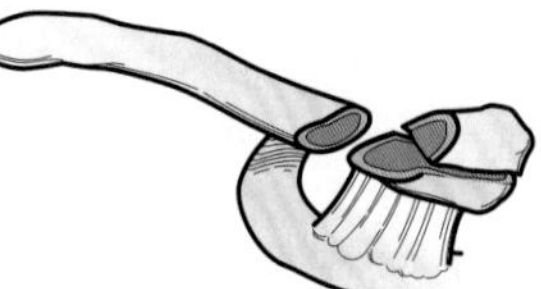

Extra-articular (Type 1B2)
Craig Type V

Allman Group III
Craig Group III

FIGURE 32-11 Clavicle fracture classification.

2. It includes prognostically important variables such as intra-articular extent, degree of displacement, and degree of comminution.
3. It is based on a simple to recall number scheme.

As with all systems, it also has its disadvantages. As has been discussed by Jupiter and Ring, division of the clavicle into thirds is somewhat arbitrary and is based more on convenience than true fracture distribution (9). Also, the unusual fracture types included by Craig (39,42) are not specifically mentioned here, although they would be included in the classification based on their location. Finally, and probably most important, the number scheme does not correspond to that used by Allman, Craig, and Neer (19,36,37,39,42). Because the term "Type II fracture" has become synonymous with distal clavicle fracture, the numbering system proposed by Robinson not only confuses our fracture "language" but would render many prior studies difficult to comprehend.

The incidence of each fracture type is somewhat unclear because there are few well-controlled epidemiologic studies and each study seems to rely on a different classification scheme. Some generalizations, however, can be made. Midshaft clavicular fractures are clearly the most common, with an incidence of 69.2% in Robinson's work and 76.2% in the study by Nordqvist and Petersson (40,41). Although the definitions of displacement differed between the studies, 47.5% of the midshaft fractures in the Malmo, Sweden review, and 72.7% of those seen by Robinson were felt to be displaced (40,41). This discrepancy may reflect differences in the classification systems. Alternatively, there may be differences in the patient populations seen at the two centers. Finally, the increased incidence seen by Robinson may be secondary to his review of a more contemporary patient population. Regardless, the most important conclusions are that midshaft clavicular fractures occur commonly and are often displaced and/or comminuted.

Other important data can be gleaned from these studies. Distal fractures were seen between 21% and 28% of the time, with an approximate nondisplaced rate of 3:1 (40,41). Medial fractures were extremely rare. Both studies found these injuries in less than 3% of the study population, the bulk of which were nondisplaced.

DIAGNOSIS

History

Most patients with a clavicle fracture, particularly young adults, will give a history of a fall directly onto the shoulder. The majority will give a history of injury of a simple fall, fall from a height, fall during sporting activity, or a motor vehicle accident (41). In the adult population, the incidence of clavicular fracture decreases from age 20 to 50 years, increasing again for age more than 70 years (41). For the older age groups, lower energy injuries become more common (19,20,37,43,44). Fracture is more common in men than women up to approximately age 50 years, at which point the incidence between the two genders approximately equilibrates (40,41).

Examination

Given its subcutaneous position, fractures of the clavicle are easily diagnosed by examination. Initial observation often reveals the diagnosis. Abrasions marking the site of application of the traumatic force are present in approximately 10% of patients (20). Ecchymosis and deformity are usually apparent. Open fractures of the clavicle are extremely rare (45,46,47), but skin tenting is common and should be identified (Fig. 32-12).

Examination for associated injuries is a must, particularly in the setting of a high-velocity injury. Associated fracture of the ipsilateral scapula and upper ribs can occur and, in the high-energy setting, a chest radiograph is mandatory (Fig. 32-13A,B) (48–54). The prevalence of pneumothorax in association with a clavicle fracture is 3% (44). This incidence, however, depends on the rate of low versus high velocity trauma seen by each individual physician. The finding of ipsilateral rib or scapula fracture on a screening supine chest film mandates an upright chest radiograph to evaluate for pneumothorax.

A case report of a not-so-subtle pulmonary injury associated with a clavicle injury secondary to a motorcycle accident was recently published (55). A traumatic extrathoracic lung herniation through a large anteroapical chest wall defect created by multiple rib fractures and a fracture dislocation of the clavicle. The medial third was apparently missing and left at the scene. High-velocity injuries can create a myriad of associated and likely more serious injuries than the clavicle fracture.

Injury to the brachial plexus in conjunction with a clavicle fracture has also been reported. Although a displaced fracture fragment can result in neurologic insult (56), more typically plexus injuries are secondary to traction (57,58) and may occur in the setting of scapulothoracic dissociation. In the awake pa-

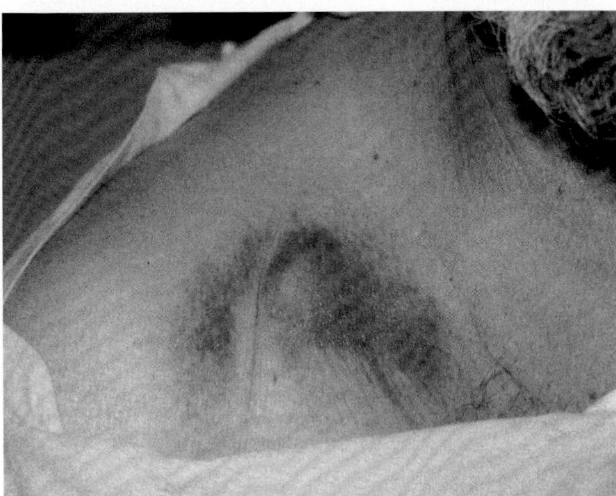

FIGURE 32-12 Skin ecchymosis and tenting are common in displaced midclavicle fractures and may alter treatment.

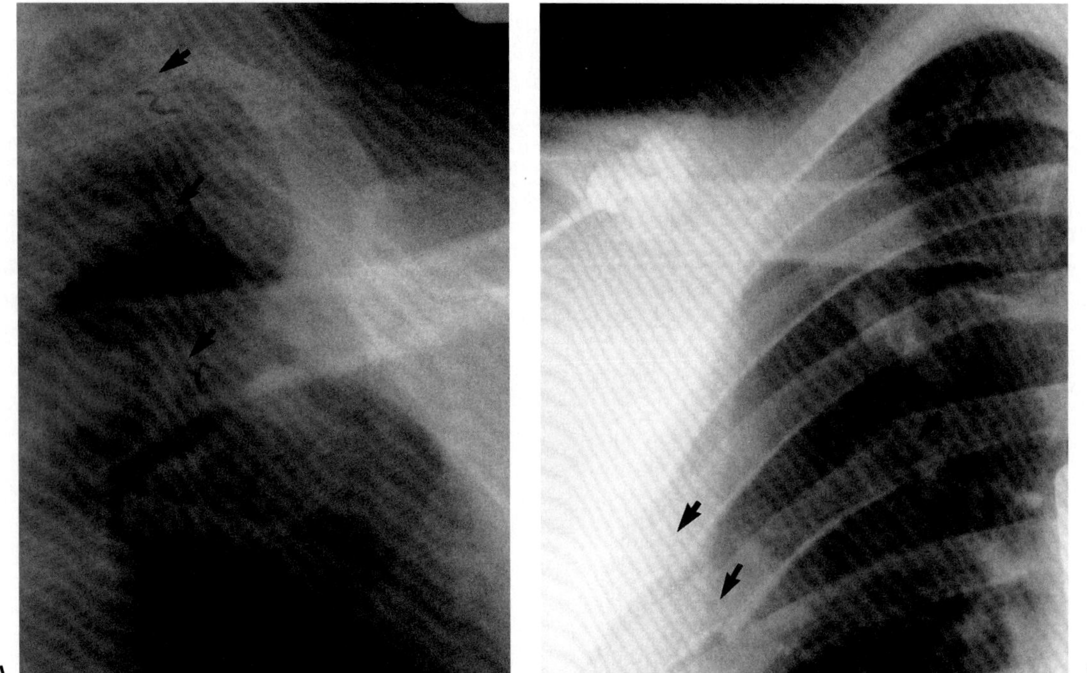

FIGURE 32-13 Rib fractures can occur in conjunction with a clavicle fracture secondary to high-energy injury. Fractures most commonly involve the upper ribs **(A)** but can be seen lower **(B)**. These findings necessitate an upright chest radiograph to identify a pneumothorax.

tient, the diagnosis is made by neurologic examination. Radiographic hints in the comatose or uncooperative patient are associated displaced scapula fracture or a wide separation of the clavicle fracture ends (Fig. 32-14), typically greater than 1 cm (51).

Vascular injuries associated with clavicle fracture, although rare, have also been reported (59–66). These lesions may be life or limb threatening. Costa and Robbs treated 167 patients with subclavian artery injury (59). All lesions involving the third part of the subclavian artery were accompanied by fractures of the clavicle. Natali and colleagues treated 10 cases, all associated with clavicle fracture, by excision of the clavicle and subclavian artery repair (64). More often, vascular injury is an intimal tear, and initial clinical findings may be minimal. In these cases, the diagnosis is usually made after late arterial thrombosis (67,68). However, even a seemingly innocuous event such as a fall during roller-blading has been reported to cause a fatal subclavian artery transection associated with a clavicle fracture (66). If initial vascular examination leaves doubt, comparison of blood pressure in the ipsilateral and contralateral extremity is necessary. If uncertainty still exists, angiography is required.

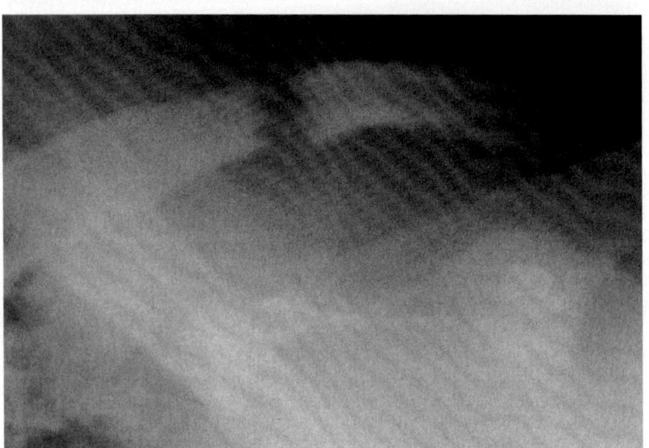

FIGURE 32-14 Clavicular diastasis, specifically greater than 1 cm, hints at the possibility of scapulothoracic dissociation and/or brachial plexus traction injury.

Radiographic Studies

The diagnosis of clavicle fracture is typically made on a single AP radiograph. In the trauma situation, the surgeon may be given a supine AP chest radiograph as the only diagnostic study. To better visualize the fracture pattern and displacement, an apical oblique radiograph is helpful (Fig. 32-15A,B) (44,69,70). To obtain this view, a bump or roll is placed under the contralateral scapula, which places the involved scapula flat against the radiographic cassette (a true AP). The beam is then angled 20 degrees cephalad, which brings the clavicular image away from the thoracic cage. For evaluation of the internally fixed clavicle, the abduction-lordotic view (the arm abducted 135 degrees and the beam angled 25 degrees cephalad) is extremely helpful (71).

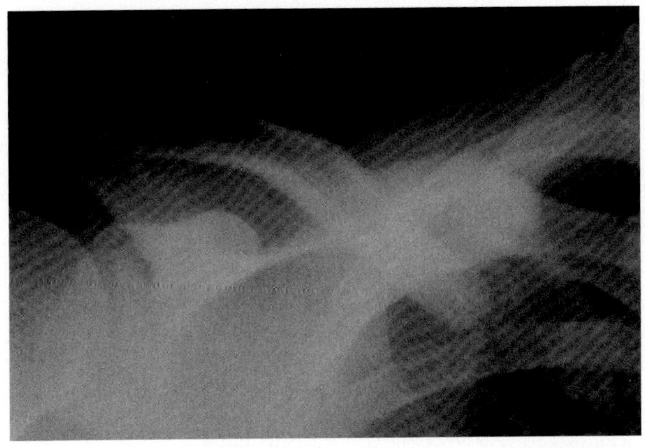

A

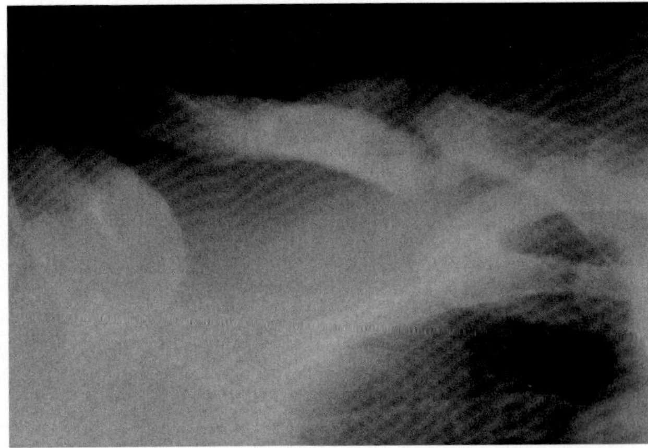

B

FIGURE 32-15 A true anteroposterior (AP) radiograph **(A)** commonly obscures the fracture pattern. An apical oblique view **(B)** is helpful to better demonstrate the fracture pattern.

Although sometimes difficult to obtain in the setting of high-velocity trauma, because the major displacing force on the midshaft clavicle fracture is gravity, standing radiographs with the affected arm left unsupported are required to determine displacement.

Fractures of the medial and lateral ends are more difficult to visualize. For the rare medial fractures, particularly those that extend into the sternoclavicular joint, a serendipity view is helpful to view anterior or posterior displacement (72). Ultimately, medial fractures in doubt require a computed tomography (CT) scan for adequate visualization (Fig. 32-16). For lateral fractures, a Zanca radiograph (AP of the acromioclavicular joint with a 15-degree cephalic tilt and soft-tissue technique) is most helpful. As with midshaft fractures, because the major displacing force is the weight of the arm, radiographs should be performed with the patient standing and the arm unsupported. A 10-pound stress view to analyze for integrity of the coracoclavicular ligaments may be necessary. An axillary radiograph may be useful to adequately define intra-articular Type III fractures and, if surgical intervention is planned, is essential to ensure integrity of the coracoid process.

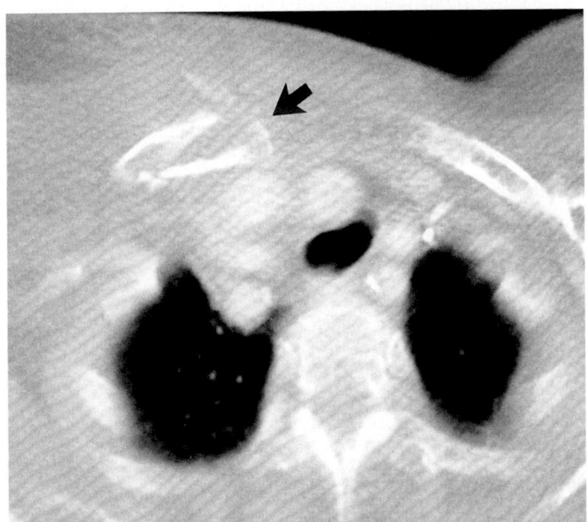

FIGURE 32-16 A computed tomography (CT) scan is useful in defining medial clavicular fractures, as in this comminuted, intra-articular fracture (*arrow*).

TREATMENT

Before contemporary improvements in fixation technique, this section would have been the shortest of the chapter. Essentially, past authors recommended immobilization for all clavicle fractures. Yet, we now know that all clavicle fractures do not heal uneventfully, and treatment recommendations should be based on these potential outcomes.

Medial Fractures

Definitive treatment recommendations for medial clavicle fractures are difficult to produce because the injury is too uncommon to provide for treatment comparisons (19,73–78). Most case reports in the literature involve Craig Group III Type IV, medial epiphyseal separations (see "Unusual Lesions") (73,76–78). Most authors report good results after nonoperative treatment, and this method is the recommended one for most medial clavicle fractures (9,19,35,39,42,73–81). Posterior displacement that threatens neurovascular structures should be managed surgically (73,77). Any concern of possible posterior displacement should be evaluated with a serendipity view and CT scan.

The medial clavicle is also the most frequent site of pathologic fracture, owing to its proximity to the head and neck. In cases of fracture displacement combined with spinal accessory palsy, operative fixation of the clavicle should be considered (Fig. 32-9B).

Midshaft Fractures

Midclavicular fractures are the most common type. Throughout history, there have been numerous devices applied to perform or maintain a reduction and to promote healing (1,21,43, 79–107). There have also been multiple recommendations for surgical intervention with various techniques described (74,108–111). These contradictory statements, combined with the extensive (abbreviated) reference list, provide evidence that this fracture remains somewhat problematic.

Immobilization

Clearly there is no need for a recommendation for nonoperative management of most midshaft clavicle fractures. Anyone who has treated this injury intuitively knows that most of these patients do extremely well, even when patient compliance may not be optimal. There are even several authors who proposed that, in the initial 3 months after injury, an orthopedic surgeon is not necessary (93,112,113). Yet, for most of us, our initial impression of a patient who had an excellent result after closed treatment of a midshaft clavicle fracture will be that of a child. Although results in adults are also good, certain injuries remain difficult.

Most authors who have reported nonoperative treatment of clavicular fractures have found superb union rates. Neer evaluated 2235 patients with midshaft fractures and determined that the nonunion rate was 0.13% (114). Rowe found a nonunion rate of 0.8% in his series of 566 fractures (44). Analysis of these data is confusing because of the addition of pediatric patients. However, other studies have confirmed excellent rates of healing even in an isolated adult population (80,84,104).

A recent study of 225 nonoperatively treated midclavicle fractures examined results at an average of 17 years of follow-up (104). Of the 225 fractures, 197 were treated in a figure-of-eight splint for an average of 3 weeks without attempted reduction, whereas 24 were allowed immediate free shoulder motion. According to this study, 185 shoulders were asymptomatic and only one patient was considered to have a poor result secondary to symptoms from thoracic outlet syndrome (TOS) that did subsequently require neurolysis. The authors state that according to their results, comminuted fractures did not fare worse than noncomminuted fractures. Also, 77% of displaced fractures were pain free with normal function at the time of follow-up.

There is some evidence, however, that not all midshaft clavicle fractures inevitably proceed to uneventful healing. White et al discovered a nonunion rate of 13%, with the rate of nonunion directly related to the degree of initial trauma (115). Hill et al (116) identified 242 consecutive patients with clavicle fractures, of which 66 (27%) were displaced, midclavicle. Of these patients, 52 were available for follow-up. All were adults. The rate of nonunion in this select group was 15%. Thirty-one percent of patients had an unsatisfactory result, and 25% of patients had mild to moderate pain. Twenty-eight of 52 patients had cosmetic complaints. Initial fracture shortening equal to or greater than 20 mm was strongly associated with nonunion; all six patients who fit this criterion had nonunion.

The findings of Wick et al (117) support the notion that clavicle fractures with greater than 20 mm of shortening were highly predisposed to develop a nonunion. Of middle third clavicle nonunions in their series, 91% (30/33) were shortened by at least 2 cm.

Recently, a large consecutive series of more than 500 diaphyseal fractures identified several independent factors predictive for the increased likelihood of nonunion. These included advancing age, female gender, absence of residual cortical contact between fracture ends, and comminution (118). Although another study did not support a difference between sexes, the authors confirmed that no bony contact on radiographs, older patients, and comminution were strong predictors of long-term sequelae (119).

More than 200 different methods of clavicle immobilization have been described (101). Various authors have opined as to the best method (9,39,42–44,80,93,95,96,105,120–122). These treatment options can be summarized as a sling, strapping, or a combination of the two (Fig. 32-17).

There are, however, no well-controlled studies that demonstrate a difference in outcome with any specific technique of immobilization. Andersen et al (84) performed a prospective, randomized study of 79 patients with midclavicle fractures treated with either a figure-of-eight bandage for 3 weeks or a simple sling to be discontinued when the patient felt ready. All fractures went on to union. The only difference between the groups was a higher rate of treatment dissatisfaction in the figure-of-eight bandage cohort. Stanley and Norris (123) reviewed a consecutive series of 140 patients with fractures of the clavicle. All had been treated with either a figure-of-eight bandage or a sling. There was no difference in either the rate or speed of recovery between the groups. Other studies have also failed to demonstrate any differences in outcome between these treatments (22,44,102).

A figure-of-eight splint may have an important role in a specialized setting. According to the experience of one group of anesthesiologists, a loss of intravenous access was seen when a patient had to be placed in the ipsilateral lateral position with a clavicle fracture. The placement of figure-of-eight splint restored the intravenous drip (124).

To summarize the literature, most midshaft clavicle fractures will go on to healing with any method of immobilization. The choice of immobilization, then, should reflect patient comfort and function issues rather than anticipated healing rates.

Closed Reduction

Hippocrates commented on the difficulty of permanently altering fracture position with manipulation of the shoulder (1). Yet, this recommendation still exists today (42,92,125–128). There are two methods commonly described. In the supine technique, a pillow is placed between the scapulae while the shoulders are manipulated superiorly and laterally (92,128). In the sitting

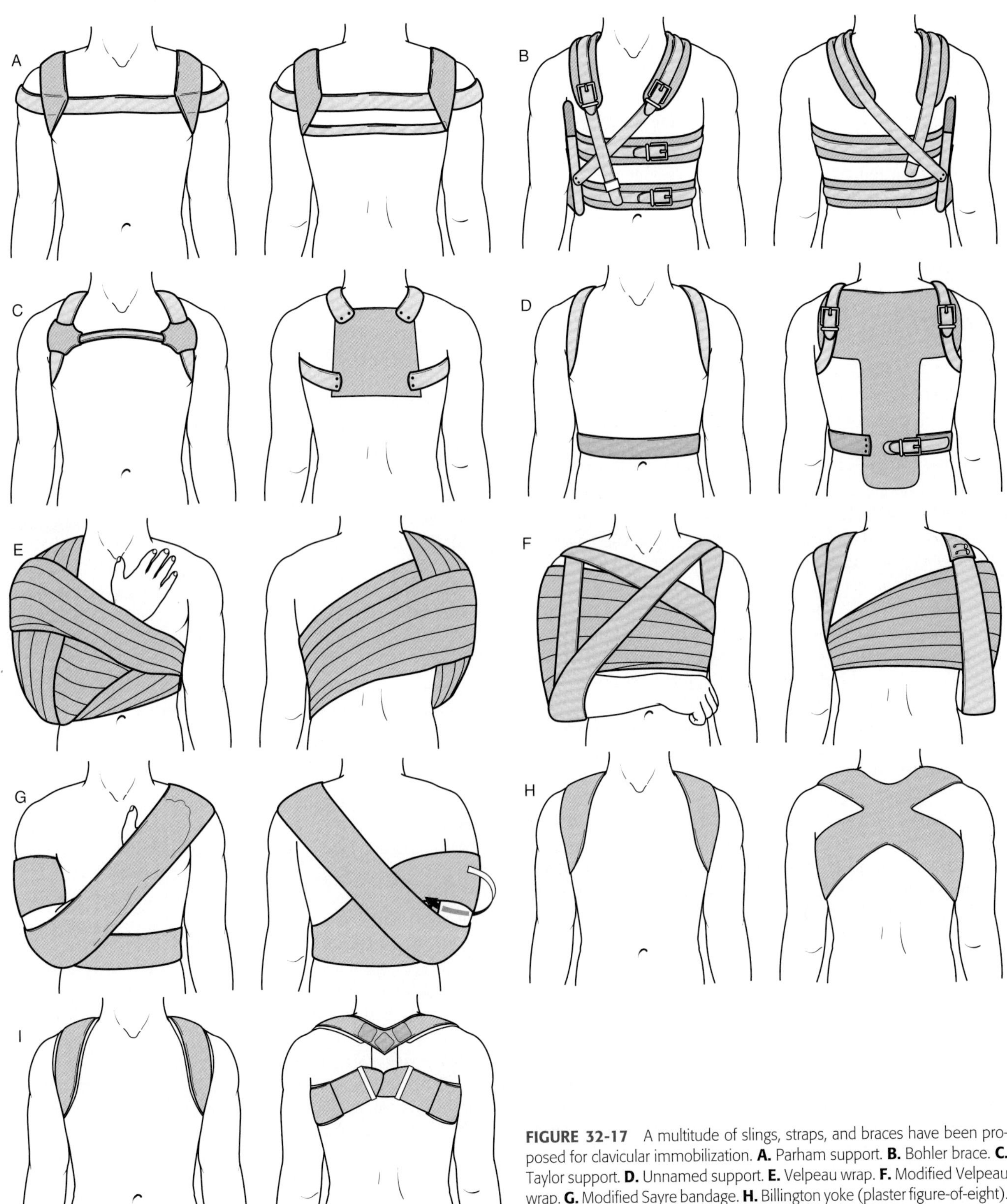

FIGURE 32-17 A multitude of slings, straps, and braces have been proposed for clavicular immobilization. **A.** Parham support. **B.** Bohler brace. **C.** Taylor support. **D.** Unnamed support. **E.** Velpeau wrap. **F.** Modified Velpeau wrap. **G.** Modified Sayre bandage. **H.** Billington yoke (plaster figure-of-eight). **I.** Commercial figure-of-eight.

technique, a knee is placed between the scapulae and a sheet is used, in configuration similar to a figure-of-eight bandage, to pull the scapulae outward (42,125–127). The use of a hematoma block aids in the technique (9,42,125). Closed reduction before immobilization has not been clearly demonstrated to aid in fracture healing (116).

External Fixation

Reports in the literature on the use of external fixation in the treatment of displaced midshaft clavicular fractures are scarce. Schuind and colleagues applied a Hoffmann fixator to the clavicle in 20 patients (129). Fifteen of these patients had acute injuries. The best indication was open fracture or severe bruising and displacement with risk of soft-tissue necrosis. All fractures united at an average of 51 days.

Open Reduction, Internal Fixation

In the past, open reduction and internal fixation (ORIF) of midclavicle fractures was deemed the surest way to *develop* a nonunion (81,114). Specifically, Neer analyzed 18 clavicular nonunions, and in 10 of these, he believed that the primary cause appeared to be ORIF (114). Nicholl (130) even questioned "Why then have they (clavicular fractures) been the target of so much surgical virtuosity?" when treatment with a sling gave consistently good results.

Several surgeons, however, have recommended primary open treatment of midshaft fractures for certain situations. These treatments fall into two main groups: intramedullary devices (131–142) and plate fixation (80,111,143–152). The surgical indications and results vary among the studies.

Advocates for intramedullary fixation report several advantages, including ease of procedure, limited exposure with minimal soft-tissue disruption, and satisfactory rates of healing (131–142). The procedure has even been described performed closed (134). Paffen and Jansen reviewed the treatment of 1400 clavicular fractures, 73 of which required open reduction and Kirschner-wire fixation (139). The rate of union was 97%, which is excellent considering that only the worst cases were fixed. Neviaser et al (137) reported their results of intramedullary fixation using Knowles pins, demonstrating a healing rate of 100%. Zenni and colleagues (142) evaluated 24 cases of clavicle fracture treated by open reduction and intramedullary wire or pin fixation, 21 of which were midshaft fractures. Indications for fixation of midclavicle fractures were neurovascular compromise caused by posterior displacement, severe angulation or comminution, and underlying neuromuscular condition (Parkinson's disease or seizure disorder) that prohibited immobilization. All fractures went on to heal in anatomic or near anatomic position. One threaded wire broke 4 weeks postoperatively. The lateral half was removed with the medial half left in situ, and the patient healed uneventfully. One patient had a refracture after a motor vehicle accident. The exact definition of "severe angulation or comminution" was not provided.

Jubel et al (133) recently published their results of treating 58 midshaft clavicle fractures in 58 patients with an elastic titanium intramedullary nail. Inclusion criteria included shortening greater than 2 cm, multiple trauma, additional lower extremity trauma that did not allow full weight bearing, concomitant neurovascular injury, or a floating shoulder. Hardware was removed at an average of 8 weeks postoperatively. No infections or refracture after hardware removal occurred. One nonunion resulted, which was treated with bone grafting and plating.

A recent retrospective review compared 40 patients who underwent open reduction and intramedullary fixation using a 2.5-mm threaded pin versus 40 patients who were treated with a figure-of-eight bandage for an average of 6 weeks (151). Those who were treated with only immobilization had a low rate of complications. Three patients experienced paresthesias that resolved with loosening of the bandage. One patient did have shoulder stiffness. The intramedullary fixation group had a much higher rate of complications (35%). This included eight superficial infections (the lateral end of the pin was cut 2 cm outside the skin), three refractures after pin removal, two cases of delayed union with pin breakage, and two nonunions. There was no significant difference in the type of fracture (simple, butterfly fragment, or comminuted) between groups. The authors concluded that given the high rate of complications, intramedullary pin fixation be reserved for those fractures that were severely displaced.

Advocates for open reduction and plate fixation argue that rigid fixation, cortical compression, and rotational control are worth the cost of increased soft-tissue stripping (80,111, 143–150). Ali Kahn and Lucas (143) reported all of 19 clavicles united after plate fixation. Poigenfurst and associates (153) reported a nonunion rate of 4.1% in 122 patients after plating of displaced clavicle fractures. All of the patients with nonunion healed with secondary plating. There were four refractures after plate removal. In a larger, more recent series, Shen et al (151) followed up on 232 acute, displaced, midshaft clavicle fractures that were fixed with an AO/Association for the Study of Internal Fixation 3.5-mm reconstruction plate or a Mizuho C-type plate. The time to radiographic union averaged 10 weeks with a 3% nonunion rate. Listed as complications were one deep infection, four superficial infections, and numbness inferior to the skin incision in 28 patients; 171 patients had their plate removed, and only two patients had refracture afterward. Ninety-four percent of patients were satisfied with the results.

Schwarz and Hocker (149) used 2.7-mm plates to repair displaced midshaft fractures. There was a fairly high failure rate of 12%, which the authors related to inadequate fixation. The rate of nonunion appeared to be critically dependent on the number of cortices secured on either side of the fracture. Specifically, if less than six cortices were traversed, three of seven fractures failed to unite. If more than six cortices were purchased, the union rate was 100%. Also, the fracture pattern was related to failure. Simple or comminuted fractures all united. For fractures with one or two small butterfly fragments (buttress type), 3 of 17 failed.

Recent advances in plate technology have added to the treatment choices for midshaft clavicle fractures. The development of locking plate technology has specific advantages for clavicular fixation. Specifically, having the plate and screws as a single construct may enhance the ability of the plate to resist the large inferiorly directed torque on the outer segment and therefore may limit the potential for plate pull-out. Alternatively, clavicular plates are now available in an s-shape, to better follow the axial course of the clavicle when they are placed in a superior position.

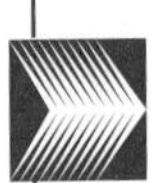

MIDSHAFT FRACTURES: AUTHORS' PREFERRED TREATMENT

Nonoperative Treatment

The most important aspect of nonoperative treatment of midshaft clavicle fractures is ensuring that the fracture is indeed nondisplaced or minimally displaced. Often, emergency department radiographs are performed with the patient in the supine position. Before proceeding with nonoperative treatment, true clavicular AP radiographs with and without a 20-degree cephalic tilt and with the patient in the standing position (arm hanging to gravity) are needed to ensure that the fracture is not significantly displaced.

Review of the literature reveals two points to be clear: (a) most midshaft clavicle fractures are effectively treated nonoperatively (Fig. 32-18A,B), and (b) the exact immobilization method does not appear to influence outcome. My treatment protocol, therefore, is based more on patient comfort and need for return to activities than it is on rates of healing. First, I explain the two treatment options that I normally use, namely, a figure-of-eight harness versus a simple sling. Often, patients will have an immediate preference simply after hearing the two choices. If not, I usually encourage patients who have fractured the clavicle of the dominant shoulder toward treatment with a figure-of-eight brace. In this way, the dominant hand can remain free for writing, keyboarding, and other activities that will allow the patient quick return to work. In addition, for fractures that demonstrate minimal shortening, I usually recommend a figure-of-eight splint as an attempt to retract the scapula and gain clavicular length. For fractures in the nondominant extremity, I often recommend a simple sling because I have found this treatment to be more comfortable and tolerable. In addition, because the main displacing force on the lateral clavicle is gravity, a simple sling will help support the weight of the arm. Treatment is maintained for 4 to 6 weeks. I counsel all patients that there will likely be some deformity to the shoulder girdle but that function will typically be normal.

Immobilization is discontinued when there is no pain or palpable fracture motion on scapular elevation and retraction. Usually, no subsequent therapy is necessary. Because the glenohumeral and humeroscapular spaces have not been violated, motion restriction is uncommon. Rarely, a patient will require some simple home stretching exercise to regain lost motion. These should be forward elevation and external rotation stretches performed supine to negate the displacing effects of gravity. Although most surgeons consider Codman pendulum exercises (154) to be a benign method of regaining motion, because the major displacing force for this injury is the weight of the arm, pendulum exercises will magnify the displacing moment and should be avoided. Unless the athlete is in the middle of his season, I usually restrict contact sports for 3 months after injury. For midseason injuries, this restriction is negotiable. Heavy laborers are returned to light-duty lifting 6 weeks after injury with return to full duty by 12 weeks.

Operative Treatment

Indications for operative intervention are listed in Table 32-3. It is clear that many of the indications are somewhat arbitrary and approached on a case-by-case basis. My preferred

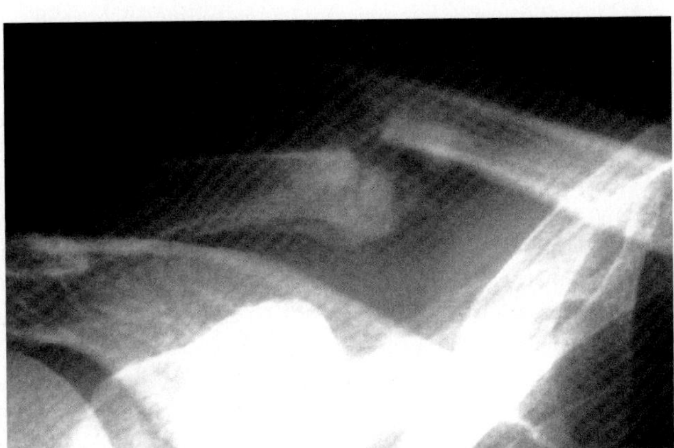
A

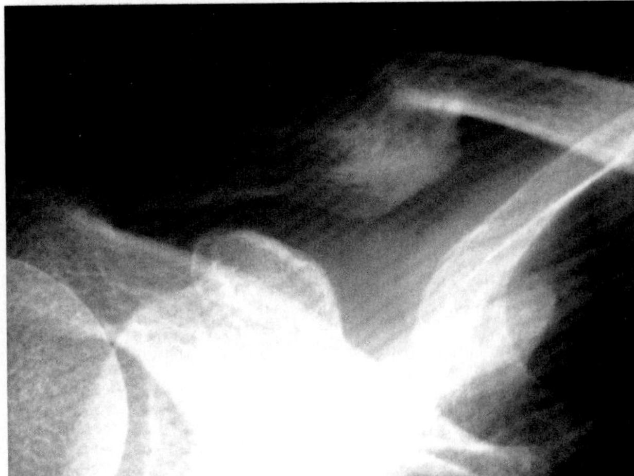
B

FIGURE 32-18 Typical midclavicle fracture **(A)** that went on to uneventful healing with closed treatment **(B)**.

TABLE 32-3 Indications for Open Reduction and Internal Fixation of Displaced Midshaft Fractures

Absolute
- Shortening of ≥20 mm
- Open injury
- Impending skin disruption and irreducible fracture
- Vascular compromise
- Progressive neurologic loss
- Displaced pathologic fracture with associated trapezial paralysis
- Scapulothoracic dissociation

Relative
- Displacement of >20 mm
- Neurologic disorder
  - Parkinson's
  - Seizures
  - Head injury
- Multitrauma
- Expected prolonged recumbency
- Floating shoulder
- Intolerance to immobilization
- Bilateral fractures
- Ipsilateral upper extremity fracture
- Cosmesis

operative approach is open reduction and plate fixation, using either a 3.5-mm locking dynamic compression plate or, less desirably, a 3.5-mm reconstruction plate. There are several advantages to this type of fixation over intramedullary:

1. For transverse fractures, compression across the fracture site is achieved.
2. For oblique fractures or butterfly fragments, lag screw fixation is possible with the plate functioning in neutralization mode.
3. Secure rotational control of the fracture is achieved.
4. Fixation is rigid enough to allow the patient to minimally weight-bear on the extremity or to use the arm for activities of daily living, if necessary.
5. Minimal soft-tissue disruption is necessary. Often, the injury itself has caused fairly extensive local soft-tissue stripping. For plate application, only soft-tissue along the superior aspect of the clavicle need be elevated.

Techniques

The patient is positioned in the beach-chair position. A Mayfield or McConnell headrest is used to provide complete access for use of instruments superior to the clavicle. Placing the cervical spine in slight extension and contralateral tilt will aid in medial clavicular access. A 10″ × 12″ radiographic cassette is placed under the padding of the operative table and positioned optimally for intraoperative radiographs. The entire shoulder girdle is prepped including the sternum, in case emergency proximal vascular access becomes necessary. The arm is draped free for intraoperative manipulation. For comminuted fractures, the contralateral iliac crest is prepared for potential bone graft. The contralateral crest is preferred for two reasons. First, operative setup is facilitated. More important, if the patient has difficulty ambulating postoperatively because of pain, it is preferable that an ambulatory aid be used in the nonoperative hand.

There are two potential incisions for approach to the clavicular midshaft. For simple transverse fractures, a longitudinal incision in Langer's lines will provide excellent access and good cosmesis. For oblique or comminuted fractures (where extensile exposure may be needed) or for fractures toward the medial extent of the central third of the clavicle (where the skin lines change to curvilinear), a transverse incision along the clavicular length is preferred. I recommend sharply carrying the incision through the subcutaneous tissue and platysma, leaving the skin flaps thick. I do not dissect the supraclavicular nerves. I have not found any detrimental effects from cutting these nerves, and because wound dehiscence is a fear, I have concerns about potentially thinning soft-tissue flaps to search for them. The overlying fascia and periosteum are next divided, in line with the clavicle. This step is performed sharply and down to bone, again leaving thick flaps for later closure. The division is started medial and lateral to the fracture site and then proceeds to the site, in case important neurovascular structures have been displaced toward the fracture. The osseous ends are freed from surrounding tissues. Soft-tissue is circumferentially removed only from the osseous ends. Periosteum is then elevated from the superior aspect of the clavicle for a length sufficient to place a plate with three holes in intact bone proximal and distal to the fracture site. At the junction of the medial and middle thirds of the clavicle, the inferior surface is exposed so that a protective instrument can be inserted during drilling. The remaining soft tissue sleeve is left intact.

At this point, the "character" of the fracture is assessed. For transverse fractures, anatomic reduction is performed and fixation is with a 3.5-mm locking DC plate placed superiorly (Fig. 32-19A–E). Attempt is made to achieve compression across the fracture site. A minimum of six intact cortices medial and lateral to the fracture site are purchased. For more oblique fractures, a 3.5-mm cortical lag screw is placed across the fracture site. Usually, the fracture obliquity will be in the axial plane so the lag screw can be placed through the plate (Fig. 32-20). If the obliquity is in the sagittal plane, direction of the lag screw will be anterior to posterior and the plate will serve as a neutralization plate (Fig. 32-21A,B). In this case, the plate may be either a 3.5-mm locking DC plate or a 3.5-mm reconstruction plate. The reconstruction plate is easier to mold in the axial plane so that it may better conform to the serpentine clavicular shape.

For large butterfly fragments or extensive comminution,

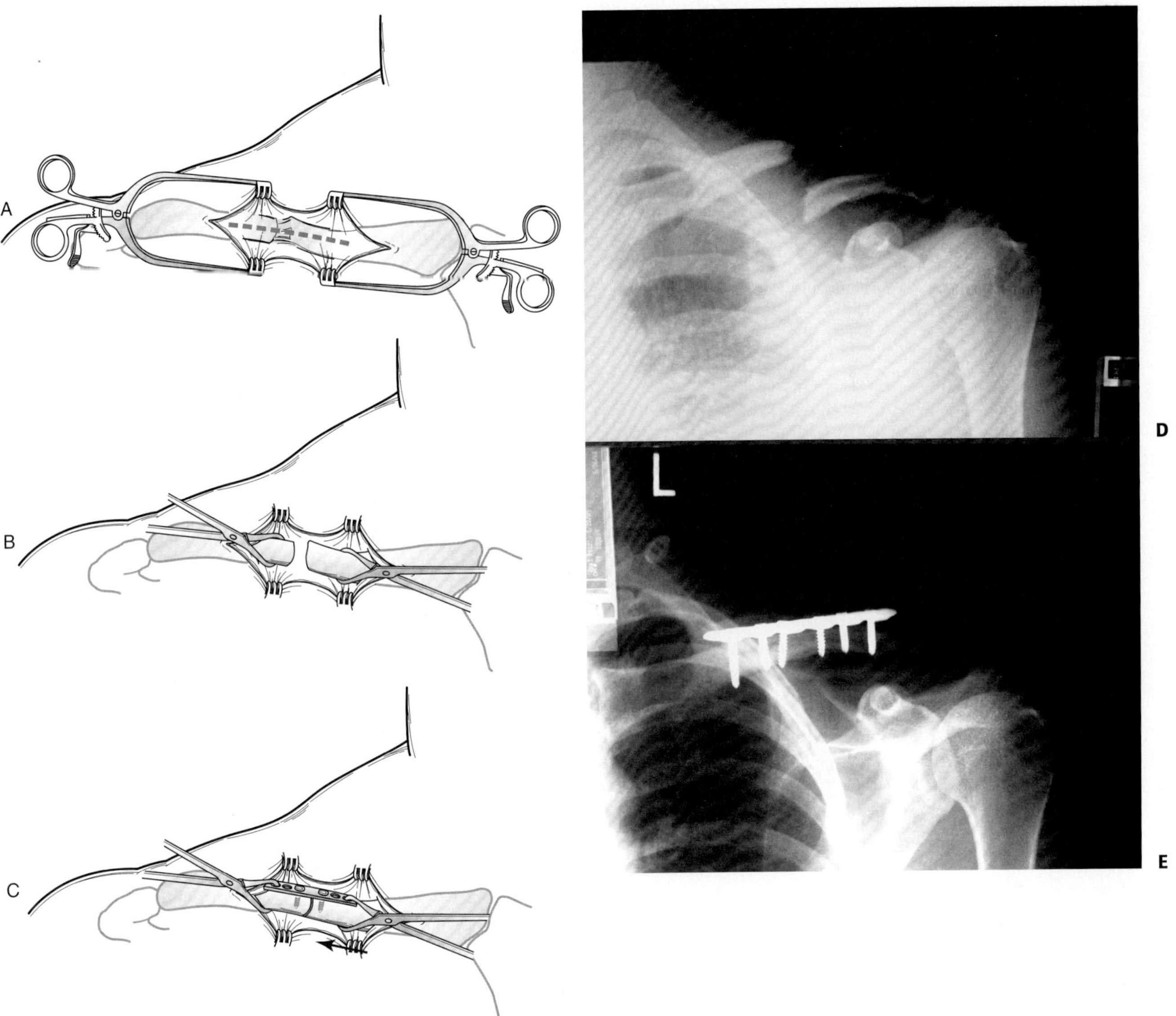

FIGURE 32-19 **A–E.** Open reduction and internal fixation (ORIF) of a transverse midclavicle fractures. **A.** Surgical exposure is achieved through a transverse incision through skin and soft-tissues. **B.** Fracture reduction is accomplished by direct manipulation, assisted with upward displacement of the arm. **C.** Fixation is performed with a 3.5-mm locking DC plate placed superiorly and in compression mode. Displaced transverse fracture in a 21-year-old man **(D)** is effectively treated with this technique **(E)**.

each case needs to be approached individually. Often, large fragments can either be lagged into the hole or fixed with a cortical position screw. Alternatively, suture or Dacron tapes can be circumferentially passed around the clavicle to secure small fragments. For extensively comminuted fractures, a 3.5-mm locking DC plate is the preferred fixation because of its strength. However, for longer fractures, the plate will have to encompass more of the s-shape of the clavicle. Therefore, it becomes difficult to fit a DC plate to this shape. Occasionally, the plate is placed obliquely along the superior surface. Also, the DC plate can be twisted such that it is placed on the anterior clavicular surface medially and then carried superiorly over the fracture site. Alternatives are a reconstruction plate, specially designed s-shaped clavicular plates (Accumed Inc., Lawrenceville, NJ), or double plating. For comminuted fractures, I will usually supplement with autologous cancellous graft from the iliac crest. Care is taken to pack graft into the fracture lines, not to leave a mass of graft. If abundant callous forms, it could later impinge on neurovascular structures.

One disadvantage of clavicular plating is that the clavicle's subcutaneous position makes all hardware extremely promi-

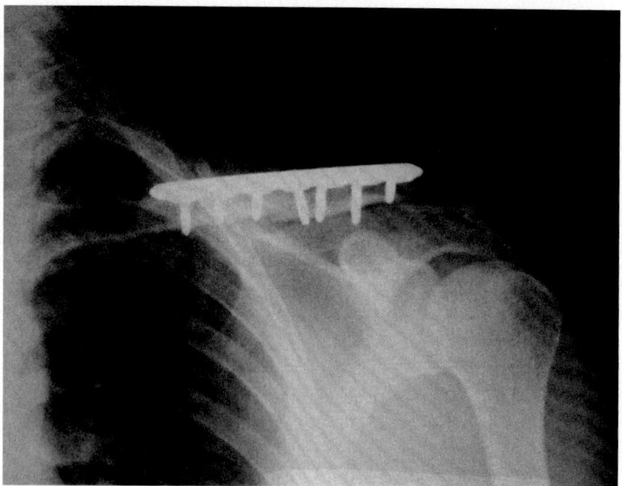

FIGURE 32-20 For fracture obliquity in the axial plane, fixation is achieved through a superior plate, either 3.5-mm DC or reconstruction plate, with lag screw fixation through the plate.

nent. Therefore, secure wound closure is vital. The periosteum and fascial layer are closed with a heavy absorbable suture in interrupted fashion. The subcutaneous tissue is also closed with interrupted suture. The skin is closed with a pullout, monofilament, subcuticular suture. The wound edges are infiltrated with 0.25% bupivacaine before closure.

Postoperatively, patients are maintained in a sling for comfort for 1 to 2 weeks. Patients may then use the arm for lightweight activities of daily living. Typically, therapy or formal exercises are not needed because the glenohumeral and humeroscapular interfaces have not been violated. If patients demonstrate some early loss of motion, a supine stretching program is begun. As with nonoperative treatment, pendulum exercises are avoided.

Patients are followed radiographically, and evidence of healing usually becomes apparent by approximately 6 to 12 weeks postoperatively. Heavy lifting is restricted until radiographic healing is noted.

Routine plate removal is somewhat controversial. In my experience, most patients will request plate removal because it is usually prominent and potentially uncomfortable as the result of its subcutaneous position. During plate removal, I will usually place allogeneic cancellous graft into the screw holes to promote consolidation. Contact sports and heavy lifting are restricted for a minimum of 3 months postoperatively from plate removal to protect against refracture. Patients understand, however, that refracture is a risk for months after plate removal (153). For those patients who retain the plate, I warn them of the risk of fracture at the plate ends.

Lateral Clavicular Fractures

Nonoperative Treatment

Neer recognized and classified distal clavicular fractures as an entity distinct from other clavicle fractures because of their unique behavior (36,37,114). Treatment recommendations for this fracture, therefore, do not necessarily mirror those of the midshaft fracture. Yet, the literature is more controversial for this fracture type than for the midclavicle.

In Neer's original series of clavicle nonunions, he discovered that, although distal clavicular fractures were uncommon, they accounted for one-half of the nonunions (114). He later classified distal clavicle fractures into three types, two of which are important in displacement terms: Type I, coracoclavicular ligaments attached to medial segment (Fig. 32-10A), and Type II, coracoclavicular ligaments detached from medial segment, trapezoid ligament attached to distal segment (Fig. 32-10B).

A

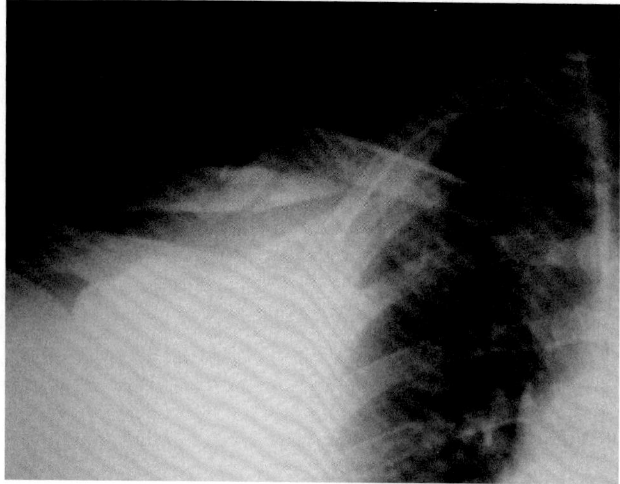

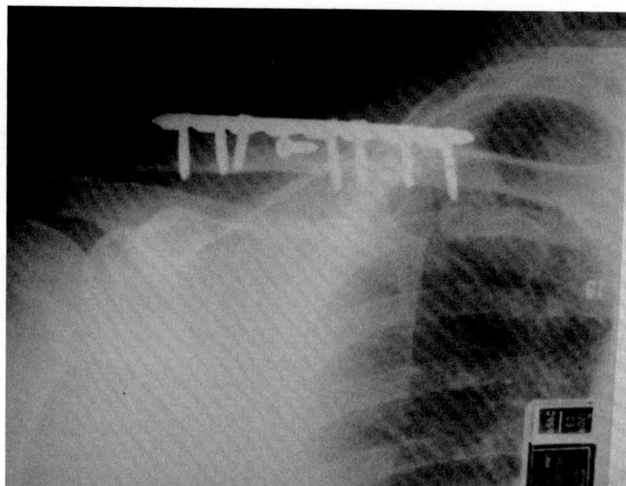

B

FIGURE 32-21 A,B. For sagittal plane obliquity or fracture comminution, AP lag screws are used with a superior plate placed in neutralization mode.

He found that the Type I fracture was more common by 3: 1, resulted from more trivial trauma, and usually healed readily. If late symptoms developed, they were usually secondary to fracture extension into the acromioclavicular joint (Type III) and subsequent posttraumatic arthrosis.

Type II fractures, alternatively, are unstable injuries, secondary to four displacing forces (Fig. 32-5):

1. the weight of the arm
2. the pull of the pectoralis major, pectoralis minor, and latissimus dorsi
3. scapular rotation, which affects the distal segment but not the proximal
4. the trapezius muscle, which draws the medial segment posterior and superior

Neer found that these lesions usually resulted from more significant trauma and had a high rate of associated injuries to the adjacent ribs and coracoid, a delayed time until union, and a high rate of nonunion. Specifically, of the 12 patients treated with closed reduction, none of the fractures were united by 16 weeks and four went on to nonunion. Other authors have commented on the high rate of *symptomatic* nonunion for the Type II distal clavicle fracture (108,155–157).

There are, however, opposing data. Nordqvist and associates (10) reviewed the outcome of 110 patients who had a lateral clavicle fracture, with a mean follow-up of 15 years. Seventy-three of the patients had Type I, 23 had Type II, and 14 had Type III injuries. All patients were treated with figure-of-eight immobilization. Outcome for pain was measured as none, slight or moderate, or severe. Outcome for function was measured as normal, slight or moderate disability, or severe disability. In the group as a whole, there were 10 nonunions, with Type II fracture and older age at presentation being significant predictors of nonunion. For Type II fractures, 22% had a nonunion. No patient, however, had severe disability. In 8 of the 10 patients the nonunion was asymptomatic. Deformity was present, but fracture instability was not found on examination. In summary, 17 of 23 Type II fractures were asymptomatic and in no patient was severe disability noted.

Robinson and Cairns (158) concluded that nonoperative treatment of most displaced lateral fractures did well. The authors based this on Short Form (SF)-36 and Constant scores of 120 patients treated nonoperatively. Only 14% had residual symptoms severe enough to require surgical intervention.

Rokito and colleagues (11) recently published a retrospective review of the results of operative and nonoperative treatment of Type II fractures. Sixteen patients were treated nonoperatively, and 14 patients were treated with coracoclavicular stabilization. All surgically treated patients healed, whereas 7 of 16 patients treated nonoperatively went on to nonunion. However, five of these seven were asymptomatic, and functional outcome was similar between the two groups.

How then do we make sense of these data? It is clear that there is a high rate of delayed union, nonunion, and deformity with closed treatment of Type II distal clavicle fractures. Exactly how the data taken from Malmo, Sweden relates to the average orthopedic practice is not clear. Also, how the patient population decided between "moderate" and "severe" pain and disability is ambiguous. However, we can deduce that many patients with Type II distal clavicle fractures will have reasonable function after closed treatment, even in the presence of nonunion (Fig. 32-22).

Operative Treatment

Several authors have recommended initial operative treatment for the displaced Type II distal clavicle fracture (36,37,108, 155–157,159–164). In his original article, Neer recommended transacromial wire fixation and reported that seven of seven fractures treated with this technique healed at an average of 6 weeks postoperatively (37). Similarly, good results were achieved in a recent study in all 32 patients treated with a transacromial Knowles pin (165). Kona et al (166), however, reported six nonunions and five deep infections in 13 patients treated by transacromial fixation and recommended against this approach. Neviaser recommended direct internal fixation using a cerclage wire (163). Yamaguchi and colleagues (164) used a temporary coracoclavicular screw to indirectly reduce the fracture and reported healing in all 11 of their patients.

Ballmer and Gerber (159) reviewed their technique of closed, indirect fracture reduction and placement of a coracoclavicular screw. With this technique, only the base of the coracoid is exposed, the fracture site itself remaining undisturbed. All five of their patients went on to complete union within 6 to 9 weeks after surgery. There were no complications. Transfer of the tip of the coracoid with attached conjoined tendon to the unstable segment has also been described, with good results (162).

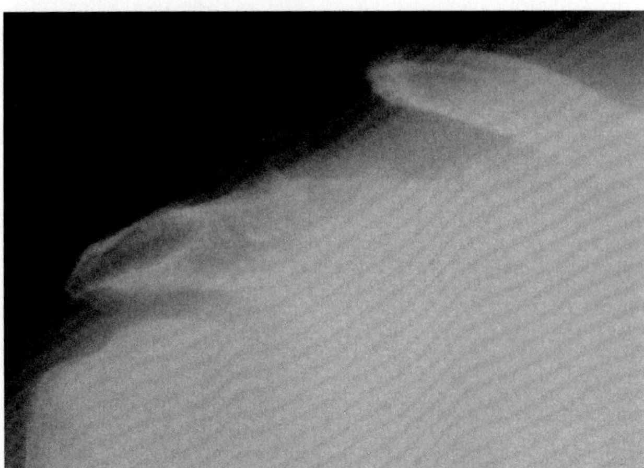

FIGURE 32-22 A patient with an established nonunion of a Type II distal clavicle fracture. Although she had obvious deformity, she felt no symptoms or functional disturbance.

Twelve patients with a Neer Type II a fracture were treated by Kao et al (167) with two 1.8-mm K-wires and tension band. The K-wires did not penetrate the acromioclavicular joint and were bent under the skin. Eleven of the 12 fractures united. The fractures united between 3 and 6 months, at which time the implants were removed. The twelfth patient fell postoperatively and required revision surgery consisting of a distal clavicle excision and coracoclavicular reconstruction. No implants were reported to have migrated.

Chen et al (168) used Mersilene tape and repair of the coracoclavicular ligaments along with number 7 tension band wire spanning the fracture to treat 13 patients with Neer Type II fractures. Eleven were available for follow-up at an average of 27 months. Ten of the 11 fractures united at 3 months, whereas the last patient's fracture united at 6 months. Nine of 11 patients were deemed to have an excellent outcome, one patient had a good outcome, and one patient had a fair outcome.

Goldberg and colleagues (161) reported their technique of reduction of the coracoclavicular interval using Dacron tape passed around the base of the coracoid and medial clavicular segment combined with suture fixation of the distal clavicular fragment to the proximal. In their nine patients, all fractures went on to union. The average time until union was 16 weeks, with all but one patient obtaining union by 18 weeks. All patients were symptom free at the most recent follow-up. Similarly, Webber and Haines (169) treated 11 acute and 4 Neer Type II lateral clavicle fractures with a Dacron arterial sling placed around the base of the coracoid over the clavicle. Those patients with nonunions were supplemented with iliac crest bone graft and an AO small fragment lag screw fixation. All fractures united, and all patients were reported to achieve full range of motion of the treated shoulder. Complications included one case of hardware irritation in the nonunion group. Two of the Dacron grafts required removal, one for infection and one for a sterile sinus.

Mall et al (170) described using a 10-mm band of absorbable suture (polydioxanone) placed through a drill hole in the distal aspect of the proximal fragment and around the coracoid in a figure-of-eight fashion. Twelve patients were treated at an average of 6 hours post-injury. All patients achieved an excellent rating according to the Constant and Murley score. All fractures united, and only one hypertrophic scar was listed as a complication.

One comparative study in the literature is worth noting. Flinkkila et al (171) contrasted the results of 22 Neer Type II fractures treated with K-wire fixation with 17 patients treated with a clavicular hook plate (Stratec Medical, Oberdorf, Switzerland). Both groups did well according to the Constant and L'Insalata scores, but the K-wire group had a much higher complication rate. This included 12 cases of wire migration resulting in loss of fixation in seven, infection in three, and nonunion in two. The clavicular hook plate group had one fractured clavicle at the medial end of the plate secondary to a new injury and two nonunions. The authors recommended the use of the plate over the K-wires.

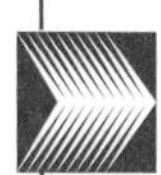

AUTHORS' PREFERRED TREATMENT

Lateral Clavicular Fractures

The first step in treatment is to ensure the diagnosis. The typical supine trauma radiographic series is inappropriate for the evaluation of this injury. A Zanca radiograph taken with the patient standing and the affected arm hanging to gravity is a must. Although medial segment instability can often be determined by fracture pattern and physical examination, I have found stress radiographs with a 10-pound weight to be helpful. For maximum sensitivity, the weight needs to be hung from the patient's wrist, not held by the patient. Finally, an axillary radiograph is essential to ensure integrity of the coracoid process before any attempted ORIF.

Type I and Type III distal clavicle fractures are treated nonoperatively. As opposed to the several available options for closed treatment of midshaft fractures, I treat these injuries in a simple sling. The main deforming force and source of discomfort is the weight of the arm, and a simple sling is more effective than a figure-of-eight brace or shoulder immobilizer at countering this force. The sling is continued until pain resolves and there is no crepitance at the fracture site during scapular elevation and retraction. Usually, this occurs by 3 to 6 weeks after injury. Both groups, but particularly those with Type III injuries, are warned of the possibility of late acromioclavicular arthrosis with the possible need for subsequent distal clavicle excision (Fig. 32-23).

For Type II fractures, my preference is operative fixation. I usually will explain the treatment options and results to the patient. When patients learn of the high nonunion rate, most choose operative fixation, even when they understand that nonunion may be asymptomatic.

My preferred technique of operative fixation will depend on the exact fracture pattern. The general choices for surgical goals are as follows:

1. direct fixation of the fracture site without coracoclavicular stabilization

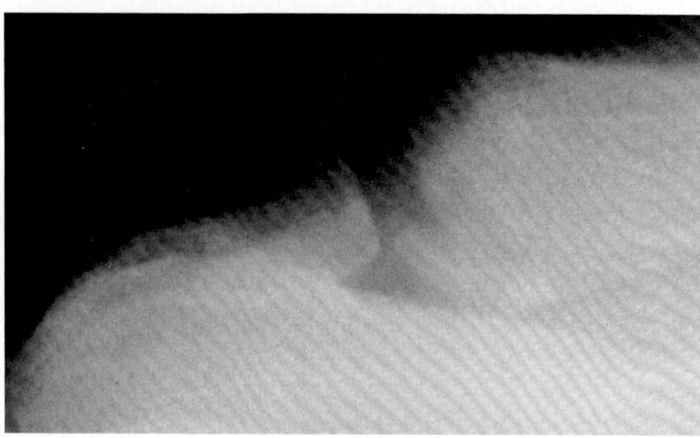

FIGURE 32-23 Acromioclavicular spur formation after a displaced intra-articular fracture.

2. direct fixation of the fracture site with coracoclavicular stabilization
3. coracoclavicular stabilization with or without excision of the lateral clavicular segment

Which surgical goal is used will depend on the pattern of fracture, quality of bone, and level of patient demand. The surgical goal chosen will dictate the technique.

Techniques

Direct Fixation of the Fracture Without Coracoclavicular Stabilization. Indications for this technique are (a) good bone quality and (b) noncomminuted fracture pattern.

The patient is placed in the beach-chair position. A Mayfield or McConnell head holder is helpful to allow superior access to the shoulder. C-arm fluoroscopic image intensifier is brought in from the opposite side of the operative table and positioned for a true scapular AP image with a 15-degree cephalic tilt. The shoulder is prepped and draped with the arm free. An incision is made in Langer's lines, positioned midway between the coracoid process and the acromioclavicular joint to permit access to both locations. The incision extends from the posterior aspect of the clavicle down to the coracoid. Large subcutaneous flaps are raised superficial to the deltotrapezial fascia. The fascia is then sharply divided along the length of the exposed clavicle, over the fracture site, and to the acromioclavicular joint. Care is taken to leave the incised fascia thick for closure. The fracture site is exposed and cleaned of debris. The acromioclavicular joint is inspected. If the intra-articular disc is torn, it is excised.

Fracture reduction is usually easily accomplished by simple elevation of the arm. Direct fixation is achieved by means of a specialized distal clavicular plate (Accumed Inc.). These plates come in left and right configurations to match the serpentine shape of the clavicle. In addition, the plate expands laterally to provide multiple screw holes, permitting rigid fixation within the distal segment (Fig. 32-24A,B)

Direct Fixation of the Fracture with Coracoclavicular Stabilization. Indications for this technique are (a) very distal fracture in a young individual and (b) fractures that involve the clavicular insertion of the coracoclavicular ligaments.

The patient is placed in the beach-chair position. A Mayfield or McConnell head holder is helpful to allow superior access to the shoulder. The C-arm fluoroscopic image intensifier is brought in from the opposite side of the operative table and positioned for a true scapular AP image with a 15-degree cephalic tilt. The shoulder is prepped and draped with the arm free. An incision is made in Langer's lines, positioned midway between the coracoid process and the acromioclavicular joint to permit access to both locations. The incision extends from the posterior aspect of the clavicle down to the coracoid. Large subcutaneous flaps are raised superficial to the deltotrapezial fascia. The fascia is then sharply divided along the length of the exposed clavicle, over the fracture site, and to the acromioclavicular joint (Fig. 32-25A). Care is taken to leave the incised fascia thick for closure. The fracture site is exposed and cleaned of debris. The acromioclavicular joint is inspected. If the intra-articular disc is torn, it is excised. Typically the joint surface is undisturbed. The anterior deltoid is raised as a flap off the medial segment. Mobilizing the deltoid will usually allow access to the base of the coracoid process. If not, the deltoid can be split longitudinally toward the base of the coracoid process. Adequate exposure of the base of the coracoid is essential.

A right-angle or cardiac C clamp is used to pass a 3-mm Dacron tape around the base of the coracoid process and

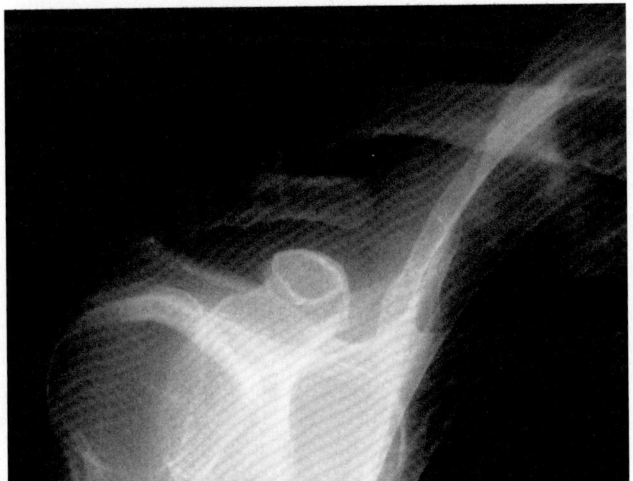
A

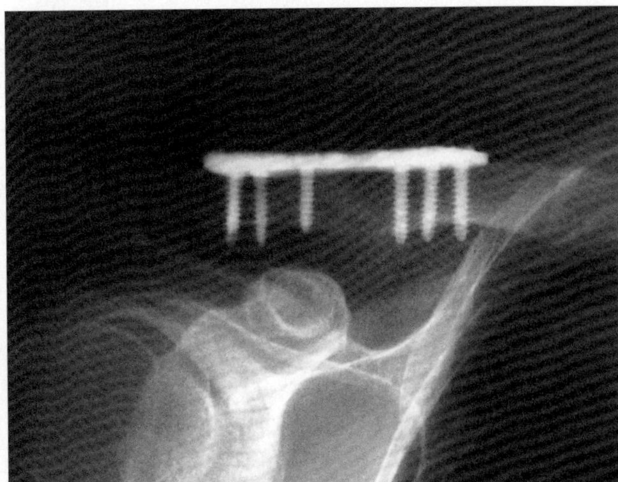
B

FIGURE 32-24 **A.** Displaced Type II distal clavicle fracture. **B.** The transverse fracture pattern and good bone quality permitted direct ORIF using a specially designed distal clavicular plate.

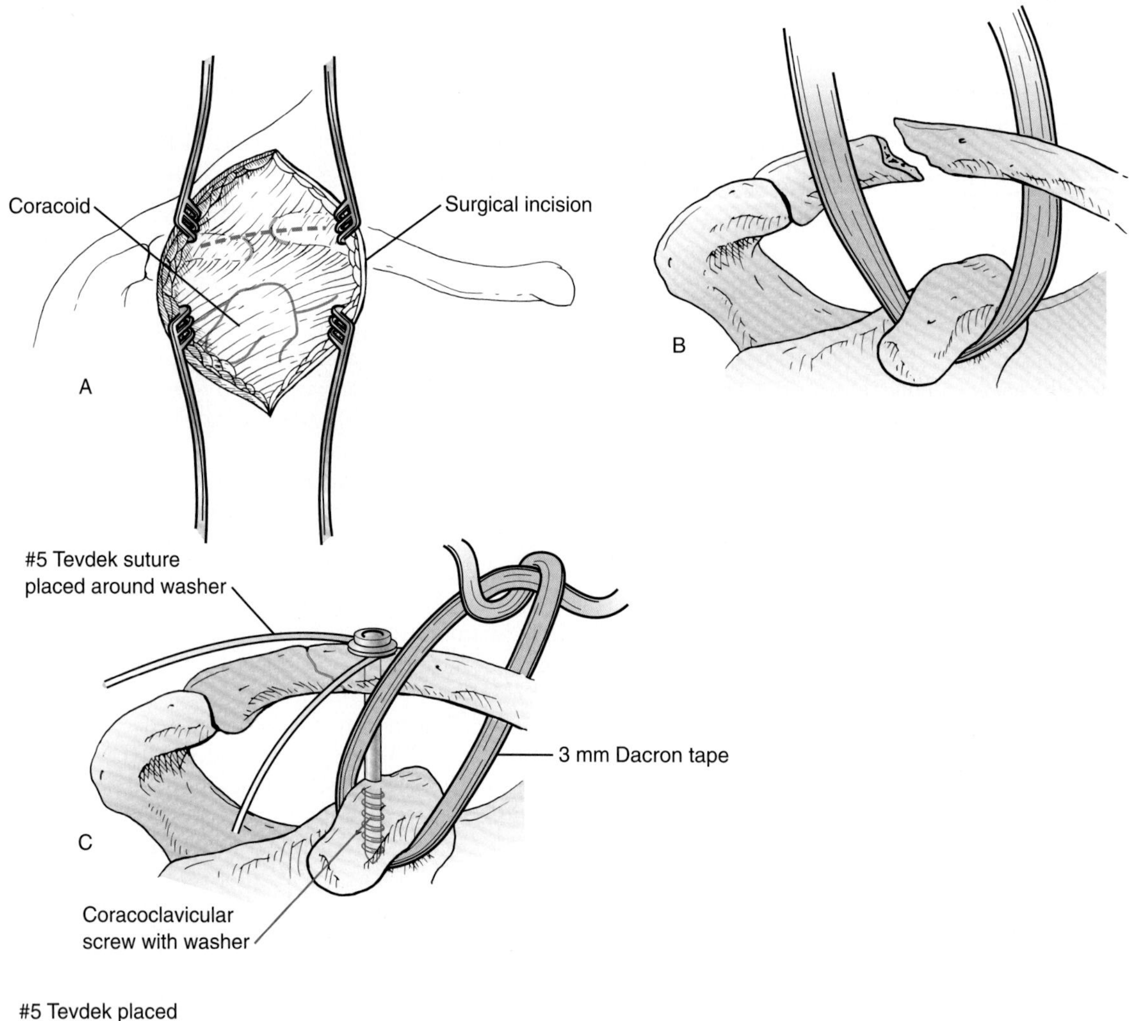

FIGURE 32-25 **A.** For fixation of a distal clavicle fracture, the incision is made in Langer's lines with the deltotrapezial fascia split laterally. If necessary for further exposure, the deltoid is split longitudinally. **B.** A 3-mm Dacron tape is passed around the base of the coracoid and around the medial clavicular segment. **C.** While the reduction is held, a coracoclavicular stabilization screw is placed. **D.** The fracture is directly fixed with a number 5 Tevdek suture placed in tension band fashion.

around the medial clavicular segment (Fig. 32-25B). By displacing the arm superiorly, the fracture is reduced. While the reduction is held, a coracoclavicular stabilization screw with washer is placed (Fig. 32-25C). I prefer a 6.5-mm partially threaded cancellous screw with washer. Typically, the clavicle is drilled with a 4.5-mm drill bit, but the coracoid is only drilled with a 3.2-mm drill. As the screw is placed, the fracture is held reduced with upward force on the arm. Before fully seating the screw, a number 5 Tevdek suture is placed under the washer. I do not make any attempt to suture the remnants of coracoclavicular ligament. An anterior to posterior bone tunnel is created in the most lateral aspect of the lateral fracture fragment, without violating the articular surface of the acromioclavicular joint. The number 5 Tevdek

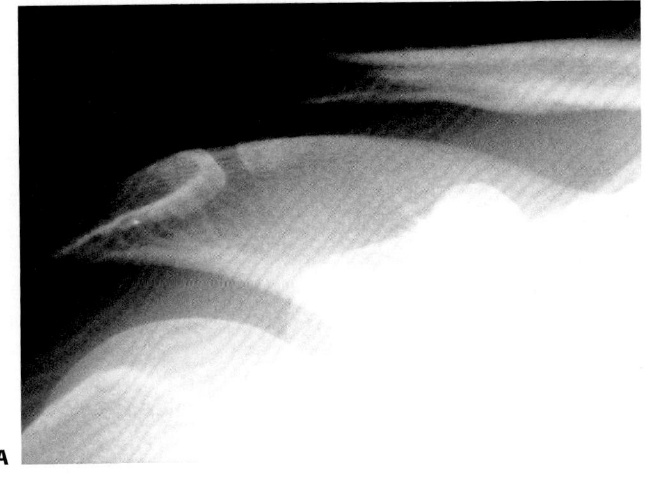

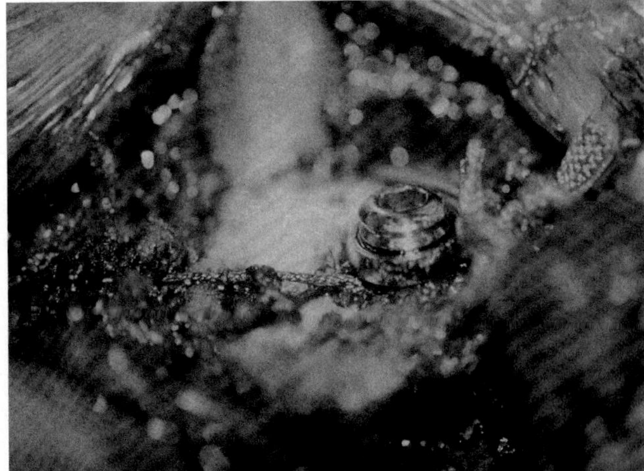

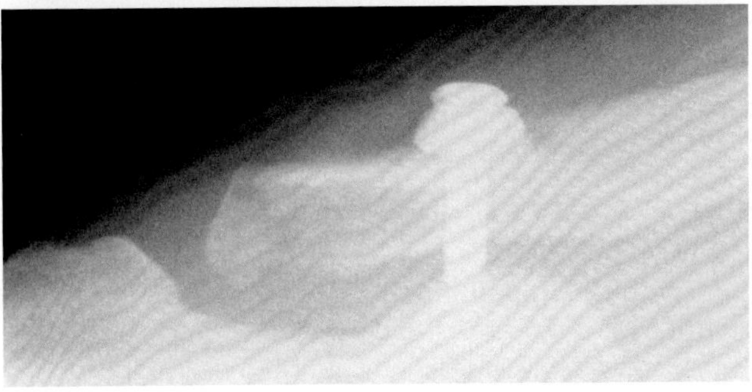

FIGURE 32-26 **A.** A 23-year-old man with a displaced Type II distal clavicle fracture. **B.** Intraoperative photograph of fixation technique. **C.** Postoperative radiograph of repaired Type II fracture.

is then crossed in tension-band fashion and passed through the bone tunnel (Fig. 32-25D). The suture is tied, and the Dacron tape is tied over the clavicle (Fig. 32-26 A–C).

Fractures that involve the coracoclavicular ligament origin require special treatment. Direct fixation of the fracture fragment to the remainder of the clavicle is essential and is usually achieved with either a simple 3.5-mm cortical lag screw or a circumferential 3-mm Dacron tape. To remove tension from the repair, I recommend supplementing the fixation with a coracoclavicular screw, as above (Fig. 32-27A,B).

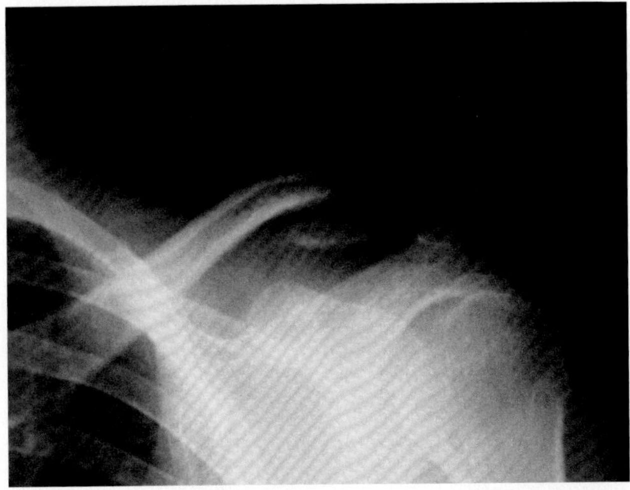

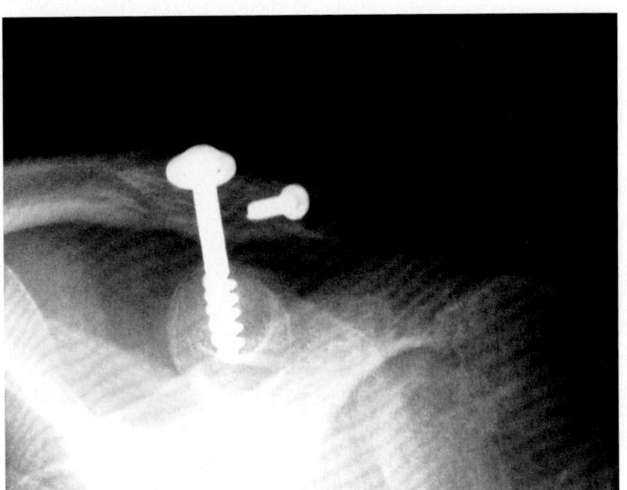

FIGURE 32-27 **A.** A 25-year-old-man with a displaced distal clavicle fracture involving the coracoclavicular ligament origin. **B.** Treatment included lag screw fixation of the fracture fragment. Tension on the repair was removed by placement of a temporary coracoclavicular lag screw.

The deltotrapezial fascia is then closed with braided, nonabsorbable suture. Toward the fracture and acromioclavicular joint, attempt is made to oversew and imbricate this closure because this tissue will help restore AP stability to the acromioclavicular joint. The subcutaneous tissue is closed with absorbable suture, and the skin is closed with a running, nonabsorbable, monofilament subcuticular suture. A simple sling is preferred over an immobilizer because the goal of postoperative protection is support not immobilization.

Postoperatively, the sling is maintained for 3 weeks. Typically, no therapy is needed. If the patient shows some minimal stiffness, a supine stretching program is begun. Pendulum exercises are avoided because these simply accentuate the displacing force. Use of the arm for light activities of daily living is permitted. The coracoclavicular screw is removed under local anesthesia 3 months postoperatively. Heavy lifting and contact sports are restricted for 6 months.

Coracoclavicular Stabilization With or Without Excision of the Lateral Clavicular Segment. Indications for this technique are (a) comminuted lateral clavicular segment; (b) older patients in whom potential healing of a small lateral clavicular segment would be difficult; (c) underlying acromioclavicular arthropathy; (d) fractures lateral to the trapezoid origin; and (e) fractures that involve the coracoclavicular ligament origin as an inferiorly displaced fragment.

The patient is placed in the beach-chair position. A Mayfield or McConnell head holder is helpful to allow superior access to the shoulder. The C-arm fluoroscopic image intensifier is brought in from the opposite side of the operative table and positioned for a true scapular AP image with a 15-degree cephalic tilt. The shoulder is prepped and draped with the arm free. An incision is made in Langer's lines, positioned midway between the coracoid process and the acromioclavicular joint to permit access to both locations. The incision extends from the posterior aspect of the clavicle down to the coracoid. Large subcutaneous flaps are raised superficial to the deltotrapezial fascia. The fascia is then sharply divided along the length of the exposed clavicle, over the fracture site, and to the acromioclavicular joint. Care is taken to leave the incised fascia thick for closure. The fracture site is exposed and cleaned of debris. The acromioclavicular joint is inspected. If the intra-articular disc is torn, it is excised. Typically the joint surface is undisturbed. The anterior deltoid is raised as a flap off the medial segment. Mobilizing the deltoid will usually allow access to the base of the coracoid process. If not, the deltoid can be split longitudinally toward the base of the coracoid process. Adequate exposure of the base of the coracoid is essential.

If the lateral fracture segment is not comminuted and the patient is a good candidate for fracture healing, the fracture is reduced. Otherwise, the fractured lateral segment is completely excised. Roughened edges are smoothed with a rasp. By displacing the arm superiorly, the coracoclavicular interval is reduced in a superoinferior direction. The anterior border of the remaining clavicle is then held in line with the anterior acromion. The horizontal distance between the clavicle and acromion should approximate the width of the excised clavicular segment. While the reduction is held, a coracoclavicular stabilization screw with washer is placed. I prefer a 6.5-mm partially threaded cancellous screw with washer. Typically, the clavicle is drilled with a 4.5-mm drill bit, but the coracoid is only drilled with a 3.2-mm drill. As the screw is placed, the fracture is held reduced with upward force on the arm (Fig. 32-28A,B).

The deltotrapezial fascia is then closed with braided, nonabsorbable suture. Toward the fracture and acromioclavicular joint, attempt is made to oversew and imbricate this closure because this tissue will help restore AP stability to the

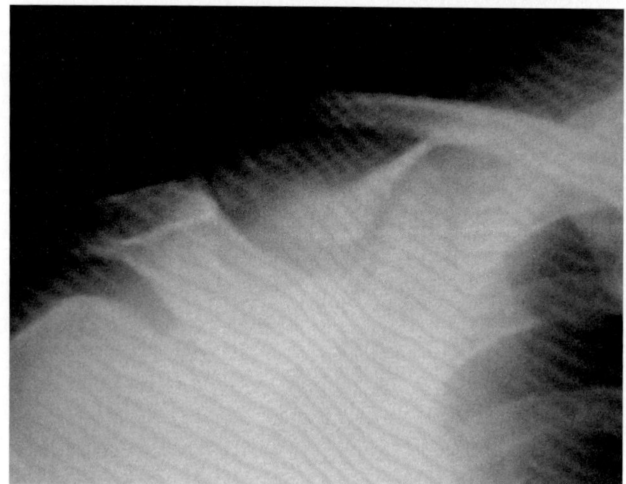

A

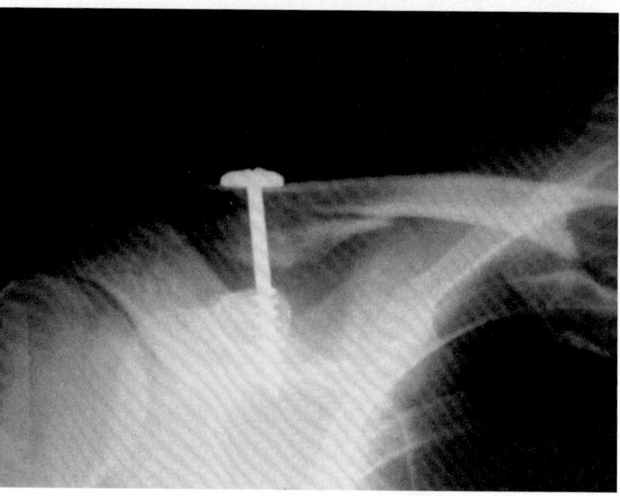

B

FIGURE 32-28 **A.** A 55-year-old woman with a history of osteoporosis had a Type II distal clavicle fracture. **B.** The patient was treated surgically with excision of the distal clavicle and coracoclavicular stabilization.

acromioclavicular joint. The subcutaneous tissue is closed with absorbable suture, and the skin is closed with a running, nonabsorbable, monofilament subcuticular suture. A simple sling is preferred over an immobilizer because the goal of postoperative protection is support not immobilization.

Postoperatively, the sling is maintained for 3 weeks. Typically, no therapy is needed. If the patient shows some minimal stiffness, a supine stretching program is begun. Pendulum exercises are avoided because these simply accentuate the displacing force. Use of the arm for light activities of daily living is permitted. The coracoclavicular screw is removed under local anesthesia 3 months postoperatively. Heavy lifting and contact sports are restricted for 6 months.

UNUSUAL FRACTURE PATTERNS

Medial Physeal Separation

It seems strange to discuss "pediatric" injuries in a chapter on clavicle fractures in adults. However, closure of the medial clavicular physis can occur as late as age 25 years, well into adulthood (76). Therefore, medial clavicular fractures or fracture dislocations are often medial physeal separations, even in young adulthood (73,76–78). This fracture is classified by Craig as the Group III, Type IV injury (Fig. 32-11) (39,42,125). The diagnosis should be considered in any medial injury in a patient less than age 25 years. A CT scan is usually needed to adequately clarify fracture displacement. Because epiphyseal injuries have remodeling ability, and considering the potential risks of open treatment adjacent to the mediastinum, most authors have recommended closed treatment for this injury (9,73,76,78). The only absolute indication for surgical treatment is acute vascular or laryngeal compromise secondary to posterior displacement (Fig. 32-29).

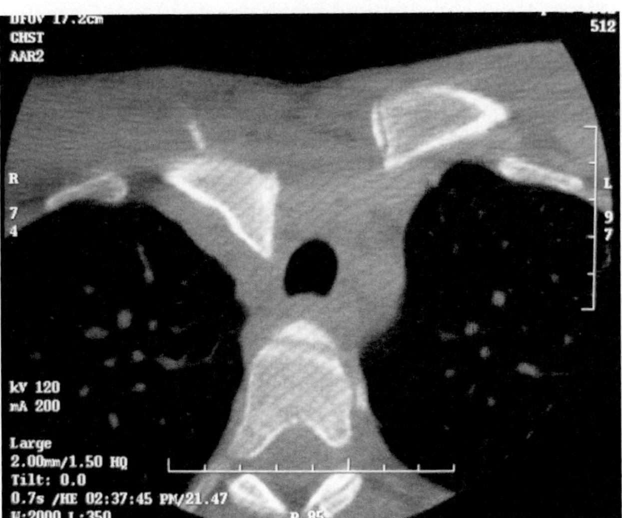

FIGURE 32-29 CT scan of a posterior medial clavicular physeal fracture dislocation in a 17-year-old patient. The treatment was immediate open reduction and stabilization by sternoclavicular capsular reconstruction.

A recent case report of an associated midshaft clavicle fracture and a medial physeal fracture was reported in a 16-year-old lacrosse player (172). This highlights the need to palpate the acromioclavicular, the entire length of the clavicle, and the sternoclavicular joint to avoid concomitant injuries.

Periosteal Sleeve Fractures

Similar to the medial physeal separation, the distal clavicle can become separated from its periosteal sleeve (173,174). This injury has been named "pseudodislocation" of the acromioclavicular joint. In the Craig classification scheme, this fracture is classified as Group II, Type IV (Fig. 32-11) (39,42,125). For this chapter, its importance arises from the fact that it can occur into the third decade of life. Ogden reported 14 cases (174). Most were treated closed, but closed reduction and pinning were performed for severely displaced injuries. Remodeling was universal and the results were good.

Midshaft Fractures with AC Separation

Wurtz and associates reported four cases of middle third clavicle fracture with concomitant acromioclavicular separation (175). In three of these patients, the acromioclavicular separation was displaced enough to require operative treatment. The clavicle fracture itself was treated closed. Other authors have provided case reports of this combination injury (176,177). Good results have been reported after surgical (177) or nonsurgical (176) treatment. Juhn and Simonian (178) reported a Type VI (clavicle-inferior) acromioclavicular dislocation associated with a midshaft clavicle fracture in a 21-year-old hockey player. Apparently the patient returned to hockey with nonoperative treatment. The authors cite conservative treatment was likely effective because the acromioclavicular dislocation was only subacromial and not subcoracoid.

Elliot reported a case of clavicle fracture with acromioclavicular separation and sternoclavicular dislocation (179). Case reports of these so-called bipolar injuries, dislocations at both ends of the clavicle or fracture at one end and a dislocation at the other, continue to be reported (180,181). An unusual pattern of injury was recently described by Pearsall and Russell (182). A 16-year-old wrestler had a midshaft clavicle fracture and ipsilateral sternoclavicular subluxation. According to the authors, a CT scan confirmed the sternoclavicular joint injury without medial physeal displacement. The patient also developed a long thoracic nerve palsy manifested by scapular winging 3 weeks after injury. Treatment included a Thoraco-Lumbo-Sacral-Orthosis brace to maintain the scapula against the chest wall and limit traction of the nerve during recovery and therapy. The authors stated that outcome was excellent.

Given the infrequency of this fracture pattern, individualized treatment is needed. First and most important is recognizing the injury (Fig. 32-30A). In this situation, consideration should be given to operative fixation of either or both sites (Fig. 32-30B). Given the severity of injury, late problems may develop (Fig. 32-30C).

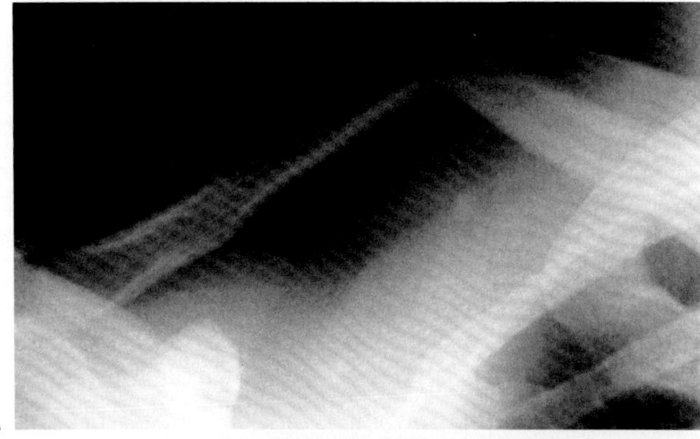

A

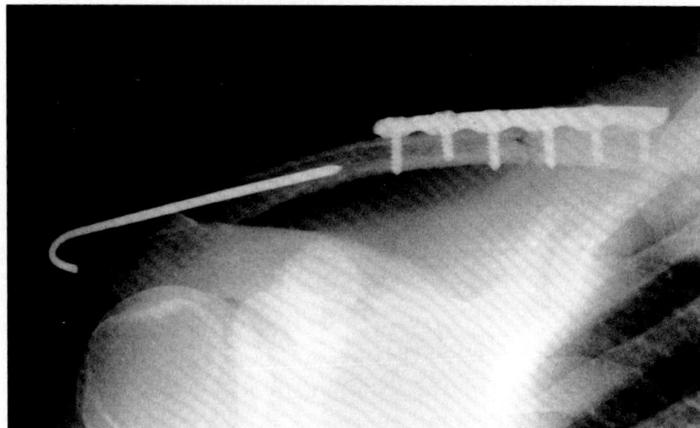

B

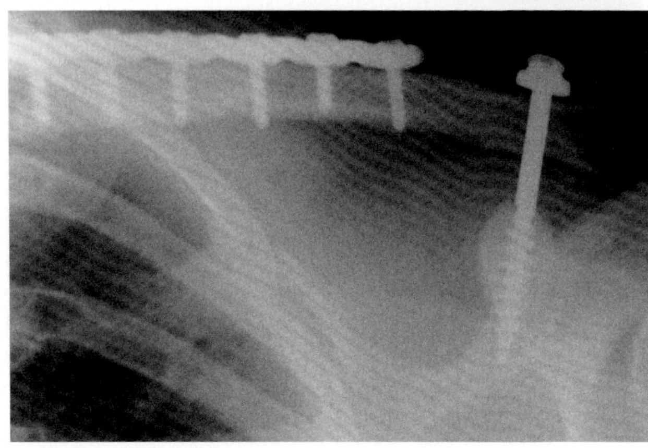

C

FIGURE 32-30 **A.** Midshaft clavicle fracture with concomitant acromioclavicular separation. **B.** The injury was treated by open plating of the clavicle with open transacromial pinning of the acromioclavicular joint. **C.** The patient later required distal clavicle excision and formal acromioclavicular stabilization and coracoacromial ligament transfer.

Floating Shoulder

Combined fracture of the clavicle and glenoid neck has been referred to as a floating shoulder. In a simple scapular neck fracture, the glenoid may still be held in appropriate orientation through the coracoacromial and coracoclavicular attachments to the intact clavicle. For the combined injury, that stability was thought to be lost (Fig. 32-31). Herscovici and colleagues reported this combination injury in seven patients (50). Treatment was plate fixation of the clavicle and closed treatment of the glenoid neck fracture. In all seven of their patients excellent functional results were achieved, without residual deformity. Hashiguchi and Ito also reported good results with clavicle fixation alone with either plate or Kirschner wires (183).

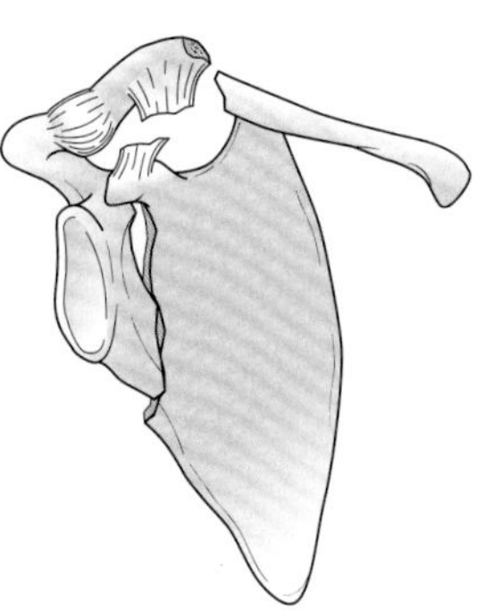

FIGURE 32-31 Stability to the glenoid may be lost for combined fractures of the glenoid neck and clavicle.

Leung and Lam recommended ORIF of both the scapular neck and clavicle fractures in the presence of a floating shoulder (52). Of the clavicle fractures in this group, 10 were located in the middle third, four in the lateral third, and one in the medial third. Five fractures were comminuted, demonstrating the significant trauma associated with this injury. The authors reported good or excellent functional results in 14 of 15 patients treated in this manner.

In contrast, Ramos et al reported nonoperative treatment for ipsilateral fracture of the scapula and clavicle (184). Their study included 16 patients, with a distribution of clavicular fracture pattern similar to that described by Leung and Lam (52). All fractures healed. Eleven of their patients were pain free and returned to vigorous activity. Even a patient who had a malunion of a glenoid neck fracture had an excellent functional outcome. Three patients, however, had significant asymmetry of the shoulder girdle. Similarly, Williams et al presented an evaluation of 9 of 11 patients who had ipsilateral clavicle and glenoid neck fractures and were treated nonoperatively (185). Results were five excellent, one good, and three fair. There was a statistically significant inverse relationship between medial glenoid displacement and functional outcome, with displacement of less than 3.0 cm associated with a better result. The authors recommended nonoperative treatment for those patients with less than 3.0 cm of medial glenoid displacement.

Egol et al (186) retrospectively examined 19 patients with a displaced clavicle fracture or acromioclavicular injury complex and displaced glenoid neck fracture. Twelve patients were treated nonoperatively, and seven patients were treated with ORIF of both disruptions. Both treatment groups were deemed to have done well. The mean forward flexion in the operative group was better (176 degrees) than the nonoperative group (153 degrees). There was a trend for better external and internal rotation strength in the nonsurgically treated group. This disappeared when normalization for hand dominance was done. The authors concluded they could advocate surgical or nonoperative treatment for displaced floating shoulder injuries. No description of the amount of displacement individual fractures exhibited was provided.

Edwards and colleagues reported on 20 floating shoulder injuries, all of which were treated nonoperatively (187). Included in the study were 11 clavicle fractures that were displaced 10 mm or more and five scapular fractures displaced greater than 5 mm. Nine patients were pleased, seven were satisfied, three were dissatisfied, and one was unhappy with their outcome. One of the three dissatisfied patients and the sole unhappy patient had clavicular displacement greater than 10 mm. The authors concluded that nonoperative treatment was certainly the treatment of choice for minimally displaced floating shoulders.

The same authors published a subsequent study examining the factors associated with the SF-36 outcome of the same group of patients (188). Only 40% of the patients had good or excellent results in terms of the SF-36 form despite 20 of 20 and 17 of 20 scoring good or excellent according to the rating system of Herscovici and Rowe, respectively. Edwards et al (188) found that so-called nonphysical factors such as emotion and mental health seemed more closely associated with the injury itself. They commented that the SF-36 form questions were probably too broad for an isolated condition such as a floating shoulder.

Recently, several articles have helped in elucidating those floating shoulder injuries that will do well with nonsurgical management from those that should be stabilized. A biomechanical cadaver study performed by Williams et al (189) examined Goss's concept of the superior shoulder suspensory complex. This ring, consisting in part of soft tissue and in part bone (glenoid, coracoid, coracoclavicular ligaments, distal clavicle, acromioclavicular joint, and acromion), was theorized to become unstable if it was disrupted at two points. Case reports of even triple disruptions of the superior shoulder suspensory complex exist (190,191). The authors performed a serial sectioning study of human cadavers. Instability judged by medial displacement of the glenoid, or a true floating shoulder, did not occur unless both the coracoacromial and coracoclavicular ligaments were disrupted. In other words, all connections, bony and ligamentous, are disrupted between the glenoid and glenohumeral joint to the rest of the scapula and axial skeleton.

van Noort et al (192) retrospectively reviewed 35 patients who had been treated for a floating shoulder; 31 of the 35 of the injuries were initially treated nonsurgically and four by plate fixation of solely the clavicle. Three patients who were treated conservatively required later ORIF of the clavicle, one for nonunion and two for malunion. Good outcome was seen for the nonoperative group unless caudal dislocation of the glenoid was observed. Less than optimal functional result occurred in three of four patients who underwent surgery despite anatomic fixation of the clavicle. These patients all had malunion of their scapular fracture. This prompted the authors to state that ligamentous injuries may preclude the achievement of indirect reduction of the scapula fracture by ORIF of the clavicle.

The pendulum seems to have swung from one extreme to the other and now rests somewhere in the middle. The early contention that all floating shoulder injuries needed to be stabilized was later disproved by multiple reports of good results with conservative treatment. The most recent evidence aided by a biomechanical study state that the truly unstable floating shoulder injuries in which both the coracoclavicular and coracoacromial ligaments are torn would benefit from stabilization. Unfortunately, it is difficult to assess and no clear consensus exists on how to judge radiographically when this occurs.

For displaced fractures (Fig. 32-32B), operative intervention should be considered for the following:

1. medial glenoid displacement of greater than 3.0 cm
2. clavicle displacement that meets indications for open reduction
3. multiple trauma with the need for upper extremity weightbearing as soon as possible
4. greater than 40 degrees of abnormal glenoid version

It is apparent that, if operative intervention is needed, patients can often do well with clavicular fixation alone (Fig. 32-33A,B). However, a recent case report of failure of fixation of a floating shoulder after plate fixation alone in two patients was described. Oh et al (193) recommended that if the scapular fracture remains unreduced after ORIF of the clavicle, fixation of the surgical neck may also be required to prevent failure of fixation. If anatomic reconstruction of the clavicle fails to reorient the glenoid, fixation of the scapular neck fracture may also be necessary.

FRACTURE COMPLICATIONS

There are several important complications related to both clavicle fractures and treatments. A thorough understanding of these potential maladies is needed to effectively manage these injuries.

Skin or Soft Tissue Compromise

As with any fracture, the overlying soft tissue envelope must be thoroughly evaluated. As mentioned previously, abrasions

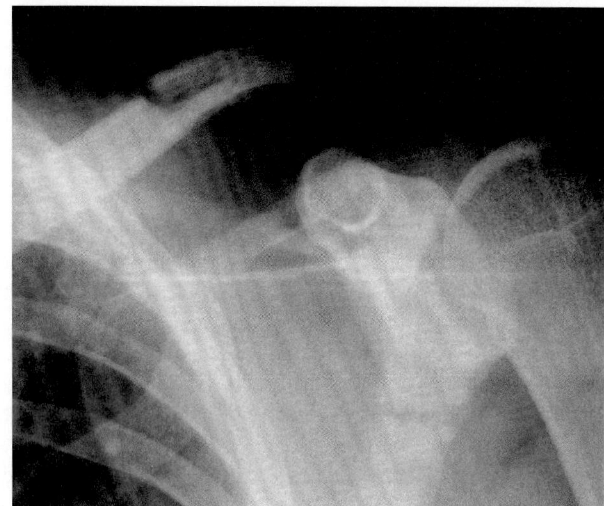

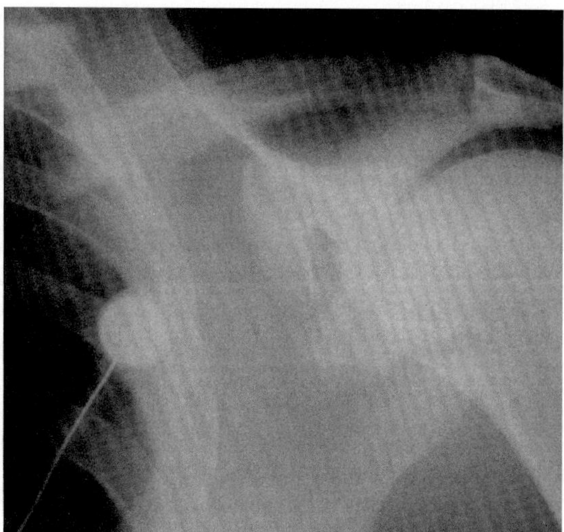

FIGURE 32-32 **A.** Nondisplaced fractures through the clavicle and scapular neck. **B.** Displaced "floating shoulder."

are commonly seen in clavicle fractures. A bump or tenting is commonly seen. What would be more of a concern is actual blanching of the skin that may signal impending skin compromise. Mandalia et al (194) recently reported a case in which impending skin compromise secondary to a displaced, comminuted midshaft clavicle fracture was treated with extraperiosteal excision of a bony spike.

Neurovascular Compromise

Clavicle fractures are often the result of high-energy trauma. Similarly, brachial plexus traction injuries also result from high energy. It would not be unexpected for the two diagnoses to occur simultaneously, without the fracture being the cause of plexopathy (58). However, the clavicle along with the first rib and the scalene muscles comprise the borders of the thoracic outlet. Therefore, it is not surprising there are instances when the clavicle fracture is clearly the cause of the brachial plexus lesion. Barbier and colleagues (56) reported a posteriorly displaced fracture fragment that resulted in a lesion of the posterior cord. The diagnosis was confirmed by magnetic resonance imaging and electromyography. On exploration, a fracture fragment was found to be pressing against the posterior cord. Similar cases were described by other authors (57,195).

Late brachial plexus lesions have been more commonly seen after clavicle fracture.

Miller and Boswick (196) described four cases of brachial plexopathy that were not present immediately after the traumatic event but developed later related to exuberant callous formation. Della Santa and associates (195) also noted brachial plexus irritation secondary to abundant fracture callous. The

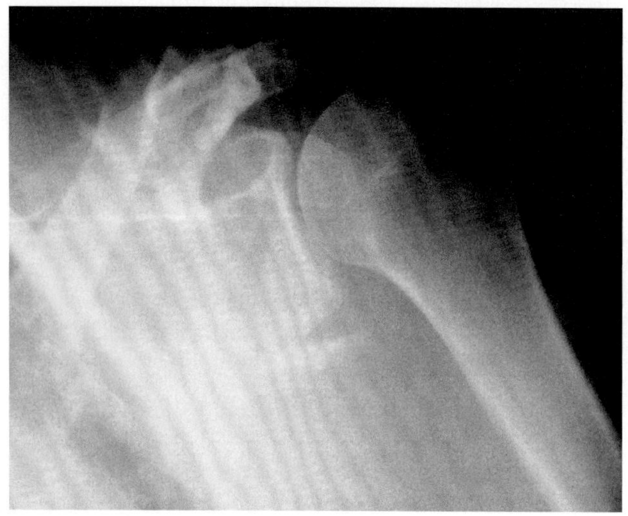

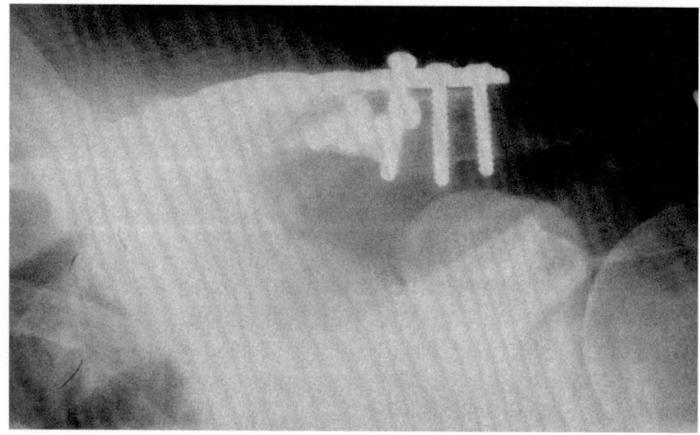

FIGURE 32-33 **A.** Displaced, comminuted clavicle and glenoid neck fractures. **B.** Treatment was by restoration of clavicular length and rigid fixation.

lesion most commonly occurred at the posterior and medial cords and prognosis after surgical excision of excess callous was favorable (195,196).

Several cases of thoracic outlet syndrome (TOS) have recently been reported as a complication of clavicle fracture. Chen and colleagues (197) presented five cases of TOS that began 1 week to 3 years from injury. Two instances of TOS were caused by hypertrophic callous, two by malunion after ORIF of the clavicle fracture, and one by bony fragments. All patients improved after decompression of the neurovascular structures.

Fujita and associates (198) treated a professional bicycle racer with a malunited midshaft clavicle fracture causing severe numbness in the involved upper extremity. The diagnosis of TOS was made on the basis of physical examination, digital subtraction arteriography, nerve conduction velocity tests, and fingertip wave pulse measurements. Decompression was done by resecting a portion of the malunion so that intraoperative wave pulse measurements became normal.

Chen and Liu (199) reported a case of delayed brachial plexus neurapraxia without hypertrophic callous. Nerve irritation was caused by malunited distal clavicle prominence. The diagnosis was confirmed by electromyographic and nerve conduction velocity tests. Symptoms resolved with corrective osteotomy.

An interesting case of TOS after middle third clavicle fracture was presented by Connolly and Ganjianpour (200). The patient underwent a first rib resection that failed to resolve his symptoms. A double osteotomy that consisted of removing the segment of clavicle and reshaping it to a more normal contour was performed. The segment was then returned and fixed with an eight-hole reconstruction plate. The authors caution that a hypertrophic malunion caused by bayonet opposition at the junction of the medial and middle thirds would unlikely be decompressed by a first rib resection alone.

Refracture

The rate of refracture after successful healing of a clavicle fracture is unclear. There are a few reports, particularly in reference to the subsequent increased risk of nonunion after refracture (156,9,201,202). However, an actual incidence of this complication is impossible to determine.

Posttraumatic Arthritis

The development of symptomatic arthritis in the acromioclavicular or sternoclavicular joints after a clavicle fracture is controversial. Clearly, intra-articular fractures can result in arthritic degeneration. The incidence of arthritis related to midshaft fractures, however, is less apparent. Edelson (203) examined 300 clavicle preparations and found nine with healed midclavicle fractures. None of these had any signs of acromioclavicular degeneration, even when the contralateral shoulder demonstrated age-related acromioclavicular changes. He postulated that the shortening associated with a clavicle fracture provided a "physiologic arthroplasty," unloading the acromioclavicular joint (203). Yet, there are times that patients develop acromioclavicular symptoms after midshaft clavicle fractures. These symptoms may be related to disruption of the intra-articular disk at the moment of initial trauma; therefore, radiographs may fail to reveal significant pathology. If a selective injection of the acromioclavicular joint provides temporary complete symptomatic relief, distal clavicle excision is curative.

Malunion

For years, the phrases "clavicle fracture" and "malunion" would have been considered an oxymoron if combined. The goal of treatment was to obtain fracture union. More recent investigators, however, have commented on malunion of clavicle fractures and the subsequent negative functional effects on the shoulder. Hill et al (126), looking only at fractures that healed, found that 2 cm or more of shortening was associated with a poor symptomatic and functional result. On the other hand, Oroko et al (204) examined 41 patients available for follow-up after healing of a clavicle fracture. A Constant and Murley score was tabulated for each patient. The authors could not establish 15 mm as critical value for a low score based on their small patient population.

Bosch and colleagues (205) performed extension osteotomy of the clavicle in four patients who had clavicle malunions. All surgeries were performed for painful shortening, with the range of shortening being 0.9 to 2.2 cm. Patients underwent extension osteotomy and placement of an iliac crest interposition graft. All healed, all had symptomatic improvement, and all had functional improvement. Simpson and Jupiter (201) also reported four cases of clavicular osteotomy for painful shortening, with good functional results. Jupiter et al (9) and Mullaji and Jupiter (147) have discussed this technique elsewhere as well. Wilkes and Halawa (206) reported a case of combined clavicle and scapula fracture in which the clavicle healed with a 60-degree superior bow. Scapular and clavicular osteotomy resulted in improved function and cosmesis. McKee et al (207) treated 15 symptomatic midshaft clavicle malunions with a corrective osteotomy and limited contact dynamic compression plate fixation without bone graft. It is interesting that 11 of the 15 patients had symptoms of TOS. Fourteen of 15 patients had union; one failure of fixation occurred. A significant improvement in DASH scores was observed.

Clearly, although commonly discussed separately, there is a correlation between clavicular malalignment and symptoms of TOS (Fig. 32-34A,B). Several of the reports discussed in the section on TOS involve patients who did not develop excessive callous. Further research into the changes in scapular position and brachial plexus tension that occur with clavicular malposition will hopefully better define this important association.

Nonunion

A fairly extensive discussion of the risk of nonunion has been given in the treatment section. To review, clavicle nonunion is defined as lack of evidence of healing 4 to 6 months after injury (Fig. 32-35) (39,42,202,208,209). The incidence of nonunion has been reported to be between 0.13% and 15% for midshaft

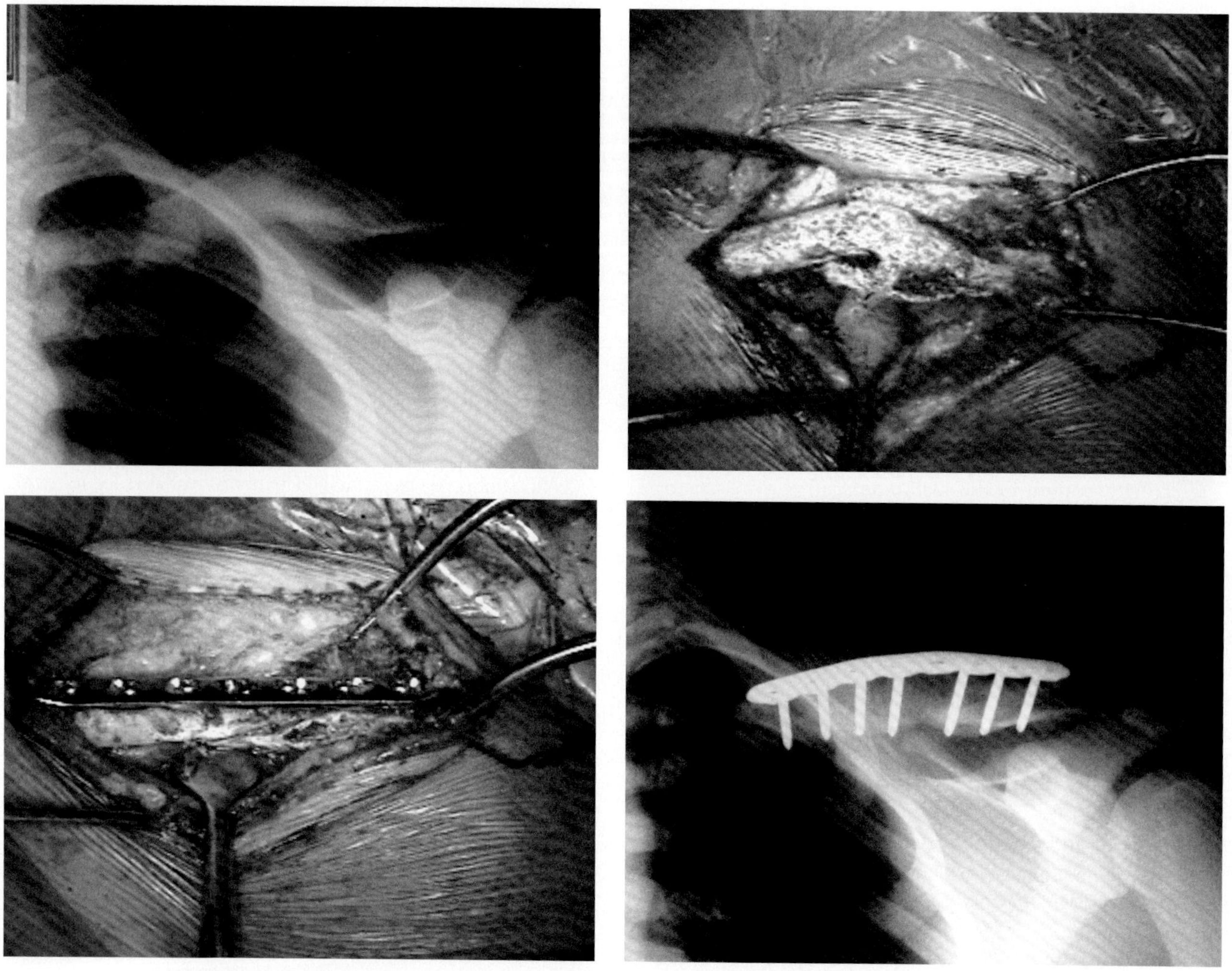

A B C D

FIGURE 32-34 **A.** Clavicular malunion in a young laborer. Initial treatment of excision of excessive fracture callous left the patient with persistent scapular pain and upper extremity paresthesias. **B.** Symptoms were successfully relieved with extension osteotomy of the clavicle. **C.** Intraoperative stabilization of osteotomy with low-contact dynamic compression plate. **D.** Postoperative radiograph showing correction of clavicular malunion.

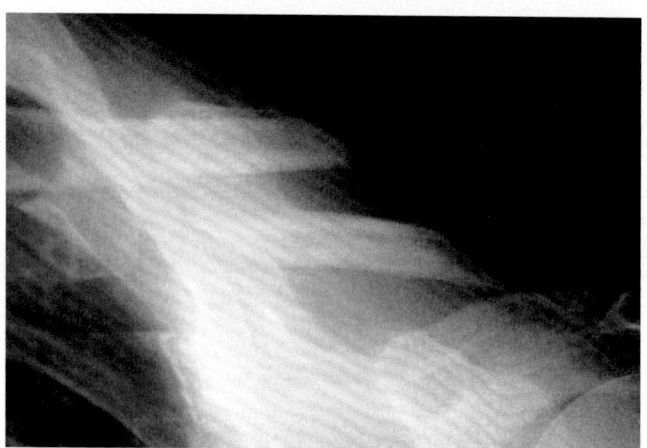

FIGURE 32-35 Established midclavicle nonunion.

fractures (114,210). The rate of nonunion for a Type II distal fracture is higher, as high as 30% or more (10,11,36,37). For midclavicular nonunions, hypertrophic nonunions seem to be more symptomatic than atrophic nonunions (202).

There are several proven and hypothetic causes of nonunion (Table 32-4). Some of these and other potential causes warrant further discussion:

Type II Fracture

Type II distal clavicle fracture has clearly been shown to be a risk factor for nonunion (10,11,36,37,160). Although nonunion may be radiographically present, many nonunions are asymptomatic (10,202). Nordqvist and associates (40) found that as many as 80% of Type II distal clavicle nonunions may be only minimally symptomatic. Rokito et al (11) found that five of seven Type II nonunions in their study were asymptomatic.

TABLE 32-4 Factors Associated with Development of Nonunion

Type II fracture
Fracture shortening of ≥20 mm
Fracture displacement of >20 mm
Increasing patient age
Increasing severity of trauma
Refracture
Primary open reduction?

Degree of Displacement

Shortening (116,117) or displacement (156) of 2 cm or more is associated with subsequent nonunion. Displacement to the point of potential soft-tissue interposition may be an important variable (208). Given the connection between the variables of displacement, shortening, and soft-tissue interposition, it is impossible to quantify which of these are the more significant independent predictors of nonunion.

Severity of Trauma

The more severe the initial trauma the higher the rate of subsequent nonunion (115,202). Although retrospectively quantifying the amount of initial trauma may be difficult when faced with a nonunion, Wilkins and Johnston (202) demonstrated a significant relationship between these factors.

Refracture

Refracture has clearly been demonstrated as an independent risk factor for nonunion (156,202). In the review of Wilkins and Johnston (202), 7 of their 31 patients had a midshaft nonunion that occurred after refracture. The length of time from initial to second fracture did not appear to be a significant prognostic factor.

Duration/Type of Immobilization

The duration of immobilization has long been considered a causative factor for the development of nonunion. Rowe (44) believed that immobilization should be continued for 4 to 6 weeks or longer, but absolutely until there was clear evidence of healing. Yet, neither the duration (202) nor the method (84) of immobilization has been clearly demonstrated to be a causative factor in the development of nonunion. Given the results of the controlled study of Andersen et al (84), as well as the great difficulty in immobilizing a clavicle with any technique, duration and type of immobilization are likely not significant contributors to nonunion.

Closed Reduction

Logically, a treating physician would think that closed reduction of a displaced fracture, particularly in the face of soft-tissue interposition, would result in an improved rate of healing. A manipulative closed reduction before immobilization has, however, not been found to alter the healing course in midshaft fractures (116,210).

Primary Open Reduction

Although some investigators postulated that open reduction was a risk factor for nonunion (44,111), there was clearly a bias toward more displaced fractures requiring open treatment; therefore, the relationship between open treatment as an independent variable and development of nonunion is still unclear. A more recent report of a relatively low nonunion rate of 3% in the acute plating of 232 completely displaced midshaft clavicle fractures has been published (151). This may highlight the fact that with modern fixation techniques, the nonunion rates may be relatively low.

TREATMENT OF NONUNION

The primary indications for treatment of an established nonunion are pain and functional impairment. There is no indication for the treatment of an asymptomatic nonunion. There are several treatment options. Each has vocal advocates and opponents. Each has clear advantages and disadvantages.

Electrical Stimulation and Low-Intensity Pulse Ultrasound

The literature contains few reports on the use of electrical stimulation in the treatment of established clavicle nonunion (211–213). Given the excellent results of surgical reconstruction, however, there are currently few indications for the use of electrical stimulation over other methods of achieving union (9,39,42). Similarly, scant evidence exists for the use of low-intensity pulsed ultrasound in clavicular nonunions (214). These techniques should be considered only when surgical intervention is impossible.

Open Bone Graft and Immobilization

There are few reports of bone grafting without fixation. Wilkins and Johnston (202) discussed three patients who had undergone this treatment method. Two of three patients failed to have union after this procedure. Given the severe deforming forces present in a nonunion setting, it seems unlikely that this technique would be associated with a significant degree of success.

Open Bone Graft and Screw Fixation

In the past, screw fixation of corticocancellous grafts was viewed as an effective technique for the treatment of midshaft nonunions (108,215). Advances in fixation technique make this

ing group and none in the intramedullary fixation group. The authors recommend intramedullary fixation as the better technique. However, the two nonunions in the intramedullary group were subsequently treated with plate fixation and both achieved solid union.

Clavicular Excision. The final treatment option for an established nonunion is clavicle excision (13,14,110,202,240). In the review by Wilkins and Johnston (202), five midshaft nonunions were treated with partial excision of the nonunion. Three of them had only minor pain, two being fully functional. Middleton and colleagues (240), in a procedure derived from that of Gurd (16), excised the clavicle lateral to the fracture in six National Hunt Jockeys who had a nonunion. All six were pleased and returned to competition. Wood discussed total claviculectomy for several indications, one of which was nonunion (14), and demonstrated good functional results. If we accept the important biomechanical functions of the clavicle (see "Biomechanics"), then partial or complete clavicle excision should be considered a salvage procedure.

Free-Fibular Vascularized Transfer. For recalcitrant midshaft clavicular nonunions, the use of a free-fibular vascularized graft is a surgical option. Momberger and colleagues reported on three cases treated in this manner, all going on to union. On average, each patient had 3.7 prior surgical attempts at obtaining union. Clearly, this would be an option to be used in rare circumstances and after failure of other fixation techniques.

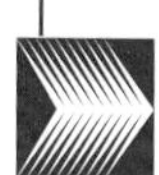

AUTHORS' PREFERRED TREATMENT

Midshaft Nonunion

My preferred technique for the treatment of a midshaft nonunion is open bone-grafting and plate fixation. This method is favored over intramedullary fixation for several reasons:

1. improved rotational stability
2. ability to incorporate an intercalary graft
3. no fear of implant migration

In my experience, there have been two near-universal findings during surgical treatment of this lesion. First, in either atrophic or hypertrophic nonunion, the clavicular ends are usually sclerotic and require some degree of resection. Second, even without resection, there is usually a degree of shortening that, with the clavicle brought out to normal length, results in a fracture gap that requires an intercalary graft. This pathology is better approached by open plating, incorporating an intercalary corticocancellous graft, than by intramedullary methods.

The patient is positioned in the beach-chair position. A Mayfield or McConnell headrest is used to provide complete access for use of instruments superior to the clavicle. A 10″ × 12″ radiographic cassette is placed under the padding of the operative table and positioned optimally for intraoperative radiographs. Before draping, an umbilical tape is used to measure the distance from the jugular notch of the manubrium to the acromioclavicular joint of the normal shoulder (Fig. 32-39A,B). Knots are tied in the tape at the appropriate

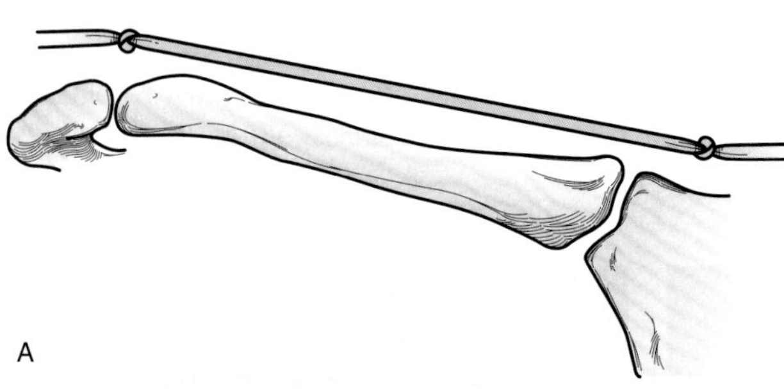

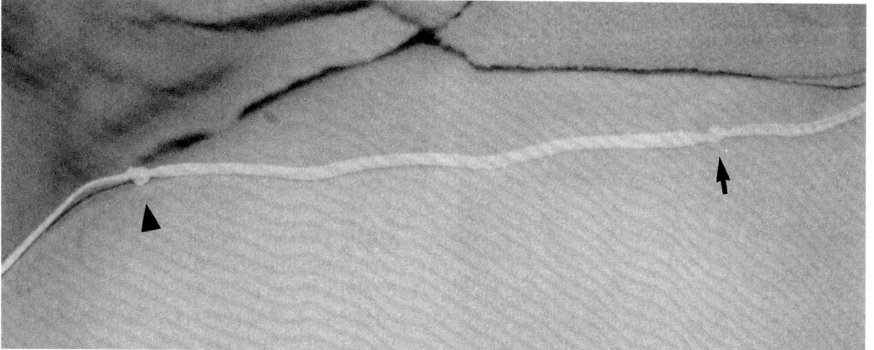

FIGURE 32-39 A,B. An umbilical tape is used to measure the length from the jugular notch of the manubrium (*arrow*) to the acromioclavicular joint (*arrowhead*) of the normal shoulder. The tape is then sterilized for intraoperative use.

measurements, and the umbilical tape is sterilized. The entire shoulder girdle is prepped including the sternum, in case emergency proximal vascular access becomes necessary. The arm is draped free for intraoperative manipulation.

Incision is made along the length of the clavicle, centered on the nonunion site. I recommend sharply carrying the incision through the subcutaneous tissue and platysma, leaving the skin flaps thick. I do not dissect the supraclavicular nerves. I have not found any detrimental effects from cutting these nerves, and because soft tissue disruption is a major postoperative risk, I have concerns about potentially thinning these tissues to search for the supraclavicular nerves. The overlying fascia and periosteum are next divided. This step is performed sharply and down to bone, again leaving thick flaps for later closure. The division is started medial and lateral to the nonunion site and then proceeds to the nonunion. Occasionally, particularly in hypertrophic nonunions, the fracture line may be difficult to locate (Fig. 32-40A). A scalpel is useful in probing the callous mass until the nonunion site is entered (Fig. 32-40B). The osseous ends are then circumferentially freed from surrounding tissues. At the junction of the medial and middle thirds of the clavicle, the inferior surface is exposed so a protective instrument can be inserted during drilling.

Once the nonunion is taken down, the character and pattern of the osseous configuration are identified. There are two choices for operative fixation, and the technique depends on the character of the clavicular ends. If the fracture ends are relatively flat, resection of atrophic bone is performed in a manner to preserve this flat surface, the operative goal being intercalary grafting and 3.5-mm DC locking plate fixation, similar to the method of Jupiter and Ring (9) (Fig. 32-36). If there is some obliquity to the fracture ends, that pattern leads toward lag-screw fixation. Although further resection of the atrophic and sclerotic bone may be necessary, the oblique pattern is maintained (Fig. 32-41A,B). Once the atrophic bone is resected, vascular channels are drilled in the cortical ends (Fig. 32-41C). Although the clavicle normally lacks a true medullary canal, one is drilled to promote vascular invasion.

Once the nonunion site is prepared, the previously sterilized umbilical tape is used to determine the true clavicular length. One knot is placed at the jugular notch. The scapula is then displaced laterally until the lateral knot lies at the acromioclavicular joint. The resultant separation in the fracture ends is measured. If choosing lag screw fixation, remember that, although the fracture ends are oblique, the graft will be rectangular. Therefore, the distance must be measured from the furthest points of obliquity, not the closest. Also, the graft must be 1 cm longer than the defect because it is beneficial to create cancellous "plugs" in the graft to lock into the created intramedullary canals of the host clavicle. A tri-cortical graft is then harvested from the contralateral iliac crest, and cancellous graft is also removed. The contralateral crest is harvested so that if the patient requires an ambulatory aid secondary to discomfort at the crest, he or she will have a weight-bearing upper extremity available.

Although any number of bony configurations are possible, there are three consistent patterns. These patterns are not fracture specific but "end" specific. That is, either fracture end may have any pattern. I make every attempt to "fit" the nonunion ends into one of these configurations, which then guides graft sculpting and plate and screw configuration.

The first pattern is simple longitudinal. With this configuration, the fracture ends are relatively straight in both the sagittal and coronal planes. As such, the pattern best fits intercalary graft placement and superior plate fixation as per the technique of Jupiter and Ring (9). A rectangular graft is fashioned

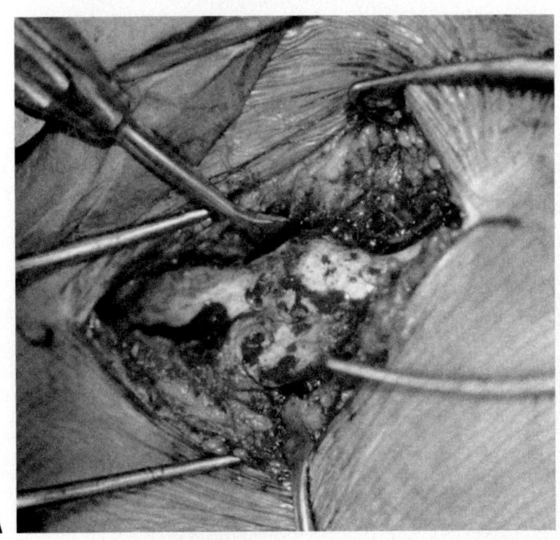
A

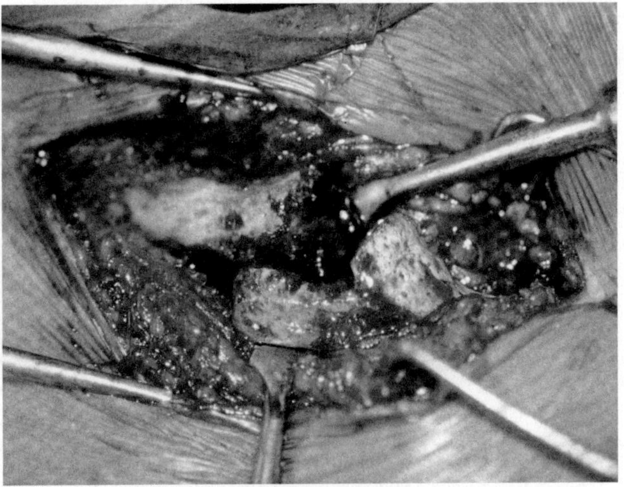
B

FIGURE 32-40 **A.** In a hypertrophic nonunion, identifying the true nonunion site may be difficult. **B.** A scalpel is helpful to probe the osseous mass and locate the site of separation.

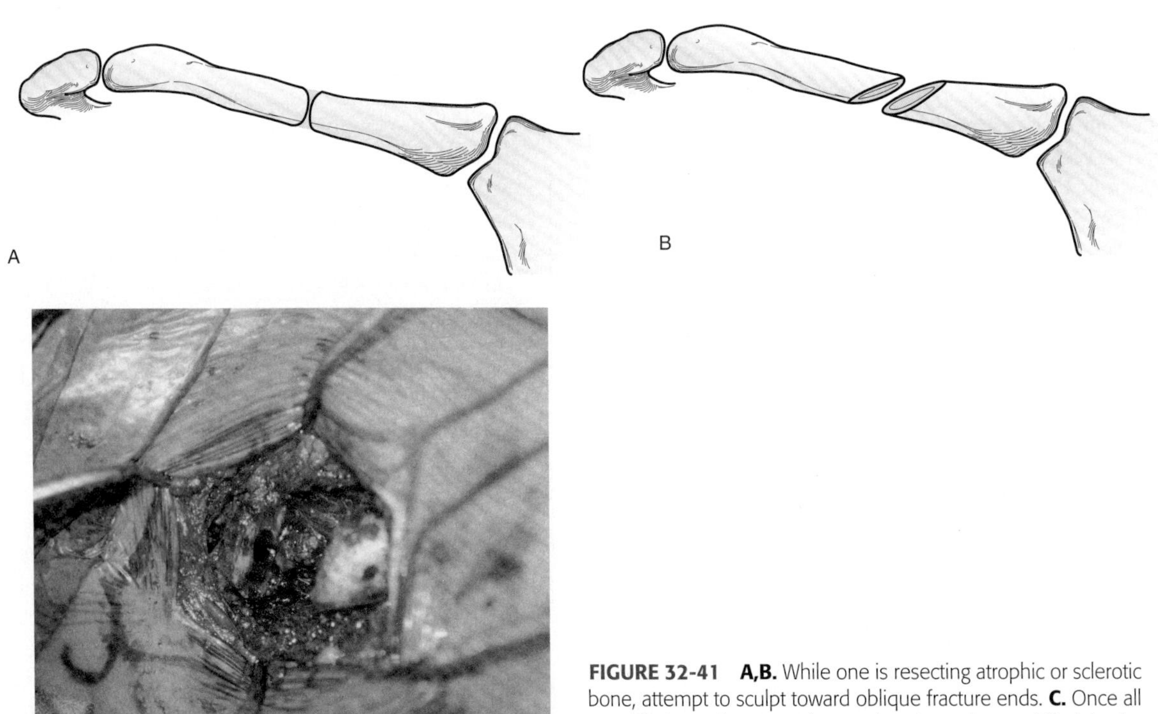

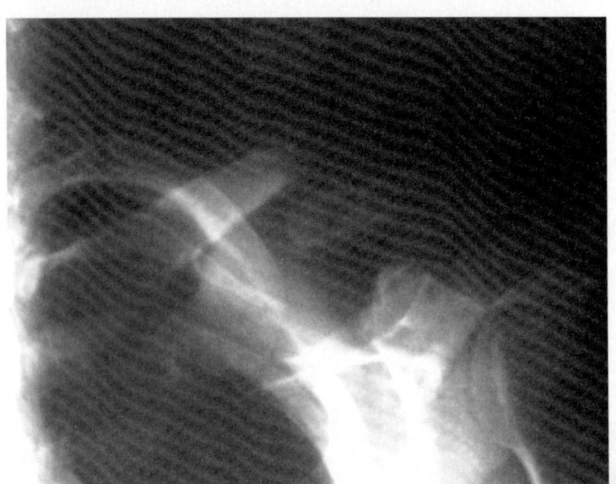

FIGURE 32-41 A,B. While one is resecting atrophic or sclerotic bone, attempt to sculpt toward oblique fracture ends. **C.** Once all atrophic bone is resected, vascular channels are drilled in the fracture ends.

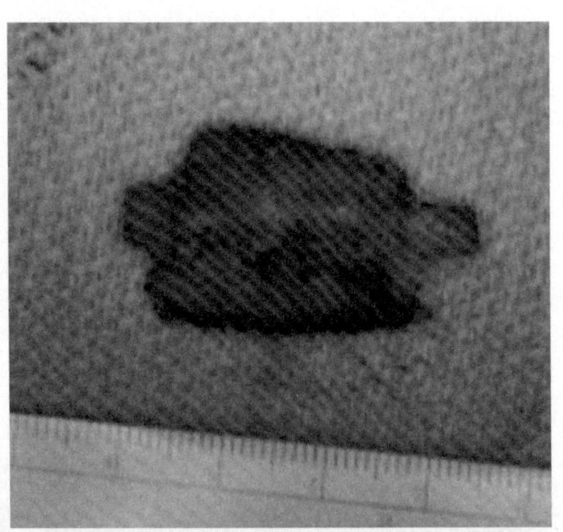

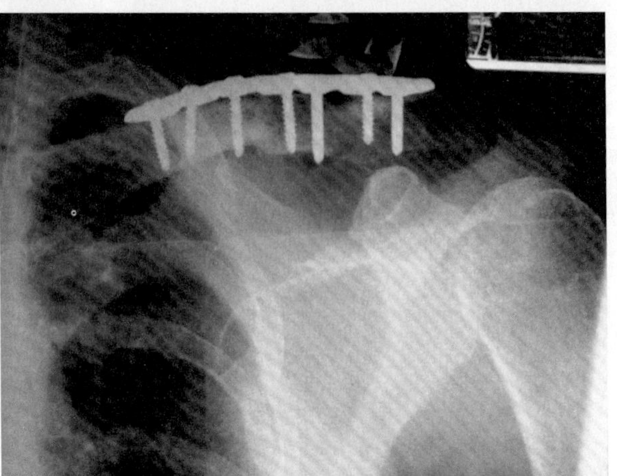

FIGURE 32-42 A. Established atrophic clavicular nonunion. **B,C.** The patient underwent open reduction, placement of an intercalary corticocancellous autograft, and fixation with a superiorly placed 3.5-mm DC locking plate.

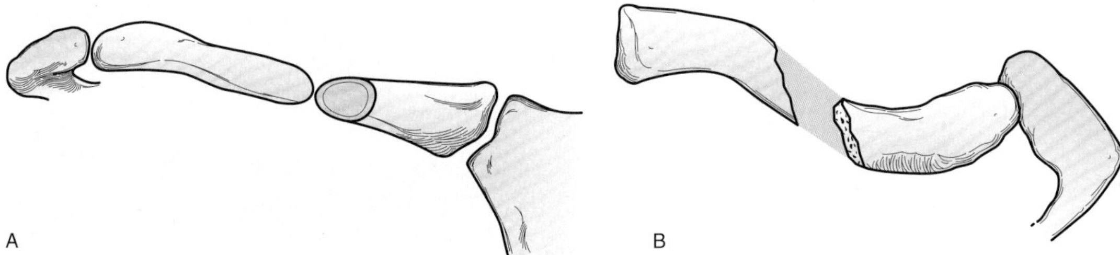

FIGURE 32-43 AP **(A)** and axial **(B)** views of a coronal oblique nonunion pattern.

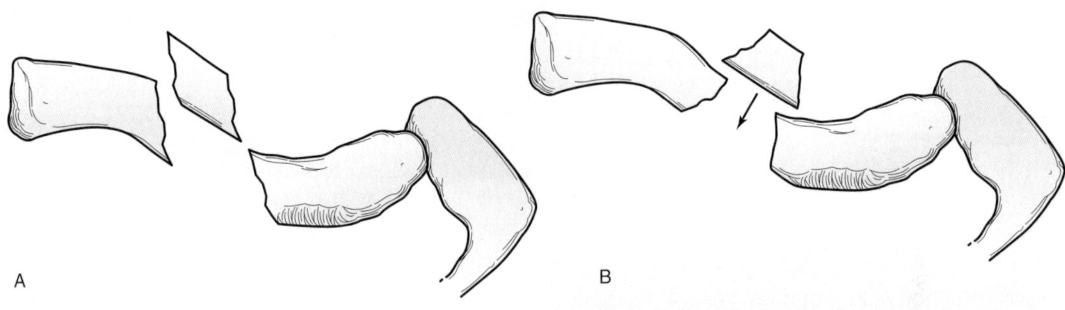

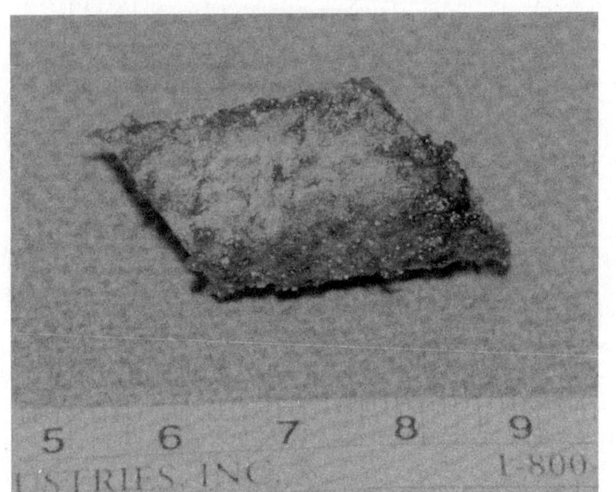

FIGURE 32-44 **A–C.** Depending on the direction of obliquity, a corticocancellous graft is fashioned in either a parallelogram or keystone configuration.

with ½-cm cancellous bone plugs at either end. The graft should be oriented with a cortical surface inferiorly. This provides a cortical surface for screw fixation and places a cortical surface on the compression side of the bone. Once the graft is keyed into the nonunion site, the construct will already attain a provisional stability. A 3.5-mm DC locking plate is placed along the superior clavicular surface. The plate should be positioned in such a way as to permit at least one locking screw in the intercalary graft (Fig. 32-42A,B).

The second pattern is coronal plane obliquity (Figs. 32-43 and Fig. 32-44A,B). For this shape, the tricortical graft is fashioned as either a parallelogram or keystone, depending on the direction of obliquity. Orientation of the graft is extremely important. The graft must be placed in a configuration such that there will be cortical surfaces available for lag screw placement and a cortical surface inferiorly on the compression side of the bone (Fig. 32-45). The graft is fashioned and fixed with bicortical lag screws (Fig. 32-46A,B).

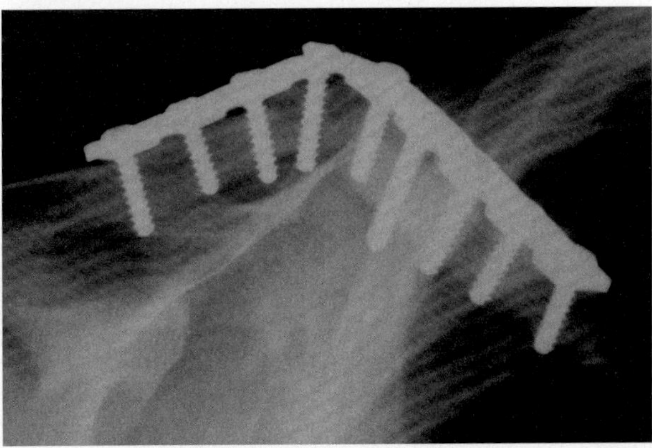

FIGURE 32-45 The intercalary graft must be fashioned such that a cortical surface is placed inferiorly on the compression side of the clavicle. Failure to sculpt the graft in this configuration may lead to graft collapse and hardware failure.

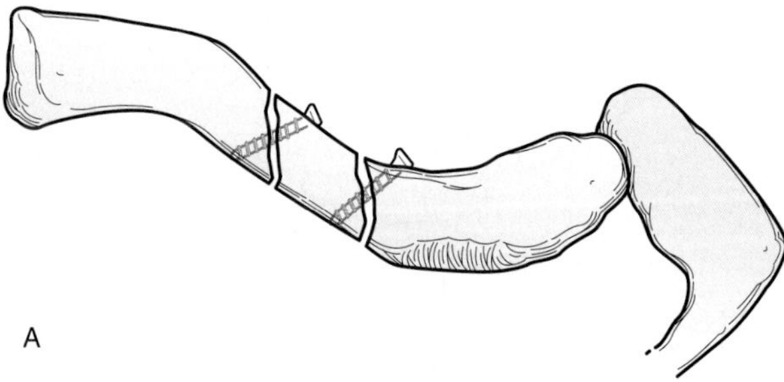

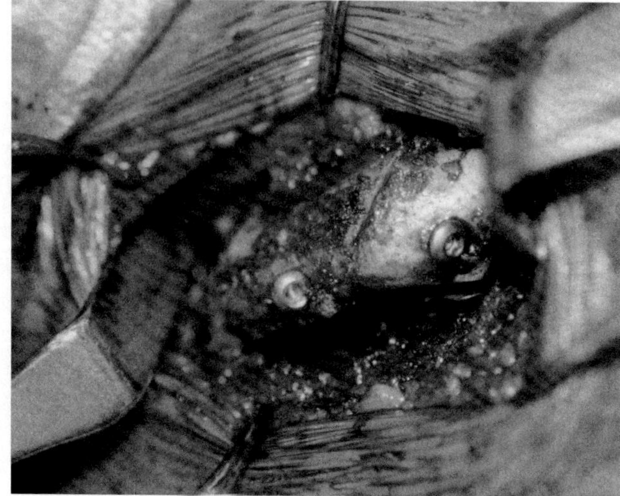

FIGURE 32-46 A,B. Once the graft is fashioned, it is fixed in place with bi-cortical lag screws.

In this pattern, a superior neutralization plate placed on the tension side of the bone is appropriate. For shorter nonunions, a 3.5-mm DC locking plate can be placed. Usually, to fit the s-shaped axial curve of the clavicle, the plate will be prominent anteromedially and posterolaterally or twisted such that it is more anterior than superior on the medial segment. Alternatively, a 3.5-mm reconstruction plate is easier to fit and, in combination with lag screw fixation, is mechanically sound (Fig. 32-47A–D). Cancellous bone is then placed into the host-graft interfaces and along the plate-graft surface.

The third pattern is axial plane obliquity (Fig. 32-

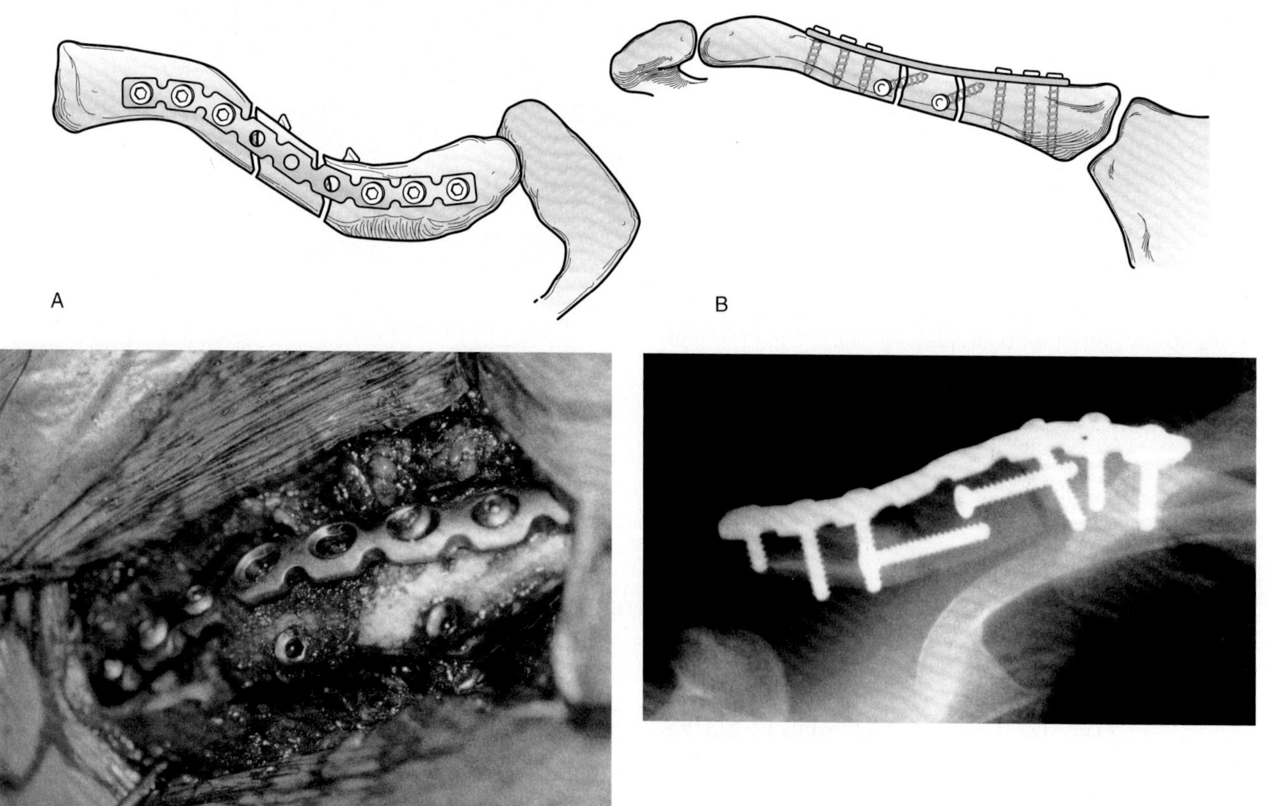

FIGURE 32-47 A–D. Fixation is completed with a superior neutralization plate, either 3.5-mm DC or reconstruction.

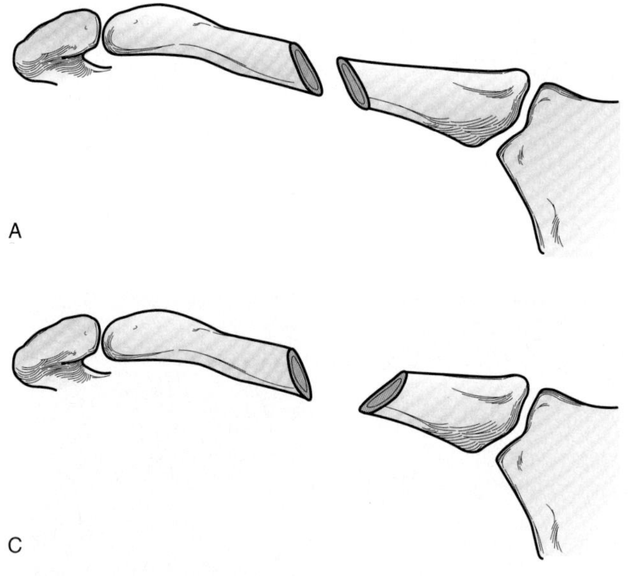

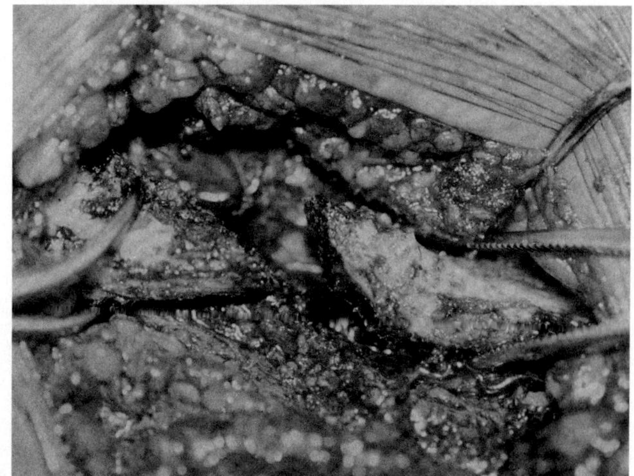

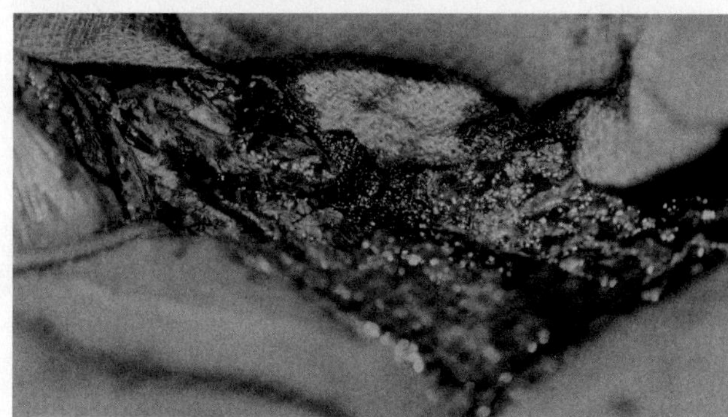

FIGURE 32-48 **A–D.** Axial plane oblique pattern of nonunion.

48A–D). Graft configuration for this pattern is easier, because the inferior cortical surface will suffice for lag screw fixation as well. The graft is fashioned and lagged through the superior plate (Fig. 32-49A–D), and cancellous bone is placed (Fig. 32-49E). Again, for shorter nonunions, a 3.5-mm DC locking plate is preferred. For longer nonunions, the plate is placed obliquely on the bone or it is twisted such that medially the plate is applied more anteriorly on the clavicle with the plate placed on the superior surface laterally. Alternatively, a reconstruction plate is used and molded in the axial plane. Occasionally, I have found it necessary to fix the clavicle straighter in the axial plane than is anatomic to fit a DC plate and lengthy intercalary graft.

Postoperatively, the patient is placed in a simple sling. Shoulder immobilizers are not as effective because the goal of postoperative protection is to assist in elevation, not to hold the arm against the body. After 3 weeks, the sling is removed and gentle, supine, active-assisted forward elevation and external rotation exercises are begun. As discussed earlier, pendulum exercises are contraindicated because downward traction is a major displacing force. After 6 weeks, gentle isometric strengthening is begun with a progressive resistance program beginning 2 months postoperatively. Patients return to light lifting 3 months postoperatively. Heavy lifting is restricted for 6 months, as are contact sports. Patients are advised of a risk of fracture at the ends of the plate should they return to contact athletics.

Most patients who undergo plate fixation of a clavicle nonunion are interested in plate removal. In its subcutaneous position, the plate is often palpable, occasionally visible, and usually bothersome to the patient. Plate removal does offer a good look at graft integration, which is usually substantial and impressive (Fig. 32-50A,B). I wait a minimum of 12 months for plate removal, which lessens the risk of refracture. Contact sports are restricted for 3 months after plate removal.

TREATMENT COMPLICATIONS

Hardware Problems

Almost any imaginable complication from migrating pins has in fact been reported. Pins used to treat clavicle fractures have been found in the aorta (109,241), the mediastinum (242), the lung (243,244), and around and in the spinal canal (242–246). A Kirschner wire used to fix a midshaft clavicle fracture was reported to have passed through the pharynx into the contralateral orbit, causing acute exophthalmos (247). A smooth Steinman pin used to fix a medial clavicle fracture was reportedly expectorated by the patient 1 month after implantation

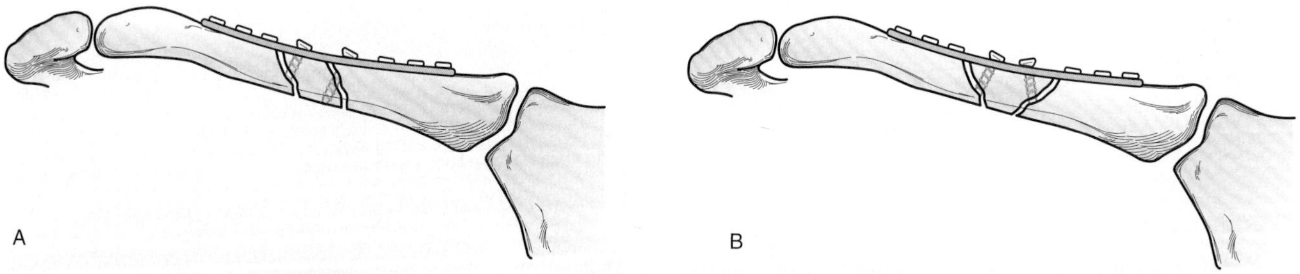

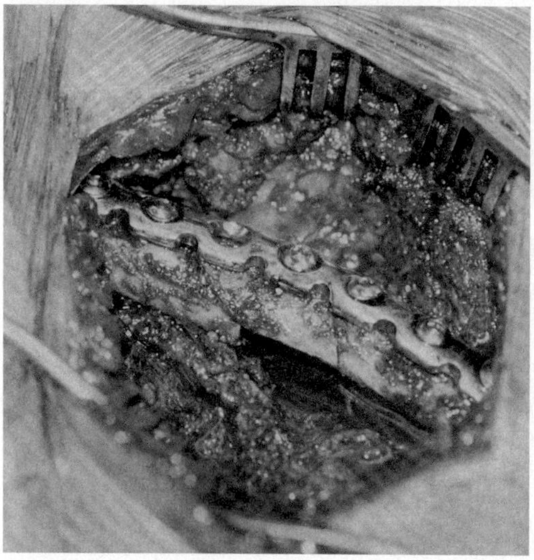

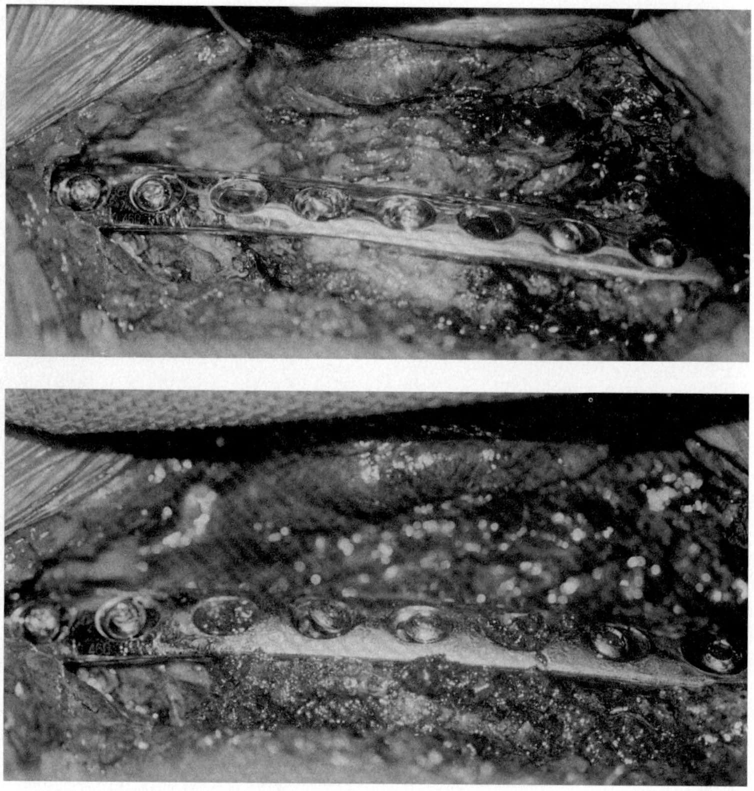

FIGURE 32-49 A–D. For the axial oblique nonunion pattern, the intercalary graft is secured by lag screw fixation to the superior plate. **E.** Cancellous bone is then packed into the graft-host interfaces.

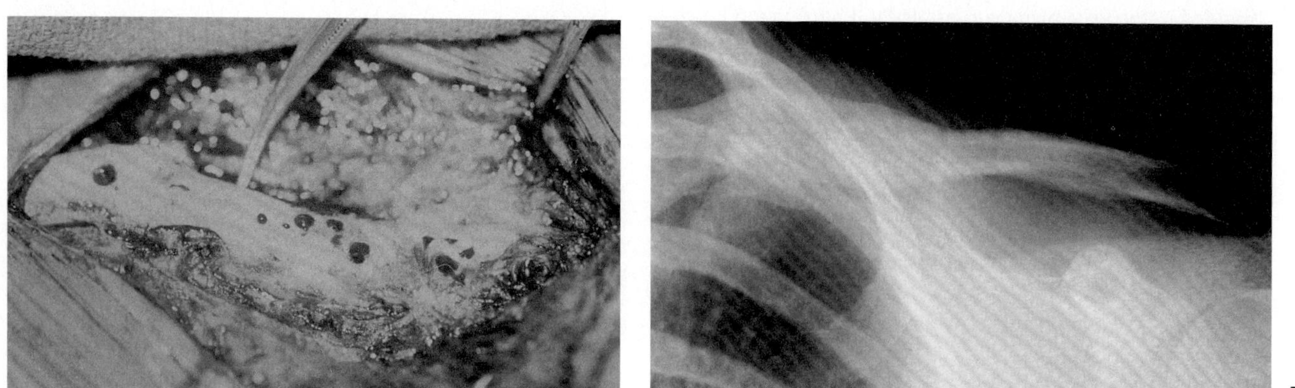

FIGURE 32-50 Complete incorporation of the intercalary graft, as seen during **(A)** and after **(B)** plate removal.

(248). These cases have obvious medical and medicolegal implications (249), and some authors have strongly cautioned against the use of smooth pins about the clavicle (247,250).

Plate failure can also occur (Figs. 32-37B and 32-40). As with fresh fracture fixation, inadequate purchase and plate size are important predictors of failure. Also, collapse of the intercalary graft will ultimately result in hardware failure.

Infection

Infection after operative treatment for fracture or nonunion can be a devastating complication. Bostman et al (251) reported an infection rate of 7.8% after clavicular plating, although most surgeons would consider that rate high. Poigenfurst (153) reported a deep infection rate of 1.2% in his series of 122 plated fractures.

Reconstruction for deep infection or osteomyelitis, particularly in the nonunion situation in which bone loss may be extensive, is often difficult. Initial treatment should include operative debridement. Although consideration can be given to retaining a stable graft-hardware configuration, given the large segment of bone graft often present, typical treatment should include removal of all graft and hardware followed by 6 weeks of intravenous antibiotics. Revision can then be undertaken, aborting surgery for any clinically apparent infection found on operative exploration (Fig. 32-51A–C). Soft tissue coverage is essential (see "Wound Dehiscence"). If major bone loss is encountered, a vascularized graft may be necessary (252).

Wound Dehiscence

Despite its subcutaneous and potentially vulnerable position, soft-tissue loss over the clavicle is rare. In cases of wound dehiscence after clavicular fixation, local adipofascial flap coverage has been described as being successful (253). A recent cadaveric study examined the possibility of using a rotational clavicular portion of pectoralis major flap for soft tissue coverage of the clavicle (254). This flap was used on a patient who had undergone multiple previous operations and had complications of a nonunion and infection. The authors stated the anatomy was consistent and could be harvested without damaging the sternocostal head.

Hypertrophic Scar

In a location as visible as the midclavicle, unsightly scars are a great concern. The potential for a hypertrophic, uncosmetic scar after open plating has been reported (9,143) and is not uncommon (Fig. 32-52). The remedy is scar excision at the time of plate removal.

Refracture

Poigenfurst and associates reported on 122 patients who underwent clavicular plating (153). After plate removal, there were

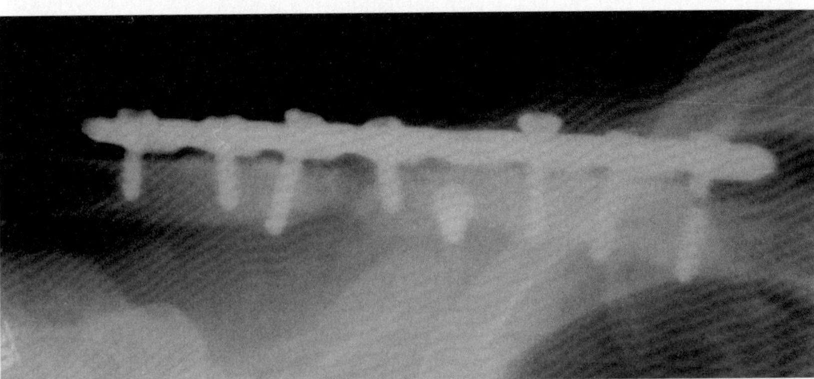

A

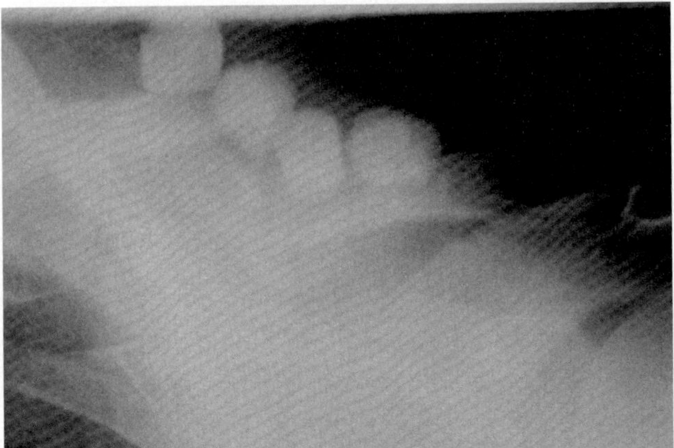

B

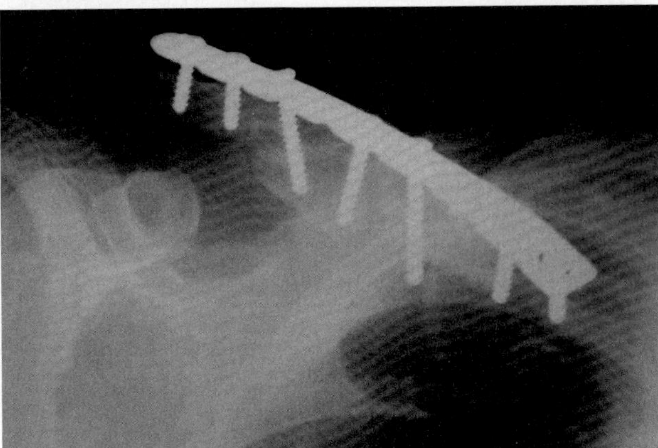

C

FIGURE 32-51 **A.** Deep infection after grafting of a midclavicle nonunion. Notice erosion of the intercalary graft, hardware loosening, and screw breakage. **B.** Initial treatment with hardware removal, extensive debridement, placement of antibiotic beads, and 6 weeks of intravenous antibiotics. **C.** Secondary reconstruction again using a corticocancellous graft harvested from the iliac crest was successful.

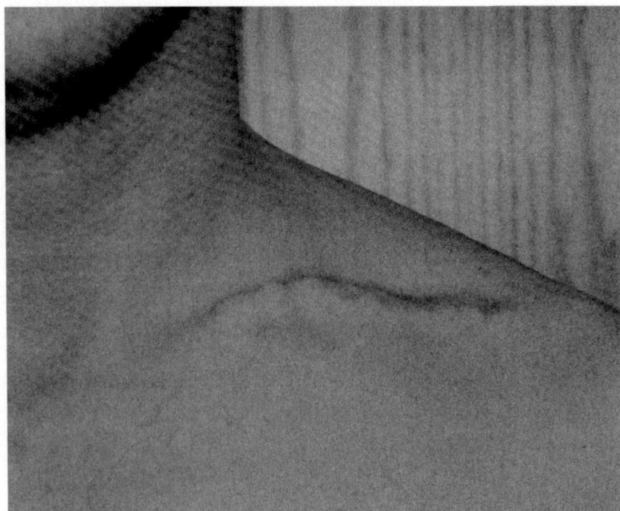

FIGURE 32-52 Hypertrophic scar and visible hardware after plating of a midclavicle nonunion.

four cases of refracture. Schwarz and Hocker (149) reported 1 of 19 patients who underwent plate removal had a refracture. Zenni and associates (142) reported refracture of a patient who had undergone successful intramedullary pinning 21 months prior. Bostman et al (251) found that initial comminuted fracture and alcohol intoxication were risk factors for subsequent refracture. It seems that the best recommendation is to leave a plate in place for 12 to 18 months and to place restrictions against contact sports for 2 to 3 months after plate removal (9,153).

CONCLUSION

Clavicle fractures usually heal uneventfully, even in the presence of treatment noncompliance. For most of these fractures, initial patient counseling as to the expected result is probably the most important aspect of treatment. In contrast, certain fracture types, such as the displaced and shortened midshaft fracture or the Type II distal clavicle fracture, require special attention. When necessary, operative intervention should be based on counterbalancing the deforming forces, specifically the weight of the arm. In the face of symptomatic nonunion, bone grafting and plate fixation are effective options.

REFERENCES

1. Adams F. *The genuine works of Hippocrates*. New York, NY: William Wood and Co., 1886.
2. Moseley HF. The clavicle: its anatomy and function. *Clin Orthop* 1968;17–27.
3. Harrington MA Jr, Keller TS, Seiler JGD, et al. Geometric properties and the predicted mechanical behavior of adult human clavicles. *J Biomech* 1993;26:417–426.
4. Bearn JG. Observations on the function of the capsule of the sternoclavicular joint in the clavicular support. *J Anat* 1967;101:159–170.
5. Spencer EE, Kuhn JE. Biomechanical analysis of reconstructions for sternoclavicular joint instability. *J Bone Joint Surg Am* 2004:86–A(1):98–105.
6. Cave AJE. The nature and morphology of the costoclavicular ligament. *J Anat* 1961; 95:170–179.
7. Salter EG, Nasca RJ, Shelley BS. Anatomical observations on the acromioclavicular joint and supporting ligaments. *Am J Sports Med* 1987;15:199–206.
8. Debski RE, Parsons IM, Woo SL, et al. Effect of capsular injury on acromioclavicular joint mechanics. *J Bone Joint Surg Am* 2001;83(9):1344–1351.
9. Jupiter JB, Ring D. Fractures of the clavicle. In: Iannotti JP, Williams GR, eds. *Disorders of the shoulder: diagnosis and management*. Philadelphia: Lippincott Williams & Wilkins, 1999.
10. Nordqvist A, Petersson C, Redlund-Johnell I. The natural course of lateral clavicle fracture. 15 (11-21) year follow-up of 110 cases. *Acta Orthop Scand* 1993;64:87–91.
11. Rokito AS, Eisenberg DP, Gallagher MA, et al. A comparison of nonoperative and operative treatment of type II distal clavicle fractures. *Bull Hosp Joint Dis* 2003;61(1–2): 32–39.
12. Copeland SM. Total resection of the clavicle. *Am J Surg* 1946;72:280–281.
13. Spar I. Total claviculectomy for pathological fractures. *Clin Orthop* 1977;236–237.
14. Wood VE. The results of total claviculectomy. *Clin Orthop* 1986;186–190.
15. Elkin DC, Cooper FW. Resection of the clavicle in vascular surgery. *J Bone Joint Surg Am* 1946;28:117.
16. Gurd FB. The treatment of complete dislocation of the outer end of the clavicle: a hitherto undescribed operation. *Ann Surg* 1941;113:1094–1098.
17. Moseley HF. *Shoulder lesions*. Edinburgh: Churchill Livingstone, 1972.
18. Dambrain R, Raphael B, Dhem A, et al. Radiation osteitis of the clavicle following radiotherapy and radical neck dissection of head and neck cancer. *Bull Group Int Rech Sci Stomatol Odontol* 1990;33:65–70.
19. Allman FL Jr. Fractures and ligamentous injuries of the clavicle and its articulation. *J Bone Joint Surg [Am]* 1967;49:774–784.
20. Stanley D, Trowbridge EA, Norris SH. The mechanism of clavicular fracture. A clinical and biomechanical analysis. *J Bone Joint Surg Br* 1988;70:461–464.
21. Fowler AW. Treatment of fractured clavicle. *Lancet* 1968;1:46–47.
22. Sankarankutty M, Turner BW. Fractures of the clavicle. *Injury* 1975;7:101–106.
23. Nowak J, Mallmin H, Larson S. The aetiology and epidemiology of clavicular fractures. A prospective study during a two-year period in Uppsala, Sweden. *Injury* 2000;35(5): 353–358.
24. Matsumoto K, Miyamoto K, Sumi H, et al. Upper extremity injuries in snowboarding and skiing: a comparative study. *Clin J Sport Med* 2002;12(6):354–359.
25. Bernard RN Jr, Haddad RJ Jr. Enchondroma of the proximal clavicle. An unusual cause of pathologic fracture-dislocation of the sternoclavicular joint. *Clin Orthop* 1982; 239–241.
26. Cummings CW, First R. Stress fracture of the clavicle after a radical neck dissection; case report. *Plast Reconstr Surg* 1975;55:366–367.
27. Fini-Storchi O, Lo Russo D, Agostini V. 'Pseudotumors' of the clavicle subsequent to radical neck dissection. *J Laryngol Otol* 1985;99:73–83.
28. Ord RA, Langdon JD. Stress fracture of the clavicle. A rare late complication of radical neck dissection. *J Maxillofac Surg* 1986;14:281–284.
29. Seo GS, Aoki J, Karakida O, et al. Case report: nonunion of a medial clavicular fracture following radical neck dissection: MRI diagnosis. *Orthopedics* 1999;22(10):985–986.
30. Kaye JJ, Nance EP, Green NE. Fatigue fracture of the medial aspect of the clavicle: an academic rather than athletic injury. *Radiology* 1982;144:89–90.
31. Shellhaas JS, Glaser DL, Drezner JA. Distal clavicular stress fracture in a female weight lifter: a case report. *Am J Sports Med* 2004:32(7):1755–1758.
32. Abbot AE, Hannafin JA. Stress fracture of the clavicle in a female lightweight rower. A case report and review of the literature. *Am J Sports Med* 2001;29(3):370–372.
33. Peebles CR, Sulkin T, Sampson MA. 'Cable maker's clavicle': stress fracture of the medial clavicle. *Skeletal Radiol* 2000;29(7):412–413.
34. Fallon KE, Fricker PA. Stress fracture of the clavicle in a young female gymnast. *Br J Sports Med* 2001;35(6):448–449.
35. Roset-Llobet J, Sala-Orfila JM. Sports-related stress fracture of the clavicle: a case report. *Int Orthop* 1998;22(4):266–268.
36. Neer CS. Fractures of the distal clavicle with detachment of the coracoclavicular ligaments in adults. *J Trauma* 1963;3:99–110.
37. Neer CS. Fractures of the distal third of the clavicle. *Clin Orthop* 1968;58:43–50.
38. Rockwood CA. Fractures of the outer clavicle in children and adults. *J Bone Joint Surg Br* 1982;64:642.
39. Craig EV. Fractures of the clavicle. In: Rockwood, CA and Matsen, FA, eds. *The shoulder*. Philadelphia: WB Saunders, 1990:367–412.
40. Nordqvist A, Petersson, C. The incidence of fractures of the clavicle. *Clin Orthop* 1994; 127–132.
41. Robinson CM. Fractures of the clavicle in the adult. Epidemiology and classification. *J Bone Joint Surg Br* 1998;80:476–484.
42. Craig EV. Fractures of the clavicle. In: Rockwood CA, Matsen FA, eds. *The shoulder*. Philadelphia: WB Saunders, 1998:428–482.
43. Heppenstall RB. Fractures and dislocations of the distal clavicle. *Orthop Clin North Am* 1975;6:477–486.
44. Rowe CR. An atlas of anatomy and treatment of midclavicular fractures. *Clin Orthop* 1968;58:29–42.
45. Gustilo R, Anderson J. Prevention of infection in the treatment of one thousand and twenty-five open fractures of long bones. *J Bone Joint Surg Am* 1976;58:453–458.
46. Simon RG, Lutz B. Open clavicle fractures: a case report. *Am J Orthop* 1999;28: 301–303.
47. Yokoyama K, Shindo M, Itoman M, et al. Immediate internal fixation for open fractures of the long bones of the upper and lower extremities. *J Trauma* 1994;37:230–236.
48. Ebraheim NA, An HS, Jackson WT, et al. Scapulothoracic dissociation. *J Bone Joint Surg Am* 1988;70:428–432.

49. Herscovici D Jr. Open reduction and internal fixation of ipsilateral fractures of the scapular neck and clavicle [letter; comment]. *J Bone Joint Surg Am* 1994;76:1112–1113.
50. Herscovici D Jr, Fiennes AG, Allgower M, et al. The floating shoulder: ipsilateral clavicle and scapular neck fractures. *J Bone Joint Surg Br* 1992;74:362–364.
51. Lange RH, Noel SH. Traumatic lateral scapular displacement: an expanded spectrum of associated neurovascular injury. *J Orthop Trauma* 1993;7:361–366.
52. Leung KS, Lam TP. Open reduction and internal fixation of ipsilateral fractures of the scapular neck and clavicle. *J Bone Joint Surg Am* 1993;75:1015–1018.
53. Rikli D, Regazzoni P, Renner N. The unstable shoulder girdle: early functional treatment utilizing open reduction and internal fixation. *J Orthop Trauma* 1995;9:93–97.
54. Weiner DS, O'Dell, HW. Fractures of the first rib associated with injuries to the clavicle. *J Trauma* 1969;9:412–422.
55. Lang-Lazdunski L, Bonnet PM, Pons F, et al. Traumatic extrathoracic lung herniation. *Ann Thorac Surg* 2002;74(3):927–929.
56. Barbier O, Malghem J, Delaere O, et al. Injury to the brachial plexus by a fragment of bone after fracture of the clavicle. *J Bone Joint Surg Br* 1997;79:534–536.
57. Reichenbacher D, Siebler G. [Early secondary lesions of the brachial plexus—a rare complication following clavicular fracture]. *Unfallchirurgie* 1987;13:91–92.
58. Rumball KM, Da Silva VF, Preston DN, et al. Brachial-plexus injury after clavicular fracture: case report and literature review. *Can J Surg* 1991;34:264–266.
59. Costa MC, Robbs JV. Nonpenetrating subclavian artery trauma. *J Vasc Surg* 1988;8:71–75.
60. DeBakey ME, Beall AC, Wukasch DC. Recent developments in vascular surgery with particular reference to orthopedics. *Am J Surg* 1965;109:134–142.
61. Dickson JW. Death following fractured clavicle. *Br Med J* 1952;2:666.
62. Howard FM, Shafer SJ. Injuries to the clavicle with neurovascular complications. A study of fourteen cases. *J Bone Joint Surg Am* 1965;47:1335–1346.
63. Javid H. Vascular injuries of the neck. *Clin Orthop* 1963;28:70–78.
64. Natali J, Maraval M, Kieffer E, et al. Fractures of the clavicle and injuries of the subclavian artery. Report of 10 cases. *J Cardiovasc Surg (Torino)* 1975;16:541–547.
65. Penn I. The vascular complications of fractures of the clavicle. *J Trauma* 1964;4:819.
66. Kendall KM, Burton JH, Cushing B. Fatal subclavian artery transection from isolated clavicle fracture. *J Trauma* 2000;48(2):316–318.
67. Leese G, Belch JJ, Rickhuss P, et al. Post-traumatic axillary artery thrombosis dissolution with low-dose intra-arterial streptokinase. *Injury* 1993;24:212–213.
68. Tse DH, Slabaugh PB, Carlson PA. Injury to the axillary artery by a closed fracture of the clavicle. A case report. *J Bone Joint Surg Am* 1980;62:1372–1374.
69. Quesada F. Technique for the roentgen diagnosis of fractures of the clavicle. *Surg Gynecol Obstet* 1926;42:424–428.
70. Weinberg B, Seife B, Alonso, P. The apical oblique view of the clavicle: its usefulness in neonatal and childhood trauma. *Skeletal Radiol* 1991;20:201–203.
71. Riemer BL, Butterfield SL, Daffner RH, et al. The abduction lordotic view of the clavicle: a new technique for radiographic visualization. *J Orthop Trauma* 1991;5:392–394.
72. Wirth MA, Rockwood CA Jr. Disorders of the sternoclavicular joint: pathophysiology, diagnosis, and management. In: Iannotti JP, Williams GR Jr, eds. *Disorders of the shoulder: diagnosis and management*. Philadelphia: Lippincott Williams & Wilkins, 1999: 783–785.
73. Brooks AL, Henning GD. Injury to the proximal clavicular epiphysis. *J Bone Joint Surg Am* 1972;54:1347–1348.
74. Herscovici D Jr, Sanders R, DiPasquale T, et al. Injuries of the shoulder girdle. *Clin Orthop* 1995;54–60.
75. Kanoksikarin S, Wearne WM. Fracture and retrosternal dislocation of the clavicle. *Aust N Z J Surg* 1978;48:95–96.
76. Lewonowski K, Bassett GS. Complete posterior sternoclavicular epiphyseal separation. A case report and review of the literature. *Clin Orthop* 1992;84–88.
77. Prime HT, Doig SG, Hooper JC. Retrosternal dislocation of the clavicle. A case report. *Am J Sports Med* 1991;19:92–93.
78. Zaslav KR, Ray S, Neer CS 2nd. Conservative management of a displaced medial clavicular physeal injury in an adolescent athlete. A case report and literature review. *Am J Sports Med* 1989;17:833–836.
79. Conwell HE. Fractures of the clavicle. A simple fixation dressing with a summary of the treatment and results attained in ninety-two cases. *JAMA* 1928;90:838–839.
80. Eskola A, Vainionpaa S, Myllynen P, et al. Outcome of clavicular fracture in 89 patients. *Arch Orthop Trauma Surg* 1986;105:337–338.
81. Post M. Current concepts in the treatment of fractures of the clavicle. *Clin Orthop* 1989; 89–101.
82. Albrecht HU, Bamert P. [The clavicular fracture: therapy and complications]. *Helv Chir Acta* 1982;48:571–583.
83. Aliev VM, Gornik AA, Makhanov SM. [A variant of Desault's bandage]. *Khirurgiia (Mosk)* 1985;143.
84. Andersen K, Jensen PO, Lauritzen J. Treatment of clavicular fractures. Figure-of-eight bandage versus a simple sling. *Acta Orthop Scand* 1987;58:71–74.
85. Bailey MM, Michalski J. Close-up on clavicle fracture. *Nursing* 1992;22:41.
86. Bar HW. [What is the proper position for the back dressing?]. *Sportverletz Sportschaden* 1992;6:182–183.
87. Bauer J, Blasko V, Kerolyi J. [Proceedings: Treatment of fresh clavicular fractures]. *Hefte Unfallheilkd* 1973;114:273–274.
88. Billington RW. A new (plaster yoke) dressing for fracture of the clavicle. *South J Med* 1931;24:667–670.
89. Bonnet J. Fracture of the clavicle. *Arch Chir Neerl* 1975;27:143–151.
90. Carley S. Towards evidence based emergency medicine: best BETS from the Manchester Royal Infirmary. Collar and cuff or sling after fracture of the clavicle. *J Accid Emerg Med* 1999;16:140.
91. Chiarelli GM, Ferretti M. [Indications for the use of "O" soft bandages in fractures of the clavicle]. *Chir Organi Mov* 1984;69:181–184.
92. Cook TW. Reduction and external fixation of fracture of the clavicle in recumbency. *J Bone Joint Surg Am* 1954;36:878–879.
93. Eiff MP. Management of clavicle fractures. *Am Fam Physician* 1997;55:121–128.
94. Everke H, Kinj K. [Results of conservative and surgical treatment of clavicular fractures]. *Chirurg* 1969;40:129–132.
95. Fedotov VK. [Comparative characteristics of some methods of conservative therapy in clavicular fractures in children]. *Vestn Khir* 1972;107:109–111.
96. Gaidukov VI. [Reposition and external immobilization in fractures of the clavicle, humerus and malleoli]. *Ortop Travmatol Protez* 1990;38–39.
97. Geyman JP, Gordon MJ. Orthopedic problems in family practice: incidence, distribution, and curricular implications. *J Fam Pract* 1979;8:759–765.
98. Hawley GW. A method of treating fracture of the clavicle. *J Bone Joint Surg Am* 1937; 19:232.
99. Hoofwijk AG, van der Werken C. [Conservative treatment of clavicular fractures]. *Z Unfallchir Versicherungsmed Berufskr* 1988;81:151–156.
100. Kempf FK, Schultze R. [Functional treatment of fractures of the shoulder girdle]. *Arch Orthop Unfallchir* 1968;64:252–267.
101. Lester CW. The treatment of fractures of the clavicle. *Ann Surg* 1929;89:600–606.
102. McCandless DN, Mowbray MA. Treatment of displaced fractures of the clavicle. Sling versus figure-of-eight bandage. *Practitioner* 1979;223:266–7.
103. Noczynski L. [Orthopedic splints in treatment of fractures of the clavicle and scapula]. *Pol Przegl Chir* 1973;45:367–370.
104. Nordqvist A, Petersson CJ, Redlund-Johnell I. Mid-clavicle fractures in adults: end result study after conservative treatment. *J Orthop Trauma* 1998;12:572–576.
105. Oneda T, Takahashi E, Sakurai S. The treatment of clavicle fractures in supine position. *Nippon Seikeigeka Gakkai Zasshi* 1965;38:1121–1125.
106. Pedersen MS, Kristiansen B, Thomsen F, et al. [Conservative treatment of clavicular fractures]. *Ugeskr Laeger* 1993;155:3832–3834.
107. Petracic B. [Efficiency of a rucksack bandage in the treatment of clavicle fractures]. *Unfallchirurgie* 1983;9:41–43.
108. Ghormley RK, Black JR, Cherry JH. Ununited fractures of the clavicle. *Am J Surg* 1941; 51:343–349.
109. Nordback I, Markkula H. Migration of Kirschner pin from clavicle into ascending aorta. *Acta Chir Scand* 1985;151:177–179.
110. Pilon L, Perreault JP, Jean G, et al. [La claviculectomy: a treatment still current]. *Union Med Can* 1977;106:743–745.
111. Poigenfurst J, Reiler T, Fischer W. [Plating of fresh clavicular fractures. Experience with 60 operations]. *Unfallchirurgie* 1988;14:26–37.
112. Eiff MP, Saultz JW. Fracture care by family physicians. *J Am Board Fam Pract* 1993;6: 179–181.
113. Hatch RL, Rosenbaum CI. Fracture care by family physicians. A review of 295 cases. *J Fam Pract* 1994;38:238–244.
114. Neer CS. Nonunion of the clavicle. *JAMA* 1960;172:1006–1011.
115. White RR, Anson PS, Kristiansen T, et al. Adult clavicle fractures: relationship between mechanism of injury and healing. *Orthop Trans* 1989;13:514–515.
116. Hill JM, McGuire MH, Crosby LA. Closed treatment of displaced middle-third fractures of the clavicle gives poor results. *J Bone Joint Surg Br* 1997;79:537–539.
117. Wick M, Muller EJ, Kollig E, et al. Midshaft fractures of the clavicle with a shortening of more than 2 cm predispose to nonunion. *Arch Orthop Trauma Surg* 2001;121(4): 207–211.
118. Robinson CM, Court-Brown CM, McQueen MM, et al. Estimating the risk of nonunion following nonoperative treatment of a clavicle fracture. *J Bone Joint Surg Am* 2004: 86(7):1359–1365.
119. Nowak J, Holgersson M, Larsson S. Can we predict long-term sequelae after fractures of the clavicle based on initial findings? A prospective study with nine to ten years of follow-up. *J Shoulder Elbow Surg* 2004:13(5):479–486.
120. Bottiglieri G, Zorzi R, Brocchetta F, et al. [Bloodless treatment of fractures of the clavicle using O-shaped soft bandages]. *Chir Ital* 1983;35:794–804.
121. Gaidukov VM, Dedushkin VS. [Immobilization in fractures of the clavicle]. *Ortop Travmatol Protez* 1991;35.
122. Malakhov VL, Kruglov AS. [Treatment of clavicular fractures]. *Voen Med Zh* 1975; 26–27.
123. Stanley D, Norris SH. Recovery following fractures of the clavicle treated conservatively. *Injury* 1988;19:162–164.
124. Dutta A, Malhotra SK, Kumar V. A fractured clavicle and vascular compression: a nonorthopedic indication of figure-of-eight bandage. *Anesth Analg* 200396:910.
125. Craig EV. Fractures of the clavicle. In: Rockwood, CA, Green, DP, Bucholz RW, Heckman JD, eds. *Rockwood and Green's fractures in adults*. Philadelphia: Lippincott-Raven, 1996:1109–1161.
126. DePalma A. *Surgery of the shoulder*. Philadelphia: Lippincott, 1983.
127. Packer BD. Conservative treatment of fracture of the clavicle. *J Bone Joint Surg* 1944; 26A:770–774.
128. Quigley TB. The management of simple fractures of the clavicle. *N Engl J Med* 1950; 243:286–290.
129. Schuind F, Pay-Pay E, Andrianne Y, et al. External fixation of the clavicle for fracture or non-union in adults. *J Bone Joint Surg Am* 1988;70:692–695.
130. Nicholl EA. Annotation. Miners and mannequins. *J Bone and Joint Surg Br* 1954;36: 171–172.
131. Breck L. Partially threaded round pins with oversized threads for intramedullary fixation of the clavicle and the forearm bones. *Clin Orthop* 1958;11:227–229.
132. Connolly JF, Dehne R. Nonunion of the clavicle and thoracic outlet syndrome. *J Trauma* 1989;29:1127–1132; discussion 1132–1133.

INDEX

Note: Page numbers followed by an "f" indicate figures; page numbers followed by a "t" indicate tables.

B

C

L

N

R